# *TRAUMA*
# *Anesthesia and Intensive Care*

# *TRAUMA*
# *Anesthesia and Intensive Care*

Edited by


**Levon M. Capan, M.D.**
*Associate Professor of Clinical Anesthesiology*
*New York University School of Medicine*
*Associate Director*
*Department of Anesthesiology*
*Bellevue Hospital Center*
*New York, New York*

**Sanford M. Miller, M.D.**
*Assistant Professor of Anesthesiology*
*New York University School of Medicine*
*New York, New York*

**Herman Turndorf, M.D.**
*Professor and Chairman*
*Department of Anesthesiology*
*New York University School of Medicine*
*Director*
*Department of Anesthesiology*
*Bellevue Hospital Center*
*New York, New York*


With 37 additional contributors

J. B. Lippincott Company Philadelphia
New York St. Louis London Sydney Tokyo

Acquisitions Editor: Nancy Mullins
Production: Bermedica Production, Ltd.
Project Coordinator: Lori J. Bainbridge
Compositor: Maryland Composition Company, Inc.
Printer/Binder: Arcata Graphics Halliday



1 3 5 6 4 2

**Library of Congress Cataloging-in-Publication Data**

Trauma : anesthesia and intensive care / [edited by] Levon M. Capan,
Sanford M. Miller, Herman Turndorf.
p. cm.
Includes bibliographical references.
Includes index.
ISBN 0-397-50618-X
1. Wounds and injuries—Surgery. 2. Anesthesia. 3. Surgical
intensive care. I. Capan, Levon M. II. Miller, Sanford M.
III. Turndorf, Herman.
[DNLM: 1. Anesthesia. 2. Critical Care. 3. Wounds and Injuries.
WO 200 T7774]
RD93.T674 1991
617.1—dc20
DNLM/DLC
for Library of Congress 91-6548
CIP

The authors and publisher have exerted every effort to ensure that drug selection and dosage set forth in this text are in accord with current recommendations and practice at the time of publication. However, in view of ongoing research, changes in government regulations, and the constant flow of information relating to drug therapy and drug reactions, the reader is urged to check the package insert for each drug for any change in indications and dosage and for added warnings and precautions. This is particularly important when the recommended agent is a new or infrequently employed drug.

*Dedicated to*

*My Father-in-Law, Keğam Shahinian*
Levon M. Capan

*My Family*
Sanford M. Miller

*My Wife, Sietske, and my sons,*
*David and Michael Pieter*
Herman Turndorf

# Contributors

**R. David Bauer, M.D.**
*Staff Physician*
*Department of Orthopedic Surgery*
*Davis-Monthan Air Force Base*
*Tucson, Arizona*

**Donald P. Bernstein, M.D.**
*Staff Anesthesiologist*
*Palomar Medical Center*
*Escondido, California*

**Vimala P. Bhatt, M.D.**
*Assistant Professor of Anesthesiology*
*New York Medical College*
*Westchester County Medical Center*
*Valhalla, New York*

**Edwin A. Bowe, M.D.**
*Professor*
*Department of Surgery/Anesthesiology*
*University of South Carolina School of Medicine*
*Columbia, South Carolina*

**Levon M. Capan, M.D.**
*Associate Professor of Clinical Anesthesiology*
*New York University School of Medicine;*
*Associate Director*
*Department of Anesthesiology*
*Bellevue Hospital Center*
*New York, New York*

**William M. Eisenberg, M.D.**
*Assistant Professor of Ophthalmology*
*New York University School of Medicine*
*New York, New York*

**Thomas J. Errico, M.D.**
*Assistant Professor of Orthopedic Surgery*
*New York University School of Medicine*
*New York, New York*

**Robert Glickman, D.M.D.**
*Assistant Professor*
*Oral and Maxillofacial Surgery*
*New York University College of Dentistry;*
*Director*
*Oral and Maxillofacial Surgery*
*Bellevue Hospital Center and Tisch Hospital*
*New York, New York*

**Gregory Gottlieb, M.D.**
*Staff Anesthesiologist*
*Swedish Hospital Medical Center*
*Seattle, Washington*

**Christopher Grande, M.D.**
*Special Consultant and Chief—Special Projects Branch*
*Department of Anesthesiology*
*Shock Trauma Center*
*Maryland Institute for Emergency Medical Services Systems*
*University of Maryland Medical Systems*
*Baltimore, Maryland*

**Gilbert J. Grant, M.D.**
*Assistant Professor of Anesthesiology*
*Associate Director, Obstetric Anesthesia*
*New York University School of Medicine*
*New York, New York*

**Craig Hartrick, M.D.**
*Staff Anesthesiologist*
*William Beaumont Hospital*
*Royal Oak, Michigan*

**John Jackson, M.D.**
*Assistant Professor of Anesthesiology*
*University of Minnesota Hospital and Clinic*
*Minneapolis, Minnesota*

**Roberta C. Kahn, M.D.**
*Associate Professor of Clinical Anesthesiology*
*New York University School of Medicine;*
*Co-Director-Neurosurgical Intensive Care Unit*
*Bellevue Hospital Center*
*New York, New York*

**Brian Kaufman, M.D.**
*Assistant Professor of Anesthesiology and Medicine*
*New York University School of Medicine;*
*Medical Director-Respiratory Therapy and Neurosurgical Intensive Care Unit*
*Tisch Hospital*
*New York, New York*

**Elmer F. Klein, Jr., M.D.**
*Professor and Chief of Anesthesia*
*Department of Surgery/Anesthesia*
*University of South Carolina*
*School of Medicine*
*Columbia, South Carolina*

**Neal Kurtti, M.D.**
*Fellow–Department of Anesthesiology*
*New York University School of Medicine*
*New York, New York*

**Anna M. Ledgerwood, M.D.**
*Professor of Surgery*
*Wayne State University*
*School of Medicine*
*Detroit, Michigan*

**Charles E. Lucas, M.D.**
*Professor of Surgery*
*Wayne State University*
*School of Medicine*
*Detroit, Michigan*

**Durgesh Mankikar, M.D.**
*Staff Anesthesiologist*
*Mountainside Hospital*
*Montclair, New Jersey*

**Robert E. Markison, M.D.**
*Associate Clinical Professor of Surgery*
*University of California, San Francisco*
*School of Medicine;*
*Chief of Hand Surgery*
*San Francisco Veterans Administration Medical Center;*
*Hand Surgeon*
*San Francisco Hand Specialists*
*San Francisco, California*

**M. Donald McGoldrick, M.D.**
*Professor of Medicine*
*Albany Medical College;*
*Head-Division of Nephrology*
*Albany Medical Center*
*Albany, New York*

**Paul Mesnick, M.D.**
*Assistant Professor of Clinical Anesthesia*
*Northwestern University School of Medicine;*
*Medical Director*
*Chicago Police Department*
*Chicago, Illinois*

**Sanford M. Miller, M.D.**
*Assistant Professor of Anesthesiology*
*New York University School of Medicine*
*New York, New York*

**Alexander Nacht, M.D.**
*Assistant Professor of Anesthesiology*
*New York University School of Medicine*
*New York, New York*

**Robert Pascucci, M.D.**
*Instructor in Anesthesia (Pediatrics)*
*Harvard Medical School;*
*Associate Director–Multidisciplinary ICU*
*The Childrens Hospital in Boston*
*Boston, Massachusetts*

**Alison Pataky, M.D.**
*Assistant Professor*
*Department of Anesthesiology*
*Yale University School of Medicine*
*New Haven, Connecticut*

**Katie P. Patel, M.D.**
*Assistant Professor of Anesthesiology*
*New York University School of Medicine;*
*Associate Director*
*Department of Anesthesiology*
*Bellevue Hospital Center*
*New York, New York*

**Charles E. Pither, MB**
*Consultant in Anesthesia and Pain Control*
*St. Thomas' Hospital*
*London, England*

**Robert M. Porges, M.D.**
*Professor and Acting Chairman*
*Department of Obstetrics and Gynecology*
*New York University School of Medicine*
*New York, New York*

**P. Prithvi Raj, M.D.**
*Professor of Anesthesiology*
*University of Texas;*
*Director, University Center for Pain Medicine at Hermann*
*Houston, Texas*

**Sivam Ramanathan, M.D.**
*Professor and Vice Chairman of Academic Affairs*
*Director of Obstetric Anesthesia*
*New York University School of Medicine*
*New York, New York*

**Mark Rivlin, M.D.**
*Staff Anesthesiologist*
*Wilson Memorial Hospital*
*Binghamton, New York*

**Andrew Rosenberg, M.D.**
*Instructor in Anesthesiology*
*New York University School of Medicine*
*New York, New York;*
*Associate Chairman*
*Department of Anesthesiology*
*Hospital for Joint Diseases*
*Orthopedic Institute*
*New York, New York*

**Richard M. Sommer, M.D.**
*Assistant Professor of Anesthesiology*
*New York University School of Medicine;*
*Chief, Anesthesiology*
*New York Veterans Administration Medical Center*
*New York, New York*

**Marc Tissot, M.D.**
*Assistant Professor of Anesthesiology*
*New York University School of Medicine*
*New York, New York*

**Donald D. Trunkey, M.D.**
*Professor and Chairman*
*Department of Surgery*
*Oregon Health Science University*
*Portland, Oregon*

**Herman Turndorf, M.D.**
*Professor and Chairman*
*Department of Anesthesiology*
*New York University School of Medicine;*
*Director*
*Department of Anesthesiology*
*Bellevue Hospital Center*
*New York, New York*

**James Walsh, M.D.**
*Clinical Instructor Cornell Medical School*
*Assistant Attending Northshore University Hospital*
*New York, New York*

**Gary W. Welch, M.D., Ph.D., J.D.**
*Professor and Chairman*
*Department of Anesthesiology*
*University of Massachusetts Medical School and Teaching Hospital*
*Worcester, Massachusetts*

# Preface

Trauma is likely to remain the most common cause of premature mortality and a prominent cause of disability for the foreseeable future. Measures to prevent injury, such as improved product design, seat-belt laws, and education, have decreased the incidence of many types of injuries. Unfortunately, these gains have been somewhat offset by injuries associated with increasing mechanization and criminal activities.

Improvements in prehospital care have been effective in lowering the immediate mortality from trauma. Many victims who previously would have succumbed in the field are now rapidly transported to hospitals, requiring physicians, including anesthesiologists, to deal with ever more severe injuries and their consequences.

Of the many texts available describing current trauma management, few are directed to the needs of anesthesiologists. *Trauma: Anesthesia and Intensive Care* is a comprehensive summary of the issues of importance to the anesthetic and general management of the injured patient. This book is divided into four sections. The opening chapter summarizes the historic, epidemiologic, and economic aspects of trauma and describes the anesthesiologist's role in trauma care. The next eight chapters discuss basic considerations of importance to clinicians treating the major trauma victim. The twelve chapters of the second section detail the management of specific injuries. The third section focuses on complications of the postinjury and postoperative period. Because victims of trauma frequently require surgery, often more than once, within the first few weeks of injury, anesthetic management of these complications is also described. The single chapter of the last section discusses the organizational aspects of emergency medical services, trauma systems, and disaster planning. Whenever necessary, the pathophysiology and consequences of injury have been discussed. Since trauma creates a wide variety of clinical states, it is not feasible to recommend specific approaches to each. For this reason understanding of basic pathophysiology is essential in order to formulate and prioritize management objectives.

Since successful outcome in trauma care depends on the efforts of many specialists, and thus on familiarity of each member of the team with the various diagnostic and therapeutic approaches to injury management, this information has been included in virtually all our chapters. This should facilitate coordination of care between anesthesiologists and other specialists, and should therefore make this book useful to any physician involved in trauma care. It has been our objective to provide the reader with a complete book on trauma anesthesia in a clear, well-illustrated, and well-referenced manner.

Although every chapter has been subjected to extensive review and editing by each of us and by the publisher, some interchapter overlap has been allowed to facilitate understanding or improve the flow of text, and to provide illustrations of varied approaches to controversial issues.

Even though trauma care in general has been evolving continuously, progress in anesthetic management of the injured patient has been relatively slow. The enormous literature on the subject contains few documents focusing specifically on anesthesia. We hope this text will stimulate interest in those who, by their attempts to answer the many remaining questions, will contribute to expansion of research in this field and improve the quality of anesthesia and all care for the injured patient.

Levon M. Capan, M.D.
Sanford M. Miller, M.D.
Herman Turndorf, M.D.

# Acknowledgments

Without the encouragement and help of many individuals it would have been impossible to produce this text. The understanding, sacrifices, and encouragement of our wives Ani, Marcia, and Sietske and of our children Natalie Capan, Kevin and Douglas Miller, and David and Michael Turndorf were the most crucial factors in making the book a reality. The initiative and encouragement of the editorial staff of the Lippincott Company, especially Stuart Freeman, Nancy Mullins, and Peter Nalle, and the assistance of the staff of Bermedica Production, Ltd. were also essential.

We are deeply appreciative of the efforts of Keğam Shahinian, the father-in-law of our senior editor, who, with endless patience and devotion, organized the references and proofread the multiple drafts of each chapter. The help of our departmental librarian, Joseph Ehrlich, in providing us with masses of necessary reading material deserves special thanks. We are also indebted to Janice Rothermel who personally and by mobilizing her secretarial staff, expedited the project. Of the departmental secretarial staff, the efforts of Eileen Krane-Fruchter, John Glen, Alma Campbell, Charles Quintyne, and Geraldine Hedling were especially notable.

The first two editors are indebted to their coeditor and department Chairman, Herman Turndorf, M.D., who for many years created the academic environment and provided the support necessary to make this and many other publications possible.

The senior editor expresses his appreciation to his wife, Ani, and daughter, Natalie, who, apart from not having a single day of vacation for 5 years, willingly and cheerfully prepared most of the illustrations and typed the many manuscripts of the book. This editor is also deeply indebted to his long-time friend and coworker, Katie P. Patel, M.D., for taking over a substantial portion of his clinical and administrative responsibilities at the Bellevue Hospital Center during the preparation of this book.

# Contents

## Section One: Basic Considerations



## Section Two: Specific Injuries

## Section Three: Complications



## Section Four: Organizational Aspects

# *TRAUMA*
# *Anesthesia and Intensive Care*

# Section One

# Basic Considerations

# Chapter One

Levon M. Capan
Sanford M. Miller
Herman Turndorf

# Trauma Overview

Traumatic injuries are among the most serious health problems facing the United States and many other countries, in terms of the morbidity and mortality they produce and also of their socioeconomic costs. Every year more than 20 million hospital days are consumed by trauma victims in the United States.[61] This represents more hospital days than are utilized by patients with cardiac disease and four times those used by cancer patients.[131] This chapter will discuss general aspects of trauma including its history, epidemiology, economic impact, and care systems. A brief discussion of the anesthesiologist's role in trauma care together with injury severity assessment will be offered in the final section.

## HISTORICAL NOTES

Trauma has undoubtedly plagued mankind for as long as the species has existed on this planet. The surgeons of ancient Egypt are reported to have performed amputations, extractions of foreign bodies, and wound dressings as early as 6000 BC.[43] The Edwin Smith papyrus, written about 1600 BC, describes many traumatic injuries.[26] Perhaps the only beneficial effect of trauma, especially that sustained in wars, is on medical knowledge; almost every specialty of medicine has realized major advances from the experience gained in the management of injuries.

Among the advances in surgery have been those in wound care. As early as 1545, Ambroise Paré managed wounds with clean dressings without medication or cauterization. Advances in experimental and surgical pathology, comparative physiology, and experimental morphology were also realized during the 18th century. John Hunter's "A Treatise on the Blood, Inflammation, and Gunshot Wounds" was inspired by his military experience and remains a surgical classic.[65]

Treatment of fractures and dislocations was described by Hippocrates around 500 BC. Management principles for open extremity wounds were established in the American Civil War, when the importance of early definitive treatment of fractures was demonstrated.[22] During this war it was also realized that optimal results from major operative procedures such as amputations could be obtained by performing them within 24 hours of injury.[22] Many techniques of vascular surgery have their roots in World War II and in the Korean and Vietnam Wars.

War surgery also led to the development of inpatient care. The concept of a hospital system was first developed by the Romans to care for wounded soldiers. These small hospitals later served as prototypes for the civilian hospitals established in the fifth century AD.[43]

The modern principles of military medicine were established by Sir John Pringle, a great epidemiologist and the Surgeon General of the English army from 1742 to 1758. His idea of considering both English and French hospitals as sanctuaries for wounded soldiers during the Battle of Dettingen in 1743, and thus his request for protection of these hospitals by both sides, formed the basis for the official agreement on this issue in the Geneva Convention of 1864.

The ambulance, one of the responsibilities of emergency medicine physicians today, was introduced by Dominique Jean Lairey, a French army surgeon during the Napoleonic

Wars. These so-called "flying ambulances" were drawn by horses and served to transport injured soldiers from the battlefield to areas behind the front for definitive care. During World War I horse-drawn ambulances were replaced with motorized ones. The air transport system utilized by many modern civilian trauma centers was first developed during the Korean War to evacuate wounded soldiers in the mountainous terrain. An air evacuation system was also used during the war in Vietnam.

Infection, particularly of wounds, was the nemesis of surgeons in the days before asepsis. During the Civil War, many physicians gained familiarity with prevention and treatment of infectious diseases.[22] However, antiseptic surgery was not developed until the second half of the 19th century when Joseph Lister recommended the use of carbolic acid spray into the wound after the demonstration of bacteria in wound cultures by Louis Pasteur.[43]

Trauma surgery also helped advance the field of anesthesiology. Shortly after the use of ether by William Morton in Boston in 1846, the Mexican-American War broke out. Although the general opinion is that the first widespread use of ether occurred during either the Crimean or German-Danish conflicts after 1848, recent information suggests that it was first used during the Mexican-American War in the spring of 1847.[1] During World War I the use of nitrous oxide on the western front marked an important advance in acceptance of this anesthetic.[41]

Intravenous fluid therapy, which is now essential for management of a wide variety of diseases, was initiated during World War I by George Crile of Cleveland. He used seawater to resuscitate hypovolemic injured soldiers.[43] Interestingly, 80 years later, the effectiveness of hypertonic saline in various types of traumatic injuries is again being evaluated.

The need for blood transfusion was recognized as early as the 17th century when non–cross-matched animal blood was given to patients.[43] In the early years of the 20th century, the principles of cross-matching and preparation of whole blood were developed. During the Second World War, large amounts of whole blood were prepared and shipped under refrigeration to the battlefield.

Recognition of the endocrine-metabolic response to trauma should also be credited to Crile who, during the First World War, realized that the nervous system must be intact for the metabolic response to occur.[42] His finding is thus the basis of the debate on whether regional anesthesia improves outcome.

Contemporary civilian trauma care also contributes to understanding of the mechanisms of various disease states which resemble those seen in injuries. Acute respiratory distress syndrome, fat embolism syndrome, thromboembolism, septic shock, acute renal failure, stress states, and many other disorders may occur in major trauma victims. Experience gained in treating these complications certainly helps improve the care of injured patients and also helps those patients who suffer these problems from nontraumatic causes.

## EPIDEMIOLOGY OF TRAUMA

Statistical data related to injury epidemiology are compiled by various agencies: the National Center for Health Statistics (NCHS), the National Highway Traffic Safety Administration (NHTSA) with its Fatal Accident Reporting System (FARS), the National Safety Council (NSC), and many others. Data from these agencies do not always correspond because they are collected and analyzed using different methodologies. In addition, research on the epidemiology of trauma has been sparse because of inadequate funds. In 1985, the National Academy of Sciences, with the collaboration of several of its committees, published a booklet entitled "Injury in America, A Continuing Public Health Problem," which discussed not only the insufficient knowledge of trauma epidemiology but also the impact of injuries on the health of the American public and the economic status of the nation.[38] Recommendations were made about future injury prevention, treatment, rehabilitation, and research strategies. This report provided a major impetus to evaluation and expansion of injury-control activities. Congress responded to its recommendations and charged the Centers for Disease Control (CDC) with conducting a pilot program for injury prevention research by creating a center for injury control at CDC. This resulted in the creation of the Center for Environmental Health and Injury Control (CEHIC). A $10 million fund was appropriated in 1986 and again in 1987 for this project. CEHIC is charged with (1) establishing surveillance systems and conducting and fostering prevention programs; (2) improving and expanding professional education and training; (3) collecting and analyzing data; and (4) serving as the lead federal agency in injury prevention and research. Establishment of this center is a major step toward improving data collection and coordination of research activities among various governmental agencies, academic institutions, and other sectors. There has already been an improvement in our understanding of the current situation. Nevertheless, further research is necessary.

The epidemiologic information presented in this section has been collected by various agencies including academic institutions. It should be pointed out that these data have a few years' lag; we have based this section on the most recent statistics, which, in most instances are 3 or 4 years old. Epidemiology of trauma will be discussed in two parts: general aspects and aspects of each type of injury.

### GENERAL ASPECTS

It is unusual for any individual not to remember involvement in at least one accident that resulted, or might have resulted, in a moderate or severe injury. In an interesting study from Sweden, 89% of men interviewed reported at least one injury that restricted their activity for 1 day or more, necessitated medical attendance, or, in the case of head injury, resulted in unconsciousness.[30] In the Northeastern Ohio Trauma Study, nearly one fifth of the population of the region sustained some sort of trauma requiring an emergency room visit during 1977. Trauma that year accounted for one half of all visits to the area's hospital emergency departments.[19]

The causes of injury, poisoning, and other adverse experiences vary widely and are classified under the E800 to E999 codes of the International Classification of Diseases (ICD)[132] (see Appendix 1). For practical purposes, however, injuries are divided into two major categories: intentional and unintentional. Suicide, homicide, assault, and war fall into the intentional category. Trauma sustained in motor vehicle colli-

TABLE 1-1. Mortality Rates Per 100,000 Population by Cause of Death in 1985 and 1987*

| CAUSES OF DEATH | MORTALITY RATE 1985 | 1987 |
|---|---|---|
| All causes | 874.8 | 874.0 |
| Heart diseases | 325.0 | 313.4 |
| Malignant neoplasms | 191.7 | 196.1 |
| Cerebrovascular disease | 64.0 | 61.3 |
| Unintentional injuries | 38.6 {58.7 | 39.0 {60.2 |
| Suicide/homicide | 20.1 | 21.2 |
| COPD† | 31.2 | 32.2 |
| Pneumonia and influenza | 27.9 | 28.8 |
| Diabetes mellitus | 16.2 | 15.6 |
| Chronic liver disease and cirrhosis | 11.2 | 10.7 |
| Congenital anomalies | 5.5 | 5.0 |
| AIDS‡ | 2.3 | 5.4 |
| Prematurity | 2.9 | 2.7 |
| Sudden infant death syndrome | 2.0 | 1.8 |

* Only major causes of death are tabulated. (Data were obtained from the National Center for Health Statistics.)
† COPD, chronic obstructive pulmonary disease.
‡ AIDS, acquired immunodeficiency syndrome.

sions; falls; fires; drowning; industrial or farm accidents; air, water, rail, and other vehicle accidents; and all other accidents are categorized as unintentional injuries. Of course, many injuries in the unintentional category may be inflicted intentionally, while firearm injuries, which in general fall in the intentional category, may be produced unintentionally.

The most accurate statistical data available in the United States on trauma relate to the injury fatality rate. Mortality figures provided by these surveys encompass deaths within 30 days of trauma, including hospital mortality. Every year approximately 140,000 people die from intentional and unintentional injuries in this country, representing an overall death rate of 60 per 100,000 population.[38] The cause-specific mortality rates for 1985[73] and 1987[80] are shown in Table 1-1, from which it is evident that trauma kills almost the same number of patients as cerebrovascular disease, the third most common cause of fatality. Heart disease and cancer remain the two most common causes of death in the United States. Trauma, however, attacks a younger population and is the most common cause of mortality in the population between the ages of 1 and 38. Thus, years of potential life lost (YPLL) from trauma exceed those of any other disease[73,80] (Table 1-2). YPLL is the number of years lost before age 65 (age 70 according to some statistics). As shown in Table-2, during each of the past several years injuries have caused between 3.5 and 4 million YPLL, which is slightly greater than those caused by cancer and heart disease combined. Although the death rate from acquired immunodeficiency syndrome (AIDS) has increased rapidly in recent years, in 1987, this disease caused only one tenth of the YPLL caused by trauma. A gradual decrease in the number of deaths from trauma occurred between 1979 and 1985.[73,98,141] With this came a decline in YPLL which was most notable between 1984 and 1985: 4.2% for unintentional injuries and 1.5% for intentional injuries[73] (Fig 1-1). However, from 1985 to 1987 mortality rate and YPLL increased by 1.5 per 100,000 population and 108,181 years, respectively.[73,80] A decline in motor-vehicle-related mortality resulting from increased use of seat belts and measures against driving while intoxicated is expected to bring about a reduction in the trauma-related death rate and thus YPLL by the end of 1990.

Death after trauma occurs at three distinct time periods.[7,129] Approximately 50% of deaths occur within 1 hour of the traumatic event; these are usually caused by central nervous system, heart, and great vessel injuries. Airway obstruction contributes to many of the deaths in this phase; however, aspiration of gastric and pharyngeal secretions and blood is considered a more important factor, even in patients with maxillofacial injuries.[5] Smoke inhalation and carbon monoxide toxicity are the major causative factors in early mortality from fires; in most of these, the burns themselves do not cause immediate death. A second rise in mortality occurs 1 to 4

TABLE 1-2. Estimated Years of Potential Life Lost before Age 65 from Diseases Associated with High Mortality Rate in 1984, 1985, 1986, and 1987*

| CAUSES OF DEATH | YPLL FOR PERSONS DYING IN 1984 | 1985 | 1986 | 1987 |
|---|---|---|---|---|
| All causes | 11,788,125 | 11,844,475 | 12,093,486 | 12,045,778 |
| Unintentional injuries | 2,313,048 | 2,235,064 | 2,358,426 | 2,295,710 |
| Suicide/homicide | 1,250,642 | 1,241,688 | 1,360,508 | 1,289,223 |
| Malignant neoplasms | 1,804,809 | 1,813,245 | 1,832,210 | 1,837,742 |
| Heart disease | 1,564,522 | 1,600,265 | 1,557,041 | 1,494,227 |
| Congenital anomalies | 685,315 | 694,715 | 661,117 | 642,551 |
| Prematurity | 474,290 | 444,931 | 428,796 | 422,813 |
| Sudden infant death syndrome | 316,909 | 313,386 | 340,431 | 286,733 |
| Cerebrovascular disease | 266,486 | 253,044 | 246,131 | 246,479 |
| Chronic liver disease | 233,099 | 235,629 | 231,558 | 228,145 |
| Pneumonia and influenza | 163,474 | 168,949 | 175,386 | 166,775 |
| AIDS† | 82,885 | 152,595 | 246,823 | 357,536 |
| COPD‡ | 123,275 | 129,815 | 128,590 | 123,260 |
| Diabetes mellitus | 119,555 | 128,229 | 121,117 | 119,155 |

* Only major causes of death are tabulated. (Data were obtained from the National Center for Health Statistics.)
† AIDS, acquired immunodeficiency syndrome.
‡ COPD, chronic obstructive pulmonary disease.

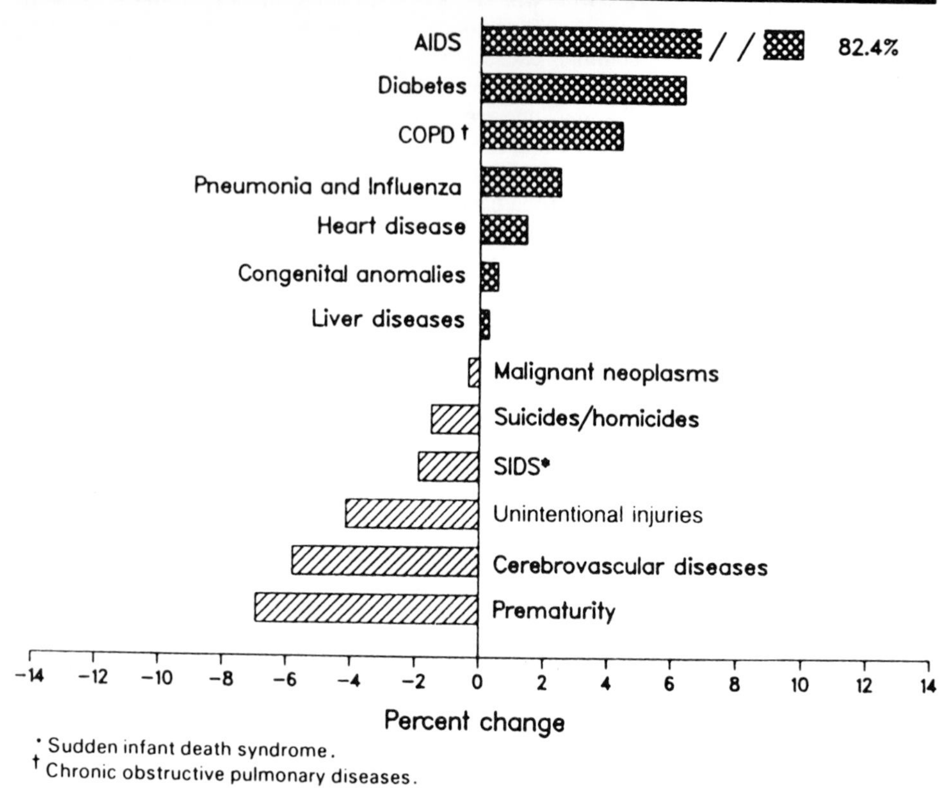


FIG. 1-1. Percentage change in years of potential life lost before age 65 from unintentional and intentional injuries in relation to other diseases in the United States between 1984 and 1985. (Reproduced with permission from American Medical Association. JAMA 257:1161,1987.)

hours after trauma, thus generally in the emergency department or in the operating or recovery rooms. Uncontrollable hemorrhage from the heart, major vessels, or vascular organs is the principal cause of death in this phase, accounting for 30% of fatalities from trauma. The remaining 20% of trauma-related deaths occur more than 1 week following injury from infection and/or multiorgan failure (Fig 1-2).

More than half of trauma deaths result from accidental injuries. Motor vehicle accidents and falls are responsible for the majority of these deaths. In the non-accidental injury category suicides and homicides together account for 30 to 40% of traumatic deaths. A small fraction of traumatic deaths results from unspecified mechanisms (Fig 1-3).

Sex and age are important determinants of trauma-related mortality. The incidences of both serious injury and death from trauma are almost three times higher in males than in females.[15,54] Injured individuals between 55 and 75 years are 4 to 6 and those above 84 are 10 to 15 times more likely to die than their younger counterparts.[15,54] In the aged, injury rates decline, but the fraction of injuries requiring hospital admission or causing fatality rises sharply. The death rate from unintentional trauma is highest in the 15- to 24-year-old group, and that for intentional injuries is greatest between 24 and 35 years. Fig 1-4 shows age-specific injury death rates in the United States for the year 1983. The graph is essentially similar to that obtained for the period between 1977 and 1979,[15] confirming the strong association of injury deaths with age. That females die at a lower rate than males is probably related to a lower rate of involvement in injury-prone activities, greater caution, and a smaller incidence of alcohol or other substance abuse. In an interesting study, the risk of fatality from physical trauma in relation to sex and age was determined for 10 categories of vehicle occupants (eg, drivers, passengers, helmeted motorcyclists, unbelted occupants) from available FARS data using a double-pair comparison

FIG. 1-2. Diagrammatic representation of characteristic phasic pattern of trauma deaths.

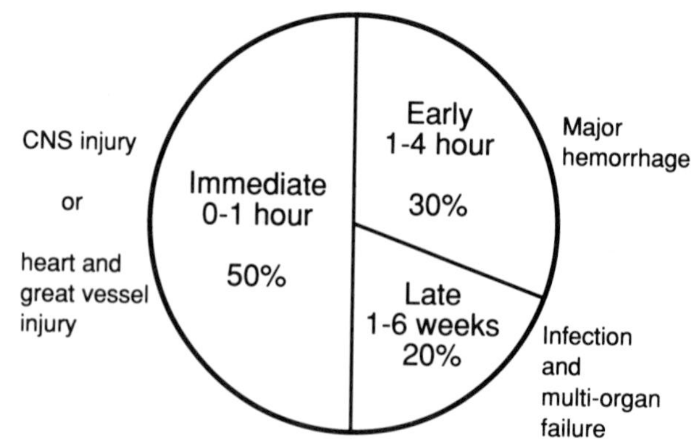

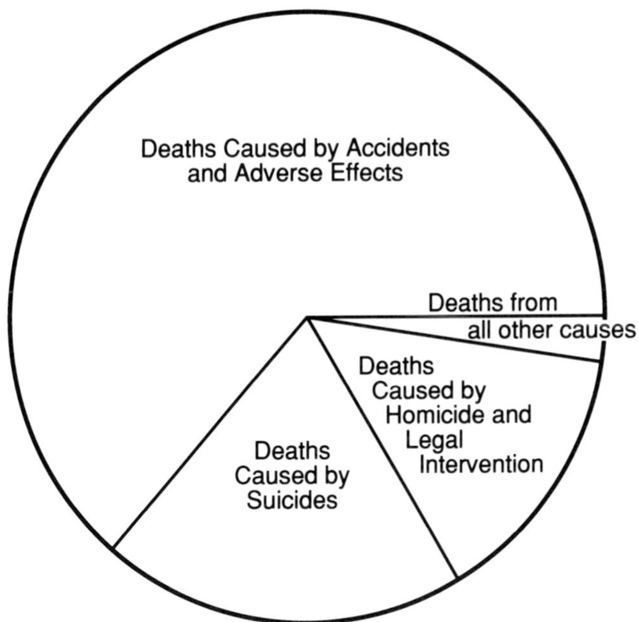


FIG. 1-3. Fraction of deaths caused by accidents, suicides, homicides and other mechanisms of trauma. This pattern remained unchanged between 1980 and 1990.

FIG. 1-4. Age-specific death rates in 1983 from unintentional and intentional injuries, from other mechanisms of trauma, and from all causes combined.

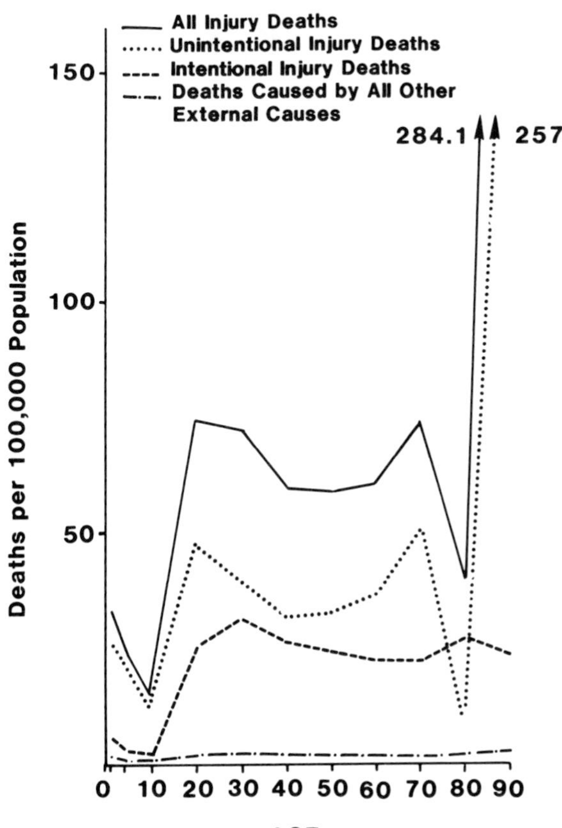


method. Females between 15 and 45 years were found to be at approximately 25% higher risk of death after injury than males of the same age group. Males at younger and older ages were at greater risk. The risk of fatality after injury was least at age 20; at age 70 the risk increased threefold.[51]

The injury-related mortality rate is higher in blacks, and probably in Hispanics as well, than in whites. Blacks represent 12% of the US population but sustain 15.3% of deaths from trauma. Homicides, pedestrian mishaps, residential fires, and drownings cause more deaths in blacks than in whites.[74] Deaths from motor vehicle accidents, although common in blacks, occur at about the same rate as in whites.[74] Death from homicide is five times more common in blacks than in whites (Fig 1-5). This prompted Trunkey[129] to conclude that in large cities black males have a 1 in 20 chance of being murdered before the age of 30. Blacks are three times more likely to die from residential fires than are whites.[74] This discrepancy probably results from a lack of smoke detectors and use of inappropriate heating devices in inner-city houses, combined with smoking in bed and slower fire department response.[17] The black to white ratio for deaths from drowning is 1.8:1,[74] but white children between 1 and 4 years old die from drowning twice as frequently as comparable age black children.[134] In whites, children are at higher risk than adolescents, but black individuals between 15 and 19 years of age are at higher risk than children, probably because few black children are exposed to private pools, and black adolescents swim with minimal instruction in poorly guarded water such as lakes, rivers, and ponds.[17] Pedestrian mishaps are more frequent in rural blacks whereas deaths from this type of injury occur more commonly in whites living in urban areas. Several theories have been advanced to explain the 50% higher incidence of pedestrian injuries in blacks: for instance,

FIG. 1-5. Age- and race-specific homicide rates in the United States in 1983. (Reproduced with permission from American Medical Association. JAMA 261:214,1989.)

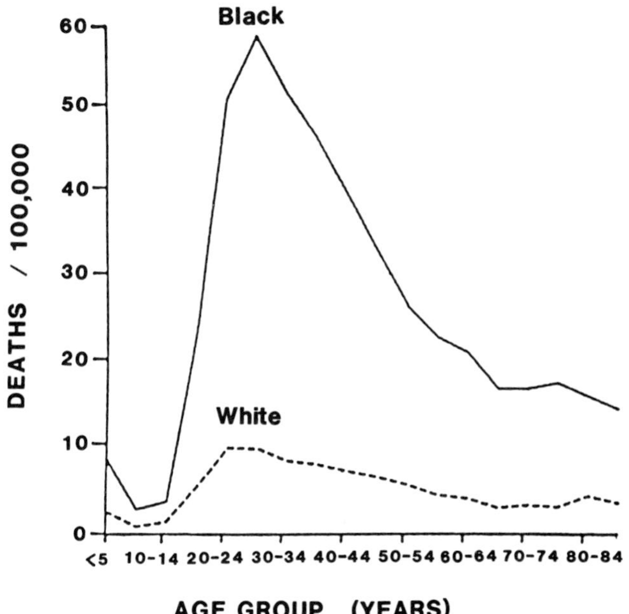

fewer blacks drive cars; and more blacks live in rural areas where driving laws are less strictly enforced, thus there is a higher average vehicle speed on impact. The racial difference in injury death rates seems to be related to socioeconomic factors; statistical data suggest that the discrepancy between blacks and whites disappears when rates are adjusted for income levels.[8]

There is also a geographical variation in injury-related deaths in the United States. For all types of injuries, death rate varies from 49 per 100,000 population in Connecticut and Rhode Island to 131 per 100,000 population in Alaska.[15] However, Baker and colleagues[16,17] hypothesized that comparisons made in this manner may lead to erroneous results because a very high or very low death rate in a small region of these states could not only alter overall mortality statistics but also prevent recognition of areas that have a higher than normal rate of mortality. They studied injury-specific trauma-related death rates for each county in the United States and concluded that the mortality from unintentional injuries is inversely related to the area's population density[16] (Fig 1-6). This is especially true for deaths of motor vehicle occupants.[17] For example, whereas the overall death rate from motor vehicle accidents is 18.7 per 100,000 population for the entire country, it is 2.5 per 100,000 in Manhattan, and 558 per 100,000 in Esmeralda County, Nev, which has 777 residents spread over 3587 square miles.[17] Population density has little influence on suicide rates which are high in Florida, the Appalachian Mountains, Nevada, New Mexico, and Wyoming.[16] The geographical distribution of homicides is affected by the income level of the region's population. These deaths are common in low-income areas, especially in the South, and in large cities.[16] Likewise, house fire deaths are common in low-income southern counties.[16] Drowning in childhood is most prevalent in Florida, the Pacific Coast region, Arizona, and northern New Mexico.[16,100] For other ages, death from this injury occurs most commonly in the vicinity of the Mississippi delta.[16]

Epidemiological data about nonfatal injuries are scarce. The trauma incidence in the Northeastern Ohio Trauma Study, a survey of a population of 2.2 million, was 197 per 1000 population.[19] Falls were the leading cause of injury (24.4%). Cutting or piercing (14.2%), striking with an object (13.8%), motor vehicle collisions (11.6%), overexertion/strain (8.2%), and assault (4.3%) were other common etiologies of

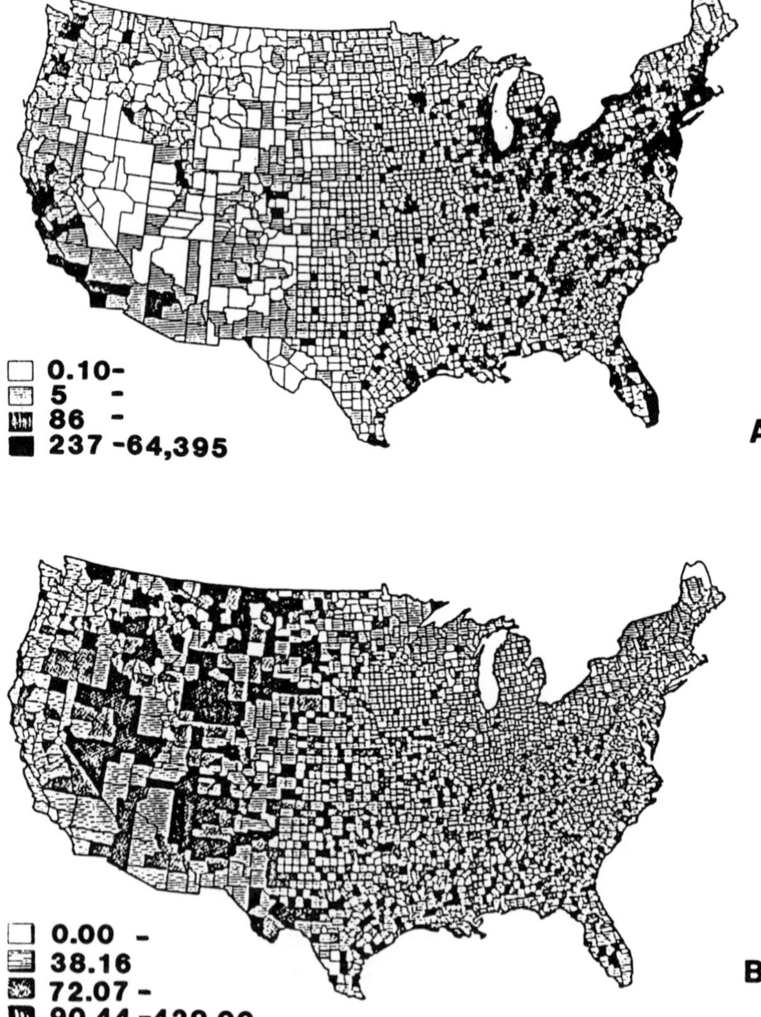


FIG. 1-6. A, Population density (per square mile) in each county of the United States; B, Unintentional injury death rates per 100,000 population in each county (1980). Note the increased rate of unintentional injury deaths in sparsely populated counties. (From Baker et al[16,17] with permission.)

trauma. Other mechanisms such as foreign bodies, nonmotorized road vehicles, poisoning, fires and flames accounted for 23.5% of the injuries. Not all of these mechanisms produced significant trauma morbidity and mortality. Falls, motor vehicle accidents, and assaults were the leading causes of serious injury and death.[19,54] Indeed, most trauma victims who require anesthetic management fall into these categories, along with firearm injuries, which have increased markedly in inner cities during recent years. The injury rates in the Northeastern Ohio Trauma Study were conservative estimates since this study considered only emergency department visits and ignored cases managed in other locations such as doctors' offices. Despite this underestimation, the rates of motor vehicle collisions and assaults were higher than those noted in official statistics.

Statistical data compiled by the NSC on the number of disabling injuries from motor vehicle, work, home, and public accidents during 1987 are shown in Table 1-3.[98] These figures do not include nonfatal intentional injuries. If it is assumed conservatively that disabling intentional injuries amount to one third of the 9 million produced by unintentional trauma, approximately 12 million disabling injuries occur in the United States every year. This figure is nearly one fifth of the estimated total of 62 million injuries that occur annually in the United States.[93]

If a total of 62 million people sustain injury every year,[93] and approximately 150,000 persons die from this cause, then for each injury-related death, there are 400 nonfatal injuries annually. Since one fifth of these injuries are disabling, for each injury-related death approximately 80 to 100 disabling injuries occur. Individuals between ages 15 and 34 are at highest risk of major injury because in this age range two major injury-producing mechanisms, motor vehicle accidents and assaults, are 2.5 and 4.4 times, respectively, more likely to occur than in the remaining age groups.[55] Between 18 and 24, the likelihood of sustaining major injury is even greater; injury from motor vehicles is 3.1 times and from assaults 4.8 times greater than in the low-risk population.[55] Until age 55, injury rates are higher in males than in females. Above this age the difference disappears.[54] About 5% of injured patients seen in the emergency department require admission to the hospital for further care, although this rate increases in the elderly; the rate is 21% in persons between ages 65 and 74 and 34% in those older than 75.[54]

In the Northeastern Ohio Trauma Study, the overall hospital admission rate for motor vehicle trauma was higher than that for nontransport injuries. This difference, however, disappeared for patients between age 34 and 65, and in fact, in those above age 65 the admission rate from nontransport injuries was higher. Although there are no large-scale data about what percentage of patients admitted to trauma services requires emergency surgery, and some variation exists among surgical departments in selection of operative versus conservative management, it is our experience that no more than 40 to 50% of admitted trauma patients require emergency surgery. The introduction of computed tomography (CT) scanning into clinical practice has reduced the rate of exploratory surgery for trauma. Of course, any conservative management policy applies only to hemodynamically stable patients with clinically equivocal injuries in certain anatomic regions (eg, neck or abdomen). Patients with hemodynamic instability generally need immediate operations.

It is difficult to predict how the epidemiology of trauma will change during the last decade of 20th century. During the past few years some governmental efforts to identify and prevent the principal causes of trauma have developed. In addition, important changes in trauma demographics are likely to occur by 1995. By the middle of the 1990s a population increase of 21 million (about 8%) compared with 1980 is expected.[55] This will almost certainly result in an increase in the absolute number of traumatic injuries even though no change or a decrease in the trauma rate may be noted. A more important change in demographics is that the size of the high-injury risk cohort (15 to 34 years) will decrease by 8.2%, and that of individuals above 65 years old will increase 18.5% by 1995 and will continue to increase for at least 25 more years.[55] The fraction of children less than 13 years old will transiently increase by 10% toward the middle of 1995 but will decrease to below its current size after that.[55] These demographic changes, together with active accident prevention measures, may make it safe to predict that the occurrence of trauma, and especially of major injury, will decrease. However, there are other forces that may prove these predictions inaccurate. As will be discussed below, the incidence of firearm injuries in inner cities has been increasing steadily over the past decade. The majority of these injuries is sustained by 15- to 24-year-old blacks and Hispanics who live below the poverty level. The size of this group is increasing at a higher rate than the rest of the population. In fact it has been estimated that in 1990 30% of the population under the age of 20 will be black or Hispanic, and 20% of youth will live at or below the poverty level.[23] If measures for prevention of firearm injuries are not taken, the increase in injuries in this population may offset or even exceed the decrease due to the expected decline

TABLE 1-3 The Number of Disabling Injuries That Occurred in Motor Vehicle, Work, Home, and Public Accidents in 1987*

| SEVERITY OF DISABLING INJURY | MOTOR VEHICLE | WORK | HOME | PUBLIC | TOTAL |
|---|---|---|---|---|---|
| Permanent impairment | 150,000 | 70,000 | 80,000 | 60,000 | 350,000 |
| Temporary total disability | 1,700,000 | 1,700,000 | 3,000,000 | 2,200,000 | 8,400,000 |
| Total | 1,800,000 | 1,800,000 | 3,100,000 | 2,300,000 | 8,800,000 |

* Totals do not add up because of rounding of figures. (From the National Safety Council.[95–98])

in the size of the high-risk age groups. A constant increase in terrorism-related injuries has also been noted throughout the world. It is likely that terrorist attacks may take place in the United States and increase traumatic injuries and death. The impact of an increasing population of elderly on the incidence of traumatic injuries is also difficult to predict. Currently this group comprises 12% of the population but accounts for only 3 to 4% of trauma admissions. Thus, this demographic change is likely to reduce traumatic injuries. However, the rate of decline may be less than that predicted from current rates. Falls and motor vehicle-related injuries are not uncommon in the elderly and may be an important source of trauma when the expected increase in this age group occurs. One important effect of an increased number of elderly trauma victims will be on health care economics, which is discussed in a later section.

## THE EPIDEMIOLOGY OF SPECIFIC MECHANISMS OF INJURY

The epidemiology of specific types of injury varies from the general aspects discussed above. In 1979 the nation's health was reviewed, and goals for 1990 were established for prevention and control of various diseases.[106] Nine of these objectives addressed specific injuries. In this section we will discuss injuries that are not only of public health importance but also, because of their prevalence, are encountered frequently by anesthesiologists.

### *Motor Vehicle Accidents*

Despite the recent increase in firearm injuries, motor vehicle accidents remain the leading mechanism of fatal trauma and the fourth most common cause of nonfatal injury in the United States; they produce 40,000 to 45,000 deaths and 4 to 5 million injuries every year.[15,19,38] Motor-vehicle-related mortality represents nearly 35% of all deaths from injury.[15] The 1978 motor vehicle fatality rate of 23.6 per 100,000 decreased to 19.6 per 100,000 in 1984. The objective of an 18.0 per 100,000 fatality rate in 1990 is expected to be met[78] (Fig 1-7, A). In children under age 15, motor vehicle accidents (MVAs) claimed 4209 lives in 1978 (9.0 per 100,000 children) but only 3106 (6.6 per 100,000 children) in 1985.[94,134] The 1990 goal of 5.5 per 100,000 should thus be attainable[78] (Fig 1-7, B). Males between 15 and 44 years are at highest risk of motor vehicle-related injury. Injury and fatality rates per passenger mile are highest between ages 16 and 24 and above 70.[8,74] Approximately 60% of MVA-related deaths occur during the night and 40% during the day. Many MVAs cause pedestrian injuries, which are included in MVA statistics. Automobiles are the principal cause of MVAs and constitute 60% of all vehicles involved in fatal crashes and 75% of those in nonfatal crashes.[67] The second most common vehicles in-

FIG. 1-7. Death rates by various types of injury from 1970 to 1984. The horizontal line on each graph represents the national 1990 objective for mortality rate from each mechanism of trauma. (Reproduced with permission from American Medical Association. JAMA 259:2069,1988.)

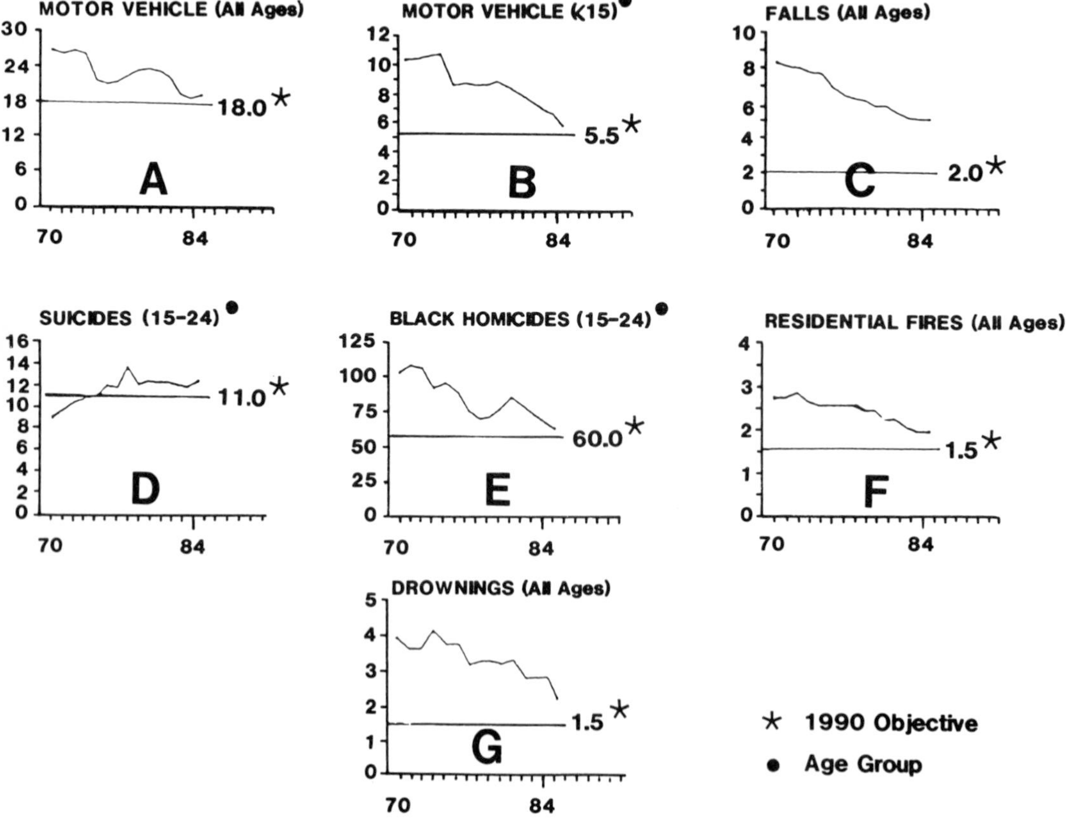

volved in both fatal and nonfatal accidents are trucks, accounting for 17% of MVA-related deaths and 19% of nonfatal injuries.[67] Motorcycles offer little protection to their riders; therefore the likelihood of sustaining major injury and death from motorcycle accidents is far greater than that caused by other vehicles. The death rate from motorcycle accidents is 35 per 100 million miles of travel, whereas that from all motor vehicles is 2.5 per 100 million miles of travel.[59,67] The number of patients who died in motorcycle accidents was 4423 in 1985[52]: nearly one motorcycle-related death for every 10 MVA fatalities. In addition there are approximately 90 frequently serious nonfatal injuries from motorcycle accidents for every fatality caused by this mechanism.[18] Mopeds are becoming increasingly popular; in 1979 the US Department of Transportation predicted that an estimated 2.5 million mopeds would result in approximately 1000 fatalities and 10,000 serious injuries every year[81] since these vehicles are no safer than motorcycles.[87] Although they are nonmotorized, bicycles cannot be ignored. It is estimated that over 78 million people and over 90% of children between the ages of 6 and 16 ride a bicycle.[72] More than half of the 1000 to 1300 deaths that result each year from injuries sustained by bicycle riders occur in children.[72,137] In the Northeastern Ohio Trauma Study pedal cycle injuries occurred primarily among youngsters and teenagers, raising the hospital admission rate of this population.[18] Head injury is the most common cause of death in bicycle accidents; its occurrence can be reduced by enforcing the use of helmets.[72,127,137]

Three predisposing factors—human, vehicular, and environmental—determine the severity of injuries from MVAs.[105] Each of these factors has a different implication during the precrash, crash, and postcrash phases of the accident. For instance, we have discussed the regional variation in incidence and mortality rate: the mortality from motor vehicle accidents is highest in areas in which the density of population is low and lowest in regions in which the density of population is high.[17] The significance of this fact for the precrash phase is that in low-density areas, poor road conditions and high travel speeds may predispose to the high rate of MVAs. In the crash phase, a low rate of seat belt use is common. Following the accident, the lack of a nearby trauma center may result in delay of acute care and thus a greater possibility of mortality. In this discussion we will review only the human factors, which we feel are the ones most relevant to anesthetic practice.

Preaccident alcohol use not only by the motor vehicle driver but also by involved pedestrians or cyclists is an important risk factor in MVA. In NHTSA statistics, a fatal accident is considered alcohol related if the blood alcohol concentration (BAC) of the person(s) primarily responsible for the accident is greater than 0.01% (10 mg/dL) and alcohol intoxication related if the BAC is greater than 0.1% (100 mg/dL).[75] Blood alcohol levels above 0.01% predispose to crash involvement by impairing driving ability; the risk of accidents increases with increasing BAC.[105] In 1987 23,360 persons, three quarters of whom were males, died from alcohol-related or alcohol intoxication-related MVAs, resulting in 783,304 YPLL.[75] In 1986 44.5% of all MVA-related YPLL occurred in alcohol-intoxicated persons; this, together with alcohol-related MVA YPLL, accounted for 6.8% of the total YPLL in the United States.[75] Alcohol use may also increase the severity of damage, particularly in central nervous system injury.[40,136] In the postcrash phase, alcohol may contribute to increasing the risks of injury because it adds diagnostic and treatment problems.[105]

Several measures have been taken during the past decade to reduce alcohol-related or alcohol intoxication-related MVAs and thus the resulting injuries and fatalities. These include raising the minimum drinking age to 21, active search for drunk drivers by traffic departments, applying severe penalties, and campaigns against drunk driving by various groups (eg, Students Against Drunk Driving, Mothers Against Drunk Driving, television programs). Many states have participated in these programs and note a significant reduction in MVA fatalities.[45] Nationally an overall 17% reduction in alcohol-related MVA fatalities and a 34% reduction in teenage MVA fatalities have been recorded between 1982 and 1987.[75] However, in certain groups such as motorcycle drivers, pedestrians, and drivers of ages 25 to 34, the reduction in alcohol use has had little effect on the incidence of fatal crashes.[75] Anesthetic problems in alcohol-intoxicated trauma victims are discussed in chapter 8.

Apart from alcohol, various drugs including minor tranquilizers, narcotics, amphetamines, barbiturates, marijuana, and cocaine are also likely to be detected in the blood of MVA crash victims. Whether these drugs contribute to the occurrence of MVAs is not clearly established.[105] Postcrash phase adverse effects of these drugs are also discussed in Chapter 8.

It is reasonable to assume that drivers with certain chronic conditions such as diabetes, epilepsy, cardiovascular disease, or visual field loss are more likely to be involved in MVAs. The available data suggest some contribution of these conditions to fatal and nonfatal MVAs, but the magnitude of the problem appears to be much less than that caused by alcohol.[105]

Since 1985, many states have implemented safety belt and child restraint laws, resulting in a reduction in fatality, injury severity, and child mortality from this measure alone.[29,34,64,103,120,133] Injuries of the abdominal aorta and cervical spine, for instance, may result from the safety belt itself, particularly when it is used improperly, but the number of persons saved from death and severe injuries far outweighs those suffering safety belt-specific trauma.[114] As we mentioned earlier, national statistical data for 1988 and 1989 are expected to show a reduction of MVA fatalities on the order of 20 to 25% as a result of more effective restraints in vehicles. Not all restraint systems work equally well. In order of increasing effectiveness, front seat occupant restraint systems can be ranked as follows: lap belts, air bags, automatic belts, lap/shoulder belts, air bags with lap belts, and air bags with lap/shoulder belts.[105] Although some European automobile manufacturers have included air bags in their products, resistance by American companies has delayed their use in this country. Some new models of American cars are now equipped with this safety system.

Among postcrash risk factors, advanced age has been proven to increase morbidity and mortality. However, this is not specific for MVA-related trauma and, as we mentioned, age affects the results of all types of injuries. Shock, head injury, age of 80 or older, cardiac and pulmonary complications, and ventilator dependence further increase risk in the elderly and are predictors of mortality.[46,63,104] Of course preexisting chronic diseases also increase postcrash morbidity and mortality as they do after other types of trauma (see Chapter 8).

### *Falls*

In the Northeastern Ohio Trauma Study, 25% of those who required emergency department care after trauma sustained their injuries because of falls.[19] Approximately 12 million persons are injured annually by falling. In 1978 falls accounted for a death rate of 6.2 per 100,000 population.[78] A decrease to 5.1 per 100,000 was noted in 1984 (11,600 deaths nationally),[78] but with such a slow rate of decline, it will be impossible to meet the 1990 objective of no more than 2 deaths per 100,000 population for this type of trauma (Fig 1-7, C). The death rate for persons under 65 was 1.5 per 100,000 in 1984, well under the 1990 goal.[78] In elderly persons mortality from falls is much higher, 10.2 per 100,000 for 65- to 74-year-olds and 147 per 100,000 for persons 85 years of age or older.[78] The overall rate of death and disability from falls will probably remain unchanged or increase in the future because of the expected 18% increase in the elderly population between 1995 and 2025.[55]

### *Suicides*

Suicide is the 10th leading cause of death in the United States, claiming nearly 30,000 lives annually since 1980.[14] The suicide rate varies significantly with age, sex, and race. It is very low under age 15, but a doubling of the suicide rate in the 10- to 14-year-old age group was noted between 1980 and 1985.[134] In males the rate increases from 15 to 24 years of age, followed by a slight decline until age 34. Between the ages of 15 and 34 suicide is the third leading cause of death, following unintentional injury and homicide.[14] A second increase results in the highest male suicide rate between ages 50 and 75. In females the rate increases until age 45 to 50 and then gradually declines. White males have the highest suicide rates at all ages; suicide is the seventh leading cause of death in this population.[14] They are followed by black and other males, white females, and black and other females. The suicide rate is 3 times greater in males (white or black) than in females.[75] Interestingly females, despite attempting suicide 4 to 5 times more frequently, are 4 times less likely to die than males.[23] Overall less than 10% of suicide attempts actually result in death,[23] meaning that a significant number of patients injured from this cause require anesthetic care. Baker et al[16] determined injury-related death rates in each county of the United States and found that suicide was most common in Florida, the Appalachian Mountains, and many counties of Nevada, New Mexico, and Wyoming.

In 1984 suicide accounted for 645,680 YPLL before age 65.[77] Eighty-nine percent of this YPLL was attributable to suicide in white males (70%) and white females (19%).[77] It is disturbing that the death rate increased three times (from 4.06 per 100,000 to 12.9 per 100,000 population) in 15- to 24-year-olds between 1955 and 1985, and there is no reason to anticipate a decline in the forseeable future.[23,78] Thus, the 1990 objective of 11 per 100,000 population will obviously not be realized[78] (Fig 1-7, D).

The methods used in suicide attempts have changed since 1950. Poisons, which were used frequently for this purpose in the 1950s, have been replaced by firearms, which now account for about 60% of suicides in both males and females between 15 and 24 years of age.[77] The increase in the rate of successful suicides over the past 30 years is attributed to the use of guns, which are more lethal than any other method.[27] Another factor that may contribute to the increase in suicide rates in young adults is alcohol. Between 15 and 64% of attempts are associated with alcohol consumption, and 30 to 80% of suicide victims ingest alcohol before the attempt.[138] A threefold increase in the proportion of suicide victims with detectable blood alcohol concentrations was noted between the early 1970s and the 1980s in one region of Pennsylvania.[27]

### *Homicides*

In 1980 24,000 homicides and legal intervention deaths occurred in the United States.[13] Since then the number of homicides has been increasing steadily. Recent Federal Bureau of Investigation (FBI) data demonstrate a 5.9% increase in homicides between 1985 and 1987.[53] Although data for more recent years are not available, our experience in a large city trauma center indicates that a 10% increase in crime-related injury occurred from 1987 to the middle of 1989. Illicit drug-related disputes seem to be the major underlying reason for these homicides. It also appears that the military weapons now used by civilians in many regions of the country cause more severe and more often lethal injuries. In 1985 YPLL from homicides was 612,556, 5.2% of total YPLL in the United States.[76] This figure represents an increase of 44% in homicide attributable YPLL since 1968. Combined with a 25% decline in total YPLL during the same period, this increase resulted in doubling of homicide-caused YPLL as a proportion of total YPLL (from 2.7 to 5.2%) in the 18-year period[76] (Fig 1-8). Although reliable data regarding the incidence of nonfatal intentional interpersonal violence are lacking, it has been estimated that for each homicide, 100 persons have been injured.[76]

Homicides occur in low-income areas, especially in the southern states, and in large cities. In addition to the large southern cities, New York, Washington, DC, Baltimore, Philadelphia, Cleveland, Detroit, Los Angeles, and San Francisco have the highest homicide rates.[16] Baker at al[16] have noted that 10 low-population density, low-income New Mexico counties also had high homicide rates. Approximately three quarters of homicides occur among males. Homicide is the leading cause of injury deaths in children under 1 year of age.[134] In the group between 15 and 24 years of age homicide is the second leading cause of death, resulting in a death rate of 15.5 per 100,000 in 1980.[23] Among black males in this age group homicide is the leading cause of death and claimed 70.7 lives per 100,000 in 1978 and 61.5 lives per 100,000 in 1984.[78] Based on these figures the 1990 national objective of homicide-related death rate in 15- to 24-year-old blacks of 60 per 100,000 will probably be met[78] (Fig. 1-7, E). Overall, blacks have a 5.2 times greater chance of dying from homicide than

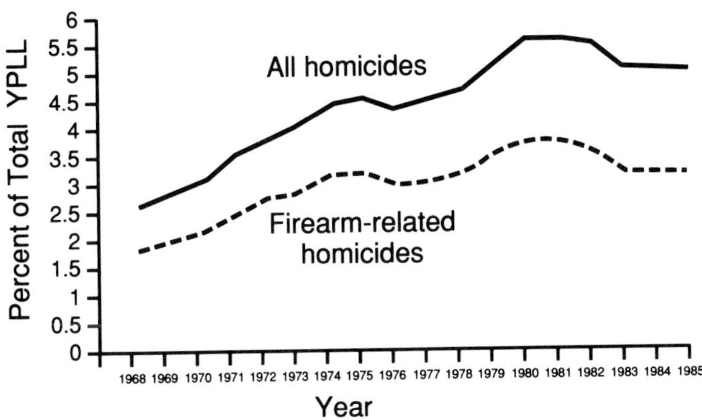


FIG. 1-8. Percent of total years of potential life lost before age 65 from homicides and firearm-related homicides in the United States between 1968 and 1985. (Reproduced with permission from American Medical Association. JAMA 260:2021,1988.)

whites.[74] Alcohol intake is a contributing factor in the occurrence of homicides.[138]

Firearms are the principal weapons used in homicides; 60% of murders are committed by firearms and explosives.[77] Sharp instruments, which in general produce less damage than firearms, are used less frequently and mainly by females.[77] Firearms are second only to motor vehicles as a cause of traumatic death. Annually about 32,000 deaths from suicide (17,000), homicide (12,000), unintentional injury (2000), legal intervention (250), or undetermined intent (500) are caused by these weapons.[78,140]

The easy access to guns in the United States appears to contribute to the high rate of homicide. An interesting study analyzing the risk of robberies, burglaries, assaults, and homicides found that the risk of death from homicide was 4.8 times higher in Seattle, Wash. than in Vancouver, British Columbia, despite similar occurrence rates of other criminal activities.[121] In terms of demographic makeup, enforcement of firearm regulations, and, as demonstrated, criminal activity rate, these two cities are fairly comparable, but in Vancouver ownership and use of handguns are regulated more strictly, and gun ownership is thus less prevalent than in Seattle.[121] The results of this scientifically rigorous although preliminary study suggest that restrictive gun control laws may be effective in reducing homicide rates. This measure may also help reduce the nearly 2000 deaths, including those of 300 children, that occur annually from unintentional firearm injuries.[78]

### *Burns*

In 1978 6000 persons died from fires and burns in the United States.[11] This number decreased gradually to 5010 in 1984.[79] However, the actual number of deaths from this cause is higher since these figures do not include fatalities from 500 arsons and numerous fires following motor vehicle and airplane accidents.[11] It is estimated that for each fatal burn, 200 nonfatal injuries occur every year.[11] Although most of these injuries are minor, nearly 10% of these patients (approximately 100,000) require prolonged hospital admission and costly medical-surgical care.[11] House fires are responsible for about 90% of burn mortality and morbidity.[79] In 1978 5401 deaths from burns resulted from this mechanism. In 1984 this number decreased 20% to 4461. The 1990 goal of 4500 annual deaths from fires in the home was thus reached by 1984 (Fig 1-7, F). Southern states have the highest rate of residential fire deaths; lower rates occur, respectively, in the Midwest, Northeast and West.[8,16,79] For all geographical areas, deaths from fires are most common in the winter and least common in summer.[79] Children and elderly individuals sustain burn injuries more frequently than individuals in the remaining age groups. Males are at higher risk than females, and mortality is higher in blacks than in whites.[74] Death from residential fires is twice as common in black males as in black females, and three and five times more common than in white males and white females, respectively.[74] Reference has already been made in the general epidemiology section to some of the factors involved in these differences. Cigarettes and alcohol are also important causes of house fires[8]; in the most common scenario an inebriated male falls asleep in bed while smoking. This mechanism is responsible for over 1500 deaths and 7000 injuries annually in the United States.[25]

The decreased mortality from this injury results mainly from the increased use of residential smoke detectors during the past decade. Recently a 3-year study by the federal government demonstrated the feasibility of a fire-safe cigarette,[25] which may help reduce cigarette-related injuries in the future. Advances in medical management of major thermal injury may also have contributed to this increase in survival rates. In 1458 patients with comparable burn size and severity, Merrell et al[88] reported a survival rate of 59% in the period between 1978 and 1981 and of 77% between 1982 and 1986.

### *Drowning and Near-drowning*

Drowning is the third most common cause of unintentional traumatic mortality in the general population and the second leading cause of death and YPLL in children.[12,102] In 1978, 1242 persons drowned in boating accidents, and 5784 persons during non–boating-related activities.[78] This was reduced to a total of 5316 by 1985.[98] The overall death rate from this cause was 3.2 per 100,000 population in 1978 and decreased to 2.3 per 100,000 in 1984, a rate that is unfortunately not expected to improve to the 1990 objective of 1.5 per 100,000 for this injury[78] (Fig 1-7 G). Alcohol intoxication is a frequent predisposing factor in boating-related drownings; 30 to 60% of victims have blood alcohol concentrations above 100 mg/dL.[128] It is estimated that near-drowning is 500 to 600 times more frequent than drowning.[102] About 60% of adolescent and adult drownings occur in public places such as lakes, ponds, and the sea.[98] For children less than 5 years old, private swimming pools represent a major hazard. Approximately 300 to 450 children die every year in this setting.[78,98] In Los Angeles alone, 1587 drownings occurred between 1976 and 1984; 44.5% of these deaths, mostly of children, occurred in private pools.[100] Almost one third of near-drowning survivors and most of those who ultimately die sustain moderate to severe neurological damage.[102]

### *Occupational Injuries*

There is considerable discrepancy among the estimates issued by various agencies regarding work-related injuries and deaths. Of the three agencies that collect and analyze statistical data on occupational fatalities, the Bureau of Labor Statistics estimated 3740; the National Center for Health Statistics (NCHS), 4960; and the National Safety Council (NSC), 11,500 deaths from workplace accidents during 1984.[123] These differences are attributable to differences in definitions and methodologies used by each agency. At any rate, according to NSC statistics, there were 1.8 million work-related disabling injuries in 1987, resulting in 70,000 people with permanent disability.[98] Most of these unintentional injuries and deaths result from accidents in agriculture, mining, construction, transportation, and public utilities.[98,123]

## ECONOMIC IMPACT OF TRAUMA

The economic cost of trauma is enormous and increasing steadily. Munoz,[92] after making some assumptions and adjustments, estimated that in 1982 trauma cost the nation $61 billion—6.9% of the total health care cost and 2.3% of the gross national product for that year. Data from the NSC, however, suggest that total cost of trauma to the nation far exceeds this estimate: even excluding the cost of intentional injuries, which comprises a significant portion of the total, the bill resulting from accidents alone was $96.9 billion in 1984 and 133.2 billion in 1987[95–98] (Table 1-4). However, these figures overestimate the costs of traumatic injury and death since they include the cost of property damage from motor vehicle accidents and fires.

When estimating the economic effect of a disease it is important to separate direct and indirect costs. Direct expenditures are treatment related: hospital charges; professional fees; rehabilitation expenses; and expenses of home health care, special aids, prostheses, medical equipment, and prescribed drugs. Indirect cost mainly includes wage loss and property damage. The insurance administration cost, the difference between premiums paid to insurance companies and claims paid out by them, may be considered either indirect or direct. It is largely the direct costs of trauma which can be affected by physicians. Therefore, the remaining discussion will focus on this component.

According to Rice et al,[110] direct health care expenses resulting from injuries and poisoning totaled $19 billion in 1980, ranking fourth behind expenditures for cardiovascular diseases ($32 billion), gastrointestinal diseases ($32 billion), and psychiatric disorders ($20 billion). Analyzing only the cost of motor vehicle accident-related injuries, Hartunian et al[60] showed that direct personal health care costs for this type of trauma ($6 billion) ranked just behind the cost of cancer ($10 billion) in 1980. These studies, however, calculated only the immediate direct costs of trauma. Many injured patients require prolonged care eg, rehabilitation, rehospitalization, and outpatient follow-up. MacKenzie et al[83] took these costs into consideration for 487 surviving trauma patients over a 1-year period. They demonstrated that the cost per patient is proportional to the severity of injury and varies between $8100 and $105,000. Severe head and/or spinal cord injuries involved the highest expense per patient, but extremity injuries, although incurring a relatively low per capita cost, consumed 43% of total expenditure because of their frequency.[83] Extrapolating their data to all 15- to 45-year-old trauma patients discharged from Maryland acute care hospitals within a 1-year period, these authors[83] estimated that the total direct cost of trauma in Maryland in 1983 was $109 million. Every year the NSC estimates the nationwide direct costs of accidental injuries and fatalities. Although these figures do not include the cost of intentional injuries, they do reflect the rate of increase in medical expenditure for trauma over the years[95–98] (Table 1-5).

There seems to be a difference between the direct costs of unintentional and of intentional injuries. MacKenzie et al[83] concluded that the average charges associated with intentional injuries were considerably less per patient ($17,600) than those resulting from unintentional trauma ($30,000 to 40,000). Although population-based data comparing medical costs of intentional and unintentional injuries are lacking, it has become clear that while intentional injuries may be less

TABLE 1-4. Total Cost of Accidents from 1984 through 1987

| YEAR | TYPE OF ACCIDENT | COST ($ BILLION)* | |
|---|---|---|---|
| 1984 | All accidents | 96.9 | |
| | Motor vehicle accidents | | 47.6 |
| | Work accidents | | 33.0 |
| | Home accidents | | 10.8 |
| | Public accidents | | 7.2 |
| 1985 | All accidents | 107.3 | |
| | Motor vehicle accidents | | 48.6 |
| | Work accidents | | 37.3 |
| | Home accidents | | 14.0 |
| | Public accidents | | 9.4 |
| 1986 | All accidents | 118.0 | |
| | Motor vehicle accidents | | 57.8 |
| | Work accidents | | 34.8 |
| | Home accidents | | 16.0 |
| | Public accidents | | 11.3 |
| 1987 | All accidents | 133.2 | |
| | Motor vehicle accidents | | 64.7 |
| | Work accidents | | 42.4 |
| | Home accidents | | 16.7 |
| | Public accidents | | 11.5 |

* Dollar figures include the cost of death and disabling injuries as well as property damage from vehicular accidents and fires. (From the National Safety Council.[95–98])

TABLE 1-5. Direct Costs (Medical Expenses) of Accidents from 1984 through 1987 in the United States*

| YEAR | DIRECT COST ($ BILLION) |
|---|---|
| 1984 | 13.8 |
| 1985 | 17.8 |
| 1986 | 20.5 |
| 1987 | 23.2 |

* Estimated cost includes only the medical cost of accidental (unintentional) injuries. (From the National Safety Council.[95–98])

costly, they incur a great economic burden on hospitals, physicians, and society. Analyzing the cost of hospitalization for firearm injuries in San Francisco, Martin and coworkers[86] estimated a yearly expenditure of $429 million nationwide, which may actually approach $1 billion when the other direct costs are added—ambulance services, physician fees, readmissions, ambulatory follow-up visits, physical therapy, rehabilitation services, and long-term care. More importantly, nearly 85% of this cost is paid by public sources, that is, by taxpayers' money. In an analysis from Seattle, Wash. Luna and coworkers[82] calculated that the average charge for a victim of nonaccidental injury was $13,000. Nearly 75% of these patients were unemployed, 70% did not have private insurance, and over 35% had no government coverage at the time of injury. Thus, even 6 months after hospitalization, 35% of all expenditures had not been reimbursed. A similar situation is also common in certain victims of unintentional injury. For instance, motorcycle trauma victims require prolonged and intensive medical services and consume a disproportionately high fraction of medical resources.[6,111] Yet in 1986 46% of the motorcycle accident victims admitted to one medical center were uninsured.[6] In a more recent analysis, 65% of the charges for hospitalized motorcycle injury victims were paid by public funds, Medicaid being the primary third-party payer.[111] These figures underscore the importance of reducing both the incidence and the severity of these injuries by passage of gun control and helmet laws, for which substantial reluctance and resistance have been expressed by lawmakers and a certain segment of the public.

Another financial disadvantage for hospitals and physicians caring for trauma victims has been created by the prospective payment system in which Medicare reimbursement is made according to diagnosis-related group (DRG) methodology. Since many trauma victims require prolonged hospitalization and expensive medical services, reimbursement by this method often falls far short of actual cost, resulting in financial losses.[47,71,126] The negative financial impact of this system, however, is not critical in most centers because most trauma victims are young, and their costs are not borne by Medicare. A severe economic crisis would be inflicted on all trauma centers in the future if other third-party payers would base their reimbursement rate on DRGs. In some states, for instance, New Jersey, all reimbursement for inpatient care is administered by DRG methodology; this has produced a severe drain on the financial resources of trauma centers.[116] The financial disincentives associated with this system can thus potentially reduce the quality and availability of trauma care.

## CURRENT STATUS OF TRAUMA CARE

Trauma is a multisystem disease, and as such its overall care requires a team effort involving not only physicians from various disciplines but also a large variety of nonphysicians including nurses, technicians, engineers, legislators, scientists, and laymen. A rapid and continuing improvement in the medical aspects of trauma care over the past 3 decades should without doubt be credited largely to surgeons. The efforts of the Committee on Trauma of the American College of Surgeons (ACS), the American Association for the Surgery of Trauma (AAST), and the American Burn Association (ABA) have contributed greatly to the organizational, educational, research, and patient care aspects of trauma. Regionalization of trauma care, continually updated guidelines for prehospital and hospital care of the injured, and development of trauma severity scores are only some of the areas in which these organizations and their members have contributed. It is also important to realize that two important publications during the past 25 years have played a key role in improvement of trauma care in this country. The first is the white paper, "Accidental Death and Disability: The Neglected Disease Of Modern Society," by the National Research Council committees on shock, on trauma, and on anesthesia, published in 1966.[37] This document, the details of which are discussed in Chapter 29, identified several problem areas such as lack of public awareness, neglect of emergency medical services, a lack of research and thus inadequate data, inadequate medical facilities, and an absence of organized trauma care systems. Some of the recommendations made in this document were implemented to varying degrees in the 1970s. The second publication was "Injury in America" by the National Research Council/National Academy of Sciences, issued in 1985.[38] This document, with many similarities to the one published 20 years before, enumerated existing problems in trauma care but focused on the need for research in five principal areas; epidemiology, prevention, biomechanics, treatment, and rehabilitation. As we mentioned earlier, the recommendation to establish an injury control center within the CDC was realized shortly after publication of this document. It is obvious that despite rapid progress there is an urgent need for further improvement in various areas of trauma care if the unacceptably high morbidity and mortality from injuries are to be reduced. It is appropriate to discuss the current status of each of these areas and point out briefly where and how these improvements can be made.

### ACCESS TO CARE

In any accident for which witnesses are available to call for help, access to care is generally prompt. Usually police and an ambulance are dispatched concomitantly so that care delays do not occur. The problem arises when the accident occurs in places where it is not witnessed, such as rural highways, or in areas in which telephones are sparsely placed. In West Germany this problem is partly solved by placement of special telephones on the autobahns. A better system is used in Australia where a signal is broadcast automatically immediately after a crash from a transmitter located in the vehicle.[130]

## PREHOSPITAL CARE AND TRANSPORT

Improvements in vehicle design, in training of paramedics, and in medical control of ambulances are among the important factors that help save the lives of many trauma victims. However, there is continuing controversy as to whether advanced trauma life support should be administered on the scene or whether the victim should be transported to the nearest hospital immediately without these measures. There are data supporting both of these views. It appears, however, that in urban areas in which transport time is less than 10 minutes, lengthy on-the-scene measures are not warranted.

Helicopters have proven useful in transport of trauma patients from remote areas. Inspired by the benefits of helicopter transport in the Korean and Vietnam Wars, Neel[99] suggested in 1968 that helicopters could also be used in civilian emergency health care. In many regions of the country hospital-based and public helicopter services are now established as an integral part of the emergency medical service (EMS). They are equipped with necessary equipment, supplies, and drugs; and their medical team, which may consist of two nurses, one nurse and one physician, or one nurse and one paramedic, is capable of performing resuscitative procedures. Most physicians feel that the quality of care delivered by the helicopter crew is superior to that given by most ground transport teams.[90] Air transport may be used to carry patients from the accident scene to a trauma center or between hospitals.[90] In areas far from a trauma center, the victim is first transported to a nearby hospital for stabilization and then transferred to the regional trauma center.[91,119] There is no doubt that air ambulances have substantial value in warfare, natural disasters, rural and wilderness rescues, and in interhospital transport of critically ill or injured patients, especially in rural areas. The better survival rates noted with air than with ground transfers may be a result not of shorter travel times but of more effective resuscitation.[91] The cost of aeromedical services is higher than that of ground transport; thus, the latter is preferable for transportation of patients with minor injuries.[90] Controversy surrounds the use of air ambulances in urban areas. Although some early studies demonstrated their value, it appears that the advantage gained in this setting is small except where traffic congestion delays the transfer unduly.[115] There has been ongoing publicity about the excessive number of fatal air ambulance accidents. With time and experience the number of these crashes will probably decrease.

## HOSPITAL CARE

As will be discussed in Chapter 29 the concept of regionalization of trauma care was born in the mid-1970s. Subsequently, certain hospitals in many states were designated as level I trauma centers, capable of optimal care of severely injured patients. Significant improvement in patient management and survival has been noted following implementation of these systems.[112,117,118] However, as of 1987, 29 states lacked a formal trauma center, and an additional 20 states had only certain components of a fully developed regionalized system.[130,139] This situation remained virtually unchanged in 1989. Numerous studies conducted before or in the beginning of the regionalization era demonstrated a preventable death rate of 30 to 35%.[28] It is quite possible that unnecessary mortality continues at this rate where proper regionalization is lacking.[130]

## RESEARCH IN TRAUMA

Trauma-related research is surrounded by several difficulties not present in most other areas of medicine. Most prominent of these is the paucity of available research funds despite the fact that trauma causes a greater loss of productive years of life than virtually any other disease. The 1983 federal expenditure for this purpose amounted to only about 10% of that allocated for cancer and less than 20% of that provided for cardiovascular diseases[8,38] (Fig 1-9). Although some efforts have been made to increase funds for trauma research, this discrepancy has remained essentially unchanged. In spite of this, the medical literature is saturated with trauma-related research papers. Most of this work, however, consists of surveys of small populations, retrospective reviews, and heavily biased patient comparisons. Scientifically rigorous and appropriately randomized multicenter clinical trials are rarely encountered. Restriction of funds is not the only factor creating this situation. The type and severity of injuries vary widely so that control of variables in the small number of patients treated in each institution is difficult.[130] The development of injury severity scoring systems has helped in making meaningful comparisons among patient groups in hospital-based injury research. However, the involvement of alcohol in nearly half of trauma patients introduces errors in patient assessment with these criteria.[135]

Hospital-based research is also hampered by other factors such as lack of appropriate technical personnel at night when the trauma service is most active and the difficulty of obtaining consent for a clinical study from severely injured patients. Laboratory research is also lacking because of inadequate funds and the scarcity of basic scientists among clinicians engaged in trauma care.[130] Clearly there is an urgent need for prioritized, well guided, organized, and meaningful trauma research. Reference has already been made to the five priority areas of research determined by the National Academy of Sciences Committee on Trauma in its 1985 report. In one of these areas—treatment—studies providing insight into shock, brain edema, injuries to various parts of the body, and testing of new therapeutic modalities should carry a high priority.[130]

Research on anesthesia for the injured patient has been long neglected. The vast majority of available data pertains to the pre- and postoperative phases; intraoperative anesthetic care has been virtually ignored. The effects of anesthetic agents and techniques, resuscitation methods, and patient monitoring on physiological parameters, complications, and outcome in various trauma states have been studied and documented inadequately at best. Encouragement by state and federal government agencies and determination and strong commitment by academic institutions are necessary to overcome these deficiencies in trauma research in the last decade of the 20th century.

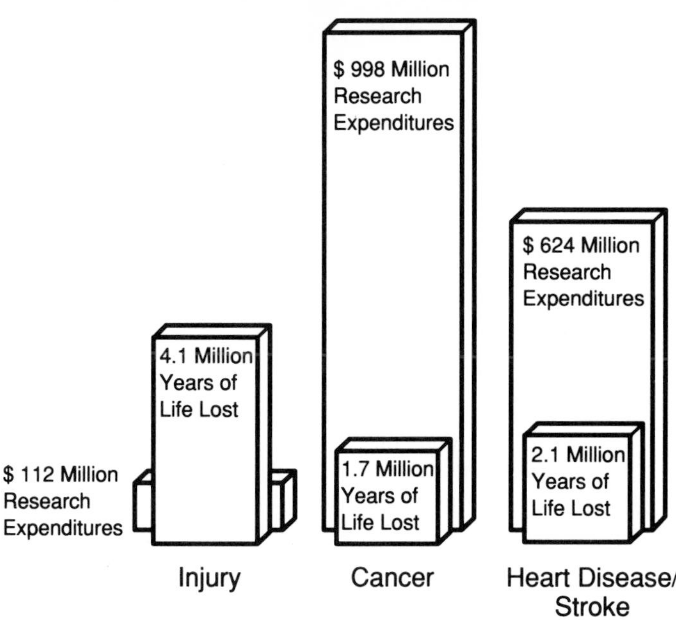


FIG. 1-9. Discrepancy between preretirement years of life lost and federal research expenditures for injury, cancer, and heart disease. (From the Committee on Trauma Research, National Research Council[38] with permission.)

## LONG-TERM CARE

Until recently little was known about the long-term quality of life after major trauma, and most evaluations of trauma care have been based on mortality rather than morbidity. In survivors, trauma can cause both physical and psychological impairment of long duration. In centers that manage injuries to all organ systems, approximately 6 to 27% of major trauma victims are restricted in their daily activities, and 25 to 40% cannot return to their usual work within 1 year[84,109] (Table 1-6). Head and spinal cord injuries result in the greatest functional impairment, followed by injuries of the extremities, especially the lower limbs.[84,109] Thoracoabdominal injuries, although producing severe physiological abnormalities and high mortality in the initial stages of trauma, do not usually cause long-term disability. The severity of injury also influences the ultimate degree of functional impairment.[84,109]

Factors that appear to have a positive effect on patients' return to their pretrauma employment are: higher level of education, white collar employment, higher preinjury income, and support from family and friends.[84] Intensive postinjury patient care was once thought to result in an increase in comatose patients who would potentially be a substantial burden on society. Experience proves otherwise. Most patients comatose from brain injury or hypoxia usually follow one of two paths: death within 6 months after being vegetative, or regaining conciousness within 6 months and returning to some sort of productive lives by 1 year.[84,109] Thus, their negative impact on health care costs is less than once anticipated. Unfortunately, the number of rehabilitation beds available for patients who may potentially recover from central nervous system or orthopedic injuries is substantially less than the actual need.[130] This is unfortunate because self-care and deinstitutionalization of these patients following rehabilitation and training can save 75 to 90% of the money spent for custodial care.[38] Some authors recommend establishment of centralized rehabilitation facilities for patients with central nervous system injuries, a system that is operating successfully in Israel.[130]

The long-term psychological consequences of trauma have also been studied during the past decade. One prospective trial from Sweden demonstrated a 22.4% incidence of psychiatric disorders after trauma.[85] Even when organic psychiatric disorders produced by head injury, alcoholism, and other causes were excluded, the incidence of mental disturbance was 16.4%. Depressive disorders were the most common abnormalities noted. Interestingly, however, many patients recovered with time so that the incidence of depression a few years after injury was only 9.6%, a rate similar to that following elective surgery for conditions other than trauma.[85] However, the incidence of psychiatric morbidity in individuals who experience the terror of combat or disasters is high, probably because the emotional stress in this situation lasts longer than in simple accidental injury.[108] Patients with head injuries have a high incidence of long-term behavioral abnormalities. In one retrospective study, 80% of head-injured patients had

TABLE 1-6. Percent of Patients with Various Degrees of Long-term Functional Recovery after Trauma in Two Recent Series

| | | ACTIVITY RESTRICTION AT 1 YEAR | | | FULL-TIME WORK | |
|---|---|---|---|---|---|---|
| AUTHOR | N* | *None* | *Moderate* | *Severe* | *1 year* | *3–4 years* |
| MacKenzie et al[84] | 479 | 57% | 16% | 27% | 57% | |
| Rhodes et al[109] | 302 | 83.1% | 11.3% | 5.6% | 75.3% | 85% |

* N represents number of patients.

borderline or abnormal neuropsychological testing that showed some correlation with the severity of injury. Associated spinal fracture, pupillary dysfunction, and signs of increased intracranial pressure after trauma were associated with long-term abnormalities in test results.[56]

Posttraumatic stress disorder is manifested by reexperiencing the trauma in dreams or thoughts, decreased or abolished responsiveness to events (numbing of responsiveness), and at least two of the following symptoms: sleep disturbance, hyperalertness, guilt, avoidance of activities prompting recall of the original stressful event, trouble in concentration, and worsening of symptoms by exposure to events resembling the original event. It was first recognized after the Vietnam War.[62,85] In fact the disorder is also called "the post-Vietnam syndrome." A presumption that this syndrome might also occur frequently after civilian accidents prompted an investigation of its prevalence in the general population and in individuals involved in various types of accidents. According to Helzer and his colleagues,[62] a history of posttraumatic stress disorder occurs in 1% of the general population. Civilians exposed to physical attack and those who were in the Vietnam War but were not wounded show a prevalence of 3.5%. The rate reaches 20% in veterans wounded in Vietnam. In a separate study, Malt[85] tested for this syndrome in patients who had been involved in accidents. Only 1 patient in a series of 107 suffered from the syndrome during a follow-up of 28 months, and its intensity had been reduced during a second examination 6 months later. In this group, anxiety disorders occurred in 4 patients, however they did not meet the criteria for posttraumatic stress disorder delineated in the *Diagnostic and Statistical Manual of Mental Disorders* (*DSM-III*) of the American Psychiatric Association.[4] Patients with posttraumatic stress disorder may occasionally present a challenge to the anesthesiologist; an anecdotal report described acute exacerbation of the syndrome after sedation with diazepam.[39] Aminophylline (1 mg/kg) can reverse this reaction, although a benzodiazepine antagonist (imidazopine, flumazenil) may be more effective.[39]

### PREVENTION

The principles of prevention of accidental injury and of anesthetic mishaps are similar; they both require establishment of automatic safety measures. Education is important but not as effective as built-in protection against hazards.[8] Significant progress has been made in this means of injury prevention during the past 50 years. Elevator accidents, which killed many people in the 1930s, rarely cause injuries today because of built-in safeguards and strict regulations. The carbon monoxide content of consumer natural gas is now below the lethal level; thus the number of intentional (suicide) and unintentional deaths from this cause has significantly decreased. Postcrash fires, which formerly caused significant mortality in potentially survivable helicopter accidents, now rarely occur because of a change in fuel systems in the 1970s. A long list of beneficial effects of automatic protection could be enumerated, including those developed with physician participation, for instance, spinal cord injury prevention, improvements in headgear, use of safety belts, and measures against drunk driving.

## THE ROLE OF THE ANESTHESIOLOGIST IN TRAUMA CARE

The anesthesiologist, with knowledge and skills in cardiovascular, respiratory, and central nervous system physiology; resuscitation techniques and critical care; and acute pain management, has a large role to play in the care of the injured patient. This is reflected in both local and nationwide health agencies' guidelines which require 24-hour in-house anesthesia coverage for level I trauma centers. The anesthesiologist's tasks are not limited to the operating room but begin in the emergency department and may continue well into the postoperative period. In fact, in some leading trauma centers, the anesthesiologist is charged with receiving the trauma patient from the ambulance.[58] In some localities, the responsibility of the anesthesiologist and intensivist extends to interhospital transport of the injured victim.[50] In many European countries, where physicians are involved in on-the-scene intervention and patient transport, anesthesiologists take an active part in prehospital care.[48,49,122] Within the hospital, the trauma victim is frequently taken to the radiology suite for CT scanning, arteriography, or embolization. Airway obstruction, hemodynamic abnormalities, or deterioration of cerebral function are not uncommon in this area and necessitate prompt intervention. Thus, in many centers, an anesthesiologist is in attendance while these procedures are performed.

Most patients who present with drug overdose, poisoning, accidental hypothermia, drowning, or burns and smoke inhalation do not require immediate surgery unless they have associated injuries. Yet an anesthesiologist is required for airway and ventilatory management in the emergency department or in the intensive care unit. Pain is a common complaint of the trauma victim and in some instances, such as chest injuries, it interferes with normal respiratory function. Many of these patients do not need surgery but do require effective pain control with techniques that the anesthesiologist is best able to manage.

Although many acute injuries require emergency intervention, definitive surgical treatment of some—for instance, maxillofacial and closed musculoskeletal injuries—can be delayed. This is especially true if there are concomitant injuries to vital organs, which require immediate surgery. Thus, prioritization, not only in management of injuries to individual organ systems but also in all other aspects of care, is a hallmark of trauma anesthesia and surgery. It must be emphasized that delay in surgical treatment of vital organ injuries due to lack of recognition or other reasons is the most important cause of preventable deaths from trauma.[28,44,112,117]

The terms *trauma anesthesia* and *emergency anesthesia* are often used interchangeably. This is appropriate only to a certain extent. In a busy trauma center a significant number of anesthetics are administered for elective surgical interventions. Some of these electively scheduled patients have underlying trauma-related complications such as acute respiratory distress syndrome, myocardial contusion, pericardial blood or effusion, deep vein thrombosis, fat embolism syndrome, sepsis, or renal failure, which require careful evaluation and optimization within a relatively short time before surgery. As emphasized in some of the chapters in this book, the anesthesiologist, as a consultant, has much to contribute to the perioperative care of these patients.

Specialization in this field of anesthesiology requires dedication, devotion, and sacrifice. As we have mentioned, a significant number of trauma patients are indigent and unable to pay for the medical services they receive. The description of trauma surgery by a surgeon several years ago is also true of anesthesia in this field: "Trauma anesthesia is no place for fat cats." Except for children, who are usually injured during the day, the majority of both intentional and unintentional injuries occur at night. Statistically, weekend and holiday nights are the busiest times in trauma centers. Although the incidence of intentional injuries does not generally vary with the seasons, unintentional injuries peak between June and January. Appropriate arrangements for additional anesthesia manpower based on this workload pattern may be necessary in some trauma centers. The demanding nature of anesthetic care for trauma requires assignment to each patient of at least two and sometimes three members of the anesthesia department. This, together with the shortage of anesthesia staff interested in trauma care, creates occasional manpower gaps in some centers. In many institutions, certified registered nurse anesthetists who are trained in trauma care are filling this need.

Two important subjects deserve mention in this section because they relate to anesthetic management of trauma: assessment of injury severity; and diagnostic, technical, and therapeutic challenges.

## ASSESSMENT OF INJURY SEVERITY

As a rule the type and severity of injury are the principal factors predicting morbidity and mortality. For instance, in one study the mortality rate of patients with severe head trauma was as high as 30% compared with a rate of 1% in those without severe brain injury.[20] Improvement in care seems to have had only a limited effect in reducing mortality following head injury.[20] Short- and long-term morbidity and mortality also increase with increasing severity of injuries to other body regions.[109] Although not clearly demonstrated, it is logical to expect that perianesthetic complications increase with increasing injury severity. Thus, an injury severity classification system may be expected to facilitate initial assessment of, and outcome prediction in, the traumatized patient.

Several scoring systems designed for this purpose correlate well with mortality. The Major Trauma Outcome Study collected data (severity scores, age, outcome, and length of hospital stay) from more than 100 institutions and periodically examined the relation between severity score and outcome in order to improve predictive ability of these indices. The data base currently includes information from more than 80,000 patients and the study is near completion according to Wayne S. Copes, PhD, director of the study. Several preliminary analyses of data show good correlation between injury severity and outcome.[31]

Depending on the criteria used, the various severity indices can be divided into two major categories: anatomically oriented and physiologically oriented. Anatomically oriented severity scales score each organ injury whereas physiologically oriented scales measure various physiological parameters (eg, pulse, blood pressure, motor response, and respiratory rate). In all systems the sum of assigned scores determines severity. It must be emphasized that the scaling systems, although capable of estimating probability of outcome, may not be accurate predictors in the individual patient. Neither type of system is designed as an assessment tool for individual patients. It is not known, for instance, whether a strong correlation exists between severity scores and perioperative complications. These scales were originally designed as research tools to provide meaningful comparisons between patient populations and for triage at the scene of a major accident, during a mass casualty, or possibly in the emergency department. Later, with pressing needs for evaluating trauma care both in and outside the hospital, they became important in quality assurance studies.[31]

Of the existing scoring systems, those based on anatomical location of the injury can be used only rarely during initial assessment of the trauma victim, since they are calculated retrospectively, after identification of the injury by surgery or autopsy, unless only superficial structures are involved. Some injuries may be identified by CT scanning or arteriography, but in severely injured patients time constraints may preclude these studies. The scoring systems based on physiological abnormalities are more amenable to initial assessment of the trauma victim.

Table 1-7 lists various scales designed during the past 20 years. In addition to these systems there are others designed to measure injury severity in specific populations, anatomical regions, or organs. These include the pediatric trauma score,[107,125] the penetrating abdominal trauma index (PATI),[89] and the penetrating cardiac trauma index (PCTI).[66] Of all these indices, the abbreviated injury scale (AIS),[2] injury severity score (ISS),[9,10] Glasgow coma scale (GCS),[124] and trauma score (TS)[42] are the most widely used.

### *Abbreviated Injury Scale*

This anatomical scale is derived by assigning a score of 1 through 6 to each of six body areas: head/neck, including the central nervous system; face; thorax; abdomen; extremities; and external. A score of 1 is assigned for a minor injury, 2 for a moderate, 3 for a severe but not life-threatening, 4 for a severe life-threatening, 5 for a critical, and 6 for a fatal injury to the specific region. Criteria for grading are defined in the AIS booklet first published by the American Association for Automotive Medicine in 1976 and revised in 1980 and 1985.[2] The AIS scale was initially applied only to blunt trauma, but it has since been expanded to include penetrating injuries. This scale, apart from being useless for preoperative assessment of injury severity, has several other drawbacks. First, it is time consuming. The AIS dictionary contains more than 1200 descriptions of injuries. This difficulty, however, has been overcome by the development of two condensed charts; one for blunt and another for penetrating trauma (Appendices 2 and 3).[35] Second, the AIS scores do not correlate well with disability or overall recovery.[31] Third, the scores assigned to each body system do not carry the same mortality risk. For instance, a score of 4 assigned to a head/neck injury is associated with a higher mortality than a score of 4 for external trauma.[31] Nevertheless, this scale is the basis for calculating

TABLE 1-7. Trauma Severity Scales Designed to Measure Injury Severity by Anatomical, Physiological, and Both Criteria*

| SCALE | TYPE OF CRITERIA | REFERENCE |
|---|---|---|
| Abbreviated injury scale (AIS) | A | American Association for Automotive Medicine[2] |
| Injury severity score (ISS) | A | Baker et al[9,10] |
| Anatomic index (AI) | A | Champion et al[33] |
| Glasgow coma scale (GCS) | P | Teasdale and Jennet[124] |
| Trauma score (TS) | P | Champion et al[32] |
| CRAMS scale | P | Gormican[57] |
| Trauma index | AP | Kirkpatrick and Youmans[69] |
| Modified trauma index | AP | Ogawa and Sugimoto[101] |
| Illness injury severity index (IISI) | AP | Bever and Veenker[21] |
| Hospital trauma index | AP | ACS[3] |

* The abbreviations used are: A, anatomical criteria; P, physiological criteria; AP, anatomical and physiological criteria.

the injury severity score, another anatomical scoring system.[9,10]

### *Injury Severity Score*

Described first by Baker and colleagues[9,10] in 1974, this system assigns a numerical value based on the number and severity of anatomical injuries. The score ranges from 1 to 75 with 1 denoting minimal injury and 75 representing maximal anatomic injury. ISS greater than 16 is considered serious injury, and greater than 25 is critical. The score is derived by summing the squares of each of the three highest single AIS ratings (Appendices 2 and 3). For example, if the AIS ratings of each of four injured anatomical regions are 2, 4, 3, and 1, the ISS score is $2^2 + 4^2 + 3^2 = 4 + 16 + 9 = 29$. A good correlation between ISS and mortality rate has been shown in the preliminary Major Trauma Outcome Study (Fig 1-10).[31] Although widely used in epidemiological studies, the ISS also has no pathological or physiological basis. This aspect of the system, together with its retrospective nature, makes it a poor preoperative indicator of injury severity.

### *Glasgow Coma Scale*

This physiological index is a highly effective tool for assessing the severity of brain dysfunction and, with repeated evaluations, the progress of the head-injured patient.[124] In this system, scores are assigned to three behavioral responses: eye opening, best motor response, and best verbal response. Criteria for assigning the scores are described in Chapter 10. The GCS correlates very well with the Glasgow Outcome Scale,[68] although its value and sensitivity as an indicator of mild brain injury have been questioned.[70] In this system the highest achievable score is 15, and the lowest is 3. A score of 5 or less after 6 hours indicates poor outcome.[68,124]

### *Trauma Score*

This physiologically based system was developed by Champion et al.[32] and is probably the most useful of all available systems for preoperative injury severity assessment. It combines the GCS with assessments of cardiovascular status (capillary return and systolic blood pressure) and respiratory rate and effort. The score is derived by summing weighted values of each variable as shown in Table 4 of Chapter 29. The highest achievable score is 16 (best prognosis), and the lowest is 1 (worst prognosis). As a predictor of survival, the trauma score correlated well with the outcome of 821 patients with blunt injury and 888 with penetrating injury.[31] It is important to repeat assessments since physiological scores change rapidly with treatment. Thus, physicians generally specify the timing of the trauma score, eg, field trauma score or hospital trauma score. The CRAMS Scale is a simplified version of the trauma score; it is based on measurement of physiologic variables in five systems: *c*irculation, *r*espiration, *a*bdomen, *m*otor, and *s*peech.[57] Its accuracy and ease of applicability for triaging trauma patients in the field have been shown in a prospective evaluation.[36]

FIG. 1-10. Mortality rates by ISS groups in the first part of the Major Trauma Outcome Study of the American College of Surgeons.

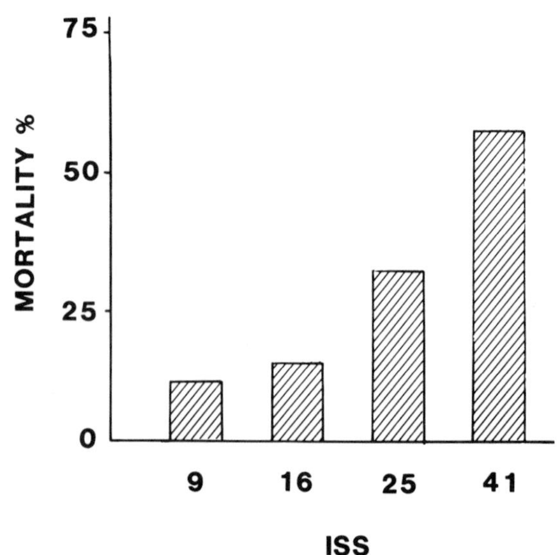

### *New Dimensions in Injury Severity Assessment*

Ongoing evaluations of both anatomical and physiological severity indices have demonstrated that none of them can predict outcome with absolute reliability. This prompted a combination of the physiologically oriented trauma score and the anatomically oriented injury severity score and the resultant development of the TRISS (Trauma-Injury Severity Scoring) system during the early 1980s.[31] This method combines physiological and anatomical indices of injury severity with patient age to characterize the injured patient; it has been applied to the Major Trauma Outcome Study.[31] More recently Sacco et al[113] have described a seven-dimensional severity profile that includes three physiological and four anatomical assessments from the trauma score and AIS values. This profile method, by virtue of its higher predictive value and lower false-negative rate, may replace TRISS in the future.

As can be inferred from the above discussion, numerical characterization of injury severity, although possibly useful, can by no means replace ongoing clinical assessment. Evaluation of the acute trauma victim varies significantly from that of other patients in that the amount of time available for history taking, physical examination, and radiographic studies is heavily influenced by the clinical condition. Although a detailed examination is justified in a stable patient, in the unstable victim evaluation should be limited to a few areas of vital importance and conducted simultaneously with therapeutic efforts. The dynamic nature of events in the injured patient also necessitates continuous updating of diagnostic and therapeutic activities.

## DIAGNOSTIC, TECHNICAL, AND THERAPEUTIC CHALLENGES

Some injuries, if unrecognized, may become life threatening under anesthesia. A small asymptomatic intracranial hematoma may enlarge during the stress of anesthesia and surgery. The contents of an open eye under swollen and closed eyelids, which preclude adequate examination, may be extruded at any time during the perioperative period. An undiagnosed basilar skull fracture may permit an intended nasotracheal intubation to become a nasocranial tube insertion. A clinically and radiographically undetected cervical spine injury may leave the patient quadriplegic following airway management or overzealous manipulation of the head and neck for whatever reason. An unrecognized bilateral condylar fracture, which causes severe restriction of mouth opening, may lead to disaster after administration of intravenous anesthetics and muscle relaxants. Pericardial tamponade and/or myocardial contusion may be missed and then become clinically obvious during the course of anesthesia. The murmur of a cardiac septal or valvular defect may not be heard in a noisy emergency department, only to produce acute myocardial failure during surgery. The list of such pitfalls for anesthesiologists is much longer than presented here; they will be discussed in various chapters of the book. The wide variability in clinical manifestations of these injuries requires not only diagnostic knowledge and expertise but also suspicion and a systematic search.

During prolonged surgery on a major trauma victim, treatment of shock, hypothermia, hypoxemia, hypercarbia, metabolic acidosis, and coagulopathy are the principal tasks of the anesthesiologist. Administration of anesthesia, if any, often becomes a secondary consideration, although it should be realized that recall of operative events by these patients is not infrequent.[24]

Technical skill, more than that required for other subspecialties of anesthesia, is an important component of trauma care. The ability to perform expeditious venous and arterial cut-downs in poorly exposed regions of the body can be extremely valuable when surgeons are in the midst of controlling an exsanguinating hemorrhage. The likelihood of an occasion to perform cricothyroidotomy, thoracostomy, or pericardiocentesis is also high for the anesthesiologist engaged in trauma care. The use of a variety of specialized equipment and techniques—rapid infusion, autotransfusion, jet ventilator, independent lung ventilation, warming devices, hyperbaric oxygen chamber, MAST trousers—in trauma care requires that the anesthesiologist be well versed in their use. It is all of these unique challenges that make caring for the injured patient as exciting and rewarding a field as any in the entire specialty of anesthesiology.

## REFERENCES

1. Aldrete JA, Marron GM, Wright AJ. The first administration of anesthesia in military surgery: on occasion of the Mexican-American War. Anesthesiology 1984;61:585.
2. American Association for Automotive Medicine. The Abbreviated Injury Scale (AIS): 1985 revision. Des Plaines,: American Association for Automotive Medicine, 1985.
3. American College of Surgeons Committee on Trauma: Field categorization of trauma patients and hospital trauma index. Bull Am Coll Surg 1980;2:28.
4. American Psychiatric Association Task Force on Nomenclature and Statistics. Diagnostic and statistical manual of mental disorders. 3rd ed. Washington, DC: American Psychiatric Press, 1980.
5. Arajarvi B, Lindqvist C, Santavirta S, et al. Maxillofacial trauma in fatally injured victims of motor vehicle accidents. Br J Oral Maxillofac Surg 1986;24:251.
6. Bach BR, Wyman ET. Financial charges of hospitalized motorcyclists at the Massachussets General Hospital. J Trauma 1986; 26:343.
7. Baker CC. Epidemiology of trauma: the civilian practice. Ann Emerg Med 1986;15:1389.
8. Baker SP. Injuries: the neglected epidemic. J Trauma 1987; 27:343.
9. Baker SP, O'Neill B. The injury severity score: an update. J Trauma 1976;16:882.
10. Baker SP, O'Neill B, Haddon W, et al. The injury severity score: a method of describing patients with multiple injuries and evaluating emergency care. J Trauma 1974;14:187.
11. Baker SP, O'Neill B, Karpf RS. Burns and fire deaths. In: Baker SP, O'Neill B, Karpf RS, eds. The injury fact book. Lexington, Mass: Lexington Books, 1984:139.
12. Baker SP, O'Neill B, Karpf RS. Drowning. In: Baker SP, O'Neill B, Karpf RS, eds. The injury fact book. Lexington, Mass: Lexington Books, 1984:155.
13. Baker SP, O'Neill B, Karpf RS. Homicide. In: Baker SP, O'Neill B, Karpf RS, eds. The injury fact book. Lexington, Mass: Lexington Books; 1984:81.

14. Baker SP, O'Neill B, Karpf RS. Suicide. In: Baker SP, O'Neill B, Karpf RS, eds. The injury fact book. Lexington, Mass: Lexington Books,1984:67.
15. Baker SP, O'Neill B, Karpf RS. Overview of injury mortality. In: Baker SP, O'Neill B, Karpf RS, eds. The injury fact book. Lexington, Mass: Lexington Books, 1984:17.
16. Baker SP, Whitfield RA, O'Neill B. County mapping of injury mortality. J Trauma 1988;28:741.
17. Baker SP, Whitfield RA, O'Neill B. Geographic variations in mortality from motor vehicle crashes. N Engl J Med 1987;316:1384.
18. Barancik JI, Chatterjee BF, Greene-Cradden YC, et al. Motor vehicle trauma in Northeastern Ohio, I: incidence and outcome by age, sex, and road-use category. Am J Epidemiol 1986; 123:846.
19. Barancik JI, Chatterjee BF, Greene-Cradden YC, et al. Northeastern Ohio Trauma Study, I. magnitude of the problem. Am J Public Health 1983;73:746.
20. Baxt WG, Moody P. The differential survival of trauma patients. J Trauma 1987;27:602.
21. Bever DG, Veenker CH. An illness-injury severity index for nonphysician emergency medical personnel. EMT J 1979;3:45.
22. Blaisdell FW. Medical advances during the Civil War. Arch Surg 1988;123:1045.
23. Blum R. Contemporary threats to adolescent health in the United States. JAMA 1987;257:3390.
24. Bogetz MS, Katz JA. Recall of surgery from major trauma. Anesthesiology 1984;60:214.
25. Botkin JR. The fire-safe cigarette. JAMA 1988;260:226.
26. Breasted JH. The Edwin Smith surgical papyrus. Chicago: University of Chicago Press, 1930.
27. Brent DA, Perper JA, Allman CJ. Alcohol, firearms, and suicide among youth: temporal trends in Allegheny County, Pennsylvania, 1960 to 1983. JAMA 1987;257:3369.
28. Cales RH, Trunkey DD. Preventable trauma deaths: a review of trauma care systems development. JAMA 1985;254:1059.
29. Campbell BJ. Safety belt injury reduction related to crash severity and front seated position. J Trauma 1987;27:733.
30. Carlsson GS, Svardsudd K, Carlsson S, Tibblin G. A study of injuries during life in three male populations. J Trauma 1986; 26:364.
31. Champion HR, Sacco WJ. Trauma severity scales. In: Maull KI, Cleveland HC, Strauch GO, Wolferth CC, eds. Advances in trauma. Chicago: Year Book Medical Publishers, 1986:1.
32. Champion HR, Sacco WJ, Carnazzo AJ, et al. The trauma score. Crit Care Med 1981;9:672.
33. Champion HR, Sacco WJ, Lepper RL, et al. An anatomic index of injury severity. J Trauma 1980;20:197.
34. Chorba TL, Reinfurt D, Hulka BS. Efficacy of mandatory seatbelt use legislation: the North Carolina experience from 1983 through 1987. JAMA 1988;260:3593.
35. Civil ID, Schwab CW. The abbreviated injury scale, 1985 revision: a condensed chart for clinical use. J Trauma 1988;28:87.
36. Clemmer TP, Orme JF, Thomas F, Brooks KA. Prospective evaluation of the CRAMS scale for triaging major trauma. J Trauma 1988;25:188.
37. Committee on Shock, Committee on Trauma, Committee on Anesthesia of National Research Council. Accidental death and disability: the neglected disease of modern society. Washington, DC: National Academy of Sciences Press, 1966.
38. Committee on Trauma Research, Commission on Life Sciences, National Research Council, Institute of Medicine. Injury in America, a continuing health problem. Washington, DC: National Academy Press, 1985.
39. Cope DK, Haynes DF, Slonaker JL, Fontanelle LJ. Diazepam-associated posttraumatic stress reaction. Anesth Analg 1987; 66:666.
40. Council on Scientific Affairs. Alcohol and the driver. JAMA 1986;255:522.
41. Courington FW, Calverley RK. Anesthesia on the western front: the Anglo-American experience of World War I. Anesthesiology 1986;65:642.
42. Crile GW. Phylogenetic association in relation to certain medical problems. Boston Med Surg J 1910;103:893.
43. Davis JH. History of trauma. In: Mattox KL, Moore EE, Feliciano DV, eds. Trauma. Norwalk, Conn: Appleton, 1988:3.
44. Deane SA, Goudry PL, Woods P, et al. The management of injuries: review of deaths in hospital. Aust NZ J Surg 1988;58:463.
45. Decker MD, Graitcer PL, Schaffner W. Reduction in motor vehicle fatalities associated with an increase in the minimum drinking age. JAMA 1988;260:3604.
46. DeMaria E, Kenney PR, Merriam MA, et al. Survival after trauma in geriatric patients. Ann Surg 1987;206:738.
47. DeMaria EJ, Merriam MA, Casanova LA, et al. Do DRG payments adequately reimburse the costs of trauma care in geriatric patients? J Trauma 1988;28:1244.
48. Drovet N. Mobile medical emergency units in France, part 1. Br Med J 1982;284:1924.
49. Drovet N. Mobile medical emergency units in France, part 2. Br Med J 1982;284:1926.
50. Ehrenwerth J, Sorbo S, Hackel A. Transport of critically ill adults. Crit Care Med 1986;14:543.
51. Evans L. Risk of fatality from physical trauma versus sex and age. J Trauma 1988;28:368.
52. Fatal accident reporting system, 1985.Washington, DC: National Highway Traffic Safety Administration, 1987. US Dept of Transportation publication DOT HS 807-071.
53. Federal Bureau of Investigation: Uniform crime reports for the United States. Washington, DC: US Dept of Justice, Federal Bureau of Investigation, 1987.
54. Fife D, Barancik JI, Chatterjee BF. Northeastern Ohio Trauma Study, II: injury rates by age, sex, and cause. Am J Public Health 1984;74:473.
55. Fischer RP, Miles DL. The demographics of trauma in 1995. J Trauma 1987;27:1233.
56. Gensemer IB, McMurry FG, Walker JC, et al. Behavioral consequences of trauma. J Trauma 1988;28:44.
57. Gormican SP. CRAMS scale: field triage of trauma victims. Ann Emerg Med 1982;11;132.
58. Grande CM, Stene JK, Barton CR. The trauma anesthesiologist. Maryland Med J 1988;37:531.
59. Gunby P. No change indicated in traffic fatality rate. JAMA 1987;258:744.
60. Hartunian NS, Smart CN, Thompson MS. The incidence and economic costs of major health impairments. Lexington, Mass: Lexington Books, 1981.
61. Haupt BJ, Graves E. Detailed diagnoses and procedures for patients discharged from short-stay hospitals: United States, 1979. Washington, DC: US Dept of Health and Human Services, 1982. DHHS publication PHS 82-1274-1.
62. Helzer JE, Robins LN, McEvoy L. Post-traumatic stress disorder in the general population: findings of the epidemiologic catchment area survey. N Engl J Med 1987;317:1630.
63. Horst HM, Obeid FN, Sorensen VJ, Bivins BA. Factors influencing survival of elderly trauma patients. Crit Care Med 1986; 14;681.
64. Huelke DF, Sherman HW. Seat belt effectiveness: case examples from real-world crash investigations. J Trauma 1987; 27:750.
65. Hunter J. A treatise on the blood, inflammation, and gunshot wounds. London: George Nicol, 1794.
66. Ivatury RR, Nallathambi MN, Rohman M, Stahl WM. Pene-

trating cardiac trauma: quantifying the severity of anatomic and physiologic injury. Ann Surg 1987;205:61.
67. Jacobs LM, Jacobs BB. Injuries: statistics, prevention and costs. In: Mattox KL, Moore EE, Feliciano DV, eds. Trauma. Norwalk, Conn. Appleton, 1988:15.
68. Jennet B, Teasdale G, Braakman R, et al. Predicting outcome in individual patients after severe head injury. Lancet 1976; 1:1031.
69. Kirkpatrick JR, Youmans RL. Trauma index: an aid in the evaluation of injury victims. J Trauma 1971;11;711.
70. Krauss JF, Nourjah P. The epidemiology of mild, uncomplicated brain injury. J Trauma 1988;28:1637.
71. Kreis DJ, Augenstein D, Civetta JM, et al. Diagnosis related groups and the critically injured. Surg Gynecol Obstet 1987; 165:317.
72. Leads from epidemiology notes: bicycle safety. NY State J Med 1988;86:505.
73. Leads from the MMWR: Changes in premature mortality: United States 1984–1985. JAMA 1987;257:1161.
74. Leads from the MMWR: Differences in death rates due to injury among blacks and whites, 1984. JAMA 1989;261:214.
75. Leads from the MMWR. Premature mortality due to alcohol-related motor vehicle traffic fatalities: United States, 1987. JAMA 1989;261:357.
76. Leads from the MMWR: Premature mortality due to homicides: United States, 1968–1985. JAMA 1988;260:2021.
77. Leads from the MMWR: Premature mortality due to suicide and homicide: United States, 1984. JAMA 1987;258:1711.
78. Leads from the MMWR: Progress toward achieving the national 1990 objectives for injury prevention and control. JAMA 1988; 259:2069.
79. Leads from the MMWR: Regional distribution of deaths from residential fires: United States, 1978–1984. JAMA 1987; 258:2355.
80. Leads from the MMWR: Years of potential life lost before age 65: United States, 1987. JAMA 1989;261:823.
81. Look out for the mopeds (medical news): JAMA 1979;242:1457.
82. Luna GK, Kendall K, Pilcher S, et al. The medical and social impact of nonaccidental injury. Arch Surg 1988;123:825.
83. MacKenzie EJ, Shapiro S, Siegel JH. The economic impact of traumatic injuries: one-year treatment-related expenditures. JAMA 1988;260:3290.
84. MacKenzie EJ, Siegel JH, Shapiro S, et al. Functional recovery and medical costs of trauma: an analysis by type and severity of injury. J Trauma 1988;28:281.
85. Malt U. The long-term psychiatric consequences of accidental injury: a longitudinal study of 107 adults. Br J Psychiatry 1988; 153:810.
86. Martin MJ, Hunt TK, Hulley SB. The cost of hospitalization for firearm injuries. JAMA 1988;260:3048.
87. Matzsch T, Karlsson B. Moped and motorcycle accidents: similarities and discrepancies. J Trauma 1986;26:538.
88. Merrell SW, Saffie JR, Sullivan JJ, et al. Increased survival after major thermal injury: a nine year review. Am J Surg 1987; 154:623.
89. Moore EE, Dunn EL, Moore JB, et al. Penetrating abdominal trauma index. J Trauma 1981;21:439.
90. Moylan JA. Impact of helicopters on trauma care and clinical results. Ann Surg 1988;208:673.
91. Moylan JA, Fitzpatric KT, Beyer AJ, Georgiade GS. Factors improving survival in multisystem trauma patients. Ann Surg 1988;207:679.
92. Munoz E. Economic cost of trauma: United States, 1982. J Trauma 1984;24:237.
93. National Center for Health Statistics, Dawson DA, Adams PF. Current estimates from the National Health Interview Survey, United States, 1986. Washington, DC, US Government Printing Office, 1987. Vital and Health Statistics Series 10, No. 164. DHHS Publication PHS 87-1592. Public Health Service.
94. National Highway Traffic Safety Administration: Fatal accident reporting system 1985: a review of information on fatal accidents in the US in 1985. Washington, DC: US Department of Transportation, National Highway Traffic Safety Administration, 1987. Dept of Transportation publication HS 807–071.
95. National Safety Council. Accident facts. 1985 ed. Chicago: National Safety Council.
96. National Safety Council. Accident facts. 1986 ed. Chicago: National Safety Council.
97. National Safety Council. Accident facts. 1987 ed. Chicago: National Safety Council.
98. National Safety Council. Accident facts. 1988 ed. Chicago: National Safety Council.
99. Neel SH. Army aeromedical evacuation procedures in Vietnam. JAMA 1968;204:99.
100. O'Carroll PW, Alkon E, Weiss B. Drowning mortality in Los Angeles County: 1976 to 1984. JAMA 1988; 260:380.
101. Ogawa M, Sugimoto T. Rating severity of the injured by ambulance attendants. J Trauma 1974;14:934.
102. Orlowski JP. Drowning, near-drowning and ice-water drowning. JAMA 1988;260:390.
103. Orsay EM, Turnbull TL, Dunne M, et al. Prospective study of the effect of safety belts on morbidity and health care costs in motor-vehicle accidents. JAMA 1988;260:3598.
104. Osler T, Hales K, Baack B, et al. Trauma in the elderly. Am J Surg 1988;156;537.
105. Polen MR, Friedman GD. Automobile injury: selected risk factors and prevention in the health care setting. JAMA 1988; 259:77.
106. Public Health Service. The 1990 health objectives for the nation: a midcourse review. Washington, DC: US Dept of Health and Human Services, Public Health Service, 1986.
107. Ramenofsky ML, Ramenofsky MB, Jurkovich GJ, et al. The predictive validity of the pediatric trauma score. J Trauma 1988; 28:1038.
108. Raphael B. When disaster strikes. London: Hutchinson, 1986.
109. Rhodes M, Aronson J, Moerkirk G, Petrash E. Quality of life after the trauma center. J Trauma 1988;28:931.
110. Rice DP, Hodgson TA, Kopstein AN. The economic costs of illness: a replication and update. Health Care Financing Rev 1985;7:61.
111. Rivara FP, Dicker BG, Bergman AB, et al. The public cost of motorcycle trauma. JAMA 1988;260:221.
112. Rivara FP, Maier RV, Mueller BA, et al. Evaluation of potentially preventable deaths among pedestrian and bycyclist fatalities. JAMA 1989;261:566.
113. Sacco WJ, Jameson JW, Copes WS, et al. Progress toward a new injury severity characterization: severity profiles. Comput Biol Med 1988;18:419.
114. Sato TB. Effects of seat belts and injuries resulting from improper use. J Trauma 1987;27:754.
115. Schiller WR, Knox R, Zinnecker H, et al. Effect of helicopter transport of trauma victims on survival in an urban trauma center. J Trauma 1988;28:1127.
116. Schwab CW, Young G, Civil I, et al. DRG reimbursement for trauma: the demise of the trauma center (the use of ISS grouping as a early predictor of total hospital cost). J Trauma 1988; 28:939.
117. Shackford SR, Hollingsworth—Fridlund P, Cooper GF, Eastman AB. The effect of regionalization upon the quality of trauma care as assessed by concurrent audit before and after institution of a trauma system: a preliminary report. J Trauma 1986;26:812.
118. Shackford SR, Mackersie RC, Hoyt DB, et al. Impact of a trauma

system on outcome of severely injured patients. Arch Surg 1989;122:523.

119. Sharar SR, Luna GK, Rice CL, et al. Air transport following surgical stabilization: an extension of regionalized trauma care. J Trauma 1988;28:794.
120. Sleet DA. Motor vehicle trauma and safety belt use in the context of public health priorities. J Trauma 1987;27:695.
121. Sloan JH, Kellerman AL, Reay DT, et al. Handgun regulations, crime, assaults, and homicide: a tale of two cities. N Engl J Med 1988;319:1256.
122. Stoddart JC. Transporting the injured patient. In: Stoddart JC, ed. Trauma and the anaesthetist. Philadelphia: Bailliere Tindall, 1984:176.
123. Stout-Wiegand N. Fatal occupational injuries in US industries, 1984: comparison of two national surveillance systems. Am J Public Health 1988;78:1215.
124. Teasdale G, Jennet B: Assessment of coma and impaired consciousness: a practical scale. Lancet 1974;2:81.
125. Tepas JJ, Ramenofsky ML, Mollitt DL, et al. The pediatric trauma score as a predictor of injury severity: an objective assessment. J Trauma 1988;28:425.
126. Thomas F, Clemmer TP, Larsen KG, et al. The economic impact of DRG payment policies on air evacuated trauma patients. J Trauma 1988;28:446.
127. Thompson RS, Rivara FP, Thompson DC. A case-control study of the effectiveness of bicycle safety helmets. N Engl J Med 1989;320:1361.
128. Transportation Research Board: Proceedings of workshop on alcohol-related accidents in recreational boating. Washington, DC: National Academy of Sciences, National Research Council, 1986.
129. Trunkey DD. Trauma. Sci Am 1983;249:28.
130. Trunkey DD. Trauma care at mid-passage: a personal viewpoint, 1987 AAST presidential address. J Trauma 1988;28:889.
131. Trunkey DD. Organization of trauma care. In: Burke JF, Boyd RJ, McCabe CJ, eds. Trauma management: early management of visceral, nervous system, and musculoskeletal injuries. Chicago: Year Book Medical Publishers, 1988:1.
132. US Dept of Health and Human Services, Public Health Service, Health Care Financing Administration. The international classification of diseases, 9th rev. clinical modification, ICD-9-CM, vol 1: disease tabular, list 2nd ed. Ann Arbor: Commission on Professional Hospital Activities. 1980. DHHS publication PHS 80-1260.
133. Wagenaar AC, Webster DW, Maybee RG. Effect of child restraint laws on traffic fatalities in 11 states. J Trauma 1987; 27:726.
134. Waller AE, Baker SP, Szocka A. Childhood injury deaths: national analysis and geographic variations. Am J Public Health 1989;79:310.
135. Waller JA. Methodologic issues in hospital-based injury research. J Trauma 1988;28:1632.
136. Waller PF, Stewart JR, Hansen AR, et al. The potentiating effects of alcohol on driver injury. JAMA 1986;256:1461.
137. Weiss BD. Preventing bicycle-related head injuries. NY State Med J 1987;87:319.
138. West LJ. Alcoholism and related problems. Englewood Cliffs, NJ: Prentice-Hall, 1984.
139. West JG, Williams MJ, Trunkey DD, Wolferth CC, Jr. Trauma systems. JAMA 1988;259:3597.
140. Wintemute GJ. Firearms as a cause of death in the United States: 1920–1982. J Trauma 1987;27:532.
141. Wise RP. Progress against cancer. N Engl J Med 1986;315:967.

## APPENDIX 1. Classification of External Causes of Injuries in the International Classification of Diseases (ICD) System

| Code | Cause |
|---|---|
| E800–807 | Railway accidents |
| E810–819 | Motor vehicle traffic accidents |
| E820–825 | Motor vehicle nontraffic accidents |
| E826–829 | Other road vehicle accidents |
| E830–838 | Water transport accidents |
| E840–845 | Air and space transport accidents |
| E845–848 | Vehicle accidents not elsewhere classifiable, eg, cable cars not on rails |
| E849 | Place of occurrence (to be used with E850–E869, E880–923 to denote place) |
| 849.0 | Home |
| 849.1 | Farm |
| 849.2 | Mine and quarry |
| 849.3 | Industrial place and premise |
| 849.4 | Place for recreation or sport |
| 849.5 | Street or highway |
| 849.6 | Public building |
| 849.7 | Residential institution |
| 849.8 | Other (eg, forest, beach, parking lot) |
| E850–858 | Accidental poisonings by drug, medicinal substances, and biologicals |
| E860–869 | Accidental poisonings by other solid and liquid substances, bases, and vapors |
| E870–876 | Misadventures to patients during surgical and medical care |
| E878–879 | Surgical and medical procedures as the cause of abnormal reaction of patient or later complication without mention of misadventure at the time of procedure |
| E880–888 | Accidental falls |
| E890–899 | Accidents caused by fire and flames |
| E900–909 | Accidents due to natural and environmental factors |
| E910–915 | Accidents caused by submersion, suffocation, and foreign bodies |
| E916–928 | Other accidents |
| E929 | Late effects of accidental injury |
| E930–949 | Drugs, medicinal, and biological substances causing adverse effects in therapeutic use |
| E950–959 | Suicide and self-inflicted injury |
| E960–969 | Homicide and injury purposely inflicted by other persons |
| E970–978 | Legal intervention |
| E980–989 | Injury undetermined whether accidentally or purposely inflicted |
| E990–999 | Injury resulting from operations of war |

APPENDIX 2. Condensed Chart Prepared by Civil and Schwab for Abbreviated Injury Scale 1985 Version (Blunt Trauma)†

| AIS SCORE | 1<br>MINOR | 2<br>MODERATE | 3<br>SEVERE: NOT LIFE THREATENING | 4<br>SEVERE: LIFE THREATENING | 5<br>CRITICAL: SURVIVAL UNCERTAIN |
|---|---|---|---|---|---|
| HEAD/NECK | Headache/dizziness 2° to head trauma<br>Cervical spine strain with no fracture or dislocation | Amnesia from accident<br>Lethargic/stuporous/ obtunded; can be roused by verbal stimuli<br>Unconsciousness <1 h<br>Simple vault fracture<br>Thyroid contusion<br>Brachial plexus injury<br>Dislocation or fracture, spinous or transverse process of C-spine<br>Minor compression fracture (≤20%) C-spine | Unconsciousness 1–6 h<br>Unconsciousness <1 h with neurological deficit<br>Fracture base of skull<br>Comminuted compound or depressed vault fracture<br>Cerebral contusion/ subarachnoid hemorrhage<br>Intimal tear/thrombosis carotid artery<br>Contusion larynx, pharynx<br>Cervical cord contusion<br>Dislocation or fracture of lamina, body, pedicle, or facet of C-spine<br>Compression fracture >1 vertebra or >20% anterior height | Unconsciousness 1–6 h with neuro deficit<br>Unconsciousness 6–24 h<br>Appropriate response only to painful stimuli<br>Fractured skull with depression >2 cm, torn dura, or tissue loss<br>Intracranial hematoma ≤100 cc<br>Incomplete cervical cord lesion<br>Laryngeal crush<br>Intimal tear/thrombosis carotid artery with neuro. deficit | Unconsciousness with inappropriate movement<br>Unconscious >24 h<br>Brain stem injury<br>Intracranial hematoma >100 cc<br>Complete cervical cord lesion C4 or below |
| FACE | Corneal abrasion<br>Sup. tongue laceration<br>Nasal or mandibular ramus* fracture<br>Tooth fracture/avulsion or dislocation | Zygoma, orbit*, body* or subcondylar mandible* fracture<br>LeFort I fracture<br>Scleral/corneal laceration | Optic nerve laceration<br>LeFort II fracture | LeFort III fracture | |
| THORAX | Rib fracture*<br>Thoracic spine strain<br>Rib cage contusion<br>Sternal contusion<br><br>* Add AIS 1 if associated with h'thorax, p'thorax or h'p'-mediastinum | 2–3 rib fractures*<br>Sternum fracture<br>Dislocation or fracture spinous or transverse process T-spine<br>Minor compression fracture (≤20%) T-spine | Lung contusion/lac. ≤ 1 lobe<br>Unilateral h' or p'thorax<br>Diaphragm rupture<br>≥4 rib fractures*<br>Intimal tear/minor lac/ thrombosis subclavian or innominate artery<br>Inhalation burn, minor<br>Dislocation or fracture of lamina, body, pedicle or facet of T-spine<br>Compression fracture >1 vertebra or more than 20% height<br>Cord contusion with transient neurological signs | Multilobar lung contusion or laceration<br>H'p'mediastinum<br>Bilat-h'p' thorax<br>Flail chest<br>Myocardial contusion<br>Tension p'thorax<br>Hemothorax >1000 cc<br>Tracheal fracture<br>Intimal aortic tear<br>Major lac-subclavian or innominate artery<br>Incomplete cord syndrome | Major aortic laceration<br>Cardiac laceration<br>Ruptured bronchus/ trachea<br>Flail chest/inhal. burn requiring mechanical support<br>Laryngotrach. separation<br>Multilobar lung laceration with tension p'thorax h'p'mediastinum, or >1000 cc hemothorax<br>Cord laceration or complete cord lesion |
| ABDOMEN | Abrasion/contusion superficial lac, scrotum, vagina, vulva, perineum<br>Lumbar spine strain<br>Hematuria | Contusion/sup. laceration stomach, mesentery, SB, bladder, ureter, urethra<br>Minor contusion/lac. kidney, liver, spleen, pancreas<br>Contusion duodenum/colon<br>Dislocation or fracture spinous or transverse process L-spine<br>Minor compression fracture (≤20%) L-spine<br>Nerve root injury | Sup. lac. duodenum, colon, rectum<br>Perforation SB/mesentery, bladder ureter, urethra<br>Major contusion, or minor lac. with major vessel invol, or h'periton.<br>>1000 cc of kidney/liver/ spleen/panc.<br>Minor iliac A. or V. laceration<br>Retroperitoneal hematoma<br>Dislocation or fracture of lamina body, facet, or pedicle of L-spine<br>Compression fracture >1 vertebra or >20% anterior height<br>Cord contus. with trans neuro signs | Perforation stomach duodenum, colon, rectum<br>Perforation with tissue loss stomach, bladder SB/ureter, urethra<br>Major liver laceration<br>Major iliac A or V lac<br>Incomplete cord syndrome<br>Placental abruption | Major lac with tissue loss or gross contamination of duodenum, colon, rectum<br>Complex rupture liver, spleen, kidney, pancreas<br>Complete cord lesion |

*(continued)*

APPENDIX 2. Condensed Chart Prepared by Civil and Schwab for Abbreviated Injury Scale 1985 Version (Blunt Trauma)† *(continued)*

| | 1<br>MINOR | 2<br>MODERATE | 3<br>SEVERE: NOT LIFE THREATENING | 4<br>SEVERE: LIFE THREATENING | 5<br>CRITICAL: SURVIVAL UNCERTAIN |
|---|---|---|---|---|---|
| EXTREMITIES | Contusion elbow, shoulder, wrist, ankle<br>Fracture/dislocation finger, toe<br>Sprain A–C joint, shoulder, elbow, finger, wrist, hip, ankle, toe | Fracture humerus*, radius* ulna*, fibula, tibia*, clavicle, scapula, carpals metacarpals, calcaneus tarsals, metatarsals, pubic rami or simple pelvic fracture<br>Dislocation elbow, hand, shoulder, A-C joint<br>Major muscle/tendon lac<br>Intimal tear/minor lac. axillary, brachial, popliteal A; axillary, femoral, popliteal V | Comminuted pelvic fracture<br>Fractured femur<br>Dislocation wrist/ankle/ knee/hip<br>Below knee or upper extremity amputation<br>Rupture knee ligaments<br>Sciatic nerve laceration<br>Intimal tear/minor lac femoral A<br>Major lac ± thrombosis axillary or popliteal A; axillary, popliteal or femoral V | Pelvic crush fracture<br>Traumatic above knee amputation/crush injury<br>Major laceration femoral or brachial artery | Open pelvic crush fracture<br><br>* Add AIS 1 to these fractures if open, displaced or comminuted |
| EXTERNAL | Abrasions/contusions ≤25 cm on face/hand ≤50 cm on body<br>Superficial lacs. ≤5 cm on face/hand ≤10 cm on body<br>1° burn up to 100%<br>2° or 3° burn/deglov. injury <10% tot. body | Abrasions/contusions >25 cm on face or hand >50 cm on body<br>Laceration >5 cm on face or hand >10 cm on body<br>2° or 3° burn or degloving injury 10–19% of total body | 2° or 3° burn or degloving injury 20–29% of total body | 2° or 3° burn or degloving injury 30–39% total body | 2° or 3° burn or degloving injury 40–89% total body |

AIS = 6 Maximum injury automatically assigned ISS = 75

| | |
|---|---|
| Head/neck | Crush fracture, crush/laceration brain stem<br>Decapitation<br>Cord crush/laceration or total transection with or without fracture C3 or above |
| Thorax | Total severance aorta<br>Chest massively crushed |
| Abdomen | Torso transection |
| External | 2° or 3° burn or degloving injury ≥90% TBS |

*Injury severity score*

| *ISS body region* | *AIS score* | *Squared* |
|---|---|---|
| Head/neck | _____ | _____ |
| Face | _____ | _____ |
| Thorax | _____ | _____ |
| Abd/pelvic contents | _____ | _____ |
| Extremities/pelvic girdle | _____ | _____ |
| External | _____ | _____ |
| ISS (sum of squares of 3 most severe only) | | _____ |

† From Civil and Schwab[35] with permission.

APPENDIX 3. Condensed Chart Prepared by Civil and Schwab for Abbreviated Injury Scale 1985 Version (Penetrating Trauma)†

| AIS SCORE | 1<br>MINOR | 2<br>MODERATE | 3<br>SEVERE: NOT LIFE THREATENING | 4<br>SEVERE: LIFE THREATENING | 5<br>CRITICAL: SURVIVAL UNCERTAIN |
|---|---|---|---|---|---|
| HEAD/NECK | | PI to neck with no organ involvement<br>PI = Penetrating injury | Complex PI to neck with tissue loss, organ involvement<br>Minor lac. carotid, vertebral A; internal jugular V<br>Transection ± segmental loss jugular V<br>Thyroid laceration<br>Superficial lac. larynx, pharynx<br>Cord contusion with transient neurological signs | Minor lac carotid, vertebral A with neurological deficit<br>Transection carotid, vertebral A; int jugular V<br>Segmental loss int jugular vein<br>Perforation larynx, pharynx<br>Cord contusion with incomplete cord syndrome | PI with entrance and exit wounds<br>PI of cerebrum, cerebellum<br>Segmental loss carotid, vertebral A<br>Complex laceration larynx, pharynx<br>Cord laceration<br>Complete cord lesion |
| FACE | PI with no tissue loss | PI with superficial tissue loss<br>Corneal/scleral lac. | PI with major tissue loss | | |
| THORAX | PI with no violation of pleural cavity | Thoracic duct laceration<br>Pleural laceration | Complex PI but no violation of the pleural cavity<br>Sup. lac. innominate, pulmonary, subclavian and other named smaller veins<br>Sup. lac. trachea, bronchus, esophagus<br>Lung laceration ≤1 lobe<br>Unilateral h' or p'thorax<br>Diaphragmatic laceration<br>Cord contusion with transient neurological signs | Sup aortic laceration<br>Major lac innominate, pulmonary, subclavian and other named smaller art; vena cava, brachiocephalic pulmonary, subclavian and other named smaller veins<br>Transection/tissue loss other named smaller veins<br>Perforation trachea, bronchus esophagus<br>Multilobar lung laceration<br>H'p'mediastinum<br>Bilateral h'p'thorax<br>Tension p'thorax<br>H'thorax >1000 cc<br>Cardiac tamponade<br>Cord contusion with incomplete cord syndrome | Major aortic laceration<br>Transection/segmental loss vena cava/ pulmonary/ brachiocephalic V & other named smaller arteries<br>Lac. trachea/bronchus/ esophagus with tissue loss<br>Multilobar lung lac with tension p'thorax, >1000 cc<br>Myocardium/valve laceration<br>Cord laceration<br>Complete cord lesion |
| ABDOMEN | PI with no peritoneal penetration | PI with superficial tissue loss but no peritoneal penetration<br>Sup lac stomach/SB/ mesentery/bladder/ureter/ kidney/liver/spleen/ pancreas<br>Laceration through peritoneum | PI with significant tissue loss but no peritoneal penetration<br>Sup lac vena cava/iliac and other named smaller arteries and veins<br>Sup lac duodenum/colon/ rectum<br>Full thickness laceration SB/mesentery/bladder/ ureter<br>Major lac or minor lac with major vessel injury/ >1000 cc h'peritoneum; kidney/liver/spleen/ pancreas<br>Cord contusion with transient neruological signs | Minor aortic laceration<br>Major lac. vena cava, iliac A & V and other named smaller arteries and veins<br>Transection/segmental loss iliac and other named smaller veins<br>Full thickness lac stomach/ colon/duodenum/rectum<br>Tissue loss/gross contamination stomach/ SB/mesentery bladder/ ureter<br>Cord contusion with incomplete cord syndrome | Major aortic laceration<br>Transection/segmental loss vena cava/iliac and other named smaller arteries<br>Tissue loss/gross contamination duodenum/colon/ rectum<br>Tissue loss kidney/liver spleen pancreas<br>Cord laceration |

(*continued*)

APPENDIX 3. Condensed Chart Prepared by Civil and Schwab for Abbreviated Injury Scale 1985 Version (Penetrating Trauma)† (*continued*)

| | 1<br>MINOR | 2<br>MODERATE | 3<br>SEVERE: NOT LIFE THREATENING | 4<br>SEVERE: LIFE THREATENING | 5<br>CRITICAL: SURVIVAL UNCERTAIN |
|---|---|---|---|---|---|
| EXTREMITIES | Sup. lac. brachial and other named veins | Simple PI with no internal structure involvement<br>Sup. lac axillary, brachial, popliteal A; axillary, femoral, popliteal V<br>Major lac ± segmental loss brachial vein and other named smaller arteries and veins<br>Lac median, radial, ulnar, femoral, tibial, peroneal N<br>Major tendon/muscle lac | Complex PI with internal structure involvement<br>Sup. laceration femoral A<br>Major lac axillary, popliteal A; axillary, femoral, popliteal V<br>Segmental loss axillary, femoral popliteal V<br>Sciatic nerve laceration<br>>1 nerve lac in same extremity<br>Multiple tendon, muscle lacerations in same extremity | Major lac brachial, femoral artery<br>Segmental loss brachial, axillary, popliteal artery | Segmental loss femoral A |
| EXTERNAL | Superficial laceration ≤5 cm on face or hand, ≤10 cm on body<br>PI with no tissue loss | Laceration >5 cm on face, hand or >10 cm on body<br>PI with superficial tissue loss | | | |

| | |
|---|---|
| AIS = 6 | Maximum injury automatically assigned ISS = 75 |
| Head/neck | Brainstem laceration |
| Thorax | Aortic transection<br>Segmental loss aorta, innominate, pulmonary, subclavian arteries<br>Complex myocardial laceration |
| Abdomen | Aortic transection/segmental loss |

*Injury severity score*

| *ISS body region* | *AIS score* | *Squared* |
|---|---|---|
| Head/neck | _____ | _____ |
| Face | _____ | _____ |
| Thorax | _____ | _____ |
| Abd/pelvic contents | _____ | _____ |
| Extremities/pelvic girdle | _____ | _____ |
| External | _____ | _____ |
| ISS (sum of squares of 3 most severe only) | | |

† From Civil and Schwab[35] with permission.

# Chapter Two

*Robert E. Markison*
*Donald D. Trunkey*

# *Establishment of Care Priorities*

Trauma is the leading cause of death among Americans between the ages of 1 and 36 and costs more than $130 billion annually.[2] Shocking statistics have evolved from regional studies comparing patient salvage rates between locales with and without trauma centers. Such reviews indicated that an average of 60 to 70% of trauma patients who died in conventional hospitals could have been saved in trauma centers.[11,65] Presently those regions that lack formal trauma systems still have a 30 to 35% preventable death rate.[64,71] The success of an integrated approach to care of the injured patient rests on proper, efficacious management of time.

Much of the current literature contains a mind-boggling array of dense and difficult-to-follow algorithms. Such linear, lockstep displays do not conform to human perceptual and cognitive processes, which are based more upon pattern perception and storage in what learning theorists refer to as *program structures.* The sophistication and accessibility of the mind's programs are a function of steady development and frequent use, ie, experience.[24] Since trauma care involves clusters of concerns from moment to moment rather than the individual tracks portrayed by algorithms, a pattern approach will be used here which consists of circled central concepts with radiating lines to associated concerns. For example, this introduction may be characterized by the pattern shown in Fig 2-1.

This chapter will focus on (1) rapid patient overview; (2) primary survey; (3) secondary survey; and (4) proper utilization of diagnostic and therapeutic techniques related to resuscitation and the formulation of a care plan.

## RAPID OVERVIEW

The importance of overview in the care of a multiply injured patient cannot be overemphasized. Formation of this initial impression occupies the first 3 to 5 seconds that the patient is in the trauma room; during this time a few preselected medical personnel are present, the room should be very quiet, and one single individual is in charge. Great restraint is practiced during these critical initial moments, and the focus is on the total patient, as the natural tendency to overwhelm him/her physically is held in check. Obvious visual content, including means of ventilatory and cardiac support, the patient's color, gross asymmetries, and the presence or absence of body movement, will suggest whether the patient is stable, unstable, dead, or dying (Fig 2-2). This overview will determine the tempo and direction of subsequent events. If, for

FIG. 2-1. Pattern approach used to define trauma-related facts in the United States. Preventable death rate (30 to 35%) represents the estimated figures in areas without trauma systems.

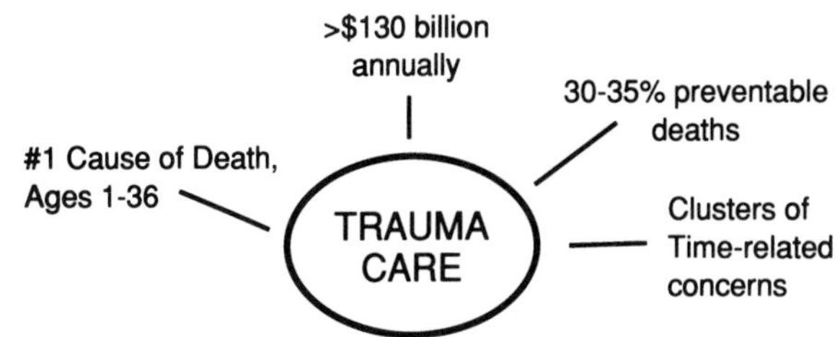

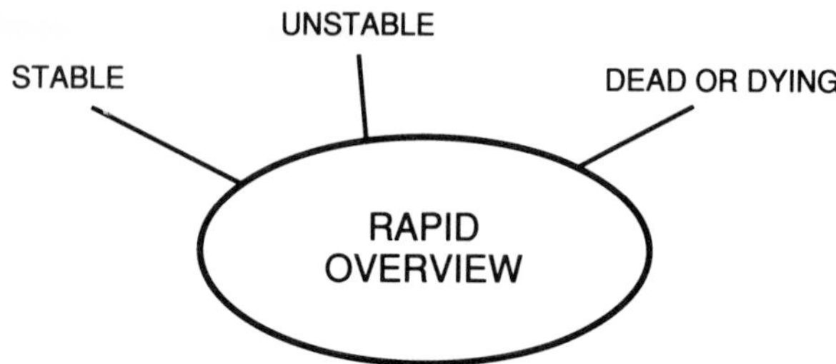


FIG. 2-2. Trauma patient presents to the emergency room in three possible conditions: stable, unstable, or dead or dying.

example, an ashen-colored patient of advanced age is wheeled into the room with cardiopulmonary resuscitation in progress, no signs of life, and multiple abrasions, the patient is most likely dead or dying from blunt trauma and will not benefit from full-scale resuscitation attempts. Conversely, an unconscious teenage motorcyclist with facial abrasions and normal color evokes the need for airway and cervical spine control in addition to early neurosurgical consultation in order to limit disability. Once the tone is set by an overview, the examiner proceeds to the primary survey.

## PRIMARY SURVEY

Development of the advanced trauma life support (ATLS) course by the committee on trauma of the American College of Surgeons has expanded the traditional ABCs to ABCDE (Fig 2-3). The letters *D* and *E* stand for *d*isability, as indicated by neurological status, and *e*xposure, which refers to complete undress of the patient to allow full evaluation.[16] The primary survey, requiring no more than several minutes, is best accomplished by the single individual who is directing the patient's emergency room care. Delegation of this responsibility to other team members should be avoided at this time because it would obscure points of improvement or deterioration as time passes.

### AIRWAY

Establishment or assurance of airway patency and maintenance head this set of priorities. One begins the assessment by attempting verbal contact with the conscious or semiconscious patient by asking his name. Clear phonation from the patient establishes that the airway is patent, and, if that is the case, the need for additional ventilatory support will depend upon neurological stability and adequacy of gas exchange. On the other hand, the unconscious patient or the

FIG. 2-3. ABCDE of primary survey for trauma victim.

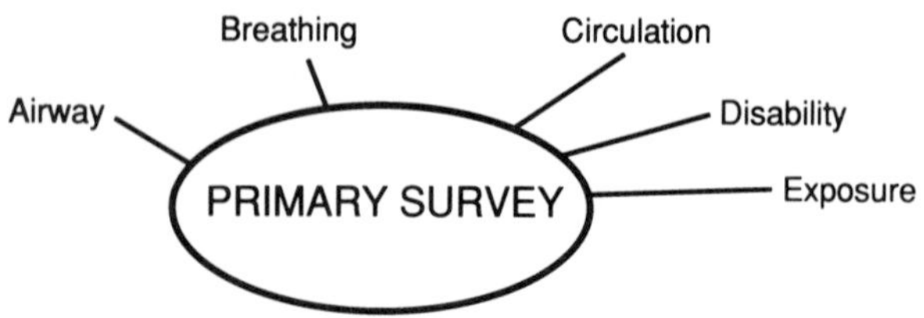


patient with massive maxillofacial trauma will require ventilatory assistance from the start.[38,60,70] In these cases, one must assume cervical spine fracture until proven otherwise and proceed accordingly[59] (see also Chapter 14). Airway always takes precedence over cervical spine injury, but the neck can be protected during airway placement. Tonsil suckers serve the purpose of blood and clot evacuation and are also useful in the detection of dentures (sometimes in fragments) by the tapping of metal on plastic. A sweep of the physician's finger around the oral cavity of the unconscious patient provides information about the bony integrity of the upper airway, the possibility of obstructing retropharyngeal hematoma, presence of foreign bodies, and airway closure by the tongue.

Once the need for intubation is clear, the patient should be preoxygenated by ambu-bag and mask, using 100% oxygen. If mask fit is not possible, use of a high-flow face mask or nasal cannula is worthwhile during the brief period prior to tube insertion. Nasotracheal intubation is only occasionally required, since orotracheal intubation is possible in most trauma patients. No more than 60 seconds is given to each oro- or nasotracheal intubation attempt, and if all attempts fail, one must proceed expeditiously to cricothyroidotomy or tracheostomy. Cricothyroidotomy is accomplished by incising the cricothyroid membrane with a No. 11 blade and using the knife handle to widen and maintain the opening, while a No. 5 or 6 cuffed tracheostomy tube is inserted.[9] Complete laryngotracheal separation from blunt trauma is the single contraindication to cricothyroidotomy and mandates tracheostomy. Further details of airway management are provided in Chapter 3.

### BREATHING

Breathing is the second priority in the primary survey following establishment of a secure airway. Observations include respiratory rate, recruitment of accessory muscles, presence of flail chest, listening for sucking chest wounds, auscultation for evidence of bowel sounds in the chest (diaphragmatic rupture or herniation), and palpation for tracheal shift (pneumo- or hemopneumothorax). If the alert patient can take a deep breath without discomfort, the chance of significant respiratory compromise is nil. Flail chest segments are stabilized by application of sandbags or, cervical spine permitting, by turning the patient flail side down. Sucking wounds of the chest are dressed occlusively, and the thorax is drained of air and blood via thoracostomy tube, at a separate site.[28,33] Chest tubes are inserted without prior chest X-ray to drain hemo- and pneumothoraces if the patient is having respiratory distress.

### CIRCULATION

Circulation is the third priority, and three concerns require prompt attention (Fig 2-4): (1) rapid control of external bleeding; (2) the pump; and (3) volume.

External bleeding is generally controlled by paramedics in the field. Occasionally, however, significant hemorrhage is present on arrival or commences shortly thereafter. Direct pressure will control even the most troublesome bleeding and should be applied to wounds at the same time that the airway

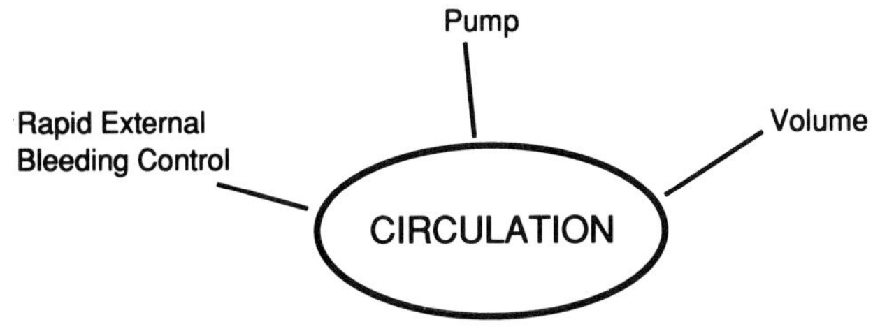


FIG. 2-4. Three areas of assessment for circulation during primary survey.

is being established. Rolled gauze is held directly on the wound, and then a circumferential bandage is wrapped around the extremity, or tape is applied over the roll to a wounded torso. Tourniquets should not be used except in the rare instance of uncontrolled hemorrhage from the stump of a traumatic amputation. Probing of rapidly bleeding wounds with blind application of clamps causes substantial tissue injury that may preclude primary vascular repair and result in permanent disability from nerve injury.

It is usually fairly easy to differentiate pump failure from volume problems in the primary survey. Once it has been ascertained that the patient is in clinical shock, the neck veins should be noted (Fig 2-5). Empty or collapsed neck veins suggest hypovolemia, and distended neck veins suggest a pump problem. There is a constellation of six factors which may hinder or halt cardiac function (Fig 2-6).

### *Cardiac Arrest*

Cardiac arrest is assumed in the patient who has no palpable pulse or blood pressure. Cardiopulmonary resuscitation, if in progress at the time of the patient's arrival, should be stopped for an interval sufficient to allow palpation of carotid and femoral pulses, then restarted. Rapid application of electrocardiographic (ECG) leads for monitoring will support the findings but is not essential to taking immediate, proper action in most instances. Emergency room thoracotomy provides the best chance for survival in this patient. The objectives of this procedure are: (1) to control great vessel and cardiac bleeding; (2) to release cardiac tamponade; (3) to optimize cardiac output; and (4) to redistribute the available blood to vital organs (brain, heart) by cross-clamping the descending aorta.

FIG. 2-5. Examination of neck veins will differentiate pump failure from hypovolemia during the primary survey.

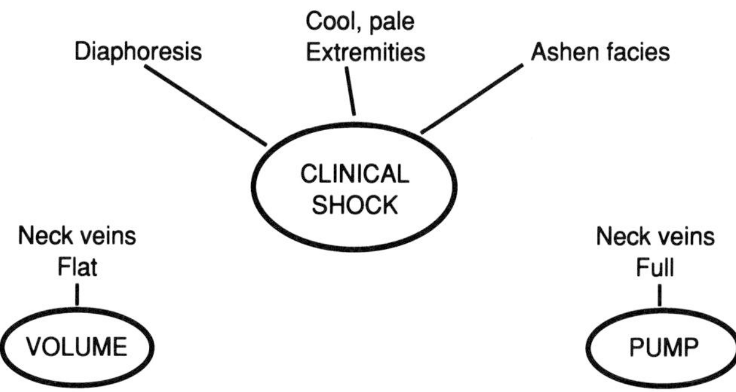


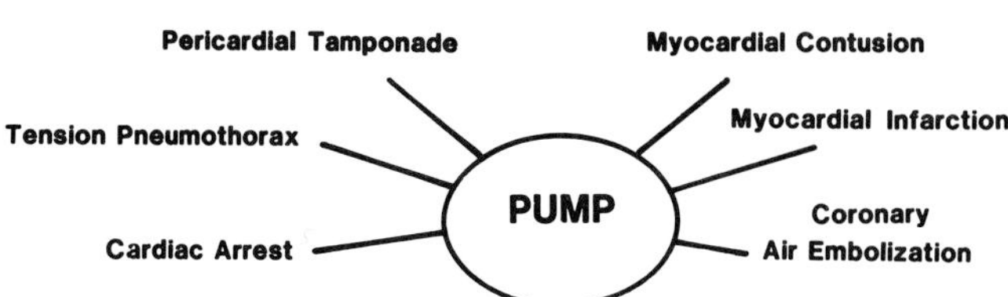


FIG. 2-6. Causes of pump failure in the injured.

However, enthusiasm for the use of emergency room thoracotomy must be tempered by several considerations.[48] If blunt trauma to the chest or abdomen is the cause of cardiac arrest in a patient of any age, the chance of salvage by thoracotomy is less than 5%. Further, a combination of massive head injury and cardiac arrest from blunt injury contraindicates thoracotomy. Figures from a series of 175 patients at San Francisco General Hospital who underwent emergency room thoracotomy included a single survivor (1.7%) among the subgroup (36%) who had blunt injury.[6] This patient was agonal upon admission and arrested in the emergency room. More recently, survivors have been reported following air embolism secondary to blunt trauma.[13]

Resources are the second issue in deciding whether or not to perform a thoracotomy for a patient in cardiac arrest. Optimal results can be achieved in an emergency department where: (1) a surgeon opens the chest; (2) proper lighting and instrument trays are available at all times; and (3) a full-scale operating room is always held open for use without delay to provide definitive care. Such circumstances existed at San Francisco General during the study period cited above and resulted in a 6.7% survival rate among 175 victims of blunt and penetrating trauma.[6] The highest salvage rate with emergency room thoracotomy occurs in patients with acute penetrating cardiac wounds.[25,41,48,58]

Experience is the third consideration in deciding whether to open the chest of a patient with arrest. The technique consists of a transverse incision involving the anterior wall of both hemithoraces including the sternum or, more commonly, of an incision from the left sternal border to the left midaxillary line through the fourth or fifth intercostal space (Fig 2-7). Exposure is broadened by parasternal division of the costal cartilages above and below the incision and insertion of a rib-spreading retractor. Immediately following entry into the thorax, the pericardium is opened by a long vertical incision on its anterior surface. Phrenic nerves are preserved as a knife nick is made; scissors are then run upward to the aortic root and downward to the level of the cardiac apex to complete the pericardiotomy. Cardiac compression is started with one hand while the other occludes the descending thoracic aorta as needed. Manual compression of the aorta is simpler and safer than using clamps. Once internal massage has begun, the assisting surgeon takes over, freeing the surgeon in charge to treat accessible lesions and assess the patient's chances of survival. Since considerable thoracic trauma experience is necessary to ensure proper management once the chest is open, the procedure should not be performed unless done frequently with acceptable rates of salvage. Further discussion in this section will assume that this expertise is available in the hospital on a 24-hour basis.

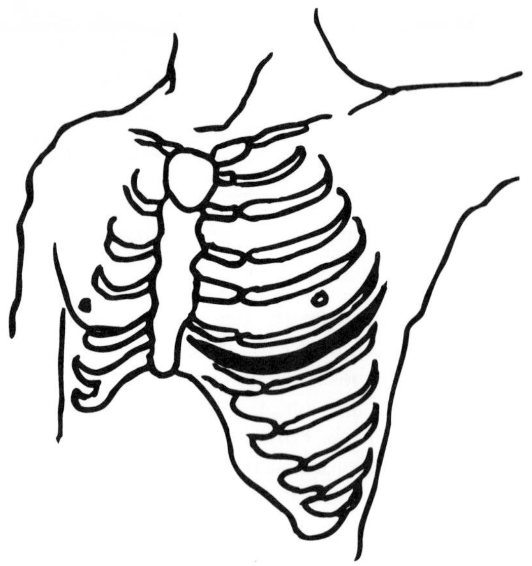

FIG. 2-7. Emergency room thoracotomy is performed by an incision on the left chest from the sternal border to the midaxillary line between the fourth and fifth ribs.

### *Tension Pneumothorax*

Tension pneumothorax is suspected in the patient who has respiratory distress, tracheal shift, distended neck veins, unilateral thoracic hyperresonance, and/or shock. Preload compromise due to mediastinal shift with venous obstruction may lead to cardiac arrest unless treatment is instituted immediately. Temporary relief is provided by inserting a 14-gauge angiocatheter in the second intercostal space at the midclavicular line of the involved side. Time should not be spent obtaining a chest X-ray prior to treatment if the patient is in distress. Definitive care then consists of insertion of a large-bore chest tube through the fifth or sixth intercostal space at the mid-to-posterior axillary line. This lateral thoracic approach permits better drainage of blood and air than an anterior tube provides. Meticulous sterile technique must be observed to avoid empyema.[19] Another safety measure is the avoidance of trocar tubes because they may cause lung lacerations. Connections are secured with tape, and the tube is immediately connected to 20 cm $H_2O$ suction. The volume of blood in the collecting system is noted at the moment of insertion and at regular intervals thereafter, as long as bleeding continues. If blood output is massive (greater than 500 mL) and continuous, autotransfusion is begun. Generally, this involves passive collection of thoracic blood via chest tube into a bottle containing citrated anticoagulant. The bottle is agitated continuously to prevent clot formation and then hung for reinfusion through a filter. Following massive autotransfusion, platelet defects may occur, but these generally resolve within 24 hours[47] (see also Chapter 6).

### *Pericardial Tamponade*

Pericardial tamponade must be considered in all patients who have shock, distended neck veins, and cool extremities with capillary filling time greater than 2 seconds in whom pneumothorax has been first ruled out or treated. Pericardiocentesis in this circumstance is the first step and may be quite beneficial, but it is seldom definitive therapy.[52] The technique consists of subxiphoid insertion of an 18-gauge spinal needle directed toward the left shoulder (Fig 2-8). Monitoring of a V-lead connected to this needle is useful in avoiding cardiac puncture, since the noisy QRS complex inverts when the epicardium is contacted. Relief of hypotension may be dramatic and allows further time for transporting the patient to the operating room. If, on the other hand, as in 50% of patients, blood is clotted and withdrawn with difficulty through the needle and the patient is failing,[63] the pericardial sac should be opened immediately through a subxiphoid incision or a left anterior thoracotomy. A long vertical pericardiotomy is used to evacuate blood and clots, and cardiac wounds are occluded by hand. Cardiorrhaphy is considered part of the resuscitation and should be performed in the emergency room whenever possible. Excellent survival rates have been achieved under these circumstances.[41] If cardiac activity has stopped, massage is continued, intravenous or intratracheal epinephrine (5 to 10 mL of a 1:10,000 solution) is given, sterile warm saline is poured into the mediastinum, and defibrillation is attempted. Internal paddles are used at a current of 20 to 40 watt-seconds or external paddles may be used at 300 watt-seconds.[3,32] The best results are obtained when coarse fibrillation is present at the time of countershock. Repeated attempts at defibrillation are often necessary.

### *Myocardial Contusion*

Myocardial contusion is particularly common after deceleration injuries.[56,61] Death from arrhythmias generally occurs in the first hour. Therefore, careful ECG monitoring is essential. This is best accomplished in an intensive care unit, but the patient should remain in the emergency room until primary and secondary surveys as well as necessary diagnostic studies have been completed.

Lidocaine (1 mg/kg bolus followed by 2 to 4 mg/min) is

FIG. 2-8. Technique of pericardiocentesis.

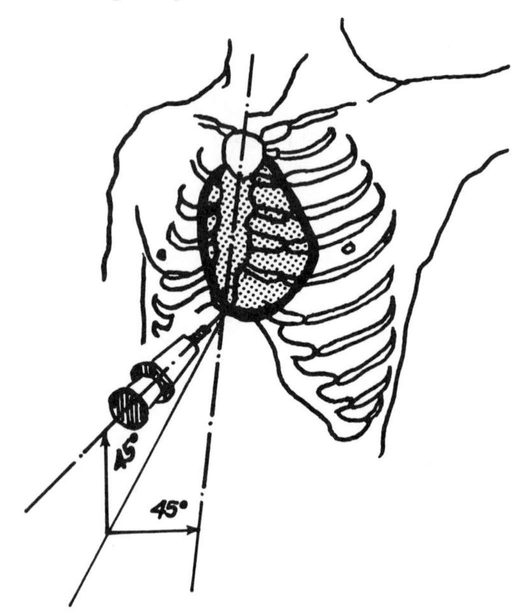

often of immediate value for arrhythmias,[3] but vasopressors should not be used until other causes of hypotension have been diagnosed.

### Myocardial Infarction

Myocardial infarction may precede the traumatic event or occur as a result of coronary hypoperfusion after injury.[31] A history obtained from the patient, relatives, and current family physicians is often valuable in determining the possibility of antecedent cardiac disease. As in myocardial contusion, treatment is directed at arrhythmias and reversal of cardiogenic shock.

### Air Embolization

Air embolization is the fistulization of air into the pulmonary circulation after parenchymal disruption of the lung. This may be the result of blunt or penetrating chest injury and must be considered early to permit any possibility of salvage. Common manifestations of air embolization are shown in Fig 2-9. If froth is obtained when arteries are punctured for blood gas determination, passage of large volumes of air into the left side of the circulation has already occurred, and salvage is not possible. In these instances air in the coronary circulation may be one of the major causes of pump failure. Early treatment consists of immediate thoracotomy on the injured side and hilar cross-clamping of the lung. Occasionally, air embolization occurs after intubation and ventilation in a previously stable patient who has major thoracic injuries. Prevention may be possible by avoiding excessive positive pressure ventilation during resuscitation. The use of high-frequency jet ventilation, if available, may be of value in these circumstances not only by reducing the chance and severity of air embolism but also in the long term by decreasing the size of the air leak and improving the pulmonary healing process.[56]

### Volume

Volume restoration begins by assessing the deficit[35] (Fig 2-10). Clinical signs will suggest whether the degree of shock is mild (10 to 20% volume loss), moderate (20 to 40%), or severe (more than 40%). The appropriate level of support can then be instituted (see Chapter 4).

Mild shock is present in the patient who has cool skin with delayed capillary filling (greater than 2 seconds) and who complains of being cold and thirsty. Tachycardia and sweating signal the upper limits of this category.

In moderate shock, maintenance of cerebral and cardiac perfusion is achieved at the expense of other organs. Since the kidney is affected early, urine output reveals this by dropping below 0.5 mL/kg per hour. Early insertion of a urinary catheter provides the ideal guide to fluid therapy for these patients.

Severe shock threatens cerebral and cardiac perfusion and is evidenced clinically by agitation that may progress to coma and arrhythmias, or ischemic changes on the electrocardiogram. Shock classification must be altered in elderly and cardiac-compromised patients because fixed peripheral resistance and/or low cardiac output states permit circulatory failure at lesser degrees of volume loss.[15]

Access to the circulation should provide diagnostic information, restore volume, and anticipate further losses. The first access in most patients is via a 14-gauge angiocatheter inserted into a forearm vein. Blood is withdrawn immediately and sent for type, cross-match, and complete blood count. Additional blood is reserved for electrolytes, glucose, blood urea nitrogen, amylase, and toxicology and is sent to the laboratory when clinically indicated. The moderately severe shock patient also has an antecubital venous cutdown simultaneously placed in the contralateral upper extremity and threaded centrally for monitoring. A premeasured 5 or 8 French feeding tube or adult size pulmonary artery catheter introducer serves this purpose well. The presence of severe shock requires a third venous access via distal saphenous cutdown or (rarely) via the femoral vein. Internal jugular and subclavian vein catheterization is fraught with complications such as pneumothorax, hemothorax, and carotid artery injury in seriously volume-depleted patients and should be avoided if possible.[1]

The choice of fluid should be limited to balanced salt solutions, such as Ringer's lactate or acetate, and blood. Newer crystalloids, for instance, Plasmalyte, may be more compatible with simultaneous infusion of blood through the same tubing. Two liters of balanced salt solution should be infused immediately, and its effect observed.[35] During infusion, goals include central venous pressure (CVP) 0 to 5, urine output of 0.5 mL/kg per hour, improved level of consciousness, better peripheral perfusion, and improved cardiac output. Without question, in the acute phase of trauma the best indications of satisfactory resuscitation are maintenance of adequate systemic blood pressure and urine output. Initial hematocrit is usually available at this time, and a decision about whether or not to transfuse blood can be made. If the patient is unstable, hematocrit is less than 25, and ongoing major losses are anticipated, transfusion of type-specific blood should begin.[17] The risk of transfusion reaction is 1% in men and 2% in women who have had children.[32] A blood warmer should be used to minimize the hypothermia already present in most trauma victims. Hematocrit should be maintained above 30%.

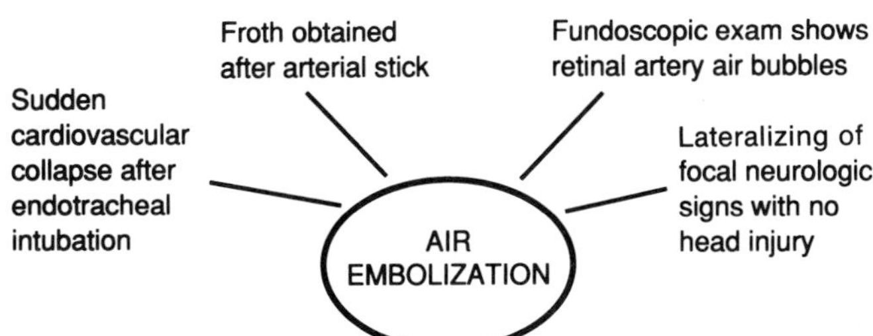


FIG. 2-9. Diagnosis of air embolization following pulmonary laceration.

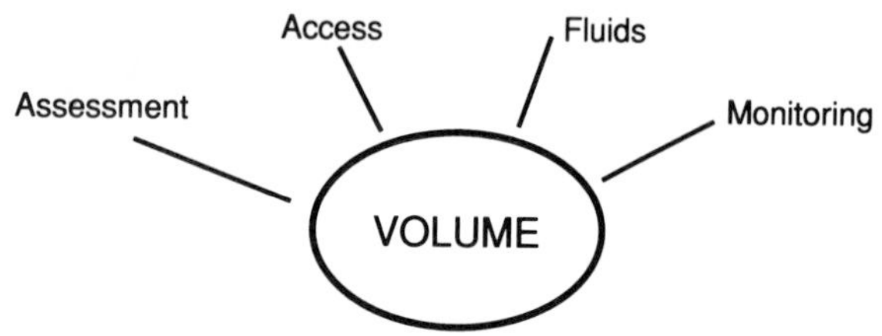


FIG. 2-10. Intravascular volume restoration requires four important considerations during the initial phase of resuscitation.

### DISABILITY

Disability within the primary survey refers to neurological evaluation. Following the guidelines of the ATLS course, the AVPU method is used:

A = *a*lert

V = respond to *v*erbal stimuli

P = respond to *p*ainful stimuli

U = *u*nresponsive

This early assessment provides a simple baseline pending more complete evaluation during the secondary survey. It should be remembered that there are other factors apart from head injury which may result in coma: alcohol and drug intoxication, hypotension, and hypoxia. Thus, a contribution from one or more of these factors should be considered during the evaluation.

### EXPOSURE

All of the patient's clothing must be removed for complete assessment. Excessive motion is avoided by the use of shears to cut away garments.

Primary survey, ie, rapid assessment of airway, breathing, circulation, disability, and exposure, is now complete. At this time it is best to overview again for several seconds because, despite the best efforts of an experienced team, the patient may be moribund. Resuscitation is stopped if no cardiac activity can be obtained over a period of 15 to 20 minutes. Patients presenting with cardiac arrest following drowning should be resuscitated for a longer period of time, since hypothermia commonly associated with this injury may be protective for the brain (see Chapter 21).

## SECONDARY SURVEY

The major difference between primary and secondary surveys is that the first aims at basic physiological support, whereas the second is directed toward formulation of a complete problem list, which in turn leads to an orderly diagnostic plan. Secondary survey requires 5 to 10 minutes and proceeds without pause from head to toe. Placement of a nasogastric tube and Foley catheter often accompanies this sequence, but major breaks in activity should be avoided since they disturb concentration and lead to omissions. Dictation of findings to a team member, who notes them, is very helpful. What follows is a brief survey outline (Fig 2-11). Regional concerns will be discussed in detail in subsequent chapters.

The head examination begins with observation and palpation of the scalp. Pupillary sizes are recorded, and ocular abnormalities are noted. It is also useful to have the patient read print if he is alert, which will reveal more subtle eye problems. Auditory canals and tympanic membranes are inspected for blood and/or cerebrospinal fluid egress. Cranial base fractures are commonly associated with blood and cerebrospinal fluid discharge from the ears and ecchymosis overlying the mastoid bone (Battle's sign) and in the periorbital soft tissue (raccoon eyes).

Maxillofacial trauma patients are assumed to have significant cervical spine injury until proven otherwise by X-ray.[38] In the meantime, the head must be steadied by sandbags and tape. This is a good time to note mentally the need for cervical spine films, but no X-rays should be ordered until the entire secondary survey has been completed.

Neck examination includes inspection and gentle palpation. In awake and alert patients, significant spine injuries are rare in the absence of pain. Penetrating wounds, crepitance, tracheal position, and neck vein appearance are all considered during this examination.

Chest examination begun during primary survey is completed here and includes palpation of clavicles and all ribs as well as auscultation of breath sounds and heart tones. Anterior-posterior sternal compression will often direct attention to the site of a fractured or flail segment. If an ECG monitor is not in place, it should be added at this time.

Abdominal examination is geared to discerning whether a surgical condition exists. Penetrating wounds of the abdomen require local exploration at a minimum. Blunt trauma requires peritoneal lavage or computerized tomographic (CT) scan (see below). A nasogastric tube should be inserted after abdominal examination unless the presence of a cribriform fracture contraindicates its use.[54]

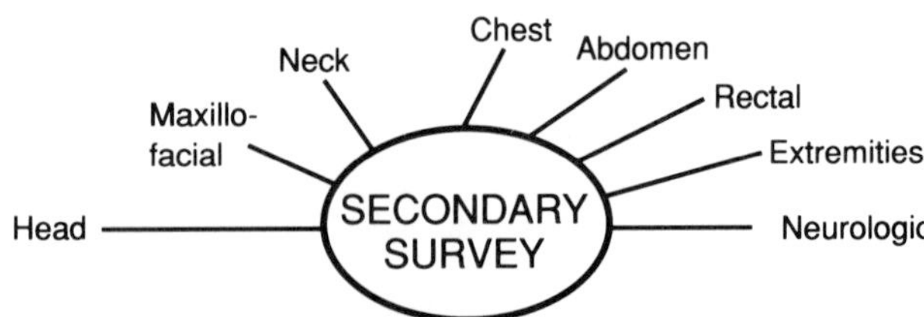


FIG. 2-11. Secondary survey requires examination of eight areas.

Rectal examination seeks to determine the presence of blood, high-riding prostate, rectal disruption, lax sphincter tone, and pelvic fractures. At this point, it is safe to insert a urinary catheter, assuming there is no blood from the urethral meatus and the prostate is in normal position.

Extremities are inspected and palpated for assessment of circulation, major soft tissue injuries, hematoma, and dislocations. Appropriate splints are applied after cultures are taken from open fracture wounds.

Neurological examination should include assessment of hemispheric function, brainstem function, spinal cord motor activity, sensation, and bulbocavernosus reflex. Early neurosurgical consultation will guide proper imaging studies in the patient who has serious head or spinal injury.

Resuscitation is well underway after the 5 to 15 minutes of primary and secondary survey has passed. Patient stability will define the amount of time that can safely be taken for further problem definition. One individual must remain in charge during this process of data gathering.

## DIAGNOSTIC STUDIES

### HISTORY

History is included in our discussion of diagnostic studies because it is informational. Material provided by the ambulance crew is very valuable in reference to actual events. Details of difficult extrications, steering column injuries, vehicle condition, downtime at the scene prior to ambulance arrival, activities in the field, transport time, status changes en route, and the existence of friends or relatives are all important pieces of information. Occasionally, patients give their past medical history at the scene prior to mental status decline from severe shock. Friends and relatives are asked to remain in a waiting room and questioned *after* primary and secondary surveys have been completed. In this way, the problem list can sometimes be abbreviated by such input as: "Yes, he is under treatment for irregular heartbeat, blood in the urine. . . . " (Fig. 2-12). Early consultation is the rule in trauma care, since it serves to reduce time and expense by focusing on essential elements of workup.

### LABORATORY DETERMINATIONS

The laboratory has clear responsibilities in the early care of an injured patient, which consist of rapid reporting of blood counts, arterial blood gases (when needed), urinalysis, and status of blood type and cross-match. Major decisions are made without immediate need for electrolytes, amylase, or hepatic enzymes, for example. In fact, serial hematocrit determinations alone set the tempo of most resuscitations in which significant shock is present. Victims with major burns should have carboxyhemoglobin determinations, and, as noted in the discussion of volume, blood should be drawn and reserved for special tests as needed.

### LAVAGE

Peritoneal lavage remains a valuable step in evaluating blunt abdominal trauma, but its use has diminished in centers where CT scanning is readily available. Lavage is often misleading when pelvic fracture or retroperitoneal hemorrhage is present because red cells from lesions that might not require surgery may transude through membranes into the free peritoneal cavity and give a positive result.[69] In the absence of such coincidental problems, the test is 97% accurate.[4,21] It is also inexpensive, rapid, and simple. The technique consists of incising into the lower midline of the abdomen one third the distance from the umbilicus to the pubis and inserting a lavage catheter that is directed caudally under direct vision into the peritoneal cavity. One liter of balanced salt solution is instilled into the abdominal cavity while the patient's flanks are gently agitated. Then the bottle is set on the floor to siphon out the lavage fluid. Although controversy exists in defining criteria to separate a positive from a negative test,[45,46] generally a positive result is indicated by a rose color, a hematocrit of 1% or greater, 75,000 red blood cells per milliliter, more than 500 white blood cells per milliliter; or the presence of bile or intestinal contents in the drainage fluid. The test requires that a urinary catheter be in place to avoid bladder injury. Previous abdominal surgery contraindicates the use of lavage. The best use of peritoneal lavage is in the unstable head-injured patient who must proceed rapidly to the operating room without time for CT scan.[53,69]

### X-RAYS

X-rays should be ordered selectively in the emergency room since each study takes time, is expensive, and may require patient movement. Chest X-ray and cervical spine films are often the only films obtained before transporting an unstable patient to the operating room.[5] The importance of routine anteroposterior pelvic and long-bone X-rays for patients who have had blunt trauma and are unconscious or obtunded has been emphasized recently.[36] All seven cervical vertebrae should be read by a radiologist as free from abnormalities prior to moving a patient who has suspected neck trauma. Plain films of the rest of the spine are worth the time if spinal cord injury is suspected. Generally, however, CT scanning provides more complete information under such circumstances. Skull X-rays are useful for finding fractures when significant

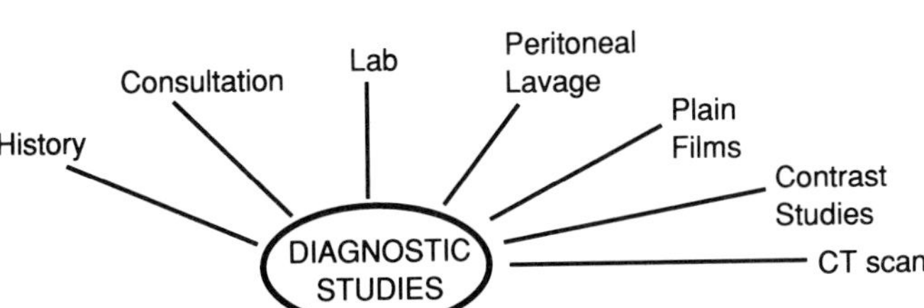


FIG. 2-12. Areas to be considered for diagnostic studies.

head injury is present in the absence of focal neurological deficit.[40] However, in the presence of such deficits, a CT scan is required for accurate diagnosis.[40] The indications for obtaining skull X-rays after head trauma have been reviewed by a multidisciplinary panel and their recommendations validated in a prospective study[40] (Table 2-1). Abdominal plain films without contrast materials are useful primarily in assessing the course and location of penetrating foreign bodies such as bullets. As mentioned, films of the pelvis provide essential information early and should therefore be obtained rapidly to direct the course of further imaging and therapy. However, unstable patients should not be detained for extremity films since these may be obtained in the operating room. The same principle applies to maxillofacial films if time is short. The precise number and sequence of X-rays to be obtained are determined by the secondary survey problem list and the patient's stability.

## CONTRAST STUDIES

Contrast studies permit assessment of the vascular tree, gastrointestinal tract, and urinary tract. Indications for angiography are: (1) neck injuries above the angle of the jaw; (2) chest injuries with mediastinal widening, first rib fracture, or deviation of the trachea to the right; (3) abdominal injuries with nonvisualization of the kidney by intravenous pyelogram (IVP); (4) pelvic fractures with massive hemorrhage; (5) all penetrating extremity injuries in proximity to major vessels; (6) dislocation of the knee; and (7) all fractures associated with abnormal pulses. Each milliliter of contrast medium injected for arteriogram may cause up to 7 mL of diuresis. Thus, the volume lost by this route should be calculated and replaced.

Contrast studies also include intravenous dye injections, the most valuable of which is the IVP. A patient with gross hematuria after blunt abdominal trauma should have an IVP.[29] Victims of major blunt or penetrating abdominal trauma should also have an IVP to confirm the presence of two promptly visualizing kidneys. A "single-shot" IVP provides adequate information in most cases; this involves injection of 100 mL of contrast material intravenously during the secondary survey and an abdominal plain film 5 minutes later. When time permits, abnormalities present on the 5-minute film should be assessed by a complete study, including

TABLE 2-1. Management Strategy for Radiographic Imaging in Patients with Head Trauma*

| LOW-RISK GROUP | MODERATE-RISK GROUP | HIGH-RISK GROUP |
|---|---|---|
| *Possible findings*<br>Asymptomatic<br>Headache<br>Dizziness<br>Scalp hematoma<br>Scalp laceration<br>Scalp contusion or abrasion<br>Absence of moderate-risk or high-risk criteria | *Possible findings*<br>History of change of consciousness at the time of injury or subsequently<br>History of progressive headache<br>Alcohol or drug intoxication<br>Unreliable or inadequate history of injury<br>Age less than 2 years (unless injury very trivial)<br>Posttraumatic seizure<br>Vomiting<br>Posttraumatic amnesia<br>Multiple trauma<br>Serious facial injury<br>Signs of basilar fracture†<br>Possible skull penetration or depressed fracture‡<br>Suspected physical child abuse | *Possible findings*<br>Depressed level of consciousness not clearly due to alcohol, drugs, or other cause (eg, metabolic and seizure disorders)<br>Focal neurological signs<br>Decreasing level of consciousness<br>Penetrating skull injury or palpable depressed fracture |
| *Recommendations*<br>Observation alone: discharge patients with head-injury information sheet (listing subdural precautions) and a second person to observe them | *Recommendations*<br>Extended close observation (watch for signs of high-risk group).<br>Consider CT examination and neurosurgical consultation<br>Skull series may (rarely) be helpful, if positive, but do not exclude intracranial injury if normal | *Recommendations*<br>Patient is a candidate for neurosurgical consultation or emergency CT examination or both |

* Physician assessment of the severity of injury may warrant reassignment to a higher risk group. Any single criterion from a higher risk group warrants assignment of the patient to the highest risk group applicable. (From Masters et al[40] with permission.)

† Signs of basilar fracture include drainage from ear, drainage of cerebrospinal fluid from nose, hematotympanum, Battle's sign, and raccoon eyes.

‡ Factors associated with open and depressed fracture include gunshot, missile, or shrapnel wounds; scalp injury from firm, pointed object (including animal teeth); penetrating injury of eyelid or globe; object stuck in the head; assault (definite or suspected) with any object; leakage of cerebrospinal fluid; and sign of basilar fracture.

nephrotomograms.[14] Nonvisualizing kidneys require examination by angiography or CT scan.[43]

Gastrointestinal tract contrast studies are generally performed with gastrografin for proximal gut assessment. Penetrating mediastinal wounds and severe blunt chest injuries require an esophogram for early diagnosis of esophageal wounds, which are devastating if overlooked. Gastroduodenal contrast studies are seldom necessary if laparotomy is planned but may be useful in cases in which the need for exploration is less certain. An important caveat pertains here: since gut contrast is a routine element of abdominal CT scanning, none should be given if a CT will soon follow because it may interfere with organ imaging. Rectal contrast studies are occasionally helpful after penetrating rectal trauma but are generally preceded by sigmoidoscopy. If sigmoidoscopy is inconclusive, a contrast film is often definitive.

## CYSTOGRAMS AND URETHROGRAMS

The bladder and urethra are well imaged by cystogram and urethrogram, respectively. All instances of bleeding from the urethral meatus require evaluation by urethrogram prior to urinary catheter insertion.[42] Patients with disrupted urethras require cystostomy for urinary drainage. A biplane cystogram is essential to the workup of all patients who have major pelvic fractures or who have sustained severe lower abdominal blunt trauma with hematuria. Inebriated individuals are particularly prone to bladder rupture since their bladders are often full at the time of injury.

## COMPUTED TOMOGRAPHY

CT scanning is a vital link in the care sequence of many trauma patients. Several cautionary points bear consideration prior to discussion of its capabilities. Location of the scanner is very important to proper use of time and the flow of activity. Ideally, the scanner should be in the emergency department as near as possible to the trauma rooms. This ensures proximity to the resources necessary for acceleration of care should the need arise. Emergency thoracotomy, for example, would be necessary in case of sudden cardiac arrest while the patient is under the scanner. Salvage would be difficult if this occurred in an isolated location. Time is another concern in the decision to include a scan in the evaluation. Combined scanning of head and abdomen requires 30 to 60 minutes under optimal circumstances. Burr holes and laparotomy for cranial decompression and control of hemorrhage may be near completion during that same period. Therefore, the desire for extensive imaging must not eclipse the clinical impression that operative intervention must proceed without delay. A third consideration is survey and resuscitation completeness prior to the scan. No scan should be performed until primary and secondary surveys are complete, resuscitation lines and appropriate monitors are in place, and a clearly articulated set of care priorities is understood by all. Finally, surveillance of the patient during the scan is of obvious importance. At our institutions, all patients undergoing CT scanning for trauma are accompanied by surgeons—and respiratory therapists, when intubated—throughout the examination. Hematocrits and blood gases are sent at appropriate intervals, and the study is terminated immediately if status is declining. Anesthesiologists and surgeons capable of rendering definitive care are always present in the hospital at the start of any scan for trauma. Surveillance in the broadest sense includes interpretation of results, which requires 24-hour availability of radiologists to interpret scans with the surgeons who are present.

The diagnostic capabilities of CT scanning in the injured are remarkable (Fig 2-13). Since each body region has its own special time and image-spacing requirements, it is best to review pertinent plain films and the secondary survey problem list with the radiologist before the study in order to avoid overscanning.

Serious head injury is best diagnosed by CT scan.[50] The study should be performed without delay in any hemodynamically stable patient suspected of having a depressed skull fracture, in patients who have severe or worsening neurological deficits, and in inebriated patients without focal deficits who are not improving with hydration and observation following head injury. The combination of modern high-resolution scanners and the administration of intravenous contrast provides assistance in discerning lesions such as subdural hematomas which in earlier times were read as isodense. Other lesions well imaged by CT scan include epidural hematoma, hemorrhagic contusion, intracerebral hematoma, subarachnoid hemorrhage, intraventricular hemorrhage, brain swelling, and traumatic hydrocephalus.[22,50] The importance of speed in evaluation of head injury and institution of treatment cannot be overemphasized. Irreversible neurological damage can occur rapidly due to expansion of an intracranial mass, increasing mortality and morbidity if treatment is delayed.[7,10,39,55]

Maxillofacial trauma is best evaluated in conjunction with plain films. This CT scan requires 15 to 30 minutes and therefore is seldom undertaken in the unstable patient. Its principal diagnostic value is in the evaluation of patients with orbital floor disruptions, midface (Le Fort) fractures, frontoethmoidal fractures, and facial gunshot wounds.[22]

CT scan of the neck is particularly useful for evaluation of soft tissue problems and also provides good resolution of supraglottic, glottic, subglottic, and tracheal injuries. The information gathered is best correlated with the findings of direct laryngoscopy.[22]

Assessment of spinal trauma is aided by the multiplane imaging capabilities of CT scanning. Metrizamide dye may be injected by cervical or lumbar approach; this provides useful data about cord encroachment as well as nerve root disruption.

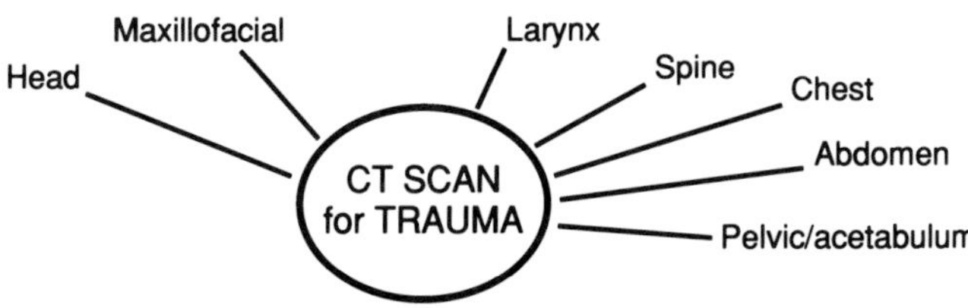


FIG. 2-13. Anatomical areas in which CT scanning is a useful diagnostic measure in the injured.

Three-dimensional reformation of images can localize precisely foreign bodies such as bullets relative to neural and osseous structures. As with other body regions, correlation with plain X-rays is important. The prime advantage of CT scanning for spinal evaluation is the amount of information gained without moving the patient.[22]

Chest evaluation by CT scan has limited value at present since plain radiographs supplemented by esophogram, angiography, and bronchoscopy when indicated give excellent definition of most problems. Particular strengths of the scan are the ability to include esophageal contrast to avoid a separate fluoroscopic study, recognition of pneumothorax and/or hemothorax, which might not be evident on initial supine chest X-ray, and visualization of diaphragmatic rupture[44,62] (see Fig 15-2). An occasional thoracic aortic injury may be noted, but in most cases, there are sufficient plain radiographic signs to indicate directly the need for aortography.[22]

Abdominal CT scanning has dramatically improved the ability to define problems preoperatively. The primary advantages of abdominal CT over peritoneal lavage are: (1) it is noninvasive; (2) it shows the organs injured including the retroperitoneal structures; and (3) its accuracy is close to 100% in distinguishing surgical from nonsurgical abdominal injury.[22,27,49] However, it takes a longer time than peritoneal lavage to elucidate intra-abdominal injury in the preoperative period. Since the findings may be obscured by peritoneal lavage fluid, one should decide which study to perform after the secondary survey is complete. This will be based mainly on the availability of time prior to surgery and the type of injury.[67] For example, many marginally stable head-injured patients are best treated by rapid lavage, head CT scan, and transport to the operating room without delay. On the other hand, stable patients with equivocal neurological and abdominal exams are best scanned thoroughly (head and abdominal scan) to determine the presence or absence of surgical lesions.

The indications for abdominal CT in the traumatized patient are[49,67]: (1) equivocal abdominal examination in a stable patient; (2) presence of head or spinal cord injury in association with suspicious abdominal trauma; (3) hematuria; (4) pelvic fractures with significant bleeding, necessitating the ruling out of associated abdominal injuries; (5) presence of associated injuries requiring surgery, with general or spinal anesthesia precluding clinical observation of the abdomen; and (6) presence of diminished mental function due to chronic cerebral disease, alcohol, or drugs.

CT scanning also has significant value in patients with pelvic fractures, 25% of whom have significant intra-abdominal injury.[66] If laparotomy can be avoided in these individuals, outcomes relative to costs and morbidity are much better. The diagnostic power of CT scanning is greatest in evaluating splenic, hepatic, duodenal (with contrast), and renal injuries as well as pelvic and retroperitoneal hematomas.[12,68] Rarely, pancreatic injuries may not be apparent for several hours until sufficient tissue reaction or blood extravasation has occurred. Therefore, a high degree of clinical suspicion must be maintained and correlated with serial abdominal examinations.[57] A final caveat; whenever a decision not to operate is based on CT scan, there is no substitute for repeated physical examination by observers capable of rendering definitive care should a change be manifest. A report of 200 cases of acute blunt abdominal trauma evaluated by CT at San Francisco General Hospital revealed one false-positive due to residual peritoneal lavage solution and no false-negatives.[23]

CT scan may be useful in demonstrating the presence or absence of peritoneal involvement in penetrating flank or back injuries. Although relatively few of these injuries involve the peritoneum, their misdiagnosis may result in significant morbidity. Reliance on peritoneal lavage in this group of patients may be misleading.[18] Thus, laparotomy is considered mandatory in some centers. Diagnosis of these injuries with contrast-enhanced CT scanning is now possible with reasonable accuracy, thereby reducing the risks of surgery and medical costs.[51]

Pelvic and acetabular CT scanning, when correlated with plain film findings, aids in orthopedic planning of hip surgery. Instillation of contrast into the bladder and rectum provides additional simultaneous organ definition. As noted above, all major pelvic fracture patients, except those who are exsanguinating, should have abdominal CT scans to sequence care of abdominal and extraabdominal injuries properly.[22]

## GENERAL APPROACH TO THE INJURED PATIENT

### PROPHYLAXIS AGAINST INFECTION

Preoperative antibiotics are useful adjuncts in the management of (1) compound fractures, particularly grade 3; (2) dirty soft tissue wounds; (3) suspected small bowel or colon injuries; and (4) exposure of tendon and/or joint cartilage.[26] The efficacy of antibiotics in other injuries has not been demonstrated. The value of antimicrobial prophylaxis in chest trauma is controversial. Although some reports support the use of routine antibiotic prophylaxis in thoracic injuries,[34] there is probably little to gain from these agents unless esophageal perforation or contamination of the chest cavity with intestinal contents occurs.[37] Suggested antibiotics are shown in Table 2-2. If antibiotics have been started for a suspected intestinal injury that is not found at surgery, the agents should be stopped in the immediate postoperative period. Otherwise, antibiotics should be given for a total of 48 to 72 hours.

Prophylaxis against tetanus should be considered for all open wounds. Guidelines have been developed by the American College of Surgeons (Table 2-3).

### ASSIGNMENT OF PRIORITIES

The preservation of life in severe multiple injury requires clear recognition of management priorities. This is especially true during the first few hours of the injury when, in most instances, time is an extremely important factor in determining the outcome. The goal at this stage is not to treat individual injuries as they present but to recognize and manage those that threaten the patient's life or function.[20,30] It is important to remember that the most striking injuries such as those involving the external genitalia or face (without airway compromise) are not always the most urgent or life threatening.

As mentioned above, airway obstruction, severe external

TABLE 2-2. Antimicrobial Prophylaxis: 72 Hours or Less

*Suspected small or large bowel injury*
- Cefoxitin,* 150 mg/kg per day intravenously in four to six divided doses†
  or
- Clindamycin‡ 40 mg/kg per day intravenously, in three to four divided doses plus tobramycin or gentamicin, 5 mg/kg per day intravenously or intramuscularly in three divided doses*

*Traumatic wound (compound fractures, extensive soft tissue injury)*
- Methicillin, nafcillin, or oxacillin, 1 g intravenously, three to four times a day
  or
- Cefazolin, cephalothin, or cephapirin, 1 g intramuscularly or intravenously preoperatively and three to four times a day thereafter. Treatment should continue for 10 days postoperatively

* Cefoxitin should not be used in patients with β-lactam allergy. More recent data suggest antibiotic combinations (metronidazole-penicillin-gentamycin or metronidazole-ampicillin-mecillinam) to be more effective in patients undergoing emergency abdominal surgery with suspected hollow viscous perforation. Prophylactic antibiotics may not be needed in penetrating thoracic trauma and in placement of chest tubes in trauma management unless there is an associated hollow viscus injury (eg, esophagus) or contamination from an associated abdominal injury.

† Penicillin, 200,000 units/kg per day in divided doses may be added.

‡ Metronidazole may be substituted for clindamycin. Give 15 mg/kg over 1 hour (loading dose), then 7.5 mg/kg every 6 hours.

bleeding, chest injuries causing cardiorespiratory embarrassment, head injuries with significant increase in intracranial pressure (ICP), and cervical spine injuries are immediate threats to life or function and must be treated immediately. Of these, airway management takes the highest priority. For instance, in the presence of both airway obstruction and cervical spine injury, the former should be treated immediately while measures to prevent damage to the spinal cord are used.

TABLE 2-3. Tetanus Prophylaxis

*Persons previously immunized*
- When the attending physician has determined that the patient has been previously fully immunized and the last dose of toxoid was given within 10 years:
  - For non–tetanus-prone wounds, no booster dose of toxoid is indicated
  - For tetanus-prone wounds and if more than 5 years has elapsed since the last dose, give 0.5 ml of absorbed toxoid. If excessive prior toxoid injections have been given, this booster may be omitted
- When the patient has had two or more prior injections of toxoid and received the last dose more than 10 years previously, give 0.5 ml of absorbed toxoid for both tetanus-prone and non–tetanus-prone wounds. Passive immunization not considered necessary

*Persons not adequately immunized*
- When the patient has had no prior injection of toxoid or has received only one prior injection of toxoid or when the immunization history is unknown:
- For non–tetanus-prone wounds, give 0.5 ml of absorbed toxoids
  - For tetanus-prone wounds,
    - Give 0.5 ml absorbed toxoid
    - Give 250 units (or more) of human tetanus antitoxin
    - Consider providing antibiotics, although the effectiveness of antibiotics for prophylaxis of tetanus remains unproved

A similar principle applies to combined airway and cerebral injuries.

Bleeding from solid intra-abdominal organs or retroperitoneal structures, stable craniocerebral injuries, burns, and extensive soft tissue injuries also threaten life, but their treatment, depending on their severity, can be delayed for a few minutes until more precarious injuries are managed.

A third group of patients includes those who will have complications or loss of function if diagnosis or treatment is delayed more than a few hours. Peripheral vascular, tendon and nerve injuries, eye injuries, and partial amputation of limbs are some of the examples.

Closed fractures, dislocations, and relatively small soft tissue injuries are those for which treatment can be delayed for several hours if necessary.

A frequently occurring situation is the combination of multiple injuries and head injury. In these instances diagnostic and therapeutic priorities depend on the hemodynamic and neurological condition of the patient. Guidelines to aid in decision making in this group of patients are shown in Fig 2-14.

A team approach is often appropriate in the patient with multiple injuries and may include simultaneous decompression of a space-occupying intracranial lesion by neurosurgeons while general surgeons explore the abdomen. In the patient with massive abdominal injuries and associated widened mediastinum, exploration of the abdomen with repair of injuries is indicated first.[8] Following laparotomy, an aortogram can be carried out and thoracic aortic rupture, if present, treated.[8] If the patient has associated major vascular injuries in the extremities, these must be controlled prior to, or at least simultaneously with, abdominal exploration. If the patient remains unstable, exploratory laparotomy should be carried out before definitive treatment of the peripheral vascular injuries.

## SURGICAL PREPARATION AND EXPOSURE

The trauma patient must be prepared and draped widely so that the surgeon can gain access to any body cavity expeditiously and can properly place drains and chest tubes, if needed. The entire torso should be prepared with iodine paint and draped so that the surgeon can work in a sterile field from the neck and clavicles to the groins, and laterally from table top to table top. Prepping should not involve more than a few minutes and is preferably carried out prior to induction of anesthesia so that should deterioration occur, immediate laparotomy or thoracotomy can be carried out. If craniotomy is anticipated in the emergency room, the hair can be cut and scalp shaved during resuscitation to expedite decompression.

For rapid access and wide exposure of the abdomen, the midline incision is the one of choice. Only rarely will transverse or oblique incisions be appropriate for trauma. Surgeons should be prepared to extend the midline incision up the sternum as a sternal splitting incision or into the right or left chest if necessary.

When the presence of abdominal injury is questionable or the site of pathology uncertain, it is usually best to start with an upper midline incision extending from just below the xiphoid to just above the umbilicus. The incision can be centered on the umbilicus if the injury is presumed to be in the lower

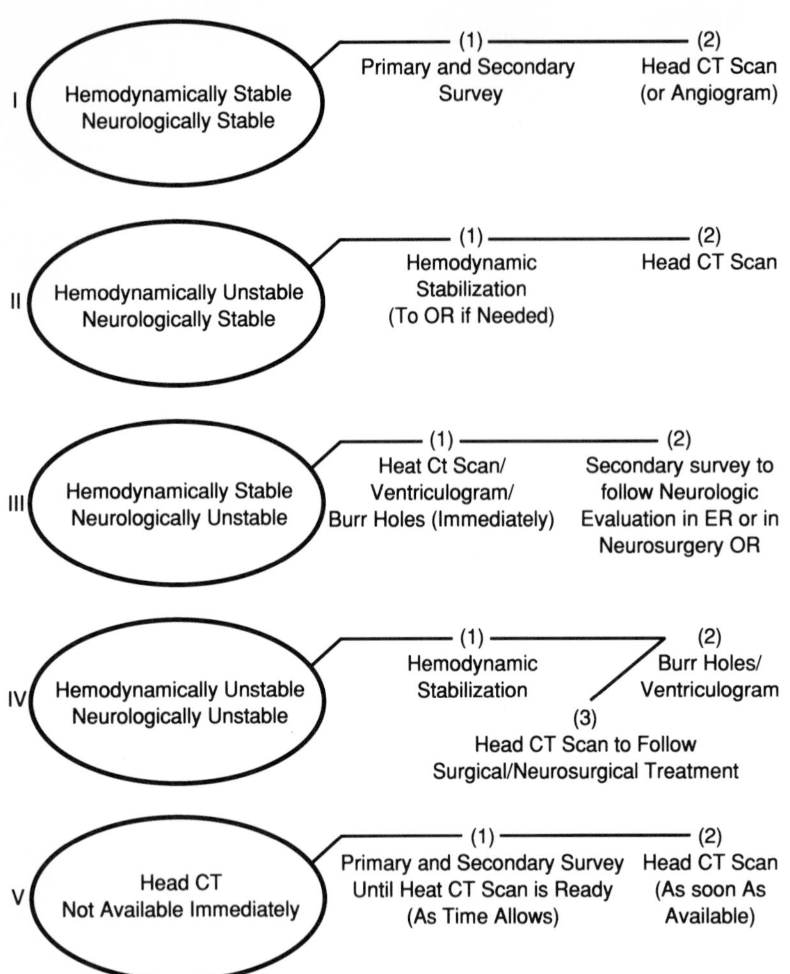


FIG. 2-14. Care priorities in five possible conditions (demonstrated by roman numerals) during management of multiple trauma patients with head injuries. Priorities follow a numerical sequence. For instance, in condition I, primary and secondary survey (1) precedes head CT scan (2).

abdomen. Most complicated problems, however, lie in the upper abdomen, hence the xiphoid-to-umbilical exploratory incision.

When intra-abdominal pathology is encountered, the incision should routinely be extended below the umbilicus to the pubis if the injuries appear major.

An abdomen filled with bright red blood indicates an arterial injury. The patient should be eviscerated, each corner of the abdomen rapidly inspected, and packs placed temporarily to absorb the free blood. All quadrants of the abdomen and the mesentery should be inspected on the first pass. This can be done within a minute or 2 so that the most major source of hemorrhage can be located and dealt with first. The application of packs will control bleeding from many arterial injuries, and, if the injury can be controlled by pack or direct pressure, this should be done while volume is restored. The injury should not be initially exposed directly because the vascular system may suddenly decompress; rapid bleeding in a previously hypovolemic patient frequently leads to cardiac arrest.

If the injury appears to be arterial and in the upper abdomen, the possibility of injury to the visceral portion of the aorta or one of its major upper abdominal branches should be considered, and proximal control must be ensured. If a hematoma extends to the level of the diaphragm, the left chest should be opened and the aorta encircled. If the aortic hiatus is free of hematoma, the gastrohepatic ligament should be divided and the aorta encircled as it emerges through the crura of the diaphragm.

Minor injuries and minor sources of bleeding should not distract the surgeon from dealing with major ongoing hemorrhage, particularly venous hemorrhage. Venous bleeding may not be obvious, unless looked for, since it is low pressure and may not be as dramatic or as evident as arterial hemorrhage. Almost all venous bleeding can be controlled by the judicious application of packs, permitting time for restoration of volume. If, during the initial exploration, retraction of the dome of the liver downward results in massive venous hemorrhage, injury to the hepatic veins or intrahepatic vena cava should be strongly suspected. Consideration of intracaval shunt should be entertained.[72]

After initial control of hemorrhage has been achieved with clamps or packs, an attempt should be made to control fecal soilage prior to definitive surgery. Obvious holes in the small bowel or colon can be temporarily controlled by running suture or Babcock clamps.

In general the supine position is preferred for all trauma. One exception is the patient with demonstrated injury to the left subclavian artery between its origin and the vertebral artery. In this injury, a right lateral decubitus position and left posterolateral thoracotomy is preferred.

After neurosurgical, thoracic, and abdominal injuries have been treated, maxillofacial and orthopedic injuries are treated, in that order, and often during the initial anesthetic. Exceptions to this general prioritization may occur.

## CONCLUSION

Trauma care is more dependent upon proper use of time than any other medical discipline. Evaluation of the multiply injured patient begins with a rapid overview consisting of a moment of quiet visual inspection. This will reveal whether the patient is stable or unstable, dead, or dying and will set the tempo of resuscitation. Primary survey follows, with the goal of basic physiological support. At the completion of the first survey, viability is again evaluated, after which the secondary survey begins. Head-to-toe examination generates a problem list to be imaged, as time permits. Priority is then given to greater definition of cervical spine, chest, head, and abdominal injuries.

Special imaging procedures must be interrupted in the rapidly deteriorating patient, who might benefit most directly from burr holes, thoracotomy, or laparotomy. The ongoing balance between definition and intervention should be directed by one single responsible individual throughout the care sequence.

## REFERENCES


1. Abraham E, Shapiro M, Podolsky S. Central venous catheterization in the emergency setting. Crit Care Med 1983;11:515.
2. Accident Facts. Chicago: National Safety Council; 1988:4.
3. Adult advanced cardiac life support, part III. JAMA 1986; 255:2933.
4. Alyono D, Morrow CE, Perry JF. Reappraisal of diagnostic peritoneal lavage criteria for operation in penetrating and blunt trauma. Surgery 1982;92:751.
5. Aronchick J, Epstein D, Gefter WB, Miller WB. Evaluation of the chest radiograph in the emergency department patient. Emerg Med Clin North Am 1985;3:491.
6. Baker CC, Thomas AN, Trunkey DD. The role of emergency room thoracotomy in trauma. J Trauma 1980;20:848.
7. Baker DP, Miller JD, Ward JD, et al. The outcome from severe head injury with early diagnosis and intensive management. J Neurosurg 1977;47:491.
8. Borman KR, Aurbakken CM, Weigelt JA. Treatment priorities in combined blunt abdominal and aortic trauma. Am J Surg 1982; 144;728.
9. Boyd AD. Tracheostomy and cricothyroidotomy. In: Worth M, ed. Principles and practice of trauma care. Baltimore: Williams and Wilkins, 1982:32.
10. Bricolo AP, Pasut LM. Extradural hematoma: toward zero mortality, a prospective study. Neurosurgery 1984;14:8.
11. Cales RH, Trunkey DD. Preventable trauma deaths: a review of trauma care systems development. JAMA 1985;254:1059.
12. Carroll PR, McAninch JW. Operative indications in penetrating renal trauma. J Trauma 1985;25:587.
13. Carveth S, Reese HE, Buchman RJ, Gangahar DM. The place for open chest cardiac compression. In: Donegan JH, ed. Cardiopulmonary resuscitation. Springfield, Ill.: Charles C Thomas, 1982:180.
14. Cass AS. Immediate radiological evaluation and early surgical management of genitourinary injuries from external trauma. J Urol 1979;122:772.
15. Coath A. Physiologic processes of aging in the cardiovascular system. In: Krechel SW, ed. Anesthesia and the geriatric patient. New York: Grune and Stratton, 1984:11.
16. Committee on Trauma, American College of Surgeons. Advanced trauma life support course: initial assessment. Washington DC: ACS, 1984:139.
17. Committee on Trauma, American College of Surgeons. Blood and fluid replacement in shock. In: Walt AJ, ed. Early care of the injured patient. Philadelphia: WB Saunders, 1982:144.
18. Coppa GF, Davalle M, Pachter HL, Hofstetter SR. Management of penetrating wounds of the back and flank. Surg Gynecol Obstet 1984;159:514.
19. Daly RC, Mucha P, Pairolero PC, et al. The risk of percutaneous chest tube thoracostomy for blunt thoracic trauma. Ann Emerg Med 1985;14:865.
20. Evans RF. The patient with multiple injuries. Br J Hosp Med 1979;22:329.
21. Fabian TC, Mangiante EC, White TJ, et al. A prospective study of 91 patients undergoing both computed tomography and peritoneal lavage following blunt abdominal trauma. J Trauma 1986; 26:602.
22. Federle MP, Brant-Zawadzki M, eds. Computed tomography in the evaluation of trauma. Baltimore: Williams and Wilkins, 1982:1–170, 235–262.
23. Federle MP, Crass RA, Jeffrey RB, Trunkey DD. Computed tomography in blunt abdominal trauma. Arch Surg 1982;117:645.
24. Hart LA. Human brain and human learning. New York: Longman, 1983:92.
25. Ivatury RR, Shah PM, Ito K, et al. Emergency room thoracotomy for the resuscitation of patients with "fatal" penetrating injuries of the heart. Ann Thorac Surg 1981;32:377.
26. Kaiser AB. Antimicrobial prophylaxis in surgery. N Engl J Med 1986;315:1129.
27. Kaufman RA, Towbin R, Babcock DS, et al. Upper abdominal trauma in children: imaging evaluation. Am J Roentgenol 1984; 142:449.
28. Kirsh MM, Sloan H. Blunt chest trauma. Boston: Little Brown, 1977:1.
29. Kisa E, Schenk WG. Indications for emergency intravenous pyelography (IVP) in blunt abdominal trauma: a reappraisal. J Trauma 1986;26:1086.
30. Larkin J, Moylan J. Priorities in management of trauma victims. Crit Care Med 1975;3:192.
31. Lau OJ, Shabbo FP, Smyllie J. Acute left anterior descending coronary artery occlusion following blunt chest injury. Injury 1984;16:55.
32. Levison M, Trunkey DD. Initial assessment and resuscitation. Surg Clin North Am 1982;62:11.
33. Lewis FR. Thoracic trauma. Surg Clin North Am 1982;62:97.
34. LoCurto JJ, Tischler CD, Swan KG, et al. Tube thoracostomy and trauma: antibiotics or not. J Trauma 1986;26:1067.
35. Lucas CE. Resuscitation of the injured patient: the three phases of treatment. Surg Clin North Am 1977;57:3.
36. Mackersie RC, Shackford SR, Garfin SR, Hoyt DB. Major skeletal injuries in the obtunded blunt trauma patient: a case for routine radiologic survey. J Trauma 1988;28:1450.
37. Mandal AK, Montano J, Thadepalli H. Prophylactic antibiotics

and no antibiotics compared in penetrating chest trauma. J Trauma 1985;25:639.

38. Manson PN. Maxillofacial injuries. Emerg Med Clin North Am 1984;2:761.
39. Marshall LF, Toole BM, Bowers SA. The National Traumatic Data Bank, II: patients who talk and deteriorate; implications for treatment. J Neurosurg 1983;59:285.
40. Masters SJ, McClean PM, Arcarese JS, et al. Skull x-ray examinations after head trauma: recommendations by a multidisciplinary panel and validation study. N Engl J Med 1987;316:84.
41. Mattox KL, Beall AC, Jordan GL, DeBakey ME. Cardiorrhaphy in the emergency center. J Thorac Cardiovasc Surg 1974;68:886.
42. McAninch JW. Traumatic injuries to the urethra. J Trauma 1981; 21:291.
43. McAninch JW, Carroll PR. Renal trauma: kidney preservation through improved vascular control, a refined approach. J Trauma 1982;22:285.
44. McLean AS. Computed tomography scanning in acute pulmonary problems. Anaesth Intensive Care 1986;14:84.
45. McLellan BA, Hanna SS, Montoya DR, et al. Analysis of peritoneal lavage parameters in blunt abdominal trauma. J Trauma 1985;25:393.
46. Merlotti GJ, Marcet E, Sheaff CM, et al. Use of peritoneal lavage to evaluate abdominal penetration. J Trauma 1985;25:228.
47. Moore EE, Dunn EL, Breslich DJ, Galloway AC. Platelet abnormalities associated with massive autotransfusion. J Trauma 1980; 10:1052.
48. Moore EE, Moore JB, Galloway AC, Eiseman B. Postinjury thoracotomy in the emergency department. Surgery 1979;86:590.
49. Peitzman AB, Makaroun MS, Slasky BS, Ritter P. Prospective study of computed tomography in initial management of blunt abdominal trauma. J Trauma 1986;26:585.
50. Peyster RG, Hoover ED. CT in head trauma. J Trauma 1982; 22:25.
51. Phillips T, Scalfani SJA, Goldstein A, et al. Use of the contrast-enhanced CT enema in the management of penetrating trauma to the flank and back. J Trauma 1986;26:593.
52. Ramp JM, Hankins JR, Mason GR. Cardiac tamponade secondary to blunt trauma: a report of two cases and review of literature. J Trauma 1974;14:767.
53. Reiner DS, Hurd R, Smith K, Kaminski DL. Selective peritoneal lavage in the management of comatose blunt trauma patients. J Trauma 1986;26:255.
54. Seebacher J, Nozik D, Mathieux A. Inadvertent intracranial introduction of a nasogastric tube: a complication of severe maxillofacial trauma. Anesthesiology 1975;42:100.
55. Seelig JM, Becker DP, Miller JD, et al. Traumatic acute subdural hematoma. N Engl J Med 1981;304:1511.
56. Shackford SR. Blunt chest trauma: the intensivist's perspective. J Intensive Care Med 1986;1;125.
57. Sherck JP, McCort JJ, Oakes DD. Computed tomography in thoracoabdominal trauma. 1984;24:1015.
58. Sherman MM, Saini VK, Yarnoz MD, et al. Management of penetrating heart wounds. Am J Surg 1978;135:553.
59. Silver JR, Morris WR, Otfinowski JS. Associated injuries in patients with spinal injury. Injury 1980;12:219.
60. Stevenson BE. Initial management of acute head injury. Otolaryngol Clin North Am 1979;12:279.
61. Tenzer ML. The spectrum of myocardial contusion: a review. J Trauma 1985;25:620.
62. Tocino IM, Miller MH, Federic PR, et al. CT detection of occult pneumothorax in head trauma. Am J Roentgenol 1984;143:987.
63. Trinkle JK, Marcos J, Grover FL, Cuello LM. Management of wounded heart. Ann Thorac Surg 1974;17:230.
64. Trunkey DD. Trauma care at mid-passage: a personal viewpoint, 1987 AAST presidential address. J Trauma 1988;28:889.
65. Trunkey DD. Trauma. Sci Am 1983;249:28.
66. Trunkey DD, Chapman MW, Lim RC Jr, Dunphy JE. Management of pelvic fractures in blunt trauma injury. J Trauma 1974; 14:912.
67. Trunkey DD, Federle MP. Computed tomography in perspective. J Trauma 1986;26:660.
68. Trunkey DD, Federle MP, Cello J. Special diagnostic procedures. In: Blaisdell FW, Trunkey DD, eds. Trauma management, 1: abdominal trauma. New York: Thieme-Stratton, 1982:19.
69. van Dongen LM, de Boer HHM. Peritoneal lavage in closed abdominal injury. Injury 1985;16:227.
70. Walton RL, Hagan KF, Parry SH, Deluchi S. Maxillofacial trauma. Surg Clin North Am 1982;62:73.
71. West JG, Williams MJ, Trunkey DD, Wolferth CC. Trauma systems: current status, future challenges. JAMA 1988;259:3597.
72. Wiencek RG, Wilson RF. Abdominal venous injuries. J Trauma 1986;26:771.

# Chapter Three

Levon M. Capan

# Airway Management

Airway management is of prime importance during all phases of priority-oriented trauma care. Many problems, shown in Fig 3-1, may complicate this aspect of care, rendering airway management a formidable challenge. Often more than one compromising condition is present, a fact that may not be recognized until attempts are made to secure the airway. Anticipating these pitfalls is as important as the skill required for intervention. Accurate diagnosis of the compromising condition is important not only for adding appropriate safety measures to the management plan, but also for avoiding unnecessarily elaborate maneuvers that may be time consuming and themselves associated with complications.

This chapter considers three aspects of airway management: (1) management of the full stomach, the most common compromising condition in the acute trauma victim; (2) initial assessment and management; and (3) postintubation management. Since detailed information on direct airway injuries is provided in forthcoming chapters, discussion of this type of trauma will be limited only to the general approach.

## THE FULL STOMACH

Aspiration of gastric and pharyngeal contents following trauma remains an important cause of airway and pulmonary complications. Although aspiration can occur any time after injury, patients are at particular risk immediately following the accident, during transportation to hospital, in the emergency department, and during the perioperative period. The incidence of pulmonary aspiration following acute trauma is not known. A clear determination of frequency is impossible, both because some patients show no clinical or radiographic signs following aspiration and because some have preexisting or trauma-induced pulmonary pathology that may mimic or mask the problem. Nevertheless, aspiration is a common occurrence if tracheobronchial protective reflexes are absent or diminished by head injury, alcohol intoxication, drug overdose, anesthesia, or impaired laryngeal function secondary to direct trauma or cranial nerve (IX to XII) injury.[45,48]

The incidence of perianesthetic aspiration in the trauma patient is also unknown. In general, silent or small-volume regurgitation occurs in approximately 10 to 20% of all patients undergoing general anesthesia; upper abdominal surgery, prone and head-down positions, and emergency surgery increase the risk of this complication.[33,51,259] However, lung damage is unlikely with aspiration of such a small volume of gastric fluid. The incidence of perioperative aspiration pneumonitis as determined by three recent large studies is lower than reported previously and varies between 1.4 and 6.4 per 10,000 anesthetics.[61,190,254] Data from a few studies suggest a higher incidence of aspiration pneumonitis associated with emergency surgery, but how many of these operations were performed on trauma victims was not specified.[45,190] Parallel to the overall decrease in incidence of aspiration pneumonitis, a reduction in mortality from this complication has also been noted. In 1973 Cameron and coworkers[47] reported an overall mortality rate of 62%: 41% if one lobe was involved, and 90% if two or more lobes were affected. More recent reports give much lower overall mortality rates from perioperative aspi-

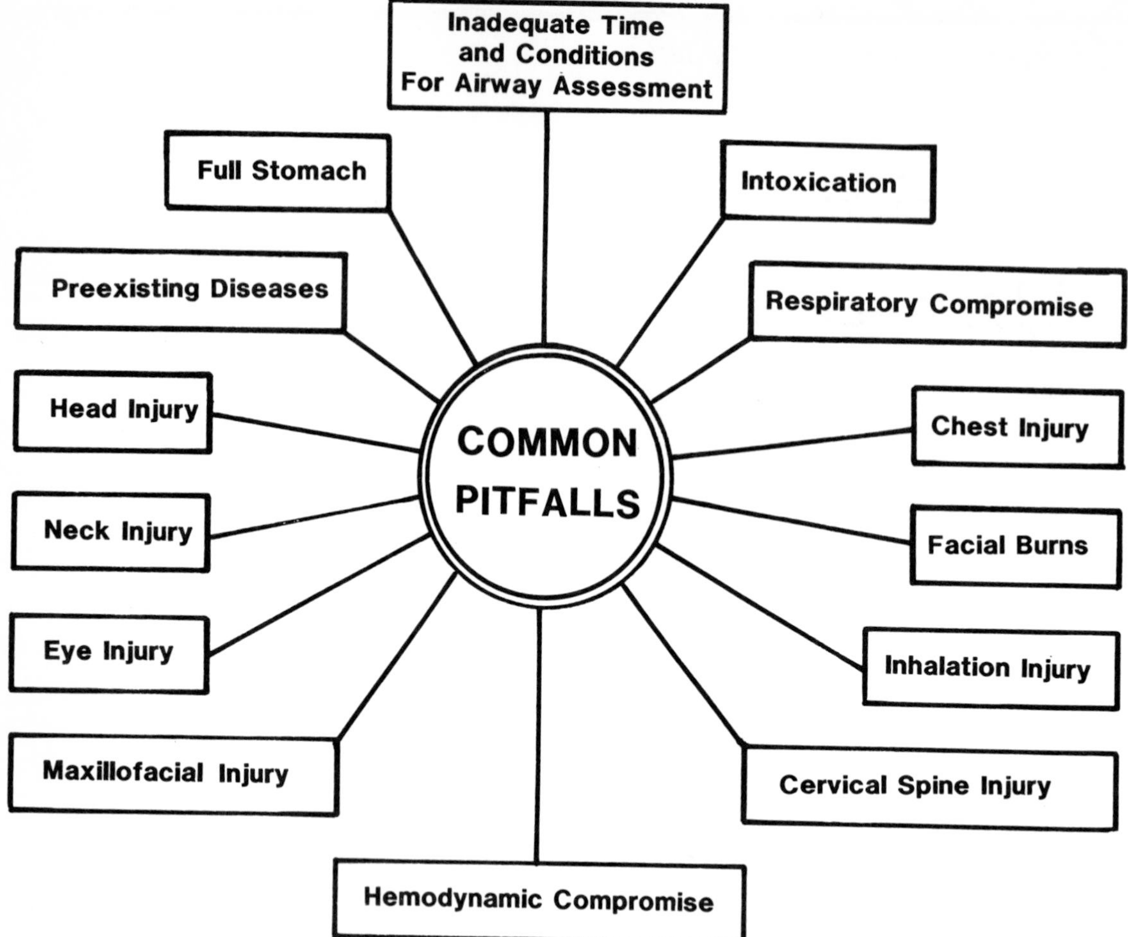


FIG. 3-1. Common pitfalls requiring modification of airway management in acute trauma.

ration pneumonitis, ranging between 5 and 25%.[190,254] Although decreased incidence, morbidity, and mortality are probably a result of more effective prevention and management, the severity of lung damage after aspiration of a large volume of gastric contents is determined by the nature of the material aspirated, the age of the patient, and the extent of organ failure following the event. Trauma victims, in whom prevention may not be possible, who aspirate a large quantity of gastric contents including food particles, and who develop multiorgan failure may have a higher mortality rate.

## FACTORS PREDISPOSING TO REGURGITATION, ASPIRATION, AND PULMONARY PATHOLOGY

In the trauma victim gastric emptying may be delayed because of pain, fear, anxiety, alcohol intoxication, narcotics, sedatives, shock, impaired consciousness, and the trauma itself.[88,235,255,285] In addition acute gastric dilatation is a well-recognized complication of multiple trauma, particularly when transport to the hospital and nasogastric tube placement are delayed.[60] These factors, coupled with elevated intra-abdominal pressure produced by intestinal distention, intraperitoneal blood, and/or increased muscular activity, result in elevated intragastric pressure and a predisposition to regurgitation. Intraabdominal pressure is directly transmitted to the stomach; normally there is no pressure gradient between the two cavities. It is the difference between lower esophageal sphincter and intragastric pressures, the barrier pressure, which determines whether regurgitation will occur. Although not documented, trauma per se, unless it involves the brain, upper abdominal organs, or the diaphragm, does not seem to interfere with lower esophageal sphincter competence; however most drugs used for anesthesia, with the exception of succinylcholine, pancuronium, and neostigmine, diminish its tone. Thus, the net result of recent trauma and anesthesia is decreased barrier pressure, which predisposes the patient to aspiration during the period when the airway is not protected. Fig 3-2 depicts the factors that predispose the trauma patient to regurgitation, aspiration, and aspiration pneumonitis.

As described by Mendelson[173] 4 decades ago, airway obstruction by particulate or solid material and chemical injury from the acid content of gastric fluid are the most common causes of pulmonary morbidity from aspiration. Obstruction of large airways by pieces of food can, of course, produce pulmonary collapse, which may be severe enough to result in asphyxiation. Small food particles, on the other hand, produce hypoxemia not only by obstructing small conducting airways

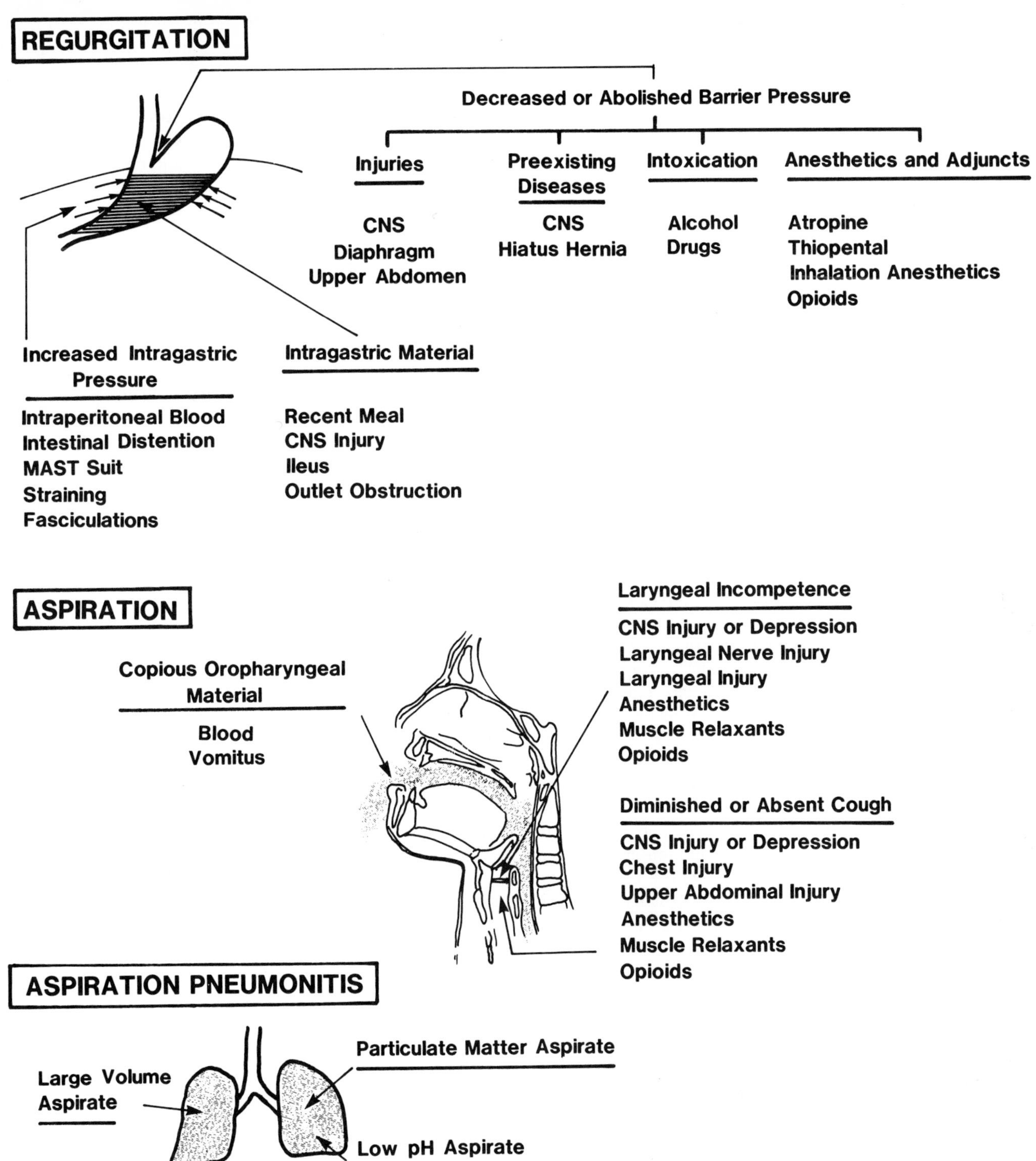


FIG. 3-2. Factors predisposing the trauma patient to regurgitation (upper panel), aspiration (middle panel), and aspiration pneumonitis (lower panel). Low aspirate pH is not a necessity for development of pneumonitis in the trauma setting.

and causing various degrees of pulmonary ventilation-perfusion abnormality, but also by causing a prolonged inflammatory reaction in the lung.[251,282] For instance, severe pulmonary exudation and bronchopneumonia can occur after aspirating milk.[179,251] This mechanism is likely to play an important role in the morbidity of the trauma victim, who often sustains the accident shortly after a meal.

The extent of chemical injury is determined by the acidity and the volume of the aspirated material. Based on unpublished data on Rhesus monkeys, pneumonitis has long been considered a risk if patients aspirate 25 mL or 0.4 mL/kg of stomach contents at a pH below 2.5.[212] More recent data on rats suggest that the critical volume of the aspirate is much lower than 0.4 mL/kg if the pH is less than 1.4. Conversely, aspirates with pH greater than 1.8 were associated with significantly fewer deaths even at volumes much higher than described previously (1.0 to 2.0 mL/kg).[131] It is important to emphasize that aspiration of gastric material with a pH greater than 2.5 cannot be considered benign. Other substances such as particulate matter in gastric contents may damage the lung even at much higher pH levels.[229]

Apart from gastric contents, the trauma victim is likely to aspirate blood if the face, neck, or chest is injured. Depending on the volume, aspiration of blood can cause a severe increase in pulmonary shunt, but these changes are of short duration; the lung is usually cleared within 6 to 24 hours, especially when artificial ventilation is administered.[204,279]

## MANAGEMENT OBJECTIVES

Although delay in gastric emptying appears to correlate with the severity of injury, pain, and shock,[189,285] any acutely traumatized patient must be considered to have a full stomach.[273] No time interval can be relied upon for complete gastric emptying, although there is probably an increased chance of "full stomach" and its consequences within the first 24 hours after injury if trauma occurred within 6 to 8 hours after oral intake. Thus, delay of urgent surgery for less than 24 hours is not likely to decrease the chance of aspiration during induction of or emergence from anesthesia. Obviously, emergent surgery cannot be delayed and must proceed using appropriate intraoperative preventive measures of aspiration.

In the emergency department unconscious individuals should not be allowed to lie supine if the trachea is not intubated. Although the head-down position can reduce the incidence of aspiration,[9] this is not always possible in the acute trauma victim and may be hazardous in the presence of head injury. Rapid intubation of the trachea with a cuffed endotracheal tube is the most reliable method of reducing the chance of aspiration in these patients, provided regurgitation does not occur during the period of laryngoscopy and intubation. In the presence of head, eye, neck, and facial injuries; nontraumatic anatomic variations of the face and neck; and preexisting coronary or cerebrovascular disease this procedure must be planned carefully to prevent aspiration, other airway complications, and exacerbation of underlying pathologic conditions. Information on these problems is provided later in this chapter and in Chapters 9, 10, 11, 12, 13, and 14.

If surgery is required in conscious individuals, including older children, regional anesthesia is preferable whenever it can be used appropriately. If this technique is chosen, great care must be taken to avoid oversedation with narcotics, tranquilizers, or sedatives since these drugs also increase the likelihood of regurgitation and aspiration. A mask for supplementary oxygen should be used with great care as copious vomiting under the mask may jeopardize the respiratory tract.

The airway must be protected if general anesthesia is administered. Preoperative pharmacologic measures advocated for aspiration prophylaxis in surgical or obstetrical patients offer little or no advantage to the major trauma victim who must be anesthetized shortly after arrival in the emergency department. The time required for these drugs to take effect usually exceeds the short period within which surgery must commence. Additionally, some of these drugs, such as sodium citrate, can only be given orally; most major trauma victims with shock, impaired consciousness, and respiratory distress are not in a condition to take oral medications. On the other hand, selected trauma victims whose surgery may be delayed for a few hours because of radiologic evaluation or for other reasons, may benefit from pharmacologic prophylaxis, although there are few data to support this supposition.[134] Thus delaying surgery merely in order to allow time for these drugs to work cannot be justified. Although well known, it cannot be overemphasized that preoperative prophylaxis of any type cannot guarantee reliable protection against aspiration; thus, proper maneuvers must still be utilized to control the airway.

Of all preoperative prophylactic measures, evacuation of the stomach with a nasogastric Salem sump tube is the most effective. Although the nasogastric tube cannot evacuate the stomach completely,[2,273] it can empty the gas bubble along with some of the fluid, reducing intragastric pressure and thus the likelihood of regurgitation. If possible the nasogastric tube should be placed preoperatively, especially if a gas bubble is detected on the abdominal radiogram. Intraoperative placement of this tube should be considered, if for any reason it is not introduced preoperatively, to protect the airway during or after extubation. Although early reports suggested that a preoperatively introduced nasogastric tube may act as a wick and thus enhance regurgitation by interfering with the competence of the esophageal sphincter,[232] passage of gastric content into the pharynx is actually less frequent with a firm tube in place if effective cricoid pressure is applied[219,223]; a firm tube is not occluded by cricoid pressure and remains capable of decompressing the stomach and thereby preventing regurgitation.[219] Thus, there is no need to remove the nasogastric tube prior to induction of anesthesia.

Over the past few decades several investigators have designed modified gastric tubes with an integral balloon near the distal end. They propose that inflation of the balloon in the stomach and applying gentle traction to the tube immediately after induction of anesthesia impact the tube against the gastroesophageal junction and prevent reflux.[103,149] As with ordinary nasogastric tubes, the lumen of the tube acts as a "blow-off" valve, equalizing intragastric and atmospheric pressures. We have demonstrated in animals that one of these tubes allows the gastroesophageal junction to withstand intragastric pressures twice that observed without the balloon inflated or without the tube.[215] There is little experience in humans with these tubes; therefore, their routine clinical use cannot be recommended at this time.

Metoclopramide, a substituted benzamide, has powerful effects on the lower esophageal sphincter, gastrointestinal motility, and the vomiting center of the brainstem.[228] It increases antegrade gastric motility, synchronizes gastric and duodenal movements, and increases lower esophageal barrier pressure.[228] At intravenous doses of 10 or 20 mg it reduces gastric volume within about 20 to 30 minutes. In two small groups of trauma patients, one of children and another of adults, metoclopramide produced moderate reduction in gastric volume but did not provide complete protection against aspiration pneumonitis.[76,189] This drug has no effect on gastric acidity, and its effects are antagonized by simultaneously administered anticholinergics, narcotics, and diazepam.[40,186,227] Although usually without untoward side effects, metoclopramide may produce irritability, flushing, dizziness, extrapyramidal symptoms, and hypotension.[46,200,226,228]

In three separate trials, cimetidine (200 to 300 mg intravenously) increased the gastric fluid pH of many, but not all, trauma patients undergoing emergency surgery.[66,80,247] It takes at least 1 hour for this drug to produce a response, and it has little effect on the volume and acidity of fluid already in the stomach. Thus its value in acute trauma, where the goal is to reduce volume as well as acidity in a short period of time, is questionable.[86,134] Rapid intravenous administration of cimetidine can result in cardiac dysrhythmias, occasionally asystole, or at least a transient but significant decrease in arterial blood pressure[128,161,237] as a result of systemic vasodilation[68,237]; it should be administered slowly over a period of at least 15 to 20 minutes.[134] Cimetidine may also interact with anticoagulants, propranolol, and benzodiazepines because of reduction of hepatic blood flow and inhibition of microsomal enzyme activity.[93,144] An interesting report, however, demonstrated no significant change in hepatic blood flow after a single 600-mg dose of cimetidine in multiple trauma victims.[130] Intravenous ranitidine (50–100 mg), although it has important advantages such as long duration, lack of drug interactions, and minimal cardiovascular effects,[68,237] is probably less desirable than cimetidine in trauma patients because of its longer onset of action. Although not very useful preoperatively, these $H_2$ receptor antagonists given during surgery may provide some protection in the early postoperative period after tracheal extubation.

Nonparticulate antacid solutions are probably more suitable than $H_2$-receptor antagonists in the trauma patient who must be anesthetized within 15 to 60 minutes after preoperative aspiration prophylaxis. Their neutralizing effect on gastric acidity is increased if the stomach is full, as in the trauma patient, because they mix well with stomach contents without passing rapidly into the duodenum. Thus, in most trauma patients, they can elevate gastric pH above dangerous levels within 15 to 30 minutes and maintain this level for about 3 hours.[55,92,266,267] Unlike particulate antacids, clear solutions do not result in significant lung damage if aspirated, provided they are not mixed with particulate matter.[90] Available clear antacids, their characteristics, and modes of administration are shown in Table 3-1. Two important disadvantages of these agents are that they increase gastric volume and that they are ineffective in preventing aspiration of solid food. Sodium bicarbonate (8.4%) seems to increase gastric pH with smaller volumes (2 to 5 mL) than other antacids[92]; therefore it may be preferable.

As mentioned above, intubation of the trachea with a cuffed tube is the only reliable way to protect the airway from pharyngeal contents when airway reflexes are lost. The choice between the two available techniques, *awake intubation* and *rapid sequence induction with cricoid pressure,* depends on the probable ease of mask ventilation and intubation. Possible indications for each of these techniques are shown in Table 3-2. However, these recommendations should not be considered absolute because the presence of more than one condition often affects the decision. For instance, although acute head injury is an indication for rapid sequence induction, awake intubation may be selected if the patient is also in shock. In this situation, increasing systemic blood pressure with awake intubation is less hazardous than the severe hypotension which may be produced by intravenous anesthetics or some muscle relaxants, despite the fact that the former technique may also increase intracranial pressure (ICP). Thus, the widely varied problems with which these patients present require individualization in selection of intubation techniques.

### *Awake Intubation*

Skillful awake tracheal intubation is the preferred approach in a patient with anticipated airway problems. Patients with extensive maxillofacial, cervical, and thoracic injuries; extreme obesity; and decreased patency of the airway due to cervicofacial edema or hematoma are good candidates for this technique. The untoward hemodynamic effects of intravenous anesthetics used during rapid sequence induction are avoided with this approach. Awake intubation is more easily accomplished in obtunded than in vigorous and agitated patients. However, the patient must be able to follow simple commands such as to open his mouth or to take a deep breath.

TABLE 3-1. Clinically Used Nonparticulate Antacids

| ANTACID | pH | CONTENT | DOSE | ONSET | DURATION | REFERENCES |
|---|---|---|---|---|---|---|
| Sodium citrate (0.34 mol/L) | 8.4 | Sodium citrate | 15 to 30 mL | 10 to 30 minutes | >180 minutes | 266,267 |
| Bicitra | 4.5 | Sodium citrate, citric acid | 30 mL | 10 to 60 minutes | >180 minutes | 100 |
| Polycitra | 5.2 | Potassium citrate monohydrate, sodium citrate dehydrate, citric acid monohydrate | 15 mL diluted in 15 mL of water | 10 to 45 minutes | >180 minutes | 64 |
| Alka-seltzer effervescent | 6.8 | Sodium and potassium bicarbonate, citric acid | Two tablets in 30 mL of water taken after effervescence is passed | 5 to 40 minutes | >120 minutes | 55 |
| Sodium bicarbonate (8.4%) | 7.5 to 8.0 | Sodium bicarbonate | 2.0 to 5.0 mL | 10 minutes | >120 minutes | 92 |

TABLE 3-2. Possible Indications for Awake Intubation and Rapid Sequence Induction Techniques in the Trauma Patient with Full Stomach

| AWAKE INTUBATION | RAPID SEQUENCE INDUCTION |
|---|---|
| Obstructed or compromised airway | Uncooperative patient |
| Anatomical variations of the face, neck, and upper airway with the potential of causing difficult intubation | Head injury<br>Open-eye injury |
| Suspected difficulty of mask ventilation and intubation | Ischemic heart disease |
| Severe maxillofacial and mandibular injuries | Reactive airway disease |
| Neck injuries that are not evaluated adequately | Asthma |
| Active upper airway bleeding | Suspected major vessel injury without active bleeding |
| Cardiac tamponade | |
| Shock | |

The oral route using direct laryngoscopy is preferred because it is usually easier and faster than nasotracheal intubation and is indicated in the moribund or apneic patient.

The clinical problem and the management contemplated must be explained to conscious patients prior to attempting intubation in order to secure their cooperation. Sedation and analgesia with appropriate agents are often necessary to facilitate airway management, but excessive doses of opioids may depress airway reflexes and interfere with glottic competence, increasing the risk of aspiration.[59,79,147] Although protective reflexes remain more active with benzodiazepines than with opioids, these agents alone are usually not sufficient to maintain patient cooperation during airway instrumentation.

Although we adjust the dose of these drugs according to the patient's response, a combination of diazepam (0.05 mg/kg) or midazolam (0.03 mg/kg) and fentanyl (1.5 μg/kg) provides satisfactory results in most patients. Topical anesthesia of the mucous membranes must be limited to the base of the tongue, vallecula, and epiglottis while sensation in the aryepiglottic fold, the vocal cords, and the trachea is preserved in order to maintain airway reactivity. Thus, translaryngeal and superior laryngeal nerve blocks should not be performed when full stomach is suspected.[79,110,252,268] Local anesthetics injected into the trachea through the cricothyroid membrane not only blunt or abolish the cough reflex but also spread to the superior surface of the true or even the false cords, interfering with protective reflexes.[268,270] Superior laryngeal nerve block leaves the cough reflex intact but prevents reflex glottic closure in response to laryngeal contact with regurgitated material.[110] Admittedly, awake endotracheal intubation without these two blocks, especially translaryngeal injection, is often difficult and uncomfortable for the patient to a degree that some clinicians have actually recommended anesthetizing the trachea topically before attempting intubation of the patient with full stomach.[74,81] The author feels that such a recommendation is unjustifiable.

Topical anesthesia can be accomplished by various techniques; we spray 4% or 10% lidocaine (160 to 200 mg) on the gums, palate, tongue, and lateral pharyngeal walls, after which lidocaine jelly is spread on the tongue, and the patient is asked to gargle. The oral cavity must be suctioned and atropine (0.6 mg) should be administered to dry the mucous membranes and thus ensure adequate surface anesthesia. A laryngoscope blade is then introduced into the mouth and the epiglottis lifted gently. If the patient gags or complains of pain, the laryngoscope is withdrawn immediately and the patient is asked to gargle with additional local anesthetic jelly. When the larynx has finally been exposed, a lubricated cuffed endotracheal tube is introduced. One or two suctions with Yankauer tip must be available for immediate removal of pharyngeal contents should vomiting occur.

The nasal route is rarely selected for tracheal intubation if airway management is complicated only by the presence of full stomach. If, however, there are associated injuries such as cervical spine fracture-dislocations, precluding neck extension, nasotracheal intubation may be required. Blind nasal intubation, once very popular, has been used infrequently during the past decade mainly because the use of the fiberoptic bronchoscope provides a more precise technique. Blind nasal intubation may, however, sometimes be extremely useful in the acute trauma setting in which time constraints, lack of patient cooperation, and soiling of the upper airway with secretions and blood make endoscopic techniques difficult or impossible.[74] On the other hand, bleeding from dilated nasal vessels during insertion of these tubes particularly in the hypoxic and hypercarbic patient, may aggravate airway compromise. The nasal route should not be used when nasal, cranial base, Le Fort II, or Le Fort III fractures are suspected; the possibility exists that the tube may enter the cranial vault.

Various solutions have been used to provide anesthesia and vasoconstriction of the nasal mucosa, including 4 to 6% cocaine, 3% lidocaine-0.25% phenylephrine mixture, 4% lidocaine-0.5% phenylephrine mixture, and oxymetazoline.[116,138,233] A few milliliters of these solutions sprayed or applied with cotton applicators on the nasal mucosa prevent nasal bleeding, especially if a prewarmed nasotracheal tube is used. It is, however, important to remember that the analgesic effect of cocaine precedes its vasoconstrictive effect by about 5 minutes. Neither cocaine nor other sympathomimetic solutions applied in this manner appear to exert clinically significant adverse effects.[14,116] Although Maltby et al[165] report that nasotracheal intubation is easily accomplished in 70% and successfully in 91% of apneic electively operated patients with an empty stomach, adequate spontaneous ventilation and intact airway reflexes should be maintained when this technique is used in patients with a full stomach. If cervical spine injury is ruled out, atlantooccipital extension and lower cervical spine flexion, the so-called *sniffing position*, facilitates blind intubation. Following this maneuver, the endotracheal tube is introduced through the nostril and advanced to the level of the vocal cords while ventilatory exchange through the tube is auscultated. An increase in air flow through the tube suggests that it is approaching the laryngeal inlet, and with further advancement the trachea will be entered. On the other hand, cessation of air flow suggests that the tip of the tube has either entered the esophagus, lodged against the wall of the pharynx, or has induced laryngeal closure. In this situation, the tube is withdrawn slightly and redirected toward the larynx. Careful inspection of the neck is often helpful in determining the location of the tube. A bulge seen or palpated laterally in the neck suggests entry of the tube into the pyriform fossa. Slight tracheal elevation anteriorly is often a sign of entry into the esophagus. Supralaryngeal bulging suggests that the tube is located between the epiglottis and the base of the tongue.[74]

If the tube is on the vocal cords but not entering the larynx, a difficulty that occurs frequently in the absence of laryngeal anesthesia, gentle rotation and sometimes spraying of the cords through the tube with local anesthetics may be useful. The use of a small-size tube (6.5- or 7.0-mm inner diameter) and extrusion of the tongue may facilitate the intubation.[1a] Passage of a firm suction catheter into the larynx and then "railroading" the endotracheal tube over the catheter has also been said to facilitate intubation and minimize trauma to the larynx and nasal passages.[41,203] Berry[24] recommends directing the endotracheal tube toward the laryngeal inlet by introducing a stylet with a sharp anterior angle at its tip. A different technique involves inflation of the endotracheal tube cuff with air once it reaches the oropharynx. This maneuver elevates the tip of the tube away from the posterior pharyngeal wall and directs it toward the laryngeal inlet, increasing the chance of success[109] (Fig 3-3). The tube can also be manipulated by using directional tip control tubes (Endotrol). When all measures fail, and the mouth can be opened, direct laryngoscopy can be performed and a Magill forceps used for appropriate positioning of the tube in patients with stable or stabilized cervical spine.

FIG. 3-3. A technique to facilitate awake, blind, nasotracheal intubation. 1, The distal tip of the tube tends to lodge against the pharynx or enter the esophagus; 2, the tube tip is redirected into the larynx by inflation of the tube cuff against the posterior wall of the oropharynx; 3, the distal portion of the tube is in the larynx; 4, the cuff is deflated to advance the tube into the trachea; 5, the cuff is below the vocal cords ready to be inflated.

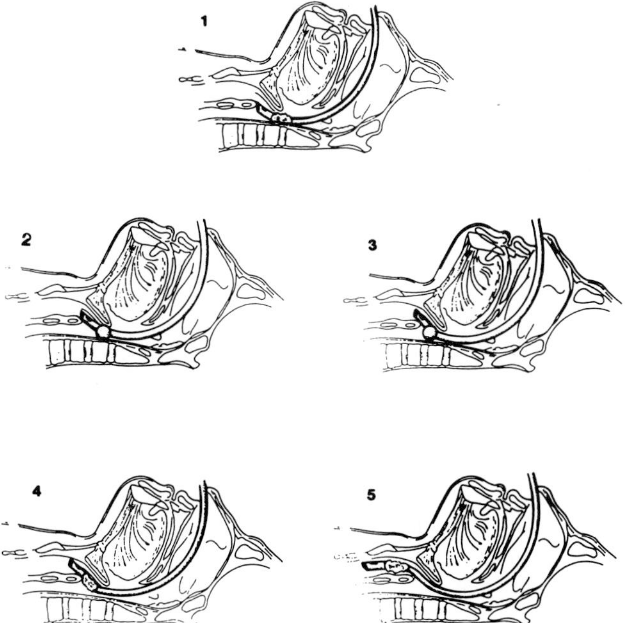


The success rate of blind nasal intubation varies between 80 and 95% in reported series in which the larynx and trachea were anesthetized.[74,105,146,165,197] Without the use of laryngeal anesthesia the success rate is probably less. Further, in only 10 to 35% of instances is intubation successful on the first attempt.[105,197] Multiple attempts may result in trauma to the airway. In one series, epistaxis, sinusitis, nasal necrosis, or retropharyngeal lacerations occurred in 3% of patients.[74] If epistaxis from excessive pressure is significant, the nasotracheal tube should be left in place to tamponade the bleeding. Of course, the nasal route should not be selected if coagulation abnormalities exist.

Some of the disadvantages of the blind technique can be overcome by use of a fiberoptic bronchoscope for either oro- or nasotracheal intubation, although this technique requires experience and may be associated with prolonged intubation time. Nevertheless a fiberoptic technique may be a safe alternative for the patient with a full stomach who is likely to be difficult to intubate or in whom there is serious limitation of mouth opening. The technique described by Ovassapian et al[194] for awake fiberoptic intubation of the patient with full stomach is as follows. After sedation with intravenous diazepam (70 to 100 μg/kg) and fentanyl (1.5 to 2.5 μg/kg), the mouth is sprayed with 14% benzocaine/tetracaine mixture (Cetacaine), and additional 20% benzocaine lubricant is applied to the base of the tongue. One of the available special oropharyngeal airways (Patil-Syracuse, Williams, or Ovassapian) is placed in the mouth after the pharynx is suctioned. The endotracheal tube is introduced and advanced with the aid of the fiberoptic bronchoscope until its tip is positioned just proximal to the vocal cords. At this stage the cords are sprayed with a few milliliters of lidocaine (4%) injected through the suction port of the bronchoscope, and after 30 to 45 seconds, the instrument is advanced through the glottis, and an additional 2 mL of lidocaine is sprayed within the trachea. The endotracheal tube is then threaded over the bronchoscope into the trachea and its cuff inflated. During the period between local anesthetic injection and tracheal intubation the airway is left unprotected; however, this period is usually short in experienced hands, making aspiration unlikely.[193,194,195]

Nasotracheal fiberoptic intubation is easier to perform than orotracheal fiberoptic technique because the larynx is visualized from a distance, and the bronchoscope can be directed easily without being shifted laterally. In elective cases, the failure rate of fiberoptic guided intubation is less than 1.5%.[193,195] The major causes of failure are poor laryngeal anesthesia and blockage of the view by secretions, pharyngeal tissues, and blood, conditions that are likely to be present in the acute trauma victim; thus the failure rate is probably higher in this group of patients. In elective situations, 30% of orotracheal and 16% of nasotracheal fiberoptic intubations are difficult.[193] The problems, however, are different from those of difficult direct laryngoscopy. Apart from the problems described, a decreased distance between the tip of the epiglottis and the posterior pharyngeal wall may increase the difficulty of intubation.[193,195] Elevation of the floor of the mouth with edema or hematoma, as in patients with maxillofacial injuries, can produce this situation. Several technical problems may contribute to difficulty in withdrawing the bronchoscope after tracheal intubation: inadvertent advancement of the instrument through the Murphy eye of the tracheal tube; leaving the tip of the scope in flexed position; inserting the tracheal tube into the esophagus while the fiberscope is in the trachea; using a poorly lubricated scope in a tight-fitting tracheal tube; and many others.[193] Hypoxemia secondary to hypoventilation, laryngospasm, or excessive suctioning during fiberoptic intubation can be prevented by insufflating high-flow oxygen via the suction channel, by appropriate ventilatory support, or by administration of high- or low-frequency jet ventilation either through the suction channel or percutaneously.[37,224]

### *Rapid Sequence Induction with Cricoid Pressure*

This is the most desirable method of anesthetic induction, if one can be sure that mask ventilation and tracheal intubation can be accomplished without difficulty. There is a high risk of pulmonary aspiration if repeated attempts at tracheal intubation are made; thus if the possibility of difficult intubation exists, an awake technique is preferred. Likewise, the presence of partial airway obstruction of unidentified cause is a contraindication to this approach; muscle relaxation may lead to total airway obstruction.

With the introduction of modern drugs and development of new techniques, the traditionally described rapid sequence induction technique[71] has been considerably altered over the past few decades (Table 3-3). The head-up position, while reducing the incidence of regurgitation from the stomach, also intensifies the depressant hemodynamic effects of intravenous anesthetics. As application of cricoid pressure obviates the need for this maneuver, head-up tilt has either been abandoned or limited to no more than 10 to 15°. The traditional preoxygenation involving breathing of 100% oxygen for 3 to 5 minutes has been replaced in some centers by the patient taking four deep breaths over a period of 30 seconds,[106] although the efficacy of the latter method is dependent on the patient's pulmonary function. Thus, pain, analgesics, brain and/or thoracoabdominal wall injury, pulmonary dysfunction, and partial airway obstruction may reduce the effectiveness of this method of preoxygenation in the acute trauma victim. Further, the decline in oxygen saturation during the apneic period following induction of anesthesia is more rapid in patients oxygenated with four breaths compared with those preoxygenated for 3 minutes or longer.[98]

Many clinicians now do not utilize precurarization prior to succinylcholine since the fasciculation-induced increase in intragastric pressure is accompanied by a simultaneous increase in lower esophageal sphincter pressure, preventing regurgitation,[238] and since nondepolarizing agents may delay the onset time of succinylcholine.[73] The first reason applies to patients with a normal gastroesophageal junction and not necessarily to persons with intraabdominal pathology or hiatus hernia. Since the limited preoperative time in many trauma victims prevents clear determination of such conditions, precurarization may have a place in this setting, especially since the finding of delay in succinylcholine effect produced by precurarization[73] has been refuted by several authors.[32,65,269] In addition, precurarization attenuates succinylcholine-induced increases in intraocular and intracranial pressures, which could be deleterious in the head- and/or eye-injured patient.[117,160,176,245] Of course, the dose of succinylcholine must be increased by 50 to 70% if this technique is used.[96] The optimal pretreatment doses and timing of the various nondepolarizing muscle relaxants and their side effects are shown in Table 3-4. Ventilation should be monitored closely following pretreatment with these agents since dyspnea and aspiration of pharyngeal contents occasionally occur because of altered respiratory mechanics and laryngeal dysfunction. Further discussion of this subject is provided in Chapter 9.

In hemodynamically stable trauma patients, rapid sequence induction is likely to produce an exaggerated hypertensive and tachycardic response that may be associated with increased myocardial oxygen consumption and decreased left ventricular ejection fraction, representing a serious additional burden for the poorly perfused heart of a patient with ischemic heart disease.[15,57] In addition, this technique results in elevation of intracranial and intraocular pressures, which is not desirable in head- and eye-injured patients. Measures designed to prevent these untoward effects are shown in Table 3-5. Opioid agents should be administered slowly over a period

TABLE 3-3. Originally Described Procedures for Rapid Sequence Induction and the Alternatives or Modifications Developed During the Past 20 Years

| ORIGINAL DESCRIPTION | ALTERNATIVES OR MODIFICATIONS |
|---|---|
| 30° to 40° head-up tilt | Often applied but not considered essential if cricoid pressure is applied |
| Evacuation of the stomach with a nasogastric tube | Unchanged |
| Removal of the nasogastric tube after evacuation of the stomach contents | The nasogastric tube is left in place in most instances |
| Preoxygenation with 100% $O_2$ for 3 to 5 minutes | Preoxygenation with four deep breaths for 30 seconds |
| Pretreatment with dTc* (3 to 6 mg) | No pretreatment<br>Pretreatment with newer nondepolarizers |
| No measure to attenuate hemodynamic response | Various measures to attenuate hemodynamic response |
| Intravenous injection of thiopental (2 to 4 mg/kg), diazepam (5 to 20 mg), ketamine (1 to 2 mg/kg) | Intravenous injection of midazolam (0.2 to 0.3 mg/kg), etomidate (0.2 to 0.25 mg/kg), or high-dose alfentanil (80 to 100 μg/kg) |
| Application of cricoid pressure | Unchanged<br>Cricoid yoke |
| Succinylcholine (1.5 to 2 mg/kg, intravenously) | Mivacurium (0.3 mg/kg intravenously)<br>Vecuronium (0.2 to 0.25 mg/kg intravenously)<br>Vecuronium priming (0.01 mg/kg + 0.1 mg/kg)<br>Pancuronium (0.2 mg/kg) |
| Maintenance of apnea after intravenous anesthetic and muscle relaxants | Ventilation by mask with cricoid pressure in selected patients |
| Intubation of the larynx | Unchanged |
| Inflation of the endotracheal tube cuff | Unchanged |

* d-Tubocurarine.

TABLE 3-4. Doses, Optimal Time of Administration, and Side Effects of Various Nondepolarizing Muscle Relaxants Used for Pretreatment to Prevent Succinylcholine Fasciculations in Adults*

| MUSCLE RELAXANT | DOSE (mg/kg) | TIME OF ADMINISTRATION (MINUTES BEFORE SUCCINYLCHOLINE) | SIDE EFFECTS |
|---|---|---|---|
| Gallamine | 0.20 to 0.25 | 2 to 3 | HR and BP increase by gallamine |
| D-Tubocurarine | 0.05 to 0.7 | 3 to 5 | Occasional dyspnea caused by diminished respiratory mechanical strength and possible luminal narrowing of the laryngeal inlet |
| Metocurine | 0.02 to 0.03 | 3 to 5 | |
| Pancuronium | 0.01 to 0.015 | 3 to 5 | |
| Atracurium | 0.05 | 3 to 5 | |
| Vecuronium | 0.01 | 2 to 3 | |

* The abbreviations used are: HR, heart rate; BP, blood pressure. (Adapted from Bruce et al[43], Horrow and Lambert[125], Kingsley et al[140], Manchikanti et al[166], Motsch et al[180] and Rao and Jacobs.[207])

of 5 minutes with constant monitoring of hemodynamics and observation of the patient;[67,70,143] apnea, chest wall rigidity, hypotension, and seizure-like tonic-clonic movements may occur with these agents. Ventilation with potent inhalational agents before intubation should be performed only when effective cricoid pressure is applied. Intravenous lidocaine (1.5 to 2 mg/kg) administered 2 to 3 minutes before intubation is a weak measure at best and prevents the stress response only in some patients.[56,250] Topical lidocaine is likewise unreliable in ameliorating these responses even when the larynx and trachea are anesthetized.[78]

Propranolol (0.01 mg/kg), given 5 minutes before rapid sequence induction, attenuates heart rate and systolic blood pressure responses to laryngoscopy and intubation.[217] Of the newer adrenergic blockers, labetalol effectively blocks the tachycardic response at doses of 0.1 to 0.2 mg/kg; however, attenuation of the hypertensive response may require doses as large as 0.75 mg/kg.[23,159] Esmolol, at doses described in Table 3-5, appears to be more effective than labetalol in controlling hemodynamic responses to laryngoscopy and intubation.[104,120] Nitroglycerine intravenously or intranasally (0.8 mg), can also be used to attenuate the pressor response to anesthetic induction.

A large variety of intravenous anesthetics is available for rapid induction of anesthesia (Table 3-3), but with the possible exception of ketamine, they all are cardiovascular depressants and should be administered to hypovolemic trauma patients with great caution at doses reduced by 40 to 50%[272] (see also

TABLE 3-5. Available Measures to Attenuate the Hypertensive and Tachycardic Response to Rapid Sequence Induction in Hemodynamically Stable Patients

| MEASURE | DRUGS AND THEIR DOSES | TIMING OF ADMINISTRATION | CONTRAINDICATIONS |
|---|---|---|---|
| Opioid preloading | Fentanyl (4 to 5 μg/kg)<br>Alfentanil (10 μg/kg)<br>Sufentanil (1 to 2 μg/kg) | Over a period of 5 minutes before anesthetic induction | Hypovolemia?<br>Increased ICP |
| Controlled ventilation with potent inhalation agents | Halothane (1 to 2% insp. concentration)<br>Enflurane (0.75 to 1% insp. concentration)<br>Isoflurane (1 to 2% insp. concentration) titrated to blood pressure | After induction with intravenous anesthetic and muscle relaxants and application of cricoid pressure | Hypovolemia<br>Head injury |
| Topical anesthesia of the oropharynx | Lidocaine 4% spray and jelly (300 to 400 mg) | Prior to anesthetic induction | |
| Intravenous lidocaine | Lidocaine (1.5 to 2 mg/kg) | 3 minutes before intubation | |
| α and β adrenergic blockers | Propranolol (0.01 mg/kg intravenously) | 5 minutes before induction and intubation | Hypovolemia<br>History of asthma |
| | Labetalol (0.1 to 0.2 mg/kg intravenously) | 2 to 3 minutes before induction and intubation | Cardiac conduction block<br>Cardiac failure |
| | Esmolol (500 μg/kg + 200 to 300 μg/kg per minute intravenously) for 15 minutes | Over a period of 15 minutes, starting the loading dose 4 minuts before induction and continuing with maintenance dose during induction | |
| Vasodilators | Nitroglycerine (5 to 10 μg/minutes intravenously) | Over a period of 3 to 5 minutes starting before intubation and titrated to hemodynamic response | Hypovolemia<br>Atelectasis<br>Increased ICP |

Chapter 9). In severely hypovolemic patients or in those with cardiac injury these agents may have to be omitted altogether.

Cricoid pressure, which was used as early as 1774 to prevent inflation of the stomach during resuscitation of near-drowning victims,[220] was introduced into anesthetic practice by Sellick in 1961[232] and is probably the most effective component of the rapid sequence induction technique. In Sellick's original description cricoid pressure was designed to serve two purposes: provision of a line of defense at the cricopharyngeal level against entry of stomach contents into the pharynx, and prevention of gastric inflation during bag-mask ventilation.[232] The efficacy of the first effect has been well proven in animals, human cadavers, adults, and children; gastric contents cannot reach the pharynx even against distal esophageal pressure gradients as high as 50 to 60 cm $H_2O$.[91,219,221] The second purpose of the maneuver was not tested in clinical conditions until recently because bag-mask ventilation has not been a part of this technique. Now, it has been demonstrated that cricoid pressure effectively prevents gastric distention if the airway is not obstructed.[151,205] This salutary effect of cricoid pressure gains particular importance during induction of patients with closed-head injuries in whom maintenance of hypocapnia is vital or of patients with acute traumatic lung pathology where even short periods of apnea are fraught with the danger of severe hypoxemia. Too often cricoid pressure is applied incorrectly; improper force is applied, or the cricoid cartilage is deviated laterally.[126] A force of 44 N (~4.5 kg or 10 lb) is estimated to protect 50% of adult patients from aspiration of passively regurgitated material.[280] Greater force may be more effective but is also likely to reduce the diameter of the larynx, especially in older persons, and thus make intubation difficult. In England a device called a *cricoid yoke* has been designed to provide consistent and reproducible cricoid pressure, enabling even inexperienced individuals to apply the maneuver correctly.[150,152] There are several contraindications to the use of cricoid pressure in the trauma victim: cervical spine fracture-dislocation, especially at the C5-C6 level; laryngeal or cricoid cartilage fracture; and the presence of a foreign body in the esophagus or airway at the C5-C6 level[114]; additional damage to the cervical spine, the vocal cords or airway, or distal or proximal migration of foreign bodies may result from this maneuver.[5] Cricoid pressure should also not be applied during awake intubation or to lightly anesthetized unparalyzed or partially paralyzed individuals; esophageal rupture may result during vigorous active vomiting in these circumstances.

Many alternatives to the use of succinylcholine for muscle relaxation in the patient with full stomach have emerged during the past 10 years. Although it remains the fastest acting muscle relaxant, succinylcholine has the drawbacks of increasing intragastric, intracranial, and intraocular pressures; producing hyperkalemia if administered more than 3 days after central nervous system trauma or extensive muscle and/or burn injury; and occasionally, of causing dysrhythmias (see also Chapter 9). Parenthetically, succinylcholine-induced dysrhythmias are especially common and may be life threatening in the presence of hypoxia and hypercarbia, frequent occurrences in the major trauma victim. Hyperkalemia, from both the direct activity of succinylcholine and acidosis, has been implicated as a mechanism of this effect, but more recent data suggest that an elevated norepinephrine level from stimulation of sympathetic ganglia and postganglionic sympathetic terminals has an important role in the production of these arrhythmias.[156] As is well known, concomitantly administered halothane exacerbates myocardial dysrhythmias, whereas enflurane suppresses them.[156] In any case, of the three alternatives to succinylcholine, mivacurium (BW B1090U) appears to be the most desirable. Metabolized by human plasma cholinesterase, mivacurium provides satisfactory relaxation for direct laryngoscopy and tracheal intubation within 60 seconds if a total dose of 0.3 mg/kg is given in two divided doses immediately before and after the intravenous anesthetic.[225] The second alternative to succinylcholine is high-dose vecuronium (0.20 to 0.25 mg/kg) or pancuronium (0.20 to 0.25 mg/kg) which provides muscle relaxation within 60 to 90 seconds.[21,42,158] The third alternative, priming with vecuronium or atracurium,[249] does not seem to provide as good intubating conditions as succinylcholine and has other important drawbacks that are described in Chapter 9.[58,167,240,241] The use of this technique will probably decrease once mivacurium becomes commercially available.

Rapid laryngoscopy and tracheal intubation after induction require proper positioning of the head and neck—atlantooccipital extension and lower cervical flexion (the sniffing position)—to align pharyngeal, esophageal, and tracheal planes. This position is different from that required for optimal cricoid pressure, which involves extension of both head and neck to increase the convexity of the cervical spine, stretch the esophagus, and thus prevent its lateral displacement by cricoid pressure.[107,232] However, despite this conflict, the sniffing position remains the correct head and neck position for rapid sequence induction for two reasons. First, in both positions the anterior convexity of the cervical spine is about the same; second, the esophagus is attached to the posterior wall of the cricoid cartilage by the longitudinal fibers of its muscular coat. Thus, it is not likely to be displaced laterally with incomplete extension of the cervical spine.[257]

The technique of cricoid pressure may have to be modified in a patient who presents with an impaling object in the back (Fig 3-4). The anesthetic induction is performed in the left lateral decubitus position. Cricoid pressure is applied using two hands: one hand applies force to the back of the neck, and the other compresses the cricoid against the cervical spine. Alternatively the patient is placed in supine position on two operating tables between which the impaling object remains undisturbed.

### *Management of Regurgitation and Aspiration*

If regurgitation occurs during laryngoscopy, a well-functioning Yankauer suction should be utilized and the patient tilted head-down to prevent pulmonary aspiration. An endotracheal tube can be inserted into the esophagus and its cuff inflated to allow the stomach contents to bypass the pharynx and to flow out of the tube while laryngeal visualization proceeds.[72]

Despite these measures, aspiration may still occur, and often, especially if the amount of aspirated material is small, the characteristic early signs—bronchospasm, hypoxemia, and diffuse mottled appearance of the lung on chest radiogram (Fig 3-5)—may not develop for several hours.[45] At this

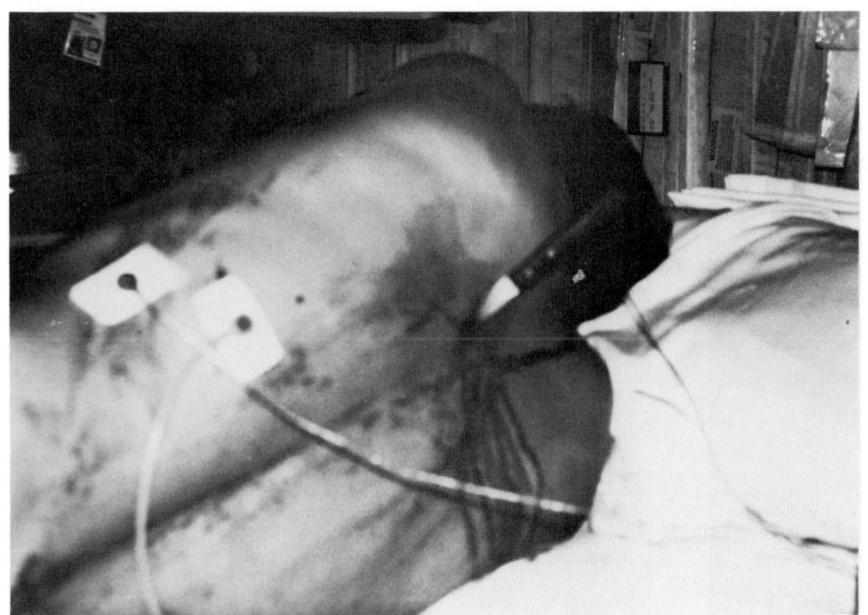

FIG. 3-4. A patient with an impaling knife in his back. The knife should be left in place until surgical exposure and control of injured vessels in deep tissues are attained. Cricoid pressure during anesthetic induction in the left lateral decubitus position can be applied using two-hand technique.

stage the presence of vomitus or gastric secretion in the tracheobronchial tree is the most valuable diagnostic finding. Early fiberoptic bronchoscopy, or rigid bronchoscopy if solid food is aspirated, should be performed and may show aspirated material, thick purulent secretions, and erythematous swelling in the trachea, large bronchi, and subsegmental airways.[50] Data from animal experiments suggest that release of tachykinin family of neuropeptides (substance P, neurokinin A, neuropeptide K) and calcitonin gene-related peptide (CGRP) in afferent neurons in the lower airways contribute to protein extravasation and airway edema after aspiration. Capsaicin, which depletes CGRP and tachykinins in the airways, reduces the edema and protein extravasation in animals.[168] Aspiration-induced mucosal changes progress over several hours to increased swelling accompanied by hemorrhage, necrosis, and ulceration. Thus, fiberoptic bronchoscopy should be repeated every few hours to observe the progress of the pathology, although by this time the chest radiogram will also become positive. Experimentally, the survival rate following aspiration is closely related to the degree of irreversible pulmonary vascular change.[36] Early initiation of controlled ventilation with positive end-expiratory pressure (PEEP) may reduce these changes. Alternatively, intermittent mandatory ventilation (IMV) with continuous positive pressure breathing (CPPB) in patients who are not hypoventilating may be used in the postoperative period, since this method is associated with lower mean intrathoracic pressure and thus less cardiac output depression. Tracheobronchial lavage with neutral or alkaline solutions does little good and may actually be harmful as it disseminates the aspirated material.[281]

### *Management of Failed Intubation*

Failure to intubate the trachea of the trauma victim during rapid sequence induction creates major difficulties for the anesthesiologist, especially when ventilation of the patient is also impossible. Although careful preoperative airway evaluation usually helps predict difficult intubation and indicates alternative airway management strategies, in some instances this assessment may not arouse suspicion of possible problems. Pulmonary aspiration often occurs during poorly planned repeated attempts to intubate a difficult airway; therefore a clear management plan in conjunction with adequate equipment and manpower must be available before embarking on a rapid sequence induction. A suggested management plan is shown in Fig 3-6.

When difficulty in intubation occurs in a setting in which adequate mask ventilation and oxygenation, as determined by clinical signs, pulse oximeter, and $CO_2$ analyzer, are possible, the further course of action will depend on laryngoscopy findings. Obviously, difficulty arises when the glottis and arytenoids cannot be visualized; but if the epiglottis is seen, the trachea can often be intubated with special techniques. A simple maneuver to facilitate intubation is described by Salem et al.[218] It consists of cephalad displacement of the larynx during laryngoscopy by an assistant. Further improvement can be provided with a leader (a flexible stylet) introduced into the trachea by sliding it behind the posterior wall of the epiglottis.[208] The endotracheal tube is then advanced over it. The LTA kit (Abbott Laboratories) can be particularly useful for this purpose[214] (Fig 3-7). The lubricated cannula is introduced through the Murphy hole of the endotracheal tube from outside and advanced to its junction with the syringe so that the tube and syringe can easily be held in one hand. After laryngoscopy, the cannula is introduced into the larynx, and the tube is then slid over it into the trachea. The cannula is thin enough not to obstruct the view during laryngoscopy and stiff enough to lift the epiglottis. In experienced hands an appropriate sized rigid bronchoscope or an optical stylet can be utilized to obtain a direct view of the larynx.[137,211] A straight laryngoscope blade may also facilitate intubation by lifting the epiglottis. An important modification of the straight

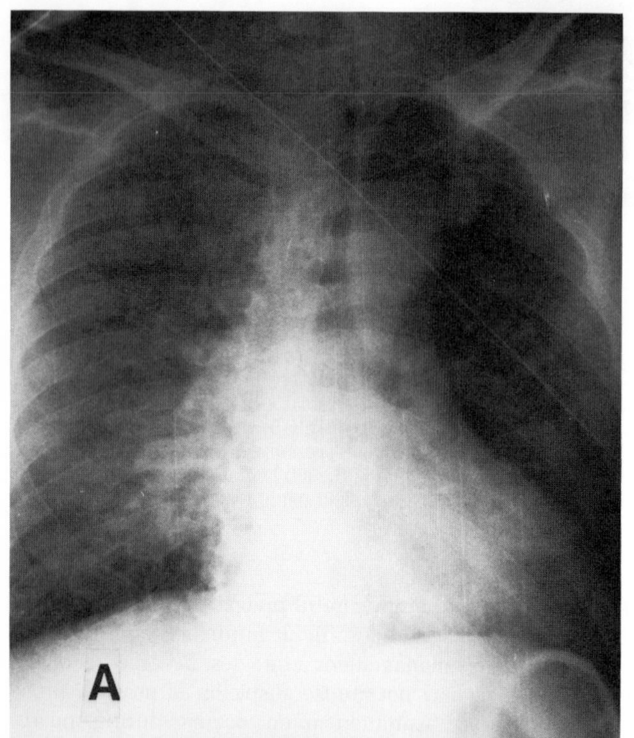


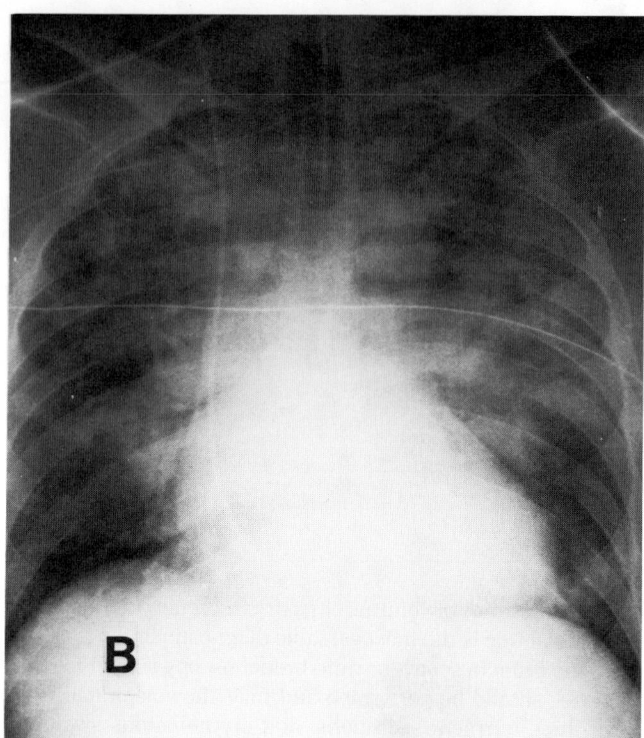


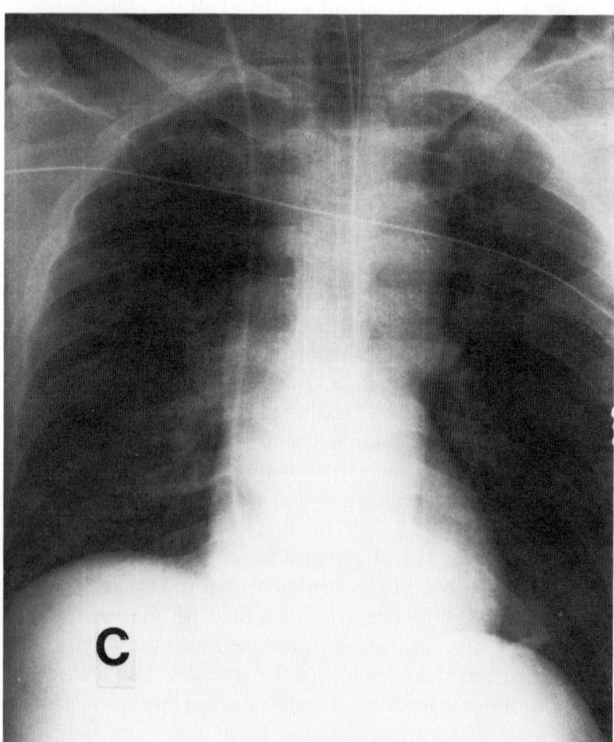


FIG. 3-5. Chest X-rays of a patient with upper extremity injury. Aspiration of gastric contents occurred shortly after extubation resulting in minimal clinical and radiographic signs for a few hours. A, chest X-ray obtained 3 hours after aspiration shows relatively mild changes; B, diffuse mottling of both lungs and hypoxemia necessitated positive pressure ventilation with PEEP 6 hours after aspiration; C, lung fields cleared after 4 days of ventilatory therapy.

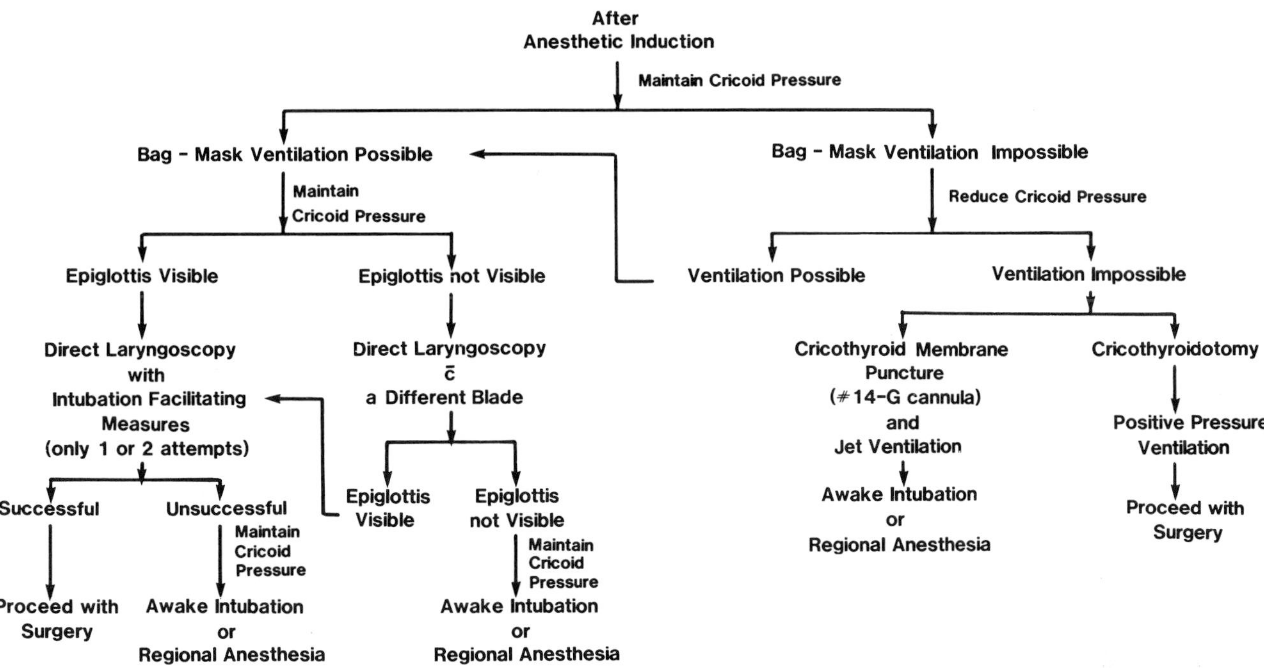


FIG. 3-6. A decision tree to manage failed intubation after rapid sequence anesthetic induction.

blade has been designed by Bellhouse;[19] it has a 45° angle at the midpoint with a prism incorporated on the posterior surface. This laryngoscope may provide visualization when other methods fail[19] (Fig 3-8).

It is important that the anesthesiologist select the technique or techniques most familiar to him/her and make no more than one or two attempts at intubation. If these attempts fail, the patient should be awakened while cricoid pressure is maintained and the airway secured using a blind or fiberoptic-guided technique or, if appropriate, the surgery should be performed using regional anesthesia.

When ventilation of the patient by mask becomes impossible during airway manipulation or from the beginning of anesthetic induction, the cause of obstruction should be determined and corrected as expeditiously as possible. The com-

FIG. 3-7. The use of LTA kit (Abbott Laboratories) as a leader to facilitate endotracheal intubation. See text for further detail. (From Rosenberg et al[214] with permission.)

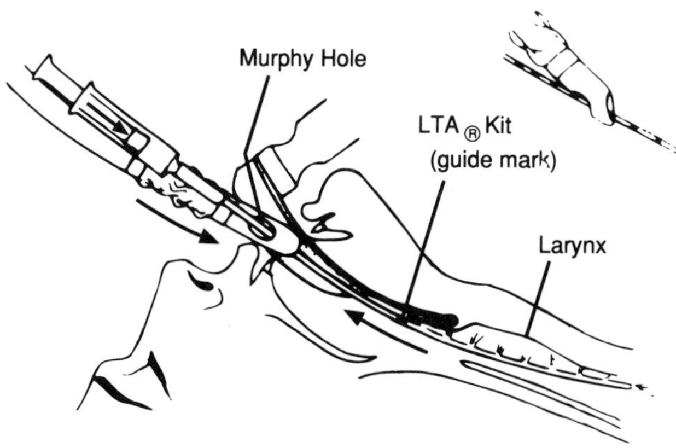


FIG. 3-8. Bellhouse laryngoscope with an attached prism. The laryngoscope can be used without the prism if it can be pulled forward sufficiently to obtain direct visualization of the larynx. The anatomical configuration of the orofacial structures depicted in the figure precludes this maneuver, necessitating the use of prism to provide indirect view of the larynx. (From Bellhouse[19] with permission.)

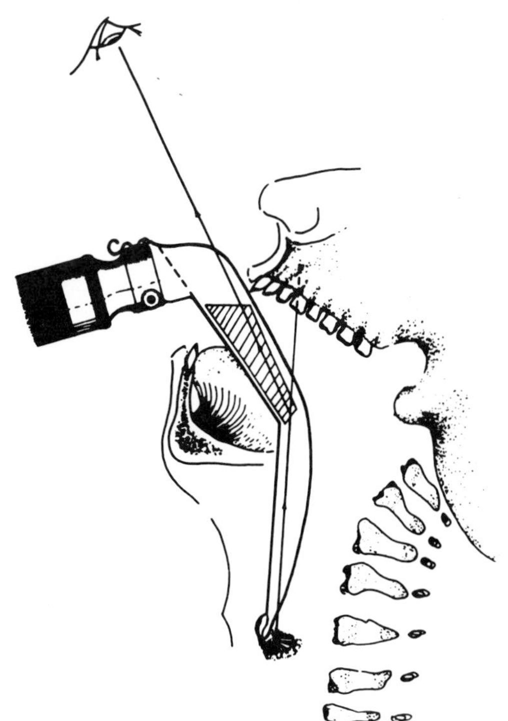

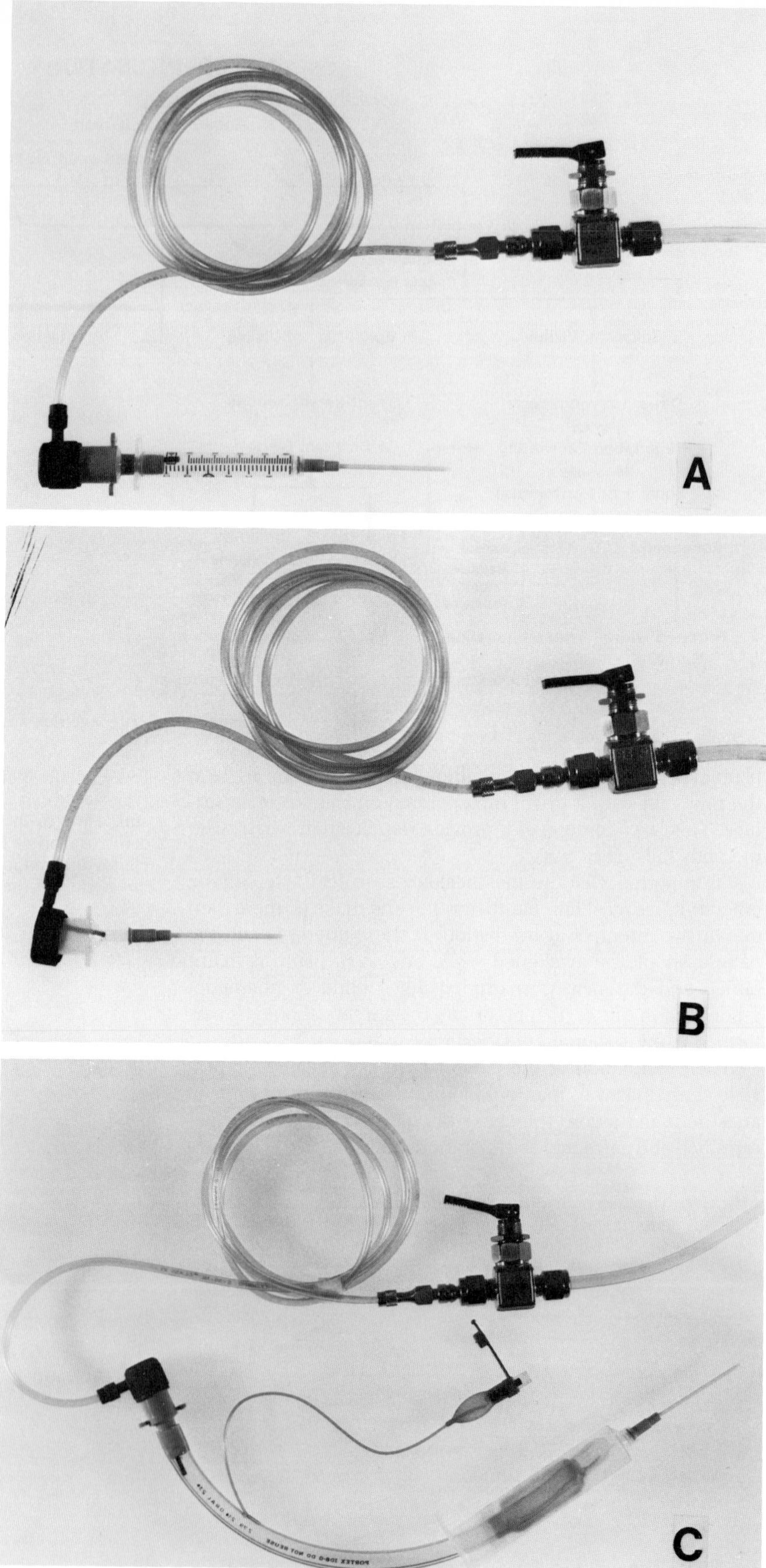


FIG. 3-9. Possible ways to connect the Sander's jet attachment to a cricothyroidotomy cannula. A, via a 7.5 ET tube adapter connected to a 3-ml syringe barrel; B, via a 3.5 ET tube adapter connected directly to the cannula; and C, via a 7.0 ET tube introduced into the barrel of a 10-ml syringe.

mon causes of difficult ventilation following injury include excessive cricoid pressure[152,280]; soft tissue and epiglottic encroachment on the larynx[35]; pharyngeal blood, secretions, and foreign bodies; inappropriately placed oral airway; light anesthesia; inadequate muscle relaxation; laryngeal edema; bronchospasm; and tension pneumothorax. If rapid amelioration of airway obstruction is not possible by reducing cricoid pressure, repositioning the head and neck, suctioning the oropharynx, or other pertinent measures, the next course of action is to establish adequate oxygenation, either by insufflation or jet ventilation via a 14-guage or larger cannula inserted through the cricothyroid membrane or to perform a cricothyroidotomy and start positive pressure ventilation. Some clinicians also recommend the use of recently described airway protection and ventilation devices: the esophageal gastric tube airway, the laryngeal mask airway, and the pharyngotracheal lumen airway or esophageal tracheal combitube.[95,258] These devices are designed to replace the esophageal obturator tube, which was associated with a high rate of complications and questionable efficacy, and are primarily used during prehospital airway management. The efficacy of these devices must be tested further before they can be recommended for the operating room or emergency department.

NEEDLE CRICOTHYROIDOTOMY AND JET VENTILATION. A 14-gauge or larger cannula is inserted percutaneously through the cricothyroid membrane in a caudad direction. After securing the cannula adequately, its hub is connected to an oxygen source,[10] a jet ventilator,[248] a self-inflating resuscitation bag,[184] or the anesthesia machine[230] by means of one of the following easily constructed adapters: (1) a 7.5-mm endotracheal tube adapter fitted tightly into a 3-mL disposable syringe barrel (Fig 3-9, A); (2) a 3.5-mm endotracheal tube adapter (Fig 3-9, B); or (3) a 7.0-mm endotracheal tube with its inflated cuff fitted inside a 10-mL disposable syringe barrel[102,210] (Fig 3-9, C). Of all these ventilation devices, the Sanders jet ventilator provides the best oxygenation and ventilation.[253,286] Oxygen flushed through the fresh gas outlet of the anesthesia machine and connected directly to the patient via high pressure tubing can also provide adequate ventilation and oxygenation, although it is less effective than the jet ventilator. Oxygen insufflation and manual ventilation with the anesthesia machine bag through the circle system or a self-inflating resuscitation bag, although capable of reversing preexisting hypoxemia, cannot provide adequate ventilation even with airway pressures as high as 80 cm $H_2O$[10,253,286] (Fig 3-10). Ventilation via a transtracheal catheter requires extreme caution in the presence of complete upper airway obstruction; tension pneumothorax, pneumomediastinum, subcutaneous emphysema, or abdominal distention may result.[53,188] Fortunately, airway obstruction is usually only inspiratory; air from the lung can be exhaled easily unless the larynx is almost completely blocked by edema, hematoma, blood clot, or foreign body. Nevertheless, careful observation for adequate chest descent after each inspiration, elevation of the jaw, and proper head positioning are crucial to facilitate exhalation.

It is wise to start jet ventilation with a low driving pressure (20 to 30 psi) and carefully increase it until adequate chest

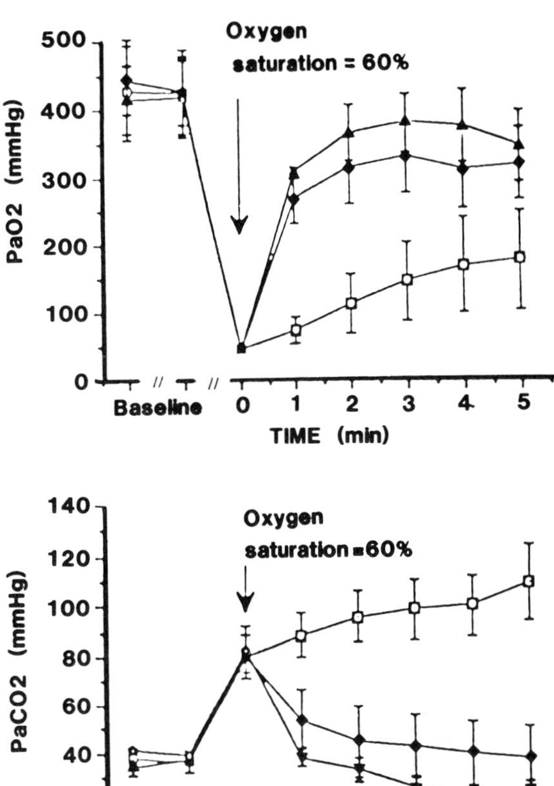


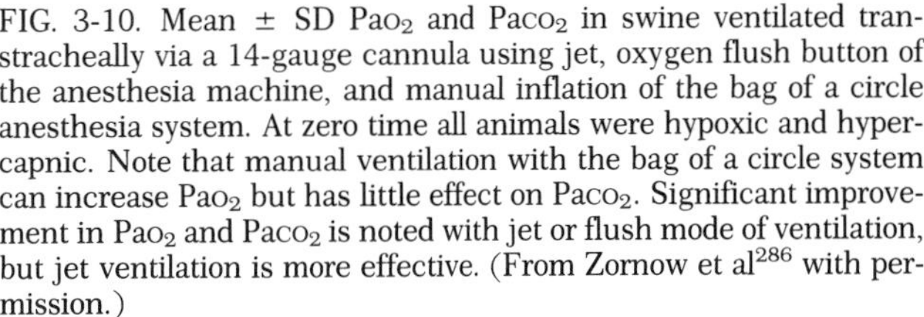


FIG. 3-10. Mean ± SD $Pa_{O_2}$ and $Pa_{CO_2}$ in swine ventilated transtracheally via a 14-gauge cannula using jet, oxygen flush button of the anesthesia machine, and manual inflation of the bag of a circle anesthesia system. At zero time all animals were hypoxic and hypercapnic. Note that manual ventilation with the bag of a circle system can increase $Pa_{O_2}$ but has little effect on $Pa_{CO_2}$. Significant improvement in $Pa_{O_2}$ and $Pa_{CO_2}$ is noted with jet or flush mode of ventilation, but jet ventilation is more effective. (From Zornow et al[286] with permission.)

excursions are noted. The translaryngeal cannula must be checked constantly; kinking, disconnection, and displacement are common complications. If complete airway obstruction is present, a cannula with an orifice of at least 3.0 mm, if an Ambu bag is used, or 2.4 mm (10-gauge), if a portable oscillatory pressure device is used, is mandatory to assist or control ventilation without barotrauma.[108,184] A 3.5-mm (inner diameter) percutaneous cannula (Abelson cricothyroidotomy system) is available.[184]

CRICOTHYROIDOTOMY. Emergency cricothyroidotomy can be performed in two other ways: with a cricothyrotome or as a formal surgical procedure. Several types of cricothyrotomes are available on the market, but the Nu-trake set is used most frequently. This set consists of a knife for skin incision; a housing unit that contains a ventilating system adapter and a two-part expanding needle with a removable sharp needle stylet inside; and three tracheal cannulas (4.5,

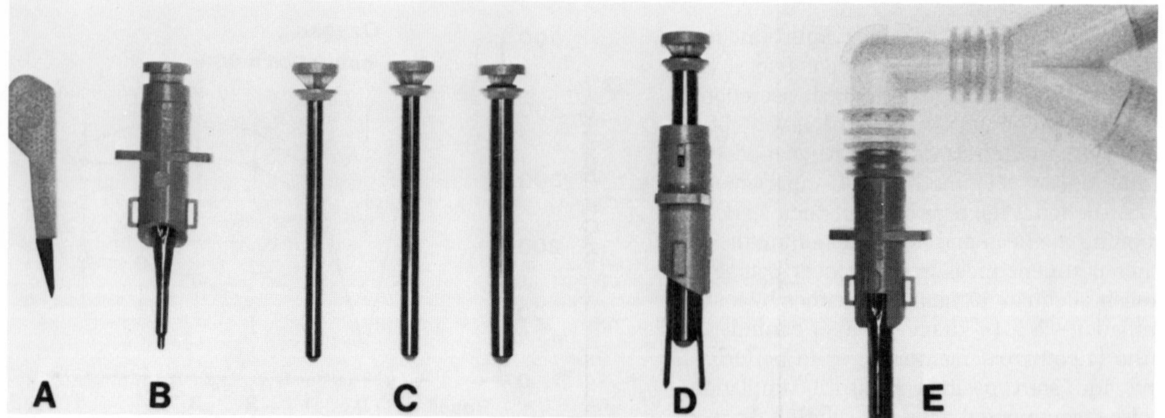


FIG. 3-11. Nu-trake cricothyroidotomy kit consisting of A, the knife blade to incise the skin; B, the housing unit with needle stylet that serves to puncture the cricothyroid membrane; C, three different size airways (4.5, 6.0, and 7.2 mm) with obturators to be introduced into the housing unit after removing the needle stylet; D, the housing unit accommodating airway with obturator inserted halfway. (Note the longitudinally split distal part of the housing unit which remains in the trachea to accommodate the airways); E, the airway completely inserted into the housing unit and, therefore, the trachea. A universal adapter may be fitted to the top of the housing to provide ventilation.

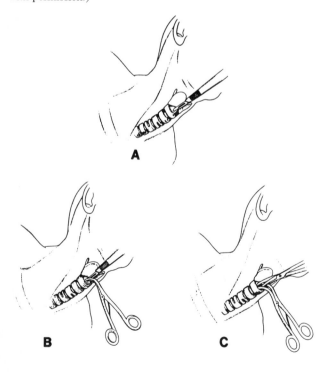

6, and 7.2 mm) with obturators (Fig 3-11). The skin over the cricothyroid membrane is incised, and the needle stylet is inserted into the trachea. The stylet is then removed, leaving the two-part blunt housing inside the trachea. The selected airway, which fits into the housing, is introduced and its obturator removed. The procedure takes approximately 1 minute.[209] Although the procedure is easy, familiarity with the device and some operator training are necessary.[209] Occasionally the larynx may be injured during the procedure, resulting in submucosal emphysema and/or posterior wall perforation.[30]

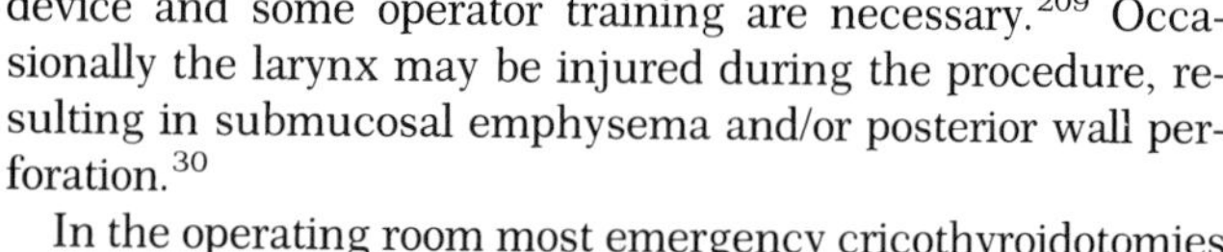

FIG. 3-12. Surgical technique of emergency cricothyroidotomy. Following a transverse or vertical skin incision (vertical incision preferred) the cricothyroid membrane is divided horizontally by a scalpel (A); opened longitudinally by a Trousseau tracheostomy dilator (B); and the opening enlarged transversely with heavy scissors (C) to insert a cuffed tracheostomy cannula with external diameter no greater than 10 mm to avoid excessive laryngeal trauma. (From Boyd et al[38] with permission.)

In the operating room most emergency cricothyroidotomies are performed by dividing the cricothyroid membrane, inserting a dilator into the larynx and opening it longitudinally, opening the cricothyroid membrane transversely with heavy scissors, and inserting the cannula[38] (Fig 3-12). Although this procedure is easy and uncomplicated in most instances, cricoid laceration, hemorrhage, esophageal perforation, disruption of laryngeal cartilages, and subglottic and glottic stenosis can occur.

## EMERGENCY AIRWAY ASSESSMENT AND INTERVENTION

In about 15 to 20% of severely traumatized patients time constraints preclude formal airway assessment; only a brief evaluation can be performed before it is necessary to secure the airway.[82] In the remaining patients some time is available for assessment of the respiratory and other systems before airway intervention. This time should be used effectively with ample consideration of care priorities. The extent of evaluation, then, largely depends on how soon resuscitative measures or surgery is indicated.

As we have already mentioned, all patients presenting within 24 hours after trauma are considered to have a full stomach for which appropriate airway intervention should be planned. In addition, assessment and management of the airway should be based on answers to the following questions.

1. Is there overt airway obstruction?
2. Is there airway compromise other than airway obstruction?
3. Is there a potential for difficult tracheal intubation and/or ventilation following anesthetic induction?
4. Is there an indication for therapeutic intubation?

5. Does the contemplated airway management technique have potential deleterious effects on other systems?

In this section recognition and management strategies for each of these conditions will be discussed.

## OVERT AIRWAY OBSTRUCTION

### *Airway Assessment*

Although improved prehospital care has reduced the number of trauma patients reaching the emergency department with obstructed airways, this complication is not infrequent. It is usually caused by relaxation and posterior displacement of the tongue, epiglottis, and periglottic soft tissue into the airway[35] secondary to unconsciousness caused by head injury, alcohol and/or drug intoxication, or severe hypotension. Airway obstruction may also occur after facial, neck, and chest injuries in which lacerated soft tissues, hematoma, bleeding, secretions, foreign bodies, dental fragments, or displaced bone or cartilage fragments reduce airway size. Bleeding into cervical fascial planes produces airway obstruction not only by bulging of the hematoma into the pharynx but also by compressing the neck veins, thus producing venous congestion and upper airway edema.[192] Subcutaneous emphysema from tracheobronchial or esophageal injury is rarely a cause of airway obstruction unless it is massive; dissects the submucosal planes of the pharynx, larynx, and trachea; or causes airway edema by compressing major veins of the neck and chest.[101,202] Loss of upper pharyngeal muscle control in rarely occurring bilateral hypoglossal nerve injuries and midline shift of the vocal cords in bilateral recurrent laryngeal nerve injuries may also result in airway obstruction. The respiratory tract may be obstructed by foreign bodies, teeth, or dental prostheses inhaled into the trachea and bronchi. Blood, either from the lungs or the upper airway, may enter the trachea and cause varying degrees of obstruction in both small and large airways. Suffocation may occur with as little as 150 mL of blood in the tracheobronchial tree of an obtunded patient. However, even massive hemoptysis—generally defined as more than 600 mL of blood loss from the tracheobronchial tree over a period of 24 hours—even though resulting in dramatic reduction in arterial oxygenation, may not be associated with major airway obstruction in conscious patients.[279] Approximately 5% of major trauma victims arrive in the emergency department with an endotracheal tube or other airway protection devices such as esophageal-gastric-tube-airway (EGTA) or pharyngeal-tracheal lumen airway (also called esophageal-tracheal combitube) (Fig 3-13). These tubes may be misplaced, kinked, or obstructed by blood, secretions, or foreign bodies, or aspiration may occur upon their removal, causing serious airway obstruction.

A grading system that correlates the severity of upper airway obstruction with the resulting signs and symptoms was described by Verrill in 1963[264] (Table 3-6). Stridor, which is inspiratory in lesions above the vocal cords, expiratory in those below the vocal cords and both in severe tracheal obstruction, may not be apparent in a quietly breathing patient even when the luminal diameter of the airway is seriously reduced. Chest retraction, noisy breathing, use of accessory respiratory muscles, dilatation of alae nasi, and dyspnea must be recognized early to prevent serious complications. Cyanosis, unless the airway obstruction is nearly complete, is a relatively late sign and is difficult to recognize in the presence of coexisting ane-

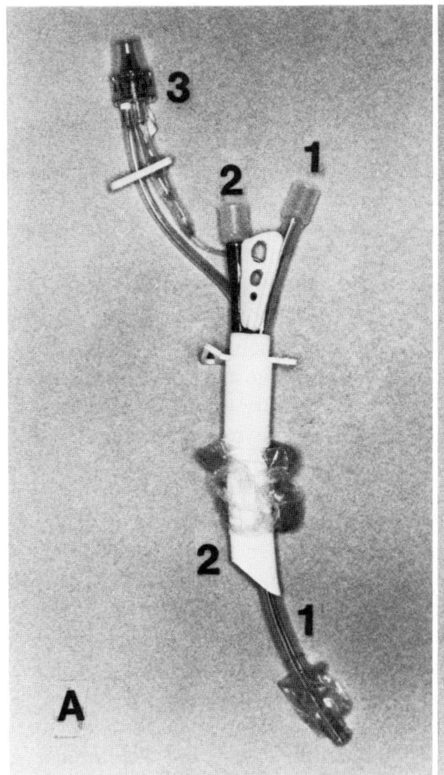


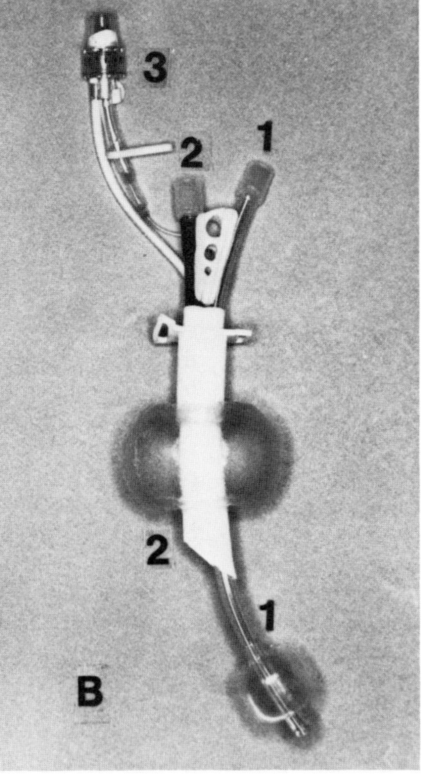


FIG. 3-13. Pharyngeal-tracheal lumen (PtL) airway with its distal and proximal cuffs deflated (A) and inflated (B). The device has a long clear tube (1) and a short white tube (2) connected proximally to endotracheal tube adapters. The small distal cuff is attached to 1 and the large proximal cuff to 2. Both cuffs can be inflated simultaneously by blowing into 3. The tube is inserted into the mouth without a laryngoscope and advanced until the strap touches the patient's teeth. Both cuffs are inflated, and an Ambu bag is attached to 2 and ventilation attempted. If the chest rises, the short tube (2) is in the pharynx and the long tube in the esophagus. If the chest does not rise, the long tube (1) is in the trachea. The large proximal cuff impacts the pharynx and prevents air leak when the long tube (1) is in the esophagus.

TABLE 3-6. A Grading System Correlating the Severity of Upper Respiratory Obstruction and the Resulting Signs and Symptoms*

| STAGE OF OBSTRUCTION | SIGNS AND SYMPTOMS |
|---|---|
| I<br>Mild or potential obstruction | No stridor at rest<br>Cough<br>Hoarseness |
| II<br>Moderate obstruction | Stridor on slight exertion<br>Rib retraction on inspiration<br>Dilatation of alae nasi on inspiration<br>Use of accessory respiratory muscles<br>Indrawing of cervical soft tissues<br>Tugging of jaw and trachea on inspiration<br>Dyspnea |
| III<br>Severe obstruction | Stridor at rest<br>Apprehension<br>Restlessness<br>Sweating<br>Pallor<br>Increase in pulse rate and blood pressure<br>Exaggerated excursion of neck veins |
| IV<br>Very severe obstruction | Slowed respiration<br>Hypotension<br>Cyanosis<br>Impaired consciousness |

* (Adapted from Verrill.[264])

mia, low-flow state, and skin pigmentation,[264] conditions not infrequently seen in acute trauma patients. Asphyxia, a combination of hypoxia and carbon dioxide retention, by affecting the central nervous system, produces apprehension and restlessness that may easily be attributed to fear and anxiety caused by trauma. The quality of voice should be assessed. Intraoral traumatic lesions, besides interfering with articulation, may also cause a guttural voice if they are located in the pharynx or hoarseness if they involve the larynx.

### *Airway Intervention*

Although further radiologic and endoscopic evaluation may be necessary before intervention in patients with partial upper airway obstruction, the pharynx should be cleared and secured immediately in patients with near-total obstruction. Chin lift, jaw thrust, placement of oropharyngeal or nasopharyngeal airway, and positioning the patient in upright or lateral decubitus position may improve the airway. A 23% increase in cross-sectional area of the pharynx occurs when awake persons move from supine to sitting position.[94] Tongue traction by means of a towel clip or a suture on the tip of the tongue may be necessary to displace obstructing soft tissues. An effective suction device is necessary to remove blood clots, foreign bodies, or dental fragments from the airway. Occasionally solid particles must be removed by inserting a finger into the patient's mouth.

In the presence of overt airway obstruction the trachea should be intubated without benefit of anesthetic or narcotic agents, despite the anxiety and agitation of the patient. The respiratory depressant effects of these drugs abolish accessory respiratory muscle activity and produce total airway obstruction in a marginally open airway. Mask oxygenation is required prior to intubation to prevent further hypoxemia during airway intervention. Helium in concentrations of 60 to 80% in oxygen may facilitate air flow through the obstruction[178,216] but prevents the use of high inspired oxygen concentrations. Thus, it is seldom indicated in the hypoxic patient with airway obstruction.

The technique by which the airway is secured depends on many factors including the level of obstruction, the type of injury, and the nature of associated injuries. As a rule, personnel and equipment capable of providing a surgical airway must be available at all times. Continuous monitoring of oxygenation with a pulse oximeter is also essential.

When clenching of the jaws, masseter spasm, or mechanical causes render mouth opening impossible, the nasal route can be selected provided that the nasal bones and the cranial base are intact. If not ruled out by careful radiographic evaluation, cervical spine injury precautions must be taken; the neck should be immobilized during airway manipulation. If possible, direct oral laryngoscopy is preferred to blind nasotracheal intubation, which may be associated with epistaxis. In severe maxillofacial trauma when both the mouth and the nose are involved, cricothyroidotomy is the only choice to relieve airway obstruction.

Following neck trauma if the airway obstruction is secondary to bleeding into the oropharyngeal cavity or to bilateral injury of the hypoglossal, vagus, and/or recurrent laryngeal nerves, oral intubation can easily be accomplished via direct laryngoscopy. When obstruction is caused by a pharyngeal wall hematoma, visualization of the vocal cords with standard laryngoscope blades is impossible because of the restricted view. Tubular laryngoscopes, such as those used by otorhinolaryngologists, can overcome this problem by creating an unobstructed space within the pharynx. However, attempting to insert an endotracheal tube through one of these laryngoscopes will result only in total obstruction of the view of the larynx. A special laryngoscope blade designed by Bainton,[12] which is tubular only in the distal 7 cm of its length, may permit introduction of the endotracheal tube with adequate visualization when the pharyngeal space is obliterated by edema or hematoma (Fig 3-14). Although preliminary results from animal and human studies suggest the usefulness of this blade, further experience is necessary to prove its efficacy in a trauma setting. Until then cricothyroidotomy remains the safest method of providing an emergency airway for these patients.

In some penetrating neck injuries, airway obstruction is caused by a flail epiglottis produced by injury of the laryngeal trapezium. Air flow through the neck wound in these instances indicates that the airway is damaged. Introduction of a tracheostomy cannula through the wound may relieve obstruction in these patients.[75] In asphyxiating neck injuries in which a midline neck wound is not present, tracheostomy is the best choice to relieve the occlusion. Cricothyroidotomy is contraindicated in laryngeal injuries because the cannula may not only further damage the larynx, but also, by creating a false passage, may produce total airway obstruction, especially

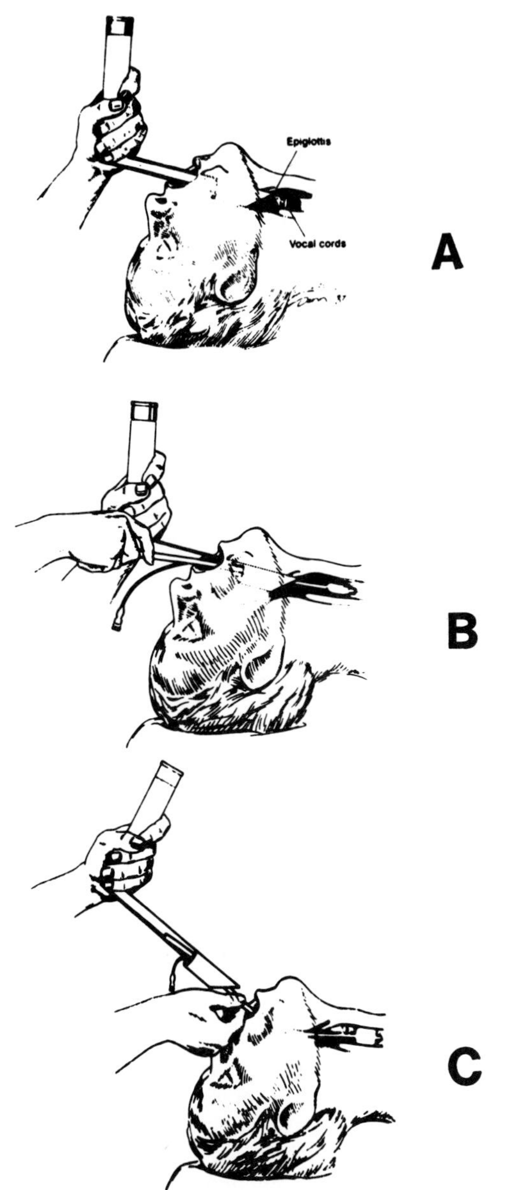


FIG. 3-14. Intubation of the trachea with the tubular blade designed by Bainton. A, the tubular portion of the blade in the pharynx lifting the epiglottis; B, an endotracheal tube without adapter is introduced into the trachea through the tubular portion of the blade; C, the blade is carefully removed from the mouth while the tube is stabilized by the right hand of the operator. (From Bainton[12] with permission.)

in cricotracheal separation injuries. Tracheostomy also may be difficult in the latter injuries since the distal part of the trachea may retract retrosternally or behind the clavicles, preventing its identification by the surgeon[49,239] (see Chapter 13).

Airway obstruction by a foreign body in the laryngeal inlet is caused both by the direct effect of the object and by the resulting edema. In adults the foreign body is removed with a Magill forceps under direct laryngoscopy. If time permits, adequate topical anesthesia of the mouth, pharynx, and epiglottis should be provided. The residual obstruction caused by glottic edema is treated expectantly with steroids (dexamethasone, 8 mg every 8 hours), nebulized racemic epinephrine (0.3 ml in 3 to 5 ml of saline), and/or intubation of the trachea with a small endotracheal tube. If the glottic foreign body is not recognized preoperatively, airway obstruction developing after induction of anesthesia[172] may necessitate expeditious direct laryngoscopy and removal of the object with a Magill forceps. If the obstruction is complete, emergency cricothyroidotomy is the only choice. In uncooperative children laryngoscopy under topical anesthesia may not be feasible, and in rare instances tracheostomy under local anesthesia may be necessary.

Foreign bodies located below the vocal cords require direct visualization of the airway with a rigid bronchoscope. In adults the intraoral and pharyngeal structures are anesthetized topically, and the bronchoscope is then introduced into the larynx. A local anesthetic solution is instilled through the bronchoscope to anesthetize the tracheal mucosa. The bronchoscope is advanced while searching for the foreign body within the trachea or the bronchi. If the aspirated body is small and unlikely to cause significant airway obstruction, the bronchoscope is introduced after rapid sequence induction of general anesthesia. This technique may be especially useful in children who may not tolerate introduction of a rigid bronchoscope without anesthesia. A fiberoptic bronchoscope may be substituted in both adults and children if the foreign body is small and the airway is not contaminated with blood.

Total or partial obstruction of the intrathoracic portion of the airway results from transsection and distal or lateral displacement of the trachea compounded by aspiration of blood and intrapulmonary hemorrhage. Death at the accident site is unavoidable if this type of injury produces total occlusion. However, the obstruction may be partial in some patients because displacement is limited by peritracheal connective tissue. Ideally, endotracheal intubation should be performed under direct vision using a fiberoptic bronchoscope in order to determine the site of injury and to prevent entry of the endotracheal tube into a false passage. With this approach the tip of the endotracheal tube is placed below the obstruction. However, fiberoptic bronchoscopes have severe drawbacks in this setting; blood in the tracheobronchial tree obstructs the view, suctioning through their small port is inadequate, and ventilation, although possible by using a jet through the suction port, is often insufficient. These problems can be overcome by using a rigid bronchoscope, but the large size of these instruments precludes passage of an endotracheal tube over them. Thus, tracheal intubation is often performed without direct vision albeit after prior endoscopic evaluation of the airway.[141] During initial bronchoscopy, if the obstruction or the injury is severe, the rigid bronchoscope can be left in the trachea so that its distal tip remains below the lesion to provide ventilation until surgical control is obtained.

## AIRWAY COMPROMISE

### *Airway Assessment*

Airway compromise may be defined for our purposes as a condition in which the patency and/or protection of the airway is likely to be jeopardized with passage of time or manipulation of the airway, although little or no obstruction or aspiration is present during initial evaluation. For instance, the airway may be compromised in an obtunded head-injured patient, since absent or diminished laryngeal reflexes may potentially result in aspiration of gastric and pharyngeal contents. Laryngeal reflexes are usually intact if the patient is able to respond to painful stimuli with purposeful movements. Pharyngeal stimulation to evaluate these reflexes is unwarranted because this maneuver, by provoking retching and vomiting, may increase intracranial pressure. In addition, an intact gag reflex may not necessarily indicate that laryngeal reflexes are also competent enough to protect against pulmonary aspiration.[34]

The edema and hematoma that develop in cervicofacial soft tissues after trauma are dynamic, not static, in nature. A variable degree of expansion of the swelling occurs over a relatively short period of time and has the potential of causing airway obstruction.[54] Thus, the airway is compromised for a period of about 6 to 12 hours after major facial and neck injuries. Bleeding from cervical or maxillofacial vessels may stop early because of hypotension and clot formation. After successful resuscitation injured vessels may rebleed, causing either a large hematoma encroaching on the pharynx and larynx or, if there is communication between the injured vessel and the airway lumen, flooding of the entire airway with blood. Careful and gentle examination of the neck and oropharynx for hematoma or entry and exit sites of penetrating objects may help in recognition of such possibilities.

Blunt trauma to the neck compromises the airway, yet recognition of this condition requires a high index of suspicion because the patient may be asymptomatic or show only nonspecific signs and symptoms.[49,239] Hoarseness, muffled voice, dyspnea, stridor, dysphagia, odynophagia, cervical pain and tenderness, cervical ecchymosis, subcutaneous emphysema, absence of thyroid prominence, signs of vocal cord paralysis, and hemoptysis, although nonspecific, suggest laryngotracheal injury in a patient with direct impact to the anterior neck.[49,239] Upper and lower airway edema following facial and cervical burns and smoke inhalation, although asymptomatic or showing few symptoms of airway obstruction initially, may increase with time because of progressive inflammation and large volume fluid administration and thereby cause airway obstruction.[119]

Traumatic rupture of the trachea and bronchi may be associated with few clinical signs if the air leak is small. Upon institution of positive pressure ventilation, the leak may enlarge and produce pneumothorax or subcutaneous, mediastinal, and pericardial emphysema. Tracheobronchial injuries present in two clinical and pathological patterns, although some overlap exists between these categories.[175] In the first pattern, the injury is intrapleural and is manifested by massive pneumothorax and continuous leak from the thoracostomy tube. Dyspnea may worsen with suction, and the affected lung may not expand. In the second pattern the airway leak is extrapleural, causing little or no pneumothorax but resulting in dissection of air into the mediastinum, pericardium, and fascial planes. The quantity of air contained in these spaces depends on the size of the laceration and the presence or absence of positive pressure ventilation. These manifestations of intrathoracic airway injury are not always obvious and may be missed during initial evaluation[31] only to be recognized during surgery or even later.[163] Complete airway obstruction may result in these patients from disruption of the injured airway by the endotracheal tube during or following airway manipulation.

Identification of this rare group of patients requires adequate awareness of these injuries and their pattern of progression and also appropriate radiological and endoscopic evaluation. Cervical soft tissue films demonstrate soft tissue swelling, airway deviation, and interruption or narrowing of the laryngotracheal air column. Routine chest films may reveal tracheal deviation and compression by a cervical hematoma. Pneumothorax, pneumomediastinum, and pneumopericardium also suggest the possibility of airway injury. In acute tracheobronchial injuries the following chest X-ray findings may be observed: deep cervical emphysema, peribronchial air, sudden obstruction in the course of an air-filled bronchus, and dropped lung. Deep cervical emphysema is characterized by a radiolucent line along the prevertebral fascia due to air tracking up from the mediastinum. Peribronchial air and sudden interruption of the bronchial air column are diagnostic of bronchial rupture. Dropped lung is characterized by descent of the apex of the collapsed lung to the level of the hilum because of loss of bronchial support.[87,145]

Patients with tracheal rupture are often intubated during initial resuscitation without awareness of the injury. In these patients attention to the subsequently obtained chest radiogram may help in diagnosis of the tracheal disruption before classic signs such as subcutaneous emphysema and pneumomediastinum develop. An overdistended cuff (diameter greater than 2.8 cm) and reduced distance between the cuff and the distal end of the tube suggest intrathoracic airway injury and indicate further diagnostic studies such as computed tomography (CT) and/or bronchoscopy[213] (Fig 3-15).

Of the more sophisticated diagnostic studies, CT scanning is an excellent method of delineating the location and severity of laryngeal injuries.[242] Indirect laryngoscopy, once very popular for diagnosis of blunt laryngeal injury, has been used rarely since the introduction of CT scanning into clinical practice, although fiberoptic bronchoscopy remains an important diagnostic method.[182] Bronchoscopy should be performed prior to endotracheal intubation if tracheobronchial injury is suspected. Angiography is useful in demonstrating the location of cervical arterial injuries and thus helps in recognition of associated airway shift and distortion.

Serial respiratory flow-volume curves and fiberoptic nasopharyngoscopy or bronchoscopy have been used successfully to identify those burn victims who develop progressive airway obstruction and require endotracheal intubation.[119] Flow-volume curves must be interpreted carefully; preexisting disease states, anxiety, and apprehension may complicate the picture. Since many burns involve the upper airway, serial nasopharyngoscopic examinations suffice to evaluate these patients. If a lower airway burn is suspected, fiberoptic bronchoscopy, although not effective in indicating the level of required respiratory support or predicting its duration,[25] provides information about the type, anatomic extent, and severity of damage and permits tracheobronchial suctioning under direct vision.[127] Fiberoptic bronchoscopy may not identify burn injury in hypotensive patients, presumably because the characteristic mucosal changes do not occur.[127] Examination of

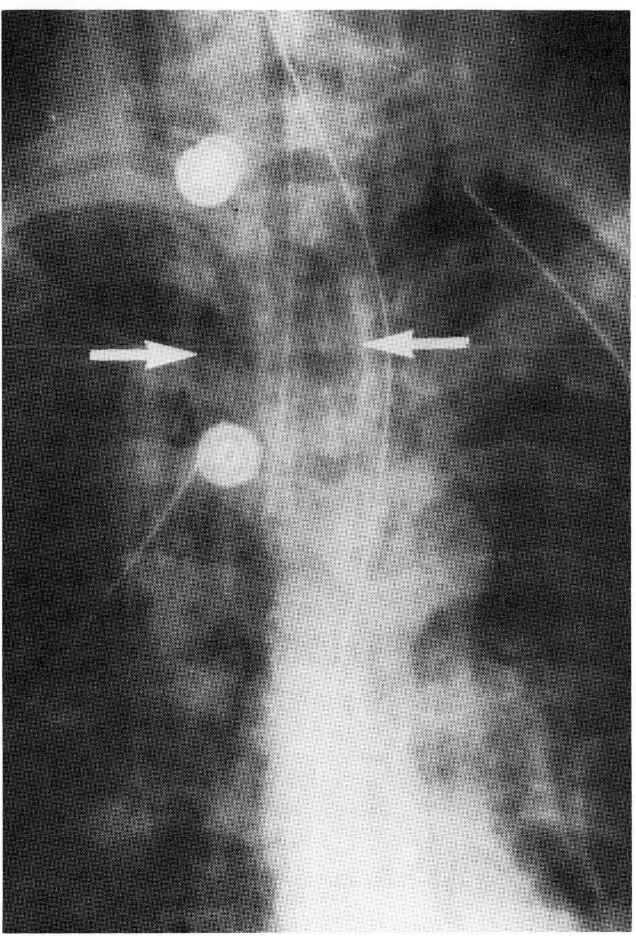

FIG. 3-15. Initial chest X-ray of a blunt chest trauma patient after intubation, showing A, excessive distention of the endotracheal tube cuff; B, no distance between the cuff and tube tip; C, pneumothorax, pneumomediastinum and subcutaneous emphysema. (From Rollins and Tocino[213] with permission.)

the lower airway with this device should be performed through an endotracheal tube to prevent upper airway obstruction including laryngeal spasm.

### *Airway Intervention*

In most patients with respiratory compromise the airway should be secured under controlled conditions soon after trauma, before severe complications such as airway obstruction, pulmonary aspiration, or increasing airway leak develop. In the presence of acute head injury airway intervention should take into account two important possibilities: coexisting cervical spine injury, and elevation of intracranial pressure during endotracheal intubation. Airway management principles for these patients will be discussed later in this chapter and are thus not elaborated in this section.

In patients with acute maxillofacial and neck injuries endotracheal intubation is preferably performed with the patient awake and breathing spontaneously unless airway compromise is ruled out by adequate airway evaluation. The technique selected for intubation depends on the type and degree of airway occlusion. Direct laryngoscopy after topical anesthesia of the oropharynx is selected if the mouth can be opened. Oro- or nasotracheal intubation with the aid of a fiberoptic bronchoscope may be selected if the view is not obstructed by blood, if direct laryngoscopy is difficult, or if associated cervical spine injury is present.[182]

Translaryngeal guided (retrograde) intubation may be required if standard techniques fail or are likely to fail, the larynx is intact, coagulation profile is normal, and the mouth can be opened to allow recovery of the catheter or wire from the pharynx.[16] Tracheostomy or cricothyroidotomy may be necessary if the mouth cannot be opened; nasotracheal intubation is contraindicated or impossible; airway obstruction is progressing rapidly; and multiple injuries involving the head, face, and neck preclude utilization of any of the other airway management techniques described.

Translaryngeal (retrograde) intubation is performed in the following fashion. After preparation with an antiseptic, the skin over the cricothyroid membrane is infiltrated with 2 to 3 mL of 1% lidocaine solution, and a 14-gauge Angiocath attached to a 10 mL syringe filled with a few milliliters of saline is inserted through the cricothyroid membrane in a slightly cephalad direction while gentle traction is applied to the plunger of the syringe. Upon entry of the Angiocath into the larynx, which is manifested by withdrawal of air bubbles into the syringe, the cannula of the Angiocath is advanced while the needle is removed. A guide wire (0.8 to 1.0-mm external diameter and 75 cm long) or a long central venous or epidural catheter is introduced through the cannula and advanced cephalad for approximately 15 to 20 cm. After opening the patient's mouth, the catheter or wire is located in the posterior pharynx and pulled out. If a nasotracheal intubation is planned, a small rubber uncuffed urinary catheter is introduced through the nostril and advanced until it is recovered from the mouth. The wire or catheter and the urinary catheter are then tied together and pulled out through the nose until the tie appears outside the nostril. After cutting the rubber catheter, an endotracheal tube is passed over the wire and advanced until it enters the larynx.

Difficulty in passage of the tube may arise at the laryngeal inlet. The tube tip tends to lodge anteriorly where it is caught by the anterior commissure of the vocal cords. This difficulty is more common during oro- rather than nasotracheal intubation. Three techniques have been described to overcome this problem. In the first approach, after the guide wire is recovered from the nose or the mouth, it is passed retrograde through the suction/biopsy port of a fiberoptic bronchoscope over which an endotracheal tube has been placed. The bronchoscope is then advanced over the wire to the laryngeal inlet. The anterior commissure may then be visualized. Bending the flexible tip of the bronchoscope posteriorly at this point permits a full view of the larynx and introduction of the bronchoscope into the trachea. The endotracheal tube is then passed over the bronchoscope through the vocal cords[154] (Fig 3-16). In the second approach the plastic protector of the guide wire is substituted for the bronchoscope[139] (Fig 3-17). The third approach is designed to be used with an epidural or a central venous catheter. It involves fixing a gliding knot around the side hole of the tracheal tube with the nasal end of the catheter, and then pulling the catheter down from its

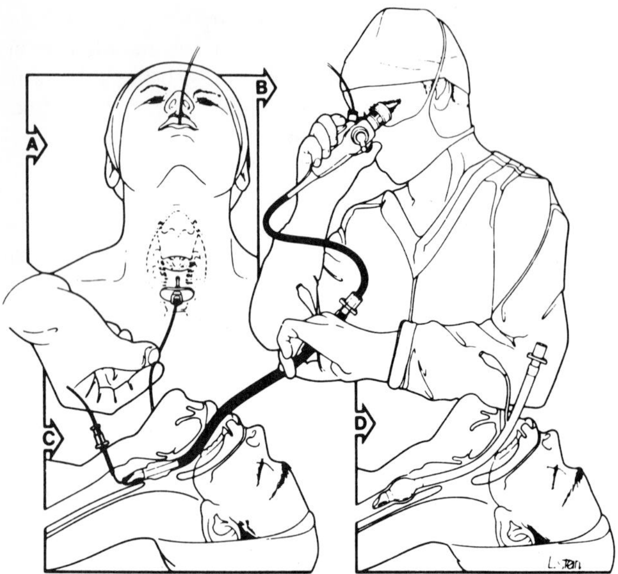


FIG. 3-16. Translaryngeal (retrograde) intubation with the aid of a fiberoptic bronchoscope. A, a translaryngeally passed guide wire is retrieved from the mouth; B and C, the guidewire is passed retrograde through the suction channel of a fiberoptic bronchoscope over which an endotracheal tube is passed. The tip of the fiberoptic bronchoscope is introduced into the larynx under direct vision by manipulating its flexible tip. D, the endotracheal tube is passed into the trachea, and the guide wire, needle, and bronchoscope have been removed. (From Lechman et al[154] with permission.)

distal end to guide the endotracheal tube into the larynx. After the tube enters the larynx the catheter is cut outside the cricotracheal membrane and its remaining part is removed by pulling it proximally.[1]

Because of the likelihood of progressive upper airway edema and the risk of delayed airway obstruction, early prophylactic endotracheal intubation is routine in many institutions involved in the care of burn victims.[263] Intubation may be extremely difficult if upper airway edema is allowed to progress. Tracheostomy may be required for some severely obstructed patients, although this procedure may be associated with an increased incidence of complications in burn victims. Direct contamination of the airway from the tracheostomy site and resulting pneumonia, tracheoesophageal fistula, and tracheal stenosis are the major causes of morbidity.[181] Endotracheal intubation in these patients can be accomplished using direct laryngoscopy while the patient is awake. Alternatively, oro- or nasotracheal intubation can be performed with the aid of a fiberoptic bronchoscope. Pharyngeal and laryngeal edema usually preclude introduction of a large endotracheal tube into the larynx. Persistence in attempts to insert a large-size tube in these circumstances may produce additional laryngeal trauma. Transient pulmonary edema beginning within 5 minutes after endotracheal intubation has been reported in burn patients and is ascribed to loss of glottic end-expiratory pressure in the face of small lung volumes.[170] Early use of continuous positive pressure following intubation is thus recommended. Many burn victims develop bronchospasm and wheezing. Intravenous aminophylline (5.6 mg/kg) over a 30-minute period followed by a maintenance dose of 0.7 mg/kg per hour infusion ameliorates this complication. Serum aminophylline levels should be monitored closely in order to achieve an effective therapeutic level (10 to 15 μg/mL) and avoid toxicity. β-2 adrenergic agonists can also be used alone or in combination with aminophylline therapy.

The management principles of airway compromise caused by intrathoracic tracheal and bronchial injuries are similar to those described for trauma to the cervical airway. All airway manipulations should be performed under direct vision; at least, a bronchoscopic examination should precede any airway intervention below the larynx.[141] Since the majority of intrathoracic tracheal lacerations occur within 2.5 cm of the carina (most commonly at the membranous portion of the trachea), the endotracheal tube or ventilating bronchoscope may have to be advanced into the intact bronchus to provide adequate ventilation without airway leak. In bronchial injuries placement of a double-lumen endobronchial tube, with its distal end inserted into the intact bronchus, may prevent air leak, and contamination of the intact lung with blood from the injured side[183] (Fig 3-18). However, this method is often in-

FIG. 3-17. Translaryngeal (retrograde) intubation with the aid of the protective sheath of the guide wire. Top, the guidewire passed translaryngeally and retrieved from the mouth; middle, the protective plastic sheath passed over the guide wire is introduced into the trachea; bottom, after removing the guide wire an endotracheal tube is introduced into the trachea by railroading it over the sheath of the guide wire. (From King et al[139] with permission.)

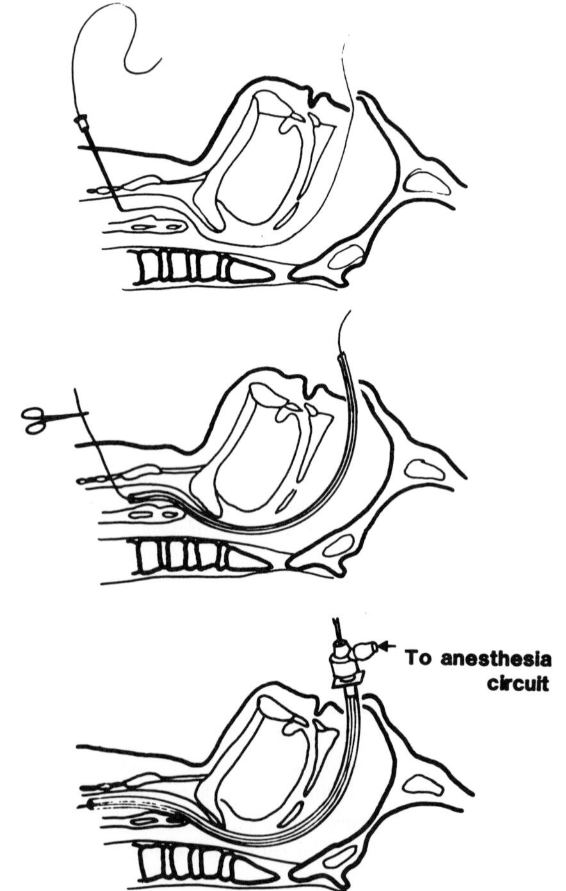

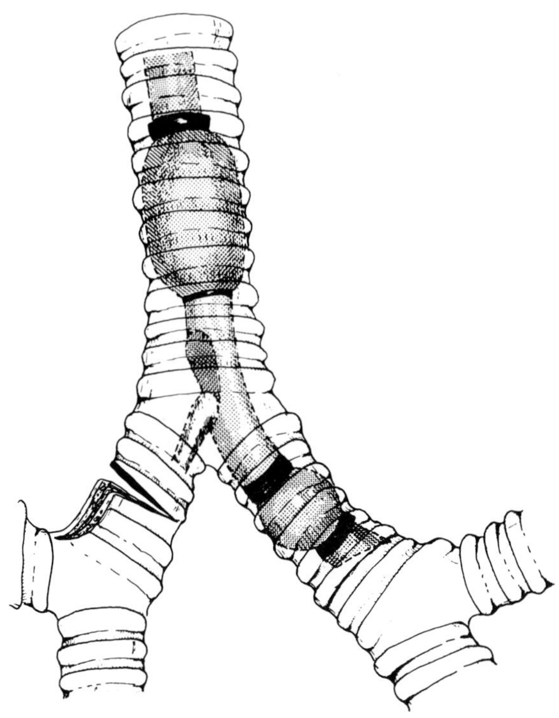

FIG. 3-18. Prevention of air leak from the injured bronchus and isolation of the intact lung by a double-lumen endobronchial tube. (From Capan LM, Turndorf H. Airway management. In Worth MH, ed. Principles and Practice of Trauma Care. Baltimore: Williams & Wilkins, 1982:19, with permission.)

effective because of frequent malposition of the endobronchial tube. Correct positioning of these tubes under fiberoptic bronchoscopic guidance is usually hindered by blood in the tracheobronchial tree. Selective intubation of the intact bronchus with an ordinary uncut 7-mm (inner diameter) endotracheal tube under direct vision is usually an easier and a more viable option,[169,279] although it may not always be successful. A few uncut sterile endotracheal tubes should be made available for placement into the intact bronchus under direct vision during thoracotomy in case of ineffective lung isolation with the initially placed tube.

Another alternative is to use an endotracheal tube with a built-in movable bronchial blocker (Univent tube)[129] (Fig 3-19). After intubation of the trachea the blocker can be advanced into the injured bronchus with the aid of a fiberoptic bronchoscope and its cuff inflated proximal to the injured site. Although isolation of the lungs with this tube is easier than with a double-lumen tube, it cannot be used when severe tracheobronchial bleeding precludes the use of a fiberoptic bronchoscope to place the blocker properly. In addition inflation of the cuff within the injured bronchus may exacerbate the bronchial damage. Thus, this tube should be used only in desperate conditions in which airway leak prevents adequate ventilation and oxygenation even with the use of a jet ventilator.

Intraoperatively, surgical repair of an injured distal trachea or bronchus may, depending on the site of injury, occasionally necessitate withdrawal of the tube from the trachea and ventilation of the intact lung with an endotracheal tube placed by the surgeon through the tracheal wound.[169] The proximal end of the tube is brought out through the surgical incision and connected to the anesthetic system. This maneuver requires a sterile endotracheal tube that is at least twice the length of an ordinary tube. Such long tubes can be prepared in advance by connecting two endotracheal tubes with an appropriate adapter.[169]

Occasionally, concomitant laceration of the trachea and esophagus leads to formation of a tracheoesophageal fistula, which usually develops 3 to 5 days after trauma.[153] Intubation of the trachea in these patients should also be done under direct vision with the aid of a fiberoptic bronchoscope to prevent inadvertent esophageal intubation through the fistula, airway obstruction, or placement of the tube above the lesion.

In most patients with tracheobronchial injury conventional positive pressure ventilation maintains satisfactory gas exchange, provided an effective seal is achieved below the laceration. Anecdotal reports have described adequate gas exchange with high-frequency jet ventilation in situations in which such conditions could not be attained.[206] However, it is not clear at this time whether high-frequency jet ventilation

FIG. 3-19. The movable blocker of a Univent tube is placed proximal to a bronchial injury to prevent air leak, and contamination of the contralateral lung.

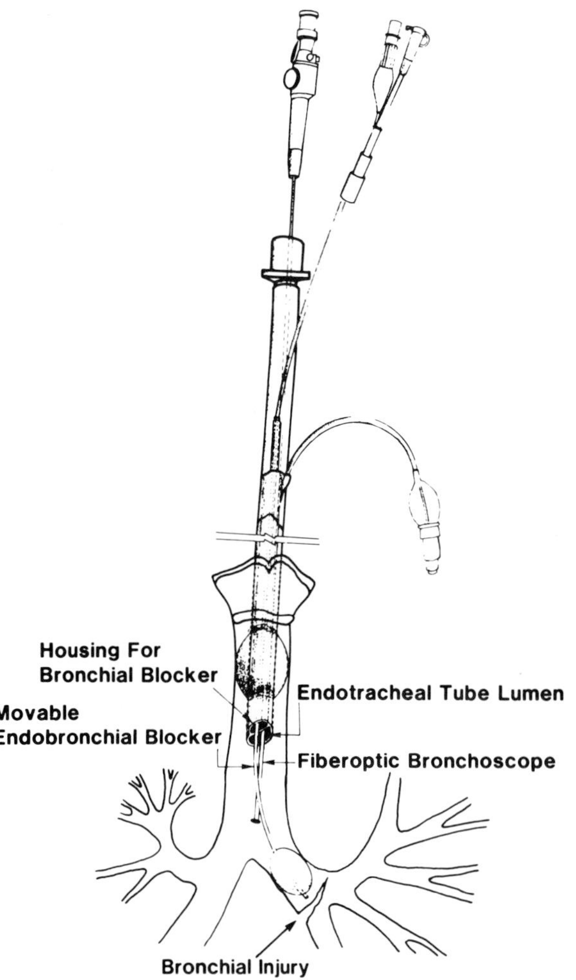

is actually beneficial in these instances since substantial reduction of air leak and improvement of gas exchange, as compared with conventional ventilation, could not be demonstrated in a group of patients with bronchopleural fistula.[27]

## POTENTIAL OF DIFFICULT VENTILATION OR INTUBATION AFTER ANESTHESIA

### *Airway Assessment*

Reference has already been made to the possibility of unrelievable airway obstruction after administration of anesthetics to patients with acute maxillofacial and cervical injuries. Acute airway obstruction and difficult intubation are also frequent in the early or late postburn period because of severe facial and cervical edema or scar contractures.[271]

Most trauma victims, however, do not have these problems, and preoperative airway assessment is the same as that for electively operated patients. Certain rare preexisting diseases, which are often characterized by cervicofacial anatomic variations, can render ventilation and tracheal intubation difficult after administration of anesthetics and muscle relaxants.[171] A list of these diseases and syndromes, most of which are congenital and encountered in children, is given in Table 3-7. The likelihood that a trauma victim is afflicted by these abnormalities is small. Obesity, body weight 30% or more over the predicted value, is common in trauma patients and may result in airway management difficulties after anesthetic induction. On the other hand, morbid obesity, which is defined as body weight greater than twice normal is infrequent in this population.

There remains another group of patients with few or no obvious preoperative signs in whom airway difficulty may arise after administration of anesthetics. The majority of these patients can be ventilated by mask, but direct laryngoscopy and tracheal intubation are unusually difficult because of physiognomical anomalies. In a small fraction of the population mask ventilation becomes impossible once anesthetic and/or muscle relaxant agents are administered. Usually such airway obstruction is produced by unrecognized hypertrophic pharyngeal soft tissues, intraoral neoplasms, large tonsils, or congenital deformities.

There has been increasing interest during the past decade in elucidation of signs that enable preoperative recognition of these patients. It should be emphasized that these signs, although to some extent capable of predicting difficult intubation, have little value in predicting problems of mask ventilation. Nevertheless, to err on the safe side, most clinicians consider that ventilation may also be troublesome in patients in whom intubation may be difficult and manage the airway with the patient awake. Adherence to this philosophy is particularly rewarding in the acute trauma victim with full stomach, who is prone to develop regurgitation and pulmonary aspiration during repeated attempts at laryngoscopy and intubation.

The airway must be thoroughly evaluated whenever possible. If available, previous anesthetic records and airway examination reports should be reviewed. Questioning the patient about previous airway management problems, changes of voice quality, difficulty in articulating words, stridor, dysphagia, inability to handle secretions, previous head and neck surgery or radiation, abnormal neck mobility, and temporomandibular joint arthritis aids in anticipation of airway management difficulties. Obviously, the yield from this type of evaluation is negligible in a trauma victim when head injury, alcohol intoxication, or anxiety precludes obtaining satisfactory information. Occasionally, valuable information can be obtained from the patient's relatives or friends. Physical examination should focus on the ability of the patient to open his/her mouth; the patency of the nares; the size and mobility of the tongue; the state and fragility of dentition; masses in the tongue base; the extent of head and neck mobility; visible or palpable masses of the neck; the shape of the face; and the presence of macrognathia, macroglossia, and/or microstomia. Atlantooccipital joint motion is assessed by asking the patient to extend the neck. Patients with limited motion of this joint tend to move the entire cervical spine posteriorly which, in the supine position, results in elevation of the shoulders. If the patient is able to extend the neck without lifting the shoulders he/she probably has a normal range of atlantooccipital motion. Of course, head and neck motion should not be evaluated if cervical spine injury may be present.

The reliable and classic predictors of difficult intubation are considered to be small mouth, short muscular neck with full set of teeth, receding mandible with obtuse mandibular angles, protruding maxillary incisors with relative maxillary overgrowth, increased alveolar-mental distance, long arched palate with a long narrow mouth, and deformed external ears.[52] White and Kander[274] concluded, after making measurements on lateral radiographs of the face and jaw, that a reduced atlantooccipital distance and/or a ratio of effective mandibular length (distance between the lower incisor teeth and the temporomandibular joint) to posterior mandibular depth (distance from the lower border of the mandible to the alveolus immediately behind the third molar tooth) less than 3.6 suggests the possibility of difficult intubation. These measurements are easy to obtain when time permits; however, more recent findings have refuted their predictive value.[20,261]

In a separate study of neck X-rays of patients who were difficult to intubate, Nichol and Zuck[185] found that contact between the posterior tubercle of the atlas and the occiput with the head and neck in neutral position prevents atlantooccipital extension and causes anterior bowing of the lower cervical spine. The resulting anterior displacement of the larynx may thus hinder laryngeal visualization during direct laryngoscopy (Fig 3-20). This sign, the predictive value of which

TABLE 3-7. Diseases and Syndromes That Are Likely to Render Mask Ventilation and Tracheal Intubation Difficult

| | |
|---|---|
| Acromegaly | Fetal alcohol syndrome |
| Stylohyoid ligament calcification | Mucopolysaccharidoses |
| Severe cervical osteoarthritis | Pierre-Robin syndrome |
| Cockayne's syndrome | Pseudoxanthoma "protein" |
| Cystic hygroma | Rheumatoid arthritis |
| Cherubism | Temporomandibular joint dysfunction |
| Goldenhar syndrome | |
| Still's disease | Tracheal agenesis |
| Klippel-Feil syndrome | |
| Ankylosing spondylitis | Treacher-Collins syndrome |

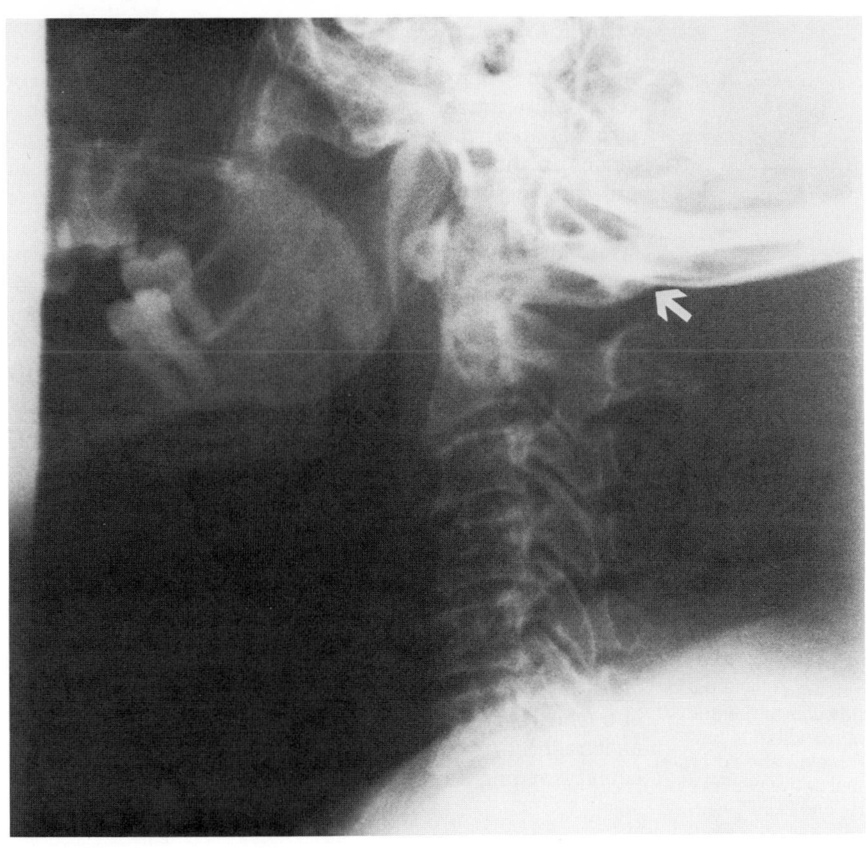

FIG. 3-20. In neutral head and neck position the spinous process of the atlas (arrow) is in contact with the occiput. This sign suggests possible difficulty in visualization of the larynx during direct laryngoscopy.

is also confirmed by others,[20] may be easy to detect in blunt trauma victims in whom a lateral cervical spine X-ray is obtained routinely to rule out fracture-dislocations of the neck.

More recently two simple clinical signs have been proposed as important predictors of difficult laryngoscopy and intubation. The first involves the distance between the lower border of the chin and the thyroid notch with the neck fully extended.[201] A distance less than 6 cm suggests the possibility of difficult laryngoscopy and intubation because of limited visibility of the vocal cords. The second sign is based on the degree of visibility of posterior intraoral structures in the sitting patient with maximally protruded tongue. Described originally by Mallampati and coworkers,[164] and later by Samsoon and Young,[222] this test is easy to perform but may have limited applicability in acute trauma when hypovolemia, shock, or cervical spine and other injuries preclude placement of the patient in a sitting position. In any case, they suggest that laryngoscopy and intubation will be easy if the soft palate, fauces, uvula, and tonsillar pillars can be seen readily. Inability to see the pillars suggests partial visibility of the vocal cords and slight difficulty of intubation. If only the soft palate and the base of the uvula are seen, the glottis will be difficult to visualize, but the arytenoid and/or corniculate cartilages may still be seen. Inability to see any of these structures suggests that laryngoscopy will be very difficult because even the arytenoids will not be exposed by direct laryngoscopy.[8,164,222]

Bellhouse and Dore,[20] in a study similar to that of White and Kander,[274] made various measurements on lateral head and neck radiograms of patients with or without difficult intubation and confirmed the predictive ability of both of these tests and of the presence of atlantooccipital extension reduced by more than one third of the normal 35°. They also pointed out the importance of a recessed chin, which leaves little space for the tongue to be maneuvered anteriorly by the Macintosh laryngoscope, as a predictive sign. Without using X-ray examination, this condition is diagnosed if the length of a perpendicular line from the lower genial tubercle of the mandible to the line of vision is less than 2.5 cm[20] (Fig 3-21). The line of vision is an imaginary line from the upper incisor teeth to the corniculate cartilage, with the head in maximally extended position.[20] According to Bellhouse and Dore,[20] the corniculate cartilage is located topographically 1.5 cm posterior to the laryngeal prominence of the thyroid cartilage (Fig 3-21).

It is important to emphasize that the difficulty of direct laryngoscopy and tracheal intubation is determined by many interacting factors. Therefore the existing predictive signs, tests, and measurements are capable of defining probabilities but cannot identify the ease or difficulty of intubation in an individual patient with complete certainty. This conclusion is supported by the work of Wilson and coworkers[278] who have identified five risk factors predictive of difficult laryngoscopy and intubation: obesity, restricted head and neck movement, receding mandible, protruding teeth, and limited motility of the jaw. Using objective criteria they designed a scoring system that graded the severity of each risk factor into three classes. After calculating the sum of the scores and subjecting the data to statistical analysis, difficult laryngoscopy, which

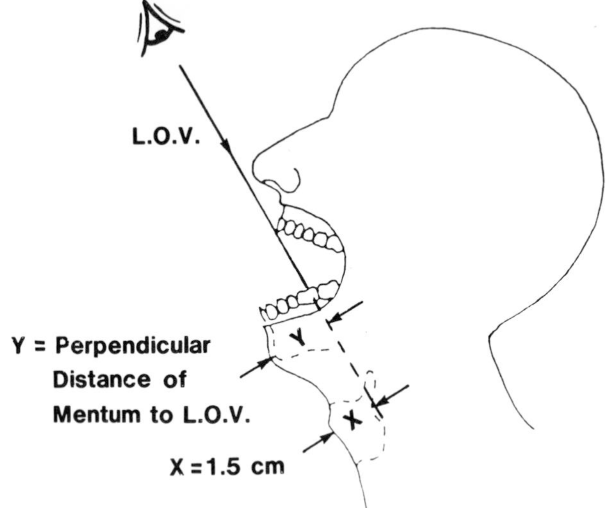


FIG. 3-21. A small distance (Y) between the mentum and the line of vision (L.O.V.) leaves a small space for the tongue which cannot be displaced anteriorly by the laryngoscope blade, rendering laryngeal visualization difficult. The line of vision is an imaginary line between the upper incisors and the corniculate cartilages, which are topographically located 1.5 cm posterior to the anterior prominence of the thyroid cartilage (X). If the length of a line perpendicular to the line of vision from the mentum is less than 2.5 cm, the mandible is considered receding, and difficulty in visualizing the larynx should be anticipated. This assessment can be easily performed at the patient's bedside without the need of X-rays. (From Bellhouse and Dore[20] with permission.)

was present in 1.5% of patients, could be predicted at best in only 75 to 92% of instances. There was also a high rate (12 to 26%) of false-positives.

### *Airway Intervention*

If a difficult intubation is suspected, gentle direct laryngoscopy ("awake look") can be performed before administration of anesthetics, using topical anesthesia of the tongue, pharynx, hypopharynx, and epiglottis. Indirect laryngoscopy, although an acceptable method for determining the severity of laryngeal damage and edema, cannot provide reliable information in this situation. Once tracheal intubation is judged to be straightforward, anesthetic induction can proceed with a rapid sequence technique as described in the section on the full stomach. Inability to visualize the larynx during the "awake look" dictates tracheal intubation while the patient is awake and breathing spontaneously. Oro- or nasotracheal intubation using a fiberoptic bronchoscope is the method of choice in these circumstances. Blind nasotracheal or orotracheal intubation using direct laryngoscopy after topical anesthesia can also be attempted. Another alternative is translaryngeal guided intubation as discussed above. The trachea can be intubated in almost all instances with one of these techniques; therefore cricothyroidotomy is almost never required unless other complicating conditions coexist. The approach to an unsuspected difficult intubation after anesthetics and muscle relaxants has already been discussed in the section on full stomach.

## OTHER INDICATIONS FOR TRACHEAL INTUBATION

Apart from surgery and management of airway obstruction or compromise, tracheal intubation may be needed to treat hypoxemia and hypercarbia caused by a variety of other conditions in the trauma patient. Chest injury, by causing an unstable chest, pulmonary contusion, or both, can interfere with oxygenation and ventilation. Acute respiratory distress syndrome may develop because of aspiration of gastric contents and/or other mechanisms. Approximately 20% of head-injured patients are hypoxic on admission to the emergency department; they may deteriorate during the ensuing 48 hours if not treated.[174,236,284] Hypercarbia with or without hypoxia may also develop in head-injured patients because of hypoventilation. Endotracheal intubation may be required in some of these patients not only to optimize ventilation but also to induce hypocarbia as a means of reducing elevated intracranial pressure. Oxygen delivery to the vital organs may be compromised by hemorrhagic or cardiogenic shock caused by bleeding, cardiac contusion, and/or pericardial tamponade. Hypoxemia and diminished oxygen delivery in these circumstances may be partly ameliorated by simply administering oxygen without securing the airway, but in many cases tracheal intubation is necessary. Frequently, effective removal of tracheal secretions and blood is also impossible without an endotracheal tube. Thus, in many instances, tracheal intubation is required despite the presence of a clear airway.

### *Airway Intervention*

Hypoxemic patients with acute pulmonary abnormalities do not tolerate prolonged periods of apnea. In severely hypoxemic patients awake endotracheal intubation under topical anesthesia with supplemental oxygen is preferred to a rapid sequence technique, especially when problems in airway management are anticipated. If a rapid induction sequence is selected, a high arterial oxygen tension should be maintained during the apneic period. Continuous monitoring of oxygen saturation is essential.

## POTENTIAL DELETERIOUS EFFECTS OF AIRWAY MANAGEMENT ON OTHER SYSTEMS

The existence of multiple injuries, hypovolemia, and preexisting diseases must be taken into account when an airway management strategy is planned for the trauma victim. Among many possible injuries, those of the head, cervical spine and cord, eye, and chest—particularly pericardial tamponade, pulmonary laceration, and aortic rupture—should be given special consideration since the effects of the injury may be exacerbated by the process of securing the airway if appropriate precautions are not taken. Definitive diagnosis of these injuries before airway intervention is desirable but not always possible. When time constraints or other conditions preclude diagnosis, the airway should be managed as if these injuries exist. Difficulties increase if more than one of these injuries are present; the technique selected to prevent making one injury worse may produce deleterious effects on the other. Intravascular volume and cardiac performance should be assessed carefully since severe shock or even cardiac arrest may occur in hypovolemic patients or in those with cardiac injuries after administration of anesthetics or as a result of airway intervention. Preexisting cardiovascular and/or cerebrovascular diseases may also be exacerbated by anesthetics and the stress of endotracheal intubation; they should be evaluated prior to intubation whenever possible.

### *Airway Intervention*

HEAD AND EYE INJURY. Intracranial pressure (ICP) elevation and decreased cerebral perfusion pressure (CPP) occur during airway manipulation[275] and can be attenuated by abolition of cough and hypertensive responses and by hyperventilation with oxygen during the apneic preintubation period. Coughing during airway stimulation appears to be the primary cause of increased ICP,[275] but even in the absence of cough, a rise in ICP may follow blood pressure elevation. On the other hand, reduction in systemic blood pressure by anesthetics causes a decrease in CPP if a simultaneous decrease in ICP does not occur.[34] A precurarizing dose of a nondepolarizing muscle relaxant followed by thiopental (2 to 4 mg/kg) and succinylcholine (1.5 mg/kg) is the usual sequence employed to blunt the response to laryngoscopy and endotracheal intubation.[234] Intravenous lidocaine (1.5 mg/kg) 3 minutes before tracheal intubation is also said to help attenuate the rise of ICP,[17] although the beneficial effect of this drug is not universally acknowledged.[275] A second dose of thiopental, half that of the first dose, given immediately prior to intubation, provides better ICP control than a single dose,[260] but also produces a significant decrease in mean arterial pressure and CPP in some patients.[260] Thiopental should not be given to hypotensive patients; the reduction in arterial pressure overrides its benefits. Many clinicians use vecuronium (0.2 mg/kg) instead of succinylcholine to avoid a fasciculation-induced ICP increase, even though available data suggest that pretreatment doses of nondepolarizing agents suffice to mitigate or abolish this effect.[117,176,245] Hyperventilation by mask with cricoid pressure to maintain $Paco_2$ between 25 and 30 mm Hg and prevent aspiration during the interval between administration of drugs and intubation is of utmost importance. Continuous monitoring of patients with a pulse oximeter, end-tidal $CO_2$ analyzer, and nerve stimulator is necessary to ensure adequate oxygenation, hypocapnia, and an appropriate degree of paralysis.

Similar principles apply during airway management of patients with open-eye injuries. Large doses of any of the available intravenous anesthetics combined with either atracurium or vecuronium prevent extrusion of intraocular contents during intubation of lightly anesthetized patients.[11] Even succinylcholine, which is known to increase intraocular pressure (IOP), is unlikely to produce deleterious effects on the eye provided it is administered after precurarization and a large dose of an intravenous anesthetic.[160]

CERVICAL SPINE INJURY. This should be suspected in all blunt trauma and some penetrating trauma victims, and if possible, tracheal intubation should be delayed until the cervical spine is evaluated. If time to obtain X-rays is not available, airway intervention must be performed only after immobilizing the head and neck.

Patients with cervical spine injury present in a variety of conditions each of which requires a somewhat different airway management strategy. An algorithm recommended by the Advanced Trauma Life Support (ATLS) Committee generalizes these conditions and facilitates decision making.[4] The algorithms presented in Fig 3-22 and Fig 3-23 are a slightly modified version of ATLS recommendations.[4] In this protocol, the airway management method is selected according to answers to three basic questions: (1) Is there a need for immediate airway management? (2) Is the patient breathing adequately? and (3) Is there any associated condition that will make airway management difficult? Not all institutions agree with this protocol, in which the importance of nasal intubation to prevent neck movement is stressed, and cricothyroidotomy is recommended if nasal intubation fails after a few attempts. The most frequently emphasized disadvantages of this protocol are the risks of nasal bleeding and of endotracheal tube entry into the cranial vault when coexisting head and/or facial injuries have caused cranial base fractures.[111] Data from a large trauma center at which 711 of 720 acute blunt trauma victims with suspected unstable cervical spine were intubated orally after administration of intravenous anesthetics and muscle relaxants showed that cricoid pressure and immobilization of the neck were sufficient to prevent deterioration of neurological function in all patients.[82,111]

Induction of anesthesia and muscle relaxation in these patients are associated with some disadvantages. The success of orotracheal intubation diminishes when cervical spine in-

FIG. 3-22. An airway management algorithm for patients with suspected cervical spine injury who require immediate airway intervention.

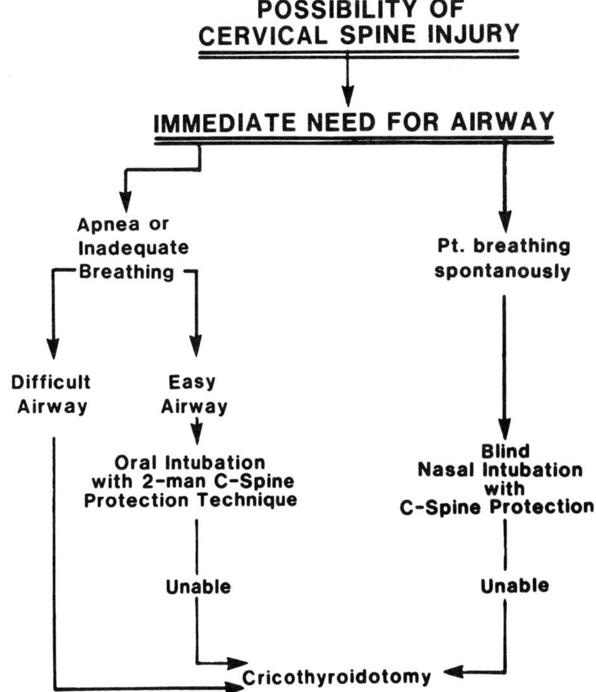

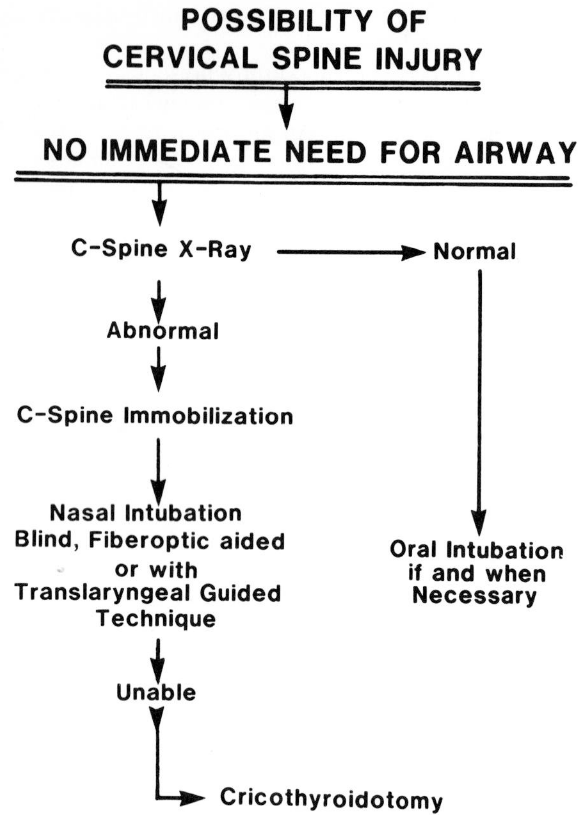


FIG. 3-23. An airway management algorithm for patients with suspected cervical spine injury without an immediate need for airway intervention.

jury precludes positioning of the head and neck in sniffing position.[13] Subsequent multiple attempts at endotracheal intubation may predispose the patient with abolished airway reflexes to aspiration and airway obstruction. Application of cricoid pressure may cause further displacement of vertebral fragments.[5] This is especially important since cervical fracture-dislocations occur frequently at C5 and C6, the area at which the pressure is applied.[44] Nevertheless, in patients with coexisting head or eye injuries, induction of general anesthesia and/or muscle relaxation are necessary to prevent ICP and IOP increases during orotracheal intubation.

If the cervical spine injury is associated with severe facial injuries, the selection of an airway management method depends on whether the oral route is available for tracheal intubation. Since nasotracheal intubation in these patients, especially those with Le Fort II and Le Fort III fractures, is associated with the risk of endotracheal tube entry into the cranial vault, cricothyroidotomy is selected if orotracheal intubation cannot be accomplished. Administration of anesthetics and muscle relaxants before intubation is fraught with the danger of airway obstruction in some of these patients and should be avoided in the early postinjury phase when adequate evaluation of the facial fracture is not possible. Further discussion of cervical spine injury is provided in Chapters 10 and 14.

THORACIC MAJOR VESSEL INJURY. Avoidance of hypertension and large swings of blood pressure are the hallmarks of airway management in thoracic aortic injuries. In most of these injuries intravascular volume can be restored by aggressive fluid resuscitation before anesthetic induction. Fentanyl (4 to 5 μg/kg), sufentanil (1 to 2 μg/kg), or alfentanil (10 μg/kg) administered over a period of 5 minutes can be followed by moderate doses of any of the available intravenous anesthetics except ketamine. Sodium nitroprusside infusion must be prepared before anesthetic induction in case the blood pressure increases more than 10% over the baseline value. Similar principles apply to the management of other major thoracic vessel injuries. In addition, excessive head and neck extension during laryngoscopy and intubation may result in a massive hemorrhage in sealed aortic arch vessel, superior vena cava or jugular system injuries.

PERICARDIAL TAMPONADE. Whenever possible, pericardial blood should be evacuated before anesthetic induction, although this may be impossible because of clotting. Ketamine is preferred to other intravenous agents since it augments myocardial contractility, providing adequate filling and emptying of the heart.

HYPOVOLEMIA. Anesthetic induction of hypovolemic patients is discussed in Chapter 9. Intravascular volume should be restored before induction of anesthesia whenever possible. In severely hypovolemic patients, intubation, if needed immediately, should be performed without anesthesia. In moderately hypovolemic patients, if there is no time for intravascular volume restoration, ketamine is the drug of choice. The dose of ketamine or any other agent should be reduced by 40 to 50% in these patients.[272]

## POSTINTUBATION AIRWAY CARE

A variety of complications may occur after the airway is secured, necessitating not only timely intervention but prevention. Prolonged intubation, which is common after multiple trauma, is associated with its own problems and requires special and meticulous care. This section summarizes management aspects of early and late postintubation problems.

### EARLY POSTINTUBATION PROBLEMS

The airway of the trauma victim is managed by individuals of different backgrounds and training depending on the time and location of care. Often the intubation is performed by a member of one discipline and subsequent airway care managed by another. It is crucial that proper endotracheal tube position and patency are ensured by both people. The diagnostic methods commonly employed to ensure proper tube placement are generally capable of detecting esophageal intubation. However, with the exception of direct cord visualization and end-tidal $CO_2$ measurement, all have the potential of giving a false impression that the tube is in the trachea when it is actually in the esophagus.[26] This is especially true in the patient with a diaphragmatic injury that permits entry of a significant portion of the stomach into the thoracic cavity, resulting in near-normal chest excursion and "breath" sounds during ventilation through an intraesophageal tube.[123] It is also possible to attribute sounds from the esophagus, which imitate breath sounds, to trauma- or aspiration-induced pulmonary abnormality.

Since it may not be possible to visualize the vocal cords in some patients during direct laryngoscopy, it is prudent to measure end-tidal $CO_2$ after intubation, even in areas outside the operating room.[26] In fact, an endotracheal tube that changes its color with $CO_2$ has been designed for use in prehospital care. Unless cardiac arrest or severe hypotension brings the pulmonary circulation to a halt, normal end-tidal $CO_2$ values and curves should be obtained if the tube is in the trachea. Ventilation by mask prior to intubation may force some expired $CO_2$ into the stomach to be detected after esophageal intubation by the analyzer, but the $CO_2$ concentration in these instances is low, has an irregular wave pattern, and diminishes quite rapidly after a few breaths.

Endobronchial intubation may occur either during intubation or with later movement of the head. Decreased breath sounds on the contralateral side may be attributed to pneumothorax and lead to unnecessary thoracostomy. Sometimes hyperinflation of the intubated lung may result in tension pneumothorax which, together with an unventilated contralateral lung, results in severe hypoxemia and cardiac arrest. It has been suggested that securing oral endotracheal tubes with the 23-cm mark in males and the 21-cm in females at the level of the upper incisors reduces the likelihood of this complication.[196] Relying only on this guideline may result in improper tube placement in some patients. The position of the tube in relation to the carina should be evaluated with a chest radiogram whenever there is doubt about proper placement.

Airway obstruction remains a major problem in the trauma victim even after intubation of the airway. Besides well-known problems such as kinking, cuff protrusion, and occlusion by the tracheal wall, blood clots from maxillofacial or airway injuries may obstruct the tracheal tube and/or the bronchi.[148,199] Foreign substances, teeth, tissue fragments, and dried secretions may produce similar results and may be pushed down the airway during intubation or positive pressure ventilation.[231] Occasionally a ball-valve effect from these bodies prevents expiration, eventually resulting in tension pneumothorax.[148] A suction catheter or fiberoptic bronchoscope should be passed into the trachea to assess the nature of the obstruction, whether tube related, lower airway related, or bronchospastic. If obstruction is secondary to tube-related factors, manipulation of the tube, deflating its cuff, or suctioning may correct the problem. The tube should be replaced if these measures are not successful. Suctioning alone may not be effective in withdrawing semisolid materials such as blood or thick secretions. Extraction of these materials with a balloon catheter (Fogarty No. 6) removes more secretions with less hypoxia, produces minimal mucosal damage, and permits continuation of positive pressure ventilation.[3,155,157]

A variety of conditions necessitate replacement of the endotracheal tube in the trauma patient. Changing a tube is a challenging task if initial airway management was difficult. An Eschmann endotracheal tube changer (manufactured by Eschmann, Lansing, Sussex, England), a 60-cm-long, 4-mm-wide hollow tube with sealed ends, can be passed through the endotracheal tube. After ensuring proper oxygenation, the endotracheal tube is removed and replaced by sliding the new tube over the stylet. Difficulty may arise during introduction of the tube into the larynx as it may be caught by the anterior comissure or by the periglottic tissues, resulting in hypoxemia in marginally oxygenated patients. Several modifications of this technique which allow oxygen insufflation or jet ventilation through the stylet during tube replacement have been described. Cutting off the sealed ends of the Eschmann stylet and fitting an adapter to its proximal end allow oxygen delivery.[6] Alternatively, a 4-mm (external diameter) polyethylene tube[18] or an 18 French Salem sump nasogastric tube with its proximal end cut off can be connected to a high-pressure oxygen source such as a Sander's jet attachment[69] (Fig 3-24).

## LATE POSTINTUBATION PROBLEMS

### *Airway Injury*

Direct injury may occur during manipulation of the airway or by prolonged pressure from the endotracheal or tracheostomy tube. Hematoma; avulsion of the vocal cords; dislocation of the arytenoid cartilage; pharyngeal, esophageal, or tracheal perforations; or vocal cord palsies can be produced during intubation of the larynx.[99,124,133,135,177] During cricothyroidotomy and tracheostomy, the airway trauma may exceed that expected from surgery. Posterior tracheal wall laceration, injury of the cricoid and/or thyroid cartilages, and incisions above the tracheal cartilage can occur. With the introduction of high-volume low-pressure cuffs and maintenance of low intracuff pressures, cuff-induced complications have decreased during the past decade. Tube-induced complications, however, occur regularly despite the use of thermolabile plastic tubes that soften at body temperature and tend to conform to the shape of the airway. The types of injuries produced by endotracheal, cricothyroidotomy, and tracheostomy tubes differ significantly, although the cuff-related complications produced by these tubes are similar.

ENDOTRACHEAL TUBE-RELATED INJURIES. These lesions are observed mainly at the posterior part of the larynx over the medial aspect of the arytenoid, the posterolateral aspect of the cricoid, and the vocal processes.[29,85,283] The tracheal mucosa at the tip of the tube is also injured.[283] The pressure required to bring the curved tube into conformation with the upper airway is primarily responsible for this distribution of injury sites.[244] Friction in these areas produced by head and laryngeal motion augments the damage. The major pathological problems are edema, ulceration, granuloma formation, membrane deposition, fibrinous adhesions, fibrous tissue formation, and stricture.[256] Occasionally an abscess may form on the wall of the larynx and trachea, and cartilage resorption may occur.

TRACHEOSTOMY TUBE-RELATED INJURIES. The stoma is the primary site at which the tracheostomy tube causes its damage.[22] Inadequate incision, infection, large tubes, and excess tube motion at the stoma site contribute to the severity of damage.[122]

CRICOTHYROIDOTOMY TUBE-RELATED INJURIES. The average height of the cricothyroid membrane is 10 mm, rang-

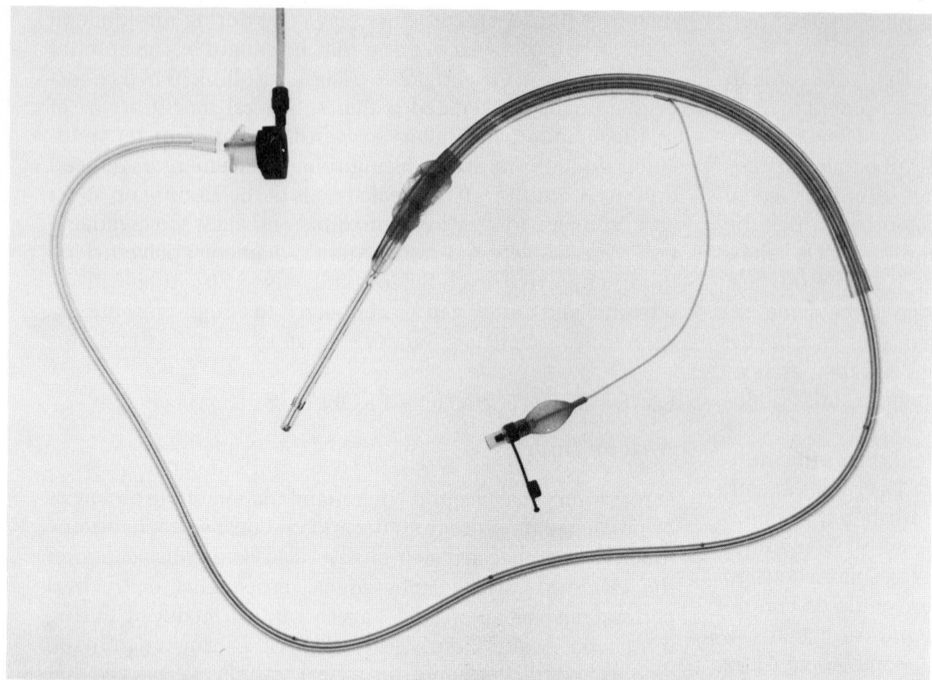

FIG. 3-24. An 18 French Salem sump nasogastric tube connected to a high-pressure oxygen source (Sander's attachment) ready to be used as a tube changer.

ing between 9 and 12 mm.[89] The cricothyroid membrane is about 15 to 20 mm below the vocal folds.[89] Thus, injury to the larynx and vocal cords after cricothyroidotomy is unlikely. However, if cricothyroidotomy cannulas with external diameter greater than 10 mm are used, damage to the thyroid and cricoid cartilages and, therefore, to the larynx may occur.[89]

CUFF-RELATED INJURIES. Tracheal tube cuffs cause damage by exerting pressure on the tracheal wall above capillary perfusion pressure, about 30 mm Hg.[84,132,187] Not all of the cuff pressure is transmitted to the tracheal wall. The approximate wall pressure can be calculated by using the equation described by Joh and coworkers[132]: $Y = 1.2X + 2.4$, where Y is the intracuff pressure, and X is the tracheal wall pressure. Using a hydrogen clearance method in dogs, Joh et al[132] demonstrated that tracheal wall pressures of 10 and 20 mm Hg caused an increase in mucosal blood flow, probably because of irritation-induced release of vasoactive substances. A tracheal wall pressure of 30 mm Hg or above was associated with reduction of mucosal blood flow. Based on these findings they concluded that intracuff pressures should not exceed 43 mm Hg, which corresponds to an approximate tracheal wall pressure of 20 mm Hg. In clinical practice, however, it is generally accepted that intracuff pressure should be kept below 30 mm Hg. Modern floppy cuffs are capable of occluding the trachea at 20 mm Hg. Even with these low pressures, however, tracheal damage may occur in hypotensive patients.[63] High airway pressures during PEEP ventilation may also cause decreased mucosal blood flow because of the need for a higher than usual cuff pressure to seal the trachea.[136] The extent and severity of the lesions are also related to the time during which tracheal wall ischemia is allowed to persist.[7,84,187] Destruction of columnar epithelium occurs within 15 minutes when tracheal wall pressure is maintained in excess of 50 mm Hg.[187]

Ciliary denudation of the tracheal mucosa is an early pathological finding of cuff-induced tracheal injury.[142] Squamous metaplasia may develop as an adaptive response. These changes interfere with clearance of particulate matter from the respiratory tree and thus may be responsible for an increased incidence of postextubation pulmonary complications.[198] Persistence of excessive tracheal wall pressure results in submucosal necrosis which, depending on the degree and duration of pressure, can extend to the cartilages, causing exposure of cartilage and infection. The tracheal cartilages soften, become fragmented, and finally disappear, resulting in tracheal enlargement or tracheomalacia.[97] Occasionally, the tracheal wall destruction extends to adjacent structures, resulting in tracheoesophageal fistula or peritracheal vascular damage.[162] During the healing process contracture of the injured tissue may result in stenotic lesions which usually become clinically obvious several weeks to months after the tracheal tube is removed (Fig 3-25). This complication, however, is more common at the stoma than at the cuff site following tracheostomy.

Short-term clinical findings from these pathologic processes are postextubation airway obstruction and laryngeal incompetence.[29] Among milder symptoms, hoarseness is a frequent complaint. Long-term complications of prolonged intubation include laryngeal stenosis, granuloma formation, and persistent hoarseness.[29] It must be emphasized that clinical symptoms associated with both short- and long-term laryngotracheal sequelae correlate poorly with pathologic changes. A significant degree of laryngeal edema, ulceration, or stenosis may produce few clinical signs and symptoms.[63] Nevertheless, frequent endoscopic examination of the laryngotra-

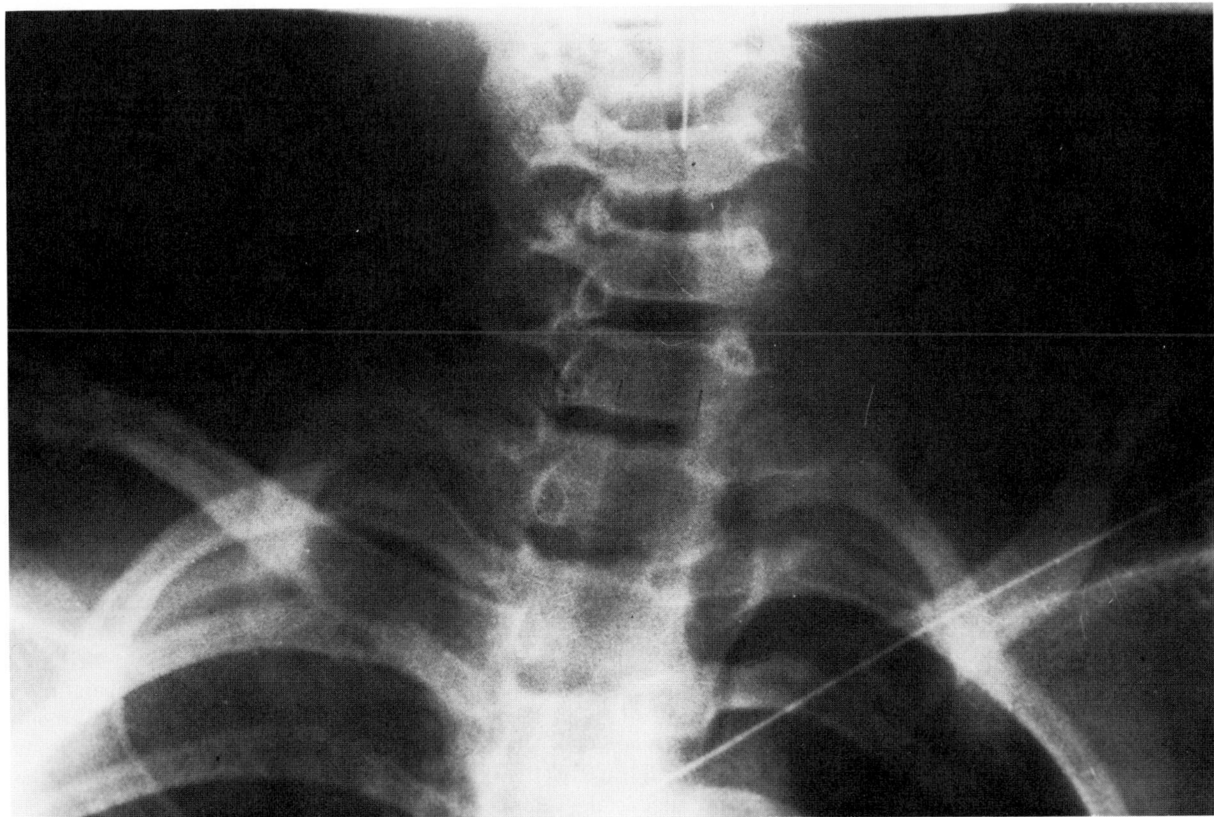

FIG. 3-25. Laryngotracheal stenosis that became clinically manifest 4 months after a 2-week period of intubation. Note the radiopaque line of the endotracheal tube above the stenotic segment. Only tubes with an inner diameter of 4 mm or smaller could be passed through the lesion.

cheal structures following prolonged intubation has been recommended by some authors to detect these lesions and predict clinical abnormalities.[136]

Several measures can prevent tube- and cuff-induced airway injury. Since motion of the tube within the larynx augments the damage, proper patient sedation may diminish the extent of injury. The use of small tubes may also decrease the incidence and severity of laryngotracheal damage. Since nasotracheal tubes are smaller than orotracheal tubes and are associated with less movement against the laryngeal mucosa, they may produce less severe injury. Nevertheless, these tubes may damage other areas of the respiratory tract such as the nose and paranasal sinuses.[115,118,277] Efforts to design endotracheal tubes that conform to the contour of the airway are promising. In a postmortem study; Lindholm's group[85] demonstrated significantly less cricoid injury with these tubes than with conventional tubes, although the rate and severity of injury of the arytenoid cartilage and the tracheal mucosa were similar. It has been suggested that the favorable effects of these tubes at the sites that are usually injured are counteracted by increased damage to other regions of airway. No such effect could be demonstrated in Lindholm's study.[85] When used improperly, high-volume low-pressure cuffs act like low-volume high-pressure cuffs. Not all cuffs have the same compliance characteristics; in some, the intracuff pressure may increase substantially upon addition of only a small amount of air beyond the sealing point. Periodic measurement of intracuff pressure remains the most reliable way to avoid cuff-related complications.

One important question has generated substantial discussion in the past 2 decades: what is the maximum safe length of endotracheal intubation? There is little controversy that with proper care, an endotracheal tube can be safely left in place for 5 days. Controversy exists about prolongation of intubation beyond this time. Whited,[276] after comparing the rate and severity of laryngeal complications in three groups of patients intubated for different time periods, concluded that "the increasing incidence as well as the changed nature of stenotic sequelae, make intubation beyond 10 days unacceptable as a routine policy" (Table 3-8). He considered the period between 7 and 10 days a "gray zone" and suggested conversion to tracheostomy during this period in patients with predisposing factors for laryngeal injury. Dunham and LaMonica[83] compared early (3 to 4 days after endotracheal intubation) and late (14 days after endotracheal intubation) tracheostomy in trauma patients who required an extended period of artificial ventilation. Although laryngeal complications occurred more frequently in head injury victims maintained in rigid positions than in other trauma victims, the incidence was similar in early and late tracheostomy groups. They concluded that ven-

TABLE 3-8. Short- and Long-Term Laryngotracheal Sequelae After Prolonged Intubation*

| LENGTH OF INTUBATION | PATIENTS N | SHORT-TERM SEQUELAE N | % | Type | LONG-TERM SEQUELAE N | % | Type |
|---|---|---|---|---|---|---|---|
| 2 to 5 days | 50 | 3 | 6 | Acute reversible laryngeal stenosis (3) | 1 | 2 | Chronic posterior commissure stenosis |
| 5 to 10 days | 100 | 5 | 5 | Laryngospasm-edema (2)<br>Limited cord abduction (3) | 5 | 5 | Isolated posterior commissure stenosis (1)<br>Extended complex stenosis (4) |
| 11 to 24 days | 50 | 5 | 10 | Stridor due to limited cord abduction (3)<br>Posterior glottic incompetence with aspiration (2) | 7 | 14 | Subclinical posterior commissure (1)<br>Extended complex stenosis (6) |

* Numbers in parentheses represent number of patients with that particular sequela. (From Whited.[276])

tilation via an endotracheal tube for up to 2 weeks is safe in trauma victims. After analyzing the data from 150 critically ill patients, Stauffer et al[243] suggested that endotracheal intubation for up to 22 days was well tolerated. Evidence from animal studies also suggests that severity of laryngeal injury increases little after the first week of intubation.[28] Stauffer et al[243] showed that the incidence of tracheal stenosis increased when tracheostomy followed prolonged tracheal intubation. This point also has been emphasized by Bishop and coworkers,[29] who feel that tracheostomy permits adhesion and thus apposition of inflamed vocal cords. There remain anecdotal reports showing that endotracheal intubation for more than a month was associated with few laryngeal complications.[265] In view of these diverse findings it is difficult to make a firm recommendation. However, it is probably safe to consider establishment of a transtracheal airway after 7 days and certainly after 10 days of intubation if a possibility of removing the endotracheal tube within a few days does not exist.[121] In the pediatric age group, however, every effort should be made to avoid tracheostomy, since morbidity and mortality from tracheostomy in children are twice those from endotracheal intubation.[191] Endotracheal tubes have been left in place for up to 3 weeks in children.[112]

Unlike establishment of a surgical airway under emergency conditions, for which cricothyroidotomy is the usual technique, tracheostomy at the second and third tracheal rings is the elective procedure of choice.[121,122] Perioperative morbidity following tracheostomy in published series varies significantly (between 6 and 51%), but more recent work demonstrates operative complication rate of only 6%.[246] Common perioperative complications include bleeding from the thyroid isthmus or anterior neck vessels, subcutaneous emphysema, pneumothorax, aspiration of blood and pharyngeal secretions, airway obstruction, and tube displacement.[121] The procedure can be performed safely in the intensive care unit over an endotracheal tube if appropriate monitoring and experienced medical and nursing personnel are available. Transport of the critically ill trauma patient to the operating room probably carries a higher risk than performing the tracheostomy in the patient's bed.[246] Long-term complications of tracheostomy include pneumonia, tracheal stenosis, tracheoinnominate fistula, tracheoesophageal fistula, aspiration, swallowing dysfunction, and stomal infection.[122] Of these, tracheoinnominate fistula is a rare but devastating complication. A low incision (at the fourth tracheal ring) predisposes the patient to this complication; the tracheostomy tube erodes directly into the artery.[122] Synchronous motion of the tube with arterial pulse may be a predictive sign of this complication. Bleeding from the trachea should be evaluated under controlled conditions, preferably in the operating room, even if it is mild. Not infrequently, an initial small amount of bleeding stops only to be followed sometime later by sudden massive hemorrhage. If massive bleeding occurs, the tracheostomy tube should be replaced with an endotracheal tube introduced either orally or through the stoma site to tamponade the bleeding artery with its inflated, or hyperinflated, cuff. Introduction of a finger through an incision over the jugular notch and anterior compression of the innominate artery against the sternum until the patient is moved to the operating room can also be helpful.[122]

Aspiration of pharyngeal secretions around the tracheostomy tube was reported to be extremely common (69%),[1] but with use of cuffed tubes this complication now occurs infrequently.

After the famous 1976 report of Brantigan and Grow[39] on the advantages and low complication rate (6% in their series) of cricothyroidotomy, and subsequent reports confirming their findings,[38,113,262] many surgeons prefer to perform elective cricothyroidotomy or leave the emergency cricothyroidotomy cannula in place when prolonged ventilatory support is required. The overall rate of subglottic stenosis from this procedure is 2%, and varying degrees of dysphonia can occur in up to 32% of patients.[62] Factors that predispose the patient to these complications and present absolute contraindications to this procedure are: (1) performing the procedure after prolonged (more than 7 days)[38] endotracheal intubation; (2) preexisting laryngeal pathology of any kind; and (3) airway obstruction following removal of the endotracheal tube.[62,89] Comparative data about the overall outcome of elective tracheostomy and cricothyroidotomy in trauma patients, or in any other patient population, are not yet available. However, it appears that conversion of the cricothyoidotomy into a tracheostomy within 24 to 48 hours and selecting tracheostomy instead of cricothyroidotomy even when endotracheal intubation has not been prolonged may decrease tne incidence and severity of laryngeal complications.

### *Paranasal Sinusitis*

A nasotracheal tube should be replaced with an orotracheal or tracheostomy tube to avoid paranasal sinusitis. This complication may occur within 3 days after nasotracheal intubation because obstruction of the sinus ducts by the tube and nasal mucosal edema prevent sinus drainage.[118] Paranasal sinusitis may occur in up to 100% of nasotracheally intubated patients.[118] Pain, fever, purulent nasal drainage, and, in severe cases, erythema of the skin over the frontal and maxillary sinuses may occur. In comatose patients who cannot complain of sinus pain, unexplained fever may be the first manifestation of this complication. It appears that the frequency of sinusitis from nasotracheal intubation after head trauma increases with the severity of head injury.[115] After removal of the nasotracheal tube, oxygenation should be monitored carefully because aspiration of purulent nasopharyngeal secretions may result in pneumonitis.[277]

### *Extubation after Prolonged Intubation*

Standard weaning protocols and extubation criteria are generally designed to evaluate pulmonary rather than airway function. Using standard criteria, Demling et al[77] noted overall extubation failure in 3% of trauma patients within 7 days of tube removal. The incidence of extubation failure in two groups of trauma patients was substantially higher than this, being 13% in a group with smoke inhalation and 5% in head injury patients. The reason for reintubation in patients with smoke inhalation was a requirement for airway maintainence and pulmonary toilet. In the head injury group the most common reason for reintubation was airway protection. Premature extubation was practically nonexistent in other trauma patients. Extubation failure is associated with significant morbidity (60%) and mortality (10%) mainly because of aspiration and severe atelectasis developing during the period of extubation. Thus, the airway should be evaluated carefully at frequent intervals prior to and following extubation, particularly in patients who have sustained head injury or smoke inhalation.

## REFERENCES


1. Abou-Madi MN, Trop D. Pulling versus guiding: a modification of retrograde guided intubation. Can J Anaesth 1989;36:336.

1a. Adams AL, Cane RD, Shapiro BA. Tongue extrusion as an aid to blind nasal intubation. Crit Care Med 1982;10:335.

2. Adelhoj B, Petring OU, Hagelsten JO. Inaccuracy of preanesthetic gastric intubation for emptying liquid stomach contents. Acta Anaesthesiol Scand 1986;30:41.
3. Allen RP, Siefkin AD. Emergency airway clot removal in acute hemorrhagic respiratory failure. Crit Care Med 1987;15:987.
4. American College of Surgeons Committee on Trauma. Advanced Trauma Life Support Course, Instructor Manual. Chicago: American College of Surgeons 1984:157–160.
5. Aprahamian C, Thompson BM, Finger WA, Darin JC. Experimental cervical spine injury model: evaluation of airway management and splinting techniques. Ann Emerg Med 1984;13:584.
6. Arndt GA, Ghani GA. A modification of an Eschmann endotracheal tube changer for insufflation. Anesthesiology 1988;69:282.
7. Arola MK, Anttinen J. Post mortem findings of tracheal injury after cuffed intubation and tracheostomy. Acta Anaesthesiol Scand 1979;23:57.
8. Arora RD, Patterson L, Hagen JF, Pinchak AC. Prediction of difficult intubation. Anesthesiology 1987;67:A472.
9. Atkinson WJ. Posture of the unconcious patient. Lancet 1970;1:404.
10. Attia RR, Battit GE, Murphy JD. Transtracheal ventilation. JAMA 1975;234:1152.
11. Badrinath SK, Vazeery A, McCarthy RJ, Ivankovich AD. The effect of different methods of inducing anesthesia on intraocular pressure. Anesthesiology 1986;65:431.
12. Bainton CR. A new laryngoscope blade to overcome pharyngeal obstruction. Anesthesiology 1987;67:767.
13. Bannister FB, Macbeth RG. Direct laryngoscopy and tracheal intubation. Lancet 1944;2:651.
14. Barash PG, Kopriva CJ, Langou R, et al. Is cocaine a sympathetic stimulant during general anesthesia? JAMA 1980;243:1437.
15. Barr AM, Thornley BA. Thiopentone and suxamethonium crash induction. Anaesthesia 1976;31:23.
16. Barriot P, Riou B. Retrograde technique for tracheal intubation in trauma patients. Crit Care Med 1988;16:712.
17. Bedford RF, Persing JA, Poberskin L, Butler A. Lidocaine or thiopental for rapid control of intracranial hypertension. Anesth Analg 1980;59:435.
18. Bedger RC Jr, Chang JL. A jet-stylet endotracheal catheter for difficult airway management. Anesthesiology 1987;66:221.
19. Bellhouse CP. An angulated laryngoscope for routine and difficult tracheal intubation. Anesthesiology 1988;69:126.
20. Bellhouse CP, Dore C. Criteria for estimating likelihood of difficulty of endotracheal intubation with the Macintosh laryngoscope. Anaesth Intensive Care 1988;16:329.
21. Bencini A, Newton DEF. Rate of onset of good intubating conditions, respiratory depression and hand muscle paralysis after vecuronium. Br J Anaesth 1984;56:959.
22. Berlauk JF. Prolonged endotracheal intubation versus tracheostomy. Crit Care Med 1986;14:742.
23. Bernstein JS, Nelson MA, Ebert TJ, et al. Beat-by-beat cardiovascular responses to rapid sequence induction in humans: effects of labetalol. Anesthesiology 1987;67:A32.
24. Berry FA. The use of a stylet in blind nasotracheal intubation. Anesthesiology 1984;61:469.
25. Bingham HG, Gallagher TJ, Powell MD. Early bronchoscopy as a predictor of ventilatory support for burned patients. J Trauma 1987;27:1286.
26. Birmingham PK, Cheney FW, Ward RJ. Esophageal intubation: a review of detection techniques. Anesth Analg 1986;65:886.
27. Bishop MJ, Benson MS, Sato P, Pierson DJ. Comparison of high-frequency jet ventilation with conventional mechanical ventilation for bronchopleural fistula. Anesth Analg 1987;66:833.
28. Bishop MJ, Hibbard AJ, Fink BR, et al. Laryngeal injury in a dog model of prolonged endotracheal intubation. Anesthesiology 1985;62:770.
29. Bishop MJ, Weymuller EA, Fink BR. Laryngeal effects of prolonged intubation. Anesth Analg 1984;63:335.
30. Bjoraker DG, Kumar NB, Brown ACD. Evaluation of an emergency cricothyroidotomy instrument. Crit Care Med 1987;15:157.
31. Blair E, Topuzlu C, Davis JH. Delayed or missed diagnosis in blunt chest trauma. J Trauma 1971;11:129.
32. Blitt CD, Carlson GL, Rolling GD, et al. A comparative evaluation of pretreatment with nondepolarizing neuromuscular blockers prior to administration of succinycholine. Anesthesiology 1981;55:687.

33. Blitt CD, Gutman HL, Cohen DD, et al. "Silent" regurgitation and aspiration during general anesthesia. Anesth Analg 1970;49:707.
34. Bogetz MS, Katz JA. Airway management of the trauma patient. Semin Anesth 1985;4:114.
35. Boidin MP. Airway patency in the unconscious patient. Br J Anaesth 1985;57:306.
36. Booth DJ, Zuidema GD, Cameron JL. Aspiration pneumonia: pulmonary arteriography after experimental aspiration. J Surg Res 1972;12:48.
37. Boucek CD, Gunnerson HB, Tullock WC. Percutaneous transtracheal high-frequency jet ventilation as an aid to fiberoptic intubation. Anesthesiology 1987;67:247.
38. Boyd AD, Romita MD, Conlan AA, et al. A clinical evaluation of cricothyroidotomy. Surg Gynecol Obstet 1979;149:365.
39. Brantigan CO, Grow JB. Cricothyroidotomy: elective use in respiratory problems requiring tracheotomy. J Thorac Cardiovasc Surg 1976;71:72.
40. Brock-Utne JG, Dimopoulos GE, Downing JW, Moshal MG. Effect of metoclopramide given before atropine sulphate on lower oesophageal spincter tone. S Afr Med J 1982;61:465.
41. Brodman E, Duncalf D. Avoiding the trauma of nasotracheal intubation. Anesth Analg 1981;60:618.
42. Brown EM, Kirshnaprasad D, Smiler BG. Pancuronium for rapid induction technique for tracheal intubation. Can Anaesth Soc J 1979;26:489.
43. Bruce DL, Downs JB, Kulkarni PS, Capan L. Precurarization inhibits maximal ventilatory effort. Anesthesiology 1984; 61:618.
44. Bunegin L, Hung TK, Chang GL. Biomechanics of spinal cord injury. Crit Care Clin 1987;3:453.
45. Bynum LJ, Pierce AK. Pulmonary aspiration of gastric contents. Am Rev Respir Dis 1976;114:1129.
46. Caldwell C, Rains G, McKiterick K. An unusual reaction to preoperative metoclopramide. Anesthesiology 1987;67:854.
47. Cameron JL, Mitchell WH, Zuidema GD. Aspiration pneumonia: clinical outcome following documented aspiration. Arch Surg 1973;106:49.
48. Cameron JL, Zuidema GD. Aspiration pneumonia: magnitude and frequency of the problem. JAMA 1972;219:1194.
49. Camnitz PS, Shepherd SM, Henderson RA. Acute blunt laryngeal and tracheal trauma. Am J Emerg Med 1987;5:157.
50. Campinos L, Duval G, Couturier M, et al. The value of early fiberoptic bronchoscopy after aspiration of gastric contents. Br J Anaesth 1983;55:1103.
51. Carlsson C, Islander G. Silent gastropharyngeal regurgitation during anesthesia. Anesth Analg 1981;60:655.
52. Cass NM, James NR, Lines V. Difficult direct laryngoscopy complicating intubation for anaesthesia. Br Med J 1956;1:488.
53. Chang JL, Meeuwis H, Bleyaert A, et al. Severe abdominal distention following jet ventilation during general anesthesia. Anesthesiology 1978;49:216.
54. Chase CR, Hebert JC, Farnham JE. Post-traumatic upper airway obstruction secondary to a lingual artery hematoma. J Trauma 1987;27:953.
55. Chen CT, Toung TJK, Haupt HM, et al. Evaluation of the efficacy of Alka-seltzer effervescent in gastric acid neutralization. Anesth Analg 1984;63:325.
56. Chraemmer-Jorgensen B, Hoilund-Carlsen PF, Marving J, Christensen V. Lack of effect of intravenous lidocaine on hemodynamic responses to rapid sequence induction of general anesthesia: a double-blind controlled clinical trial. Anesth Analg 1986;65:1037.
57. Chraemmer-Jorgensen B, Hoilund-Carlsen PF, Marving J, Christensen V. Left ventricular ejection fraction during anaesthetic induction: comparison of rapid-sequence and elective induction. Can Anaesth Soc J 1986;33:754.
58. Cicala R, Westbrook L. An alternative method of paralysis for rapid-sequence induction. Anesthesiology 1988;69:983.
59. Claeys DW, Lockhart CH, Hinkle JE. The effects of translaryngeal block and innovar on glottic competence. Anesthesiology 1973;38:485.
60. Cogbill TH, Bintz M, Johnson JA, Strutt PJ. Acute gastric dilatation after trauma. J Trauma 1987;27:1113.
61. Cohen MM, Duncan PG, Pope WDB, Wolkenstein C. A survey of 112,000 anaesthetics at one teaching hospital (1975–83). Can Anaesth Soc J 1986;33:22.
62. Cole RR, Aguilar EA. Cricothyroidotomy versus tracheotomy: an otolaryngologist's perspective. Laryngoscope 1988;98:131.
63. Colice GL. Prolonged intubation versus tracheostomy in the adult. J Intensive Care Med 1987;2:85.
64. Conklin KA, Ziadlou-Rad F. Buffering capacity of citrate antacids. Anesthesiology 1983;58:391.
65. Cook WP, Schultetus RR, Caton D. A comparison of D-tubocurarine pretreatment and no pretreatment in obstetric patients. Anesth Analg 1987;66:756.
66. Coombs D, Hooper D, Pageau M. Emergency cimetidine prophylaxis against acid aspiration. Ann Emerg Med 1982;11:252.
67. Cork RC, Weiss JL, Hameroff SR, Bentley J. Fentanyl preloading for rapid-sequence induction of anesthesia. Anesth Analg 1984;63:60.
68. Coursin DB, Farin-Rusk C, Springman SR, Goelzer SL. The hemodynamic effects of intravenous cimetidine versus ranitidine in intensive care unit patients: a double-blind, prospective, cross-over study. Anesthesiology 1988;69:975.
69. Coveler LA. More on management of the difficult airway. Anesthesiology 1987;67:154.
70. Crawford DC, Fell D, Achola KJ, Smith G. Effects of alfentanil on the pressor and catecholamine responses to tracheal intubation. Br J Anaesth 1987;59:707.
71. Cromartie RS III. Rapid anesthesia induction in combat casualties with full stomachs. Anesth Analg 1976;55:74.
72. Cucchiara RF. A simple technic to minimize tracheal aspiration. Anesth Analg 1976;55:816.
73. Cullen DJ. The effect of pretreatment with nondepolarizing muscle relaxants on the neuromuscular blocking action of succinylcholine. Anesthesiology 1971;35:572.
74. Danzl DF, Thomas DM. Nasotracheal intubations in the emergency department. Crit Care Med 1980;8:677.
75. Davies JR. The fiberoptic laryngoscope in the management of cut throat injuries. Br J Anaesth 1978;50:511.
76. Davies JAH, Howells TH. Management of anaesthesia for the full stomach case in the casualty department. Postgrad Med J 1973;(July Suppl):58.
77. Demling RH, Read T, Lind LJ, Flanagan HL. Incidence and morbidity of extubation failure in surgical intensive care patients. Crit Care Med 1988;16:573.
78. Derbyshire DR, Smith G, Achola KJ. Effect of topical lignocaine on the sympathodrenal responses to tracheal intubation. Br J Anaesth 1987;59:300.
79. D'Hollander AA, Monteny E, Dewachter B, et al. Intubation under topical supra-glottic analgesia in unpremedicated and non-fasting patients: amnesic effects of sub-hypnotic doses of diazepam and Innovar. Can Anaesth Soc J 1974;21:467.
80. Dobb G, Jordan MJ, Williams JG. Cimetidine in the prevention of the pulmonary acid aspiration (Mendelson's) syndrome. Br J Anaesth 1979;51:967.
81. Duncan JAT. Intubation of the trachea in the conscious patient. Br J Anaesth 1977;49:619.
82. Dunham CM, Britt LD, Stene JK. Emergency tracheal intu-

bation in the blunt injured patient. Paper from the Maryland Institute Emergency Medical Services Systems. Presented at the Eastern Association of Trauma Surgeons, 1987.
83. Dunham CM, LaMonica C. Prolonged tracheal intubation in the trauma patient. J Trauma 1984;24:120.
84. Dunn CR, Cunn DL, Moser KM. Determinants of tracheal injury by cuffed tracheostomy tubes. Chest 1974;65:128.
85. Eckerbom B, Lindholm CE, Alexopoulos C. Airway lesions caused by prolonged intubation with standard and with anatomically shaped tracheal tubes: a post-mortem study. Acta Anaesthesiol Scand 1986;30:366.
86. Editorial. Cimetidine and the acid aspiration syndrome. Lancet 1980;1:465.
87. Eijgelaar A, Homan V, Heide JW. A reliable early sign of bronchial and tracheal rupture. Thorax 1970;25:116.
88. England DW, Davis IJ, Timmins AE, et al. Gastric emptying: a study to compare the effects of intrathecal morphine and IM papaveretum analgesia. Br J Anaesth 1987;59:1403.
89. Esses BA, Jafek BW. Cricothyroidotomy: a decade of experience in Denver. Ann Otol Rhinol Laryngol 1987;96:519.
90. Eyler SW, Cullen BF, Murphy ME, Welch WD. Antacid aspiration in rabbits: a comparison of Mylanta and Bicitra. Anesth Analg 1982;61:288.
91. Fanning GL. The efficacy of cricoid pressure in preventing regurgitation of gastric contents. Anesthesiology 1970;32:553.
92. Faure EAM, Lim HS, Block BS, et al. Sodium bicarbonate buffers gastric acid during surgery in obstetric and gynecologic patients. Anesthesiology 1987;67:274.
93. Feely J, Wilkinson GR, Wood AJJ. Reduction of liver blood flow and propranolol metabolism by cimetidine. N Engl J Med 1981;304:692.
94. Fouke JM, Stohl KP. Effect of position and lung volume on upper airway geometry. J Appl Physiol 1987;63:375.
95. Frass M, Frenzer R, Zahler J, et al. Ventilation via the esophageal tracheal combitube in a case of difficult intubation. J Cardiothorac Anesth 1987;1:565.
96. Freund F, Rubin A. The need for additional succinylcholine after D-tubocurarine. Anesthesiology 1972;36:185.
97. Fryer ME, Marshall RD. Tracheal dilatation. Anaesthesia 1976;31:470.
98. Gambee AM, Hertzka RE, Fisher DM. Preoxygenation techniques: comparison of three minutes and four breaths. Anesth Analg 1987;66:468.
99. Gibbin KP, Egginton MJ. Bilateral vocal cord paralysis following endotracheal intubation. Br J Anaesth 1981;53:1091.
100. Gibbs CP, Banner TC. Effectiveness of Bicitra® as a preoperative anatacid. Anesthesiology 1984;61:97.
101. Gibney RTH, Finnegan B, FitzGerald MX, Lynch V. Upper airway obstruction caused by massive subcutaneous emphysema. Intensive Care Med 1984;10:43.
102. Gildar JS. A simple system for transtracheal ventilation. Anesthesiology 1983;58:106.
103. Gilman S, Abrams AL. Prevention of aspiration of gastric contents during general anesthesia. N Engl J Med 1956;255:508.
104. Gold MI, Brown M, Coverman S, Herrington C. Heart rate and blood pressure effects of esmolol after ketamine induction and intubation. Anesthesiology 1986;64:718.
105. Gold MI, Buechel DR. Translaryngeal anesthesia: a review. Anesthesiology 1959;20:181.
106. Gold MI, Duarte I, Muravchick S. Arterial oxygenation in conscious patients after 5 minutes and after 30 seconds of oxygen breathing. Anesth Analg 1981;60:313.
107. Goldberg JS. What is the correct position of the neck for rapid sequence induction in the patient with a "full stomach"? Anesthesiology 1987;66:588.
108. Goldman E, McDonald JS, Peterson SS, et al. Transtracheal ventilation with oscillatory pressure for complete upper airway obstruction. J Trauma 1988;28:611.
109. Gorback MS. Inflation of the endotracheal tube cuff as an aid to blind nasal endotracheal intubation. Anesth Analg 1987; 66:913.
110. Gotta AW, Sullivan CA. Anaesthesia of the upper airway using topical anaesthetic and superior laryngeal nerve block. Br J Anaesth 1981;53:1055.
111. Grande CM, Barton CR, Stene JK. Appropriate techniques for airway management of emergency patients with suspected spinal cord injury. Anesth Analg 1988;67:714.
112. Gregory G. Respiratory care of the child. Crit Care Med 1980;8:582.
113. Greisz H, Qvarnström O, Willen R. Elective cricothyroidotomy: a clinical and histopathological study. Crit Care Med 1982; 10:387.
114. Greschner M, Devitt JH. Unexpected migration of an esophageal foreign body. Anesthesiology 1987;67:565.
115. Grindlinger GA, Niehoff J, Hughes SL, et al. Acute paranasal sinusitis related to nasotracheal intubation of head-injured patients. Crit Care Med 1987;15:214.
116. Gross JB, Hartigan ML, Schaffer DW. A suitable substitute for 4% cocaine before blind nasotracheal intubation: 3% lidocaine-0.25% phenylephrine nasal spray. Anesth Analg 1984;63: 915.
117. Haigh JD, Nemoto EM, DeWolf AM, Bleyaert AL. Comparison of the effects of succinylcholine and atracurium on intracranial pressure in monkeys with intracranial hypertension. Can Anaesth Soc J 1986;33:421.
118. Hansen M, Poulsen MR, Bendixen DK, Hartmann-Andersen F. Incidence of sinusitis in patients with nasotracheal intubation. Br J Anaesth 1988;61:231.
119. Haponik EF, Meyers DA, Munster AM, et al. Acute upper airway injury in burn patients: serial changes of flow-volume curves and nasopharyngoscopy. Am Rev Respir Dis 1987; 135:360.
120. Harrison L, Ralley FE, Wynands JE, et al. The role of an ultra short-acting adrenergic blocker (esmolol) in patients undergoing coronary artery bypass surgery. Anesthesiology 1987; 66:413.
121. Heffner JE, Miller KS, Sahn SA. Tracheostomy in the intensive care unit; part 1: indications, technique, management. Chest 1986;90:269.
122. Heffner JE, Miller KS, Sahn SA. Tracheostomy in the intensive care unit, part 2: complications. Chest 1986;90:430.
123. Heiselman D, Polacek DJ, Snyder JV, Grenvik A. Detection of esophageal intubation in patients with intrathoracic stomach. Crit Care Med 1985;13:1069.
124. Holley HS, Gildea JE. Vocal cord paralysis after tracheal intubation. JAMA 1971;215:281.
125. Horrow JC, Lambert DH. The search for an optimal interval between pretreatment dose of D-tubocurarine and succinylcholine. Can Anaesth Soc J 1984;31:528.
126. Howells TH, Chamney AR, Wraight WJ, Simons RS. The application of cricoid pressure: an assessment and a survey of its practice. Anaesthesia 1983;38:457.
127. Hunt JL, Agee RN, Pruitt BA. Fiberoptic bronchoscopy in acute inhalation injury. J Trauma 1975;15:641.
128. Iberti TJ, Paluch TA, Helmer L, et al. The hemodynamic effects of intravenous cimetidine in intensive care unit patients: a double-blind, prospective study. Anesthesiology 1986;64:87.
129. Inoue H, Shohtsu A, Ogawa J, et al. Endotracheal tube with movable blocker to prevent aspiration of intratracheal bleeding. Ann Thorac Surg 1984;37:497.

130. Ivatury RR, Khan MB, Nallathambi M, et al. Cimetidine and hepatic blood flow in polytrauma patients. Crit Care Med 1985;13:436.
131. James CF, Modell JH, Gibbs CP, et al. Pulmonary aspiration: effects of volume and pH in the rat. Anesth Analg 1984;63:665.
132. Joh S, Matsuura H, Kotani Y, et al. Change in tracheal blood flow during endotracheal intubation. Acta Anaesthesiol Scand 1987;31:300.
133. Johnson KG, Hood DD. Espophageal perforation associated with endotracheal intubation. Anesthesiology 1986;64:281.
134. Joyce T III. Prophylaxis for pulmonary acid aspiration. Am J Med 1987;83:46.
135. Kambic V, Radsel Z. Intubation lesions of the larynx. Br J Anaesth 1978;50:587.
136. Kastanos N, Miro RE, Perez AM, et al. Laryngotracheal injury due to endotracheal intubation: incidence, evolution, and predisposing factors, a prospective long-term study. Crit Care Med 1983;11:362.
137. Katz RL, Berci G. The optical stylet: a new intubation technique for adults and children with specific reference to teaching. Anesthesiology 1979;51:251.
138. Katz RI, Hovagim AR, Finkelstein H, et al. A comparison of cocaine, lidocaine with epinephrine and oxymetazoline for prevention of epistaxis on nasal intubation. Anesth Analg 1988;67:S110.
139. King HK, Wang LF, Khan AK, Wooten DJ. Translaryngeal guided intubation for difficult intubation. Crit Care Med 1987;15:869.
140. Kingsley BP, Vaughan S, Vaughan RW. Cardiovascular effects of nondepolarizing relaxants employed for pretreatment prior to succinylcholine. Can Anaesth Soc J 1984;31:13.
141. Kirsh MM, Orringer MB, Behrendt DM, Sloan H. Management of tracheobronchial disruption secondary to nonpenetrating trauma. Ann Thorac Surg 1976;22:93.
142. Klainer AS, Turndorf H, Wu WH, et al. Surface alterations due to endotracheal intubation. Am J Med 1975;58:674.
143. Kleinman J, Marlar K, Silva DA, et al. Sufentanil attenuation of the stress response during rapid sequence induction. Anesthesiology 1985;63:A379.
144. Klotz U, Reimann I. Delayed clearance of diazepam due to cimetidine. N Engl J Med 1980;302:1012.
145. Klumpe DH, Sang OHK, Wayman SA. A characteristic finding in unilateral complete bronchial transection. Am J Roentgenol Radium Ther Nucl Med 1970;110:704.
146. Kopman AF, Wollman SB, Ross K, et al. Awake endotracheal intubation: a review of 267 cases. Anesth Analg 1975;54:323.
147. Kopriva CJ, Eltringham RJ, Siebert PE. A comparison of the effects of intravenous Innovar and topical spray on the laryngeal closure reflex. Anesthesiology 1974;40:596.
148. Kruczek ME, Hoff BH, Keszler BR, Smith RB. Blood clot resulting in ball-valve obstruction in the airway. Crit Care Med 1982;10:122.
149. Lahiri SK. Preventing gastric regurgitation with a ballooned nasogastric tube. Ann R Coll Surg Engl 1987;69:122.
150. Lawes EG. Cricoid pressure with or without the "cricoid yoke." Br J Anaesth 1986;58:1376.
151. Lawes EG, Campbell I, Mercer D. Inflation pressure, gastric insufflation and rapid sequence induction. Br J Anaesth 1987;59:315.
152. Lawes EG, Duncan PW, Bland B, et al. The cricoid yoke: a device for providing consistent and reproducible cricoid pressure. Br J Anaesth 1986;58:925.
153. Layton TR, DiMarco RF, Pellegrini RV. Tracheoesophageal fistula from nonpenetrating trauma. J Trauma 1980;20:802.
154. Lechman MJ, Donahoo JS, MacVauch H III. Endotracheal intubation using percutaneous retrograde guide wire insertion followed by antegrade fiberoptic bronchoscopy. Crit Care Med 1986;14:589.
155. Leiman BC, Hall ID, Stanley TH. Extirpation of endotracheal tube secretions with a Fogarty arterial embolectomy catheter. Anesthesiology 1985;62:847.
156. Leiman BC, Katz J, Butler BD. Mechanisms of succinylcholine-induced arrhythmias in hypoxic or hypoxic hypercarbic dogs. Anesth Analg 1987;66:1292.
157. Leiman BC, Katz J, Stanley TH, Butler BD. Removal of tracheal secretions in anesthetized dogs. Anesth Analg 1987;66:529.
158. Lennon RL, Olson RA, Gronert GA. Atracurium or vecuronium for rapid sequence endotracheal intubation. Anesthesiology 1986;64:510.
159. Leslie JB, Kalayjian RW, McLoughlin TM, et al. Ablation of the hemodynamic responses to tracheal intubation with preinduction intravenous labetalol. Anesthesiology 1987;67:A30.
160. Libonati MM, Leahy JJ, Ellison N. The use of succinylcholine in open-eye surgery. Anesthesiology 1985;62:637.
161. Lineberger AS III, Sprague DH, Battaglini JW. Sinus arrest associated with cimetidine. Anesth Analg 1985;64:554.
162. LoCicero J III: Tracheo-carotid artery erosion following endotracheal intubation. J Trauma 1984;24:907.
163. Lynn RB, Iyengar K. Traumatic rupture of the bronchus. Chest 1972;61:81.
164. Mallampati SR, Gatt SP, Gugino LD, et al. A clinical sign to predict difficult tracheal intubation: a prospective study. Can Anaesth Soc J 1985;32:429.
165. Maltby JR, Cassidy M, Nanji GM. Blind nasotracheal intubation using succinylcholine. Anesthesiology 1988;69:946.
166. Manchikanti L, Grow JB, Colliver JA, et al. Atracurium pretreatment for succinylcholine-induced fasciculations and postoperative myalgia. Anesth Analg 1985;64:1010.
167. Martin C, Bonneru JJ, Brun JP, et al. Vecuronium or suxamethonium for rapid sequence intubation: which is better? Br J Anaesth 1987;59:1240.
168. Martling CR, Lundberg JM. Capsaicin sensitive afferents contribute to acute airway edema following tracheal instillation of hydrochloric acid or gastric juice in the rat. Anesthesiology 1988;68:350.
169. Mathisen DJ, Grillo H. Laryngotracheal trauma. Ann Thorac Surg 1987;43:254.
170. Mathru M, Venus B, Rao TL, Matsuda T. Noncardiac pulmonary edema precipitated by tracheal intubation in patients with inhalation injury. Crit Care Med 1983;11:804.
171. McIntyre JWR. The difficult tracheal intubation. Can J Anaesth 1987;34:204.
172. Mehta RM, Pathak PN. A foreign body in the larynx: case report. Br J Anaesth 1973;45:755.
173. Mendelson CL. The aspiration of stomach contents into the lungs during obstetric anesthesia. Am J Obstet Gynecol 1946;52:191.
174. Miller JD, Butterworth JF, Gudeman SK, et al. Further experience in the management of severe head injury. J Neurosurg 1981;54:289.
175. Mills SA, Johnston FR, Hudstpeth AS, et al. Clinical spectrum of blunt tracheobronchial disruption illustrated by seven cases. J Thorac Cardiovasc Surg 1982;84:49.
176. Minton MD, Grosslight K, Stirt JA, Bedford RF. Increases in intracranial pressure from succinylcholine: prevention by prior nondepolarizing blockade. Anesthesiology 1986;65:165.
177. Minuck M. Unilateral vocal-cord paralysis following endotracheal intubation. Anesthesiology 1976;45:448.
178. Mizrahi S, Yaari Y, Lugassy G, Cotev S. Major airway obstruction relieved by helium/oxygen breathing. Crit Care Med 1986;14:986.

179. Moran TJ. Milk-aspiration pneumonia in human and animal subjects. Arch Pathol 1953;55:286.
180. Motsch J, Fuchs W, Hoch P, et al. Side effects and changes in pulmonary function after fixed dose precurarization with alcuronium, pancuronium or vecuronium. Br J Anaesth 1987;59:1528.
181. Moylan JA, West JT, Nash G, et al. Tracheostomy in thermally injured patients: a review of five years' experience. Am Surg 1972;38:119.
182. Mulder DS, Wallace DH, Woolhouse FM. The use of the fiberoptic bronchoscope to facilitate endotracheal intubation following head and neck trauma. J Trauma 1975;15:638.
183. Murray JF. A case of total rupture of the right main bronchus after closed chest injury. Br J Anaesth 1971;43:407.
184. Neff CC, Pfister RC, Van Sonnenberg E. Percutaneous transtracheal ventilation: experimental and practical aspects. J Trauma 1983;23:84.
185. Nichol HC, Zuck D. Difficult laryngoscopy: the "anterior" larynx and the atlanto-occipital gap. Br J Anaesth 1983;55: 141.
186. Nimmo WS, Wilson J, Prescott LF. Narcotic analgesics and delayed gastric emptying during labour. Lancet 1975;1:890.
187. Nordin U. The trachea and cuff-induced tracheal injury. Acta Oto-Laryngol (Stockholm) 1977;345(suppl.):7.
188. Oliverio R Jr, Ruder CB, Fermon C, Cura A. Pneumothorax secondary to ball-valve obstruction during jet ventilation. Anesthesiology 1979;51:255.
189. Olsson GL, Hallen B. Pharmacological evacuation of the stomach with metoclopramide. Acta Anaesth Scand 1982;26:417.
190. Olsson GL, Hallen B, Hambraeus-Jonzon K. Aspiration during anaesthesia: a computer-aided study of 185,358 anaesthetics. Acta Anaesthesiol Scand 1986;30:84.
191. Orlowski JP, Ellis NG, Amir NP, Crumrine RS. Complications of airway intrusion in 100 consecutive cases in a pediatric ICU. Crit Care Med 1980;8:324.
192. O'Sullivan JC, Wells DG, Wells GR. Difficult airway management with neck swelling after carotid endarterectomy. Anaesth Intensive Care 1986;14:460.
193. Ovassapian A, Dykes MHM. The role of fiber-optic endoscopy in airway management. Semin Anesth 1987;6:93.
194. Ovassapian A, Krejcie T, Yelich SJ, Dykes MHM. Awake fiberoptic intubation in the patient at high risk of aspiration. Br J Anaesth 1989;62:13.
195. Ovassapian A, Yelich SJ, Dykes MHM, Brunner EE. Fiberoptic nasotracheal intubation: incidence and causes of failure. Anesth Analg 1983;62:692.
196. Owen RL, Cheney FW. Endobronchial intubation: a preventable complication. Anesthesiology 1987;67:255.
197. Oyegunle AO. The use of propanidid for blind nasotracheal intubation. Br J Anaesth 1975;47:379.
198. Paegle R, Bernhard W. Squamous metaplasia of tracheal epithelium associated with high-volume low-pressure airway cuffs. Anesth Analg 1975;54:340.
199. Papovich J Jr, Babcock R. Intraluminal blood clot casts causing obstructive emphysema and recurrent pneumothorax. Crit Care Med 1982;10:482.
200. Park GR. Hypotension following metoclopramide administration during hypotensive anaesthesia for intracranial aneurysm. Br J Anaesth 1978;50:1268.
201. Patil V, Stehling L, Zauder H. Techniques of endotracheal intubation. In: Patil V, Stehling L, Zauder H, eds. Fiberoptic Endoscopy in Anesthesia. Chicago: Year Book Medical Publishers, 1983:75.
202. Peatfield RC, Edwards PR, Johnson MN. Two unexpected deaths from pneumothorax. Lancet 1979;1:356.
203. Pedersen B. Blind nasotracheal intubation: a review and new guided technique. Acta Anaesthesiol Scand 1971;15:107.
204. Perel A, Downs JB, Crawford CA, et al. Continuous positive airway pressure improves oxygenation in dogs after the aspiration of blood. Crit Care Med 1983;11:868.
205. Petito SP, Russell WJ. The prevention of gastric inflation: a neglected benefit of cricoid pressure. Anaesth Intensive Care 1988;16:139.
206. Pizov R, Shir Y, Eimerl D, et al. One-lung high-frequency ventilation in the management of traumatic tear of bronchus in a child. Crit Care Med 1987;15:1160.
207. Rao TLK, Jacobs HK. Pulmonary function following "pretreatment" dose of pancuronium in volunteers. Anesth Analg 1980;59:659.
208. Rao TLK, Mathru M, Gorski DW, Salem MR. Experience with a new intubation guide for difficult tracheal intubation. Crit Care Med 1982;10:882.
209. Ravlo O, Bach V, Lybecker H, et al. A comparison between two emergency cricothyroidotomy instruments. Acta Anaesthesiol Scand 1987;31:317.
210. Reich DL, Schwartz N. An easily assembled device for transtracheal oxygenation. Anesthesiology 1987;66:437.
211. Rigg D, Dwyer B. The use of the rigid bronchoscope for difficult intubations. Anaesth Intensive Care 1985;13:431.
212. Roberts RB, Shirley MA. Reducing the risk of acid aspiration during cesarean section. Anesth Analg 1974;53:859.
213. Rollins RJ, Tocino I. Early radiographic signs of tracheal rupture. AJR 1987;148:695.
214. Rosenberg MB, Levesque PR, Bourke DL. Use of the LTA® kit as a guide for endotracheal intubation. Anesth Analg 1977;56:287.
215. Rosenberg AD, Sommer RM, Capan L, et al. Efficacy of gastroesophageal balloon occlusion in preventing passive regurgitation in dogs. Anesthesiology 1983;59:A155.
216. Rudow M, Hill AB, Thompson NW, Finch JS. Helium-oxygen mixtures in airway obstruction due to thyroid carcinoma. Can Anaesth Soc J 1986;33:498.
217. Safwat AM, Fung DL, Bilton DC. The use of propranolol in rapid sequence anaesthetic induction: optimal time interval for pretreatment. Can Anaesth Soc J 1984;31:638.
218. Salem MR, Heyman HJ, Livschutz V, Mahdi M. Cephalad displacement of the larynx facilitates tracheal intubation. Anesthesiology 1987;67:A453.
219. Salem MR, Joseph NJ, Heyman HJ, et al. Cricoid compression is effective in obliterating the esophageal lumen in the presence of a nasogastric tube. Anesthesiology 1985;63:443.
220. Salem MR, Sellick BA, Elam JO. The historical background of cricoid pressure in anesthesia and resuscitation. Anesth Analg 1974;53:230.
221. Salem MR, Wong AY, Fizzotti GF. Efficacy of cricoid pressure in preventing aspiration of gastric contents in pediatric patients. Br J Anaesth 1972;44:401.
222. Samsoon GLT, Young JRB. Difficult tracheal intubation: a retrospective study. Anaesthesia 1987;42:487.
223. Satiani M, Bonner JT, Stone HH. Factors influencing intraoperative gastric regurgitation. Arch Surg 1978;113:721.
224. Satyanarayana T, Capan L, Ramanathan S, et al. Bronchofiberscopic jet ventilation. Anesth Analg 1980;59:350.
225. Savarese JJ, Ali HH, Basta SJ, et al. Sixty-second tracheal intubation with BW B109OU after fentanyl-thiopental induction. Anesthesiology 1987;67:A351.
226. Scheller MS, Sears KL. Postoperative neurologic dysfunction associated with preoperative administration of metoclopramide. Anesth Analg 1987;66:274.
227. Schmidt JF, Jorgensen BC. The effect of metoclopramide on

gastric contents after preoperative ingestion of sodium citrate. Anesth Analg 1984;63:841.
228. Schulze-Delrieu K. Metoclopramide. N Engl J Med 1981;305:28.
229. Schwatz DJ, Wynne JW, Gibbs CP, et al. The pulmonary consequences of aspiration of gastric contents at pH values greater than 2.5. Am Rev Respir Dis 1980;121:119.
230. Scuderi PE, McLeskey CH, Comer PB. Emergency percutaneous transtracheal ventilation during anesthesia using readily available equipment. Anesth Analg 1982;61:867.
231. Seifert RD, Starsnic M, Zwillenberg D. Acute obstruction of the left mainstem bronchus following an attempted nasotracheal intubation: an unusual case report. Anesthesiology 1985;62:799.
232. Sellick BA. Cricoid pressure to control regurgitation of stomach contents during induction of anaesthesia. Lancet 1961;2:404.
233. Sessler CN, Vitaliti JC, Cooper KR, et al. Comparison of 4% lidocaine/0.5% phenylephrine with 5% cocaine: which dilates the nasal passage better? Anesthesiology 1986;64:274.
234. Shapiro HM, Galindo A, Wyte SR, Harris AB. Rapid intraoperative reduction of intracranial pressure with thiopentone. Br J Anaesth 1973;45:1057.
235. Simpson KH, Stakes AF. Effect of anxiety on gastric emptying in preoperative patients. Br J Anaesth 1987;59:540.
236. Sinha RP, Ducker TB, Periot PL Jr. Arterial oxygenation findings and its significance in central nervous system trauma patients. JAMA 1973;224:1258.
237. Smith CL, Bardgett DM, Hunter JM. Haemodynamic effects of the IV administration of cimetidine or ranitidine in the critically ill patient: a double-blind prospective study. Br J Anaesth 1987;59:1397.
238. Smith G, Dalling R, Williams TIR. Gastro-oesophageal pressure gradient changes produced by induction of anaesthesia and suxamethonium. Br J Anaesth 1978;50:1137.
239. Sofferman RA. Management of laryngotracheal trauma. Am J Surg 1981;141:412.
240. Sosis M, Larijani GE, Marr AT. Priming with atracurium. Anesth Analg 1987;66:329.
241. Sosis M, Stiner A, Larijani GE, Marr AT. An evaluation of priming with vecuronium. Br J Anaesth 1987;59:1236.
242. Stanley RB. Value of computed tomography in the management of acute laryngeal injury. J Trauma 1984;24:359.
243. Stauffer JL, Olson DE, Petty TL. Complications and consequences of endotracheal intubation and tracheotomy: a prospective study in 150 critically ill patients. Am J Med 1981;70:65.
244. Steen JA, Lindholm GE, Brdlik GC, Foster CA. Tracheal tube forces on the posterior larynx: index of laryngeal loading. Crit Care Med 1982;10:186.
245. Stirt JA, Grosslight KR, Bedford RF, Vollmer D. "Defasciculation" with metocurine prevents succinylcholine-induced increases in intracranial pressure. Anesthesiology 1987;67:50.
246. Stock MC, Woodward CG, Shapiro BA, et al. Perioperative complications of elective tracheostomy in critically ill patients. Crit Care Med 1986;14:861.
247. Strain JD, Moore EE, Markovchick VJ, Van Duzer-Moore S. Cimetidine for the prophylaxis of potential gastric acid aspiration pneumonitis in trauma patients. J Trauma 1981;21:49.
248. Swartzman S, Wilson MA, Hoff BH, et al. Percutaneous transtracheal jet ventilation for cardiopulmonary resuscitation: evaluation of a new jet ventilator. Crit Care Med 1984;12:8.
249. Taboada JA, Rupp SM, Miller RD. Refining the priming principle for vecuronium during rapid-sequence induction of anesthesia. Anesthesiology 1986;64:243.
250. Tam S, Chung F, Campbell M. Intravenous lidocaine: optimal time of injection before tracheal intubation. Anesth Analg 1987;66:1036.
251. Teabeaut JR. Aspiration of gastric contents: an experimental study. Am J Pathol 1952;28:51.
252. Thomas JL. Awake intubation: indications, techniques and a review of 25 patients. Anaesthesia 1969;24:28.
253. Thomas TC, Zornow MH, Scheller MS, Unger RJ. The efficacy of three different modes of percutaneous trans-tracheal ventilation in hypoxic, hypercarbic swine. Can J Anaesth 1988;35:561.
254. Tiret L, Desmonts JM, Hatton F, Vourch G. Complications associated with anaesthesia: a prospective survey in France. Can Anaesth Soc J 1986;33:336.
255. Todd JG, Nimmo WS. Effect of premedication on drug absorption and gastric emptying. Br J Anaesth 1983;55:1189.
256. Tonkin JP, Harrison GA. The surgical management of the laryngeal complications of prolonged intubation. Laryngoscope 1970;81:297.
257. Tran DO. The correct position of the head and neck for rapid sequence induction. Anesthesiology 1987;67:861.
258. Tunstall ME, Geddes C. "Failed intubation" in obstetric anaesthesia: an indication for use of the "esophageal gastric tube airway." Br J Anaesth 1984;56:659.
259. Turndorf H, Rodis ID, Clark TS. "Silent" regurgitation during general anesthesia. Anesth Analg 1974;53:700.
260. Unni VKN, Johnston RA, Young HSA, McBride RJ. Prevention of intracranial hypertension during laryngoscopy and endotracheal intubation. Br J Anaesth 1984;56:1219.
261. Van der Linde JC, Roelofse JA, Steenkamp EC. Anatomical factors relating to difficult intubation. S Afr Med J 1983;63:976.
262. van Hasselt EJ, Bruining HA, Hoeve LJ. Elective cricothyroidotomy. Intensive Care Med 1985;11:207.
263. Venus B, Matsuda T, Copiozo JB, Mathru M. Prophylactic intubation and continuous positive airway pressure in the management of inhalation injury in burn victims. Crit Care Med 1981;9:519.
264. Verrill PJ. Anaesthesia in upper respiratory obstruction. Br J Anaesth 1963;35:237.
265. Via-Reque E, Rattenborg CC. Prolonged oro- or nasotracheal intubation. Crit Care Med 1981;9:637.
266. Viegas OJ, Ravindran RS, Shumacker CA. Gastric fluid pH in patients receiving sodium citrate. Anesth Analg 1981;60:521.
267. Viegas OJ, Ravindran RS, Stoops CA. Duration of action of sodium citrate as an antacid. Anesth Analg 1982;61:624.
268. Walts LF. Anesthesia of the larynx in the patient with a full stomach. JAMA 1965;192:121.
269. Walts LF, Dillon JB. Clinical studies of the interaction between D-tubocurarine and succinylcholine. Anesthesiology 1969; 31:39.
270. Walts LF, Kassity KJ. Spread of local anesthesia after upper airway block. Arch Otolaryngol 1965;81:77.
271. Waymack JP, Law E, Park R, et al. Acute upper airway obstruction in the postburn period. Arch Surg 1985;120:1042.
272. Weiskopf RB, Bogetz MS. Haemorrhage decreases the anaesthetic requirement for ketamine and thiopentone in the pig. Br J Anaesth 1985;57:1022.
273. White FA, Clark RB, Thompson DS. Preoperative oral antacid therapy for patients requiring emergency surgery. South Med J 1978;71:177.
274. White A, Kander PL. Anatomical factors in difficult direct laryngoscopy. Br J Anaesth 1975;47:468.
275. White PF, Schlobohm RM, Pitts LH, Lindauer JM. A randomized study of drugs for preventing increases in intracranial pressure during endotracheal suctioning. Anesthesiology 1982;57:242.

276. Whited RE. A prospective study of laryngotracheal sequelae in long-term intubation. Laryngoscope 1984;94:367.
277. Willatts SM, Cochrane DF. Paranasal sinusitis: a complication of nasotracheal intubation; two case reports. Br J Anaesth 1985;57:1026.
278. Wilson ME, Spiegelhalter D, Robertson JA, Lesser P. Predicting difficult intubation. Br J Anaesth 1988;61:211.
279. Wilson RF, Soullier GW, Wiencek RG. Hemoptysis in trauma. J Trauma 1987;27:1123.
280. Wraight WJ, Chamney AR, Howells TH. The determination of an effective cricoid pressure. Anaesthesia 1983;38:461.
281. Wynne JW, Modell JH. Respiratory aspiration of stomach contents. Ann Intern Med 1977;87:466.
282. Wynne JW, Reynolds JC, Hood I, et al. Steroid therapy for pneumonitis induced in rabbits by aspiration of foodstuff. Anesthesiology 1979;51:11.
283. Yates WG, Shaap RN, McGill LD. An evaluation of tracheal damage test method for cuffed tracheal tubes (final report). Task order No. 6, October 27, 1979.
284. Yen JK, Rhodes GR, Bourke RS, et al. Delayed impairment of arterial blood oxygenation in patients with severe head injury: preliminary report. Surg Neurol 1978;9:323.
285. Zaricznyj B, Rockwood CA Jr, O'Donaghue DH, Ridings GR. Relationship between trauma to the extremities and stomach motility. J Trauma 1977;17:920.
286. Zornow MH, Thomas TC, Scheller MS. The efficacy of three different methods of transtracheal ventilation. Can J Anaesth 1989;36:624.

# Chapter Four

Charles E. Lucas
Anna M. Ledgerwood

# Hemodynamic Management of the Injured

During treatment of the trauma patient it is not uncommon for anesthesiologists to be involved in more than one aspect of care. Hemodynamic management is among the most important problems facing them. Although not as immediately life threatening as airway obstruction, for instance, severe hemorrhage is a more common result of trauma and accounts for a significant proportion of injury-related morbidity and mortality. Optimal treatment of severe hemorrhage and shock has been a controversial topic for many years. However, experience has provided a better understanding of some of the issues involved. This chapter will deal with these issues and identify the priorities of hemodynamic management of the trauma patient during the various phases of his or her care.

## ETIOLOGY OF SHOCK IN THE INJURED

In the traumatized patient, circulatory shock may be due to the following causes (Table 4-1).[225,256,259]

### HYPOVOLEMIA

Hemorrhage, internally or externally, is the most common cause of shock in the injured. In one series intraperitoneal bleeding was present in almost half the patients arriving to the emergency room in shock after blunt trauma[128]; pelvic and long bone fractures accounted for 37% and thoracic bleeding for 13% of the cases in this group of patients.[128] Hemorrhage from noncavitary body regions—fractures, lacerations, muscle contusions—is a frequent etiology of hypovolemic shock in the trauma population, and its severity should not be underestimated.[189] Death is almost unavoidable when hemorrhagic shock is associated with head injury.[101,128] Hypovolemic shock also may occur in the acutely traumatized patient from translocation of fluids within burned or contaminated tissues (eg, the peritoneum). Hypovolemia is a common finding in almost all forms of shock in the injured, and its timely diagnosis and treatment are essential for a successful outcome.

### CHEST TRAUMA

These injuries are particularly important as they may induce shock by hemorrhage, malignant arrhythmias, pericardial tamponade, or cardiac failure caused by myocardial infarction or contusion.

### DILATATION OF CAPACITANCE OR RESISTANCE VESSELS

Hypotension caused by this mechanism may result from spinal cord injuries. Sepsis may lead to shock by causing vasodilatation, hypovolemia, and cardiac dysfunction. Intoxication with alcohol or other drugs may worsen shock by a similar mechanism. Anaphylactic reactions from various medications, transfusions, or toxins cause severe vasodilatation and hypotension.

TABLE 4-1. Etiology of Circulatory Shock in the Injured

| TYPE OF SHOCK | ETIOLOGY |
|---|---|
| Hypovolemic | Blood loss due to hemorrhage<br>Plasma loss due to burns, surgery, and/or infections |
| Cardiogenic | Myocardial contusion<br>Myocardial infarction<br>Congestive heart failure<br>Arrhythmia |
| Distributive (increased venous capacitance and/or decreased vascular resistance) | Spinal cord injury<br>Septic shock<br>Intoxication<br>Anaphylactic reaction |
| Obstructive | Pericardial tamponade<br>Pulmonary embolism<br>Pneumothorax; hemothorax<br>Air embolism<br>Fat embolism |

### EMBOLISM

Various types of embolism including air, fat, and thromboembolisms may result in sudden, frequently unexplained shock and even cardiac arrest after severe injury.

### MISCELLANEOUS

Chemical or biologic agents such as toxic gases or "biowarfare" agents, venom stings, or bites are rare causes of shock in the injured.

Proper recognition of these causes of shock will greatly affect the type of treatment instituted and thus the outcome. For instance, hypotension due to cardiac tamponade will improve little and only transiently with fluid resuscitation but will respond to pericardial drainage.

## HEMODYNAMIC CHANGES DURING HEMORRHAGIC SHOCK

Shock, regardless of its cause, is characterized by suboptimal tissue oxygenation that leads to inefficient energy utilization by anaerobic metabolism. Normally, oxygen delivery to tissues is affected by both blood flow and oxygen content (see Chapter 5). In traumatic shock, both of these factors are altered, compromising tissue oxygen supply. During hemorrhagic shock, the imbalance between circulating blood volume and vascular capacity initiates complex homeostatic events that involve both the macrocirculation and microcirculation. On the macrocirculatory level, diminished venous return is the prime hemodynamic abnormality.[105] Normally, the amount of blood returning to the right atrium is determined by three important factors: mean systemic venous pressure, venous resistance, and intrapleural pressure.[89,105,140] In order for venous blood to flow toward the right atrium, a pressure gradient must exist between the distal veins and the heart. The greater the gradient, the greater will be the venous return. Thus, mean systemic venous pressure and right atrial pressure determine the volume of venous return. Resistance to blood flow occurs at the superior and inferior venae cavae because the cross-section of each vessel is smaller than the sum of the areas of the small, distal veins. Thus, any reduction in vena caval diameter by increased intrathoracic or intraabdominal pressures results in increased resistance to venous return.

In hemorrhagic shock, decreased mean systemic venous pressure leads to decreased venous return.[90] When intrapleural pressure increases, the resistance to venous return increases. Tension pneumothorax, pericardial tamponade, closed-chest cardiopulmonary resuscitation, and positive pressure ventilation cause a decrease in venous return by this mechanism.[105] Increased intraabdominal pressure caused by intraperitoneal bleeding or military antishock (MAS) trousers may also reduce venous return by increasing venous resistance.[66,118] Additionally, sudden changes in intraabdominal pressure may cause hemodynamic changes by altering left ventricular afterload, diaphragmatic position, and regional distribution of cardiac output.[210]

Myocardial contractility during the early stages of hemorrhagic shock is usually well maintained. However, during the late stages it may be reduced because of decreased coronary perfusion, lactic acidosis, myocardial depressant polypeptides, lysozomal enzymes, and "passive transferable lethal factor" which is produced by the reticuloendothelial system.[136]

## PHYSIOLOGIC RESPONSES TO HEMORRHAGIC SHOCK

Hemorrhagic shock leads to several well-defined physiologic responses that act to preserve venous return, cardiac output, and tissue perfusion. These responses are effective in mild or moderate shock, but in severe or prolonged shock the compensatory mechanisms are overwhelmed.

### INCREASED SYMPATHETIC ACTIVITY

Reduction of blood volume and blood pressure inhibits baroreceptor reflexes and stimulates chemoreceptor discharge.[70] At systolic blood pressures below 70 mm Hg there is no baroreceptor discharge and normal inhibition of endogenous vasoactive hormone secretion does not occur.[213] Also impulses from chemoreceptors, that are stimulated by low tissue $PO_2$, are relayed to the hypothalamus where cardiac and vascular components of the sympathetic system are stimulated.[126] A highly complex series of events leads to stimulation of the peripheral sympathetic system and adrenal medulla.[18] Circulating catecholamines may increase 10- to 40-fold.[11] Elevation of serum noradrenaline is caused by spillover from sympathetic synapses, whereas adrenaline is released from the adrenal medulla.[213] The elevated serum catecholamines potentiate the effects of increased sympathetic nervous system activity. However, their effects may be modulated by various mechanisms. For instance, they act on three separate vascular adrenergic receptors (postsynaptic $\alpha_1$, presynaptic $\alpha_2$, and extrasynaptic $\alpha_2$) which not only have different vascular activities (vasoconstriction and vasodilatation) but have significant interactions with each other.[18]

Other humoral agents may modify sympathetic activity, including adrenocorticotropic hormone (ACTH),[86] angiotensin II,[8,55] vasopressin (antidiuretic hormone),[38] aldosterone,[213] enkephalins,[129] and β-endorphins.[129] Histamine, plasma kinins, complement components, and arachidonic acid metabolites are also released in shock. These substances act primarily on the microcirculation and may have important effects that lead to pulmonary pathology following shock.[135] Increased sympathetic activity affects almost all elements of the cardiovascular system.

### *Effects on the Heart*

In mild or moderate shock, increased sympathetic discharge leads to increases in heart rate and contractility.[213] However, reversible decreases of heart rate may occur in up to 7% of conscious hypotensive patients during rapid hemorrhage.[9,215] Bradycardia in severe and prolonged shock is refractory to fluid infusion. Tachycardia, especially in elderly patients, may be absent in the supine position even when blood loss is greater than 10% of the blood volume.[225] In contrast, tachycardia may be present with minimal bleeding in young injured patients because of pain, fear, and anxiety.[225] Despite increased contractility and heart rate, cardiac output falls progressively once blood loss exceeds 15% of the normal blood volume.[262] In dogs, a 50 to 60% reduction of blood volume causes a significant decrease in stroke work, dP/dt, and myocardial efficiency because of a progressive decrease in coronary blood flow and shunting of endocardial blood flow toward the epicardium.[108]

### *Effects on Venous Return*

As mentioned earlier, the primary hemodynamic abnormality in hemorrhagic shock is decreased venous return. The compensatory increase in sympathetic activity in early mild or moderate shock causes venoconstriction, increasing mean systemic venous pressure and thus venous return. As blood loss reaches 15% of the blood volume, this compensatory mechanism begins to fail, and preload progressively decreases.[262] In the injured patient, pain-induced muscular rigidity of the extremities may compress the small veins and venules, increasing mean systemic venous pressure and augmenting venous return.[105,134] Administration of narcotics, sedatives, muscle relaxants, and/or general, spinal, or epidural anesthesia may decrease this compression and thus venous return. On the other hand, the mild to moderate hypothermia frequently observed in injured patients may constrict the venules and increase venous return.[81] Rewarming prior to volume restoration, therefore, may be counterproductive. The use of diuretics and vasodilators also counteracts this compensatory hemodynamic effect of sympathetic stimulation.[105]

### *Effects on Peripheral and Pulmonary Vascular Resistances*

The total peripheral resistance (TPR) initially increases during bleeding.[187] This increase persists after cardiac output falls and helps maintain the arterial blood pressure.[88,187] Thus, blood pressure decreases only after a significant reduction in cardiac output (Fig 4-1). There is a close correlation between pulmonary artery pressure and cardiac output during the initial stage of hemorrhage.[186] With further bleeding (up

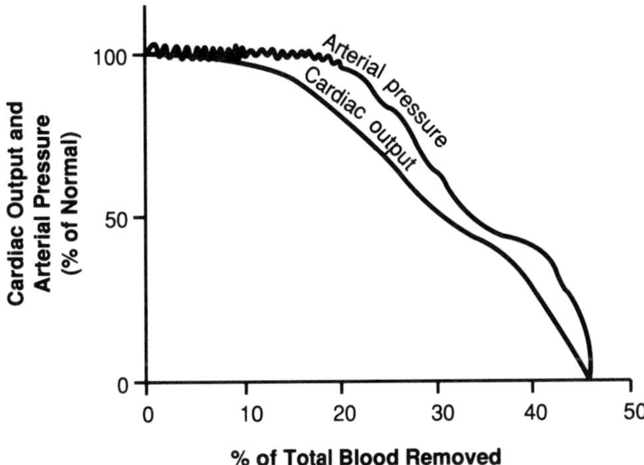


FIG. 4-1. Relationship between cardiac output and arterial blood pressure during graded hemorrhage. Note that the arterial pressure is well maintained to a 20% reduction in blood volume, but cardiac output begins to decline when blood loss is less than 10%. (From Guyton AC[88] with permission.)

to 15 to 20% of blood volume), the increase in pulmonary vascular resistance exceeds that of the TPR.[100,187]

## REPLENISHMENT OF INTRAVASCULAR VOLUME (TRANSCAPILLARY REFILL)

A second compensatory response to hemorrhage is restitution of intravascular volume. Normally, the total body water of a 70-kg individual is 42 L or 60% of body weight (Fig 4-2). The intracellular space contains 28 L (40% of total body weight) and the extracellular space, 14 L (20% of total body weight).[26,150] The intracellular fluid (ICF) is subdivided into the extravascular volume of 26 L within muscle and parenchymal cells, and the intravascular component, the red cell volume, which contains 2 L. The extracellular fluid (ECF)

FIG. 4-2. Normal volume of fluid compartments in a 70-kg man. RBCV, red blood cell volume; PV, plasma volume.

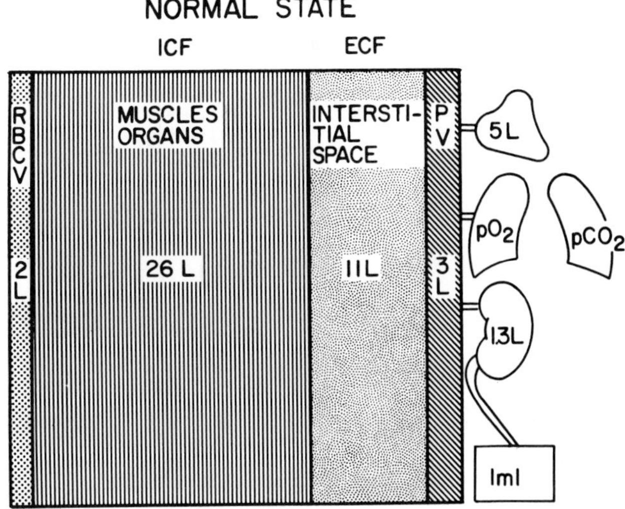

consists of the interstitial fluid containing 11 L and the plasma volume of 3 L. Thus, total blood volume averages about 5 L.

The initial loss following injury comes from the intravascular volume; however, the body's protective mechanisms facilitate restoration of the plasma volume from extravascular stores.[23] When a patient presents with hypovolemic shock, the red cell mass may be reduced by 50%, whereas the plasma, which is replenished by interstitial fluid, may be reduced less than 35%.

Refilling of the plasma volume from the interstitial space occurs by several mechanisms. Decreased systemic blood pressure decreases capillary pressure.[53] Reflex constriction of the nutrient capillary beds and precapillary sphincters further reduces intracapillary hydrostatic pressure.[91] Water flux across the biologic membranes is governed by the Starling equation[238]: $FH_2O = K_c \times SA (P_c - P_i) - (OP_i - OP_c)$, where $FH_2O$ is the amount of water crossing the tissue-capillary interface, $K_c$ is the capillary permeability, SA is the capillary surface area, $P_c$ and $P_i$ are the capillary and interstitial hydrostatic pressures, and $OP_c$ and $OP_i$ are the capillary and interstitial oncotic pressures, respectively. A decrease in $P_c - P_i$ results in a net fluid flux into the intravascular space (transcapillary refill).[47,150] Most of this movement takes place at the venous end of the capillary because hydrostatic pressure is lower there than at the arterial end. An interplay between α-adrenergic vasoconstrictor and β-adrenergic vasodilator activities causes intermittent opening and closure of pre- and postcapillary sphincters and may also be an important mechanism of transcapillary refill during hemorrhagic shock.[92]

Protein shift by way of lymphatic channels from the interstitial space into the tissue capillaries also aids in replenishment of the intravascular space (Figs 4-3 and 4-4).[47,150] During hemorrhage, plasma protein (mostly albumin) concentration in the intravascular space decreases.[5] As a compensatory mechanism, the flux of albumin from intravascular to interstitial space (normally 7% of intravascular albumin enters the interstitial space hourly) decreases. In addition, augmented lymphatic flow from the interstitium to the intravascular space results in some albumin and water replenishment.[35] During this process the interstitial space is contracted further (Fig 4-4).

FIG. 4-3. A patient in hypovolemic shock has a large deficit in the red blood cell (RBC) volume, plasma volume (PV), and interstitial volume, which actively replenishes the plasma volume. This leads to flow reduced cardiac output, renal blood flow (RBF), glomerular filtration rate (GFR), and urine output.

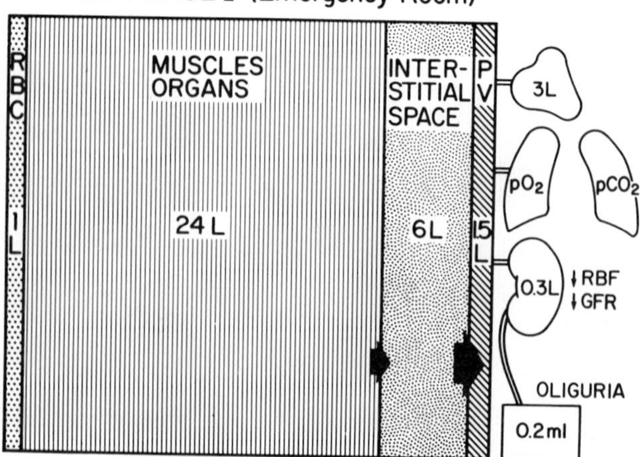


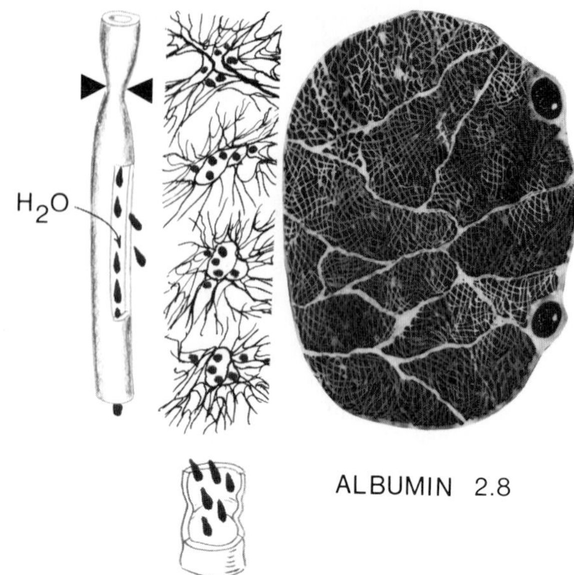


FIG. 4-4. Hypotension as a result of hypovolemia is associated with precapillary vasoconstriction and reduced efflux of salt and water into the interstitial fluid space, reduced extracapillary albumin (dark dots) movement, a contracted interstitial fluid space, and increased lymphatic flow from the interstitial space.

Intravascular water flux is augmented further by an increased plasma osmolality caused by release into the bloodstream of glucose, lactate, pyruvate, urea, electrolytes, and amino acids, mainly from the muscles and liver. The extent of these biochemical changes parallels the severity of injury.[25,121,185,241] Increased plasma osmolality in the capillaries results in a stepwise osmotic gradient increasing from the intracellular to the interstitial, to the intravascular compartments.[69,193] Thus, a fluid shift occurs from the intracellular space into the interstitial space. Increasing the volume of interstitial space increases the pressure in this compartment, causing water and proteins to move into the capillaries.[176,192]

Capillary refill cannot fully compensate for severe hemorrhage. Animal studies suggest that capillary refill can replace a 10% blood loss at most.[71] Larger hemorrhage leads to reduction of intravascular volume, decreased venous return, and decreased cardiac output with associated reduction of blood pressure.

During shock, resting skeletal muscle membrane potentials increase from −90 to −50 mV,[42,43,48,150,227] resulting in electrolyte and fluid movement across the cell membrane. Although this fluid moves in both directions, at times most of the flow may be into the cells. As a result, the intracellular space expands at the expense of the other compartments. Several liters of fluid can be lost by this mechanism, causing severe intravascular and interstitial volume depletion following acute hemorrhage.

The intravascular space is the only compartment that is readily accessible to therapy. Thus, fluid administration is often guided by changes in plasma volume without consideration of concomitant changes in the interstitial and intracellular spaces. Within limits, serial determinations of hemoglobin or hematocrit aid in assessment of blood loss whereas changes in vital signs provide guidance to changes in plasma volume.

### OPENING OF PERIPHERAL ARTERIOVENOUS SHUNTS

During the normovolemic state little blood flows through the arteriovenous shunts in the peripheral tissues.[74] With hemorrhage, increased vasomotor tone results in closure of the precapillary and postcapillary sphincters, increasing both total peripheral resistance and mean systemic venous pressure. A significant portion of the cardiac output then reaches the venous side through the newly opened shunts.[105,240] This mechanism improves venous return and prevents severe preload reduction in the heart. However, the shunted blood bypasses the tissues, resulting in tissue hypoxia. If tissue hypoxia persists, the precapillary sphincters relax, and capillary permeability increases. In addition to hypoxia, locally released enzymes such as histamine, prostaglandins, kinins, and lysozomes may also produce increased capillary permeability.[135] During this stage fluid shift from the intravascular to the interstitial space causes further hypovolemia.

### SELECTIVE ORGAN PERFUSION

Selective perfusion of vital organs is a major compensatory mechanism during hemorrhage. Even with severe blood loss, blood flow to the heart and brain is maintained.[62,124,234] Hypotension-induced tissue hypoxia causes vasodilatation in the brain and myocardium, permitting a significant portion of the cardiac output to be diverted to these organs. For instance, a 50% reduction in blood volume, which produces a mean arterial pressure of 35 mm Hg and a 70% reduction in cardiac output, will cause only a 20% decrease in coronary blood flow.[108] Depending on the extent of hemorrhage, varying degrees of vasoconstriction occur in muscles, skin, and gut.[62] Blood flow to the liver and kidney is also reduced (see Chapter 5).

## THE THREE PHASES OF SHOCK

Most patients with severe injury and hypotension present with large intravascular and extravascular fluid deficits.[26,150] These reflect both blood loss from the injured sites and blood and serum loss into contused soft tissues. Patients with hollow viscus perforation also have significant fluid translocation due to localized sepsis. These fluid shifts continue into the postoperative period. Thus, treatment of hypovolemic shock must not be limited to the initial restoration of blood volume and vital signs in the emergency room. The body's physiologic responses to hypovolemic shock may be divided into three phases.[147] Although the transition from one phase into the next may be indistinct, the stages themselves are clearly different (Table 4-2). Each has its own characteristics and its own treatment objectives.[147,150] Phase 1 reflects the period of shock and active hemorrhage; this stage extends from initial treatment to the termination of resuscitation or surgery for control of internal bleeding. Based on our experience, in most patients with serious injury requiring operative intervention phase 1 averages 7 to 8 hours; the first 60 to 150 minutes is utilized for preoperative management, and the remaining 4 to 7 hours is the intraoperative period.

Phase 2 is the period of extravascular fluid sequestration beginning when bleeding is controlled and lasting until the time of maximum weight gain. Our own data indicate that phase 2 averages 24 to 36 hours in patients receiving 15 U of blood during phase 1.[152] The extravascular fluid sequestration seen during phase 2 is obligatory; it cannot be safely prevented by limiting fluid infusion. Indeed, fluid restriction, particularly early in phase 2 leads to increased hypotension, renal failure, and cardiovascular collapse. The expansion of the extravascular space appears to include both interstitial and intracellular compartments. The obligatory nature of this "third-space" expansion is comparable to that seen in the burn patient, with the prime difference being the mechanism of injury—that is, cellular ischemia rather than direct tissue damage. Cellular ischemia is associated with an increase in the cell membrane potential from −90 mV to about −50 mV in the experimental animal in severe shock, resulting in intracellular accumulation of sodium and water as depression of the sodium pump reduces the quantity of these substances removed from the cell.[42,43,48,150,227] Studies indicate that the volume of the interstitial space also increases during phase 2.[151] Thus, interstitial volume may double to 11 L, while total extravascular fluid increase during phase 2 may exceed 20 L in some patients. Intracellular swelling after shock has been confirmed in rodents by electron microscopy of both hepatocytes and myocytes.[4] The severity of this obligatory extravascular expansion appears to be directly related to the degree and duration of cellular insult as reflected by shock time and the number of transfusions needed to restore blood loss.[150]

Phase 3 is the mobilization and diuretic period. It extends from the time of maximum weight gain until the end of diuresis as reflected by maximal weight loss. Although there is no precise moment when one phase ends and the next one begins, most patients appear to reach a steady state of blood pressure and pulse toward the end of phase 2 in which only small volumes of fluid are needed to maintain vital signs and urine output. During phase 3, salt and water exit from the

TABLE 4-2. Three Phases of Shock and Resuscitation

| | |
|---|---|
| Phase 1 | Active hemorrhage and acute hypovolemia<br>From admission to end of operation |
| Phase 2 | Extravascular fluid sequestration<br>From end of operation until maximal weight gain |
| Phase 3 | Fluid mobilization and diuresis<br>From maximal weight gain until restoration of positive fluid balance |

interstitial and intracellular spaces back into the lymphatic channels and plasma.[47] This reverse movement is thought to reflect the restoration of cell membrane potential and normal cellular function.[42,43,48,227]

## GRADE OF SHOCK

The severity of the physiologic derangement produced by shock correlates with both the volume deficit and the duration of hypotension. Although shock is a continuum progressing from mild hemorrhage to death, categorization of different grades of severity is helpful in organizing and implementing treatment.[150] Patients with mild (class I) hemorrhage—on the order of 750 mL—present with normal blood pressure, tachycardia, and little fluid shift. Urine output may be minimally reduced and readily responds to infusion of balanced electrolyte solution (Table 4-3).[144] Moderate or class II hemorrhage, associated with a 1000- to 1250-mL deficit, is characterized by a fall in systolic blood pressure, a narrowed pulse pressure, and tachycardia. Compensatory transfer of 2 or 3 L of extravascular fluid into the bloodstream occurs, and urine output falls to less than 0.3 mL/min. Severe (class III) hemorrhage—1500 to 1750 mL of blood loss—is associated with profound hypotension, narrowed pulse pressure, and severe tachycardia. In class III hemorrhage compensatory fluid shift into the intravascular space may exceed 5 L, while urine output is usually less than 0.1 mL/min. Catastrophic acute loss of 2000 to 2500 mL of blood (class IV) causes severe shock, at times to the point where the blood pressure can be recorded only with a direct intraarterial line or a Doppler sphygmomanometer. Marked narrowing of the pulse pressure, or even absence of a recordable diastolic pressure, profound tachycardia (although preterminal bradycardia may be present), and anuria occur. The compensatory fluid shifts may exceed safe limits, and the patient will soon die unless resuscitative measures are implemented immediately.

## ORGAN RESPONSE TO SHOCK

With a reduction in circulating blood volume and cardiac output, organ response correlates directly with the severity of injury and degree of hypovolemia. Since the kidneys perform vital cardiovascular regulatory functions, their response to shock has been studied extensively.[26,99,145] Normally, approximately 25% of the cardiac output or 1250 mL/min flows through the kidneys; the normal effective renal plasma flow thus averages about 650 mL/min. The volume of protein-free fluid filtered into the glomerulae (glomerular filtration rate, GFR) averages 125 mL/min. Class I hemorrhagic shock causes a reduction in renal plasma flow (RPF), but there is little or no change in GFR. Consequently, excretion of electrolytes and water and urine specific gravity remain normal. This phenomenon, known as autoregulation, is due to isolated postglomerular (efferent arteriolar) vasoconstriction, which maintains glomerular hydrostatic pressure. Class II hemorrhagic shock exceeds the autoregulatory capacity; the kidneys respond with both pre- and postglomerular vasoconstriction, resulting in a reduction in RPF to about 30% of normal and a 40 to 50% fall in GFR. Excretion of electrolytes and urine output also fall below 50% of normal (Table 4-3). Severe hemorrhage (class III) leads to a reduction of RPF to less than 10% of normal and of GFR to less than 20% of normal. Excretion of urine is less than 0.1 mL/min. Class IV hemorrhage is characterized by impending cardiac arrest with very low systemic pressure, tachycardia, and anuria, reflecting extreme renal vasoconstriction with absence of measurable perfusion or filtration.

The physiologic control mechanisms producing these renal responses to hypovolemic shock are intricate.[145] The most sensitive is the renin-angiotensin axis. The juxtaglomerular apparatus (JGA) functions as part of a feedback loop for each nephron. Three factors that stimulate renin release from the JGA are perfusion pressure in the renal arterioles, sodium concentration in the JGA blood vessels, and catecholamine perfusion of the nephrons. Once released, renin causes the conversion of angiotensin I, a decapeptide, to angiotensin II, an octapeptide. Angiotensin II is a very potent vasoconstrictor and contributes to a further reduction in renal perfusion and filtration. Renin also stimulates aldosterone secretion, which augments sodium reabsorption from the distal convoluted tubules. Water excretion is controlled by antidiuretic hormone (ADH) which is released from the pituitary gland in response to hyperosmolemia and activation of baroreceptors within the cardiovascular system. Antidiuretic hormone promotes increased water reabsorption from the distal tubule and collecting ducts depending on the osmolar gradient between these sites and the inner medullary interstitium (Fig. 4-5). In response to shock, blood flow to the kidneys may decrease from a normal of 1300 mL/min to less than 100 mL/min. Despite the severity of this vasoconstriction, the kidneys are still able to respond to replacement therapy with restoration of function.

Other organs also contribute to the preservation of vital organ perfusion.[26] The brain has essentially a dual-flow system, with one component supplying the cortex, and the other, the brain stem. During hypovolemic shock, cortical flow decreases while brain stem flow is maintained.[146] Little change

TABLE 4-3. Adaptation to Hypovolemic Shock

| SEVERITY OF HEMORRHAGE | BLOOD PRESSURE (mm Hg) | PLASMA VOLUME (L) | INTERSTITIAL SPACE (L) | CRYSTALLOID NEEDS (L) | URINE OUTPUT (ml/min) |
|---|---|---|---|---|---|
| Normal | 120/80 | 5000 | 11 | | 1.0 |
| Class I | 120/80 | 4600 | 10 | 2 | 1.0 |
| Class II | 115/80 | 3800 | 9 | 4 | 0.3 |
| Class III | 90/70 | 3200 | 7.5 | 7 | 0.1 |
| Class IV | 60/40 | 2500 | 6 | 10 | 0 |

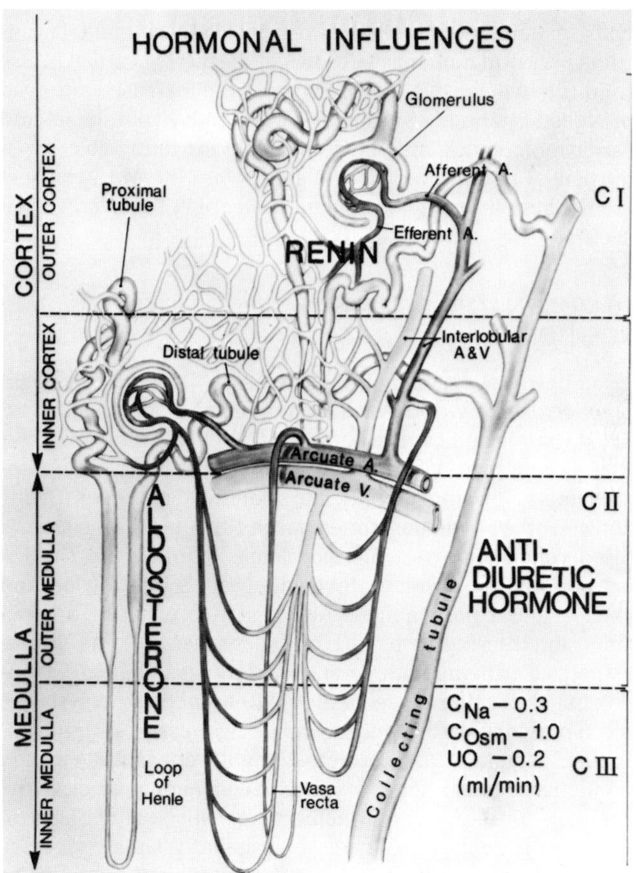


FIG. 4-5. The humoral response to acute hemorrhagic shock includes increased circulating catecholamines that promote renin release from the kidney which, in turn, leads to aldosterone secretion from the adrenal glands. Combined with antidiuretic hormone release there is a marked decrease in renal perfusion, filtration, and excretion of sodium and water.

in brain function is seen if the low cardiac output state is temporary.

The splanchnic circulation exhibits increased vascular resistance and decreased perfusion in response to hemorrhagic shock. Although this may contribute to postshock adynamic ileus, the immediate result is preservation of cardiac output for perfusion of the brain, heart, and lungs. The liver may contain up to 500 mL of blood that is redistributed to the central circulation during the acute phase of hemorrhagic shock. The blood flow to the liver is supplied by hepatic arteries (30%) and the portal vein (70%). During acute hemorrhage, blood flow to the liver from both sources decreases because of increased sympathetic activity.[37] Portal venous pressure in excess of central venous pressure is commonly observed early in hemorrhagic shock.[37] The decreased hepatic blood flow accompanying hemorrhage may cause elevation of liver function tests, reticuloendothelial system dysfunction, and rarely acute liver failure resulting in death.[213]

The severity of organ dysfunction tends to parallel the degree and duration of shock. The number of transfusions administered and the time during which the patient's systolic pressure is below 80 mm Hg correlate directly with fall in RPF and GFR, the incidence of renal failure, the elevation of liver enzymes, the degree of pulmonary dysfunction, and the postresuscitation confusion caused by reduced cerebral blood flow.[150]

## THERAPEUTIC INTERVENTION

Assuming that the patient has an adequate airway and cardiac activity, the initial therapeutic objective must be to restore volume deficit and stop further blood loss. While this primary treatment is in progress, steps are taken to diagnose and manage internal injuries that may be responsible for additional blood loss or fluid relocation consequent to sepsis.

### CONTROL OF EXTERNAL BLEEDING

Although the major emphasis of this chapter is volume restoration, immediate control of external bleeding followed by early control of internal bleeding are obvious concurrent needs. External bleeding from small wounds is best controlled by direct pressure. Digital pressure with a gloved finger stops bleeding from most wounds, particularly neck wounds with injury of the carotid artery or internal jugular vein. Extremity wounds are also best controlled by direct pressure. When hemorrhage comes from a partially severed artery in the extremity, one must resist the temptation to stop the bleeding by blind application of a hemostat. Such hurried attempts at hemostasis may result in irreparable damage to the bleeding artery, necessitating either ligation or complicated vascular reconstruction.

Bleeding from larger wounds is best contained by a sterile dressing secured by a compressive wrap and, if necessary, reinforced by an Ace bandage. Bleeding that continues despite proper application of such a dressing is best controlled by a proximal tourniquet inflated above systolic pressure. During transit to the emergency facility, bleeding from an underlying fracture is controlled by pneumatic splints over the site of the injury. When long distances are involved, MAS trousers applied with low pressures (20 to 40 mm Hg) may help reduce venous bleeding from both fractures and soft tissues and also splint lower-extremity fractures.[61,117,190,237]

### MILITARY ANTISHOCK TROUSERS

MAS trousers raise the systemic blood pressure.[29,61,114,167] However, controversy exists regarding their effect on cardiac output, venous return, and peripheral vascular resistance. Although early studies suggested an elevation of central blood volume of 750 to 1000 mL, Bivins and coworkers[17] found less than a 5% rise with MAS trousers. Both increased and decreased cardiac output and stroke volume have been reported.[10,59,66,255] In animal studies, improvement was noted in cardiac output and blood flow to vital organs, but these results may not apply to hypotensive humans.[10,212] In baboons, Holcroft and coworkers[106] noted that venous return could be both augmented and impeded. In volunteers, Jennings et al[114] showed that with 50 mm Hg inflation pressures, blood pressure increase was mainly caused by increased peripheral vascular resistance. At pressures of 100 mm Hg the rise in arterial pressure was mediated by increased cardiac output as well as elevated peripheral vascular resistance.[66]

Factors other than inflation pressure also influence the hemodynamic effects of MAS trousers. Blood volume prior to the inflation is important. Bellamy and coworkers[10] found that MAS trousers caused little improvement in cardiac output in normovolemic swine but increased cardiac output by 41% in the face of hypovolemia. They hypothesized that preload increase by MAS trousers-induced autotransfusion would have little effect on cardiac output in normovolemic states since the left ventricle operates on the flat portion of the Starling curve. In hypovolemic animals, however, ventricular filling is on the steep portion of the curve; thus, an increased preload is more likely to produce a significantly increased cardiac output. Positive pressure ventilation may alter the hemodynamic response to antishock trousers. Burchard and coworkers[22] demonstrated that MAS trousers-induced augmentation of right and left ventricular filling pressures and the left ventricular response to these changes were blunted by mechanical ventilation.

The value of MAS trousers in prehospital hemodynamic management of the trauma victim has been questioned recently. At least two prospective randomized studies have demonstrated that MAS trousers provide no advantage with regard to survival, length of hospital stay, or reduced hospital costs for injured patients with prehospital times of 30 minutes or less.[15,165]

Current recommendations of Committee on Trauma[32] for the use of MAS trousers are as follows: (1) splinting and control of hemorrhage in pelvic fractures during transport; (2) tamponading hemorrhage in soft tissue; (3) stabilizing multiple fractures of the leg; (4) stabilizing the circulation for long-distance transport; and (5) maintaining perfusion of the upper torso when intravenous therapy cannot be initiated or when volume replacement is inadequate.

When the patient arrives at the emergency facility or the operating room, all compartments of the MAS trousers should be left inflated until the systolic pressure has been restored to above 100 mm Hg. The most cephalad segment of the MAS trousers should be deflated first and the blood pressure rechecked. Each time a segment is deflated, volume replacement should be maintained and the blood pressure checked frequently to ensure that systolic pressure remains at least 100 mm Hg. When the MAS trousers are kept inflated until the end of surgery for control of bleeding, deflation of the device and examination of the areas exposed must be done in the operating room prior to closure of the incision in order to locate hidden injuries of the perineum, rectum, or scrotum.

Restoration of blood pressure may be difficult during deflation of the MAS trousers in spite of infusion of large amounts of fluid and blood. There may be several reasons for this. Low inflation pressures cannot control arterial bleeding. Thus, significant blood loss may be present even when the MAS trousers are inflated. Deflation of the garment in the presence of such bleeding may cause further deterioration of blood pressure despite fluid resuscitation. As we have discussed, the increase in systemic blood pressure is due to elevation of systemic vascular resistance (SVR). Deflation of the garment may result in a sudden reduction of SVR which cannot be rapidly compensated for with fluid administration. Finally, patients with limited coronary blood flow and left ventricular dysfunction may sustain significant myocardial injury from the hypotensive episode or from the increased afterload produced by the MAS trousers. Thus, both hypovolemic and cardiogenic shock may be responsible for intractable hypotension. A pump must be available before the MAS trousers are deflated in order to reinflate the garment if hypotension occurs.

## HEMODYNAMIC EFFECTS OF TRENDELENBURG POSITION

Head-down positioning of hypovolemic patients has been practiced since World War I in an attempt to improve central blood volume and cardiac output.[87,258] Recent studies suggest that as much as 35° of tilt provides little hemodynamic improvement.[34] Using radionuclide scanning techniques, Bivins and coworkers[16] demonstrated only a 1.8% increase in central blood volume in awake normovolemic volunteers in the 15° Trendelenburg position. Sibbald et al[231] and Taylor and Weil[243] found no beneficial hemodynamic effect of this position in either normotensive or hypotensive patients. In anesthetized patients with coronary artery disease, a 20° Trendelenburg position caused a slight (10%) increase in systemic blood pressure, cardiac index, and filling pressures; right ventricular dilatation and decreased right ventricular ejection fraction were also noted.[206] The hemodynamic effect of the Trendelenburg position in hemorrhagic shock is not known, but these patients probably respond similarly. Greater degrees of head-down tilt (up to 75°) cause a significant reduction in right atrial pressure, probably because of drainage of blood from the heart toward the head.[34] Thus, it appears that the Trendelenburg position offers little, if any, beneficial hemodynamic effect during management of shock. In addition, in normal individuals, this position has been shown to decrease cerebral blood flow, probably by increasing the jugular vein pressure and impeding venous drainage.[220] In patients with increased intracranial pressure, Trendelenburg position further increases the ICP and may reduce the cerebral perfusion pressure. The head-down position may also cause respiratory embarrassment because cephalad displacement of intraabdominal contents and the diaphragm reduces lung volumes.[34] The hemodynamic effects of passive leg raising are similar to those of the Trendelenburg position.[206]

## VOLUME RESTORATION

Replenishment of the plasma volume by transcapillary refill occurs both during and following active hemorrhage and continues until the intravascular volume has been fully restored. Adequate resuscitation therefore requires restoration not only of the plasma volume but also of the interstitial fluid space (IFS) and the intracellular volume. Since plasma and interstitial fluids differ only in protein content, the best vehicle to achieve this expansion is a balanced electrolyte solution (BES). Addition of carbohydrate to the infusion is not indicated since the normal endocrine response to hypovolemic shock includes catecholamine release, which promotes hepatic glycogenolysis and consequent hyperglycemia.[26] Furthermore, this effect is augmented by simultaneous release of growth hormone, corticosteroids, and glucagon. Addition of carbohydrate to the resuscitation fluid may exaggerate this hyperglycemia and lead to an inappropriate osmotic diuresis while the patient is still in a volume-depleted state.[150] Since the IFS is the milieu between the cell and the vascular space, it assumes an important role in cell nutrition. Failure to replenish this space with fluid may result in cell death. Theoretically, one could monitor the ongoing changes in interstitial space compliance and intracellular movement of sodium and water, but this is impossible in the clinical setting. Therefore, the efficacy of resuscitation must be based upon careful assessment of changes in clinical parameters.

Although measurement of third-space volume is impractical, clinical guidelines provide a basis for fluid replacement during early resuscitation. The optimal ratio of BES replacement to blood loss should be approximately 3:1 during the early resuscitation period. Consequently, a patient with 1500 mL of acute blood loss should require about 5 L of BES during emergency resuscitation. This guideline is crude, however, and some patients with acute blood loss and severe shock require an even greater volume of fluid to restore vital signs. Our own data indicate that patients who receive multiple blood transfusions require approximately 2 L of BES for each liter of whole blood transfused by the time operative intervention is completed.[133] Patients receiving primarily packed red cells during an operation require approximately 2.5 L of BES per liter of packed red cells in order to maintain adequate circulatory volume, vital signs, renal function, and urine output by the end of the surgical procedure (Table 4-4).[153]

Initial resuscitation should include 2 L of BES given over a period of 15 to 30 minutes through at least two large-bore intravenous lines.[145] Most injured patients will respond to administration of fluid alone. Consequently, blood replacement can usually be deferred until blood typing and cross-matching have been completed. Occasionally a patient will not respond to rapid infusion of BES. Such patients are candidates for additional BES and transfusion of type-specific, non–cross-matched blood that should be available within 15 minutes after their arrival in the emergency facility. Despite many years of frequent use, the transfusion of type-specific blood has been associated with no recognized complications at our institution.

Rarely, the patient is moribund despite rapid infusion of BES, and there is no time to obtain type-specific blood. In this situation, low-titer, type O-negative, non–cross-matched blood may be lifesaving. Fortunately, this circumstance is quite rare, even in a very busy urban trauma center. More commonly, a patient with an unusual blood type requires massive replacement, which can be done only with low-titer, type O Rh negative transfusions. Even in this setting, the incidence of transfusion reaction has been rare. Our experiences suggest that the ability to respond to a foreign antigen is impaired during severe hypovolemic shock and in the period immediately following its correction. One patient with B-negative blood received more than 10 U of mismatched blood during his first operation and over 40 mismatched U 2 weeks later when an emergency right hepatectomy was performed. Incompatibility to the foreign antigen did not appear until 8 weeks later at about the time he became responsive to an antigen skin test (see also Chapter 6).

TABLE 4-4. Guidelines to Fluid Volume Replacement

| | |
|---|---|
| Emergency room | Three liters of crystalloid solution for each liter of estimated blood loss |
| Operating room | Two liters of crystalloid solution for each liter of *whole* blood replacement<br>Two and one-half liters of crystalloid solution for each liter of packed red cells |
| Recovery room | Crystalloid solution to maintain vital signs and urine flow, blood to maintain hemoglobin level and adequate tissue oxygenation |

The use of blood alone without BES for resuscitation has long been known to reduce the survival rate from hemorrhagic shock in experimental animals.[225,226] Likewise, administration of only Ringer's lactate solution to dogs bled to 40% of their blood volume is associated with high mortality. Thus, initial resuscitation of patients with class II or greater hemorrhagic shock should utilize both blood and crystalloid solution.[180,214,225,226,264]

## HEMODYNAMIC MONITORING OF THE INJURED DURING PHASE 1

Patients presenting with class I hypovolemic shock usually do not have a life-threatening injury and can be resuscitated before surgery with infusion of fluids via two intravenous lines. Noninvasive blood pressure measurement, an ECG, and a Foley catheter to monitor urine output usually are sufficient. The vast majority of such patients require no sophisticated pre- or postoperative hemodynamic monitoring. However, it is important to remember that in previously young and healthy individuals loss of as much as 25% of the blood volume may not be associated with significant arterial hypotension.[95] In the clinical setting the blood pressure response to hemorrhage depends on numerous factors such as the rate, severity, duration, and nature of bleeding; the patient's age, medical status, and position; and the rate and adequacy of fluid resuscitation. However, it is generally agreed that reduction of stroke volume and cardiac output occurs earlier than the decrease in blood pressure[88,104] (Fig 4-1). Thus, normal arterial blood pressure in a bleeding trauma patient may be associated with significant intravascular volume depletion and decreased cardiac output. Pulse pressure is generally believed to correlate with stroke volume.[261] Many clinicians monitor the changes in pulse pressure along with the systolic and diastolic pressures as an index of adequacy of fluid resuscitation.[261] However, Cullen[41] observed no correlation between stroke volume and pulse pressure in both anesthetized and awake patients.

During hemorrhage, reduced glomerular filtration and increased water and sodium reabsorption result in decreased urine output.[205] Careful monitoring of urine output helps guide volume replacement during resuscitation. In diabetic patients with high serum glucose levels and in those who have received radiocontrast dye or diuretics, urine output does not reflect the status of renal perfusion because of the osmotic diuresis.

Patients presenting with class II hemorrhage and hypotension that stabilizes with early resuscitation require two large intravenous lines, one of which should function as a central venous pressure (CVP) monitor. Placement of an indwelling arterial catheter provides beat-to-beat arterial pressure monitoring and intermittent sampling of blood for blood gas analysis.

Monitoring of the CVP may be useful in previously healthy hypovolemic trauma victims, since it reflects the interplay among blood volume, venous capacitance, and cardiac function.[110] Thus, in injured patients with normal hearts and reflex capacitance vessel constriction, a low CVP is a signal of hypovolemia. Increase of the CVP during fluid resuscitation should suggest restoration of intravascular volume. Moreover, CVP data together with systemic arterial pressure changes during a so-called "fluid challenge" may provide useful information regarding the patient's overall cardiovascular dynamics. For instance, after fluid administration, an increase of CVP to approximately 15 mm Hg associated with a declining arterial pressure may indicate cardiac failure. However, it should be remembered that the CVP monitors primarily right heart function. Patients with isolated left ventricular failure may develop hypotension or even pulmonary edema with normal CVP.[28] Also, changes in intrathoracic pressure caused by spontaneous breathing or positive pressure ventilation; coughing; Valsalva maneuver; or accumulation of thoracic or mediastinal air, blood, and fluid are all reflected in the CVP.[110] Traditionally, during volume replacement, a normal CVP (7 to 8 mm Hg) in the presence of a normal blood pressure suggests adequate blood volume restoration. However, data from several studies comparing CVP and blood volume measurements during fluid resuscitation indicate that a 20 to 30% blood volume deficit may still be present at the time that CVP and systemic blood pressure return to normal.[166,219,232] Surprisingly, similar results have been reported for pulmonary artery wedge pressure during fluid resuscitation.[223] In summary, the CVP may be useful, provided that factors affecting it are recognized and its limitations in indicating normovolemia during fluid resuscitation are understood.

Direct arterial pressure monitoring provides beat-to-beat information, allowing rapid intervention when hypotension occurs. Furthermore, an exaggerated respirophasic variation in systolic blood pressure during mechanical ventilation indicates hypovolemia.[36,191,194] The difference between the highest and the lowest systolic pressure exceeds 10 mm Hg in the hypovolemic patient; the magnitude of the variation correlates with the severity of volume loss[36,191,194] (Fig 4-6). The magnitude of the decrease in systolic pressure from that recorded during end expiration also correlates with the degree of hypovolemia.[191,194] In animals, respirophasic variations correlate better with hypovolemia than the CVP does.[191] Respirophasic changes have also been observed on pulse oximetry recordings from hypovolemic patients, but the accuracy of this variation as an indicator of hypovolemia remains to be determined.

Obviously changes in systolic blood pressure correspond to alterations in left ventricular output which are affected primarily by the venous return. There is some evidence to suggest that systolic pressure variation during hypovolemia is due to squeezing of pulmonary capillary blood into the left ventricle,[209] resulting in increased left ventricular preload and

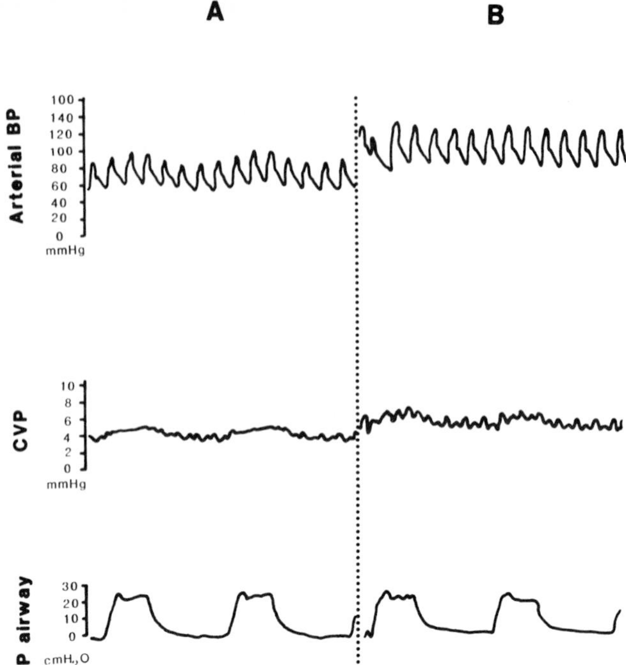


FIG. 4-6. Simultaneously obtained arterial (above), central venous (middle), and airway (below) pressure traces in a mechanically ventilated patient during hypovolemia (A); and after restoration of blood volume (B). Note the exaggerated decrease of arterial blood pressure after inspiration. Also note a minimal respirophasic change of systolic pressure during normovolemic state.

thus increased stroke volume during early inspiration. This phenomenon does not occur in normovolemic animals probably because in these instances zone III conditions ($P_{pa} > P_{LA} > P_{alv}$) predominate, and significant increase in pulmonary outflow does not occur. Whatever the mechanism, the information obtained by this phenomenon is very useful in detecting hypovolemia in normotensive patients. With fluid resuscitation and restoration of normovolemia, this response disappears.[36]

The arterial pressure trace may also provide information about myocardial contractility, stroke volume, and the systemic vascular resistance.[110] It is generally accepted that a steep upstroke of the pressure wave indicates a vigorous left ventricular contraction, the area under the systolic ejection period (from the beginning of systolic upstroke to the dicrotic notch) correlates with the stroke volume, and the location of the dicrotic notch and the steepness of the downstroke are proportional to the SVR. Thus, a low dicrotic notch and steep downstroke suggest low SVR.[110] Recently, however, the value of the contour of the arterial waveform as an indicator of SVR and stroke volume has been questioned. In a small number of patients no correlation could be found between the height of the dicrotic notch and systemic vascular resistance, diastolic run-off, or cardiac output.[75]

Patients with class III, life-threatening injuries require three large-bore intravenous lines including a central venous line. During the operative procedure, replacement of blood and BES should be guided by serial hemoglobin or hematocrit measurements and careful observation of changes in direct arterial and central venous pressures and urine output. When circumstances permit, placement of a pulmonary artery (PA) catheter may help measure filling pressures, cardiac output, oxygen transport variables, and systemic and pulmonary vascular resistances. A PA catheter may be useful during the operative procedure, but the old adage "hypotension in the seriously injured patient requires more blood and fluid replacement" still holds. The major benefit of a PA catheter is usually realized during the postoperative period. In general, pulmonary capillary wedge pressure ($P_{pw}$) is a reliable index of left ventricular end-diastolic pressure (normal $P_{pw}$ = 10 to 15 mm Hg). Values below 10 mm Hg in the injured hemorrhaging patient indicate hypovolemia, whereas $P_{pw}$ above 15 mm Hg suggests hypervolemia or left ventricular dysfunction. However, interpretation of $P_{pw}$ may be difficult during hypovolemia, since pulmonary vascular pressure may decrease below alveolar pressure, and thus $P_{pw}$ measures alveolar rather than vascular pressure. Many patients with a $P_{pw}$ greater than 15 mm Hg after resuscitation from severe shock will respond to a fluid challenge with a steep rise in cardiac output and little change in $P_{pw}$, thus indicating normal left ventricular function. On the other hand, increased $P_{pw}$ without an increase in stroke volume suggests exhaustion of cardiac reserve.[135]

Absolute levels of hemoglobin or hematocrit during phase 1, when only acellular fluids are administered, are not reliable indices of blood loss because restoration of plasma volume by transcapillary refill and fluid infusion results in hemodilution. Restoration of the red cell mass may take several hours; thus, the measured hematocrit is the result of both blood loss and hemodilution. However, during administration of blood, serial hemoglobin or hematocrit measurements are useful indicators of the adequacy of blood transfusion.

Patients presenting in class IV shock require at least three intravenous lines to restore intravascular volume. Thoracotomy and placement of a right atrial line may be necessary in some of these patients to improve the rate of fluid infusion. Invasive monitoring and continuous measurement of arterial blood pressure, CVP, pulmonary artery pressure, $P_{pw}$, $S\bar{v}O_2$ and periodic determinations of cardiac output, blood gases, and electrolytes may be necessary. Frequently, placement of central intravascular catheters is not possible during initial resuscitation. Low jugular or subclavian venous pressures may make insertion of these lines difficult. One must remember that delaying treatment of a severely hypotensive patient in order to insert a central venous catheter will result in disaster. Many physicians feel that the first 30 to 60 minutes after shock is the golden period of treatment. Complications will arise if this period is not used appropriately. Hypotension in the presence of bleeding is almost always due to significant plasma volume depletion, and rapid fluid and blood administration is mandatory. Thus, estimation of intravascular volume during the initial stage should be based on blood pressure, heart rate, and urine output.

Aggressive resuscitation with Ringer's lactate does not increase an existing lactic acidosis when shock is reversible. Each liter of Ringer's lactate solution contains 28 mEq of lactate, about half of which is metabolized in the liver. The remaining lactate is cleared rapidly from the plasma once tissue perfusion is improved by fluid infusion.[259] Thus, the past concerns expressed by some clinicians seem to be unwarranted.[225]

## POSTOPERATIVE HOMEOSTASIS

The greatest therapeutic challenge of hemorrhagic shock occurs after resuscitation with the development of significant extravascular fluid sequestration. Expansion of the intracellular space because of disruption of cell membrane function plus expansion of the interstitial space because of structural and functional changes in its matrix cause an obligatory efflux of sodium and water from the blood vessels.[26,150] Although this fluid shift is often referred to as organ dysfunction, these changes probably reflect a protective response to insult.[47,76] Regardless of the underlying mechanism, the end result is plasma volume depletion, often associated with derangement in oxygenation as reflected by changes in the ratio of arterial oxygen tension to the percent inspired oxygen ($PO_2/FIO_2$), the amount of physiologic shunting in the lungs, and the alveolar-arterial oxygen tension difference.[150]

Since this extravascular expansion occurs at the expense of plasma volume, the patient develops signs of inadequate perfusion, reduced cardiac output, tachycardia, marginal blood pressure, narrowed pulse pressure, and oliguria. The combination of increased total body water, deranged oxygenation, hyperventilation, marginal perfusion pressure, and oliguria raises the specter of combined failure of the kidneys, heart, and lungs. Should therapy be directed toward the inadequate circulatory volume, as reflected by low blood pressure and oliguria, or to the so-called vascular overload, as reflected by the edema, weight gain, increased filling pressure, and decreased oxygenation? The use of diuretics at this time often leads to profound diuresis and reduction in plasma volume.[157] The underlying problem in these patients, however, is not cardiac failure; the postdiuretic fall in plasma volume reduces perfusion pressure, RPF, GFR, and urine output, which in turn may require treatment by vasopressors. If the underlying problem is cardiac decompensation, the resultant reduction in cardiac work after diuretic therapy is beneficial. However, as we have said, heart failure in this setting is very uncommon.[157,159] Since precise definition of the cause for oliguria at this time is often difficult, therapy should be adjusted to organ response.

### LEFT HEART WORK/CENTRAL FILLING PRESSURE RESPONSE TO THERAPY

Left ventricular stroke work index is calculated according to the following formula:

$$LVSWI = \frac{CO \times (MAP - P_{pw})}{HR \times BSA} \times 13.6$$

where LVSWI is left ventricular stroke work index; CO, cardiac output; MAP, mean arterial pressure; $P_{pw}$, pulmonary capillary wedge pressure; HR, heart rate; and BSA, body surface area. The normal value for LVSWI is between 40 and 60 $g \cdot m/m^2$.

The response of the LVSWI to changes in central filling

pressures helps define the cardiac component of these changes.[2,26,44,159] After resuscitation from severe hypovolemic shock, extravascular sequestration of sodium and water leads to swelling of the pulmonary interstices. Consequently, a marked rise in $P_{pw}$ to above 20 mm Hg concomitant with a reduction in LVSWI to below 40 g·m/m$^2$ may be because of either lung or heart failure[116,159] (Fig 4-7). Rather than assuming cardiac compromise, the patient should receive a bolus infusion of 500 mL of BES over 20 minutes to monitor the response of both LVSWI and $P_{pw}$.[116,150] A sharp rise in heart work with little change in wedge pressure (steep slope) clearly indicates normal myocardial reserve; a flat slope indicates cardiac compromise (Fig 4-8). Oliguria and marginal perfusion pressure in a patient with a steep slope should be treated with volume replacement rather than exogenous diuresis. When the patient enters phase 3, the central filling pressure will fall.

Sequential monitoring of the LVSWI/$P_{pw}$ ratio thus provides a rational basis for deciding whether inotropic support and diuretic therapy is indicated in oliguric patients with elevated central filling pressures. Clearly, the assumption that an elevated wedge pressure after resuscitation from shock results from heart failure is hazardous when the slope of this ratio in response to a fluid challenge has not been measured.[150,159] Patients with low perfusion as reflected by low blood pressure and cardiac output in conjunction with a low central filling pressure obviously require volume replacement; loop diuretics are contraindicated in this setting (Table 4-5). Patients with poor perfusion, marginal blood pressure, and a high central filling pressure need serial monitoring of left heart work and wedge pressures in response to a bolus infusion of BES. When this challenge produces a steep slope on the LVSWI/$P_{pw}$ diagram, loop diuretics are hazardous; volume replacement is the treatment of choice despite the elevated $P_{pw}$. When a patient has a low perfusion state plus a high central filling pressure, and the bolus infusion of BES results in a flat LVSWI/$P_{pw}$ curve, heart compromise exists. Such patients are candidates for reduction in preload with diuretic agents and possibly appropriate inotropic support as well.[145,150] Afterload reduction with vasodilators (nitroglycerin, sodium nitroprusside) may also be indicated if the systemic blood pressure is normal.

FIG. 4-7. After large volumes of fluid have sequestered in an extravascular location, this fluid overload may be inappropriately attributed to cardiac compromise. A fluid bolus in a patient with a high central filling pressure (solid dots) leads to a prompt rise in left heart work with little change in central filling pressure, producing a slope parallel to the normal slope of the Frank-Starling curve.

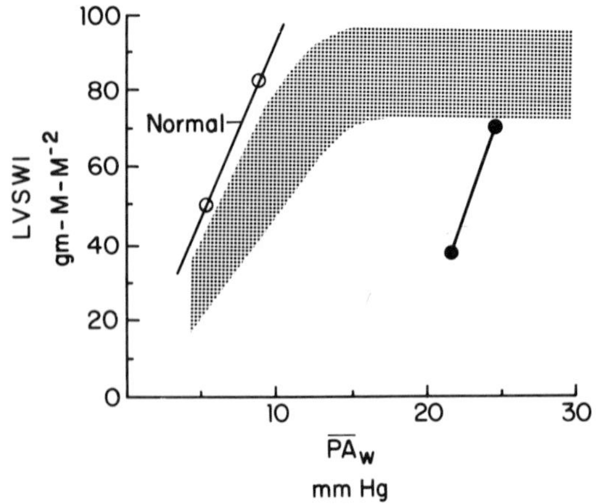


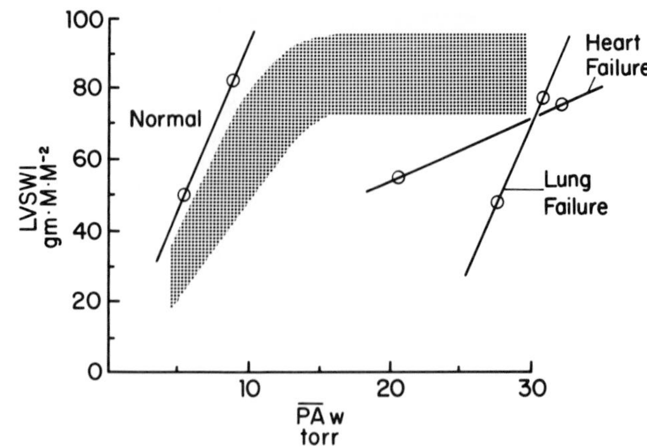


FIG. 4-8. When a patient with a high central filling pressure receives a bolus of balanced electrolyte solution, a sharp rise in left heart work with little change in central filling pressure indicates normal cardiac reserve and probable pulmonary failure. A sharp rise in the central filling pressure with little rise in left heart work indicates cardiac compromise with or without associated pulmonary failure.

## GUIDELINES FOR PHASE 2 TREATMENT

During the extravascular fluid sequestration phase, the hemoglobin should be maintained at approximately 10 to 12 g % by means of transfusion of packed red cells. Early in phase 2, when movement of salt and water out of the plasma is rapid, BES is used to maintain effective plasma volume. During this time weight gain will occur due to extravascular volume expansion. This finding should not lead to reducing the fluid infusion rate, which should be based, as we have discussed, on central filling pressures and their relationship with LVSWI (Table 4-6).

During phase 2, cardiac compromise as manifested by a flat and right-shifted LVSWI/$P_{pw}$ curve, may be treated by one or a combination of the following therapeutic modalities.[150]

TABLE 4-5. Guidelines to Diuretic Therapy for Oliguria after Hemorrhagic Shock

| |
|---|
| Low perfusion pressure, low central filling pressure<br>*Contraindicated* |
| Low perfusion pressure, *high* central filling pressure<br>1. Good response (steep slope) of LVSWI/$P_{pw}$ to fluid bolus<br>*Very dangerous*<br>2. Poor response (flat slope) of LVSWI/$P_{pw}$ to fluid bolus<br>*Helpful to reduce preload* |
| High perfusion pressure, *low* central filling pressure<br>*Helpful to define prerenal problem* |
| High perfusion pressure, high central filling pressure<br>*Helpful to define prerenal problem; helpful to "break" oliguric renal failure as part of "shotgun" therapy* |

TABLE 4-6. Guidelines to Therapy During Sequestration Phase

| |
|---|
| Correct ongoing volume deficit |
| Use balanced salt solution |
| Restore blood pressure, pulse pressure, urine output |
| Must replace plasma and interstitial volume deficits |
| Must accommodate to cellular swelling |
| Ignore weight gain |
| Correct postoperative anemia |
| Maintain hemoglobin at 12 g % |
| Use packed cells |
| Carefully observe coagulation status |
| Correct with fresh frozen plasma and platelet transfusion if necessary |
| Concomitant support of heart and lungs as needed |

### *Diuretic Agents*

Furosemide (5 to 10 mg intravenously) usually induces diuresis and reduces left ventricular preload. If a diuretic response is not obtained within 30 minutes following this dose, higher doses (40 to 100 mg) may be administered. Osmotic diuretics (eg, mannitol) are contraindicated in this stage as they produce an initial increase of intravascular volume by shifting intracellular fluid into the intravascular space and may precipitate cardiac failure.

### *Digitalization*

If satisfactory diuresis does not occur with furosemide or if in spite of this diuresis the central filling pressures remain elevated, digoxin (0.25 mg intravenously) twice within a period of 30 to 60 minutes can be administered. This is followed by a 0.25-mg dose every 4 to 6 hours to a total dose of 1.5 mg. With the availability of rapidly acting potent inotropic agents, this form of therapy is used infrequently. During digitalization, the ECG should be monitored carefully to prevent toxicity.[236] The use of digitalis may allow a decrease in the doses of other vasoactive drugs required for cardiovascular stability.

### *Supplemental Calcium Administration*

This type of therapy may be considered when serum ionized calcium ($Ca^{2+}$) levels are low. An excellent review by Drop[52] summarizes the characteristics and hemodynamic effects of ionized calcium. The dose of intravenous $CaCl_2$ varies from 3 to 15 mg/kg of body weight. The drug is administered as a bolus over a period of 60 seconds. The calcium content of the chloride salt is 27% and of the gluconate only 9%. Thus, when equal volumes are administered, a greater response can be obtained with $CaCl_2$ than with calcium gluconate.[52] Bolus administration of $CaCl_2$ (15 mg/kg) results in a 60 to 70% increase of serum ionized calcium within 2 minutes.[54] After this, the serum $Ca^{2+}$ concentration drops rapidly over the next 10 minutes. However, at the end of this time, serum $Ca^{2+}$ levels are still 10 to 15% higher than those obtained before the infusion.[54] The increased blood pressure observed after calcium administration is a result of both the myocardial and the vascular effects of the drug.[52] The improvement in myocardial contractility is dose dependent, varying from 10% following 5 mg/kg to 20% with a 15-mg/kg dose.[52] An increase in serum $Ca^{2+}$ concentration improves left ventricular function in both ischemic and normal areas of the myocardium.[73] Increased peripheral vasoconstriction is due both to a direct effect of calcium on vascular smooth muscle and to its effect on the autonomic nervous system.[73] Calcium causes catecholamine release from adrenal medulla and sympathetic nerve endings. Experimentally, stimulation of both α- and β-adrenergic receptors by calcium is also suggested.[73] The extent of hemodynamic effects after calcium injection depends on the initial functional state of the myocardium and on sympathetic nervous system activity.[109] Theoretically, patients whose sympathetic activity is already maximal may have little beneficial effect from calcium administration. Injection of calcium is not without hazards; major arrhythmias including sinus bradyarrhythmia, atrioventricular (A-V) dissociation, and junctional rhythms have been reported.[27] Patients receiving digitalis are particularly vulnerable to the arrhythmic effects of calcium.[130] Another undesirable effect of calcium infusion is augmentation of myocardial oxygen consumption not associated with increased myocardial blood flow.[73] Thus, in patients with a marginal myocardial supply/demand ratio the drug should be used carefully. In summary, a bolus infusion of calcium causes a prompt increase in cardiac output and left ventricular work. The increase in blood pressure is due to both improved myocardial function and peripheral vasoconstriction. The hemodynamic response to bolus calcium infusion is transient and lasts no more than 30 minutes.

### *Inotropic Agents*

As mentioned earlier, inotropic support may be necessary to improve tissue perfusion during phase 2.[149] Apart from digitalization this can be best achieved by dopamine and dobutamine infusion.[143,159] Newer inotropic agents such as amrinone, a phosphodiesterase inhibitor, may also be useful.

Dopamine acts on α, β, and dopaminergic receptors.[79] It also causes release of endogenous norepinephrine. In the trauma patient in the second phase of hemorrhagic shock, dopamine, through its cardiac β-receptor and renal dopaminergic receptor activities, can provide improved left ventricular function and urine output. Its renal dopamine receptor-stimulating activity occurs at low doses (1 to 3 μg/kg of body weight/min). At this dose dopamine has been shown to increase cardiac output and renal cortical blood flow and to improve diuresis, natriuresis, and kaliuresis.[78,80] According to a more recent report[103] the diuretic effect of dopamine may also be due to a direct inhibitory effect of this drug on tubular solute reabsorption. It should be remembered that the diuretic effect of dopamine may not be observed in severely hypovolemic patients. The severe reduction of renal blood flow prevents redistribution of blood from the inner to the outer cortex.

Administration of higher doses of dopamine (5 to 10 μg/kg of body weight/min) results in significant improvement of left ventricular function without causing a significant increase in systemic vascular resistance. However, doses greater than 10 to 15 μg/kg/min may defeat the beneficial effects of positive inotropism, since tachycardia and increased systemic vascular resistance seen at this dose level may augment the myocardial oxygen demand.[78] This effect can be modified by concomitant use of vasodilator agents (nitroglycerin or sodium nitroprusside).[141,172]

Dobutamine is a synthetic β-1 receptor agonist. Unlike dopamine, dobutamine does not cause endogenous norepinephrine release. At low concentrations it increases myocardial contractile force and causes mild tachycardia. Originally, dobutamine was thought to cause a profound inotropic effect without accelerating the heart rate. However, it has become apparent that it may cause mild tachycardia at doses up to 15 μg/kg/min and moderate tachycardia above this dose.[138] The smaller effect on heart rate of dobutamine than of other sympathomimetic agents is ascribed to the α-2 agonist activity of the drug.[120] Dobutamine has no effect on renal dopaminergic receptors. Thus, improvement of renal function with this agent is primarily because of improved cardiac output and not to renal vasodilatation. When an increase in renal cortical blood flow is desired, a low-dose infusion of dopamine may be added.[207] In summary, when improved inotropy with the least possible tachycardia and systemic vasoconstriction is desired, dobutamine appears to be the drug of choice.

The search for improved cardiotonic agents has provided a new family of drugs: the phosphodiesterase inhibitors. Their clinical pharmacology and use have been reviewed by Colucci et al.[31] These agents produce powerful positive inotropic effects with moderate peripheral vasodilatation. Although their mechanism of action is not known clearly, they appear to inhibit cardiac phosphodiesterase (F-III) selectively. Amrinone is the only agent in this family which is approved by the Food and Drug Administration. It is used intravenously in patients with congestive heart failure refractory to other inotropic agents. The hemodynamic effects of amrinone resemble those of a combination of dobutamine and nitroprusside, and it does not increase heart rate or peripheral vascular resistance. Amrinone dilates both resistance and capacitance vessels.[31] Thus, its use in hypovolemic patients may result in significant hypotension. The drug is administered as an initial bolus dose of 0.75 mg/kg, infused over a period of 3 to 5 minutes. The maintenance dose is 5 to 10 μg/kg/min titrated to the hemodynamic response. The recommended total dose for a 24-hour period is about 7 to 10 mg/kg. Because of the potential for this drug to cause hypotension, its use should be guided by careful hemodynamic monitoring.

## GUIDELINES FOR PHASE 3 TREATMENT

Eventually, although there is no clear end point to phase 2, the patient reaches a plateau at which no further weight gain occurs and vital signs and urine output can be maintained with a slower rate of fluid administration. Electrolytes and water move from the nonfunctional third space into the vascular space.[76] Renal excretion is the most effective mechanism for eliminating this autoinfusion. Occasionally, renal parenchymal damage leads to impairment of renal excretion. If the rate of autoinfusion is greater than that which can be eliminated by the kidney, acute hypervolemia and hypertension will result.[47,76] This impairment of excretion coincides with increased renal vascular resistance and a decrease in RPF. The guidelines to therapy in phase 3, therefore, are to maintain the hemoglobin level with packed red cell replacement and to reduce effective plasma volume by decreasing exogenous fluid intake and augmenting diuresis. While slowing fluid replacement to a "keep open" rate, one must recognize that supplemental drug and antibiotic therapy requires fluid so that often the minimal infusion rate will total 3 L/day. Careful, judicious use of antibiotics and other drugs helps keep the daily infusion to below 700 mL. The change from BES to one-third normal saline or 5% dextrose/water further reduces the intravascular sodium load.

When a patient develops hypertension at the beginning of phase 3, a small dose of a loop diuretic, such as 5 or 10 mg of furosemide, will often "open the tap" and initiate a prompt and prolonged diuresis. Avoidance of multiple doses of the diuretic will protect against a sudden fall in circulatory volume and urine output and deterioration of renal function.

A syndrome of postresuscitative hypertension may occur early in phase 3; it is associated with hypervolemia and an increase in the ratio of plasma volume to interstitial fluid volume.[76] Consequently, the interstitial space compliance is reduced so that its capacity to compensate for alteration of plasma volume is compromised. The margin of safety between postresuscitative hypertension and hypovolemia is thus narrowed. As the patient continues to mobilize third-space fluid and excrete it through the kidneys, blood pressure gradually returns to normal. Thus, if antihypertensive agents are used during this stage, cardiovascular function should be monitored carefully to avoid hypotension. Incremental intravenous doses of labetalol (5 to 20 mg, up to a total of 60 to 80 mg) usually provide adequate blood pressure and heart rate control without causing hypotension. In some patients a total labetalol dose up to 220 mg may be required to control the hypertension.[179]

## THE ROLE OF VASOPRESSOR AND INOTROPIC AGENTS

Vasoactive drugs are useful in maintaining cardiac support and urine output.[145] The use of low-dose dopamine or dobutamine infusion (5 to 10 μg/kg/min) may help increase peripheral perfusion pressure, cardiac output, and oxygen delivery even when the fluid infusion rate is reduced. Although infusion of a vasoactive drug has theoretic appeal in injured patients with cardiac insufficiency, abuse of this regimen may all too frequently lead to drug tachyphylaxis and subsequent death. A low-dose infusion (8 μg of dopamine or less per minute) augments cardiac output without increasing peripheral vascular resistance or reducing flow to vital organs. The increase in blood flow also increases urine output. Although this diuretic effect has been attributed to renal vasodilatation, our own studies (unpublished) indicate that RPF and distribution of renal blood flow remain constant or else fluctuate in proportion to the change in cardiac output after low-dosage dopamine infusion. These findings have been corroborated by Hilberman et al[103] who suggest that the diuresis and natriuresis caused by dopamine may occur independently of any effects on renal blood flow. As we have mentioned, it is possible that dopamine directly inhibits tubular solute reabsorption and thus causes diuresis[103] or that it causes a decrease in ADH release. Ultimately, the place for infusion of vasoactive drugs to reduce fluid needs in the critically ill patient will be determined by careful monitoring of cardiopulmonary function, oxygen delivery, oxygen consumption, and multiple organ function. Part of this monitoring, in the future, should be directed to measurement of cell and interstitial space fluid balance.

## THE EFFECTS OF ARTIFICIAL VENTILATION ON FLUID THERAPY

Patients with severe hemorrhage may develop varying degrees of respiratory embarrassment, requiring ventilatory support. Controlled mechanical ventilation (CMV) with zero end-expiratory pressure (ZEEP) has been shown to produce changes in renal function.[77,233] With the addition of positive end-expiratory pressure (PEEP), alteration of renal function is even more pronounced.[112,119,125] In one study in head-injured patients, addition of 10 cm $H_2O$ of PEEP to CMV reduced urine output by 34%, GFR by 19%, renal blood flow (RBF) by 32%, and sodum excretion by 33%.[3] Decreased water and sodium excretion results in water retention; weight gain; tissue edema; and decreased hematocrit, plasma osmolality, and plasma sodium concentration.[12] Thus, ventilatory adjustments designed to improve arterial oxygen content may significantly alter fluid therapy.

Respirator-induced changes of renal function have been attributed to several mechanisms.[60] Experimentally, it has been suggested that increases in inferior vena cava (IVC), hepatic, and renal vein pressures, which accompany administration of PEEP, contribute to the altered renal function.[162,221] However, release of hepatic congestion by means of a vena cava to jugular venous shunt during PEEP does not improve renal function.[196] In addition, despite significant increases in IVC pressure during PEEP, deterioration of renal function has been shown to occur only in hypovolemic and normovolemic but not in hypervolemic animals.[252] Thus, renal congestion secondary to increased IVC pressure by PEEP appears to contribute little to altered renal function. Hall et al[93] suggested that redistribution of RBF from cortical to juxtamedullary nephrons could cause impairment of renal function; however, a more recent study by the same group using radioactive microspheres failed to demonstrate any blood flow redistribution.[197]

At present, available evidence suggests that the impaired cardiovascular function induced by PEEP and to a lesser extent by CMV is the primary cause of the renal effects. Both high tidal volumes and PEEP reduce venous return and cardiac output,[82,96] probably as a result of diminished left ventricular end-diastolic volume caused by elevated intrathoracic pressure, autonomic reflex alterations, and decreased venous return.[51,203] Increased pulmonary vascular resistance[51,203] and altered ventricular geometry with cardiac septal or lateral free wall shifting[111,173] caused by PEEP may also result in reduced cardiac output. The improvement in oxygenation, therefore, may be offset by the reduction in cardiac output, and thus, tissue oxygen delivery may decrease (Fig 4-9).[163] Furthermore, the frequently associated decrease in arterial blood pressure inhibits baroreceptor discharge, which in turn enhances sympathetic tone, catecholamine secretion, and renin-angiotensin-aldosterone activity.[188] These acute compensations maintain circulatory homeostasis and minimize further decreases in blood pressure but also produce severe hemodynamic changes in the kidney. As described by Berry,[12] the extent and severity of renal and cardiovascular changes caused by PEEP are dependent on the pulmonary, cardiac, and intravascular volume status of the patient, the amount of PEEP applied, and the type of anesthetic and sedative drugs used. For instance, in patients with decreased lung compliance, elevated airway pressures may not be transmitted to the intrapleural space, thus the elevation of intrathoracic pressure may be relatively small.[12,244,254] This, of course, results in minimal reduction in venous return, blood pressure, and renal function. Likewise, patients with adequate intravascular volume are little affected by the deleterious renal and hemodynamic effects of PEEP.[196,251,252]

Although elevated plasma ADH levels have been demonstrated during the initial phases of PEEP therapy, corresponding decreases in free water clearance have been observed only

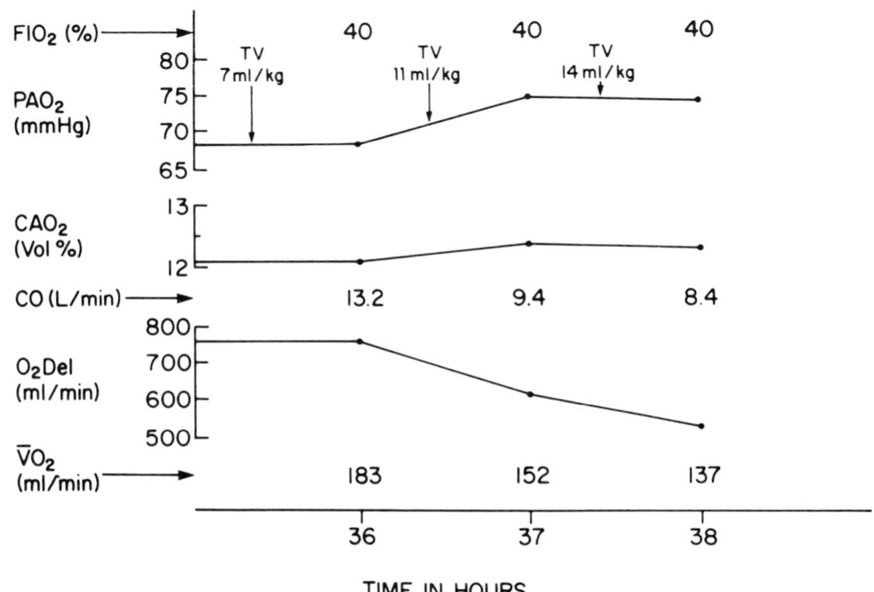


FIG. 4-9. A severely injured patient requiring multiple transfusions was monitored for total oxygen dynamics at tidal volumes of 7, 11, and 14 mL/kg. Oxygen tension and oxygen content rose with higher tidal volumes, but a concomitant fall in cardiac output resulted in oxygen delivery and oxygen consumption being greatest at the lowest tidal volume.

infrequently.[12] This suggests that ADH acts as a vasoconstrictor rather than an antidiuretic. Furthermore, Payen et al[188] showed recently in a small number of patients that ADH was not involved in the antidiuretic effect of PEEP. Several mechanisms may be responsible for the ADH elevation during ventilation with PEEP: stimulation of low- (atrial) and high-pressure (left atrial and arterial) baroreceptors by decreased central blood volume,[168,217] angiotensin release,[3] and increased plasma osmolality.

Recently, atrial natriuretic factor (ANF) has been shown to contribute to the development of PEEP-induced antidiuresis.[122,139] ANF is secreted from the atrial wall in response to increased atrial transmural pressure. The physiologic role of ANF is to activate homeostatic mechanisms that restore normal blood volume and pressure, and electrolyte levels. The sites of action of ANF are the kidneys, the adrenals, vascular smooth muscle, and possibly the central nervous system. ANF levels increase in congestive failure and volume overload to induce diuresis. During ventilation with PEEP the increase in intrathoracic pressure tends to decrease transmural pressures within the heart and results in decreased ANF secretion, which in turn results in antidiuresis.[122,139]

After a period of mechanical ventilation, the retained water and exogenously administered fluids cause an increase in intravascular and total body water. Increased intravascular volume improves cardiac filling pressures and thus cardiac output.[13] Diminished sympathetic tone, reduced ADH and renin-angiotensin activity, and probably increased ANF secretion result in improved hemodynamics and thus in increased urine output and sodium excretion. The possible mechanisms of ventilator-induced renal dysfunction and its reversal are summarized in Fig 4-10.

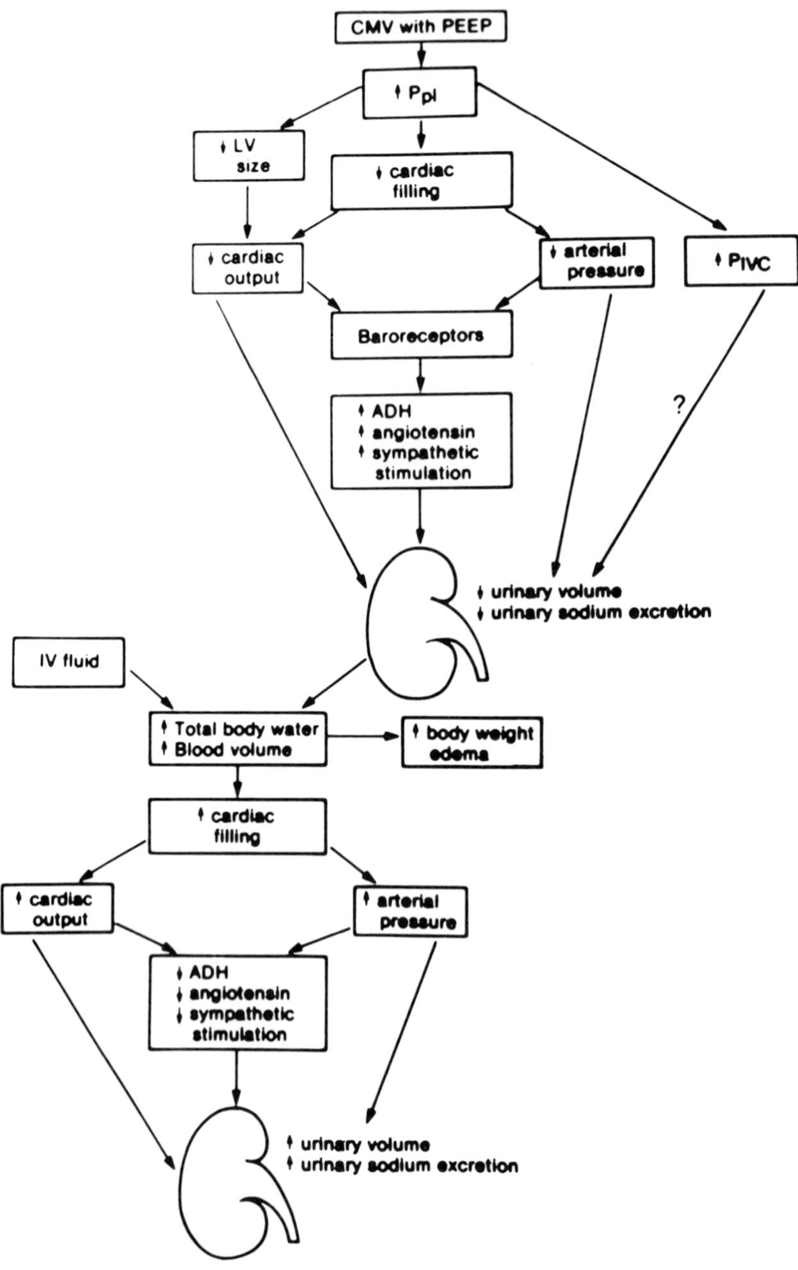


FIG. 4-10. Possible mechanisms of altered renal function during mechanical ventilation with PEEP and its reversal with restoration of the blood volume. $p_{pl}$, pleural pressure; LV, left ventricle; $P_{IVC}$, inferior vena cava pressure. (From Berry[12] with permission.)

Data relative to the long-term effects of mechanical ventilation on kidney function in humans are not available. Animal studies have shown that mechanical ventilation of dogs with 10 cm of $H_2O$ PEEP resulted in twice as much water retention as ventilation without PEEP.[13] The urine output eventually increased during long-term ventilation. However, improvement was slower in PEEP-treated dogs (46 hours) than in those treated with only CMV (27 hours). Thus, renal dysfunction and fluid and electrolyte imbalance with ventilatory therapy eventually improve with optimization of intravascular volume, but this occurs slowly in PEEP-treated animals.

Hemodynamic management of the multiple trauma patient, who is almost invariably on ventilator therapy during the early postoperative period, requires sound clinical judgment. The clinician is usually faced with the dilemma of optimizing ventilatory, hemodynamic, and renal functions. At times this goal may be difficult to achieve because therapeutic maneuvers designed to improve the function of one system may produce derangements in another. Furthermore, adverse interactions may take place among these organs in such a way that functional and/or morphologic deterioration may occur in the organ that was treated primarily. For instance, institution of CMV with PEEP to treat respiratory failure of the multiple trauma patient may result in water retention and increased lung water, which may further impair lung function. The treatment of this edema with diuretics may result in decreased intravascular volume, decreased cardiac function, and abnormal renal function.[12] Optimization of oxygen delivery and utilization rather than concentration on each individual organ's function should form the mainstay of therapy. Thus, frequent monitoring of hemodynamic and oxygen transport parameters and appropriately adjusting tidal volume, PEEP, fluid infusion rate, and inotropic therapy will probably result in the most favorable treatment (see Chapter 5).

Maintenance of normal intravascular volume is necessary to prevent ventilator-induced disturbances in cardiac, renal, and pulmonary function. As mentioned earlier, normovolemia or hypervolemia minimizes the adverse effects of positive pressure ventilation on cardiac and renal function.[196,251,252]

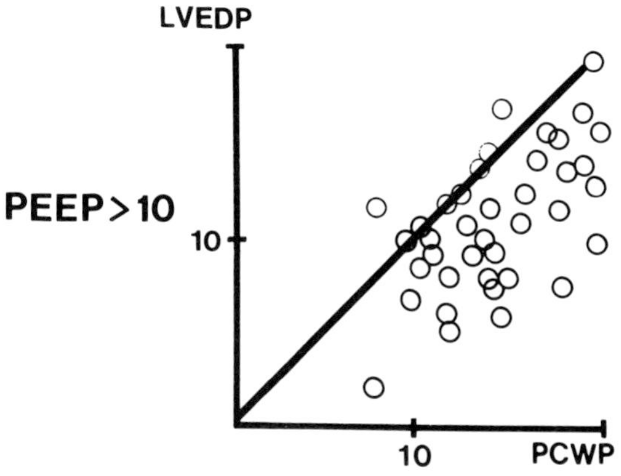


FIG. 4-11. Relationship between left ventricular end-diastolic pressure (LVEDP) and pulmonary capillary wedge pressure (PCWP) during PEEP > 10 cm of $H_2O$. Note that in most instances PCWP overestimated LVEDP. (From Jardin et al[111] with permission.)

However, in patients with severe pulmonary abnormalities accompanied by increased lung water, dopamine infusion (5 μg/kg/min) may be used. This agent has been shown to improve cardiac output, oxygen transport, and renal function of normovolemic patients with respiratory failure treated with CMV and PEEP.[102] The use of diuretics in this setting may be considered; however, they should be administered carefully with appropriate monitoring. Reduction in blood volume and cardiac output by these drugs may cause further renal dysfunction. Finally, the need for elevated airway pressures should be assessed frequently by monitoring oxygen transport variables to define the most optimal setting. High-frequency jet ventilation may provide some hemodynamic advantages in patients with circulatory shock and respiratory failure,[65] but its beneficial effect on renal function in humans remains to be determined. Likewise, the effect of intermittent mandatory ventilation (IMV) on renal function should be determined in humans since it produces less water and salt retention in animals than CMV.[239]

### INTERPRETATION OF PULMONARY ARTERY WEDGE PRESSURE DURING TREATMENT WITH PEEP

When patients are ventilated with PEEP greater than 10 cm of $H_2O$, interpretation of $P_{pw}$ should be given special consideration.[111,204] The increased intrathoracic pressure produced by PEEP may result in a $P_{pw}$ reading higher than the actual left ventricular end-diastolic pressure (LVEDP) (Fig 4-11). This discrepancy is a function of compressive forces of increased intrathoracic or pericardial pressure upon the heart as well as transmission of alveolar pressure to the pulmonary artery catheter. Increased extracardiac pressure alters the left ventricular pressure-volume relationship.[111,204,259] Because the discrepancy between $P_{pw}$ and LVEDP is least during end expiration, $P_{pw}$ measurements should be performed at this time.[14] The extent of PEEP transmitted to the heart is dependent upon the lung compliance.[254] The greater the pulmonary compliance, the greater the effect of applied PEEP on the discrepancy between $P_{pw}$ and transmural LVEDP.[111] In patients with low pulmonary compliance caused by acute respiratory distress syndrome (ARDS), for example, the measured $P_{pw}$ corresponds closely to the LVEDP.[244] For rough estimation of LVEDP from $P_{pw}$ in patients with normal or slightly decreased lung compliance, half of the applied PEEP may be subtracted from the $P_{pw}$.[20] The measurement of intrapleural or esophageal pressure may allow more accurate estimation of actual LVEDP.[111] A brief cessation of PEEP may also permit estimation of LVEDP, although this may result in a precipitous drop in $Pa_{O_2}$.[6,204]

## RESUSCITATION FLUIDS

### ALBUMIN VERSUS CRYSTALLOID (TABLES 4-7 AND 4-8)

Despite the recognition in 1959 that colloid, especially albumin, would have little effect on the pulmonary plasma to interstitial oncotic pressure ratio after certain insults,[178] the 1960s and 1970s saw a phenomenal rise in supplemental albumin therapy for patients with ARDS after shock and sep-

TABLE 4-7. Characteristics of Various Colloid Solutions*

| | SODIUM CONTENT (g/L) | $Na^+$ (mEq/L) | $Cl^-$ (mEq/L) | ALBUMIN (g/L) | DEXTRAN (g/L) | HES (g/L) | COP (mm/Hg) |
|---|---|---|---|---|---|---|---|
| Human serum albumin (5%) | 9 | 154 | 154 | 50 | | | 20 |
| Plasmanate (heat-treated plasma protein fraction) | 9 | 130–160 | 130 | 42 | | | 18 |
| Human serum albumin (25%) Salt-poor albumin | 9 | 154 | 154 | 12.5g/50 mL | | | 100 |
| Dextran 40 in dextrose | | | | | 100 | | 68 |
| Dextran 40 in normal saline | 9 | 154 | 154 | | 100 | | 68 |
| Dextran 70 | 9 | 154 | 154 | | 60 | | 70 |
| Hydroxyethyl starch | 9 | 154 | 154 | | | 60 | 70 |

* The abbreviations used are: PL, plasma volume; ARF, acute renal failure; HES, hydroxyethyl-substituted amylopectin; COP, colloid oncotic pressure.
† Cost represents contract prices for a large metropolitan hospital.

TABLE 4-8. Characteristics of Various Crystalloid Solutions*

| | SODIUM CONTENT (g/L) | $Na^+$ (mEq/L) | $K^+$ (mEq/L) | $Ca^{2+}$ (mEq/L) | $Mg^{2+}$ (mEq/L) | $Cl^-$ (mEq/L) | LACTATE (mEq/L) | ACETATE (mEq/L) |
|---|---|---|---|---|---|---|---|---|
| Lactated Ringer's | 6 | 130 | 4 | 3 | | 109 | 28 | |
| Lactated Ringer's with D5 | 6 | 130 | 4 | 3 | | 109 | 28 | |
| Normal saline | 9 | 154 | | | | 154 | | |
| 5% Dextrose, ⅓ normal saline | 3.3 | 56 | | | | 56 | | |
| Hypertonic lactated saline | 14.5 | 250 to 300 | | | | 100 to 150 | 100 to 200 racemic | |
| Plasma-lyte A | 8 | 140 | 5 | | 3 | 98 | | 27 |
| Normosol-R (pH 7.4) | 8 | 140 | 5 | | 3 | 98 | | |
| $D_5W$ | | | | | | | | |

* The abbreviations used are: PL, plasma volume; D5, five percent dextrose; $D_5W$, five percent dextrose solution in water.
† Cost represents contract prices for a large metropolitan hospital.

| DEXTROSE (g/L) | pH | OSMOLALITY (mOsm/L) | INCREASE IN PLASMA VOLUME (per 100 mL) | DISTRIBUTION | COST† ($/L) | COMPLICATIONS |
|---|---|---|---|---|---|---|
| | 6.6 | 290 | 50 to 100, unpredictable | PL (IFS) | 150 | Urticaria, fever, chills (0.05%) |
| | 6.9 | 290 | 50 to 100, unpredictable | PL (IFS) | 37.65/ 250 mL | |
| | 6.9 | 310 | 100 to 450 in 60′ | PL (IFS) | 36.50/ 50-ml vial | Urticaria, fever, chills (0.05%) |
| 50 | 6.7 | 320 | 50 to 70, short-lived | PL (IFS) | 29.33 | ARF<br>Anaphylaxis (0.008%)<br>Anaphylactoid reactions (0.035%)<br>Clotting defect at doses >20 ml/kg/ 24 h |
| | 6.7 | 320 | 50 to 70, short-lived | PL (IFS) | 29.33 | ARF<br>Anaphylaxis (0.008%)<br>Anaphylactoid reactions (0.035%)<br>Clotting defect at doses >20 ml/kg/ 24 h |
| | 6.3 | 320 | 80 to 100 | PL | 169.82 | Anaphylaxis (0.008%)<br>Anaphylactoid reactions (0.035%)<br>Clotting defect at doses >20 ml/kg/ 24 h |
| | 5.5 | 310 | 70, long-lasting | PL | 71.70 | Clotting defect? (dose related)<br>Interference with immune system?? |

| GLUCONATE (mEq/L) | DEXTROSE (g/L) | pH | OSMOLARITY (mOsm/L) | DISTRIBUTION | COST† ($/L) | COMPLICATIONS |
|---|---|---|---|---|---|---|
| | | 5.1 | 273 | PL, IFS | 1 | Peripheral edema<br>↑ Lactate?<br>Lactic acidosis?? |
| | 50 | 4.6 | 525 | PL, IFS, ICF, dextrose | 0.92 | Peripheral edema<br>↑ Lactate?<br>Lactic acidosis?? |
| | | 6.0 | 308 | PL, IFS | 0.78 | Peripheral edema<br>↑ Serum $Cl^-$?<br>Metabolic acidosis?? |
| | 50 | 4.0 | 365 | PL, IFS, ICF, dextrose | 0.82 | Peripheral edema |
| | | | 550 | PL, IFS | 1.29 | Hypernatremia<br>Hyperosmolality |
| 23 | | 7.4 | 294 | PL, IFS | 2.19 | Hypocalcemia?<br>Peripheral edema? |
| | | 7.4 | 295 | PL, IFS | 1.92 | Peripheral edema<br>Hypocalcemia? |
| | 50 | 4.0 | 252 | PL, IFS, ICF | 0.81 | Peripheral edema<br>Unable to augment plasma volume |

sis.[152] In 1896, when Starling[238] published his now-famous equation describing transcapillary albumin flux, he emphasized that capillary hydraulic conductivity would likely be altered by changes in venular pressure and interstitial space dynamics. Pulmonary failure after hemorrhagic shock is associated with increased transcapillary albumin flux; albumin can be detected in the airway secretions. The use of supplemental albumin to restore intravascular oncotic pressure and thereby to reduce the net transcapillary loss of salt and water is based on the assumption that this added albumin will remain within the blood vessels. This theoretical objective of supplemental albumin therapy is frustrated by two generally unrecognized facts: (1) most of the total body albumin is normally located within the interstitial space; and (2) 7% of intravascular albumin leaves the plasma volume each hour.[152,242] Interestingly, supplemental albumin therapy for hemorrhagic shock actually increases the rate of extravascular flux to 10%/h.[150,152] The factors leading to this increased flux are not known, but its effects on extravascular oncotic pressure do not help and may aggravate ARDS. Changes in extravascular albumin flux may be related in part to an alteration in the IFS matrix and a reapportionment of fluid between the sol and the gel portions of the IFS.[47,183,242] When the gel portion excludes albumin, the effective oncotic pressure within the sol portion is elevated.[183] Thus, albumin returns more quickly to the plasma via the lymphatic system. Supplemental albumin therapy may permit incorporation of more albumin in the matrix, thereby increasing the IFS oncotic pressure and augmenting transcapillary albumin leak. Virgilio and coworkers[253] demonstrated that albumin-depleted baboons have a marked increase in pulmonary lymphatic albumin efflux, reducing the pulmonary interstitial oncotic pressure and helping to maintain an optimal plasma to interstitial oncotic ratio. Starling's equation assumed a closed system with no albumin leak and no lymphatic system. The dynamic interactions between the plasma and IFS preclude the blind application of Starling's equation in a situation in which the complex interactions within the interstitial space cannot be measured. Because of this restriction, the only meaningful way to evaluate the therapeutic merits of albumin is by clinical trial.

During a 2-year period, 94 trauma patients treated by the Emergency Surgery Service at Detroit General Hospital were randomized and prospectively studied. The resuscitation regimen used for all patients included BES and blood upon the patients' arrival at the emergency room. Approximately 1 U of fresh frozen plasma (FFP) was given for every 7 U of transfused blood to restore deficiencies in coagulation factors. These 94 patients were in shock (systolic pressure below 80 mm Hg) for an average of 33 minutes and received an average of 14.5 U of blood, 9 L of BES, and 2.7 U of FFP while they were in the emergency and operating rooms. Forty-six patients also received an average of 31 g of supplemental albumin during the operation and 150 g/day for the next 3 to 5 days. This regimen was chosen to restore serum albumin levels to normal and was based upon previous retrospective studies. Following the operation, serial measurements were made in order to monitor the effects of supplemental albumin on individual organ function.

The combination of hypovolemic shock and treatment with the standard nonalbumin regimen produced a decrease in both total serum protein (TSP) and serum albumin (SA) concentrations. The TSP and SA averaged, at the time of the first postoperative study, 5.4 and 2.9 g/dL, respectively. The SA concentration in nonalbumin patients remained below 3 g/dL throughout the first 5 postoperative days. The mean TSP and SA concentrations in the albumin-treated patients averaged 6.04 and 4.2 g/dL, respectively. The SA concentration rose from 3.4 g/dL immediately following the operation to 4.7 g/dL by 4 days. The increased SA concentration was associated with an increased plasma volume (3895 versus 3579 mL), whereas red cell volumes were equal between the two groups. This increased plasma volume in the albumin-treated patients was associated with an increase in renal plasma flow but, paradoxically, a decrease in GFR, sodium clearance, osmolar clearance, and urine output.[145] These changes were present throughout the first 5 postoperative days; 21 of the albumin-treated patients required loop diuretics compared with only 10 of the non–albumin-treated patients. Furthermore, 13 of the albumin-treated patients developed acute renal insufficiency compared with only one of the non–albumin-treated patients. Renal insufficiency was considered present when the GFR fell below 30 mL/min or the serum creatinine exceeded 3.0 mg/dL.

The impaired salt and water excretion in the albumin patients led to increased weight gain during the fluid sequestration phase (8 versus 6.1 kg) and was associated with a significant increase in central filling pressures.[152] The CVP and the $P_{pw}$ were both significantly elevated in the albumin-treated patients; this led to impaired oxygenation as reflected by the $FIO_2/PO_2$ ratio. At the time of the first postoperative study, the average $FIO_2/PO_2$ ratio was 0.62 in the albumin-treated patients and 0.33 in the non–albumin-treated patients.[152] This impaired oxygenation was also reflected in an increased physiologic shunting in the lungs, which averaged 29% in the albumin patients compared with 19% in the nonalbumin patients. The albumin-treated patients required ventilator therapy for an average of 7.7 days, and the nonalbumin patients, for 2.9 days.[152]

After analyzing the changes in pulmonary oxygenation, central filling pressures, and the need for diuresis, it became apparent that albumin may also interfere with left ventricular function and exert a negative inotropic effect in the heart.[45] This possibility was analyzed by noting the ratio of left ventricular work to central filling pressure as monitored by either the LVSWI/$P_{pw}$ ratio or a calculated index of left ventricular work/central venous pressure.[45] All of these ratios were reduced in the albumin patients compared with the nonalbumin patients. The compromise in left ventricular function indicated by these findings resulted in an increased need for inotropic support of the heart. Twenty-four of the 46 albumin patients were digitalized for congestive heart failure, whereas only 11 of the 48 nonalbumin patients required digitalization. The mechanism whereby supplemental albumin might cause ventricular dysfunction is unclear. Myocardial depression has been reported after shock, and a myocardial depressant factor, possibly of pancreatic origin, has been postulated.[45] Albumin might potentiate the release of such a factor although no evidence for this phenomenon is available. Alternatively, albumin might impair cardiac function by altering calcium dynamics. The albumin patients had an increase in total serum calcium concentration but a reduction in both the level of ionized calcium and the ratio of ionized to total calcium.[149] Hypocalcemia is known to decrease the excitability of myocardial cells and to inhibit intracellular enzyme function including oxidative phosphorylation. Clearly, the detrimental effects of albumin on myocardial, renal, and respiratory functions are interrelated and mitigate against the use of albumin supplementation for hypovolemic shock.

Other potential hazards relate to the effects of albumin on the immunoglobulin system, the coagulation system, and the intrahepatic production of needed proteins. The albumin-treated patients had a uniform reduction in all nonalbumin proteins.[115] Therefore, patients resuscitated with albumin have decreased levels of immunoglobulins associated with a reduction in immunoglobulin activity as judged by the immune response to tetanus toxoid.[30,56] Albumin-treated patients also had a reduction in coagulation activity as reflected by increased prothrombin times and decreased fibrinogen activity.[154] These alterations correlated with an increased need for transfusion after the operation.[115] These findings have been confirmed in a canine model of hemorrhagic shock in which one group was resuscitated with shed blood and crystalloid whereas the other received blood, crystalloid, and albumin.[137] Confirmation of these adverse effects of albumin supplementation in a controlled animal study indicates that the clinical findings were not spurious.

Several criticisms of this trial relate to the amount of supplemental albumin infusion and the duration of therapy (3 to 5 days). Both the amount and duration of albumin therapy were designed to restore serum oncotic pressure to a normal level of 22 mOsm/L both during the operation and in the early postresuscitation period when volume needs are large and pulmonary failure is anticipated. Despite this regimen, these objectives were not reached: the average serum oncotic pressure was only 19 mOsm/L by day 2 in the albumin-supplemented patients compared with 14.5 mOsm/L in the crystalloid group. Our findings demonstrating the superiority of crystalloids over albumin have been reflected in the results of a recent metaanalysis that compared mortality following resuscitation with crystalloid and colloid solutions: the overall mortality of trauma patients treated with crystalloids was 12.3% less than those treated with colloids.[249]

Controversy still exists regarding the use of albumin versus crystalloids. The proponents of albumin[19,98,113,202,228,229,230] contend that volume resuscitation can be accomplished faster and with much smaller volumes of colloid than of crystalloid solutions. Such studies place little emphasis on restoration of function to organs such as the kidney. Another argument involves the severe reduction of colloid oncotic pressure (COP) and the decreased gradient between COP and $P_{pw}$ (COP − $P_{pw}$) seen with crystalloids; this is said to favor the development of pulmonary edema.[202] Reduction in COP is a common occurrence with large-volume crystalloid resuscitation. Interstitial COP, however, changes with the intravascular COP; thus, the effective oncotic pressure is not altered after crystalloid resuscitation. Furthermore, it has been shown in both animals and humans that this reduction during crystalloid infusion is not associated with increased pulmonary extravascular lung water.[67,68,247] The use of the COP − $P_{pw}$ gradient[257] as an index of pulmonary interstitial water content or as a predictor of pulmonary edema may be erroneous.[247] Pulmonary artery wedge pressure is not equal to pulmonary capillary pressure. Thus, it cannot be used in Starling's law. Furthermore, Starling's law does not take into account the balance between fluid flux into the interstitium and the evacuation of this fluid by the lymphatic vessels. Although Rackow et al[202] demonstrated that crystalloid infusion was associated with a greater incidence of pulmonary edema than albumin, the majority of their patients were septic, and their mean age was 79. Tranbaugh and coworkers[247] showed that the primary determinants of pulmonary interstitial fluid accumulation in trauma patients were sepsis and lung contusion and not the type of fluid administered. A final argument of albumin proponents is that the increased peripheral edema caused by crystalloid solutions delays wound healing and interferes with tissue oxygen exchange.[248] Preliminary unpublished data from this unit deny this effect.

Crystalloid proponents argue that (1) the contracted extracellular compartment can be expanded more effectively by crystalloid solutions than by albumin;[224,253] (2) increased $P_{pw}$ is less likely with this solution than with albumin because of rapid equilibration;[253] (3) crystalloid solutions are considerably less expensive than the albumin or synthetic colloid solutions;[144,181] (4) better postoperative organ function can be maintained with crystalloid solutions than with albumin;[30,45,145,152,154] and (5) the risk of anaphylactoid reactions is eliminated by the use of crystalloid solutions.[169]

There is yet a third group of clinicians who believe that a successful outcome can be achieved using either approach[135] or by combining both crystalloid and colloid solutions.[235] Although we believe strongly that Ringer's lactate and blood are far superior to albumin solutions for volume resuscitation of multiple trauma patients, other studies may be needed to explore this issue further.

## HYPERTONIC SALT SOLUTIONS

There has been a growing interest in the use of hypertonic salt solutions for resuscitation of various shock states. The efficacy of these solutions in improving hemodynamic status has been shown experimentally in thermal burn,[161] hemorrhage,[33,131,170,184,250] and endotoxic shock[199] models. The results of several clinical studies also suggest that hypertonic saline solutions may be beneficial during resuscitation of the injured.[24,39,40,49,107,160,182,216] The advantages of these solutions include a smaller water load to achieve the same hemodynamic end point as lactated Ringer's solution,[184,198,199] less peripheral edema after resuscitation,[24,177,182] and more sustained hemodynamic effect than that obtained with isotonic crystalloid solutions[250] although there has been no universal agreement about the last.[198,199] Various hypertonic solutions including glucose, mannitol, NaCl, and $NaHCO_3$ have been used experimentally, but only NaCl has gained acceptance for clinical use.[250] The hemodynamic effects of both glucose and mannitol are evanescent because of their osmotic diuretic properties, and $NaHCO_3$ may result in a severe hyperosmotic state, metabolic alkalosis, and hypokalemia. Hypertonic saline has been used in two different concentrations: hypertonic lactated saline with a sodium content of 250 to

300 mEq/L (Table 4-8) and 7.5% NaCl, with a sodium concentration of 1200 mEq/L. Table 4-9 shows the osmolarity, sodium content, molar concentration, and osmotic pressure of these solutions. Recently Cross et al[39,40] also described the postoperative use of 1.8% NaCl in cardiac surgical patients. Each mOsm of an osmotically active substance produces an osmotic pressure of 19 mm Hg. Thus, hypertonic solutions with osmolarity between 550 and 2400 mOsm can generate osmotic pressure many times normal. In the hospital, only solutions containing sodium within the range of 250 to 300 mEq/L have been used[24,177,182,216] although deFelippe et al[49] used 7.5% saline solution (4 mL/kg) in hemorrhagic shock patients without any apparent adverse effects.

The use of 7.5% saline solution is favored in the prehospital setting in which the constricted veins of the trauma victim may make large bore intravenous cannula insertion difficult and thereby preclude infusion of adequate fluid volume. Although 7.5% NaCl allows rapid improvement of hemodynamics with small volumes (4 mL/kg) of fluid, the beneficial effect of this solution is evanescent, lasting only 15 minutes. Addition of 6% dextran 70 to this solution prolongs the effect to 30 or more minutes. This hypertonic/hyperoncotic solution has already been shown to be superior to lactated Ringer's or Plasma-lyte A for resuscitation of trauma victims in the field.[107,160]

Hypertonic saline solutions improve the hemodynamic status of hypovolemic patients primarily by restoring extracellular fluid volume with intracellular water.[50] Since sodium enters the cell slowly, an osmotic gradient is created between the extracellular and intracellular spaces with subsequent efflux of water from the cell. In addition, hyperosmotic solutions improve myocardial contractility,[122,260] constrict capacitance vessels, and induce precapillary dilatation in both systemic and pulmonary vasculature.[72,155,158,184] The pulmonary vasodilator effect of hypertonic saline results in improvement of right ventricular function and augmentation of the cardiac output. Lopes et al[142] have suggested that the cardiac effects of hypertonic saline are mediated, at least in part, by pulmonary or peripheral osmoreceptors, since infusion of 7.5% NaCl into the aortas of dogs or intravenously to vagotomized dogs produced little hemodynamic improvement. More recent data suggest that increased contractility is a direct response of the myocardium to increased osmolarity.[123]

The extent of reduction in resuscitative volume with hypertonic saline, as compared with isotonic solutions, depends on the osmotic concentration of the fluid used. Solutions with relatively low osmolarity (550 mOsm) may allow a 15 to 20% volume reduction as compared with lactated Ringer's infusion.[184] It is notable that the sodium load during resuscitation with hypertonic saline solution may be the same as that administered with lactated Ringer's solution.[198] Urine output increases with all hypertonic saline solutions, probably because of osmotic diuresis.[156] Likewise, urinary sodium excretion increases when the serum sodium level exceeds 150 mEq/L. The net loss from the intracellular space during acute resuscitation with hypertonic fluids usually amounts to 2 to 3 L, which is not likely to cause significant cell dehydration.[184] However, the optimal volume of intracellular water after severe shock is not known, and continued infusion of hypertonic solutions may lead to cell dehydration and injury.

Except for burn resuscitation, hypertonic saline has not yet been used routinely for intrahospital management of the trauma victim. In a small group of trauma patients, Holcroft and coworkers[107] showed that intraoperative use of 3% NaCl restored blood pressure, pH, and urine output with 50% of the fluid volume required by a comparable group of patients treated with balanced salt solution. The advantage offered by hypertonic saline during the operation was less obvious than that observed in the prehospital setting. However, hypertonic saline may prove useful during the initial resuscitation of drug addicts or small children who have limited venous access. In this situation hypertonic saline can be infused through a small-gauge cannula until a large cannula is inserted for isotonic solutions.

Hypertonic saline may offer other benefits. Cross and coworkers,[39,40] using 1.8% NaCl in the postoperative period, demonstrated an early negative fluid balance and attenuation of hormonal response to injury. The mechanism whereby the stress response is suppressed by hypertonic saline is not known. These authors also showed less postoperative chest tube drainage than was seen in patients treated with isotonic solutions, probably because of decreased edema formation. This suggests that interstitial hydrostatic pressure after hypertonic saline is also lower than that produced by balanced electrolyte solutions. Consequently the inference can be made that the morbidity and mortality associated with edema and compartment syndrome after extremity trauma may be reduced by using hypertonic saline. For the same reason these solutions may be useful in the resuscitation of multiple trauma patients with closed-head injury and hemorrhagic shock.

Resuscitation of brain-injured animals with crystalloids results in transient elevation of ICP.[195,246,263] Hyperoncotic volume expanders also increase brain water or may augment the cerebral blood flow, resulting in increased ICP[1,63,222,263] al-

TABLE 4-9. Characteristics of Hypertonic Fluids

| | OSMOLARITY (mOsm/L) | SODIUM CONTENT (mEq/L) | MOLAR CONCENTRATION (M) | OSMOTIC PRESSURE (mm Hg) |
|---|---|---|---|---|
| 0.9% NaCl | 310 | 155 | 0.15 | 5,900 |
| Hypertonic lactated saline | 550 | 250 | 0.25 | 10,450 |
| 8.4% $NaHCO_3$ | 1,800 | 900 | 0.9 | 34,200 |
| 7.5% NaCl | 2,400 | 1,200 | 1.2 | 45,600 |

though generally the extent of increase is less than that produced by crystalloids.[195,246] By shifting fluids from intracellular and interstitial compartments into the vascular space, hypertonic saline may reduce the brain volume and minimize ICP elevation. There has been no human study to substantiate this hypothesis. However, in animals with intact or injured brain, ICP increase is less with hypertonic than with isotonic crystalloid solutions.[198,265] Conversely, reduction of ICP with highly concentrated saline solutions may possibly produce a subdural hematoma by causing disruption of intracranial veins.[7] Further studies are obviously needed.

Several complications may arise from the use of hypertonic saline solutions. An elevated serum sodium level may lead to seizures, especially in pediatric and elderly patients. Thus, serum $Na^+$ should be monitored frequently. The serum $Na^+$ concentration is considered safe up to 155 to 160 mEq/L. If values are above that level, volume replacement should be continued with isotonic solutions.[50] A hyperosmolar state may arise not only from an elevated serum sodium level but also from the concomitant elevation of serum glucose which is frequently seen in acutely traumatized patients. Thus, serum glucose and osmolality should also be monitored. Concern has also been expressed about the rapid increase of blood pressure produced by hypertonic solutions in the presence of uncontrolled hemorrhagic shock. Elevation of blood pressure before surgical control of intraabdominal and thoracic injuries can increase bleeding and thus precipitate irreversible shock.[83,84] In addition a rapid expansion of the extracellular space may produce hypokalemia and arrhythmias. Hypertonic solutions also cause venous irritation and phlebitis. Dextran-containing solutions may also cause bleeding abnormalities and interference with cross-matching of blood.

## DEXTRAN SOLUTIONS (TABLE 4-7)

Dextrans, commonly used in the 1960s and 1970s as volume expanders, have lost their popularity in recent years, probably because of their potential to cause allergic reactions and the availability of other synthetic colloids. Dextrans are produced by enzymatic conversion of sucrose by lactobacilli or a special bacterial strain, *Leuconostoc mesenteroides* B-512. Dextrans are long-chain linear polysaccharide molecules with a high molecular weight; they behave as colloids. Dextran 70 (Macrodex) and dextran 40 (Rheomacrodex) are the preparations available on the market. Dextran 70 is supplied as a 6% solution in normal saline. It is composed of molecules with an average molecular weight of 70,000, comparable to that of albumin (65,000). However, dextran 70 is more hyperoncotic than albumin. Each gram of dextran 70 retains approximately 25 mL of water within the intravascular space, whereas each gram of plasma proteins can retain only 13 mL.[57] Dextran 70 produces an 80 to 120% increase in plasma volume[127,228] and has an intravascular retention of 30% 24 hours after infusion.[57,171]

Dextran 40 is supplied as a 10% solution in either normal saline or 5% dextrose. Its average molecular weight is 40,000. Shortly after infusion, small molecules either enter the interstitial space or are excreted by the kidney; therefore, the effect of dextran 40 on intravascular volume is shorter in duration than that of dextran 70. Dextran 40 has an intravascular retention of less than 60% at 4 hours after infusion.[57]

Because of their high oncotic pressures (two to eight times that of plasma proteins), both dextran 70 and dextran 40 cause a transient diminution in interstitial fluid volume.[164] Therefore, they should be administered with large amounts of crystalloids, preferably lactated Ringer's solution. The adverse effects of dextrans are not limited to early interstitial volume depletion. Most dextran 40 molecules are filtered by the kidney; few are reabsorbed by the tubules. In hypovolemic patients with reduced renal blood flow and urine formation, these molecules may block the renal tubules and produce renal failure.[58] This complication, however, does not occur with dextran 70 (or hetastarch) probably because the molecular weights of most particles in these solutions are above the renal threshold.

Both dextran 40 and dextran 70 solutions, when given at a dose greater than 1.5 g/kg/day (ie, greater than 1500 mL in an average adult), can cause coagulation abnormalities and produce bleeding. The mechanism of this clotting defect is not known definitely. Coating of the platelets with a dextran film and dilution of coagulation factors with intravascular volume expansion are thought to contribute to this complication.[57] Prolonged prothrombin time (PT), partial thromboplastin time (PTT), and bleeding time and reduced platelet counts have been reported following large amounts of dextran infusion.[57] Perhaps because of these effects on coagulation, dextran 40 but not dextran 70 improves blood rheology in the microcirculation. Erythrocyte sludging, frequently seen in hemorrhagic shock, is minimized by dextran 40 infusion.[57] The mechanism is thought to be a reduction of intercellular binding forces by the formation of a dextran film over the erythrocytes. However, hemodilution by the saline solvent may also be responsible for the improved microcirculatory blood flow.[57] Dextran infusion also interferes with subsequent cross-matching or sedimentation rate measurements. Thus, prior to these studies, erythrocytes must be washed.[21] Perioperative administration of dextran 40 is shown to reduce the incidence of postoperative thromboembolic complications.[85]

Anaphylactoid reactions occur with dextran at a frequency of 0.032%.[208] Severe, life-threatening complications are less frequent (0.008%).[208] These reactions appear to be more pronounced in anesthetized or unconscious patients.[64] Based on the above-mentioned disadvantages, many clinicians believe that dextrans should not be used in trauma patients as intravascular volume expanders and that their use should be reserved for preventing thrombotic or thromboembolic complications.[21,248] However, Modig[174] showed that early aggressive treatment of traumatic shock with dextran 70 and continuation of this therapy in the posttrauma period for 1 week resulted in a significantly lower incidence of ARDS than was observed with Ringer's acetate solution. We no longer use dextran in resuscitation of injured patients with hemorrhagic shock.

## RESUSCITATION WITH HYDROXYETHYL-SUBSTITUTED AMYLOPECTIN (HES) (TABLE 4-7)

Currently, the most popular form of HES is a 6% solution of hetastarch in 0.9% sodium chloride, Hespan. HES is formed by selectively substituting hydroxyethyl starch radicals onto the amylopectin moiety of starch, thus yielding a heterogenous group of molecules with a molecular weight ranging from 10,000 to over one million (average, 450,000). Its osmolarity is approximately 310 mOsm/L, pH is 5.5, and colloid oncotic pressure is 30 mm Hg. In animals, HES has been shown to stay within the vascular space for days and augment plasma volume as effectively as human serum albumin. Thompson and Walton[243] showed that HES, when compared with dextran, remained within the vascular system longer, was less toxic, and caused fewer adverse reactions or effects on the coagulation system. More recently, Shatney and coworkers[218] prospectively compared HES with 5% plasma protein fraction (PPF) in 32 patients with traumatic shock. They concluded that HES leads to plasma volume restoration equivalent to that with PPF and affects organ function, including that of the liver, lungs, and kidneys as does PPF. The PTT, however, was significantly prolonged after HES, whereas the PT and platelet counts were similar for two groups. In this study an average of 3600 mL of HES was administered within a short period of time. The elevated PTT lasted 48 hours and then returned to normal (Fig 4-12). Despite a prolongation in PTT, none of the patients showed clinically significant bleeding abnormalities. The recommended safe dose of HES as a component therapy for surgical blood loss is 20 mL/kg.[94]

FIG. 4-12. Platelet count, partial thromboplastin time, prothrombin time, and hematocrit following hydroxyethyl starch and albumin infusion in traumatized patients. (From Shatney et al[218] with permission.)

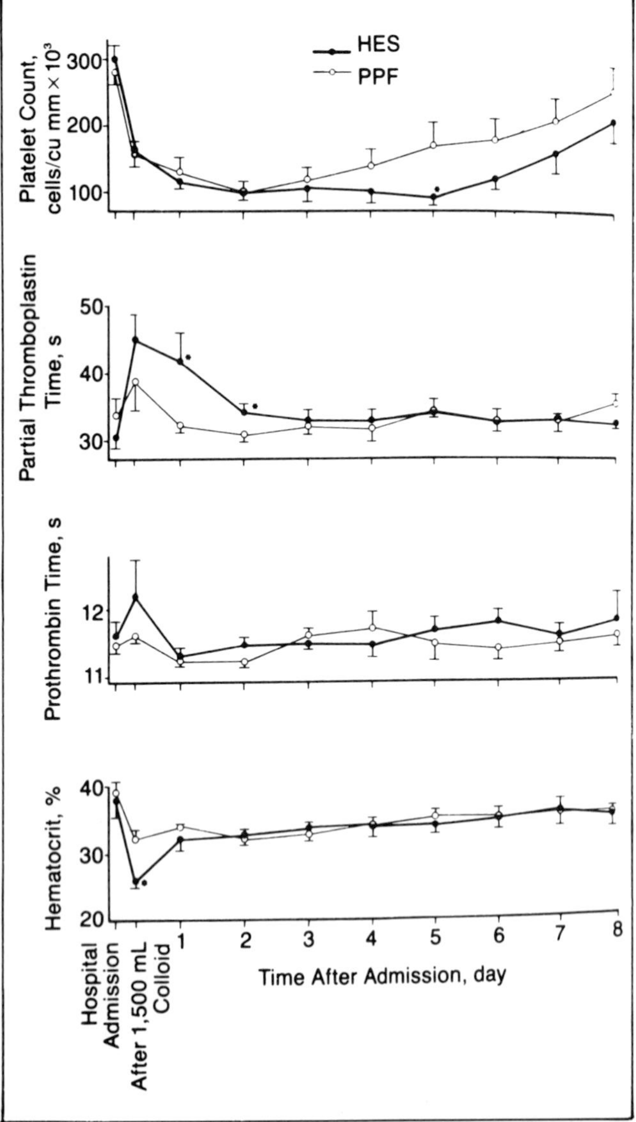


Rock and Wise[211] noted that the rise in the PTT after HES therapy was additive when HES was given daily for 4 days. Coagulation abnormalities after HES result primarily from dilution of platelets and coagulant proteins. However, we have demonstrated recently in dogs that HES, like albumin, induces relocation of serum proteins into the IFS and from there to the lymphatic system.[148] This oncotically driven protein shift probably serves to maintain a specific lymph to plasma oncotic balance. The end result is a decrease in all serum protein levels and functions including procoagulant activity. Hemodilution with HES should be done carefully in head-injured patients, since coagulopathy caused by this agent may result in fatal intracranial hemorrhage.[46] The potential adverse effects of HES on the coagulation system and other plasma protein functions need further prospective analysis in both man and animals. The effect of HES on other physiologic responses including pulmonary function, inotropic effectiveness, immune function, and liver and kidney function should also be evaluated, although available human studies suggest remarkable safety with this agent.[97,132,175,200,201] Anaphylactoid reactions have been reported with hydroxyethyl starch at a frequency of about 0.006%.[208]

## CONCLUSION

Care of the injured patient begins at the time of injury and involves a well-established communication system, emergency medical service system, and strategically located trauma centers designed and prepared to care for the injured patient. Initial therapy for the patient should maintain cardiovascular function, secure the airway, and stop the bleeding. Once these are accomplished, treatment of hemorrhagic shock takes priority. This treatment should limit the duration of the body's natural compensatory responses to hemorrhagic shock—responses such as peripheral vasoconstriction, reduced renal blood flow and urinary excretion, and the release of humoral agents designed to maintain perfusion of the heart and brain while decreasing the amount of blood and fluid in the extravascular spaces. Part of this action includes a relocation of electrolytes and water from the interstitial space into the plasma.

Severe hemorrhagic shock therefore requires rapid resuscitation with blood and balanced electrolyte solution. The end points of this resuscitation should be restoration of peripheral perfusion, as shown by blood pressure, pulse, and urine output, and also of extravascular volume. When such restoration is accomplished, oxygen delivery is provided for maintenance of organ function. Currently, red cell replacement is provided by packed red cells since most trauma centers do not have ready access to large volumes of whole blood when the patient first arrives. Ringer's lactate solution may be used as the balanced electrolyte solution to restore intravascular and extravascular volume deficits. During the period of active hemorrhage neither fresh frozen plasma nor platelet transfusion is indicated unless the patient shows evidence of unexplained nonmechanical bleeding.

Various colloid supplements have been advocated for treatment of hypovolemia. The most popular of these has been human serum albumin. Based upon the effects of albumin on organ function, its cost, and a lack of demonstrated benefit, albumin supplementation is not recommended by the authors. Other colloids such as the dextrans are less useful during active hemorrhage because of problems related to coagulopathy, expense, and lack of effectiveness. Hetastarch appears to be effective and safe in fluid resuscitation of the injured. Crystalloid solutions advocated for resuscitation from hemorrhagic shock include normal saline, hypertonic saline, Plasma-lyte A, and Normosol-R. Although much study remains to be done with these agents the authors advocate a balanced electrolyte solution that mimics plasma concentrations.

Following restoration of circulatory volume and surgical control of bleeding, the patient typically enters into a period of extravascular fluid sequestration characterized by total body weight gain caused by expansion of the intracellular and interstitial spaces. This phase lasts an average of 24 to 36 hours in patients who require an average of 15 U of blood during the period of acute bleeding. This extravascular fluid sequestration occurs at the expense of the plasma volume; thus, rational therapy requires large volumes of balanced electrolyte solution in order to maintain effective plasma volume and peripheral perfusion. The use of supplemental colloid such as albumin at this time does not prevent extravascular fluid sequestration since 55% of the normal extravascular albumin is located within the interstitial space, and administration of supplemental albumin equilibrates in the same ratio between the plasma and the interstitial space. During this period diuretic therapy for oliguria aggravates the hypovolemic state. Concomitant support of the heart and lungs may be required.

Following stabilization, the patient enters into a fluid mobilization period when the previously sequestered fluid is returned to the plasma and excreted by the kidneys. During the early portion of this phase the patient may develop acute expansion of the plasma volume; diuretic therapy may be helpful in augmenting excretion of the excess fluid if renal function has been depressed by the episode of shock. During this period fluids should be restricted, and sodium load should be reduced since the patient is in a transient period of hypervolemia and occasionally of hypertension. Once diuresis occurs the various body compartments will return toward normal as will organ function. Whenever sepsis supervenes during the extravascular sequestration phase, the mobilization phase is delayed and morbidity and mortality from the combined insults rise. Appropriate antibiotic therapy and organ system support are necessary throughout this time.

## REFERENCES


1. Albright AL, Phillips JW. Oncotic therapy of experimental cerebral oedema. Acta Neuro Chir 1982;60:257.
2. Alyono D, Ring WS, Chao RY, et al. Characteristics of ventricular function in severe hemorrhagic shock. Surgery 1983; 94:250.
3. Annat G, Viale JP, Bui-Xuan B, et al. Effect of PEEP ventilation on renal function, plasma renin, aldosterone, neurophysins and urinary ADH, and prostaglandins. Anesthesiology 1983;58:136.
4. Antonenko DR. Early structural changes in mitochondria in response to acute reductions in capillary flow on oxygen transport to tissues. Adv Med Biol 1976;75:165.
5. Aono K, Tanaka T, Urakami H, et al. Physicochemical changes during hemorrhage and following infusion. Br J Anaesth 1981; 53:973.
6. Archer G, Cobb A. Long-term pulmonary artery pressure monitoring in the management of the critically ill. Ann Surg 1974; 180:747.
7. Arvidsson S, Haggendal E, Winso I. Effect on cerebral blood flow of infusion of hyperosmolar saline during cerebral vasodilation in the dog. Acta Anaesthesiol Scand 1981;25:153.
8. Averill DB, Scherr AM, Feigl ED. Angiotension causes vasoconstriction during hemorrhage in baroreceptor denervated dogs. Am J Physiol 1983;245:H667.
9. Barriot P, Riou B. Hemorrhagic shock with paradoxical bradycardia. Intensive Care Med 1987;13:203.
10. Bellamy RF, DeGuzman LR, Pedersen DC. Immediate hemodynamic consequences of MAST inflation in normal and hypovolemic anesthetized swine. J Trauma 1984;24:889.
11. Benedict CR, Grahame-Smith DG. Plasma noradrenaline and adrenaline concentrations and dopamine hydroxylase activity in patients with shock due to septicemia, trauma and hemorrhage. Q J Med 1978;47:1.
12. Berry AJ. Respiratory support and renal function. Anesthesiology 1981;55:655.
13. Berry AJ, Geer RT, Marshall C, et al. The effect of long-term controlled mechanical ventilation with positive end-expiratory pressure on renal function in dogs. Anesthesiology 1984;61:406.
14. Berryhill RE, Benumof JL, Rauscher LA. Pulmonary venous pressure reading at the end of exhalation. Anesthesiology 1978; 49:365.
15. Bickell WH, Pepe PE, Bailey ML, et al. Randomized trial of pneumatic antishock garments in the prehospital management of penetrating abdominal injuries. Ann Emerg Med 1987; 16:653.
16. Bivins HG, Knopp R, dos Santos PAL. Blood volume distribution in the Trendelenburg position. Ann Emerg Med 1985;14:641.
17. Bivins HG, Knopp R, Tiernan C, et al. Blood volume displacement with inflation of anti-shock trousers. Ann Emerg Med 1982;11;409.
18. Bond RF, Johnson GJ. Vascular adrenergic interactions during hemorrhagic shock. Fed Proc 1985;44:281.
19. Boutros AR, Ruess R, Olson L, et al. Comparison of hemodynamic, pulmonary and renal effects of use of three types of fluids following major surgical procedures on the abdominal aorta. Crit Care Med 1979;7:9.
20. Boysen PG. Hemodynamic monitoring in the adult respiratory distress syndrome. Clin Chest Med 1982;3:157.
21. Bristow A, Giesecke AH. Fluid therapy of trauma. Semin Anesth 1985;4:124.
22. Burchard KW, Slotman GJ, Jed E, et al. Positive pressure respirators and pneumatic anti-shock garment application: hemodynamic response. J Trauma 1985;25:83.
23. Byrnes GJ, Pirkle JC Jr, Gann DS. Cardiovascular stabilization

after hemorrhage depends upon restitution of blood volume. J Trauma 1978;18:623.
24. Caldwell FT, Bowser BH. Critical evaluation of hypertonic and hypotonic solutions to resuscitate severely burned children: a prospective study. Ann Surg 1979;189:546.
25. Carey LC, Lowery BD, Cloutier CT. Blood sugar and insulin response in human shock. Ann Surg 1970;172:342.
26. Carey LD, Lowery BD, Cloutier CT. Hemorrhagic shock. Curr Prob Surg 1971;8:1048.
27. Carlon GC, Howland WS, Goldiner PS, et al. Adverse effects of calcium administration. Arch Surg 1978;113:882.
28. Civetta JM, Gabel JC, Laver MB. Disparate ventricular function in surgical patients. Surg Forum 1971;22;136.
29. Civetta JM, Nussenfeld SR, Rowe TR, et al. Prehospital use of military anti-shock trouser (MAST). JACEP 1976;5:581.
30. Clift DR, Lucas CE, Ledgerwood AM, et al. The effect of albumin resuscitation for shock on immunoglobulin activity. J Surg Res 1982;32:449.
31. Colucci WS, Wright RF, Braunwald E. New positive inotropic agents in the treatment of congestive heart failure: mechanisms of action and recent clinical developments. N Engl J Med 1986; 314:349.
32. Committee on Trauma, American College of Surgeons. Advanced trauma life support course, instructor's manual. Chicago: American College of Surgeons, 1984:189.
33. Cone JB, Wallace BH, Caldwell FT, et al. Beneficial effects of a hypertonic solution for resuscitation in the presence of acute hemorrhage. Am J Surg 1987;154:585.
34. Coonan TJ, Hope CE. Cardiorespiratory effects of change of body position. Can Anaesth Soc J 1983;30:424.
35. Cope O, Litwin SB. Contribution of the lymphatic system to the replenishment of plasma volume following hemorrhage. Ann Surg 1962;156:655.
36. Coyle JP, Teplick RS, Long MC, et al. Respiratory variations in systemic arterial pressure as an indicator of volume status. Anesthesiology 1983;59:A53.
37. Cowley RA, Hankins JR, Jones RT, et al. Pathology and pathophysiology of the liver. In: Cowley RA, Trump BF, eds. Pathophysiology of shock, anoxia and ischemia. Baltimore: Williams and Wilkins, 1982:285.
38. Cowley AW, Quillen EW, Skelton MM. Role of vasopressin in cardiovascular regulation. Fed Proc. 1983;42:3170.
39. Cross JS, Gruber DP, Burchard KW, et al. Hypertonic saline fluid therapy following surgery: a prospective study. J Trauma 1989;29:817.
40. Cross JS, Gruber DP, Gann DS, et al. Hypertonic saline attenuates the hormonal response to injury. Ann Surg 1989;209:684.
41. Cullen DJ. Interpretation of blood pressure measurements in anesthesia. Anesthesiology 1974;40:6.
42. Cunningham JN, Shires GT, Wagner Y. Cellular transport defects in hemorrhagic shock. Surgery 1971;70:215.
43. Cunningham JN, Shires GT, Wagner Y. Changes in intracellular sodium and potassium content of red blood cells in trauma and shock. Am J Surg 1971;70:215.
44. Czer LS, Shoemaker W. Myocardial performance in critically ill patients: response to whole blood transfusions as a prognostic measure. Crit Care Med 1980;8:710.
45. Dahn MS, Lucas CE, Ledgerwood AM. Negative inotropic effect of albumin resuscitation for shock. Surgery 1979;86:235.
46. Damon L, Adams M, Stricker RB, Ries C. Intracranial bleeding during treatment with hydroxyethyl starch. N Engl J Med 1987; 317:964.
47. Dawson CW, Lucas CE, Ledgerwod AM. Altered interstitial fluid space dynamics and postresuscitation hypertension. Arch Surg 1981;116:657.
48. Day B, Friedman SM. Red cell sodium and potassium in hemorrhagic shock measured by lithium substitution analysis. J Trauma 1980;20:52.
49. deFelippe J, Timoner J, Velasco IT, et al. Treatment of refractory hypovolemic shock by 7.5% sodium chloride injections. Lancet 1980;2:1002.
50. Demling RH. Colloid or crystalloid resuscitation in sepsis. In: Sibbald W, Sprung C, eds. Perspectives on sepsis and septic shock. Los Angeles: Society of Critical Care Medicine, 1986:275.
51. Dorinsky PM, Whitcomb ME. The effect of PEEP on cardiac output. Chest 1983;84:210.
52. Drop LJ, Ionized calcium: the heart and hemodynamic function. Anesth Analg 1985;64:432.
53. Drucker WR, Chadwick CDJ, Gann DS. Transcapillary refill in hemorrhage and shock. Arch Surg 1981;116:1344.
54. Eriksen C, Sorensen MB, Bille-Brahe NE, et al. Hemodynamic effects of calcium chloride administered intravenously to patients with and without cardiac disease during neuroleptanaesthesia. Acta Anaesthesiol Scand 1983;27:13.
55. Errington, ML, Silva R. On the role of vasopressin and angiotensin in the development of irreversible hemorrhagic shock. J Physiol (London) 1974;242:119.
56. Faillace DF, Ledgerwood AM, Lucas CE, et al. Immunoglobulin changes after varied resuscitation regimens. J Trauma 1982; 22:1.
57. Falk, JL, Rackow EC, Weil MH. Colloid and crystalloid fluid resuscitation. Acute Care 1983–1984;10:59.
58. Feest TG. Low molecular weight dextran: a continuing cause of acute renal failure. Br Med J 1976;2:1300.
59. Ferrario CM, Nadzam G, Fernandez LA, et al. Effects of pneumatic compression on the cardiovascular dynamics in the dog after hemorrhage. Aerosp Med 1970;41:411.
60. Fewell JE, Bond GC. Role of sinoaortic baroreceptors in initiating the renal response to continuous positive pressure ventilation in the dog. Anesthesiology 1980;52:408.
61. Flint LM, Brown A, Richardson JF, et al. Definitive control of bleeding from severe pelvic fractures. Ann Surg 1979;189:709.
62. Forsyth, BP. Redistribution of cardiac output during hemorrhage in the unanesthetized monkey. Circ Res 1970;27:311.
63. Fujimoto S, Roccaforte P, Patel AR, et al. Intravascular aggregation after acute intracranial hypertension by epidural balloon compression in cats. J Neurosurg 1982;57:210.
64. Furhaff AK. Anaphylactoid reaction to dextran: a report of 133 cases. Acta Anaesthesiol Scand 1977;21:161.
65. Fusciardi J, Rouby JJ, Barakat T, et al. Hemodynamic effects of high-frequency jet ventilation in patients with and without circulatory shock. Anesthesiology 1986;65:485.
66. Gaffney FA, Thal ER, Taylor WF, et al. Hemodynamic effects of medical antishock trousers (MAST garment). J Trauma 1981; 21:931.
67. Gallagher TJ, Banner MJ, Barnes P. Large volume crystalloid resuscitation does not increase extravascular lung water. Anesth Analg 1985;64:323.
68. Gallagher JD, Moore RA, Kerns D, et al. Effects of colloid or crystalloid administration on pulmonary extravascular water in the postoperative period after coronary artery bypass grafting. Anesth Analg 1985;64:753.
69. Gann DS: Endocrine control of plasma protein and volume. Surg Clin North Am 1976;56:1135.
70. Gann DS, Amarall JF. Pathophysiology of trauma and shock. In: Zuidema GD, Rutherford RB, Ballinger WF, eds. The management of trauma. 4th ed. Philadelphia: WB Saunders, 1985:37.
71. Gann DS, Carlson DE, Byrnes GJ, et al. Impaired restitution of blood volume after large hemorrhage. J Trauma 1981;21:598.

72. Gazitua SJB, Scott JB, Chou CC, et al. Effect of osmolarity on canine renal vascular resistance. Am J Physiol 1969;217:1216.
73. Geffin GA, Drop LJ, O'Keefe DD, et al. Global and regional function in the regionally ischemic left ventricle related to plasma ionized calcium. Cardiovasc Res 1983;17:415.
74. George RJD, Tinker J. The pathophysiology of shock. In: Tinker J, Rapin M, eds. Care of the critically ill patient. Berlin: Springer Verlag, 1983:163.
75. Gerber MJ, Hines RL, Barash PG. Arterial waveforms and systemic vascular resistance: is there a correlation? Anesthesiology 1987;66:823.
76. Gerrick SJ, Ledgerwood AM, Lucas CE. Postresuscitative hypertension: a reappraisal. Arch Surg 1980;115:1486.
77. Gett PM, Jones ES, Shepherd GF. Pulmonary edema associated with sodium retention during ventilator treatment. Br J Anaesth 1971;43:460.
78. Goldberg LI. Dopamine: clinical uses of an endogenous catecholamine. N Engl J Med 1974;291:707.
79. Goldberg LI, Hsieh YY, Resnekov L. Newer catecholamines for treatment of heart failure and shock: an update on dopamine and a first look at dobutamine. Prog Cardiovasc Dis 1977;19:327.
80. Goldberg LI, McDonald RH, Zimmerman AM. Sodium diuresis produced by dopamine in patients with congestive heart failure. N Engl J Med 1961;269:1060.
81. Green JF, Jackman AP. Mechanism of increased vascular capacity produced by mild perfusion hypothermia in the dog. Circ Res 1979;44:411.
82. Grindlinger GA, Manny J, Justice R, et al. Presence of negative inotropic agents in canine plasma during positive end-expiratory pressure. Circ Res 1979;45;460.
83. Gross DG, Landau EH, Assalia A, Krausz MM. Is hypertonic saline resuscitation safe in "uncontrolled" hemorrhagic shock? J Trauma 1988;28:751.
84. Gross D, Landau EH, Klin B, Krausz MM. Quantitative measurement of bleeding following hypertonic saline therapy in "uncontrolled" hemorrhagic shock. J Trauma 1989;29:79.
85. Gruber UF, Sturm V, Rem J, et al. The present state of prevention of postoperative thromboembolic complications. Bibl Haematol 1975;41;98.
86. Guillemin R, Vargo T, Rossier J, et al. Beta-endorphin and adrenocorticotropin are secreted concomitantly by the pituitary gland. Science 1977;197:1367.
87. Gunteroth WG, Abel FL, Mullins GL. The effect of Trendelenburg's position on blood pressure and carotid flow. Surg Gynecol Obstet 1964;119:345.
88. Guyton AC. Circulatory shock and physiology of its treatment. Textbook of medical physiology. Philadelphia: WB Saunders, 1981:332, 337.
89. Guyton AC. Determination of cardiac output by equating venous return curves with cardiac response curves. Physiol Rev 1955; 35:123.
90. Guyton AC, Lindsey AW, Kaufmann BN. Effect of blood transfusion and hemorrhage on cardiac output and on the venous return curve. Am J Physiol 1958;194:263.
91. Haddy FJ, Scott JB, Molnar JJ. Mechanisms of volume replacement and vascular constriction following hemorrhage. Am J Physiol 1965;208:169.
92. Haljamae H. Microcirculation and hemorrhagic shock. Am J Emerg Med 1984;2:100.
93. Hall SV, Johnson EE, Headley-Whyte J. Renal hemodynamics and function with continuous positive-pressure ventilation in dogs. Anesthesiology 1974;41:452.
94. Halonen P, Linko K, Myllyla G. A study of haemostasis following the use of high doses of hydroxyethyl starch 120 and dextran in major laparotomies. Acta Anaesthesiol Scand 1987;31:320.
95. Hardaway RM. Monitoring of the patient in a state of shock. Surg Gynecol Obstet 1979;148:339.
96. Harrigan C. Optimization of oxygen delivery and utilization in patients with Laennec's cirrhosis and respiratory failure. Master's thesis, Wayne State University, Department of Physiology. January 9, 1978.
97. Haupt MT, Rackow EC. Colloid osmotic pressure and fluid resuscitation with hetastarch, albumin and saline solutions. Crit Care Med 1982;10:159.
98. Hauser CJ, Shoemaker WC, Turpin I, et al. Oxygen transport responses to colloids and crystalloids in critically ill surgical patients. Surg Gynecol Obstet 1980;150:811.
99. Hayes DF, Werner MH, Rosenberg IK, et al. Effects of traumatic hypovolemic shock on renal function. J Surg Res 1974;16: 490.
100. Hechtman HB, Lonergan EA, Staunton PG, et al. Pulmonary entrapment of platelets during acute respiratory failure. Surgery 1978;83:277.
101. Hekmatpanah J. The management of head trauma. Surg Clin North Am 1973;53:47.
102. Hemmer M, Suter PM. Treatment of cardiac and renal effects of PEEP with dopamine in patients with acute respiratory failure. Anesthesiology 1979;50:399.
103. Hilberman M, Maseda J, Stinson EB, et al. The diuretic properties of dopamine in patients after open heart operation. Anesthesiology 1984;61:489.
104. Hinshaw LB, Peterson M, Huse WM, et al. Regional blood flow in hemorrhagic shock. Am J Surg 1961;102:224.
105. Holcroft JW. Impairment of venous return in hemorrhagic shock. Surg Clin North Am 1982;62:17.
106. Holcroft JW, Link DP, Lantz BMT, et al. Venous return and the pneumatic antishock garment in hypovolemic baboons. J Trauma 1984;24:928.
107. Holcroft JW, Vassar MJ, Turner JE, et al. 3% NaCl and 7% NaCl/dextran 70 in the resuscitation of severely injured patients. Ann Surg 1987;206:279.
108. Horton J, Landrenau R, Tuggle D. Cardiac response to fluid resuscitation from hemorrhagic shock. Surg Gynecol Obstet 1985;160:444.
109. Horwitz LD, Lifschitz MD. Role of the autonomic nervous system in the pressure response to calcium in conscious dogs. Cardiovasc Res 1980;14:522.
110. Hug CC. Monitoring. In: Miller RD, ed. Anesthesia. 2nd ed. New York: Churchill Livingstone, 1986;411.
111. Jardin F, Farcot JC, Boisante L, et al. Influence of positive end-expiratory pressure on left ventricular performance. N Engl J Med 1981;304:387.
112. Jarnberg PO, Dominguez de Villota E, Eklund J, et al. Effects of positive end-expiratory pressure on renal function. Acta Anaesthesiol Scand 1978;22:508.
113. Jelenko C III, Williams JB, Wheeler ML, et al. Studies in shock and resuscitation, I: use of a hypertonic, albumin containing, fluid demand regimen (HALFD) resuscitation. Crit Care Med 1979;7:157.
114. Jennings TJ, Usaf C, Seaworth JF, et al. The effects of inflation of antishock trousers on hemodynamics in normovolemic subjects. J Trauma 1986;26:544.
115. Johnson SD, Lucas CE, Gerrick SJ, et al. Altered coagulation after albumin supplements for treatment of oligemic shock. Arch Surg 1979;114:379.
116. Johnston WE, Prough DS, Royster RL, et al. Pulmonary artery wedge pressure may fail to reflect left ventricular end-diastolic pressure in dogs with oleic acid-induced pulmonary edema. Crit Care Med 1985;13;487.
117. Kaplan BC, Civetta JM, Nagel EL. The military anti-shock trou-

ser in civilian prehospital emergency care. J Trauma 1973; 13:843.
118. Kashtan J, Green JF, Parsons EQ, et al. Hemodynamic effects of increased abdominal pressure. J Surg Res 1981;30:249.
119. Kaukinen S, Eerola R. Positive end-expiratory pressure ventilation, renal function and renin. Ann Clin Res 1979;11:58.
120. Kenakin TP. An in vitro quantitative analysis of the alpha adrenocreceptor partial agonist activity of dobutamine and its relevance to inotropic selectivity. J Pharmacol Exp Ther 1981; 216:210.
121. Kenney PR, Allen-Rowlands CF, Gann DS. Glucose and osmolality as predictors of injury severity. J Trauma 1983;23:712.
122. Kharasch ED, Yeo KT, Kenny MA, Buffington CW. Atrial natriuretic factor may mediate the renal effects of PEEP ventilation. Anesthesiology 1988;69:862.
123. Kien ND, Kramer GC. Cardiac performance following hypertonic saline. Braz J Med Biol Res 1989;22:245.
124. Kovach AGB, Sandor P. Cerebral blood flow and brain function during hypotension and shock. Annu Rev Physiol 1976;38:571.
125. Kumar A, Pontoppidan H, Baratz RA, et al. Inappropriate response to increased plasma ADH during mechanical ventilation in acute respiratory failure. Anesthesiology 1974;40:215.
126. Lambertson CJ. Neural control of respiration. In: Mountcastle VB, ed. Medical physiology. 14th ed. St Louis: CV Mosby, 1980:1749.
127. Lamke LO, Liljedahl SO. Plasma volume changes after infusion of various plasma expanders. Resuscitation 1976;5:93.
128. Lane PL, McLellan BA, Johns PD. Etiology of shock in blunt trauma. Can Med Assoc J 1985;133:199.
129. Lang RE, Bzuckner UB, Hexmann K, et al. Effect of hemorrhagic shock on the concomitant release of endorphin and enkephalin-like peptides from the pituitary and adrenal gland in the dog. In: Costa E, Trabucci M, eds. Regulatory peptides: from molecular biology to function. New York: Raven Press, 1982:363.
130. Lawn B, Black H, Moore FD. Digitalis, electrolytes and the surgical patient. Am J Cardiol 1960;6:309.
131. Layon J, Duncan D, Gallagher TJ, Banner MJ. Hypertonic saline as a resuscitation solution in hemorrhagic shock: effects on extravascular lung water and cardiopulmonary function. Anesth Analg 1987;66:154.
132. Lazrove S, Waxman K, Shippy C, et al. Hemodynamic, blood volume, and oxygen transport responses to albumin and hydroxyethyl starch infusions in critically ill postoperative patients. Crit Care Med 1980;8:302.
133. Ledgerwood AM, Lucas CE. Postresuscitation hypertension: etiology, morbidity, and treatment. Arch Surg 1974;108:531.
134. Ledingham IMcA. The pathophysiology of shock. Br J Hosp Med 1979;22:472.
135. Ledingham IMcA, Ramsay G. Hypovolemic shock. Br J Anaesth 1986;58:169.
136. Lefer AM. Properties of cardioinhibitory factors produced in shock. Fed Proc 1978;37:2734.
137. Leibold W, Lucas CE, Ledgerwood AM, et al. Effect of albumin resuscitation on canine coagulation activity and content. Ann Surg 1983;198:630.
138. Leier CV, Unverferth DV. Dobutamine. Ann Intern Med 1983; 99:490.
139. Leithner C, Frass M, Pacher R, et al. Mechanical ventilation with positive end-expiratory pressure decreases release of alpha-atrial natriuretic peptide. Crit Care Med 1987;15:484.
140. Levy MN. The cardiac and vascular factors that determine systemic blood flow. Circ Res 1979;44:739.
141. Loeb HS, Ostrenga JP, Gaul W, et al. Beneficial effects of dopamine combined with intravenous nitroglycerin on hemodynamics in patients with severe left ventricular failure. Circulation 1983;68:813.
142. Lopes OU, Pontieri V, Roche E, et al. Hyperosmotic NaCl and severe hemorrhagic shock: role of the innervated lung. Am J Physiol 1981;241:H883.
143. Lovett WM, Wangensteen SL, Gleen TM, et al. Presence of a myocardial depressant factor in patients with circulatory shock. Surgery 1981;70:223.
144. Lowe RJ, Moss GS, Jilek J, et al. Crystalloid versus colloid in the etiology of pulmonary failure after trauma: a randomized trial in man. Crit Care Med 1979;7:107.
145. Lucas CE. Renal considerations in the injured patient. Surg Clin North Am 1982;62:133.
146. Lucas CE. The renal response to acute injury and sepsis. Surg Clin North Am 1976;56:953.
147. Lucas CE. Resuscitation of the injured patient: the three phases of treatment. Surg Clin North Am 1977;57:3.
148. Lucas CE, Denis R, Ledgerwood AM, Grabow D. The effects of hespan on serum and lymphatic albumin, globulin, and coagulant protein. Ann Surg 1988;207:416.
149. Lucas CE, Kovalik SG, Ledgerwood AM, et al. The cardiac effect of altered calcium homeostasis after albumin resuscitation. J Trauma 1981;21:275.
150. Lucas CE, Ledgerwood AM. The fluid problem in the critically ill. Surg Clin North Am 1983;63:439.
151. Lucas CE, Ledgerwood AM, Benishek DJ. Reduced oncotic pressure after shock. Arch Surg 1982;117:675.
152. Lucas CE, Ledgerwood AM, Higgins RF, et al. Impaired pulmonary function after albumin resuscitation from shock. J Trauma 1980;20:446.
153. Lucas CE, Ledgerwood AM, Higgins RF. Impaired salt and water excretion after albumin resuscitation for hypovolemic shock. Surgery 1979;86:544.
154. Lucas CE, Ledgerwood AM, Mammen EF. Altered coagulation protein content after albumin resuscitation. Ann Surg 1982; 196:198.
155. Lucas CE, Read RC. Red cell crenation and the renal hemodynamic effect of mannitol. Surgery 1966;59:408.
156. Lucas CE, Read RC. Vascular hypertensity: a mechanism for vasodilation in the dumping syndrome. Surgery 1966;60: 395.
157. Lucas CE, Zito JG, Carter KM, et al. Questionable value of furosemide in preventing renal failure. Surgery 1977;82:315.
158. Lundvall J, Mellander S, White T. Hyperosmolarity and vasodilation in human skeletal muscle. Acta Physiol Scand 1969; 77:224.
159. Mammana RB, Hiro S, Levitsky S, et al. Inaccuracy of pulmonary capillary wedge pressure when compared to left atrial pressure in the early postsurgical period. J Thorac Cardiovasc Surg 1982;84:420.
160. Maningas PA, Mattox KL, Pepe PE, et al. Hypertonic saline-dextran solutions for the prehospital management of traumatic hypotension. Am J Surg 1989;157:528.
161. Markley K, Smallman E, Millican RC. The efficacy and toxicity of iso-, hypo-, and hypertonic sodium solutions in the treatment of burn shock in mice. Surgery 1965;57:698.
162. Marquez JM, Douglas ME, Downs JB, et al. Renal function and cardiovascular responses during positive airway pressure. Anesthesiology 1979;50:393.
163. Marquez J, Guntupalli K, Sladen A, et al. Renal function and renin secretion during high frequency ventilation and varying levels of airway pressure. Crit Care Med 1983;11:930.
164. Marty AT, Zweifach BW. The high oncotic pressure effects of dextrans. Arch Surg 1970;101:421.
165. Mattox KL, Bickell W, Pepe P, Mangelsdorff AD. Prospective

randomized evaluation of antishock "MAST." J Trauma 1986; 26:779.
166. McNamara JJ, Suehiro GT, Suehiro A, et al. Resuscitation from hemorrhagic shock. J Trauma 1983;23:552.
167. McSwain NE. Pneumatic trousers and the management of shock. J Trauma 1977;17:719.
168. Menninger RP. Response of supraoptic neurosecretory cells to changes in left atrial distension. Am J Physiol 1979;236:R261.
169. Messmer K. Blood substitutes in shock therapy. In: Shires GT III, ed. Clinical surgery international, vol. 9: shock and related problems, Edinburgh: Churchill Livingstone, 1984:192.
170. Messmer K, Mokry G, Jeseh F. The protective effect of hypertonic solutions in shock. Br J Surg 1969;56:626.
171. Metcalf W, Dargan EI, Hehre D, et al. Clinical physiological characterization of a new dextran. Surg Gynecol Obstet 1962; 115:199.
172. Miller RR, Awan NA, Joge JA, et al. Combined dopamine and nitroprusside therapy in congestive heart failure: greater augmentation of cardiac performance by addition of inotropic stimulation to afterload reduction. Circulation 1977;55:881.
173. Mitaka C, Nagura T, Sakanishi N, et al. Two-dimensional echocardiographic evaluation of inferior vena cava, right ventricle, and left ventricle during positive-pressure ventilation with varying levels of positive end-expiratory pressure. Crit Care Med 1989;17:205.
174. Modig J. Effectiveness of dextran 70 versus Ringer's acetate in traumatic shock and adult respiratory distress syndrome. Crit Care Med 1986;14:454.
175. Moggio RA, Somberg ED, Praeger PI, et al. Hemodynamic comparison of albumin and hydroxyethyl starch in postoperative cardiac surgery. Crit Care Med 1983;11:943.
176. Mohsemin V, Dubois AB. Intercompartmental fluid shifts due to glucose release during hemorrhage in rabbits. Am J Physiol 1983;245:H143.
177. Monafo WW, Chuntrasakul C, Ayvazian VH. Hypertonic sodium solutions in the treatment of burn shock. Am J Surg 1973; 126:778.
178. Moore, FD. Metabolic care of the surgical patient. Philadelphia: WB Saunders, 1959.
179. Morel DR, Forster A, Suter PM. Evaluation of IV labetalol for treatment of posttraumatic hyperdynamic state. Intensive Care Med 1984;10:133.
180. Moss GS. An argument in favor of electrolyte solution for early resuscitation. Surg Clin North Am 1972;52:3.
181. Moss GS, Lowe RJ, Jilek J, et al. Colloid or crystalloid in the resuscitation of hemorrhagic shock. Surgery 1981;89:434.
182. Moylan JA, Reckler JM, Mason AD. Resuscitation with hypertonic lactate saline in thermal injury. Am J Surg 1973;125:580.
183. Mullins RJ, Bell DR. Permeability of rabbit skin and muscle microvasculature after saline expansion. J Surg Res 1982; 32:390.
184. Nerlich M, Gunther R, Demling RH. Resuscitation from hemorrhagic shock with hypertonic saline or lactated Ringer's: effect on the pulmonary and systemic microcirculations. Circ Shock 1983;10:179.
185. Oppenheim W, Williamson D, Smith R. Early biochemical changes and severity of injury in man. J Trauma 1980;20:135.
186. Pardy BJ, Dudley HAF. Comparison of pulmonary artery pressures and mixed venous oxygen tension with other indices in acute hemorrhage: an experimental study. Br J Surg 1977; 64:1.
187. Pardy BJ, Dudley HAF. Sequential patterns of haemodynamic and metabolic changes in experimental hypovolemic shock: responses to acute hemorrhage. Br J Surg 1979;66:84.
188. Payen DM, Farge D, Beloucif S, et al. No involvement of antidiuretic hormone in acute antidiuresis during PEEP ventilation in humans. Anesthesiology 1987;66:17.
189. Pedowitz RA, Shackford SR. Non-cavitary hemorrhage producing shock in trauma patients: incidence and severity. J Trauma 1989;29:219.
190. Pelligra R, Sandberg EC. Control of intractable abdominal bleeding by external counterpressure. JAMA 1979;241:708.
191. Perel A, Pizov R, Cotev S. Systolic blood pressure variation is a sensitive indicator of hypovolemia in ventilated dogs subjected to graded hemorrhage. Anesthesiology 1987;67:498.
192. Pirkle JC Jr, Gann DS. Expansion of interstitial fluid is required for full restoration of blood volume after hemorrhage. J Trauma 1976;16:937.
193. Pirkle JC Jr, Gann DS. Restitution of blood volume after hemorrhage: mathematical description. Am J Physiol 1975;228:821.
194. Pizov R, Ya'ari Y, Perel A. Systolic pressure variation is greater during hemorrhage than during sodium nitroprusside-induced hypotension in ventilated dogs. Anesth Analg 1988;67:170.
195. Poole GV, Prough DS, Johnson JC, et al. Effects of resuscitation from hemorrhagic shock on cerebral hemodynamics in the presence of an intracranial mass. J Trauma 1987;27:18.
196. Priebe HJ, Heimann JC, Headley-Whyte J. Effects of renal and hepatic venous congestion on renal function in the presence of low and normal cardiac output in dogs. Circ Res 1980;47:883.
197. Priebe HJ, Heimann JC, Headley-Whyte J. Mechanisms of renal dysfunction during positive end-expiratory pressure ventilation. J Appl Physiol 1981;50:643.
198. Prough DS, Johnson JC, Poole GV, et al. Effects on intracranial pressure of resuscitation from hemorrhagic shock with hypertonic saline versus lactated Ringer's solution. Crit Care Med 1985;13:407.
199. Prough DS, Johnson JC, Stullken EH, et al. Effects on cerebral hemodynamics of resuscitation from endotoxic shock with hypertonic saline versus lactated Ringer's solution. Crit Care Med 1985;13:1040.
200. Puri VK, Howard M, Paidipaty BB. Resuscitation in hypovolemia and shock: a prospective study of hydroxyethyl starch and albumin. Crit Care Med 1983;11:518.
201. Puri VK, Paidipaty B, White L. Hydroxyethyl starch for resuscitation of patients with hypovolemia and shock. Crit Care Med 1981;9:833.
202. Rackow EC, Falk JL, Fein IA, et al. Fluid resuscitation in circulatory shock: a comparison of the cardiorespiratory effects of albumin, heta-starch, and saline solutions in patients with hypovolemic and septic shock. Crit Care Med 1983;11:839.
203. Rankin JS, Olsen CO, Arentzen CE, et al. The effects of airway pressure on cardiac function in intact dogs and man. Circulation 1982;66:108.
204. Raper R, Sibbald WJ. Misled by wedge? The Swan-Ganz catheter and left ventricular preload. Chest 1986;89:427.
205. Rector JB, Stein JH, Bay WH, et al. Effects of hemorrhage and vasopressor agents on distribution of blood flow. Am J Physiol 1972;222:1125.
206. Reich DL, Konstadt SN, Raissi S, et al. Trendelenburg position and passive leg raising do not significantly improve cardiopulmonary performance in the anesthetized patient with coronary artery disease. Crit Care Med 1989;17:313.
207. Richard C, Ricome JL, Rimailko A, et al. Combined hemodynamic effects of dopamine and dobutamine in cardiogenic shock. Circulation 1983;67:620.
208. Ring J, Messmer K. Incidence and severity of anaphylactoid reactions to colloid volume substitutes. Lancet 1977;1:466.
209. Robotham JL, Bell RL, Badke FR, et al. Left ventricular geometry during positive end-expiratory pressure in dogs. Crit Care Med 1985;13:617.

210. Robotham JL, Wise RA, Bromberger B, et al. Effects of changes in abdominal pressure on left ventricular performance and regional blood flow. Crit Care Med 1985;13:803.
211. Rock G, Wise P. Plasma expansion during granulocyte procurement: cumulative effects of hydroxyethyl starch. Blood 1979;53:1156.
212. Roth JA, Rutherford RB. Regional blood flow effects of G suit application during hemorrhagic shock. Surg Gynecol Obstet 1971;133:637.
213. Runciman WB, Skowronski GA. Pathophysiology of hemorrhagic shock. Anaesth Intensive Care 1984;12:193.
214. Scholten DJ. Electrolytes and plasma volume regulation in hypovolemic shock. Am J Emerg Med 1984;2:86.
215. Secher NH, Jensen KS, Werner C, et al. Bradycardia during severe but reversible hypovolemic shock in man. Circ Shock 1984;14:267.
216. Shackford SR, Sise MJ, Fridlund PH, et al. Hypertonic sodium lactate versus lactated Ringer's solution for intravenous fluid therapy in operations on the abdominal aorta. Surgery 1983; 94:41.
217. Share L. Role of cardiovascular receptors in the control of ADH release. Cardiology 1976;61(suppl 3):51.
218. Shatney CH, Deepika K, Millitello PR, et al. Efficacy of hetastarch in the resuscitation of patients with multisystem trauma and shock. Arch Surg 1983;118:804.
219. Sheldon CA, Cerra FB, Bohnhoff N. Peripheral postcapillary venous pressure: a new, more sensitive monitor of effective blood volume during hemorrhagic shock and resuscitation. Surgery 1983;94:399.
220. Shenkin HA, Scheuerman EB, Spitz EB, et al. Effect of change of posture upon cerebral circulation of man. J Appl Physiol 1949; 2:317.
221. Shinozaki M, Muteki T, Kaku N, Tsuda H. Hemodynamic relationship between renal venous pressure and blood flow regulation during positive end-expiratory pressure. Crit Care Med 1988;16:144.
222. Shinozuka T, Nemoto EM, Bleyaert AL. Cerebral cortical oxygenation and perfusion during hetastarch hemodilution. Surg Forum 1981;32:502.
223. Shippy CR, Appel PL, Shoemaker WC. Reliability of clinical monitoring to assess blood volume in critically ill patients. Crit Care Med 1984;12:107.
224. Shires GT, Braun FT, Canizaro PC, et al. Distributional changes in extracellular fluid during acute hemorrhagic shock. Surg Forum 1960;11:115.
225. Shires GT, Canizaro PC, Carrico CJ. Shock. In: Schwartz SI, Shires GT, Spencer FC, Storer EH, eds. Principles of Surgery. 4th ed. New York: McGraw-Hill, 1984:116.
226. Shires GT, Carrico CJ, Canizaro PC. Response of the extracellular fluid. In: Shires GT, ed. Shock: major problems in clinical surgery. vol 13. Philadelphia: WB Saunders, 1973:15.
227. Shires T, Cunningham JN, Barke CRE, et al. Alterations in cellular membrane function during hemorrhagic shock. Ann Surg 1972;176:288.
228. Shoemaker WC. Comparison of the relative effectiveness of whole blood transfusions and various types of fluid therapy in resuscitation. Crit Care Med 1976;4;71.
229. Shoemaker WC, Hauser CJ. Critique of crystalloid versus colloid therapy in shock and shock lung. Crit Care Med 1979;7:117.
230. Shoemaker WC, Schluchter M, Hopkins JA, et al. Comparison of the relative effectiveness of colloids and crystalloids in emergency resuscitation. Am J Surg 1981;142:73.
231. Sibbald WJ, Paterson NAM, Holliday RL, et al. The Trendelenburg position: hemodynamic effects in hypotensive and normotensive patients. Crit Care Med 1979;7:218.
232. Simmons RL, Heisterkamp CA, Moseley RV, et al. Postresuscitative blood volumes in combat casualties. Surg Gynecol Obstet 1969;128:1193.
233. Sladen A, Laver MB, Pontoppidan H. Pulmonary complications and water retention in prolonged mechanical ventilation. N Engl J Med 1968;279:448.
234. Slater GI, Vladeck BC, Bassin R, et al. Sequential changes in distribution of cardiac output in hemorrhagic shock. Surgery 1973;73:714.
235. Smith JAR, Norman JN. The fluid of choice for resuscitation of severe shock. Br J Surg 1982;69:702.
236. Smith TW, Braunwald E. The management of heart failure. In: Braunwald E, ed. Heart disease: a textbook of cardiovascular medicine. Philadelphia: WB Saunders, 1984:503.
237. Soler T, Muller H, Kennedy TJ. Clinical use of G suit. JACEP 1976;5:609.
238. Starling EH. On the absorption of fluids from the connective tissue spaces. J Physiol (London) 1896;19:312.
239. Steinhoff HH, Kohlhoff RJ, Falke KJ. Facilitation of renal function by intermittent mandatory ventilation. Intensive Care Med 1984;10:59.
240. Stoddart JC. Shock: acute cardiocirculatory failure. In: Stoddart JC, ed. Trauma and the anaesthetist. London: Bailliere Tindall, 1984:13.
241. Stoner HB, Frayn KN, Barton RN, et al. The relationship between plasma substrates and hormones and the severity of injury in 277 recently injured patients. Clin Sci 1979;56:563.
242. Taylor AE, Granger DN. A model of protein and fluid exchange between plasma and interstitium. In: Squoris JT, Rene A, eds. Proceedings of the workshop on albumin. Bethesda: National Institutes of Health, 1976:93.
243. Taylor J, Weil MH. Failure of the Trendelenburg position to improve circulation during clinical shock. Surg Gynecol Obstet 1967;124:1005.
244. Teboul JL, Zapol WM, Brun-Buisson C, et al. A comparison of pulmonary artery occlusion pressure and left ventricular end-diastolic pressure during mechanical ventilation with PEEP in patients with severe ARDS. Anesthesiology 1989;70:261.
245. Thompson WL, Walton RF. Blood changes, renal function, and tissue storage following massive infusion of hydroxyethyl starch. Fed Proc 1963;22:640.
246. Tommasino C, Moore S, Todd MM. Cerebral effects of isovolemic hemodilution with crystalloid or colloid solutions. Crit Care Med 1988;16:862.
247. Tranbaugh RF, Elings VB, Christensen J, et al. Determinants of pulmonary interstitial fluid accumulation after trauma. J Trauma 1982;22;820.
248. Twigley AJ, Hillman KM. The end of crystalloid era? A new approach to peri-operative fluid administration. Anaesthesia 1985;40:860.
249. Velanovich V. Crystalloid versus colloid fluid resuscitation: a meta-analysis of mortality. Surgery 1989;105:65.
250. Velasco IT, Pontieri V, Rocha E, et al. Hyperosmotic NaCl and severe hemorrhagic shock. Am J Physiol 1980;239:H664.
251. Venus B, Jacobs HK, Lim L. Treatment of the adult respiratory distress syndrome with continuous positive airway pressure. Chest 1979;76:257.
252. Venus B, Mathru M, Smith RA, et al. Renal function during application of positive end-expiratory pressure in swine: effects of hydration. Anesthesiology 1985;62:765.
253. Virgilio RW, Rice CL, Smith DE, et al. Crystalloid versus colloid resuscitation: is one better? Surgery 1979;85:129.
254. Wallis TW, Robotham JL, Compean R, et al. Mechanical heart-lung interaction with positive end-expiratory pressure. J Appl Physiol 1983;54:1039.
255. Wangensteen SL, Ludewig RM, Eddy DM. The effect of ex-

ternal counterpressure on the intact circulation. Surg Gynecol Obstet 1968;127:253.

256. Weil MH, Henning RJ. New concepts in the diagnosis and fluid treatment of circulatory shock. Anesth Analg 1979;58:124.

257. Weil MH, Henning RJ, Puri VK. Colloid oncotic pressure: clinical significance. Crit Care Med 1979;7:113.

258. Weil MH, Udhoji VN, Allen KS. The head-down position in treatment of shock. Surg Gynecol Obstet 1963;116:669.

259. Wiener S, Barrett S. Hypovolemic shock and resuscitation. In: Wiener S, Barrett S, eds. Trauma management for civilian and military physicians. Philadelphia: WB Saunders, 1986:37.

260. Wildenthal K, Mierzwiak DS, Mitchell JH. Acute effects of increased serum osmolality on left ventricular performance. Am J Physiol 1969;216:898.

261. Wilson RF. Science and shock: a clinical perspective. Ann Emerg Med 1985;14;714.

262. Wilson RF. The pathophysiology of shock. Intensive Care Med 1980;6:89.

263. Wisner D, Busche F, Sturm J, et al. Traumatic shock and head injury: effects of fluid resuscitation on the brain. J Surg Res 1989;46:49.

264. Wolfman EF, Neil SA, Heaps DK, et al. Donor blood and isotonic salt solution. Arch Surg 1963;86:869.

265. Zornow MH, Scheller MS, Shackford SR. Effect of a hypertonic lactated Ringer's solution on intracranial pressure and cerebral water content in a model of traumatic brain injury. J Trauma 1989;29:484.

# Chapter Five

Donald P. Bernstein

# Oxygen Transport and Utilization in Trauma

## With Special Reference to Hemorrhagic Shock and Rationale for Transfusion

The red blood cell is merely a courier in the biologic scheme of life's metabolic processes. Its major function is to bind oxygen to the hemoglobin molecule at the alveolar-pulmonary capillary interface and then deliver it to the cells of every organ and tissue of the body. After $O_2$ delivery, the biologic waste gas, $CO_2$, enters the red cell and is transported either in combination with hemoglobin (carbamino-$CO_2$) or is converted to hydrogen ions and bicarbonate. The red cell then traverses the venous system back to the lungs where carbamino-bound $CO_2$ is discharged, $O_2$ is loaded, and the cycle repeats itself. The mature red cell is simple when compared with other biologically active cells in that it has no nucleus or mitochondria. It is also unique in that it does not itself require oxygen to survive. Due to its basic morphologic design and the trauma caused by repeated collisions within the circulation, the erythrocyte's life span is relatively short (120 days).

This chapter does not concern itself with the red cell per se but rather with its cargo, oxygen. The quantity of oxygen arriving at the sites of intracellular utilization will be used as the goal in treatment of the trauma victim. Moreover, the archaic notions that adequacy of transfusion therapy may be inferred by static, unidimensional determination of hematocrit or hemoglobin concentration will be dispelled. The oxygen transport system is dynamic; it involves the integrated modulation of the ambient oxygen tension, pulmonary and cardiovascular function, blood volume and red cell mass, the functional quality of the hemoglobin contained within the red cells, and physical status of the microcirculation. Finally, adequacy of oxygen transport as a therapeutic goal will be shown to be pivotal in optimization of regional and global cellular function: life.

### THE OXYGEN TRANSPORT SYSTEM

Oxygen transport is a multifaceted dynamic process whereby $O_2$ is extracted from the environment and delivered via several organ systems to sites of intracellular utilization.[97,346] Systemic oxygen transport ($SO_2T$) or oxygen delivery ($\dot{D}O_2$) is defined as the product of cardiac output ($\dot{Q}_t$) and the arterial oxygen content ($CaO_2$).[236] Thus,

$$\dot{D}O_2 = \dot{Q}_t(CaO_2)$$

where $\dot{D}O_2$ is the volume of $O_2$ delivered to the systemic circulation in 1 minute (mL of $O_2$ per minute). It represents the bulk movement of $O_2$ to potential sites of uptake, the systemic capillary-cellular interface. $\dot{Q}_t$ is the cardiac output or total body flood flow expressed in liters per min. Cardiac output is multidimensional. It is most simply defined as the product of stroke volume and heart rate (ie, $\dot{Q}_t = SV \times f$) but may also be expressed as follows.[161]
If

$$TPR = \frac{MAP - CVP}{\dot{Q}_t}$$

where

$$\text{TPR} = \text{total peripheral resistance;}$$
$$\text{MAP} = \text{mean arterial pressure;}$$
$$\text{CVP} = \text{central venous pressure,}$$

then

$$\dot{Q}_t = \frac{\text{MAP} - \text{CVP}}{\text{TPR}}.$$

Thus, $\dot{Q}_t$ may be expressed as a product of volume and frequency or as a ratio of pressure to resistance.

$Cao_2$ is arterial oxygen content in mL of $O_2$ per liter of blood. It is the quantity of $O_2$ in the arterial blood and, like $\dot{Q}_t$, $Cao_2$ is determined by several mutually exclusive but interdependent variables.[96,297]

$Cao_2$ is the sum of the volume of $O_2$ bound to hemoglobin and the volume of $O_2$ dissolved in the blood plasma, and is computed by the following formula.

$$Cao_2 = [Hb](Sao_2 \times 1.34) + (0.03 \times Pao_2)$$

where

[Hb] = the hemoglobin concentration in g/L;
1.34 = the number of mililiters of $O_2$ that 1 g of normal hemoglobin can carry when fully saturated;
$Sao_2$ = the percent saturation of arterial hemoglobin; it is the ratio of oxyhemoglobin to total hemoglobin,

$$\frac{[O_2\ Hb]}{[\text{total Hb}]} \times 100$$

and is dictated by the partial pressure of arterial oxygen ($Pao_2$) mainly via:
The alveolar partial pressure of oxygen ($P_{AO_2}$), which is determined by the $F_{IO_2}$ and $\dot{V}_A$
The total intrapulmonary shunt, $\dot{Q}_{sp}/\dot{Q}_t$
The mixed venous oxygen content ($C\bar{v}o_2$) (only when $\dot{Q}_{sp}/\dot{Q}_t$ increases).

Dissolved oxygen is the amount of $O_2$ dissolved in the plasma in mL/L. It is the product of $O_2$ partial pressure and a solubility coefficient, which is 0.03 at 38°C. The quantity of dissolved oxygen usually contributes little to tissue oxygenation. For instance, if $Pao_2$ = 95 mm Hg, the dissolved $O_2$ contributing to $Cao_2$ would be

$$0.03 \times 95 = 2.85 \text{ mL/L of blood.}$$

If we assume the following:

$$[Hb] = 150 \text{ g/L}, Pao_2 = 95 \text{ mm Hg}$$
$$Sao_2 = 97\%$$

then

$$Hbo_2 = [Hb] \times Sao_2 \times 1.34$$
$$= 150 \times 0.97 \times 1.34$$
$$= \text{approximately 195 mL of } O_2 \text{ per liter of blood.}$$

If

$$Cao_2 = Hbo_2 + \text{dissolved } O_2$$

then

$$Cao_2 = 195 \text{ mL} + 2.9 \text{ mL}$$
$$= \text{approximately 198 mL of } O_2 \text{ per liter of blood.}$$

This is the normal value for an adult male; the contribution of dissolved $O_2$ is thus only 1.5% of total $Cao_2$ under normal conditions. However, if $Pao_2$ is raised to 500 mm Hg, the contribution of dissolved $O_2$ to $Cao_2$ may be of major importance.

If we assume the following:

$$[Hb] = 150 \text{ g/L}$$
$$Pao_2 = 500 \text{ mm Hg}$$
$$Sao_2 = 100\%$$

then

$$Cao_2 = (150 \times 1.00 \times 1.34) + (0.03 \times 500)$$
$$= 201 \text{ mL/L} + 15 \text{ mL/L}$$
$$= 216 \text{ mL/L}.$$

Dissolved $O_2$ now represents approximately 7% of $Cao_2$. Dissolved $O_2$ may contribute up to 40% of tissue oxygen requirement in severely anemic patients.[108]

## VARIABLES AFFECTING $Cao_2$

### *Arterial Saturation of Hemoglobin with Oxygen ($Sao_2$)*

Arterial saturation of hemoglobin with oxygen ($Sao_2$) is related to and dependent upon $Pao_2$ by the familiar hemoglobin-oxygen dissociation curve (Fig 5-1). Hemoglobin is approximately 97% saturated with $O_2$ at a $Pao_2$ of 100 mm Hg. Thus, intraerythrocytic $O_2$, the primary determinant of $Cao_2$, is maximized at a $Pao_2$ of 100 mm Hg. Any increase in $Pao_2$ beyond this level contributes more to dissolved $O_2$ than to that carried by hemoglobin.

The curve defines the $Sao_2$ at any given $Pao_2$. As can be seen on the upper flat portion of the curve, a drop in $Pao_2$ from 100 to 40 mm Hg produces only a 25% reduction in $Sao_2$. Thus, considerable arterial hypoxemia can occur before significant arterial desaturation ensues. However, when the steep portion of the curve is encountered, further reductions in $Pao_2$ are associated with rapid deterioration of arterial saturation. For example, when $Pao_2$ drops only 13 mm Hg from 40 to 27 mm Hg, arterial saturation drops another 25%.

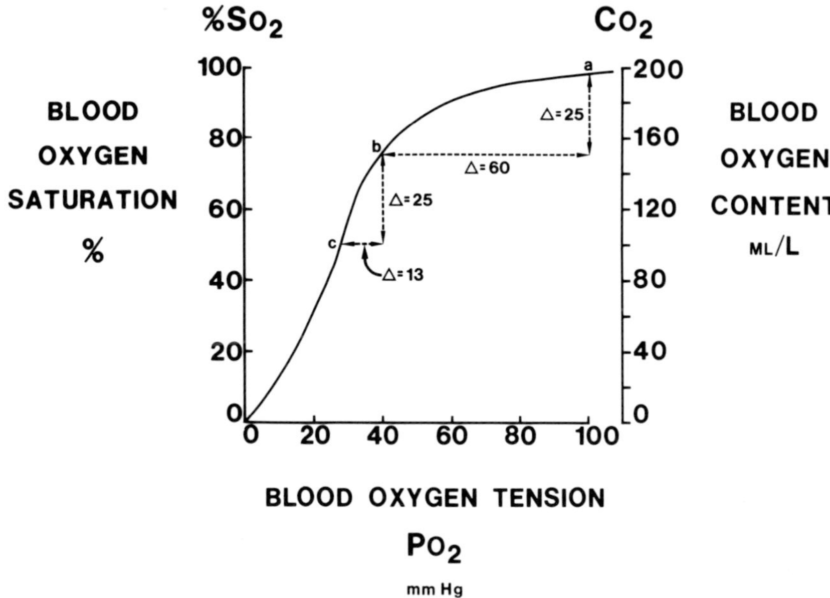


FIG. 5-1. Normal oxyhemoglobin dissociation curve. *Conditions:* [Hb] = 150 g/L, pH = 7.40, temperature = 37°C, $Pco_2$ = 40 mm Hg. Note that a reduction in $Po_2$ from 100 to 40 mm Hg produces only a 25% reduction in $So_2$, but on the steep portion of the curve, a mere 13-mm Hg reduction in $Po_2$, from 40 to 27 mm Hg, also produces a 25% decrease in $So_2$.

### *Hemoglobin Concentration*

The effect of reduction in [Hb] on $Cao_2$ is shown in Fig 5-2 and in the following example in which contribution of dissolved $O_2$ is neglected:

$$[Hb] = 100 \text{ g/L}$$
$$Sao_2 = 100\%$$
$$\therefore Cao_2 = [Hb] \times Sao_2 \times 1.34$$
$$= 100 \times 1.00 \times 1.34$$
$$= 134 \text{ mL of } O_2 \text{ per liter.}$$

Thus, a 33% reduction in [Hb] from the normal 150 g/L produces a concurrent decrease in $Cao_2$ of 33%.

### *Arterial Oxygen Tension*

The effect of low $Pao_2$ with arterial desaturation is shown in Fig 5-3 and in the following example (contribution of dissolved $O_2$ is neglected).

$$[Hb] = 150 \text{ g/L}$$
$$Pao_2 = 40 \text{ mm Hg}$$
$$Sao_2 = 75\%$$
$$\therefore Cao_2 = 150 \times 0.75 \times 1.34$$
$$= \text{approximately } 150 \text{ mL of } O_2 \text{ per liter of blood.}$$

Thus, a $Pao_2$ reduction of 60% (from 100 mm Hg to 40) produces an arterial $O_2$ content reduction of only 25% (from 200 mL to 150 mL of $O_2$ per liter).

### *Combined $Pao_2$ and [Hb] Reduction*

The effect of combined hypoxemia and anemia on $Cao_2$ is shown in Fig 5-2 and the following example.

$$[Hb] = 100 \text{ g/L}$$
$$Sao_2 = 75\%$$
$$Pao_2 = 40 \text{ mm Hg (contribution of dissolved } O_2 \text{ is neglected)}$$
$$\therefore Cao_2 = 100 \times 0.75 \times 1.34$$
$$= \text{approximately } 100 \text{ mL of } O_2 \text{ per liter.}$$

Hence, a reduction of [Hb] by 33% added to a reduction in $Sao_2$ of 25% produces a 50% reduction in $CaO_2$ (from 200 mL to 100 mL of $O_2$ per liter).

In summary, moderate degrees of arterial hypoxemia have a smaller effect on arterial $O_2$ content than reduction in hemoglobin concentration.

## OXYGEN DELIVERY ($\dot{D}o_2$)

Adequate oxygen delivery cannot be assessed by isolated sampling of [Hb], $Sao_2$, or $Pao_2$. These variables are merely elements of the arterial oxygen content, $Cao_2$, which, in turn, determines only the static unit volume of oxygen carried in the blood. Thus, $Cao_2$ in and of itself does not convey any information as to the adequacy of oxygen delivery.[80] The bulk

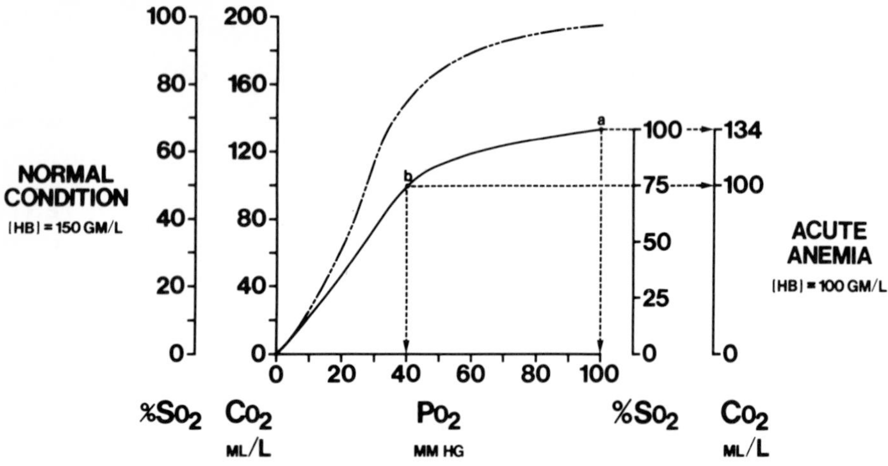


FIG. 5-2. Effect of acute anemia and anemia with hypoxemia on $CaO_2$. *Conditions:* pH = 7.40, temperature = 37°C, $P_{CO_2}$ = 40 mm Hg. Reducing [Hb] from 150 g/L (upper curve) to 100 g/L (lower curve) produces a $Ca_{O_2}$ of 134 mL/L (point a) at 100% saturation. If $Sa_{O_2}$ is reduced to 75% ($Pa_{O_2}$ = 40 mm Hg, point b), $Ca_{O_2}$ decreases to 100 mL/L.

movement or flux of oxygen can be determined only by multiplying cardiac output $\dot{Q}_t$ by $Ca_{O_2}$, ie, $\dot{D}_{O_2} = \dot{Q}_t \times Ca_{O_2}$.[239] If we assume that a normal adult male has a 6 L/min cardiac output and a normal arterial oxygen content of 200 mL/L, then normal systemic oxygen transport, or oxygen delivery ($\dot{D}_{O_2}$), should be

$$\dot{D}_{O_2} = \dot{Q}_t \times Ca_{O_2}$$
$$= 6 \times 200$$
$$= 1200 \text{ mL of } O_2 \text{ per minute.}$$

If this individual's body surface area is 1.7 $m^2$, then the $\dot{D}_{O_2}$ index will be 705 mL/min/$m^2$. The normal range of $\dot{D}_{O_2}$ is 520 to 720 mL/min/$m^2$.[2,318]

FIG. 5-3. Arterial hypoxemia. *Conditions:* [Hb] = 150 g/L, pH = 7.40, temperature = 37°C, $P_{CO_2}$ = 40 mm Hg. When $Pa_{O_2}$ = 40 mm Hg (point a), $Sa_{O_2}$ is 75%. Consequently, $Ca_{O_2}$ = 150 mL/L. Dissolved oxygen is neglected.

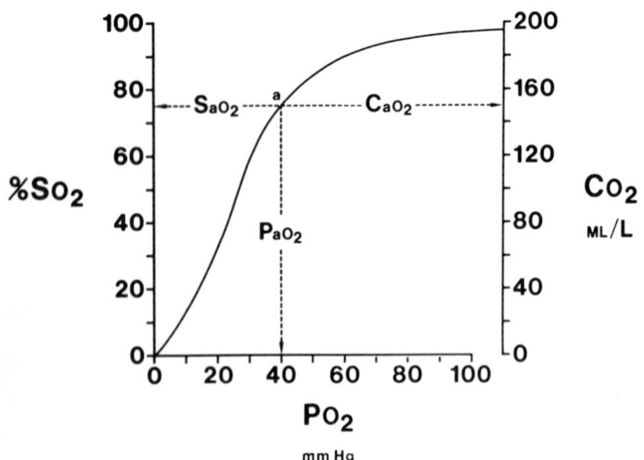


## *Distribution of $\dot{D}_{O_2}$*

Although $Ca_{O_2}$ is uniform throughout the systemic circulation, the distribution of $\dot{Q}_t$ is not (Table 5-1). Thus, $\dot{D}_{O_2}$ partition among the various organs is based on regional blood flow.

It is apparent from Table 1 that blood flow varies greatly from organ to organ and that in the healthy individual, at steady state, regional oxygen delivery parallels the distribution of cardiac output, ie, $\dot{D}_{O_2} \alpha \dot{Q}_t$. The oxygen delivery system subserves the oxygen requirements of all the aerobic metabolic processes of the organism. Adequacy of $\dot{D}_{O_2}$ is assured if these requirements are met.

## OXYGEN CONSUMPTION ($\dot{V}_{O_2}$) AND TISSUE OXYGENATION

Oxygen consumption or uptake ($\dot{V}_{O_2}$) is the total body utilization of $O_2$. $\dot{V}_{O_2}$ subserves oxygen demand, which is the total amount of oxygen required to satisfy the aerobic metabolic needs of the organism.[160] In the steady state, oxygen consumption equals oxygen demand:

$$\dot{V}_{O_2} \text{ (consumed)} = \dot{V}_{O_2} \text{ (demanded).}$$

Mean steady-state oxygen consumption at rest in the awake state is approximately 140 mL/min/$m^2$ (range, 100 to 180).[74,113,318] Hence, the average 70-kg adult male of 1.7-$m^2$ body surface area consumes approximately 240 to 250 mL of $O_2$ per minute. In the steady state, for every 1000 to 1200 mL of $\dot{D}_{O_2}$, only 250 mL undergoes cellular uptake ($\dot{V}_{O_2}$). The *extraction ratio*, or *utilization coefficient*, is thus normally 0.25 (ie, 25%).[123]

$$\text{Extraction ratio} = \dot{V}_{O_2}/\dot{D}_{O_2}$$
$$= \text{approximately 0.25 (range, 0.22 to 0.30)}$$

TABLE 5-1. Distribution of $\dot{Q}_t$ and $\dot{D}O_2$ in a Normal Adult Male[97,279,333,373] (70 kg; BSA, 1.7 $m^2$)

| CIRCULATION | REGIONAL BLOOD FLOW *mL/min* | REGIONAL BLOOD FLOW *mL/100 gm/min* | % TOTAL $Q_t$ | REGIONAL $\dot{D}O_2$ (mL $O_2$/min) | % TOTAL $\dot{D}O_2$ |
|---|---|---|---|---|---|
| Splanchnic | 1400 | ~100 | 24 | 280 | 24 |
| Renal | 1100 | ~370 | 19 | 220 | 19 |
| Cerebral | 750 | ~60 | 13 | 150 | 13 |
| Coronary | 250 | ~85 | 4 | 50 | 4 |
| Skeletal muscle* | 1200 | ~4 | 21 | 240 | 21 |
| Skin† | 500 | ~25 | 9 | 100 | 9 |
| Other organs | 600 | | 10 | 120 | 10 |
| Totals | $\dot{Q}_t$ = 5800 ≅6000 mL | | 100 | $\dot{D}O_2$ = 1160 ≅1200 mL | 100 |

* Skeletal muscle assumed to be 40% of ideal body weight.
† Assumes total weight of skin to be 2 kg.

This concept is more easily understood by analysis of the oxyhemoglobin dissociation curve in Fig 5-4 and the following example.

$[Hb]$ = 150 g/L

$SaO_2$ = 100%

$PaO_2$ = 100 mm Hg at approximately 100% saturation

$\dot{Q}_t$ = 5 L/min

Extraction ratio = 0.25.

Here, $\dot{D}O_2$ = 1000 mL/min (5 L/min × 200 ML/L of $O_2$). If only 250 mL of $O_2$ per minute is consumed by tissues, then the mixed venous effluent in the pulmonary artery must contain the $O_2$ not used (ie, 1000 − 250 = 750 mL of $O_2$). Since arterial $O_2$ content ($CaO_2$) is expressed in mL of $O_2$ per liter, and $\dot{D}O_2 = \dot{Q}_t \times CaO_2$, then

$$\dot{D}O_2/\dot{Q}_t = CaO_2$$

thus

$$CaO_2 = 1000/5 = 200 \text{ mL of } O_2 \text{ per liter.}$$

On the oxyhemoglobin dissociation curve this represents the arterial point (point a) (Fig 5-4). If 750 mL of $O_2$/min is unused, then 750/5 = 150 mL/L represents the mixed venous

FIG. 5-4. Normal oxygen consumption. *Conditions:* 70-kg male, 1.7 $m^2$ BSA, awake and at rest. [Hb] = 150 g/L, pH = 7.40, temperature = 37°C, $PCO_2$ = 40 mm Hg, $\dot{Q}_t$ = 5 L/min. $CaO_2$ = 200 mL/L (point a). Hence, $\dot{D}O_2$ = 1000 mL/min, $C\bar{v}O_2$ = 150 mL/L (point V). Therefore, the arteriovenous oxygen content difference, ($CaO_2 - C\bar{v}O_2$) = 50 mL/L. Thus, $\dot{V}O_2$ = 250 mL/min.

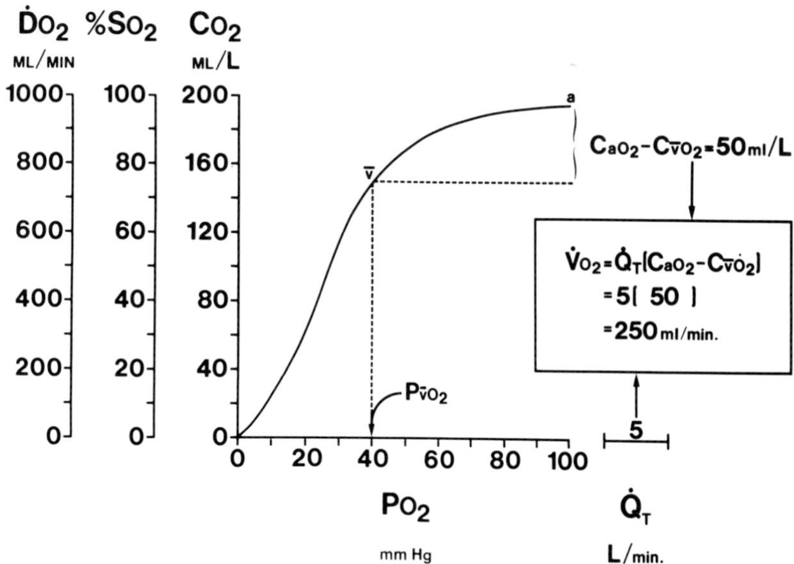

oxygen content, $C\bar{v}O_2$. Point $\bar{v}$ on the curve will then represent $C\bar{v}O_2$[20] (Fig. 5-4),

$$C\bar{v}O_2 = [Hb](S\bar{v}O_2 \times 1.34) + 0.03 \times P\bar{v}O_2),$$

where

$[Hb]$ = hemoglobin concentration in g/L;

$S\bar{v}O_2$ = mixed venous oxygen saturation (percent);

$P\bar{v}O_2$ = mixed venous oxygen tension (in mm Hg).

The calculation of $C\bar{v}O_2$ is thus analogous to that of $CaO_2$ except for $C\bar{v}O_2$, $S\bar{v}O_2$ is dependent on $P\bar{v}O_2$. Normally, a $C\bar{v}O_2$ of 150 mL/L corresponds to an $S\bar{v}O_2 = 75\%$ at a $P\bar{v}O_2 = 40$ mm Hg. Thus, if $C\bar{v}O_2 = 150$ mL of $O_2$ per liter, and $CaO_2 = 200$ mL/L, then the arterial-mixed venous oxygen content difference equals

$$(CaO_2 - C\bar{v}O_2) = 200 \text{ mL/L} - 150 \text{ mL/L}$$
$$= 50 \text{ mL/L}.$$

The extraction ratio may thus also be expressed as

$$\frac{CaO_2 - C\bar{v}O_2}{CaO_2}$$

In this example the extraction ratio $= \frac{50}{200} = 0.25$, which is normal.

If the arterial-mixed venous oxygen content difference is 50 mL of $O_2$ per liter, and the cardiac output is 5 L/min, then $\dot{V}O_2 = 5 \times 50 = 250$ mL/min. Stated another way, oxygen consumption is equal to the difference between the total oxygen delivered and that which is unused and returned to the pulmonary artery,[110] ie,

$$\dot{V}O_2 = \dot{D}O_2 - \text{unused } O_2$$
$$\therefore \dot{V}O_2 = (\dot{Q}_t \times CaO_2) - (\dot{Q}_t \times C\bar{v}O_2)$$
$$\dot{V}O_2 = \dot{Q}_t(CaO_2 - C\bar{v}O_2).$$

This is the familiar Fick equation, which relates arterial oxygen delivery ($\dot{Q}_t \times CaO_2$) to that portion of the delivered $O_2$ which is not consumed ($\dot{Q}_t \times C\bar{v}O_2$).

Viewed slightly differently, global oxygen uptake is equal to that fraction of total oxygen delivery which undergoes extraction by the tissues.[39] Thus

$$\dot{V}O_2 = (\dot{Q}_t \times CaO_2) \times \frac{(CaO_2 - C\bar{v}O_2)}{CaO_2}$$

that is, uptake = delivery × extraction ratio.

Oxygen delivery ($\dot{D}O_2$) to the various organ systems is contingent upon each organ's share of the total cardiac output ($\dot{Q}_t$) at any level of arterial oxygen content ($CaO_2$). Under physiologic conditions, oxygen extraction is determined by cellular metabolic oxygen requirements. Vasoregulation at the arteriolar and metarteriolar level controls distribution of regional $\dot{D}O_2$; these resistance vessels dilate and contract to modulate flow, as a function of oxygen need. At the organ level, then[39]

$O_2$ uptake (organ) = delivery (resistance vessels)

× extraction (exchange vessels, ie, capillaries)

Where extraction is normally high (eg, in the heart), augmented oxygen requirements are satisfied only by enhanced delivery ($\dot{Q}$, $\dot{D}O_2$). Changes in global $\dot{Q}_t$ are thus accompanied by regional alterations in exchange and resistance vessels. When $CaO_2$ is low, either flow, extraction, or both must increase. When the extremes of delivery and/or extraction are met and exceeded, anaerobiosis ensues, with attendant cellular hypoxia.

Table 5-2 summarizes the normal values of $O_2$ related variables.

## THE DISTRIBUTION OF TOTAL BODY OXYGEN CONSUMPTION

Unlike arterial oxygen, which is uniformly distributed among the various organ systems, the regional venous oxygen contents, tensions, and saturations differ from one organ to another. To complicate matters, the various regional venous effluents do not, in general, parallel or reflect their respective arterial blood flows or rates of oxygen delivery. More specifically, in the awake and resting state, there exists a mismatching of regional blood flow and regional oxygen delivery with respect to regional oxygen demands (see Tables 5-1 and 5-3). Rather, the regional venous effluents mirror each system's efficiency in extracting delivered oxygen. Table 5-3 and Fig 5-5 summarize these concepts.

From Table 5-3, it is readily apparent that measurement of the total body oxygen-related variables gives little insight into

TABLE 5-2. Summary of Normal Total Body Oxygen-related Variables

| | mL $O_2$/min | mL $O_2$/min | mL/L | mL/L | mL/L | mm Hg | % | EXTRACTION RATIO |
|---|---|---|---|---|---|---|---|---|
| Variable | $\dot{D}O_2$ | $\dot{V}O_2$ | $CaO_2$ | $C\bar{v}O_2$ | $CaO_2 - C\bar{v}O_2$ | $P\bar{v}O^2$ | $S\bar{v}O_2$ | |
| Average | 1000 | 250 | 200 | 150 | 50 | 40 | 75 | 0.25 |
| Range (mL/min/m$^2$)* | 880 to 1225 | 170 to 300 | 160 to 214 | 120 to 160 | 40 to 55 | 33 to 53 | 70 to 78 | 0.22 to 0.30 |

* $\dot{D}O_2$ and $\dot{V}O_2$ only

TABLE 5-3. Summary of Normal $O_2$ and Flow-related Variables of the Various Organ Systems (Resting State)*[220,298,333,349,373]

| | $\dot{Q}$ (mL/min) | $\dot{D}O_2$ (mL/min) | $CaO_2$ (mL/L) | $C\bar{v}O_2$ (mL/L) | $CaO_2 - C\dot{v}O_2$ (mL/L) | $\dot{V}O_2$ (mL/min) | $\dot{V}O_2$ (% of total) | $P\bar{v}O_2$ (mm Hg) | $S\bar{v}O_2$ | EXTRACTION RATIO |
|---|---|---|---|---|---|---|---|---|---|---|
| Splanchnic | 1400 | 280 | 200 | 159 | 41 | 57 | 22 | 45 | 80 | 0.20 |
| Renal | 1100 | 220 | 200 | 187 | 13 | 14 | 5 | 74 | 94 | 0.06 |
| Cerebral | 750 | 150 | 200 | 137 | 63 | 47 | 18 | 35 | 69 | 0.31 |
| Coronary | 250 | 50 | 200 | 86 | 114 | 29 | 11 | 23 to 27 | 37 to 50 | 0.58 |
| Skeletal muscle | 1200 | 240 | 200 | 120 | 80 | 96 | 36 | 32 | 60 | 0.40 |
| Skin | 500 | 100 | 200 | 190 | 10 | 5 | 2 | 75 | 95 | 0.05 |
| Other organs | 600 | 120 | 200 | 170 | 30 | 18 | 6 | 55 | 85 | 0.15 |
| Totals | 5800 | 1160 | Mean 200 | Mean 155 | Mean 45 | 266 | 100 | Mean 40 | Mean 77 | Mean 0.23 |

* 70-kg male, BSA = 1.7 $m^2$; [Hb] = 150 g/L; $SaO_2$ = 100%; $Q_t$ = 5.80 L/min.

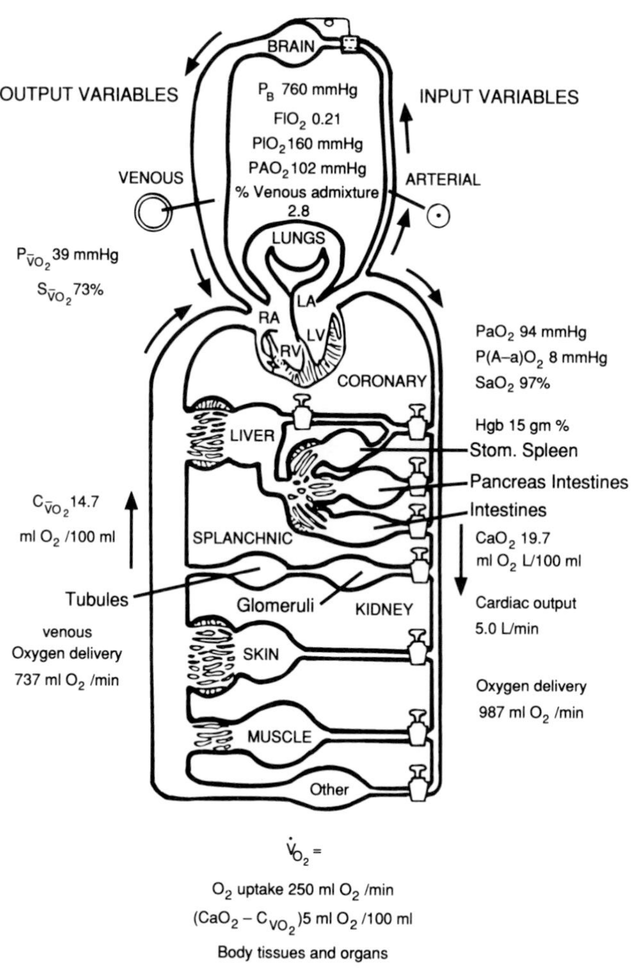


FIG. 5-5. Oxygen transport system. (Modified from Rowell LB. Human circulation. New York: Oxford University Press, 1986;10. Representative normal oxygen transport data taken from Martin L. Pulmonary physiology in clinical practice. St. Louis: CV Mosby, 1987;114.

the metabolic demands of different organs. It is convenient to discuss the efficiency of oxygen extraction of each organ by comparing their respective extraction ratios. For instance, the heart extracts approximately 60% of its total delivered $O_2$,[11,40,65,341,353] ie,

$$\frac{\text{coronary arterial } O_2 \text{ content} - \text{coronary sinus venous } O_2 \text{ content}}{\text{coronary arterial } O_2 \text{ content}} = \frac{M\dot{V}O_2}{M\dot{D}O_2}$$

$$= \text{approximately } 60\%.$$

where $M\dot{V}O_2$ and $M\dot{D}O_2$ are the myocardial oxygen consumption and delivery, respectively. The kidneys, on the other hand, extract only 6% of delivered $O_2$, and the extraction ratios of brain and splanchnic viscera are similar to that of the body as a whole, 0.31 and 0.20, respectively.

Table 5-4 shows the metabolic $O_2$ demands ($\dot{V}O_2$) of various organs. Thus, when the major vital organs are compared on a weight-to-weight basis, the heart maintains an oxygen consumption roughly twice that of the kidney and liver and two and one half times that of the brain.

Extraction ratios may also be computed by comparing regional $\dot{V}O_2$ with regional $\dot{D}O_2$. The mismatching of supply and demand is obvious when analyzed in this way[349] (Table 5-5). Thus, organs with high extraction ratios (heart, brain) require increased blood flow if oxygen demands increase (supply dependent), whereas those with low extraction ratios (kidney, liver, skin) can simply extract more oxygen from the same blood supply (supply independent). As a result, simple bedside measurement of global $\dot{V}O_2$, ($CaO_2 - C\bar{v}O_2$), $S\bar{v}O_2$, and $\dot{Q}_t$ are poor indicators of the metabolic activity of regional tissue beds. As emphasized by Taylor et al,[349] "total body $\dot{V}O_2$ will be an insensitive indicator of the oxygen demands of individual organs, such as the brain and heart, because the total body $\dot{V}O_2$ is weighted toward the supply-independent organs, and the small amount of blood flowing through these supply-dependent organs will have little effect on (global) $\dot{V}O_2$." As a corollary, the global extraction ratio is not always an accurate predictor of tissue hypoxia. Capillary recruitment, capillary transit time, changes in $O_2$ diffusivity, and alterations in mi-

TABLE 5-4. $\dot{V}O_2$/100 g of Heart, Brain, Kidney, and Liver per Minute

| | AVERAGE WEIGHT (g) | $\dot{V}O_2$/100 g of TISSUE (MEAN) |
|---|---|---|
| Heart | 300 | 9.7 |
| Brain | 1300 | 3.6 |
| Kidney | 150 × 2 | 4.7 |
| Liver | 1350 | 4.2 |

crovascular control can diminish the amount of $O_2$ extracted from the blood and can result in low extraction ratios even though tissue oxygen requirements are enhanced.[118]

## ACUTE COMPENSATIONS IN OXYGEN DELIVERY ($\dot{D}O_2$) AND EXTRACTION TO MAINTAIN ADEQUATE TISSUE OXYGENATION (MAINTENANCE OF $\dot{V}O_2$)

The Fick equation allows us to analyze what alternatives exist when pathologic derangements in blood flow ($\dot{Q}_t$) or arterial oxygen content ($CaO_2$) occur. If $\dot{V}O_2$ is to remain constant, a reduction in one variable in this equation should produce a corresponding but opposite alteration in the other. Specifically, a critical reduction in flow is compensated for by increasing oxygen extraction. Conversely, reduction of $CaO_2$ to critical levels is compensated for by augmentation of regional and global blood flow.[37,291]

### REDUCTION IN TOTAL BODY BLOOD FLOW (LOW CARDIAC OUTPUT STATE)

In compensated low cardiac output states, total body oxygen consumption is preserved by augmentation of oxygen extraction from hemoglobin and by redistribution of blood flow from areas of lesser importance to survival to the vital organs (ie, heart and brain).[97,330,331,335,383] Specifically, if $\dot{V}O_2$ is constant and $\dot{Q}_t$ decreases, then ($CaO_2 - C\bar{v}O_2$) increases.[137,166,187,279,280,291,299,303,326,343,366,381,383]

TABLE 5-5. $\dot{V}O_2$, $\dot{D}O_2$ and $\dot{V}O_2/\dot{D}O_2$ Values of Heart, Brain, Kidney, Liver, and Skeletal Muscle per 100 g of Tissue per Minute

| | $\dot{V}O_2$ (mL of $O_2$ per 100 g/min) | $\dot{D}O_2$ (mL of $O_2$ per 100 g/min) | EXTRACTION RATIO $\dot{V}O_2$/$\dot{D}O_2$ |
|---|---|---|---|
| Heart | 9.7 | 16.6 | 0.58 |
| Brain | 3.3 | 10.7 | 0.31 |
| Kidney | 4.7 | 73.3 | 0.06 |
| Liver | 4.2 | 20.7 | 0.20 |
| Skeletal muscle | 0.34 | 0.86 | 0.40 |

### ACUTE REDUCTION IN ARTERIAL OXYGEN CONTENT

When $CaO_2$ decreases, $\dot{V}O_2$ can be maintained only by augmentation of cardiac output and regional blood flow to the vital organs. The causes of decreased $CaO_2$ are hypoxemia, anemia, or both.

#### *Arterial Hypoxemia*

In the face of life-threatening arterial hypoxemia, the body increases cardiac output in order to maintain oxygen delivery to the tissues.[45,56,85,267] In the normal heart, the coronary vessels dilate almost immediately. Compensatory increases in coronary blood flow, which are seen at $SaO_2$ = 90 to 92%, are adequate until $SaO_2$ decreases to approximately 30%.[278] The cerebral circulation is not as responsive to arterial hypoxemia as are the coronary vessels; they begin to dilate only when $PaO_2$ falls below 50 mm Hg and are maximally dilated at $PaO_2$ = 30 mm Hg.[171,183] In nonacclimatized dogs, arterial hypoxemia ($PaO_2$ = 34 mm Hg) is associated with hyperlactatemia.[327] Normocapnic dogs subjected to arterial hypoxemia ($PaO_2$ = 29 to 34 mm Hg) during halothane anesthesia (1 Minimum Alveolar Concentration (MAC)) show enhancement in $\dot{Q}_t$ of approximately 50% primarily because of an increase in heart rate.[64,289] Thus, reduction in $SaO_2$, one of the two major components of $CaO_2$, produces a compensatory increase in $\dot{Q}_t$ and regional blood flow in order to preserve $\dot{V}O_2$.

#### *Acute Dilutional Anemia*

During acute normovolemic hemodilution, hemoglobin concentration decreases.[156] Compensation for mild to moderate hemodilution is accomplished by a reciprocal increase in cardiac output[110,124,207,270,271,291] primarily because of an increase in stroke volume mediated by enhanced venous return (ie, increased preload),[125,208] which, in turn, results from decreased blood viscosity and total peripheral resistance.[154] The arteriovenous oxygen content difference during acute dilutional anemia is unchanged or slightly diminished.[92,110,182,271] Thus, if $CaO_2$ decreases due to a mild to moderate decrease in [Hb], oxygen delivery is maintained by an increase in $\dot{Q}_t$ to support $\dot{V}O_2$.

The theoretical, experimental, and clinical evidence suggesting that mild to moderate degrees of induced intraoperative normovolemic hemodilution may be safe and even beneficial in the treatment of hemorrhage will be presented later in this chapter.[24,49,155,195]

## TISSUE HYPOXIA, INADEQUATE $\dot{V}O_2$, OR SHOCK

In basic terms, tissue hypoxia or dysoxia may be defined as a biochemical state in which there is insufficient intracellular (mitochondrial and extramitochondrial) oxygen to maintain aerobic metabolism.[40,45,110,238,267] Tissue hypoxia results when the oxygen delivery system or the capillary-cellular interface fails to supply sufficient $O_2$ to the organism or to one or more of its parts.[110,280] Hypoxia in one isolated organ may be responsible for subsequent hypoxia of the whole organism. For example, during an acute myocardial infarction, there is first regional myocardial hypoxia distal to the obstructed coronary artery. When extensive, this may result in left ventricular failure which, in turn, may lead to pulmonary edema, arterial hypoxemia,[181] and finally generalized hypoxia. In this condition both elements of $\dot{D}O_2$ are reduced, threatening total body $\dot{V}O_2$. Cardiac output is depressed by left ventricular failure, and $CaO_2$ is reduced by a fall in $SaO_2$. When $\dot{D}O_2$ is severely reduced, compensatory mechanisms (autoregulation of blood flow, increased $O_2$ extraction) ultimately fail.[280,335,383] As $\dot{D}O_2$ approaches $\dot{V}O_2$, lethal hypoxic limits are exceeded, and death ensues.

Tissue hypoxia may be caused by inadequate hemoglobin concentration, inadequate saturation of hemoglobin because of low $PaO_2$, and/or insufficient cardiac output or regional blood flow.[110] Deficiencies in these keystones of life were categorized in 1920 by Barcroft[12] into three subsets: (1) stagnant hypoxia (decreased flow); (2) anoxic hypoxia (decreased arterial oxygen); and (3) anemic hypoxia (decreased hemoglobin). Each of these mechanisms alone or in combination may be responsible for suboptimal oxygenation of trauma patients during the perioperative period.

## STAGNANT HYPOXIA

Hypoxia is stagnant when diminished blood flow with normal $CaO_2$ causes local or generalized tissue oxygen deficiency. During anesthesia this situation may be caused by reduction in circulating blood volume (hemorrhage, dehydration, third-space fluid sequestration), or low cardiac output states with normal blood volume (primary pump failure, bradyarrhythmia,[276] hypothermia,[223] overdose of anesthetic agents). If a low cardiac output state is present and the preceding causes have been ruled out in a previously healthy injured patient, myocardial contusion, tension pneumothorax, and/or pericardial tamponade should be suspected.[98,130,198,295,376]

## ANOXIC HYPOXIA

Insufficient oxygenation of blood by the lungs results in anoxic hypoxia. In healthy man, sudden bradycardia and cardiac arrest occur at an $FIO_2$ of 0.09.[267] When normothermic dogs are subjected to acute graded reductions of $FIO_2$, a $PaO_2$ of 24 to 27 mm Hg is generally associated with the beginning of terminal events.[117,291] Moreover, the EEG has been noted to become flat when $PaO_2$ is reduced acutely to 25 to 30 mm Hg.[300] In routine anesthetic practice, anoxic hypoxia usually results from physician inattentiveness, equipment failure, or both.[75,95,126,141,157,168,199,247,265,266,387] In trauma, however, acute life-threatening anoxic arterial hypoxemia is usually caused by the following:[98,295,377]

1. Obstruction of a bronchus by aspirated gastric contents or blood clots
2. Pneumothorax with atelectasis
3. Severe pulmonary contusion
4. Endotracheal tube placement into the right mainstem bronchus during initial resuscitation
5. Intrapulmonary hemorrhage
6. Flail chest secondary to rib fractures
7. Hemothorax
8. Tracheal and bronchial injuries
9. Diaphragmatic rupture
10. Neurogenic pulmonary edema[91]
11. Transfusion-induced noncardiogenic pulmonary edema[85,184]
12. Volume overload or cardiogenic pulmonary edema[181]
13. Esophageal intubation

In each situation, or combination thereof, the end result is decreased $PaO_2$ and $SaO_2$ due to increased right to left intrapulmonary shunting. The arterial desaturation can be properly treated only by recognition of the problem and institution of appropriate therapy.

## ANEMIC HYPOXIA

During acute reduction in hemoglobin concentration with normal circulating blood volume, limits may be reached which are no longer compatible with regional and total body aerobic metabolism.[45,136,154] As we have discussed, compensatory increases in $\dot{Q}_t$ initially supply adequate levels of $\dot{D}O_2$. However, this mechanism ultimately reaches a maximum and, with further decreases in [Hb], fails to compensate for the decreasing $CaO_2$.[136,154] Below a critical concentration hemoglobin can no longer supply the voracious myocardial $O_2$ demand.[33,154,291] As a result, $M\dot{V}O_2$ falls with a concomitant drop in $\dot{Q}_t$.

In normothermic dogs, whose myocardial glycolytic enzymes and metabolism are similar to those of man,[180] whole body $\dot{V}O_2$ and $\dot{Q}_t$ drop precipitously during acute normovolemic hemodilution when hematocrit is less than 20% ([Hb] $< 70$ g/L).[154] Excess lactate production and an acute drop in $M\dot{V}O_2$ have been documented when hematocrit is reduced to this level.[44,154] Clearly then, anemic hypoxia is present regionally and probably globally at hematocrit levels of less than 20%.[110] More recent experimental data even suggest that in healthy canine hearts with a stable work requirement, hematocrits as low as 10% ([Hb] $=$ 30 g/L) support normal resting $M\dot{V}O_2$. However, when coronary insufficiency was simulated, $M\dot{V}O_2$ was maintained only by hematocrit greater than 17%.[63] A detailed discussion of acceptable or optimal intraoperative and postoperative hemoglobin concentration is presented in the section on oxygen transport in hemorrhage.

In summary, the organism's response to alterations of oxygen delivery may be viewed sequentially and temporally. Deviation from normal oxygen delivery values results in appropriate changes of $\dot{Q}_t$ and/or $CaO_2 - C\bar{v}O_2$ in order to preserve $\dot{V}O_2$. If adequate alteration of the elements of $\dot{D}O_2$ ($\dot{Q}_t$ and $CaO_2$) is possible, compensation is achieved.[280,291] However, if progressive deterioration of one or both of these elements persists, one or more organ systems will become starved for oxygen,[110] and anaerobic metabolism will ensue. If this sequence is allowed to continue, irreversible damage and cell death will occur regionally or globally.[280] Optimization of $\dot{D}O_2$ and extraction to preserve $\dot{V}O_2$ require identification of the problem ($\dot{Q}_t$, [Hb], or $SaO_2$). Institution of appropriate therapy is then based on the etiologic deficiencies.

## LIMITING FACTORS IN TISSUE OXYGEN EXTRACTION

### CONSUMABLE OR AVAILABLE OXYGEN

The oxyhemoglobin dissociation curve does not provide quantitative information about the amount of oxygen that can actually be extracted for utilization. Oxygen delivered to the capillaries at a $Po_2$ of 20 mm Hg or less under normothermic conditions is unavailable for diffusion into certain tissues.[40,41,42,72,99,121,194,214] At this level, most tissues will take up oxygen only in amounts less than needed for oxidative metabolism.[41,72,309] Thus, these tissues must resort to anaerobic glycolysis with lactic acid production. The concept of *critical* $Po_2$ is based on the observation that unconsciousness ensues and the EEG becomes flat when cerebral venous (jugular) $Po_2$ falls below 20 mm Hg.[214,238,300]
Thus, since

$$\text{total } \dot{D}o_2 = \dot{Q}_t \times Cao_2$$

then *consumable* $O_2$ or the oxygen actually *available* for aerobic metabolism equals

$\dot{D}o_2$ (consumable or available) approximately

$$= \dot{Q}_t(Cao_2 - C\bar{v}o_2) \text{ at } P\bar{v}o_2 = 20 \text{ mm Hg}$$

or

$\dot{D}o_2$ (consumable or available) approximately

$$= \dot{Q}_t(Cao_2 - [S_{20}\bar{v}o_2 \times 1.34 \times Hb])$$

where $S_{20}\bar{v}o_2$ is the derived $O_2$ saturation of blood calculated for $Po_2$ at 20 mm Hg under mixed venous conditions at 37°C.[41,42]

Thus, the oxyhemoglobin dissociation curve may be redrawn showing the intersect of the sigmoidal curve with a vertical line drawn at $Po_2$ = 20 mm Hg (Fig 5-6). The saturation corresponding to this point is called $S_{20}\bar{v}o_2$. For the normal oxyhemoglobin curve, $S_{20}\bar{v}_2$ is 32%.[238] This point correlates with the minimum hemoglobin saturation at which tissue can extract oxygen and aerobic metabolism can occur without tissue hypoxia.[72,383] Based on clinical[167] and experimental[327] data demonstrating that hyperlactatemia routinely supervenes at a $P\bar{v}o_2$ of 27 to 28 mm Hg, Snyder[337] proposes that the blood oxygen saturation corresponding to this critical $P\bar{v}o_2$ be used in consumable oxygen calculations (ie, $S_{28}\bar{v}o_2$). Assuming a normal $P_{50}$, $P\bar{v}o_2$ at 27 to 28 mm Hg corresponds to $S\bar{v}o_2$ = 50 to 53%. Others have confirmed this higher anaerobic threshold in normothermic animals.[287,288] Thus, whereas $P\bar{v}o_2 \leq 20$ mm Hg is indicative of exhaustion of all metabolic reserves and imminent death of the organism, $P\bar{v}o_2 \leq 27$ to 28 mm Hg is pathognomonic of severe metabolic disruption, which, if left untreated, will lead to multisystem organ failure and death. As a consequence of these considerations, the extraction ratios for the various organ systems (Table 5-3) should be recalculated taking into account the actual consumable or available $O_2$.

For example, the extraction ratio for the myocardium, $M\dot{V}o_2/M\dot{D}o_2$, is approximately 60% when compared with total oxygen delivery, $\dot{D}o_2 = Q_{CBF} \times Cao_2$ (see Tables 5-3 and 5-5)[11] but when referenced to $S_{20}\bar{v}o_2$, the extraction ratio

$$= \frac{M\dot{V}o_2}{\text{consumable } O_2}$$

FIG. 5-6. Consumable oxygen. *Conditions:* [Hb] = 150 g/L, pH = 7.40, temperature = 37°C, $Pco_2$ = 40 mm Hg. Although total oxygen delivery ($\dot{D}o_2$) to tissues is 1000 mL/min at $\dot{Q}_t$ = 5 L/min, the amount available for aerobic utilization is only 680 mL/min, or roughly two thirds of the total amount delivered. Oxygen delivered to end capillaries at $Po_2$ less than 20 mm Hg is, in general, considered to be unavailable for aerobic metabolism.

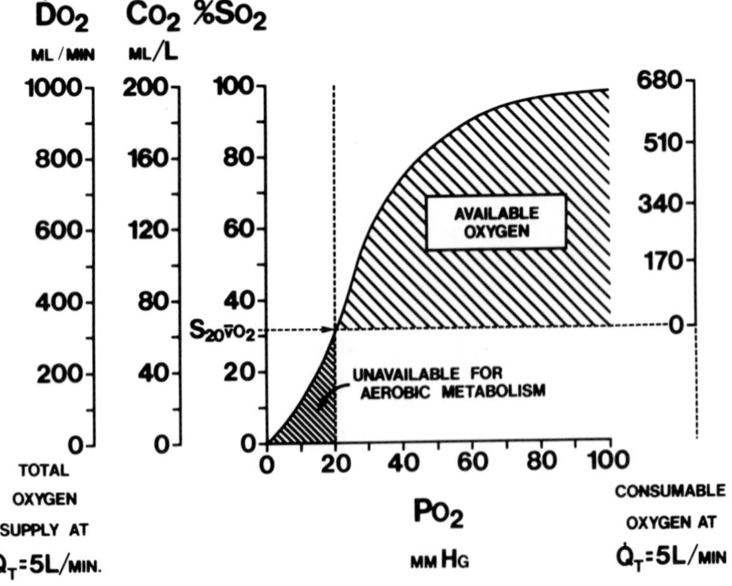

$$= \frac{M\dot{V}O_2}{Q_{CBF}\,(CaO_2 - S_{20}\bar{v}O_2 \times 1.34\,[Hb])}$$

$$= \frac{29 \text{ mL of } O_2 \text{ per minute}}{34 \text{ mL of } O_2 \text{ per minute}}$$

$$= 85\%$$

Thus, if steady-state $M\dot{V}O_2$ (myocardial $O_2$ consumption) is 29 mL of $O_2$ per minute and consumable $O_2$ approximately 34 ml/min, then the effective extraction ratio is 85%. Hence, the heart does, in fact, strip most of the available oxygen from hemoglobin.

Similarly, if this analysis is applied to the total body, the average effective extraction ratio for the organism referenced to consumable $O_2$ (available $O_2$) equals

$$\frac{\dot{V}O_2}{\text{consumable } O_2} \cong 35\%$$

During anesthesia, the critical $PO_2$ may be lower because the cerebral metabolic rate for oxygen ($CMRO_2$) is markedly reduced by most anesthetics,[224] indicating a potential protective effect of these drugs.[132] The concept of critical $P\bar{v}O_2$ or the critical flow-weighted mean $PO_2$, which represents the mean tissue oxygen tension needed to maintain aerobic metabolism, needs further clarification. In an elegant review, Willford et al have shown that the critical $P\bar{v}O_2$ is reduced by hypothermia.[390] Their human values, extrapolated from animal studies, have been verified by others.[117] For example, in humans, consumable oxygen at normothermia is calculated using $S_{20}\bar{v}O_2$, whereas at 30°C, consumable oxygen is calculated using $S\bar{v}O_2$ at ≈ 14 mm Hg (ie, $S_{14}\bar{v}O_2$).[390] In spite of this, the concepts of critical $PO_2$ and consumable or available $O_2$ are important for estimating the amount of $O_2$ which can actually be utilized for aerobic metabolism.

## AFFINITY OF HEMOGLOBIN FOR OXYGEN ($P_{50}$)[110]

Acting independently, but in concert with consumable $O_2$, alterations in the affinity of hemoglobin for $O_2$ theoretically determine the amount that can be aerobically extracted by tissues.[139,304,351,395,397] The affinity or tenacity with which hemoglobin binds $O_2$ has been quantitatively defined as the partial pressure of oxygen at which 50% of the binding sites of hemoglobin are saturated with $O_2$ ($P_{50}$). The $P_{50}$ of normal hemoglobin at pH = 7.40, $PCO_2$ = 40 mm Hg, and 37°C is 26 to 27 mm Hg.[296]

Graphically, this value is determined by locating the point on the sigmoid curve which corresponds to 50% hemoglobin saturation (Fig 5-7). $P_{50}$ is extrapolated by dropping a vertical line from this point. In Fig 5-7, curve 1 is the normal curve. At 50% saturation, its $P_{50}$ = 26 to 27 mm Hg. Curve 2 is shifted to the right of the normal curve. The $P_{50}$ of this curve is 40 mm Hg. Curve 3 is shifted to the left; its $P_{50}$ is approximately 16 mm Hg.

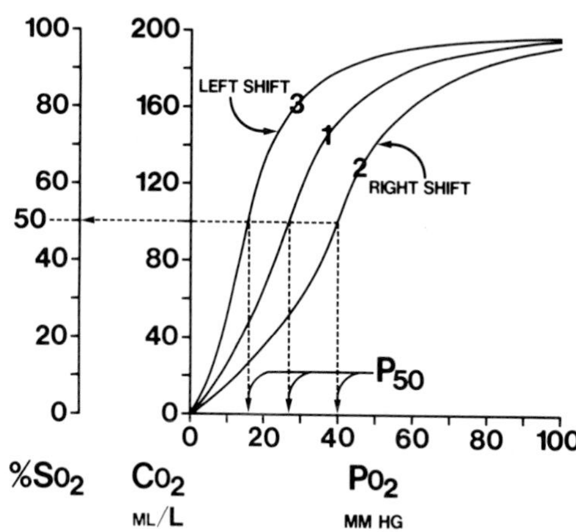


FIG. 5-7. Affinity of hemoglobin for oxygen. Altered affinity of hemoglobin for oxygen may be depicted graphically as alteration in the position and shape of the oxyhemoglobin dissociation curve. Changes in the position of the curve are quantitated by analysis of the $P_{50}$, that $PO_2$ which produces 50% saturation of hemoglobin. A right-shifted curve indicates decreased affinity and a higher $P_{50}$ (curve 2); a left-shifted curve indicates increased affinity and a lower $P_{50}$. (curve 3).

### *Decreased Oxygen Affinity of Hemoglobin (Shift to the Right)*

When the curve is shifted to the right, at any given hemoglobin saturation $O_2$ is delivered to tissues at a higher $PO_2$.[301] Thus, a greater pressure gradient exists, as compared with the normal curve, for oxygen's diffusion into the cells. A shift to the right (decreased affinity) also implies that at any given capillary $PO_2$, less $O_2$ is bound to hemoglobin; it is therefore more available to tissues for uptake and utilization.[351] Decreased blood (hemoglobin) oxygen affinity may be caused by the following:

1. Elevated levels of 2,3-DPG (2,3-diphosphoglycerate)
2. Acidosis (eg, in hemorrhagic shock, capillary acidosis acutely induces decreased affinity and increased $P_{50}$)[142]
3. Hypercapnia
4. Hyperthermia

### *Increased Oxygen Affinity of Hemoglobin (Shift to the Left)*

A left-shifted oxyhemoglobin dissociation curve implies increased affinity of hemoglobin for $O_2$.[301] At any given saturation of hemoglobin, a lower than normal capillary $PO_2$ exists. This means that the tissues are exposed to a smaller end capillary-tissue gradient for $O_2$ diffusion. Further analysis of the left-shifted curve reveals that at any specified capillary $PO_2$, more $O_2$ is bound to hemoglobin (ie, higher percent saturation), and thus less is available for uptake and utilization. Increased blood oxygen affinity and left shift of the oxyhemoglobin dissociation curve are caused by

1. Decreased levels of 2,3-DPG
2. Alkalosis
3. Hypocapnia
4. Hypothermia[117]

### *Clinical Significance of Alterations in Hemoglobin's Affinity for Oxygen*

In discussing the effects of changes in oxygen affinity, it would seem relevant to emphasize the organs that normally function in a virtually pure aerobic environment. One such organ is the heart, which is a net consumer, rather than producer, of lactate.[110,223,278,279] Because the heart muscle cannot maintain itself by anaerobic metabolism, total deprivation of $O_2$ for more than 2 minutes results in cessation of mechanical activity.[107] The average intramyocardial cellular $Po_2$ is approximately 20 mm Hg.[278] Thus, when the intramyocardial $Po_2$ falls below this value, lactate production in excess of consumption begins. Although the critical $Po_2$ of the heart is said to be between 5 and 10 mm Hg,[278] anaerobic metabolism and net lactate production begin at a coronary sinus $So_2$ of 30% (or $Po_2$ = 20 mm Hg).[278,279] In the following three examples, the effects produced by altered $O_2$ affinity of hemoglobin upon myocardial tissue oxygenation are examined (Fig. 5-8). For the sake of simplicity, we will assume a steady state in which $M\dot{V}o_2$ and coronary blood flow (250 mL/min) remain constant. Also [Hb] = 150 g/L, temperature = 37°C, pH = 7.40, $Sao_2$ = 100%, and critical $Po_2$ of the heart = 20 mm Hg.

EXAMPLE 1 (CURVE B). This represents a decreased $O_2$ affinity or a shift to the right of the oxyhemoglobin dissociation curve ($P_{50}$ = 35 mm Hg). Deliverable or consumable $O_2$ within the confines of aerobic metabolism is defined as

$$\dot{Q}_t(Cao_2 - [S_{20}\bar{v}o_2 \times [Hb] \times 1.34]).$$

For curve B, $S_{20}\bar{v}o_2$ is approximately 25%; therefore, consumable $O_2$ = 38 mL of $O_2$ per 250 mL/min or approximately 150 mL of $O_2$ per liter per minute.

EXAMPLE 2 (CURVE A). This is an example of normal hemoglobin $O_2$ affinity; $P_{50}$ = 27 mm Hg; no shift; $S_{20}\bar{v}o_2$ approximately = 32%; therefore, total consumable or available $O_2$

$$= 0.25(200 - [0.32 \times 150 \times 1.34])$$

$$= 34 \text{ mL of } O_2 \text{ per 250 mL/min}$$

$$= 136 \text{ mL of } O_2 \text{ per liter/min.}$$

EXAMPLE 3 (CURVE C). Left shift of the oxyhemoglobin dissociation curve (ie, increased affinity of hemoglobin for $O_2$); $P_{50}$ = 18 mm Hg; $S_{20}\bar{v}o_2$ = 55%; therefore, total available $O_2$

$$= \dot{Q}_t(Cao_2 - [S_{20}\bar{v}o_2 \times [Hb] \times 1.34])$$

$$= 22 \text{ mL of } O_2 \text{ per 250 mL/min (total available } O_2)$$

$$= 88 \text{ mL of } O_2 \text{ per liter/min}$$

It is self evident from these examples that consumable or available $O_2$ to the heart may be considerably affected by changes in hemoglobin's affinity for oxygen.

## RESERVE OXYGEN, OXYGEN DEFICIT, AND AFFINITY HYPOXIA

The computation of consumable $O_2$, the $O_2$ actually available for aerobic metabolism, permits a clearer understanding of the effects of altered affinity. In the case of hemoglobin with a normal $P_{50}$, 34 mL of $O_2$ per minute are available for consumption by the heart, and 29 mL is actually consumed

FIG. 5-8. Reserve oxygen, oxygen deficit, and affinity hypoxia of the heart. *Conditions:* Coronary blood flow = 250 mL/min, [Hb] = 150 g/L, $Sao_2$ = 100%. The normal coronary arterial-coronary sinus oxygen content difference = 114 mL/L. When consumable oxygen exceeds 114 mL/L, an oxygen reserve exists (curves A and B). When consumable oxygen is less than 114 mL/L, an oxygen deficit is generated (curve C), and affinity hypoxia results.

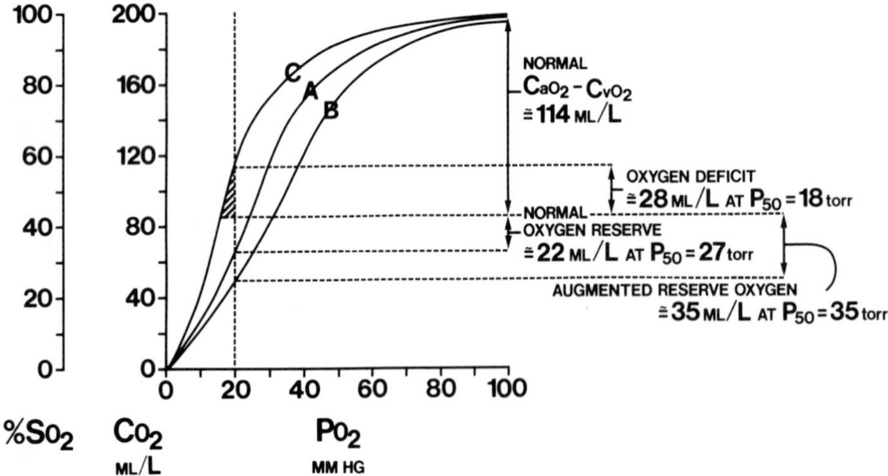

(Table 5-3), giving a net excess of 5 mL of $O_2$ per minute. This excess is called the *oxygen reserve.*[19] For hemoglobin with decreased $O_2$ affinity, the reserve $O_2$ amounts to 9 mL of $O_2$ per minute, an increase of 4 mL of $O_2$ per minute over normal (Fig 5-8).

Analysis of the low $P_{50}$ (18 mm Hg), high $O_2$ affinity, left-shifted curve reveals consumable or available $O_2$ of only 22 mL of $O_2$ per minute. If basal consumption of the heart requires 29 mL of $O_2$ per minute, the minimum aerobic requirements are not met, and hypoxia results. When aerobic demands exceed available or consumable oxygen, an oxygen deficit (debt) exists. A deficit caused by low $P_{50}$ blood is defined as affinity hypoxia[42,84,139] (Fig 5-8).

Fortunately, oxygen demand is generally met by an autoregulatory increase in coronary blood flow[84,394,396] (Fig 5-9). Likewise, the brain, an obligatory aerobic organ, increases cerebral blood flow when $P_{50}$ is reduced.[396] Thus, moderate to severe reductions in $P_{50}$ are usually well compensated for by autoregulation in the coronary and cerebral circulations.[55,395,394] However, if severe coronary or cerebrovascular stenosis is present, the fixed flow distal to the obstruction may result in myocardial or cerebral hypoxia if consumable $O_2$ is reduced by increased affinity to hemoglobin.[84,139,397] The controversial area of affinity hypoxia and low 2,3-DPG levels in old banked blood is discussed in the section on storage lesions of banked blood in Chapter 6.

Other clinical implications of altered blood oxygen affinity on tissue oxygenation are more obvious. Affinity hypoxia may occur in flow-limited areas of various organs (especially the brain and heart) because of respiratory and metabolic alkalosis caused by overzealous positive pressure ventilation and sodium bicarbonate administration.[59,76,139,215,217,395] Moderate to extreme hypothermia from environmental causes as well as from rapid administration of cold resuscitation fluids or blood may have the same effect.[87,216,304]

FIG. 5-9. Effect of change in hemoglobin oxygen affinity on myocardial oxygen delivery and consumption in a beating isolated rat heart perfused with blood. In this experiment the $P_{50}$ of control blood was 21.5 mm Hg. A decrease of $P_{50}$ to 9.0 mm Hg was achieved by use of an abnormal hemoglobin. Note that with perfusion of high oxygen affinity blood ($P_{50}$ = 9 mm Hg), the coronary arterial-coronary sinus oxygen content difference decreased, but there was an associated rise in coronary blood flow (Q). When $P_{50}$ was restored to control levels, the ($CaO_2 - CcsO_2$) difference rose, and Q fell to control levels. Thus, augmentation of coronary blood flow compensated for high oxygen affinity blood, and myocardial oxygen delivery ($M\dot{D}O_2$) remained adequate to preserve $M\dot{V}O_2$ (myocardial oxygen consumption). (Ccs = coronary sinus oxygen content) (From Duvelleroy et al[84] with permission.)

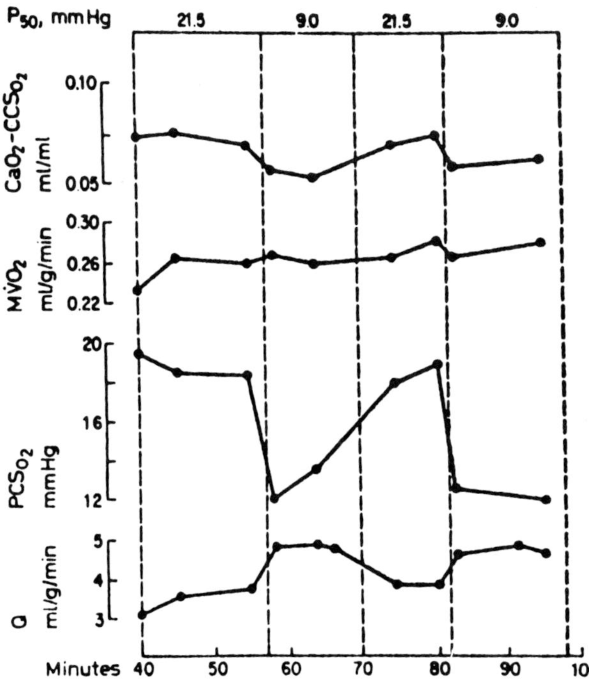


## OTHER DETERMINANTS OF OXYGEN EXTRACTION AND UTILIZATION

### CELLULAR RESPIRATION (INTRINSIC METABOLIC OXYGEN NEEDS)

Mitochondrial and extramitochondrial oxygen requirements change dramatically in the unsteady state. Tissue oxygen uptake ($\dot{V}O_2$) is governed by these requirements. Virtually any physical event or therapeutic intervention can change $\dot{V}O_2$. Common causes are:

1. Trauma
2. Surgery
3. Temperature change
4. Drug therapy (including anesthetic agents)
5. Mechanical ventilation
6. Major burns
7. Neurologic injuries
8. Postoperative shivering.

### PHYSICAL STATUS OF THE MICROCIRCULATION (DIFFUSIONAL INTERFACE)

Transport of oxygen from the capillary to the tissue cells is a direct function of tissue oxygen needs and the distances across which oxygen must diffuse. Diffusion distance depends on the number of perfused capillaries and their architecture. Microvascular oxygen transport is also dependent on[118]:

1. Relative distribution of cardiac output
2. Microvascular control mechanisms (both neurogenic and metabolic vasoregulation)
3. Capillary red cell transit time
4. Microcirculatory hematocrit
5. Capillary recruitment
6. Peripheral vascular shunts (anatomic or functional).

In addition, other factors that could limit oxygen delivery or utilization at the cell level include[349]:

1. Presence of metabolites or conditions in damaged organs which interfere with mitochondrial utilization of oxygen (eg, complement activation, arachidonic acid metabolites, oxygen radical damage, acidosis)
2. Physical impediments to microcirculatory flow such as

microemboli, edema, or platelet and white cell thrombi, which increase diffusion distance from the capillary to the tissue cell.

In conclusion, oxygen transport is a corporate affair involving the harmonic interaction of the lungs, heart, blood, and microcirculation.[38,268] Reduction in the efficiency of the lungs or heart, deficiencies in the quantity or quality of blood, or disruption of the functional integrity of the microcirculation will induce compensatory mechanisms to maintain oxygen delivery. When these fail, hypoxia and ultimately cell death ensue. Vigilant maintenance of these four variables will ensure adequate cardiac output, arterial oxygen content, and tissue oxygen extraction. In order to achieve optimal fractional unloading of oxygen at the capillary level, maintenance of normal or moderately decreased blood oxygen affinity is important and desirable.[60,351]

Oxygen delivery, $\dot{D}o_2$, subserves oxygen consumption, $\dot{V}o_2$.[46,245,280] The anesthesiologist's task is to maintain an adequate buffer zone between these dynamic entities. $\dot{V}o_2$ is the marker of all aerobic life, and it rises and falls according to aerobic metabolic demands. Consequently, $\dot{D}o_2$ must rise and fall in parallel with these demands.[390] Failure to maintain $\dot{D}o_2$ will end either in regional system failure[230] or in death of the organism.[83,86,164,242,280,392]

## SYSTEMIC OXYGEN TRANSPORT ($\dot{D}o_2$) IN HEMORRHAGE

Untreated hemorrhage and its sequel, hemorrhagic shock, may be viewed as a progressive failure of the oxygen delivery system. More specifically, continuing loss of circulating blood volume sets in motion certain compensatory physiologic adjustments that seek to preserve oxygen delivery to vital organs at the expense of biologically less significant tissues.[316,317,330,331]

A reduction in circulating blood volume produces a drop in cardiac output.[82,291,303,324] The acute compensations for this include the following:[3,82,197,316,317,334,382]

1. Arteriolar and metarteriolar vasoconstriction
2. Venoconstriction and reduced capacitance of the great veins
3. Tachycardia and increased myocardial contractility
4. Pulmonary vasoconstriction
5. Progressive increase in arterial-mixed venous oxygen content difference (ie, increased extraction of $O_2$ resulting from slowing of the blood flow)
6. Systemic arteriovenous shunting through non-nutrient microvascular channels
7. Shift of the oxyhemoglobin dissociation curve to the right[137,142]
8. Transcapillary refill (endogenous autotransfusion)
9. Redistribution of cardiac output within and between organs.

The essence of compensation in hemorrhage is the redistribution of a progressively diminishing total oxygen delivery in an attempt to maintain oxygen consumption ($\dot{V}o_2$) in vital organs. This process includes diverting $\dot{D}o_2$ from areas of lesser biologic survival significance and lower extraction ratios, which function relatively well under anaerobic conditions, to areas vital to survival (heart, brain), which have relatively high extraction ratios and function poorly, or not at all, in the absence of sufficient oxygen (Fig 5-10).[97,331]

Fig 5-11 depicts alterations in hemodynamic and oxygen transport variables in hemorrhage, normovolemic anemia, and arterial hypoxemia in the dog. Compensations in the early and middle periods of exsanguination include a dramatic rise in total peripheral resistance (arteriolar and metarteriolar vasoconstriction) and an augmentation of the arteriovenous oxygen content difference (increased extraction of oxygen). With increasing blood loss, compensation begins to fail; there is a marked drop in TPR and oxygen extraction. Coincident with these events, $\dot{V}o_2$ plummets, and death ultimately follows. It should be noted that $\dot{V}o_2$ is well maintained until decompensation occurs at a blood volume approximately 50% of control. The maintenance of normal total body $\dot{V}o_2$ by no means implies that all is well.[112] During the early phase of compensation, some organs such as muscle, skin, bone, kidney, and intestines may be rendered ischemic by arteriolar and metarteriolar vasoconstriction, while the heart may have increased oxygen demand and consumption because of increased contractility and tachycardia.

Since the primary pathophysiologic defect in hemorrhagic shock is impaired $O_2$ transport,[316,317] the oxygen delivery equation and its close relative, the Fick equation, may be useful as guides to diagnosis and treatment of the syndrome.

$$\dot{D}o_2 = \dot{Q}_t \times Cao_2 = \text{delivery}$$

$$\dot{V}o_2 = \dot{Q}_t(Cao_2 - C\bar{v}o_2) = \text{consumption}$$

If

$$TPR = \frac{MAP - CVP}{\dot{Q}_t}$$ [105,162]

and

$$TPR = SVR \times \eta$$

where

SVR = systemic vascular resistance (vascular hindrance)[94,154]

and

$$\eta = \text{viscosity},$$

then

$$\dot{Q}_t = \frac{MAP - CVP}{SVR \times \eta}.$$

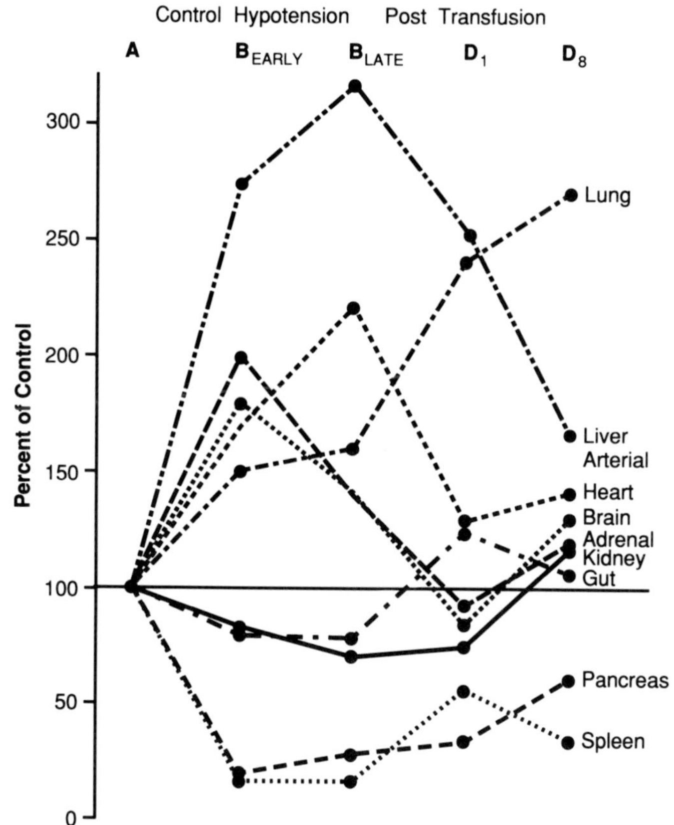


FIG. 5-10. Distribution of cardiac output in hemorrhagic shock. When unanesthetized dogs are hemorrhaged to 50% of control blood volume and mean arterial pressure, redistribution of cardiac output occurs. During hemorrhagic hypotension (cardiac output 50% of control) regional blood flow, expressed as percentage of normal, increased markedly to the heart, brain, adrenal glands, and liver, while flow to the gut, kidney, pancreas, and spleen decreased. (From Slater et al[331] with permission.)

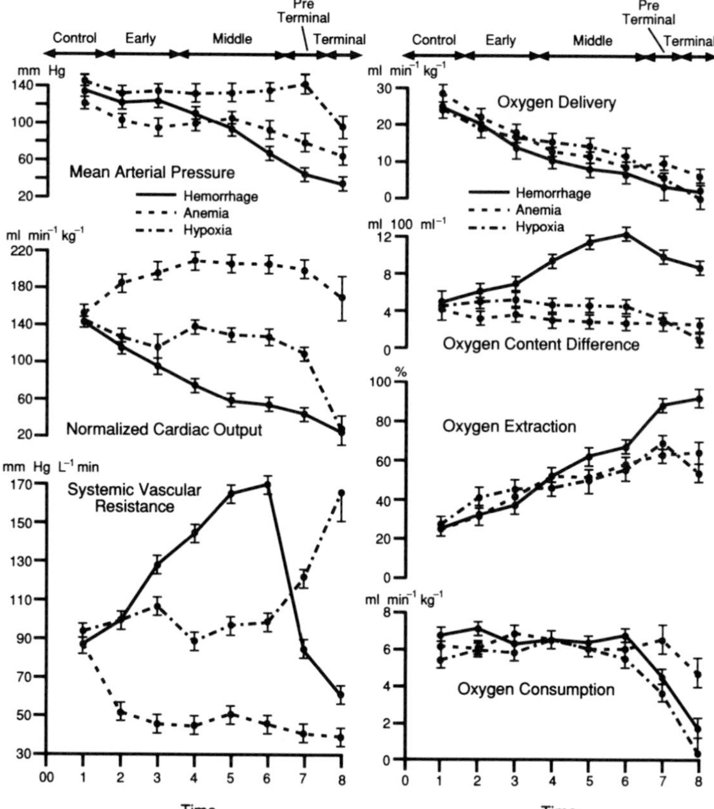


FIG. 5-11. Representative hemodynamic (left) and oxygen transport (right) variables during progressive hemorrhage, acute normovolemic anemia, and arterial hypoxemia. (From Schwartz et al[291] with permission.)

and

$$\dot{D}O_2 = \frac{MAP - CVP}{SVR \times \eta} \times CaO_2$$

$$\dot{D}O_2 = \frac{MAP - CVP}{SVR \times \eta} \times ([Hb] \times SaO_2 \times 1.34).$$

(dissolved $O_2$ omitted)

Furthermore,

consumable $O_2$

$$= \frac{MAP - CVP}{SVR \times \eta} \times [CaO_2 - ([Hb] \times S_{20}\bar{v}O_2 \times 1.34)]$$

The oxygen delivery equation in its various modifications allows analysis of the hemorrhagic syndrome temporally and sequentially. Early clinical descriptions of the hemorrhagic state characterized it as being one of tachycardia, low flow, high resistance, low blood pressure, and reduced central venous pressure. These notions are simplistic since moderate deficiencies in blood volume may occur without hypotension, significant drop in CVP, or significant elevation in heart rate.[17,291,293,303,315,328,381]

In the so-called normotensive phase of hemorrhagic shock, MAP may be entirely normal[138] because of a compensatory increase in TPR and ultimately increased heart rate to offset the progressively diminishing stroke volume, ie, MAP = HR × SV × TPR (see Fig 5-11). Likewise, CVP may give no clue as to the severity of hemorrhage in its early phases, if sufficient peripheral venoconstriction and contraction of the great veins have taken place.[194,328] Central venous pressure is multidimensional and is determined primarily by right ventricular function, blood volume, and venous tone.[162,315] A moderate reduction in blood volume may be well compensated for by reduced venous capacitance, which may not reflect itself as a reduced CVP.[120,205]

Hemoglobin concentration may be entirely normal if hemorrhage has been sufficiently rapid and effective transcapillary refill has not occurred.[82,398,315,381] Thus, a gross reduction in red cell mass may not be reflected in reduced hematocrit. Likewise, if supplemental oxygen is given, arterial oxygen saturation ($SaO_2$) may be normal.[164,166,187,230,234,303,324,360,363,365,381]

Despite normal MAP, CVP, and $CaO_2$, oxygen delivery is reduced in early hemorrhage because of a drop in $\dot{Q}_t$ mediated primarily by decreased preload and increased TPR.[291] Attempts to maintain $\dot{Q}_t$ include venoconstriction to enhance venous return and thus ventricular preload.[120] A marked rise in TPR in the presence of mild changes of MAP, CVP, and $CaO_2$ in either direction leads to a decline in $\dot{D}O_2$, ie,

$$\frac{MAP(\pm) - CVP(\pm)}{TPR(+++)} \times CaO_2\,(\pm) \text{ results in decreased } \dot{D}O_2.$$

However, certain physiologic compensatory responses take place to preserve $\dot{D}O_2$ to vital organs.[3,316,317,331] For instance, there is progressive augmentation of heart rate to compensate for the declining stroke volume.

As hemorrhage continues, blood flows more slowly through nonvital areas of the microcirculation. In addition, the declining blood volume becomes progressively maldistributed to the extent that some tissues are almost completely deprived of blood flow, eg, skin, muscle, bone, kidney, and intestine (Fig 5-10).[331] These and other organs are then obliged to extract a greater percentage of oxygen from less blood, causing progressive widening of the arterial-mixed venous oxygen content difference.[166,291,303] When oxygen extraction proceeds beyond the limits of the critical $PO_2$ values of the various tissues, anaerobiosis—first regional, then global—ensues.[230] This physiologic event marks the beginning of stagnant hypoxia and decompensation.

Decompensated hemorrhagic shock is characterized by the following[3]:

1. Rapid fading of arteriolar and metarteriolar vasoconstriction, with decreasing systemic vascular resistance
2. Sustained venoconstriction
3. Progressive decline in venous return
4. Inexorable fall in MAP
5. Progressive decline in $\dot{Q}_t$
6. Increasing lactic acidosis.

Thus, TPR drops, reducing effective perfusion through systemic arteriovenous shunts and severely decreasing venous return to the central circulation. Concurrently, consumable oxygen rapidly approaches total body oxygen consumption. Physiologically and temporally, this stage of shock is a preterminal phase in which virtually all compensatory mechanisms have failed. In the splenectomized, lightly anesthetized dog, this occurs when blood volume has been reduced 40 to 50%.[291]

The foregoing discussion is based on findings during controlled hemorrhage in dogs; this model is too simplistic to be applied to humans involved in trauma.[316,317] The physiologic responses to blunt trauma without hemorrhage are quite different from those seen in hemorrhage without tissue injury. Trauma, per se, produces an immediate response characterized by[316]

1. Increased $\dot{Q}_t$ with increased heart rate and stroke volume
2. Increased $\dot{D}O_2$
3. Decreased MAP
4. Decreased TPR
5. Decreased arterial-mixed venous oxygen content difference
6. Decreased oxygen extraction
7. Decreased $\dot{V}O_2$.

After trauma, there is a generalized increase in autonomic activity with release of neurohormones and stimulation of the cardiac and respiratory centers of the brain. This results in tachycardia, increased myocardial contractility, and augmented alveolar ventilation. If the victim is normovolemic, stroke volume and thus $\dot{Q}_t$ increase because of increased venous return. Thus, patients who are involved in massive trauma with little or no hemorrhage present a totally different clinical picture from those who are hemorrhaging briskly from relatively minimal trauma. When trauma and hemorrhage coexist, vital signs and cardiorespiratory variables may result from both entities and not be truly representative of either. Eventually, however, after sufficient blood loss, the physiologic hallmarks of hemorrhage become obvious.

## GOALS OF RESUSCITATION IN HEMORRHAGIC SHOCK

1. Augmentation, restoration, and proper redistribution of the oxygen transport by asanguinous fluid infusion
2. Optimization of the arterial oxygen content by transfusion of red blood cells or whole blood and augmentation of $Sa_{O_2}$ if arterial hypoxemia is present. Restoration of a fully saturated critical red cell mass
3. Improvement of nutrient microcirculatory flow
4. Assessment and optimization of blood oxygen affinity to ensure adequate fractional unloading of oxygen at the capillary-tissue interface.

The principal goal of resuscitation is restoration of overall oxygen delivery by rapid augmentation of cardiac output.[86,391] Since hemorrhage produces an absolute reduction in circulating blood volume and red cell mass, one could simply administer blood and, since $Ca_{O_2}$ does not change during rapid hemorrhage, increase $\dot{D}_{O_2}$ by improving venous return, stroke volume, and thus $\dot{Q}_t$. However, it has been found that splenectomized dogs subjected to a lethal hemorrhagic shock protocol were found to have a 20% survival when resuscitated with blood replacement alone compared with a 70% survival when lactated Ringer's plus blood was administered[148,250,310,393] (see also Chapter 4). This improvement is attributed to replenishment of the functional interstitial fluid space as well as to restoration of microcirculatory flow.[24,47,195,208,231,309]

Thus, initial therapeutic efforts should be directed toward increasing the circulating blood volume and cardiac output and restoration of interstitial fluid space by infusion of balanced salt solutions.[16,48,57,58,93,148,201,338,339,340] Administration of acellular fluids will lead to an increase in $\dot{Q}_t$, a more equitable distribution of $\dot{D}_{O_2}$, and, if acellular infusion is sufficient to restore the circulating blood volume, to normovolemic hemodilution.

### OXYGEN TRANSPORT IN TRANSITION FROM HEMORRHAGIC HYPOVOLEMIA TO ACUTE NORMOVOLEMIC HEMODILUTION

As we have discussed, compensation for rapid hemorrhage basically entails a progressive redistribution of the diminishing blood volume to vital organs by increases in TPR and augmented extraction of $O_2$ from the reduced blood flow to the nonvital but biologically essential tissues.[197,291,331] In other words, the rate of decrease in $\dot{D}_{O_2}$ is less for the heart and brain than for any other organ in the body. As a corollary, $\dot{V}_{O_2}$ values of vasoconstricted tissues fall more rapidly than those of the heart and brain.[112,316] These changes most probably parallel the redistribution and maldistribution of cardiac output.[331]

Restoration of the circulating blood volume, and thus $\dot{Q}_t$, by rapid acellular fluid administration is in a sense a rapid iatrogenic acceleration of the normal transcapillary refill seen in slow hemorrhage.[82,222] During fluid resuscitation, effective replenishment of the functional extracellular fluid space (FECFS) requires administration of a volume of balanced salt solution three to four times that of the blood lost.[250,251,272,273] Furthermore, since crystalloid solutions are lost so rapidly from the intravascular space,[138,314] normovolemia can be maintained only by continued infusion even after blood volume and FECFS have been normalized.

Although unreplaced loss of 30 to 40% of blood volume (1500 to 2000 mL in a 70-kg man) produces shock and possibly death, the red cell mass remaining after hemorrhage may be sufficient to sustain life if rapidly and properly distributed. Thus, the goal of rapid volume expansion with acellular fluids during initial resuscitation is to redistribute the remaining red cell mass to those areas deprived of oxygen during hemorrhagic compensation. This will, in effect, produce acute normovolemic (dilutional) anemia. Once the blood volume is restored with asanguinous fluids the [Hb] or hematocrit levels may give a rough approximation of the extent of blood loss.

## HEMORHEOLOGY (THE STUDY OF BLOOD FLOW)

Blood flow, $\dot{Q}$, is equal to the pressure differential, $\Delta P$, between the two measured points in the circulation, divided by the flow resistance, R.[122] That is,

$$\dot{Q} = \frac{\Delta P}{R}$$

The major resistance to flow occurs in the microcirculation. Resistance at this level is directly proportional to the length of the microvascular segment, l, and the viscosity of the blood, $\eta$, and inversely proportional to the fourth power of the radius of the vessel, $r^4$. Viscosity may be simply defined as the inherent resistance of a liquid to flow. Specifically,

$$R = \frac{8 \cdot l \cdot \eta}{\pi \cdot r^4}$$

The subject of blood viscosity is at best complex; only those aspects that apply to hemorrhage will be discussed here. Blood viscosity is dependent on[24,49,50,105,175,177,208]

1. Hematocrit
2. Flow velocity (shear rate)
3. Red cell deformability
4. Rouleaux formation (red cell aggregation)
5. Plasma proteins (mainly fibrinogen and $\alpha_2$ globulins)
6. Temperature.

From Fig 5-12, it is evident that alterations in hematocrit are followed by disproportionate changes in blood viscosity. It is

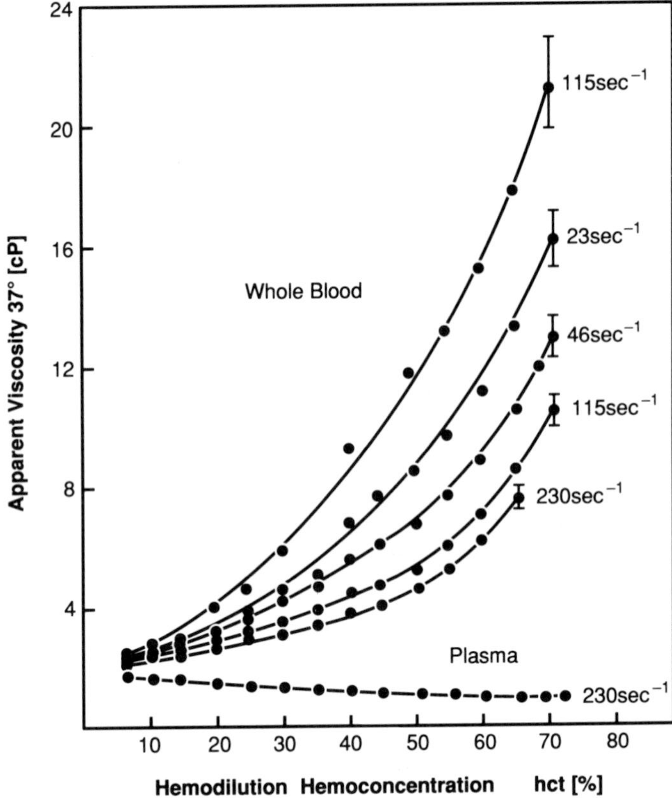


FIG. 5-12. The hematocrit-viscosity relationship at different shear rates. (From Messmer K, et al. Prog Surg 1974;13:208, with permission.)

also apparent that as hematocrit increases, viscosity is inversely related to the shear rate or velocity of flow; that is, the higher the shear rate at any given hematocrit, the lower the viscosity. This property of blood defines it as a non-Newtonian fluid, since Newtonian fluids do not change their viscosity with changes in shear rate. The relationship of flow velocity to viscosity becomes progressively less important as hematocrit decreases to 30% with hemodilution.[208] It may be seen from Fig 5-13 that changes in viscosity at any given hematocrit are most marked in the postcapillary venules where shear rates are lowest.[49,195,208] Hence, rouleaux formation and stasis are most likely to occur in this area of the microvasculature. Thus, the rheologic alterations of moderate hemodilution have their most prominent effects in the postcapillary venules.

Hypothermia increases the viscosity of a fluid by increasing its density.[177] For instance, decreasing a patient's temperature from 37 to 25°C with hematocrit = 45% increases viscosity by 50%.[105] In order to keep viscosity constant, a reduction in hematocrit to 20% would be necessary.

If

$$\dot{Q} = \frac{\Delta P}{R},$$

and

$$R = \frac{8 \cdot 1 \cdot \eta}{\pi \cdot r^4},$$

then

$$\dot{Q} = \frac{\Delta P}{\frac{8 \cdot 1 \cdot \eta}{\pi \cdot r^4}} = \frac{\Delta P \cdot \pi \cdot r^4}{8 \cdot 1 \cdot \eta},$$

which is Poiseuille's Law.[49,122,218,332]

FIG. 5-13. Effect of hemodilution on blood viscosity, related to changes in shear rate *in vivo*. (From Messmer K et al. Prog Surg 1974;13:208, with permission.)

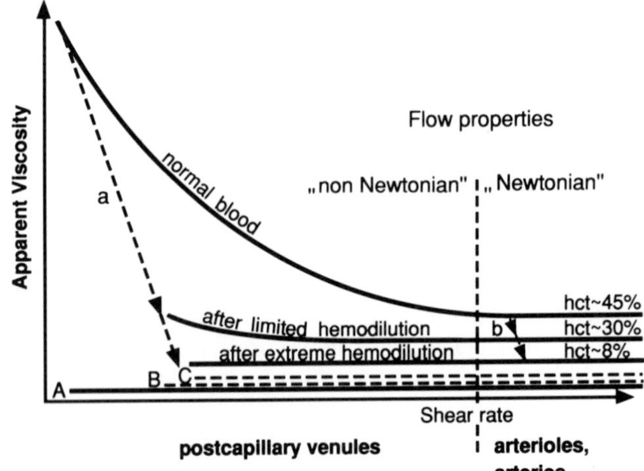

Poiseuille's Law was originally designed to determine flow of Newtonian fluids through cylindric tubes.[218,332] Since the normal hematocrit in the true capillaries is approximately 8.5%[170,190] (ie, 91.5% plasma) and plasma is nearly Newtonian[208] (Fig 5-12), Poiseuille's Law may be used qualitatively to describe blood flow through the microcirculation[51] (Shu Chien, personal communication).

It is obvious from this relationship that blood flow is enhanced by an augmented pressure gradient across the vessel bed and by an increase in radius of the vessel. In fact, a doubling of vessel radius, all other factors constant, produces a 16-fold increase in blood flow.[241] Conversely, if the radius is reduced by 50%, flow is reduced to $\frac{1}{16}$th. Moreover, flow rate through a microvessel is inversely related to viscosity, $\eta$. As viscosity increases due to increasing hematocrit, reduced velocity of flow, hypothermia, or rouleaux formation, flow rate decreases.[175]

The Poiseuille equation may thus be used qualitatively to analyze the pathophysiologic derangements of flow in the microcirculation resulting from hemorrhagic hypovolemia.[49] During untreated brisk hemorrhage, intense arteriolar, metarteriolar, and venous constriction occur,[3,316,317,382] and thus $\dot{Q}$ and flow velocity decrease.[122] At very low velocity, intense aggregation and rouleaux formation, alteration in red cell shape, and decrease in red cell deformability occur.[49,203] Indeed, frank plugging of the microcirculation not only with red cells but with white blood cells and platelets has been observed microscopically.[115,140,203]

During the course of progressive vasoconstriction in some microvascular beds, the remaining blood is shunted through systemic arteriovenous anastomoses[3,140,214]; thus, arterialized blood flows away from the nutrient vessel beds of nonvital tissues into the systemic venous circulation where it enhances venous return and ventricular preload.[3]

If regional microcirculatory flow is

$$\dot{Q}r = \frac{\Delta P \cdot \pi \cdot r^4}{8 \cdot 1 \cdot \eta}$$

then total body microcirculatory blood flow will be

$$\dot{Q}_{r1} + \dot{Q}_{r2} + \dot{Q}_{r3} \ldots + \dot{Q}_{rn} = Q_{r\text{total}}.$$

If

$$\dot{Q}r_1 = \left(\frac{\Delta P \cdot \pi \cdot r^4}{8 \cdot 1 \cdot \eta}\right) r_1$$

Then

$$\dot{Q}_{r\text{total}} = \left(\frac{\Delta P \cdot \pi \cdot r^4}{8 \cdot 1 \cdot \eta}\right) r_{\text{total}}$$

If the entire cardiac output, $\dot{Q}_t$, traverses the microcirculation, then[52,119,122]

$$\dot{Q}_t = \left(\frac{\Delta P \cdot \pi \cdot r^4}{8 \cdot 1 \cdot \eta}\right) r_{\text{total}} = \frac{\text{MAP} - \text{CVP}}{\text{SVR} \cdot \eta}$$

Thus, cardiac output is directly proportional to pressure gradients across the microvascular beds and the geometry of the microvessels ($r^4$) and inversely proportional to capillary and postcapillary venular viscosity. Furthermore, if $\dot{Q}_t = \dot{Q}_c + \dot{Q}_s$, where $\dot{Q}_c$ = the fraction of $\dot{Q}_t$ traversing nutrient capillaries, and $\dot{Q}_s$ = the fraction of $\dot{Q}_t$ traversing systemic arteriovenous shunts, then

$$\dot{Q}_t = \sum\left(\frac{\Delta P \cdot \pi \cdot r^4}{8 \cdot 1 \cdot \eta}\right) r_c + \sum\left(\frac{\Delta P \cdot \pi \cdot r^4}{8 \cdot 1 \cdot \eta}\right) r_s$$

In early hemorrhagic hypovolemia, $\dot{Q}_t$ declines progressively with a relatively larger proportion of the diminishing total output represented as $\dot{Q}_s$. Compensatory mechanisms ensuring perfusion to the heart and brain (ie, $\dot{Q}_c$) thus rely on a functional $\dot{Q}_s$ through nonvital tissues in early shock to augment venous return.[3]

As arteriolar and metarteriolar vasoconstriction progressively fade and venoconstriction persists in early decompensation, relatively more of the further reduced $\dot{Q}_t$ is directed to $\dot{Q}_c$ (in nonvital tissues) and away from $\dot{Q}_s$. Since velocity and pressure gradients are already very low, stagnation and a no-flow phenomenon evolve in nutrient capillaries because of persistent venoconstriction. Thus, venous return to the heart is further reduced by the diminished $\dot{Q}_s$.[3]

If $\dot{V}O_2 = \dot{Q}_t(CaO_2 - C\bar{v}O_2)$, and all oxygen consumption occurs via nutrient capillaries (not via shunts), then $\dot{V}O_2 = \dot{Q}_c(CaO_2 - C\bar{v}O_2)$. As $\dot{Q}_c$ falls early in hemorrhage, $\dot{V}O_2$ in vasoconstricted tissue beds declines as oxygen extraction reaches its maximum. The proportion of $\dot{Q}_t$ reaching the heart and brain, whose vessels dilate because of autoregulation, may maintain a satisfactory $O_2$ supply-demand ratio ($\dot{D}O_2$ versus $\dot{V}O_2$) in these organs during early moderate hemorrhage.[30,79,186,330] This is accomplished by a combination of increased extraction of available oxygen (which is limited in the case of the heart)[94,154,155] and decreased oxygen demand. Indeed, myocardial $O_2$ requirements ($M\dot{V}O_2$) per beat are considerably reduced immediately after hemorrhage because of decreased ventricular volume and lower intracavitary pressure in both systole and diastole. As hemorrhage progresses, however, the reduced $M\dot{V}O_2$ is offset by a disproportionate drop in coronary blood flow.[7,78,148] Hence, lactate accumulation occurs (anaerobiosis).

Since multisystem organ failure determines survival or death after initial resuscitation in hemorrhagic shock, primary therapy must be directed at the microcirculatory flow.[102,114,296] The objectives are:

1. Prevention and amelioration of stagnation in nutrient capillaries and postcapillary venules
2. Global augmentation of $\dot{D}O_2$ to nutrient microvascular beds
3. Reestablishment of $\dot{V}O_2$ consistent with $O_2$ demand in vasoconstricted anaerobically metabolizing tissues.

Thus, rapid hemodilution with acellular fluids is again unquestionably the initial treatment of choice.[102,155,372]

## SYSTEMIC OXYGEN TRANSPORT IN HEMODILUTION

Clinical and experimental studies have consistently shown a marked increase in $\dot{Q}_t$ during progressive acute normovolemic hemodilution (Fig 5-11).[92,94,104,110,125,136,154,182,207,271,385] The rise in $\dot{Q}_t$ is attributed almost solely to enhanced venous return to the right heart (ie, increased preload),[207] resulting in augmented stroke volume with little or no change in heart rate compared with controls.[92,182,271] The increase in venous return is mediated by the enhanced fluidity of hemodiluted blood[94,154]; that is, viscosity, $\eta$, is diminished with a resulting drop in total peripheral resistance although systemic vascular resistance may remain high.[94,136,154,175,177] Left ventricular afterload is also reduced by decreased TPR, minimizing myocardial oxygen demand.[136] Thus, with hemodilution, myocardial work progressively shifts from a pressure to a volume mode.[207]

$\dot{D}O_2$ is maximal at hematocrit levels of 40 to 45% and decreases during normovolemic hemodilution.[110,136,154,182,291] When hypervolemia is induced, $\dot{D}O_2$ has been reported to be maximal at a hematocrit of 30%.[207] In dogs, normovolemic hemodilution to a hematocrit of 20%, ie, 50% reduction of red cell mass, produces a $\dot{D}O_2$ reduction of only 35%.[94,136,154] Hemodilution to 30% hematocrit, that is, a one-third reduction in hemoglobin concentration, diminishes $\dot{D}O_2$ by only 15% (Fig 5-14). Although systemic oxygen transport falls at hematocrit levels below normal, coronary oxygen transport (myocardial oxygen delivery) remains unchanged at hematocrits down to a level of 20%[154] (Fig 5-14).

Since $\dot{D}O_2$ subserves $\dot{V}O_2$, it is relevant to ask at what hematocrit level total body and myocardial oxygen consumption decline. Remarkably, both $\dot{V}O_2$ and $M\dot{V}O_2$ are shown to be constant in the normothermic dog from control hematocrit down to 20%, below which they both fall precipitously[154] (Fig 5-15). This is virtually identical to the hematocrit below which

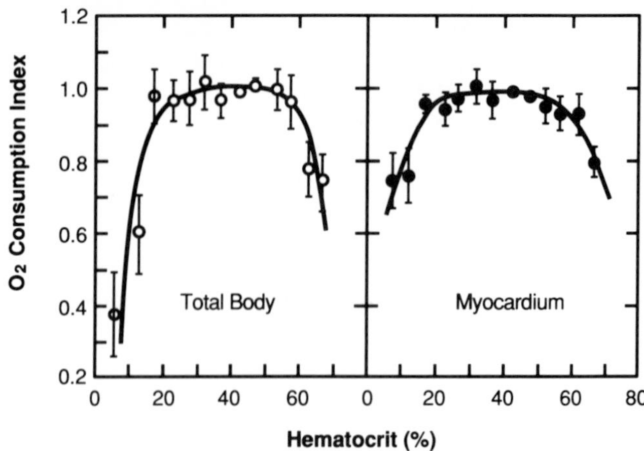


FIG. 5-15. Effects of hematocrit variation on oxygen consumption in the whole body (left) and myocardium (right). Oxygen consumption index is calculated by dividing oxygen consumption value by that obtained at hematocrit of 45%. (From Jan and Chien[154] with permission.)

coronary oxygen transport rapidly decreases. Selective isolated coronary hemodilution in healthy dogs suggests that $M\dot{V}O_2$ is supported to a critical hematocrit of 10%.[63] Maintenance of $M\dot{V}O_2$ in the presence of coronary insufficiency requires a hematocrit >17%.

Thus, in the dog, which has an $M\dot{V}O_2$ index nearly identical to that of the human, maintenance of normal total body $\dot{V}O_2$ and $M\dot{V}O_2$ seems dependent on coronary oxygen transport rather than on systemic oxygen delivery ($\dot{D}O_2$).[154] Since coronary oxygen transport is not measured clinically, the minimum systemic oxygen transport value ($\dot{Q}_t \times CaO_2$), which coincides with the minimum coronary oxygen transport value capable of supporting $M\dot{V}O_2$, should be the lower limit of acceptability in acute normovolemic hemodilution. This value of $\dot{D}O_2$ in the lightly anesthetized, normothermic dog appears to be 65% of control.[154] The hematocrit value at which this is achieved appears to be approximately 20% ([Hb] 70 g/L),[110,111,156,207] although Wilkerson et al[389] have shown in a baboon model that strictly normovolemic hemodilution is safe to a hematocrit of approximately 10%. Their data suggest that total body $\dot{V}O_2$ and myocardial aerobic metabolism are maintained at control levels down to 10% hematocrit and 50% whole body extraction ratio.

When normovolemia is maintained with moderate hemodilution, heart rate, MAP, CVP, and ($CaO_2 - C\bar{v}O_2$) remain essentially unchanged while $\dot{Q}_t$ increases and TPR decreases[156,182,207,208,271] (Fig. 5-11). Tachycardia in the presence of decreased MAP, $S\bar{v}O_2$, or $P\bar{v}O_2$ during hemodilution indicates a diminished $\dot{Q}_t$ and $\dot{D}O_2$, which, in all probability, is due to hypovolemia.[207,385]

During hemodilution to a hematocrit of 20 to 25%, tissue $PO_2$ values of skeletal muscle, liver, pancreas, small intestine, and kidney remain normal[209] (Fig 5-16). Coronary sinus $PO_2$, likewise, remains unchanged at hemodilution to 20% hematocrit.[62,207] However, at hematocrit of 15%, a redistribution of flow away from the subendocardium has been noted and

FIG. 5-14. Effects of hematocrit variation on oxygen transport rates in systemic (left) and coronary (right) circulations. Oxygen transport index is calculated by dividing oxygen transport value by that obtained at hematocrit of 45%. (From Jan and Chien[154] with permission.)

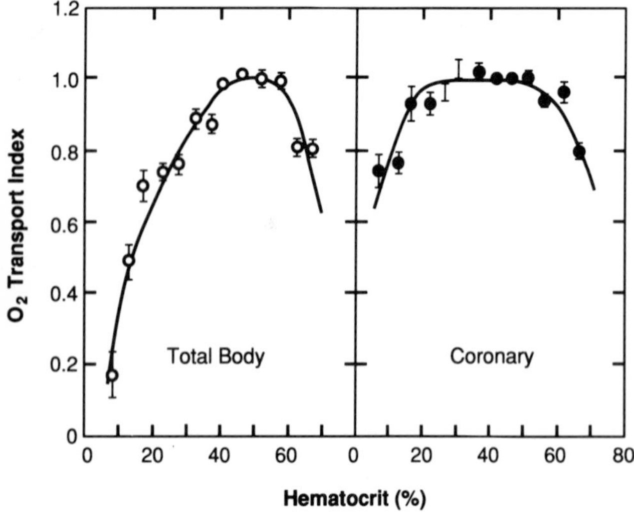

is associated with an ischemic ECG pattern and myocardial failure.[32,33,208]

Blood flow to the brain is increased during hemodilution[94,307,394,396] to the extent that $CMRo_2$ is maintained.[211] However, when hemodilution is associated with hyperventilation-induced hypocapnia to a $Paco_2$ less than 20 mm Hg, brain hypoxia may result from the combined effects of cerebral vasoconstriction, reduced arterial oxygen content, and leftward shift of the oxyhemoglobin dissociation curve.[127,133,395,397] At hematocrits between 16 and 20%, EEG changes consistent with hypoxia have been described.[226] These findings correlate with the observation that at a hematocrit of approximately 20%, brain tissue oxygen tension falls precipitously.[307]

In summary, rapid normovolemic hemodilution during resuscitation of the patient with hemorrhagic hypovolemia is unquestionably the initial goal of therapy.[155,195] If the red cell mass remaining after resuscitation is sufficient to maintain a hematocrit of 20% or greater ([Hb] 70 g/L), tissue perfusion and oxygenation will remain adequate.[110,169,216a] It must be emphasized, however, that $\dot{D}o_2$ at a hematocrit of 20% in acute hemodilution produces only borderline tissue oxygenation; thus, volume restoration when hematocrit is this low should be augmented by increased $Cao_2$ (ie, transfusion) and not by further increase in $\dot{Q}_t$.[193] Maintenance of adequate $\dot{D}o_2$ to support aerobic metabolism during hemodilution requires augmentation of $\dot{Q}_t$, which can be achieved only by maintenance of normovolemia.[207] However, if left ventricular function has been compromised by shock, rapid hemodilution may result in frank left ventricular failure and pulmonary edema rather than restoration of systemic oxygen transport. Some elderly individuals may be unable to increase $\dot{Q}_t$ by increasing stroke volume, and thus this group of patients may not tolerate even moderate hemodilution.[90,193,269,367] This may be especially true in patients who are being treated with β-adrenergic or calcium channel-blocking agents.[54,90] Thus, successful fluid resuscitation depends upon the patient's ability to increase cardiac output in order to optimize $\dot{D}o_2$ at a decreased hematocrit.

## OXYGEN TRANSPORT AND CONSUMPTION IN HEMORRHAGIC HYPOVOLEMIA WITH VARIATIONS IN HEMATOCRIT (HYPOVOLEMIC HEMODILUTION)

During hemorrhage in dogs when the blood volume is maintained to yield a constant MAP of 50 mm Hg, coronary oxygen transport (ie, coronary blood flow × $Cao_2$) is maximal at a hematocrit of 25%. In fact, coronary oxygen transport in hemorrhagic hypovolemia at this hematocrit is similar to that of prehemorrhage levels[155] (Fig 5-17). Increasing the hematocrit to 45% reduces coronary oxygen transport to 75% of normal in hypovolemic dogs. Systemic oxygen transport ($\dot{D}o_2$) during hemorrhage, although grossly depressed at normal hematocrit, is only slighty more reduced with hemodilution to a hematocrit of 25%.[155] Myocardial oxygen consumption ($M\dot{V}o_2$) in hemorrhagic hypotension is normal at hemodilution to a hematocrit of 25% but only 80% of normal at a hematocrit of 45%. Whole body oxygen consumption ($\dot{V}o_2$), however, is at a constant 60% of normal in hemorrhagic hypotension at hematocrits ranging from 45 to 25% (Fig 5-18). From these results it seems obvious that intentional he-

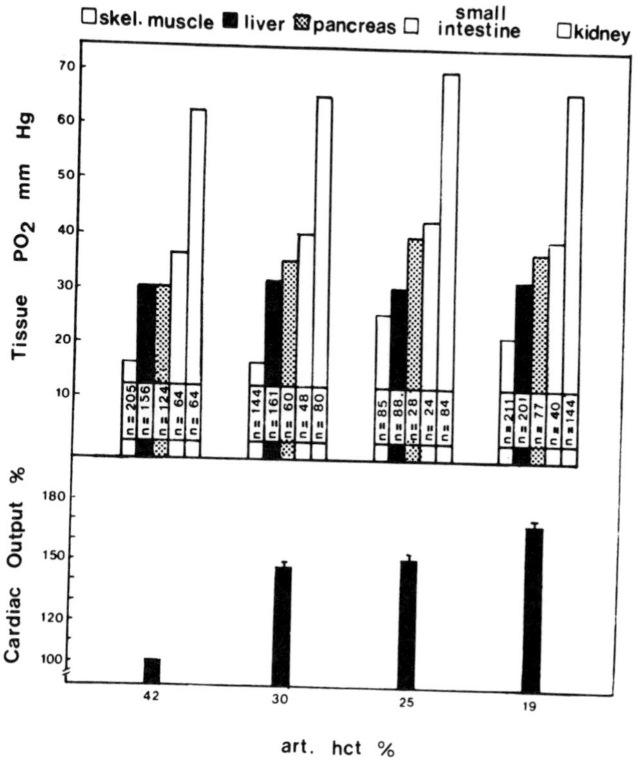

FIG. 5-16. Changes in local tissue $Po_2$ of different organs at varying cardiac outputs in relation to arterial hematocrit during acute normovolemic hemodilution with dextran 60 in dogs. (From Messmer et al.[209] with permission.)

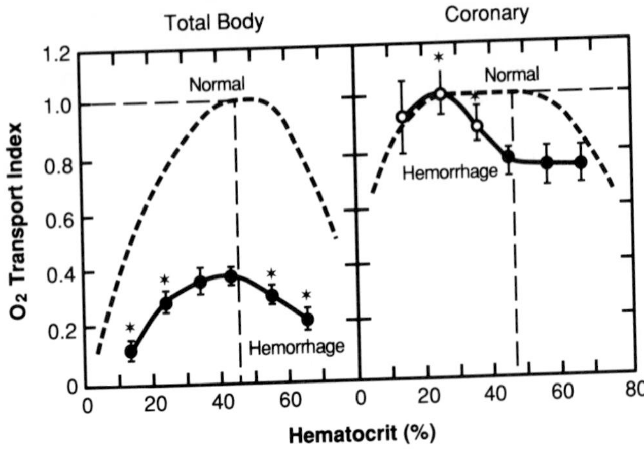


FIG. 5-17. Effects of hematocrit variation on oxygen transport rates in systemic (left) and coronary (right) circulations at arterial pressure of 50 mm Hg (hemorrhage). Normovolemic control data are shown as dashed curves (normal). Oxygen tranport index is calculated by dividing $O_2$ transport value by that obtained at hemotocrit = 45%. (From Jan et al[155] with permission.)

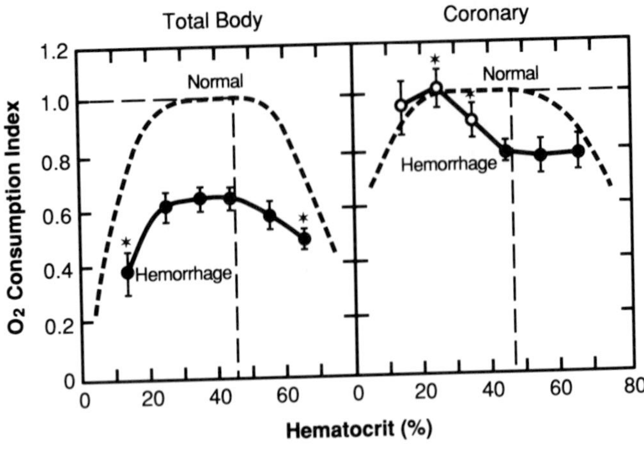


FIG. 5-18. Effects of hematocrit variation on $O_2$ consumption in total body (left) and in coronary (right) circulation at arterial pressure = 50 mm Hg (hemorrhage). Data previously obtained under normovolemic conditions are shown as dashed curves (normal). $O_2$ consumption index is calculated by dividing $O_2$ consumption value by that obtained at hematocrit = 45%. (From Jan et al[155] with permission.)

modilution is not only desirable but virtually mandatory in hemorrhagic hypovolemia in order to maintain normal myocardial metabolism.

Thus, the systemic oxygen transport adaptations to acute hypovolemic oligemia and acute normovolemic anemia are completely opposite.[137] In acute hypovolemia, compensation depends on preferential redistribution of less, slower flowing, near normally concentrated blood to vital organs and tissues that extract increasing percentages of oxygen. In acute normovolemic anemia, compensation depends on global redistribution of more, rapidly flowing, less concentrated blood to organs or tissues where normal or slightly reduced extraction occurs.[136]

Table 5-6 summarizes these changes during transition from hemorrhagic hypovolemia to acute normovolemic hemodilution.

## THE CRITICAL LEVEL OF OXYGEN DELIVERY IN ANESTHETIZED MAN

Shibutani et al[174,176,290,306] have found that the critical $\dot{D}O_2$ level in nearly normothermic, anesthetized man is 330 mL/min/m$^2$ or roughly 560 mL/min/70 kg. The mean steady-state $\dot{V}O_2$ of their 58 patients during anesthesia, and before surgery, was 109 mL/min/m$^2$ (ie, 80% of normal). $\dot{D}O_2 > 330$ mL/min/m$^2$ was not associated with a rise in $\dot{V}O_2$ (Fig 5-19). Lactate levels rose 50% when $\dot{D}O_2$ was $< 330$ mL/min/m$^2$, indicating anaerobiosis. When $\dot{D}O_2$ increased beyond the critical level of 330 mL/min/m$^2$, $P\bar{v}O_2$ and $S\bar{v}O_2$ rose linearly toward normal, and arterial-mixed venous oxygen content difference decreased as $S\bar{v}O_2$ approached normal.

No correlation could be found between $\dot{D}O_2$ and $S\bar{v}O_2$ when $\dot{D}O_2$ was below the critical value (Fig 5-20). The scatter of $S\bar{v}O_2$ and $P\bar{v}O_2$ when $\dot{D}O_2$ is $< 330$ mL/min/m$^2$ is probably due to maldistribution of flow caused by the effects of anesthetics upon the microcirculation. It is likely that anesthesia causes systemic arteriovenous shunting and reduces $\dot{V}O_2$ in the nutrient capillary beds deprived of adequate flow. If it is assumed that during anesthesia under normothermic conditions, the lowest level of $\dot{D}O_2$ consistent with aerobic metabolism is 330 mL/min/m$^2$ and that a maximal $\dot{Q}_t$ of 130% of normal is achievable[182] by acute normovolemic hemodilution, then the minimum hemoglobin concentration for adequate $\dot{D}O_2$ is roughly 70 to 80 g/L at $SaO_2$ of 95%. This level of oxygen delivery should support $\dot{V}O_2$ in normothermic anesthetized man. It should be noted, as one would expect, that like the critical $P\bar{v}O_2$, the critical level of $\dot{D}O_2$ is reduced by hypothermia,[118,390] anesthetic agents,[143] and other factors.[191]

$\dot{V}O_2$ during anesthesia and surgery is generally reduced

TABLE 5-6. Systemic Oxygen Transport Adaptations During Hemorrhagic Hypovolemia and Acute Normovolemic Hemodilution

| | BLOOD VOLUME | $CaO_2$ Hct and Hb | $\dot{Q}_t$ | $\dot{D}O_2$ | TPR | $CaO_2 - C\bar{v}O_2$ | $\dot{V}O_2$ |
|---|---|---|---|---|---|---|---|
| Hemorrhagic hypovolemia | ↓↓ | Normal or slight ↓ | ↓↓ | ↓↓ | ↑ During compensation | ↑↑↑ | ↓ |
| Acute normovolemic hemodilution | ± Normal | ↓↓ | ↑ | ↓ | ↓ | Normal or ↓ | Normalized with successful resuscitation (if Hct >20%) |

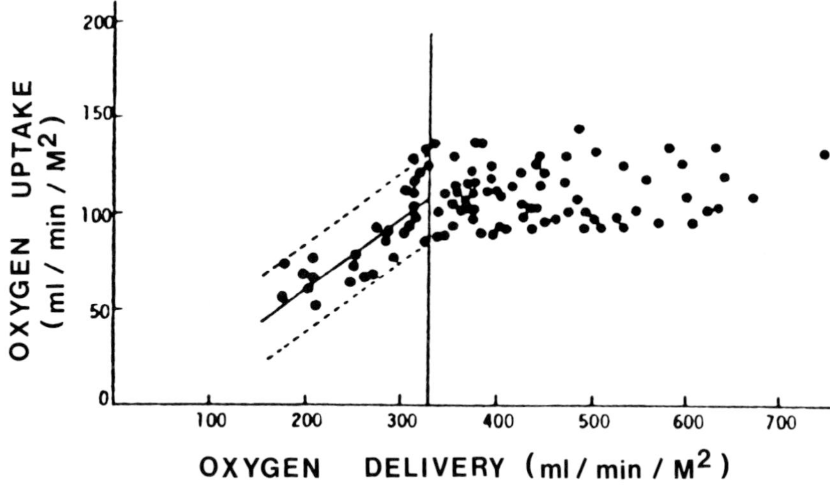


FIG. 5-19. Relationship between oxygen delivery ($\dot{D}O_2$) and oxygen consumption under anesthesia. Note that the critical level of oxygen delivery is approximately 330 mL/min/m$^2$, below which $\dot{V}O_2$ falls linearly. (From Komatsu et al[176] and Shibutani et al[306] with permission.)

from the awake resting state by 20 to 25%.[213,237,252,306,379] This has been ascribed to the effects of anesthetics and inadvertent hypothermia, which decrease oxygen demand by reducing cellular metabolism.[34,118,227,233,390] In addition, as discussed previously, significant hemorrhage, in and of itself, reduces oxygen consumption even in the presence of normal or increased oxygen demand. The cause of diminished $\dot{V}O_2$ after hemorrhage is not reduced demand. Instead, it is insufficient and maldistributed oxygen delivery, which results in anaerobiosis.[164] Recently it has been postulated that anesthetics may not only reduce demand but may contribute to maldistribution of blood flow in the microcirculation.[306,379,380,381] This may then cause oxygen deficits predisposing to anaerobic metabolism and excess lactate production. Intraoperative oxygen deficit equals the duration of surgery × (preoperative − intraoperative $\dot{V}O_2$).[379,380]

Indeed, the combined $O_2$ deficits caused by trauma, surgery, hemorrhage, and anesthetic agents evoke an elevation in $\dot{V}O_2$ of 20% to 25% during the first postoperative day. This cannot be accounted for by reduced preoperative or intraoperative $\dot{D}O_2$.[379] Regardless of how well $\dot{D}O_2$ is maintained during anesthesia, surgery, and hemorrhage, the postoperative rise in $\dot{V}O_2$ is accompanied by an augmentation in $\dot{D}O_2$ of 20 to 25%, mediated by a rise in $\dot{Q}_t$[324,379] (Fig 5-21).

Although intraoperative normovolemic hemodilution produces a maximal rise in $\dot{Q}_t$ at a hematocrit of 20 to 25%, the obligatory postoperative increase in $\dot{D}O_2$ may not be possible at this hematocrit level. Accordingly, blood transfusion is in-

FIG. 5-20. Relationship between $S\bar{v}O_2$ and $\dot{D}O_2$ under anesthesia. Note that at $\dot{D}O_2$ less than 330 mL/min/m$^2$, no correlation exists. (From Shibutani et al[306] with permission.)

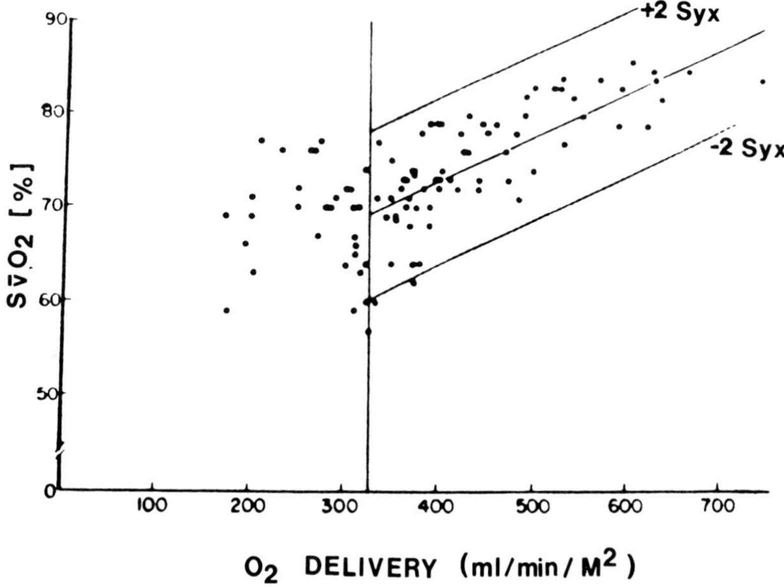

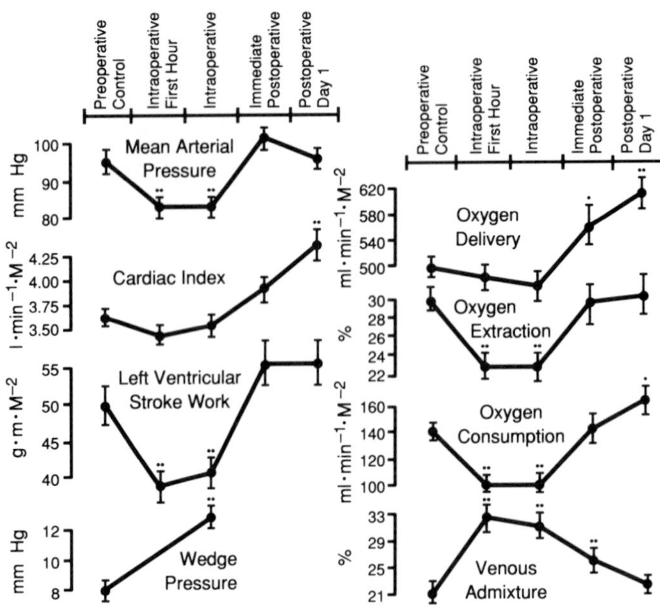


FIG. 5-21. Hemodynamic (left) and oxygen transport variables (right) of 53 high-risk surgical patients. Although cardiac index and oxygen delivery were held relatively constant throughout surgery, oxygen consumption and extraction decreased. In the postoperative period, oxygen consumption rose to above preoperative control levels. This rise was accompanied by a parallel increase in $\dot{D}O_2$. (From Waxman et al[379] with permission.)

dicated to augment $CaO_2$ and thus to support the elevated oxygen demand and consumption. If the average first postoperative day $\dot{D}O_2$, $\dot{Q}_t$, and $SaO_2$ values are 620 mL/min/m$^2$, 4.5 L/min/m$^2$, and 95%,[379] respectively, a hemoglobin concentration of at least 110 g/L (ie, hematocrit = 33%) is required.

## IN SEARCH OF THE OPTIMAL PERIOPERATIVE HEMATOCRIT AND HEMOGLOBIN CONCENTRATION

The optimal perioperative hemoglobin concentration and hematocrit has been a disputed topic for years. It is obvious from the preceding discussion that the optimal level varies from patient to patient.[111,210] Moreover, as discussed, this so-called "optimal" level changes from the initial phase of the hemorrhagic insult through complete recovery and is dictated by the interdependent variables of systemic oxygen delivery, oxygen demand, and oxygen consumption. In addition, the static, unidimensional hemoglobin concentration must be correlated to its more dynamic counterparts, red cell mass (RCM) and blood volume.[308,315]

In a prospective randomized study, Shoemaker et al[318] evaluated the importance to survival of 32 cardiorespiratory variables in critically ill postoperative patients. Their results showed that the preferred hemoglobin concentration of greater than 12 g/dL was present in only 66% of surviving patients. However, when they investigated the optimal red cell mass (blood volume − plasma volume), the correlation in surviving patients was 85%. Of all the cardiorespiratory variables measured, optimal efficiency of tissue oxygen extraction

$$\text{ETOE} = \frac{CaO_2 - C\bar{v}O_2}{\text{RCM}}$$

was present in 91% of survivors. Thus, they concluded that some of the most commonly monitored variables such as hematocrit have low capacities to predict survival and hence have little importance in therapeutic decision making.

On the other hand, in an earlier retrospective study of 94 critically ill postoperative patients, Czer and Shoemaker[66] determined an optimal postoperative hematocrit of 32% or [Hb] of approximately 11 g/dL. Survival in the hematocrit range of 27 to 33% was 87%, whereas survival with a hematocrit of 21 to 27% was 60%. Interestingly, hematocrits greater than 33% were associated with only 62% survival (Fig 5-22). These results are supported by Fortune et al[100] and McCormick et al[202].

Unquestionably, hematocrits in the 20s and even much lower[188] have been tolerated by countless patients.[66,110,111,227] Posttrauma hemodilution to this level, however, will be successful only if the patient has the ability to augment $\dot{Q}_t$, and normovolemia or slight hypervolemia is maintained.[156,200,207] Since $\dot{D}O_2$ is the product of $\dot{Q}_t$ and $CaO_2$, any precipitous drop in $CaO_2$ below critical levels must be compensated for by a rise in $\dot{Q}_t$. In aged patients with limited cardiac reserve or in patients treated with negative inotropic drugs, this compen-

FIG. 5-22. Relationship between survival rate and hematocrit values after major surgery. (From Czer and Shoemaker[66] with permission.)

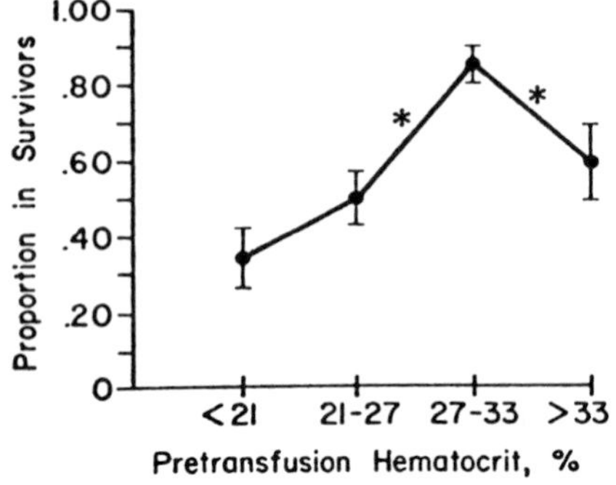

satory increase in $\dot{Q}_t$ may not be safe or even possible.[193,269] Moreover, the effects of hemorrhagic shock, per se, on the heart may include reduced compliance and overall performance.[4,5,65,78]

In summary, the decisions of when and how much blood to transfuse are largely determined by the physician's assessment of the oxygen transport system.[268] Barcroft's original description of the anoxemias is as valid today as it was in 1920. If severe pulmonary insufficiency exists (hypoxic anoxia), therapeutic intervention should be directed at augmenting $Sa_{O_2}$ by whatever means necessary. If postoperative, severe, intractable arterial desaturation is present, obviously a higher hemoglobin concentration is necessary to augment and optimize $Ca_{O_2}$.[286] If cardiac output ($\dot{Q}_t$) is severely depressed (stagnant anoxia), volume, inotropic support, and/or appropriate afterload reduction are indicated.[268,280] In pure hemorrhagic shock, if the pulmonary and cardiac components have been optimized, and signs, symptoms and laboratory data suggest insufficient tissue oxygenation despite attainment of normovolemia, then transfusion of red cells is indicated.

In the final analysis, optimal oxygen delivery is the only immediate perioperative therapeutic goal.[26,86,268,322] The quest for an optimal hematocrit as a goal in transfusion therapy is obviously simplistic and naïve. From the preceding discussion it must be apparent that the optimal hemoglobin concentration and hematocrit will change with time through the hemorrhagic insult and into the postoperative period.

The physician's goal in transfusion therapy is thus to establish a safe buffer zone between $\dot{V}_{O_2}$ (a marker of aerobic life) and $\dot{D}_{O_2}$ (the deliverer of life's fuel, $O_2$).

## MONITORING FLUID AND TRANSFUSION THERAPY IN THE INJURED (MONITORING TISSUE OXYGENATION)

As discussed previously, many factors, in addition to transfusion, impact on the adequacy of tissue oxygen utilization. Thus, monitoring of blood and volume replacement should be directed toward obtaining information about, and identifying the causes of, suboptimal total body and tissue oxygenation. This will allow institution of proper treatment during the perioperative period. Numerous monitoring methods are available for this purpose. Although many of them are capable of providing important information, they may be sophisticated, invasive, and time consuming. Thus, their use may have to be reserved for the relatively stable patient. An apprehensive, pallid, cadaveric, blood-stained auto accident victim needs immediate resuscitation with fluids and blood and surgical control of bleeding sites before institution of any sophisticated monitoring. Wasting time by placing a pulmonary artery catheter to measure cardiac output and calculate $\dot{D}_{O_2}$ or $\dot{V}_{O_2}$ will certainly result in catastrophe. Thus, priorities must be recognized and care rendered accordingly. Likewise, clinical signs and symptoms must be observed carefully, especially during the acute phase of management. The patient's color, heart rate, blood pressure, respiratory rate, breath sounds, heart sounds, capillary filling, and urine output are all essential for institution of proper treatment and should be monitored continuously.[244] Immediate resuscitation requires measurement of only the basic, but crucially important, cardiorespiratory variables. Once the clinical situation is under control, one should plan for more complex techniques. The following discussion reviews the available monitoring methods, their rationale, and their appropriateness.

### INTRAVASCULAR PRESSURE MONITORING

#### *Central Venous and Pulmonary Artery Pressures*

Resuscitative goals are, in general, centered around optimal replenishment of the circulating blood volume with fluids and blood. Assessment of blood volume replacement, in turn, has focused on the monitoring of intravascular pressures in systemic arterial, central venous, and pulmonary arterial circulations.[48,302,303,308] Optimization of these pressures is assumed to imply that blood volume, cardiac output, and tissue oxygenation must be satisfactory; hence, they may be used inappropriately as end points of therapy.

Simmons et al[328] reported that despite stable mean arterial pressure, central venous pressure, and adequate urinary output, the ratio of measured to predicted total blood volume ranged from 0.59 to 0.82 (mean, 0.71). More recently, McNamara et al,[205] in a hemorrhagic shock model, verified in baboons these human findings from Vietnam. The results of these studies have led to the conclusion that despite massive replacement, in some instances, a contracted blood volume cannot be rapidly expanded to normal levels. In the baboon study, maintenance of normal left atrial pressure after resuscitation with blood and lactated Ringer's solution led to massive diuresis without complete expansion of the circulating blood volume. Another animal study demonstrated normal pulmonary artery occluded pressure (PAOP) at only 65% of returned shed blood volume during resuscitation from hemorrhagic shock.[302,303] At full volume replacement with shed blood, PAOP was 140% of baseline when cardiac output and $S\bar{v}_{O_2}$ had returned to normal. In these studies, CVP was normal after only 50% of the hemorrhaged volume had been reinfused. These observations and others imply that CVP and PAOP cannot predict hypovolemia accurately after severe hemorrhagic shock.[189,244,274,364] Indeed, when carefully performed postoperative blood volume studies are compared with MAP, CVP, PAOP, hematocrit, and even cardiac index, little correlation is noted (Figs 5-23 through 5-25).[308,317]

The value of PAOP as a reflection of left ventricular end-diastolic volume (LVEDV) (left ventricular preload) has been questioned in a variety of critical illnesses.[18,47,77,88,89,129,153,257] Preliminary studies in patients with complex vascular surgery, systemic sepsis, and acute myocardial infarction show little or no correlation between PAOP and LVEDV (Fig. 5-26)[47,77,88,128] probably because sepsis and myocardial infarction may cause major changes in left ventricular compliance. Experimentally, severe and/or prolonged hemorrhagic shock also has been shown to reduce left ventricular compliance.[4,5] Thus, the PAOP may not reflect LVEDV in the presence of hemorrhagic shock.[244,355,391]

Following cardiopulmonary bypass, the correlation between PAOP and direct left atrial pressure (LAP) is reported to be poor for at least 12 hours following surgery[196] (Fig 5-27). The

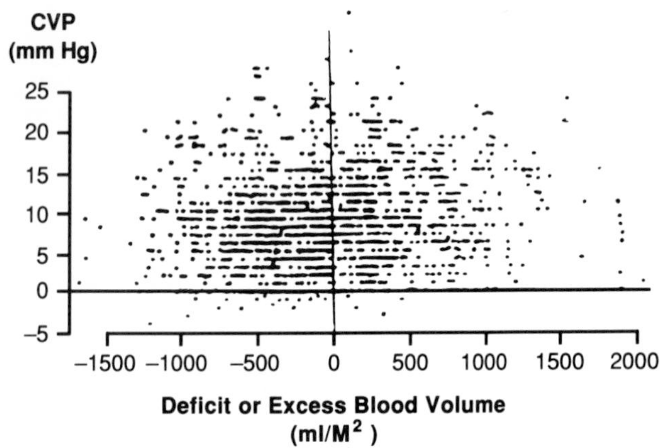


FIG. 5-23. Individually measured blood volume excess or deficit plotted against corresponding CVP values. Note complete lack of correlation. (From Shippy et al[108] with permission.)

inordinate elevation of PAOP postoperatively is thought to be related to mechanical pulmonary venoconstriction resulting from the increased interstitial lung water caused by hemodilution, although these results have been refuted recently.[144] Since intentional normovolemic hemodilution is integral to resuscitation from hemorrhagic shock, caution must be exercised in interpretation of PAOP as an indicator of left heart end-diastolic pressure. Studies involving acute blood loss of greater than 1000 mL within a 10-minute period have demonstrated a 40% reduction in baseline PAOP.[381] After apparent volume restoration, MAP, heart rate, and PAOP returned to baseline. However, at this time, deficits in cardiac output, approximating 25% of control values, remained. Compensation for hemorrhage included marked elevation in both systemic and pulmonary vascular resistance.[381] Thus, it appears that PAOP is moderately reflective of hypovolemia; however, restoration of intravascular volume based on this value may lead to an inaccurate estimate of blood volume.

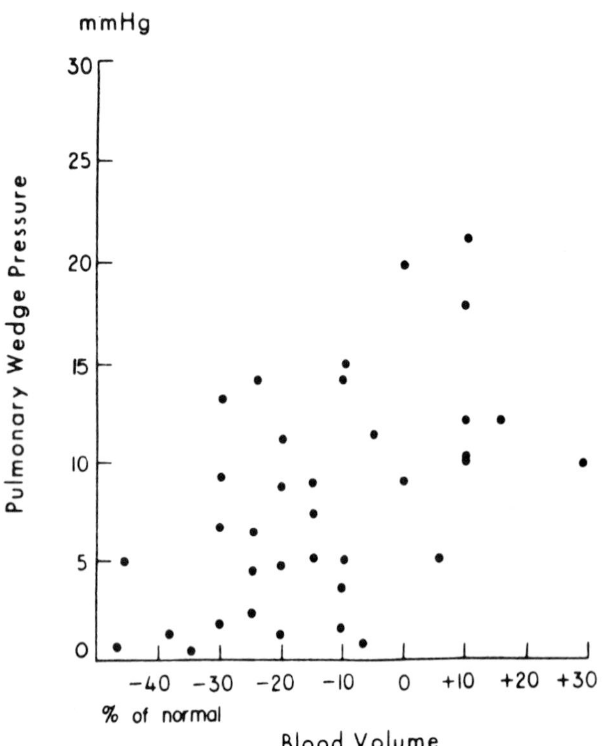


FIG. 5-24. Pulmonary wedge pressure values plotted against corresponding measured blood volumes in a series of unselected consecutive ICU patients. There is a slight tendency toward reduced wedge pressures with reduced blood volume, but the correlation is not statistically significant. Wedge pressures, by themselves, are *not* an adequate basis for blood volume assessment. (From Shoemaker WC, Ayres S, Grenvik A, Thompson WL, Hobrock PR, eds. Textbook of critical care medicine. Philadelphia: WB Saunders, 1984;117, with permission.)

## *MEAN ARTERIAL PRESSURE*

The fact that MAP is a poor indicator of blood volume and cardiac output should come as no surprise.[93,193,205,308,315,328] Fig 5-28 depicts the determinants of MAP. Since MAP is the product of $\dot{Q}_t$ and TPR, a reduction in $\dot{Q}_t$ accompanied by an appropriate rise in TPR produces little or no change in MAP. Critical analysis of Fig 5-28 further reveals the dynamic factors in MAP. In early moderate hemorrhage, volume deficits may be masked by a normal MAP. During progressive hemorrhage, preload diminishes with consequent reduction in stroke volume despite increased myocardial contractility. Additionally, compensatory augmentation of afterload results in further stroke volume reduction. Usually an increase in heart rate partially buffers the decrease in cardiac output. Ultimately, TPR reaches a critical value at which MAP decreases with further reductions in flow ($\dot{Q}_t$). MAP is usually reduced when blood loss approximates 20 to 30% of blood volume.[244] At this point, cardiac output is about 50% of normal[120,291,303] (Fig 5-11). Thus, a significantly reduced MAP in the presence of hemorrhage reflects deterioration of previously maximized compensatory cardiovascular reflexes (reduction in venous capacitance, TPR, PVR, tachycardia). It follows then that a normal MAP in the face of hemorrhage implies only that compensatory reflexes are functional. Hence, large deficits in blood volume and cardiac output may coexist with an acceptable MAP.[244,336] MAP itself, then, should *not* be used as an end point during volume restoration.[244,391] Finally, and possibly more importantly, it should not be used as an indicator of cardiac output.[391] Specifically, little useful information about oxygen delivery or consumption is encoded in MAP[234,244,291,360,379,380,381] (Fig 5-29).

It must be stated, however, that initial resuscitation from hemorrhagic shock must include arterial and central venous pressure monitoring as early trend indicators to the adequacy of volume replacement.[151,246,248,308,323,391] Attainment of a normal MAP from critically depressed levels implies at least that compensatory reflexes are intact and that the heart and brain are adequately perfused.[151] In addition, initial fluid and blood replacement probably should be guided by a rational protocol using MAP and CVP, as proposed by Hopkins et al[146] and Shoemaker et al.[323]

Monitoring techniques discussed so far pertain to the immediate resuscitation phase after trauma. Additional more sophisticated techniques can be used to assess systemic and tissue oxygenation after this phase. Table 5-7 lists those tech-

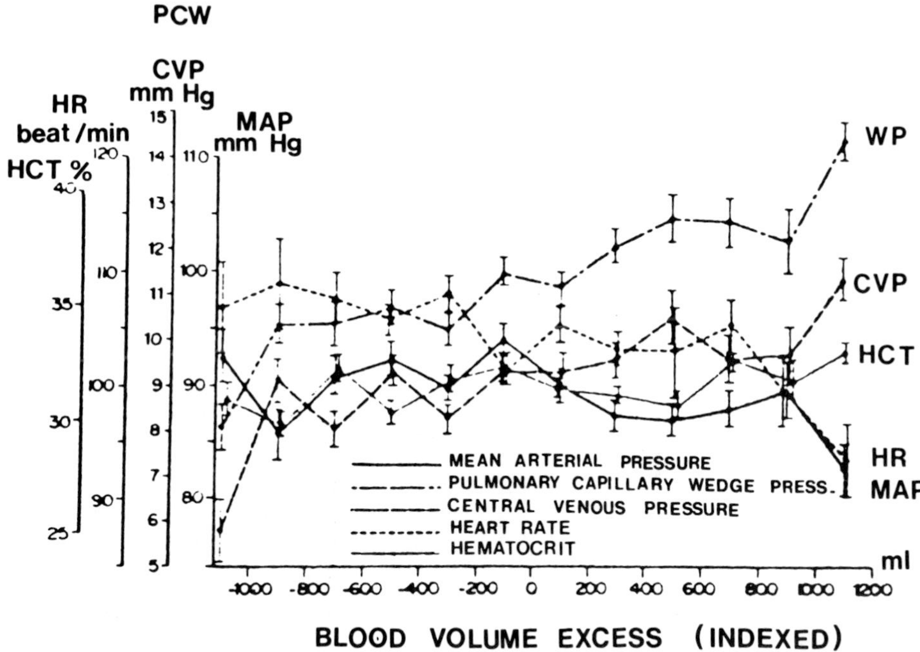


FIG. 5-25. Mean ± SD of commonly measured variables as a function of the corresponding blood volume excess (+) or deficit (−). Note the poor correlation of pulmonary capillary wedge (PCW) pressure and CVP except in extremes of blood volume excess or deficit. (From Shippy et al[108] with permission.)

niques that are available clinically, whereas the techniques listed in Table 5-8, although very useful, are not yet clinically available, except transcutaneous oxygen tension monitoring ($Ptco_2$).

FIG. 5-26. The relationship of left ventricular end-diastolic volume as measured by radionuclide angiography and pulmonary capillary wedge pressure. Note the lack of significant correlation. (From Calvin et al[47] with permission.)

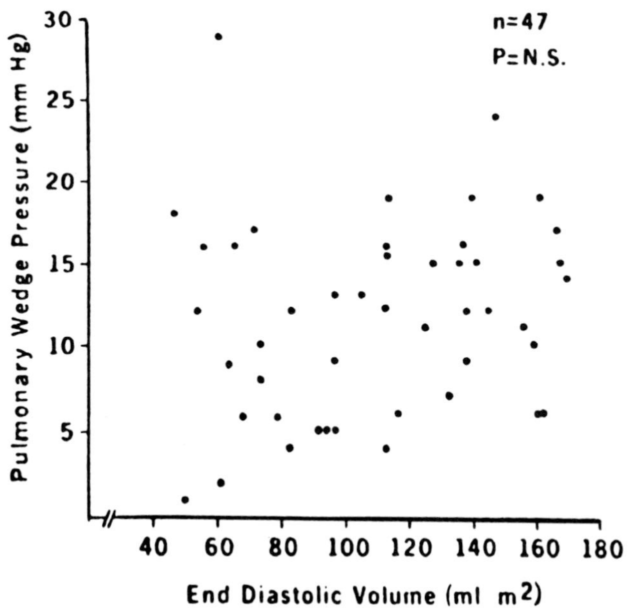


## MONITORING CARDIAC OUTPUT, BULK MOVEMENT OF OXYGEN, AND OXYGEN CONSUMPTION

After initial resuscitation, seriously injured patients may require a pulmonary artery catheter to monitor cardiac output and mixed venous blood gases. Currently, cardiac output determination by the thermodilution technique is standard.[145] As discussed earlier, cardiac output, although vitally important, is only one component of a far more important cardiorespiratory variable: oxygen delivery.[365] Standing by itself, it yields insufficient information about the quantity of oxy-

TABLE 5-7. Clinically Available Measured and Derived Global Variables Indicating Adequate Blood and Tissue Oxygenation

| Variable | |
|---|---|
| *Input variables* | |
| Oxygen delivery ($\dot{D}O_2$) | |
| Cardiac output ($\dot{Q}_t$) | |
| Arterial oxygen content ($CaO_2$) | |
| % $SaO_2$ | Major Determinants |
| [Hb] | Major Determinants |
| $PaO_2$ | Minor determinant except in extreme anemia or hypothermia |
| *Utilization variables* | |
| Oxygen consumption ($\dot{V}O_2$) | |
| Extraction Ratio $\left(\frac{\dot{V}O_2}{\dot{D}O_2}\right)$ | |
| *Output variables* | |
| $S\bar{v}O_2$ and $P\bar{v}O_2$ | |
| Lactate | |

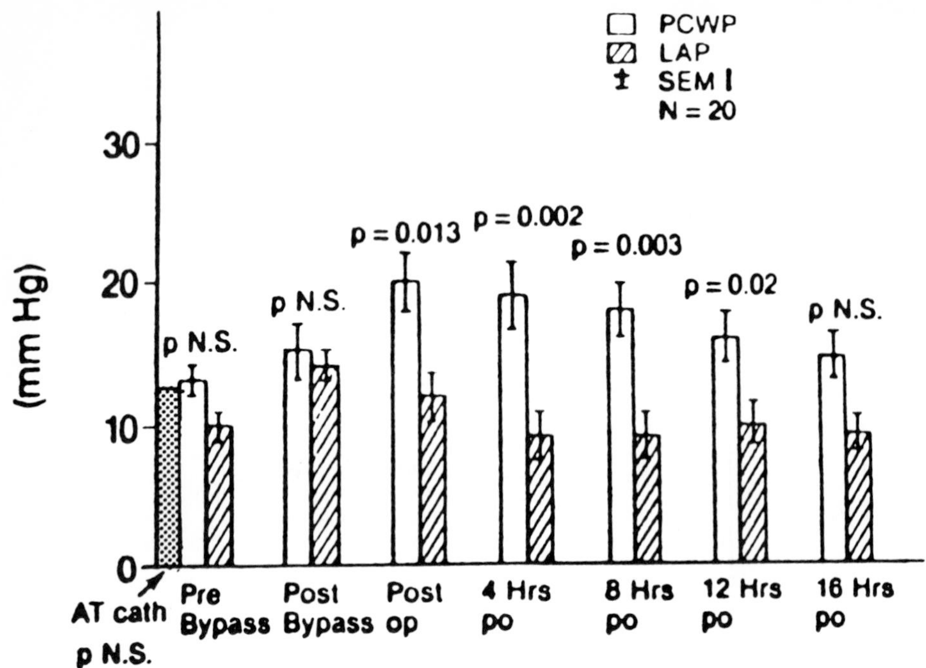


FIG. 5-27. Pulmonary capillary wedge pressure (PCWP) compared with left atrial pressure (LAP) from the pre-bypass period to 16 hours postoperatively. Note the lack of statistical correlation between PCWP and LAP from the immediate postoperative period to 12 hours postoperatively. (From Mammana et al[196] with permission.)

gen delivered to the intended tissues.[26,46,118,245,268,313,317,324,379,390] For instance, a cardiac output of 6 L/min in a 70-kg resting normovolemic male with a body surface area (BSA) of 1.7 $m^2$, [Hb] = 150 g/L, and $Sa_{O_2}$ = 97% is normal and appropriate. If this individual incurs chest injuries (pulmonary and myocardial contusions) and suffers significant hemorrhage, the following values may be obtained under anesthesia: $\dot{Q}_t$ = 6 L/min (CI = 3.5 L/min/$m^2$), [Hb] = 70 g/L, hematocrit = 20%, and $Sa_{O_2}$ = 70%. In this situation, calculated oxygen delivery is only 232 mL/min/$m^2$. The critical $\dot{D}_{O_2}$ in stable anesthetized patients appears to be approximately 330 mL/min/$m^2$, and therefore, in this example, a $\dot{Q}_t$ of 6 L/min is too low to maintain adequate tissue oxygenation.[174,176,290,305,306] An appropriate physiologic response to normovolemic hemodilution under light anesthesia is augmentation of cardiac output to 130% of normal or even greater.[182] The effect of the shock episode on the heart has prevented a rise in $\dot{Q}_t$ to compensate for the severely reduced $Ca_{O_2}$ and thus to provide the minimum required $\dot{D}_{O_2}$. If this patient's cardiac output were viewed without regard to oxygen delivery ($\dot{Q}_t \times Ca_{O_2}$), physiologic catastrophe and probably death might follow.[268]

The appropriateness of indexed cardiac output must also be questioned in the postoperative period. If, in our present hypothetical situation, the patient is noted to have a cardiac output of approximately 6 L/min (CI = 3.5 L/min/$m^2$), [Hb] = 110 g/L, and $Sa_{O_2}$ = 95%, then calculated $\dot{D}_{O_2}$ is 490 mL/min/$m^2$. This level of $\dot{D}_{O_2}$ intraoperatively would be satisfactory to maintain aerobic metabolism. However, in the postoperative period, $\dot{D}_{O_2}$ levels between 550 and 620 mL/min/$m^2$ are required to supply the augmented oxygen demand and consumption[26,27,317,324,379,381] (Fig 5-21). Thus, if hemoglobin

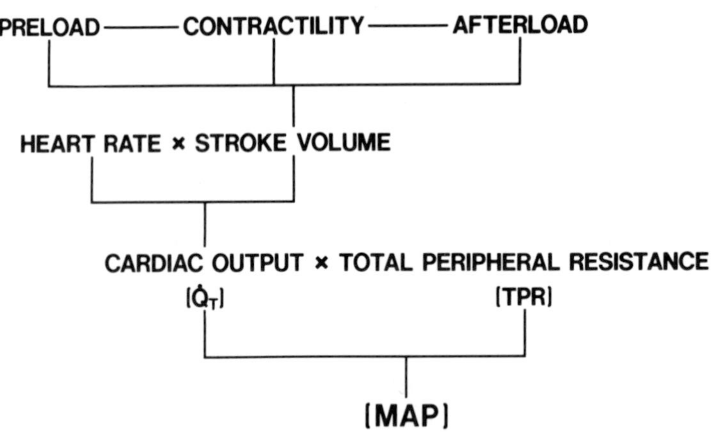


FIG. 5-28. Determinants of mean arterial pressure.

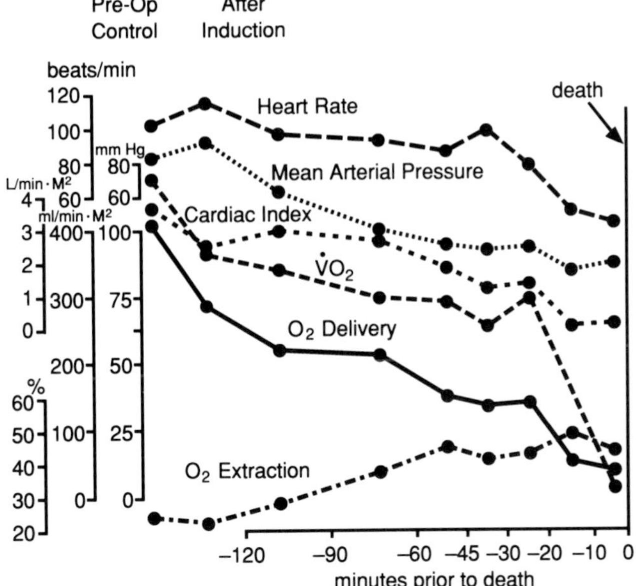


FIG. 5-29. Hemodynamic and oxygen transport variables during intraoperative monitoring of three patients who died during surgery. Note the fall in cardiac index after induction, with similar changes in $\dot{D}O_2$ and $\dot{V}O_2$ shortly thereafter. The change in MAP occurred later. (From Nolan and Shoemaker[234] with permission.)

concentration and $SaO_2$ remain constant, cardiac output should increase. In fact, it has been shown in a large series of critically ill postoperative patients that cardiac indices between 4.5 and 5.5 L/min/m$^2$ are necessary for survival[25,27,315,317,379] (Fig 5-21). Optimization of cardiac output may be accomplished by judicious infusion of blood and acellular fluids, inotropic therapy, and on some occasions, by afterload reduction.[268,280,317] During treatment preload (PAOP, CVP), contractility (left ventricular stroke work; LVSW),[65] afterload (TPR, SVR), cardiac rhythm, cardiac rate, and acid-base and electrolyte status should be monitored carefully.[101,305]

## OXYGEN CONSUMPTION

Oxygen consumption ($\dot{V}O_2$) reflects the body's global state of aerobic metabolism.[110,112,280,312] Prolonged depression of oxygen consumption in patients with circulatory shock correlates well with mortality.[25,26,245,311,313,317,318,324,329] Thus, in critically ill trauma patients, $\dot{V}O_2$ should be determined frequently during the perioperative period as a guide to diagnosis and treatment.[46,86,205,313,315,317,318,322,324,329,365] In common with cardiac output and oxygen delivery, proper assessment of oxygen consumption requires appraisal of oxygen demand.[390] Despite the shortcomings of global $\dot{V}O_2$ measurement,[43,69,116,349] as a predictor of individual organ function, $\dot{V}O_2$ optimization remains an important goal of trauma management.[26,86,311,319,321]

TABLE 5-8. Desirable, but Clinically Unavailable, Tissue Oxygenation Variables

| |
|---|
| *Input Variables* |
| Regional oxygen delivery (except skin: $PtcO_2$) |
| Physical status of the microcirculatory-diffusional interface |
| *Utilization variables* |
| Regional oxygen demand |
| Regional oxygen uptake |
| Regional extraction ratios |
| ATP generation and utilization: may be measured by positron emission tomography (PET scan) or magnetic resonance spectroscopy[117] |
| *Output variables* |
| Regional $PvO_2$ and $SvO_2$ |
| ATP and toxic metabolites |

### *Reduced Demand and Reduced Consumption*

During anesthesia a 20 to 25% reduction in $\dot{V}O_2$ (from 140 mL/min/m$^2$, to 105 to 110 mL/min/m$^2$) is not unusual[306] and is probably secondary to reduced oxygen demand induced by anesthesia, muscle relaxation, and mild hypothermia.[34,188,227,386] This reduction of $\dot{V}O_2$ is observed even when oxygen delivery is kept at preoperative levels.[379] A grossly reduced $\dot{V}O_2$ (greater than 30%) during anesthesia should arouse the suspicion of anaerobiosis.[306]

### *Reduced Consumption with Increased or Normal Demand*

This situation is frequently encountered during hypovolemic shock.[7,164,317] Treatment includes rapid optimization of $\dot{D}O_2$ with acellular fluids and blood to augment oxygen consumption at the nutrient capillary beds.[268] Anesthetic agents with the least potential of causing myocardial depression should be chosen to prevent reductions in $\dot{Q}_t$ and thus $\dot{D}O_2$.[29,386] Interpretation of $\dot{V}O_2$ in these instances requires caution and thoughtful consideration of its components. Since $\dot{V}O_2 = \dot{Q}_t (CaO_2 - C\bar{v}O_2)$, a reduction in $\dot{Q}_t$ of up to 33% with an appropriate compensatory increase in oxygen extraction (25 to 50%) may not result in a significant reduction of $\dot{V}O_2$.[86,371] This relatively normal $\dot{V}O_2$ may imply only that supranormal $O_2$ extraction is taking place in the perfused tissues. Thus, interpretation of $\dot{V}O_2$ should include simultaneous evaluation of $\dot{Q}_t$, $CaO_2$, and $C\bar{v}O_2$. As described earlier, poorly perfused or unperfused tissues do not participate in $\dot{V}O_2$; they contribute to anaerobiosis and cause lactic acidosis.[164] Thus, ultimately, sufficient contraction of blood volume will produce a gross reduction in $\dot{V}O_2$ at the critical level of $\dot{D}O_2$ which may not be reversible if aggressive therapeutic intervention is delayed.[26,291,296,381]

### *Increased Consumption with Increased Demand*

In the postoperative period oxygen consumption rises to pay back the intraoperative oxygen debt.[26,380] Moreover, this increased level of $\dot{V}O_2$ is compounded by the augmented oxygen demand of the posttrauma or postsurgical metabolic state.[110,311,379] Following surgery, $\dot{V}O_2$ values equal to or in excess of 167 mL/min/m$^2$ have been recorded[26,316,317,318,324,379] (Fig 5-21). Multiple trauma with hemorrhagic shock and surgical intervention often results in doubling of the normal steady-state $\dot{V}O_2$ (ie, to approximately 280 mL/min/m$^2$).[315] Thus, a "normal" $\dot{V}O_2$ of 140 mL/min/m$^2$

in these patients should be considered inappropriately low and hence, abnormal.

## EVALUATION OF THERAPY DIRECTED AT IMPROVEMENT OF $\dot{V}O_2$

An enhanced $\dot{V}O_2$ after therapy implies[135,317]

1. Improved tissue perfusion as a result of therapy
2. Spontaneous improvement of tissue perfusion, or
3. Therapy-induced increase in oxygen demand and thus, obligatory increase of oxygen consumption. This must be avoided.

No change in $\dot{V}O_2$ after therapy implies

1. Ineffective therapy[159]
2. Presence of irreversible circulatory shock[296] or
3. Optimal oxygen delivery before therapy.

Reduced $\dot{V}O_2$ after therapy implies

1. Circulatory deterioration at the time of therapeutic intervention[7] or
2. Wrong therapy.

In a study of critically ill postoperative intensive care unit (ICU) patients, Shoemaker et al[320,321,322] evaluated the efficacy of therapy directed toward optimal values of CVP, PAOP, $\dot{Q}_t$, $\dot{D}O_2$, and $\dot{V}O_2$. Mortality in group I, in whom CVP was optimized, was 23%. Group II patients had therapy directed to optimization of PAOP. Mortality in this group was 35%. When cardiac output and oxygen delivery were manipulated to optimize oxygen consumption ($\dot{V}O_2$), mortality decreased to 4%.[320,321]

Morbidity and mortality in critically ill patients are due either to single-system or multisystem organ failure.[46] Organ system failure and ultimately death, in turn, are due to dysoxia, defined by Robin[268] as abnormal $O_2$ utilization by the cell.[296] Hypoxic dysoxia is evoked by decreased systemic oxygen transport or inadequate (or abnormal) cellular utilization of oxygen in the presence of seemingly adequate $\dot{D}O_2$.[46,60a,296,381] This is exactly the condition in treatment-resistant, or irreversible, hemorrhagic shock. It follows, then, that therapy of hemorrhagic shock should be directed toward prevention and reversal of hypoxic dysoxia and its sequelae.[60a] Thus, treatment must include augmentation and optimization of the flow-related cardiorespiratory variables ($\dot{Q}_t$, $\dot{D}O_2$, and $\dot{V}O_2$) since oxygen transport and utilization are flow and not pressure dependent. It is no wonder then that CVP and even PAOP values are not very precise predictors of survival, even when therapeutically optimized.

## MONITORING OF BLOOD GASES

### *Arterial Blood Gases*

All critically injured patients should have an intraarterial catheter in place to allow for continuous blood pressure measurement and ready access for arterial blood gas sampling. However, most patients suffering from significant hemorrhage without concurrent respiratory system derangement have normal $Sa_{O_2}$ and $Pa_{O_2}$ when supplemental oxygen is administered. These values have been consistently noted up to the point of circulatory collapse and death.[164,166,187,230,234,317,318,324,360,363,366] Despite their shortcomings as predictors of $\dot{D}O_2$, $Pa_{O_2}$ and $Sa_{O_2}$ should be monitored repeatedly in critically injured patients to obtain information about pulmonary gas exchange (see also the next section). In isolation, however, these values convey only incomplete information regarding the overall state of tissue oxygenation ($\dot{D}O_2$ and $\dot{V}O_2$).

NONINVASIVE, CONTINUOUS ARTERIAL BLOOD OXYGEN SATURATION MONITORING. Arterial oxygen saturation ($Sa_{O_2}$) is one of the three major components of oxygen delivery. Although incomplete, it provides some information regarding the bulk oxygen flux to the tissues. $Sa_{O_2}$ is affected by the inspired oxygen fraction ($F_{IO_2}$), alveolar ventilation ($V_A$), intrapulmonary shunt ($\dot{Q}_{sp}/\dot{Q}_t$), and mixed venous oxygen saturation ($S\bar{v}_{O_2}$). Any permutation of diminished $F_{IO_2}$, $V_A$, and $S\bar{v}_{O_2}$ and augmented $\dot{Q}_{sp}/\dot{Q}_t$ may produce a significant and potentially life-threatening drop in $Sa_{O_2}$.[35] A significant reduction in $Sa_{O_2}$ can occur in traumatized patients when gross derangement of the respiratory system occurs.[31] In addition, $Sa_{O_2}$ may be affected by the varying levels of $F_{IO_2}$ and airway pressure administered during anesthetic and ICU management. Thus, continuous measurement of $Sa_{O_2}$ is desirable, if not mandatory.

$Sa_{O_2}$ can be measured noninvasively, continuously, and accurately within the 22 to 100% range with pulse oximetry.[35,158,206,212,294,350,398] As in classic oximetry, discrete wavelengths of light are used to measure the optical density of hemoglobin. However, with pulse oximetry, arterial blood is distinguished from venous blood, skin, connective tissue, and bone. The proper functioning of the pulse oximeter depends on measurement of light absorbance changes during arterial pulsation. Multiple arteriolar beds (eg, fingers, toes, nasal septum) may be selected as monitoring sites. The device is simple to use and requires no warm-up time or calibration.

Pulse oximeters may not be accurate under certain clinical conditions such as hypothermia, increased sympathetic tone, hypovolemia with mean arterial pressure less than 50 mm Hg, severe anemia, severe right heart failure, tricuspid regurgitation, obstructed venous return, administration of positive end-expiratory pressure (PEEP), patient movement, and cardiopulmonary resuscitation.[232,358] Dyshemoglobinemias also may affect the accuracy of these monitors.[14,15,357]

Since the most common cause of anesthetic morbidity and mortality is undiagnosed arterial hypoxemia,[160] pulse oximeters should be used in all anesthetized patients. However, in the severely hypoxic, hypotensive, and hypothermic trauma victim, their accuracy and reliability remain dubious.

### *Venous Blood Gases*

MONITORING OF MIXED VENOUS OXYGEN SATURATION ($S\bar{v}_{O_2}$). In general, $S\bar{v}_{O_2}$ reflects the overall state of $O_2$ extraction by the tissues. Increased global $O_2$ extraction, usually caused by inadequate $O_2$ delivery (to be distinguished from exercise), results in decreased $S\bar{v}_{O_2}$.[228] Thus, $S\bar{v}_{O_2}$ monitoring should provide information about the existence and extent of such deficiencies and allow appropriate treatment. To appreciate fully the significance of $S\bar{v}O_2$, we again refer to the Fick equation.

If

$$\dot{V}O_2 = \dot{Q}_t \times (CaO_2 - C\bar{v}O_2)$$

Then

$$C\bar{v}O_2 = CaO_2 - \frac{\dot{V}O_2}{\dot{Q}_t}$$

Since

$$C\bar{v}O_2 = [Hb] \times 1.34 \times S\bar{v}O_2 \text{ (neglecting dissolved oxygen)}$$

Then

$$S\bar{v}O_2 \propto CaO_2 - \frac{\dot{V}O_2}{\dot{Q}_t}$$

This relationship thus allows us to analyze, within limits, the degree of oxygen extraction by the body as a whole.[228,282,283] Mixed venous oxygen saturation ($S\bar{v}O_2$) is the result of dynamic interactions between $CaO_2$ ([Hb] and $SaO_2$), $\dot{V}O_2$, and $\dot{Q}_t$.[72,283] Analysis of the variables comprising $S\bar{v}O_2$ permits a clear understanding of the difficulties of interpretation. Moreover, proper interpretation of $S\bar{v}O_2$ requires awareness of the fact that physiologically, few parameters change in isolation.[134,228] Generally, alteration of one variable will produce a change in another, and the sum of these changes is consequently a composite; so it is with $S\bar{v}O_2$.[228,283]

This discussion of $S\bar{v}O_2$ in hemorrhage will be presented in a hypothetical clinical situation. Let us assume that a 70-kg man of 1.7-$m^2$ body surface area has sustained significant hemorrhage. With a pulmonary artery catheter, his measured $\dot{Q}_t$ is 1.75 L/min (ie, 25 to 30% of normal), and $S\bar{v}O_2$ is 32% ($P\bar{v}O_2$ approximately 20 mm Hg). If the average normal total body oxygen extraction is roughly 25% (ie, $S\bar{v}O_2$ = 75%), then the patient's $O_2$ extraction is roughly 2.5 times normal. If, in this hypothetical patient, it is also known that [Hb] = 150 g/L (15 g %), $SaO_2$ = 100%, and arterial pH = 7.25, then his oxyhemoglobin dissociation curve would be as depicted in Fig 5-30. His calculated $\dot{V}O_2$ is 238 mL/min, which is within normal range. Thus, oxygen extraction at the aerobic limits yields a normal total body $\dot{V}O_2$ just equal to consumable oxygen (Fig 5-6). As demonstrated by this example, during hemorrhagic shock, $S\bar{v}O_2$ is severely depressed because of increased $O_2$ extraction in preferentially perfused nutrient capillary beds[164,166,187,303] (Table 5-9). Although global $\dot{V}O_2$ is normal, regional $\dot{V}O_2$ values of nonvital tissues (muscle, skin, kidney) are probably depressed due to redistribution of $\dot{Q}_t$ and $\dot{D}O_2$. Thus, normal global $\dot{V}O_2$ can mask regional depression of $\dot{V}O_2$ and, consequently, tissue hypoxia.

$S\bar{v}O_2$ DURING RESUSCITATION WITH ACELLULAR FLUIDS AND BLOOD. If

$$S\bar{v}O_2 \propto CaO_2 - \frac{\dot{V}O_2}{\dot{Q}_t}$$

then infusion of acellular fluids (crystalloid or colloid) will have a triple effect on $S\bar{v}O_2$. Rapid administration of acellular fluids increases $\dot{Q}_t$ and thus $\dot{D}O_2$.[164] At the same time, however, because of a progressive dilution of the intravascular red cell mass and reduction in [Hb], $CaO_2$ decreases.[154] In addition, during rapid acellular fluid resuscitation, poorly perfused or nonperfused anaerobically metabolizing tissues begin to participate in $\dot{V}O_2$. Therefore, $\dot{V}O_2$ rises. If hemodilution with acellular fluids proceeds to normovolemia so that the effective

FIG. 5-30. Oxygen delivery and consumption in hemorrhagic shock. *Conditions:* [Hb] = 150 g/L, pH = 7.25, temperature = 34°C, $PCO_2$ = 40 mm Hg. Even though oxygen consumption appears to be normal, $\dot{V}O_2$ equals consumable oxygen. More specifically, although $\dot{D}O_2$ = 350 mL/min, only 238 mL/min is available for aerobic consumption. Compare with Fig 5-6.

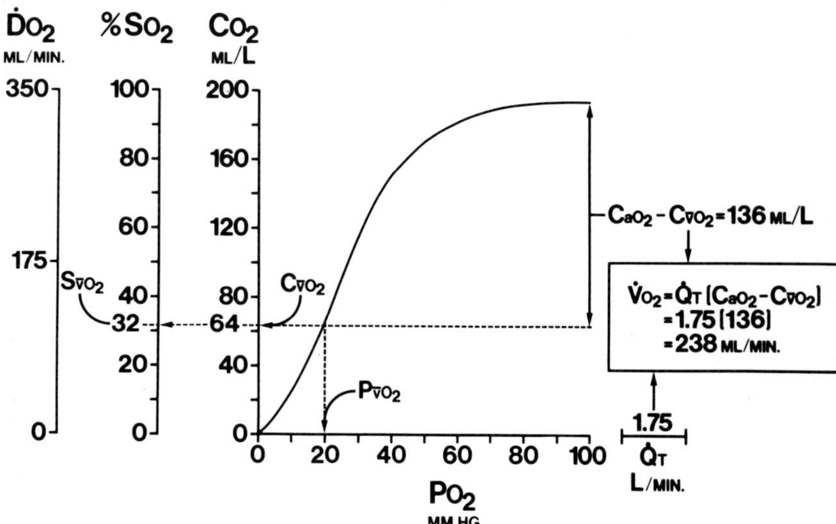

TABLE 5-9. Initial Arterial and Mixed Venous Blood Gas Studies in Patients with Traumatic Shock. Note that in the vast majority of patients, $Pa{O_2}$ and $Sa{O_2}$ are satisfactory. However, survivors usually displayed higher initial $S\bar{v}{O_2}$ values.*

| | | ARTERIAL BLOOD GASES | | | | MIXED VENOUS GASES | | | | A-V $O_2$ DIFFERENCE | UTILIZATION COEFFICIENT |
|---|---|---|---|---|---|---|---|---|---|---|---|
| GROUP | PATIENT | $Pa{O_2}$ | $Pa{CO_2}$ | pH | $Sa{O_2}$ | $P\bar{v}{O_2}$ | $P\bar{v}{CO_2}$ | pH | $S\bar{v}{O_2}$ | ($Ca{O_2}$ − $C\bar{v}{O_2}$) | (%) |
| Survivors | 1 | 74 | 33 | 7.301 | 92.0 | 16 | 51 | 7.287 | <30 | 8.757 | 69.7 |
| | 2 | 138 | 42 | 7.358 | 98.7 | 26 | 55 | 7.283 | 40 | 8.214 | 59.0 |
| | 3 | 120 | 32 | 7.234 | 97.7 | 33 | 46 | 7.360 | 61 | 5.107 | 38.1 |
| | 4 | 134 | 28 | 7.479 | 99.3 | 30 | 37 | 7.438 | 58 | 5.610 | 42.6 |
| Average | | 117 | 34 | 7.343 | 96.8 | 26 ± 6.5 | 47 | 7.341 | 46 ± 13.4 | 6.982 | 52.3 |
| Nonsurvivors | 1 | 164 | 47 | 7.078 | 98.0 | 9 | 55 | 7.122 | <30 | 9.859 | 72.2 |
| | 2 | 250 | 50 | 7.290 | 99.3 | 20 | 55 | 6.860 | <30 | 10.266 | 72.9 |
| | 3 | 455 | 60 | 7.070 | 99.9 | 47 | 39 | 6.914 | <30 | 10.904 | 73.7 |
| | 4 | 124 | 47 | 7.072 | 95.8 | 67 | 55 | 7.034 | 81 | 2.159 | 16.3 |
| | 5 | 52 | 39 | 7.299 | 82.0 | 13 | 43 | 7.278 | <30 | 7.358 | 66.0 |
| | 6 | 99 | 52 | 7.140 | 90.0 | 30 | 60 | 7.100 | 37 | 7.316 | 59.2 |
| Average | | 191 | 49 | 7.158 | 94.2 | 31 ± 20 | 51 | 7.051 | 36 ± 19 | 7.977 | 60.4 |

* (From Kazarian and DelGuercio[166] with permission.)

[Hb] is 75 g/L and the measured $\dot{Q}_t$ is 8 L/min, then the oxyhemoglobin dissociation curve at the end of initial fluid resuscitation would be as depicted in Fig 5-31.

In this example, although the $Ca{O_2}$ is decreased, the arterial-mixed venous oxygen content difference is reduced considerably from 136 to 30 mL/L after fluid resuscitation. Compensation involving rapid elevation of $\dot{Q}_t$ to 8 L/min produces an $S\bar{v}{O_2}$ within the normal range, 70%. After stabilization and during normovolemic hemodilution, any drop in $S\bar{v}{O_2}$ (ie, increased $O_2$ extraction) may indicate increased $\dot{V}{O_2}$, additional bleeding causing hypovolemia and reduction in $\dot{Q}_t$, primary cardiac pump failure, or further reduction in [Hb] if $\dot{Q}_t$ is at maximum.[207] The foregoing conclusions, of course, assume an optimal $Sa{O_2}$ (ie, 95 to 100%). The effect of crystalloid infusion on $S\bar{v}{O_2}$ is depicted in Fig 5-32.

After blood transfusion, $Ca{O_2}$ increases as a function of enhanced [Hb]. As hematocrit and [Hb] increase following maximal hemodilution, a reduction in $\dot{Q}_t$ may be observed as a function of the efficacy of transfusion therapy. As an end point of transfusion therapy, $S\bar{v}{O_2}$, in this stage, should be within the acceptable range of 60 to 80%.[9,166] Fig 5-33 and Fig 5-34 depict sequential changes in $S\bar{v}{O_2}$ as functions of crystalloid infusion and blood transfusion. It should be noted that all survivors had acceptable $S\bar{v}{O_2}$ after volume resuscitation, and nonsurvivors did not. Also to be noted is that four of the six nonsurvivors had initial $S\bar{v}{O_2}$ values less than 30%, whereas in only one of four survivors was $S\bar{v}{O_2}$ at this level. Thus, an $S\bar{v}{O_2} < 30\%$, in the presence of hemorrhagic shock, seems to carry a grim prognosis.

From the foregoing discussion it can be seen that $S\bar{v}{O_2}$ is a barometer of the entire oxygen transport system.[160,228,283] It represents a composite of changes mediated by alterations

FIG. 5-31. Oxygen consumption in acute normovolemic hemodilution. *Conditions:* Upper curve (dots and dashes) is the same as the oxyhemoglobin dissociation curve in Fig 5-30. Lower curve ([Hb] = 75 g/L, pH = 7.40, $P{CO_2}$ = 40 mm Hg, temperature = 36°C) represents oxyhemoglobin dissociation curve after aggressive accellular fluid resuscitation. This illustrates the improvement in oxygen transport from hemorrhagic hypovolemia to acute normovolemic hemodilution (compare with Fig 5-30). $\dot{D}{O_2}$ has risen from 350 to 800 mL/min, $P\bar{v}{O_2}$ and $S\bar{v}{O_2}$ are now within the normal range, and $\dot{V}{O_2}$ is normal.

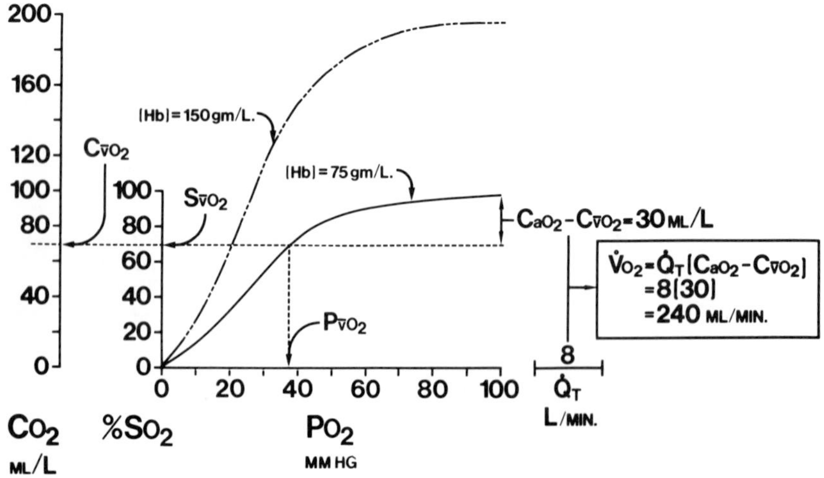

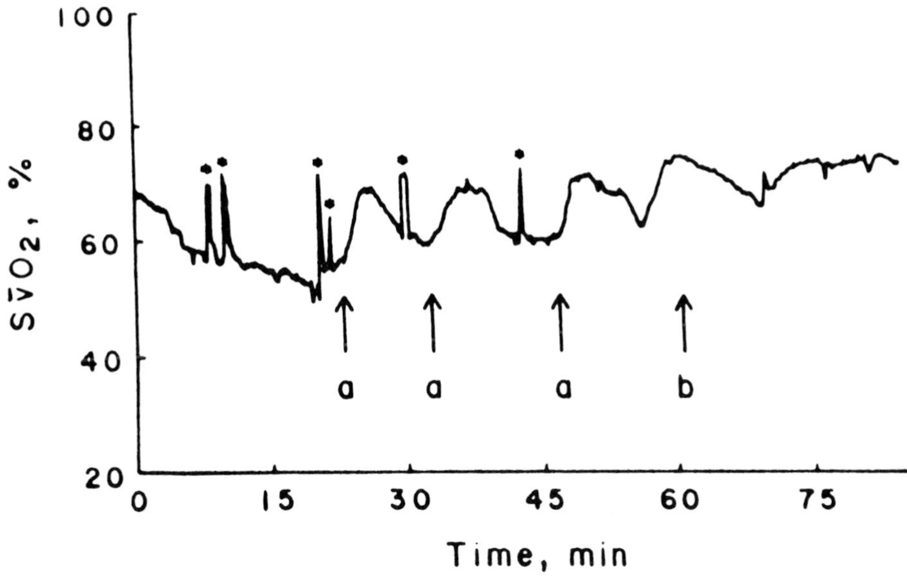


FIG. 5-32. Ability of successive 100-mL intravenous bolus doses of lactated Ringer's (LR) solution (arrow a) to reverse downward trend in $S\bar{v}O_2$, and subsequent maintenance of normal $S\bar{v}O_2$ by increased rate of LR infusion (arrow b). * indicates catheter balloon inflation to measure PCWP. (From Baele et al[9] with permission.)

in oxygen delivery, oxygen consumption, and oxygen demand.

CAUSES OF HIGH $S\bar{v}O_2$ (>80%)

### *Decreased Oxygen Consumption Due to Decreased Oxygen Demand*

This condition is common during anesthesia. If $\dot{Q}_t$ and $CaO_2$ remain relatively constant and $\dot{V}O_2$ drops, $S\bar{v}O_2$ must rise, reflecting oxygen delivery in excess of demand. The reduced oxygen demand is augmented by mild to moderate hypothermia[118,233,390] and skeletal muscle paralysis.[227] Flow maldistribution from functional systemic arteriovenous shunting may also cause elevation of $S\bar{v}O_2$ and reduced nutrient capillary $O_2$ extraction.[192,306,379,380,381] Elevation of $S\bar{v}O_2$ during anesthesia is magnified in the presence of hyperoxia.

### *Normal or Increased Oxygen Demand with Reduced Oxygen Consumption*

1. Sepsis syndrome: whether systemic arteriovenous shunting, poor uptake of oxygen at the nutrient capillary-cellular interface, or reduced intracellular $O_2$ uti-

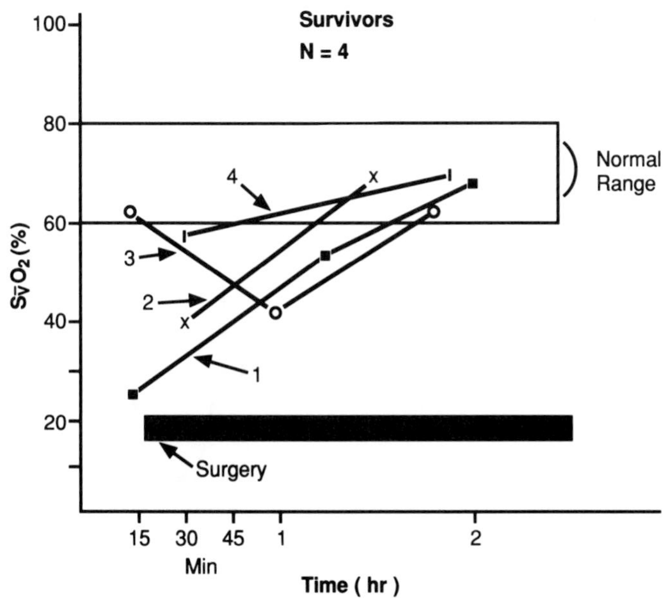


FIG. 5-33. Hemorrhagic shock, $S\bar{v}O_2$, and survival. The effect of volume replacement, tracheal intubation, oxygenation, and operative control of hemorrhage is improvement of $S\bar{v}O_2$ to normal range. (From Kazarian and Del Guercio[166] with permission.)

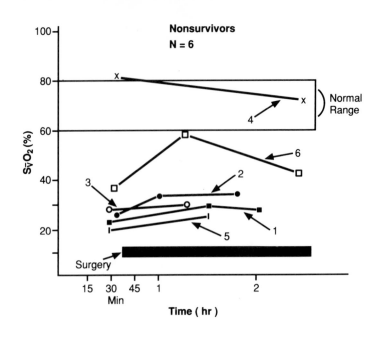

FIG. 5-34. Hemorrhagic shock, $S\bar{v}O_2$, and nonsurvival. The effect of failed resuscitation with accellular fluids, blood, and operative intervention is a failure of $S\bar{v}O_2$ to rise. In patient 4, the high initial $S\bar{v}O_2$ probably represents severe systemic arteriovenous shunting and/or histotoxic hypoxia. $S\bar{v}O_2$ fell into the normal range with therapy, but this final value is still inappropriately high. (From Kazarian and Del Guercio[166] with permission.)

lization is the cause of the elevated or inappropriately normal $S\bar{v}O_2$ values seen in septic shock is not known.[72,106,149,160,164,214,388] Regardless of the cause, elevated or inappropriately normal $S\bar{v}O_2$ values with reduced $O_2$ extraction ratio and metabolic (lactic) acidosis imply poor tissue oxygenation and poor prognosis.[8,249]

2. Cyanide poisoning[354]: uncoupling of oxidative phosphorylation
3. Maldistribution of microcirculatory flow[8,68,173,178,296]
4. Adult respiratory distress syndrome (ARDS)[68,245]

### *Normal or Reduced Oxygen Demand and Consumption with Increased Oxygen Delivery: Excessive Inotropic Therapy[204]*

If $CaO_2$ and $\dot{V}O_2$ remain relatively constant in the presence of iatrogenic increase in $\dot{Q}_t$, the $O_2$ supply may exceed demand, and $S\bar{v}O_2$ rises.

## CAUSES OF LOW $S\bar{v}O_2$ (<60%)

### *Decreased Oxygen Delivery*

HEMORRHAGIC SHOCK. As discussed earlier, hemorrhagic shock with an associated fall in $\dot{Q}_t$ and blood volume causes a reduction in $S\bar{v}O_2$[86,164,166,255,274,302,303] because of more complete extraction of oxygen from hemoglobin traversing nutrient capillary beds.[291] Tending to offset this fall in $S\bar{v}O_2$ is anatomic and/or functional shunting of arterialized blood into the mixed venous effluent.[3,140,214]

PRIMARY CARDIAC FAILURE. Left ventricular failure with attendant reduction in $\dot{Q}_t$, in the presence of stable $CaO_2$ and $\dot{V}O_2$, produces a reduction in $S\bar{v}O_2$.[23,106,134,187,277,280,383] Treatment of the failure may then be tracked by improvement in $S\bar{v}O_2$[23,72,106,134,280,281,342,374,375,383] (Fig 5-35). Some studies have shown poor correlation between $S\bar{v}O_2$ (and $P\bar{v}O_2$) and $\dot{Q}_t$, probably because of simultaneous $\dot{D}O_2$-dependent changes in $\dot{V}O_2$.[134,221,368]

REDUCTION IN $CaO_2$. Hypovolemia in the presence of reduction in hemoglobin concentration inhibits the compensatory rise in $\dot{Q}_t$.[207] Even when normovolemia is maintained and an appropriate rise in $\dot{Q}_t$ occurs, $S\bar{v}O_2$ falls slowly with progressive hemodilution.[154] If a precipitous reduction in $S\bar{v}O_2$ is noted, then hypovolemia and diminishing $\dot{Q}_t$ should be suspected. If normovolemia is present, frank cardiac failure may be the cause. Alternatively, a rise in $\dot{V}O_2$ mediated by increased demand might be instrumental.[91,110] Needless to say, if $SaO_2$ drops for any reason without adequate cardiovascular compensation, $S\bar{v}O_2$ falls.[72,91] Improvement of $S\bar{v}O_2$ after respi-

FIG. 5-35. Gradual decline in $S\bar{v}O_2$ over 20 minutes heralded onset of cardiac arrest (arrow). Resuscitation was successful and paralleled by a rise in $S\bar{v}O_2$ to control levels. (From Baele et al[9] with permission.)

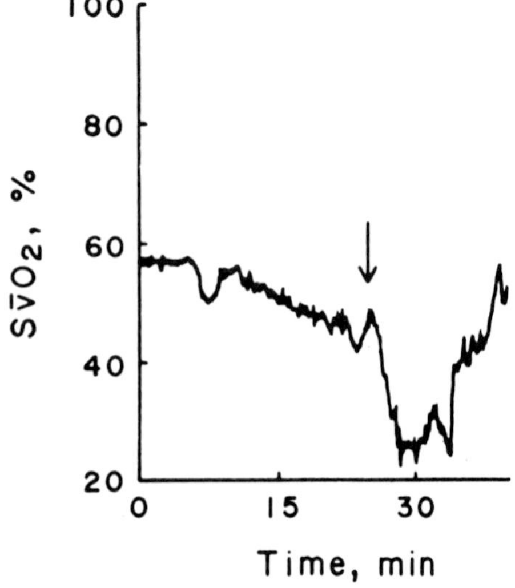

ratory therapy such as PEEP implies improvement of $Sa_{O_2}$, $\dot{Q}_t$, and tissue oxygenation.[91,165,185] In fact, in most nonseptic patients with hypoxemic respiratory failure, the PEEP level that produces the highest $S\bar{v}_{O_2}$ is associated with optimal oxygen delivery, and changes in $S\bar{v}_{O_2}$ correlate with changes in $\dot{D}_{O_2}$.[91]

### *Increased Oxygen Demand*

In the postoperative period, a fall in $S\bar{v}_{O_2}$ may be expected if increased metabolic demands are not met by appropriate enhancement in $\dot{Q}_t$.[110,163,243,256,288,378] Likewise, postoperative fever mandates increased $\dot{V}_{O_2}$.[292] If appropriate increases in $\dot{Q}_t$ are not realized, $S\bar{v}_{O_2}$ will fall.[163]

It is obvious that proper assessment of tissue oxygenation based on $S\bar{v}_{O_2}$ analysis requires thoughtful consideration.[235] Any therapy based on $S\bar{v}_{O_2}$ changes requires knowledge of which variable (or variables) is the primary cause. Moreover, the delicate oxygen supply-demand ratio must be appraised in order to institute rational therapy.

As mentioned earlier, $S\bar{v}_{O_2}$ is the composite index of oxygenation variables and reflects the overall status of tissue oxygenation—the balance between $O_2$ demand and supply ($\dot{V}_{O_2}/\dot{D}_{O_2}$ or $O_2$ extraction ratio). Since $\dot{V}_{O_2}$ can be expressed as $(Ca_{O_2} - C\bar{v}_{O_2}) \times \dot{Q}_t$, and $\dot{D}_{O_2}$ as $Ca_{O_2} \times \dot{Q}_t$, then the $O_2$ extraction ratio

$$\dot{V}_{O_2}/\dot{D}_{O_2} = \frac{(Ca_{O_2} - C\bar{v}_{O_2})\dot{Q}_t}{Ca_{O_2} \times \dot{Q}_t} = 1 - \frac{C\bar{v}_{O_2}}{Ca_{O_2}}$$

If $Sa_{O_2} = 1.0$, then $C\bar{v}_{O_2}/Ca_{O_2} = S\bar{v}_{O_2}$. Thus, $\dot{V}_{O_2}/\dot{D}_{O_2} = 1 - S\bar{v}_{O_2}$, or, by rearranging the equation, $S\bar{v}_{O_2} = 1 - \dot{V}_{O_2}/\dot{D}_{O_2}$ (see Table 5-3). It is obvious that the $O_2$ extraction ratio, $\dot{V}_{O_2}/\dot{D}_{O_2}$, can be calculated easily from $S\bar{v}_{O_2}$. In fact, Nelson[228] demonstrated, in critically ill surgical patients, an excellent correlation ($r = 0.96$) between $S\bar{v}_{O_2}$ and the $O_2$ extraction ratio, corroborating the results of earlier work by Schmidt et al[283] (Fig 5-36). These results demonstrated little correlation between $S\bar{v}_{O_2}$ and the individual determinants of $O_2$ transport ($\dot{Q}_t$, $\dot{V}_{O_2}$, and $\dot{D}_{O_2}$), confirming that $S\bar{v}_{O_2}$ is an indicator of the overall balance between oxygen consumption and delivery. Others have arrived at the same conclusions.[134,178,221,368]

Using simultaneous noninvasive continuous pulse oximetry and continuous mixed venous oximetry, Rasanen et al[259] have shown that the extraction ratio can be calculated, using the formula

$$\frac{Sa_{O_2} - S\bar{v}_{O_2}}{Sa_{O_2}}.$$

Compared with the approximation $1 - S\bar{v}_{O_2}$, this formula demonstrates a smaller overall difference in absolute values

FIG. 5-36. Correlation between $S\bar{v}_{O_2}$ and cardiac output (A), oxygen delivery (B), oxygen consumption (C), and oxygen utilization (D). Note the poor correlation with A, B, and C and the excellent correlation with D. (From Nelson[228] with permission.)

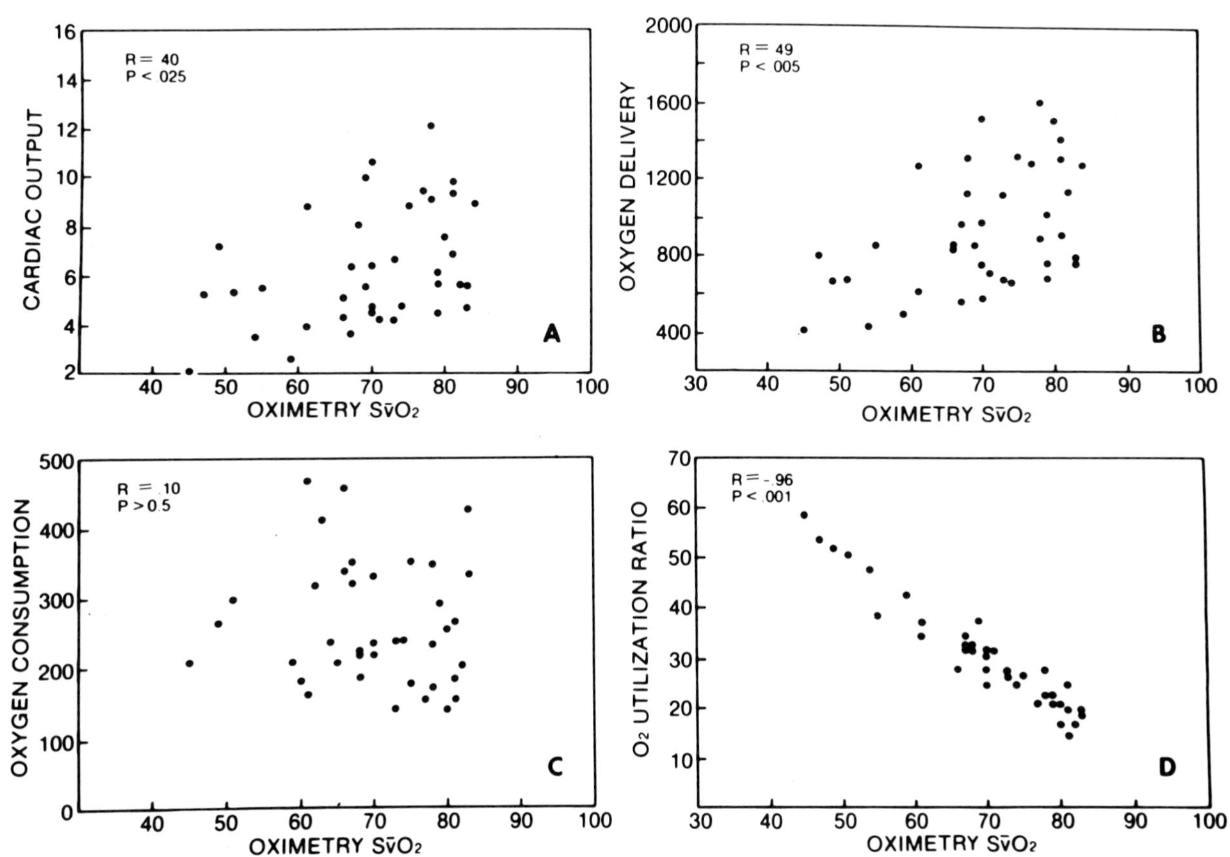

from the calculated extraction ratio. Furthermore, assuming that pulmonary end-capillary blood is fully saturated with oxygen and neglecting the effect of dissolved oxygen, the equation for venous admixture (shunt) can be simplified as follows.[258,260]

$$\dot{Q}_{sp}/\dot{Q}_t \approx \frac{(1 - SaO_2)}{(1 - S\bar{v}O_2)}$$

Special pulmonary artery catheters equipped with a fiberoptic photometric cable are capable of measuring thermodilution cardiac output and continuous $S\bar{v}O_2$. They are reliable and accurate over wide ranges of $S\bar{v}O_2$[9,10,91,228,284,375]; catheters with a three-wavelength system provide more accurate measurement than those using a two wave-length system.[28,103,263] Equipped with such sophisticated technology, which is readily available to even the modest community hospital, physicians are now capable of monitoring all the variables in the oxygen transport system with the exception of the status of the microcirculation and the regional distribution of $\dot{D}O_2$ and $\dot{V}O_2$.

If a pulmonary artery catheter is contraindicated or otherwise found unnecessary for successful management of the patient, there are other reasonable alternatives to the measurement of $S\bar{v}O_2$.[70,187,225,277] Right atrial blood oxygen saturation ($SRAO_2$) has been found to reflect changes in cardiac output and $S\bar{v}O_2$ accurately in the absence of intracardiac shunts as patients in clinical shock improve with therapy.[187,225,262,274,277,303,391] However, superior vena caval oxygen saturation ($SsvcO_2$), is less accurate.[264] If only trends in improvement of oxygen extraction are required, $SsvcO_2$ may be satisfactory.[264,348] However, exact quantitation of $\dot{V}O_2$ or intrapulmonary shunt can be made only with a pulmonary artery catheter.[53] The decreased reliability of $SsvcO_2$ results primarily from the venous effluent of the kidney (Table 5-3). Blood returning from the kidney is approximately 95% saturated with oxygen and comprises roughly 20% of the $\dot{Q}_t$. During low-flow shock due to redistribution of blood flow away from the kidney and gut toward the brain and heart, the $O_2$ saturation and relative contribution to venous return of blood from the superior vena cava are higher than those of the inferior vena cava.[187,229,277] Therefore, $SsvcO_2$ does not closely parallel $S\bar{v}O_2$, although $SRAO_2$ does (Table 5-10).[262] Thus, if a reflection of pulmonary artery oxygen saturation is desired, placement of a long CVP catheter (right atrial) and monitoring of $SRAO_2$ may be appropriate.

## PITFALLS IN INTERPRETATION OF $S\bar{v}O_2$

Because of maldistribution of flow between and within different organs and tissues in severe hemorrhagic shock, systemic arteriovenous admixture occurs,[3,140,160,166,214] resulting in varying degrees of arterialization of the mixed venous effluent. As a consequence, in many instances, $S\bar{v}O_2$, $C\bar{v}O_2$, and $P\bar{v}O_2$ do not truly reflect the flow-weighted means of individual organ and total body oxygen extraction.[235] This physiologic shunting (anatomic and/or functional) is diagrammatically depicted in Fig 5-37. Obviously, as all oxygen consumption

TABLE 5-10. Oxygen Saturation and Hemodynamic Data from Patients in Shock. Right Atrial, but Not Superior Vena Caval, Blood Oxygen Saturation Closely Approximates Pulmonary Artery Blood Oxygen Saturation ($S\bar{v}O_2$).*

| | | $O_2$ SATURATION (%) | | | | | | PULMONARY ARTERY PRESSURE | | | |
|---|---|---|---|---|---|---|---|---|---|---|---|
| AGE (years) | TYPE OF SHOCK | *Central Venous* | *Right Atrium* | *Right Ventricle* | *Pulmonary Artery* | *Systemic Artery* | *Inferior Vena Cava* | *mm Hg* | *Mean* | $\dot{Q}$ (L/min) | CARDIAC INDEX |
| 53 | Septic | 59.0 | 51.5 | 53.0 | 51.5 | 96.5 | 44.7 | 26/10 | 15 | 2.9 2.7(F†) | 1.58 |
| 61 | Septic | 68.7 | 58.0 | 63.0 | 60.0 | 96.0 | 53.9 | 28/16 | 21 | 3.9 | 1.90 |
| | | 68.0 | | 56.0 | 56.5 | 93.5 | | 30/17 | 22 | 3.3 | 1.62 |
| 45 | Hemorrhagic | 68.5 | 61.0 | 60.5 | 60.0 | 96.8 | | 27/12 | 19 | 3.9 3.8(F) | 1.36 |
| 63 | Neurogenic | 78.8 | 69.0 | 67.5 | 68.0 | 99.4 | | 26/10 | 17 | 3.1 | 1.62 |
| | | 72.3 | | 62.0 | 63.5 | 97.8 | | 25/12 | 16 | 3.9 | 2.04 |
| 35 | Hemorrhagic | 71.2 | 63.5 | 62.0 | 61.2 | 100.0 | | 34/18 | 24 | 3.5 | 1.82 |
| 33 | Hemorrhagic | 71.0 | 62.5 | 60.5 | 60.5 | 98.9 | 52.4 | 18/9 | 14 | 3.3 | 1.65 |
| 31 | Hemorrhagic | 67.0 | 56.0 | 57.5 | 54.5 | 97.2 | 43.7 | 25/14 | 18 | 3.3 | 1.58 |
| 78 | Septic | 58.5 | 52.0 | 51.0 | 50.0 | 99.5 | | 55/20 | 38 | 2.7 | 1.51 |
| 57 | Septic | 60.0 | | 52.0 | 48.0 | 100.0 | | 38/15 | 24 | 2.9 3.2(F) | 1.61 |
| 60 | Hemorrhagic | 63.2 | 53.5 | 56.0 | 54.5 | 99.6 | 48.9 | 26/10 | 17 | 3.2 | 1.65 |
| 59 | Hemorrhagic | 59.5 | 53.0 | 50.5 | 51.0 | 100.0 | | 18/8 | 12 | 2.7 | 1.43 |
| | | 62.5 | | 46.0 | 44.5 | 100.0 | | 20/8 | 12 | 2.6 | 1.35 |
| 51 | Neurogenic | 65.5 | 49.0 | 56.5 | 53.0 | 98.7 | | 16/8 | 12 | 3.7 | 1.95 |
| 57 | Septic | 63.3 | 57.0 | 56.5 | 58.5 | 99.4 | | 26/15 | 19 | 3.3 2.9(F) | 1.89 |
| 67 | Septic | 69.0 | 60.3 | 58.0 | 56.0 | 100.0 | | 38/14 | 23 | 4.0 3.9(F) | 1.93 |
| | | 67.8 | | 61.4 | 59.5 | 97.7 | | 35/10 | 20 | 3.7 4.0(F) | 1.71 |
| 39 | Septic | 61.5 | | 54.5 | 53.0 | 90.8 | | 35/17 | 24 | 3.0 2.8(F) | 1.76 |

* From Lee et al[187] with permission.
† F = determined by the Fick principle.

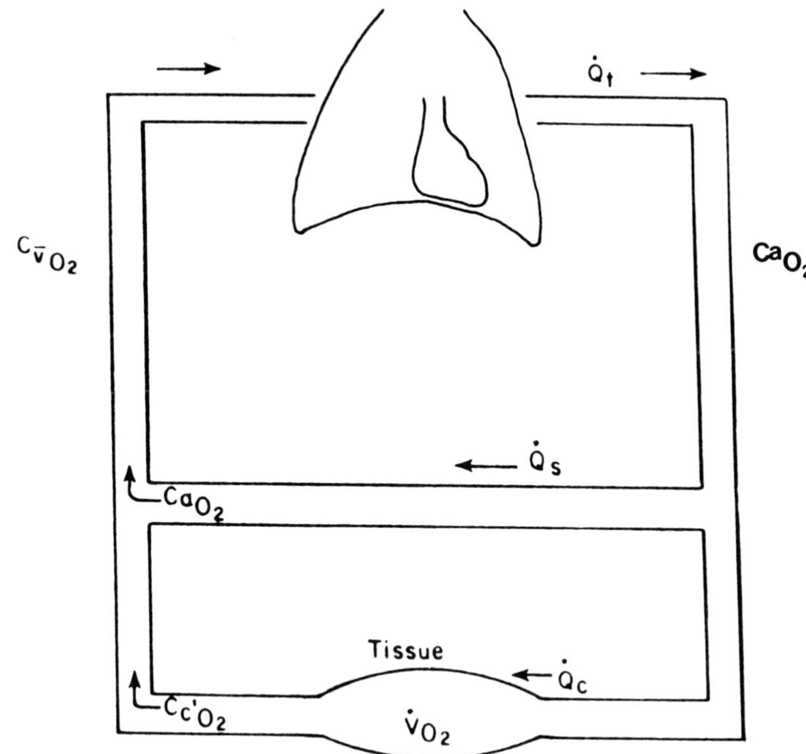


FIG. 5-37. Two-compartment model of the systemic circulation, $\dot{Q}_t$, cardiac output; $\dot{Q}_s$, blood flow shunted from arterial to venous circulation; $\dot{Q}_c$, tissue capillary blood flow; $Cao_2$, arterial oxygen content; $C\bar{v}o_2$, mixed venous oxygen content; $Cc'o_2$, oxygen content of blood leaving nutrient capillaries. As all $\dot{V}o_2$ occurs in tissues perfused by nutrient capillaries ($\dot{Q}_c$), blood leaving the shunt compartment ($\dot{Q}_s$) has the composition of systemic arterial blood. (From Miller[214] with permission.)

occurs in the tissues, the arterial blood that is shunted away from nutrient capillaries to the systemic venous circulation will be unavailable for overall $\dot{V}o_2$. Even when cardiac indices are 50% of normal and profound lactic acidosis is present, extraction ratios of only 42% have been noted ($S\bar{v}o_2$ of approximately 58%).[164] It is probable that within the confines of aerobic metabolism, maximal extraction ratios of 66 to 70% ($S\bar{v}o_2$ of approximately 32%) are possible.[160,287,288,383] Thus, during hypoperfusion and systemic arteriovenous shunting, arterialized blood may be present in the mixed venous effluent, spuriously increasing the $S\bar{v}o_2$. This, of course, results in an underestimation of actual $O_2$ extraction ratios in those capillary beds that are perfused. Recently, however, Schlichtig et al.[280] have reported sustained $S\bar{v}o_2$ values in the 22 to 26% range in three patients with chronic low cardiac output syndromes. These episodes were associated with extraction ratios of 70 to 80%, normal $\dot{V}o_2$ indices, and no signs of clinical decompensation. The mechanisms explaining these phenomena and other nuances of $S\bar{v}o_2$ are discussed in their review.

As $\dot{Q}_t \times Cao_2$ represents systemic oxygen delivery to tissues, $\dot{Q}_t \times C\bar{v}o_2$ accurately represents the oxygen transported from the capillary beds to the right heart if no arteriovenous shunting, maldistribution, or abnormal utilization is present. However, as discussed, in severe hemorrhagic shock, as in ARDS[68,245] and sepsis,[8] maldistribution and abnormal $O_2$ utilization are present and may seriously affect the proper interpretation of $C\bar{v}o_2$ and, hence, $S\bar{v}o_2$.[67,296]

Algebraically,

If

$$\dot{Q}_t \times C\bar{v}o_2 = (\dot{Q}_c \times Cc'o_2) + (\dot{Q}_s \times Cao_2)$$

where

$$\dot{Q}_s = \text{shunt flow}$$

$$\dot{Q}_c = \text{nutrient capillary flow}$$

$$Cc'o_2 = \text{tissue end-capillary oxygen content,}$$

then

$$C\bar{v}o_2 = \frac{(\dot{Q}_c \times Cc'o_2) + (\dot{Q}_s \times Cao_2)}{\dot{Q}_t}$$

and

$$S\bar{v}o_2 \propto \frac{(\dot{Q}_c \times Cc'o_2) + (\dot{Q}_s \times Cao_2)}{\dot{Q}_t}$$

Hence, in hemorrhagic shock, where $\dot{Q}_s \times Cao_2$ ($\dot{D}o_2$ through the shunt) increases, $S\bar{v}o_2$ may be higher than predicted in the face of a critically reduced cardiac output and diminished $\dot{V}o_2$.[166,296] In a broader sense, in the presence of gross hypovolemic shock, a minimally reduced or normal $S\bar{v}o_2$ implies shunting, poor oxygen utilization, tissue anaerobiosis, and lactic acidosis[166] (Fig 5-34, patient 4).

To summarize, if $\dot{Q}_t$ is severely maldistributed within and between organs in patients with hemorrhagic shock, oxygen supply to a particular nonvital organ may be insufficient to meet its demand. Vital tissues receive a relatively abundant flow through redistribution and extract greater amounts of oxygen. Nonvital tissues with poor nutrient capillary blood flow then exhibit lactic acidosis, shunting, and inappropriately high $Svo_2$, while the venous effluents of vital organs with adequate nutrient capillary flow have $Svo_2$ and $Cvo_2$ values appropriately lower than normal. Thus, $S\bar{v}o_2$ does not always represent a constant proportion, flow-weighted mean of different tissues, contributing to the total venous drainage[68,235] (see Table 5-3); rather, it may reflect only adequately perfused, high oxygen-extracting, vital organ tissues plus shunt flow from nonvital, low oxygen-extracting organs and tissues.[164,214] In these instances, metabolic acidosis with elevated lactate levels may confirm the existence of overall inadequate tissue oxygenation and anaerobiosis.[8,167,179]

## LACTIC ACIDOSIS

The complex metabolic changes that follow trauma include dramatic rises in blood lactate.[384] In some instances, lactic acid level and base deficit correlate directly with the degree of injury[240] and mortality.[61,71,109,167,219] It must be appreciated, however, that elevated serum lactic acid may be caused by increased synthesis of lactate in anaerobic glycolysis and also by its decreased metabolism by the liver. The interpretation of elevated lactic acid, therefore, is not necessarily unequivocal.[2] Perhaps more important than serum lactic acid level is the lactate/pyruvate ratio which clearly shows anaerobiosis when its value exceeds 10/1.[150] Allen et al[2] have shown that elevated lactic acid and pyruvate levels with a normal lactate/pyruvate ratio are not associated with anaerobiosis. Thus, caution is advised when instituting therapy based upon isolated serum lactate determinations.

Regardless of the mechanism of lactic acidemia, both Waxman et al[380] and Vincent et al[370] found regular decreases in serum lactate levels during resuscitation. Furthermore, a direct correlation between increased lactate and decreased $\dot{V}O_2$ has been found during anesthesia and surgery.[380] Serum lactate elevation does not correlate with decreased MAP or CI, but only with reduction in $\dot{V}O_2$ (Fig 5-38). In addition, postoperative lactic acidosis is directly proportional to the calculated intraoperative oxygen deficit (Fig 5-39). Lactic acidosis caused by hemorrhagic shock is best treated by enhancement of oxygen delivery[109] via infusion of acellular fluids and blood.

It has been shown experimentally that administration of sodium bicarbonate in the face of hemorrhagic shock results in no significant increase in pH or serum bicarbonate, or improvement of hemodynamic parameters or respiratory gases.[152] Controlled, prospective clinical studies in patients with stable but severe congestive heart failure and in other critically ill patients with lactic acidosis demonstrate no apparent benefit from sodium bicarbonate administration.[22a,60b] Administration of sodium bicarbonate to patients with metabolic acidosis due to excess lactate results in impaired arterial oxygenation, decreased or unchanged systemic $\dot{D}O_2$ and $\dot{V}O_2$, and decreased $M\dot{V}O_2$ with unchanged myocardial oxygen demand.[22a] Moreover, sodium bicarbonate appears to decrease serum ionized calcium and increase $PaCO_2$.[60b] Normalization of arterial pH by sodium bicarbonate infusion does not appear to improve the cardiovascular response to infused catecholamines as purported. Any transient increase in $\dot{Q}_t$ observed with sodium bicarbonate administration is probably due to increased preload from translocation of extravascular fluid in response to the infused hyperosmolar sodium load and not to enhanced intrinsic cardiac performance from normalization of pH. Despite these observations, the use of bicarbonate until

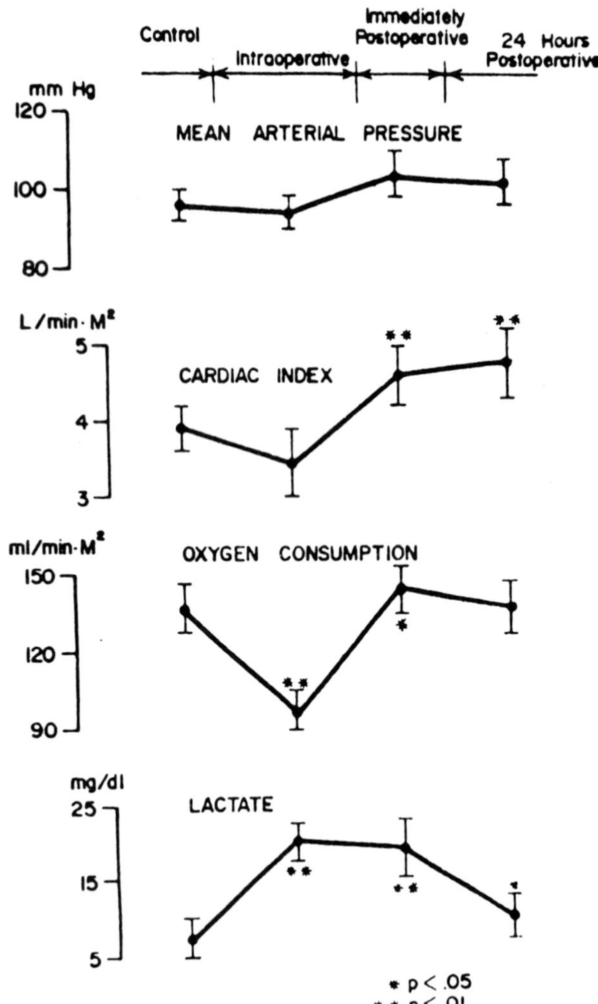


FIG. 5-38. Elevated lactate levels and decreased oxygen consumption during anesthesia and surgery. Note that regardless of maintenance of cardiac index (CI) and mean arterial pressure (MAP), serum lactate levels rise with decreasing $\dot{V}O_2$ and return to baseline values when $\dot{V}O_2$ returns to control levels. (From Waxman et al[380] with permission.)

recently was still advocated whenever arterial pH decreased below 7.20 or the bicarbonate level below 10 to 12 mEq/L.[219] It must be emphasized that on balance, bicarbonate therapy has not been shown to enhance survival in lactic acidosis associated with tissue hypoxia. Other drug therapies are currently under investigation.[22]

## NONINVASIVE MONITORING OF TISSUE OXYGENATION

### *Transcutaneous Oxygen Tension*

Ideally monitoring of critically ill patients should include assessment of the quantity of oxygen delivered directly to the tissues. The ultimate purpose of fluid infusion and blood transfusion is restoration and maintenance of global tissue oxygenation. Teleologically, the skin and other nonvital tis-

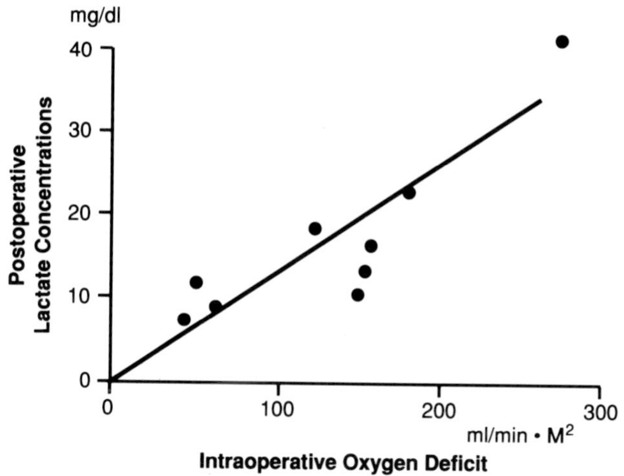


FIG. 5-39. Postoperative arterial blood lactate levels plotted against corresponding intraoperative $\dot{V}o_2$ deficits. Note the strong positive correlation between these two variables (r = 0.83). (From Waxman[380] with permission.)

sues are secondary or perhaps tertiary organs in the biologic hierarchy of preferential blood flow distribution.[335,383] This is especially true in the hemorrhagic shock syndrome, in which perfusion of the heart and brain is well maintained after other tissues have been rendered ischemic.[330,331] Consequently, adverse changes in oxygen delivery to the skin may be an early warning to the clinician that additions to or alterations of therapy are required.[356]

Transcutaneous oxygen tension ($Ptco_2$) monitoring involves placement of a heated Clark polarographic electrode to the skin. The effects of heating the skin are as follows.[360]

1. Heating the stratum corneum beyond 40°C changes its structure, which permits more rapid diffusion of $O_2$.
2. Heating the dermal capillary blood increases local $O_2$ tension by shifting the oxyhemoglobin dissociation curve to the right.
3. Heat causes dermal capillary hyperemia, which arterializes capillary blood.

To obtain measurable $Ptco_2$ values from the skin, the skin sensor must be heated to between 43 and 45°C.

Since its first clinical use, the proper interpretation of derived $Ptco_2$ values has been shrouded in confusion and misunderstanding.[6,13,325,356,361] Upon its application to neonatal monitoring it was noted that $Ptco_2$ was equal or nearly equal to $Pao_2$.[147] However, in critically ill, hemodynamically unstable neonates, $Ptco_2$ and $Pao_2$ values showed great divergence. This led some neonatologists to conclude that since $Ptco_2$ did not always equal $Pao_2$, the technology was unreliable.[369]

Ironically, the poor correlation between $Ptco_2$ and $Pao_2$ during hemodynamic instability is a strength of the technique.[325,356] Simply stated, $Ptco_2$ tracks oxygen delivery to the skin.[234,345,359,360,363] For instance, the observations shown in Fig 5-40 were made when thermodilution cardiac output, $Ptco_2$, and $Pao_2$ were monitored in anesthetized dogs.[363] During induction and maintenance of arterial hypoxemia, $Ptco_2$ tracked $Pao_2$ and $\dot{D}o_2$. When hypovolemic shock was produced, $Ptco_2$ tracked both $\dot{Q}_t$ and $\dot{D}o_2$ but not $Pao_2$. In summary, $Ptco_2$ tracks the components of oxygen delivery, $\dot{Q}_t$ and $Cao_2$. $Ptco_2$ tracks $Pao_2$ only when $\dot{Q}_t$ and [Hb] remain stable.[131] Thus, since $Ptco_2$ closely follows changes in $\dot{D}o_2$, its value as a sensitive indicator of tissue perfusion in hypovolemic shock is obvious.[13,261,356]

Clinically, $Ptco_2$ values in adults are always lower than $Pao_2$, even during optimal levels of oxygen delivery.[346,360] This is to be expected since $O_2$ transport is a first-order rate reaction, and thus a diffusion gradient must exist from arterialized capillary blood through the skin to the oxygen sensor. During periods of hemodynamic stability (CI > 2.2 L/min/m$^2$ and normal $Cao_2$), $Ptco_2$ values approximate 80% of $Pao_2$ (range = 79 ± 12%). In these circumstances $Ptco_2$ tracks $Pao_2$[131,254] (Fig 5-41). This relationship of $Ptco_2$ to $Pao_2$ is known as the transcutaneous oxygen tension index.

FIG. 5-40. Relation of $Pao_2$, cardiac output, and $O_2$ delivery with $Ptco_2$. Note that during induction and maintenance of arterial hypoxemia, $Ptco_2$ tracks $Pao_2$ and $\dot{D}o_2$ but not $\dot{Q}_t$. During hemorrhagic shock, $Ptco_2$ tracks $\dot{Q}_t$ and $\dot{D}o_2$ but not $Pao_2$. Thus, $Ptco_2$ tracks oxygen delivery to skin, per se, and not its components: $\dot{Q}_t$ and $Cao_2$. (From Tremper et al[363] with permission.)

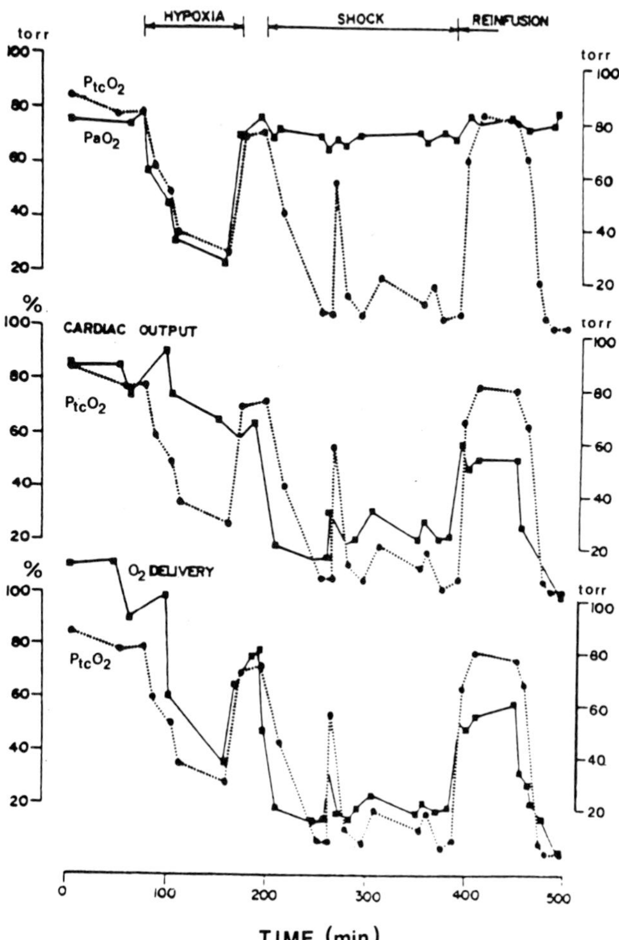

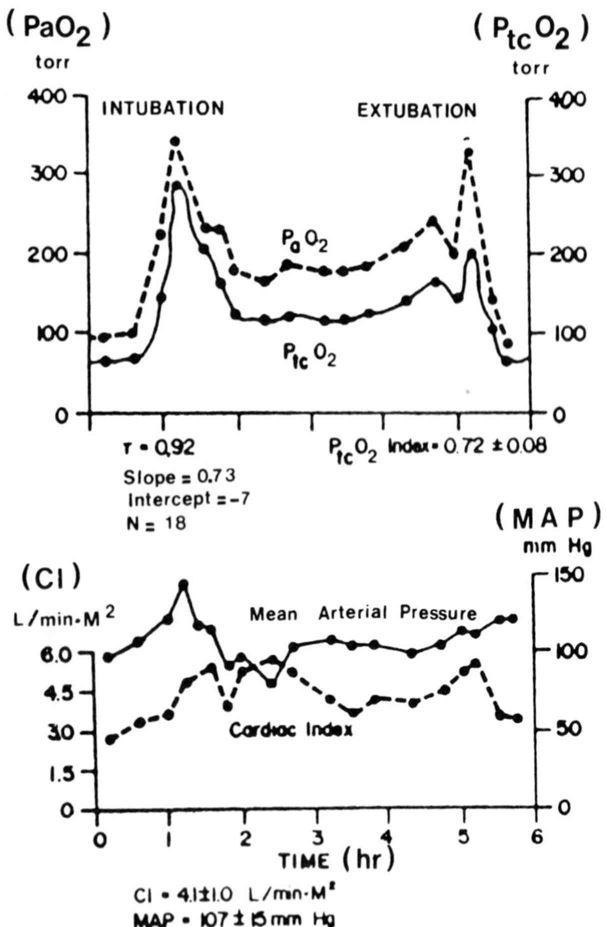


FIG. 5-41. Transcutaneous oxygen tension (Ptco$_2$) and Ptco$_2$ index during hemodynamic stability. Note that Ptco$_2$ tracks Pao$_2$ (r = 0.92); the Ptco$_2$ index = 72 ± 8%. (From Tremper and Shoemaker[360] with permission.)

$$\text{Ptco}_2 \text{ index} = \frac{\text{Ptco}_2}{\text{Pao}_2}^{13,360}$$

When there is a moderate degree of low-flow shock (CI > 1.5 L/min/m$^2$ but < 2.2 L/min/m$^2$), Ptco$_2$ still tracks Pao$_2$, but the Ptco$_2$ index is reduced to 50% (48 ± 7%) (Fig 5-42). Severe low-flow shock (CI < 1.5 L/min/m$^2$) is characterized by a gross divergence of Ptco$_2$ and Pao$_2$ values, with a resulting Ptco$_2$ index of only 12% (12 ± 12%). The Ptco$_2$ index in severe shock correlates closely with the cardiac index (Fig 5-43).

If one refers to the idealized formula for oxygen delivery through the microcirculation,

$$\text{Do}_{2\text{skin}} = (\dot{Q}_c \times \text{Cc}'\text{o}_2) + (\dot{Q}_s \times \text{Cao}_2), \text{ or}$$

$$\text{Do}_{2\text{skin}} = \frac{\Delta P \pi r^4}{81\eta} \times \text{Cc}'\text{o}_2 + (\text{shunt flow}),$$

it is easy to comprehend how a reduction in metarteriolar and precapillary sphincter radius (r) will affect Do$_2$ to the skin; it

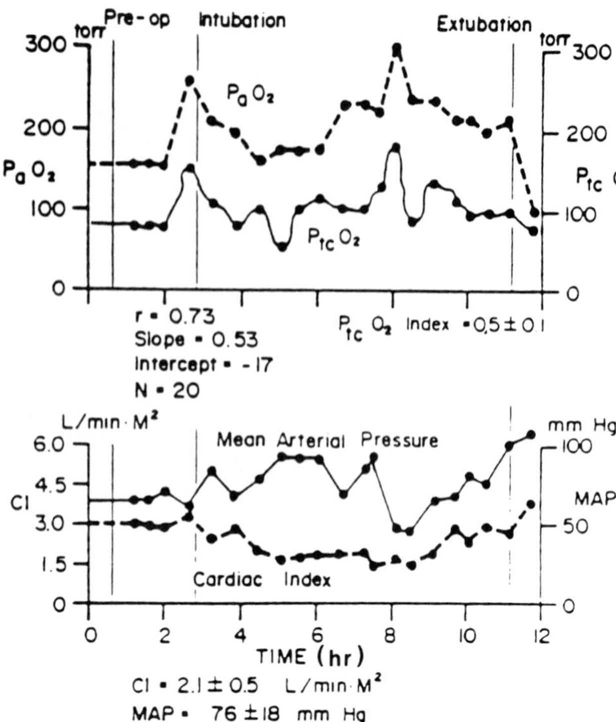


FIG. 5-42. Ptco$_2$ and Ptco$_2$ index in moderate low-flow shock. Note that Ptco$_2$ tracks Pao$_2$ (r = 0.73), but the Ptco$_2$ index is only 50 ± 10%. (From Tremper and Shoemaker[360] with permission.)

FIG. 5-43. Ptco$_2$ and Ptco$_2$ index in severe low-flow shock. Note the gross disparity between Pao$_2$ and Ptco$_2$ (Ptco$_2$ index = 8 ± 11%). However, the correlation between cardiac index and the Ptco$_2$ index is excellent (r = 0.90). (From Tremper and Shoemaker[360] with permission.)

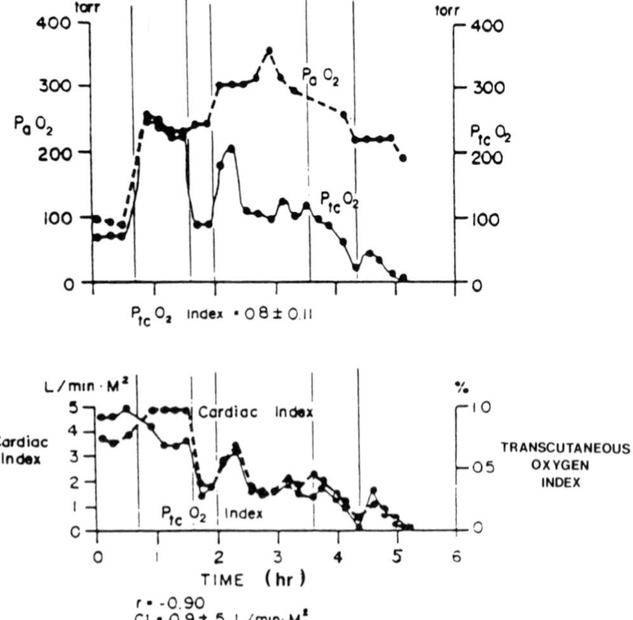

will fall. Likewise, reduction in flow velocity (shear rate) in the capillary circulation by vasoconstriction together with aggregation of blood cells increases viscosity ($\eta$). These hemorheologic abnormalities further reduce oxygen delivery to the dermal capillaries. The disparity between $P_{tcO_2}$ and $P_{aO_2}$ as low-flow shock evolves may thus be explained by functional and anatomic systemic arteriovenous shunting. Thus, as skin oxygen delivery decreases, $P_{tcO_2}$ and $P_{tcO_2}$ index fall.[13,360]

The technique of $P_{tcO_2}$ monitoring is relatively simple. After calibrating the Clark oxygen sensor, the skin is prepared with alcohol, and the electrode is placed on the skin. Following a short period of equilibration, the transcutaneous $O_2$ tension value is obtained. Baseline arterial blood gases are then drawn, and the initial value of $P_{tcO_2}$ is compared with the $P_{aO_2}$.

Interpretation of the data is the key to understanding the technology. The following examples are offered to familiarize the reader with this aspect of $P_{tcO_2}$.

EXAMPLE 1 *Derived Values.* $F_{IO_2} = 0.5$. If $P_{aO_2} = 300$ mm Hg and $P_{tcO_2} = 240$ mm Hg, then the $P_{tcO_2}$ index = 0.8.

*Interpretation.* The patient is hemodynamically stable, and oxygen delivery is adequate (ie, $\dot{D}O_2$ is within normal limits).

*Therapy.* None needed.

EXAMPLE 2. $F_{IO_2} = 0.5$. If $P_{aO_2} = 300$ mm Hg and $P_{tcO_2} = 150$ mm Hg, then the $P_{tcO_2}$ index = 0.5.

*Interpretation.* Moderate low-flow shock.

*Evaluation.*

1. Volume status.
2. Cardiac performance.

*Therapy.*

1. Crystalloids, colloids, and blood if the patient is hypovolemic.
2. Inotropic support and/or afterload reduction if necessary.

EXAMPLE 3. $F_{IO_2} = 0.5$. If $P_{aO_2} = 300$ mm Hg and $P_{tcO_2} = 40$ mm Hg, then the $P_{tcO_2}$ index = 0.13.

*Interpretation.* Severe low-flow shock.

*Evaluation.* Same as in Example 2.

*Therapy.* Same as in Example 2, but more aggressive.

EXAMPLE 4.[131,356] $F_{IO_2} = 0.5$. If $P_{aO_2} = 60$ mm Hg and $P_{tcO_2} = 50$ mm Hg, then the $P_{tcO_2}$ index = 0.83.

*Interpretation.*

1. Cardiac output adequate.
2. Arterial hypoxemia present.

*Evaluation.*

1. Assess adequacy of $F_{IO_2}$, alveolar ventilation.
2. If these are adequate, evaluate ventilatory apparatus for malfunction or kinking of tubing.
3. If 1 and 2 are ruled out, assess the reason for grossly abnormal intrapulmonary shunt, including endobronchial intubation, pneumothorax, excessive vasodilator therapy.[362]

*Therapy.* Correction of above parameters to increase $P_{aO_2}$.

In summary, transcutaneous oxygen monitoring measures oxygenation of the skin as a function of oxygen delivery ($\dot{D}O_2$).[1,356] Perturbations in oxygen delivery will thus be reflected in the $P_{tcO_2}$ index.[13] This technology does not replace measurement of flow and cardiac performance; it complements them.[81,356] If a stable clinical situation deteriorates, continuous $P_{tcO_2}$ monitoring will detect downward trends in $\dot{D}O_2$.[1,13,81,172,275] Logically, therapeutic interventions that improve oxygen delivery will be reflected as improvement in $P_{tcO_2}$ and its index. The severity of the clinical situation will then dictate the necessity for quantitative invasive cardiorespiratory monitoring. $P_{tcO_2}$, however, may also be affected by local vasoconstriction, for instance, that caused by hypothermia, without changes in central hemodynamics. This should be excluded before initiating therapy.

### *Pulse Oximetry Versus Transcutaneous Oxygen Monitoring: A Comparison*

Both pulse oximetry and $P_{tcO_2}$ measure cardiorespiratory variables, but this is the only similarity between them. Arterial oxygen saturation is an independent component of $C_{aO_2}$, and thus, $\dot{D}O_2$. Specifically, a decrease in hemoglobin concentration or cardiac output which causes a reduction in $\dot{D}O_2$ may not change $S_{aO_2}$. In hemorrhagic shock, intrapulmonary shunt decreases due to decreased perfusion of the dependent portions of the lungs. If $V_A$ is adequate and $F_{IO_2}$ increased with supplemental oxygen, even profound reductions in $S_{\bar{v}O_2}$ do not usually reduce $S_{aO_2}$ to dangerously low levels unless thoracic trauma or insult to the upper airway has occurred[166] (Table 5-9). Hence, using $S_{aO_2}$, as interpreted by pulse oximetry, to judge the adequacy of $\dot{D}O_2$ is misleading and inappropriate.[13] Moreover, because of the shape of the oxyhemoglobin dissociation curve, arterial saturation of 100% implies only that all the hemoglobin present is fully saturated. Thus, a hypovolemic patient with reduced cardiac output, arterial oxygen content, and $\dot{D}O_2$ may still have $S_{aO_2} = 100\%$ (see Table 5-9).

Despite its technical and theoretical limitations, pulse oximetry is a mandatory adjunct to patient care. Its most valuable attribute is in the detection of downward trends in $S_{aO_2}$.[352] Any reduction in $S_{aO_2}$ should alert the anesthesiologist that $F_{IO_2}$ and/or $V_A$ may be inadequate or that total intrapulmonary shunt has increased. Proper diagnosis of the offending variables will lead to rational therapy and improvement of $S_{aO_2}$.[36]

As discussed, transcutaneous oxygen ($P_{tcO_2}$) monitoring provides information about the overall adequacy of oxygen delivery. Periodic arterial blood gas determinations allow calculation of the $Ptco_2$ index which enables the physician to differentiate between perturbations of blood flow, ventilation, or both. Therapeutic intervention targeted at improvement of oxygen delivery will be reflected as augmentation of $Ptco_2$ and its index if $\dot{Q}_t$ is inadequate, or by increased $Ptco_2$ and $Pao_2$, if flow is adequate but hypoxemia is present. Thus, monitoring of $Ptco_2$, in conjunction with intermittent $Pao_2$ analysis, gives both quantitative and qualitative information regarding oxygen transport. On the other hand, $Ptco_2$ monitoring is not as easy to use as pulse oximetry. It requires calibration of the instrument, warm-up time, electrode and skin preparation, and periodic changing of sensor sites to prevent skin burns. The sensor frequently becomes displaced, leading to erroneous information.[261] As a consequence, this monitoring technique has not been used widely in adult clinical practice.

## CONCLUSIONS

In the context of trauma it serves us well to remember that the ultimate goal of therapy is to restore and maintain an adequate intracellular partial pressure of oxygen in all tissues.[60a,230] Insufficiency of aerobic respiration causes anaerobiosis—an inefficient short-term solution to cellular survival. This is especially true for the brain and heart. Therapeutic optimization of aerobic metabolism involves manipulation and modulation of those cardiorespiratory variables comprising systemic oxygen transport ($\dot{D}o_2$).[245] Failure to improve $\dot{D}o_2$ rapidly when it is near the critical level will inevitably lead to irreversible shock. Stated differently, sustained levels of oxygen transport below critical levels of $\dot{D}o_2$ will lead to hypoxic dysoxia (regional then global) that manifests itself as an inability to maintain or reestablish adequate levels of oxygen consumption ($\dot{V}o_2$) for basic cellular demands.[68,117,230,245,280,285,291,306]

As emphasized in this chapter, basal, steady-state ("normal") values of $\dot{D}o_2$ and $\dot{V}o_2$ are not appropriate therapeutic goals in the critically ill patient. The augmented metabolic $O_2$ demands in severe illness mandates higher levels of $\dot{D}o_2$ to subserve $\dot{V}o_2$. Thus, the critical $\dot{D}o_2$ of otherwise unperturbed individuals under anesthesia, reported by Shibutani et al[306] as 330 mL/min/$m^2$, may be inappropriately low in the face of trauma and hemorrhagic shock. Likewise, the hypermetabolic $O_2$ demands of the postoperative period require higher than basal values of $\dot{D}o_2$ to support the required $\dot{V}o_2$ in excess of 170 mL/min/$m^2$. With the exceptions of sepsis and severe ARDS, or when $\dot{V}o_2$ becomes supply ($\dot{D}o_2$) dependent, the overall adequacy of global tissue oxygenation may be reasonably assessed by the $O_2$ extraction (demand-supply) ratio, $\dot{V}o_2/\dot{D}o_2 = Cao_2 - C\bar{v}o_2/Cao_2$.[285] With the stipulations discussed in the text, $S\bar{v}o_2$ analysis yields similar information.[228]

Clinically, oxygen transport is therapeutically optimized by assessing the adequacy of $\dot{Q}_t$, $Sao_2$, and [Hb]. Insufficient levels of one or more of these variables will inevitably lead to regional or global tissue hypoxia. Major trauma usually produces derangement of one or more of the components of $\dot{D}o_2$. Treatment, therefore, depends primarily upon identification of deficiencies: contracted blood volume, suboptimal cardiac contractility, pulmonary insufficiency, or inadequate red cell mass. Specific therapy thus involves acellular fluid infusion, inotropic therapy, restoration of ventilatory parameters, and appropriate transfusion.

Volume replacement should be guided initially by monitoring of MAP, pulse rate, CVP, urine flow, and $Sao_2$. Restoration of these values to acceptable levels implies gross cardiorespiratory compensation. In the young, healthy individual requiring minimal surgical intervention, optimization of these physiologic parameters will usually suffice. It must be reemphasized, however, that large deficits in blood volume, $\dot{Q}_t$, $\dot{D}o_2$, and $\dot{V}o_2$ may coexist with normal values of MAP, CVP, heart rate, $Sao_2$, and even PAOP. With certain limitations, noninvasive assessment of the oxygen transport system may be made through employment of $Ptco_2$ monitoring, pulse oximetry, and possibly noninvasive cardiac output measurement.[21,73] In conjunction with intermittent sampling of [Hb] and $S_{RA}o_2$, quasi-quantitative measurements of $\dot{D}o_2$, $\dot{V}o_2$, and their directional changes may be derived. In the critically injured trauma victim who has sustained profound and/or prolonged periods of oxygen deprivation, invasively derived cardiorespiratory measurements are indicated. Quantitative, frequently repeated measurement of $\dot{Q}_t$, [Hb], and $Sao_2$ in conjunction with continuous monitoring of $S\bar{v}o_2$ permits calculation of $\dot{V}o_2$, $\dot{D}o_2$, and the oxygen extraction ratio. These complex variables should be optimized to achieve the end point of therapy: survival. In the future, magnetic resonance spectroscopy and positron emission tomography may be available for clinical assessment of tissue hypoxia. For now, the techniques and concepts discussed, although flawed, will have to suffice.[117]

## REFERENCES


1. Abraham E, Smith M, Silver L. Continuous monitoring of critically ill patients with transcutaneous oxygen and carbon dioxide and conjunctival oxygen sensors. Ann Emerg Med 1984;13:1021.
2. Allen SHG, Rahm R, Shah DM. Metabolic alterations in trauma: lactate and pyruvate levels after aortic surgery. Circ Shock 1983;11:13.
3. Altura BM. Endothelium, reticuloendothelial cells and microvascular integrity: roles in host defense. In: Altura BM, Lefer AM, Shumer W, eds. Handbook of shock and trauma: basic science. New York: Raven Press, 1983;1:51.
4. Alyono D, Ring WS, Anderson RY. The effects of hemorrhagic shock on the diastolic properties of the left ventricle in the conscious dog. Surgery 1978;83:691.
5. Alyono D, Ring WS, Chao RY. Characteristics of ventricular function in severe hemorrhagic shock. Surgery 1983;94:250.
6. Andriano KP, Pace NL, Wiebrink J, et al. Intraoperative transcutaneous $Po_2$ ($TcPo_2$) monitoring quantitates $Pao_2$: fact or fiction? Anesth Analg 1984;63:178.
7. Archie JP, Mertz WR. Myocardial oxygen delivery after experimental hemorrhagic shock. Ann Surg 1978;187:205.
8. Astiz ME, Rackow EC, Kaufman B, et al. Relationship of oxygen delivery and mixed venous oxygenation to lactic acidosis in patients with sepsis and acute myocardial infarction. Crit Care Med 1988;16:655.
9. Baele PL, McMichan JC, Marsh HM, et al. Continuous monitoring of mixed venous oxygen saturation in critically ill patients. Anesth Analg 1982;61:513.
10. Baele PL, McMichan JC, Marsh HM, et al. Continuous moni-

toring of mixed venous saturation in critically ill patients. Anesthesiology 1981;55:A113.
11. Baim DS, Rothman MT, Harrison DC. Simultaneous measurement of coronary venous blood flow and oxygen saturation during transient alterations in myocardial oxygen supply and demand. Am J Cardiol 1982;49:743.
12. Barcroft J. On anoxaemia. Lancet 1920;2:485.
13. Barker SJ, Tremper KK. Transcutaneous oxygen tension: a physiologic variable for monitoring oxygenation. J Clin Monit 1985;1:130.
14. Barker SJ, Tremper KK, Hufstedler S, et al. The effects of carbon monoxide inhalation on noninvasive oxygen monitoring. Anesth Analg 1986;65:S12.
15. Barker SJ, Tremper KK, Hyatt J. Effects of methemoglobinemia on pulse oximetry and mixed venous oximetry. Anesthesiology 1989;70:112.
16. Barnes A. The blood bank in hemotherapy for trauma and surgery. In: Barnes A, ed. Hemotherapy in trauma and surgery. Washington DC: American Association of Blood Banks, 1979:77.
17. Barriot P, Riou B. Hemorrhagic shock with paradoxical bradycardia. Intensive Care Med 1987;13:203.
18. Beaupre PN, Cahalan MK, Kremer PF, et al. Does pulmonary artery occlusion pressure adequately reflect left ventricular filling during anesthesia and surgery? Anesthesiology 1983;59:A3.
19. Bendixen H, Laver M. Hypoxia in anesthesia: a review. Clin Pharmacol Ther 1965;6:510.
20. Benumof JL. Respiratory physiology and respiratory function during anesthesia. In: Miller RD, ed. Anesthesia. 2nd ed. New York: Churchill Livingstone, 1986;2:1115.
21. Bernstein DP. Noninvasive cardiac output measurement. In: Shoemaker WC, Ayres S, Grenvik A, Thompson WL, Holbrook PR, eds. Textbook of critical care. Philadelphia: WB Saunders, 1989:159.
22. Bersin RM, Arieff AI. Recent advances in the therapy of lactic acidosis. Intensive Care World 1987;4:128.
22a. Bersin RM, Chatterjee K, Arieff AI. Metabolic and hemodynamic consequences of sodium bicarbonate administration in patients with heart disease. Am J Med 1989;87:7.
23. Birman H, Hag A, Hew E, et al. Continuous monitoring of mixed venous oxygen saturation in hemodynamically unstable patients. Chest 1984;86:753.
24. Biro GP. Anaemia and haemodilution. In: Prys-Roberts C, ed. The circulation in anaesthesia: applied physiology and pharmacology. 1st ed. Oxford: Blackwell, 1980:327.
25. Bland RD, Shoemaker WC. Probability of survival as a prognostic and severity of illness score in critically ill surgical patients. Crit Care Med 1985;13:91.
26. Bland RD, Shoemaker WC, Abraham E, et al. Hemodynamics and oxygen transport patterns in surviving and nonsurviving postoperative patients. Crit Care Med 1985;13:85.
27. Bland R, Shoemaker WC, Shabot MM. Physiologic monitoring goals for the critically ill patient. Surg Gynecol Obstet 1978;147:833.
28. Bodin L, Rouby JJ, Mezzaroba P, et al. An evaluation of two mixed venous saturation catheters in patients with circulatory shock and respiratory failure. Anesthesiology 1988;69:A190.
29. Bogetz NS, Weiskopf RB. Cardiovascular effects of volatile anesthetics during hypovolemia. Anesthesiology 1984;61:A51.
30. Bond RF, Manning ES, Gonzalez NM, et al. Myocardial and skeletal muscle responses to hemorrhage and shock during alpha-adrenergic blockage. Am J Physiol 1973;225:247.
31. Bowe EA, Klein EF. Pulmonary contusion. Semin Anesth 1985;4:145.
32. Brazier JN, Cooper N, Buckberg GD. The adequacy of subendocardial oxygen delivery: the interaction of determinants of flow, arterial oxygen content and myocardial oxygen need. Circulation 1974;49:968.
33. Brazier J, Cooper N, Maloney JV, et al. The adequacy of myocardial oxygen delivery in acute normovolemic anemia. Surgery 1974;75:508.
34. Brismar B, Hedenstierna G, Lundh R, Tokics L. Oxygen uptake, plasma catecholamines and cardiac output during neurolept-nitrous oxide and halothane anesthesias. Acta Anaesthesiol Scand 1982;26:541.
35. Brodsky JB, Shulman MS, Swan M, et al. Pulse oximetry during one lung anesthesia. Anesthesiology 1985;63:212.
36. Brooks TD, Gravenstein N. Pulse oximetry for early detection of hypoxemia in anesthetized infants. J Clin Monit 1985;1:135.
37. Bruns FJ, Fraley DS, Haigh J, et al. Control of organ blood flow. In: Snyder JV, Pinsky MR, eds. Oxygen transport in the critically ill. Chicago: Year Book, 1987:87.
38. Bryan-Brown CW. Blood flow to organs: parameters for function and survival in critical illness. Crit Care Med 1988;16:170.
39. Bryan-Brown CW. Overview of chapters and presentations. In: Bryan-Brown CW, Ayres SM, eds. Oxygen transport and utilization. Fullerton: Society of Critical Care Medicine, 1987:327.
40. Bryan-Brown CW. Tissue blood flow and oxygen transport in critically ill patients. Crit Care Med 1975;3:103.
41. Bryan-Brown CW, Baek SM, Makabali G, et al. Consumable oxygen: availability of oxygen in relation to oxyhemoglobin dissociation. Crit Care Med 1973;1:17.
42. Bryan-Brown CW, Gutierrez G. Gas transport and delivery. In: Shoemaker WC, Ayres S, Grenvik A, Thompson WL, Holbrook PR, eds. Textbook of critical care. 2nd ed. Philadelphia: WB Saunders, 1989:491.
43. Buran MJ. Oxygen consumption. In: Snyder JV, Pinsky MR, eds. Oxygen transport in the critically ill. Chicago: Year Book, 1987:16.
44. Cain SM. Appearance of excess lactate in anesthetized dogs during anemic and hypoxic hypoxia. Am J Physiol 1965; 209:604.
45. Cain SM. Peripheral oxygen uptake and delivery in health and disease. Clin Chest Med 1983;4:139.
46. Cain SM. Supply dependency of oxygen uptake in ARDS: myth or reality. Am J Med Sci 1984;288:119.
47. Calvin E, Drieger AA, Sibbald WJ. Does the pulmonary capillary wedge pressure predict left ventricular preload in critically ill patients? Crit Care Med 1981;9:437.
48. Carrico CJ, Maier RV. Balanced salt solutions in massive trauma. In: Brown BR, ed. Fluid and blood therapy in anesthesia: contemporary anesthesia practice. Philadelphia: FA Davis, 1983:57.
49. Chien S. Biophysical behavior of red cells in suspensions. In: Surgenor DM, ed. The red blood cell. 2nd ed. New York: Academic Press, 1975;2:1031.
50. Chien S. Hemorheology in clinical medicine. Clin Hemorheol 1982;2:137.
51. Chien S. Role of blood cells in microcirculatory regulation. Microvasc Res 1985;29:129.
52. Chien S, Lipowsky HH. Correlation of hemodynamics in macrocirculation and microcirculation. Int J Microcirc Clin Exp 1982;1:351.
53. Civetta JM. Invasive catheterization. In: Shoemaker WC, ed. Critical care: state of the art. Fullerton: Society of Critical Care Medicine, 1980;1:B.
54. Clark TN, Foex P, Roberts JG, et al. Circulatory responses of the dog to acute isovolemic anemia in the presence of high grade adrenergic beta-receptor blockade. Br J Anaesth 1980;52:337.
55. Coetzee A, Holland D, Foex P, et al. The effect of hypocapnia on coronary blood flow and myocardial function in the dog. Anesth Analg 1984;63:991.

56. Cohen PJ, Alexander SC, Smith TC, et al. Effects of hypoxia and normocarbia on cerebral blood flow and metabolism in conscious man. J Appl Physiol 1967;23:183.
57. Collins JA. Hemorrhage, shock and burns. In: Petz LD, Swisher SN, eds. Clinical practice of blood transfusion. New York: Churchill Livingstone, 1981:425.
58. Collins JA, moderator. Transfusion practices in emergencies. In: Collins JA, Murawski K, Shafer AW, eds. Massive transfusion in surgery and trauma. New York: Alan R Liss, 1982:285.
59. Collins JA, Simmons RL, James PM, et al. Acid-base status of seriously wounded combat casualties, II: resuscitation with stored blood. Ann Surg 1971;173:6.
60. Collins JA, Stechenberg L. The effects of the concentration and function of hemoglobin on the survival of rats after hemorrhage. Surgery 1979;85:412.
60a. Connett RJ, Honig CR, Gayeski TEJ, et al. Defining hypoxia: A system view of $\dot{V}O_2$, glycolysis, energetics and cell $PO_2$. J Appl Physiol 1990;68:833.
60b. Cooper DJ, Walley KR, Wiggs BR, et al. Bicarbonate does not improve hemodynamics in critically ill patients who have lactic acidosis. Ann Intern Med 1990;112:492.
61. Cowley RA, Hankins JR, Jones RT, et al. Pathology and pathophysiology of the liver. In: Cowley RA, Trump BF, eds. Pathophysiology of shock, anoxia and ischemia. Baltimore: Williams and Wilkins, 1982:285.
62. Crystal GJ, Rooney MW, Salem MR. Myocardial blood flow and oxygen consumption during isovolemic hemodilution alone and in combination with adenosine-induced controlled hypotension. Anesth Analg 1988;67:539.
63. Crystal GJ, Salem MR. Myocardial oxygen consumption and segmental shortening during selective coronary hemodilution in dogs. Anesth Analg 1988;67:500.
64. Cullen DJ, Eger EI. The effects of hypoxia and isovolemic anemia on the halothane requirements (MAC) of dogs, I: the effects of hypoxia. Anesthesiology 1970;32:28.
65. Czer LSC, Shoemaker WC. Myocardial performance in critically ill patients: response to whole blood transfusion as a prognostic measure. Crit Care Med 1980;8:710.
66. Czer LSC, Shoemaker WC. Optimal hematocrit value in critically ill postoperative patients. Surg Gynecol Obstet 1978; 147:363.
67. Dahn MS, Lange MP, Jacobs LA. Central mixed and splanchnic venous oxygen saturation monitoring. Intensive Care Med 1988;14:373.
68. Danek SJ, Lynch JP, Weg JG, et al. The dependence of oxygen uptake on oxygen delivery in the adult repiratory distress syndrome. Am Rev Respir Dis 1980;122:387.
69. Dantzker DR. Interpretation of data in the hypoxic patient. In: Bryan-Brown CW, Ayres SM, eds. Oxygen transport and utilization. Fullerton: Society of Critical Care Medicine, 1987:93.
70. Davies GG, Mendenhall J, Symreng T. Measurement of right atrial oxygen saturation by fiberoptic oximetry accurately reflects mixed venous oxygen saturation in swine. J Clin Monit 1988;4:99.
71. Davis JW, Shackford SR, Mackersie RC, et al. Base deficit as a guide to volume resuscitation. J Trauma 1988;28:1464.
72. Divertie MB, McMichan JC. Continuous monitoring of mixed venous oxygen saturation. Chest 1984;85:423.
73. Djordjevich L, Sadove MS, Ivankovich AD. EHD: noninvasive monitoring of cardiac output. Anesthesiology 1981;55:A35.
74. Donald KW, Bishop JM, Cumming G, et al. The effect of nursing positions on the cardiac output of man. Clin Sci 1953;12:199.
75. Dorsch SE, Dorsch JA. Use of oxygen analysers should be mandatory. Anesthesiology 1983;59:161.
76. Douglas ME, Downes JB, Mantini EL, et al. Alterations of oxygen tension and oxyhemoglobin saturation: a hazard of sodium bicarbonate administration. Arch Surg 1979;114:326.
77. Douglas PS, Edmunds LH, St John Sutton M, et al. Unreliability of hemodynamic indexes of left ventricular size during cardiac surgery. Ann Thorac Surg 1987;44:31.
78. Downing SE. The heart in shock. In: Altura BM, Lefer AM, Shumer W, eds. Handbook of shock and trauma: basic science. New York: Raven Press, 1983;1:5.
79. Downing SE, Lee JC. Cardiac function and metabolism following hemorrhage in the newborn lamb. Ann Surg 1976;184:743.
80. Downs JB. Monitoring oxygen delivery in acute respiratory failure. Respir Care 1983;28:608.
81. Dronen SC, Moningas PA, Foutch R. Transcutaneous oxygen tension measurements during gradual hemorrhage and reinfusion. Ann Emerg Med 1985;14:534.
82. Drucker WR, Chadwick CDJ, Jann DS. Transcapillary refill in hemorrhage and shock. Arch Surg 1981;116:1344.
83. Duff JH, Groves AC, McLean LPH, et al. Defective oxygen consumption in septic shock. Surg Gynecol Obstet 1969;128:1051.
84. Duvelleroy MA, Martin JL, Teisseire BP, et al. Abnormal hemoglobin oxygen affinity and coronary circulation. Bibl Haematol 1980;46:70.
85. Ebert JP, Grimes B, Niemann KMW. Respiratory failure secondary to homologous blood transfusion. Anesthesiology 1985; 63:104.
86. Edwards JD, Redmond AD, Nightingale P, et al. Oxygen consumption following trauma: a reappraisal in severely injured patients requiring mechanical ventilation. Br J Surg 1988;75:690.
87. Elder PT. Accidental hypothermia. In: Shoemaker WC, Thompson WL, Holbrook PR, eds. Textbook of critical care medicine. Philadelphia: WB Saunders, 1984:85.
88. Ellis RJ, Mangano DT, Van Dyke DC. Relationship of wedge pressure to end-diastolic volume in patients undergoing myocardial revascularization. J Thorac Cardiovasc Surg 1979; 78:605.
89. Entress JJ, Dhamee MS, Olund T, et al. Pulmonary artery occlusion pressure does not accurately reflect left atrial pressure after cardiopulmonary bypass. Anesth Analg 1989;68:S81.
90. Estafanous FG, Salim W, Tarazi RC. Effects of cardiac depression on hemodynamic responses to hemodilution. Anesthesiology 1985;63:A38.
91. Fahey PJ, Harris K, Vanderwarf C. Clinical experience with continuous monitoring of mixed venous oxygen saturation in respiratory failure. Chest 1984;86:748.
92. Fahmy NR, Chandler HP, Patel DG, et al. Hemodynamics and oxygen availability during acute hemodilution in conscious man. Anesthesiology 1980;53 suppl:84.
93. Falk JL, Rackow ES, Fein IA, et al. Cardiac function during fluid challenge with albumin, hetastarch or saline in patients with circulatory shock. Anesthesiology 1982;57:A110.
94. Fan FC, Chen RYC, Schuessler GB, et al. Effects of hematocrit variations on regional hemodynamics and oxygen transport in the dog. Am J Physiol 1980;238:H545.
95. Feeley TW, Bancroft ML. Problems with mechanical ventilators. Int Anesthesiol Clin 1982;20:83.
96. Filley GF. Acid base and blood gas regulation. 1st ed. Philadelphia: Lea and Febiger, 1971:75.
97. Finch CA, Lenfant CL. Oxygen transport in man. N Engl J Med 1972;286:407.
98. Finucane BT. Thoracic trauma. In: Kaplan JA, ed. Thoracic anesthesia. 1st ed. New York: Churchill Livingstone, 1983:475.
99. Fitzpatrick JH, Gilbol DD, Drewes LR, et al. Relationship of cerebral oxygen uptake to EEG frequency in isolated canine brain. Am J Physiol 1976;231:1840.

100. Fortune JB, Feustel PJ, Saifi J, et al. Influence of hematocrit on cardiopulmonary function after acute hemorrhage. J Trauma 1987;27:243.
101. Fowles RE. Interpretation of cardiac catheterization. In: Ream AK, Fogdall RP, eds. Acute cardiovascular management: anesthesia and intensive care. Philadelphia: JB Lippincott, 1982: 69(82).
102. Gelin LE, Dawidson I. Plasma expanders and hemodilution in the treatment of hypovolemic shock. In: Cowley RA, Trump BF, eds. Pathophysiology of shock, anoxia and ischemia. Baltimore: Williams and Wilkins, 1982:454.
103. Gettinger A, De Traglia MC, Glass D. In vivo comparison of two mixed venous saturation catheters. Anesthesiology 1987; 66:373.
104. Gisselsson L, Rosberg B, Ericsson M. Myocardial blood flow, oxygen uptake and carbon dioxide release of the human heart during hemodilution. Acta Anaesthesiol Scand 1982;26:589.
105. Gordon RJ, Ravin MB. Rheology and anesthesiology. Anesth Analg 1978;57:252.
106. Gore JM, Sloan K. Use of continuous monitoring of mixed venous saturation in the coronary care unit. Chest 1984;86:757.
107. Gorlin R, Herman MV. Physiology of the coronary circulation. In: Hurst JW, Logue RB, Schlant RC, Wenger NK, eds. The heart. 4th ed. New York: McGraw-Hill, 1978:101.
108. Gould SA, Rosen AL, Sehgal LR, et al. Red cell substitutes: hemoglobin solution or fluorocarbon? J Trauma 1982;22:736.
109. Groeneveld ABJ, Kester ADM, Nauta JJP, et al. Relation of arterial blood lactate to oxygen delivery and hemodynamic variables in human shock states. Circ Shock 1987;22:35.
110. Gump FE. Anemia in surgical patients. Bibl Haematol 1980;46:105.
111. Gump FE. Trauma and hemorrhage. Surg Clin North Am 1983;63:305.
112. Gump FE. Whole body metabolism. In: Altura BM, Lefer AM, Schumer W, eds. Handbook of shock and trauma: basic science. New York: Raven Press, 1983;1:241.
113. Gump FE, Martin P, Kinney JM. Oxygen consumption and caloric expenditure in surgical patients. Surg Gynecol Obstet 1973;137:499.
114. Gustafsson L, Appelgren L, Myrvold HE. Effects of hemodilution on skeletal muscle blood flow and blood viscosity in vivo after splanchnic stasis. Eur Surg Res 1985;17:366.
115. Gustafsson L, Appelgren L, Myrvold HE. Hemoconcentration, hemodilution and apparent viscosity in vivo in experimental shock. J Surg Res 1982;33:116.
116. Gutierrez G. Peripheral delivery and utilization of oxygen. In: Dantzker DR, ed. Cardiopulmonary critical care. Orlando: Grune and Stratton, 1986:169.
117. Gutierrez G, Pohil RJ. Assessment of hypoxia by magnetic resonance spectroscopy and positron emission tomography. In: Bryan-Brown C, Ayres SM, eds. Oxygen transport and utilization. Fullerton: Society of Critical Care Medicine, 1987:171.
118. Gutierrez G, Warley AR, Dantzker DR. Oxygen delivery and utilization in hypothermic dogs. J Appl Physiol 1986; 60:751.
119. Guyton AC, ed. Cardiac output venous return and their regulation. In: Textbook of medical physiology. 6th ed. Philadelphia: WB Saunders, 1981:274.
120. Guyton AC, ed. Circulatory shock and physiology of its treatment. In: Textbook of medical physiology. 6th ed. Philadelphia: WB Saunders, 1981:332.
121. Guyton AC, ed. Muscle blood flow during exercise: cerebral splanchnic and skin blood flows. In: Textbook of medical physiology. 6th ed. Philadelphia: WB Saunders, 1981:344.
122. Guyton AC, ed. Physics of blood, blood flow and pressure: hemodynamics. In: Textbook of medical physiology. 6th ed. Philadelphia: WB Saunders, 1981.
123. Guyton AC, ed. Transport of oxygen and carbon dioxide in the blood and body fluids. In: Textbook of medical physiology. 6th ed. Philadelphia: WB Saunders, 1981:508.
124. Guyton AC, Jones EC, Coleman TG. Circulatory physiology: cardiac output and its regulation. Philadelphia: WB Saunders, 1973.
125. Guyton AC, Richardson TQ. Effect of hematocrit on venous return. Circ Res 1961;9:157.
126. Hamilton WK. Unexpected deaths during anesthesia: wherein lies the cause? Anesthesiology 1979;50:381.
127. Hansen NB, Miller R, Nowicki P, et al. Brain blood flow alterations during prolonged respiratory alkalosis. Crit Care Med 1985;13:296.
128. Hansen RM, Viguerat CE, Matthay MA, et al. Poor correlation between pulmonary arterial wedge pressure and left ventricular end-diastolic volume after coronary artery bypass graft surgery. Anesthesiology 1986;64:764.
129. Hanson FN. Right heart catheterization in the critically ill patient. N Engl J Med 1983;309:376.
130. Harley DP, Mena I, Miranda R, et al. Myocardial dysfunction following blunt chest trauma. Arch Surg 1983;118:1384.
131. Harnik E, Kulczycki L, Gomes MN. Transcutaneous oxygen monitoring during bronchoscopy and washout for cystic fibrosis. Anesth Analg 1983;62:357.
132. Harp JR, Hagerdal M. Brain oxygen consumption. In: Cottrell JE, Turndorf H, eds. Anesthesia and neurosurgery. 1st ed. St Louis: CV Mosby, 1980:25.
133. Harp JR, Wollman H. Cerebral hypoxia with hyperventilation. In: Orkin FK, Cooperman LH, eds. Complications in anesthesiology. Philadelphia, JB Lippincott, 1983:331.
134. Hassan E, Roffman DS, Applefeld MM. The value of mixed venous oxygen saturation as a therapeutic indicator in the treatment of advanced congestive heart failure. Am Heart J 1987;113:743.
135. Haupt MT, Gilbert EM, Carlson RW. Fluid loading increases oxygen consumption in septic patients with lactic acidosis. Am Rev Respir Dis 1985;131:912.
136. Hauser CJ, Kaufman C, Frantz R, et al. Use of crystalline hemoglobin as replacement of RBC mass. Arch Surg 1982;117:782.
137. Hauser CJ, Shoemaker WC. Hemoglobin solution in the treatment of hemorrhagic shock. Crit Care Med 1982;10:283.
138. Hauser CJ, Shoemaker WC, Turpin I, et al. Oxygen transport responses to colloids and crystalloids in critically ill surgical patients. Surg Gynecol Obstet 1980;150:811.
139. Hechtman HB, Grindlinger GA, Vegas AM, et al. Importance of oxygen transport in clinical medicine. Crit Care Med 1979;7:419.
140. Hengo H. Cellular metabolism in shock. In: Lewis DH, Haglund U, eds. Shock research. Amsterdam: Elsevier Science Publishers, 1983.
141. Henling CE, Diaz JH. The cluttered anesthesia machine: a cause for hypoxia. Anesthesiology 1983;58:288.
142. Herman CM, Rodkey FL, Valeri CR, et al. Changes in oxyhemoglobin dissociation curve and peripheral blood after acute red cell mass depletion and subsequent red cell mass restoration in baboons. Ann Surg 1971;174:734.
143. Hershenson MB, O'Rourke PP, Schena JA, et al. Effect of halothane on critical levels of oxygen transport in the anesthetized newborn lamb. Anesthesiology 1987;67:174.
144. Hessel EA, Bazaral MG, Stewart R, et al. Pulmonary artery wedge pressure compared to left atrial pressure in cardiac surgical patients. Anesthesiology 1984;61:A71.

145. Hillis LD, Firth BG, Winniford MD. Analysis of factors affecting the variability of Fick versus indicator dilution measurements of cardiac output. Am J Cardiol 1985;56:764.
146. Hopkins JA, Shoemaker WC, Chang PC, et al. Clinical trial of an emergency resuscitation algorithm. Crit Care Med 1983; 11:621.
147. Horber JD, Clark JT, Lucey JF. The newborn oxygram: automated processing of transcutaneous oxygen data. Pediatrics 1980;66:84.
148. Horton J, Landreneau R, Tuggle D. Cardiac response to fluid resuscitation from hemorrhagic shock. Surg Gynecol Obstet 1985;160:444.
149. Houtchens BA, Westenskow DR. Oxygen consumption in septic shock: collective review. Circ Shock 1984;13:361.
150. Huckabee WE. Relationships of pyruvate and lactate during anaerobic metabolism. J Clin Invest 1958;37:244.
151. Hug CC. Monitoring. In: Miller RD, ed. Anesthesia. 2nd ed. New York: Churchill Livingstone, 1986;1:411.
152. Iberti TJ, Kelly KM, Gentili DR, et al. Effects of sodium bicarbonate in canine hemorrhagic shock. Crit Care Med 1988;16:779.
153. Ivanov J, Weisel RD, Mickleborough M, et al. Rewarming hypovolemia after aortocoronary bypass surgery. Crit Care Med 1984;12:1049.
154. Jan KM, Chien S. Effect of hematocrit variations on coronary hemodynamics and oxygen utilization. Am J Physiol 1977;233:H106.
155. Jan KM, Heldman J, Chien S. Coronary hemodynamics and oxygen utilization after hematocrit variations in hemorrhage. Am J Physiol 1980;239:H326.
156. Jobes DR, Gallagher J. Acute normovolemic hemodilution. Int Anesthesiol Clin 1982;20:77.
157. Johnstone RE. Equipment malfunction. In: Orkin FK, Cooperman LH, ed. Complications in anesthesiology. Philadelphia: JB Lippincott, 1983:639.
158. Kagle DM, Alexander CM, Berko RS, et al. Evaluation of the Ohmeda 3700 pulse oximeter: steady state and transient response characteristics. Anesthesiology 1987;66:376.
159. Kahn RC, Zaroulis C, Howland WS, et al. Hemodynamic, oxygen delivery changes and 2,3-DPG changes after transfusion of patients in acute respiratory failure. Anesthesiology 1982; 57:A106.
160. Kandel G, Aberman A. Mixed venous oxygen saturation: its role in the assessment of the critically ill patient. Arch Intern Med 1983;143:1400.
161. Kaplan JA. Cardiac anesthesia. 1st ed. New York: Grune and Stratton, 1979;1:95.
162. Kaplan JA. Hemodynamic monitoring. In: Kaplan JA, ed. Cardiac anesthesia. New York: Grune and Stratton, 1979;1:71.
163. Kaplan JA, Guffin AV. Shivering and changes in mixed venous oxygen saturation after cardiac surgery. Anesth Analg 1985;64:235.
164. Kaufman BS, Rackow EC, Falk JJ. The relationship between oxygen delivery and consumption during fluid resuscitation of hypovolemic and septic shock. Chest 1984;85:337.
165. Kawakami Y, Kishi F, Yamamoto H, et al. Relation of oxygen delivery, mixed venous oxygenation and pulmonary hemodynamics to prognosis in chronic obstructive pulmonary disease. N Engl J Med 1983;308:1045.
166. Kazarian KK, Del Guercio LRM. The use of mixed venous blood gas determinations in traumatic shock. Ann Emerg Med 1980;9:179.
167. Kaznitz P, Druger GL, Yorra F, et al. Mixed venous oxygen tension and hyperlactatemia. JAMA 1976;236:570.
168. Keenan RL, Boyan CP. Cardiac arrest due to anesthesia: a study of incidence and causes. JAMA 1985;253:2373.
169. Kim YD, Katz NM, Ng L, et al. Effects of hypothermia and hemodilution on oxygen metabolism and hemodynamics in patients recovering from coronary artery bypass operations. J Thorac Cardiovasc Surg 1989;97:36.
170. Klitzman B, Duling BR. Microvascular hematocrit and red cell flow in resting and contracting striated muscle. Am J Physiol 1979;237:481.
171. Kogure K, Scheinberg P, Reinmuth OM, et al. Mechanisms of cerebrovasodilatation in hypoxia. J Appl Physiol 1970;29:223.
172. Komatsu T, Bhalodia R, Kubal K, et al. Monitoring of transcutaneous oxygen tension during progressive perfusion failure in dogs. Anesthesiology 1983;59:A147.
173. Komatsu T, Kubal C, Krishnamurthy U, et al. Oxygen transport to tissue during controlled hypotension with sodium nitroprusside. Anesthesiology 1983;59:A125.
174. Komatsu T, Kumar V, Sanchala V, et al. Oxygen requirement in the postbypass period. Anesthesiology 1982;57:A125.
175. Komatsu T, Kumar V, Sanchala V, et al. Systemic vascular resistance needs correction for hematocrit values. Anesthesiology 1982;57:A124.
176. Komatsu T, Shibutani K, Bizzarri DV. Critical level of oxygen delivery in anesthetized man. Anesth Analg 1982;61:196.
177. Komatsu T, Shibutani K, Bizzarri D. Systemic vascular resistance needs correction for hematocrit and temperature values. Anesthesiology 1984;61:A70.
178. Komatsu T, Shibutani K, Okamoto K, et al. Critical level of oxygen delivery after cardiopulmonary bypass. Crit Care Med 1987;15:194.
179. Kruse JA: Blood lactate and oxygen transport. Intensive Care World 1987;4:121.
180. Kubler W. Glycolytic pathways in the myocardium. In: Muir JR, ed. Prospects in the management of ischaemic heart disease. London: CIBA, 1974.
181. Kudoh I, Segawa Y, Numata K, et al. $Pa_{O_2}$ change during progressive pulmonary edema in dogs. Crit Care Med 1985; 13:1020.
182. Laks H, Pilon RN, Klovekorn WP, et al. Acute hemodilution: its effects on hemodynamics and oxygen transport in anesthetized man. Ann Surg 1974;180:103.
183. Lassen NA. Cerebral and spinal cord blood flow. In: Cottrell JE, Turndorf H, eds. Anesthesia and neurosurgery. 1st ed. St Louis: CV Mosby, 1980:1.
184. Latson TW, Kickler TS, Baumgartner WA. Pulmonary hypertension and non-cardiogenic pulmonary edema following cardiopulmonary bypass associated with an antigranulocyte antibody. Anesthesiology 1986;64:106.
185. Laughlin TP, McMichan JC. Adjustment of PEEP according to continuous measurement of mixed venous $O_2$ saturation ($S\bar{v}_{O_2}$). Anesth Analg 1984;63:242.
186. Lee JC, Downing SE. Myocardial oxygen availability and cardiac failure in hemorrhagic shock. Am Heart J 1976;92:201.
187. Lee J, Wright F, Barber R, et al. Central venous oxygen saturation in shock: a study in man. Anesthesiology 1972;36:472.
188. Lichtenstein A, Eckhart WF, Swanson KJ, et al. Unplanned intraoperative and postoperative hemodilution: oxygen transport and consumption during severe anemia. Anesthesiology 1988;69:119.
189. Lichtor JL, Ellis JE, Vitvlugt A, et al. Transesophageal echocardiography during liver transplantation. Anesth Analg 1987;66:S104.
190. Lipowsky HH, Usami S, Chien S. In vivo measurements of "apparent viscosity" and microvessel hematocrit in the mesentery of the cat. Microvasc Res 1980;19:297.
191. Lubarsky D, Kaufman B. Oxygen delivery under anesthesia: a prospective evaluation of 330 mL/min/m$^2$ as a "critical" value. Anesth Analg 1989;68:S173.

192. Lubarsky D, Kaufman BS, Sharnick S, et al. The effects of induction of anesthesia on mixed venous and peripheral venous oxygen saturations. Anesth Analg 1989;68:S172.
193. Lundsgaard-Hansen P. Hemodilution: new clothes for an anemic emperor. Vox Sang 1979;36:321.
194. Malmberg PO, Hlastala MP, Woodson RD. Effect of increased blood-oxygen affinity on oxygen transport in hemorrhagic shock. J Appl Physiol 1979;47:889.
195. Malmberg PO, Woodson RD. Effect of anemia on oxygen transport in hemorrhagic shock. J Appl Physiol 1979;47:882.
196. Mammana RB, Hiro S, Levitsky S, et al. Inaccuracy of pulmonary capillary wedge pressure when compared to left atrial pressure in the early post-surgical period. J Thorac Cardiovasc Surg 1982;84:420.
197. Maningas PA. Resuscitation with 7.5% NaCl in 6% dextran-70 during hemorrhagic shock in swine: effects on organ blood flow. Crit Care Med 1987;15:1121.
198. Mannix FL. Hemorrhagic shock. In: Rosen P, Baker FJ, Braen GR, Dailey RH, Levy RC, eds. Emergency medicine: concepts and clinical practice. St Louis: CV Mosby, 1983:129.
199. Marks WE. A plea for the routine use of oxygen analyzers. Anesthesiology 1983;59:159.
200. Martin E, Hansen E, Peter K. Acute normovolemic hemodilution: a method for avoiding homologous transfusion. World J Surg 1987;11:53.
201. Masud KZ, Masud M. Crystalloid vs colloid fluid therapy in hemorrhagic shock. Anesthesiology 1981;55:A96.
202. McCormick M, Feustel PJ, Newall JC, et al. Effect of cardiac index and hematocrit changes on oxygen consumption in resuscitated patients. J Surg Res 1988;44:499.
203. McCuskey RS. Microcirculation: basic considerations. In: Cowley RA, Trump BF, eds. Pathophysiology of shock, anoxia and ischemia. Baltimore: Williams and Wilkins, 1982:156.
204. McMichan JC. Continuous monitoring of mixed venous oxygen saturation: theory applied to practice. In: Schweiss JF, ed. Continuous measurement of blood oxygen saturation in the high risk patient. San Diego: Beach International 1983;1:27.
205. McNamara JJ, Suehiro GT, Suehiro A, et al. Resuscitation from hemorrhagic shock. J Trauma 1983;23:552.
206. Mendelson Y, Kent JC, Shahnarian A, et al. Simultaneous comparison of three noninvasive oximeters in healthy volunteers. Med Instrum 1987;21:183.
207. Messmer K. Compensatory mechanisms for acute dilutional anemia. Bibl Haematol 1981;47:31.
208. Messmer K. Hemodilution. Surg Clin North Am 1975;55:659.
209. Messmer K, Goernandt L, Jesch F, et al. Oxygen transport and tissue oxygenation during hemodilution with dextran. Adv Exp Med Biol 1973;37B:669.
210. Messmer KFW. Acceptable hematocrit levels in surgical patients. World J Surg 1987;11:41.
211. Michenfelder JD, Theye RA. The effects of profound hypothermia and dilutional anemia on canine cerebral metabolism and blood flow. Anesthesiology 1969;31:449.
212. Mihm FG, Halperin BD. Noninvasive detection of profound arterial desaturation using a pulse oximetry device. Anesthesiology 1985;62:85.
213. Mikat M, Peters J, Zindler M, et al. Whole body oxygen consumption in awake, sleeping and anesthetized dogs. Anesthesiology 1984;60:220.
214. Miller MJ. Tissue oxygenation in clinical medicine: a historical review. Anesth Analg 1982;61:527.
215. Miller RD. Complications of massive blood transfusions. Anesthesiology 1973;39:82.
216. Miller RD. Problems posed by transfusion. In: Orkin FK, Cooperman LH, eds. Complications in anesthesiology. Philadelphia: JB Lippincott, 1983:461.
216a. Miller RD. Current perspectives on blood transfusion. International Anesthesia Research Society. 1990 review course p 57.
217. Miller RD, Tong MJ, Robbins TO. Effects of massive transfusion of blood on acid-base balance. JAMA 1971;216:1762.
218. Milnor WR. Hemodynamics. Baltimore: Williams and Wilkins, 1982:12.
219. Mizock BA. Controversies in lactic acidosis: implications in critically ill patients. JAMA 1987;258:497.
220. Moffitt EA, Sethna DH. The coronary circulation and myocardial oxygenation in coronary artery disease. Anesth Analg 1986;65:395.
221. Mohsenifar Z, Amin D, Jasper AC, et al. Dependence of oxygen consumption on oxygen delivery in patients with congestive heart failure. Chest 1987;92:447.
222. Moore FD. Transcapillary refill, the unrepaired anemia, and clinical hemodilution. Surg Gynecol Obstet 1974;139:245.
223. Morris DL, Chambers HF, Morris MG, et al. Hemodynamic characteristics of patients with hypothermia due to acute infection and other causes. Ann Intern Med 1985;102:153.
224. Murkin JM, Farrar JK, Tweed WA, et al. Cerebral blood flow, oxygen consumption, and EEG during isoflurane anesthesia. Anesth Analg 1986;65:S107.
225. Musch TI, Zarach DR. $O_2$ content of blood sampled from different venous compartments of the rat. J Appl Physiol 1988;65:988.
226. Nagao S, Roccaforte P, Moody RA. The effects of isovolemic hemodilution and reinfusion of packed erythrocytes on somatosensory and visual evoked potentials. J Surg Res 1978;25:530.
227. Nearman HS, Eckhauser MI. Postoperative management of a severely anemic Jehovah's witness. Crit Care Med 1983;11:142.
228. Nelson LD. Continuous venous oximetry in surgical patients. Ann Surg 1986;203:329.
229. Nelson LD. Mixed venous oximetry. In: Snyder JV, Pinsky MR, eds. Oxygen transport in the critically ill. Chicago: Year Book, 1987:235.
230. Nelimarkka O, Niinikoski J. Renal venous oxygen tension as an indicator of tissue hypoxia in hemorrhagic shock. Crit Care Med 1986;14:128.
231. Neuhof H. Clinical problems in shock: microcirculation and peripheral gas exchange. Clin Hemorheol 1982;2:691.
232. New W. Pulse oximetry. J Clin Monit 1985;1:126.
233. Ngai SH, Papper EM. Metabolic effects of anesthesia. Springfield: Charles C Thomas, 1962.
234. Nolan LS, Shoemaker WC. Transcutaneous $O_2$ and $CO_2$ monitoring of high risk surgical patients during the perioperative period. Crit Care Med 1982;10:762.
235. Norfleet EA, Watson CB. Continuous mixed venous oxygen saturation measurement: a significant advance in hemodynamic monitoring? J Clin Monit 1985;1:245.
236. Nunn JF. Applied respiratory physiology with special reference to anesthesia. 3rd ed. London: Butterworths, 1987:256.
237. Nunn JF. Applied respiratory physiology. 3rd ed. London: Butterworths, 1987:366.
238. Nunn JF. Applied respiratory physiology with special reference to anesthesia. 3rd ed. London: Butterworths, 1987:471.
239. Nunn JF, Freeman J. Problems of oxygenation and oxygen transport during haemorrhage. Anaesthesia 1964;19:206.
240. Oppenheim WL, Williamson DH, Smith R. Early biochemical changes and severity of injury in man. J Trauma 1980; 20:135.
241. Orr MD. Hemodilution. In: Sandler SG, Silvergleid AJ, eds. Autologous transfusion. Arlington: American Association of Blood Banks, 1983:23.
242. Ozawa K, Aoyama H, Yasuda K, et al. Metabolic abnormalities associated with postoperative organ failure. Arch Surg 1983; 118:1245.

243. Pavlin EG, Yazaki S, Winn R, et al. The effect of shivering on gas exchange in goats. Anesthesiology 1983;59:A483.
244. Peitzman A. Principles of circulatory support and the treatment of hemorrhagic shock. In: Snyder JV, Pinsky MR, eds. Oxygen transport in the critically ill. Chicago: Year Book, 1987:407.
245. Pepe PE, Culver BH. Independently measured oxygen consumption during reduction of oxygen delivery by PEEP. Am Rev Respir Dis 1985;132:788.
246. Perel A, Pizov R, Cotev S. The systolic blood pressure variation is a sensitive indicator of hypovolemia in ventilated dogs subjected to graded hemorrhage. Anesthesiology 1987;67:498.
247. Peter JD, Fineberg KS, Kroll DA, et al. Anesthesiology and the law. Ann Arbor: Health Administration Press, 1983:336.
248. Pizov R, Ya'ari Y, Perel A. Systolic pressure variation is greater during hemorrhage than during sodium nitroprusside-induced hypotension in ventilated dogs. Anesth Analg 1988;67:170.
249. Pollack MM, Fields AI, Ruttimann UE. Distributions of cardiopulmonary variables in pediatric survivors and nonsurvivors of septic shock. Crit Care Med 1985;13:454.
250. Pool GV, Meredith JW, Pennell T, et al. Comparison of colloids and crystolloids in resuscitation from hemorrhagic shock. Surg Gynecol Obstet 1982;154:577.
251. Pruitt BA, Moncrief JA, Mason AD. Effect of buffered saline solution upon the blood volume of man after acute measured hemorrhage. Annual research progress report. Texas: US Army Surgical Research Unit, 1965.
252. Prys-Roberts C. The metabolic regulation of circulatory transport. In: Scurr C, Feldman S, eds. Scientific foundations of anaesthesia. 2nd ed. Chicago: Year Book, 1974:125.
253. Prys-Roberts C. Ventricular performance. In: Prys-Roberts C, ed. The circulation in anaesthesia: applied physiology and pharmacology. 1st ed. Oxford: Blackwell, 1980:115(132).
254. Rafferty TD, Marrero O, Nardi D, et al. Transcutaneous $Po_2$ as a trend indicator of arterial $Po_2$ in normal anesthetized adults. Anesth Analg 1982;61:252.
255. Rah KH, Dunwiddie WC, Lower RR. A method for continuous postoperative measurement of mixed venous oxygen saturation in infants and children after open heart procedures. Anesth Analg 1984;63:873.
256. Ralley FE, Wynands JE, Ramsay JG, et al. The effects of shivering on oxygen consumption and carbon dioxide production in patients rewarming from hypothermic cardiopulmonary bypass. Can J Anaesth 1988;35:332.
257. Raper R, Sibbald WJ. Misled by wedge? The Swan-Ganz catheter and left ventricular preload. Chest 1986;89:427.
258. Rasanen J, Downs JB, DeHaven B. Titration of continuous positive airway pressure by real-time dual oximetry. Chest 1987;92:853.
259. Rasanen J, Downs JB, Malec DJ, et al. Estimation of oxygen utilization by dual oximetry. Ann Surg 1987;206:621.
260. Rasanen J, Downs JB, Malec DJ, et al. Real-time continuous estimation of gas exchange by dual oximetry. Intensive Care Med 1988;14:118.
261. Reed RL, Maier RV, Landicho D, et al. Correlation of hemodynamic variables with transcutaneous $Po_2$ measurements in critically ill adult patients. J Trauma 1985;25:1045.
262. Reinhart K. Monitoring of oxygen transport. Anaesthesist 1988;37:1.
263. Reinhart K, Moser N, Rudolph T, et al. Accuracy of two mixed venous saturation catheters during long-term use in critically ill patients. Anesthesiology 1988;69:769.
264. Reinhart K, Rudolph T, Bredle DL, et al. Comparison of central-venous to mixed-venous oxygen saturation during changes in oxygen supply/demand. Chest 1989;95:1216.
265. Rendell-Baker L. Problems with anesthetic gas machines and their solutions. Int Anesthesiol Clin 1982;20:1.
266. Rendell-Baker L, Meyer JA. Failure to use $O_2$ analyzers to prevent hypoxic accidents. Anesthesiology 1983;58:287.
267. Roberts JG. The effects of hypoxia on the systemic circulation during anesthesia. In: Prys-Roberts C, ed. The circulation in anaesthesia: applied physiology and pharmacology. 1st ed. Oxford: Blackwell, 1980:311.
268. Robin ED: Dysoxia and the general problem of $O_2$ delivery by the blood. Bibl Haematol 1980;46:96.
269. Rosberg B, Wulff K. Hemodynamics following normovolemic hemodilution in elderly patients. Acta Anaesthesiol Scand 1981;25:402.
270. Rosberg B, Wulff K. Regional blood flow in normovolemic and hypovolemic haemodilution. Br J Anaesth 1979;51:423.
271. Rose D, Forest R, Coutsoftides M. Acute normovolemic hemodilution. Anesthesiology 1979;51:91.
272. Rush B, Eiseman B. Limits of non-colloid solution replacement in experimental hemorrhagic shock. Ann Surg 1967;165:977.
273. Rush BF. Volume replacement: when, what, and how much? In: Schumer W, Nyhus LM, eds. Treatment of shock: principles and practice. Philadelphia: Lea and Febiger, 1974.
274. Scalea TM, Holman M, Fuortes M, et al. Central venous blood oxygen saturation: an early, accurate measurement of volume during hemorrhage. J Trauma 1988;28:725.
275. Schacter EN, Rafferty TD, Knight C, et al. Transcutaneous oxygen and carbon dioxide monitoring. Arch Surg 1981;116:1193.
276. Schauble JF, Murphy V, Elliot P. Bradycardia and hemodynamic instability during anesthesia. Anesthesiology 1982;57:A72.
277. Scheinman MM, Brown BA, Rapaport E. Critical assessment of use of central venous oxygen saturation as a mirror of mixed venous oxygen in severely ill cardiac patients. Circulation 1969;40:165.
278. Schlant RC: Metabolism of the heart. In: Hurst JW, Logue RB, Schlant RC, Wenger NK, eds. The heart. 4th ed. New York: McGraw-Hill, 1978:107.
279. Schlant RC. Normal physiology of the cardiovascular system. In: Hurst JW, Logue RB, Schlant RC, Wenger NK, eds. The heart. 4th ed. New York: McGraw-Hill, 1978:71.
280. Schlichtig R, Cowden WL, Chaitman BR. Tolerance of unusually low mixed venous oxygen saturation: adaptations in the chronic low cardiac output syndrome. Am J Med 1986; 80:813.
281. Schmidt CR, Frank LP, Estafanous FB. Continuous pulmonary artery oximetry: an early warning monitor in cardiac surgery patients. Anesthesiology 1983;59:A139.
282. Schmidt CR, Frank LP, Forsythe SB, et al. Continuous $S\bar{v}o_2$ and oxygen transport patterns with cardiac surgery. Anesth Analg 1983;62:281.
283. Schmidt CR, Frank LP, Forsythe SB, et al. Continuous $S\bar{v}o_2$ measurement and oxygen transport patterns in cardiac surgery patients. Crit Care Med 1984;12:523.
284. Schmidt CR, Starr NJ. Evaluation of a continuous $S\bar{v}o_2$ monitoring system. Anesthesiology 1981;55:A125.
285. Schumacker PT, Cain SM. The concept of critical oxygen delivery. Intensive Care Med 1987;13:223.
286. Schumacker PT, Long GR, Wood LDH. Effect of increased hematocrit on the relationship between oxygen delivery and consumption in the dog. Am Rev Respir Dis 1984;129:A97.
287. Schumacker PT, Long GR, Wood LDH. Tissue oxygen extraction during hypovolemia: role of hemoglobin $P_{50}$. J Appl Physiol 1987;62:1801.
288. Schumacker PT, Rowland J, Saltz S, et al. Effects of hyperthermia and hypothermia on oxygen extraction by tissues during hypovolemia. J Appl Physiol 1987;63:1246.
289. Schumacker PT, Suggett AJ, Wagner PD. Role of hemoglobin 50 in $O_2$ transport during normoxic and hypoxic exercise in the dog. J Appl Physiol 1985;59:749.

290. Schumacker PT, Wood LDH. Limitations of aerobic metabolism in critical illness. Chest 1984;85:453.
291. Schwartz S, Frantz RA, Shoemaker WC. Sequential hemodynamic and oxygen transport responses to hypovolemia, anemia and hypoxia. Am J Physiol 1981;10:H864.
292. Schweiss JF. Use of continuous $S\bar{v}O_2$ intra and postoperatively in managing the hemodynamics of cardiac surgery patients. In: Schweiss JF, ed. Continuous measurement of blood oxygen saturation in the high risk patient. San Diego: Beach International 1983;1:81.
293. Secher NH, Jensen KS, Werner C, et al. Bradycardia during severe but reversible hypovolemic shock in man. Circ Shock 1984;14:267.
294. Sendak MJ, Harris AP, Donham RT. Accuracy of pulse oximetry during arterial oxyhemoglobin desaturation in dogs. Anesthesiology 1988;68:111.
295. Shackford SR. Blunt chest trauma: the intensivist's perspective. J Intensive Care Med 1986;1:125.
296. Shah DM, Newell JC, Saba TM. Defects in peripheral oxygen utilization following trauma and shock. Arch Surg 1981; 116:1277.
297. Shapiro BA, Harrison RA, Walton JR. Clinical application of blood gases. 3rd ed. Chicago: Year Book, 1982:77.
298. Shapiro BA, Harrison RA, Walton JR. Clinical application of blood gases. 3rd ed. Chicago: Year Book, 1982:153.
299. Shapiro BA, Harrison RA, Walton JR. Clinical application of blood gases. 3rd ed. Chicago: Year Book, 1982:206.
300. Shapiro HM. Anesthesia effects upon cerebral blood flow, cerebral metabolism electroencephalogram and the evoked potentials. In: Miller RD, ed. Anesthesia. New York: Churchill Livingstone, 1986;2:1249.
301. Shappell SD, Lenfant CJM. Adaptive, genetic and iatrogenic alterations of the oxyhemoglobin-dissociation curve. Anesthesiology 1972;37:127.
302. Sheldon CA, Belani KG, Liao, et al. Evaluation of PCVP during hemorrhage and controlled venous return: introduction of a new PCVP catheter. Anesthesiology 1983;59:A175.
303. Sheldon CA, Cerra FB, Bohnhoff N, et al. Peripheral postcapillary venous pressure: a new, more sensitive monitor of effective blood volume during hemorrhagic shock and resuscitation. Surgery 1983;94:399.
304. Sheldon GF. Diphosphoglycerate in massive transfusion and erythropoesis. Crit Care Med 1979;7:407.
305. Shibutani K, Del Guercio LRM. Preoperative hemodynamic assessment of the high risk patient. Semin Anesth 1983;2:231.
306. Shibutani K, Komatsu T, Kubal K, et al. Critical level of oxygen delivery in anesthetized man. Crit Care Med 1983;11:640.
307. Shinozuka T, Nemoto EM, Bleyaert AL. Cerebral cortical oxygenation and perfusion during progressive hydroxyethyl starch (volex) hemodilution. Anesthesiology 1981;55:A91.
308. Shippy CR, Appel PL, Shoemaker WC. Reliability of clinical monitoring to assess blood volume in critically ill patients. Crit Care Med 1984;12:107.
309. Shires GT, Carrico CJ, Canizaro PC. Alterations in oxygen transport in shock. In: Major problems in clinical surgery. Philadelphia: WB Saunders, 1973;3:97.
310. Shires GT, Carrico CJ, Canizaro PC: Response of the extracellular fluid, in shock. In: Major problems in clinical surgery. Philadelphia: WB Saunders, 1973;13:15.
311. Shoemaker WC. A new approach to physiology, monitoring, and therapy of shock states. World J Surg 1987;11:133.
312. Shoemaker WC. Cardiorespiratory patterns in complicated and uncomplicated septic shock. Ann Surg 1971;174:119.
313. Shoemaker WC. Circulatory mechanisms of shock and their mediators. Crit Care Med 1987;15:787.
314. Shoemaker WC. Evaluation of colloids, crystalloids, whole blood and red cell therapy in the critically ill patient. Clin Lab Med: Symp Blood Banking Hemother 1982;2:35.
315. Shoemaker WC. Monitoring of the critically ill. In: Shoemaker WC, Ayres S, Grenvik A, Thompson WL, Holbrook PR, eds. Textbook of critical care medicine. Philadelphia: WB Saunders, 1989:145.
316. Shoemaker WC. Pathophysiology and therapy of hemorrhage and trauma states. In: Cowley RA, Trump BF, eds. Pathophysiology of shock, anoxia and ischemia. Baltimore: Williams and Wilkins, 1982:439.
317. Shoemaker WC. Shock states: pathophysiology monitoring, outcome prediction and therapy. In: Shoemaker WC, Ayres S, Grenvik A, Thompson WL, Holbrook PR, eds. Textbook of critical care medicine. Philadelphia: WB Saunders, 1984:52.
318. Shoemaker WC, Appel PL, Bland R. Use of physiologic monitoring to predict outcome and to assist in clinical decisions in critically ill postoperative patients. Am J Surg 1983;146:43.
319. Shoemaker WC, Appel PL, Kram HB. Role of oxygen transport patterns in the pathophysiology prediction of outcome, and therapy of shock. In: Bryan-Brown CW, Ayres SM, eds. Oxygen transport and utilization. Fullerton: Society of Critical Care Medicine, 1987:65.
320. Shoemaker WC, Appel PL, Kram HB, et al. Comparison of two monitoring methods (central venous pressure versus pulmonary artery catheter) and two protocols as therapeutic goals (normal values versus values of survivors) in a prospective randomized clinical trial of critically ill surgical patients. Crit Care Med 1985;13:304.
321. Shoemaker WC, Appel PL, Kram HB, et al. Prospective trial of supranormal values of survivors as therapeutic goals in high-risk surgical patients. Chest 1988;94:1176.
322. Shoemaker WC, Bland RD, Appel PL. Therapy of critically ill postoperative patients based on outcome prediction and prospective clinical trials. Surg Clin North Am 1985;65:811.
323. Shoemaker WC, Hopkins JA. Clinical aspects of resuscitation with and without an algorithm: relative importance of various decisions. Crit Care Med 1983;11:630.
324. Shoemaker WC, Montgomery ES, Kaplan E, et al. Physiologic patterns in surviving and nonsurviving shock patients: use of sequential cardiorespiratory variables in defining criteria for therapeutic goals and early warning of death. Arch Surg 1973;106:630.
325. Shoemaker WC, Vidyasagar D. Physiological and clinical significance of $Ptco_2$ and $Ptcco_2$ measurements. Crit Care Med 1981;9:689.
326. Sibbald WJ, ed. Shock. In: Synopsis of critical care. 2nd ed. Baltimore: Williams and Wilkins, 1984:34.
327. Simmons DH, Alpas AP, Tashkin DP, et al. Hyperlactatemia due to arterial hypoxemia or reduced cardiac output, or both. J Appl Physiol 1978;45:195.
328. Simmons RL, Heisterkamp CA, Moseley RV, et al. Postresuscitative blood volumes in combat casualties. Surg Gynecol Obstet 1969;128:1193.
329. Skootsky SA, Abraham E. Continuous oxygen consumption measurement during initial emergency department resuscitation of critically ill patients. Crit Care Med 1988;16:706.
330. Slater GI, Vladeck BC, Bassin R, et al. Sequential changes in cerebral blood flow and distribution of flow within the brain during hemorrhagic shock. Ann Surg 1975;181:1.
331. Slater GI, Vladeck BC, Bassin R, et al. Sequential changes in distribution of cardiac output in hemorrhagic shock. Surgery 1973;73:714.
332. Smith JJ, Kampine JP. Circulatory physiology. 2nd ed. Baltimore: Williams and Wilkins, 1984:16.
333. Smith JJ, Kampine JP. Circulatory physiology. 2nd ed. Baltimore: Williams and Wilkins, 1984:138.

334. Smith JJ, Kampine JP: Circulatory physiology. 2nd ed. Baltimore: Williams and Wilkins, 1984:258–261.
335. Smith JJ, Kampine JP. Circulatory physiology. 2nd ed. Baltimore: Williams and Wilkins, 1984:287–289.
336. Smith JJ, Kampine JP. Circulatory physiology. 2nd ed. Baltimore: Williams and Wilkins, 1984:305.
337. Snyder JV. Assessment of systemic oxygen transport. In: Snyder JV, Pinsky MR, eds. Oxygen transport in the critically ill. Chicago: Year Book, 1987:179.
338. Sohmer PR. The pathophysiology of hemorrhagic shock. In: Barnes A, ed. Hemotherapy in trauma and surgery. Washington DC: American Association of Blood Banks, 1979:1.
339. Sohmer PR, Dawson RB. Transfusion therapy in hemorrhagic shock. In: Cowley RA, Trump BF, eds. Pathophysiology of shock, anoxia and ischemia. Baltimore: Williams and Wilkins, 1982:447.
340. Sohmer PR, Dawson RB. Transfusion therapy in trauma: a review of the principles and techniques used in the MIEMS program. Am Surg 1979;45:109.
341. Sonntag H, Merin RG, Donath W, et al. Myocardial metabolism and oxygenation in man awake and during halothane anesthesia. Anesthesiology 1979;51:204.
342. Sottile FD, Durbin CG, Hoyt JW, et al. Evaluation of pulmonary artery oximetry as a predictor of cardiac output. Anesthesiology 1982;57:A127.
343. Spann JF, Hurst JW. Etiology and clinical recognition of heart failure. In: Hurst JW, Logue RB, Schlant RC, Wenger NK, eds. The heart. 4th ed. New York: McGraw-Hill, 1978:561.
344. Stahl WM. Maintenance of organ perfusion. In: Worth MH, ed. Principles and practice of trauma care. Baltimore: Williams and Wilkins, 1982:298.
345. Steinacker CD, Spittelmeister W. Dependence of transcutaneous $O_2$ partial pressure on cutaneous blood flow. J Appl Physiol 1988;64:21.
346. Stokes CD, Blevins S, Siegel JH, et al. Prediction of arterial blood gases by transcutaneous $O_2$ and $CO_2$ in critically ill hyperdynamic trauma patients. J Trauma 1987;27:1240.
347. Sullivan SF. Oxygen transport. Anesthesiology 1972;37:140.
348. Tahvanainen J, Meretoja O, Nikki P. Can central venous blood replace mixed venous blood samples? Crit Care Med 1982;10:758.
349. Taylor AE, Hernandez L, Perry M, et al. Overview of tissue oxygen utilization. In: Bryan-Brown CW, Ayres SM, eds. Oxygen transport and utilization. Fullerton: Society of Critical Care Medicine, 1987:13.
350. Taylor MB, Whitwam JG. The accuracy of pulse oximeters: a comparative clinical evaluation of five pulse oximeters. Anaesthesia 1988;43:229.
351. Teisseire BP, Ropars C, Vallez MO, et al. Physiological effects of high-$P_{50}$ erythrocyte transfusion on piglets. J Appl Physiol 1985;58:1810.
352. Thys DM, Cohen E, Eiseinkraft JB, et al. The pulse oximeter, a non-invasive monitor of oxygenation during one-lung anesthesia. Anesth Analg 1985;64:185.
353. Tinker JH. Perioperative hypertension. In: Kaplan JA, ed. Cardiac anesthesia, cardiovascular pharmacology. New York: Grune and Stratton, 1983;2:365.
354. Tinker JH, Michenfelder JD. Cyanide toxicity induced by nitroprusside in the dog. Anesthesiology 1978;49:109.
355. Todd TRJ, Baile EM, Hogg JC. Pulmonary arterial wedge pressure in hemorrhagic shock. Am Rev Respir Dis 1978;118:613.
356. Tremper KK. Transcutaneous $Po_2$ measurement. Can Anaesth Soc J 1984;31:664.
357. Tremper KK, Barker SJ. Pulse oximetry. Anesthesiology 1989;70:98.
358. Tremper KK, Hufstedler SM, Barker SJ, et al. Accuracy of a pulse oximeter in the critically ill adult. Anesthesiology 1985;63:175.
359. Tremper KK, Katz R, Shoemaker WC. Transcutaneous $Po_2$ and $Ptco_2$ monitoring on adult ICU and intraoperative patients with and without low flow shock. Anesthesiology 1981;55:A136.
360. Tremper KK, Shoemaker WC. Transcutaneous oxygen monitoring of critically ill adults with and without low flow shock. Crit Care Med 1981;9:706.
361. Tremper KK, Shoemaker WC, Wender D. Monitoring oxygen transcutaneously in critically ill patients. N Engl J Med 1985;312:241.
362. Tremper KK, Waxman KS, Konchigeri, et al. Effects of sodium nitroprusside on the relationship between transcutaneous and arterial $Po_2$. Anesthesiology 1983;59:A158.
363. Tremper KK, Waxman K, Shoemaker WC. Effects of hypoxia and shock on transcutaneous $Po_2$ values in dogs. Crit Care Med 1979;7:526.
364. Tuchschmidt J, Mecher C, Wagers P, et al. Elevated pulmonary capillary wedge pressure in a patient with hypovolemia. J Clin Monit 1987;3:67.
365. Ulstad DR, Robbins R, Godfrey PM, et al. Transfusions and pulmonary artery catheters. Crit Care Med 1989;17:S81.
366. Vander Kleij AJ, de Koning J, Beerthuizen G, et al. Early detection of hemorrhagic hypovolemia by muscle oxygen pressure assessment: preliminary report. Surgery 1983;93:518.
367. Vara-Thorbeck R, Guerrero-Fernandez Marcote JA. Hemodynamic response of elderly patients undergoing major surgery under moderate normovolemic hemodilution. Eur Surg Res 1985;17:372.
368. Vaughn S, Puri VK. Cardiac output changes and continuous mixed venous oxygen saturation measurement in the critically ill. Crit Care Med 1988;16:495.
369. Versmold HT, Linderkamp O, Holzmann M, et al. Transcutaneous monitoring of $Po_2$ in newborn infants: where are the limits? Influences of blood pressure, blood volume, blood flow, viscosity and acid base state. The National Foundation-March of Dimes, Birth Defects 1979;15:285.
370. Vincent JL, Dufaye P, Berre J, et al. Serial lactate determinations during circulatory shock. Crit Care Med 1983;11:449.
371. Vladeck BC, Bassin R, Kark AE, et al. Rapid and slow hemorrhage in man. Ann Surg 1971;173:331.
372. Verman HJ, Groenveld AB. Blood viscosity and circulatory shock. Intensive Care Med 1989;15:72.
373. Wade OL, Bishop JM. Cardiac output and regional blood flow. Oxford: Blackwell, 1962.
374. Waller JL, Kaplan JA, Bauman DI, et al. Clinical evaluation of a new fiberoptic catheter oximeter. Anesthesiology 1981; 55:A133.
375. Waller JL, Kaplan JA, Bauman DI, et al. Clinical evaluation of a new fiberoptic catheter oximeter during cardiac surgery. Anesth Analg 1982;61:676.
376. Walt AJ, ed. Committee on Trauma, American College of Surgeons. Early care of the injured patient. 3rd ed. Philadelphia: WB Saunders, 1982:3.
377. Walt AJ, ed. Committee on Trauma, American College of Surgeons. Early care of the injured patient. 3rd ed. Philadelphia: WB Saunders, 1982:120.
378. Ward ME, Roussos C. The respiratory muscles in shock: service or disservice? Intensive Crit Care Dig (England) 1985;4:3.
379. Waxman K, Lazgrove S, Shoemaker WC. Physiologic responses to operation in high risk surgical patients. Surg Gynecol Obstet 1981;152:633.
380. Waxman K, Nolan LS, Shoemaker WC. Sequential perioperative lactate determination: physiological and clinical implications. Crit Care Med 1982;10:96.

381. Waxman K, Shoemaker WC. Physiologic responses to massive intraoperative hemorrhage. Arch Surg 1982;117:470.
382. Webb WR, Brunswick RA. Microcirculation in shock: clinical review. In: Cowley RA, Trump BF, eds. Pathophysiology of shock, anoxia and ischemia. Baltimore: Williams and Wilkins, 1982:181.
383. Weber KT, Janicki JS, Maskin CS. Pathophysiology of cardiac failure. Am J Cardiol 1985;56:3B.
384. Weil MH, Afifi AA. Experimental and clinical studies on lactate and pyruvate as indicators of the severity of acute circulatory failure (shock). Circulation 1970;41:989.
385. Weinstein ES, Hampton WW, Yokum MD, et al. Isovolemic hemodilution: correlations of mitochondrial and myocardial performance. J Trauma 1986;26:620.
386. Weiskopf RB, Townsley MI, Riordan KK, et al. Comparison of cardiopulmonary responses to graded hemorrhage during enflurane, halothane, isoflurane and ketamine anesthesia. Anesth Analg 1981;60:481.
387. Whitcher C, New W, Bacon BE. Perianesthetic oxygen saturation vs skill of the anesthetist. Anesthesiology 1982;57:A172.
388. Wiedemann HP, Mathay MA, Mathay RA. Cardiovascular-pulmonary monitoring in the intensive care unit, part 1. Chest 1984;85:537.
389. Wilkerson DK, Rosen AL, Gould SA, et al. Oxygen extraction ratio: a valid indicator of myocardial metabolism in anemia. J Surg Res 1987;42:629.
390. Willford DC, Hill EP, Moores WY. Theoretical analysis of oxygen transport during hypothermia. J Clin Monit 1986;2:30.
391. Wilson RF: Science and shock: a clinical perspective. Ann Emerg Med 1985;15:714.
392. Wilson RF, Christensen C, Leblanc LP. Oxygen consumption in critically ill surgical patients. Ann Surg 1972;176:801.
393. Wolfman EF, Neil SA, Heaps DK, et al. Donor blood and isotonic salt solution. Arch Surg 1963;86:869.
394. Woodson RD. Importance of 2,3-DPG in banked blood: new data in animal models. In: Collins JF, Murawski K, Shafer AW, eds. Massive transfusion in surgery and trauma. New York: Alan R Liss, 1982:69.
395. Woodson RD. Physiological significance of oxygen dissociation curve shifts. Crit Care Med 1979;7:368.
396. Woodson RD, Auerbach S. Effect of increased oxygen affinity and anemia on cardiac output and its distribution. J Appl Physiol 1982;53:1299.
397. Woodson RD, Fitzpatrick JH, Costello DJ, et al. Increased blood oxygen affinity decreases canine brain oxygen consumption. J Lab Clin Med 1982;100:411.
398. Yelderman M, New W. Evaluation of pulse oximetry. Anesthesiology 1983;59:349.

# Chapter Six

Donald P. Bernstein

# Transfusion Therapy in Trauma

After initial resuscitation of the hypovolemic patient with acellular fluids to restore intravascular volume and stabilize vital signs and organ perfusion, the anesthesiologist must consider the necessity for blood transfusion. The decision to transfuse homologous bank blood and its components should be weighed against the complications inherent in this form of therapy.[122] This is not to say that transfusion therapy should be withheld if indicated. Complications of inadequate tissue oxygenation due to a critically reduced red cell mass may lead to irreversible organ damage and death.[51] In the injured, coagulopathies may also arise, necessitating blood component therapy.

Rational transfusion therapy requires a knowledge of oxygen transport, oxygen consumption, and the pathophysiologic derangements to which these parameters are subjected in hemorrhage and its sequel, hemorrhagic shock. These topics are fully discussed in Chapter 5. In addition, a fundamental understanding of the immunology of blood is necessary because a homologous transfusion is a tissue transplant! Because of its unique method of preservation, banked blood undergoes metabolic and biochemical changes that may seem serious but are in general quite benign.[179] Thus, transfusion of blood is rational only when these variables are clearly understood.[318]

## COMPATIBILITY TESTING IN EMERGENCY TRANSFUSION

This section will not include an exhaustive review of the subject since space is limited, and complete discussions may be found elsewhere.[10,149,214,278] The following is offered as a distilled summary.

### BLOOD TYPE

Drawing blood for serologic typing is mandatory before any transfusion is initiated. Each of the four major blood groups (A, B, AB, and O) is characterized by specific antigens on the red cell membrane. The Caucasian population of the United States has approximately the following distribution of the major blood groups: O, 47%; A, 42%; B, 8%; AB, 3%.[10] In addition, the Rh(D) (Rhesus) antigen is present on the erythrocytes of 85% of the population. Patients whose red cells contain this antigen are categorized as Rh positive. Also, present in the serum are antibodies (anti-A and anti-B) that are formed whenever the red cell membrane is devoid of the A and/or B antigen, respectively. Patients who are Rh negative, however, do not possess Rh (D) antibodies.

### CROSS-MATCH

A complete cross-match is an in vitro "transfusion" that is designed to simulate the in vivo compatibility of donor red cell antigens with recipient serum antibodies. It requires 45 to 60 minutes to perform.

There are three phases to a complete cross-match.

#### *Phase 1: Intermediate*

Donor red cells are mixed with recipient serum at room temperature. Here gross errors in ABO typing as well as the presence of naturally occurring antibodies to the MNS, P, and Lewis systems are detected.

### *Phase 2: Incubation*

Specimens from phase 1 are incubated in albumin at 37°C, which permits detection of incomplete antibodies or those capable of reacting with specific antigens but incapable of causing agglutination in a saline suspension of red cells. Phase 2 also detects the rare antibodies to the Rh system, which may be present if previous sensitization has taken place.

### *Phase 3: Indirect Antiglobulin Test*

The addition of Coombs, or human antiglobulin serum, to phase 2 incubated test tubes detects immunoglobulin G surface antibodies on the red cells. Agglutination in this phase detects most of the incomplete antibodies capable of causing severe hemolytic reactions against the Kell, Kidd, and Duffy antigens.

### TYPE AND ANTIBODY SCREEN

This form of compatibility testing is used primarily to improve the distribution of a relatively small quantity of donor blood to the large group of potential recipients who are statistically not likely to require blood during elective surgery. The technique of "type and antibody screen" involves combining the potential recipient's serum with commercially supplied type-specific red cells[264] that contain an optimal concentration of surface antigens. Testing is carried out in the three phases described above.

It is also necessary to screen donor serum in a similar manner to ensure that it does not contain antibodies that may agglutinate recipient red cells. The time required for a type and screen is similar to that for a type and cross-match. Type and screen is used primarily to improve availability of blood and to prevent wastage. Consequently, it is inappropriate to order type and screen for any circumstance in which blood will definitely be given. Type and screen of elective patients, however, improves the availability of blood for trauma victims.[10]

### TYPE AND PARTIAL CROSS-MATCH

This involves taking typed recipient serum, combining it with donor red cells in saline at room temperature, and after centrifuging for 5 seconds, observing for macroscopic agglutination. This procedure obviates errors that may have occurred during ABO typing.

## PROTOCOL FOR EMERGENCY BLOOD TRANSFUSION

Patients identified as hypovolemic due to severe hemorrhage will ideally have several large-bore venous catheters in place.[3,65,84,136,155,197,212] Crystalloid infusion, warmed and preferably under pressure, should be initiated to restore circulating blood volume and cardiac output rapidly.[3,65,84,102,176,304,362] During the course of initial resuscitation, blood must be drawn for type and cross-match. If the patient responds to initial volume infusion, the blood should undergo complete cross-matching to ensure maximum safety. However, if hypovolemia is severe enough to compromise tissue oxygenation and acellular fluid infusion is not likely to cause any improvement, then an un–cross-matched transfusion must be considered[181,309] (see also Chapter 4).

Initially, before oxygen transport indices are measured, blood and crystalloid can be administered according to the Advanced Trauma Life Support (ATLS) guidelines, using estimated blood loss, vital signs, and other signs and symptoms as guides to treatment (Table 6-1). This should be done with care because the ATLS algorithm can occasionally result in excessive or inadequate therapy.[383]

### TYPE-SPECIFIC, PARTIALLY CROSS-MATCHED BLOOD

If time permits (5 to 10 minutes), a type and partial cross-match should be performed. If no agglutination is noted, these units should be released and transfused immediately.[10]

### TYPE-SPECIFIC, UN–CROSS-MATCHED BLOOD

If time does not permit a partial cross-match, un–cross-matched type-specific blood may be transfused with relative safety.[10,53] During a 1-year period in a nonmilitary setting, Blumberg and Bove[19] successfully transfused 49 patients with 221 U of type-specific un–cross-matched blood without apparent adverse effects. However, they cautioned against the routine use of un–cross-matched blood, as the possibility of serious hemolytic transfusion reactions still exists. In a more recent study, Gervin and Fischer[109] reported the administration of 875 U of type-specific un–cross-matched blood to 160 severely hypovolemic trauma patients. No transfusion reactions resulted, and subsequent complete cross-matching of the dispensed units failed to reveal blood incompatibility or significant antibodies. Similar results reported by others are reviewed by Barnes.[10] Approximately 1 in 800 patients (0.13%) exhibits an abnormal serum antibody during complete cross-match, and only 1 in 2500 (0.04%) has antibodies capable of causing hemolysis.[321] Therefore, although type-specific un–cross-matched blood may be necessary and is relatively safe, caution is advised, especially in pregnant or previously transfused patients.[10]

### GROUP O, Rh NEGATIVE RED CELL CONCENTRATES (PACKED CELLS) AND "UNIVERSAL DONOR" WHOLE BLOOD

Since group O, Rh negative red blood cells lack A, B, and Rh surface antigens, they may be given to the vast majority of potential recipients.[10,109,181,309] However, the absence of the major antigens does not preclude other less common groups.[262] This is important only when the recipient's serum contains antibodies to these unexpected antigens. Since most of the population lacks these antibodies, transfusion of group O Rh negative red cells is relatively safe.[181] If the gravity of the clinical situation dictates emergency transfusion and type-specific blood is not available, then group O, Rh negative cells

TABLE 6-1. Estimated Fluid and Blood Requirements in a 70-kg Male*

| | INITIAL PRESENTATIONS | | | |
|---|---|---|---|---|
| | *Class I* | *Class II* | *Class III* | *Class IV* |
| Blood loss (ml) | <750 | 750 to 1500 | 1500 to 2000 | ≥2000 |
| Blood loss (% BV) | <15% | 15 to 30% | 30 to 40% | ≥40% |
| Pulse rate | <100 | >100 | >120 | ≥140 |
| Blood pressure | Normal | Normal | Decreased | Decreased |
| Pulse pressure (mm Hg) | Normal or increased | Decreased | Decreased | Decreased |
| Capillary blanch test | Normal | Positive | Positive | Positive |
| Respiratory rate | 14 to 20 | 20 to 30 | 30 to 40 | >35 |
| Urine output (mL/h) | 30 or more | 20 to 30 | 5 to 15 | Negligible |
| CNS—mental status | Slightly anxious | Mildly anxious | Anxious and confused | Confused and lethargic |
| Fluid replacement (3:1 rule) | Crystalloid | Crystalloid | Crystalloid + blood | Crystalloid + blood |

* From the American College of Surgeons (ACS) Committee on Trauma. *Advanced Trauma Life Support Course, Instructor Manual*, 1983/1984.

(packed cells)* should be given.[10,181,309] Group O, Rh negative blood should probably not be given as whole blood.[10] The serum of blood of this type may contain high anti-A and anti-B titers that may cause hemolysis of recipient red cells. Moreover, if more than 4 U of O negative whole blood is administered, type-specific blood should not be given subsequently since the potentially high anti-A and -B titers could cause hemolysis of the donor blood.[9,10] However, anti-A, anti-B, agglutination titers of less than 1/200 in group O Rh negative whole blood identify it as true "universal donor" blood. These low antibody titers are not likely to cause hemolysis of recipient cells or of subsequently administered group-specific red blood cells. Unfortunately, anti-A, anti-B serum titers are no longer assayed; hence, potentially hemolytic donor serum may be transfused. In any event, if significant volumes of group O, Rh negative *whole blood* have been given, and it is desirable to switch to the patient's blood type, recipient anti-A and anti-B titers should be determined by the blood bank.[10] On the other hand, patients may be switched to type-specific blood even after transfusion of as much as 10 U of group O, Rh negative *red cells,* since there is an insignificant risk of hemolysis from the small volume of plasma administered with red cells.[309]

Indiscriminate use of group O, Rh negative red cells or whole blood in emergencies, however, should be condemned. During military combat, Monaghan et al.[233] found that only 157 U of group O, Rh negative blood were administered because urgency precluded the administration of type-specific blood in approximately 2900 hemorrhaging casualties over a 4-year period.

In summary, if time permits, fully typed and cross-matched blood is, without a doubt, the safest product to transfuse. In life-threatening situations, partially cross-matched or un–cross-matched type-specific blood should be administered. In the rare circumstance in which the above products are unavailable or the patient is close to exsanguination, group O, Rh negative red cells should be given.[181] If the patient has received group O, Rh negative blood, transfusion should be switched to type-specific blood as soon as possible. When universal donor whole blood has been given in large amounts, caution should be exercised in changing back to type-specific blood.[10] It should be noted that some active trauma centers use group O, Rh positive red cells in mass casualty situations,[53] probably because group O, Rh negative blood is always in short supply. Moreover, the notion that type-specific blood can be provided within 5 minutes is considered by many to be unrealistic; 20 minutes or longer may be required.[53] Following transfusion of group O, Rh positive red cells, approximately 75% of Rh negative recipients develop Rh antibodies.[53] This is an important consideration in female trauma victims of childbearing age and in individuals who may require transfusions in the future.

* In this chapter, the terms *red cells* or *red blood cells* are synonymous with the older usage of *packed cells.*

The most important principles in emergency transfusion are[233]:

1. Proper patient identification and labeling of specimens for type and cross-match
2. Proper patient identification and checking of donor units before any transfusion is started.

Most fatal hemolytic transfusion reactions (HTRs) are the result of clerical error.[249,250] In a review of transfusion-associated fatalities, Honig and Bove[143] found that of 44 HTRs reported, 38 cases (86%) were caused by transfusions of ABO-incompatible blood because of clerical error. The largest number of transfusion errors, with or without HTR, was due to administration of cross-match-compatible blood . . . *to the wrong patient!*

## BLOOD STORAGE AND PRESERVATION

Essentially, transfusion of compatible blood from one individual to another is a *graft* of living tissue. Ever since the riddle of histocompatibility was solved, new and better ways of blood preservation have been sought.[77] For transfusion to be successful (ie, to improve tissue oxygenation and hemostasis), transfused red cells or whole blood must be preserved in a storage solution that maintains red cell viability and function and prevents coagulation.

## VIABILITY AND FUNCTION

The red blood cell produces energy by anaerobically metabolizing each mol of glucose to generate 2 mol of adenosine 5′-triphosphate (ATP) and 2 mol of lactic acid. The ATP is responsible for the energy required for gas exchange, maintenance of cell shape and membrane activity, maintenance of reduced hemoglobin, and transport of ions across the cell membranes.[157] A decreased level of intraerythrocytic ATP is associated with change in shape (disc to spheroidal), reduction of membrane lipid activity, increased osmotic fragility, and increased cellular rigidity.[125] These changes are associated with decreased posttransfusion red cell survival time.[75,216,374]

Blood preservation began in 1916, when dextrose was added to the anticoagulant citrate. In 1914, it was shown that intravenous citrate was safe when given to humans. Citrate-dextrose-preserved blood was successfully given to British soldiers in 1917 and to the armies of the Spanish Civil War in 1937. During World War II, the importance of acidification of dextrose to prevent caramelization during autoclaving was demonstrated. This work resulted in the development of ACD (acid-citrate-dextrose), which allowed a shelf life of 21 days. After World War II, the U.S. federal standard for shelf life was set at 70% survival of transfused red cells 24 hours after administration.[68]

The past 3 decades have witnessed the development and clinical introduction of the preservatives citrate-phosphate-dextrose (CPD) and citrate-phosphate-dextrose-adenine-1 (CPDA-1). Addition of phosphate reduced the need for citrate by 25%, thus raising the pH. Moreover, it provided inorganic phosphate as a substrate for glycolysis and ATP production. It has been demonstrated clearly that although the standard storage time for cells in CPD is only 21 days, they actually have a posttransfusion survival of more than 75% after 28 days.[68]

The addition of 0.25 mmol/L adenine and 25% more glucose to CPD further increased the survival time of transfused red cells to 35 days (Fig 6-1). This development brings us to the present. Further addition of adenine (Adsol-AS1) has been shown to enhance 70% survival of red cells to 49 days and of whole blood to 56 days.[68] Adsol, a preservative containing mannitol in addition to saline, dextrose, and adenine, assures a 42-day shelf life. It is now used widely. The early fears of nephrotoxicity and renal failure from the metabolism of adenine to dihydroxyadenine have been dispelled. A dose of adenine equivalent to 60 U of CPDA-1 has been given to humans without permanent sequelae.[95]

Obviously, much work has been accomplished in maintaining morphologic viability; but is red cell function also preserved? Unfortunately, the decreased ability of stored red cells to release $O_2$ to the tissues has been studied, but the issue is not resolved. In 1954, Valtis and Kennedy[356] made the first observation that blood stored in ACD preservative solution had increased $O_2$ affinity. Subsequently, Benesch and Benesch[15] and Chanutin and Curnish[43] demonstrated that organic phosphates within the red cells interact with hemoglobin and reduce its affinity for $O_2$. The principal compound implicated was 2,3-diphosphoglycerate (2,3-DPG), decreasing levels of which were directly correlated to increasing $O_2$ affinity in stored blood.[37]

The depletion of red cell 2,3-DPG during storage is caused by the acidity of the preservative solution and by continued anaerobic glycolysis with production of $CO_2$ and lactate. Two enzymes control the level of 2,3-DPG. 2,3-DPG mutase controls the synthesis of 2,3-DPG, which is facilitated by a neutral pH. 2,3-DPG phosphatase catalyzes the degradation of 2,3-DPG and is most active in an acidic environment.[217] Fig 6-2 depicts the decline of 2,3-DPG levels in CPD and CPDA-1 solution. After 10 days of storage, 2,3-DPG levels are approximately 50% of normal. By 3 weeks, they are approximately 10% of normal and decline little thereafter.[238] Various attempts to maintain 2,3-DPG levels have been made.[157] Purine nucleosides, primarily inosine, have been used in Europe. Un-

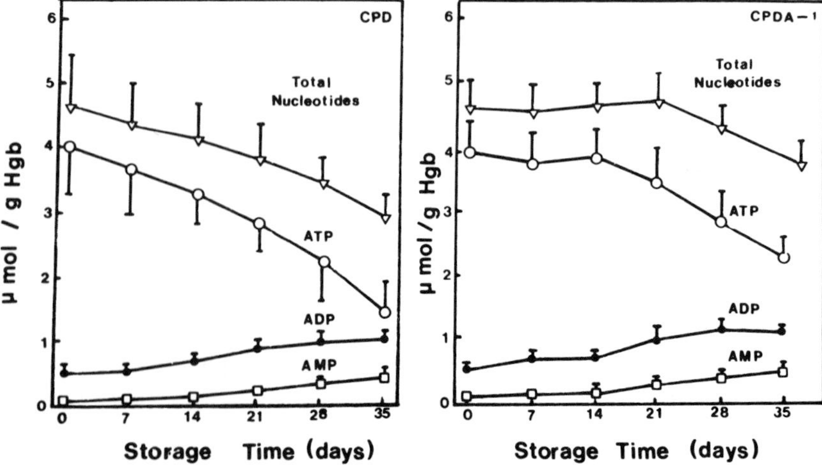


FIG. 6-1. Levels of ATP and total nucleotides contained in erythrocytes preserved in CPDA-1 (right) compared with those preserved in CPD anticoagulant (left). The higher ATP levels of cells preserved in CPDA-1 extend the morphologic viability and shelf life to 35 days. (From Moroff and Dende[238] with permission.)

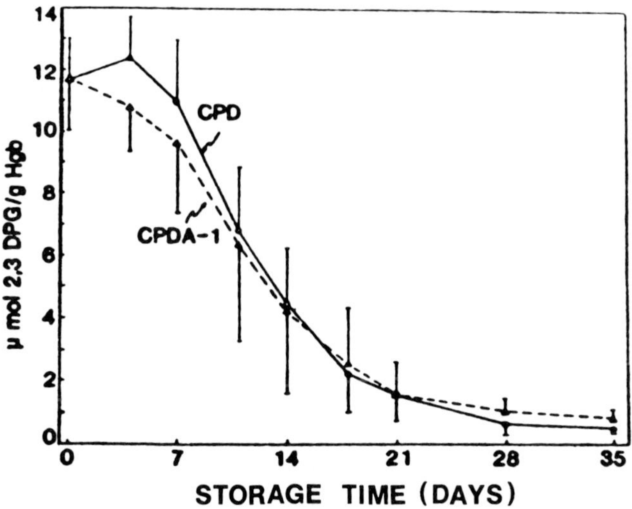


FIG. 6-2. Changes in 2,3-DPG levels during storage of red cells anticoagulated with CPD (solid line) or CPDA-1 (dashed line). The only significant difference is at 3 days ($P < 0.01$). (From Moroff and Dende[238] with permission.)

fortunately, inosine is metabolized to uric acid, which may be deposited in the kidney.[218] Other additives such as phosphoenolpyruvate,[124] dihydroxyacetone,[270] and ascorbate 2-phosphate[236] have been shown to elevate and maintain 2,3-DPG levels but usually at the expense of decreased ATP concentration and therefore, of reduced viability.[235] Present research is aimed at optimizing both viability and function; but since the clinical importance of normal levels of 2,3-DPG has yet to be established, preservation of morphologic viability has taken preference. A discussion of the significance of 2,3-DPG is presented in the section on complications of massive transfusion.

The biochemical characteristics of stored whole blood are given in Table 6-2.[238] As can be seen, there are significant elevations of plasma $K^+$ and free hemoglobin in banked blood, as well as significant increases of lactate and $CO_2$ with consequent reduction in pH.

## STORAGE LESIONS OF BLOOD

The chemical and cellular changes that result from collection, storage, and continued metabolism of preserved blood are referred to as *storage lesions*.

### *Changes in Hemostatic Components*

FACTORS V AND VIII The storage of whole blood at 4°C appears to have little effect on the plasma levels of most coagulation factors except for the labile factors V and VIII[39,254] (Figs 6-3 and 6-4, respectively). Even though its level is reduced, the factor V concentration in ACD blood 21 days after collection ranges from 20 to 60 U/dL, whereas only 10 to 15 U/dL is needed for normal hemostasis.[284,291] Likewise, factor VIII levels in ACD blood at 21 days range from 20 to 50 U/dL, whereas only 25 to 30 U/dL is required for adequate clotting.[284,291] Thus, stored whole blood contains sufficient coagulation factors to achieve hemostasis in most clinical situations.[62,205] Moreover, the stress of trauma stimulates a rise in plasma factor VIII levels.[62] Obviously, the concentrations of factor V and factor VIII are reduced significantly in stored red cells, even when the product is fresh.

PLATELETS The only true hemostatic deficiency in stored whole blood is the lack of functional platelets.[62,208,325] Storage of platelets at 4°C for 24 hours results in an irreversible loss of shape and functional ability.[219] Only 20% of platelets are viable in whole blood after 72 hours of storage.[171] For all intents and purposes, then, blood stored for longer than 2 days can be considered functionally devoid of platelets.

TABLE 6-2. Biochemical Characteristics of Stored Whole Blood

| | CPD ($N$ = 8) | | CPDA-1 ($N$ = 8) | |
|---|---|---|---|---|
| CHARACTERISTICS | *Day 0* | *Day 21* | *Day 0* | *Day 35* |
| Plasma glucose (mg/dL) | 337 ± 49* | 222 ± 32 | 388 ± 36 | 246 ± 30 |
| Total blood glucose (mg/dL) | 351 ± 24 | 210 ± 32.5 | 366 ± 16 | 227 ± 26 |
| ATP mol/(g Hgb) | 4.1 ± 0.5 | 2.5 ± 0.5 | 3.5 ± 0.3 | 1.8 ± 0.3 |
| Red cell $K^+$ (mEq/L)† | 94 ± 2 | 66 ± 3 | 93 ± 3.8 | 61 ± 3.3 |
| Red cell $Na^+$ (mEq/L)† | 12 ± 1.6 | 34 ± 4.5 | 14 ± 2 | 41 ± 3 |
| Plasma $K^+$ (mEq/L)† | 3.4 ± 0.2 | 22 ± 2 | 4 ± 0.5 | 28 ± 2. |
| Plasma $Na^+$ (mEq/L)† | 169 ± 4 | 154 ± 1.5 | 167 ± 6 | 153 ± 5. |
| Plasma hemoglobin (mg/dL) | 1.5 ± 1.5 | 18 ± 9 | 5 ± 3 | 34 ± 1 |
| % hemolysis | | 0.1 ± 0.04 | | 0.2 ± |
| pH (37°C) | 7.1 ± 0.07 | 6.86 ± 0.17 | 7.2 ± 0.05 | 6.8 ± |
| Hematocrit (%) | 39 ± 3.2 | 40 ± 3 | 39 ± 3 | 40 ± |
| Blood volume (mL) | 474 ± 6.2 | | 466 ± 13 | |

* Data are expressed as mean ± SD.
† Units were held for 4 hours at 20 to 24°C following phlebotomy. Day 0 values represen at the completion of this holding period. Units were not mixed during storage.
(From Moroff and Dende,[238] with permission.)

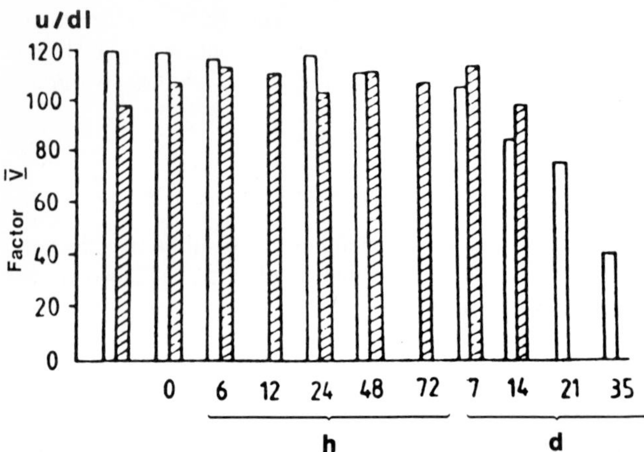


FIG. 6-3. Mean factor V activity (U/dL) in whole blood (□) and plasma (▨). Assays done immediately (0 hours) and at various time intervals after collection of blood. h, hours; d, days. (From Nilsson et al[254] with permission.)

## COMPLICATIONS OF MASSIVE TRANSFUSION RELATED TO STORAGE LESIONS

Massive transfusion may be defined as the administration of at least 1 to 1.5 times the patient's estimated blood volume during a 6- to 8-hour period. Because banked blood undergoes metabolic and degradative changes during storage, many clinicians and researchers have ascribed the complications of massive transfusion to these changes. Some of these problems are predictable, some are theoretical, and some are questionably predictable from the observed alterations during storage. In addition, some of the complications historically ascribed to massive transfusion appear to be caused by undertransfusion and hypovolemia.[49,204] Lastly, some complications may be caused by empiric treatment of suspected deficiencies or excesses.

FIG. 6-4. Mean factor VIII activity (U/dL) in whole blood (□) and plasma (▨). Mean values obtained after various storage times. h, hours; d, days. (From Nilsson et al[254] with permission.)

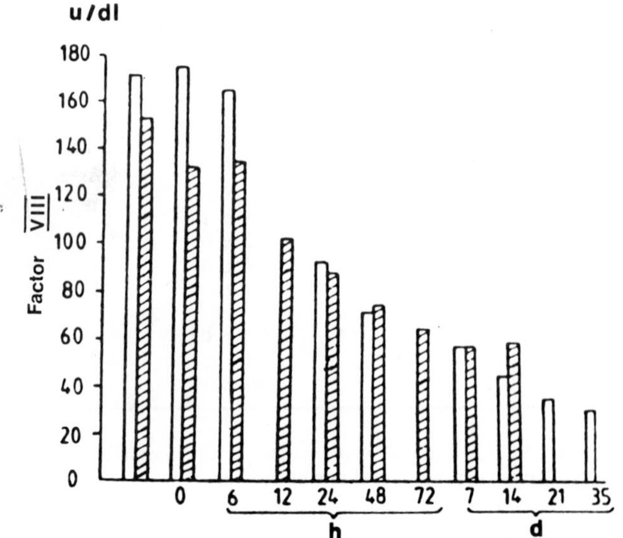


### PREDICTABLE COMPLICATIONS RELATED TO LOSS OF PLATELET FUNCTION

Dilutional thrombocytopenia occurs frequently during massive transfusion and may cause microvascular bleeding.[61,62,208,325] There is a relationship between the platelet count and the number of units transfused[61,257] (Fig 6-5). In an elegant prospective study by Counts et al[62] of 27 patients receiving a mean of 33 U of modified whole blood, 8 (24%) developed generalized "oozing," due to dilutional thrombocytopenia in 5 patients and to disseminated intravascular coagulation (DIC) in the remaining 3. They concluded that platelet counts should be monitored closely after 1.5 to 2.0 blood volumes are replaced.[276] However, the absolute platelet count is less important than the fact that functional thrombocytopenia may produce coagulopathy. Normal platelet counts have wide variations so that a platelet count of 80,000/μL may provide adequate hemostasis for one individual, whereas greater than 100,000/μL may be insufficient for another.[62,325] It should be noted that laboratory tests such as the bleeding time are useful only if the result is markedly abnormal.[62] Many patients have only moderately prolonged bleeding times, moderate thrombocytopenia, and no clinically apparent hemostatic defect following massive transfusion.[62,130,285] Thus, patients should receive platelets only if generalized oozing becomes apparent.[4] Counts's group concluded more recently that routine prophylactic platelet administration is not warranted during massive blood transfusion.[285]

In summary, if generalized oozing occurs during massive transfusion, platelets should be administered and other

FIG. 6-5. Comparison between mean observed and predicted (calculated) platelet counts during massive transfusion. It is assumed that the stored blood is platelet free. (From Miller et al[208] with permission.)

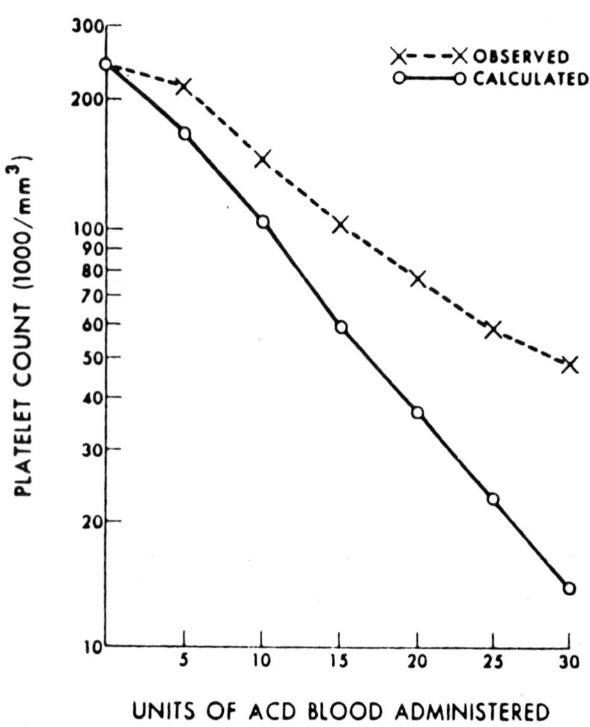

causes of the hemorrhagic diathesis investigated. Reliance on the platelet count or bleeding time will only confuse the issue. In addition, platelets should never be given empirically or prophylactically according to some cookbook recipe.[4] A platelet count above 50,000/μL is adequate in the majority of patients for primary hemostasis during massive transfusion.[62,208] However, one can never be sure of the functional quality of these platelets[184] even if their numbers exceed 100,000/μL.

## UNCOMMON COMPLICATIONS OF EQUIVOCAL SIGNIFICANCE

### *Citrate Intoxication*

This term should more aptly be *citrate-induced decrease in serum ionized calcium* ($Ca^{2+}$).[145] Since citrate binds $Ca^{2+}$ in vitro and hence acts as an anticoagulant, early concerns were that large volumes of citrated blood would cause hemostatic defects and depression of the cardiovascular system in vivo. The latter fear was compounded by Strawitz et al,[336] who demonstrated dramatic improvement in systemic blood pressure (BP), pulse pressure, and peripheral perfusion following administration of calcium after massive transfusion of soldiers with ACD blood during the Korean conflict. Moreover, Bunker et al[36] noted hemodynamic depression after infusion of sodium citrate solution in doses equivalent to blood transfused at 20 U/h. The cardiovascular effect was associated with elevated serum citrate and reduction of calculated serum $Ca^{2+}$ levels. Howland et al and others have also found decreased serum $Ca^{2+}$ with associated elevation of serum citrate during massive transfusion.[129,147,148,160,350] However, at no time did their patients exhibit significant deterioration of cardiac output ($\dot{Q}_t$), central venous pressure (CVP), pulmonary capillary wedge pressure (PCWP), or BP. A prolonged QT interval on the electrocardiogram (ECG) was the only finding associated with these alterations in serum $Ca^{2+}$ and citrate. However, there remain isolated case reports linking rapid transfusion with cardiac failure,[12,60] but prolongation of the QT interval is not a consistent observation.[178] During rapid transfusion, the decrease in serum $Ca^{2+}$ is directly related to the rate of infusion.[2,60,73,82,160] If normovolemia is maintained, serum $Ca^{2+}$ levels rise immediately after cessation of blood administration[60,73,82] (Fig 6-6 and Fig 6-7).

Citrate is a normal intermediary metabolite and is rapidly metabolized after transfusion,[49] principally in the liver, kidneys, and skeletal muscle.[129,160] Hence, blood flow reduction to these areas may result in decreased citrate breakdown. Citrate elimination in the urine is also reduced in low-flow states.[2] The metabolic degradation of citrate is retarded by hypothermia, liver disease, and acidosis.[190] Therefore, depression of serum $Ca^{2+}$ is enhanced when these conditions are present.

It should be noted that hypomagnesemia can result from elevated citrate levels and is associated with tachydysrhythmias, refractory ventricular fibrillation, and sudden death.[201] A comprehensive review of the significance of magnesium to anesthesia has appeared recently.[107]

The serum $Ca^{2+}$ level is controlled by several complicated dynamic equilibria and by the action of parathyroid hormone (PTH) on bone.[2,73,129] It has been shown that infusion of citrate elicits an almost immediate rise in serum PTH.[211] The ability of bone to mobilize $Ca^{2+}$ is largely dependent on blood flow. This effect was described by Harrigan et al[129] who found that after massive trauma with hypovolemic shock and subsequent massive transfusion, serum $Ca^{2+}$ levels remained depressed for 24 hours postoperatively, long after the termination of transfusion. However, their patients displayed no cardiovascular instability directly attributable to hypocalcemia. They concluded that the decreased $Ca^{2+}$ level seen in the massively bleeding trauma patient is due to inadequate end-organ response to PTH, redistribution of $Ca^{2+}$ to the intracellular fluid, and the $Ca^{2+}$-binding effects of citrated blood. Even following calcium administration, serum $Ca^{2+}$ levels may remain low for 24 hours postoperatively.[129]

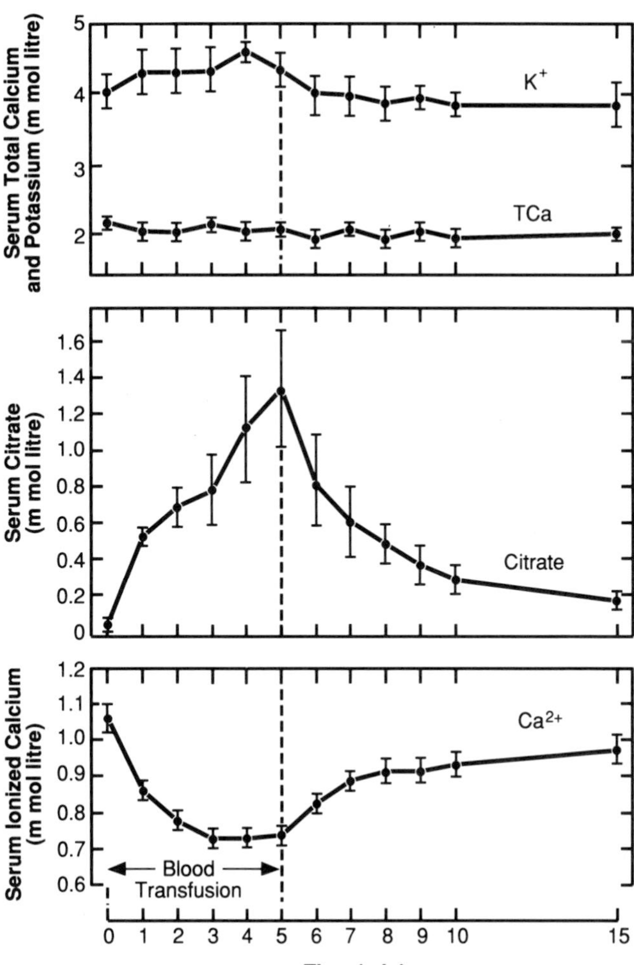


FIG. 6-6. Serum $K^+$, total calcium (TCa), serum citrate, and serum ionized calcium ($Ca^{2+}$) changes during blood transfusion at 100 mL/70 kg/min in four patients. Note that serum $K^+$ rises slightly, total serum calcium remains unchanged, but serum ionized calcium ($Ca^{2+}$) falls dramatically with the rise in serum citrate. (From Denlinger et al[73] with permission.)

It has been emphasized by Hauser et al[133] that a common thread unites most if not all of the hypocalcemias (excluding, of course, hypoparathyroidism): hypoperfusion of bone due to catecholamine release, and decreased and maldistributed systemic perfusion with subsequent end-organ unresponsive-

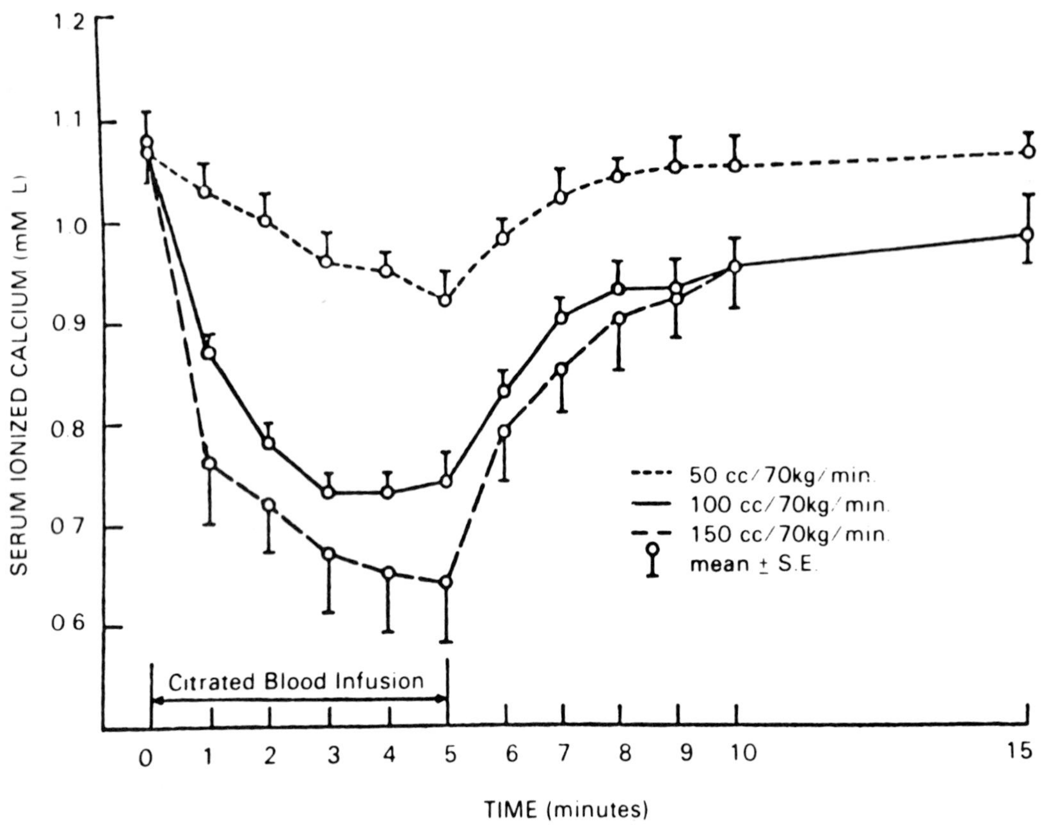


FIG. 6-7. Serum ionized calcium ($Ca^{2+}$) during and following blood transfusion at three flow rates. (From Denlinger et al[73] with permission.)

ness to elevated levels of PTH. Normal serum $Ca^{2+}$ levels are reestablished only when hypovolemia is corrected.

Is the treatment of low serum $Ca^{2+}$ necessary?[5] This question has not yet been answered clearly, but the fact remains that empiric treatment of hypocalcemia may be detrimental.[82,373] Friedman et al[106] reported several episodes of cardiac arrest immediately following administration of calcium during the transfusion of ACD blood. Routine calcium administration has probably been lethal in innumerable cases.[373] It must also be appreciated that infusion of calcium has only an evanescent inotropic effect.[82,83,314,361] In addition, intravenous $CaCl_2$ may cause systemic vasoconstriction.[82,253,314] Thus, the elevation of systemic blood pressure seen with $CaCl_2$ infusion is in part due to increased vascular resistance, which may be detrimental to the microvascular beds emerging from the reduction in blood flow induced by hemorrhagic hypovolemia. Theoretically, at least, the enhancement of oxygen consumption ($\dot{V}O_2$) during resuscitation from hemorrhagic shock may be retarded by the empiric infusion of calcium salts. Another possible hazard of empiric $CaCl_2$ administration is activation of the fibrinolytic system because of an excess of a plasminogen activator. This may result in generalized oozing.[94]

As a rule of thumb, blood transfusions not exceeding 1.4 mL/min/kg (1 U of whole blood administered to a 70-kg man in 5 minutes) should cause no citrate-related problems.[49,73] Courcy et al[63] reported a patient with hemorrhagic shock who was treated successfully with the equivalent of 173 U of whole blood given over a period of 30 hours. No calcium salts were administered, and no hemodynamic instability attributable to hypocalcemia was encountered during or after the transfusion. In this patient, blood was administered at a rate of approximately 1 U every 10 minutes.

### *Affinity Hypoxia*

As discussed previously, red blood cell storage results in significant depletion of 2,3-DPG after approximately 1 week.[238] The sole purpose of transfusing red cells to the oligemic patient is to improve $O_2$ delivery ($\dot{D}O_2$) to the tissues. The improved oxygenation augments $O_2$ utilization, reducing anaerobic metabolism and lactic acidosis. In order to reach the cells, $O_2$ must be released from hemoglobin, traverse the red cell membrane, diffuse through the plasma, and finally traverse the capillary wall and the cell membrane. If the ability to unload $O_2$ from hemoglobin is reduced, could this prevent transfused blood from improving cellular oxygenation?[161] In other words, does the leftward shift of the oxyhemoglobin dissociation curve compromise $O_2$ delivery to vital organs?[88,200]

The normal in vivo response to hemorrhage is augmented synthesis of 2,3-DPG with resulting increase in $P_{50}$ and decreased $O_2$ affinity of hemoglobin.[138] Sugerman et al[337] noted a leftward shift of the oxyhemoglobin dissociation curve and lowered $P\bar{v}O_2$ values after massive transfusion with 2,3-DPG depleted blood in a group of five patients. However, their patients suffered no complications that could be attributed to the transfusion. Reports from Vietnam on patients massively transfused with 2,3-DPG depleted ACD blood also showed no clinical evidence of impaired tissue oxygenation.[25] Metabolic studies in these patients revealed rapid clearing of lactic acidosis.[55] These combat casualties were young and in optimal physical condition. $O_2$ transport and delivery are influenced by cardiac output; regional autoregulation of the heart, brain, and other organs; hemoglobin concentration; and $Sa_{O_2}$. The ability of hemoglobin to bind, carry, and release $O_2$ is only one of the mechanisms ensuring adequate tissue oxygenation. Thus, on the basis of available data, it appears that in healthy individuals, cardiovascular and pulmonary homeostatic mechanisms adequately compensate for altered hemoglobin $O_2$ affinity.[377] In addition, 2,3-DPG is rapidly regenerated during transfusion. Valeri and Hirsch[355] found that red cell 2,3-DPG was regenerated to 25% of normal within 3 hours and 50% of normal in 24 hours. Beutler and Wood[17] found regeneration to be 50% of normal within 5 hours of transfusion. In addition, if transfused red cells (CPDA-1) have been stored for less than a week, nearly normal levels of 2,3-DPG are found.[238]

When normal compensatory mechanisms are altered by disease states such as coronary or cerebrovascular insufficiency, altered hemoglobin affinity for $O_2$ may result in impaired oxygenation of the heart and brain.[88,376,379,380] The heart has the highest $O_2$ extraction rate (11.4 volume %) and the highest $O_2$ consumption index (9.6 mL/100 g/min) of all the vital organs. Consequently, the heart utilizes approximately 85% of the available $O_2$ from red cells in the coronary circulation (see Chapter 5). In fact, the $P\bar{v}_{O_2}$ of human coronary sinus blood is only 23 to 27 mm Hg at rest. Thus, any adverse alteration in the $O_2$ supply-demand ratio may result in myocardial ischemia and reduced performance.[88,345] For instance, myocardial blood flow is reduced moderately when coronary stenosis is 60 to 70% and markedly when it is 90%.[162] In order for myocardial $O_2$ supply to at least equal demand in the face of reduced coronary blood flow, hemoglobin concentration and saturation must be optimal.[88] Moreover, the ability of hemoglobin to release $O_2$ must be optimal; ideally this hemoglobin should have a reduced affinity.[88,270] At any given venous oxygen content or saturation, a leftward shift of the oxyhemoglobin dissociation curve results in decreased consumable $O_2$,[32,88,379,380] whereas a rightward shift increases $O_2$ delivery[315,381,382] (see Fig 5-7 and Fig 5-8 in Chapter 5).

Clinical and experimental studies evaluating the effects of 2,3-DPG-depleted red cells on myocardial oxygenation are inconclusive but provocative. Dennis et al[74] evaluated 22 patients with severe coronary artery disease undergoing coronary artery bypass grafting. Postoperative cardiovascular function following transfusion with blood containing high or low levels of 2,3-DPG was evaluated. The group that received elevated 2,3-DPG blood (150% of normal) had a trend toward higher cardiac indices and improved oxygen consumption. Cardiac performance, as measured by PCWP in response to fluid challenge, was also improved in this group. In vivo indices of $P_{50}$, arterial-mixed venous oxygen content difference $(A\text{-}\bar{v})\ D_{O_2}$, and $\dot{V}_{O_2}$ were all increased in the patients treated with high 2,3-DPG blood.

Baboons resuscitated from hemorrhagic shock with 2,3-DPG-depleted blood were shown to require more hemodynamic compensation than those transfused with 2,3-DPG-rejuvenated blood.[289] The inference is that patients with severe coronary stenosis may have a protracted and even unsuccessful surgical result if old banked blood is used for resuscitation.

Pantely and associates,[270] in an experimental myocardial infarction model in dogs, have demonstrated a reduction in the extent of myocardial necrosis when high $P_{50}$ blood is used. Briefly, this study demonstrated an augmentation of myocardial tissue oxygenation with transfusion of increased $P_{50}$ blood when myocardial blood flow was restricted.

Malmberg et al[193] have noted in rats that prior normovolemic exchange transfusion of blood with high oxygen affinity reduced survival time in hemorrhagic shock as compared with controls. Moreover, when compared with control rats that were hemorrhaged and reinfused with normal 2,3-DPG blood, rats transfused with low 2,3-DPG blood experienced 20 to 35% higher mortality. Similar results were reported by Collins and Stechenberg[56] in a hemorrhagic shock model simulating clinical conditions. In another study[378] when normal rats were exchange transfused with high $O_2$ affinity blood, coronary and cerebral blood flow increased by 100 and 88%, respectively, compared with controls transfused with normal $P_{50}$ blood. If normovolemic anemia and high blood $O_2$ affinity were superimposed,[376,378] coronary and cerebral blood flow increased by 280 and 125%, respectively, compared with control rats. These data indicate that in the normal animal, compensatory autoregulatory changes in coronary and cerebral blood flow occur to prevent the fall in myocardial and cerebral tissue $P_{O_2}$.

To assess the effect of perfusion with altered $P_{50}$ blood in the presence of constant cerebral blood flow (mimicking insufficiency) on cerebral oxygenation, Woodson et al[376,379,380] utilized an isolated canine brain preparation. When the brain was perfused with low $P_{50}$ blood, oxygen consumption dropped by 25%, and the arteriovenous $O_2$ content difference decreased by 23%. In addition, the electroencephalogram (EEG) showed major abnormalities compared with controls perfused with normal blood. In this context, the reduced $(A\text{-}\bar{v})\ D_{O_2}$ was associated with an increase in $C_{V_{O_2}}$. The implication of this experiment was that cerebral cellular $O_2$ extraction at a $P_{V_{O_2}}$ of 20 mm Hg was curtailed, causing affinity hypoxia. Clinical implications are obvious: if an individual with severe cerebrovascular insufficiency is subjected to the combined insults of massive transfusion with cold 2,3-DPG-depleted blood, hyperventilation-induced respiratory alkalosis, and metabolic alkalosis from citrate metabolism, severe cerebral affinity hypoxia could ensue.

In summary, old banked blood with a high oxygen affinity is probably not harmful to healthy humans with normal compensatory mechanisms.[47,88,308,378] However, experimental data suggest deleterious effects of high oxygen affinity blood when regional blood flow is constant or restricted.[128,270,379,380] It would seem prudent, therefore, to transfuse normal or preferably high $P_{50}$ (increased 2,3-DPG) blood to older individuals with known or suspected coronary or cerebrovascular insufficiency who require extensive or massive transfusion.[50,88,137,377,378,379,380]

## PREDICTABLE COMPLICATIONS RELATED TO ACID-BASE STATUS, ELECTROLYTE IMBALANCE, AND TEMPERATURE

### *Acid-Base Imbalance*

Upon addition of CPDA-1 preservative, the pH of fresh banked blood approximates 7.0.[27] After 35 days of storage, the pH drops to 6.80,[238] mainly because of accumulation of lactate and $CO_2$, which cannot easily escape from plastic blood bags. The typical picture of banked blood is a combined respiratory ($P_{CO_2}$ = 104 to 130 mm Hg) and metabolic acidosis ($HCO_3^-$ = 8 to 12 mEq/L).[146]

Intuitively, it would appear that rapid transfusion of massive amounts of grossly acidic blood should routinely cause severe acidosis in the recipient. This is simply not the case.[7,55,81,204,205,210] The $CO_2$ in the blood bag is rapidly eliminated by the lungs. Thus, any elevation in $Pa_{CO_2}$ during massive transfusion is probably due to hypoventilation. Almost complete dissociation of citrate after transfusion also results in $H^+$ utilization and thus serum bicarbonate elevation within a few hours. Each unit of CPDA-1 blood contains 7.6 mmol of citrate, which results in generation of 22.8 mEq of $HCO_3^-$ per unit of blood, although life-threatening alkalosis does not occur because of ongoing degradation of citrate in the liver.[7,81]

In Vietnam, massive transfusion of hypotensive and acidotic patients, even with old ACD blood, was associated with improvement of acid-base balance to near-normal levels (Fig 6-8 and Fig 6-9).[55] Failure in improvement of acid-base status with blood transfusion was generally seen in victims with uncontrollable bleeding and persistent hypovolemic shock. Successful resuscitation is generally followed by mild metabolic alkalosis.[55,63,81,146] Since there is considerable variability in the acid-base response to massive transfusion,[20] empiric administration of $NaHCO_3^-$ should be abandoned.[153,210,385] Moreover, conditions that impede citrate metabolism should be prevented or corrected. As mentioned earlier, hypothermia is a potent inhibitor of citrate metabolism.[190] Therefore, warming of blood and crystalloids promotes citrate metabolism. Maintenance of optimal blood volume and cardiac output also assists citrate metabolism.

Severe metabolic alkalosis is probably as bad as or worse than metabolic acidosis. Metabolic alkalosis shifts the oxyhemoglobin dissociation curve to the left, reducing $O_2$ availability to tissues.[38,55,80,210] If the $O_2$ demand is high, compensatory increases in $\dot{Q}_t$ and local blood flow are required. If global or regional blood flow cannot increase, then oxygen extraction at a lower $P\bar{v}_{O_2}$ will result (Fig 6-10).[80] Thus, in an individual with compromised coronary or cerebral blood flow, augmentation of regional blood flow may not be possible, and subsequent affinity hypoxia may occur.[32,379,380]

If acid-base disturbance is suspected during massive transfusion, arterial blood gases should be analyzed.[55,210] As mentioned, mild alkalosis is expected during and after massive transfusion. However, if respiratory alkalosis is also present,

FIG. 6-8. Patient with multiple blast amputations and penetrating wounds in unusually severe metabolic acidemia on admission was treated with transfusion of banked blood (massive transfusion) as indicated without administration of sodium bicarbonate. Lactic acidemia was rapidly reversed, and mild metabolic alkalosis was evident 20 hours after admission. (From Collins et al[55] with permission.)

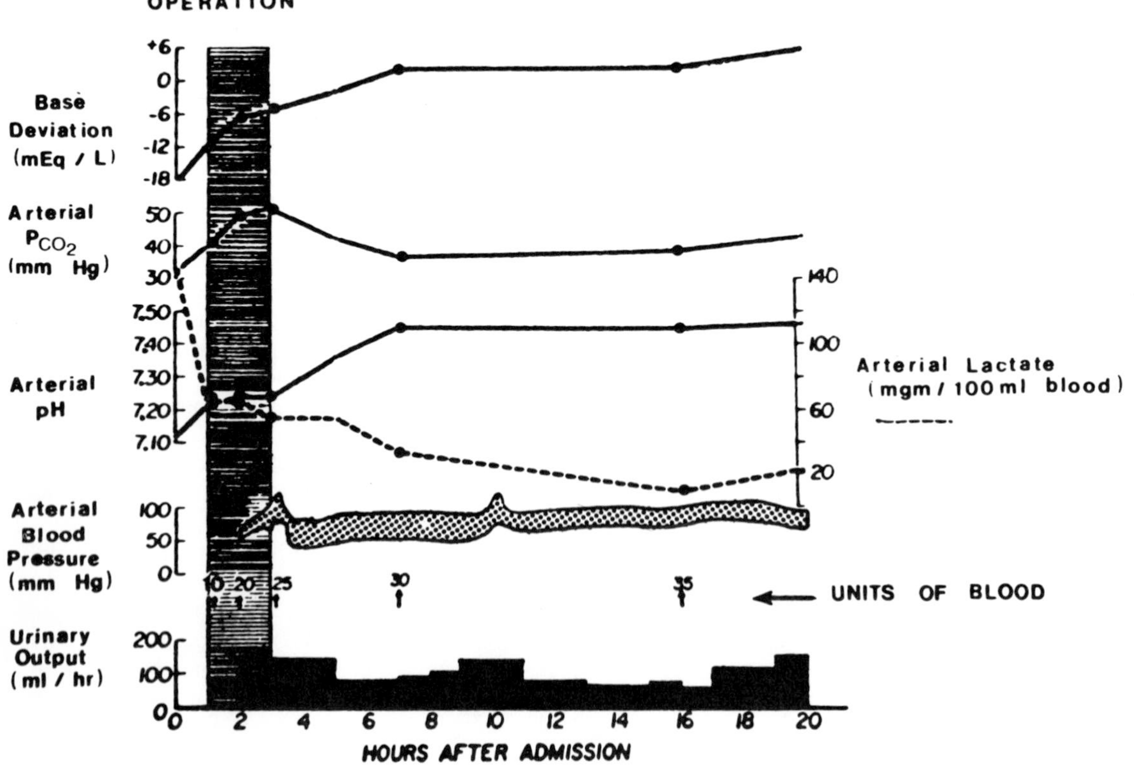

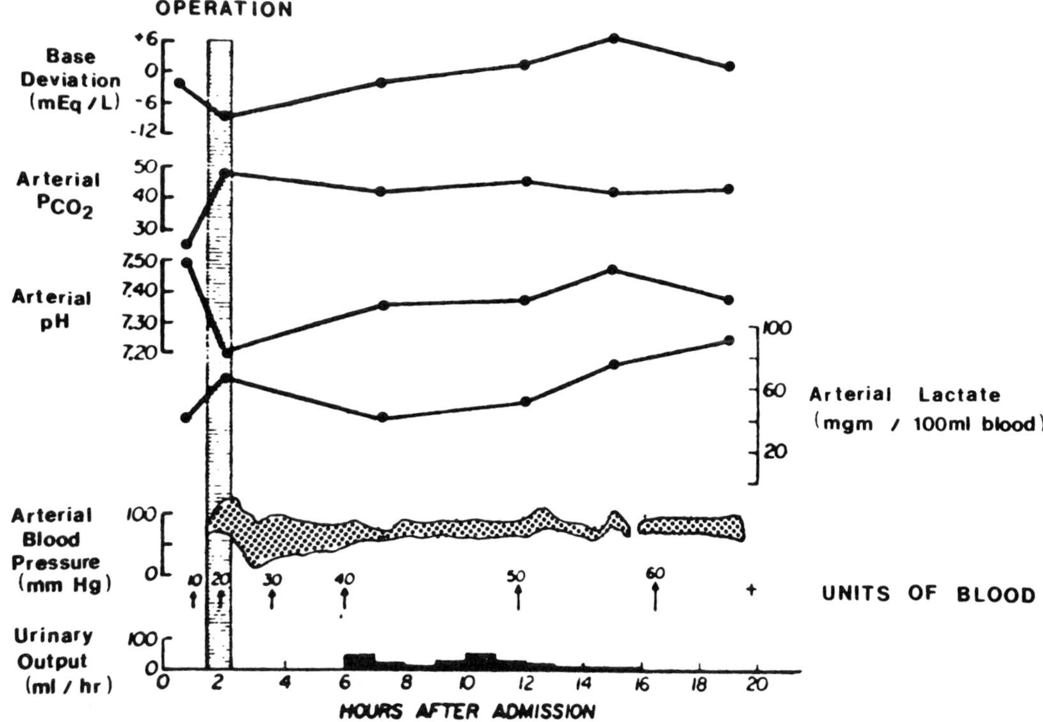


FIG. 6-9. Patient with a perfused but dead leg who developed anuria, pulmonary insufficiency, generalized bleeding, and profound clotting abnormalities. Acidosis did not develop despite prolonged hypotension and transfusion of 60 units of blood in 16 hours. The blood lactate level rose steadily after the 12th hour despite the use of fresh blood beyond that point. (From Collins et al[55] with permission.)

minute ventilation should be decreased to restore eucapnia. When metabolic acidosis is present, all efforts should be directed at optimizing the patient's temperature and systemic perfusion. These measures alone will usually correct the acidosis. Indiscriminate use of sodium bicarbonate may result in severe alkalosis with affinity hypoxia and electrolyte imbalance, most importantly, hypokalemia.[146] $CO_2$ from dissociation of bicarbonate may also enter the cell rapidly and produce intracellular acidosis if it cannot be eliminated because of severe shock, cardiac arrest, and/or inadequate ventilation. This can result in deterioration of hemodynamics and diminished response to resuscitative measures.

FIG. 6-10. Response of mixed venous oxygen tension ($P\bar{v}O_2$) after administration of $NaHCO_3$ to nearly drowned swine with reduced cardiac outputs. (From Douglas et al[80] with permission.)

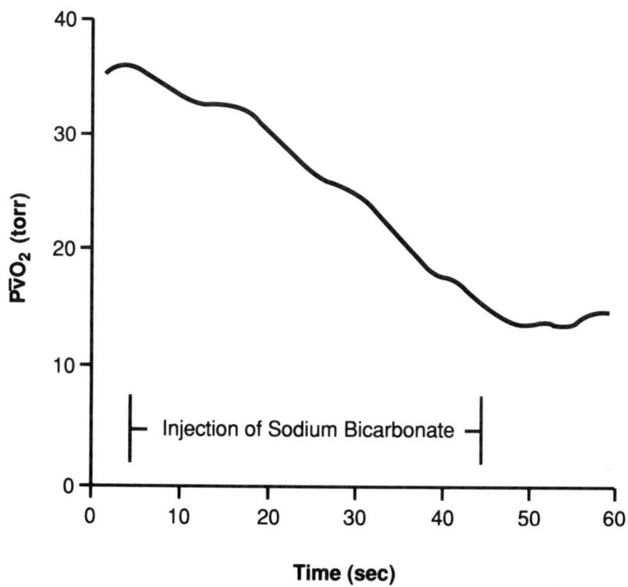


### Hyperkalemia-Hypokalemia

The plasma concentration of $K^+$ in 35-day-old CPDA-1 blood is approximately 28 mEq/L.[238] During storage, $K^+$ gradually diffuses from the red cell into the surrounding plasma. At 4°C, the ATP-dependent sodium-potassium pump is inhibited, allowing the concentration gradient to dictate the final intraerythrocytic and plasma $K^+$ concentrations.[360]

Despite the high plasma $K^+$ concentration of stored blood, the amount of potassium administered with each unit of whole blood is not great. Since only 300 mL of plasma is present in a unit of whole blood, a $K^+$ level of 28 mEq/L translates into a total plasma $K^+$ content of approximately 8.5 mEq.

Thus, in the worst possible situation, if 10 U of 35-day-old CPDA-1 whole blood is given, 85 mEq of $K^+$ will be transfused. The patient's blood loss nullifies part of this potassium load. Assuming that the normal serum $K^+$ concentration is roughly 4 to 5 mEq/L, a loss of 500 mL of blood with a hematocrit of 40% represents a $K^+$ loss of 1.2 to 1.5 mEq (4 to 5 mEq/L × 0.3). The net gain early in therapy is thus only 6 mEq of $K^+$ for each transfused unit. The final $K^+$ gain during transfusion is dependent upon the amount of blood administered and the percentage of the original blood volume replaced. If transfusion is concomitant with blood loss, 10 U of whole blood—that is, approximately 1 adult blood volume—results in a 70 to 75% replacement of the patient's blood.[52] Twenty units of whole blood (2 blood volumes) results in 90%, and 30 U, 97% replacement of the patient's own blood.[52] Net $K^+$ gain after 1 blood volume (10 U) transfusion then can be calculated as follows: 8.5 mEq/U of whole blood × 10 U × 0.75 = 65 mEq. If 2 blood volumes are transfused, the net $K^+$ gain = 8.5 × 20 × 0.9 = 150 mEq. For Adsol-preserved blood, in which supernatant $K^+$ is approximately 50 mEq/L on day 42, similar values can be calculated.[57]

If the patient's blood were completely replaced and no compensatory mechanisms existed to deal with this $K^+$ load, serum $K^+$ would ultimately equal that in the transfused blood. Fortunately, this is not usually the case.[385] To the contrary, hypokalemia is the rule after a well-conducted massive transfusion; hyperkalemia is exceptional.[57,146,319,327] The metabolic alkalosis that follows restoration of the blood volume promotes movement of $K^+$ and $Cl^-$ into the cells while the extracellular $H^+$ level rises in order to lower pH.[18,80,146] As intracellular $K^+$ levels rise, $HCO_3^-$ reabsorption by the kidney increases, further enhancing the metabolic alkalosis.[18] Thus, in addition to increased production of $HCO_3^-$ by the effects of citrate and lactate, increased reabsorption of $HCO_3^-$ in the kidney augments metabolic alkalosis during massive transfusion. Hypokalemia is further enhanced by diuresis, promoted by balanced salt solutions, and $K^+$ reentry into the transfused red cells.[355] To complicate matters, with hypothermia, an uncompensated metabolic acidosis can coexist with hypokalemia.[20] The mechanism for this is unclear.

Since the kidney is the principal route of $K^+$ excretion, it would seem that hyperkalemia would occur in a functionally anephric patient following massive transfusion. Just the opposite is true.[7] Since $HCO_3^-$ is excreted by the kidney only when its blood level is beyond a certain threshold,[18] chronic renal failure promotes accumulation of $HCO_3^-$, metabolic alkalosis, and once again, hypokalemia. Howland and associates[146] state that dialysis may be required in massively transfused patients in renal failure for malignant metabolic alkalosis with hypokalemia.

The treatment of hypokalemic, hypochloremic metabolic alkalosis consists of intravenous KCl infusion. Potassium administration is associated with increased urinary $HCO_3^-$ excretion.[18] In refractory, severe metabolic alkalosis (pH > 7.55), dilute infusions of hydrochloric acid (HCl) and acetazolamide have been recommended.[137,297,370] These agents, however, should be reserved for those cases in which renal compensatory mechanisms have failed.

Although hypokalemia is the rule, hyperkalemia occasionally occurs after massive transfusion.[29,204] Hyperkalemia may be transient if large volumes of banked blood are rapidly administered to a patient with a contracted blood volume, tissue hypoperfusion, and acidosis.[49,57,188,335] The cardiovascular response to hyperkalemia is augmented in the presence of hypothermia, which inhibits citrate metabolism, thereby decreasing serum $Ca^{2+}$ concentration.[52] Therefore, during massive transfusion of patients with severe hypovolemic shock, hypothermia, and metabolic acidosis, serum $K^+$ and $Ca^{2+}$ should be monitored closely.[29,57,188]

The amount of $K^+$ given during massive transfusion may be minimized by administering freshly prepared concentrated red cells reconstituted in normal saline. Each unit of fresh red blood cell concentrate contains only 1 to 2 mEq $K^+$.[324] Older or nearly outdated red blood cell units contain a quantity of $K^+$ equal to that of whole blood and indeed all of the other metabolic products of blood storage in a smaller volume of fluid.[29,306] It cannot be overemphasized, however, that hypokalemia is the rule after massive blood transfusion, whereas hyperkalemia is a much less frequent event.

### *Hypothermia*

Most critically injured patients have been exposed to factors that predispose them to hypothermia.[159,191,386] Low ambient temperatures, alcohol intoxication, hemorrhagic shock, and unconsciousness all cause a rapid decline of body temperature. Body heat loss is caused by various mechanisms: radiation, convection, conduction, and evaporation.[93] The factors that may increase hypothermia in the operating room include exposure of the body or body cavities to cold; infusion of fluids at room temperature; inhalation of cold, dry anesthetic gases; skeletal muscle relaxation; cutaneous vasodilatation, and loss of central temperature regulation reflexes.[300,343,346]

The presence and degree of hypothermia can be evaluated only by measurement of the core temperature. The distal esophagus, pulmonary artery, rectum, bladder, and tympanic membrane are suitable sites for temperature monitoring.[58,59,62] The severity of hypothermia is defined as follows[93,243]: mild, 33.5 to 35.5°C; moderate, 28 to 33.5°C; and deep, 17 to 27.5°C. Mild to moderate hypothermia is frequently seen in patients with traumatic injuries. Table 6-3 summarizes the adverse effects of hypothermia.

Measures to prevent heat loss in the operating room are summarized in Table 9-12 of Chapter 9. Of these, heating and

TABLE 6-3. Adverse Effects of Hypothermia

| PRIMARY EFFECTS | SECONDARY EFFECTS |
|---|---|
| Cardiac dysrhythmia | Cardiac standstill |
| Inhibition of citrate metabolism | Hypocalcemia<br>Acidosis |
| Leftward shift of oxyhemoglobin dissociation curve | Reduced tissue oxygenation with coronary or cerebrovascular insufficiency |
| Increased blood viscosity[175] | Microcirculatory stagnation<br>DIC<br>Decreased cardiac output |
| Increased sensitivity to inhalation anesthetics[92] | Decreased MAC |
| Decreased elimination of nondepolarizing muscle relaxants[209,375] | Prolonged muscle paralysis |
| Postopertive shivering[357] | Increased $O_2$ demand[163] |
| Acute renal failure[316] | |
| CNS depression[316] | |
| Peripheral vasoconstriction[239] | Decreased cardiac output |
| Thrombocytopenia, impaired platelet aggregation[118,354] | Hypocoagulability[118,192,354] |

humidifying the inspired gases and warming the intravenous fluids are under direct control of the anesthesiologist.[346] The subject of humidification is beyond the scope of this chapter, and thus, only a brief review is presented here. It is also discussed in Chapter 9.

In the average 70-kg man, the surface area of the alveolar ducts is 1.7 $m^2$ and of the alveoli, 70 $m^2$.[14] Thus, the lung functions as an efficient heat exchanger. Heat loss from the lungs is maximal during the first hour of anesthesia when a semiclosed circle system is used.[334] Since the inspired gases are administered at room temperature and at a relative humidity of only about 40%, their heating and humidification to 37°C and 100% humidity by the patient results in a loss of 21.84 kJ/h and 7.8 mL of water vapor per hour. In a 70-kg adult, 21.84 kJ/h represents 7.6% of basal heat production. Stone et al[334] determined that normothermia could be maintained during anesthesia and surgery when anesthetic gases were heated to 37°C with 100% relative humidity, regardless of the type, extent, or length of the procedure. In addition, if patients were allowed to become hypothermic, warming and humidifying the gases resulted in elevation of core temperature. If heated and humidified gases are employed, airway temperatures must be monitored closely. Temperatures in excess of 43.3°C (110°F) can produce severe tracheobronchitis.[173] A heat and moisture exchanger (HME) placed between the anesthetic circuit and the endotracheal tube may also minimize the rate of fall of core temperature although it cannot increase temperature of hypothermic patients.[42,132] The HME is simple to use and is probably free of complications. However, obstruction of the filter with excess water or secretions may possibly result in a significant increase in airway resistance. The HME also increases dead space, but this is of little clinical significance in mechanically ventilated patients. It should be noted that warming blankets alone are ineffective in maintaining normothermia in adults[240] and, in fact, may augment heat loss.[256] On the other hand, studies of rewarming from experimental hypothermia in dogs reveals that closed-system peritoneal and pleural lavage is more effective than heated, humidified aerosol administration.[269]

## HYPOTHERMIA RESULTING FROM BLOOD TRANSFUSION

Transfusion of cold blood in large quantities and at a rapid rate generally results in hypothermia.[26,52,191,205,228] Raising the temperature of 1 U of whole blood (500 mL) from 4 to 37°C requires 134.4 kJ; roughly 1260 kJ is necessary in a complete blood volume replacement. This represents approximately 50% of the basal heat production of a 70-kg person.[300] As discussed previously, hypothermia magnifies the usually benign storage lesions of bank blood.[52,335] Moreover, it predisposes the heart to altered contractility, conduction disturbances, and augmented irritability.[93,243,267,386] Indeed, the high mortality associated with massive transfusion prior to the routine use of blood warming may have been caused by hypothermia-induced malignant dysrhythmias.[228] Intractable ventricular fibrillation may result when body temperature falls below 30°C. Hypothermia-induced dysrhythmias may be heralded by the characteristic J wave (Osborn wave) on the ECG (Fig 6-11). Hypothermia causes cardiac dysrhythmias directly by its effects on the heart[26] and indirectly by inducing hypocalcemia, hyperkalemia, and acidosis.[335]

FIG. 6-11. The electrocardiogram in hypothermia. The Osborn wave (J wave) is an acute elevation of the terminal portion of the QRS which represents an acute current of injury. In the presence of moderate to severe hypothermia, the appearance of the Osborn wave is a preterminal event signaling the inevitability of hypothermic cardioplegia and treatment-resistant ventricular fibrillation. The ECG tracings are from a 19-year-old male auto accident victim admitted in profound hemorrhagic shock. Core temperature was 28.3°C at the time of cardiac arrest. (From Osborn JJ. Experimental hypothermia: respiratory and blood pH changes in relation to cardiac function. Am J Physiol 1953, 175:389.)

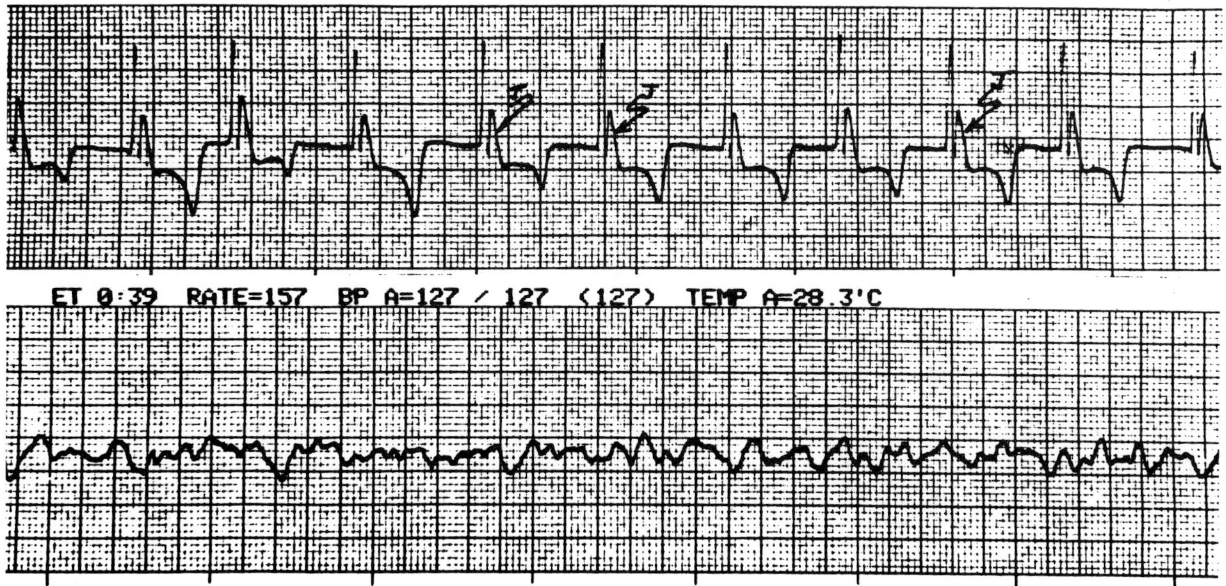

Rapid transfusion of cold blood through large CVP lines to hypovolemic trauma patients should therefore be avoided.[194,197] When peripheral venous access is unsuccessful and the central venous route is the only one available, blood must be warmed and administered at a rate no greater than 1.43 mL/kg/min (ie, 100 mL/min in a 70-kg man).[49] When both central and peripheral venous lines are in place, warmed blood should be administered through the peripheral vein and warmed crystalloid or colloid solutions through the CVP line.

Massive transfusion, even with warmed blood, ultimately results in some degree of hypothermia[303] because the maximal achievable temperature of the transfused blood with most blood warmers (32 to 33°C) is less than body temperature. A modest fall in body temperature (0.3 to 1.2°C) is associated with postoperative shivering and a resultant increase in $\dot{V}O_2$ of as much as 92%.[294] Postoperative rewarming should be done slowly.[293,294] Shivering can be terminated by small intravenous doses of meperidine (25 mg), chlorpromazine (5 to 10 mg), or nondepolarizing muscle relaxants.[163,273,283] The elimination of shivering decreases $M\dot{V}O_2$ and $O_2$ demand of the vital organs.[274,283,293,294]

As mentioned, blood warmers should be used routinely during massive blood transfusion to minimize hypothermia and its associated complications (Table 6-3). Ideally, a blood warmer must warm the transfused blood effectively, safely, rapidly, and consistently. It must be easy to use, and it should allow high flow rates with minimal tubing resistance.[303] The minimal temperature of the administered blood should be 32°C at high flow rates (150 mL/min) to prevent cardiac disturbances.[299] In a study comparing the Portex immersion coil and the DW1220 (or DW1000 and DW1000A made by Gorman Rupp Industries), the Portex coil was found to offer lower resistance and higher flow rates at any temperature above 32°C.[186] The highest infusion temperature, 34°C, was attained with the DW1220 at flow rates of approximately 85 mL/min. Thus, approximately 1 U of blood can be administered every 6 minutes using this unit, close to the recommended maximum rate of 1 U every 5 minutes.[49,207] The coil-through-bath (Hemokinetitherm) system provides lower blood infusion temperatures than are provided by the DW1000A at maximum achievable flow rates.[44] Microwave blood warmers have been largely abandoned because of the risk of hemolysis.[187,199]

In a preliminary study,[371] mixing erythrocytes at 6 to 10°C with heated saline (50 to 60°C) achieved equilibrated temperatures of 29 to 34°C without significant hemolysis. High-efficiency blood warmers have been introduced recently and promise to revolutionize massive transfusion.[102,176,304] These devices utilize large-bore, low-resistance tubing and filters interfaced with closed-flow 40°C countercurrent water bath heat exchangers. The commercially available Level-1 fluid warmer (Level 1 Technologies, Plymouth, MA) can deliver saline-reconstituted red blood cells warmed to 35°C at flow rates of 500 mL/min and to 37°C at 300 mL/min. During prolonged contact (mean, 14 min) of 42-day-old, Adsol-preserved, banked blood with the heat exchanger, no appreciable changes in plasma hemoglobin, potassium, or pH were noted compared with controls.[176] Red cell osmotic fragility and survival were also found to be acceptable.[176] Despite these advances in transfusion technique, caution is advised. Now blood can indeed be administered rapidly at normothermic or near-normothermic temperatures. However, administration of blood or reconstituted red blood cells at such high flow rates could possibly cause dangerous levels of hyperkalemia, hypocalcemia, pH reduction, and attendant cardiovascular complications *despite normothermia*. Using a prototype of the Level-1 fluid warmer, Fried et al[102] refuted these concerns in a dog model. Prospective human studies addressing these issues are necessary.

## THEORETICAL COMPLICATIONS

### *Microaggregate Infusion and Respiratory Failure: Is There a Relationship?*

Bank blood contains storage debris composed of platelets, leukocytes, and small fibrin clots, which are collectively termed *microaggregates*. These range in size from 20 to 200 μm and increase markedly in number after 5 days of storage.[206,229] Microaggregates are quantitated by measuring the screen filtration pressure (SFP), ie, the pressure required to force blood through a 20-μm micropore filter at a constant rate.[339] Microaggregates pass through the standard 170-μm transfusion filters, and the majority are able to traverse a 40-μm screen.[123] The total microaggregate volume in a 3-week-old unit of blood is less than 1 mL.[110]

Several questions are raised by the existence of these particles.[28,185]

1. Can microaggregates from transfused stored blood be found in the pulmonary vasculature?
2. To what extent do these particles contribute to pulmonary damage, specifically acute respiratory distress syndrome (ARDS)?
3. Is there a positive correlation between the volume of transfused blood and the incidence and severity of ARDS?
4. If these microaggregates do cause ARDS, does microfiltration of the transfused blood reduce its incidence and severity?

The theoretical sequence of events whereby infused microaggregates might cause ARDS is summarized in Fig 6-12.[87] Results from early studies in Vietnam supported the conclusion that infused microparticles caused ARDS.[241,323] Shortly thereafter, these observations were confirmed in civilian trauma patients. Thus, the beneficial role of microfilters in preventing ARDS was thought to have been established.[286,287]

More recent investigations, however, have shed doubt on the role of microaggregates in the pathophysiology of ARDS. In a large retrospective study of massively transfused battle casualties, Collins et al[54] found that the location and severity of injury were much more closely correlated with lung dysfunction than the volume of blood transfused. Specifically, they found that patients who had chest injuries and massive transfusion had greater hypoxemia than those who had massive transfusion for abdominal or peripheral injuries. All the patients were 18 to 22 years old, all were physically fit prior to injury, and all received nearly outdated ACD blood through standard filters (170 μm).

In a prospective randomized study, Durtschi et al[87] re-

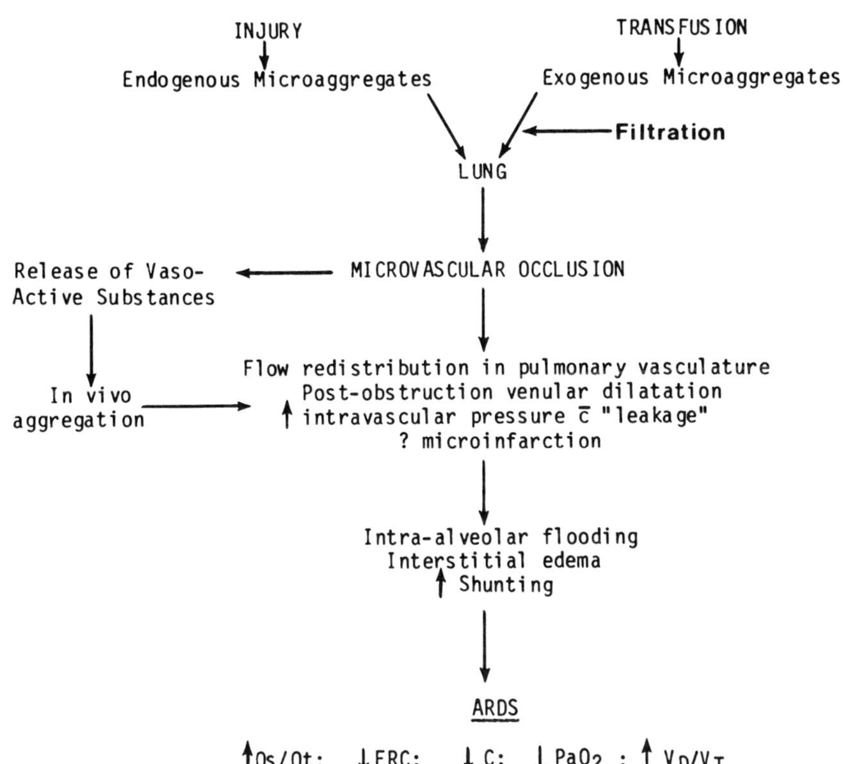


FIG. 6-12. Hypothesized development of adult respiratory distress syndrome from microaggregate infusion. (From Durtschi et al[87] with permission.)

viewed 27 dissimilar patients who received massive transfusion. The control group (14 patients) received blood through 265-μm filters, and the study group (13 patients) was transfused via 40-μm filters. Five of 14 patients (35%) in the control group and 3 of 13 (23%) in the microfiltered group developed ARDS. The authors concluded that their study failed to reveal a significant difference in either the degree of pulmonary abnormality or the development of clinically recognizable ARDS between the two groups.

In a study designed to predict the incidence of ARDS, Pepe et al[275] found that when massive transfusion was isolated as the sole risk factor, more than 22 U of blood transfusion were necessary to qualify it as a cause of ARDS. No patients who received fewer than 22 U developed ARDS in the absence of known etiologic factors for this disease.

To determine the effect of microaggregate filtration on patients with preexisting pulmonary dysfunction, Snyder et al[329] transfused their control group through 170-μm filters and the experimental group through 20-μm filters. There was no demonstrable increase in pulmonary dysfunction in either group following blood transfusion, and none of these patients developed ARDS. They concluded that the use of microaggregate filters for a 6- to 7-U blood transfusion does not provide significant benefit. A similar conclusion was reached by Virgilio[358] and by Grindlinger et al.[123]

Although these data seem to indicate a benign effect of microaggregate infusion, subtle pulmonary physiologic changes have been observed. In a study designed to detect these changes, Robinson et al[292] found small increases in both ventilation-perfusion and dead space-tidal volume ratios. These changes could not be correlated with total microaggregate load, but rather only with microaggregates more than 90 μm in diameter. These alterations were thus ascribed to pulmonary vasoconstriction and microvascular occlusion.

Implication of bank blood per se in the genesis of ARDS is difficult because transfusion is frequently performed in the presence of many other known causes of ARDS such as sepsis syndrome, aspiration of gastric contents and/or blood, pulmonary contusions, multiple major fractures, and prolonged hypotension with concomitant DIC.[275] In addition, overzealous resuscitation with acellular fluids and blood may cause circulatory overload with or without left ventricular failure. Thus, arterial hypoxemia and the clinical picture of ARDS may evolve independently of transfusion. Indeed, in both the sepsis and massive transfusion syndromes, ARDS has been linked to complement activation and the level of C3a. Patients with massive transfusion as their only risk factor for ARDS had lower levels of C3a (250 ± 80 ng/mL) and a 0% incidence of ARDS versus a 55% incidence of ARDS in patients with additional risk factors and C3a levels of 600 ± 120 ng/mL.[166]

In conclusion, based on current data, the routine use of microaggregate blood filters is not justified even during massive transfusion.[76,328] However, these filters may be useful in prevention of febrile transfusion reactions, which are caused by interactions between recipient antibodies and donor leukocyte and platelet antigens[226,307] (see also the section on nonhemolytic immunologic reactions).

## TRANSFUSION REACTIONS UNRELATED TO STORAGE CHANGES

Transfusion reactions are generally divided into two categories: immunologic and nonimmunologic.[33] Immunologic reactions are caused by antigen-antibody complex formation with or without the participation of complement. Nonimmunologic reactions do not involve antigen-antibody interaction. These reactions are classified as follows.

- I. Immunologic transfusion reactions
  - A. Hemolytic
    1. Acute hemolytic reactions
    2. Delayed hemolytic reactions
    3. Interdonor hemolytic reactions
    4. Lysis of recipient cells by antibodies in donor serum
  - B. Nonhemolytic (allergic) reactions
    1. Febrile reactions
    2. Anaphylactic reactions
    3. Urticaria
    4. Noncardiogenic pulmonary edema
    5. Posttransfusion purpura
- II. Nonimmunologic transfusion reactions

## IMMUNOLOGIC TRANSFUSION REACTIONS

### *Hemolytic*

ACUTE HEMOLYTIC TRANSFUSION REACTION. This is one of the most dreaded and disastrous complications of blood transfusion. As discussed previously, it is usually caused by clerical error,[143,249,250] but on rare occasions it may be due to an incompatibility undetected by presently available serologic testing techniques.[33,342] Acute HTR is characterized by in vivo destruction of red blood cells, caused by the interaction of donor red cell antigen and recipient serum antibody.[150] This reaction may or may not involve complement fixation. Hemolysis may occur intravascularly, in the reticuloendothelial system, or both.[222] Free hemoglobin and red cell stromal debris in the plasma produced by intravascular hemolysis results in hemoglobinuria and renal tubular damage. Clinical signs and symptoms may become apparent after the transfusion of small (10 to 30 mL) volumes of blood.[311]

The classic signs and symptoms—fever, chills, back pain, chest pain, flushing, and dyspnea—may be masked by anesthesia. Progressive, unexplained hypotension, coupled with generalized oozing from the surgical wound may be the only clues leading to diagnosis of this complication in anesthetized patients.[115,142,311] If urinary output is monitored, gross hemoglobinuria may be observed. However, this sign may be absent in patients with severe hypotension and anuria.

If HTR is suspected, transfusion should be stopped immediately. The risk of a severe reaction is much greater if more than 200 mL of red blood cells is administered.[115,142,150] Indeed, morbidity and mortality are directly proportional to the amount of incompatible blood given.[150]

Diagnostic evaluation of a suspected HTR should include the following tests.[142,342]

*Plasma Free Hemoglobin Level.* A visually perceptible red tinged plasma corresponds to 25 to 50 mg/dL of free hemoglobin. This concentration can be produced by intravascular lysis of as little as 5 to 10 mL of red blood cells. Urinary free hemoglobin also should be tested.

*Direct Antiglobin Test.* This test is used to detect circulating antibody-coated red cells.

*Serum Haptoglobin Determination.* A reduced serum haptoglobin concentration suggests increased binding to the free hemoglobin liberated by hemolysis.

*Compatibility Testing.* A recipient blood specimen should be sent to the blood bank along with the offending donor unit for compatibility testing.

SEQUELAE OF HTR. Two major sequelae of HTR are DIC and acute renal failure.

*Disseminated Intravascular Coagulation.* The hemorrhagic diathesis caused by HTR is probably initiated by the release of thromboplastic substances from lysed red cells and antigen-antibody complex activation of the coagulation system.[115] Activation of clotting by antigen-antibody complexes appears to involve primary interaction of these complexes with Hageman factor, platelets, leukocytes, and complement[115] (Fig 6-13).

Diagnosis is confirmed by the presence of hypofibrinogenemia, thrombocytopenia, and fibrin split products. Primary treatment involves stopping the transfusion, administration of platelets and fresh frozen plasma, and volume support. Chapter 7 addresses this issue more extensively.

*Acute Renal Failure.* Renal failure secondary to HTR is due primarily to deposition of fibrin thrombi in the renal microvasculature[115] (Fig 6-14). In addition, and equally important, a series of vasomotor changes mediated by vasoactive amines reduces renal cortical perfusion (Fig 6-15). The end result is reduced glomerular filtration rate (GFR) and renal tubular ischemia with subsequent oliguria or anuria. It was originally thought that renal failure secondary to HTR results from obstruction of renal tubules by hemoglobin casts or by a direct toxic effect of hemoglobin on the tubular epithelium. These notions have been dispelled by work showing that massive infusion of stroma-free hemoglobin solution is nontoxic to the kidneys.[104,115]

The most effective treatment of renal failure is prevention. Hypovolemia, if present, should be vigorously corrected. Drug therapy should include furosemide, which increases renal cortical blood flow.[13] Mannitol is probably not beneficial; it does not improve renal blood flow even though it may transiently increase intravascular volume by moving water into the intravascular space.[13] Dopamine (1 to 10 μg/kg/min) may be used to improve renal blood flow and GFR when oliguria persists despite adequate volume replacement[140,361] (see also chapter 25).

Mortality from hemolytic transfusion reaction varies between 17 and 53%.[33] Prevention of this complication rests on careful collection and labeling of blood specimens; development of safe blood bank protocols; and most important, giving properly typed and cross-matched blood to the intended recipient.[143,249,250]

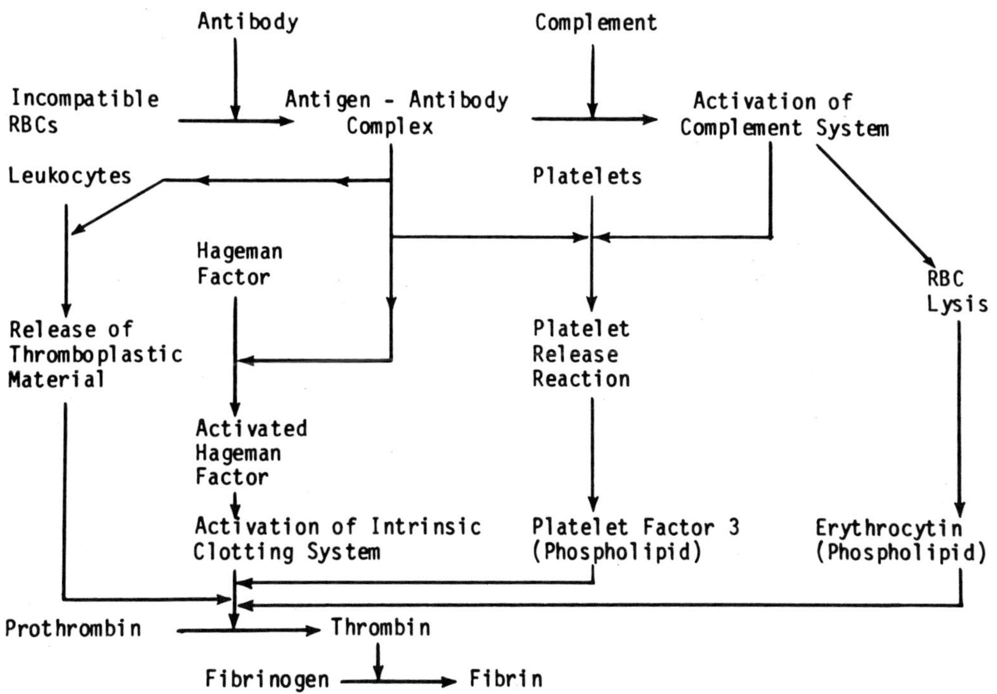


FIG. 6-13. Reactions contributing to fibrin formation and DIC. (From Goldfinger[115] with permission.)

DELAYED HEMOLYTIC TRANSFUSION REACTIONS. Delayed HTRs occur several days to 2 weeks after transfusion of seemingly compatible blood.[66] They are found mainly in patients who have been previously transfused or in women who have been sensitized to foreign red cell antigens during pregnancy.[139,224,311] After initial sensitization to red cell antigen, serum antibody levels rise and then fall. When these patients undergo subsequent compatibility testing, antibody titers are so low that they cannot be detected by current techniques.[139,282] Thus, a potentially dangerous antigen may be administered to a sensitized recipient. Following transfusion, donor red cell antigens stimulate production of antibodies in the recipient within 1 to 5 days—the so-called *booster* or *anamnestic* response.[33,66,224,282] Because a significant number of transfused donor cells are still circulating at this time, hemolysis occurs,[66,116,282] resulting in a rapid fall of hematocrit,

FIG. 6-14. Reactions contributing to acute renal failure in hemolytic transfusion reaction. (From Goldfinger[115] with permission.)

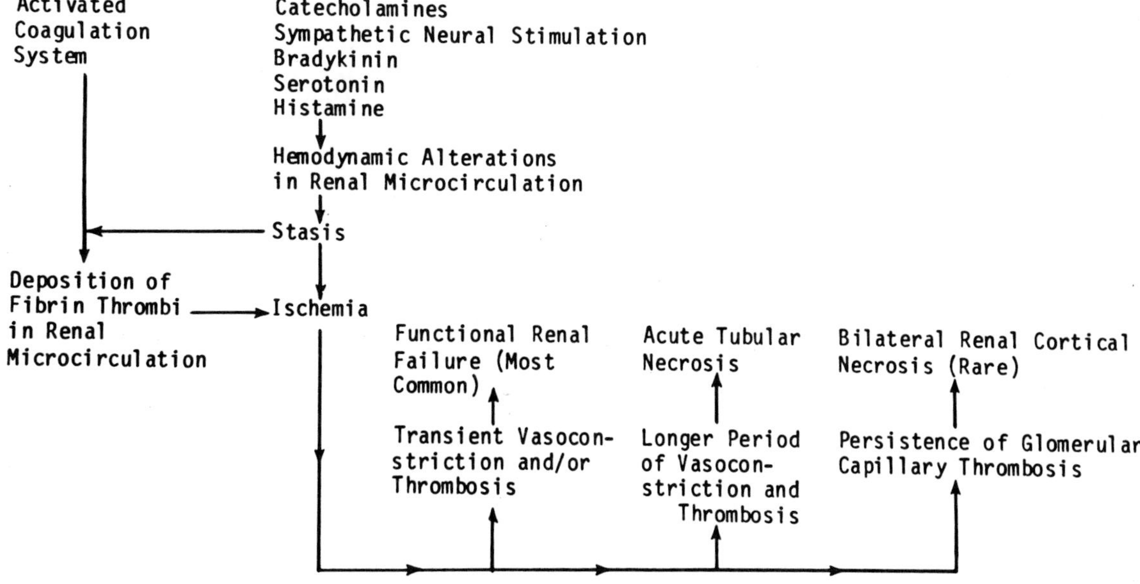

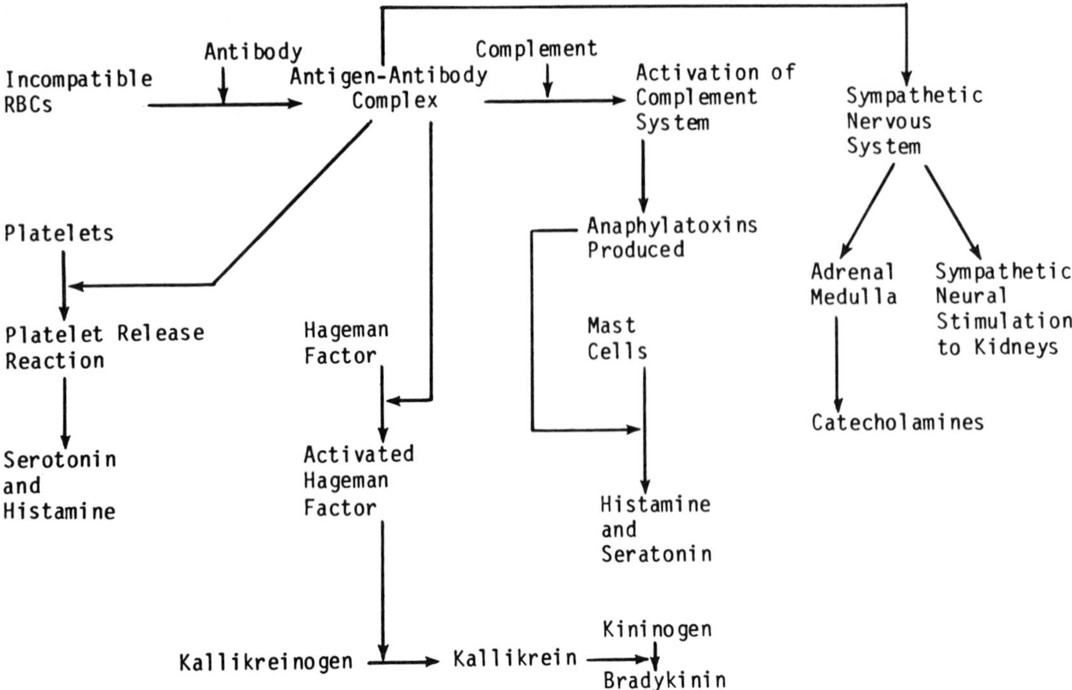


FIG. 6-15. Vasomotor alterations resulting from transfusion reaction. (From Goldfinger[115] with permission.)

FIG. 6-16. Delayed hemolytic transfusion reaction (intravascular hemolysis) occurring 25 days after blood transfusion. The patient presented with hemoglobinuria, anemia, and mild hyperbilirubinemia. The antibodies subsequently detected (anti-C + D + E + JKa) were not detected by the initial cross-match. ⊙ denotes units. (From Davis and Abbott[66] with permission.)

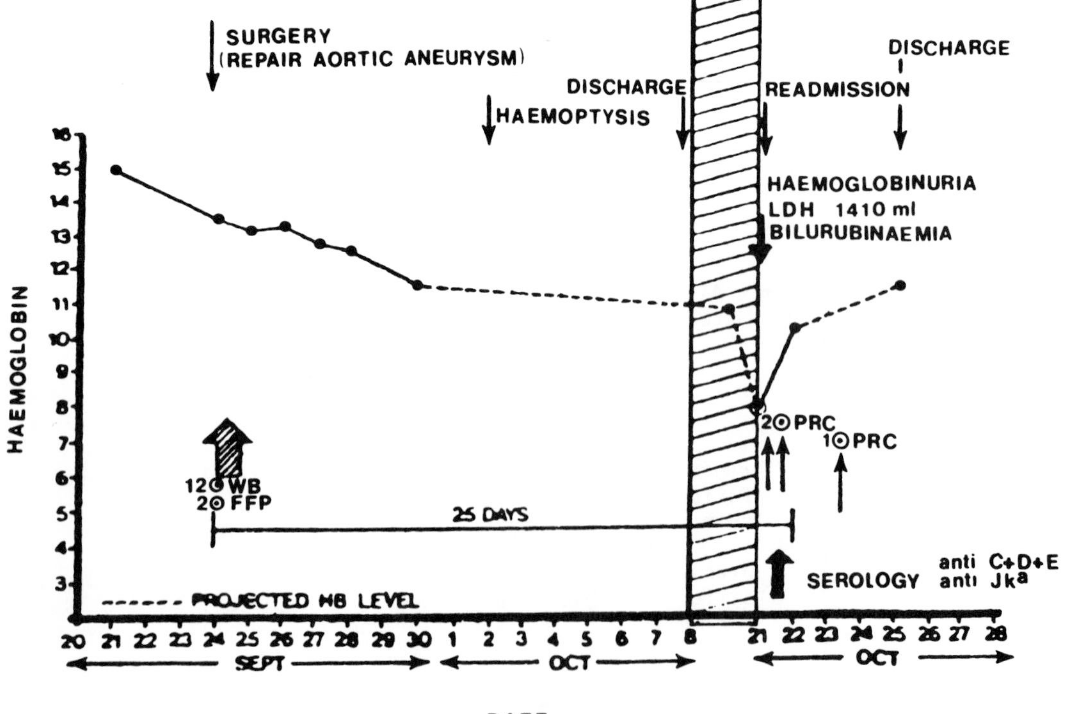

hemoglobinuria, a rise in serum bilirubin, and fever[66] (Fig 6-16). Although acute renal failure and DIC have been reported following delayed hemolytic transfusion reactions, such life-threatening sequelae are rare.[116,342]

Delayed HTRs may occur following initial antigenic exposure.[116,139] In this form, alloantibodies are produced slowly in a 10-day to 2-week period after transfusion. Since there is a gradual rise in serum antibodies, hemolysis of the transfused red cells occurs slowly, eliciting few symptoms. Laboratory studies may show a decrease in hemoglobin concentration, mild hyperbilirubinemia, and a positive direct antiglobulin (Coombs) test. Occasionally, a delayed HTR may go unnoticed.[139] Because these patients are at risk of developing acute HTR or severe delayed HTR during blood transfusion in the future, every effort must be spent to identify them.

INTERDONOR HEMOLYTIC TRANSFUSION REACTIONS. This type of reaction occurs in the course of multiple transfusions when the plasma of a donor unit contains an undetected antibody that destroys subsequently transfused red cells. Since all blood banks screen donor serum for abnormal antibodies, this situation is rare.[33]

LYSIS OF RECIPIENT CELLS BY PASSIVELY TRANSFUSED ANTIBODY IN DONOR SERUM. When group O, Rh negative blood is given for the initial transfusion, high titers of anti-A and anti-B are occasionally transfused into a type A, B, or AB recipient. This high-titer serum may cause lysis of recipient cells.[33] The volume of plasma given is usually very small, especially if concentrated red cells are given or if the number of universal donor units is less than 4. Thus, these reactions are generally quite mild.

### *Nonhemolytic Immunologic Reactions (Allergic)*

These reactions occur in approximately 3% of patients receiving properly typed and cross-matched blood.[333]

FEBRILE REACTIONS. Febrile transfusion reactions are the most common encountered. They occur during or shortly after transfusion and are most often caused by antibodies against donor leukocyte and platelet antigens.[226] Febrile reactions develop in patients who have a history of prior multiple transfusions or multiparity.[33,116] Although multiple somatic complaints are elicited in the awake state, fever, often high, may be the only sign in anesthetized patients. Febrile reactions are as a rule not dangerous, but they must be differentiated from acute hemolytic reactions and blood contamination.[33,142] The use of leukocyte-poor blood or a microfilter will generally prevent further febrile episodes.[202,226,307,328]

ANAPHYLACTIC REACTIONS. Fortunately, anaphylactic reactions are rare. Anaphylaxis develops when a patient with immunglobin A (IgA) deficiency (1 in 700 people) is transfused with plasma containing IgA. Sensitization occurs with the production of antibodies against IgA. When the patient is again exposed to IgA-containing blood, anaphylaxis is precipitated.[116,142,227,333]

Under anesthesia, signs may include flushing, wheezing, and severe hypotension. Anaphylaxis is differentiated from HTR, leukocyte incompatibility, and sepsis by the absence of fever. Treatment for any anaphylactic reaction includes stopping the transfusion, brisk crystalloid infusion with epinephrine $\frac{1}{10,000}$, (10 mL over 5 minutes), and intravenous aminophylline as dictated by assessment of bronchomotor tone.

If a known IgA-deficient patient presents for emergency transfusion, frozen or saline-washed red cells from which IgA proteins have been eliminated are safe to use. Alternatively, if time permits, blood from IgA-deficient donors may be administered.

URTICARIAL REACTIONS. Urticaria is second in frequency only to febrile reactions. If hives are the only manifestation of a reaction, the transfusion may be continued.[33,142] Detailed investigation to determine the cause is unnecessary. Recurrent hives are probably due to release of histamine from the recipient's mast cells directed against antigens on donor serum proteins. Pretreatment with an antihistamine is usually sufficient. The use of concentrated washed red cells may be considered, but this is inappropriate and unnecessary in the presence of trauma.

NONCARDIOGENIC PULMONARY EDEMA (LEUKOAGGLUTININ-INDUCED ACUTE LUNG INJURY). Very rarely, acute pulmonary edema may develop after transfusion of modest amounts of blood.[108,182,333] The syndrome is characterized by normal PCWP and increased cardiac index[91,271] and is thought to be due to a reaction of leukocyte antibodies in donor plasma with recipient leukocytes. The leukocyte-antibody complex precipitates an inflammatory reaction in the lungs which resembles pulmonary edema.[91,101,108,180,271] Bilateral pulmonary infiltrates without cardiac enlargement are seen on X-ray. In anesthetized patients, clinical signs include decreased pulmonary compliance, audible rales, and signs of poor tissue oxygenation. There is no definitive treatment. If suspected, administration of positive end-expiratory pressure (PEEP) and high-dose corticosteroids seems reasonable.[91,101,142,271] Diuretics should be given only if clear signs of volume overload or left ventricular failure are present.[182]

POSTTRANSFUSION PURPURA. This is another rare syndrome that results from the formation of antiplatelet antibodies after transfusion.[86] A recipient antibody-donor platelet antigen complex is formed which attacks the patient's platelets, resulting in severe thrombocytopenic purpura approximately 1 week after transfusion.[86] Treatment consists of high-dose prednisone therapy and/or exchange plasmapheresis to remove the antigen-antibody complex. Most of the reported cases have been in multiparous women sensitized during pregnancy.[225]

## NONIMMUNOLOGIC TRANSFUSION REACTIONS: HEMOLYSIS DUE TO PHYSICAL CAUSES

### *Mechanical Factors*

Mechanical factors affect the viability of transfused red blood cells. These factors may be categorized as intracellular and extracellular.[40,305]

INTRACELLULAR CAUSES. The primary intracellular variable affecting red cell integrity is osmotic pressure, which, in turn, is affected by the type and quantity of diluent employed to reconstitute packed red cells. Hypotonic solutions (ie, 0.45% NaCl) cause red cells to swell and lyse, whereas hypertonic solutions result in shrinkage and crenation.[305] Not only is diluent tonicity important, but its biochemical composition is as well.[90] Five percent dextrose in water causes crenation and agglutination of red cells in vitro. When they are resuspended in plasma, agglutination reverses, and the red cells appear morphologically normal. However, when transfused, only 25% of these erythrocytes survive 48 hours after administration. Exposure to a diluent medium devoid of electrolytes ($Na^+$, $K^+$) causes irreversible red cell membrane damage and hence, reduced life span. The safest diluent solution for red cell suspension remains normal saline.[305] Apart from normal saline Normosol-R (pH 7.4) may be used safely to dilute packed cells.[31] Plasmanate (plasma protein fraction), a derivative of plasma, causes hemolysis because of its low osmolality (180 mOsm) and therefore should not be used for this purpose.[31] Controversy surrounds the use of lactated Ringer's solution to reconstitute red cells, since it contains 3 mEq/L calcium. Countless anesthesiologists have noted that when blood is transfused through tubing that contains lactated Ringers, no clotting occurs if the flow is rapid. However, blood exposed to lactated Ringer's solution for 30 minutes will clot.[210,301] Available data suggest that there is no difference between normal saline and lactated Ringer's solution in clot production if dilution and transfusion are accomplished rapidly and if the amount of lactated Ringer's added is no more than half the volume of the red cells.[168,169,262,313]

EXTRACELLULAR CAUSES. The extraerythrocytic causes of hemolysis during transfusion are biophysical. Red cell hemolysis is directly proportional to shear stress,[40,305] which is the resultant of three factors: yield stress, viscosity, and shear rate. Yield stress is a function of the degree of red cell aggregation and the amount of force required to start flow. Blood viscosity, or the inherent resistance of blood to flow, is dictated by hematocrit, plasma viscosity, protein concentration, and temperature. Shear rate, or flow velocity, is a function of the velocity gradient, which in turn is determined by the characteristics of the flow: laminar or turbulent. Laminar flow increases shear rate, but turbulent flow decreases it. Concisely, measures designed to decrease shear stress during blood transfusion improve red cell survival and decrease hemolysis. It has been shown clearly that dilution of red blood cells with 200 mL of normal saline improves the flow rate at any given external pressure up to 300 mm Hg and that the degree of hemolysis is reduced as dilution proceeds from 0 to 200 mL.[40]

### *Thermal Factors*

Extremes of temperature destroy red cells. Temperatures less than −3°C or greater than 50°C are likely to cause hemolysis and denaturation of plasma proteins.[223] The current standards of the American Association of Blood Banks state that blood must not be warmed above 37°C.[331]

### *Infected Blood*

Bacterial contamination of bank blood results in hemolysis of red cells during storage. The effects of this physical alteration are dwarfed by the septic reaction that follows blood transfusion. Despite improved collection and storage techniques, blood still may become infected with bacteria.[30,116,143,230] The incidence of bacterial contamination seems to be directly related to the length of storage.[167] The offending organisms have most often been found to be cold-growing Gram-negative bacteria.[167,279] Shortly after transfusion, a septic shock syndrome ensues due to Gram-negative endotoxemia.[33] A full-blown syndrome produces signs almost identical to an acute HTR: high fever, shock, hemoglobinuria, renal failure, and DIC.[142,167,279] Under anesthesia, hypotension unresponsive to volume or drugs, tachycardia, and increased cardiac index may be the only clues.[30]

Diagnosis is confirmed when bacteria are found in Gram stains of the donor unit and both donor unit and patient develop positive cultures.[167] Sensitivity studies should not delay immediate institution of broad spectrum antibiotic coverage. Other treatment includes appropriate fluid administration and inotropic support during the period of septic shock (see also Chapter 27).

## POSTTRANSFUSION VIRAL HEPATITIS

Viral hepatitis and its sequelae remain the most common lethal complications of blood transfusion.[144,231] Three types of hepatitis virus are recognized: type A (HAV, infectious hepatitis), type B (HBV, serum hepatitis), and non-A, non-B. The last is now generally referred to as hepatitis virus type C (HCV). Hepatitis A virus is rarely, if ever, transmitted in transfused blood and therefore does not play a role in the etiology of posttransfusion hepatitis.[96,348] Despite universal serologic testing of donors for its surface antigen (HBsAg), HBV is still responsible for posttransfusion viral hepatitis in 1 to 2% of transfused patients and in 10% of all cases of transfusion-related hepatitis.[8] Between 150,000 and 300,000 non-A, non-B hepatitis infections occur in the United States each year.[144] Of these, 5 to 10% (7500 to 30,000) is associated with transfusion. Non-A, non-B hepatitis accounts for roughly 90% of posttransfusion viral hepatitis.[1,320,341] Before 1986 the incidence of posttransfusion viral hepatitis due to non-A, non-B was between 4 and 14% in patients receiving 1 to 9 U of volunteer HBsAg-negative donor blood.[348,368] When more than 10 U was transfused, the incidence increased to nearly 30%. When combinations of volunteer donor and paid donor units were utilized, the incidence of posttransfusion viral hepatitis increased to as much as 60 to 65%.[348] The prevalence of non-A, non-B infection in volunteer blood donors is still high. An epidemiologic study conducted in volunteer blood donors from 1985 through 1986 by the Greater New York Blood Program demonstrated that the overall prevalence of anti-HCV was 0.9 to 1.4%; black and hispanic donors had a higher prevalence than whites.[332a] The risk of hepatitis increases not only with the number of units transfused but also with the amount of pooled plasma derivatives, especially factor VIII, factor IX, and fibrinogen (no longer available in the US). In one study in which commercial pooled clotting factor concentrates were used, 57% of patients developed posttransfusion viral hepatitis.[348] (Fig 6-17)

Donor screening and testing policies that were developed in 1986 have reduced the incidence of posttransfusion viral hepatitis by approximately 30%.[24,332a] Based on these policies, blood from donors with elevated alanine aminotransferase (ALT) levels and from those who test positive for hepatitis B core antigen (anti-HBc) is discarded. The anti-HCV test for blood donors, which became available in May 1990, is expected to detect 60 to 80% of blood infected with a non-A, non-B hepatitis virus (HCV).[3a,241a,332a] This test is now used routinely in addition to surrogate testing that involves measurement of ALT and anti-HBc assay of the donor blood. Although combined use of surrogate and anti-HCV testing can reduce posttransfusion hepatitis substantially, some donors with hepatitis infection may remain undetected because of the long window period before HCV seroconversion, disappearance of the HCV antibody with time (especially when the infection is transient), and/or possible presence of another unidentified hepatitis virus as an etiologic agent.[3a,3b,241a,332a] Thus, treatment with blood and its components should be based on sound clinical and laboratory criteria, not intuitive feelings or rote formulas.

## ACQUIRED IMMUNODEFICIENCY SYNDROME (AIDS) AND THE RISK OF BLOOD TRANSFUSION[6,24,103,177,213,277,363]

Acquired immunodeficiency syndrome (AIDS), a disease of the immune system, is a result of infection with a human retrovirus, the human immunodeficiency virus, HIV. HIV infection can present 6 to 13 days after exposure as an acute viral syndrome resembling infectious mononucleosis, with sore throat, headache, fever, nausea, myalgia, macular rash, malaise, lymphadenopathy, and diarrhea lasting about 2 weeks.

FIG. 6-17. Incidence of posttransfusion hepatitis in two groups of cardiac surgery patients receiving only blood or blood and blood products. (From Tremolada F et al[348] with permission.)

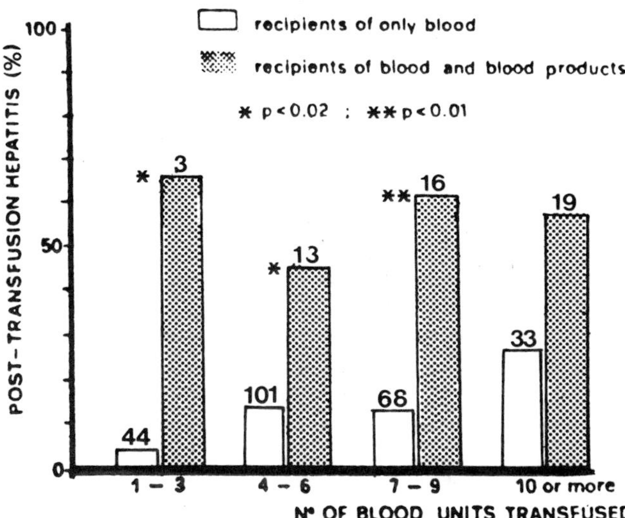


Seroconversion to HIV antibody positivity usually occurs within 3 to 12 weeks of exposure to the virus and is diagnosed by positive ELISA (enzyme-linked immunosorbent assay) and Western blot immunofluorescence assay. Because of the 3- to 12-week window of seronegativity after infection, a small fraction of donors with HIV infection may not be identified by these tests. Thus, present screening tests are only 96 to 98% accurate. The false-negatives are important because they are the source of HIV contamination of the blood supply. Individuals who are identified as being in high-risk groups for HIV infection should be vigorously excluded from the donor pool.

Prior to routine serotesting of blood donors in April 1985, it was estimated that about 3 to 4 blood U per 10,000 were positive for HIV. This has been extrapolated into an estimate of 2000 transfusion-related AIDS cases and 12,000 persons infected with HIV. Since the mean incubation period for transfusion-associated AIDS may be 54 months or longer, the number of reported transfusion-related AIDS cases will probably rise until 1990 and then decline.

Despite predonation information about high-risk behavior disqualifying a potential donor, the incidence of detected positive donations is now 100 per million (1:10,000). If the available screening tests are 96% correct in predicting infection, then at worst 4 of 100 infected persons eludes detection. Their HIV-infected blood, then, represents 4 U/1,000,000, an incidence of approximately 1/250,000. Thus, the current incidence of transfusion-related HIV infection is probably between 1/250,000 and 1/500,000. If 18 million U of blood components (red blood cells, platelets, plasma) are transfused per year, between 72 and 90 persons are infected annually with HIV by transfusion of seronegative blood. A pessimistic estimate puts this figure as high as 460 HIV-infected units from otherwise seronegative donors. At present, in addition to serologic testing, all blood donors are screened to exclude those in high-risk groups: male homosexuals, intravenous drug abusers, bisexual males, sex partners of people at high risk for AIDS, and promiscuous heterosexuals.

Thus, by any measure, the blood supply in the United States is reasonably safe. The risk of transfusion-acquired HIV infection and AIDS has been unnecessarily sensationalized. Current donor exclusion policies, public education about HIV transmission, and better tests for HIV will ultimately eradicate HIV from the blood supply. Of perhaps greater concern than transmission of HIV via blood transfusion is the transmission of human T-cell leukemia virus type 1 (HTLV-1) by this mode. HTLV-1 results in adult T-cell leukemia and progressive myelopathy, although only progressive myelopathy has so far been reported after transfusion. Currently donated units have not been screened for HTLV-1 antibody, and it appears that transfusion-related risk of HTLV-1 seropositivity is approximately 10 times greater than that of HIV (0.024%/U).[46]

For trauma victims, especially those involved in motor vehicle accidents, there remains the possibility of acquiring these infections during the accident, not by transfusion, but by contamination of the blood of similarly injured and hemorrhaging infected accident victims. This is more likely to occur in areas in which these infections are endemic (central

Africa, Caribbean basin),[141] but it can also occur in the United States, since one study reported a 16% incidence of HIV seropositivity in actively bleeding "inner-city" trauma victims between the ages 25 and 34.[6]

## WHOLE BLOOD AND COMPONENT THERAPY IN TRAUMA

There are four major reasons for transfusion of blood and its components in the hemorrhaging patient[298,306].

1. Improvement of systemic $O_2$ transport
2. Restoration of critical red cell mass
3. Correction of bleeding caused by dilutional thrombocytopenia, platelet dysfunction, or pathologic platelet consumption
4. Correction of bleeding caused by factor deficiency or pathologic consumption of coagulation proteins (procoagulants).

The keystone of successful hemotherapy is rational use of these lifesaving, but potentially dangerous, blood products. This section reviews only those products that may benefit the actively bleeding trauma patient and that are found in most hospital blood banks in the United States. Also, this section offers a rational approach to this rather controversial, ambiguous, and misunderstood area.

### WHOLE BLOOD

Whole blood is the product from which all components derive. Approximately 450 mL of blood is withdrawn from the donor and collected in a plastic bag containing approximately 63 mL of CPDA-1 solution, for a total volume of approximately 513 mL. A unit of whole blood initially contains all of the cellular and hemostatic constituents found in donor blood. Over time, storage lesions, as discussed previously, occur. A unit of whole blood in CPDA-1 may be stored 35 days, after which it must, according to Federal regulations, be discarded if unused. Adsol-preserved blood may be legally stored for 42 days.

The prime indication for whole blood transfusion in an actively bleeding patient is severe and continuing reduction in red cell mass and $DO_2$.[48,154,194,215,260,306,317] In addition, whole blood has the advantage of supplying all hemostatic factors except for viable platelets; levels of factors V and VIII are reduced but hemostatically adequate.[62,126,127,254]

### MODIFIED WHOLE BLOOD

Modified whole blood is prepared by removing platelets and cryoprecipitate (fibrinogen and factor VIII) for component use.[326] The major application of this product is in the treatment of massive hemorrhage, where it has been shown to be as effective in its hemostatic capacity as unmodified whole blood.[62]

### RED BLOOD CELLS (PACKED RED CELLS, CONCENTRATED RED CELLS)

Red blood cells are merely concentrates of whole blood prepared by removing roughly two thirds of the plasma after sedimentation or centrifugation. Thus, a unit of red cells contains approximately 200 mL of cells and 100 mL of plasma. This component may be prepared immediately after whole blood donation or at any time during the legal storage period. The storage lesions of whole blood are present in red blood cells even if separation occurs immediately after donation. The final hematocrit of red blood cells depends upon the donor's hematocrit, the volume of anticoagulant added, and the volume of plasma removed during the concentration process. Consequently, hematocrit varies widely in this product, but 65 to 70% is usual.

Reduced arterial oxygen content ($Cao_2$) with compromise of the systemic $O_2$ transport capacity is the primary indication for administration of red blood cells. Thus, red blood cells are most appropriately used in situations of insufficient tissue oxygenation caused by chronic anemias or during surgery in which hemorrhage is well controlled and not expected to exceed 30 to 40% of blood volume (1500 to 2000 mL/70 kg).[39,207,215] One unit of red blood cells may be expected to raise the recipient's hemoglobin concentration by approximately 1 g/dL if hemorrhage has been controlled and relative normovolemia maintained. Indeed, young, healthy patients may not need red blood cell transfusion even at this level of blood loss if circulating blood volume is replaced by acellular fluids. As mentioned in the section on emergency transfusion, type-specific, or group O, Rh negative red blood cells may be issued by the blood bank as the initial units of a potential massive transfusion. Coupled with acellular fluids, red cells represent appropriate initial care. In fact, in the hypovolemic, hemorrhaging trauma victim, crystalloid reconstituted red blood cells may be preferable to whole blood initially, because room temperature or warmed saline raises the temperature of 4°C bank blood, improving its flow characteristics and reducing the magnitude of hypothermia if a blood warmer is not in place. Finally, although citrate-induced hypocalcemia is seldom a problem, it probably does occasionally cause ventricular dysrhythmias when whole blood is administered to a patient with acute hyperkalemia, hypothermia, and hypovolemia.[335] Since red blood cells contain one third the amount of citrate preservative solution contained in whole blood, they are less likely to cause hypocalcemia and its consequences and thus they may be preferable to whole blood as initial resuscitation units on this basis.

The major objection to the use of red blood cells is their slow flow rate even when external pressure is applied.[189] This increased viscosity is caused by both high hematocrit and low temperature. As we have already discussed, augmented flow and reduced hemolysis may be achieved by reconstituting each unit of red cells in 100 to 250 mL of warmed normal saline[40,387] or other electrolyte solutions.[31,168,169,313]

Increased utilization of red blood cells has permitted greater availability of platelet and procoagulant concentrates. Thus, blood products are now widely available for patients suffering from congenital deficiency or abnormality of procoagulants (eg, hemophilia). Likewise, surgical patients who need platelet transfusion for dilutional thrombocytopenia, or coagulation factors to treat DIC are now well served by most community blood banks. Again, it must be emphasized that red blood cells are the product of choice when hemorrhage is not massive.

## FRESH FROZEN PLASMA

Fresh frozen plasma (FFP) is extracted from whole blood and frozen to −34°C within 6 hours of blood collection. It must be used within 6 hours after thawing or discarded.[246] FFP contains all of the coagulation proteins in at least 70% of normal levels. If stored for 3 months, it will retain approximately 60% of its original factor VIII activity.[290,291] In all respects, except for the absence of platelets, it mirrors the coagulation capability of fresh blood. FFP is supplied in 200- to 250-mL units.

Although FFP does not require cross-matching, it must be compatible with the recipient's ABO blood type. Hemolysis will occur because of alloantibodies if the donor plasma is incompatible with recipient red cells.[41] Rh typing of FFP is unnecessary since red cell contamination rarely occurs.

### *Indications for Fresh Frozen Plasma*

The use of FFP in massive transfusion has been controversial ever since it became widely available.[64] In accordance with the early notions that banked blood lacked sufficient quantities of labile coagulation factors V and VIII to correct hemostatic deficiencies, empirical formulas were promulgated using FFP as a cure-all for intraoperative coagulopathies.[27] Consequently, FFP has generally been administered when not needed, which only adds to the very real problems of needless viral exposure and wasted money.[8,99,232,306,348,351] As indicated earlier, Rapaport et al[284] showed that levels of factor V in 3-week-old ACD blood were 20 to 60 U/dL. Rizza[291] subsequently demonstrated that only 10 to 15 U/dL is required for hemostasis. In the same 3-week-old ACD blood, measured factor VIII levels were 20 to 50 U/dL, with hemostatic levels of only 25 to 30 U/dL required.[284,291] These studies have been corroborated more recently in CPD-banked blood by Nilsson et al,[254] who concluded, "Storage of blood at 4°C appears to have little effect on the levels and function of various coagulation factors, including those considered labile (factor VIII and factor V)." In addition, Counts et al[62] found that factor VIII levels were rarely below 50% of normal even in patients massively transfused (average, 33 U) with modified whole blood (cryoprecipitate removed). Their data suggest a large physiologic reserve of factor VIII (approximately 200% of normal immediately after trauma) and that the empiric administration of FFP should be considered wasteful and unnecessary when whole or modified whole blood is transfused.

In a prospective, randomized study of 36 trauma patients, Harke and Rahman[126,127] have addressed clearly the issues of banked blood, massive transfusion, and hemorrhagic shock in the genesis of DIC, and inferentially, the need for FFP. The only independent variable in their study was the trauma victim's time in shock. Each group contained the same number of patients (seven or eight), had similar quantities of blood replacement (2.5 blood volumes), and all were transfused with banked blood averaging 9 days of storage. No components were administered. Their results may be summarized as follows.

1. If shock time was 40 to 90 minutes (mean, 65 minutes) (group III), platelet counts remained within the hemostatic range (75,000 to 100,000/mm³) (Fig 6-18).
2. Partial thromboplastin time (PTT) remained within the normal range if the mean shock time did not exceed 90 minutes (group III). In contrast, trauma victims in groups IV and V with mean shock times of 150 and 300 minutes, respectively, showed significant elevations of PTT, well out of the hemostatic range (Fig 6-19).
3. Thrombin coagulase time, a sensitive index of fibrinolytic activity, showed a significant prolongation from group IV (150-minute shock time) to group V (300-minute shock time). This change is a typical sign of advanced DIC (Fig 6-20).

FIG. 6-18. Platelet concentration and function (collagen-induced aggregation) during massive transfusion in five groups of patients with different shock duration. (From Harke and Rahman[127] with permission.)

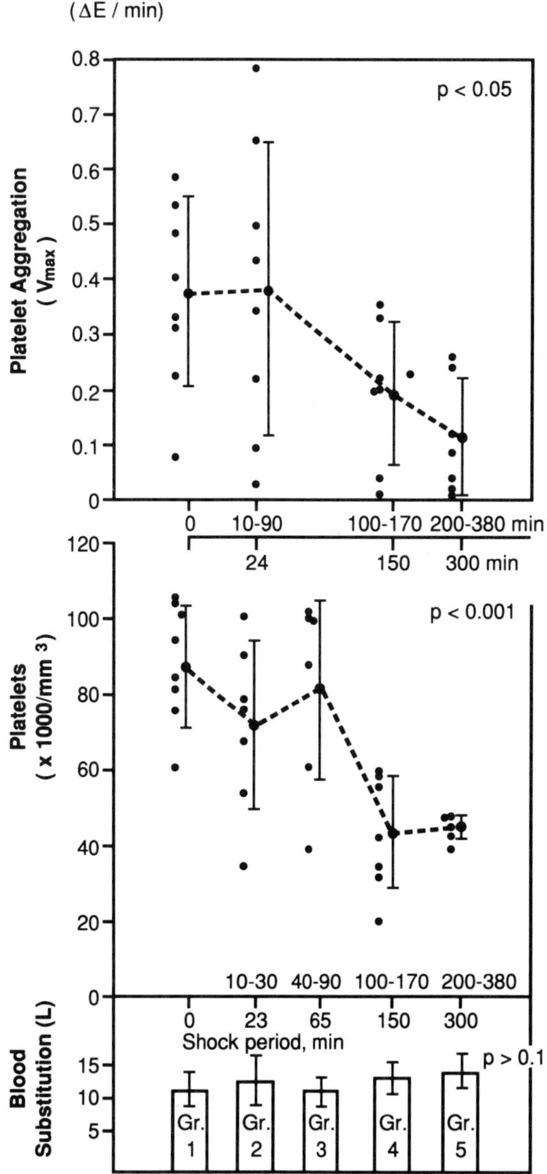

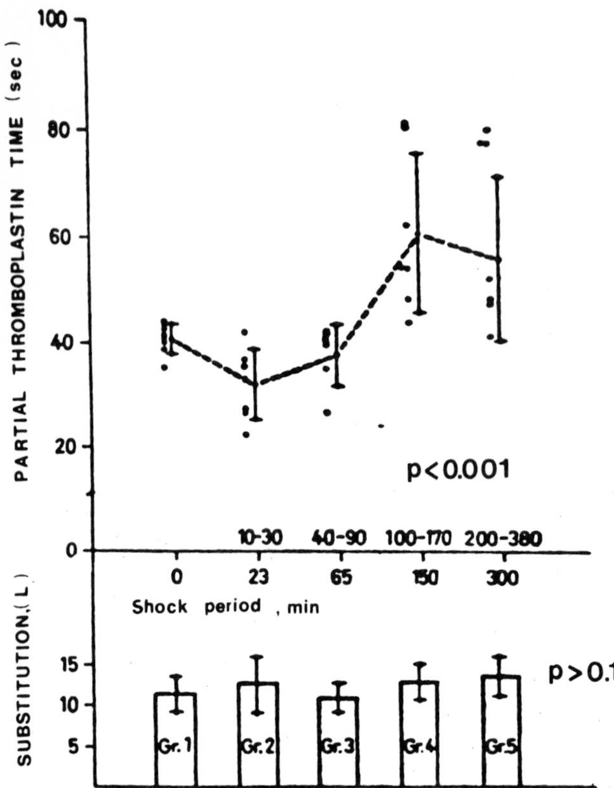


FIG. 6-19. PTT during massive transfusion in the same five groups of patients as in Fig. 6-18. (From Harke and Rahman[127] with permission.)

4. Time in shock correlated directly with the incidence of DIC.
5. Time in shock before definitive blood volume repletion correlated directly with mortality (Fig 6-21).
6. Factor V activity was decreased once the shock time exceeded 65 minutes. There were, however, two patients, one in group III and another in group IV, in whom factor V activity remained within the hemostatic range despite a shock time longer than 65 minutes (Fig 6-20).

Their conclusions were:

1. Massive transfusion of 9-day-old banked blood does not cause DIC.
2. DIC and death are directly linked to time in shock, not to massive transfusion.

These findings have been validated by others.[204,265,266]

If these conclusions are true, how can routine, empiric administration of FFP be justified? On the basis of a large retrospective study by Mannucci et al,[195] a review by Braunstein and Oberman,[27] the NIH consensus conference,[351] prospective hemorrhagic shock studies in dogs by Martin et al,[196] and the study of Counts et al,[62] it seems unlikely that empiric treatment with FFP has a place in massive transfusion therapy if whole blood, modified whole blood, or even packed red cells are employed.[247] Accordingly, a recent survey suggests

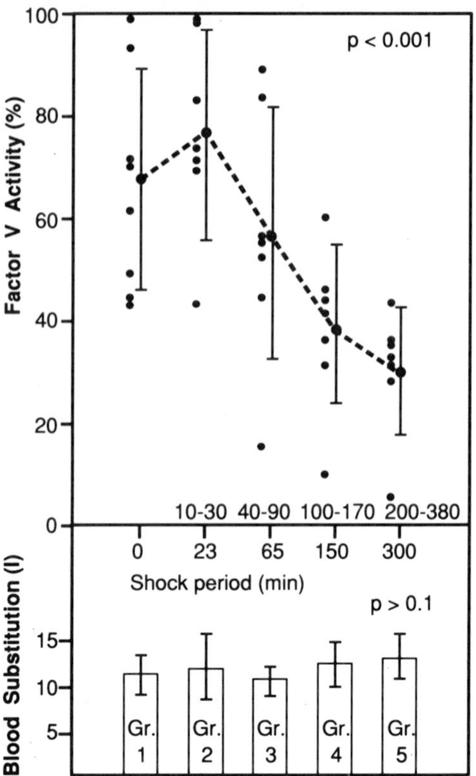


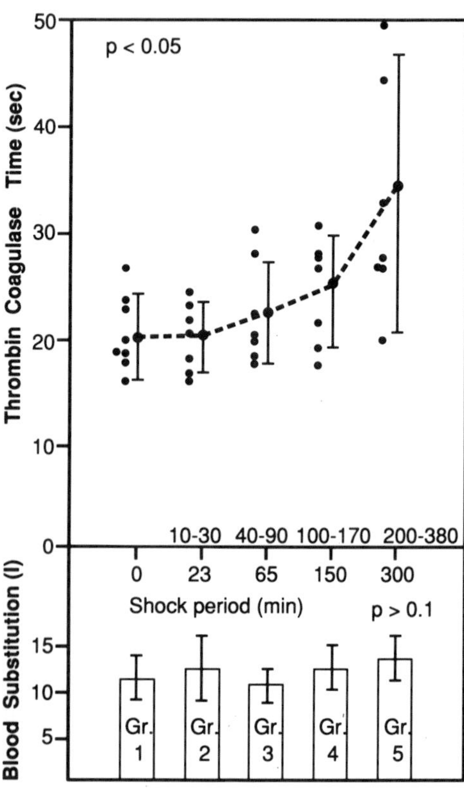


FIG. 6-20. Factor V activity and thrombin coagulase time during massive transfusion in the same five groups of patients as in Fig. 6-18. (From Harke and Rahman[127] with permission.)

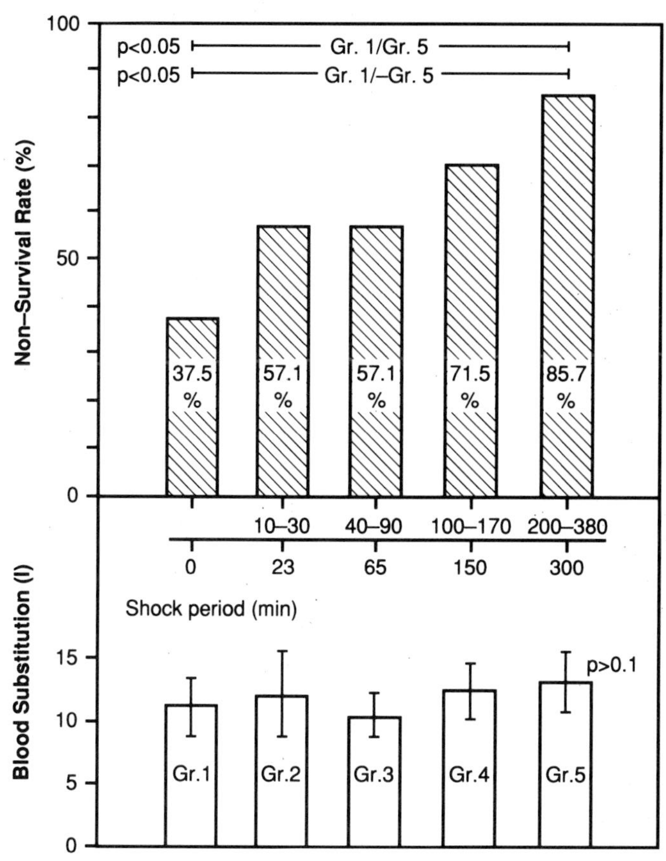


FIG. 6-21. Death rate after massive transfusion in the five groups of patients in Fig. 6-18. (From Harke and Rahman[127] with permission.)

that use of FFP peaked in 1982 and thereafter has remained constant.[338] Despite these trends, changing attitudes, and scientific data condemning prophylactic FFP administration during massive transfusion, some writers still advocate its use.[280]

Unquestionably, if whole or modified whole blood is unavailable and, as currently practiced, red blood cells are the only product the blood bank can issue, administration of FFP is fully justified if clinical coagulopathies appear during massive transfusion.[248,352] Although correct, the last statement is bothersome. Why should hypovolemic, massively transfused patients be deprived of whole blood?[64,251] The addition of multiple units of FFP adds a significant risk of hepatitis over and above the risk of each unit of red blood cells.[320,348,351] This author believes, as does Schmidt,[306] that the blood bankers of this country have been overzealous in their condemnation of whole blood and in the promotion of red blood cells as the universally ideal product. Undoubtedly, whole blood or modified whole blood is the ideal product to use in the massively bleeding trauma patient.

FFP is clearly indicated in the rare hemorrhaging trauma victim who has been receiving long-acting anticoagulants.[27,351] Also, in well established DIC, FFP may be necessary in addition to platelets to replete consumed factors even after the inciting cause has been identified.[22] FFP should be given in this context only when generalized oozing, hypofibrinogenemia, thrombocytopenia, and fibrin split products are present. In addition, FFP may be administered justifiably to patients with severe hepatic insufficiency in whom gross abnormalities in the coagulation profile have been documented and in whom surgery is anticipated.[22,351] "Liver disease," per se, without grossly prolonged PTT and prothrombin time (PT) is not an indication for FFP.[27]

All previous studies assessing the hemostatic qualities of banked blood have been performed on ACD and CPD blood stored for no more than 2 to 3 weeks. The possibility does exist that individuals in whom massive transfusion is carried out mainly with nearly outdated CPDA-1 or Adsol units might develop borderline or even frank deficiencies of factor VIII and possibly of factor V.[247] In the very rare instance in which platelet concentrates do not correct generalized oozing and DIC has been ruled out, FFP may be given. If the patient is only factor VIII deficient, only the PTT will be prolonged. If both factor V and VIII are subnormal, then both PT and PTT will be prolonged. It must be emphasized again that the most recent literature does not support routine use of prophylactic FFP if whole or modified whole blood is given, even during massive transfusion.[22,23,27,41,62,208,248,261,352] If red blood cells are used, the likelihood of coagulopathy caused by factor deficiency increases after 1- to 1.5-blood volume replacement in conjunction with a measured fibrinogen level of 75 mg/dL or less.[247,248] Even in this situation *prophylactic* FFP administration does not seem to be warranted.[247,248]

## PLATELET CONCENTRATES

Platelet concentrates are generally prepared by differential centrifugation of fresh plasma, although plasmapheresis is sometimes used.[322] Because of the wide variability of normal platelet counts (140,000 to 440,000/μL),[372] there may be a threefold difference in the number of platelets supplied in different units of platelet concentrate. However, federal law requires a minimum of $5.5 \times 10^{10}$ platelets in 75% of the units collected.[151] The optimal storage temperature of platelets has been a controversial issue for years, but it has been firmly established recently that platelet function and survival are superior at 22°C, if gentle agitation is applied, than at 4°C.[4,98,174,310] Storage time is limited to 5 days after which the platelets must be discarded.[4,245] Platelet concentrate is supplied in 50-mL bags diluted in citrated plasma. Transfusion of a single unit of platelet concentrate should be expected to raise the platelet count of a 75-kg individual by approximately 10,000/μL.[220,325] Thus, the usual dose of 6 to 8 U of platelet concentrates should raise the platelet count by 60,000 to 80,000/μL, well within the hemostatic range.

A platelet count should be performed approximately 1 hour after completion of platelet infusion to confirm an adequate response to therapy.[322] Platelet counts may be reduced following massive transfusion by rapid utilization, splenic sequestration, fever, and infection.[207,285,322]

During preparation of platelet concentrates a variable degree of red cell contamination occurs.[117,220] Transfusion of even small numbers of Rh positive red cells to an Rh negative female of childbearing age may stimulate production of Rh negative antibodies. $Rh_o$ (D) immune globulin should be given to these patients during subsequent pregnancy to avoid the possibility of erythroblastosis. If possible, these individuals should receive platelets from Rh negative donors.[220] Furthermore, when possible, platelets from ABO-compatible donors should be given since fatal hemolytic transfusion reactions have been reported from transfusion of group O platelet concentrates.[244,281]

Dilutional thrombocytopenia is the most common cause of hemorrhagic diathesis during and after massive transfusion[62,205,208]; it generally presents as oozing from the surgical incision, venipuncture sites, and gingiva. As stated earlier, dilutional thrombocytopenia may manifest as a hemorrhagic diathesis at various platelet concentrations and is usual below 60,000 to 75,000/μL.[205,208] In general, mild dilutional thrombocytopenia need not be treated if it does not cause abnormal bleeding.[4,130,131,285] However, if thrombocytopenia is associated with diffuse oozing, platelets should be given. This is usually, but not always, sufficient as sole treatment.[62,285] The timing of platelet administration is also important.[347] If active surgical bleeding is occurring, it should be controlled prior to platelet infusion, otherwise many donor platelets will be wasted on the operative field. In addition, the temperature of the severely hypothermic patient should be raised to a euthermic or mildly hypothermic level in order for platelets to become hemostatically active.[354] As is true of all components, platelets should not be administered according to some predetermined scheme.[131,285] They are expensive, and each donor unit carries a risk of hepatitis.[306]

### CRYOPRECIPITATE (CONCENTRATED FACTOR VIII)

In the occasional hemorrhaging hemophiliac patient who presents for emergency surgery after trauma, cryoprecipitate will have to be given.[221]

Cryoprecipitate is derived from the proteins that precipitate during thawing of FFP. After removal of nearly all the supernatant plasma, the precipitate is refrozen and may be stored for as long as 2 years with preservation of factor VIII activity. In addition to factor VIII (antihemophilic factor), cryoprecipitate contains about 30 to 50% of the fibrinogen contained in the original unit of blood.[221] Cryoprecipitate is supplied as 10- to 25-mL volume U.

Cryoprecipitate may also be used effectively in patients with von Willebrand's disease,[221] characterized by reduction of factor VIII to a much lesser extent than that seen in hemophilia A. These patients may have no prior history of a bleeding disorder but may ooze diffusely during minor surgery when only modest amounts of blood are usually lost. In general, there are few bona fide uses for cryoprecipitate in the general surgical population.[306] An exception may be the volume-overloaded patient with confirmed DIC. These patients require both factor VIII and fibrinogen and cannot tolerate the volume load of FFP.

## INTRAOPERATIVE AUTOTRANSFUSION

Although it has only recently become popular in busy trauma centers, the concept of intraoperative salvage and reinfusion of shed blood is not new. In 1818 Blundell was credited with performing the first autotransfusion.[263] The technique was never practical in the 19th century because of lack of adequate technology, poor results, and the skepticism of the majority of the medical profession. Early in the 20th century, transfusion of homologous banked blood became practical[77] and with this, autotransfusion all but died.

With time, however, it became apparent that homologous banked blood was less than ideal and was frequently in too short supply for massive transfusions. Advances in biomedical engineering during the latter half of the 20th century have allowed contemporary proponents of autotransfusion to demonstrate its lifesaving capabilities, general safety, and ability to conserve scarce blood resources.[100]

Autotransfusion is the collection and reinfusion of a patient's own blood for intravascular volume replacement. Ideally, then, it may be lifesaving for an individual who has sequestered a significant proportion of the circulating blood volume in the thoracic or abdominal cavities.

Emergency autotransfusion has three general indications[111,288,384]:

1. Thoracic trauma with acute blood loss of 1000 to 5000 mL through the thoracostomy. This blood may be salvaged and reinfused.
2. Profound abdominal or thoracic blood loss when bank blood is unavailable immediately and augmented $O_2$-carrying capacity is essential to survival (ie, when the alternative is exsanguination and death).
3. Supplementation of homologous blood in massive transfusions.

A fourth category is those individuals whose religious beliefs preclude administration of homologous blood or products. Not uncommonly, a Jehovah's Witness will accept fresh autologous blood and not interpret this as a scriptural violation.[100,111,165,183,198] Many of these individuals believe that $O_2$-

carrying blood substitutes are commercially available and are as efficacious as blood. They should be informed that this is not true and given the option of autotransfusion when excessive blood loss is expected.

According to Orr[268] and Symbas[340] the ideal autotransfusion system must possess the following nine characteristics.

1. *Rapid Assembly*. If the apparatus cannot be assembled with reasonable speed, its raison d'être is lost. Rapid bleeding must be rapidly controlled. If blood obscures the bleeding site(s), the surgeon will usually reach for any available suction. If the autotransfusion suction is not on the field, blood will be lost in the wall suction.
2. *Ease of Operation*. Any machine that distracts surgeons, anesthesiologists, and nurses from direct patient care defeats its own purpose.
3. *Relatively Low Cost of Hardware and Software*. Any technology that has limited use and requires a high initial expenditure will be frowned upon by most hospital budget committees. Moreover, the cost-benefit ratio must be favorable.[152,165,330]
4. *In-line Filtration*. The ideal scavenging device should have in-line filtration so that tissue particles are separated from the blood.[165]
5. *Minimal Air-Blood Interface*. The less the contact between air and blood, especially under pressure, the smaller the chance of fatal air embolism.[85] Ideally, there should be no air in the system.[165]
6. *Simple Nonsystemic Anticoagulation*. Obviously, systemic anticoagulation with heparin, as used in cardiopulmonary bypass, does not make sense in the treatment of trauma victims with multiple injuries until surgical hemostasis is achieved. The ideal system should use agents such as citrate anticoagulants, which are inactivated in the systemic circulation.[111,156,384] Nevertheless, heparin has been used during intraoperative autotransfusion.
7. *Red Cell Concentrating Capability*. The ability to concentrate red cells protects the patient from inadvertent volume overload once hemorrhage is controlled.
8. *Removal of Cellular and Fluid Contaminants and Other Extraneous Debris*. Along with in-line filtration, washing and concentration of red cells help remove small particles including the debris of hemolyzed red cells, platelet and leukocyte aggregates, and free hemoglobin.[165]
9. *Minimal Destruction of Cellular Elements or Induction of Coagulopathy*. Retrieval, processing, and reinfusion should not be associated with an appreciable degree of red cell hemolysis. In addition, the processed infusate should not induce coagulopathy.

## EQUIPMENT FOR AUTOTRANSFUSION

### *Bentley ATS-100*

This was the first commercially available autotransfusion device in the United States. It enjoyed great popularity in the 1970s because of its rapid scavenging and reinfusion flow rates.[100,364] Unfortunately, because of several episodes of fatal air embolism,[85,258] it was withdrawn from the market. The Bentley system consisted of a roller pump, a blood reservoir with a filter and air release line at the apex, and two large-caliber infusion lines. Blood was aspirated from the surgical field by the roller pump. It was then delivered to the reservoir, where pressure generated by a large compressed air-blood interface forced the blood into the infusion lines. Air embolism was generally the result of technician inattentiveness, tampering with the built-in fail-safe mechanism,[268] or small films of clot occluding the photoelectric sensing device.[111]

### *Sorenson Receptal*

This system consists of suction tubing in which CPD anticoagulant is added to the salvaged blood in a ratio of 1 to 7 (the standard ratio in banked blood). Thus, anticoagulated blood suctioned at 30 to 60 mm Hg pressure is deposited into sterile 500- to 1900-mL soft plastic bags attached to a rigid plastic outer canister. When full, the inner bag is removed, and its contents may be reinfused by gravity flow or under pressure. Micropore filtration is recommended to remove particulate debris suctioned from the operating field. The manufacturer, however, recommends that the salvaged blood be washed and concentrated prior to reinfusion. Since there is no contact of the blood with air, the possibility of air embolism is eliminated. Utilizing the Sorenson autotransfusion system, Noon et al[259] have successfully salvaged up to 10,000 mL of blood during vascular procedures.

### *Haemonetics Cell Saver*

In this system (Fig 6-22), red cells are retrieved, washed, and concentrated in one continuous process. Blood is suctioned from the surgical field, anticoagulated in the suction tubing as in the Sorenson device, and temporarily stored in a cardiotomy reservoir. It is then delivered via roller pump into a centrifuge bowl in which the red cells are washed in saline and concentrated. During the washing process, virtually all plasma, tissue, cell debris, and anticoagulant are eliminated and deposited in a waste receptacle. The remaining suspension consists of approximately 225 to 500 mL of salvaged blood with a hematocrit over 50%.[165,364] The processed cells are then transferred to a blood bag where they are reinfused by gravity or external pressure. The whole process requires 8 to 10 minutes from initial salvage to reinfusion, and although it is slow, it is adequate for most situations in which blood loss is not massive.[364]

A modification of this system permits bypassing the washing and concentrating stage and direct reinfusion at high flow rates via the roller pump.[364] Thus, shed blood may be reinfused rapidly when massive hemorrhage occurs. With this modification, an air-blood interface exists which requires an antiembolism device and the constant attention of a trained technician. The latest Haemonetics devices (Haemonetics-4, Haemonetics-plus) are totally automated and require less supervision.

### *IBM Blood Cell Processor*

The IBM 2991 blood cell processor is primarily a red blood cell washing system that is in theory analogous to the Haemonetics system. It was originally designed for washing and

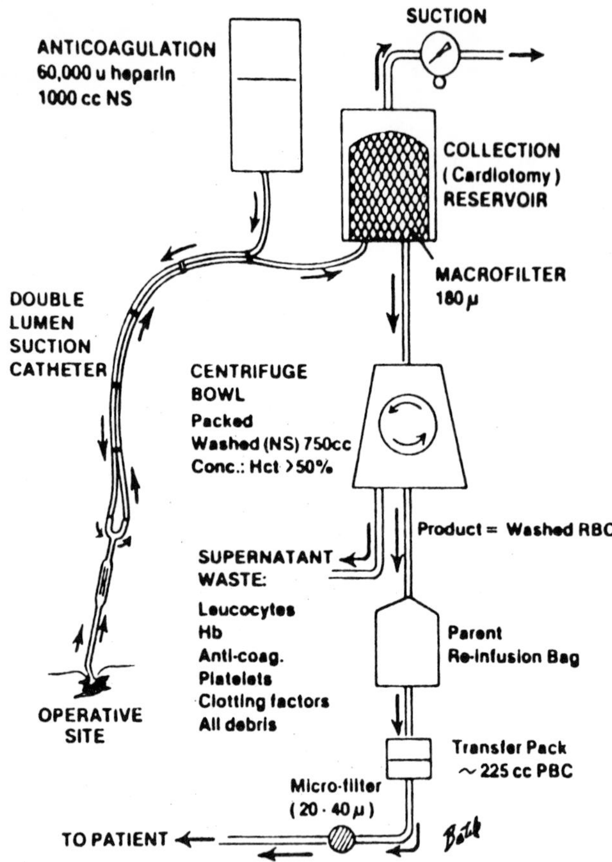


FIG. 6-22. Haemonetics Cell Saver with modifications. (From Keeling et al[165] with permission.)

deglycerolization of frozen red cells and is usually kept in the hospital blood bank rather than in the operating room. The IBM blood cell processor can be interfaced with the Sorenson scavenging system, and used successfully if massive autotransfusion is not required. A complete washing and concentration cycle requires approximately 15 minutes, limiting its use in cases of massive blood loss.

## COMPLICATIONS OF AUTOTRANSFUSION

The complications of autotransfusion are classified into two categories, hematologic and nonhematologic.[384]

### *Hematologic Complications*

Obviously, suctioning, pumping, washing, concentrating, turbulent flow, and reinfusion under pressure take their toll on formed elements and clotting factors. The following hematologic abnormalities have been noted[156,165,234,237,252,302,384]:

1. Thrombocytopenia
2. Hemolysis with hemoglobinemia
3. Decreased hematocrit
4. Increased fibrin split products
5. Prolonged PT and activated PTT
6. Hypofibrinogenemia.

The possibility that tissue thromboplastins may play a role in initiating DIC in autotransfused patients was investigated by Kingsley et al.[170] They found that if scavenged blood is washed with a continuous flow centrifuge to remove thromboplastic substances, DIC can largely be avoided. It should be remembered that in massive transfusion, DIC is probably not due to the transfused blood but rather to the primary problem that makes the transfusion necessary.[111] In any event, whether a coagulopathy is due to dilution, primary fibrinolysis or DIC, platelets and/or FFP may be required.

### *Nonhematologic*

SEPSIS. Various studies have shown that bacteremia may be reduced but not eliminated by red cell washing and antibiotic therapy.[21,100,113,114,172,344,384] A contaminated wound is only a relative contraindication to autotransfusion[112,344]: if little or no banked blood is available and the alternative is exsanguination and death, autotransfusion is indicated.[100,112,156,344] Administration of broad-spectrum antibiotics and maintenance of adequate hemodynamics and oxygenation will reduce morbidity in these circumstances.[344] Postoperative sepsis is more easily explained than exsanguination in the operating room when an autotransfuser is available and ready to function.[21]

AIR EMBOLISM. Any system with a significant air-blood interface under pressure is capable of causing fatal air embolism.[85] If this complication does occur, immediate recognition is mandatory. The treatment consists of turning the patient to a left lateral Trendelenberg position and aspirating through a large-bore central venous or right atrial catheter until air no longer returns.[164] Additionally, nitrous oxide, if in use, should be discontinued.

MICROEMBOLISM. Infusion of small particles of bone, fat, and other tissue is possible but is largely eliminated by microfiltration and cell washing.[165] Although autotransfusion devices should remove all cellular elements other than red cells, some leukocyte and platelet adherence to the centrifuge bowl can occur and results in their subsequent return to the patient. This can cause not only coagulopathy but also severe posttransfusion pulmonary pathology.[35] These complications can be minimized by avoiding excessive dilution of the salvaged blood with saline, by preventing contamination of the blood with thrombin, and by maintaining citrate concentration of the blood during the initial processing, since all of these factors promote leukocyte adhesion to the centrifuge bowl.[34,35] Administration of calcium salts during massive transfusion to compensate for the citrate anticoagulant may thus be deleterious if autotransfusion is being used.[34]

## CONTRAINDICATIONS

There are no absolute contraindications to autotransfusion in emergency situations if blood is unavailable or in short supply. However, in grossly contaminated abdominal wounds and wounds older than 4 to 6 hours, the use of homologous blood, if available, is preferred.[21]

ADVANTAGES OF EMERGENCY INTRAOPERATIVE AUTOTRANSFUSION

The purported benefits of intraoperative blood salvage are as follows[89,100,165,384]:

1. Provides blood immediately
2. Reduces incompatibility problems
3. Conserves blood bank resources
4. Reduces the risk of viral transmission
5. Fresh, minimally hypothermic red cells with normal 2,3-DPG levels are administered
6. Cost effective in moderate to massive transfusions
7. Reduces blood bank workload
8. Is acceptable to many Jehovah's Witnesses.

Although it is true that emergency intraoperative autotransfusion reduces the risks of hepatitis and immunologic incompatibility, these are weak arguments for its use.[111] In massive hemorrhage, patients still require homologous blood despite efficient scavenging.[89,112,152] In a study of 224 trauma victims, Glover and Broadie[111] found that when blood loss was approximately 2500 mL, the ratio of homologous to autotransfused blood was roughly 1:1. As total blood loss approached 23,000 mL, this ratio decreased to approximately 1:3. Obviously, autotransfusion reduces the necessity for banked blood, but its real virtue probably rests in saving at least a few lives when homologous blood is not immediately available and exsanguination is imminent.

## FRONTIERS OF HEMOTHERAPY

OXYGEN-CARRYING SOLUTIONS

Blood is an expensive, relatively scarce resource with certain undesirable properties. Consequently, recent research has focused on attempting to develop asanguinous $O_2$-carrying solutions with the following characteristics[71,312,353]:

1. Ability to load, transport, and unload oxygen
2. Sufficient vascular retention to maintain blood volume
3. Freedom from antigenicity and pyrogenicity
4. Lack of organ toxicity
5. Favorable rheologic properties in order to augment and improve microcirculatory flow, thereby maintaining organ function
6. Reasonable biologic half-life
7. Prolonged storage capability
8. Freedom from induction of coagulopathy
9. Cost effective and readily available in mass casualties.

Extensive research has produced two alternatives to red cells, stroma-free hemoglobin and perfluorochemical emulsions.

STROMA-FREE HEMOGLOBIN (SFH)

Human hemoglobin solution may ultimately be useful as an oxygen-carrying resuscitation fluid.[69,367] The following advantages of SFH are given by De Venuto[69,70,71]:

1. Component of normal blood
2. Transports and exchanges $O_2$
3. Adequate oncotic activity
4. No typing or cross-matching necessary
5. No antigenicity
6. Soluble in physiologic solutions
7. Low viscosity
8. Prepared from outdated red cells
9. Long-term storage
10. Little direct toxicity.

These advantages seem to match the characteristics of an ideal asanguinous solution. However, two major problems have been encountered,[67,70,158,296,353] high $O_2$ affinity and poor vascular retention.

The oxygen-binding capacities of free and intracellular hemoglobin are equivalent,[69,70,242] approximately 1.34 mL of $O_2$ per gram of hemoglobin. However, free hemoglobin has a much greater affinity for $O_2$. $P_{50}$ values for SFH and normal erythrocytes at 37°C and pH 7.40 are 12 to 16 and 26 to 27 mm Hg, respectively.[70] Thus, at any given $O_2$ saturation SFH releases less $O_2$ to the cells (Fig 6-23).[70,134,242,295] By comparison, 2,3-DPG-depleted red cells have a $P_{50}$ of approximately 18 mm Hg.[47,125] The factors responsible for the increased $O_2$ affinity of SFH include lack of 2,3-DPG, lower concentration than intraerythrocytic hemoglobin, and pH elevation of as much as 0.2 units resulting in a Bohr effect.[70] The left-shifted oxyhemoglobin dissociation curve of SFH results in decreased tissue oxygenation.[135,242] Sequential hemodilution with SFH is characterized by lack of augmentation of cardiac output despite reduced viscosity[72,120,134] because of increased systemic vascular resistance with this agent. Thus, hemodilution with SFH results in decreased $P\bar{v}O_2$ without increased $O_2$ extraction.[134,135,242,295]

Despite its molecular weight of 68,000, the hemoglobin molecule's osmotic properties and volume effect are inadequate because the tetrameric molecule dissociates into two dimers that are metabolized in the reticuloendothelial system by com-

FIG. 6-23. Oxyhemoglobin dissociation curves of human blood (....), unmodified hemoglobin solutions (---), and pyridoxylated-polymerized hemoglobin (——) at pH 7.40 and 37°C. Note the leftward shifts of modified and unmodified hemoglobin solutions compared with whole blood. (From De Venuto F[70] with permission.)

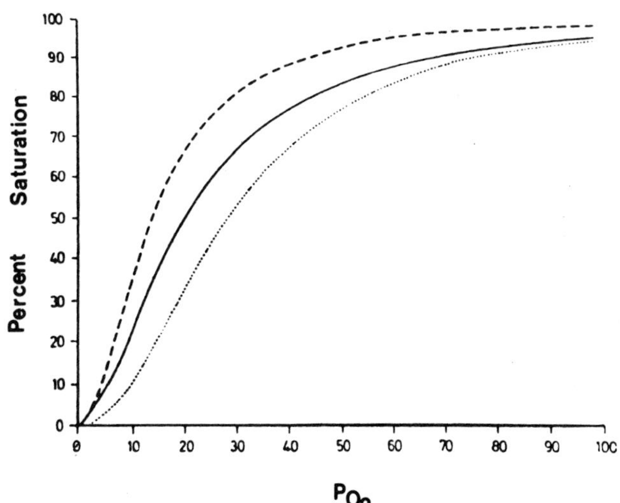

plex formation with haptoglobin or excreted by the kidney.[203,353] The biologic half-life of unmodified SFH is 2 to 4 hours,[69] coinciding with osmotic diuresis and a rapid intravascular volume decline of 42% after exchange transfusion with this agent.[104]

Since unmodified SFH is a less than ideal resuscitation fluid, biochemical modifications have been attempted in order to improve its high $O_2$ affinity and poor intravascular retention.[70,121] Pyridoxylation and polymerization of the hemoglobin molecule is one possible answer. When the hemoglobin molecule reacts with pyridoxal 5-phosphate—an analog of 2,3-DPG which increases its $P_{50}$—and is polymerized with glutaraldehyde to improve its vascular retention, the resulting hemoglobin solution has a $P_{50}$ of 19.6 ± 0.4 mm Hg and is retained 6 to 10 times longer than unmodified SFH.[70,119] Pyridoxylated, polymerized SFH solution has been shown to support normal $\dot{V}O_2$ at an otherwise lethal hematocrit following exchange transfusion.[119]

Recent research has attempted to encapsulate the hemoglobin molecule in phospholipid-cholesterol membranes. The resulting synthetic erythrocytes are called hemosomes and are capable of transporting $CO_2$ and $O_2$ at a $P_{50}$ of 28 mm Hg.[78,79]

### PERFLUOROCHEMICALS

The perfluorochemicals are a group of aliphatic compounds in which all the C-H groups are replaced by C-F.[45,353] These organic derivatives have a much greater capacity for $O_2$ and $CO_2$ than plasma.[45,353] Consequently, there has been much research into their usefulness.

In contrast to hemoglobin, the oxygen dissociation curve of perfluorochemicals is linear rather than sigmoidal[45,120,203] (Fig 6-24). Hence, even though oxygen is several times more soluble in fluorocarbons than in plasma,[45,203] the oxygen-carrying capacity of these compounds is appreciable only when the inspired $O_2$ concentration is very high. With an $FIO_2$ of 1.0 at 37°C, only 5.6 mL of $O_2$ per deciliter is transported by Fluosol DA-20% (perfluoro chemical-emulsion).[120] Even though this is a small amount of $O_2$, it has been shown to support and sustain life down to a hematocrit less than 2% in baboons. Moreover, during progressive hemodilution with Fluosol DA-20%, no significant changes were noted in oxygen consumption, cardiac output, or arteriovenous $O_2$ content despite a precipitous reduction of total $O_2$ delivery.[120] In assessing the efficacy of Fluosol, it has been observed that its contribution to oxygen delivery and consumption becomes significant only when the recipient's hematocrit is below 10%.[120] For this reason, it is unlikely that Fluosol DA can contribute much to tissue $O_2$ supply in patients suffering mild to moderate blood loss.[203] Its potential usefulness in resuscitation is thus dubious. In addition to its meager contribution to $\dot{D}O_2$ and $\dot{V}O_2$ at hematocrits greater than 10%, several potentially disastrous complications have been noted. Perhaps due to complement activation, 0.5-mL test doses of Fluosol DA-20% have been followed by profound bradycardia and dramatic elevation of pulmonary artery systolic and diastolic pressures.[349] Even when a negative response to a test dose is elicited, profound hypotension has been observed when infusion rates exceed 20 mL/min.[255,365,366] Other complications associated with the use of Fluosol DA-20% include alterations of liver function tests—increased serum glutamic-pyruvic transaminase (SGPT), -oxaloacetic transaminase (SGOT), lactate dehydrogenase (LDH) and alkaline phosphatase—bilateral pulmonary infiltration with arterial hypoxemia, transient circulating leukocyte depression, and cytotoxic changes with cell growth inhibition.[359] Because of these complications research on Fluosol DA-20% was discontinued several years ago in the United States.

FIG. 6-24. Oxygen content curves for whole blood (WB), stroma-free hemoglobin (SFH), and Fluosol DA-20% (FL-DA). Note that optimization of oxygen content for WB and SFH occurs at an oxygen tension of approximately 100 mm Hg, whereas the maximal but small contribution to oxygen content of Fluosol occurs only at very high $PO_2$ (500 to 600 mm Hg). (From Gould et al[120] with permission.)

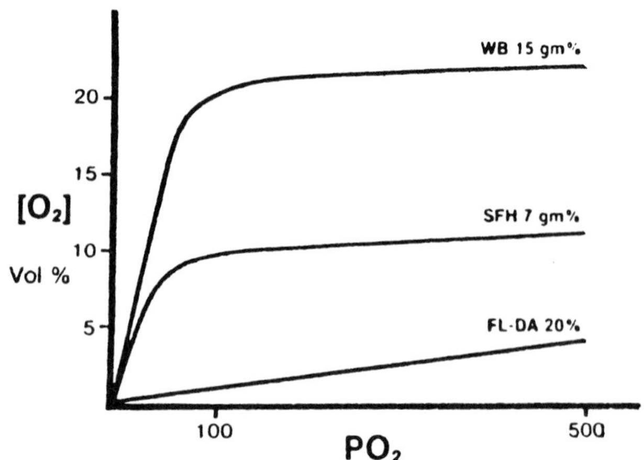


## CONCLUSION

Administration of blood and its components to the injured patient may be approached rationally and safely if basic principles are clearly understood.[272,332] The decision to administer emergency group O, Rh negative concentrated red cells instead of fully typed and cross-matched blood depends on the gravity of the clinical situation. If total red cell volume is judged to be inadequate to support life, then immediate transfusion with type O cells is indicated. If, however, global oxygen transport is deemed adequate after volume replacement with acellular fluids, there is time to cross-match or at least to order type-specific blood if it is required. Whole blood is indicated only in the presence of massive ongoing and/or uncontrollable blood loss; whereas red cells are indicated in situations in which loss of red cell mass is moderate, massive transfusion is not contemplated, and surgical hemostasis is secured.

Although stored blood undergoes progressive biophysical and biochemical deterioration, storage lesions, although seemingly significant, are in general not clinically harmful. Maintenance of normovolemia and normothermia, by whatever means, will prevent many of the complications formerly thought to be caused by storage changes. Warming of all administered fluids and heating and humidifying of inspiratory gases cannot be overemphasized.[16,159]

Dilutional thrombocytopenia may occur with massive transfusion, however empiric or prophylactic administration of platelets is to be condemned.[51] Cookbook administration of FFP is also to be avoided; whole blood is indicated in massive transfusion rather than packed red cells and colloid in the form of FFP.

Microaggregate blood filters also have no place in massive transfusion therapy. Unless proven otherwise, use of these filters should be considered wasteful and unscientific.

Life-threatening transfusion reactions are largely avoided by proper patient and donor identification and by stringent blood bank protocol. Minor transfusion reactions such as febrile episodes or urticaria may not be avoidable, but fortunately they are of little consequence.

Emergency autotransfusion capability should be available in any active trauma center. Effective employment of this technology should save lives, reduce the incidence of viral infection, and avoid depletion of the blood supply.

In conclusion, emergency transfusion can be a lifesaving procedure. Moreover, failure to recognize the hazards of insufficient transfusion of blood or its components may result in coagulopathies, multisystem organ dysfunction, and death.[51]

## REFERENCES


1. Aach RD, Szmuness W, Mosley JW, et al. Serum alanine aminotransferase of donors in relation to the risk of non-A, non-B hepatitis in recipients: the transfusion transmitted viruses study. N Engl J Med 1981;304:989.
2. Abbott TR. Changes in serum calcium fractions and citrate concentrations during massive blood transfusions and cardiopulmonary bypass. Br J Anaesth 1983;55:753.
3. Aeder MI, Crowe JP, Rhodes RS, et al. Technical limitations in the rapid infusion of intravenous fluids. Ann Emerg Med 1985;14:307.

3a. Alter HJ, Purcell RH, Shih JW, et al. Detection of antibody to hepatitis C virus in prospectively followed transfusion recipients with acute and chronic non-A, non-B hepatitis. N Engl J Med 1989;321:1494.

3b. Alter MJ, Sampliner RE (Editorial). Hepatitis C and miles to go before we sleep. N Eng J Med 1989;321:1538.

4. Aster RH (chairperson). Platelet transfusion therapy: consensus conference. JAMA 1987;257:1777.
5. Auffant RA, Downs JB, Amick R. Ionized calcium concentration and cardiovascular function after cardiopulmonary bypass. Arch Surg 1981;116:1072.
6. Baker JL, Kelen GD, Sivertson KT, et al. Unsuspected human immunodeficiency virus in critically ill emergency patients. JAMA 1987;257:2609.
7. Barcenas CG, Fuller TJ, Knochel JP. Metabolic alkalosis after massive blood transfusion: correction by hemodialysis. JAMA 1976;236:953.
8. Barker LF. Viral hepatitis and other infections transmitted by transfusion: use of active and passive immunization. In: Petz LD, Swisher SN, eds. Clinical practice of blood transfusion. New York: Churchill Livingstone, 1981:757.
9. Barnes A. The blood bank in hemotherapy for trauma and surgery. In: Barnes A, Umlas J, eds. Hemotherapy in trauma and surgery. Washington DC: American Association of Blood Banks, 1979:77.
10. Barnes A. Transfusion of universal donor and uncrossmatched blood. Bibl Haematol 1980;46:132.
11. Barnette RE, Fish DJ, Eisenstaedt RS. Impact of physician education on perioperative utilization of FFP. Anesth Analg 1988;67:S7.
12. Bashour TT, Ryan C, Kabbani S, et al. Hypocalcemic acute myocardial failure secondary to rapid transfusion of citrated blood. Am Heart J 1984;108:1040.
13. Bastron RD. Diuretics. In: Kaplan JA, ed. Cardiac anesthesia, cardiovascular pharmacology. New York: Grune and Stratton, 1983:325.
14. Bates DV, Macklem PT, Christie RV. Respiratory function in disease. 2nd ed. Philadelphia: WB Saunders, 1973:3.
15. Benesch R, Benesch RE. The effect of organic phosphates from the human erythrocyte on the allosteric properties of hemoglobin. Biochem Biophys Res Commun 1967;26:162.
16. Bernard JM, Pinaud M, Souron R. Perioperative hypothermia prevention. Acta Anaesthesiol Scand 1987;31:521.
17. Beutler E, Wood L. The in vivo regeneration of red cell 2,3-diphosphoglyceric acid (DPG) after transfusion of stored blood. J Lab Clin Med 1969;74:300.
18. Bevan DR. Renal function in anaesthesia and surgery. New York: Grune and Stratton, 1979:57.
19. Blumberg N, Bove JR. Uncrossmatched blood for emergency transfusion. JAMA 1978;240:2057.
20. Boelhouwer RU, Bruining HA, Giok GL. Correlations of serum potassium fluctuations with body temperature after major surgery. Crit Care Med 1987;15:310.
21. Boudreaux JP, Bornside GH, Cohn I. Emergency autotransfusion: partial cleansing of bacteria-laden blood by cell washing. J Trauma 1983;23:31.
22. Bove JR. Fresh frozen plasma: too few indications—too much use. Anesth Analg 1985;64:849.
23. Bove JR. International forum: which is the factual basis, in theory and clinical practice, for the use of fresh frozen plasma? Vox Sang 1978;35:428.
24. Bove JR. Transfusion-associated hepatitis and AIDS: what is the risk? N Engl J Med 1987;317:242.
25. Bowen JC, Fleming WH. Increased oxyhemoglobin affinity after transfusion. Ann Surg 1974;180:760.
26. Boyan CP. Cold or warm blood for massive transfusion. Ann Surg 1964;160:282.
27. Braunstein AH, Oberman HA. Transfusion of plasma components. Transfusion 1984;24:281.
28. Bredenberg CE. Microaggregate filters. Int Anesthesiol Clin 1982;20:195.
29. Brown K, Bissonnette B, Poon AO. Hyperkalemia during massive blood transfusion in pediatric craniofacial surgery. Anesth Analg 1989;68:S40.
30. Brown SE, White SE. *Yersinia enterocolitica* and transfusion-induced septicemia. Anesth Analg 1988;67:415.
31. Brown WJ, Kim BS, Weeks DB, et al. Physiologic saline solution, Normosol-R pH 7.4 and Plasmanate as reconstituents of packed human erythrocytes. Anesthesiology 1978;49:99.
32. Bryan-Brown CW, Baek SM, Makabali G, et al. Consumable oxygen: availability of oxygen in relation to oxyhemoglobin dissociation. Crit Care Med 1973;1:17.
33. Brzica SM. Complications of transfusion. Int Anesthesiol Clin 1982;20:171.
34. Bull BS, Bull MH. Enhancing the safety of intraoperative RBC salvage. J Trauma 1989;29:320.
35. Bull MH, Bull BS, Van Arsdell GS, et al. Clinical implications of procoagulant and leukoattractant formation during intraoperative blood salvage. Arch Surg 1988;123:1073.
36. Bunker JP, Bendixen HH, Murphy AJ. Hemodynamic effects of intravenously administered sodium citrate. N Engl J Med 1962;266:372.

37. Bunn HF, May MH, Kocholaty WF, et al. Hemoglobin function in stored blood. J Clin Invest 1969;48:311.
38. Bureau MA, Begin R, Berthiaume Y, et al. Cerebral hypoxia from bicarbonate infusion in diabetic acidosis. J Pediatr 1980;96:968.
39. Caggiano V. Red blood cell transfusions. In: Silver H, ed, Blood, blood components and derivatives in transfusion therapy. Washington DC: American Association of Blood Banks, 1980:1.
40. Calkins JM, Vaughan RW, Cork RC, et al. Effects of dilution, pressure and apparatus on hemolysis and flow rate in transfusion of packed erythrocytes. Anesth Analg 1982;61:776.
41. Cederbaum AI. The appropriate use of plasma and plasma components in clinical medicine. In: Silver H, ed. Blood, blood components and derivatives in transfusion therapy. Washington DC: American Association of Blood Banks, 1980:105.
42. Chalon F, Markham FP, Ali MM, et al. The pall ultipor breathing filter: an efficient heat and moisture exchanger. Anesth Analg 1984;63:566.
43. Chanutin A, Curnish RR. Effect of organic and inorganic phosphates on oxygen equilibrium of human erythrocytes. Arch Biochem 1967;96:121.
44. Cherry MS, Hodgson GH, Notiebrock H. Comparison of two in-line blood warmers. Can Anaesth Soc J 1981;28:180.
45. Clark LC. Theoretical and practical considerations of fluorocarbon emulsions in the treatment of shock. In: Cowley RA, Trump BF, eds. Pathophysiology of shock, anoxia and ischemia. Baltimore: Williams and Wilkins, 1982:507.
46. Cohen ND, Munoz A, Reitz BA, et al. Transmission of retroviruses by transfusion of screened blood in patients undergoing cardiac surgery. N Engl J Med 1989;320:1172.
47. Collins JA. Abnormal hemoglobin-oxygen affinity and surgical hemotherapy. Bibl Haematol 1980;46:59.
48. Collins JA. Blood transfusions and disorders of surgical bleeding. In: Sabiston DC, ed, Davis-Christopher textbook of surgery. 11th ed. Philadelphia: WB Saunders, 1981:128.
49. Collins JA. Massive transfusion: what is current and important? In: Nusbacher J, ed. Massive transfusion 1978. Washington DC: American Association of Blood Banks, 1978:1.
50. Collins JA. Pertinent recent developments in blood banking: symposium on critical illness. Surg Clin North Am 1983;63:483.
51. Collins JA. Recent developments in the area of massive transfusion. World J Surg 1987;11:75.
52. Collins JA. Surgical problems of transfusion therapy, including cardiopulmonary bypass. In: Petz LD, Swisher SN, eds. Clinical practice of blood transfusion. New York: Churchill Livingstone, 1981:455.
53. Collins JA (moderator). Transfusion practices in emergencies. In: Collins JA, Murawski K, Shafer AW, eds. Massive transfusion in surgery and trauma. New York: Alan R Liss, 1982:285.
54. Collins JA, James PM, Bredenberg CE, et al. The relationship between transfusion and hypoxemia in combat casualties. Ann Surg 1978;188:513.
55. Collins JA, Simmons RL, James PM, et al. Acid-base status of seriously wounded combat casualties, II: resuscitation with stored blood. Ann Surg 1971;173:6.
56. Collins JA, Stechenberg L. The effects of the concentration and function of hemoglobin on the survival of rats after hemorrhage. Surgery 1979;85:412.
57. Conroy JM, Baker JD, Cooke JE. Supernatant potassium levels in stored blood. Anesth Analg 1988;67:S38.
58. Cork RC, Vaughan RW, Humphrey LS. Precision and accuracy of intraoperative temperature monitoring. Anesth Analg 1983;62:211.
59. Cork RC, Vaughan RW, Rothrock L. Effect of site and time on temperature assessment. Anesthesiology 1981;55:A135.
60. Coté CJ, Drop LI, Hoaglin DC. Ionized hypocalcemia after fresh frozen plasma administration to thermally injured children: effects of infusion rate, duration and treatment with calcium chloride. Anesth Analg 1988;67:152.
61. Coté CJ, Liu LMP, Szyfelbein SK, et al. Changes in serial platelet counts following massive blood transfusion in pediatric patients. Anesthesiology 1985;62:197.
62. Counts RB, Haisch C, Simon TL, et al. Hemostasis in massively transfused trauma patients. Ann Surg 1979;190:91.
63. Courcy PA, Brotman S, Dawson B. Massive blood transfusion in acute trauma. Transfusion 1983;23:404.
64. Crowley JP, Guadagnoli E, Pezzullo J, et al. Changes in hospital component therapy in response to reduced availability of whole blood. Transfusion 1988;28:4.
65. Dailey RH. "Code red" protocol for resuscitation of the exsanguinated patient. J Emerg Med 1985;2:373.
66. Davis KG, Abbott RL. Delayed haemolytic transfusion reactions: review of three cases. Med J Aust 1982;Apr 17:335.
67. Dawidson I, Drukker S, Hedlund B, et al. Deleterious effects of stroma-free hemoglobin used as resuscitative fluid for rats with ischemic intestinal shock. Crit Care Med 1988;16:606.
68. Dawson RB. Historical perspective. In: Sohmer PR, Schiffer CA, eds. Blood storage and preservation. Anaheim: American Association of Blood Banks, 1982:1.
69. De Venuto F. Hemoglobin solutions as oxygen-delivering resuscitation fluids. Crit Care Med 1982;10:238.
70. De Venuto F. Modified hemoglobin solution as a resuscitation fluid. Vox Sang 1983;44:129.
71. De Venuto F. Oxygen-carrying resuscitation solutions. Crit Care Med 1982;10:237.
72. De Venuto F, Busse KR, Zegna AI. Viscosity of human blood hemodiluted with crystalline hemoglobin solution. Transfusion 1981;21:752.
73. Denlinger JK, Nahrwold ML, Gibbs PS, et al. Hypocalcemia during rapid blood transfusion in anesthetized man. Br J Anaesth 1976;48:995.
74. Dennis RC, Vito L, Weisel RD, et al. Improved myocardial performance following high 2,3-diphosphoglycerate red cell transfusions. Surgery 1975;77:741.
75. Dern RJ, Brewer GJ, Wiorkowski JJ. Studies on the preservation of human blood, II: the relationship of erythrocyte adenosine triphosphate levels and other in vitro measures to red cell storageability. J Lab Clin Med 1967;69:968.
76. Derrington MC. The present status of blood filtration. Anaesthesia 1985;40:334.
77. Dixon B. Of different bloods. Science 1984;Nov:65.
78. Djordjevich L, Mayoral J, Miller IF, et al. Cardiorespiratory effects of exchange transfusions with synthetic erythrocytes in rats. Crit Care Med 1987;15:318.
79. Djordjevich L, Miller IF. Synthetic erythrocytes from lipid encapsulated hemoglobin. Exp Hematol 1980;8:584.
80. Douglas ME, Downs JB, Mantini EL, et al. Alteration of oxygen tension and oxyhemoglobin saturation: a hazard of sodium bicarbonate administration. Arch Surg 1979;114:326.
81. Driscoll DF, Bistrian BR, Jenkins RL, et al. Development of metabolic alkalosis after massive transfusion during orthotopic liver transplantation. Crit Care Med 1987;15:905.
82. Drop LJ. Ionized calcium, the heart, and hemodynamic function. Anesth Analg 1985;64:432.
83. Drop LJ, Laver MB. Low plasma ionized calcium and response to calcium therapy in critically ill man. Anesthesiology 1975;43:300.
84. Dula DJ, Lutz P, Vogel MF, et al. Rapid flow rates for resuscitation of hypovolemic shock. Ann Emerg Med 1985;14:303.
85. Duncan SE, Klebanoff G, Rogers W. A clinical experience with intraoperative autotransfusion. Ann Surg 1974;180:296.
86. Dunstan RA, Rosse WF. Posttransfusion purpura. Transfusion 1985;25:219.

87. Durtschi MB, Haisch CE, Reynolds L, et al. Effect of micropore filtration on pulmonary function after massive transfusion. Am J Surg 1979;138:8.
88. Duvelleroy MA, Martin JL, Teisseire B, et al. Abnormal hemoglobin oxygen affinity and the coronary circulation. Bibl Haematol, 1980;46:70.
89. Dzik WH, Jenkins R. Use of intraoperative blood salvage during orthotopic liver transplantation. Arch Surg 1985;120:946.
90. Easton DJ, Ternoey CM. Hemolysis of donor cells in "two thirds-one third" solution. Transfusion 1985;25:85.
91. Ebert JP, Grimes B, Niemann KMW. Respiratory failure secondary to homologous blood transfusion. Anesthesiology 1985;63:104.
92. Eger EI. Anesthetic uptake and action. Baltimore: Williams and Wilkins, 1974:11.
93. Elder PT. Accidental hypothermia. In: Shoemaker WC, Ayres S, Grenvik A, Holbrook PR, Thompson WL, eds. Textbook of critical care. Philadelphia: WB Saunders, 1989;101.
94. Fahmy NR, Demetrios G, Lappas G. Intravenous calcium chloride and the coagulation-fibrinolytic system. Anesthesiology 1979;51:S117.
95. Falk JS, Linglad GTO, Westman BJM. Histopathological studies on kidneys from patients treated with large amounts of blood preserved with ACD-adenine. Transfusion 1972;12:376.
96. Feinstone SM, Kapikian AZ, Purcell RH, et al. Transfusion-associated hepatitis not due to viral hepatitis type A or B. N Engl J Med 1975;292:767.
97. Feola M, Gonzalez H, Canizaro PC, et al. Development of bovine stroma-free hemoglobin solution as a blood substitute. Surg Gynecol Obstet 1983;157:399.
98. Filip DJ, Aster RH. Relative hemostatic effectiveness of human platelets stored at 4°C and 22°C. J Lab Clin Med 1978;91:618.
99. Fish DJ, Barnette RE, Eisenstaedt RS. Fresh frozen plasma: justification of perioperative use. Anesth Analg 1987;66:S57.
100. Fleming AW. Intraoperative salvage. In: Sandler SG, Silvergleid AJ, eds. Autologous transfusion. Arlington: American Association of Blood Banks, 1983:41.
101. Freysz M, Kobtane R, Isnardon JP, et al. Syndrome de detresse respiratoire aigue de l'adulte aprés transfusion sanguine: rôle possible des anticorps antileucocytaires et, en particulier, des anticorps antigranulocytaires. Nouv Presse Méd 1982;11:3658.
102. Fried SJ, Satiani B, Zeeb P. Normothermic rapid volume replacement for hypovolemic shock: an in vivo and in vitro study utilizing a new technique. J Trauma 1986;26:183.
103. Friedland GH, Klein RS. Transmission of the human immunodeficiency virus. N Engl J Med 1987;317:1125.
104. Friedman HI, De Venuto F. Morphological effects of transfusions with hemoglobin solutions. Crit Care Med 1982;10: 288.
105. Friedman HI, De Venuto F, Schwartz BD, et al. *In vivo* evaluation of pyridoxalated-polymerized hemoglobin solution. Surg Gynecol Obstet 1984;159:429.
106. Friedman Z, Hanley WB, Radde JC. Ionized calcium in exchange transfusion with tham-buffered ACD blood. J Can Med Assoc 1972;107:742.
107. Gambling DR, Birmingham CL, Jenkins LC. Magnesium and the anaesthetist. Can J Anaesth 1988;35:644.
108. Gans RO, Duurkens VA, van Zunder AA, et al. Transfusion-related acute lung injury. Intensive Care Med 1988;14:654.
109. Gervin AS, Fischer RP. Resuscitation of trauma patients with type specific uncrossmatched blood. J Trauma 1984;24:327.
110. Gervin AS, Mason KG, Wright CB. Microaggregate volumes in stored human blood. Surg Gynecol Obstet 1974;139:519.
111. Glover JL, Broadie TA. Intraoperative autotransfusion. In: Collins JA, Murawski K, Shafer AW, eds. Massive transfusion in surgery and trauma. New York: Alan R Liss, 1982:51.
112. Glover JL, Broadie TA. Intraoperative autotransfusion. World J Surg 1987;11:60.
113. Glover JL, Smith R, Yaw PB, et al. Autotransfusion of blood contaminated by intestinal contents. J Coll Emerg Phys 1978;7:142.
114. Glover JL, Smith R, Yaw PB, et al. Intraoperative autotransfusion: an underutilized technique. Surgery 1976;80:474.
115. Goldfinger D. Acute hemolytic transfusion reactions: a fresh look at pathogenesis and considerations regarding therapy. Transfusion 1977;17:85.
116. Goldfinger D. Adverse reactions to blood transfusion. In: Transfusion reactions. Arlington: American Association of Blood Banks, 1982:29.
117. Goldfinger D, McGinnis MH. Rh-incompatible platelet transfusions: risks and consequences of sensitizing immunosuppressed patients. N Engl J Med 1971;284:942.
118. Goto H, Nonami R, Hamasaki Y, et al. Effect of hypothermia on coagulation. Anesthesiology 1985;63:A107.
119. Gould SA, Rosen AL, Sehgal LR, et al. Polymerized pyridoxylated hemoglobin: efficacy as an $O_2$ carrier. J Trauma 1986;26:903.
120. Gould SA, Rosen AI, Sehgal LR, et al. Red cell substitutes: hemoglobin solution or fluorocarbon? J Trauma 1982;22:736.
121. Greenburg AG, Hayashi R, Siefert I, et al. Intravascular persistence and oxygen delivery of pyridoxalated, stroma-free hemoglobin during gradations of hypotension. Surgery 1979;86:13.
122. Greenwalt TJ (conference and panel chairperson). Perioperative red blood cell transfusion: consensus conference. JAMA 1988;260:2700.
123. Grindlinger GA, Vegas AM, Churchill WH, et al. Is respiratory failure a consequence of blood transfusion? J Trauma 1980;20:627.
124. Hamasaki N, Hirota-Chigita C. Acid-citrate-dextrose-phosphoenolpyruvate medium as a rejuvenant for blood storage. Transfusion 1983;23:1.
125. Haradin RI, Weed RI, Reed CF. Changes in physical properties of stored erythrocytes: relationship to survival in vivo. Transfusion 1969;9:229.
126. Harke H, Rahman S. Coagulation disorders in massively transfused patients. In: Collins JA, Murawski K, Shafer AW, eds. Massive transfusion in surgery and trauma. New York: Alan R Liss, 1982:213.
127. Harke H, Rahman S. Haemostatic disorders in massive transfusion. Bibl Haematol 1980;46:179.
128. Harken AH, Woods M. The influence of oxyhemoglobin affinity on tissue oxygen consumption. Ann Surg 1976;183:130.
129. Harrigan C, Lucas CE, Ledgerwood AM. Significance of hypocalcemia following hypovolemic shock. J Trauma 1983;23:488.
130. Harrigan C, Lucas CE, Ledgerwood AM, et al. Primary hemostasis after massive transfusion for injury. Am Surg 1982;48:393.
131. Harrigan C, Lucas CE, Ledgerwood AM, et al. Serial changes in primary hemostasis after massive transfusion. Surgery 1985;98:836.
132. Haslam KR, Nielsen CH. Do passive heat and moisture exchangers keep the patient warm? Anesthesiology 1986;64:379.
133. Hauser CJ, Kamrath RO, Sparks J, et al. Calcium homeostasis in patients with acute pancreatitis. Surgery 1983;94:830.
134. Hauser CJ, Kaufman C, Frantz R, et al. Use of crystalline hemoglobin as replacement of RBC mass. Arch Surg 1982;117:782.
135. Hauser CJ, Shoemaker WC. Hemoglobin solution in the treatment of hemorrhagic shock. Crit Care Med 1982;10:283.
136. Haynes BE, Carr FJ, Niemann JT. Catheter introducers for rapid fluid resuscitation. Ann Emerg Med 1983;12:606.

137. Hechtman HB, Grindlinger GA, Vegas AM, et al. Importance of oxygen transport in clinical medicine. Crit Care Med 1979;7:419.
138. Herman CM, Rodkey FL, Valeri CR, et al. Changes in oxyhemoglobin dissociation curve and peripheral blood after acute red cell mass depletion and subsequent red cell mass restoration in baboons. Ann Surg 1971;174:734.
139. Hewitt PE, Macintyre EA, Devenish A, et al. A prospective study of the incidence of delayed haemolytic transfusion reactions following peri-operative blood transfusion. Br J Haematol 1988;69:541.
140. Hilberman M, Maseda J, Stinson EB, et al. The diuretic properties of dopamine in patients after open-heart operation. Anesthesiology 1984;61:489.
141. Hill DR. HIV infection following motor vehicle trauma in central Africa. JAMA 1989;261:3282.
142. Holland PV. Other adverse effects of transfusion. In: Petz LD, Swisher SN, eds. Clinical practice of blood transfusion. New York: Churchill Livingstone, 1981:783.
143. Honig CL, Bove JR. Transfusion-associated fatalities: review of bureau of biologics reports 1976–1978. Transfusion 1980;20:653.
144. Hornbrook MC, Dodd RY, Jacobs P, et al. Reducing the incidence of non-A, non-B post-transfusion hepatitis by testing donor blood for alanine amino transferase. N Engl J Med 1982;307:1315.
145. Howland WS. Anesthesiologic perspectives of blood transfusion. In: Petz LD, Swisher SN, eds. Clinical practice of blood transfusion. New York: Churchill Livingstone, 1981:471.
146. Howland WS. Calcium, potassium and pH changes during massive transfusion. In: Nusbacher J, ed. Massive transfusion. Washington DC: American Association of Blood Banks, 1978:17.
147. Howland WS, Bellville JW, Zucker MB, et al. Massive blood transfusion: failure to demonstrate citrate intoxication, V. Surg Gynecol Obstet 1957;105:529.
148. Howland WS, Schweizer O, Carlon GC, et al. The cardiovascular effects of low levels of ionized calcium during massive transfusion. Surg Gynecol Obstet 1977;145:581.
149. Huestis DW, Bove JR, Busch S. Practical blood transfusion. 3rd ed. Boston: Little, Brown, 1981.
150. Huestis DW, Bove JR, Busch S. Practical blood transfusion. 3rd ed. Boston: Little, Brown, 1981:249.
151. Huestis DW, Bove JR, Busch S. Practical blood transfusion. 3rd ed. Boston: Little, Brown, 1981:302.
152. Huth JF, Maier RV, Pavlin EG, et al. Utilization of blood recycling in nonelective surgery. Arch Surg 1983;118:626.
153. Iberti TJ, Kelly KM, Gentili DR, et al. Effects of sodium bicarbonate in canine hemorrhagic shock. Crit Care Med 1988;16:779.
154. Iserson KV. Whole blood in trauma resuscitation. Am J Emerg Med 1985;3:358.
155. Iserson KV, Reeter AK, Criss E. Comparison of flow rates for standard and large-bore blood tubing. West J Med 1985;143:183.
156. Jacobs LM, Hsieh JW. A clinical review of autotransfusion and its role in trauma. JAMA 1984;251:3283.
157. Jaffe ER. Erythrocyte metabolism and its relation to the liquid preservation of human blood. In: Petz LD, Swisher SN, eds. Clinical practice of blood transfusion. New York: Churchill Livingstone, 1981:265.
158. Jesch FH, Peters W, Hobbhahn J, et al. Oxygen-transporting fluids and oxygen delivery with hemodilution. Crit Care Med 1982;10:270.
159. Jurkovich GJ, Greiser WB, Luterman A, et al. Hypothermia in trauma victims: an ominous predictor of survival. J Trauma 1987;27:1019.
160. Kahn RC, Jascott D, Carlon GC, et al. Massive blood replacement: correlation of ionized calcium, citrate and hydrogen ion concentration. Anesth Analg 1979;58:274.
161. Kahn RC, Zaroulis C, Howland WS, et al. Hemodynamic, oxygen delivery changes after transfusion of patients in acute respiratory failure. Anesthesiology 1982;S57:A106.
162. Kaplan JA. Hemodynamic monitoring. In: Kaplan JA, ed. Cardiac anesthesia. New York: Grune and Stratton, 1987;179.
163. Kaplan JA, Griffin AV. Shivering and changes in mixed venous oxygen saturation after cardiac surgery. Anesth Analg 1985;64:235.
164. Kashuk JL, Penn I. Air embolism after central venous catheterization. Surg Gynecol Obstet 1984;159:249.
165. Keeling MM, Gray LA, Brink MA, et al. Intraoperative autotransfusion: experience in 725 consecutive cases. Ann Surg 1983;197:536.
166. Ketai LH, Grum CM. C3a and adult respiratory distress syndrome after massive transfusion. Crit Care Med 1986;14:1001.
167. Khabbaz RF, Arnow PM, Highsmith AK, et al. *Pseudomonas fluorescens* bacteremia from blood transfusion. Am J Med 1984;76:62.
168. King WH, Gloyna DF, Patten EV, et al. Dilution of packed red blood cells: saline or Ringer's lactate. Anesth Analg 1984;63:A234.
169. King WH, Patten ED, Bee DE. In vitro evaluation of ionized calcium levels and clotting in red blood cells diluted with lactated Ringer's solution. Anesthesiology 1988;68:115.
170. Kingsley JR, Valeri CR, Peters H. Citrate anticoagulants and online cell washing in intraoperative autotransfusion in the baboon. Surg Forum 1973;24:258.
171. Kissmeyer-Nielsen F, Madsen CB. Platelets in blood stored in untreated and silicone glass bottles and plastic bags, II: survival studies. J Clin Pathol 1961;14:630.
172. Klebanoff G, Phillips J, Evans W. Use of a disposable autotransfusion unit under varying conditions of contamination. Am J Surg 1970;120:351.
173. Klein EF, Graves SA. "Hot pot" tracheitis. Chest 1974;65:225.
174. Koerner K. Platelet function after shipment of room temperature platelet concentrates. Vox Sang 1983;44:37.
175. Komatsu T, Shibutani K, Bizzarri D. Systemic vascular resistance needs correction for hematocrit and temperature values. Anesthesiology 1984;61:A70.
176. Kruskall MS, Pacini DG, Ryan E, et al. Evaluation of a new high-efficiency blood warmer. Transfusion 1987;27:518(S46).
177. Kunkel SE, Warner MA. Human T-cell lymphotropic virus type III (HTLV-III) infection: how it can affect you, your patients, and your anesthesia practice. Anesthesiology 1987;66:195.
178. Ladenson JH, Miller WV, Sherman LA. Relationship of physical symptoms, ECG, free calcium and other blood chemistries in reinfusion with citrated blood. Transfusion 1978;18:670.
179. Latham JT, Bove JR, Weirich FL. Chemical and hematologic changes in stored CPDA-1 blood. Transfusion 1982;22:158.
180. Latson TW, Kickler TS, Baumgartner WA. Pulmonary hypertension and noncardiogenic pulmonary edema following cardiopulmonary bypass associated with an antigranulocyte. Anesthesiology 1986;64:106.
181. Lefebre J, McClellon BA, Coovadia AS. Seven years experience with group O unmatched packed red blood cells in a regional trauma unit. Ann Emerg Med 1987;16:1344.
182. Levy GL, Shabot MM, Hart ME, et al. Transfusion-associated noncardiogenic pulmonary edema: report of a case and a warning regarding treatment. Transfusion 1986;26:278.
183. Lichtiger B, Dupuis JF, Seski J. Hemotherapy during surgery

for Jehovah's witnesses: a new method. Anesth Analg 1982;61:618.
184. Lim RC, Olcott C, Robinson AJ, et al. Platelet response and coagulation changes following massive blood replacement. J Trauma 1973;13:577.
185. Linko K. Does blood transfusion cause respiratory failure? Ann Chir Gynaecol 1982;71 (Suppl 196):37.
186. Linko K. Testing of a new in-line blood warmer. Anesthesiology 1980;52:445.
187. Linko K, Hynynen K. Erythrocyte damage caused by the haemotherm microwave blood warmer. Acta Anaesthesiol Scand 1979;23:320.
188. Linko K, Tigerstedt I. Hyperpotassemia during massive blood transfusions. Acta Anaesthesiol Scand 1984;28:220.
189. Lovric VA, Schuller M, Rose G, et al. Flow properties of modified packed red cells. Anaesth Intensive Care 1987;15:407.
190. Ludbrook J, Wynn V. Citrate intoxication. Br Med J 1958;2:523.
191. Luna GK, Maier RV, Pavlin EG, et al. Incidence and effect of hypothermia in seriously injured patients. J Trauma 1987;27:1014.
192. Mahajan SL, Myers TJ, Baldini MG. Disseminated intravascular coagulation during rewarming following hypothermia. JAMA 1981;245:2517.
193. Malmberg PO, Hlastala MP, Woodson RD. Effect of increased blood-oxygen affinity on oxygen transport in hemorrhagic shock. J Appl Physiol 1979;47:889.
194. Mannix FL. Hemorrhagic shock. In: Rosen P, Baker FJ, Braen GR, Dailey RH, Levy RC, eds. Emergency medicine: concepts and clinical practice. St Louis: CV Mosby, 1983;1:129.
195. Mannucci PM, Federici AB, Sirchia G. Hemostasis testing during massive blood replacement. Vox Sang 1982;42:113.
196. Martin DJ, Lucas CE, Ledgerwood AM, et al. Fresh frozen plasma supplement to massive red blood cell transfusion. Ann Surg 1985;202:505.
197. Mateer JR, Thompson BM, Aprahamian C, et al. Rapid fluid resuscitation with central venous catheters. Ann Emerg Med 1983;12:149.
198. Mattox KL. Comparison of techniques of autotransfusion. Surgery 1978;84:700.
199. McCollough J, Polesky HF, Nelson C, et al. Iatrogenic hemolysis: a complication of blood warmed by a microwave device. Anesth Analg 1972;51:102.
200. McConn R. Massive transfusion and its effect on hemodynamic function in the recipient. In: Nusbacher J, ed. Massive transfusion. Washington DC: American Association of Blood Banks, 1978:25.
201. McLellan BA, Reid SR, Lane PL. Massive blood transfusion causing hypomagnesemia. Crit Care Med 1984;12:146.
202. Menitove JE, McElligott MC, Aster RH. Febrile transfusion reaction: what blood component should be given next? Vox Sang 1982;42:318.
203. Messmer K. Hemoglobins, chelates and perfluorochemical emulsions. In: Shoemaker WC, Thompson WL, Holbrook PR, eds. Textbook of critical care. Philadelphia: WB Saunders, 1984:775.
204. Michaelson T, Salmela L, Tigersted I, et al. Massive blood transfusion: is there a limit? Crit Care Med 1989;17:699.
205. Miller RD. Complications of massive blood transfusions. Anesthesiology 1973;39:82.
206. Miller RD. Problems posed by transfusion. In: Orkin FK, Cooperman LH, eds. Complications in anesthesiology. Philadelphia: JB Lippincott, 1983:461.
207. Miller RD, Brzica SM. Blood, blood components, colloids and autotransfusion therapy. In: Miller RD, ed. Anesthesia. 2nd ed. New York: Churchill Livingstone, 1986;1329.
208. Miller RD, Robbins TO, Tong M, et al. Coagulation defects associated with massive blood transfusion. Ann Surg 1971;174:794.
209. Miller RD, Rupp SM, Fisher DM, et al. Clinical pharmacology of vecuronium and atracurium. Anesthesiology 1984;61:444.
210. Miller RD, Tong MJ, Robbins TO. Effects of massive transfusion of blood on acid-base balance. JAMA 1971;216:1762.
211. Miller RN, Engelhardt R, Collins JA, et al. Observations on the biochemical effects of transfusion of citrate-phosphate-dextrose stored blood in man. Laryngoscope 1976;86:1272.
212. Millikan JS, Cain TL, Hansbrough J. Rapid volume replacement for hypovolemic shock: a comparison of techniques and equipment. J Trauma 1984;24:428.
213. MMWR update. HIV infections in health-care workers exposed to blood of infected patients. JAMA 1987;257:3032.
214. Mollison PL. Blood transfusion in clinical medicine. 7th ed. Oxford: Blackwell Scientific Publications, 1983.
215. Mollison PL: Blood Transfusion in Clinical Medicine. 7th Edition, Oxford, Blackwell, 1983:46.
216. Mollison PL. Blood transfusion in clinical medicine. 7th ed. Oxford: Blackwell, 1983:133.
217. Mollison PL. Blood transfusion in clinical medicine. 7th ed. Oxford: Blackwell, 1983:142.
218. Mollison PL. Blood transfusion in clinical medicine. 7th ed. Oxford: Blackwell, 1983:144.
219. Mollison PL. Blood transfusion in clinical medicine. 7th ed. Oxford: Blackwell, 1983:164.
220. Mollison PL. Blood transfusion in clinical medicine. 7th ed. Oxford: Blackwell, 1983:167.
221. Mollison PL. Blood transfusion in clinical medicine. 7th ed. Oxford: Blackwell, 1983:181.
222. Mollison PL. Blood transfusion in clinical medicine. 7th ed. Oxford: Blackwell, 1983:628.
223. Mollison PL. Blood transfusion in clinical medicine. 7th ed. Oxford: Blackwell, 1983:640.
224. Mollison PL. Blood transfusion in clinical medicine. 7th ed. Oxford: Blackwell, 1983:659.
225. Mollison PL. Blood transfusion in clinical medicine. 7th ed. Oxford: Blackwell, 1983:713.
226. Mollison PL. Blood transfusion in clinical medicine. 7th ed. Oxford: Blackwell, 1983:730.
227. Mollison PL. Blood transfusion in clinical medicine. 7th ed. Oxford: Blackwell, 1983:738.
228. Mollison PL. Blood transfusion in clinical medicine. 7th ed. Oxford: Blackwell, 1983:748.
229. Mollison PL. Blood transfusion in clinical medicine. 7th ed. Oxford: Blackwell, 1983:755.
230. Mollison PL. Blood transfusion in clinical medicine. 7th ed. Oxford: Blackwell, 1983:760.
231. Mollison PL. Blood Transfusion in clinical medicine. 7th ed. Oxford: Blackwell, 1983:768.
232. Mollison PL. Blood transfusion in clinical medicine. 7th ed. Oxford: Blackwell, 1983:769.
233. Monaghan WP, Levan DR, Camp FR. Blood transfusion aboard a naval hospital ship receiving multiple casualties in a combat zone, a controlled medical environment. Transfusion 1977;17:473.
234. Moore EE, Dunn EL, Breslick DJ, et al. Platelet abnormalities associated with massive autotransfusion. J Trauma 1980;20:1052.
235. Moore GL. Red blood cell preservation: a survey of recent research. In: Sohmer PR, Schiffer CA, eds. Blood storage and preservation. Anaheim: American Association of Blood Banks, 1982:9.
236. Moore GL, Ledford ME. Development of an optimized additive

solution containing ascorbate 2-phosphate for the preservation of red cells with retention of 2,3-diphosphoglycerate. Transfusion 1985;25:319.
237. Moore KL, Bendick PL, Broadie TA, et al. Systemic effects of intraoperative autotransfusion. Med Instrum 1983;17:85.
238. Moroff G, Dende D. Characterization of biochemical changes occurring during storage of red cells: comparative studies with CPD and CPDA-1 anticoagulant-preservative solutions. Transfusion 1983;23:484.
239. Morris DL, Chambers HF, Morris MG, et al. Hemodynamic characteristics of patients with hypothermia due to occult infection and other causes. Ann Intern Med 1985;102:153.
240. Morris RH, Kumar A. The effect of warming blankets on maintenance of body temperature of the anesthetized paralyzed adult patient. Anesthesiology 1972;36:408.
241. Moseley RV, Doty DB. Death associated with multiple pulmonary emboli soon after battle injury. Ann Surg 1970;171:336.
241a. Mosley JW, Aach RD, Hollinger FB, et al. Non-A, non-B hepatitis and antibody to hepatitis C virus. JAMA 1990;263:77.
242. Moss GS, Gould SA, Sehgal LR, et al. Hemoglobin solution: from tetramer to polymer. Surgery 1984;95:249.
243. Moss J. Accidental severe hypothermia. Surg Gynecol Obstet 1986;162:501.
244. Murphy S. ABO blood groups and platelet transfusion. Transfusion 1988;28:401.
245. Murphy S, Simon T. Characteristics of prolonged platelet storage in a new container. Transfusion 1981;21:637.
246. Murray C, Tishkoff GH. Preparation of components and their characteristics: plasmapheresis and cytopheresis. In: Petz LD, Swisher SN, eds. Clinical practice of blood transfusion. New York: Churchill Livingstone, 1981:213.
247. Murray DJ, Olson J, Strauss R, et al. Coagulation changes during packed red cell replacement of major blood loss. Anesthesiology 1988;69:839.
248. Murray DJ, Olson J, Strauss R. Packed red cells for blood replacement: when is FFP required? Anesth Analg 1988;67:S155.
249. Myhre BA. Fatalities from blood transfusion. JAMA 1980;244:1333.
250. Myhre BA, Bove JR, Schmidt PJ: Wrong blood: a needless cause of surgical deaths. Anesth Analg 1981;60:777.
251. Napier JA. Whole blood transfusion (letter). Transfusion 1986;26:398.
252. Napoli VM, Symbas PJ, Vroon DH, et al. Autotransfusion from experimental hemothorax: levels of coagulation factors. J Trauma 1987;27:296.
253. Nerothin DD, Kane PB. Calcium-vasodilator or vasoconstrictor? Anesth Analg 1984;63:A255.
254. Nilsson L, Hedner U, Nilsson IM, et al. Shelf-life of bank blood and stored plasma with special reference to coagulation factors. Transfusion 1983;23:377.
255. Nishimura N, Takahiro S. Changes of hemodynamics and $O_2$ transport associated with the perfluorochemical blood substitute, Fluosol-DA. Crit Care Med 1984;12:36.
256. Noback CR, Tinker JH. Efficacy of warming blankets in cardiovascular surgery. Anesthesiology 1981;55:A118.
257. Noe DA, Graham SM, Luff R, et al. Platelet counts during rapid massive transfusion. Transfusion 1982;22:392.
258. Noon GP. Intraoperative autotransfusion. Surgery 1978;84:719.
259. Noon GP, Solis RT, Natelson FA. A simple method of intraoperative autotransfusion. Surg Gynecol Obstet 1976;143:65.
260. Nusbacher JN. Transfusion of red blood cell products. In: Petz LD, Swisher SN, eds. Clinical practice of blood transfusion. New York: Churchill Livingstone, 1981:289.
261. Oberman HA. Inappropriate use of fresh-frozen plasma. JAMA 1985;253:556.
262. Oberman HA. Surgical blood ordering, blood shortage situations and emergency transfusion. In: Petz LD, Swisher SN, eds. Clinical practice of blood transfusion. New York: Churchill Livingstone, 1981:393.
263. Oberman HA. The history of blood transfusion. In: Petz LD, Swisher SN, eds. Clinical practice of blood transfusion. New York: Churchill Livingstone, 1981:9.
264. Oberman HA, Barnes BA, Friedman BA. The risk of abbreviating the major crossmatch in urgent or massive transfusion. Transfusion 1978;18:137.
265. Ordog GL, Wasserberger J. Coagulation abnormalities in traumatic shock (letter). Crit Care Med 1986;14:519.
266. Ordog GL, Wasserberger J, Balasubramaniam S. Coagulation abnormalities in traumatic shock. Ann Emerg Med 1985;14:650.
267. Orkin FK. Physiologic disturbances associated with induced hypothermia. In: Orkin FK, Cooperman LH, eds. Complications in anesthesiology. Philadelphia: JB Lippincott, 1983:624.
268. Orr MD. Autotransfusion: intraoperative scavenging. Int Anesthesiol Clin 1982;20:97.
269. Otto RJ, Metzler MH. Rewarming from experimental hypothermia: comparison of heated aerosol inhalation, peritoneal lavage and pleural lavage. Crit Care Med 1988;16:869.
270. Pantely GA, Oyama AA, Metcalfe J, et al. Improvement in the relationship between flow to ischemic myocardium and the extent of myocardial necrosis with glycolytic intermediates that decrease blood oxygen affinity in dogs. Circ Res 1981;49:395.
271. Papovsky MA, Abel MD, Moore SB. Transfusion-related acute lung injury associated with massive transfer of antileukocyte antibodies. Am Rev Respir Dis 1983;128:185.
272. Patterson A. Massive transfusion. Int Anesthesiol Clin 1987;25:61.
273. Pauca AL, Savage RT, Simpson S, et al. Effect of pethidine, fentanyl and morphine on post-operative shivering in man. Acta Anaesthesiol Scand 1984;28:138.
274. Pavlin EG, Yazaki S, Winn R, et al. The effect of shivering on gas exchange in goats. Anesthesiology 1983;59:A483.
275. Pepe PE, Potkin RT, Reus DH, et al. Clinical predictors of the adult respiratory distress syndrome. Am J Surg 1982;144:124.
276. Perkins HA. Strategies for massive transfusion. In: Petz LD, Swisher SN, eds. Clinical practice of blood transfusion. New York: Churchill Livingstone, 1981:485.
277. Peterman TA, Stoneburner RL, Allen JR, et al. Risk of human immunodeficiency virus transmission from heterosexual adults with transfusion-associated infection. JAMA 1988;259:55.
278. Petz LD, Swisher SN, eds. Clinical practice of blood transfusion. New York: Churchill Livingstone, 1981.
279. Phillips P, Grayson L, Stockman K, et al. Transfusion-related *Pseudomonas* sepsis. Lancet 1984;2:879.
280. Phillips TF, Soulier G, Wilson RF. Outcome of massive transfusion exceeding two blood volumes in trauma and emergency. J Trauma 1987;27:903.
281. Pierce RN, Reich LM, Mayer K. Hemolysis following platelet transfusions from ABO-incompatible donors. Transfusion 1985;25:60.
282. Pineda AA, Taswell HF, Brzica SM. Delayed hemolytic transfusion reaction: an immunologic hazard of blood transfusion. Transfusion 1978;18:1.
283. Ralley FE, Wynands E, Ramsay JG, et al. The effects of shivering on oxygen consumption and carbon dioxide production in patients rewarming from hypothermic cardiopulmonary bypass. Can J Anaesth 1988;35:4.
284. Rapaport SI, Ames SB, Mikkelsen S. The levels of antihemophiliac globulin and proaccelerin in fresh and bank blood. Am J Clin Pathol 1959;31:297.

285. Reed RL, Ciavarella D, Heimbach DM, et al. Proplylactic platelet administration during massive transfusion: prospective, randomized, double-blind clinical study. Ann Surg 1986;203:40.
286. Reul GJ, Beall AC, Greenberg SD. Protection of the pulmonary microvasculature by fine screen blood filtration. Chest 1974;66:4.
287. Reul GJ, Greenberg SD, Lefrak EA, et al. Prevention of posttraumatic pulmonary insufficiency: fine screen filtration of blood. Arch Surg 1973;106:386.
288. Reul GJ, Solis RT, Greenberg SD, et al. Experience with autotransfusion in the surgical management of trauma. Surgery 1974;76:546.
289. Rice CL, Herman CM, Kiesow LA, et al. Benefits from improved oxygen delivery of blood in shock therapy. J Surg Res 1975;19:193.
290. Rizza CR. Coagulation factor therapy. Clin Haematol 1976;5:113.
291. Rizza CR. Management of patients with coagulation factor deficiencies. In: Biggs R, ed. Human blood coagulation, haemostasis and thrombosis. Oxford: Blackwell, 1976:392.
292. Robinson NB, Heimbach DM, Reynolds LO, et al. Ventilation and perfusion alterations following homologous blood transfusion. Surgery 1982;92:183.
293. Rodriguez J, Weissman C, Askanazi J, et al. Suppression of the physiologic stress to postoperative rewarming. Anesthesiology 1982;57:A120.
294. Rodriguez JL, Weissman C, Damask MC, et al. Physiologic requirements during rewarming: suppression of the shivering response. Crit Care Med 1983;11:49.
295. Rosen AL, Gould S, Sehgal LR, et al. Cardiac response to extreme hemodilution with hemoglobin solutions of various $P_{50}$ values. Crit Care Med 1979;7:380.
296. Rosen AL, Gould SA, Sehgal LR, et al. Hemoglobin solutions as red cell substitutes. Crit Care Med 1982;10:275.
297. Rothe KF, Heisler N. Correction of metabolic alkalosis by HCl and acetazolamide: effects on extracellular and intracellular acid-base status in rats in vivo. Acta Anaesthesiol Scand 1986;30:566.
298. Rudowski WJ. Blood transfusion: yesterday, today and tomorrow. World J Surg 1987;11:86.
299. Russell WJ: A review of blood warmers for massive transfusion. Anaesth Intensive Care 1974;2:109.
300. Ryan JF. Unintentional hypothermia. In: Orkin FK, Cooperman LH, eds. Complications in anesthesiology. Philadelphia: JB Lippincott, 1983:284.
301. Ryden SE, Oberman HA. Compatibility of common intravenous solutions with CPD blood. Transfusion 1975;15:250.
302. Saarela E. Autotransfusion: a review. Ann Clin Res 1981;13(Suppl. 33):48.
303. Sassano JJ, Waterman PM, Marquez J, et al. Limitations of conventional transfusion systems. Anesthesiology 1985;63:A152.
304. Satiani B, Fried SJ, Zeeb P, et al. Normothermic rapid volume replacement in traumatic hypovolemia. Arch Surg 1987;122:1044.
305. Saunders RJ, Calkins JM. Practical considerations in transfusion techniques during anesthesia. In: Brown BR, ed. Fluid and blood therapy in anesthesia. Philadelphia: FA Davis, 1983:169.
306. Schmidt PL. Component therapy. Int Anesthesiol Clin 1982;20:23.
307. Schned AR, Silver H. Use of microaggregate filtration in prevention of febrile transfusion reactions. Transfusion 1981;21:675.
308. Schumacker PT, Suggett AJ, Wagner PP, et al. Role of hemoglobin $P_{50}$ in $O_2$ transport during normoxic and hypoxic exercise in the dog. J Appl Physiol 1985;59:749.
309. Schwab CW, Shayne JP, Turner J. Immediate trauma resuscitation with type O uncrossmatched blood: a two-year prospective experience. J Trauma 1986;26:897.
310. Scott NJ, Harris JR, Bolton AE. Effect of storage on platelet release and aggregation responses. Vox Sang 1983;45:359.
311. Seyfried H, Walewska I. Immune hemolytic transfusion reactions. World J Surg 1987;11:25.
312. Shackford SR. Fluid resuscitation: theory and practice. In: Trauma management 1984 (a symposium). San Diego: University of California School of Medicine, 1984:92.
313. Shackford SR, Virgilio RW, Peters RM. Whole blood versus packed-cell transfusions: physiologic comparison. Ann Surg 1981;193:337.
314. Shapira N, White RD, Schaff HV, et al. Peripheral vascular versus cardiac response to $CaCl_2$ injection immediately following cardiopulmonary bypass in man. Anesthesiology 1982;57:A63.
315. Shappell SD, Murray JA, Nasser MG, et al. Acute changes in hemoglobin affinity for oxygen during angina pectoris. N Engl J Med 1970;282:1219.
316. Sheehy TW, Navari RM. Hypothermia. Ala J Med Sci 1984;21:374.
317. Sheldon GF, Watkins GM, Glover JL, et al. Panel: present use of blood and blood products. J Trauma 1981;21:1005.
318. Sherman LA. The implications of trends in transfusion (editorial). Transfusion 1988;28:511.
319. Shin B, MacKenzie CF, Helrich M. Hypokalemia in trauma patients. Anesthesiology 1986;65:90.
320. Shorey J. The current status of non-A, non-B viral hepatitis. Am J Med Sci 1985;289:251.
321. Shulman IA, Nelson JM, Soxena S, et al. Experience with the routine use of an abbreviated crossmatch. Am J Clin Pathol 1984;82:178.
322. Silvergleid AJ. Clinical platelet transfusions. In: Silver H, ed. Blood, blood components and derivatives in transfusion therapy. Washington DC: American Association of Blood Banks, 1980:45.
323. Simmons RL, Heisterkamp CA, Collins JA, et al. Respiratory insufficiency in combat casualties, IV: hypoxemia during convalescence. Ann Surg 1969;170:53.
324. Simon GE, Bove JR. The potassium load from blood transfusion. Postgrad Med 1971;49:61.
325. Slichter SJ. Identification and management of defects in platelet hemostasis in massively transfused patients. In: Collins JA, Murawski K, Shafer AW, eds. Massive transfusion in surgery and trauma. New York: Alan R Liss, 1982:225.
326. Slichter SJ, Counts RB, Henderson R, et al. Preparation of cryoprecipitated factor VIII concentrates. Transfusion 1976;16:616.
327. Smith SJ. Hypokalemia in resuscitation from multiple trauma. Surg Gynecol Obstet 1978;147:18.
328. Snyder EL, Bookbinder M. Role of microaggregate blood filtration in clinical medicine. Transfusion 1983;23:460.
329. Snyder EL, Hezzey A, Barash PG, et al. Microaggregate blood filtration in patients with compromised pulmonary function. Transfusion 1982;22:21.
330. Solomon MD, Rutledge ML, Kane LE, et al. Cost comparison of intraoperative autologous versus homologous transfusion. Transfusion 1988;28:379.
331. Standards for Blood Banks and Transfusion Services. 10th ed. American Associations of Blood Banks. 1981:32.
332. Stehling L, Esposito B. An analysis of the appropriateness of intraoperative transfusion. Anesth Analg 1989;68:S278.
332a. Stevens CE, Taylor PE, Pindyck J, et al. Epidemiology of hepatitis C virus. A preliminary study in volunteer blood donors. JAMA 1990;263:49.

333. Stoelting RK. Allergic reactions during anesthesia. Anesth Analg 1983;62:341.
334. Stone DR, Downs JB, Paul WL, et al. Adult body temperature and heated humidification of anesthetic gases during general anesthesia. Anesth Analg 1981;60:736.
335. Stoops CM. Acute hyperkalemia associated with massive blood replacement. Anesth Analg 1983;62:1044.
336. Strawitz JG, Howard JM, Artz CP. Effect of intravenous calcium gluconate on post-transfusion hypotension: clinical observations. Arch Surg 1955;70:223.
337. Sugerman HJ, Davidson DT, Vibul S, et al. The basis of defective oxygen delivery from stored blood. Surg Gynecol Obstet 1970;131:733.
338. Surgenor DM, Wallace EL, Hale SG, et al. Changing patterns of blood transfusions in four sets of United States hospitals, 1980–1985. Transfusion 1988;28:513.
339. Swank RL. Alteration of blood on storage: measurement of adhesiveness of "aging" platelets and leukocytes and their removal by filtration. N Engl J Med 1961;265:728.
340. Symbas PN. Autotransfusion in thoracic trauma. In: Hauer JM, Thurer RL, Dawson RB, eds. Autotransfusion. New York: Elsevier North Holland, 1981:83.
341. Tabor E, Gerety RJ. Non-A, non-B hepatitis: new findings and prospects for prevention. Transfusion 1979;19:669.
342. Taswell HF, Pineda AA, Moore SM. Hemolytic transfusion reactions: frequency and clinical and laboratory aspects. In: Transfusion reactions. Arlington: American Association of Blood Banks, 1982:47.
343. Tausk HC, Miller R, Roberts RB. Maintenance of body temperature by heated humidification. Anesth Analg 1976;55:719.
344. Timberlake GA, McSwain NE. Autotransfusion of blood contaminated by enteric contents: a potentially life-saving measure in the massively hemorrhaging trauma patient? J Trauma 1988;28:855.
345. Tinker JH. Perioperative hypertension. In: Kaplan JA, ed. Cardiac anesthesia. New York: Grune and Stratton, 1983:363.
346. Tollofsrud SG, Gunderson Y, Andersen R. Perioperative hypothermia. Acta Anaesthesiol Scand 1984;28:511.
347. Tomasulo PA. Platelet transfusion for nonmalignant diseases. In: Petz LD, Swisher SN, eds. Clinical practice of blood transfusion. New York: Churchill Livingstone, 1981:527.
348. Tremolada F, Chiappetta F, Noventa F, et al. Prospective study of posttransfusion hepatitis in cardiac surgery patients receiving only blood or blood products. Vox Sang 1983;44:25.
349. Tremper KK, Vercellotti GM, Hammerschmidt DE. Hemodynamic profile of adverse clinical reactions to Fluosol DA-20%. Crit Care Med 1984;12:428.
350. Trunkey D, Holcroft J, Carpenter MA. Calcium flux during hemorrhagic shock in baboons. J Trauma 1976;16:633.
351. Tullis JL, Alving B, Bove JR, et al (consensus development panel). Fresh frozen plasma indications and risks. JAMA 1985;253:551.
352. Tuman KJ, Spiess BD, McCarthy RJ, et al. Effects of progressive blood loss on coagulation as measured by thrombelastography. Anesth Analg 1987;66:856.
353. Tye RW. Blood substitutes as therapy in massive surgery and trauma. In: Collins JA, Murawski K, Shafer AW, eds. Massive transfusion in surgery and trauma. New York: Alan R Liss, 1982:79.
354. Valeri CR, Feingold H, Cassidy G, et al. Hypothermia-induced reversible platelet dysfunction. Ann Surg 1987;205:175.
355. Valeri CR, Hirsch NM. Restoration in vivo of erythrocyte adenosine triphosphate, 2, 3-diphosphoglycerate, potassium ion and sodium ion concentrations following transfusion of acid-citrate-dextrose-stored human red blood cells. J Lab Clin Med 1969;73:722.
356. Valtis DJ, Kennedy AC. Defective gas transport function of stored red blood cells. Lancet 1954;1:119.
357. Vaughan MS, Vaughan RW, Cork RC. Postoperative hypothermia in adults: relationship of age, anesthesia and shivering to rewarming. Anesth Analg 1981;60:746.
358. Virgilio RW. Blood filters and postoperative pulmonary dysfunction: weekly anesthesiology update. Princeton: Weekly Anesthesiology Update, Inc, 1979;2 (lesson 14):1.
359. Wake EJ, Studzinski GP, Bhandal A. Changes in human cultured cells exposed to a perfluorocarbon emulsion. Transfusion 1985;25:73.
360. Wallas CH. Sodium and potassium in blood bank-stored human erythrocytes. Transfusion 1979;19:210.
361. Waller JL. Inotropes and vasopressors. In: Kaplan JA, ed. Cardiac anesthesia, cardiovascular pharmacology. New York: Grune and Stratton, 1983:273.
362. Ward CF, Ozaki GT. Pressure-augmented fluid administration: modified system and general results. Crit Care Med 1989;17:70.
363. Ward JW, Holmberg SD, Allen JR, et al. Transmission of HIV by blood transfusions screened as negative for HIV antibody. N Engl J Med 1988;318:473.
364. Warnock DF, Davison JK, Brewster DC, et al. Modification of the haemonetics cell saver for optional high flow rate autotransfusion. Am J Surg 1982;143:765.
365. Waxman K, Cheung CK, Mason R. Hypotensive reaction after a perfluorochemical emulsion. Crit Care Med 1984;12:609.
366. Waxman K, Tremper KK, Cullen BF, et al. Perfluorocarbon infusion in bleeding patients refusing blood transfusions. Arch Surg 1984;119:721.
367. Waxman K, Tremper KK, Mason GR. Blood and plasma substitutes: plasma expansion and oxygen transport properties. West J Med 1985;143:202.
368. Wick MR, Moore S, Taswell HF. Non-A, non-B hepatitis associated with blood transfusion. Transfusion 1985;25:93.
369. Wiley JF, Koepke JA. Changes in serum potassium in premature infants receiving packed red blood cells. Clin Lab Haematol 1985;7:27.
370. Williams DB, Lyons JH. Treatment of severe metabolic alkalosis with intravenous infusion of hydrochloric acid. Surg Gynecol Obstet 1980;150:315.
371. Wilson EB, Iserson KV. Admixture bloodwarming: a technique for rapid warming of erythrocytes. Ann Emerg Med 1987;16:413.
372. Wintrobe MM. Clinical hematology. 6th ed. Philadelphia: Lea and Febiger, 1967:304.
373. Wolf PL, McCarthy LJ, Hafleigh B. Extreme hypercalcemia following blood transfusions combined with intravenous calcium. Vox Sang 1970;19:544.
374. Wolfe LC. The membrane and the lesions of storage in preserved red cells. Transfusion 1985;25:185.
375. Wood M. Neuromuscular blocking agents. In: Wood M, Wood AJJ, eds. Drugs and anesthesia: pharmacology for anesthesiologists. Baltimore: Williams and Wilkins, 1982:299.
376. Woodson RD. Importance of 2,3-DPG in banked blood: new data in animal models. In: Collins JA, Murawski K, Shafer AW, eds. Massive transfusion in surgery and trauma. New York: Alan R Liss, 1982:69.
377. Woodson RD. Physiological significance of oxygen dissociation curve shifts. Crit Care Med 1979;7:368.
378. Woodson RD, Auerbach S. Effect of increased oxygen affinity and anemia on cardiac output and its distribution. J Appl Physiol 1982;53:1299.

379. Woodson RD, Costello DJ, Gilboe DD. Increased blood oxygen affinity decreases brain $O_2$ consumption. Clin Res 1979;27:405A.
380. Woodson RD, Fitzpatrick JH, Costello DJ, et al. Increased blood oxygen affinity decreases canine brain oxygen consumption. J Lab Clin Med 1982;100:411.
381. Yang SC, Puri VK, Raheja R. Oxygen delivery and consumption and $P_{50}$ in patients with acute myocardial infarction. Circulation 1986;73:1183.
382. Yang SC, Puri VK, Raheja R, et al. Effects of $P_{50}$ on oxygen consumption in patients with low cardiac output due to acute myocardial infarction. Crit Care Med 1985;13:318.
383. Yeston NS, Niehoff JM, Dennis RC. Transfusion therapy. In: Civetta JM, Taylor RW, Kirby RR, eds. Critical care. Philadelphia: JB Lippincott, 1988:1481.
384. Young GP, Purcell TB. Emergency autotransfusion. Ann Emerg Med 1983;12:182.
385. Zauder HL. Massive transfusion. Int Anesthesiol Clin 1982;20:157.
386. Zell SC, Kurtz KJ. Severe exposure hypothermia: a resuscitation protocol. Ann Emerg Med 1985;14:339.
387. Zorko MF, Polsky SS. Rapid warming and infusion of packed red blood cells. Ann Emerg Med 1986;15:907.

Chapter Seven

Roberta C. Kahn

# Coagulation Abnormalities and Their Management in the Injured

The trauma patient's survival may depend on support of vital systems and control of hemorrhage. Bleeding disorders that complicate resuscitation may defeat efforts to preserve the patient's life or may worsen organ dysfunction. Although it is possible that coagulation disorders may preexist or develop in the injured patient prior to treatment,[50,54] and efforts should be made to identify such disorders, the overwhelming majority of cases of bleeding are due to structural injuries that require surgical hemostasis. This chapter will review briefly normal coagulation and will consider disorders of hemostasis which may arise during the course of management of traumatic injuries.

## PHYSIOLOGY OF COAGULATION

Normally, thrombosis is initiated by the cooperative action of platelets and coagulation factors in response to disruption of the vascular endothelial surface. The fact that clot formation is normally localized to the area of injury reflects the remarkable mechanisms of intravascular regulation of clot formation, arrest of coagulation, and eventual clot dissolution, a series of processes that are still incompletely elucidated.

The classic representation of coagulation is presented schematically in Fig 7-1. Following adhesion and aggregation of platelets at a disrupted vessel site, a series of enzymatic reactions is initiated in which activation of procoagulant proteins results in generation of thrombin, a proteolytic enzyme that catalyzes formation of fibrinopeptides from fibrinogen. These peptides then polymerize to form a fibrin mesh. Thrombin also stimulates platelets to release vasoactive products and adenosine 5′-diphosphate (ADP), which attract more platelets to the injured site. Coagulation proceeds even more rapidly outside the blood vessels, since tissue thromboplastin, found in brain, lung, liver, spleen, kidney, and placenta, as well as leukocytes and endothelial cells powerfully activate factors VII and X to generate thrombin.

Arrest of coagulation is mediated by conversion of plasminogen to plasmin, a reaction that is controlled by activated factor XII. The action of plasmin on fibrin limits propagation of the clot. Large molecular weight fibrin degradation products that are generated by the action of plasmin on both fibrin and fibrinogen compete with fibrinogen for the active binding sites of the thrombin molecule, thus slowing further progress of clot formation. Activated coagulation factors and the products of fibrinogen and fibrin degradation are cleared from the bloodstream by the reticuloendothelial system. The fibrinolytic sequence is depicted in Fig 7-2.

Spontaneous bleeding is not a risk unless severe deficiencies of platelets ($<20,000/\mu L$) or coagulation factors (10 to 30%) exist. The recommendations for control of bleeding in patients with congenital clotting factor deficiencies are very secure; however, the same precision cannot be relied on when dealing with patients who may have shock or sepsis, who have received multiple blood volume transfusions or large quantities of acellular fluids, or who are actively bleeding from the site of injury.

The nomenclature of in vitro clotting studies is based on their historical development and does not necessarily indicate specific factor deficiencies or the technique utilized for the

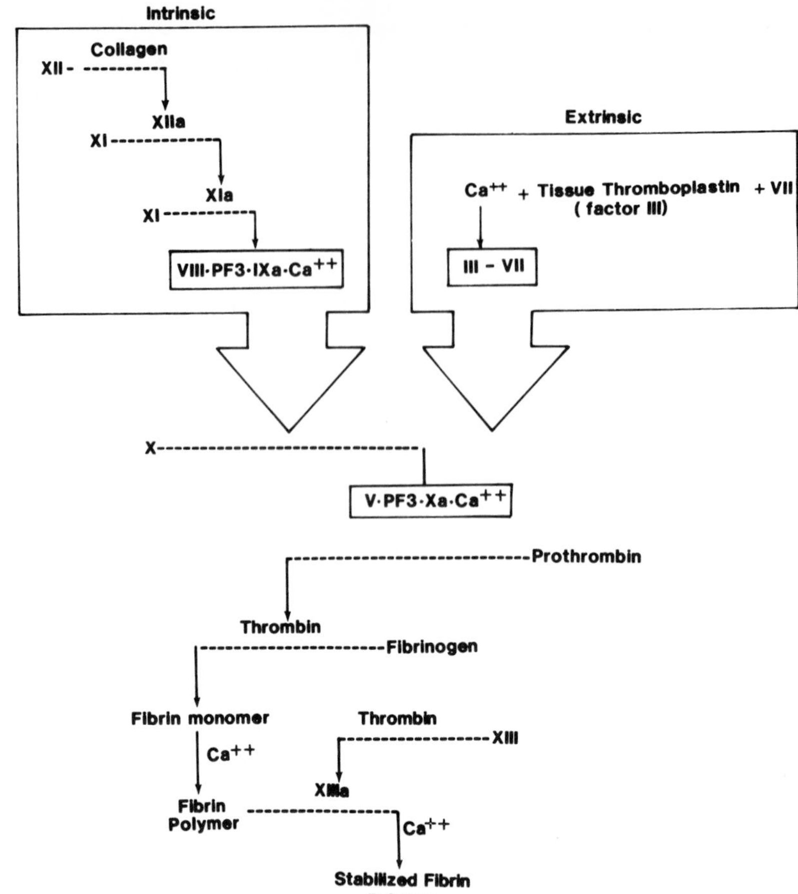


FIG. 7-1. Classic coagulation pathways, demonstrating the sequential activation of coagulation factors (Roman numerals). The generation of thrombin induces several reactions responsible for the formation of a stable, insoluble fibrin clot, as well as incorporation of platelets.

analyses. The major tests available for evaluation of clotting and hemostasis are listed in Table 7-1. It is appropriate to emphasize that laboratory evidence of clotting abnormalities does not necessarily correlate with clinical bleeding, particularly in critically ill trauma patients.[49,52] Furthermore, results are not always available as quickly as the clinician managing a hemorrhaging patient might desire. This does not imply that rapid evaluation in the clinical setting cannot be done; indeed, an understanding of fundamental clotting mechanisms, alert clinical observation, and laboratory test results can direct management much more specifically and appropriately than standardized protocols for transfusion therapy.

## COAGULATION ABNORMALITIES IN THE INJURED

For a review of management of congenital bleeding disorders, the reader is referred to Chapter 8, and other sources.[1,61,73] This section will discuss the acquired coagulation defects likely to be encountered in the injured patient, including medications and disease states that may coexist with acute injury.

### TRAUMA AND ITS EFFECT ON COAGULATION

The widespread distribution of tissue thromboplastin in the body would lead one to expect that trauma to various sites induces an acceleration of clotting.[2] Experimental evidence has demonstrated that this is the case.[8,30,47] The extent of soft tissue damage in animals can be directly correlated with depression of fibrinogen levels within 6 hours, followed by rebound hyperfibrinogenemia.[30] Others have found hypercoagulability and increased fibrinogen activity within 9.5 hours after experimental soft tissue trauma.[47] Trauma to both femurs in dogs caused increased fibrinolytic activity and consumption of coagulation factors, which could be prevented by administration of heparin, indicating that coagulation was taking place.[7] This was followed in 24 hours by inhibition of fibrinolysis and a rebound increase in fibrinogen levels. Clinical studies in human injuries indicate the same response.[3,4,31,44,45,57] Biphasic changes in factor levels and clotting function are seen:[3,57] a decrease in fibrinogen and clotting factors is followed by sustained hyperfibrinogenemia.[27a,54] Factors II, V, VII, and X are generally 70 to 90% of normal after trauma. Factor VIII and von Willebrand's factor are also decreased. The decrease in von Willebrand's factor may contribute to increased bleeding after major injury or surgery since desmopressin (DDAVP), which causes elevation of von Willbrand's factor, has been shown to reduce blood loss in this situation.[37] In addition, increased fibrinolytic activity due to increased plasminogen activation is noted.[3,30,31,54] These changes are indicative of a consumptive process rapidly followed, in survivors, by accelerated production of coagulation factors. The severity of coagulation abnormalities appears to increase with increasing severity of in-

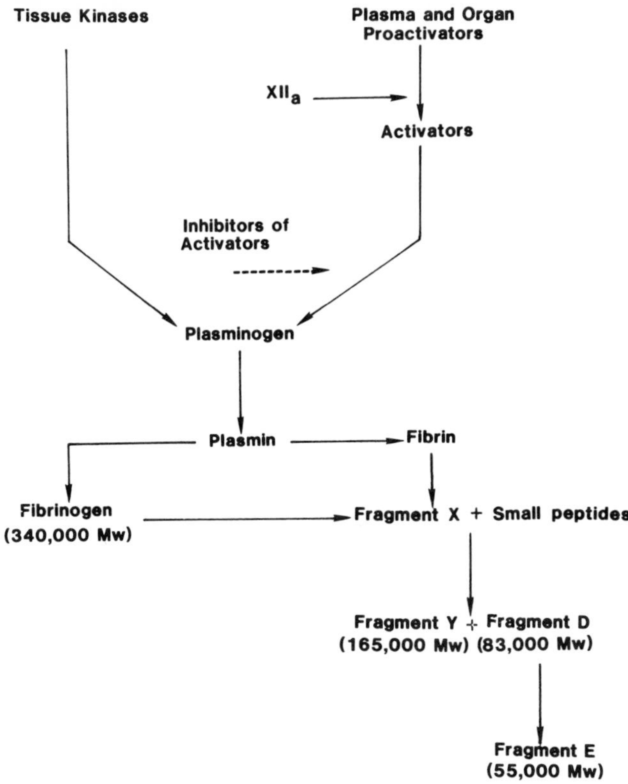


FIG. 7-2. The fibrinolytic sequence. Note that plasmin is capable of generating FDP/fdp from a fibrin clot or from circulating fibrinogen.

jury. For example, the levels of two powerful inhibitors of coagulation, antithrombin III and antiprotease $\alpha_2$-antiplasmin, decrease more in more severely injured patients.[54,55] Septic patients and those in shock show severe and sustained consumption because of decreased ability to produce clotting factors.[4,15,44] Nevertheless, coagulation abnormalities are, in general, more severe after septic than after traumatic shock.[5] Clearly, much of this response results from utilization of platelets and clotting factors for hemostasis at the site of injury.[58] The ability of the organism to respond by increasing circulating coagulation factors determines whether a hypercoagulable state is observed; if production cannot compensate, a decrease in factor levels is seen.

TABLE 7-1. Major Laboratory Tests for Coagulation

| TEST NAME | ABNORMALITY (PROLONGED/ POSITIVE TEST) INDICATES |
|---|---|
| Prothombin time | V, VII, X, II deficiency |
| Activated partial thromboplastin time | XII, XI, X, IX, VIII, V, II, I deficiency |
| Thrombin time | I (fibrinogen) deficiency, heparin, fibrinolytics, FDP/fdp |
| Reptilase time | Heparin effect on TT |
| Fibrin degradation products assay | Circulating FDP/fdp |
| Paracoagulation tests: Ethanol gelation Protamine sulfate serial dilution | Circulating fibrin monomer |
| Antithrombin III assay | Depressed in DIC and hypercoagulable states |
| Euglobulin lysis time | Activators of plasminogen |
| Factor assays | Specific deficiencies |
| Bleeding time | Platelet deficiency or abnormality |
| Platelet aggregation | Intrinsic or acquired functional deficit |

Hypercoagulability may also be caused by other mechanisms. As already noted, many tissues contain thromboplastin, which is released into the bloodstream when tissue injury occurs.[2,7,9,44] Epinephrine released during stress decreases clotting time.[7,12,18,23] A striking hypercoagulation response is also observed after electric stimulation of the hypothalamus.[18] These nonspecific mechanisms are undoubtedly responsible for the spectrum of clinical clotting conditions that may be seen in trauma patients. The importance of the reticuloendothelial system as a compensatory factor in coagulation will be discussed below.

### HEAD INJURY

In view of the fact that intracranial blood loss is never substantial enough to compromise circulating blood volume in adults, and shock is not a likely complication of head injury, the extensive literature documenting derangement of clotting after head injuries provides compelling evidence for the importance of nonspecific mechanisms in the initiation of widespread coagulation.[3,18,64,65,67] Both minor and severe head injury can be followed by evidence of hypercoagulation.[64,65] Head-injured patients have shorter clotting times, greater utilization of coagulation factors, and lower platelet counts than patients with extracranial trauma.[3] The severity of the brain injury may be correlated with the severity of the coagulopathy observed, with the appearance of circulating fibrin monomer and fibrin degradation products as well as thrombocytopenia and abnormal coagulation studies.[65]

The brain has the highest tissue thromboplastin concentration of any of the body's organs.[2] As already noted, release of thromboplastin into the bloodstream after cerebral damage initiates coagulation. Although gunshot wounds to the brain initiate defibrination, injuries to the skull alone do not.[65]

The mediation of epinephrine as a procoagulant has already been mentioned, as has the importance of the anterior hypothalamus in this response. It is well known that head injury induces a dramatic catecholamine release from the adrenals which causes a variety of complications in addition to hypercoagulability, including arrhythmias, electrocardiographic abnormalities, noncardiogenic pulmonary edema, hypertension, and myocardial necrosis.[20,22,28] Although this response is thought to be primarily from activation of the adrenal medulla, stimulation of the anterior hypothalamus induces hypercoagulability in adrenalectomized animals, suggesting that other mediators may also be involved.[18]

## PREEXISTING CONDITIONS THAT CAUSE BLEEDING

### CIRRHOSIS OF THE LIVER

A multiplicity of causes is involved in bleeding diatheses of the patient with end-stage liver disease[61] or of the patient with liver trauma[13a] or severe shock. The liver produces all of the coagulation factors except the bulk of factor VIII. The liver also produces the inhibitors of plasminogen activators. The inadequately functioning liver fails to clear activated factors and plasminogen activators from the circulation. In addition, hyperbilirubinemia alters platelet function,[62] and portal hypertension may allow sequestration of platelets in an enlarged spleen.

Assessment of the patient with end-stage liver disease is summarized in Fig 7-3. Basic coagulation studies provide some indication of specific deficiencies. If all of the coagulation studies are abnormal, specific assays for factors V, VIII, and X are helpful. Since factor V is produced in the liver but factor VIII is not (up to 80% is made in the reticuloendothelial system), a finding of factor V depression with normal factor VIII levels is indicative of inadequate liver function. If both levels are depressed, consumption of factors is the most likely cause.

Factor X is vitamin K dependent but has a relatively long half-life, so that if prothrombin time (PT) is prolonged and factor X activity is normal, assay of factor VII is indicated. Thrombin time (TT) may be prolonged due to hypofibrinogenemia, but tests to identify circulating antithrombin should be performed, including an assay for fibrin degradation products and ethanol gelation or protamine sulfate serial dilution for the presence of soluble fibrin monomer. Vitamin K therapy should be instituted, but this will not be reflected in the PT for at least 4 hours. Therefore, acute bleeding should be treated with fresh frozen plasma (FFP) where indicated by the specific factor deficiencies present. Since factor VII has the shortest half-life (6 hours), the amount of FFP necessary to restore minimally adequate levels of this factor as well as of all the others will be 10 mL/kg every 6 hours, if the patient has no endogenous factor production. This may represent an intolerable fluid load for a cirrhotic patient; prothrombin complex concentrates (Konyne, Proplex, FEIBA) may be suitable alternatives, but their use should be undertaken with great caution, since these agents are prepared from pooled plasma and have the risk of hepatitis transmission, as well as a risk of causing disseminated intravascular coagulation (DIC) because of the administration of activated factors.

If the principal clotting defect in the cirrhotic patient is found to be hypofibrinogenemia, especially if this is caused by excessive destruction by plasmin, therapy with ϵ-aminocaproic acid (Amicar) may be tried.

Appropriate therapy should be continued to maintain control of bleeding and improvement of coagulation studies.

## RENAL FAILURE

Platelet dysfunction, which causes impaired platelet adhesiveness, aggregation, and abnormal bleeding time, is a well-known consequence of both acute and chronic renal failure. There is no reliable correlation between blood urea nitrogen concentration and bleeding tendency; however, a prolonged bleeding time may return to normal with dialysis.[32] The abnormality, not fully elucidated, involves failure of in vivo activation of platelet factor 3, since these patients' platelets behave normally in vitro. Cryoprecipitate infusions may improve platelet function, supporting the belief that platelet factor 3 inactivation is the significant coagulation abnormality in uremia.[32] More recently, intravenous infusion of DDAVP (0.3 μg per kg) has been shown to be helpful in decreasing bleeding problems in these patients.[70]

## VITAMIN K DEFICIENCY

Vitamin K deficiency is produced by a variety of mechanisms, but parenteral alimentation and intake of newer broad-spectrum antibiotics such as cefoperazone, moxalactam, cefa-

FIG. 7-3. Evaluation of the cirrhotic patient. Initial diagnostic steps □ are performed simultaneously. Subsequent studies lead to both therapy ◇ and diagnosis.

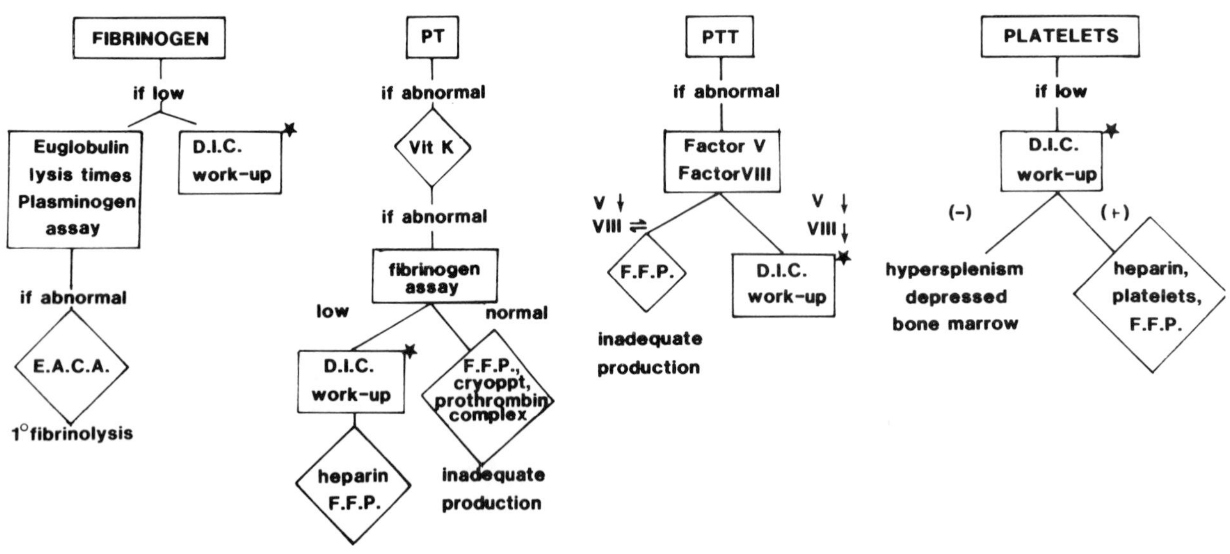

mandole, or ceftizoxime are the most likely causes in the trauma patient. Vitamin K is a cofactor of the hepatic microsomal carboxylase, which is also the site of action of the coumarin anticoagulants. Purified vitamin K administered intravenously (5 mg) produces correction of clotting time within 6 to 12 hours. The drug should be administered slowly; anaphylaxis and death may occur. The intramuscular dose is 25 mg; administration for 3 days results in total body vitamin K repletion. These regimens are ineffective in the bleeding vitamin K-deficient patient in whom only the rapid administration of FFP will correct the coagulopathy in a timely manner.

## COMMON MEDICATIONS

Significant disorders of hemostasis may be caused by the medications listed in Table 7-2.

### *Aspirin and Nonsteroidal Antiinflammatory Drugs*

These drugs inhibit synthesis in the platelets of prostaglandins generated by the cyclooxygenase pathway which are necessary for aggregation.[48] In addition, aspirin is known to acetylate platelet protein and interfere with platelet adhesion to collagen. Aspirin's effects are cell bound and thus irreversible.[71] As little as 600 mg of aspirin can cause depression of platelet aggregation and prolongation of bleeding time for 72 hours. Simultaneous alcohol ingestion has a profound potentiating effect on the platelet dysfunction caused by aspirin. Nonsteroidal antiinflammatory agents (NSAIDs) have a reversible effect on platelet aggregation, but emergency surgery may not allow enough time for spontaneous reversal of the hemostatic deficit after cessation of the drug.[71] Patients who have ingested aspirin or NSAIDs within 72 hours before surgery should probably have a bleeding time performed. If abnormal, the urgency of surgery will dictate whether delay is advisable until the bleeding time returns to normal. Platelet transfusion is indicated in those patients who develop abnormal bleeding during emergency surgery.

### *Dextran and Hydroxyethyl Starch*

Dextran binds a plasma protein necessary for normal platelet aggregation, making it useful as an antithromboembolic agent. If administered to replace hemorrhagic losses, large volumes of dextran (greater than 20 mL/kg) may produce bleeding since dilutional hypofibrinogenemia and depletion of coagulation factors may occur.[25] Dilutional coagulopathy may also occur after doses of hydroxyethyl starch greater than 20 mL/kg.[25] This agent has also been shown to deplete coagulant proteins by shifting them into the interstitial space[42] (see also Chapter 4).

TABLE 7-2. Commonly Used Medications Associated with Clinically Significant Disorders of Hemostasis

| |
|---|
| Aspirin |
| Phenylbutazone |
| Indomethacin |
| Dipyridamole |
| Sulfinpyrazone |
| Dextran |
| Hydroxyethyl starch |
| Heparin |
| Dicumarol and warfarin |

### *Heparin*

Heparin has multiple effects on hemostasis.

1. It acts as an antithrombin and inhibits activation of factor X. This is its most sensitive and immediate effect and is the basis for current "minidose" therapy. This effect requires the presence of antithrombin III, an intrinsic factor. Prolongation of thrombin time is seen before any effect on partial thromboplastin time (PTT) occurs.
2. It blocks factor IXa, causing prolongation of PTT.
3. Its anionic charges increase the net negative charge and hydration of fibrinogen, making the molecule more soluble.
4. It decreases platelet adhesiveness (generally not at therapeutic doses).

Heparin is extensively bound to α-globulins and has a mean half-life of approximately 1.5 hours. Twenty-five percent of administered heparin is excreted unchanged in the urine. The effect of heparin on TT should be distinguished from other causes of coagulopathy such as circulating fibrin degradation products. If thrombin time is prolonged, a reptilase time should be performed. A normal reptilase time indicates heparin effect, whereas a prolonged value indicates antithrombin activity. Alternatively, some laboratories add toluidine blue or protamine to the blood sample before repeating the TT in order to inactivate any heparin that may be present.

When urgent reversal is necessary, protamine sulfate (0.5 to 1 mg/100 U of administered heparin) should be given slowly. The patient should be monitored carefully to avoid hypotension or excessive dosage of protamine, which can itself cause bleeding. An activated clotting time (ACT) value of 80 to 150 seconds indicates adequate reversal of heparin effect.

### *Dicumarol and Warfarin*

These oral anticoagulants interfere with vitamin K-dependent synthesis of the prothrombin complex (II, VII, IX, X). Prolongation of PT is used to monitor therapeutic efficacy.

Dicumarol has a half-life of 36 hours. A number of drugs can potentiate or interfere with its effects. Dicumarol therapy should be stopped at least 48 hours before surgery, which should be performed only when PT has returned to normal. In acute situations, both vitamin K and FFP reverse the effects of dicumarol. The required dose of vitamin K ranges from 2.5 to 25 mg; it takes 2 to 4 hours to be effective.

### *Fibrinolytic Agents*

Streptokinase, urokinase, and tissue type plasminogen activator are administered directly into the circulation to accelerate conversion of plasminogen to plasmin, producing lysis of a fresh fibrin clot.[33] In the trauma setting, these agents may be used rarely to treat pulmonary embolism. Their use in patients with fresh surgical wounds is contraindicated. More extensive information about these drugs may be found in the literature.[14,36,60,66,68]

## HYPOTHERMIA AND COAGULATION

Hypothermia below 34°C is probably the most common cause of coagulopathy in the trauma patient, although its importance has been appreciated only recently. The effects of decreased body temperature on clotting function result from several mechanisms.[51] Hypothermia alters platelet number, morphology, function, and sequestration, resulting in prolonged bleeding and clotting times. These changes are reversible and return to normal upon rewarming. The fibrinolytic activity of plasma is also enhanced by hypothermia, and primary fibrinolysis may be the mechanism of coagulopathy in some patients. A third mechanism involves retardation of enzyme function which results in delay in initiation and propagation of clot formation. Hypothermia may also induce DIC by producing cell injury and subsequent thromboplastin release and by causing tissue hypoxia because it depresses cardiac output.

Shock, alcohol intoxication, massive fluid and blood infusion, exposure to cold, and prolonged surgery predispose the patient to hypothermia. Chapters 6 and 9 provide detailed information about means of preventing hypothermia and its complications.

## DISSEMINATED INTRAVASCULAR COAGULATION

This syndrome results from an accentuation of the normal processes of induction and cessation of coagulation. The mechanism of DIC is presumed to be widespread activation of the intrinsic coagulation pathway, although diffuse thrombus deposition is not consistently found.[56] Activation of coagulation in a localized area initiates a process of consumption of platelets, fibrinogen, and coagulation factors, with resultant generation of fibrin degradation products (FDP/fdp) which exert anticoagulant effects. In its most severe expression, diffuse bleeding occurs. A nonspecific stress to the entire organism may set off the same process.[4,12,34,56] There are multiple reasons for this. As mentioned earlier, catecholamine output stimulates coagulation; vasoconstriction causes slowing of peripheral blood flow, allowing clotting to take place; loss of blood flow through the splanchnic bed impairs the function of the reticuloendothelial system, which is responsible for clearance of circulating tissue debris, fibrin, bacteria, and other material that otherwise promote microthrombosis[44]; decreased liver perfusion prevents the liver from clearing and eliminating activated coagulation factors from the circulation[61]; and endotoxin stimulates coagulation.[44] Table 7-3 lists many of the most commonly described trauma-related causes of disseminated intravascular coagulation. Although many authors stress that treatment of the underlying etiology is the only therapy necessary to arrest DIC, clearly the patient who is injured, bleeding, and requires surgery needs vigorous replacement therapy with blood, FFP, and platelets to reverse the bleeding diathesis. Also, the rapid efficacy of these blood products in expanding the intravascular volume is extremely helpful, since a major inciting factor of DIC in trauma patients is the shock state. The degree to which endogenous compensation is capable of restoring coagulation factors and platelets to the circulation varies with the individual patient and with the rapidity of evolution of DIC. Also, underlying unsuspected hypercoagulability may predispose to the development of DIC when an inciting stress arises.[56]

TABLE 7-3. Major Predisposing Conditions Associated with Disseminated Intravascular Coagulation in Trauma

| |
|---|
| Shock |
| Hypothermia |
| Hyperthermia |
| Major blood type incompatibility |
| Massive transfusion |
| Autotransfusion |
| Hepatic cirrhosis |
| Liver injury |
| Head injury |
| Near-drowning |
| Burns |
| Inhalation injury |
| Pulmonary embolism |
| Fat embolism |
| Air embolism |
| Acute renal failure |
| Pregnancy |

Acute DIC is diagnosed by:

1. Presence of a predisposing condition
2. Prolongation of TT, PT, and PTT
3. Demonstration of soluble fibrin monomers and/or monomer-FDP complexes by ethanol gelation or protamine sulfate serial dilution
4. Depletion of fibrinogen, platelets, and coagulation factors (II, V, VIII, XII)
5. Demonstration of circulating FDP/fdp
6. Depressed antithrombin III level
7. Fragmented red cells on peripheral smear, a characteristic of microangiopathic anemia.

It is worthwhile to emphasize that obtaining normal values of some of these laboratory tests does not rule out DIC. An excellent study of 38 patients with acute DIC showed that PT was prolonged in 76% and elevated PTT was present in only 63%.[8] The most reliable results, both from the standpoint of aiding the diagnosis before therapy and of demonstrating normalization after therapy, were found to be the presence of FDP/fdp, depletion of antithrombin III, and reduced platelet count followed by the presence of soluble fibrin monomers and prolonged TT.[8] These tests should be available to the clinician at all times to maximize the specificity of the diagnosis.

The diffuse bleeding from venipunctures, membranes, and wound sites characteristic of DIC should not be confused with inadequately controlled surgical bleeding. Astute clinical observation is as important as laboratory results and usually yields information more rapidly. The reliability of the diagnosis may become clouded in situations in which coagulation studies are drawn too soon after the patient has received a large volume of crystalloids during resuscitation.[40,59,63] Obviously, appropriate component therapy in a bleeding patient should not be withheld in order to clarify the diagnosis.

There is an extensive literature demonstrating that low-dose heparin therapy is specific for reversing the DIC process.[7,8,34,56] Although heparin has been used successfully in postsurgical patients,[3,41] many clinicians are unwilling to risk starting anticoagulant therapy even at low doses in an acutely bleeding patient. ε-Aminocaproic acid is not generally recommended except as adjunctive therapy for a patient who is already receiving heparin,[34] since it accentuates rather than reverses the underlying thrombotic process of DIC.

The first approach to the treatment of any case of DIC is to reverse the underlying cause.[3,15,29,34,57] Rapid and aggressive treatment of shock, hypovolemia, and sepsis, is crucial to reduce both immediate morbidity and secondary mortality from organ failure.[44] As many as 53% of patients with acute DIC have evidence of renal microvascular thrombosis[8]; the resultant acute renal failure in association with traumatic or septic shock carries a high mortality. DIC has also been implicated as a cause of adult respiratory distress syndrome,[44,65] although this association is not as obvious as it previously appeared.

Replacement of coagulation factors and platelets should be guided by clinical response to therapy and by laboratory findings, especially the TT. FFP replaces depleted antithrombin III, the most important endogenous anticoagulant substance, as well as coagulation factors; its replenishment helps control the hypercoagulable state.[8] Vitamin K should probably be given to all patients because of its frequent association with DIC.

A recently introduced technique can be effective in controlling coagulopathy-induced intraoperative bleeding from solid organs. This involves surface or intraparenchymal application of fibrin glue. This material consists of four components: (1) highly concentrated fibrinogen; (2) trypsin inhibitor aprotinin; (3) dried thrombin; and (4) calcium chloride. Preliminary results suggest that fibrin glue achieves remarkable local hemostasis and may be lifesaving in patients with coagulation disorders, including DIC.[38]

The differentiation between DIC and primary fibrinolysis is less important than was thought previously since the latter is a rare disorder.[27a,34] Primary fibrinolysis is generally associated with prostatic carcinoma and liver failure, but it can also occur in the trauma setting, for example during intraoperative autotransfusion. The treatment involves correction of underlying cause and administration of ε-aminocaproic acid (5 gm followed by 1 gm per hour) and blood products.[34,61]

Euglobulin lysis time is positive in primary lytic states and negative in DIC, but the test takes a relatively long time to perform. The demonstration of soluble fibrin monomer by ethanol gelation was originally introduced as a rapid, easy bedside test to differentiate between DIC and fibrinolysis.[8] The transformation of fibrinogen to fibrin polymer generates fibrin monomers as an intermediary step. These monomers are present in soluble form in the plasma and can also form soluble complexes with FDP/fdp. The generation of soluble fibrin monomer and fibrin complexes occurs only when the coagulation process is proceeding normally and is thus termed the *paracoagulation process*.[8,56] Primary fibrinolysis (or fibrinogenolysis) generates FDP/fdp but not soluble fibrin monomer. Consequently, tests that demonstrate the presence of the monomer distinguish between these two conditions.[34] In practical terms, tests of paracoagulation are important as sensitive indicators of DIC and should be performed whenever the diagnosis is entertained.[8] The available tests are performed easily in the laboratory and use either ethanol or protamine added to the plasma sample. Soluble fibrin monomer becomes insoluble in the presence of either of these reagents and precipitates out of the sample as a characteristic gel.

## COAGULATION AND MASSIVE TRANSFUSION

Coagulopathies associated with massive blood replacement, excluding consumption, have often been ascribed to blood banking techniques in which coagulation factors and platelets are depleted during storage or which isolate blood components for different uses. Substantial differences in results of coagulation tests are encountered in different studies when diffuse or abnormal bleeding has been observed during massive transfusion.[10,19,24,29,39,46,57,59,72,74] We will next consider some of the many reasons for these discrepancies.

### DIFFERENCES IN COMPONENTS GIVEN

Investigations in which packed red cells[46] are transfused cannot be readily compared with studies which have used whole blood[10,24,39,57] or modified whole blood (platelets and/or cryoprecipitate removed).[19] The latter two products contain substantially greater amounts of fibrinogen and coagulation factors than packed red cells. In addition, the differences in volume of units between these blood products imply differences in intravascular volume restoration which are not accounted for by some investigators.

### TIMING OF CLOTTING STUDIES

Studies of changes in coagulation assays after trauma demonstrate cyclic patterns of depression and recovery of clotting factor levels.[3,15,27a,57] Since the timing of coagulation tests during clinical investigations of transfused patients is generally arbitrary, eg, after every 10 U of blood, the normal oscillatory patterns in coagulation may be unwittingly superimposed on the results obtained, explaining why some studies demonstrate significant changes in coagulation studies and others do not.

### DURATION OF SHOCK AND TIMING OF VOLUME REPLACEMENT

This consideration is perhaps the most crucial cause of the discrepancies among the results of different studies. Fig 7-4 and its accompanying table demonstrate theoretical exchange transfusions. It can be seen that normovolemic exchange (patient A) retains the greatest percentage of the original blood

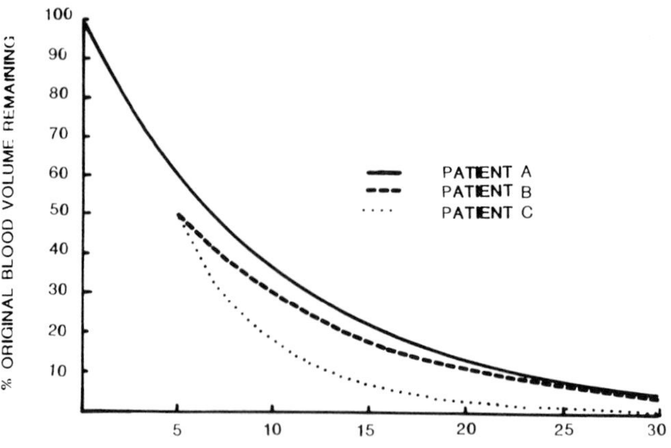


| Patient | *Percent of original blood volume remaining** | | |
|---|---|---|---|
| | *1 blood volume (10 units)* | *2 blood volumes (20 units)* | *3 blood volumes (30 units)* |
| A | 36.8 (34.9) | 13.5 (12.2) | 5 (4.2) |
| B | 30.4 (29.5) | 11.2 (10.3) | 4.1 (3.6) |
| C | 18.4 (16.4) | 2.5 (1.8) | 0.4 (0.2) |

* Computations based on continuous exchange formula; results with incremental exchange formula indicated in parentheses.

FIG. 7-4. Replacement of initial blood volume, based on timing of intervention. Normovolemic exchange results in the greatest preservation of blood volume. (From Collins[15] with permission.)

volume, whereas the patient who is transfused late in the course of hemorrhage (patient B) or with incomplete restoration of volume (patient C) will suffer greater dilution of his own blood volume and its components. Since it is impossible to control the timing of intervention in the acutely hemorrhaging patient, the degree of dilution cannot be predicted in the individual case. The impact of the duration of hemorrhage and shock on subsequent alterations in coagulation is not accounted for in some studies, nor is the effectiveness of resuscitation as judged by other clinical indicators.[19,46] In fact, many clinical studies show that abnormal bleeding secondary to multiple coagulation defects develops while the patients are in shock.[15,29,39,45,57] Studies of normovolemic hemodilution demonstrate only mild alterations in factor levels and platelet counts,[40,59,63] indicating that effective maintenance of blood volume has an important impact on subsequent clotting function; even when coagulation abnormalities are seen, they are transient and unaccompanied by bleeding problems.

One study has investigated precisely the effect of duration of shock on subsequent coagulopathy in patients who were massively transfused with red cell concentrate and crystalloids.[29] Although the volume of fluid administered at given time intervals after hemorrhage was unrelated to subsequent prolongation of PTT, the duration of hypotension correlated very strongly with PTT elevation during the interval immediately following hemorrhage as well as during all subsequent time intervals observed.

Thus, although fluid resuscitation may temporarily dilute clotting factors, it is hypotension which impairs the patient's ability to correct this depression of coagulation factors because shock decreases factor production,[6] reduces or reverses mobilization of factors from tissue spaces,[29] and/or induces consumption.[3,15,44,53,57]

## PLATELET NUMBER AND FUNCTION

Several articles have ascribed bleeding after massive transfusion to dilutional thrombocytopenia.[19,39,45] The studies which demonstrate changes in platelet count are variable in their findings. During hemorrhage and replacement with bank blood (which has no viable platelets), platelet counts drop with volume replaced, and an exponential "washout" curve is observed. The level at which platelet count stabilizes has been identified as 100,000/μL in some studies[24,57] and approximately 50,000/μL in others.[19,39,53] Two studies identify the level of thrombocytopenia below which bleeding occurs as approximately 65,000/μL.[13,46] Other authors describe the minimal platelet count for hemostasis following trauma to be 50,000/μL,[39,72] 70,000/μL,[1,13] or 100,000/μL.[69] All these values are, of course, substantially higher than are necessary for hemostatic function in other thrombocytopenic conditions. A study that concluded that platelet transfusions are necessary to restore hemostasis demonstrated no difference between the platelet counts of those patients who bled abnormally and those who did not.[19] Other studies that came to similar conclusions ascribed bleeding to multiple causes.[10,24,57,72,74]

Because of these inconsistencies, some attempt has been made to identify a transfusion-induced functional platelet defect that would explain why some but not all patients with diffuse bleeding have abnormal platelet counts. Lim et al[41] claimed that there were aggregation abnormalities of circulating platelets during massive blood replacement. However, this hypothesis has not been investigated further.

More recently, a well-designed double-blind randomized study was performed to investigate the value of prophylactic platelet transfusion in patients receiving massive blood replacement.[53] Particular attention was paid to the volumes administered, since patients received either platelet concentrate or an equivalent volume of FFP, a standardization not used in previous studies. It was found that there was no difference in platelet counts or in the incidence of bleeding between the two groups. Only one patient with diffuse bleeding had thrombocytopenia. The authors concluded that dilutional thrombocytopenia is an uncommon cause of abnormal bleeding. The decrease of platelet numbers seen during massive transfusion was less than predicted from the appropriate washout equation. This observation has been made in other studies as well,[19,24,35,59] and implies that an individual is capable of mobilizing reserves of platelets acutely.[40] Since splanchnic perfusion must be preserved to enable platelets sequestered in the spleen to enter the circulation, the importance of restoring and maintaining blood volume during resuscitation is again emphasized. Indeed, in Miller's series[46] in which dilutional thrombocytopenia was identified as the cause of bleeding, "transfusion of 3 to 4 units of fresh blood resulted in marked increases in platelet counts." This rise cannot be explained by the number of platelets present in the blood transfused[13] but is consistent with platelet mobilization resulting from effective restoration of splanchnic blood flow. Other studies in which fresh blood was given in a similar fashion but an increased platelet count did not result noted that shock was still present.[39,57]

Thus, there are few absolute indications for platelet transfusion in the trauma patient and, from the recommendations of the 1987 consensus conference, they can be summarized as follows.[17]

1. Platelet count less than 20,000/μL
2. Diffuse bleeding (oozing) during or after massive transfusion
3. Platelet count less than 50,000/μL in an actively bleeding patient who needs urgent or emergent surgery requiring massive transfusion
4. Bleeding time greater than 15 minutes in a patient who is actively bleeding and who will undergo major surgery.

In order to be effective, platelets should preferably be administered after control of surgical bleeding, otherwise they will be lost in the suction bottle. Platelets are supplied as either a single-unit random-donor concentrate, or multiple-unit single-donor concentrate. The former is produced from conventional whole blood donations within 6 hours of collection, whereas the latter is collected by mechanical apheresis from one donor. Each multiple unit collection has as many platelets as 6 to 10 single units. Each unit of platelet concentrate increases blood platelet concentration by 10,000/μL; thus, for a therapeutic effect, 6 to 7 U must be transfused. Single-donor platelet concentrate may be obtained from donors of known HLA type to yield HLA-matched platelets or from the patient's family members. The effect of the transfusion should be evaluated by clinical observation and platelet counts obtained 1, 12, and 24 hours after administration, if possible. A platelet count increase of at least 5000/μL should be achieved per unit transfused. An increase of less than this value suggests immunization—unless the patient is rapidly consuming platelets by bleeding, fever, or as a result of DIC.

There is some evidence to suggest that platelet adhesion to the vascular endothelium and platelet aggregation are decreased in anemic patients. Thus, low hematocrit values that are considered adequate for tissue oxygenation may be inadequate for hemostasis in thrombocytopenic patients.[21] However, the clinical importance of this finding and the optimal hematocrit value for a given platelet count in the trauma patient remain to be determined.

## FRESH FROZEN PLASMA

It is now clear that FFP transfusion is unjustifiable for intravascular volume expansion or for nutritional purposes.[11,16] It is also clear that there is no indication for prophylactic FFP administration if whole blood or modified whole blood, which are the preferred products in severe trauma patients, are used for massive transfusion.[11,16,27,43] Patients who receive packed red cells may require FFP after a 1.5 to 2 blood volume replacement.[49] However, even in these patients, prophylactic administration of this product, despite being recommended by some authors,[27a,52] appears unwarranted[11,16,43,49] (see also Chapter 6). If nonsurgical bleeding (oozing) occurs, and it is believed to be caused by factor deficiency, FFP is indicated. In these patients FFP should be administered in large volumes (600 to 2000 mL) and rapidly, in order to correct coagulation abnormalities and possibly bleeding.[11] Reference has already been made in previous sections to other indications for FFP in the trauma patient (severe liver injury, cirrhosis, vitamin K deficiency, dicumarol and warfarin therapy, and DIC).

## RECOMMENDATIONS FOR MANAGEMENT OF MASSIVE TRANSFUSION

It would appear that the best approach to the hemorrhaging patient depends on rapid, aggressive restoration of blood volume. Satisfactory volume repletion requires a goal-directed approach toward normalization of acidosis, urinary output, tissue perfusion, and oxygen delivery and consumption. These are better indicators of adequacy of volume status than are vital signs; resuscitation should emphasize these goals even after blood pressure is stable. Whole blood or modified whole blood appears to be preferable to packed red blood cells for patients requiring acute massive transfusion[19] but possibly only because more rapid blood volume restoration can be achieved, and FFP, which carries the risk of viral disease transmission, may not be necessary.

Coagulation studies within the first half-hour of the resuscitation period are not very helpful for management purposes, especially when large volumes of crystalloids are administered,[29,40,59] but prolonged PTT values after the first 3 hours of resuscitation are significant, since this finding indicates that inadequate resuscitation, excessive dilution, or consumption has taken place. Some clinicians believe that a battery of tests including plasma fibrinogen level, platelet count, PTT, PT, and bleeding time performed before transfusion and at 2- to 3-hour intervals during transfusion may provide valuable information about overall coagulation status of the patient. Likewise a tube test, which involves drawing blood and observing it for clot formation, clot retraction, and clot lysis times, or serial thrombelastograms may be useful (See Chapter 9). In the massively bleeding trauma patient these tests are usually omitted, and management is guided by clinical observation of the type and extent of the bleeding.

No specific level of platelets appears to be ideal; thrombocytopenia may not be the primary cause of abnormal bleeding in most cases. No standard protocol for prophylactic FFP or platelet transfusion can be recommended on the basis of the information currently available[16,17]; rather, replacement of platelets and/or factors should be guided by signs of diffuse oozing or bleeding from venipuncture sites and the presumption that consumption and shock are ongoing problems. Bleeding time is not a useful study if the platelet count is already depressed. On the other hand coagulation studies, fibrinogen levels, and platelet counts may help guide replacement.

## CONCLUSION

Control of hemorrhage in the traumatized patient depends on rapid surgical control of bleeding sites and aggressive restoration of circulating volume, tissue perfusion, and oxygen delivery. Efficient accomplishment of these goals enables the patient to restore platelets and coagulation factors that are lost or consumed at wound sites by mobilization of stores and increased production. In otherwise healthy individuals this is accomplished in a matter of hours to days without complications. Indeed, it is interesting to note that the time necessary for platelet counts to return to normal is the same whether or not platelets have been transfused.[26] Inadequate resuscitation, shock, severe liver injury, and prolonged hypoperfusion of the liver and spleen interfere with these compensatory mechanisms, allowing secondary complications of consumption coagulopathy, dilutional coagulopathy, and dilutional thrombocytopenia to supervene.

In patients with head trauma and abnormal coagulation studies, immediate and aggressive replacement therapy should not be delayed, even if abnormal bleeding is not seen, since even small intracranial blood collections are not well tolerated; blood component therapy directed toward correcting abnormal coagulation should be instituted immediately.

Although the literature indicates that most patients who are massively transfused have decreased platelet counts, many thrombocytopenic patients do not bleed abnormally, and some with adequate platelet counts do. One study reports a bleeding patient with a platelet count of 140,000/μL who improved after platelet transfusion.[19] However, the possibility that functional platelet defects result from massive transfusion remains unproven. Multiple causes of bleeding are probably involved and should be sought and treated. Consumption coagulopathy should be treated by replacement of deficient coagulation factors with FFP and, if thrombocytopenia is present, with platelets.

## REFERENCES


1. Aggeler PM. Physiologic basis for transfusion therapy in hemorrhagic disorders. Transfusion 1961;1:71.
2. Astrup T. Assay and content of tissue thromboplastin in different organs. Thromb Diath Haemorrh 1965;14:401.
3. Attar S, Boyd D, Layne E, et al. Alterations in coagulation and fibrinolytic mechanisms in acute trauma. J Trauma 1969;9:939.
4. Attar S, Kirby WH Jr, Masaitis C, et al. Coagulation changes in clinical shock. Ann Surg 1966;164:34.
5. Bagge L, Haglund O, Wallin R, et al. Differences in coagulation and fibrinolysis after traumatic and septic shock in man. Scand J Clin Lab Invest 1989;49:63.
6. Benson RE, Ishister JP. Massive blood transfusion. Anaesth Crit Care 1980;8:152.
7. Bergentz SE, Nilsson IM. Effect of trauma on coagulation and fibrinolysis in dogs. Acta Chir Scand 1961;122:21.
8. Bick RL. Disseminated intravascular coagulation: a clinical/laboratory study of 48 patients. Ann NY Acad Sci 1981;370:843.
9. Biggs R, MacFarlane RG, Pilling J. Observations on fibrinolysis: experimental activity produced by exercise or adrenalin. Lancet 1947;1:402.
10. Boyan CP, Howland WS. Problems related to massive blood transfusions. Anesth Analg 1962;41:497.
11. Braunstein AH, Oberman HA. Transfusion of plasma components. Transfusion 1984;24:281.
12. Cannon WB, Gray H. Factors affecting the coagulation time of blood, II: the hastening or retarding of coagulation by adrenalin injection. Am J Physiol 1914;34:232.
13. Cavins JA, Farber S, Roy AJ. Transfusions of fresh platelet concentrates to adult patients with thrombocytopenia. Transfusion 1968;8:24.

13a. Clagett GP, Olsen WR. Non-mechanical hemorrhage in severe liver injury. 1978;187:369.

14. Collen D, Topol EJ, Tiefenbrunn AJ. Coronary thrombolysis with recombinant human tissue-type plasminogen activator: a prospective randomized placebo controlled trial. Circulation 1984;70:1012.
15. Collins JA. Problems associated with the massive tranfusion of stored blood. Surgery 1974;75:274.
16. Consensus conference. Fresh-frozen plasma: indications and risks. JAMA 1985;253:551.
17. Consensus conference. Platelet transfusion therapy. JAMA 1987;257:1777.
18. Correll JW. Central neural structures and pathways important for control of blood clotting: evidence for release of anti-heparin factor. International Conference of Microcirculation, Gothenberg, 1968:36.
19. Counts RB, Haisch C, Simon TL, et al. Hemostasis in massively transfused trauma patients. Ann Surg 1979;190:91.
20. Ducker TB. Increased intracranial pressure and pulmonary edema, 1: clinical study of 11 patients. J Neurosurg 1968;28:112.
21. Escolar G, Garrido M, Mazzara R, et al. Experimental basis for the use of red cell transfusion in the management of anemic-thrombocytopenic patients. Transfusion 1988;28:406.
22. Evans DE, Alta WA, Shatsky SA, et al. Cardiac arrhythmias resulting from experimental head injury. J Neurosurg 1976;45:609.
23. Friedman M, Uhley HN. Role of the adrenal in hastening blood coagulation after exposure to stress. Am J Physiol 1959;197:205.
24. Gollub S, Ulin AW, Winchell HS, et al. Hemorrhagic diathesis associated with massive transfusion. Surgery 1959;45:204.
25. Halonen P, Linko K, Myllyla G. A study of haemostasis following the use of high doses of hydroxyethyl starch and dextran in major laparotomies. Acta Anaesthesiol Scand 1987;31:320.
26. Harding SA, Shakoor MA, Grindon AJ. Platelet support of cardiopulmonary bypass surgery. J Thorac Cardiovasc Surg 1975;70:350.
27. Harke H, Rahman S. Haemostatic disorders in massive transfusion. Bibl Haematol 1980;46:179.

27a. Harrigan C, Lucas CE, Ledgerwood AM. The effect of hemorrhagic shock on the clotting cascade in injured patients. J Trauma 1989;29:1416.

28. Hawkins WE, Clower BR. Myocardial damage after head trauma and simulated intracranial hemorrhage in mice: the role of the autonomic nervous system. Cardiovasc Res 1971;5:524.
29. Henson JR, Neame PB, Kumar N, et al. Coagulopathy related to dilution and hypotension during massive transfusion. Crit Care Med 1985;13:387.
30. Hildago J, Fowell AH, Ralls RJ. Effect of tissue damage on the plasma fibrinogen level. Surg Gynec Obstet 1952;95:661.
31. Innes D, Sevitt S. Coagulation and fibrinolysis in injured patients. J Clin Pathol 1964;17:1.
32. Janson PA, Jubelirer SJ, Weinstein MJ. Treatment of the bleeding tendency in uremia with cryoprecipitate. N Engl J Med 1980;303:1318.
33. Kakkar VV, Scully MF. Thrombolytic therapy. Br Med Bull 1978;34:191.
34. Kazmier FJ, Bowie EJW, Hagedorn AB, et al. Treatment of intravascular coagulation and fibrinolysis (ICF) syndromes. Mayo Clin Proc 1974;49:665.
35. Keleman E, Lehoczy D, Cserhati I, et al. Demonstrability of a serum factor inducing thrombocytosis prior to acute rises of platelets in mice and men. Acta Haematol 1963;29:16.
36. Khaja F, Walton JA, Brymer JF, et al. Intracoronary fibrinolytic therapy in acute myocardial infarction: report of a prospective randomized trial. N Engl J Med 1983;308:1305.
37. Kobrinsky NL, Letts RM, Patel LR, et al. 1-Desamino-8-D-arginine vasopressin (desmopressin) decreases operative blood loss in patients having Harrington rod spinal fusion surgery. Ann Intern Med 1987;107:446.
38. Kram HB, Nathan RC, Stafford FJ, et al. Fibrin glue achieves hemostasis in patients with coagulation disorders. Arch Surg 1989;124:385.
39. Krevans JR, Jackson DP. Hemorrhagic disorders following massive whole blood transfusions. JAMA 1955;159:171.
40. Laks H, Handin RI, Martin V, et al. The effects of acute normovolemic hemodilution on coagulation and blood utilization in major surgery. J Surg Res 1976;20:225.
41. Lim RC, Olcott C, Robinson AJ, et al. Platelet response and coagulation changes following massive blood replacement. J Trauma 1973;13:577.
42. Lucas CE, Denis R, Ledgerwood AM, Grabow D. The effects of hespan on serum and lymphatic albumin, globulin, and coagulant protein. Ann Surg 1988;207:416.
43. Mannucci PM, Federici AB, Sirchia G. Hemostasis testing during massive blood replacement. Vox Sang 1982;42:113.
44. McKay DG. Trauma and disseminated intravascular coagulation. J Trauma 1969;9:646.
45. McNamara JJ, Burrau EL, Stemple JF, et al. Coagulopathy after major combat injury: occurrence, management and pathophysiology. Ann Surg 1972;176:243.
46. Miller RD, Robbins TO, Tong MJ, et al. Coagulation defects associated with massive blood transfusions. Ann Surg 1971; 174:794.
47. Miller WR, Willson JT, Elliot TS. Blood changes in the dog following trauma. Angiology 1959;10:375.
48. Moncada S. Arachidonic acid metabolites and the interactions between platelets and blood vessel walls. N Engl J Med 1979;300:1142.
49. Murray DJ, Olson J, Strauss R, Tinker JH. Coagulation changes during packed red cell replacement of major blood loss. Anesthesiology 1988;69:839.
50. Ordog GJ, Wasserberger J, Balasubramanium S. Coagulation abnormalities in traumatic shock. Ann Emerg Med 1985;14:650.
51. Patt A, McCroskey BL, Moore EE. Hypothermia-induced coagulopathies in trauma. Surg Clin North Am 1988;68:775.
52. Phillips TF, Soulier G, Wilson RF. Outcome of massive transfusion exceeding two blood volumes in trauma and emergency surgery. J Trauma 1987;27:903.
53. Reed RL, Ciavarella D, Heimbach DM, et al. Prophylactic platelet administration during massive transfusion. Ann Surg 1986; 203:40.
54. Risberg BO, Medegard ALF, Heideman M, et al. Early activation of humoral proteolytic systems in patients with multiple trauma. Crit Care Med 1986;14:917.
55. Seyfer AE, Seaber AV, Dombrose FA, Urbaniak JR. Coagulation changes in elective surgery and trauma. Ann Surg 1981;193:210.
56. Sharp AA. Diagnosis and management of disseminated intravascular coagulation. Br Med Bull 1977;33:265.
57. Simmons RL, Collins JA, Heisterkamp CA, et al. Coagulation disorders in combat casualties. Ann Surg 1969;169:455.
58. Slichter SJ, Funk DD, Leandoer LE, et al. Kinetic evaluation of haemostasis during surgery and wound healing. Br J Haematol 1974;27:115.
59. Takaori M, Safar P. Treatment of massive hemorrhage with colloid and crystalloid solutions. JAMA 1967;199:297.
60. Tennant SN, Dixon J, Venable TC, et al. Intracoronary thrombolysis in patients with acute myocardial infarction: comparison of the efficacy of urokinase with streptokinase. Circulation 1984;69:756.
61. Tullis JL. Acquired hypoprothrombinemia in the coagulant chop suey of cirrhosis. In: Tullis JL, ed. Clot. Springfield: Charles C Thomas, 1976:350.
62. Tullis JL. Acquired hypoprothrombinemia. In: Tullis JL, ed. Clot. Springfield: Charles C Thomas, 1976:354.
63. Umlas J, Sakhuja R. The effect on blood coagulation of the exclusive use of frozen red cell transfusions during and after cardiopulmonary bypass. J Thorac Cardiovasc Surg 1975;70:519.
64. Van der Sande JJ, Emels JJ, Lindeman J. Intravascular coagulation: a common phenomenon in minor experimental head injury. J Neurosurg 1981;54:21.
65. Van der Sande JJ, Veltkamp JJ, Boekhout-Mussert RJ, et al. Head injury and coagulation disorders. J Neurosurg 1978;49:357.
66. Van de Werf F, Lundbrook PA, Bergmann SR, et al. Coronary thrombolysis with tissue-type plasminogen activator in patients with evolving myocardial infarction. N Engl J Med 1984;310:609.
67. Vecht CJ, Minderhoud JM, Smiot Sibingen CTH. Platelet aggregability in relation to impaired consciousness after head injury. J Clin Pathol 1975;28:814.
68. Verstraete M, Bernard R, Bory M, et al. Randomized trial of intravenous recombinant tissue-type plasminogen activator versus intravenous streptokinase in acute myocardial infarction. Lancet 1985;1:842.
69. Voorhees AB, Elliot HE. Surgical experiences with thrombocytopenic patients. Ann NY Acad Sci 1964;115:1.
70. Watson AJ, Keogh JA. 1-Desamino-8-D-arginine vasopressin as a therapy for the bleeding diathesis or renal failure, Am J Nephrology 1984;4:49.
71. Weiss HJ. Antiplatelet therapy. N Engl J Med 1978;298:1344.
72. Wilson RF, Mammen E, Walt AJ. Eight years of experience with massive blood transfusions. J Trauma 1971;11:275.
73. Wintrobe MM. Blood coagulation. In: Wintrobe MM, ed. Clinical hematology. Philadelphia: Lea and Febiger, 1981:1267.
74. Zucker MB, Siegel M, Clifton EE, et al. Generalized excessive oozing in patients undergoing major surgery and receiving multiple blood transfusions. J Lab Clin Med 1957;50:849.

# Chapter Eight

Christopher M. Grande
Marc Tissot
Vimala P. Bhatt
Alison Pataky
Mark Rivlin
Neal Kurtti

# Preexisting Compromising Conditions

Although trauma patients are often young, many of them have concurrent diseases. In a retrospective analysis of nearly 36,000 trauma patients admitted to San Francisco General Hospital over a 10-year period, Morris and coworkers[4] found that 15,000 (41%) had one or more preexisting diseases. In a subsequent study using a large population base ($n$ = 27,029) these authors demonstrated that 19% of surviving trauma patients had one or more preexisting conditions, and 5% had two or more.[3] Of the 11 concurrent diseases isolated, hypertension was the most common and coagulation defects the least common.[3] The prevalence of associated pathology increased with age; more than 30% of patients above 55 years old had one or more diseases as compared with 8% in the 15- to 55-year-old age group[3] (Table 8-1). The most striking finding was the effect of preexisting disease on mortality and the length of hospital stay. Patients with one concurrent disease were 30% more likely to die than those without a preexisting compromising condition; those with two were 60% more likely to die. Injured patients with pulmonary disease, coagulation defects, cirrhosis, and ischemic heart disease were at highest risk of dying.[5] In addition, the length of hospitalization was prolonged by the presence of a preexisting condition. The likelihood of staying in the hospital for more than 3 weeks doubled in the presence of an associated disease.[3] This effect, however, was more pronounced in young patients with less severe injuries.[3] Since both age and severe injury increase morbidity and mortality, the effect of concurrent disease on the length of the hospital stay decreased in those trauma patients who were older than 55 years and had injury severity scores greater than 20.[3] (Table 8-2).

Does the presence of preexisting disease similarly affect anesthetic care and outcome in the trauma patient? There are no data available to answer this question with certainty. In fact there is not even clear information about the anesthetic risk of trauma surgery for healthy patients. Emergency surgery is considered a preoperative risk factor,[1,2,6] but whether the same risk applies to trauma anesthesia is not known. In any case, based on data from several risk and outcome studies,[2,6] it appears that preexisting disease should negatively affect anesthetic care and outcome. Accepting this assumption, the objective of this chapter is to review several commonly encountered medical diseases that are likely to be present in the trauma population.

## ALCOHOL AND DRUG INTOXICATION

### ACUTE ALCOHOL INTOXICATION IN TRAUMA

Alcohol is the most common intoxicating substance found in trauma victims, some of whom may be chronic alcoholics with multiorgan disease.[18,31,68,75] Table 8-3 presents the potential perioperative problems likely to be encountered in acutely intoxicated patients, their mechanisms, and recommended clinical approaches to modifying their effects. Most of these problems can be recognized during the preoperative evaluation of the trauma victim. However, the extent of alcohol-related in-

TABLE 8-1. Frequency of 11 Preexisting Diseases and Their Distribution Between Age Groups in 27,029 Adult Trauma Patients*

| PREEXISTING DISEASE | NO. OF PATIENTS WITH PREEXISTING CONDITION | % OF TOTAL† | % IN 15- TO 54-YEAR-OLD GROUP | % IN >55-YEAR-OLD GROUP |
|---|---|---|---|---|
| Hypertension | 1800 | 6.7 | 2.2 | 13.3 |
| Ischemic heart disease | 920 | 3.4 | 0.3 | 6.6 |
| Psychoses | 829 | 3.1 | 1.4 | 4.8 |
| Alcohol/drug | 813 | 3.0 | 3.4 | 3.7 |
| Diabetes | 798 | 3.0 | 1.1 | 5.8 |
| Pulmonary disease | 822 | 3.0 | 0.4 | 6.7 |
| CNS degeneration | 345 | 1.2 | 0.1 | 2.7 |
| Obesity | 203 | 0.8 | 2.7 | 1.1 |
| Epilepsy | 156 | 0.6 | 0.7 | 0.6 |
| Cirrhosis | 137 | 0.5 | 0.4 | 1.0 |
| Coagulation defects | 61 | 0.2 | 0.2 | 0.3 |

* (From MacKenzie et al[3] with permission.)
† Total is greater than 19% because some patients had more than one disease.

traoperative metabolic, cardiovascular, respiratory, and central nervous system responses to anesthetic agents is difficult to predict. Stress and hemorrhage produced by trauma and surgery, concomitant use of other self-administered drugs, preexisting diseases, and the severity of alcohol intoxication may modify these responses. Although Lee et al[54,55] in retrospective studies demonstrated that there was no increase in the rate of intraoperative hypotension or perioperative morbidity in acutely intoxicated patients with blood alcohol levels less than 250 mg/dL, a small number of patients with levels above 250 mg/dL seemed to be unfavorably affected by anesthesia and surgery. In most trauma centers a blood sample is obtained for alcohol and drug level determinations, but the results are rarely available for the anesthesiologist before surgery even though rapid methods of measuring the blood alcohol level are available.[50,83] A simple indirect method of estimating blood alcohol level involves simultaneous measurement of serum osmolality and sodium and glucose concentrations.[72] Serum osmolality values above those calculated from serum sodium and glucose concentrations,

$$\text{serum osmolality} = (2 \times \text{sodium}) + (\text{serum glucose}/18)$$

suggest that the osmotic load is produced by alcohol. A faster and simpler determination can be made by measuring nasal and/or oral breath alcohol concentration with a hand-held pocket size analyzer which correlates very well with venous alcohol concentration.[34]

As described in Table 8-3, decreased tracheobronchial reflexes and an increased incidence of vomiting and silent regurgitation in heavily intoxicated patients may necessitate additional precautions during anesthesia. The airway should be protected with an endotracheal tube as early as possible. Procedures that induce gagging may cause vomiting which, in the presence of diminished cough reflex, may easily result in aspiration pneumonitis. Whenever possible, rapid sequence induction rather than awake laryngoscopy and intubation should be chosen. The patient should be observed carefully during the oxygenation phase of this technique; silently regurgitated gastric material may find its way into the trachea.[17] Extubation should be attempted only when the patient regains his or her tracheobronchial reflexes.

The ability of the intoxicated patient to withstand hypovolemia may be diminished.[35,61] Systemic vasodilatation,[9] possible reduction in myocardial contractility,[25] possible in-

TABLE 8-2. Mean Length of Hospital Stay (LOS) Stratified According to Age, Injury Severity Score (ISS), and Presence of Preexisting Condition (PEC)*

| | AGES 15 TO 54 YEARS | | | AGES 55 AND OLDER | | |
|---|---|---|---|---|---|---|
| | *Mean LOS (Days)* | | *% Difference in LOS* | *Mean LOS (Days)* | | *% Difference in LOS* |
| ISS | *No PEC* | *≥1 PEC* | | *No PEC* | *≥1 PEC* | |
| 1 to 8 | 4.0 | 5.9 | +45 | 6.6 | 8.8 | +33 |
| 9 to 12 | 6.4 | 11.1 | +73 | 12.9 | 15.5 | +20 |
| 13 to 15 | 11.2 | 17.6 | +57 | 13.6 | 16.0 | +18 |
| 16 to 19 | 11.3 | 16.1 | +42 | 15.0 | 19.2 | +28 |
| 20+ | 21.8 | 18.2 | −20 | 28.3 | 29.8 | +5 |
| All live discharges | 5.3 | 7.8 | +47 | 9.6 | 12.5 | +30 |

* (From Mackenzie et al[3] with permission.)

TABLE 8-3. Potential Anesthetic Problems Associated with Acute Alcohol Intoxication, Their Mechanisms, and Clinical Approaches to Minimize Morbidity

| POTENTIAL PROBLEM | MECHANISM | CLINICAL APPROACH |
|---|---|---|
| Pulmonary aspiration of gastric contents | Stimulation of gastric secretion<br>Vomiting and silent regurgitation<br>Diminished tracheobronchial reflexes | Avoid inducing gag reflex<br>Observe the patient for vomiting and regurgitation during $O_2$ administration by mask<br>Induce anesthesia with rapid sequence technique whenever possible<br>Extubate patient only after the return of tracheobronchial reflexes |
| Exaggerated hemodynamic response to hypovolemia | Depressed cardiovascular reflexes<br>Peripheral vasodilatation<br>Pulmonary vasoconstriction<br>Coronary vasoconstriction<br>Myocardial depression<br>Metabolic acidosis | Monitor CVP during fluid therapy<br>Avoid sudden positional changes<br>Monitor ECG with precordial leads to diagnose myocardial ischemia<br>Treat metabolic acidosis by restoring intravascular volume |
| Hypovolemia | Increased diuresis caused by osmotic load of alcohol and alcohol-induced antidiuretic hormone inhibition | Measured urine output and replace with balanced salt solution<br>Use central venous pressure as a guide for fluid therapy |
| Hypothermia | Peripheral vasodilatation | Monitor core temperature<br>Employ all available measures to prevent heat loss. Use blood warmer, heated gas humidifiers, and temperature blanket. Elevate ambient temperature, and wrap the head and torso with clear plastic bags |
| Hypoglycemia | Depressed adenine dinucleotide (NAD)-dependent gluconeogenesis depletes liver glycogen stores. Reduction of NAD to NADH during alcohol metabolism depletes NAD. Thus, in a starved alcoholic, further alcohol consumption without food intake results in hypoglycemia | Monitor blood sugar<br>Add dextrose to intravenous fluid regimen<br>Do not rely on stress-induced increase of blood sugar to prevent this complication |
| Alcoholic ketoacidosis | Fasting-induced mild ketoacidosis and increased acetate formation by the liver during alcohol metabolism | Monitor arterial blood gases, and serum $HCO_3^-$<br>Add dextrose to intravenous fluids<br>Administer sodium bicarbonate to elevate $pH_a$ |
| Alcoholic lactic acidosis | Precise mechanism unknown<br>Lactic acidosis in this setting is due to decreased utilization of lactic acid by the liver rather than increased generation of lactate | Treat other causes of lactic acidosis (shock, cardiac arrest, convulsions) if present<br>Increase caloric intake by adding dextrose to intravenous fluids<br>Use normal saline rather than Ringer's lactate as intravenous fluid |
| Altered mental status (disorientation, combativeness, stupor, coma) | Direct CNS effect of alcohol | Rule out intracranial pathology by physical and radiologic examination |
| Decreased cerebral tolerance to hypoxia | Unclear | Ensure adequate oxygenation<br>Avoid apneic episodes<br>Monitor $O_2$ saturation |
| Augmented central nervous, cardiovascular, and respiratory system response to barbiturates, opiates, inhalational anesthetics, major and minor tranquilizers and tricyclic antidepressants | Additive or depressant effect of alcohol | Reduce doses of these drugs and monitor cardiovascular and respiratory responses carefully |
| Possible approximation of respiratory and cardiac depressant effects of inhalational agents | Unclear | Titrate inhalational anesthetics to response to pain rather than to that of blood pressure |
| Multiorgan system involvement when there is underlying chronic alcoholism (alcoholic cardiomyopathy, skeletal myopathy, hepatic dysfunction, hematologic and coagulation disturbance) | Chronic alcohol toxicity | Avoid inhalational agents<br>Avoid anesthetic techniques that reduce liver blood flow<br>Monitor response to drugs carefully; drug pharmacokinetics are altered in chronic alcoholics<br>Obtain routine coagulation profile preoperatively and repeat periodically during the intraoperative and postoperative phases<br>Treat coagulation abnormality with vitamin K, fresh frozen plasma, and platelets |

(*Table continues*)

TABLE 8-3. Potential Anesthetic Problems Associated with Acute Alcohol Intoxication, Their Mechanisms, and Clinical Approaches to Minimize Morbidity (*continued*)

| POTENTIAL PROBLEM | MECHANISM | CLINICAL APPROACH |
|---|---|---|
| Withdrawal symptoms (tremor, anxiety, tachycardia, mild hypertension, hallucination, seizures) | CNS excitation | Eliminate other causes of anxiety and disorientation (other drugs, hypoxia, hypoglycemia)<br>Postpone surgery if possible<br>Monitor fluid balance and serum electrolytes, particularly $K^+$ and $Mg^+$<br>Administer benzodiazepines (diazepam) in titrated doses until the symptoms subside |
| Potentiation of tissue injury caused by trauma | Possible alteration of cell membranes by free-radical formation | None presently<br>Experimentally, the use of free-radical scavengers such as superoxide dismutase catalase, allpurinol, and dimethyl sulfoxide |

hibition of vascular response to norepinephrine,[63] increased diuresis, and metabolic acidosis may render these patients sensitive to even minor reductions of intravascular blood volume. Appropriate fluid therapy requires continuous monitoring of arterial blood pressure and central filling pressures. Alcohol also predisposes animals to arrhythmias during the 2-hour period after a blunt chest injury.[71] Likewise, in animals alcohol intoxication has been shown to result in pulmonary and coronary artery vasoconstriction.[13,82] In patients with limited coronary blood supply or myocardial function, these effects may be detrimental. Thus, monitoring of precordial electrocardiographic (ECG) leads and pulmonary artery pressures may be indicated.

Acute ethanol intoxication has been shown to result in thrombocytopenia and platelet dysfunction in man.[32,42] In the traumatized patient, this may augment the blood loss from injured and operated sites. Obtaining a preoperative platelet count may serve to inform the clinician about such blood dyscrasias.

Hypothermia, a common intraoperative occurrence in the trauma patient, is potentiated in the presence of alcohol intoxication because of peripheral vasodilatation.[81] All available measures to preserve heat must be employed to avoid this complication and its consequences.

The blood glucose level should be measured in intoxicated patients preoperatively and at regular intervals during surgery and the early postoperative period. Gluconeogenesis is inhibited in the alcoholic patient since adenine nucleotide (NAD), a necessary substrate of glucose metabolism, is in short supply because it is reduced to NADH during alcohol metabolism.[81,84] In addition, starvation or inadequate food intake, which is not uncommon in alcoholics, causes depletion of hepatic glycogen. Thus, heavy drinking without adequate food ingestion may result in hypoglycemia (Fig 8-1). Addition of dextrose to intravenous fluids can prevent or correct this problem.

Another metabolic complication is alcoholic ketoacidosis.[20,22,84] This is seen in the starved alcoholic who is deprived of food and alcohol. Normally the starved alcoholic generates energy by lipolysis which yields large amounts of free fatty acids (FFA). If alcohol ingestion continues, conversion of FFA to ketones is inhibited (Fig 8-2, A). However, when alcohol is withdrawn, this inhibition disappears, and the excessive amount of FFA accumulated in the blood is converted to ketones in the liver, resulting in ketoacidosis (Fig 8-2, B). Furthermore, peripheral clearance of ketones is decreased because the insulin level is low in this situation. Thus, ketoacidosis results from both increased production and decreased clearance of ketone bodies. Two serum ketones, β-hydroxybutyrate and acetoacetate, are markedly elevated—the former more than the latter. Clinically, however, acetoacetate is emphasized because a dipstick test can measure it but not β-hydroxybutyrate. Serum lactate levels are normal or slightly elevated. After eliminating the possibility of diabetic ketoacidosis, these patients should be treated with vigorous fluid therapy, including intravenous glucose. In addition, thiamine (100 mg/day) and phosphate supplementation (12–15 mEq/day) may be necessary. Lactic acidosis in the alcoholic patient usually results from decreased lactate utilization by the liver and can be treated by intravenous normal saline.

Altered mental status—euphoria, anxiety, agitation, and combativeness; or disorientation, stupor, and coma—poses problems for the anesthesiologist. In hyperactive patients there may be difficulty in obtaining an adequate history, starting intravascular lines, drawing blood samples, and inserting a urinary catheter. One might expect that high doses of sedative and opioid agents would be necessary to control these symptoms. Frequently, the opposite is true; large boluses of these drugs may produce undesirable effects such as apnea and hypotension.[17] Thus, it is prudent to administer these

FIG. 8-1. Pathogenesis of alcoholic hypoglycemia.

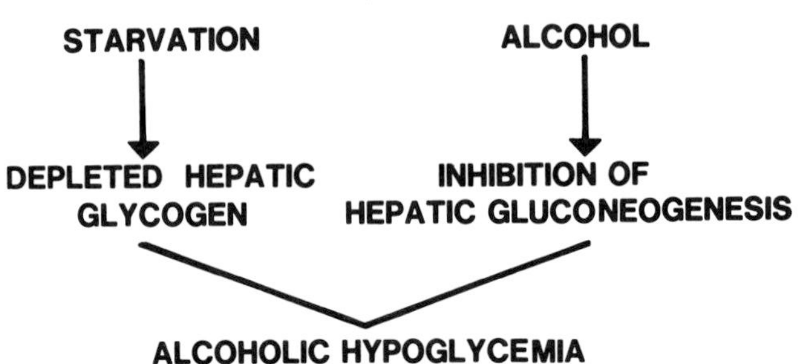

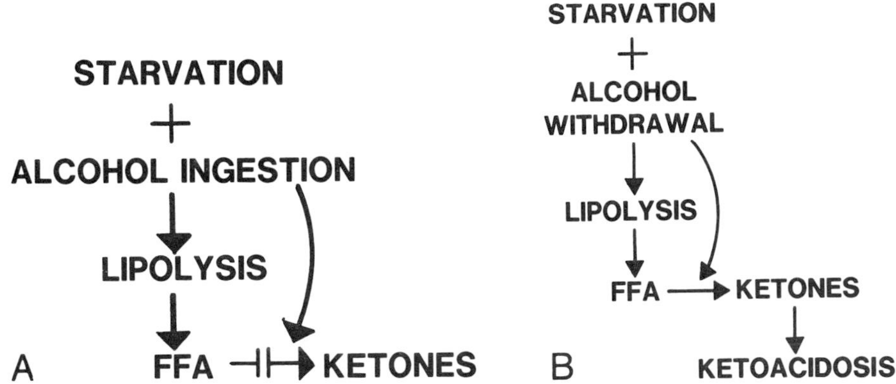


FIG. 8-2. Pathogenesis of alcoholic ketoacidosis: (A) if starvation or inadequate food intake is accompanied by alcohol ingestion, conversion of free fatty acids (FFA) to ketones is inhibited or blocked, preventing excessive accumulation of ketones; (B) if the patient is denied both food and alcohol, FFAs are freely converted to ketones, resulting in ketacidosis.

agents in small increments until the desired sedative effect is attained. Stupor and coma pose different problems; apart from being unable to obtain a history, the anesthesiologist is obliged to learn the exact cause of the mental depression, whether alcohol intoxication or injury to the central nervous system. Physical findings and neurologic status may be difficult to evaluate in these instances. Unless the patient is in severe hemorrhagic shock requiring immediate surgical control of bleeding, the possibility of intracranial pathology must be eliminated by careful physical and radiologic examination before anesthesia is administered.

On the basis of animal data, the brain of an acutely intoxicated patient is probably less tolerant of hypoxia than that of a nonintoxicated patient.[62] Thus, oxygenation should be monitored at all times during the perioperative period, and apneic episodes of even short duration should be avoided.

Although much of the available information comes from animal studies, there is little doubt that acute alcohol intoxication results in augmented central nervous system, cardiovascular, and respiratory responses to a wide variety of anesthetic, analgesic, analeptic, and antidepressant agents.[17,58,85] Thus, the doses of these agents should be reduced. Extra caution is necessary in the hemorrhaging patient in whom most of the blood flow, and thus most of the injected drug, is directed to the heart and brain. Further, Wolfson and Freed[86] showed that acute ethanol intoxication in rats results in approximation of the cardiac and respiratory depressant effects of halothane. In other words, during administration of halothane, both cardiac failure and respiratory arrest occur at virtually the same time.

Wolfson and Freed[86] measured halothane concentrations in the brains and hearts of chronically intoxicated rats in three different experimental settings: before withdrawal, after withdrawal, and after withdrawal and reintoxication with alcohol. In all of these conditions the brain halothane concentration that produced anesthesia was higher than that measured in acutely intoxicated rats. If these findings can be extrapolated to humans, the required concentration of inhalational anesthetic should be either normal or increased. However, in chronic alcoholics, these experimental findings can only provide guidelines; they are by no means absolute rules. In an individual patient, anesthetic management is influenced by many factors including the effects of the trauma itself, the severity of chronic and acute alcohol intoxication, withdrawal symptoms, and the effects on other organs of chronic alcohol use; thus, careful titration of anesthetic drugs is required under all circumstances.

According to a report from France, underlying chronic alcoholism is a common characteristic of the intoxicated polytrauma patient.[43] Multiorgan system involvement including alcoholic cardiomyopathy, hepatic dysfunction, and hematologic and coagulation abnormalities are common findings in these patients.[57,76] At times it may be difficult to recognize chronic alcoholism. Generally a patient who is coherent and does not seem to be drunk and has a blood alcohol level in excess of 200 mg % is considered a chronic drinker.[85] Likewise, a decline of more than 15%/h in blood alcohol levels suggests the same conclusion.[85] A mean corpuscular volume greater than 95 $\mu m^3$ and $\gamma$-glutamyltranspeptidase ($\gamma$-GT) greater than 18 IU in a woman or 28 IU in a man are also considered markers of chronic alcoholism.[43] However, the urgency of the surgical procedure may preclude waiting for appropriate laboratory tests. Answers to two specific questions: "Have you ever had a drinking problem?" and "Have you consumed alcohol within the past 24 hours?" can identify the chronic alcoholic with high reliability.[24]

In patients with alcoholic cardiomyopathy, inhalation agents should be avoided as they result in severe depression of myocardial contractility.[17,85] In alcoholic hepatitis, the usual approach is to postpone surgery until liver function tests are normal or stable. This is generally not possible in patients requiring emergency surgery for injuries. In these circumstances, the anesthetic technique that reduces liver blood flow least must be utilized. General anesthesia using nitrous oxide and muscle relaxant with maintenance of normocarbia has been shown to have little effect on liver blood flow.[28] However, the necessity for other anesthetic and analgesic agents and surgical manipulation in the upper abdomen can result in significant hepatic blood flow reduction.[33] In a small number of patients with mild alcoholic hepatitis undergoing peripheral surgery, Zinn et al[87] showed little difference in postoperative liver function tests following enflurane, nitrous oxide-narcotic, or spinal anesthetic techniques. None of the patients showed a significant alteration in liver function tests during the postoperative period. Mild hepatitis was defined as enlarged liver, elevated liver enzymes and/or prothrombin time greater than 50% of control. In view of these findings they suggested that general or spinal anesthesia has little deleterious effect on liver function in patients with mild alcoholic hepatitis provided surgery does not involve body cavities.

While plasma albumin concentrations are frequently reduced in patients with liver disease, globulin fractions may be increased. Although this should increase the fraction of unbound drug and reduce the required doses of intravenous anesthetics and muscle relaxants, other factors such as the type of liver disease, the distribution volume, and the extent of enzyme induction affect the pharmacokinetics of drugs and make estimation of dosages difficult. It is therefore best to titrate doses to the desired effect.

Occasionally, an acutely traumatized patient may present to the anesthesiologist with withdrawal symptoms—tremor, anxiety, tachycardia, and mild hypertension—which may develop within 6 hours of cessation of alcohol intake.[85] Thus, the problem is most likely to occur in the recovery room rather than in the emergency room. More overt withdrawal symptoms such as hallucinations and convulsions occur 24 to 48 hours after alcohol withdrawal.[85] If possible, surgery should be postponed until symptoms are controlled with benzodiazepines, thiamine, and fluid and electrolyte therapy. Some patients may require enormous doses of benzodiazepines[65]; the dose should be adjusted to effect rather than a suggested dosage regimen. It should be emphasized that seizures in alcoholics may not necessarily indicate withdrawal. A dose-dependent relationship between chronic alcohol ingestion and development of seizures has been demonstrated.[64]

There is growing evidence that ethanol has a potentiating effect on the tissue response to traumatic injury,[8,15,26,29,79] possibly as a result of free radical release with resultant damage of cell membrane lipids,[8,29] although other mechanisms may also be responsible. If the free-radical theory is established, it may be possible to control this phenomenon by use of free-radical scavengers such as superoxide dismutase, catalase, allopurinol, mannitol, or dimethyl sulfoxide.

In spite of the potential problems mentioned above, however, there is controversy about the effect of acute alcohol intoxication on the mortality rate of trauma patients. According to the results of some studies, acute alcohol intoxication increased the mortality rate[59,79]; however, others have failed to demonstrate this effect.[44,54,75,80]

## ILLICIT DRUG USE AND TRAUMA

Abuse of other self-administered drugs is another characteristic of the trauma victim, although this is probably a less common problem than alcohol abuse.[18] In the series of Giuffrida and coworkers,[37] one fourth of the 139 drug addicts who received anesthesia had emergency surgery for traumatic injuries. During a 6-month survey at Parkland Memorial Hospital in Dallas, 8.8% of 615 traumatized patients had one or more of a wide variety of drugs in their blood.[75] The true incidence of drug intake in these patients must have been higher, since no attempt was made to detect morphine, hydromorphone, cannabinoids, or cocaine. According to an earlier unpublished study by Williams and coworkers, of 400 male drivers killed in automobile accidents in California, 81% had one or more drugs, and approximately 50% had two or more drugs in their blood.[75] More recent data from the same area showed that 30% of fatally injured drivers used marijuana, cocaine, or phencyclidine shortly before the accident; narcotics were used less frequently.[18] A comparable incidence of drug use in trauma victims has also been reported from Seattle.[66]

The exact effects of drug abuse on the prognosis of injured patients have not been well documented. However, the consequences of acute and chronic drug intake may pose significant problems for the traumatized patient during the perioperative period. Sclerosis of both peripheral and deep (jugular and subclavian) veins in intravenous drug abusers may result in difficulty in placing intravascular lines. Patients with recent drug intake may be under the influence of these substances during the perioperative period. Table 8-4 lists the acute effects of various drugs. As this table shows, self-administered drugs may modify respiratory, cardiovascular, and central nervous system (CNS) responses to trauma and hemorrhage, increasing the difficulty of perioperative assessment and management of the injured. For example, opiates taken shortly before trauma may result in drowsiness, nausea, vomiting, and respiratory depression, interfering with the evaluation of possible head injury. Likewise, the sympathomimetic effects of amphetamines and lysergic acid diethylamide (LSD) may produce hypertension, causing underestimation of hypovolemia in the hemorrhaging patient.[81] The level of anesthesia is frequently estimated by heart rate and blood pressure. Significant alteration of these signs by drugs may confuse the clinician as to the depth of anesthesia and result in difficulties in adjusting the doses of anesthetic agents.

Substance abuse predisposes the individual to both acute and chronic medical problems[21,38,40,45,60] (Table 8-5). The trauma victim who is also a substance abuser may be affected by one or more of these complications and present additional difficulties for the anesthesiologist. It should be noted, however, that there are few data in the literature substantiating the impact of drug-related medical complications on the outcome of trauma or on the anesthetic management of these patients.

Interactions may occur when two or more drugs are taken together. For instance, amphetamines taken with barbiturates elevate the mood more than either drug alone.[21] Significant potentiation of the central nervous system and cardiovascular effects of alcohol may be noted when it is used with marijuana.[81] On the other hand there seems to be no interaction between marijuana and amphetamines.[81] There may also be interactions between self-administered and therapeutic drugs. For instance, the half-life of aminophylline is reduced in the marijuana smoker.[51] Likewise, the metabolic clearance rate of dexamethasone is increased by concomitant phenobarbital use; the dose of dexamethasone in barbiturate-abusing asthmatics should be increased.[16] The pharmacokinetics of digitalis, warfarin, and phenytoin are also altered in the drug addict.[60] Specific interactions between various anesthetic agents and self-administered drugs also occur and will be discussed later in this section.

TABLE 8-4. Acute Toxic Manifestations of Commonly Used Drugs in Trauma Patients

| DRUG TYPE | CENTRAL NERVOUS SYSTEM | CARDIO-VASCULAR SYSTEM | OTHER SYSTEMS |
|---|---|---|---|
| Narcotics | Drowsiness, mood changes, mental clouding, euphoria, dysphoria, nausea, vomiting, respiratory depression (slow ventilatory rate and normal or increased tidal volume; apnea in severe intoxication), miosis, mydriasis (caused by hypoxia in apneic patients). Convulsions may occur with acute meperidine toxicity | Orthostatic hypotension and syncope due to capacitance vessel dilation<br>Myocardial depression in heroin abusers from the adulterant quinine<br>Pulmonary edema may occur with severe narcotic intoxication; often after heroin | Hypothermia |
| Barbiturates and benzodiazepines | Drowsiness, somnolence, respiratory depression | Hypotension due to myocardial depression and capacitance vessel dilatation | Hypothermia with barbiturates at CNS depressant doses |
| Amphetamines | Anxiety, psychosis, hyperactivity, hyperreflexia, occasionally convulsions; mydriasis | Hypertension (subarachnoid bleeding, angina, myocardial infarction may result), tachycardia, dysrhythmias, palpitations | Sweating, hyperthermia, gastrointestinal hypomotility, hypovolemia, acidosis, ketoacidosis |
| Cocaine* | Euphoria, alertness, dysphoria, dysphoric agitation, paranoid ideation, delirium, syncope, tremors, seizures | Hypertension (may lead to cerebral hemorrhage, acute myocardial infarction, rupture of ascending aorta), tachycardia, dysrhythmias (may be the cause of sudden death observed in these patients) | Hyperpyrexia, nausea, vomiting, respiratory paralysis |
| LSD | Euphoria, hallucination, mydriasis, piloerection, tremor, hyperreflexia, hyperactivity, psychosis, alterations of mood, analgesia (may lead to inability to perceive an acute injury); convulsions and respiratory arrest may occur | Hypertension, tachycardia | Elevation of body temperature |
| Cannabis (marijuana and hashish) | Drowsiness | Increased heart rate<br>Orthostatic hypotension | |

* Manifestations of acute cocaine toxicity are rarely seen in the operating room because of its rapid metabolism.

Tolerance to self-administered drugs develops in chronic abusers, reflecting an increased rate of biotransformation by induced microsomal enzymes in the liver, adaptation of brain receptors, or both.[21,46] Often this effect is not specific to the drug used, and cross-tolerance may develop to other drugs. It is generally agreed that physical dependence has developed when normal physiologic functions cannot continue without the presence of some level of the drug in the body.[47,60,77] Failure to maintain the required tissue concentration results in a withdrawal syndrome, the severity of which depends on the type, amount, and time of drug use; the duration of abuse; and the physical and emotional condition of the patient. The withdrawal syndrome is usually mild and prolonged when the abused drug has a long elimination half-life, for instance, methadone; and pronounced and brief with drugs having a short elimination half-life.[60] Withdrawal symptoms may also occur in patients habituated to drugs that cause psychologic, but not physical, dependence; this type of withdrawal syndrome, however, is usually less intense. Amphetamines, cocaine, LSD, and cannabinoids (marijuana) are believed to cause psychologic dependence. The withdrawal syndromes of these agents are usually less troublesome than those caused by narcotics, barbiturates, benzodiazepines, and other sedative tranquilizers (glutethimide, meprobamate, methaqualone).[21,46,60]

The trauma victim who is a chronic substance abuser is particularly prone to develop withdrawal during the perioperative period because of unconsciousness, prolonged anesthesia, or a reluctance to give a true history. Whenever possible, all injured patients should be questioned about any history of drug abuse. Friends or relatives should be questioned if the patient cannot respond. The manifestations, onset time, peak intensity, duration, and treatment of withdrawal symptoms vary considerably. Characteristics of abstinence symptoms of narcotics, barbiturates, and benzodiazepines,[19] the most frequently confronted withdrawal syndromes, are shown in Table 8-6. Severe syndromes may occur with other sedative-tranquilizers such as glutethimide, meprobamate, and methaqualone, the clinical manifestations of which resemble those of barbiturate withdrawal.[2] It is important to ensure that addicts receive adequate doses of the chronically taken narcotic, barbiturate, and benzodiazepine, or of a drug within the same class, at appropriate intervals during the perioperative period. Although the withdrawal syndrome often occurs during the late phases of prolonged surgery and in the postoperative period, patients who have not

TABLE 8-5. Common Medical Complications Caused by Various Classes of Substances*

| SUBSTANCE CLASS | COMMONLY ABUSED AGENTS | MEDICAL COMPLICATIONS |
|---|---|---|
| Narcotics | Codeine<br>Methadone<br>Heroin<br>Pentazocine | Superficial infections<br>cellulitis, abscesses, gas gangrene, fasciitis |
| | | Tetanus |
| | | AIDS (disease or human immunodeficiency virus (HIV) seropositivity) |
| | | Bacterial endocarditis |
| | | Respiratory diseases<br>airway obstruction, nasal septal perforation, aspiration pneumonia, AIDS with pulmonary infection, atelectasis, bronchiectasis, bullous damage (diffusing capacity gas exchange abnormalities), pulmonary fibrosis/granulomatosis, pneumonia (bacterial), mediastinal or hilar adenopathy, pneumomediastinum, pulmonary edema, respiratory depression, pulmonary vascular involvement, pulmonary hypertension, foreign body emboli, foreign body aspiration, altered pulmonary function |
| | | Liver disease<br>hepatitis (A, B, non A, non B), enlarged liver (malnutrition) |
| | | Central nervous system<br>miosis<br>mydriasis (meperidine) |
| | | Positive VDRL (true or false) |
| | | Hematolgic system<br>anemia |
| | | Metabolic<br>hyperglycemia |
| CNS depressants | Secobarbital<br>Diazepam<br>Chlordiazepoxide<br>Glutethimide<br>Paraldehyde | Pulmonary diseases<br>atelectasis, aspiration pneumonia, pulmonary edema, respiratory depression |
| CNS stimulants | Amphetamines<br>Amphetamine<br>Dextroamphetamine<br>Methamphetamine | Necrotizing angiitis resulting in renal failure, hypertensive encephalopathy, pulmonary edema |
| | | Cardiovascular system<br>hypertension, tachycardia, dysrhythmia |
| | | Metabolic<br>hyperthermia, dehydration, acidosis, ketosis |
| | | CNS<br>irritability, psychosis, anxiety |
| | Cocaine | Cardiovascular system<br>myocardial infarction, cardiac arrhythmia, rupture of ascending aorta, pneumopericardium |
| | | Respiratory system<br>nasal septum perforation, pneumomediastinum, pulmonary edema, pulmonary hypertension, granulomatous pneumonitis, AIDS with pulmonary infections, reduced CO diffusion |
| | | Central nervous system<br>cerebrovascular accidents, hyperthermia, convulsions, fungal cerebritis |
| | | Obstetric complications<br>spontaneous abortion, abruptio placentae, fetal malformations, high perinatal mortality, neurobehavioral impairments |
| | | Gastrointestinal complications<br>intestinal ischemia and gangrene |
| | | Miscellaneous complications<br>blood glucose abnormalities, malnutrition, psychiatric complications |
| Psychedelics | LSD | No major organ system derangements<br>Physiologic changes are noted in Table 4 |
| | Cannabis (marijuana and hashish) | Respiratory system<br>pharyngitis, rhinitis, acute bronchodilatation, chronic bronchoconstriction, bronchitis, pneumomediastinum, altered pulmonary function tests, altered pulmonary defense mechanisms |
| | | Cardiovascular system<br>tachycardia (may lead to myocardial infarction in patients with angina) |
| | | Acute illness following intravenous use<br>manifested by chills, fever, nausea, vomiting, diarrhea, hypotension, glycosuria, leukocytosis, and transient thrombocytopenia |

* Information obtained from Caldwell,[21] McCammon,[60] Glassroth et al,[38] Gregler and Mark,[40] and Isner et al.[45]

TABLE 8-6. Characteristic Features, Prevention, and Treatment of Withdrawal Syndromes Caused by Narcotics, Barbiturates, and Benzodiazepines

| AGENT | EXPECTED ONSET (HOURS) | EXPECTED PEAK INTENSITY (HOURS) | EXPECTED DURATION (DAYS) | SYMPTOMS EXPERIENCED FROM INITIAL STAGES TO LATE STAGES | PREVENTION | TREATMENT |
|---|---|---|---|---|---|---|
| Narcotics | | | | | | |
| Morphine | 8 to 12 | 30 to 48 | 8 to 12 | Craving for the drug, anxiety, diaphoresis, yawning, rhinorrhea, lacrimation, restlessness, mydriasis, piloerection, tremor, hot and cold flashes, muscle and bone aches, anorexia, hypertension, tachycardia, tachypnea, hyperreflexia, abdominal cramps, diarrhea, muscle spasms, jerking and extension of the legs. Intraoperative hypotension may be caused by narcotic withdrawal. Convulsions do not occur<br>Dehydration, acidosis, and ketosis may occur in patients not receiving parenteral fluid therapy | Administration of adequate doses of narcotic agents. Avoidance of agonist-antagonist-type narcotic agents. Avoidance of narcotic antagonists | Administration of the abused narcotic at appropriate intervals<br>or<br>Administration of any narcotic at appropriate intervals<br>or<br>Administration of the long-acting narcotic methadone (10 mg intramuscularly) every 2 to 3 hours until the symptoms are aborted. The usual dose over a 24-hour period is about 49 to 60 mg<br>or<br>Clonidine (6 to 10 μg/kg by mouth), which can be repeated up to 17 μg/kg/day for several days |
| Heroin | 8 to 12 | 30 to 48 | 8 to 12 | | | |
| Meperidine | 3 to 6 | 8 to 12 | 4 to 5 | | | |
| Methadone | 1 to 2 | 4 to 6 | 14 to 21 | | | |
| Pentobarbital and secobarbital* | 12 to 36 | 48 to 72 | 15 to 20 | Anxiety, tremors, weakness, hyperreflexia, insomnia, nausea, vomiting, tachycardia, postural hypotension, hyperthermia, grand mal seizures. Barbiturate withdrawal may be life threatening and often results in neurologic and musculoseketal sequelae | Administration of barbiturates at appropriate intervals | Administration of barbiturate at regular intervals, eg, pentobarbital (300 to 600 mg every 6 hours). Administration of diazepam titrated to effect (usually 5 to 10 mg every 4 to 6 hours) |
| Benzodiazepines* | 18 to 24† | 72 to 96 | 25 to 30 | Similar to those described for barbiturates, but they are milder. Tinnitus, involuntary movement, and perceptual changes may occur | Administration of benzodiazepine agents at regular intervals | Administration of benzodiazepine agents at regular intervals |

* Withdrawal syndromes caused by other sedative-tranquilizers resemble those of barbiturates and benzodiazepines.
† Sometimes symptoms may not appear for several days because of long elimination half-life.

taken the drug for relatively long periods prior to trauma may develop symptoms preoperatively.

Intraoperative manifestations of abstinence syndrome are difficult to detect, but many reports suggest that unexplained hypotension during surgery may be due to narcotic withdrawal and that administration of narcotics alone may be effective in raising the blood pressure.[27] Presently, narcotic abstinence syndrome is rarely observed during intraoperative and postoperative periods because most patients receive opiates for anesthesia or postoperative pain relief. The situation is different for other agents such as sedative-tranquilizers which are used seldom or not at all perioperatively. It is important to remember that an agonist-antagonist opioid can precipitate a sudden withdrawal syndrome in narcotic addicts; thus, these agents should be avoided.[46]

A potential problem in narcotic addicts is the occurrence of clonidine withdrawal syndrome. Clonidine has been used successfully to detoxify opiate addicts without producing withdrawal symptoms.[39] The drug is sold illegally in some areas for self-administration. A trauma victim who is taking clonidine for this purpose may develop dysrhythmia, hypertension, congestive heart failure, and mental dysfunction from withdrawal of clonidine, opiates, or both. These patients should be given tapering doses of clonidine for at least 10 days postoperatively.

As mentioned earlier, significant interactions may occur between various self-administered drugs and anesthetic agents. Unfortunately, human studies on this subject are scarce, and knowledge is derived mostly from animal research. Extrapolation of these data to humans should be done cautiously, especially in the acutely injured patient with significant hypovolemia and metabolic and endocrine derangement. It is to be noted that interactions between these drugs and anesthetic agents differ according to whether substance abuse is acute or chronic.

There are four major categories of self-administered drugs that may produce such interactions: narcotics, central nervous system depressants (sedative-tranquilizers), central nervous system stimulants, and psychedelics.

### *Narcotic Agents*

The patient who has taken narcotics shortly before trauma and arrival in the operating room may require reduction in doses of intravenous and inhalational anesthetic agents. Dogs receiving intravenous heroin (1 mg/kg) have a highly significant and prolonged decrease in cardiac output, aortic pressure, and heart rate without change in stroke volume.[14] Pulmonary artery pressure increases only briefly following administration of heroin, but pulmonary vascular resistance remains high 1 hour after injection. The addition of intravenous and inhalational agents in the usual doses may exacerbate these hemodynamic changes, but the net result of this interaction is dependent on the degree of tolerance to the narcotic, intravascular volume, and myocardial function. Since potentiation of narcotic-induced hemodynamic changes by anesthetics is difficult (if not impossible) to predict in drug addicts, careful adjustment of the anesthetic dose is necessary. Acute use of narcotics in patients with no history of chronic drug use reduces anesthetic requirements.[23] In contrast, chronic narcotic usage has been shown to increase the minimum alveolar concentration (MAC) of halothane and to decrease analgesic response to nitrous oxide in animals.[12,41] In agreement with these experimental findings, one study showed that narcotic abusers required higher than normal doses of narcotics for preoperative medication. It was the impression of the authors of this study that the thiopental requirement was also increased in these patients.[27] An increased narcotic requirement for control of postoperative pain is a common observation.

### *Central Nervous System Depressants*

Acute administration of barbiturates, chlorpromazine, diazepam, and hydroxyzine reduces the MAC of inhalational agents in animals and humans.[23] Chronic use of barbiturates leads to induction of microsomal enzymes. Although this should result in an increased breakdown of anesthetic agents and thereby increase anesthetic requirement, controlled studies to verify this effect are lacking. However, some anecdotal reports suggest that increased doses of thiopental are required and that its duration of effect is decreased.[7,56] Unlike barbiturates, benzodiazepines do not cause significant enzyme induction. It is not known, however, whether chronic benzodiazepine intake results in increased anesthetic requirement.

### *Central Nervous System Stimulants*

In animals, acute dextroamphetamine administration in doses of 0.1, 0.5, and 1 mg/kg resulted in MAC increases of 19, 67, and 96%, respectively.[48] In contrast, chronic administration of the same drug (5 mg/kg/day) for 7 days decreased MAC by 21%.[48] Acute amphetamine administration increases catecholamine concentrations at the nerve terminals of both central and peripheral sympathetic systems. This phenomenon results from both stimulation of release from neural cells and inhibition of reuptake of catecholamines into the nerve terminals. Increased catecholamine concentration in nerve endings produces alertness and thereby an increased anesthetic requirement. In patients using amphetamine for several weeks, catecholamine stores in the body are depleted, resulting in a reduction of anesthetic requirement.

Because of its high price, cocaine was once called the "champagne of drugs," but since 1978 there has been a significant price reduction and increased use. Freebase cocaine (crack), which has been in common use since 1984, is a purified form of the drug which produces faster and higher blood levels and a higher incidence of addiction. Cocaine is a short-acting drug; blood concentration rises within 20 minutes after intranasal use, reaching a peak concentration in 1 hour.[60] Most of the administered drug is metabolized within 2 or 3 hours.[60] Thus, when surgery does not commence within 3 hours of cocaine intake, significant interaction with anesthetic agents is unlikely. Most emergency surgery for trauma, however, is performed shortly after injury and presumably shortly after the last cocaine dose. Hence, a significant amount of the drug may remain in the blood and produce a change in response to anesthetics. Stoelting et al[73] demonstrated a dose-dependent increase in the halothane requirement which lasted approximately 3 hours after acute intravenous administration of cocaine to dogs. The mechanism of increased anesthetic requirement after this drug is believed to be similar to that of amphetamines: release of norepinephrine into the CNS nerve terminals and prevention of catecholamine reuptake.[11,73] Similar increases in catecholamine level may occur at peripheral sympathetic nerve endings, explaining the cardiovascular effects of the drug: tachycardia, dysrhythmia, hypertension. Labetalol, which has both α- and β-adrenergic blocking activity, appears to control hypertension effectively. The increased catecholamine levels produced by cocaine may result in a decreased arrhythmogenic dose of exogenously administered epinephrine during halothane-$N_2O$ anesthesia.[53] Barash et al,[11] however, administering 1.5 mg/kg cocaine intranasally, could not demonstrate a significant increase in heart rate, blood pressure, or extrasystoles in men receiving 0.5% halothane and 60% $N_2O$.

### *Psychedelics*

LSD is a potent analgesic and thus may prolong the analgesic action of narcotic agents in acutely intoxicated patients.[60] The physiologic effects of LSD (mild increase of heart rate, blood pressure, and temperature; mydriasis; piloerection; tremor; hyperreflexia) last approximately 6 to 8 hours whereas psychic effects continue for 12 to 18 hours.[30] In chronic LSD abusers anesthesia may precipitate a "flashback," a panic reaction, which can be treated with diazepam.[60] LSD has anticholinesterase activity in vitro which may result in prolongation of the action of succinylcholine and ester-type local anesthetic agents.[60]

Marijuana stimulates the sympathetic nervous system while inhibiting the parasympathetics.[60] The duration of its effects depends on the mode of use, 2 to 3 hours after smoking, and 3 to 5 hours following ingestion of the drug.[46] In animal models, acute administration of marijuana reduces the MAC of halothane and cyclopropane[74,78] and prolongs sleep time following barbiturates[67] and ketamine.[70] In volunteers, it potentiates narcotic-induced respiratory depression.[49] Chronic administration of this drug to animals does not appear to alter the MAC of inhalation agents.[74,78] However, reduction in MAC has been observed after acute administration of marijuana to chronically treated animals.[78]

TABLE 8-7. Suggested Guidelines for Management of Trauma Victim Who May Be Acutely Intoxicated or Chemically Dependent

1. Wear double gloves and goggles during management of all trauma victims. A 13 to 16% incidence of HIV seropositivity in a small group of trauma victims between the ages of 28 and 34 has been demonstrated. Thirty-three percent of these patients had a history of intravenous drug abuse.[10,52] Other infections such as hepatitis may be present.
2. Expect a wide variety of medical complications associated with drug abuse (see Table 6) and act accordingly.
3. Always consider four etiologies in the comatose injured patient: diffuse cerebral pathology, focal cerebral pathology, acute drug or alcohol intoxication, and metabolic or infectious disturbances. Whenever possible obtain an exact diagnosis before administering anesthesia.
4. Include drug withdrawal and/or cocaine, amphetamine, LSD, and marijuana abuse in the differential diagnosis of perioperative hypertension, tachycardia, and dysrhythmia.
5. Be prepared at all times to treat the four most serious complications of drug abuse: respiratory arrest, seizures, acidosis, and dysrhythmia.
6. Use direct acting vasopressors rather than indirect acting ones. Longstanding use of some CNS stimulants may deplete catecholamine stores. Vasopressors should be used with caution. The presence of CNS stimulants may potentiate their effect on the heart.
7. Monitor body temperature continuously. Narcotic addicts may develop hypothermia while under the influence of amphetamines. Cocaine and LSD may result in hyperthermia.
8. Monitor blood sugar, blood gases, electrolytes, and ketone bodies. Metabolic disturbances can occur in traumatized patients.
9. Monitor the effects of various nonanesthetic drugs (theophylline, warfarin, digitalis, steroids) given during the perioperative period. Significant interaction between self-administered drugs and these agents may result in decreased bioavailability.
10. In order to prevent withdrawal syndrome, use appropriate doses of agonist narcotics and benzodiazepines during the perioperative period until the results of the toxicology screen are available.
11. Avoid narcotic antagonists and narcotics with agonist-antagonist action.
12. Titrate anesthetic, sedative, and narcotic agents to the desired effect. Avoid using preset doses of these agents.

In this discussion it is assumed that the abused drugs are known to the physician. In practice, however, unless a history is obtained, the anesthesiologist is rarely aware of the type, amount, or timing of drug intake by the patient prior to surgery. Although a toxicology screen is routinely performed in many trauma centers upon admission of the patient to the emergency room, its results are almost never available before or during surgery. In most instances, a drug history is either unavailable because the patient is in coma due to head injury, intoxication, or metabolic disorders, or it is inadequate and inaccurate because of the patient's concern about prosecution or disclosure of his addiction to friends, relatives, or employers. Clinical signs of drug abuse may be helpful in assessing the type and degree of drug intoxication, but these are frequently altered by trauma, hemorrhage, and the unpredictable degree of the patient's tolerance of a particular drug. In addition, many patients abuse more than one substance, including alcohol,[18,36,40,66,69] in which case clinical signs are not helpful at all.

Given these facts, the anesthesiologist is forced to assume that the patient presenting to surgery for repair of traumatic injuries is acutely or chronically intoxicated with alcohol and/or various other substances and to be prepared to prevent and treat a wide variety of complications associated with this condition. A summary of general principles for management of these patients is offered in Table 8-7.

## METABOLIC-ENDOCRINE DISORDERS

### DIABETES MELLITUS

Based on data collected by Melton and coworkers[101] between 1960 and 1969, the incidence of diabetes in patients below age 40 is approximately 30/100,000 population, a rate ⅟₁₃ of that of the group between 40 and 70 (Table 8-8). Thus, in the age group that is most prone to injuries, diabetes is a relatively infrequent disease. Nevertheless, both forms of diabetes mellitus may be encountered in the trauma population: type I (insulin-dependent, juvenile onset) or type II (non–

TABLE 8-8. Incidence Rates of Type I and Type II Diabetes in the First 4 Decades of Life and Between Ages 40 and 70*

| AGE | TYPE I INSULIN-DEPENDENT DIABETES (PER 100,000 PERSONS/YEAR) | TYPE II ADULT ONSET DIABETES (PER 100,000/YEAR) |
|---|---|---|
| 0 to 40 | 9 | 21 |
| 40 to 69 | 23 | 363 |

* Based on data obtained by Melton et al[101]

insulin-dependent, adult onset). Depending on its type, severity, chronicity, and the adequacy of therapeutic control, diabetes may have profound effects on many organ systems, most significantly the cardiovascular and neurologic systems.[88,91,95,100,104,105,108] The trauma patient with such complications may thus also be under treatment for his or her secondary disease.

Upon arrival of any trauma victim in the emergency room, blood glucose levels are determined routinely. Hyperglycemia is frequently observed even in previously nondiabetic patients. This so-called *diabetes of trauma* (also known as *stress diabetes* or *diabetes of surgery*) is caused by acute insulin resistance.[89,97,98] The major contributing factor is stress-induced catecholamine secretion, whose effects are amplified by endocrine mechanisms, for instance, glucagon release. This results in a catabolic hyperglycemic state. These natural responses to injury will probably be magnified in the diabetic trauma victim, whose metabolic balance is abnormal at the outset. If the diabetic trauma patient has been taking regular doses of insulin, glucose levels may rise or fall depending upon the particular insulin preparation he is receiving, the time of the last insulin dose, the time of the last meal, and the patient's ability to respond to the hyperglycemic factors induced by stress (Table 8-9).

Clinically significant hyperglycemia (blood glucose >250 mg/dL) or hypoglycemia (blood glucose < 80 mg/dL) must be treated. Hyperglycemia should be avoided especially in those trauma patients whose injury is complicated by brain ischemia or hypoxia. The best therapy for hyperglycemia is bolus doses of regular insulin. A dose of 5 to 10 U is given, and the blood glucose level is redetermined after 1 hour. If it is still high, an additional dose of intravenous insulin is administered. If the patient becomes hypoglycemic, a 25 to 50-g bolus of concentrated glucose solution ($D_{25}$ or $D_{50}$) should be injected, and a glucose-containing crystalloid solution should be infused. Subsequent therapy may consist either of sequential intravenous bolus doses or of a continuous insulin infusion, whose rate should be dictated by the results of periodic blood glucose determinations.[88–91,95,97,98,100,103–109] The degree of insulin resistance is dynamic, and it is not unusual for the patient to demonstrate wide swings in glucose levels and insulin response over the course of hours or days.

TABLE 8-9. Characteristics of Available Parenteral Insulin Preparations

| FORM | ACTION* | ONSET* (hours) | PEAK ACTION* (hours) | DURATION OF ACTION* (hours) |
|---|---|---|---|---|
| Regular | Rapid | 0.25 | 2 to 5 | 5 to 8 |
| Semilente | Rapid | 0.5 | 2 to 10 | 12 to 16 |
| Neutral protein hagedorn (NPH) | Intermediate | 1 to 2 | 6 to 12 | 18 to 28 |
| Lente | Intermediate | 1 to 2 | 6 to 12 | 18 to 28 |
| Protamine zinc (PZI) | Prolonged | 3 to 4 | 14 to 24 | 24 to >36 |
| Ultralente | Prolonged | 3 to 4 | 10 to 30 | 24 to >36 |

* After subcutaneous injection.

If time permits, patients receiving oral hypoglycemic agents should have their medications discontinued prior to major surgery. It should be noted that long-acting agents such as chlorpropamide may have effects lasting for 24 to 48 hours (Table 8-10); thus there may not be sufficient time for their activity to dissipate before emergency surgery. The patient should be observed carefully for allergic or anaphylactic reactions when standard insulin preparations (bovine, porcine) are used. These reactions are less common following administration of human-derived insulin prepared by recombinant DNA techniques.

At least four regimens are suggested for the perioperative management of the electively operated insulin-dependent diabetic.[88–91,95,97,98,100,103–109]

1. The patient remains NPO from midnight prior to surgery, and insulin is withheld. Serial blood glucose levels are determined based on clinical indicators such as the "brittleness" of the particular patient and the amount of insulin he or she normally requires. Generally, measurement every 4 hours is sufficient, although brittle diabetics may require determinations every 1 or 2 hours, particularly during a crisis such as hypo- or hyperglycemia. Insulin or glucose is given as needed to maintain normal glucose levels. Blood glucose levels are determined upon the patient's arrival in the operating room and at regular intervals during and after surgery.

2. The patient receives one third to one half of the usual morning dose of insulin subcutaneously. A 5% dextrose infusion is begun; its rate can be guided by the normal minimum glucose requirement of 2 g/kg/24 h. Since long-acting forms of insulin can create unpredictable variations in blood glucose levels perioperatively, serial blood glucose determinations are mandatory.

3. In this method, intravenous infusion of 5% dextrose is begun, blood sugar is determined on a regular schedule, and regular insulin is given subcutaneously, titrated according to a sliding scale. Intermediate and long-acting insulin are avoided. This regimen is probably optimal for providing efficacious and safe therapy during the perioperative period.

4. Insulin and dextrose are given by continuous infusion. The initial rate of insulin administration should be in the range of 1 to 2 U/h. 500 mL of 5% dextrose is administered over the first hour followed by an infusion of 125 mL/h.[107] If the initial blood glucose is high (>300 mg/dL), a small bolus dose of insulin may be given intravenously at the time the infusion is started. Once again, there is no substitute for rou-

TABLE 8-10. Characteristics of Oral Hypoglycemic Agents

| GENERIC NAME | TRADE NAME | ONSET (hours) | DURATION OF ACTION (hours) |
|---|---|---|---|
| Tolbutamide | Orinase | 0.5 to 1 | 6 to 12 |
| Chlorpropamide | Diabinese | 1 to 2 | 60 to 90 |
| Acetohexamide | Dymelor | 0.5 to 1 | 12 to 24 |
| Tolazamide | Tolinase | 4 to 6 | 10 to 24 |
| Glipizide | Glucotrol | 1 to 3 | 12 to 24 |
| Glyburide | Diabeta/ Micronase | 0.5 to 1 | 24 to 60 |

tine glucose determinations. The insulin infusion is adjusted to the glucose level.

The older, obese, diabetic trauma victim is likely to have some degree of peripheral vascular disease and/or cardiovascular atherosclerosis manifesting as hypertension and/or ischemic heart disease. Thus, optimization of cardiovascular and renal hemodynamics by volume replacement and appropriate medication is of utmost importance.

Autonomic neuropathy in diabetics may produce delayed gastric emptying, implying that they are even more likely than most trauma victims to have retained gastric contents.[94] Thus, extreme care must be taken to protect the airway. Autonomic neuropathy may also affect the cardiovascular system and may cause fatal cardiac arrhythmias.[96,110] Because of enhanced response to α- and β-adrenergic receptor-mediated drugs, vasoactive agents should be used cautiously. In hemodynamically stable patients, autonomic neuropathy can be diagnosed by ECG. On deep breathing, these patients exhibit a less than five-beat per minute variation in heart rate between maximal inspiration and expiration.[96,99,110]

Two complications of diabetes may add to the problems of management of the trauma victim: diabetic ketoacidosis (DKA) and the hyperosmolar nonacidotic, nonketotic (HHNK) state.

In the conscious patient, DKA may produce symptoms that mimic a surgical emergency, especially anorexia, nausea, and vomiting. In the unconscious patient, DKA may be diagnosed only after acidosis, hyperglycemia, and ketonemia are demonstrated by laboratory tests. Central venous pressure may be extremely low in a diabetic trauma patient with DKA since the osmotic diuretic effect of elevated levels of glucose and ketones exacerbates any fluid deficit. The severe volume depletion and lactic acidosis caused by the trauma may act additively with the effects of DKA and produce a markedly reduced pH.

Since the compromised patient may be unable to meet the demands of his respiratory system's drive to compensate for the acid-base derangement, airway control and mechanical ventilation are generally necessary. Fluid resuscitation is accomplished with crystalloid; pH, sodium, potassium, and magnesium levels should be monitored closely and treated appropriately. Regular insulin is infused at a rate of 0.1 U/kg/h until blood glucose and ketones come under control. Another approach is to administer insulin 0.3 U/kg, half by intravenous bolus and half intramuscularly, followed by hourly intramuscular injections of 7.0 U. As blood glucose levels fall, the rate of insulin infusion or the dose and interval of intramuscular injection should be reduced. The end point is a blood glucose level of 150 to 250 mg/dL. Dextrose and insulin infusions are continued at a rate sufficient to maintain the optimal glucose level, which should be monitored at regular intervals. Bicarbonate administration is not an essential therapeutic measure even when the acidosis is severe.[102]

The type I diabetic is more likely to manifest DKA. Conversely, type II diabetics are more likely to display HHNK, which is not a state of insulin deficiency but one of increased insulin resistance induced by stresses such as infection or trauma.[92,93] In fact, HHNK may be thought of as an extreme result of the diabetes of stress seen in nondiabetics (see above). Hyperglycemia and dehydration secondary to osmotic diuresis occur but not the metabolic derangements seen with DKA. However, dehydration may be additive with the hypovolemia from trauma, and lactic acidosis may cause a drop in pH. Fluid resuscitation and intravenous insulin are required. Potassium levels usually fall during treatment as insulin and glucose facilitate the diffusion of the cation into the cells. Potassium levels should thus be followed and replacement given as needed.

## OBESITY

Obesity, considered as a disease entity, may be classified as an epidemic. In a 1974 study 15% of men and 25% of women between the ages of 20 and 74 were overweight by as much as 20%. Obesity is defined as *morbid* when the subject is more than twice his or her ideal weight.[111,117,120] As with diabetes mellitus, the presence of obesity implies the likelihood of coexisting pathology. For example, cardiovascular diseases such as hypertension, and respiratory derangements such as decreased functional residual capacity (FRC), and primary hypoventilation may be present.[111,114,115,117–120] In obese people, most of the common degenerative diseases begin at an earlier age, progress more rapidly, and become life threatening more frequently.

The possibility of these derangements should be borne in mind during the acute phase of care of the obese trauma patient. The most common compromising conditions are: (1) cardiovascular problems, especially arteriosclerosis and hypertension; (2) pulmonary disease, both restrictive and obstructive; (3) cerebrovascular disease; (4) diabetes mellitus and its complications; and (5) a high incidence of smoking and its effects.[111,114,115,117–120]

Other problems are caused by obesity itself, notably increased blood volume, to perfuse the extra adipose tissue; polycythemia, to compensate for chronic hypoxemia; and elevated blood pressure, with increased cardiac output and possibly elevated left ventricular end-diastolic pressure. There is decreased respiratory compliance resulting in diminished FRC in the face of a normal closing capacity, and elevated oxygen consumption and carbon dioxide production as the work of breathing claims a greater proportion of total body metabolism.

The combination of circulatory and pulmonary derangements in obesity produces a low ventilation/perfusion ($\dot{V}/\dot{Q}$) ratio with increased intrapulmonary shunting and abnormal gas exchange, which commonly results in hypoxemia and hypercarbia. Injury, especially to the chest, or surgical compromise, eg, subdiaphragmatic packs or a high abdominal incision, may accentuate these abnormalities. Although the usual level of positive end-expiratory pressure (PEEP, 10 to 12 cm $H_2O$) may reduce $\dot{V}/\dot{Q}$ mismatch, it may also promote diversion of blood from ventilated lung regions to atelectatic sites. Thus its effect on oxygenation is unpredictable in the obese. Ventilation with large tidal volumes may be more desirable since it permits reducing the level of PEEP to 5 to 7 cm $H_2O$, thus producing less of a deleterious effect.

There may be a tendency to underestimate the amount of volume replacement needed for the obese trauma patient.[116,120] Hemodynamic resuscitation may be complicated by at least two other factors. First is the difficulty encountered when attempting to place percutaneous intravascular lines. This situation is made worse in the trauma patient by hypovolemia and hypothermia; venous cutdown may be necessary. Second, indirect methods of blood pressure measurement are often faulty in obese patients. For example, an inappropriately sized blood pressure cuff may give a spuriously high reading. It is wise, therefore, to place an intraarterial catheter early, both for accurate arterial blood pressure measurement and to monitor the adequacy of ventilation.

Technical difficulties in performing laryngoscopy may be encountered due to a heavy upper chest, stout neck, and redundant soft tissue in the facial area.[111,116,120] The importance of continuous cricoid pressure cannot be overstated. Besides the risk of a full stomach, which may be present in any trauma patient, the obese patient tends to have increased gastric volume, reduced gastric pH, increased intraabdominal pressure, and increased incidence of lower esophageal sphincter incompetence and hiatus hernia.[112] Additionally, the obese diabetic may have autonomic neuropathy and delayed gastric emptying. All of this increases the likelihood of regurgitation, vomiting, and aspiration and the severity of subsequent pneumonitis.

Obese patients metabolize inhalational anesthetic agents in a different manner from their nonobese counterparts.[116,120] Increased adipose tissue represents a large reservoir for anesthetic sequestration, which may result in prolonged recovery time and, although not well documented, may increase the availability of anesthetics for biotransformation. Some volatile anesthetics (eg, halothane, enflurane) are metabolized to inorganic fluoride to a greater extent than normal in obese patients. Obese surgical patients may fare better with a narcotic technique although none of the above considerations represents a true contraindication to inhalation agents. Decisions should thus be made, as in any trauma patient, based on the nature of the injury and surgery and on the patient's condition.

The greatest postoperative problems, generally in the form of hypoxia and carbon dioxide retention, are presented by the obese patient's pulmonary abnormalities. These may produce difficulties both in mechanical ventilation and in weaning the patient from the ventilator. Realistically it may be necessary to accept somewhat abnormal blood gas values or ventilatory parameters in order to terminate ventilation in these patients. This is almost certainly true in the rare patient with obesity hypoventilation syndrome (OHS) otherwise known as primary hypoventilation or Pickwickian syndrome. These patients demonstrate higher total pulmonary resistance than their counterparts with simple obesity. Not all of this increase is a result of decreased chest compliance secondary to the heavy chest wall since these patients may have inspiratory muscle weakness. The CNS is also thought to play a role in OHS in the form of a pathologic endogenous respiratory servocontrol mechanism. Gas exchange may be deranged, with severe hypoxemia and hypercarbia. These patients have decreased pulmonary reserve, and recovery from complications like pneumonia is markedly prolonged. Thus, ventilatory abnormalities should be expected while weaning the patient from the ventilator. Use of a ventilator with a pressure support mode during weaning may be of some value.

Long-term postoperative recovery is often complicated by wound infections.[113] Thrombophlebitis and pulmonary embolism also appear more likely in these patients than in those with normal weight.

## ASTHMA

Asthma affects more than 5% of adults and approximately 7 to 10% of children.[121,123,128] It is thus very likely to be seen in the traumatized population. Although it is possible that a trauma-induced increase in plasma catecholamines protects the injured to some extent against bronchospasm, other fac- other factors associated with the injury may precipitate asthmatic symptoms: noxious fumes, cold exposure, physiologic and emotional stress, and awake tracheal intubation may all provoke an attack. Further, the lack of an adequate history and the likelihood of inadequate anesthesia, general or topical, for tracheal intubation because of concern about the patient's hemodynamic status or the possibility of a full stomach increase the risk of bronchospasm. Therefore, an abrupt asthmatic attack may occur in any trauma patient, and one must be prepared to treat it.

If a history of asthma can be obtained on admission, the patient's current medications, if any, should be determined when possible. The serum aminophylline level is measured if the patient has been receiving this agent.

One may choose prophylactic aerosol treatment for asthmatic patients. If chest auscultation reveals wheezing, bronchodilator therapy should definitely be initiated. The choices include aminophylline, selective $\beta_2$-adrenergic agonists, epinephrine, or isoproterenol (Table 8-11). Aminophylline alone, although a potent agent, is not as effective as other bronchodilators such as epinephrine.[125] However, it remains the most commonly used treatment for asthma despite its toxicity. $\beta_2$-Agonists are more selective and thus have a reduced incidence of side effects such as tachycardia. The metabolism of these newer drugs is slower than that of epinephrine or isoproterenol, and their effects are therefore longer lasting.[127] There is some evidence that intravenous bronchodilators may have a more pronounced effect on smaller airways than inhaled agents. Thus, combined inhalational and intravenous therapy may provide maximum benefit.[127] Anticholinergics such as atropine, glycopyrrolate, or ipratropium, intravenously or endotracheally, also provide bronchodilatation but may cause tachycardia when given parenterally.

Corticosteroids are usually considered "last resort" therapy in the treatment of moderate to severe asthma. Beclomethasone (400 to 800 μg per day) is the most commonly used agent for long-term therapy. It is administered as an aerosol, but severe cases may require systemic steroids in addition to standard emergency treatment. Methylprednisolone (125 mg intravenously), in conjunction with usual therapy for acute asthma will improve bronchospasm in a significant number of patients.[126] In the absence of an adequate history, the possibility that an asthmatic patient may be steroid dependent must be considered, especially when otherwise unexplainable hypotension occurs. In this situation, hydrocortisone (100 to 200 mg intravenously q6h) or methylprednisolone (50 to 100 mg intravenously q6h) should be given.

All currently prescribed medications for the treatment of

TABLE 8-11. Pharmacologic Agents for the Treatment of Asthma*

| AGENT | ROUTE | DOSE | SIDE EFFECTS | COMMENTS |
|---|---|---|---|---|
| *Theophylline Derivative* | | | | |
| Aminophylline | IV | Load 4 to 6 mg/kg over 30 minutes<br>Maintenance 0.4 to 0.6 mg/kg/h | GI: nausea/vomiting<br>Cardiac: arrhythmias<br>CNS: seizures | May need to adjust dosage based upon smoking history, liver disease, concurrent cimetidine intake<br>Therapeutic level, 10 to 20 μg/mL |
| *Sympathomimetics* | | | | |
| Epinephrine (Adrenaline) | SC/IM | 0.2 to 0.5 mL of 1:1000 solution every 20 to 30 minutes as needed | Cardiac: arrhythmias, hypertension | Avoid in patients with atherosclerotic heart disease |
| Terbutaline (Brethine) | SC | 0.25 mg, repeat in 15 minutes, as needed (use <0.5 mg/4 h) | Same as epinephrine but less pronounced | Specific $\beta_2$-receptor agonist |
| Isoproterenol (Medihaler—ISO) | Nebulizer | 0.5 mL, 0.5% solution in 3 mL NSS over 15 to 20 minutes every 5 hours as needed | Same as epinephrine | Avoid in patients with atherosclerotic disease |
| Isoetharine (Bronkosol) | Nebulizer | 0.25 to 0.5 mL, 1% solution in 3 mL NSS every 4 h as needed | Same as epinephrine but less pronounced | Specific $\beta_2$-receptor agonist |
| Metaproterenol (Alupent) | Nebulizer | 0.3 mL, 5% solution every 4 to 6 hours, | Same as epinephrine but less pronounced | Specific $\beta_2$-receptor agonist |
| | PO | 20 mg every 6 hours | | |
| *Corticosteroids* | | | | |
| Methylprednisolone | IV | 50 to 100 mg every 6 hours | None acutely | Onset of action is delayed |
| Hydrocortisone | IV | 100 to 200 mg every 6 hours | Same as methylprednisolone | Same as methylprednisolone |

* The abbreviations used are: IV, intravenous; SC, subcutaneous; IM, intramuscular; NSS, normal saline solution; PO, by mouth.

asthma may be continued during anesthesia. In fact, if time permits, it is prudent to ensure that therapeutic levels of aminophylline (10 to 20 μg/mL) are present if the patient is receiving it. Steroid use within the previous year should raise suspicion of adrenal suppression. If time permits, a corticotropin (ACTH) stimulation test may be performed. Abnormal results have been found as long as 9 months after discontinuation of steroid therapy. If an ACTH stimulation test cannot be performed, steroids may be given empirically.

In electively operated trauma patients, preoperative medication should consist of adequate analgesics, sedatives, and anticholinergics.[121,123,128] Prior to anesthetic induction, a slow, methodical preparation of the airway with a topical anesthetic or nerve blocks may be performed. Ketamine has been recommended for induction of anesthesia in the asthmatic patient or in airway management of those in status asthmaticus because of its sympathomimetic effects[124]; but any agent, including the barbiturates, will prevent bronchospasm in response to tracheal intubation if given in adequate doses. Ventilation of the patient by mask with inhalational agents followed by intravenous lidocaine (1.5 mg/kg) 2 to 3 minutes before intubation may also be helpful in blunting airway response. Maintenance of anesthesia generally should not present a problem for the asthmatic provided that the depth of anesthesia is adequate. Frequently, initial signs and symptoms (wheezes, decreased compliance) resolve quickly once an adequate level of anesthesia is achieved, although specific bronchodilator therapy is occasionally necessary. At least two groups of agents used during maintenance of anesthesia are associated with histamine release, which in turn may induce an asthmatic attack: some narcotic analgesics (eg, morphine), and some muscle relaxants (eg, curare, atracurium). These agents should probably be avoided or, if used, they should be given in small repeated doses rather than as a large bolus. Extubation of the trachea is preferably performed while the patient is maintained under a deep level of anesthesia but is breathing adequately. If this is not possible, one must wait until the patient is fully awake and then be prepared to treat an asthmatic episode if it occurs.

Anesthetic management of the acute trauma victim undergoing emergency surgery is somewhat different. Hemodynamic instability prevents administration of large doses of barbiturates or benzodiazepines for anesthetic induction, necessitating the use of other measures. Prophylactic administration of aerosolized $\beta_2$-adrenergic agonists, but not aminophylline infusion, has been shown to prevent histamine-induced increase in airway resistance.[122] Thus, preoperative treatment with these agents may be particularly useful in the trauma patient who can tolerate only small doses of anesthetic agents. Ketamine, because of its bronchodilator action and beneficial circulatory effects, may also be more valuable in the asthmatic trauma victim than in the electively operated asthmatic. In these patients, intraoperative ketamine infusion (30 to 40 μg/kg/min) may also obviate the need for maintenance with inhalation agents, which may depress the blood pressure.[129] Postoperatively, immediate extubation of the major trauma patient is seldom possible because of a full stomach and the need for prolonged ventilation. Thus, the likelihood of a need for postoperative bronchodilator therapy is probably increased in these patients. Regional anesthesia may be useful and may be used in asthmatics with extremity injury; this technique however may be impractical for surgery in other body regions or unsafe in the hypovolemic or obtunded trauma patient.

## HEMATOLOGIC DISORDERS

### SICKLE CELL HEMOGLOBINOPATHY

Sickle cell hemoglobinopathy varies in its presentation: the homozygous form (HbSS) is most severe. There are also several heterozygous forms (eg, HbS-O, HbS-C, HBS-A). Of the heterozygous types, HbS-A—the carrier state, or sickle cell trait—occurs in 8 to 9% of black Americans.[136] The homozygous form is of greatest concern, as persons with this type of hemoglobin have a propensity to sickle cell crisis; it is commonly known as *sickle cell disease* or *sickle cell anemia*. It is much less common than the carrier state, presenting in approximately 1 out of every 600 black Americans. However, the young black American male has the greatest probability of being a victim of penetrating trauma from interpersonal violence (approximately three times that of his white male counterpart and nine times that of a young white female). Thus, it is likely that sickle cell disease will be encountered in the admitting area or operating room of a trauma center. Further, the factors that initiate sickle cell crisis—anemia, hypoxia, hypovolemia, hypothermia, acidosis, stress—are very common in acute trauma. Finally, if the patient requires a transfusion, the low levels of 2,3-diphosphoglyceride (2,3-DPG) found in stored, banked blood may also contribute to precipitation of a crisis.[130,133,136,137]

Sickle cell disease is caused by a single nucleotide substitution in the affected patient's β-globin gene. Because of intermolecular interactions, the abnormal hemoglobin molecules have a tendency to deform into the shape of a sickle. While some HbS is sickled at 100% oxygen saturation, the number of sickled cells increases as saturation falls. The sickling process is accelerated by the factors mentioned above. Sickle cells are unable to pass through the microvasculature and may become lodged in precapillary arterioles, the capillary bed, or the venules. Once vascular occlusion has occurred, ischemia and hypoxia lead to further sickling.[130,133,136,137,140]

It should be realized that sickle cell crisis is not restricted to patients with sickle cell disease (HbSS). It can occur in patients with sickle cell trait if precipitating conditions are severe enough. In fact, it has been shown that patients with sickle cell trait have a significant incidence of sudden death during exercise.[139] Davis[134] suggests that the lactic acidosis that develops during exercise has an important role in the development of this phenomenon. It is likely that the acidotic trauma victim with sickle cell trait runs a similar risk. Thus, all major trauma patients with HbS should be treated with this complication in mind.[136,137,140] As hemoglobin electrophoresis typing is not possible in the setting of acute trauma, and the conscious injured patient may be unaware of whether or not he has the sickle cell trait, the anesthesiologist should assume that any black patient is HbS positive. If possible, a Sickledex test should be performed, which requires only a few drops of blood from a finger prick.[137] It must be kept in mind that the cardiac, pulmonary, and renal systems may be compromised by infarction secondary to chronic sickling. In the acute setting, the anesthesiologist can only avoid or attempt to correct the factors that may precipitate a crisis. There is some evidence that intraoperative autotransfusion may cause a substantial amount of sickling in these patients.[132] Although in the exsanguinating patient with sickle cell trait, this technique may be lifesaving, it probably should not be used when adequate homologous blood is available.

More detailed preoperative evaluation and preparation are possible if elective surgery is performed. Of course, all black patients should be questioned regarding sickle cell disease and trait. If the history is positive, further information such as the details of previous crises and a systems review to delineate organ system compromise should be elicited. Also, a sickle cell screen should be conducted in all black patients, with the "positives" being evaluated further by hemoglobin electrophoresis for definitive diagnosis.

For both homozygous and heterozygous patients, the percentage of HbS present is an index of the severity of the disease. In sickle cell disease, HbS makes up approximately 80 to 95% of total hemoglobin. Preoperative transfusion of normal blood is thought to lower the percentage of HbS present and thus buffer the effects of a crisis should it occur. Transfusion may also decrease the incidence of those factors that may instigate a crisis. However, in a recent series of 66 patients with sickle cell hemoglobinopathy, preoperative or intraoperative transfusion did not reduce the postoperative complication rate.[131] If a decision is made to transfuse, the resultant hematocrit should not be above 35%, as the increased viscosity that accompanies a higher hematocrit increases the risk of sludging. A reasonable goal of transfusion is replacement of HbSS with HbAA to the extent that less than 50 to 60% of the original level of HbSS remains.[135,136,138] The level is confirmed either by quantitative measurement of the percentage of sickle cells present on pre- and posttransfusion smears or by hemoglobin electrophoresis.

During the immediate preoperative period sedatives should be used judiciously, and supplemental oxygen should be given. Patients should also be well hydrated; intravenous fluids should be administered as long as the patient is not eating. The operating room should be prewarmed, and the patient should be carefully positioned and padded on the table.[136,138,140]

Intraoperatively, any carefully managed anesthetic technique may be used. In addition to standard techniques, monitoring should focus on accurate observation of blood pressure, body temperature, pH, and oxygenation. Blood loss should be aggressively replaced and normal temperature maintained. One author recommends maintaining mild respiratory alkalosis.[136] This may not be beneficial since alkalosis shifts the oxygen-hemoglobin dissociation curve to the left and thus makes oxygen less available to the tissues. Vasoconstrictors should be avoided if possible.

Postoperatively, normoxemia and eucapnia should be ensured and adequate hydration maintained. Pulmonary toilet and chest physiotherapy are important, as postoperative atelectasis and pneumonia are common causes of morbidity in these patients.

## HEMOPHILIA

Classic hemophilia, hemophilia A, is characterized by factor VIII deficiency and is inherited as a sex-linked recessive disorder. It is manifested almost exclusively in males with females being the genetic carriers. The female offspring of a hemophiliac male and a carrier female has a 50% chance of manifesting the classic disease, but this is an exceedingly rare occurrence.[155] Approximately one male in 10,000 is afflicted with hemophilia A, making it the most common severe hereditary coagulation disorder.[155] Hemophilia B (Christmas disease), which is clinically indistinguishable from hemophilia A, occurs seven times less frequently and is caused by hereditary deficiency of Christmas factor (factor IX).[155] Neither hemophilia A nor hemophilia B has an ethnic or geographic predilection.

The protein complex of factor VIII consists of factor VIII:C (FVIII:C) and factor VIII:von Willebrand factor (FVIII:vWF). Patients with classic hemophilia lack procoagulant FVIII:C.[154] FVIII:vWF, which also possesses coagulant activity, is deficient in patients with von Willebrand disease, a bleeding disorder of variable severity with a prevalence of 30 to 125 per 1 million population.[155] FVIII:C deficiency in hemophiliacs may result either from low plasma factor levels or from a nonfunctional factor present in normal concentrations.

In hemophiliacs, platelet function remains intact, allowing the vascular plug to develop promptly after trauma. However, fibrin formation is limited to deposition only of thin strands at the wound periphery, preventing the central core of the thrombosis from gaining in consistency.[167] Since primary hemostasis is unaffected in hemophilia, the onset of bleeding is characteristically delayed for several hours or sometimes even for days after injury.[154,155,163] Thus bleeding into body cavities or fascial planes may not be recognized until some time after the injury, when hemorrhagic shock develops or an expanding hematoma exerts pressure on adjacent tissues or organs.

The likelihood and severity of bleeding are primarily determined by the FVIII:C level in the plasma (Table 8-12). Bleeding is unlikely in patients with FVIII:C levels above 50% of normal even after major injury or surgery. The likelihood of bleeding in those with FVIII:C levels below 50% is dependent on the severity of trauma. Plasma levels between 25 and 50%, which may be present in some carriers, are associated with increased bleeding after major trauma, whereas levels between 1 and 5% of normal predispose the patient to bleeding even after minor injury. Recurrent spontaneous bleeding, usually into muscles or weight-bearing joints, occurs in patients with FVIII:C levels below 1%.[169] Surgery or trauma may cause significant bleeding even in patients with FVIII:C levels of 5 to 25% because depletion of the marginal level of FVIII:C occurs with ongoing clotting, and activation of factor X is thus retarded.

In any trauma patient with extensive deep-tissue bleeding or prolonged oozing from wounds or sites of venipuncture, the possibility of a preexisting hemostatic defect should be considered, and if reliable information cannot be obtained from the patient, relatives or friends must be questioned. Although attention to the relation of the bleeding pattern to the extent of trauma and physical examination may provide some important clues, the diagnosis is established by laboratory tests[163] (Table 8-13). Of the routine coagulation tests, platelet count and prothrombin time (PT) are normal, and partial thromboplastin time (PTT) is prolonged.[163] However, coexisting causes of coagulopathy in the severely injured may result in a decreased platelet count and prolonged PT, complicating the diagnosis. Even the FVIII:C level, which is diagnostic of hemophilia, may be decreased in the trauma victim who is treated with massive amounts of cellular and acellular fluids. Thus, a definitive diagnosis of hemophilia may be delayed in severely injured patients. In the hemodynamically stable patient in whom the diagnosis of hemophilia can be made by FVIII:C measurement, the presence of an inhibitor as the basis of deficient factor VIII function should be excluded.

Hemorrhage in hemophilia is particularly deleterious if it is intracranial, lingual, laryngeal, retropharyngeal, pericardial, or pleural. Hematomas at these sites expand rapidly, resulting in life-threatening displacement of intracranial, cervical, or thoracic organs.[155] Although these conditions require immediate factor VIII replacement, emergency decompression of the brain or heart or establishment of airway patency may be necessary. Airway management may be associated with great difficulty and risk because distortion is caused not only by rapid extravasation of blood dissecting the fascial planes, but also by edema secondary to venous obstruction. In general, the management techniques discussed in Chapter 3 for patients with airway obstruction apply to these patients as well.

Intracranial hemorrhage occurs in 3 to 14% of hemophiliacs and is associated with a 25 to 35% risk of mortality.[143,149,151] The latter rate was 70% before the introduction of cryopre-

TABLE 8-12. Relationship between Plasma FVIII:C Levels and Severity of Bleeding in Hemophilia*

| PLASMA FVIII:C LEVEL (% normal) | BLEEDING AFTER MAJOR TRAUMA | BLEEDING AFTER MINOR TRAUMA | SPONTANEOUS BLEEDING |
|---|---|---|---|
| 50 to 100 | − | − | − |
| 25 to 50 | + | − | − |
| 5 to 25 | + + | + | − |
| 1 to 5 | + + + | + + + | + |
| <1 | + + + | + + + | + + |

* The symbols used are: −, no bleeding; +, possible bleeding; + +, moderate bleeding; + + +, severe bleeding.

TABLE 8-13. Results of Coagulation Tests in Hemophilia A

| TEST | RESULTS |
|---|---|
| Bleeding time | Normal |
| Platelet count | Normal |
| Platelet aggregation | Normal |
| Prothrombin time | Normal |
| Partial thromboplastin time | Prolonged |
| FVIII:C level | Low (diagnostic) |
| FVIII:vWF | Normal |

cipitate in the early 1960s.[160] Even minor head trauma may result in bleeding from small intracranial vessels. Symptoms occur after a symptom-free interval, most often within 24 to 48 hours after injury.[149,160] Trauma is the most common cause of intracranial bleeding in hemophiliacs; a history of injury can be elicited in 45 to 60% of patients.[149,160] The most common presenting symptoms are headache, emesis, seizures, and altered sensorium which may be accompanied by symptoms of spinal cord compression since intraspinal bleeding may also occur in hemophiliacs.[143,149,151,160] Intracerebral hematoma accounts for 40% and epidural and subdural hematoma for 60% of intracranial bleeding in hemophiliacs. Unless the hematoma is large or occupies the extradural space, conservative therapy with high-dose factor VIII concentrate and frequent evaluation with computed tomography (CT) scan is preferred by some authors.[155] They consider craniotomy only for those patients who do not improve or who deteriorate within a few hours after the start of replacement therapy.[160] If this protocol is followed, patients who present for surgery will have an increased likelihood of severe intracranial hypertension. Other authors, using operative indications similar to those used for nonhemophiliacs with CNS bleeding—evacuation of subdural and epidural hematomas and conservative treatment with steroids and other agents for intracerebral and subarachnoid bleeding—have demonstrated that the mortality rate was 64% for patients with intracerebral hematomas. The prognosis was better for those who had subdural or subarachnoid hemorrhage (mortality rate of 14%).[149]

Patients with hemophilia may show roentgenographic abnormalities of the cervical spine: increased atlanto-dens distance, end-plate irregularity, and cysts within the vertebral bodies.[164] In the hemophiliac with suspected cervical spine injury, these abnormalities may render X-ray evaluation of the cervical spine difficult. If there is doubt, the cervical spine should be immobilized before airway management.

Bleeding into joints, muscles, or interfascial spaces may occur with or without trauma and result in complications such as hypovolemia, peripheral neuropathies, and infection. Massive retroperitoneal bleeding may occur and may be complicated by subsequent rupture into the peritoneal cavity, causing a sharp drop in blood pressure and severe anemia.[161] Peptic ulceration occurs at least five times more frequently in hemophiliacs than in normal adult males and increases the likelihood of gastrointestinal bleeding.[155] Patients with hemophilia also have a high incidence of urinary tract bleeding, which occasionally leads to severe renal colic.[155] In the injured hemophiliac undergoing emergency or elective surgery, these potential bleeding sites should be examined preoperatively. Intraoperative positioning should be done carefully, and pressure points must be thickly padded to prevent hemorrhage.

In addition to the basic management principles of trauma, the injured patient with hemophilia requires rapid evaluation and prompt treatment of the hemostatic defect. Delay in treatment increases the risk of hemorrhagic complications.[153] Essentially, the treatment involves factor VIII replacement with FVIII:C concentrate or in the case of hemophilia B with factor IX concentrate. Only the treatment of hemophilia A will be discussed since it is a more common form. The dose of FVIII:C concentrate is determined by several factors: (1) the severity and site of hemorrhage; (2) the amount of FVIII:C contained in the concentrate to be administered; (3) the estimated plasma level of FVIII:C required to halt the bleeding; (4) the disappearance rate of the administered factor VIII; and (5) the presence of factor VIII inhibitor in the serum. Generally a dose of 1 U/kg factor VIII concentrate increases the plasma level by 2%. Thus, to increase plasma FVIII:C level by 30% in a 70-kg man, 1050 U of factor VIII concentrate should be administered:

$$\frac{30\%}{2\%} \times 70 = 1050 \text{ units}$$

A more precise calculation for replacement therapy is as follows[144]:

$$\text{Units needed} = (\text{desired level} - \text{initial level})$$
$$\text{Total units needed} = \text{units needed} \times 0.6 \times \text{body weight (kg)}$$
$$\text{Milliliters of concentrate needed} = \frac{\text{Total units needed}}{\text{U/mL in concentrate}}$$

Since the biologic half-life of FVIII:C is between 8 and 12 hours, many hemophiliacs require repeated perioperative doses. Adequacy of plasma levels must be ensured by quantitative assays in these patients.[144] Although hemostasis can be assured with 10 to 25% plasma FVIII:C activity in patients with hemarthrosis and intramuscular hematomas, considerably higher concentrations, ranging from 35 to 50%, are necessary after major trauma or surgery.

There are several dozen factor VIII preparations on the market, each produced by a different method and thus varying in potency, purity, and composition. However, they can be classified by three properties: (1) FVIII:C potency measured as U/mL; (2) protein concentration measured as mg/mL; and (3) specific activity, the ratio between potency and protein concentration.[142] Based on this classification, five categories of factor VIII concentrate can be discerned: high-purity concentrate, intermediate-purity concentrate, cryoprecipitate, fresh frozen plasma, and whole blood (Table 8-14). FVIII:C concentration in whole blood and fresh frozen plasma is low, and a relatively large volume of these products must be given to obtain an adequate hemostatic effect. At least 2 L of fresh whole blood are necessary to produce hemostasis. This amount of whole blood may cause serious volume overload if it is administered to a normovolemic patient. Smaller amounts of fresh frozen plasma are required, but congestive heart failure is still a possibility in the absence of ongoing bleeding.

TABLE 8-14. Specific Activity and FVIII:C Potency of Four Available Factor VIII Products

| PRODUCT | SPECIFIC ACTIVITY (unit/mg) | FVIII:C POTENCY (unit/mL) |
|---|---|---|
| High purity concentrate | >1 | 20 to 40 |
| Intermediate purity concentrate | 0.4 to 0.9 | 15 to 40 |
| Cryoprecipitate | 0.1 to 0.4 | 3 to 6 |
| Fresh frozen plasma | 0.02 | 1 |
| Fresh whole blood | 0.006 | 0.3 |

Cryoprecipitate, which contains 80 to 100 U of FVIII:C and FVIII:vWF and 200 to 300 mg of fibrinogen in 10 to 20 mL, does not carry this risk. However, its FVIII:C concentration is variable, and this product may potentially lead to renal damage because of its high fibrinogen content.[144] Both intermediate and high-purity concentrates have reliable amounts of FVIII:C and are the products of choice in severe hemophiliacs and in those who have inhibitors against FVIII:C.

Inhibitors (antibodies) to FVIII:C are present in about 10% of severe hemophiliacs and less frequently in mild cases.[155] Although previous administration of commercial FVIII:C concentrates was thought to be responsible for these antibodies, this has not been confirmed by the findings of a multicenter trial.[145] Quantitative titration of plasma FVIII:C inhibitor is necessary to determine the treatment of these patients. If the inhibitor titer is low, treatment involves increasing the dose of FVIII:C. Plasmapheresis prior to FVIII:C administration is also recommended if surgery is performed electively. Patients with high-titer FVIII:C inhibitors are treated with activated prothrombin complex concentrates (75 to 100 U/kg every 4 to 8 hours),[159,166] which are derived from standard factor IX preparations.

Other agents used in hemophiliacs include desmopressin (DDAVP), ε-aminocaproic acid (EACA), and tranexamic acid (AMCA). Although the exact mechanism of action of DDAVP is unclear, it has been postulated that it acts by releasing a second messenger, possibly from the brain, which in turn acts upon the endothelial cells to release FVIII:C and FVIII:vWF. DDAVP may also increase platelet adhesion and aggregation at the injury site. The drug is useful in patients with mild to moderate hemophilia A. In these patients, a transient but greater than two-fold increase in FVIII:C levels results from 30 to 40 μg/kg DDAVP administered intranasally.[148] The effective intravenous dose is 3 to 4 μg/kg. Tachyphylaxis, presumably as a result of depletion of factor VIII stores, occurs after repeated DDAVP administration. Thus, this drug can ensure adequate hemostasis only for minor procedures and cannot be relied upon following major trauma. EACA and AMCA are inhibitors of plasminogen activators and thus act as antifibrinolytic agents. As with DDAVP, these agents are useful in mild to moderate hemophiliacs undergoing minor surgery. They can also prevent spontaneous bleeding. However, in major trauma or surgery they can only be adjuncts to factor VIII:C replacement.[157]

## VON WILLEBRAND DISEASE

This disease results from qualitative and quantitative abnormalities of von Willebrand factor. Its severity varies widely because of the phenotypic heterogeneity of the factor protein. At least 21 subtypes of FVIII:vWF have been identified.[165] As in hemophilia, the treatment of this disease consists of replacement of deficient FVIII:vWF. Cryoprecipitate can reliably normalize the prolonged bleeding time, but commercial factor VIII concentrates seem to be ineffective because they lack most of the active forms of von Willebrand factor. DDAVP stimulates the production and release of FVIII:vWF but has variable efficacy in von Willebrand disease.[165] In the trauma patient with this disease, a combination of cryoprecipitate and DDAVP (0.4 μg/kg) may be effective. However, the serious risk of viral disease transmission with cryoprecipitate has recently directed efforts to prepare a virus-inactivated FVIII concentrate. Currently, virus sterilization is achieved either by heating (60°C for 24 hours) or by treating the product with solvent detergent. In a small number of patients, sterilized factor VIII concentrates have been shown to be hemostatically effective.[152]

## IDIOPATHIC THROMBOCYTOPENIC PURPURA

Idiopathic thrombocytopenic purpura (ITP) or, more appropriately, immune thrombocytopenic purpura is a hemorrhagic autoimmune disorder caused by antiplatelet antibodies. It occurs in acute and chronic forms. The diagnosis of this disease is made by exclusion; in the trauma patient other causes of thrombocytopenia—alcoholism, drug effect, sepsis, viral infections, uremia, posttransfusion thrombocytopenia, thrombotic thrombocytopenic purpura (TTP)—must be eliminated before the diagnosis of ITP is established.

ITP results from a series of complex autoimmune phenomena, the exact nature of which is as yet incompletely understood. According to the most accepted mechanism, an immunoglobulin, which can be an intrinsic autoantigen of the platelet membrane, a tightly bound extrinsic antigen (drug, virus, or self-antigen), or an immune complex produced by an antigen-antibody reaction is adsorbed to the platelet surface (Fig 8-3), making it susceptible to destruction by macrophages in the spleen and bone marrow (Fig 8-4).

Acute ITP is predominantly a disease of children, occurring most commonly between 2 and 9 years of age. It usually exhibits an abrupt onset, following a viral illness or upper respiratory infection by 1 to 3 weeks. Common presenting signs are petechiae and purpura. The platelet count may fall below 20,000/μL, and bleeding may occur at various sites in the body. There may be hemorrhage even when the platelet count is as high as 50,000/μL if platelet function is abnormal.[168] Acute ITP is a benign and self-limiting disease in children; more than 80% of patients recover within 6 months whether or not they are treated with steroids. Thus, steroid therapy is controversial in children. In adults, however, steroids seem to be warranted since a greater number of untreated patients develop the chronic form of the disease.[162] Platelet transfusions are reserved for patients with active or life-threatening hemorrhage; antiplatelet antibodies may shorten platelet survival to as little as a few minutes. Most patients can be treated with corticosteroids and intravenous γ-globulin with good results. However, persistent bleeding despite steroids, γ-globulin, and platelet transfusions may necessitate emergency splenectomy. Approximately 20% of patients with acute ITP do not recover in 6 months; the subsequent clinical course of these patients is indistinguishable from chronic ITP. Clinical differences between acute and chronic ITP are shown in Table 8-15.

Chronic ITP is more indolent than the acute form and is associated with prolonged remissions and episodic relapses over many years. In general, prednisone is given for 4 weeks and, if the response is inadequate, a trial of 6 weeks is recommended.[147,156] Approximately 25% of patients with chronic ITP achieve complete remission after a single course of glucocorticoids.

| PLATELET MEMBRANE AUTOANTIGEN | ADSORBED AUTO OR FOREIGN ANTIGEN | ADSORBED IMMUNE COMPLEXES AUTO OR FOREIGN ANTIGEN |
|---|---|---|
| | Foreign Molecule | Foreign Molecule |
| | Native Molecule | Native Molecule |

FIG. 8-3. Three possible antigens may be responsible for coating the platelets in idiopathic thrombocytopenic purpura (ITP). (Left) intrinsic autoantigen of platelet membrane; (center) extrinsic antigen, which may be a drug or a virus; (right) immune complex that results from the interaction of a foreign or native antigen and an antibody. (From McMillen R. The pathogenesis of immune thrombocytopenic purpura. CRC Crit Rev Clin Lab Sci 1977; 8:303, with permission.)

FIG. 8-4. Schematic representation of the mechanism of platelet destruction in ITP. A platelet-associated antigen (solid rectangle) is attached to the platelet (P) (1). Antigenic stimulation and lymphoid proliferation occur in the spleen (2) or in the bone marrow (3). Antigen-specific cells develop and cause generalized immune response (4). Antiplatelet antibody synthesis occurs in the spleen, bone marrow, or other tissues (5) and IgG antiplatelet antibody (G) binds to platelet-associated antigen (6). This results in phagocytosis by means of macrophage receptors (7) or after complement activation by C3b receptors in the macrophage (8,9). The antiplatelet antibody may also bind to the megakaryocyte (10). (From McMillan R. Immune thrombocytopenia. Clin Hematol 1983; 12/1:76, with permission.)

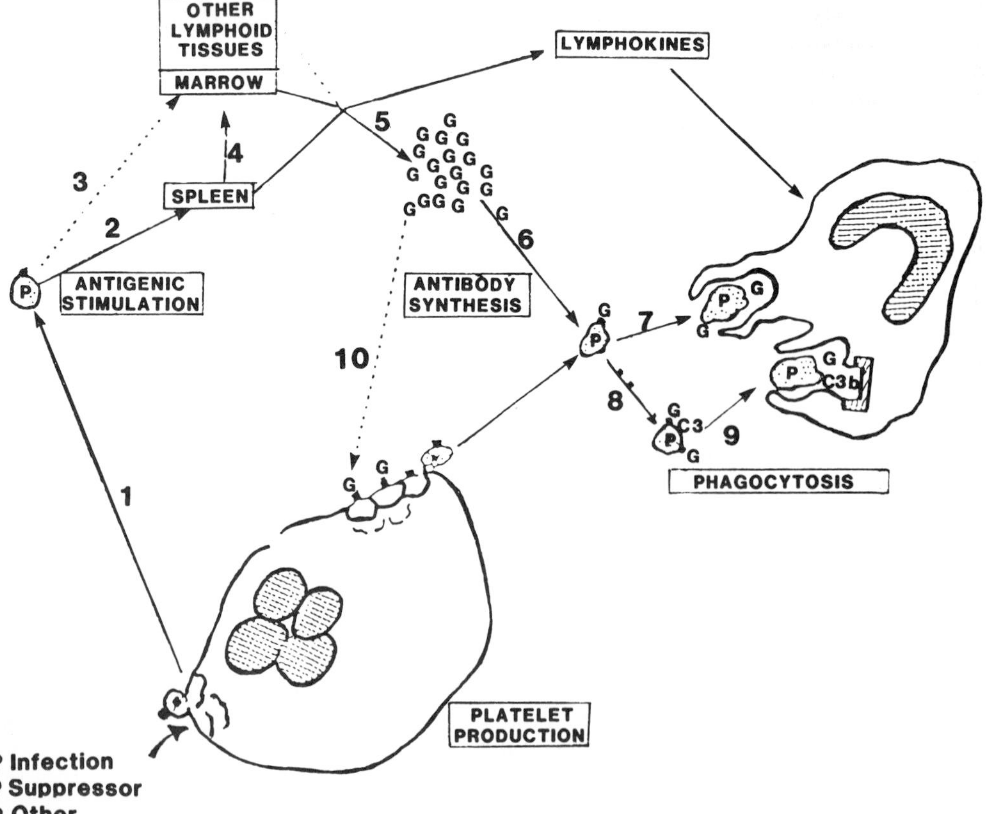

TABLE 8-15. Clinical Differences Between Acute and Chronic Idiopathic Thrombocytopenic Purpura

| | ACUTE | CHRONIC |
|---|---|---|
| Age | 2 to 9 | 20 to 50 |
| Sex ratio (M/F) | 1/1 | 1/4 |
| Previous infection | Common | Uncommon |
| Onset of symptoms | Abrupt | Gradual |
| Duration | 2 to 6 weeks | Years |
| Spontaneous remission | 80% | Uncommon |
| Platelet count | <30,000/μL | 30,000 to 100,000/μL |
| Response to steroids | Uncommon in children (adults more responsive) | Common |
| Response to splenectomy | Unpredictable | Common |

If the response to corticosteroids is inadequate or if extended (>6 to 8 weeks) treatment with high-dose prednisone (>15 mg/daily) is necessary, splenectomy is indicated.[158] Splenectomy removes the antibody source as well as the site of platelet destruction. Approximately 80% of splenectomized patients improve; 60 to 70% of these patients show permanent restoration of platelet count. Relapses occur in the remaining patients and necessitate additional steroid trials or other therapeutic measures such as intravenous γ-globulin, plasmapheresis, immunosuppressors, and the synthetic androgen danazol.[141,146,150] However, response to these measures is variable.

In most instances the injured ITP patient who presents for emergency surgery is in remission, and thus the marginally adequate number and function of his or her platelets are sufficient to prevent excessive perioperative bleeding. In some patients adequate hemostasis may result from ongoing corticosteroid treatment. An additional dose of steroid (hydrocortisone, 100 mg) may have to be administered to these patients prior to surgery to prevent hypotension secondary to adrenocortical atrophy during the stress of surgery. Emergency surgery for the rare ITP patient who is in relapse and thus has abnormal bleeding creates management difficulties because a response to corticosteroid and γ-globulin requires at least 4 to 5 days of treatment. Nevertheless high-dose γ-globulin (1 to 1.5 g/kg) followed by platelet transfusion may be effective in some patients. It has been postulated that γ-globulin saturates phagocytic receptors on the macrophages and may thus prevent destruction of subsequently administered platelets.[150,170]

## EPILEPSY

Patients with chronic epilepsy require maintenance of therapeutic levels of anticonvulsive medications at all times (Table 8-16). In the trauma patient with a seizure disorder, history is important because the results of the toxicologic screen, which is usually performed on admission to the trauma center and includes analysis of phenytoin and phenobarbital levels, will not be available soon enough to be useful. If no history is obtained, seizures should be anticipated, although they may occur after several hours, when drug levels become subtherapeutic.

Of course, a number of trauma patients develop seizures as a result of head injury.[176] Within the first week after nonpenetrating head trauma, 5% of patients (usually those with depressed skull fractures or intracranial hematoma) develop a seizure disorder. This number may be higher in pediatric trauma victims. Twelve percent of head trauma patients develop seizures after the first week.[176]

If seizures develop in the acutely injured patient, they should be controlled by judicious use of diazepam, as long as blood pressure is stable.[171,172,180] In patients who are intubated and mechanically ventilated, 5-mg increments of diazepam can be given until seizures are terminated (usually up to 30 mg, total dose). If control cannot be achieved with this or larger doses of diazepam, sodium thiopental or another short-acting barbiturate should be given.[184] A simultaneous infusion of a loading dose of another anticonvulsant, first phenytoin (50 mg/min to a total dose of 18 mg/kg), then phenobarbital, should be started.[175] Caution must be exercised when administering phenytoin, especially in hypovolemic trauma patients, because it can produce hypotension and ventricular arrhythmias.

Another important consideration is the alteration of phenytoin pharmacokinetics in trauma patients during the first week of injury. It appears that increased phenytoin clearance in this group of patients often results in subtherapeutic plasma levels.[173] The dose of this drug should thus be increased; frequent monitoring of plasma phenytoin levels is necessary to ensure effective treatment.

The acute development of seizures in the perioperative period should prompt a search for other possible causes such as hypoglycemia, uremia, or intracranial hemorrhage. As we mentioned, seizures may also result from chronic alcohol use or alcohol withdrawal in patients with delirium tremens; the latter usually occurs 12 to 36 hours after the last ingestion of alcohol.

TABLE 8-16. Characteristics of Anticonvulsive Medications

| GENERIC NAME | TRADE NAME | DAILY DOSAGE (mg/day) | THERAPEUTIC BLOOD LEVEL (μg/mL) | TOXIC BLOOD LEVEL (μg/mL) |
|---|---|---|---|---|
| Phenytoin | Dilantin | 300 | 10 to 20 | >20 |
| Phenobarbital | Luminal | 120 | 10 to 30 | >40 |
| Primidone | Mysoline | 750 | 5 to 10 | >12 |
| Carbamazepine | Tegretol | 1200 | 3 to 7 | >8 |
| Valproic acid | Depakene | 1500 | 40 to 70 | >100 |
| Ethosuximide | Zarontin | 100 | 40 to 100 | >100 |

Status epilepticus is defined as continuous seizures for more than 30 minutes or three or more grand mal seizures with brief interim periods of incomplete recovery of consciousness. Although this condition occurs in less than 5% of patients with known epilepsy, it may be the first manifestation of the disease. Head trauma is known to be a common cause of status epilepticus, but alcohol withdrawal and metabolic derangements also may be responsible.[174] The mortality and morbidity of status epilepticus are related to the duration of uncontrolled seizures. Severe neurologic damage or death may result if treatment is not instituted immediately. Treatment includes airway control and adequate ventilation. Intravenous diazepam is administered at a rate of 2 mg/min until seizures stop or until a 20-mg dose is reached.[174,177,180] Alternatively, lorazepam (4 to 8 mg, intravenously), which is a longer-acting agent than diazepam, may be used.[183] Intravenous phenytoin (50 mg/min to a total dose of 18 mg/kg) and, if necessary, phenobarbital (100 mg/min, intravenously), are administered.

If both phenytoin and phenobarbital have been given to therapeutic levels without response, administration of these agents should continue until supramaximal plasma levels of each agent are obtained (Table 8-16). Valproic acid or carbamezapine are also recommended.[181,182] If seizures continue after all of these measures, general anesthesia may be required.

Patients who are chronically treated with phenytoin for epilepsy require larger and more frequent doses of all nondepolarizing muscle relaxants except atracurium.[178,179] Resistance to nondepolarizing agents is due to an as yet undefined pharmacodynamic alteration in this group of patients.

## CARDIAC DISEASES

### ARRHYTHMIAS IN THE TRAUMA PATIENT

As in the general population, arrhythmias are not uncommon in trauma victims. Their presence may precede trauma, or they may be caused by the injury itself; trauma to the chest, eyes, neck, spinal cord or head can result in a variety of arrhythmias.[194,197,199,200,201,209,218] Resuscitative measures, by producing electrolyte disturbances or hypothermia or by a direct effect on the heart, can also cause rhythm abnormalities. The basic approach to a trauma patient with an arrhythmia is the same as that used for a patient with an elective condition: the arrhythmia must be diagnosed and categorized and its etiology determined and treated.

Trauma patients who present for surgery can be divided into two broad categories: those who need surgery urgently (in the next several hours), and those who need immediate surgery as a lifesaving procedure. In the first category a nearly complete preoperative evaluation is possible, including a 12-lead ECG; measurement of arterial blood gases, pH, and electrolytes; and determination of serum levels of antiarrhythmic agents if the patient is taking them. If the patient presents with a permanent pacemaker, its type, date of insertion, and working condition should be determined. A full cardiac history will help in planning the type of intraoperative monitoring needed. In this setting, any arrhythmia that is likely to worsen (more than five premature ventricular contractions [PVCs] per minute, R on T phenomena, short runs of ventricular tachycardia, or a second degree heart block) or is causing hemodynamic compromise (rapid atrial fibrillation or flutter; tachycardia in association with mitral stenosis, aortic stenosis, or coronary artery disease) should be treated. The trauma patient in the second category presents the problem of diagnosing and treating the arrhythmia intraoperatively whether it is acute or chronic.

Arrhythmias can be grouped into five categories: tachyarrhythmias, bradyarrhythmias, conduction defects, ectopic beats, and electromechanical dissociation.

#### *Tachyarrhythmias*

SINUS TACHYCARDIA. Sinus tachycardia is almost always a physiologic response to a primary insult or stimulus. It is perhaps the most common type of arrhythmia in the trauma patient. It has multiple etiologies: hypoxia, hypercapnia, hypovolemia, anemia, pain, inadequate anesthesia, anxiety, hypothermia, and hyperthermia. On the ECG, P waves may be lost in the preceding T waves, and at times the QRS complex may be widened due to aberrant conduction. Treatment is directed at correction of the underlying cause.[219] In the elderly with possible coronary artery disease, invasive monitoring must be considered, and the heart rate should be rapidly controlled to less than 100 per minute; at times pharmacologic intervention may be required. Care should be taken when controlling the heart rate with drugs in a hypovolemic patient since significant hypotension may result.

If the underlying etiology of sinus tachycardia cannot be determined and immediate control of the heart rate is necessary, then a β-adrenergic blocker should be used. If hypotension results, the blood pressure may be raised with an $alpha_1$-adrenergic agonist.

Esmolol is an excellent choice for treating sinus tachycardia in the trauma patient. It has a half-life of only 9 minutes, therefore if significant hypotension develops it will be of short duration. The patient is given a slow initial dose of 0.5 mg/kg, intravenously. This dose is repeated every 4 to 5 minutes until adequate control of heart rate is obtained. For continuing control after the pulse has been reduced, an esmolol infusion is administered at a rate of 25 to 300 μg/kg/min.

ATRIAL FLUTTER AND FIBRILLATION. The etiologies of atrial flutter and fibrillation include hypoxia, pulmonary embolism, ischemic heart disease, valvular heart disease, thyrotoxicosis, cardiomyopathies, and alcohol ingestion. Cardiac contusion may also result in atrial flutter and fibrillation as well as premature atrial and ventricular contractions. Atrial flutter is characterized by flutter waves; these are saw-toothed in appearance and have a regular rate of 250 to 300 beats per minute (Fig. 8-5). The ventricular response is generally regular at a rate of about 150 beats per minute with 2:1 conduction. At times, the ventricular rhythm is irregular, with varying conduction ratios or Wenckebach periodicity.

Atrial fibrillation presents as an irregular rhythm with no P waves (Fig 8-5). The ventricular rate is between 100 and 180 beats per minute depending on conduction through the atrioventricular (AV) node. The QRS complex is usually of

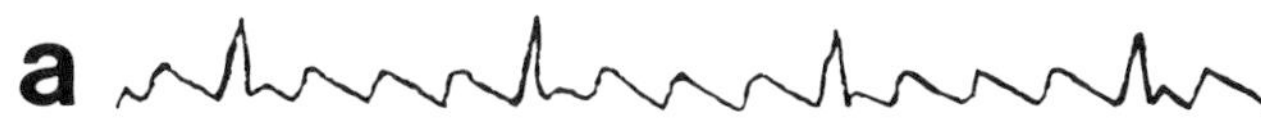


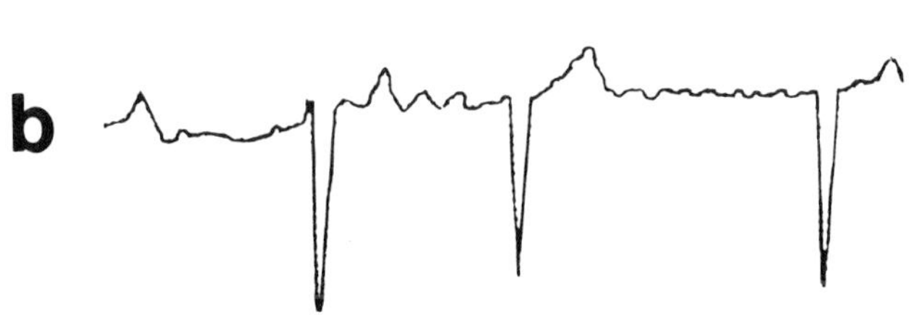


FIG. 8-5. Examples of (a) atrial flutter with its typical saw-toothed pattern and (b) atrial fibrillation.

normal duration but may be wide because of aberrant conduction. Atrial fibrillation may be paroxysmal or chronic, whereas atrial flutter is usually of short duration and converts to normal sinus rhythm or atrial fibrillation.

The choice of treatment depends on the patient's hemodynamic stability and the onset of the arrhythmia. A hemodynamically unstable patient with acute onset of atrial fibrillation or flutter should be cardioverted. Cardioversion should be synchronized to the QRS complex and initiated at 25 J for atrial flutter and 50 J for atrial fibrillation.[217] If this treatment is unsuccessful, it should be repeated at a higher energy level. If the patient's hemodynamic instability is secondary to blood loss, fluid resuscitation should be performed prior to cardioversion.

If an adequate history cannot be obtained, a rapid ventricular rate should be controlled with digoxin, β-blockers, or overapamil. Cardioversion should not be attempted because of the possibility of embolization from an atrial thrombus. Treatment with digoxin is initiated in doses of 0.25 mg, intravenously, repeated every 20 to 30 minutes.[188] The total digitalization dose is usually between 1.0 and 2.0 mg. If heart rate is still not controlled (<110 beats per minute), then verapamil (0.07 to 0.15 mg/kg, intravenously) is administered over 1 minute and repeated in 10 to 20 minutes if no response is noted. The total dose should not exceed 10 mg. Propranolol can also be used to control heart rate in the patient with atrial fibrillation/flutter and is given intravenously in 0.5-mg divided doses up to a total dose of 0.1 to 0.15 mg/kg.[191] Verapamil or β-blockers should be given cautiously to patients with congestive heart failure. In this situation, administration of calcium may greatly reduce the negative inotropic effects of verapamil, without significantly affecting its ability to slow the ventricular response.

Once the ventricular rate has been controlled, quinidine or procainamide may be used to convert the arrhythmia to a normal sinus rhythm. The interaction between quinidine and digoxin is well described; quinidine can increase the plasma concentration of digoxin and therefore increase the risk of digoxin toxicity.[198,202] If heart rate has not been controlled, quinidine and procainamide are contraindicated because of their vagolytic properties.

TABLE 8-17. Mechanisms of Paroxysmal Supraventricular Tachycardia (PSVT) with Reported Incidences*

| MECHANISM | INCIDENCE (%) |
|---|---|
| AV nodal reentry | 58 |
| AV reentry via a concealed extranodal pathway | 30 |
| SA nodal reentry | 4 |
| Intraatrial reentry | 4 |
| Automatic atrial tachycardia | 4 |

* (From Walsh et al[217] with permission.)

PAROXYSMAL SUPRAVENTRICULAR TACHYCARDIA. The causes of supraventricular tachycardia (SVT) include underlying heart disease and chronic lung disease. If the SVT is associated with AV block, digitalis toxicity must be strongly suspected. Ventricular rates with this arrhythmia are between 150 and 200 beats per minute. P waves are usually not discernible because they are lost in the QRS complex or the T wave (Fig 8-6). The QRS may be of normal duration or wide due to aberrant conduction. Five different cardiac mechanisms may produce paroxysmal supraventricular tachycardia (PSVT) (Table 8-17). AV nodal reentry and AV nodal reentry via an extranodal pathway account for 90% of cases of this arrhythmia. If the source of the PSVT is in the sinoatrial (SA) node or if it results from intraatrial reentry, P waves are seen prior to the QRS. If the source of the PSVT is AV nodal reentry via an extranodal pathway then inverted P waves are seen after the QRS. PSVT resulting from AV nodal reentry through an extranodal accessory pathway is similar to the tachycardia seen in Wolff-Parkinson-White syndrome (WPW); however, the accessory pathway is referred to as a concealed Kent bundle. This bundle can conduct only in the retrograde (orthodromic) direction (Fig 8-7). During normal sinus rhythm conduction propagates through the AV node, resulting in a normal PR interval and no delta wave. In automatic atrial tachycardia, the QRS is of normal duration because conduction travels antegrade through the AV node.

Vagal stimulation often terminates the tachycardia. If digitalis toxicity is responsible for the arrhythmia, the drug should be withheld. Digoxin toxicity is treated with phenytoin, using repeated doses of 50 to 100 mg, intravenously, over 5 minutes until a therapeutic effect is obtained; up to 15 mg/kg have been given.[189] Verapamil, (2.5 to 10 mg, intravenously) is the drug of choice in treatment of SVT. β-Blockers and digoxin are also effective in slowing conduction through the AV node.

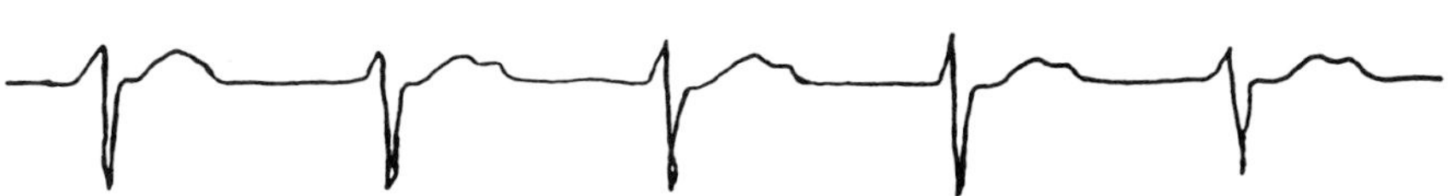

FIG. 8-6. An example of paroxysmal supraventricular tachycardia (PSVT), with normal QRS duration and a P wave lost in the QRS. Increasing the sweep speed of the monitor will help in visualizing the P wave.

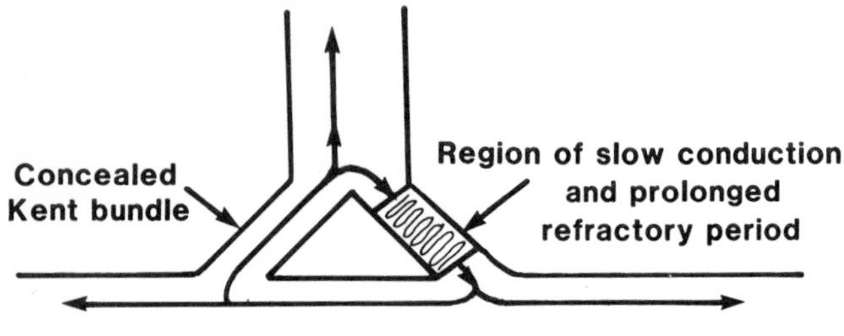


FIG. 8-7. Mechanism of paroxysmal supraventricular tachycardia (PSVT) resulting from AV nodal reentry via an extranodal accessory pathway referred to as a concealed Kent bundle. (Adapted from Bigger JT, Hoffman BF. Antiarrhythmic drugs. In: Gilman AG, Goodman LS, Roll TW, et al, eds. The Pharmacologic Basis of Therapeutics. 7th ed. New York: Macmillan, 1985:753, with permission.)

Quinidine and nifedipine block conduction in the retrograde pathway. They are the drugs of choice in the treatment of SVT resulting from intraatrial reentry or of automatic atrial tachycardia as long as the ventricular response is first controlled. Procainamide may also be used. It is given intravenously in 100-mg doses over 5 minutes and repeated until a therapeutic effect is obtained or a total dose of 1 g is reached. Administration should be discontinued if hypotension develops or if the QT interval is prolonged by 50% or more. Finally, if SVT results in hemodynamic instability, the patient should be electrically cardioverted.

WOLFF-PARKINSON-WHITE SYNDROME. WPW has an overall incidence of 0.15% in the general population.[210] The characteristic ECG findings are a PR interval of less than 0.2 second and a QRS complex wider than 0.12 second. The QRS is prolonged by a delta wave that results from early depolarization of the ventricles via an accessory bundle (Fig 8-8). Three different anomalous pathways have been identified. The classic delta wave and short PR interval are seen with a Kent bypass which connects the atrium and ventricle outside the AV node. Unlike PSVT with a concealed Kent bundle, conduction during tachycardia may be antegrade or retrograde. James fibers connect the atrium with the bundle of His, completely bypassing the AV node. As a result the PR interval is shortened. There is, however, no delta wave, and the QRS complex is therefore normal. The Mahaim pathway connects the AV node to the ventricles by a shorter pathway than the normal conducting system (Fig 8-9). This results in a normal PR interval (the AV node is not bypassed) and a QRS complex with a delta wave (Fig 8-8). Kent fibers can be divided further into type A and type B. Type A fibers originate posteriorly, resulting in an upright delta wave and QRS with early depolarization of the left ventricle, whereas type B fibers originate anteriorly and produce a negative delta wave and QRS in leads $V_1$ and $V_2$. As a result, WPW may mimic right or left bundle branch block or a posterior wall myocardial infarction.

Reentry accounts for 80% of the tachycardias associated with WPW, and atrial fibrillation and flutter account for the remaining 20%. The tachycardia is often initiated by a premature atrial contraction or by a rapid sinus rate. Therefore, a trauma patient with sinus tachycardia and an anomalous pathway may develop an extremely rapid WPW tachycardia. WPW is also associated with Epstein's anomaly (atrialization of the right ventricle) as well as atrial and ventricular septal defects, although 70% of all WPW patients have no associated cardiac defects.

When ventricular rate is above 200 and hemodynamic compromise is present, cardioversion is the treatment of choice.

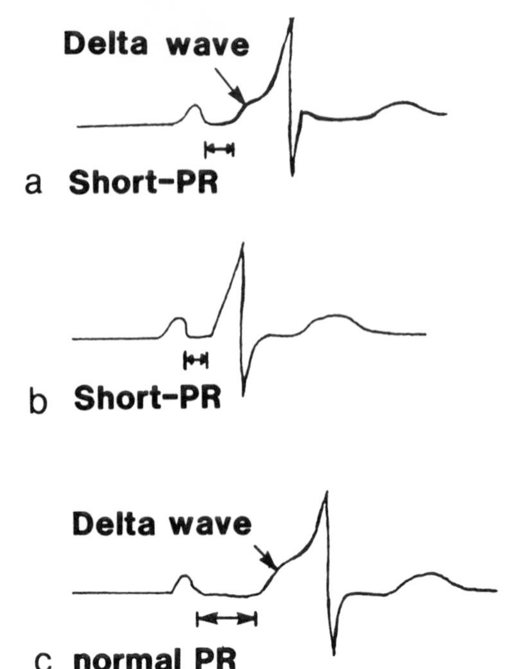


FIG. 8-8. Characteristic ECG of Wolff-Parkinson-White (WPW) syndrome utilizing (a) Kent bundle, (b) James fiber, (c) Mahaim pathway.

FIG. 8-9. A representation of the three types of pathways found in WPW: a Kent bundle, which connects the atrium to the ventricle outside the AV node; a James bundle, which bypasses the AV node by connecting the atrium with His bundle fibers; and the Mahaim pathway, which connects the distal AV node directly to the ventricles bypassing the ventricular conducting system.

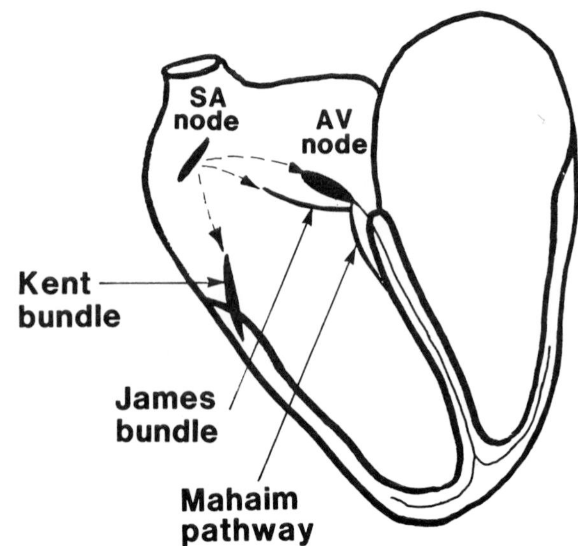

Verapamil, β-blockers, and lidocaine may all be used in the treatment of WPW. However, they are contraindicated when there is associated atrial flutter or fibrillation. All of these drugs decrease the refractory period of the accessory pathway, may increase the ventricular response, and may even precipitate ventricular fibrillation.[191] In this setting, procainamide is the treatment of choice.

VENTRICULAR TACHYCARDIA. Ventricular tachycardia is defined as three or more consecutive premature ventricular contractions. The QRS complex is wide, and there are no P waves. The ventricular rate is between 100 and 220 beats per minute. Many times it is impossible to differentiate between supraventricular and ventricular tachycardia. In hemodynamically stable patients, a vagal maneuver (eg, carotid compression) can be performed to slow the heart rate and thereby differentiate between the two. This is important because verapamil, which is frequently used in SVT, is ineffective and may even aggravate ventricular tachycardia.[207] The most common cause of ventricular tachycardia is ischemic heart disease. Other etiologies include valvular heart disease, myocarditis, cardiomyopathies, hypoxia, hypercapnia, hypokalemia, and hypomagnesemia. The underlying cause should be corrected whenever possible. Cardiac contusion may also result in ventricular tachycardia, although several series did not specifically report its occurrence.[187,195,196,209,215] The overall incidence of myocardial contusion in blunt chest trauma is between 15 and 75%,[217] and PVCs occur in some of these patients[215] (Table 8-18).

Treatment depends on the hemodynamic state of the patient. In hemodynamically stable patients, lidocaine is the treatment of choice. Intravenous procainamide or bretylium can be used if lidocaine is unsuccessful. In hemodynamically unstable patients, cardioversion is attempted.

TORSADES DE POINTES. Torsades de pointes presents as ventricular tachycardia with QRS complexes of varying amplitude and axis (Fig 8-10). It is an unstable arrhythmia, spontaneously converting to sinus rhythm or degenerating to ventricular fibrillation. It is often associated with the antiarrhythmic agents quinidine and procainamide and the presence of mitral valve prolapse, myocarditis, hypokalemia, hypomagnesemia, or hypocalcemia.[219] Torsades de pointes also occurs after ligation of the cervical sympathetic trunk and the vagus during right radical neck dissection.[205] It is thought to result from an imbalance between right and left autonomic input to the heart. Thus, disruption of the right vagus nerve by trauma to the neck or chest may theoretically result in torsades de pointes, although there have not been any reported cases. Treatment involves overdrive pacing and correction of electrolyte abnormalities; if the rhythm degenerates into ventricular fibrillation, cardioversion must be performed.

TABLE 8-18. Initial ECG Abnormalities in 36 of 300 Patients Who Presented with Blunt Chest Trauma*

| ARRHYTHMIA | NO. OF PATIENTS |
|---|---|
| Nonspecific ST and T wave changes | 18 |
| Sinus tachycardia | 17 |
| Premature atrial contractions | 2 |
| Premature ventricular contractions | 9 |
| Heart block | 11 |
| Left anterior hemiblock | 2 |
| Right bundle branch block | 3 |
| 2° atrioventricular block | 2 |
| 1° atrioventricular block | 1 |
| Intraventricular conduction defect | 2 |
| Left bundle branch block | 1 |
| Ischemic changes | 5 |

* (From Snow et al[215] with permission.)

### *Bradyarrhythmias*

Bradyarrhythmias are common in the trauma patient and can result in life-threatening hypotension. Direct trauma to the heart may cause complete heart block[215]; trauma to the neck or eyes, in particular retrobulbar hematoma, may produce vagal stimulation; while head trauma with increased intracranial pressure (ICP) may result in sinus bradycardia associated with Cushing's reflex.[197,199,200] Acute compression of the spinal cord may also result in bradyarrhythmias and even sinus arrest,[194] whereas a pacemaker may malfunction secondary to the traumatic event. Bradyarrhythmias are divided into three categories: sinus bradycardia, junctional rhythm, and complete heart block; the last will be considered in a later section.

SINUS BRADYCARDIA. Sinus bradycardia may be normal; secondary to head, neck, or chest trauma; or due to β-blockers. Severe hemorrhage immediately after trauma may also produce paradoxic bradycardia instead of tachycardia. These patients usually remain conscious but hypotensive.[186] If a slow heart rate is not associated with hypotension, no treat-

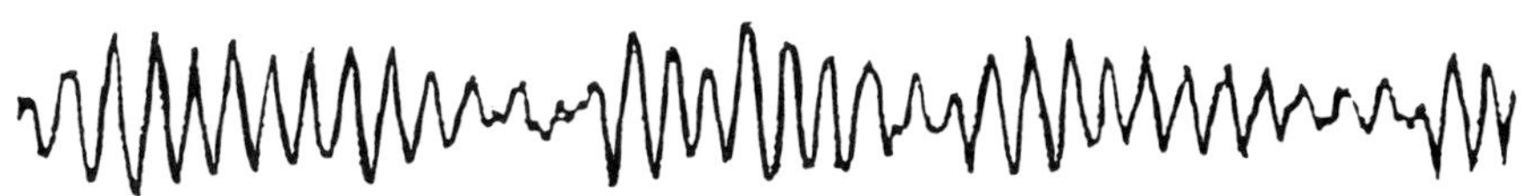

FIG. 8-10. Ventricular tachycardia (upper tracing) compared with torsades de pointes (lower tracing). Note the characteristic QRS complexes of varying amplitude and axis in torsades de pointes.

ment is required. If, however, hypotension is present, either from the bradycardia itself or secondary to blood loss, treatment is indicated. Paradoxical bradycardia should be treated with rapid and vigorous volume loading; administration of atropine may be fraught with the danger of ventricular fibrillation.[186] If the bradycardia results from causes other than severe hemorrhage, atropine (0.01 to 0.02 mg/kg) is the drug of choice. Isoproterenol or epinephrine (1 to 4 μg/min, intravenously) may be tried if atropine fails, although isoproterenol may produce vasodilatation in the hypovolemic patient, resulting in accentuated hypotension. If the heart rate fails to respond to these measures, external pacing or insertion of a temporary transvenous pacemaker is indicated.

JUNCTIONAL BRADYCARDIA. Junctional bradycardia results from suppression of the SA node with a resulting escape rhythm. Thus, the rhythm originates in the AV node or the ventricular conduction system. The resulting P waves may be lost in the QRS or occur in inverted from following the QRS. If central venous pressure (CVP) monitoring is in place, diagnostic Cannon A waves, resulting from contraction of the atrium against a closed AV valve, will be noted. Junctional bradycardia is at times a result of contusion in and around the SA node; however, this rhythm is usually caused by inhalational anesthetic agents. Treatment, if required, consists of atropine or decreasing the anesthetic concentration. If hypotension and bradycardia persist despite treatment, pacing may be required.

### *Conduction Defects*

Conduction defects in the young trauma victim are more likely to be caused by the trauma than by preexisting cardiac disease. They may be seen after chest trauma complicated by myocardial contusion or penetrating injury to the coronary arteries.[215] In one case at our institution, a 24-year-old patient who presented with a stab wound to the chest had a lacerated left anterior descending artery with a resulting ECG pattern of left bundle branch block. Autonomic dysfunction after closed-head injury may also result in acute myocardial infarction that may cause conduction defects as well as ventricular arrhythmias.[197,199,200,218] Of concern to the anesthesiologist are which conduction defects require pacing and the possible effect of pulmonary artery catheterization on the conduction defect.

FIRST-DEGREE HEART BLOCK. First-degree heart block is characterized by a PR interval greater than 0.2 second. It is caused by ischemic heart disease; chronic degenerative changes of the conduction system; myocarditis; the increased vagal tone associated with neck, eye, and head injuries; digoxin toxicity; and anesthetic agents. It is usually asymptomatic and requires no treatment; if treatment is needed, however, atropine is the drug of choice.

SECOND-DEGREE HEART BLOCK. Second-degree AV block is characterized by progressive prolongation of the PR interval or a sudden dropped beat. It is most likely to be encountered in the elderly trauma patient with chronic degenerative changes in the AV node or the His-Purkinje conduction system. Patients with acute myocardial contusion may also develop this conduction abnormality.

Second-degree heart block can be divided into type I (Wenckebach) and type II blocks (Fig 8-11). Type I block is characterized by a progressive prolongation of the PR interval and ultimately a dropped QRS complex. Wenckebach block is caused by delayed conduction through the AV node. No treatment is required since it is a stable arrhythmia and unlikely to degrade into complete heart block. Pacing is indicated only if the patient is symptomatic. Type II block, however, is caused by changes in the His-Purkinje conduction system and is a precursor of third-degree heart block. This type of second-degree heart block requires placement of a pacemaker either preoperatively or intraoperatively.

BIFASCICULAR BLOCK. A bifascicular block is defined as a left bundle branch block or a right bundle branch block associated with a block of one of the fascicles of the left bundle branch. Right bundle branch block associated with left anterior hemiblock is the most common bifascicular block, occurring in about 1% of the adult population.

Concern has arisen about the possibility of spontaneous or anesthesia- and surgery-induced conversion of bifascicular block to complete heart block. Available data suggest that conversion of any nontraumatic bifascicular block to complete heart block is unlikely.[192,204,211,212] Anesthesia or surgery also does not seem to increase this risk.[206,208] Therefore, these patients do not seem to require prophylactic pacemaker insertion unless the conduction defect is associated with a history of syncopal episodes. This statement, however, may not apply to patients with combined chronic bifascicular block and first-degree heart block, evidence of trifascicular disease, or trauma-induced acute bifascicular block. Physiologic aberrations produced by trauma and surgery may lead to complete heart block in these patients. Thus, pacing capability in the form of an external pacemaker, transvenous pacemaker, or a pacing pulmonary artery catheter must be available.

Right bundle branch block develops in 8% of patients dur-

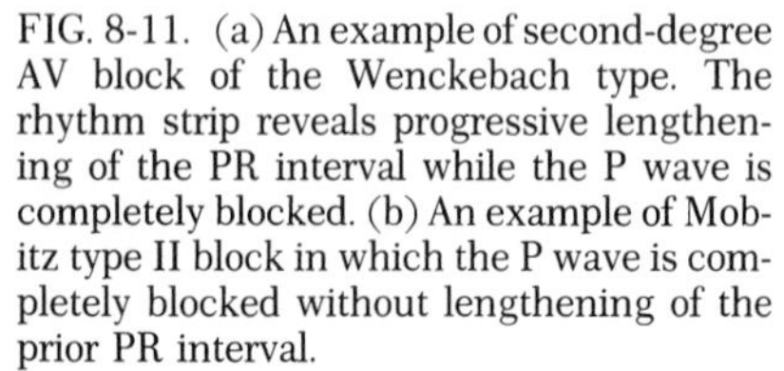

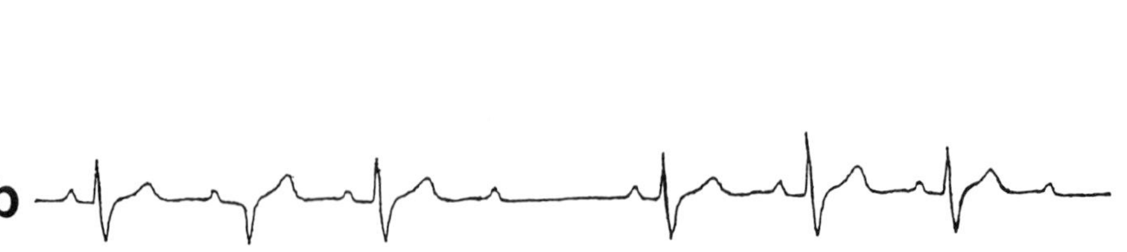


FIG. 8-11. (a) An example of second-degree AV block of the Wenckebach type. The rhythm strip reveals progressive lengthening of the PR interval while the P wave is completely blocked. (b) An example of Mobitz type II block in which the P wave is completely blocked without lengthening of the prior PR interval.

ing pulmonary artery catheterization.[216] Available data suggest that the incidence of complete heart block during passage of this catheter in patients with preexisting left bundle branch block varies between 0%[216] and 1%.[185,190,193,213] Thus, complete heart block during this procedure is rare, but its consequences are grave, necessitating prevention or capacity for immediate treatment if it occurs. Prophylactic insertion of a transvenous pacemaker prior to pulmonary artery catheterization or of a pacing pulmonary artery catheter may be considered. Another, and probably more reasonable, approach is to place an external pacemaker in order to initiate pacing if complete heart block develops. Although these pacemakers are reliable and capture at all times, it is prudent to have equipment ready for transvenous pacemaker insertion.

COMPLETE HEART BLOCK. Complete heart block is an absolute indication for pacemaker insertion. If the AV node is blocked, the QRS complexes are narrow, and the heart rate is 45 to 55 beats per minute. If the block occurs below the AV node, QRS complexes are wide, with a rate of 30 to 40 beats per minute. The causes of complete heart block include chronic degenerative changes of the conduction system, coronary heart disease, cardiomyopathies, myocarditis, increased vagal tone, digitalis toxicity, β-blockers, and hyperkalemia. It is possible that acute complete heart block can occur following trauma as a result of cardiac contusion, increased vagal tone, or hyperkalemia during massive blood transfusion in the hypovolemic and hypothermic patient. Lidocaine should not be used to treat the wide QRS complexes of a complete heart block since it will slow the rate further.

### *Ectopic Beats*

Ectopic beats are of three types: premature atrial contractions, premature junctional contractions, and premature ventricular contractions. Premature atrial contractions are usually of no significance and do not require treatment. Junctional arrhythmias have already been discussed. They usually do not require treatment unless the patient is hemodynamically unstable and requires a faster heart rate or atrial function is needed to maintain cardiac output.

Premature ventricular contractions arise from an ectopic focus below the AV node. The QRS complex is wide and often bizarre in appearance. PVCs are associated with coronary artery disease, hypoxia, hypercapnia, cardiac contusion, and inadequate anesthetic depth. Hypokalemia should be suspected in any trauma patient with PVCs since it is a common electrolyte abnormality in this setting.[214] Treatment should be started if the PVCs are multifocal in origin, if there are more than five PVCs per minute, or if they occur on the ascending aspect of the prior T wave. Lidocaine and procainamide are the drugs of choice. If the extrasystoles are escape beats resulting from a slow sinus rate, they should be treated with atropine or overdrive pacing.

### *Electrical-Mechanical Dissociation (EMD)*

EMD is characterized by normal cardiac electrical activity with no generation of blood pressure. Patients with massive trauma or seemingly minor chest injury may present with EMD. Other causes in the trauma patient are massive bleeding, hypocalcemia, tension pneumothorax, acute hemorrhagic pericardial tamponade, and inhalation anesthetic overdose. In all of these conditions venous return and ventricular output are compromised. Treatment should be initiated immediately and requires identifying the etiology. Treatment of the underlying cause may restore the cardiac output and be lifesaving. Of course, cardiopulmonary resuscitation should initiated promptly upon recognition of EMD.

## CORONARY ARTERY DISEASE

It is reasonable to assume that trauma victims older than 50 have some degree of coronary artery disease (CAD) and may develop myocardial ischemia or even infarction under the stress of trauma and surgery. Acute ischemia may lead to myocardial dysfunction and further compromise organ perfusion and oxygenation.

Myocardial function deteriorates when its $O_2$ demand exceeds its $O_2$ supply. The main determinants of $O_2$ demand are heart rate, myocardial wall tension, and contractility. Tachycardia not only increases $O_2$ demand, but also decreases left ventricular perfusion because only a short period of time is available for diastolic filling of the coronary vessels. Wall tension, a product of intraventricular pressure and ventricular radius, increases in the dilated failing ventricle and thus exacerbates myocardial ischemia; the larger the ventricle, the higher the wall tension and the $O_2$ demand. In these patients decreasing ventricular size with inotropes or reducing preload with nitroglycerine may diminish the $O_2$ requirement provided that the beneficial effect of decreased heart size outweighs the effect of the increased myocardial contractility produced by the inotropes or any decrease in perfusion pressure caused by the capacitance vessel dilator.

Myocardial $O_2$ supply also has several determinants. Overall myocardial blood flow is proportional to the driving pressure and inversely proportional to the coronary resistance. The driving pressure is often referred to as the coronary perfusion pressure and is calculated, for the subendocardium, as the difference between diastolic blood pressure and left ventricular end diastolic pressure (LVEDP) or pulmonary capillary wedge pressure (PCWP). For the calculation of intramural and epicardial coronary perfusion pressure, the right atrial pressure is subtracted from the aortic diastolic pressure. This gives only a rough estimate of the driving pressure, which actually is not constant since changes in left ventricular pressure occur throughout diastole. In addition, this calculation does not take into account changes in coronary vascular resistance during the cardiac cycle. Coronary resistance may be affected by locally released metabolic mediators such as adenosine, autoregulation, various drugs, neural factors, and the mechanical effect of ventricular contraction on myocardial blood vessels. As to the last factor, greater extraluminal compression is exerted on subendocardial than on epicardial vessels during ventricular systole.

Factors that increase the risk of myocardial ischemia in the trauma patient with CAD are anemia, tachycardia, hypertension, and hypotension. Thus, the goals of anesthetic management are as follows.

CONTROL OF THE HEART RATE. Myocardial oxygen demand can be limited by maintaining a relatively slow heart rate. Although exact values of optimal heart rate are difficult to state, and factors such as coexisting valvular heart disease may alter the "ideal" rate for a given patient, a range between 50 and 70 beats per minute in the patient with sinus rhythm is generally recommended. Pain, anxiety, light anesthesia, hypovolemia, anemia, acidosis, and hypoxia are major causes of tachycardia in the acute trauma victim and should be treated aggressively. Often, increasing anesthetic depth and/or restoring blood volume is sufficient to reduce the heart rate to normal levels, although β-adrenergic blocking agents may be used if tachycardia persists, provided the patient is otherwise hemodynamically stable. Frequently these patients may be taking medications that offset the hemodynamic response to trauma; most notably, a β-blocker may prevent tachycardia, resulting in a marked decrease in systemic blood pressure and tissue perfusion in the acutely hypovolemic and anemic patient.

ADEQUATE OXYGEN-CARRYING CAPACITY. Maximal extraction of $O_2$ by the heart and the limited period of left ventricular perfusion (only during diastole) necessitate adequate blood $O_2$-carrying capacity to prevent myocardial ischemia. In addition, anemia imposes an increased workload on the heart, since the main compensatory response to a low hematocrit is an increase in cardiac output. Although optimal tissue oxygenation occurs at a hematocrit of 30 in healthy individuals, hematocrit may be maintained between 30 and 35 if CAD is present.

MAINTENANCE OF ADEQUATE BLOOD PRESSURE. Although mean arterial pressure is an important determinant of optimal tissue perfusion, adequate diastolic blood pressure must be provided to maintain normal myocardial perfusion. Thus, hypotension, whether it is caused by hemorrhage or by ischemic myocardial dysfunction, should be treated aggressively using fluids, vasopressors, or both. The blood pressure must be maintained within the patient's normal range. It is often difficult to ascertain what the normal pressure is, especially if the trauma victim is unconscious and/or intoxicated. If reliable information cannot be obtained from the patient or his/her relatives or friends, the blood pressure should be maintained at levels appropriate for the victim's age. Alternatively, in normovolemic patients with normal pulse rate, blood pressure can be adjusted to levels that provide adequate urine output and prevent ischemic changes on the ECG (Fig 8-12).

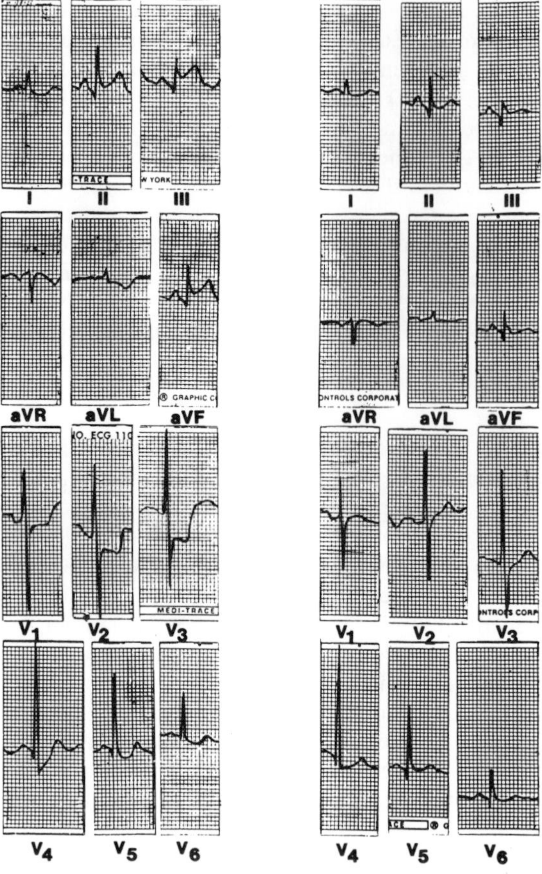


FIG. 8-12. A 47-year-old sailor with a history of previous angioplasty but continuing stable angina required exploratory laparotomy 2 days after blunt abdominal trauma. Postoperatively, he developed hypotension (90/70 mm Hg) with concomitant ischemic ST segment changes. Systemic blood pressure was raised to 110/80 mm Hg with aggressive fluid administration, but ST segment changes persisted despite adequate cardiac output ($\dot{Q}_t$) and pulmonary wedge pressure (PWP). Nitroglycerine infusion (40 μg/min) was started without significant improvement of ischemic ECG changes (left panel). Increasing blood pressure to 130/70 mm Hg with neosynephrine infusion (25 μg/min) resulted in an abrupt normalization of ST segment elevation.

Thus, detection of myocardial ischemia by ECG and/or other means is of great importance in these patients. Although optimal electrode placement may be limited by the surgical procedure, ECG monitoring with at least two simultaneous leads will permit detection of myocardial ischemia in most instances. Lead 2 provides good P wave morphology and monitors ischemic events in the inferior wall, and the $V_5$ lead detects such changes in the anterolateral wall. Of the bipolar leads, $CC_5$ is used for anterolateral and $CM_5$ for anteroinferior wall monitoring. For $CC_5$ the positive lead is placed in the $V_5$ position and the negative lead in the right $V_5$ position, whereas for $CM_5$ the positive lead is at $V_5$, and the negative lead is at the manubrium. Lead ML, which requires placement of the positive lead at the left iliac crest and the negative lead at the manubrium, may be used to monitor inferior wall ischemia. Whenever possible, three simultaneous leads (2, $V_4$, $V_5$) should be used, which appears to be superior to two-lead monitoring.[240a]

Transesophageal echocardiography has been used to detect intraoperative myocardial ischemia[226,237,250] and infarction and to assess mitral regurgitation,[247–249] chorda tendinae rupture,[247] and aortic stenosis.[233] In the trauma patient it may prove to be a useful monitor as it permits intraoperative evaluation of ventricular function and valvular disease, especially when little time is available for preoperative workup.

An ischemia-induced decrease in left ventricular compliance may cause a significant increase in PCWP. Additionally, papillary muscle dysfunction in an ischemic heart may result in the acute appearance of V waves on the PCWP trace, suggesting left ventricular abnormality. Thus, monitoring of left ventricular function with a pulmonary artery (PA) catheter offers important advantages in patients with CAD, especially in those with left ventricular dysfunction.

### *Anesthetic Techniques*

REGIONAL ANESTHESIA. Regional anesthesia enables the patient to communicate about his or her chest pain and eliminates the tachycardia, hypotension, and hypertension that may result from general anesthesia, especially during induction. Although this anesthetic technique may be preferable in patients with CAD, its indications are limited to extremity surgery. In addition, central blockade may lead to hypotension and thus decreased coronary perfusion in hypovolemic patients. Addition of a regional technique to general anesthesia may reduce the frequency of perioperative ischemic episodes,[255a] but a clear benefit from this technique has not yet been demonstrated.

GENERAL ANESTHESIA. Prospective randomized studies comparing various anesthesia techniques in trauma patients with or without CAD are lacking. Experience gained from nontrauma patients undergoing cardiac or noncardiac surgery suggests that opioids, benzodiazepines, neuroleptics, and muscle relaxants may all be used safely, provided that they are carefully titrated to patient response. Addition of titrated doses of inhalational agents, in the absence of myocardial failure or shock, prevents the hypertensive and tachycardic response to surgery and may be beneficial in patients with CAD. There are, however, some controversies about the use of isoflurane in this setting. "Coronary steal" phenomenon has been demonstrated in a dog model with this anesthetic,[222] but the significance of this phenomenon in humans is questionable. Moreover the significance of coronary steal in dogs is unclear since myocardial ischemia did not result from this phenomenon in another study.[252] In humans given 1% isoflurane there is a decrease in blood pressure and an increase in heart rate which may be associated with ECG evidence of myocardial ischemia,[246] but there is also a suggestion that this anesthetic prevents myocardial ischemia in certain situations.[231,244,251] On the other hand, in the presence of decreased blood pressure and increased heart rate, as may be seen in trauma patients, isoflurane should be avoided because the hemodynamic changes produced by this agent may increase the risk of myocardial ischemia. Although still a subject of controversy, a combination of opioids and low doses (up to 1% inspired concentration) of isoflurane probably does not increase the risk of myocardial ischemia if significant blood pressure and heart rate changes do not occur. Enflurane and halothane can be used in patients without left ventricular failure, although neither anesthetic is indicated in hypovolemic patients, and halothane is probably better avoided if β-sympathomimetic agents are infused.

Nitrous oxide limits the concentration of inspired oxygen and thus exacerbates the hypoxemia of trauma patients who have sustained pulmonary complications such as aspiration pneumonitis, lung contusion, and smoke inhalation. It has also been suggested that this agent may predispose to myocardial ischemia when combined with other inhalation agents,[241,242] although according to other findings such an effect is unlikely.[232] Nitrous oxide with high-dose fentanyl has also been shown to compromise left ventricular performance in coronary artery bypass surgery,[241] but more recent studies have failed to demonstrate impairment of left ventricular function or of myocardial oxygenation.[224]

Given the controversies over the safety of various anesthetics in CAD and the wide variability in severity of both traumatic injury and CAD and in the extent of preoperative optimization of these conditions, it is difficult to recommend a specific anesthetic technique for these patients. However, based on available knowledge, the following approach may be used as a guideline.

*Induction of Anesthesia.* Whether CAD is present or not, anesthesia should be induced only after adequate fluid resuscitation, oxygenation, and monitoring. Anesthetic induction should be modified according to the type of trauma, degree of hypovolemia, urgency of tracheal intubation, and any anticipated difficulty of airway management. In the absence of hypovolemia or airway compromise, sufficient doses of intravenous anesthetic, opioids, and muscle relaxants are necessary to prevent a hypertensive and tachycardic response to intubation. Among intravenous anesthetics, ketamine probably should be avoided in the normovolemic trauma victim with CAD, since it increases myocardial oxygen demand. On the other hand, in moderately hypovolemic patients, a ketamine-muscle relaxant combination may theoretically relieve ischemia by elevating the blood pressure. Thus, its use should be individualized based on the hemodynamic condition of the patient, the severity of CAD, and other prevailing circumstances. Some evidence obtained from patients undergoing coronary artery bypass surgery suggests that the combination of ketamine and diazepam used for induction and maintenance of anesthesia may be associated with less postoperative hypotension, less requirement for vasopressor therapy, and lower fluid requirement than a high-dose fentanyl technique.[234,238,239,254] However, it is difficult to extrapolate these results to the trauma patient with CAD.

*Maintenance of Anesthesia.* Any agent can be used for maintenance of anesthesia provided it is carefully titrated to prevent significant deviations of blood pressure and heart rate from normal. In practice, this goal is usually achieved by combined use of opioids and low concentrations of potent inhalation agents. Potent inhalation agents should be avoided if hypovolemia exists or abnormal ventricular function is suspected or documented preoperatively.

β-Adrenergic blocking agents can be used to control heart rate and thus decrease myocardial $O_2$ requirement. Calcium channel blockers may also decrease myocardial $O_2$ requirement by reducing myocardial contractility and by causing a slight decrease in heart rate. Diltiazem (0.15 mg/kg followed by 3 μg/kg/min intravenously) may protect the myocardium against myocardial ischemia.[230] However, these agents may augment the myocardial depression produced by inhalational agents.[235,255] Experimental evidence suggests that the myocardial depression produced by calcium channel blockers may be reversed by glucagon[256] or calcium.[240] Glucagon may also be used to treat β-blockade-induced hypotension, which also results from myocardial depression.[225,229,245]

Nitroglycerine is frequently used because of its vasodilator effect on both the coronary arteries and the systemic circulation. In hemodynamically stable patients, the dose of nitroglycerine which provides adequate myocardial protection is at least 1 μg/kg/min; lower doses appear to offer little benefit.[228,253] Nitroglycerine should probably be used prophylactically, as well as therapeutically, since there is a relatively high probability that evidence of myocardial ischemia may be absent or delayed on the ECG monitor and because once ischemia occurs, ventricular dysfunction may persist even after treatment.[220] Nitroglycerine has also been used to treat coronary artery spasm.[223,227] Thus it is reasonable to combine this drug with a calcium channel blocker such as nifedipine[227,236] or verapamil[243] when ischemic ECG changes occur without hemodynamic alteration and when spasm is felt to be a likely cause of ischemia. Obviously, nitroglycerine or nifedipine should be avoided if hypotension is present.

*Postoperative Course.* The trachea should be extubated after ensuring that the patient is hemodynamically stable, there is no residual muscle relaxation, and spontaneous breathing will suffice for adequate oxygenation and ventilation. A postoperative ECG is obtained and compared with the preoperative tracing to rule out ischemic myocardial changes. It should be noted that some changes in T wave morphology may develop postoperatively for reasons other than myocardial ischemia.[221] However, trauma patients who have had an unstable hemodynamic course in the operating room should probably be managed postoperatively as patients at high risk of myocardial infarction; nitrate therapy and heart rate control should be continued throughout the recovery period and for the first 3 postoperative days, and these measures should be discontinued only gradually after myocardial infarction is ruled out.

## CONGESTIVE HEART FAILURE

The stress of trauma is usually fairly well tolerated by young patients with good cardiopulmonary reserve. By comparison, patients with underlying heart failure tolerate this stress poorly. Identification of patients with underlying left ventricular dysfunction is usually difficult following acute injury. On the other hand, the early management of the major trauma patient with massive hemorrhage is the same whatever preexisting condition he or she may have: fluid resuscitation and surgical hemostasis. It is in the trauma patient with relatively stable hemodynamics that knowledge of the cardiac status helps the anesthesiologist to make appropriate changes in the anesthetic plan in order to optimize cardiac function and avoid perioperative pulmonary edema.

During preoperative assessment, the patient with congestive heart failure (CHF) may give a history of heart disease or symptoms of left ventricular dysfunction such as easy fatigability, dyspnea at rest or with minimal exertion, pulmonary edema, orthopnea, paroxysmal nocturnal dyspnea, and/or nocturia. If biventricular failure is present, signs of right ventricular dysfunction such as hepatic congestion and pedal edema may also be noted. Physical examination may demonstrate rales, heart murmur, $S_3$ or $S_4$ gallop, jugular venous distension, and a laterally displaced point of maximal impulse. These signs may be difficult to detect in the trauma patient who is tachycardic, hypovolemic, and has pulmonary abnormalities. A chest radiogram may reveal cardiomegaly, pulmonary venous congestion with Kerley B lines, and pleural effusion; but again, in the acutely injured, they may be interpreted as trauma-induced changes. The ECG may show nonspecific changes, ischemic ST or T wave abnormality, evidence of previous myocardial infarction, or a variety of dysrhythmias, conduction abnormalities, abnormal axes, or atrial enlargement. Echocardiography may be very useful as it reveals dilated cardiac chambers or ventricular wall dyskinesis, although it is rarely possible to obtain this study during the rapid preoperative assessment of the trauma victim.

CHF may be a result of valvular abnormalities or myocardial dysfunction. In some valvular lesions CHF may occur even in the absence of impaired left ventricular contractility. For example, tachycardia after trauma decreases diastolic filling time and thus may precipitate pulmonary edema in patients who have mitral stenosis with little myocardial dysfunction. Heart failure resulting from impaired myocardial contractility can be divided into two categories: diastolic dysfunction and systolic dysfunction. Each of these occurs by different mechanisms and can best be appreciated by examining the ventricular pressure-volume loops shown in Fig 8-13. CHF associated with diastolic dysfunction is characteristic of hypertrophic cardiomyopathy and pericardial disease, in which ventricular filling occurs at a high end-diastolic pressure. Systolic dysfunction occurs when ventricular contractility diminishes because of myocardial ischemia, infarction, or degeneration (myocarditis or cardiomyopathy) and results in decreased pump function. This discussion will focus mainly on the most commonly seen form of CHF, systolic dysfunction, and particularly on its effects on management of the acutely injured patient.

The ventricle with systolic dysfunction can respond to increasing preload by increasing its output although at a smaller magnitude than a normal ventricle (Fig. 8-14). The failing ventricle, however, cannot tolerate the stress of increased systemic vascular resistance (SVR), and its output decreases[262] (Fig 8-15). Thus, in acute trauma the reflex increase in afterload caused by hypovolemia, anemia, pain, hypotension, or hypertension places a major strain on the failing heart and causes a substantial decrease of its output. CHF may become clinically apparent in the trauma patient with underlying systolic dysfunction at any time from admission to the postoperative period, depending on the degree of preexisting ventricular dysfunction and the severity of the physiologic disturbances produced by the injury. Consequently, its treatment requires measures that directly affect cardiac contractility and output as well as interventions to reduce or minimize

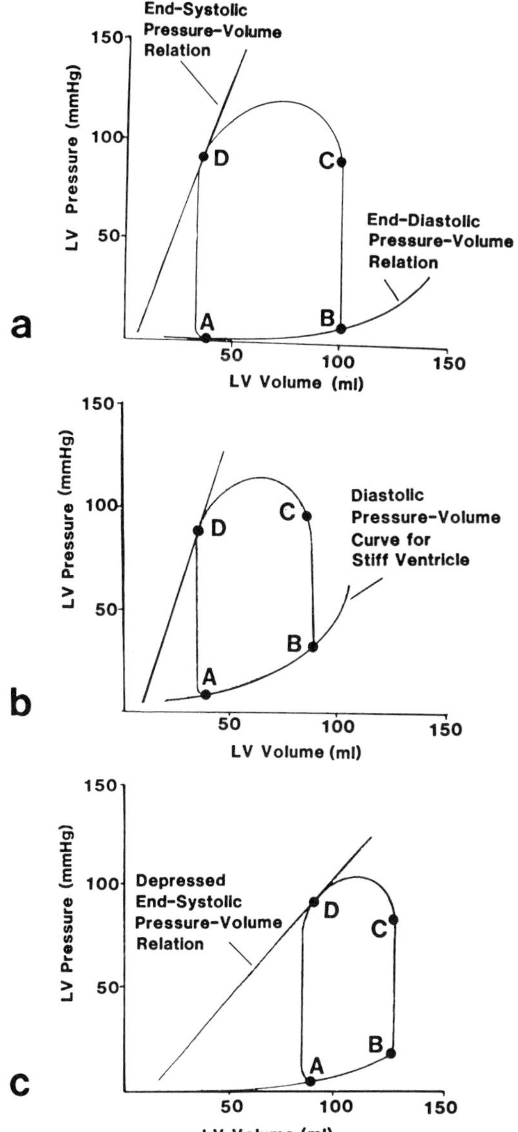


FIG. 8-13. Left ventricular pressure-volume loops in the normal heart (a), and in the heart with diastolic dysfunction (b), and systolic dysfunction (c). In the normal heart, diastolic filling begins at point A (mitral valve opening) and continues until point B (mitral valve closure), where isovolemic contraction begins. At point C, isovolemic contraction ends, the aortic valve opens, and left ventricular ejection ensues. This is accompanied by a further increase in left ventricular pressure and a steady decrease in left ventricular volume. As left ventricular volume decreases, the pressure also starts to decline (after an initial rise) to point D at which the aortic valve closes, isovolemic relaxation begins, and left ventricular pressure decreases abruptly until point A when the mitral valve reopens. In this loop, point B represents the end-diastolic pressure-volume relation. Point D (aortic valve closure) represents the end-systolic pressure-volume relation. If this loop were constructed for different end-systolic volumes, the slope of the line uniting point D of each loop would reflect contractility (normal 1.7 mm Hg/mL/m$^2$). The pressure-volume loop in diastolic dysfunction (b) differs from the normal curve in that end-diastolic pressure is elevated (point B) without a concomitant increase in the end-diastolic volume. In systolic dysfunction, diastolic filling begins at a larger ventricular volume although the volume increase is not associated with an increase in ventricular end-systolic pressure (c). The slope of the tangent to point D and thus, myocardial contractility, is decreased as compared with normal.

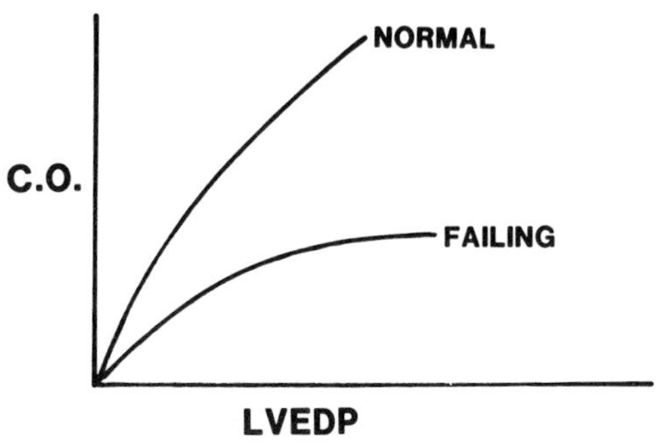


FIG. 8-14. Cardiac output (C.O.) in the failing ventricle, as in the normal ventricle, increases by increasing left ventricular end-diastolic pressure (LVEDP). The difference from the normal ventricle is the magnitude of increase. For a given LVEDP, cardiac output increases less in the failing than in the normal ventricle.

trauma-induced physiologic disturbances. For example, in a patient with multiple fractures but small blood loss, vasoconstriction and hypertension caused by pain may be the factors precipitating cardiac failure. Control of pain and/or use of vasodilators may be sufficient to decrease SVR and thus to improve cardiac function in this patient. On the other hand, in a patient with major blood loss, resuscitative efforts with acellular fluids may fail despite adequate replacement because the failing heart may be unable to increase its output, a normal compensatory response to acute anemia.

Once CHF develops, several other responses to resuscitation may be lacking. The failing heart maintains its output in part by increasing its rate. Thus, tachycardia in the trauma patient with CHF may continue despite adequate resuscitation and treatment of other causes that result in this abnormality. As a result, to base fluid resuscitation on the heart rate may lead to overt pulmonary edema. Urine output may also not increase with fluid resuscitation in these patients. Nevertheless, preexisting CHF is not the only possible reason for the trauma patient's not responding to resuscitation; inadequate volume replacement, right or left ventricular dysfunction because of direct cardiac trauma or pulmonary hypertension,[259] acute tubular necrosis, or urinary tract injury may all be responsible.

Decreased urine output in CHF results primarily from hormonal changes. Elevated levels of vasopressin,[260] renin,[258]

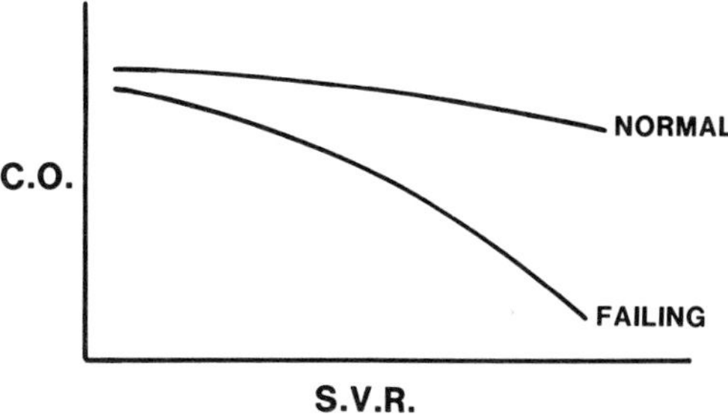


FIG. 8-15. Qualitative relationship of cardiac output (C.O.) and systemic vascular resistance (SVR). A normal heart can tolerate elevations of SVR or afterload because pump function is adequate. The failing heart has poor ability to maintain cardiac output in the face of increasing SVR.

and atrial natriuretic factor (ANF) are variably present in patients with CHF. Renin causes release of angiotensin, a vasoconstrictor that stimulates aldosterone secretion and sodium retention. Angiotensin-converting enzyme inhibitors such as captopril prevent these changes and thus decrease sodium retention. ANF is stimulated by an increase in atrial transmural pressure. Secretion of this factor promotes diuresis and decreases, to a certain extent, the ventricular preload.[257,263,264]

### Anesthetic Goals in the Trauma Patient with CHF

There are four objectives in hemodynamic optimization of the trauma victim with CHF.

PRELOAD RESTORATION. Without adequate intravascular volume neither the normal nor the failing heart can maintain cardiac output. Appropriate amounts of acellular fluids and packed cells should be administered.

AFTERLOAD CONTROL. Blood pressure control with judicious doses of appropriate vasodilators may improve blood flow by unloading the left ventricle (Table 8-19). High blood pressure or increased SVR may be caused by pain; adequate analgesia is as important as afterload manipulation with vasodilators.

HEART RATE CONTROL. As previously mentioned, tachycardia in response to stress, hypovolemia, anemia, or pain decreases diastolic filling time and thus left ventricular perfusion. Together with increased myocardial work, this results in myocardial ischemia in patients with underlying CAD. Extreme tachycardia should be avoided or treated by fluid and blood product resuscitation, appropriate anesthetic depth, and correction of hypotension and metabolic derangements. Rhythm disturbances should be treated with antiarrhythmic therapy as indicated. If tachycardia is a result of CHF, inotropic support may be indicated (Table 20). Myocardial ischemia should also be corrected as it leads to ventricular dysfunction and tachycardia.

MINIMIZING MYOCARDIAL DEPRESSION. Further myocardial depression should be avoided by selecting techniques or drug doses that have the least effect on ventricular performance.

Obviously, appropriate monitoring must be used to recognize the type and severity of failure, to detect its precipitating causes, and to gauge the response to therapy. Since coexisting CAD is frequently present, ECG monitoring should be capable of detecting ischemia (see the section on CAD). Severe blood pressure changes and the need for frequent blood gas determinations in the major trauma patient dictate direct arterial cannulation and Foley catheterization even when CHF is not suspected. Pulmonary artery catheterization enables sequential monitoring of ventricular filling pressures, cardiac output, global oxygen utilization, and titration of fluids and cardioactive drugs. Transesophageal echocardiography may be very useful in this setting since it permits evaluation of ventricular size and wall motion and detection of myocardial ischemia.

### Anesthetic Management

The varying degrees of myocardial depression produced by most anesthetics dictate careful selection and use of these agents when CHF complicates management of any surgical problem, especially severe injury. Because of their profound depressant effect on hemodynamics, inhalational agents should probably be omitted or at most used in very small concentrations. The presence of hypovolemia further complicates the use of anesthetics, particularly those administered intravenously. The doses required to anesthetize animals, and most probably humans too, are decreased by about 35 to 40%.[261,265] This probably results from decreased volume of distribution and preferential distribution of blood flow to the

TABLE 8-19. Vasodilators for Use During Intraoperative and Early Recovery Phases

| DRUG | DOSAGE | ACTION | COMMENTS |
|---|---|---|---|
| Nitroprusside | 0.25 to 10 μg/kg/min | Arterial and venous dilatation<br>Direct action on vessels | May cause reflex tachycardia<br>Tachyphylaxis may occur<br>Cyanide toxicity may occur<br>May impair thyroid uptake of iodine<br>May cause coronary steal |
| Nitroglycerine | 0.25 to 10 μg/kg/min | Mainly venodilator<br>Arteriolar dilatation<br>Direct effect | Reflex may occur<br>Does not cause coronary steal |
| Hydralazine | 2.5 to 20 mg intravenously every 4 to 6 hours<br>20 to 40 mg intramuscularly every 4 to 6 hours | Direct vasodilator<br>More prominent dilator effect on arterioles than on veins | May cause reflex tachycardia<br>Increases cerebral, coronary renal and splanchnic blood flows |
| Trimethaphan | 1 to 4 mg/min | Vasodilatation through ganglionic blockade | Histamine release<br>Tachyphylaxis may occur<br>Potentiates effects of succinylcholine |
| Phentolamine | 2 to 5 mg intravenously | Alpha blockade<br>Mainly arterial dilator | Reflex tachycardia<br>Hypoglycemia |

TABLE 8-20. Commonly Used Inotropic Agents and Their Characteristics

| DRUG | DOSAGE | ACTION | COMMENTS |
|---|---|---|---|
| Dobutamine | 2.5 to 15 μg/kg/min | $\beta_2$-Adrenergic stimulation | Tachycardia, dysrhythmias may cause myocardial ischemia |
| Dopamine | 1 to 3 μg/kg/min dopaminergic<br>5 to 10 μg/kg/min β-effect<br>10 μg/kg/min and above α- and β-stimulation | Dopaminergic stimulation at lower doses, β- and then α-stimulation at higher doses | Tachycardia, hypertension, dysrhythmias |
| Epinephrine | Start at 0.5 to 1 μg/min and increase as needed | Adrenergic stimulation $\beta > \alpha$ at lower doses | May cause dysrhythmias, tachycardia, hypertension |
| Isoproterenol | Start at 1 μg/min and increase as needed | β-Adrenergic stimulation | Dysrhythmias, tachycardia, myocardial ischemia |
| Amrinone | 0.75 to 3 mg/kg loading dose then infusion at 5 to 10 μg/kg/day (start loading dose at 0.75 mg/kg, increase if indicated)<br>Maximum dose, 10 mg/kg/day | Direct effect, possibly in part by phosphodiesterase inhibition. It also improves cardiac output by causing vasodilatation | May cause thrombocytopenia<br>Do not infuse in dextrose-containing solution |

brain. Since there is also preferential blood flow distribution to the heart in hypovolemia, normal doses of intravenous anesthetics produce excessive hemodynamic depression. Thus, they should be used in small amounts and titrated to hemodynamic response rather than giving predetermined fixed doses.

Intraoperatively, depression of cardiac output despite adequate preload can be treated with vasodilators such as nitroprusside. If the intraoperative course is complicated by high filling pressures, nitroglycerine and diuresis may be helpful. Insufficient response to these agents or decreased systemic blood pressure associated with their use is an indication for inotropic support with close hemodynamic monitoring.

Vasoactive agents should be titrated to response in each individual. However, some rough guidelines can be formulated for their use. If fluid resuscitation fails to restore cardiac and urine output despite elevation of PCWP to 15 to 20 mm Hg, sodium nitroprusside can be used to lower systemic vascular resistance and thus increase forward flow, provided that systemic blood pressure remains adequate (Table 8-19). If filling pressures are above 20 mm Hg, a trial of nitroglycerine may improve cardiac output as it reduces the preload and moves the heart to a more optimal portion of the Frank-Starling curve. Simultaneous diuretic therapy may also be instituted if urine output is low. Additional doses of nitroprusside in this situation may improve cardiac performance further by reducing the afterload. Simultaneous control of preload and afterload decreases both systolic and diastolic wall stress. This is important since wall stress is a factor in myocardial oxygen consumption, and a failing dilated heart pumping against an elevated afterload may become ischemic. Nitroglycerine may be given in addition to nitroprusside to promote dilatation of coronary vessels and thus to prevent coronary artery steal, which may be produced by nitroprusside. If response to combined preload and afterload reduction is unsatisfactory or if filling pressures are high despite low systemic blood pressure and cardiac output, an inotrope is indicated (Table 8-20).

There is another approach to fluid and electrolyte therapy in CHF. Instead of hydrating the patient to an arbitrary wedge pressure, cardiac output or left ventricular stroke work index (LVSWI) may be plotted against PCWP before and after a 250- to 500-mL fluid challenge; if the LVSWI increases with only a slight elevation in PCWP, additional fluids may produce further improvement. If, however, PCWP increases without significant LVSWI improvement, further volume repletion is unlikely to be of benefit. In this situation vasodilators and/or inotropes may be indicated.

The postoperative course may be complicated by pulmonary edema as a result of fluid reabsorption from "third-space" losses. Continued invasive monitoring with frequent assessment of hemodynamics and appropriate use of vasodilators, inotropes, and diuretics may be required during the first few postoperative days.

## REFERENCES

### INTRODUCTION

1. Cohen M, Duncan PG, Tate RB. Does anesthesia contribute to operative mortality? JAMA 1988;260:2859.
2. Derrington MC, Smith G. A review of studies of anesthetic risk, morbidity and mortality. Br J Anaesth 1987;59:815.
3. Mackenzie EJ, Morris JA, Edelstein SL. Effect of pre-existing disease on length of hospital stay in trauma patients. J Trauma 1989;29:757.
4. Morris JA, Auerbach PS, Bluth R, Trunkey DD. Pre-injury health: determinant of survival in trauma patients. J Trauma 1986;26:680 (abstr).
5. Morris JA, Mackenzie EJ, Edelstein SL. Effect of pre-existing conditions on mortality in trauma patient. Crit Care Med 1989;17:S145 (abstr).
6. Pederson T, Eliasen K, Ravnborg M, et al. Risk factors, complications and outcome in anaesthesia: a pilot study. Eur J Anaesth 1986;3:225.

### ALCOHOL AND DRUG INTOXICATION

7. Adriani J, Morton RC. Drug dependence: important considerations from the anesthesiologist's viewpoint. Anesth Analg 1968;47:472.
8. Albin MS, Bunegin L. An experimental study of craniocerebral trauma during ethanol intoxication. Crit Care Med 1986;14:841.
9. Altura BM, Altura BT. Microvascular and vascular smooth mus-

cle actions of ethanol, acetaldehyde, and acetate. Fed Proc 1982;41:2447.

10. Baker JL, Kelen GD, Sivertson KT, Quinn TC. Unsuspected human immunodeficiency virus in critically ill emergency patients. JAMA 1987;257:2609.
11. Barash PG, Kopriva CJ, Langou R, et al. Is cocaine a sympathetic stimulant during general anesthesia? JAMA 1980;243:1437.
12. Berkowitz BA, Finck AD, Hynes MD, Ngai SH. Tolerance to nitrous oxide analgesia in rats and mice. Anesthesiology 1979;51:309.
13. Blomqvist S, Thörne J, Elmer O, et al. Early post-traumatic changes in hemodynamics and pulmonary ventilation in alcohol-pretreated pigs. J Trauma 1987;27:40.
14. Brashear RE, Cornog JL, Forney RB. Cardiovascular effects of heroin in the dog. Anesth Analg 1973;52:323.
15. Brodner RA, Van Gilder JC, Collins WF. Experimental spinal cord trauma: potentiation by alcohol. J Trauma 1981;21:124.
16. Brooks SM, Werk EE, Ackerman SJ et al. Adverse effects of phenobarbitol on corticosteroid metabolism in patients with bronchial asthma. N Engl J Med 1972;286:1125.
17. Bruce DL. Alcoholism and anesthesia. Anesth Analg 1983;62:84.
18. Budd RD, Muto JJ, Wong JK. Drugs of abuse found in fatally injured drivers in Los Angeles County. Drug Alcohol Depend 1989;23:153.
19. Busto U, Sellers EM, Naranjo CA, et al. Withdrawal reaction after long-term therapeutic use of benzodiazepines. N Engl J Med 1986;315:854.
20. Cahill GF, Arky RA, Perlman AJ. Diabetes mellitus. In: Rubenstein E, Federman DD, eds. Scientific american medicine. New York: Scientific American, 1987:8.
21. Caldwell T III: Anesthesia for patients with behavioral and environmental disorders. In: Katz J, Benumof J, Kadis LB, eds. Anesthesia and uncommon diseases: pathophysiologic and clinical correlations. 2nd ed. Philadelphia: WB Saunders, 1983:672.
22. Cooperman MT, Davidoff F, Spark R, Pallotta J. Clinical studies of alcoholic ketoacidosis. Diabetes 1974;23:433.
23. Culler DJ. Anesthetic depth and MAC. In: Miller RD, ed. Anesthesia. 2nd ed. New York: Churchill Livingstone, 1986:533.
24. Cyr MG, Wartman SA. The effectiveness of routine screening questions in the detection of alcoholism. JAMA 1988;259:51.
25. Desiderio MA. Effects of acute, oral ethanol on cardiovascular performance before and after experimental blunt cardiac trauma. J Trauma 1987;27:267.
26. Desiderio MA. The potentiation of the response to blunt cardiac trauma by ethanol in dogs. J Trauma 1986;26:467.
27. Eiseman B, Lam RC, Rush B. Surgery on the narcotic addict. Ann Surg 1964;159:748.
28. Epstein RM, Wheeler HO, Frumin MJ, et al. The effect of hypercapnia on estimated hepatic blood, circulating splanchnic blood volume, and hepatic sulfobromophthalein clearance during general anesthesia in man. J Clin Invest 1961;40:592.
29. Flamm ES, Demopoulos HB, Seligman ML, et al. Ethanol potentiation of central nervous system trauma. J Neurosurg 1977;46:328.
30. Freedman DX. The psychopharmacology of hallucinogenic agents. Ann Rev Med 1969;20:409.
31. Friedman IM. Alcohol and unnatural deaths in San Francisco youths. Pediatrics 1985;76:191.
32. Galea G, Davidson RJL. Some haemorheological and haematological effects of alcohol. Scand J Haematol 1983;30:308.
33. Gelman SI. Disturbances in hepatic blood flow during anesthesia and surgery. Arch Surg 1976;111:881.
34. Gerberich SG, Gerberich BK, Fife D, et al. Analyses of the relationship between blood alcohol and nasal breath alcohol concentration: implications for assessment of trauma cases. J Trauma 1989;29:338.
35. Gettler DT, Albritten FF. Effect of alcohol intoxication on the respiratory exchange and mortality rate associated with acute hemorrhage in anesthetized dogs. Ann Surg 1963;158:151.
36. Girre C, Facy F, Lagier G, Dally S. Detection of blood benzodiazepines in injured people: relationship with alcoholism. Drug Alcohol Depend 1988;21:61.
37. Giuffrida JG, Bizzarri DV, Saure AC, Sharoff RL. Anesthetic management of drug abusers. Anesth Analg 1970;49:272.
38. Glassroth J, Adams GD, Schnoll S. The impact of substance abuse on the respiratory system. Chest 1987;91:597.
39. Gold MS, Pottash AC, Sweeney DR, Kleber HD. Opiate withdrawal using clonidine: a safe, effective, and rapid nonopiate treatment. JAMA 1980;243:343.
40. Gregler LL, Mark H. Medical complications of cocaine abuse. N Engl J Med 1986;315:1495.
41. Han YJ, Shiwaku Y, Deery A, et al. Effects of chronic morphine addiction and naloxone on halothane MAC in dogs. Abstracts of scientific papers, Annual meeting of the American Society of Anesthesiologists, New Orleans, Oct 15–19; 1977:737.
42. Haut MF, Cowan DH. The effect of ethanol on haemostatic properties of human blood platelets. Am J Med 1974;56:22.
43. Herve C, Gaillard M, Roujas F, Huguenard P. Alcoholism in polytrauma. J Trauma 1986;26:1123.
44. Huth JF, Maier RV, Simonowitz DA, Herman CM. Effect of acute ethanolism on the hospital course and outcome of injured automobile drivers. J Trauma 1983;23:494.
45. Isner JM, Estes M, Thompson PD, et al. Acute cardiac events temporally related to cocaine abuse. N Engl J Med 1986;315:1438.
46. Jaffe JH. Drug addiction and drug abuse. In: Goodman L, Gilman AG, eds. The pharmacologic basis of therapeutics. New York: Macmillan, 1985:532.
47. Jenkins LC. Anesthetic problems due to drug abuse and dependence. Can Anaesth Soc J 1972;19:461.
48. Johnston RR, Way WL, Miller RD. Alteration of anesthetic requirements by amphetamine. Anesthesiology 1972;36:357.
49. Johnstone RC, Lief PL, Kulp RA, Smith TC. Combination of delta-9-tetrahydrocannabinol with oxymorphone or pentobarbital. Anesthesiology 1975;42:674.
50. Jones D, Gerber LP, Drell W. A rapid enzymatic method for estimating ethanol in body fluids. Clin Chem 1970;16:402.
51. Jusko WJ, Schentag JJ, Clark JJ, et al. Enhanced biotransformation of theophylline in marijuana and tobacco smokers. Clin Pharm Ther 1978;24:406.
52. Kelen GD, Fritz S, Quqish B, et al. Unrecognized human immunodeficiency virus infection in emergency department patients. N Engl J Med 1988;318:1645.
53. Koehntop DE, Liao JC, Van Bergan FH. Effects of pharmacologic alteration of adrenergic mechanisms by cocaine, tropolone, aminophylline, and ketamine on epinephrine-induced arrhythmias during halothane-nitrous oxide anesthesia. Anesthesiology 1977;46:83.
54. Lee JF, Giesecke AH Jr, Jenkins MT. Anesthetic management of trauma: influence of alcohol ingestion. South Med J 1967;60:1240.
55. Lee JF, Samuelson RJ, Watson TD, Giesecke AH. Anesthesia for trauma: is blood alcohol level a factor? Tex Med 1974;70:84.
56. Lee PKY, Cho MH, Dobkin AB. Effects of alcoholism, morphinism, and barbiturate resistance on induction and maintenance of general anaesthesia. Can Anaesth Soc J 1964; 11:354.
57. Lieber CS. Biochemical and molecular basis of alcohol-induced injury to liver and other tissues. N Engl J Med 1988;319:1639.

58. Lieber CS. Metabolism of ethanol and associated interactions with other drugs, carcinogens and vitamins. NY State J Med 1986;86:297.
59. Luna GK, Maier RV, Sowder L, et al. The influence of ethanol intoxication on outcome of injured motorcyclists. J Trauma 1984;24:695.
60. McCammon RL. Anesthesia for the chemically dependent patient. International Anesthesia Research Society Review course lectures, 1986:47.
61. Moss LK, Chanault OW, Gaston EA. The effects of alcohol ingestion on experimental hemorrhagic shock. Surg Forum 1959;10:390.
62. Nettles JL, Olson RN. Effects of alcohol on hypoxia. JAMA 1965;194:1193.
63. Newsome HH. Ethanol modulation of plasma norepinephrine response to trauma and hemorrhage. J Trauma 1988;28:1.
64. Ng SKC, Hauser WA, Brust JCM, Susser M. Alcohol consumption and withdrawal in new-onset seizures. N Engl J Med 1988;319:666.
65. Nolop KB, Natow A. Unprecedented sedative requirements during delirium tremens. Crit Care Med 1985;13:246.
66. Rivara FP, Mueller BA, Fligner CL, et al. Drug use in trauma victims. J Trauma 1989;29:462.
67. Siemens AJ, Kalant H, Khanna JM, et al. Effect of cannabis on pentobarbital-induced sleeping time and pentobarbital metabolism in the rat. Biochem Pharmacol 1974;23:477.
68. Soderstrom CA, Arias JD, Carson SL, et al. Alcohol consumption among vehicular occupants injured in crashes. Alcoholism 1984;8:269.
69. Soderstrom CA, Trifillis AL, Shankar BS, et al. Marijuana and alcohol use among 1023 trauma patients: a prospective study. Arch Surg 1988;123:733.
70. Sofia RD, Knoblock LC. The effect of delta-9-tetrahydrocannabinol pretreatment on ketamine, thiopental, or CT-1341-induced loss of righting reflex in mice. Arch Int Pharmacodyn Ther 1974;207:270.
71. Stein PD, Sabbah HN, Przybylski J. Effect of alcohol upon arrhythmias following nonpenetrating cardiac impact. J Trauma 1988;28:466.
72. Stene JK. Anesthesia for the critically ill trauma patient. In: Siegel JH, ed. Trauma, emergency surgery and critical care. New York: Churchill Livingstone, 1987:843.
73. Stoelting RK, Creasser CW, Martz RC. Effect of cocaine administration on halothane MAC in dogs. Anesth Analg 1975;54:422.
74. Stoelting RK, Martz RC, Gartner J, et al. Effects of delta-9-tetrahydrocannabinol on halothane MAC in dogs. Anesthesiology 1973;38:521.
75. Thal ER, Bost RO, Anderson RJ. Effects of alcohol and other drugs on traumatized patients. Arch Surg 1985;120:708.
76. Urbano-Marquez A, Estruch R, Navarro-Lopez F, et al. The effects of alcoholism on skeletal and cardiac muscle. N Engl J Med 1989;320:409.
77. Viegas OJ. Drug abuse and overdose. In: Stoelting RK, Dierdorf SF, eds. Anesthesia and coexisting disease. New York: Churchill Livingstone, 1983:673.
78. Vitez TS, Way WL, Miller RD, Eger EI II. Effects of delta-9-tetrahydrocannabinol on cyclopropane MAC in rat. Anesthesiology 1973;38:525.
79. Waller PF, Stewart JR, Hansen AR, et al. The potentiating effects of alcohol on driver injury. JAMA 1986;256:1461.
80. Ward RE, Flynn, TC, Miller PW, Blaisdell WF. Effects of ethanol ingestion on the severity and outcome of trauma. Am J Surg 1982;144:153.
81. Watson TD, Lee JF. Intoxication and trauma. In: Giesecke AH, ed. Anesthesia for the surgery of trauma. Philadelphia: FA Davis, 1976;11:n31.
82. Webb WR, Degerli IU. Ethyl alcohol and the cardiovascular system: effects on coronary blood flow. JAMA 1965;191:77.
83. Wetmore K. Dipstick: quick quantitation of ethanol in body fluids. JAMA 1983;250:1658.
84. Williams HE. Alcoholic hypoglycemia and ketoacidosis. Med Clin North Am 1984;68:33.
85. Wolfson B. Alcohol. Semin Anesth 1984;3:242.
86. Wolfson B, Freed B. Influence of alcohol on anesthetic requirements and acute toxicity. Anesth Analg 1980;59:826.
87. Zinn SE, Fairly HB, Glenn JD. Liver function in patients with mild alcoholic hepatitis after enflurane, nitrous oxide-narcotic, and spinal anesthesia. Anesth Analg 1985;64:487.

## METABOLIC-ENDOCRINE DISORDERS

### *Diabetes Mellitus*

88. Adler AG, Merli GJ, McElwain GE, Martin JH. Diabetes Mellitus. In: Adler AG, Merli GJ, McElwain GE, Martin JH, eds. Medical evaluation of the surgical patient. Philadelphia: WB Saunders, 1985:64.
89. Alberti KGMM, Thomas DJB. The management of diabetes during surgery. Br J Anaesth 1979;51:693.
90. Barnett AH, Robinson MH, Harrison JH, Watkins PJ. Minipump: method of diabetic control during minor surgery under general anaesthesia. Br Med J 1982;280:78.
91. Blackshear PJ. Care of the diabetic patient. In: Rippe J, Csete M, eds. Manual of intensive care medicine. Boston: Little, Brown, 1983:293.
92. Blackshear PJ. Diabetic ketoacidosis. In: Rippe J, Csete M, eds. Manual of intensive care medicine. Boston: Little, Brown, 1983:296.
93. Blackshear PJ: Hyperosmolar nonketotic diabetic coma. In: Rippe J, Csete M, eds. Manual of intensive care medicine. Boston: Little, Brown, 1983:300.
94. Buysschaert M, Moulart M, Urbain JL, et al. Impaired gastric emptying in diabetic patients with cardiac autonomic neuropathy. Diabetes Care 1987;10:448.
95. Chang VD, Drucker WR. Management of diabetes mellitus in surgery and trauma. In: Siegel, JH, ed. Trauma: emergency surgery and critical care. New York: Churchill Livingstone, 1987:753.
96. Ewing DJ, Campbell IW, Clarke BF. Assessment of cardiovascular effects in diabetic autonomic neuropathy and prognostic implications. Ann Intern Med 1980;92:308.
97. Fletcher J, Langman MJS, Kellock TD. Effect of surgery on blood-sugar levels in diabetes mellitus. Lancet 1965;1:52.
98. Giesecke AH, Spier CJ, Stanley VF, Seltzer HS. Considerations in the anesthetic management of the diabetic patient. Clin Anesth 1963;3:53.
99. Hilsted J, Richter E, Madsbad S, et al. Metabolic and cardiovascular responses to epinephrine in diabetic autonomic neuropathy. N Engl J Med 1987;317:421.
100. Loughran PG, Giesecke AH. Diabetes mellitus: anesthetic considerations. Semin Anesth 1984;3:207.
101. Melton LJ III, Palumbo PJ, Chu Pin C. Incidence of diabetes mellitus by clinical type. Diabetes Care 1983;6:75.
102. Morris L, Murphy M, Kitabchi A. Bicarbonate therapy in severe diabetic ketoacidosis. Ann Intern Med 1986;105:836.
103. Murphy R, Smalley PE. Medical management of the surgical diabetic patient. Lahey Clin Bull 1963;13:5.
104. Pender JW, Basso LV. Diseases of the endocrine system. In: Katz J, Benumof J, Kadis LB, eds. Anesthesia and uncommon

diseases: pathophysiologic and clinical correlations. 2nd ed. Philadelphia: WB Saunders, 1981:155.
105. Root HF. Preoperative medical care of the diabetic patient. Postgrad Med 1966;40:439.
106. Steinke J. Management of diabetes mellitus and surgery. N Engl J Med 1970;282:1472.
107. Taitelman U, Reece EA, Bessman AN. Insulin in the management of the diabetic surgical patient: continuous intravenous infusion vs subcutaneous administration. JAMA 1977;237:658.
108. Tomkin GH: The endocrine pancreas. In: Vickers MD, ed. Medicine for anasthetists. London: Blackwell, 1977:483.
109. Walts LF, Miller J, Davidson MB, Brown J. Perioperative management of diabetes mellitus. Anesthesiology 1981;55:104.
110. Watkins PJ, Mackay JD. Cardiac denervation in diabetic neuropathy. Ann Intern Med 1980;92:304.

### *Obesity*

111. Blass NH. Morbid obesity and other nutritional disorders. In: Katz J, Benumof J, Kadis LB, eds. Anesthesia and uncommon diseases: pathophysiologic and clinical correlations. 2nd ed. Philadelphia: WB Saunders, 1981:450.
112. Mercer CD, Wren SF, DaCosta LR, Beck IT. Lower espophageal sphincter pressure and gastroesophageal pressure gradients in excessively obese patients. Can J Med 1987;18:135.
113. Pasulka PS, Bistrian BR, Benotti PN, Blackburn GL. The risks of surgery in obese patients. Ann Intern Med 1986;104:540.
114. Rochester DF, Enson Y. Current concepts in the pathogenesis of the obesity-hypoventilation syndrome: mechanical and circulatory factors. Am J Med 1974;57:402.
115. Sharp JT, Henry JP, Sweany SK, et al. The total work of breathing in normal and obese men. J Clin Invest 1964;43:728.
116. Vaughan RW. Anesthetic management of the morbidly obese patient. In: Brown BR Jr, ed. Anesthesia and the obese patient. Philadelphia: FA Davis, 1982:71.
117. Vaughan RW: Definitions and risks of obesity. In: Brown BR Jr, ed. Anesthesia and the obese patient. Philadelphia: FA Davis, 1982:1.
118. Vaughan RW. Pulmonary and cardiovascular derangements in the obese patient. In: Brown BR Jr, ed. Anesthesia and the obese patient. Philadelphia: FA Davis, 1982:19.
119. Vaughan RW, Conahan TJ III. Minireview, part I: cardiopulmonary consequences of morbid obesity. Life Sci 1980;26:2119.
120. Vaughan RW, Vaughan MS. Morbid obesity: implications for anesthetic care. Semin Anesth 1984;3:218.

## ASTHMA

121. Dueck R. Anesthesia for the asthmatic patient. Semin Anesth 1987;6:2.
122. Jones JG, Jordan C, Slavin B, Lehane JR. Prophylactic effect of aminophylline and salbutamol on histamine-induced bronchoconstriction. Br J Anaesth 1987;59:498.
123. Kingston HGG, Hirshman CA. Perioperative management of the patient with asthma. Anesth Analg 1984;63:844.
124. L'Hommedieu CS, Arens JJ. The use of ketamine for the emergency intubation of patients with status asthmaticus. Ann Emerg Med 1987;16:568.
125. Littenberg B. Aminophylline treatment in severe, acute asthma: a meta-analysis. JAMA 1988;259:1678.
126. Littenberg B, Gluck EH. A controlled trial of methylprednisolone in the emergency treatment of acute asthma. N Engl J Med 1986;314:150.
127. Marney SR Jr. Asthma: recent developments in treatment. South Med J 1985;78:1084.
128. Shnider SM, Papper EM. Anesthesia for the asthmatic patient. Anesthesiology 1961;22:886.
129. Strube PJ, Hallam PL. Ketamine by continuous infusion in status asthmaticus. Anaesthesia 1986;41:1017.

## HEMATOLOGIC DISORDERS

### *Sickle Cell Hemoglobinopathy*

130. Adler AG, Merli GJ, McElwain GE, Martin JH. Hematology: hemostatic disorders. In: Adler AG, Merli GJ, McElwain GE, Martin JH, ed. Medical evaluation of the surgical patient. Philadelphia: WB Saunders, 1985:44.
131. Bischoff RJ, Williamson A, Dalali MJ, et al. Assessment of the use of transfusion therapy perioperatively in patients with sickle cell hemoglobinopathies. Ann Surg 1988;207:434.
132. Brajtbord D, Johnson D, Ramsay W, et al. Use of the cell saver in patients with sickle cell trait. Anesthesiology 1989;70:878.
133. Burrington JD, Smith MD. Elective and emergency surgery in children with sickle cell disease. Surg Clin North Am 1976;56:55.
134. Davis AM. Sickle-cell trait as a risk factor for sudden death in physical training. N Engl J Med 1988;318:787.
135. Fullerton MW, Philippart AI, Sarnaik S, Lusher JM. Preoperative exchange transfusion in sickle cell anemia. J Pediatr Surg 1981;16:297.
136. Gibson JR Jr. Anesthesia for the sickle cell diseases and other hemoglobinopathies. Semin Anesth 1987;5:27.
137. Howells TH, Huntsman RG, Boys JE, Mahmood A. Anesthesia and sickle-cell haemoglobin. Br J Anaesth 1972;44:975.
138. Janik J, Seeler RA. Perioperative management of children with sickle hemoglobinopathy. J Pediatr Surg 1980;15:117.
139. Kark JA, Posey DM, Schumacher HR, Ruehle CJ. Sickle-cell trait as a risk factor for sudden death in physical training. N Engl J Med 1987;317:781.
140. McGarry P, Duncan C. Anesthetic risks in sickle cell trait. Pediatrics 1973;51:507.

### *Hemophilia, von Willebrand Disease, Idiopathic Thrombocytopenic Purpura*

141. Ahn YS, Harrington WJ, Simon SR, et al. Danazol for the treatment of idiopathic thrombocytopenic purpura. N Engl J Med 1983;308:23.
142. Allain JP. Transfusion support for haemophiliacs. Clin Haematol 1984;13:99.
143. Andes WA, Wulff K, Smith WB. Head trauma in hemophilia: a prospective study. Arch Intern Med 1984;144:1981.
144. Bick RL. Congenital coagulation factor defects and von Willebrand's disease (factor VIII:C defects). In: Bick RL, ed. Disorders of hemostasis and thrombosis: principles of clinical practice. 6th ed. New York: Thieme, 1985:136.
145. Biggs R. Jaundice and antibodies directed against factors VIII and IX in patients treated for haemophilia or Christmas disease in the United Kingdom. Br J Haematol 1974;26:313.
146. Blanchette VS, Hogan VA, McCombie NE, et al. Intensive plasma exchange therapy in ten patients with idiopathic thrombocytopenic purpura. Transfusion 1984;24:5.
147. Difino SM, Lachant MA, Kirshner JJ, Gottlieb AJ. Adult idiopathic thrombocytopenic purpura: clinical findings and response to therapy. Am J Med 1980;69:430.

148. Eastman JR, Nowakowski AR, Triplett DA. DDAVP: review of indications for its use in the treatment of factor VIII deficiency and report of a case. Oral Surg 1983;56:246.
149. Eyster ME, Gill FM, Blatt PM, et al. Central nervous system bleeding in hemophiliacs. Blood 1978;51:1179.
150. Fehr J, Hofmann V, Kappeler UCM. Transient reversal of thrombocytopenia in idiopathic thrombocytopenic purpura by high-dose intravenous gamma globulin. N Engl J Med 1982;306:21.
151. Frederici A, Mannucci PM, Minetti D, et al. Intracranial bleeding in haemophilia: a study of eleven cases. J Neurosurg Sci 1983;27:31.
152. Furlan M, Lammle B, Aeberhard A, et al. Virus-inactivated factor VIII concentrate prevents postoperative bleeding in a patient with von Willebrand disease. Transfusion 1988;28:489.
153. Guthrie TH Jr, Sacra JC. Emergency care of the hemophiliac patient. Ann Emerg Med 1980;9:476.
154. Hougie C. Hemophilia and related conditions: congenital deficiencies of prothrombin (factor II), factor V, and factors VII to XII. In: Williams WJ, Beutler E, Erslev AJ, Lichtman MA, eds. Hematology. 3rd ed. New York: McGraw-Hill, 1983:1381.
155. Jandl JH. Disorders of coagulation. In: Jandl JH, ed. Blood: textbook of hematology, Boston: Little, Brown, 1987:1095.
156. Jiji RM, Firozvi T, Spurling CL. Chronic idiopathic thrombocytopenic purpura: treatment with steroids and splenectomy. Arch Intern Med 1973;132:380.
157. Kasper CK, Dietrich SL. Comprehensive management of haemophilia. Clin Haematol 1985;14:489.
158. Koller CA. Immune thrombocytopenic purpura. Med Clin North Am 1980;64:4.
159. Kurezynski, EM, Penner JA. Activated prothrombin concentrate for patients with factor VIII inhibitors. N Engl J Med 1974;291:164.
160. Martinowitz U, Heim M, Tadmor R, et al. Intracranial hemorrhage in patients with hemophilia. Neurosurgery 1986;18:538.
161. Peters M, Henny CP, tenCate JW, et al. Lumbar arterial rupture secondary to iliopsoas hemorrhage in a hemophiliac patient. Acta Haematol (Basel) 1984;71:128.
162. Pizzuto J, Ambriz R. Therapeutic experience on 934 adults with idiopathic thrombocytopenic purpura: multicentric trial of the cooperative Latin American group on hemostasis and thrombosis. Blood 1984;64:1179.
163. Rifkind RA, Bank A, Marks PA, et al. Disorders of coagulation. In: Rifkind RA, Bank A, Marks PA, Kaplan KL, Ellison RR, Lindenbaum J, eds. Fundamentals of hematology. 3rd ed. Chicago: Year book, 1986:187.
164. Romeyn RL, Herkowitz HN. The cervical spine in hemophilia. Clin Orthop 1986;210:113.
165. Ruggeri ZM, Zimmerman TS. von Willebrand factor and von Willebrand disease. Blood 1987;70:895.
166. Sindet-Pedersen S, Stebjerg S, Ingerslev J. Treatment of bilateral fracture of the mandible in a hemophilic patient with inhibitor to factor VIII. J Oral Maxillofac Surg 1987;45:537.
167. Sixma JJ, Van Den Berg A. The haemostatic plug in haemophilia A: a morphological study of haemostatic plug formation in bleeding time skin wounds of patients with severe haemophilia A. Br J Haematol 1984;58:741.
168. Stuart MJ, Kelton JG, Allen JB. Abnormal platelet function and arachidonate metabolism in chronic idiopathic thrombocytopenia purpura. Blood 1981;58:2.
169. Thompson RB, Proctor SJ. The haemorrhagic disorders II: defects of coagulation. In: Thompson RB, Proctor SJ, eds. Concise textbook of hematology. Baltimore: Urban & Schwarzenberg, 1984:480.
170. Uchida T, Yui T, Umezu H, Kariyone S. Prolongation of platelet survival in idiopathic thrombocytopenic purpura by high-dose intravenous gamma globulin. Thromb Haemostas 1984;51:65.

## EPILEPSY

171. Adler AG, Merli GJ, McElwain GE, Martin JH. The nervous system: seizure disorder. In: Adler AG, Merli GJ, McElwain GE, Martin JH, eds. Medical evaluation of the surgical patient. Philadelphia: WB Saunders, 1985:195.
172. Beal F. Status epilepticus. In: Rippe J, Csete M, eds. Manual of intensive care medicine. Boston: Little, Brown, 1983:386.
173. Boucher BA, Rodman JH, Jaresko GS, et al. Phenytoin pharmacokinetics in critically ill trauma patients. Clin Pharmacol Ther 1988;44:675.
174. Celesia GG, Messert B, Murphy MJ. Status epilepticus of late adult onset. Neurology 1972;22:1047.
175. Cranford RE, Leppik IE, Patrick B, et al. Intravenous phenytoin in acute treatment of seizures. Neurology 1979;29:1474.
176. Dacey RG Jr, Dikmen SS. Mild head injury. In: Cooper PR, ed. Head injury. 2nd ed. Baltimore: Williams & Wilkins, 1987:125.
177. Nicol CF, Tutton JC, Smith BH. Parenteral diazepam in status epilepticus. Neurology 1969;19:332.
178. Ornstein E, Matteo RS, Schwartz AE, et al. The effect of phenytoin on the magnitude and duration of neuromuscular block following atracurium or vecuronium. Anesthesiology 1987;67:191.
179. Ornstein E, Matteo RS, Young WL. Resistance to metocurine-induced neuromuscular blockade in patients receiving phenytoin. Anesthesiology 1985;63:294.
180. Prensky AL, Raff MC, Moore MJ, Schwab RS. Intravenous diazepam in the treatment of prolonged seizure activity. N Engl J Med 1967;276:779.
181. Thorpy MJ. Rectal valproate syrup and status epilepticus. Neurology 1980;30:1113.
182. Vajda FJE, Mihaly GW, Miles JL, et al. Rectal administration of sodium valproate in status epilepticus. Neurology 1978;28:897.
183. Walker JE, Homan RW, Vasko MR, et al. Lorazepam in status epilepticus. Ann Neurol 1979;6:207.
184. Young GB, Blume WT, Bolton CF, Warren KG. Anesthetic barbiturates in refractory status epilepticus. Can J Neurol Sci 1980;7:291.

## CARDIAC DISEASES

### *Arrhythmias*

185. Abernathy SF. Complete heart block caused by the Swan-Ganz catheter. Chest 1974;65:349.
186. Barriot P, Riou B. Hemorrhagic shock with paradoxical bradycardia. Intensive Care Med 1987;13:203.
187. Beresky R, Klingler R, Peake J. Myocardial contusions: when does it have clinical significance? J Trauma 1988;28:64.
188. Bigger JT, Hoffman BF. Digitalis and allied cardiac glycosides. In: Gilman AG, Goodman LS, Rall TW, Murad F, ed. The pharmacological basis of therapeutics. 7th ed. New York: Macmillan, 1985:748–783.
189. Bigger JT, Schmidt DH, Kutt H. Relationship between the plasma level of diphenylhydantoin sodium and its cardiac antiarrhythmic effect. Circulation 1968;38:363.
190. Castellanos A, Ramirez AV, Mayorga-Cortez A, et al. Left fascicular blocks during right-heart catheterization using the Swan-Ganz catheter. Circulation 1981;64:1271.
191. Davis RF. Etiology and treatment of perioperative cardiac dys-

rhythmias. In: Kaplan JA, ed. Cardiac anesthesia. Orlando: Grune & Stratton, 1987:411.
192. Denes P, Dhingra RC, Wu D, et al. Sudden death in patients with chronic bifascicular block. Arch Intern Med 1977; 137:1005.
193. Engel TR, Luck JC. Transient right bundle branch block with "Swan-Ganz" catheterization. Am Heart J 1976;92:263.
194. Evans DE, Kobrine AJ, Rizzoli HV. Cardiac arrhythmias accompanying acute compression of the spinal cord. J Neurosurg 1980;52:52.
195. Fabian TC, Mangiante EC, Paterson RC, et al. Myocardial contusions in blunt trauma: clinical characteristics, means of diagnosis, and implications for patient management. J Trauma 1988;28:50.
196. Flancbaum L, Wright J, Siegel JH. Emergency surgery in patients with post-traumatic myocardial contusions. J Trauma 1986;26:745.
197. Galloon S, Rees GAD, Brisco CE, et al. Prospective study of electrocardiographic changes associated with subarachnoid haemorrhage. Br J Anaesth 1972;44:511.
198. Herre SM. Advances in the management of tachyarrhythmias. J Intensive Care Med 1987;2:65.
199. Hersch C. Electrocardiographic changes in head injuries. Circulation 1961;23:853.
200. Jackuck SJ, Ramani PS, Clark F, et al. Electrocardiographic abnormalities associated with raised intracranial pressure. Br Med J 1975;1:242.
201. Jacobson SA, Danufsky P. Marked electrocardiographic changes produced by experimental head trauma. J Neuropathol Exp Neurol 1954;13:462.
202. Leahey EB, Reiffel JA, Drusin RE, et al. Interaction between quinidine and digoxin. JAMA 1978;240:565.
203. Macander PJ, Kuhnlein JL, Buiteweg J, Cheng-Chong L. Electrode detachment: a complication of the indwelling pacing Swan-Ganz catheter. N Engl J Med 1986;314:1711.
204. McAnulty JH, Rahimtoola SH, Murphy E, et al. Natural history of "high-risk" bundle branch block: final report of a prospective study. N Engl J Med 1982;307:137.
205. Otteni JC, Pottecher T, Bronner G, et al. Prolongation of the QT interval and sudden cardiac arrest following right radical neck dissection. Anesthesiology 1983;59:358.
206. Pastore JO, Yurchak PM, Janis KM, et al. The risk of advanced heart block in surgical patients with right bundle branch block and left axis deviation. Circulation 1978;57:677.
207. Rankin AC, Rae AP, Cobbe SM. Misuse of intravenous verapamil in patients with ventricular tachycardia. Lancet 1987;2:472.
208. Rooney SM, Goldiner PL, Muss E. Relationship of right bundle branch block and marked left axis deviation to complete heart block during general anesthesia. Anesthesiology 1976;44:64.
209. Ross P, Degutis L, Baker CC. Cardiac contusion: the effect on operative management of the patient with trauma injuries. Arch Surg 1989;124:506.
210. Sazama KJ. The syndrome known as WPW: a review. JAMA 1976;31:56.
211. Schneider JF, Thomas E, Kreger BE. Newly acquired left bundle branch block: the Framingham study. Ann Intern Med 1979;90:303.
212. Schneider JF, Thomas E, Kreger BE, et al. Newly acquired right bundle branch block. Ann Intern Med 1980;92:37.
213. Shah KB, Rao TL, Laughlin S, et al. A review of pulmonary artery catheterization in 6245 patients. Anesthesiology 1984;61:271.
214. Shin B, McKenzie CF, Helrich M. Hypokalemia in trauma patients. Anesthesiology 1986;65:90.
215. Snow N, Richardson DJ, Flint LM. Myocardial contusions: implications for patients with multiple traumatic injuries. Surgery 1982;92:744.
216. Sprung CL, Elser B, Schein RMH, et al. Risk of right bundle branch block and complete heart block during pulmonary artery catheterization. Crit Care Med 1989;17:1.
217. Walsh KA, Ezri MD, Denes P. Emergency treatment of tachyarrhythmias. Med Clin North Am 1986;70:791.
218. Weilder DJ. Myocardial damage and cardiac arrythmias after intracranial hemorrhage: a critical review. Stroke 1974;5:759.
219. Zaidan JR, Curling PE. Cardiac dysrhythmias: recognition and management. In: Stoelting RK, Barash PG, Gallagher TJ, eds. Advances in anesthesia. Chicago: Year Book, 1985:207.

### *Coronary Artery Disease*

220. Braunwald E, Kloner R. The stunned myocardium: prolonged, postischemic ventricular dysfunction. Circulation 1982; 66:1146.
221. Breslow MJ, Miller CF, Parker SD, et al. Changes in T wave morphology following anesthesia and surgery: a common recovery-room phenomenon. Anesthesiology 1986;64:398.
222. Buffington CW, Romson JL, Levine A, et al. Isoflurane induces coronary steal in a canine model of chronic coronary occlusion. Anesthesiology 1987;66:280.
223. Buxton AE, Goldberg S, Harken A, et al. Coronary-artery spasm immediately after myocardial revascularization. N Engl J Med 1981;304:1249.
224. Cahalan MK, Prakash O, Rulf EN, et al. Addition of nitrous oxide to fentanyl anesthesia does not induce myocardial ischemia in patients with ischemic heart disease. Anesthesiology 1987;67:925.
225. Chernow B, Reed L, Geelhoed GW, et al. Glucagon: endocrine effects and calcium involvement in cardiovascular actions in dogs. Circ Shock 1986;19:393.
226. Clements FM, de Bruijn NP. Perioperative evaluation of regional wall motion by transesophageal two-dimensional echocardiography. Anesth Analg 1987;66:249.
227. Cohen DJ, Foley RW, Ryan JM. Intraoperative coronary artery spasm successfully treated with nitroglycerin and nifedipine. Ann Thorac Surg 1983;36:97.
228. Coriat P, Daloz M, Bousseau D, et al. Prevention of intraoperative myocardial ischemia during noncardiac surgery with intravenous nitroglycerin. Anesthesiology 1984;61:195.
229. Einzig S, Lucas RV. Glucagon: use in cardiac resuscitation of a propranolol-treated infant. Pediatr Cardiol 1980;1:219.
230. Godet G, Coriat P, Baron JF, et al. Prevention of intraoperative myocardial ischemia during noncardiac surgery with intravenous diltiazem: a randomized trial versus placebo. Anesthesiology 1987;66:241.
231. Hess W, Arnold B, Schulte-Sasse U, Tarnow J. Comparison of isoflurane and halothane when used to control intraoperative hypertension in patients undergoing coronary artery bypass surgery. Anesth Analg 1983;62:15.
232. Hilfiker O, Larsen R, Sonntag H. Myocardial blood flow and oxygen consumption during halothane-nitrous oxide anaesthesia for coronary revascularization. Br J Anaesth 1983;55:927.
233. Hofmann T, Kasper W, Meinertz T, et al. Determination of aortic valve orifice area in aortic stenosis with two-dimensional transesophageal echocardiography. Am J Cardiol 1987;59:330.
234. Jackson APF, Dhadphale PR, Callaghan ML, Alseri S. Haemodynamic studies during induction of anaesthesia for open-heart surgery using diazepam and ketamine. Br J Anaesth 1978;50:375.
235. Kapur PA, Bloor BC, Flacke WE, Olewine SK. Comparison of

cardiovascular responses to verapamil during enflurane, isoflurane, or halothane anesthesia in the dog. Anesthesiology 1984;61:156.
236. Kopf GS, Riba A, Zito R. Intraoperative use of nifedipine for hemodynamic collapse due to coronary artery spasm following myocardial revascularization. Ann Thorac Surg 1982;34:457.
237. Kremer P, Canalan MK, Beaupre P, et al. Intraoperative myocardial ischemia detected by transesophageal 2-dimensional echocardiography. Circulation 1983;68:Supp. III:332.
238. Kumar SM, Kothary SP, Zsigmond EK. Lack of cardiovascular stimulation during endotracheal intubation in cardiac surgical patients anesthetized with diazepam-ketamine-pancuronium. Clin Ther 1980;3:43.
239. Kumar SM, Kothary SP, Zsigmond EK. Plasma-free norepinephrine and epinephrine concentrations following diazepam-ketamine induction in patients undergoing cardiac surgery. Acta Anaesthesiol Scand 1978;22:593.
240. Lehot JJ, Leone BJ, Foëx P. Calcium reverses global and regional myocardial dysfunction caused by the combination of verapamil and halothane. Acta Anesthesiol Scand 1987;31:441.
240a. London MJ, Hollenberg M, Wong MG, et al. Intraoperative myocardial ischemia: Localization by continuous 12-lead electrocardiography. Anesthesiology 1988;69:232.
241. Moffitt EA, Scovil JE, Barker RA, et al. The effects of nitrous oxide on myocardial metabolism and hemodynamics during fentanyl or enflurane anesthesia in patients with coronary disease. Anesth Analg 1984;63:1071.
242. Moffitt EA, Sethna DH, Gary RJ, et al. Nitrous oxide added to halothane reduces coronary flow and myocardial oxygen consumption in patients with coronary disease. Can Anesth Soc J 1983;30:5.
243. Nussmeier NA, Slogoff S. Verapamil treatment of intraoperative coronary artery spasm. Anesthesiology 1985;62:539.
244. O'Young J, Mastrocostopoulos G, Kyritsis A, et al. The effect of isoflurane on regional and global coronary circulation during intraoperative hypertension. Anesthesiology 1986;65:A504.
245. Peterson A, Lucchesi B, Kirsh MM. The effect of glucagon in animals on chronic propranolol therapy. Ann Thorac Surg 1978;25:340.
246. Reiz S, Balfors E, Sorensen MB, et al. Isoflurane: a powerful coronary vasodilator in patients with coronary artery disease. Anesthesiology 1983;59:91.
247. Schlüter M, Kremer P, Hanrath P. Transesophageal 2-D echocardiographic feature of flail mitral leaflet due to ruptured chordae tendinae. Am Heart J 1984;108:609.
248. Schlüter M, Langenstein BA, Hanrath P et al. Assessment of transesophageal pulsed Doppler echocardiography in the detection of mitral regurgitation. Circulation 1982;66:784.
249. Shively B, Cahalan M, Benefiel D, Schiller N. Intraoperative Doppler echocardiography: intraoperative assessment of mitral valve regurgitation by transesophageal Doppler echocardiography. J Am Coll Cardiol 1986;7:228A.
250. Smith JS, Cahalan MK, Benefiel DJ, et al. Intraoperative detection of myocardial ischemia in high-risk patients: electrocardiography versus two dimensional transesophageal echocardiography. Circulation 1985;72:1015.
251. Tarnow J, Markschies-Hornung A, Schulte-Sasse V. Isoflurane improves the tolerance to pacing-induced myocardial ischemia. Anesthesiology 1986;64:147.
252. Tatekawa S, Traber KB, Hantler CB, et al. Effects of isoflurane on myocardial blood flow, function, and oxygen consumption in the presence of critical coronary stenosis in dogs. Anesth Analg 1987;66:1073.
253. Thomson IR, Mutch WAC, Culligan JD. Failure of intravenous nitroglycerin to prevent intraoperative myocardial ischemia during fentanyl-pancuronium anesthesia. Anesthesiology 1984;61:385.
254. Tuman KG, Keane DM, Speiss BD, et al. Effect of high dose fentanyl on fluid and vasopressor requirements after cardiac surgery. J Cardiothorac Anesth 1988;2:419.
255. Videcoq M, Arvieux CC, Ramsay JG, et al. The association isoflurane-verapamil causes regional left-ventricular dyssynchrony in the dog. Anesthesiology 1987;67:635.
255a. Yaeger MP, Glass DD, Neff RK, Brink-Johnsen T. Epidural anesthesia and analgesia in high-risk surgical patients. Anesthesiology 1987;66:729.
256. Zaritsky AL, Horowitz M, Chernow B. Glucagon antagonism of calcium channel blocker-induced myocardial dysfunction. Crit Care Med 1988;16:246.

## CONGESTIVE HEART FAILURE

257. Burnett JC, Kao PC, Hu DC, et al. Atrial natriuretic peptide elevation in congestive heart failure in the human. Science 1986;231:1145.
258. Curtiss G, Cohn JN, Vrobel T, et al. Role of renin-angiotensin system in the systemic vasoconstriction of congestive heart failure. Circulation 1978;58:763.
259. Eddy AC, Rice CL, Anardi DM. Right ventricular dysfunction in multiple trauma victims. Am J Surg 1988;155:712.
260. Goldsmith SR, Francis GS, Cowley AW, et al. Increased plasma arginine vasopressin in patients with congestive heart failure. J Am Coll Cardiol 1983;1:1385.
261. Klockowski P, Levy G. Kinetics of drug action in disease states: effect of experimental hypovolemia on the pharmacodynamics and pharmacokinetics of desmethyl diazepam. J Pharmacol Exp Therap 1988;245:508.
262. Mason DT, Awan NA, Joyce JA, et al. Treatment of acute and chronic congestive heart failure by vasodilator-afterload reduction. Arch Intern Med 1980;140:1577.
263. Shenker Y, Sider RS, Ostafin EA, et al. Plasma levels of immunoreactive atrial natriuretic factor in healthy subjects and in patients with edema. J Clin Invest 1985;76:1684.
264. Tikkanen I, Fyhrquist F, Metsarinne K, et al. Plasma atrial natriuretic peptide in cardiac disease and during infusion in healthy volunteers. Lancet 1985;2:66.
265. Weiskopf RB, Bogetz MJ. Hemorrhage decreases the anesthetic requirement for ketamine and thiopentone in the pig. Br J Anaesth 1985;57:1022.

# Chapter Nine

Levon M. Capan
Gregory Gottlieb
Andrew Rosenberg

# General Principles of Anesthesia for Major Acute Trauma

Experience gained during military conflicts over the past 140 years has contributed greatly to the development of anesthesia for trauma surgery. Ether was first used in military surgery by Dr. Edward H. Barton during the Mexican-American War in the spring of 1847, just 6 months after the anesthetic properties of this agent were demonstrated by Dr. William Morton.[11] During the U.S. Civil War, nearly 100,000 anesthetics were administered using chloroform, ether, or a mixture of the two.[360] As industrial accidents were rare and motor vehicle accidents were nonexistent in those days, military conflicts represented virtually the only source of experience in anesthesia and surgery for trauma. By the turn of the century, the concept of general anesthesia was well established, and many surgical procedures were performed with the benefit of ether. However, appropriate anesthesia training, anesthesia equipment, and knowledge of basic cardiorespiratory physiology and pharmacology were not available; anyone, including nonphysician personnel, was allowed to administer an anesthetic. Only regional anesthesia, mostly in the form of infiltration and peripheral nerve blocks, was administered by physicians. Nitrous oxide was available, but it was used sporadically and at high, frequently hypoxic, inspired concentrations.

In their review, "Anesthesia on the Western Front," Courington and Calverley[110] documented how the war contributed to improvement in the quality of anesthetic care. It was during this war that Crile described the benefits of nitrous oxide and oxygen for seriously wounded soldiers. Also at this time, the need for anesthesia specialists became apparent, and physicians and specially trained nursing sisters were appointed to administer anesthesia using relatively sophisticated anesthesia machines equipped with flow meters, multiple gases, and heated vaporizers. Advances in understanding the mechanisms of hemorrhagic shock were made by Crile and his colleagues, and an anesthetic technique called *anoci-association,* combining morphine, nitrous oxide, and infiltration anesthesia, was introduced to care for military trauma victims.[125] Spinal anesthesia gained popularity during this war since it required less nursing care, reduced the hospitalization period, produced fewer bronchoconstrictive complications than inhalational agents, and was not associated with pulmonary aspiration.[360]

Between World Wars I and II improvements in the organization of the anesthesia community resulted in advances in training, equipment, anesthetic and adjunct drugs, and quality of care. During this period an increase in civilian accidents paralleled the rise in the number of motor vehicles and industrial progress. By the outbreak of World War II, anesthesiologists were better equipped: intravenous anesthesia was established, advanced anesthesia machines were available, other anesthetic equipment and supplies were refined, nitrous oxide was in adequate supply, cyclopropane was available, and intraoperative monitoring of blood pressure was practiced by most physicians. World War II provided abundant experience in trauma anesthesia. It was during this war that Halford,[215] after using large doses of thiopental in victims of the Pearl Harbor attack, described the drug as "an ideal method of euthanasia in war surgery." His findings were challenged by Adams and Gray,[8] who successfully anesthetized a patient in hemorrhagic shock with small doses of thiopental. Another significant finding at this time was increased survival of hypovolemic animals given spinal anesthesia.[152,363] In fact spinal anesthesia was used successfully in 42% of surgical procedures by Clement and Elder.[94] Various regional nerve blocks also gained popularity; in one series 99% of 3050 anesthetics for wounded soldiers used these techniques.[61]

Subsequent wars in Korea, Vietnam, and the Middle East have further added to our experience of prehospital management, patient transport, fluid and cardiopulmonary resuscitation (CPR), transfusion, acute respiratory distress syndrome (ARDS—then termed *shock lung*), acute renal failure, infections, and many anesthetic and adjunct drugs.

Experience, however, did not come only from war surgery. Civilian injuries requiring surgical and anesthetic management resulted in improvement in various areas of care. For at least 25 years, trauma has been the leading cause of death during the first 4 decades of life, and as such it accounts for the greatest number of years of potential life lost (YPLL) before age 65 (see also Chapter 1). Although, in comparison with other causes of premature mortality, YPLL caused by intentional and unintentional injuries has been slightly declining in recent years,[270] trauma remains the leading cause of premature mortality. During the 1970s a number of studies demonstrated that up to 30% of trauma-related deaths could be prevented if appropriate systems for trauma care were developed.[81] Details of these systems are discussed in Chapter 29. In general, regionalization of hospitals; improvement in organization of emergency medical services; designation and verification of trauma centers based on institutional commitment, appropriate auditing, education, and research represent the basic ingredients of this system. These systems are now well in place and have reduced major trauma-related morbidity and mortality.[413,414]

Consonant with these developments, anesthetic care of the injured also has changed considerably over the years. However, few scientifically sound experimental and clinical studies of the effects of anesthesia in the traumatized patient have been performed. Much of the information available relative to anesthetic care of the injured is based on anecdotal reports, data from nontraumatized patients, or a few animal studies. We feel that research in this realm similar to that performed in other subspecialties of anesthesiology such as pediatric, obstetrical, neurosurgical, or cardiac anesthesia is needed. There are, however, certain established principles to be followed during anesthetic management of an acutely injured patient. This chapter is a summary of these principles with special emphasis on practical aspects of anesthetic care of the major trauma victim. For specific areas, the reader is referred to other chapters in the book, where more detailed information is provided.

## GENERAL CHARACTERISTICS OF THE MAJOR TRAUMA VICTIM

Available information from national statistics[6,24,339] and the Maryland Institute of Emergency Medical Systems[428] (MIEMSS) demonstrates that 75% of multiple trauma patients admitted to a trauma center are males under the age of 40; the mean age is 26. Although the incidence of major trauma due to falls, burns and motor vehicle accidents (MVA) in patients over 60 years of age has increased, this age group represents only 6.5 to 8.3% of all seriously injured patients admitted to MIEMSS.[428] Approximately 20% of all seriously injured patients admitted to MIEMSS have some type of preexisting chronic disease, suggesting that a significant number of trauma victims younger than 60 are not entirely healthy. Available data suggest that 65% of trauma patients admitted to the hospital have serious injuries.[428] The causes of these are summarized in Table 9-1. It is obvious that MVA, falls, and work-related accidents are responsible for approximately 75 to 80% of patients admitted to trauma centers. Since these types of accidents cause primarily blunt trauma, it is not surprising that the majority of patients admitted to most trauma centers present with injuries to more than one organ system. Penetrating injuries occur less often, except in inner-city trauma centers where violent crime or homicide attempts occur more frequently. Overall morbidity and mortality from blunt injuries are probably higher than those from penetrating trauma.[52] In the abdomen, penetrating weapons produce more predictable organ injury than does blunt trauma. In the penetrating trauma category, mortality is four times more likely from a gunshot wound than from a stab wound.[52] There is a seasonal variation in both incidence of and mortality from MVA-related injuries; the rate is highest during the summer months and lowest during the winter.[130] There is also a diurnal variation in the occurrence of trauma and operative treatment of its victims. In Bellevue Hospital Center, New York City, 70% of major trauma surgery is performed between the hours of 7 PM and 7 AM.

Not all major trauma victims admitted to a trauma center require surgery.[428] As shown in Table 9-2, only 16.7% of patients with injury severity scores (ISS) between 1 and 12 required emergency surgery, and only 22.2% of this group were operated on at any time during their hospitalization. The frequency of emergency or follow-up surgery more than tripled for patients with ISS between 13 and 19, and more than quadrupled for those who had ISS ≥ 20. The mortality rate of these patients also increased with increasing ISS. Emergency surgery was performed in 49.1% of patients admitted with severe brain injury, 25% of those with spinal cord injury, and 44% of patients with combined brain and spinal cord injury. Approximately 50 to 60% of these patients required surgery during their hospitalization. The mortality rate was highest, approximately 30%, in the group with severe central nervous system (CNS) injuries. These data are roughly in keeping

TABLE 9-1. Causes of Serious Injuries in Patients Admitted to Maryland Trauma Hospitals in 1984

| | % |
|---|---|
| Motor vehicle accidents | 23 |
| Falls | 35 |
| Industrial, farm, and construction accidents | 21 |
| Burns | 1 |
| Suicide attempts | 1 |
| Homicide attempts | 8 |
| Other causes | 11 |

(From Siegel et al[428] with permission.)

TABLE 9-2. Surgery and Mortality Rates of All Trauma Admissions (Excluding Admission Cardiac Arrest) to MIEMSS (1983 to 1984) by Category of Injury

| | NUMBER | % TOTAL | % EMERGENCY OPERATION | % ANY SURGERY | % MORTALITY IN CATEGORY |
|---|---|---|---|---|---|
| ISS 1–12 | 699 | 42.3 | 16.7 | 22.2 | 0.6 |
| ISS 13–19 | 209 | 12.7 | 53.1 | 63.2 | 3.4 |
| ISS ≥ 20 | 228 | 13.8 | 77.2 | 86.8 | 11.8 |
| Severe brain injury | 279 | 16.9 | 49.1 | 61.3 | 29.8* |
| Spinal cord deficit | 132 | 8.0 | 25.0 | 50.0 | 3.0 |
| Multiple neurological injury (brain and spinal cord) | 9 | 0.5 | 44.4 | 66.6 | 33.3 |

* 14.5% mortality for all brain injury (573 patients).
(From Siegel and Dunham[428] with permission.)

with those from other centers where approximately 40 to 50% of admitted patients undergo major surgery by the trauma service, an additional 25 to 30% by specialty services, and 20 to 30% are managed without surgery.[221]

Table 9-3 shows the percentages of types of surgery performed in each of the patient categories. In the group without head or spinal cord trauma, the rate of surgery for each of the anatomical areas increased with increasing severity of injury. Interestingly, patients with severe brain trauma needed almost the same number of general surgical procedures as they required for their head injury. Likewise, 53% of patients with spinal cord injury required neurosurgical intervention, and 28.8% of these patients also required general surgical procedures. This pattern is characteristic of blunt trauma in which more than one organ system is commonly injured, and surgery by different specialists is required.

Generally, all life-, organ-, and limb-saving procedures are performed during the initial emergency operation. These procedures, depending on the severity, multiplicity, and complexity of the injury, may last from 30 minutes to 12 hours. The duration of both emergency and follow-up surgery is greater in patients with severe head injury and those with high ISS than in those with spinal cord injuries or low ISS. In the MIEMSS the duration of surgery for patients who subsequently died in the hospital tended to be less, especially for the group with severe brain injury, suggesting that fatal brain injury was recognized and only palliative decompression procedures were performed.[428]

On the average, 5 to 6 hours are spent in emergency surgery for most patients who sustain multiple trauma. Occasionally, as in the case of pelvic fractures with significant arterial bleeding, the patient may have to be transported to the radiology unit and anesthesia continued there for embolization of bleeding arteries that cannot be controlled surgically.[404] Thus, the anesthesiologist must adopt a flexible approach, anticipating intraoperative events as additional injuries are discovered and helping coordinate the activity of different surgical disciplines in a priority-oriented fashion.

The overall mortality rate from trauma in major centers such as the MIEMSS approaches 12%.[428] However, this figure includes patients who arrived at the emergency room in full cardiac arrest and those with brain injuries and a Glasgow coma scale of 3. The mortality rate in this group of patients ranges between 80 and 95%. Exclusion of these patients from MIEMSS statistics results in a 5.3% mortality rate. In the younger patient, there is a strong correlation between injury severity, as determined by ISS, and mortality; there is a death rate of 2 to 3% for patients with an ISS of 20 to 29, 37.5% for an ISS of 30 to 49, and 87.5% when the ISS is 50.[23,24] The mortality rate of elderly patients is 5 times that of young patients, probably because of an increased incidence of multiple preexisting diseases; their physiological disturbances make the anatomically oriented ISS an unreliable predictor of survival.[353] The presence of CNS injury and the occurrence of hypovolemic shock even for short periods seem to increase mortality in the elderly.[353] In one study, elderly survivors of

TABLE 9-3. Frequency (%) and Types of Surgery Performed on Trauma Patients at the MIEMSS (1983 to 1984) According to Trauma Category*

| PROCEDURE TYPE | ISS 1 to 12 | ISS 13 to 19 | ISS ≥ 20 | SEVERE BRAIN INJURY | SPINAL FRACTURE WITH CORD DEFICIT |
|---|---|---|---|---|---|
| Neurosurgery | 5.4† | 12.4† | 20.2† | 65.6 | 53.0 |
| Craniofacial | 7.9 | 14.8 | 19.7 | 18.6 | 6.1 |
| Thoracic surgery | 2.0 | 15.8 | 37.3 | 18.3 | 15.9 |
| General surgery | 16.7 | 35.9 | 64.5 | 56.6 | 28.8 |
| Orthopedic surgery | 12.6 | 46.4 | 49.6 | 18.3 | 19.7 |
| Plastic reconstructive surgery, debridement (including craniofacial) | 35.1 | 45.5 | 43.0 | 28.0 | 14.4 |

* Numbers in columns represent percent of patients operated on. (From Siegel and Dunham[428] p 24, with permission.)
† Minor neurological surgery (eg, ICP bolt).

trauma had higher hemoglobin, lower systemic vascular resistance, and higher oxygen delivery than nonsurvivors.[230] Thus, utmost attention should be paid, and appropriate monitoring should be used to avoid hypovolemia, tissue hypoxia, and anemia in these patients.

A significant number of trauma deaths occurs during surgery. At the MIEMSS, 1.8% of all trauma patients died in the operating room due to uncontrollable hemorrhage, coagulation abnormalities, hypothermia, shock, and or acidosis.[428] This figure represented 15.4% of trauma deaths in this institution and was only slightly lower than the 21.3% rate of mortality in the intensive care unit (ICU) caused by ARDS, multiorgan failure, and sepsis.

Nearly every patient with major trauma presents a different set of problems, depending on the type, severity, and multiplicity of injuries; preexisting medical problems; intoxication; and resulting anatomical and physiological disturbances. Unlike elective or most other emergency surgical patients, satisfactory preoperative evaluation may be hindered by time constraints, communication difficulties, and preoccupation with immediate resuscitative measures. Thus, injuries may easily be missed, and important medical problems that would otherwise require modification of anesthetic care may go unnoticed only to be recognized when problems develop during the intraoperative or early postoperative period. In addition, the rapidly changing status of these patients requires constant observation, treatment, and documentation. Hence, during the perioperative period the anesthesiologist not only assumes the task of administering a safe anesthetic but also is committed to being an acute care specialist with both diagnostic and therapeutic responsibilities.

Caring for the major trauma patient in the operating room involves resuscitation as well as administration of anesthesia. After securing an airway and ensuring adequate ventilation, restoration of blood volume with cellular and acellular fluids is the most important aspect of resuscitative care. Shock is a frequent occurrence in the acutely traumatized patient and is most commonly caused by hemorrhage. It is suggested that both early and late fatalities can be reduced if shock is treated rapidly and effectively following trauma.[154,172,194,474] The first hour following injury is termed the *golden period* during which successful treatment of shock is associated with lower mortality.[67] Obviously, failure to maintain the restored blood volume during the ensuing hours of surgery will obviate the beneficial effect of early treatment. Appropriate fluid resuscitation in the traumatized patient can also improve, at least temporarily, the hemodynamic deterioration resulting from other causes of hypotension such as pericardial tamponade[267] and acute spinal cord trauma.[291]

The trauma victim with multiple injuries poses a difficult decision-making situation, and even minor deviations from sound judgment may result in unanticipated problems. Prioritizing both anesthetic and surgical management is of critical importance for these patients. For instance, the injured brain is sensitive to even small elevations of $Pa_{CO_2}$ caused by apnea, airway obstruction, or failure of ventilation. Thus, in a patient presenting with combined head and thoracic injuries, allowing a period of apnea or hypoventilation in order to place a double-lumen tube may result in disastrous complications. As a basic principle, immediate therapeutic intervention should be directed to the most life-threatening problems. The ABCs of CPR should be remembered at all times; airway, breathing, and circulation must be established as soon as possible before specific management of other organ systems is undertaken.

Trauma victims, especially those injured in MVAs, are frequently intoxicated with alcohol and/or other substances such as cocaine, opiates, barbiturates, marihuana tricyclic antidepressants, or phencyclidine.[182,441,461] Anesthetic management of these patients may be complicated by the effects of these agents; careful and expectant perioperative care is required. This subject is discussed in detail in Chapter 8.

As most patients who sustain major trauma are young, the presence of preexisting disease is an exception rather than a general characteristic. However, with the steadily increasing number of individuals over the age of 65 and earlier recognition of some chronic abnormalities by improved diagnostic techniques, more trauma victims are likely to present to the anesthesiologist with some type of known preexisting disease. Available data about the risk of emergency trauma surgery in the presence of preexisting disease are inconclusive but suggest that mortality is higher in these patients[157,175,382,479] (see also Chapter 8). Obesity; diabetes mellitus; sickle cell anemia; asthma; hypertension; cirrhosis; and renal, cardiovascular, and neurological diseases present special challenges to the anesthesiologist. Not infrequently, patients are on chronic drug therapy. The possible interaction of these agents with trauma, hemorrhage, and anesthetic agents should be considered.

Infection control precautions should be taken by physicians, nurses, and other personnel managing acute trauma patients. In a preliminary study in Baltimore, Baker et al[22] noted a 16% incidence of human immunodeficiency virus (HIV) seropositivity in trauma victims between the ages of 25 and 34 years. Thirty-three percent of these patients had a history of drug abuse. Precautions to prevent transmission of HIV to health care workers include provision of appropriate barriers such as gloves, gowns, and goggles to prevent skin and mucous membrane exposure to patients' blood and body fluids; washing of hands and other skin or mucous surfaces immediately after contact with patient secretions and blood; prevention of injuries by sharp contaminated objects (needles, scalpel, instruments); use of appropriate mouthpieces, resuscitation bags, or other ventilation devices to avoid mouth-to-mouth resuscitation during emergency airway management; and refraining from direct patient care when the worker has open skin lesions in exposed areas.[271]

## PREINDUCTION PHASE

### PREPARATION OF THE OPERATING ROOM

Often, after a brief period of evaluation and stabilization in the emergency department, the multiply injured patient is quickly transported to surgery. Thus, a trauma center must have operating rooms prepared in advance to receive critically injured patients on a moment's notice. Preparation of the operating room involves not only readiness of anesthetic equipment, supplies, and drugs, but also coordination, in advance, of rapid and adequate help from other departments such as nursing, blood bank, radiology, and laboratory. Table 9-4 lists the essential and occasionally needed items required for anesthetic care of the injured. All essential items must be ready for use at the time of the patient's arrival. This involves ensuring proper function of all equipment, preparation of balanced salt infusions, infusion systems and fluid warmers, setting up and calibrating transducers, and preparation of medications in labeled syringes. Drug security in the operating room must be maintained. One way of providing this is by sealing filled syringes in a transparent, nonresealable plastic bag.[70] All drugs must be dated and signed by the person preparing them. Keeping drug-filled syringes or the sealed bag in a locked anesthesia machine drawer adds further to drug security. At times, some infrequently used items may be life saving, necessitating their instant availability. Stocking and periodic checking of a special "trauma anesthesia cart" will assure easy access to these items.

## EVALUATION PRIOR TO ANESTHETIC INDUCTION

Although in most instances the anesthesiologist becomes involved in care upon the patient's arrival in the emergency department, not infrequently the severity of injuries mandates immediate transport of the patient to the operating room where a brief preanesthetic evaluation takes place. Even if the patient is examined in the emergency department, he/she must be reassessed prior to induction of anesthesia since the condition of the trauma victim changes from one moment to the next. This is especially true during patient transport to

TABLE 9-4. Anesthesia Equipment, Supplies, and Drugs Needed for Trauma Surgery

| ESSENTIAL | OCCASIONALLY NEEDED |
|---|---|
| *Equipment* | *Equipment* |
| Anesthesia machine with volume-controlled ventilator | Jet ventilator |
| Laryngoscope with different type and size blades | PEEP valves |
| Two blood warmers | Transcutaneous $O_2$ monitor |
| Rapid infusion system (Level 1, Haemonetics) | Noninvasive cardiac output monitors (bioimpedance or transesophageal doppler) |
| Warming blanket (Bair Hugger) | Fiberoptic bronchoscope |
| Heated humidifier to warm inspired gases | Additional blood and fluid bag pressurizing devices |
| Automatic blood pressure monitor with different sizes of cuffs | Autotransfusion device |
| ECG monitor | Calibrated infusion pumps to deliver vasopressors or inotropes |
| Pulse oximeter | Transesophageal Echocardiography Device |
| End-tidal $CO_2$ monitor | *Supplies* |
| Defibrillator with internal and external paddles | Material for specialized airway management: translaryngeal wire, 14-gauge intravenous catheter over a needle connected to a 3-mL syringe and appropriate endotracheal tube connector for ventilation of lung during uncorrectable airway obstruction, Magill forceps, necessary instruments for cricothyrotomy or tracheostomy, double-lumen endobronchial tube with appropriate attachments |
| Blood and fluid bag pressurizing devices | Material for pulmonary artery line placement |
| Neuromuscular function monitor | Fluid infusion sets with microdrip chamber |
| Temperature monitor | Tube thoracostomy set |
| Two-channel intravascular pressure monitor | *Drugs* |
| Multichannel recorder | Atropine |
| Inspired oxygen analyzer | Vasopressors and inotropes (ephedrine, phenylephrine dopamine, dobutamine, epinephrine) |
| Ambu bag with PEEP attachment | Calcium chloride or gluconate |
| *Supplies* | Lidocaine 4% for topical use |
| Different sizes of masks, oro- and nasopharyngeal airways, endotracheal tubes, stylets | Lidocaine 2% for intravenous use |
| Material required for intravenous, intra-arterial, and central venous line placement | |
| Two intravenous infusion sets with pumps | |
| Large clear plastic bags for covering patient's head and torso to minimize heat loss | |
| Heat and moisture exchanger to be connected between the anesthesia circuit and the endotracheal tube | |
| Yankauer suction tip | |
| Regular suction catheter | |
| Blood- and fluid-heating coils or bags | |
| *Drugs* | |
| Intravenous induction agents | |
| Muscle relaxants | |
| Inhalation agents | |
| Opiates or opioids | |

the operating room, a notorious time for occurrence of major hemodynamic and blood gas deteriation without appropriate monitoring.

Clinical evaluation before anesthetic induction should be performed rapidly, with special attention to the airway, oxygenation, hemodynamic status, level of consciousness, associated injuries, and ongoing resuscitative measures. If the patient is conscious and able to talk about the state of his/her health, medications, allergies, and previous anesthetics, a history should be obtained as time permits.

Patients may arrive in the operating room with an endotracheal or tracheostomy tube or, rarely, an esophageal obturator airway (EOA) in place. Correct position and patency of the tracheal tube must be confirmed, and the EOA should be left in the esophagus until a cuffed endotracheal tube is inserted. Removing an EOA before tracheal intubation places the patient at risk of aspiration. However, in individuals with small stature and a short neck, intubation of the trachea in the presence of an EOA may prove to be difficult.[133] Availability of a well-functioning suction device with a Yankauer tip will reduce the risk of aspiration associated with EOA removal in these patients. The use of EOA in the prehospital setting has been abandoned in most areas, and thus problems associated with this device are now rarely seen.

In patients with multiple injuries, pulmonary gas exchange is often disturbed. Pulmonary contusion, pneumothorax, hemothorax, rib fractures, aspiration of gastric contents, fluid overload, and ARDS are common causes of lung dysfunction in the injured. Oxygen should be administered to all patients immediately upon arrival in the operating room. Baseline arterial blood gases should be obtained to assess oxygenation and acid-base status. In patients with impaired gas exchange due to aspiration, ARDS, or fluid overload, distending ventilatory pressures such as positive end-expiratory pressure (PEEP) or continuous positive airway pressure (CPAP) should be applied with the level titrated according to $Pa_{O_2}$ and hemodynamic response. Auscultation of breath sounds and examination of the chest X-ray are important in order to rule out rib fractures, diaphragmatic hernia, hemothorax, and pneumothorax.

Gross estimation of intravascular volume can be made by observing central venous and arterial pressure, pulse rate, external bleeding, chest tube drainage, and the rate and amount of fluid infusion. If central venous pressure (CVP) monitoring is not available and the blood pressure is within normal range, a decrease in arterial blood pressure of more than 10 to 15% in response to 45 to 60° head-up tilt suggests mild to moderate hypovolemia. Dimensional changes of the thigh or abdomen are poor indicators of the amount of internal blood loss. From a simple principle of geometry, in a normal adult an increase of 1 cm in the radius of the thigh (considered as a cylinder) represents a blood loss of 2 L, and an increase of 2 cm amounts to a hemorrhage of 4.5 L.[475] While such small changes in thigh size are difficult to appreciate, usually swelling in the extremity after a fracture assumes a spherical rather than a cylindrical shape, making estimation even more difficult. In addition, with the passage of time, fluid accumulation in the tissues may further increase extremity size and result in overestimation of blood loss. Nevertheless, a grossly swollen extremity immediately after acute injury suggests at least 2 to 3 L of blood loss. Reliance on abdominal circumference to predict the amount of hemoperitoneum is particularly misleading because not only blood but air or fluid may accumulate in this cavity. In addition, the diaphragm can move cephalad, allowing significant blood loss without change in abdominal circumference.

Restoration of intravascular volume with colloid or crystalloid solutions before induction of anesthesia should be given a high priority during this phase. Even if the patient requires immediate surgery, rapid and vigorous fluid infusion during the brief preoperative period can reduce the hemodynamic complications of anesthetic induction.

Ongoing neurological evaluation during the preinduction phase of anesthesia includes assessment of the level of consciousness, of the size of the pupils, and monitoring of intracranial pressure (ICP) if an epidural bolt, an intracerebral fiberoptic sensor (Camino Laboratories, San Diego, CA) or a ventricular catheter, is in place. Drowsiness or disorientation may be the result of alcohol or drug intoxication, hypoglycemia, hypoxia, hypotension, intracranial pathology, and/or electrolyte abnormalities. These possibilities should be kept in mind and the exact cause determined if time permits. Patients with epidural hematomas may develop unconsciousness following a lucid interval; thus, consciousness should be monitored continuously. Important principles in patients with known intracranial pathology during the preinduction phase are hyperventilation in order to lower $Pa_{CO_2}$ to a level between 25 and 30 mm Hg, 30° elevation of the head, and prevention of bucking, coughing, and agitation.

Sometimes associated injuries are not recognized during initial evaluation of the trauma victim in the emergency department. Of these, head and cervical spine injuries, eye injuries, hemothorax, pneumothorax, airway injuries, pulmonary and cardiac contusion, hemopericardium, thoracic aortic injury, and diaphragmatic injury are particularly important for the anesthesiologist as they may require special anesthetic techniques. In all trauma victims who have been rushed to the operating room without adequate preoperative evaluation, these possibilities should be considered, and careful but rapid assessment—by obtaining information from the trauma surgeon, by clinically evaluating the patient, and by reviewing X-rays and laboratory findings—should be made.

Ongoing evaluation of resuscitative measures includes checking venous lines for proper placement, ensuring unimpeded flow of intravenous fluids, monitoring arterial and central venous pressures and waveforms on the oscilloscope, observing the amount and color of the urine, and monitoring the ECG for heart rate, dysrhythmias, and ST-T segment abnormalities. Severely hypovolemic trauma victims and those with pelvic injuries may present to the operating room with military antishock trousers (MAST) in place. Rapid deflation of the MAST may result in hypotension; thus great care and coordination between anesthetic and surgical teams are required to effect a hemodynamically smooth deflation. Patients with elevated ICP, congestive heart failure, or pulmonary edema may not tolerate MAST.[496] Thus, the device should be used with great caution and appropriate monitoring in these patients. Bleeding from perineal injuries may be hidden by MAST. A special effort must be made to evaluate the rate of bleeding from the perineum in these patients during the preinduction phase. Other major complications of MAST include ischemic skin changes, compartment syndromes, renal perfusion failure, and acidosis during reperfusion of areas under the MAST.[73,302,496]

Occasionally patients with impalement injuries of the head, face, torso, or extremities may present to the anesthesiologist. It is important to realize that the impaling object may have injured a large vessel inside the body; it should be removed only under controlled conditions after the patient is anesthetized.[234]

## PREMEDICATION

Although patients with mild injuries often benefit from analgesics or sedatives, hypovolemic patients with major trauma should not be medicated prior to their arrival in the operating room. Premedication, if desired, can be given intravenously to patients with adequate circulating blood volume. Small doses of narcotic (morphine, 1 to 2 mg; fentanyl, 25 to 50 μg) or sedative (diazepam, 2.5 mg; midazolam, 0.5 to 1 mg) are administered in the emergency room with close monitoring of blood pressure, heart rate, and respiration and repeated as required to obtain the desired degree of analgesia and sedation. The patient should then be accompanied to the operating room or to the radiology suite.

There is no indication for premedicating trauma patients with $H_2$ receptor antagonists if surgery will take place within 1 hour of administration. On the other hand, intravenous administration of cimetidine (300 mg) at least 1 hour before surgery has been shown to protect between 80 and 90% of emergency patients from acid-induced pneumonitis during intubation and extubation.[101,131,452] The drug should be given as a slow infusion over a period of 10 minutes with careful ECG and blood pressure monitoring since rapid injection may produce hypotension and sinus arrest.[235,281] Experience with ranitidine in the trauma patient is lacking, but intravenous ranitidine (50 mg) has been shown to raise the pH of gastric fluid above 5.0 within 45 to 60 minutes in all of a group of volunteers.[123] The onset of action of intravenous metoclopramide is faster (15 to 30 minutes) than that of $H_2$ receptor antagonists, but this drug cannot reduce gastric fluid volume reliably. Nevertheless, metoclopramide, 10–20 mg intravenously, has been used with success in Europe to prevent acid aspiration pneumonitis during anesthetic induction of emergency patients.[124,351] Nonparticulate antacids (30 ml of 0.3 mol/L sodium citrate, two tablets of Alka-seltzer Gold in 30 ml of water, or 5 to 10 ml of 8.4% sodium bicarbonate) given 10 to 60 minutes prior to anesthetic induction may be useful, but there is little experience with these agents in the trauma patient. Although any of these agents or their combination reduces the risk of aspiration pneumonitis, none can guarantee reliable protection. Thus, their use does not eliminate the requirement for anesthetic induction techniques designed to prevent aspiration.

## TRANSFER TO THE OPERATING TABLE

Transfer of the patient from the emergency room stretcher to the operating room or X-ray table requires care. Hypovolemic patients and those with head and spine injuries may be at particular risk. Hypovolemic patients can become hypotensive on changing position because of decreased venous return caused by gravitational pooling of blood. Many head-injured patients are intubated in the emergency room or X-ray suite prior to arrival in the operating room. Movement of the head during transfer to the operating room table may result in tracheal stimulation by the tube and coughing. In order to avoid cough-induced increase in ICP, administration of lidocaine (1.5 mg/kg), or at times, thiopental and muscle relaxant, may be indicated prior to moving these patients. Patients with cervical spine injury should be kept in constant cervical traction during transfer; it is wise to ask the surgeon to coordinate this movement since the anesthesiologist is preoccupied with maintaining the airway.

## POSITIONING

The presumption that autotransfusion of blood from the lower extremities to the central circulation would support blood pressure and aid in maintaining blood flow to vital organs led to widespread use of the Trendelenburg position in hypovolemic combat victims during the First and Second World Wars.[138] It is now established that this position not only results in little—if any—and unsustained hemodynamic improvement[372] but also has deleterious effects on respiratory function and ICP.[102]

Passive leg raising 3 minutes after changing from upright to supine position produced an 8 to 10% increase in cardiac output and stroke volume in healthy normovolemic persons, but this improvement disappeared within 7 minutes of leg elevation.[186] More importantly, leg raising after 45 minutes of supine position in normovolemic volunteers had no beneficial hemodynamic effect.[186] In a more recent study, passive leg raising improved cardiac and stroke volume indices (more in mildly hypovolemic than in normovolemic awake volunteers), but complete hemodynamic compensation for as little as 1 unit of blood loss could not be obtained.[507] The volume of blood in the lower extremities, especially in patients with compensatory vasoconstriction following acute hemorrhage, is insufficient to produce a clinically meaningful autotransfusion.[186] Thus, neither Trendelenburg position nor passive leg raising can produce hemodynamic improvement in the major trauma victim; rapid infusion of fluids provides much more effective and reliable intravascular volume repletion than either of these maneuvers.

Repair of multiple organ injuries requires prolonged surgery. Pressure on parts of the body in contact with the operating table or arm boards may result in suboptimal perfusion and decubitus ulcers. Adequate padding of the posterior aspects of the feet, elbows, and head and the use of soft mattresses will minimize these complications.

## INTRAVENOUS LINES

Establishment of immediate venous access and rapid fluid administration remain of paramount importance in the treatment of hypovolemic shock. Several large-bore intravenous catheters may be necessary to restore the traumatized patient's intravascular volume. In the majority of instances these lines have already been placed in the field and the emergency department. Many times, however, additional access may be needed in the operating room.

Vasoconstriction in the hypovolemic patient usually precludes cannulation of peripheral veins. In these circumstances a central vein may easily be cannulated with a small catheter (18- or 16-gauge), which may be rapidly converted to a large-volume infusion system by using a guide wire and vessel dilator. The femoral vein can be catheterized with an 8.5 French introducer sheath or a same size teflon catheter if vessels proximal to the infusion site are not disrupted.[292a] Thus, following pelvic or abdominal trauma this route should not be used unless venous injuries are ruled out. In patients with a palpable femoral artery pulse, the entry point to the femoral vein is 1 cm medial to the artery just below the ilioinguinal ligament. When profound shock does not allow palpation of the femoral artery, the vein may be located at a point one third of the distance from the pubic tubercle to the anterior superior iliac spine, just below the ilioinguinal ligament. This approach was used with success in the Vietnam War, even in patients with cardiac arrest.[196] Short-term femoral vein catheterization in this series did not increase the incidence of thromboembolism. Complications of this technique were accidental arterial puncture without sequelae (6.3%), local hematoma (1.3%), and local infection (1.4%).[196]

The technique of percutaneous infraclavicular subclavian vein catheterization was used by Simpson and Aitchison[430] with 95% success in 172 patients with hypovolemic shock; only one attempt was required in 70% of the patients. There was, however, a 5% complication rate including pneumothorax, hydrothorax, hemothorax, and neck hematoma. The internal jugular vein may be cannulated using an anterior approach at the junction of the sternal and clavicular heads of the sternocleidomastoid muscle or through an approach posterior to this muscle. The need for Trendelenburg position when jugular or subclavian vein cannulation is performed limits the use of these techniques in patients with head injury. If percutaneous techniques are not possible, venous access can be attained by cut-down to the brachial, external jugular, or saphenous vein. On rare occasions, in the severely hypovolemic patient who is transported to the operating room following an emergency room thoracotomy, a large-bore catheter introduced into the right, or in some instances into the left, atrium by the surgeon may serve as an effective fluid infusion line. Care should be taken to avoid air embolization via the catheter in this situation.

The flow rates of intravenously administered fluids depend on the type and temperature of the fluids; the calibers of the tubing, catheter, and the vein; and whether a micropore filter or a pressurizing system is used. Laminar flow rates are determined by Hägen-Poiseuille equation,[468]

$$F = \frac{\Delta P \pi r^4}{8 \eta L}$$

where $F$ is the flow rate (in $cm^3/s$),$\Delta P$ is the pressure drop across the tubing (in dyne/$cm^2$), $\eta$ is the viscosity of fluid (in centipoise), $L$ is the length of tubing (in centimeters), and $r$ is the internal radius of the tubing (in centimeters). Under certain circumstances laminar flow becomes turbulent and the relationship between driving pressure and flow is no longer linear.[366] The factors that increase turbulent flow (high driving pressures, high flow rates, check valve within the intravenous tubing, and stopcocks) increase resistance and thereby restrict the maximum achievable flow.[366] The rate of turbulent flow through straight tubes is determined by the following equation:

$$F^2 = \frac{\Delta P 4 \pi^2 r^5}{f L \rho}$$

where $f$ is a dimensionless friction factor that depends on tube wall roughness and somewhat on the Reynolds number, and $\rho$ is the fluid density (in g/$cm^3$).[468] Thus, the rate of laminar flow is inversely proportional to fluid viscosity whereas that of turbulent flow is inversely proportional to fluid density.[468]

It is well known that the high viscosity of packed red blood cells (PRBC) slows infusion rates by 50 to 80% as compared with crystalloid solutions. Although reducing the hematocrit of PRBC to 45—as in whole or saline-reconstituted blood—results in an improvement, infusion rates still remain 30 to 35% less than those obtained with Ringer's lactate.[137] The flow rates of albumin are similar to those of crystalloid solutions.[137] Of the several systems employed to increase driving pressure of intravenous fluids, gravity is the least effective.[137,224,313] Slow infusion rates are somewhat improved by "pushing in" blood or fluid with a 50-mL syringe and three-way stopcock assembly interposed in the infusion tubing.[137] Flow rates can be increased by this method over those obtained by a gravity system only when catheters smaller than 14 gauge are used; little advantage is obtained with larger catheters.[137] In contrast, infusion rates of blood or fluids through all sizes of catheters can be increased by the use of reservoir pumps.[137] For a given catheter size, manually inflated pressure cuffs at 200 to 300 mm Hg can triple the infusion rates obtained by gravity.[137,224,300,313] Unfortunately, long set-up time and difficulty in maintaining constant pressure are major disadvantages of hand-filled pressure cuffs. These problems are partially obviated by box-enclosed high-pressure-driven infusor pumps that allow rapid manipulation of bags and short inflation/deflation times[239,488a] (Fig 9-1). This system, when used with large-bore intravenous infusion tubing, allows infusion of 2 L of Ringer's lactate in about 3 minutes (640 mL/min); the corresponding time with a standard-bore hand-pumped device is approximately 10 minutes (190 mL/min).[239] In 1984, Philip and Philip[365] designed another pressurized infusion system that consisted of four pressure infusor cuffs inflated with compressed air distributed through a plastic manifold. Inflation pressure in this system was regulated by a pressure regulator commonly used to adjust pressure in limb tourniquets (Fig 9-2). Depending on the diameter of the intravenous tubing, this system can infuse Ringer's lactate at a rate of 500 to 600 mL/min and blood at 300 to 400 mL/min.[365] In another system advocated by Rosenblatt et al[392] rapid blood transfusion has been accomplished by using an old Bentley autotransfusion system as a single-pass infusion pump. Blood and saline solution is poured in a pitcher, suctioned, and transferred to a reservoir by a roller pump and then transfused to the patient (Fig 9-3). The fluid

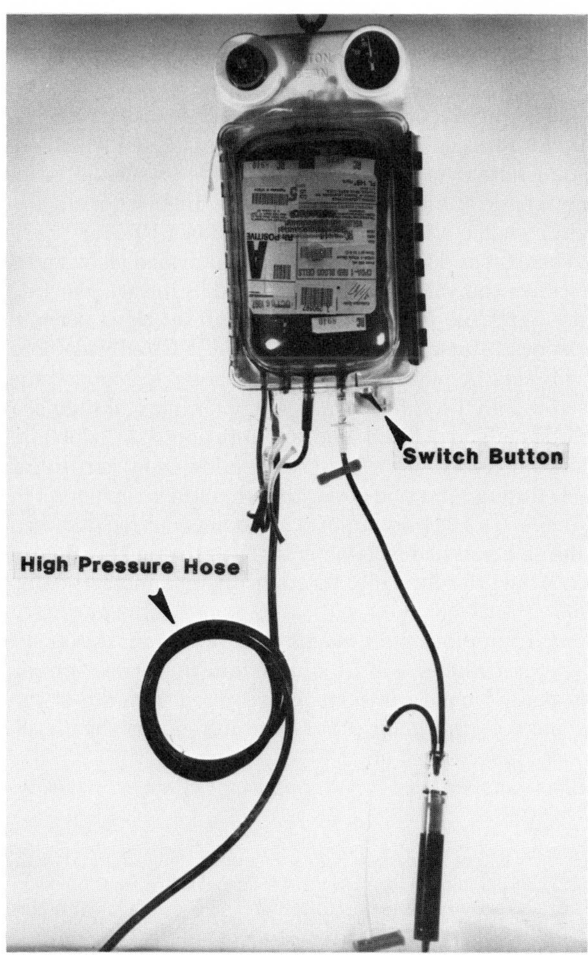


FIG. 9-1. Photograph of a box-enclosed, high-pressure-driven infusor cuff. Pressure to the system is provided by the high-pressure hose connected to a wall air source. Inflation and deflation of the cuff inside the box are achieved by switching the button indicated by the arrow.

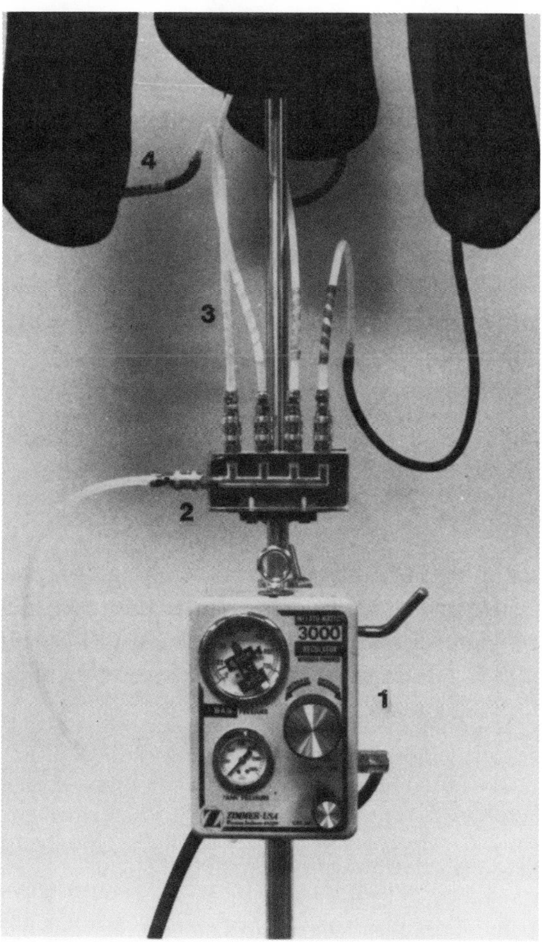


FIG. 9-2. Pressure infusor assembled by Philip and Philip. 1, Zimmer pressure regulator; 2, plastic manifold; 3, connecting tubings; 4, infusor cuffs. (From Philip and Philip[365] with permission.)

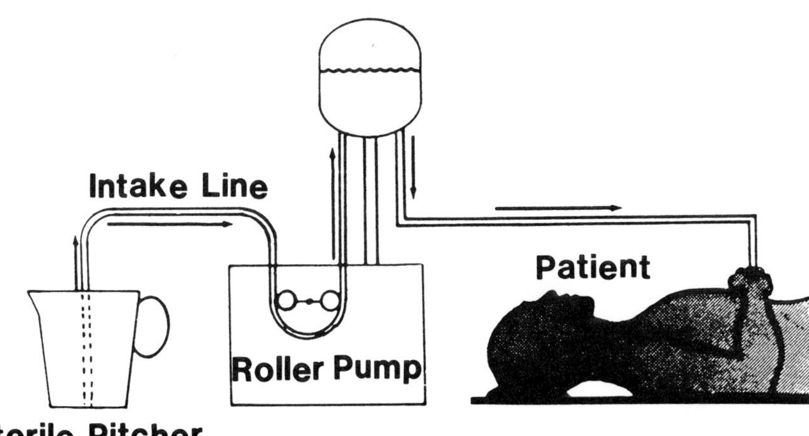


FIG. 9-3. Schematic diagram of the system used by Rosenblatt et al for rapid transfusion. See text for explanation. (From Rosenblatt et al[392] with permission.)

can be warmed to 40°C to help maintain core temperature. In the six cases reported by Rosenblatt et al,[392] 500 to 1000 mL/min blood-crystalloid mixture was infused; heparinization of blood products was not necessary. One should obviously be familiar with whatever device is used before employing it clinically. This also applies to several other rapid fluid infusion systems which have recently become available (Level-1, Marshfield, MA, Haemonetics, Braintree, MA). Infusion of fluids under high pressure may be associated with the danger of air embolism if there is excess air in the bag; elimination of air from the fluid container will decrease the danger.[364] The maximal fluid flow rate at which the air trap supplied with the Level-1 infusor is effective is 600 mL/min; above this rate air embolism is inevitable if air is allowed to enter the tubing. Another potential complication is fluid overload, which can be minimized by careful monitoring of fluid intake and hemodynamics.

A significant portion of the resistance to flow in ordinary intravenous sets comes from the small diameter (3.5 mm) of the tubing. Thus, it is not surprising that an improvement in flow rate is obtained by the use of the 6-mm tubing available in a urology set.[138a,313,336] However, the extent of improvement is dependent upon the size of the catheter in the vein. In vitro studies demonstrate that improvement of flow with urological tubing was greatest when used with a 9.5- to 10-gauge intravenous catheter or 8.5French catheter introducer; there was little improvement in flow rate through 16-gauge catheters[313,336] (Fig 9-4). Blood filters, which are now used infrequently, are another source of resistance, but their effect on flow rate is less pronounced than that produced by narrow tubing and small catheters.[336]

Of all the factors affecting infusion flow rate, the diameter and length of the intravenous catheter are probably the most important; large-bore short-length cannulas can deliver more fluid than narrow-bore long catheters[9,137,224] (Fig 9-5). In order to increase infusion rates, direct venous cannulation with feeding tubes, intravenous tubing, or pulmonary artery catheter introducers has been advocated. A short 8.5French catheter infusion system is currently marketed which allows administration of 300 to 400 mL/min crystalloid or blood (emergency infusion device, Arrow International). Hansbrough et al[218] showed that placement of a 10-gauge catheter via venous cut-down was simple and provided blood and fluid flow rates equivalent to those obtained by intravenous tubing. They were able to administer 1200 mL of blood per minute by using a 10-gauge catheter with pressurized wide-bore infusion sets. A pulmonary artery catheter introducer sheath inserted into the subclavian, femoral, or internal jugular vein provides effective blood and fluid infusion if introducer kinking is prevented.[9,138a,313] It is tempting, however, to infuse fluids through the side port rather than the main port of these catheters. In 1981 Benumof et al[45] demonstrated that the hub of the side port had a diameter equal to that of 16-gauge catheter. Thus, the flow rate through this channel is nearly the same as that obtained with a 16-gauge catheter (Fig 9-6). Although improvement in this feature was recommended, a 16-gauge catheter still fit snugly into the Arrow introducer side port. If rapid infusions are required, removal of the attachment at the main port of the introducer sheath allows direct connection of an intravenous set.

Blood temperature has an important effect on viscosity.[138a]

FIG. 9-4. Flow rates through urological set (Y-URO), urological set with blood filter (Y-URO + BF), and ordinary blood transfusion set (Y − Transfusion) with different size intravenous catheters. * No catheter used. (From Nadeau and Tousignant[336] with permission.)

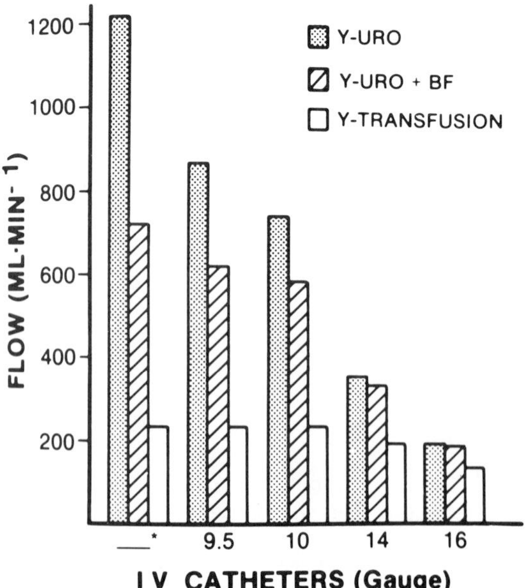


FIG. 9-5. Effect of catheter gauge (upper diagram) and catheter length (lower diagram) on flow rate of normal saline solution delivered at gravitational pressure. (From Hodge and Fleisher[224] with permission.)

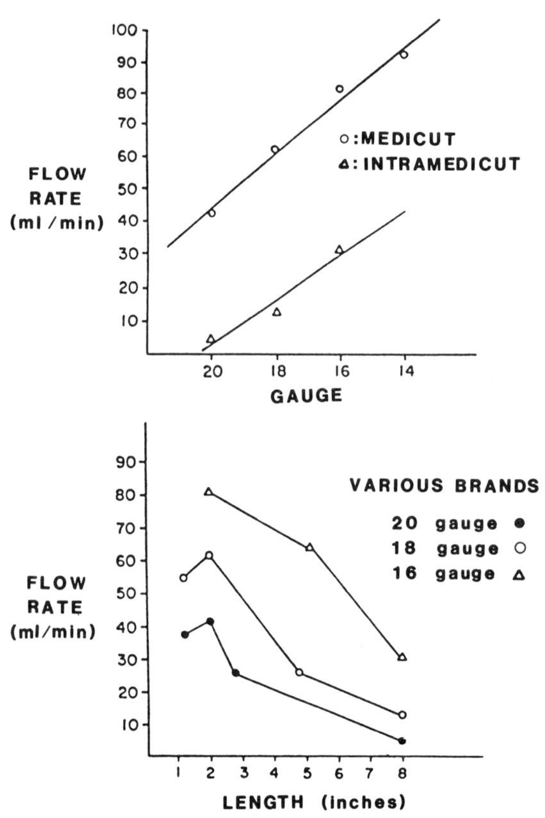

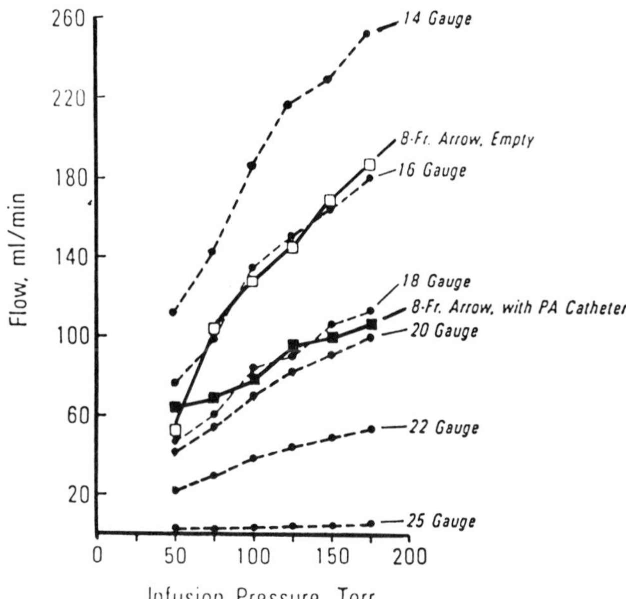


FIG. 9-6. Pressure-flow relationships of saline through various sized catheters and side port of Arrow 8French introducer with and without indwelling 7French triple lumen thermodilution pulmonary artery catheter. (From Benumof et al[45] with permission.)

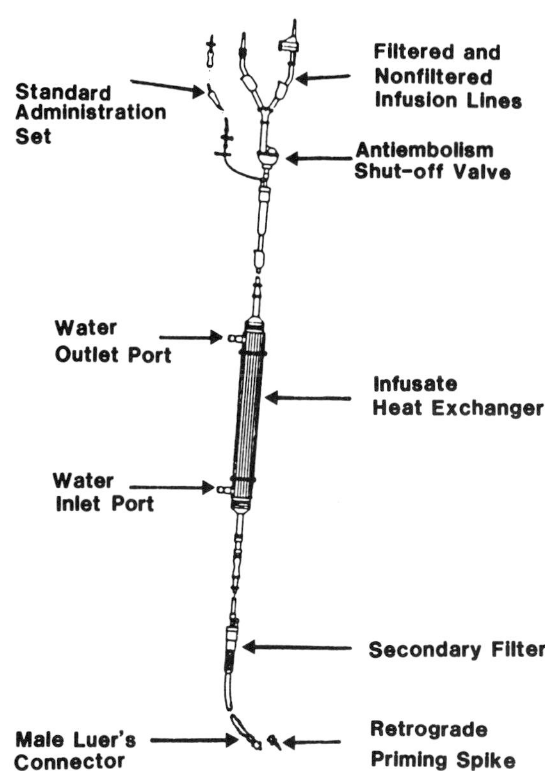


FIG. 9-7. Rapid infusion system originally designed by Fried et al[181] and with slight modifications manufactured by Level 1 Technologies Inc. Components of the system are connected by 5-mm polyvinylchloride perfusion tubing. Water ports of the infusate heat exchanger are integrated with a separate heating unit. (From Satiani et al[401] with permission.)

Knight[260] showed that warming the blood to body temperature doubles the flow compared with transfusion at 10°C. In order to improve infusion rates and maintain normothermia Fried et al[181] designed an infusion system in which high flow rates are achieved by using low-resistance filters and large-bore perfusion tubing. The administration set incorporates an extracorporeal heat exchanger maintaining infusate temperature at 37°C regardless of the infusion rate and initial fluid temperature (Fig 9-7). This system allows crystalloid, colloid, and blood flow rates of up to 1600 mL/min in animals[181] and provides massive fluid infusion in severely injured patients without significant drop in body temperature.[401] The device is commercially available (Level 1, Marshfield, MA).

## MONITORING

Although many critically injured patients are young and healthy, their physiological condition deteriorates rapidly from the time of trauma to the time of surgery because of severe impairment of vital organ functions. In addition, a small percentage of injured patients is elderly or has significant chronic diseases. Successful anesthetic management of these patients is predicated on the careful, sequential assessment of vital organ functions which can be attained by sophisticated monitoring techniques. This is not to say, however, that a full complement of invasive techniques should be utilized in all acutely traumatized patients prior to emergency surgery. Quite the contrary, the valuable time wasted in placement of intravascular monitoring lines, calculation of hemodynamic and oxygenation indices, and waiting for laboratory results in a severely hemorrhaging patient limits the effectiveness of subsequent surgical control of bleeding and, in fact, can decrease the chance of survival. Also, in many physiologically stable trauma victims careful clinical assessment and routine intraoperative monitoring may be sufficient. Thus, prioritizing diagnostic and therapeutic modalities according to prevailing circumstances, the most important principle of acute trauma management, applies to the operating room selection of monitoring techniques as well.

Basic monitoring for all traumatized patients undergoing emergency surgery includes ECG, arterial blood pressure, body temperature, urine output, inspired $O_2$ concentration, auscultation of breath and heart sounds, end-tidal $CO_2$, and pulse oximetry. In many injured patients, however, additional monitoring methods are required. Table 9-5 lists monitoring techniques currently used in the operating room and their importance in the intraoperative care of the trauma patient.

### *Electrocardiogram*

Continuous oscilloscopic monitoring of the standard lead II ECG provides detection of dysrhythmias and inferior wall ischemia.[251] Another useful lead for dysrhythmia detection is $V_1$, which can be monitored in a five-wire ECG system by placing the chest lead in the $V_1$ position at the fourth intercostal space to the right of the sternum.[251] Myocardial ischemia is best monitored with a five-lead system by placing the chest lead in the $V_5$ position, the left fifth intercostal space at or slightly anterior to the anterior axillary line. With this arrangement, displaying leads II and $V_5$ simultaneously al-

TABLE 9-5. Currently Available Techniques to Monitor Various Physiological Parameters and Their Importance in Intraoperative Management of the Trauma Patient

| PHYSIOLOGICAL PARAMETER | DEGREE OF IMPORTANCE | MONITORING EQUIPMENT | SPECIFIC INTRAOPERATIVE USES IN THE TRAUMA PATIENT |
|---|---|---|---|
| Cardiac rate, rhythm, and myocardial ischemia | Essential | Five-lead ECG system with oscilloscope, digital display, recorder and printer (three-lead system can be used) | Routine |
| Arterial blood pressure | Essential | Blood pressure cuff<br>Doppler system<br>Programmable oscillometric system<br>Pressure transducer with calibrated oscilloscope and recorder, digital display, and printer | Routine |
| Central venous pressure | Useful | Water manometer (not desirable)<br>Pressure transducer with calibrated oscilloscope and recorder, digital display and printer | Hypovolemia<br>Pericardial tamponade<br>Air embolism |
| Pulmonary artery systolic, mean, diastolic and occluded pressures | Useful in some patients | Pressure transducer with calibrated oscilloscope and recorder, digital display and printer | Blunt chest injury (myocardial contusion)<br>ARDS<br>Differentiation of low- and high-pressure pulmonary edema<br>Traumatic (cardiac contusion) or preexisting heart failure |
| Cardiac output | Useful | Noninvasive<br>Transesophageal Doppler (not tested in the trauma patient)<br>Bioimpedance device (not tested in the trauma patient)<br>Invasive<br>Thermodilution cardiac output computer with recorder and printer | Same as pulmonary artery pressure measurement |
| Cardiac wall motion abnormalities, myocardial ischemia, flow through valves or septal defects | Useful | Transesophageal echocardiograph | Cardiac contusion?<br>Coronary artery injuries?<br>Septal injuries<br>Air embolism |
| Ventilation | Essential | End-tidal $CO_2$ monitor with waveform display and recording<br>Mass spectrometer (slow response time) | Head injury<br>Air embolism |
| Arterial oxygenation | Essential | Pulse oximeter<br>Transcutaneous $Po_2$ ($Ptco_2$) monitor<br>Arterial blood gases (intermittent or continuous) | Simultaneous $Ptco_2$ and $Pao_2$ measurement may be useful in the diagnosis of shock |
| Tissue oxygenation | Useful | Arterial pH electrode<br>Transcutaneous $Po_2$ ($Ptco_2$) monitor (with $Pao_2$)<br>Oximetry pulmonary artery catheter<br>Arterial/venous lactate analyzer | Low perfusion states |
| Renal function | Essential | Foley catheter and graduated container | In all major trauma patients |
| Temperature | Essential | Esophageal or rectal probe | Routine |
| Neuromuscular function | Essential | Peripheral nerve stimulator<br>EMG? | Head injury<br>Open globe<br>Sealed major vessel injury |
| Neurological function | Useful | ICP measurement with bolt, catheter or fiberoptic sensor | Head injury |

lows detection of anterolateral and inferior wall ischemia as well as dysrhythmias. If a multiple wire system is not available, a modified $V_5$ lead may suffice to detect myocardial ischemia with reasonable accuracy. One way of obtaining this is by placing the right arm electrode just below the clavicle on the right shoulder, the left arm electrode in the $V_5$ position, and the left leg electrode in its usual position. In this system, turning the selector switch to lead I (or AVL) allows detection of anterior wall ischemia while lead II (or AVF) detects inferior wall ischemia.[250] We monitor a true or modified $V_5$ lead routinely in trauma patients over 30 years of age unless lead placement interferes with surgery. When the use of many electrodes is inconvenient, bipolar leads may be used for detection of dysrhythmia and myocardial ischemia. Modified chest lead I ($MCL_1$) can be monitored by placing the left arm lead beneath the left clavicle, the left leg lead in the $V_1$ position, and setting the lead selector switch to lead III.[251] Another useful bipolar lead is $CB_5$ which is capable of detecting both dysrhythmias and anterior wall ischemia; the left arm lead is placed over the right scapula posteriorly and the left leg lead in the $V_5$ position.[39]

With all of the above systems, myocardial ischemia is recognized by ST segment depression greater than 1 mm at a point 0.06 second from the J-point. ST segment elevation suggests significant transmural ischemia. The severity of myocardial ischemia is probably proportional to the extent of ST segment elevation or depression, but it should be remembered that these changes may also be caused by oscilloscopic artifacts. With the new generation of ECG oscilloscopes these errors are probably less frequent. Addition of an ST segment analyzer to the operating room monitor can be useful in reducing the rate of diagnostic error.

### *Arterial Blood Pressure*

Measurement of arterial blood pressure in the hypovolemic trauma victim by means of the traditional auscultatory method is both difficult and inaccurate. An automated oscillometric or Doppler blood pressure device may overcome some of these problems and should be used routinely in all trauma patients. However, there is probably no effective substitute for direct intra-arterial pressure monitoring since it permits beat-to-beat data acquisition during critical moments such as induction of anesthesia, clamping and unclamping of major vessels, or rapid hemorrhage. In addition, the arterial waveform enables the anesthesiologist to judge intravascular volume and, if pulsus paradoxus occurs, to diagnose pericardial tamponade (Fig 9-8).

The shape of arterial pressure trace, the location of the dicrotic notch, and the slope of the diastolic run-off have long been used by clinicians to derive information about systemic vascular resistance (SVR) and cardiac output. A high dicrotic notch and a slow diastolic run-off usually suggest increased SVR. These signs, however, are not always reliable; in one study no correlation could be found between the height of the dicrotic notch, SVR, cardiac output, and the slope of the diastolic run-off.[193] In contrast, the cyclical change of arterial pressure trace during positive pressure ventilation suggests hypovolemia and is a useful sign to guide fluid therapy.[112,242,361] Ventilation-dependent changes of the arterial pressure trace during hypovolemia are discussed further in Chapter 4. The presence of an arterial line also allows easy blood sampling for measurement of blood gases, electrolytes, and glucose. Thus, every effort must be made to place this line—even if it requires surgical cut-down—prior to surgery. If time constraints preclude establishment of an intra-arterial line before anesthetic induction or airway management, a high priority should be given to its insertion as soon after induction as possible, without delaying surgical control of bleeding.

The site chosen for arterial cannulation depends on the nature of the injury, the planned operation, and the anesthe-

FIG. 9-8. Arterial pressure trace of a 35-year-old man who was stabbed on the chest and developed pericardial tamponade. Upper panel shows pulsus paradoxus before drainage of pericardial tamponade. Lower panel shows normalized arterial pressure trace immediately after relief of tamponade.

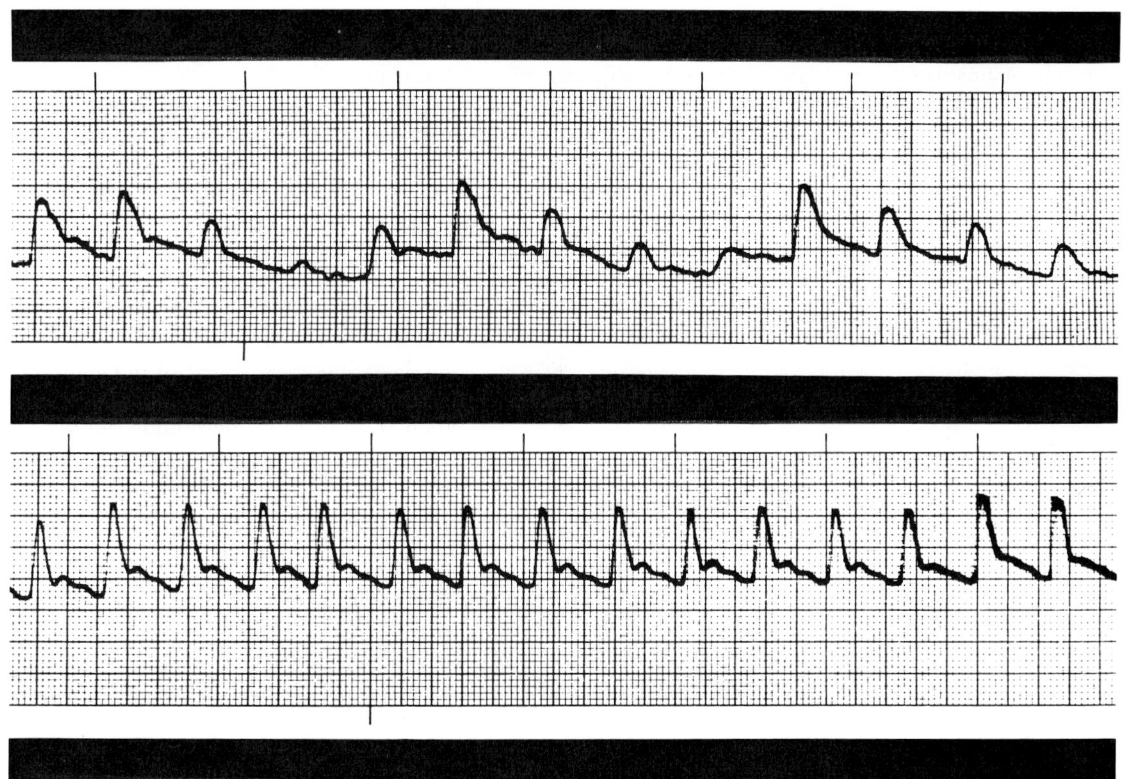

siologist's preference. The radial artery is most commonly used because it is accessible, easy to cannulate, supplies the hand which receives collateral circulation through the ulnar artery, and is relatively free from serious complications.[40,41,337,433] It is the artery of choice in abdominal or chest trauma in which the aorta may be cross-clamped, making a femoral or dorsalis pedis cannula nonfunctional. Although the artery of the nondominant hand is usually selected, the right radial artery is preferred in cases of chest trauma in which cross-clamping of the descending aorta might result in occlusion of the left subclavian artery. The dorsalis pedis and femoral vessels are safe alternatives[211,337,396,511] if the arms are injured or if the subclavian vessels are damaged, as in some penetrating wounds of the neck.

Both overdamping and underdamping of the arterial pressure trace may result in inaccurate measurement and thus inappropriate therapy. The consequences of these artifacts in the acutely traumatized patient may be detrimental since hemodynamic management of the injured is heavily based on blood pressure measurement. Overdamping is characterized by a poorly defined peak pressure and a slurred or lost dicrotic notch. The systolic blood pressure is attenuated while the diastolic pressure rises toward the mean arterial pressure. Overdamping of the arterial trace is caused by small air bubbles in the tubing or transducer, highly compliant tubing, or the use of multiple stopcocks in the system. Underdamping is characterized by narrow, highly peaked waves with a low or late dicrotic notch. It may result in a systolic blood pressure reading of as much as 50% above the true value. The diastolic portion of the curve drops below the actual pressure level, resulting in a relatively unaffected mean arterial pressure measurement. Underdamping is caused primarily by too much tubing (greater than 1 meter) between the insertion site of the catheter and the transducer and by large tubing diameter. Artifactual errors caused by overdamping and underdamping can be recognized easily by comparing the arterial pressure with that measured by cuff.[30]

### *Central Venous Pressure*

Central venous pressure should be monitored when large amounts of fluid administration are anticipated or pericardial tamponade is suspected. The catheter placed for this purpose may also serve for rapid fluid resuscitation and provides access to the central circulation if rapid response to pharmacological therapy—as in hypoperfusion or nonperfusion states—is needed.

The CVP reflects the relationship between intravascular volume and right ventricular function. It may not reflect left-sided filling pressure, especially in patients with ischemic or valvular heart disease. Caution is advised in interpreting CVP during massive fluid infusion since high CVP readings obtained at this time may drop quickly to low levels a few minutes after stopping the infusion.[359] The CVP is also usually high in the presence of pericardial tamponade, myocardial contusion, and in some patients with pneumothorax or hemothorax even when hypovolemia is present.[359] CVP should be measured with a pressure transducer since a water manometer does not have an adequate frequency response in the tachycardia patient, cannot provide continuous monitoring, and does not permit rapid verification of catheter position.

### *Pulmonary Artery Pressures and Cardiac Output*

Time constraints usually preclude preinduction placement of a pulmonary artery catheter in the massively traumatized patient. Fortunately, there is usually little need for this catheter during intraoperative management of most critical injuries. However, it may be helpful in patients with known left ventricular dysfunction, severe coronary artery disease, and/or valvular heart disease. In addition, a pulmonary artery catheter may be useful in guiding intraoperative PEEP therapy when ARDS has developed; in differentiating between high- and low-pressure pulmonary edema; and during intraoperative management of patients with spinal cord and blunt chest trauma, especially myocardial contusion.[147,169,291,440,455] When time permits, insertion of an introducer sheath before surgery via the internal jugular or subclavian vein may be extremely useful as it allows rapid fluid administration as well as later introduction of a pulmonary artery catheter, if needed.

All directly measured intravascular pressures should be displayed on a calibrated oscilloscope and a recorder. Recently introduced operating room monitors have the capability of giving a printout of the screen display including digital readings. The accuracy of digital pressure readings—even with newly introduced microprocessor algorithms—has been questioned because they are affected by positive pressure ventilation and patient movement.[490] Thus, it is important to read arterial and venous pressure values directly from a calibrated oscilloscopic screen or recording.

Measurement of cardiac output ($\dot{Q}_t$) during the acute stage of trauma may be useful in guiding fluid therapy since it is more sensitive to intravascular volume reduction than arterial blood pressure[212] (see Chapter 4). In addition, $\dot{Q}_t$ measurement may allow further refinement in therapy by permitting calculation of various hemodynamic and oxygenation indices. As we mentioned above, placement of a pulmonary artery catheter to measure $\dot{Q}_t$ is not practical and cannot be strongly recommended during the initial care of the uncomplicated trauma victim. However, two new techniques, thoracic bioimpedance[47,48] and esophageal Doppler ultrasonography,[296] measure $\dot{Q}_t$ noninvasively with reasonable accuracy and may be used as trend indicators. Although neither of these methods has been tested in the acutely traumatized patient and they both have limitations, further work may demonstrate their usefulness in the trauma setting.

Caution is advised in measurement and interpretation of $\dot{Q}_t$ by the thermodilution technique in acute trauma. The potential for error appears to be large at low flow states; thus a given cardiac output measurement must be interpreted only in conjunction with other clinical and hemodynamic parameters in the presence of hemorrhagic shock.[335]Inaccurate $\dot{Q}$ values may be obtained in patients with left-to-right shunts, right-to-left shunts, or pulmonary or tricuspid regurgitation resulting from chest injury, because of loss of injected indicator or recirculation of blood within the heart.[335] The effect of positive pressure ventilation on the accuracy of $\dot{Q}_t$ determination is well known. Results may vary up to 20% depending on the time of measurement during the respiratory cycle. At least two measurements—preferably at mid-inspiration and end-expiration—and averaging of values have been recommended to reduce this error.[350] Perhaps the most interesting error may occur during rapid administration of fluids through peripheral intravenous lines. Wetzel and Latson[503] demonstrated underestimation of $\dot{Q}_t$ by 80% when measurement was made during intermittent rapid infusion of crystalloid solutions at room temperature. This error is caused by fluctuations in baseline blood temperature because of changes in peripheral infusion rate. The rate of fluid administration should be kept constant, or the infusion should be stopped at least 30 seconds prior to cardiac output measurement.

COMPLICATIONS OF INVASIVE HEMODYNAMIC MONITORING. Invasive arterial and venous monitoring, although often useful for proper evaluation of trauma patients, is associated with problems. Complications of radial artery cannulation include limb ischemia, thrombosis, pain, hematoma formation, infection, and emboli.[54] Emboli from the cannula are the probable cause of the most serious complication—ischemia. The ability of the classic Allen's test to evaluate collateral circulation and determine the patient's risk of ischemia has been questioned. In a study of 1700 patients, 16 had an abnormal preoperative Allen's test but did not suffer sequelae while cannulated.[433] The incidence of thrombosis with partial or total occlusion of the artery in this study was 20%. Careful observation, the use of small-gauge Teflon catheters, continuous heparin flush, and dressing care all help decrease complications.[54]

The complication rate of central venous catheterization increases when cannulation is performed under emergency conditions.[4,148,376] Pneumothorax, hemothorax, hydrothorax, thrombosis, extravasation of the cannula, cardiac tamponade, arrhythmias, air embolism, and catheter embolism have all been reported following subclavian vein catheterization.[115,159,261,292,498] The internal jugular approach decreases the incidence of pneumothorax although the problem may still occur. One must also beware of carotid artery puncture with this approach.

Complications of pulmonary artery (PA) catheterization include those from central venous line insertion plus arrhythmias, right bundle branch block (RBBB), pulmonary infarction, pulmonary artery rupture, cardiac damage, catheter knotting, infections, balloon rupture, thrombosis, and thrombocytopenia.[148,357,376,498] Arrhythmias occur frequently; lidocaine and a functioning defibrillator must be available. Normally the incidence of RBBB during placement of a PA catheter is 3 to 6%, but it increases to 25% with preexisting left bundle branch block (LBBB).[445] A pacing catheter can be utilized, or preferably, a pacing wire should be available. Special catheters (Paceport, Edwards Co), which have a separate port to introduce a pacing wire, are more expensive than regular catheters but provide considerable ease and patient safety when emergency cardiac pacing is indicated. The high incidence of thrombosis associated with the original PA catheters has decreased with the use of heparin bonding.[223] Pulmonary infarction and rupture are the major complications associated with the use of PA catheters. To prevent pulmonary infarction, the pressure trace must be monitored continuously, and the balloon should be inflated only briefly for wedge pressure measurement. Overwedging and forceful catheter flushing should be avoided to prevent pulmonary artery rupture.[445]

### *Noninvasive Cardiovascular Imaging Techniques*

Of the recently developed cardiovascular imaging techniques, transesophageal two-dimensional echocardiography has become a diagnostic tool for anesthesiologists, especially those involved in cardiovascular anesthesia. The device consists of a 3.5-mHz transducer system mounted on the tip of a gastroscope, an acoustical lens to focus an ultrasound beam, and an ultrasonograph to phase the elements. All four cardiac chambers, the left ventricular outflow tract, and the cardiac valves can be imaged by this method once the gastroscope is advanced about 35 to 40 cm into the esophagus. Operator experience is a prime requisite for proper use of the technique and interpretation of the data. Insertion and positioning of the ultrasound transducer usually require less than 60 seconds, which speaks highly for the practical value of the method.[79] The capabilities of transesophageal echocardiography include real-time evaluation of cardiac morphology, ventricular function, segmental myocardial wall motion, myocardial ischemia and infarction, and detection of air embolism with high sensitivity.[79,93] At this time the device costs approximately $100,000, and few operating rooms are equipped with it.

Although there are no reports describing the use of this device during intraoperative management of acutely injured patients, it may provide valuable information in specific types of trauma, particularly in blunt chest injury, which has the potential of causing myocardial contusion, cardiac septal and/or valvular damage, coronary artery injury, pericardial tamponade, and pulmonary trauma which may in turn be complicated by air embolism upon institution of positive pressure ventilation. Myocardial contusion, apart from causing cardiac irritability, can also reduce the heart's ability to compensate for the abnormal hemodynamic states produced by other injuries. The use of a pulmonary artery catheter has been suggested in these patients as a guide for hemodynamic management.[147,169,440,455] Transesophageal echocardiography, despite its limited ability to quantitate hemodynamic variables, may eliminate the need for pulmonary artery catheterization in these patients by providing information on cardiac chamber size and wall motion. However, further experience in this area is needed to substantiate these speculations.

### *Urine Output*

Urine output is routinely monitored as an indicator of organ perfusion, hemolysis, skeletal muscle destruction, and urinary tract integrity following trauma. Although there is no doubt that urine output is a useful guide to judging intravascular volume and kidney perfusion, information obtained by this method may be misleading at times. Following hemorrhage and prolonged shock, renal failure may already be present at the time of the patient's arrival in the operating room. In these instances the rate of urine flow will be affected by the existing renal failure (high output or oliguric) as well as kidney perfusion. Also, some injured patients may receive radiopaque dye for diagnostic X-rays prior to or during surgery. Osmotic diuresis produced by these agents will eliminate the reliability of urine output as an index of tissue perfusion. Finally, the response time of urine flow to intravascular volume changes is rather slow, reducing its efficacy.

The excretion of dark, cola-colored urine in the traumatized patient suggests either hemoglobinuria or myoglobinuria. Hemoglobinuria in the traumatized patient is usually caused by incompatible blood transfusion or thermal injury. In the former case, hypotension, bronchial wheezing, and sometimes skin manifestations may be present. Myoglobinuria results from massive skeletal muscle destruction. Pink-stained serum seen following centrifugation of a blood specimen suggests hemoglobinuria, and unstained serum usually indicates myoglobinuria. Urine reacts positively to the benzidine test in both instances, thus positive identification of the pigment requires electrophoresis or immunoprecipitation. Finally, myoglobinuria, but not hemoglobinuria, is associated with a significant rise in serum creatine phosphokinase (CPK) levels. Both hemoglobinuria and myoglobinuria may cause acute renal failure, which may be prevented by promoting diuresis with mannitol. In myoglobinuria, alkalinization of the urine with sodium bicarbonate to pH levels above 5.6 may also help prevent acute renal failure. Further information on hemoglobinuria and myoglobinuria is provided in Chapter 25.

Red-colored urine usually suggests hematuria which, in the traumatized patient, usually results from urinary tract injury. Likewise, the absence of urine flow may be caused by total interruption of the urinary tract by the injury or by preexisting conditions. These possibilities should be kept in mind and discussed with the other members of the operating team. Intravenous injection of methylene blue (5 to 10 mL) may be useful in helping the surgeon locate the site of urinary tract injury during abdominal surgery.

### *End-tidal $CO_2$ Concentration*

Monitoring of ventilation by inspection of chest excursions, continuous auscultation of breath sounds, and observation of airway pressure is of prime importance during anesthesia for any type of surgery. Additional safety is provided by monitoring the end-tidal $CO_2$ concentration, either by an infrared $CO_2$ detector or a mass spectrometry system. Apart from informing the anesthesiologist about acute hypoventilation, endotracheal tube malposition, abnormal breathing patterns, and pulmonary embolism and allowing continuous estimation of $Pa_{CO_2}$, end-tidal $CO_2$ can be extremely useful during anesthetic management of patients with head and open-eye injuries in whom maintaining $Pa_{CO_2}$ below normal is of crucial importance. In this respect, infrared $CO_2$ monitors are probably preferable to mass spectrometry because they have a quicker response time. It is important to remember that a $CO_2$ sensor placed between the endotracheal tube and the Y-piece of the anesthesia breathing system may not detect partial obstruction distal to this site. Thus, careful monitoring of airway pressure is important even when expired $CO_2$ is being monitored.

The gradient between end-tidal and arterial $CO_2$ is affected by the type of ventilation used; the gradient is smallest during spontaneous breathing (1 to 2 mm Hg), slightly increased during intermittent positive pressure ventilation (3 to 5 mm Hg), and greatest during jet ventilation (10 to 25 mm Hg). Low-frequency jet ventilation results in a lower gradient than does high-frequency jet ventilation[83] (Table 9-6). As the difference between arterial and end-tidal $CO_2$ varies during jet ventilation, a fudge factor cannot be used to estimate $Pa_{CO_2}$ from end-tidal $CO_2$.[83] Thus, estimation of $Pa_{CO_2}$ from end-tidal $CO_2$ during jet ventilation requires cessation of ventilation, delivery of a large breath with a conventional breathing circuit, and recording of the waveform to determine the end-tidal point of the curve.[310] Continuous $Pa_{CO_2}$ estimation can also be provided by a transcutaneous $CO_2$ electrode. This method appears to be a good trend indicator and is not affected by anesthetic agents. However, it is less useful than end-tidal $CO_2$ monitor in measuring absolute $Pa_{CO_2}$ values.[377]

### *Oxygenation*

Hypoxemia occurs frequently in the traumatized patient from pneumothorax; hemothorax; airway disruption; pulmonary edema; aspiration of blood, foreign bodies, or gastric contents; pulmonary embolism; or problems in airway management. In addition, alterations in metabolic, circulatory, and red blood cell homeostasis—which occur frequently in the injured patient—interfere with normal oxygen transport. Hence, monitoring of oxygenation at both the arterial and tissue levels is of prime importance during management of these patients. Although this subject is discussed extensively in Chapter 5, in this section we will review briefly some aspects of oxygen monitoring which relate to the practice of the anesthesiologist involved in the care of the injured.

Intermittent analysis of blood obtained from arterial cannulas has long been the mainstay of oxygen monitoring in the injured. This method is highly reliable and, as we mentioned above, despite its invasiveness, is associated with low morbidity. However, it has the disadvantage of the inability to provide continuous real-time $Pa_{O_2}$. Recent advances in technology make continuous invasive $Pa_{O_2}$ monitoring possible with special indwelling catheters equipped with polarographic[68] or fiberoptic sensors.[33,34] Preliminary studies with these devices both in animals and in humans are en-

TABLE 9-6. $Pa_{CO_2}$-$Pet_{CO_2}$ Gradients with Four Types of Ventilation in Dogs*

| MODE | $Pa_{CO_2}$ (mmHg) | $Pet_{CO_2}$ (mmHg) | GRADIENT (mmHg) |
|---|---|---|---|
| SB | 38 ± 2 | 38 ± 2 | 0.3 ± 0.04 |
| IPPV | 36 ± 2 | 32 ± 2 | 3.7 ± 1 |
| LFJV | 37 ± 8 | 24 ± 4 | 13 ± 5 |
| HFJV | 39 ± 8 | 15 ± 5 | 24 ± 8 |

* Gradients refer to differences between $Pa_{CO_2}$ and $Pet_{CO_2}$. All $Pet_{CO_2}$ values were significantly ($p < .001$) smaller than $Pa_{CO_2}$, except during spontaneous breathing. The abbreviations used are: SB, spontaneous breathing; IPPV, intermittent positive pressure ventilation; LFJV, low-frequency jet ventilation; HFJV, high-frequency jet ventilation. (From Capan et al[83] with permission.)

couraging, although the method has not yet been used widely in clinical practice. Technical problems such as catheter clotting from improper flushing, dependence of results on body temperature, long and cumbersome calibration procedures, sensor drift,[68] and decreased accuracy at low $PO_2$ levels[34] are important disadvantages that hopefully will be resolved in the future.

Three noninvasive methods—pulse oximetry and transcutaneous and transconjunctival $PO_2$ measurements—provide continuous real-time monitoring but have limitations in the traumatized patient. Rapid, easy, and accurate determinations of $SaO_2$ between 65% and 100% are possible with pulse oximeters.[460] Some pulse oximeters (Physiocontrol 1600, Novametrix 500 version 2.2 or 3.3) are even capable of measuring accurately $SaO_2$ values as low as 40%.[410] However, the technique may become nonfunctional or inaccurate following trauma. Peripheral vasoconstriction caused by circulatory shock, hypothermia, and vasopressors[311]; elevated carboxyhemoglobin levels after burns[31] or exogenously administered dyes[257] (methylene blue, indocyanine green); bright ambient light[72,107,217]; and dyshemoglobinemias[311] interfere with proper function of the oximeter (Fig 9-9).

The transcutaneous $O_2$ ($PtcO_2$) monitor measures tissue rather than arterial gas tension, and thus the measured $PtcO_2$ in a normal adult averages 70 to 80% of $PaO_2$.[32,471,473] Inhalation anesthetics do not appear to affect measurement of $PO_2$ by this method.[398] In the presence of severely reduced cardiac output or impairment of tissue perfusion, the gradient between tissue gas tension and $PaO_2$ changes markedly and becomes blood flow dependent.[394,471,472] In the trauma patient this may be a useful characteristic since it allows early diagnosis of shock. In fact, the transcutaneous $PO_2$ index, the ratio between transcutaneous and arterial $PO_2$, helps assess peripheral perfusion[471,472] (see Chapter 5). In addition, unlike the pulse oximeter, the transcutaneous $PO_2$ monitor does not overestimate $PO_2$ in carbon monoxide poisoning and falls linearly as the carboxyhemoglobin concentration in the blood increases[31] (Fig 9-9). Unfortunately, the transcutaneous $PO_2$ monitor requires long calibration and electrode-heating times (15 to 30 minutes), the location of the sensor electrode on the skin must be changed frequently to avoid burns, and the device may continue to display $PO_2$ values when its proper function is disrupted by technical difficulties.

The transconjunctival oxygen monitor consists of a small, unheated polarographic electrode that is placed over the palpebral conjunctiva to measure directly oxygen tension in the underlying tissues. The effect of anesthetic agents on the accuracy of this technique is unknown. Several animal and human studies demonstrate that following hemorrhage, reduction in $PO_2$ measured by this method precedes any other physiological changes, including blood pressure.[3,5,437] However, the electrode—although small in size—is bulky, and we are not aware of any report describing its use during anesthesia.

Pulse oximeters, transcutaneous, and possibly transconjunctival $PO_2$ monitors can provide important information as trend indicators during anesthetic management of the injured patient and should be used in conjunction with direct arterial blood gas determination. However, they should not be used as a substitute for direct arterial monitoring until their accuracy, reliability, and practicality in the trauma setting have been confirmed by further studies.

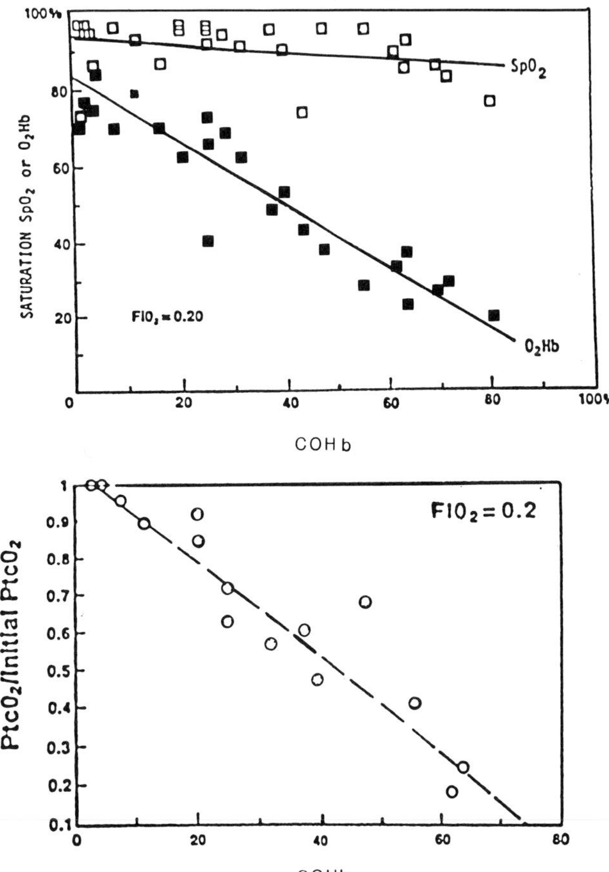


FIG. 9-9. Upper panel shows the relationship between increasing concentrations of arterial carboxyhemoglobin (COHb) and arterial oxygen saturation measured by pulse oximetry ($SPO_2$, open squares) and Cooximeter ($O_2Hb$, solid squares) at $FIO_2$ = 0.20 in dogs. Note that despite an increasing COHb and decreased actual $O_2Hb$, saturation measured by pulse oximetry remains within normal limits. Similar results were obtained at $FIO_2$ = 1.0. Lower panel shows the relationship between increasing concentrations of COHb and transcutaneous $PO_2$ ($PtcO_2$). Note the decreasing $PtcO_2$ with increasing COHb. (From Barker and Tremper[31] with permission.)

Tissue oxygen consumption ($\dot{V}O_2$) is an important predictor of survival following trauma (see Chapter 5). A $\dot{V}O_2$ below normal is associated with high mortality, and therefore every attempt should be made to increase this variable. If a pulmonary arterial line is in place, $\dot{V}O_2$ can be calculated easily using the Fick equation, $\dot{V}O_2 = \dot{Q}_t\,(CaO_2 - C\bar{v}O_2)$. When a pulmonary artery catheter with mixed venous $O_2$ saturation sensor is selected, $\dot{V}O_2$ can be measured continuously.[19] At present, mixed venous saturation catheters with three-wavelength measurement are used, because they provide more accurate information under adverse physiological conditions than those with two-wavelength function.[195]

In most instances a pulmonary artery catheter is not placed prior to or during emergency surgery for trauma. In these situations, measurement of the difference between inspired and expired $O_2$ concentration with a mass spectrometry system, if available, may permit calculation of pulmonary oxygen uptake, provided the respiratory quotient is accurately estimated and the volume of inspired and expired $O_2$ is known. This method gives only a crude estimation of $\dot{V}O_2$. Thus, the results should be interpreted with caution. In addition, it is not practical in the trauma setting because measurement of inspired and expired $O_2$ volume is difficult and time consuming. Another method of determining $\dot{V}O_2$ involves the use of closed-circuit anesthesia with 100% inspired $O_2$. With this approach, the flow rate of inspired $O_2$ is adjusted in such a way that the height of the ventilator bellows during each respiratory cycle remains constant. The oxygen flow rate will then be equal to $\dot{V}O_2$, provided there is no gas leak in the system. However, often there is not sufficient time to determine $\dot{V}O_2$ during efforts to maintain hemodynamic stability in the major trauma victim.

Blood lactate determination provides useful information about tissue oxygen utilization. Unfortunately, many operating room laboratories are not equipped with a rapid lactate analyzer. Further discussion on the importance of blood lactate determination is provided later in this chapter.

### *Temperature*

Hypothermia, a common occurrence following major injury,[246,283,287] is further aggravated during anesthesia; thus, careful monitoring of core temperature is required. The tympanic membrane is an ideal site for temperature monitoring in humans because temperature in this area closely approximates that of the blood supplying temperature-regulating centers in the hypothalamus.[46] However, technical problems such as poor sensor contact due to cerumen in the ear canal and the possibility of tympanic membrane perforation during manipulation of the thermistor limit the usefulness of this technique.[324]

In a definitive study, Cork et al[103] determined the precision and accuracy of various temperature-monitoring sites in elective surgical patients. Precision was quantitated as the correlation between the tympanic membrane temperature and the temperature measured at each of the other sites. Accuracy was defined as the difference between temperatures of the tympanic membrane and each of the other measurement sites. The nasopharynx, esophagus, and bladder were recommended as sites of intraoperative temperature monitoring as they provided the best combination of precision and accuracy. The rectum, although providing reasonable accuracy, lacked precision. Superficial sites like the axilla, forehead, and great toe did not correlate reliably with core temperature, indicating that temperature monitoring with superficially placed liquid crystal discs is not reliable (Fig 9-10 and Fig 9-11). An interesting finding in this study was that the precision of rectal and great toe sites improved with increasing duration of anesthesia (Fig 9-10). A temperature difference of up to 1°C has been demonstrated among various sites in the esophagus by Kaufman[253] in electively operated patients; the esophageal temperature is lowest where heart sounds are heard best and is highest 12 to 16 cm inferior to this location. Thus, esophageal stethoscopes that contain a temperature probe at the auscultatory cuff may underestimate core temperature. The temperature measured from the tip of a pulmonary artery catheter is considered a reliable core temperature.[324] To our knowledge, the relative reliability of temperature monitoring in these sites has not been determined in trauma patients.

### *Neuromuscular Function*

Although a nerve stimulator should be used in all patients undergoing emergency surgery for trauma, it is essential in those with head injury, sealed major vessel damage, or an open globe to avoid coughing, bucking, straining, and vomiting, which is crucial in the anesthetic care of these patients.

### *Laboratory Determinations*

Arterial and—if available—mixed venous blood gas analysis, hemoglobin, hematocrit, serum electrolytes ($Na^+$, $K^+$, $Ca^{2+}$), and blood glucose determinations must be made on admission and repeated at regular intervals intraoperatively.

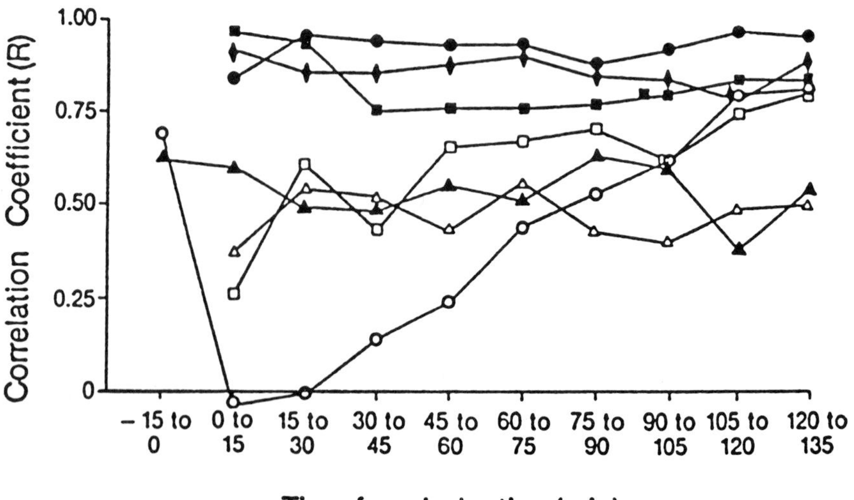


FIG. 9-10. Precision of various temperature measurement sites intraoperatively. Precision is quantitated with the correlation coefficient (R) between tympanic temperature and other temperature measurement sites: ■, bladder; ◆, esophageal; ●, nasopharyngeal; △, forehead; □, rectal; ▲, axillary; and ○, great toe. Note that temperatures measured at the bladder, esophagus and nasopharynx correlate well with tympanic temperature. There is poor correlation between tympanic membrane and forehead, rectal, axillary, and great toe temperatures. However, precision of rectal and great toe temperatures improves markedly 90 to 120 minutes after the beginning of anesthesia. (From Cork et al[103] with permission.)

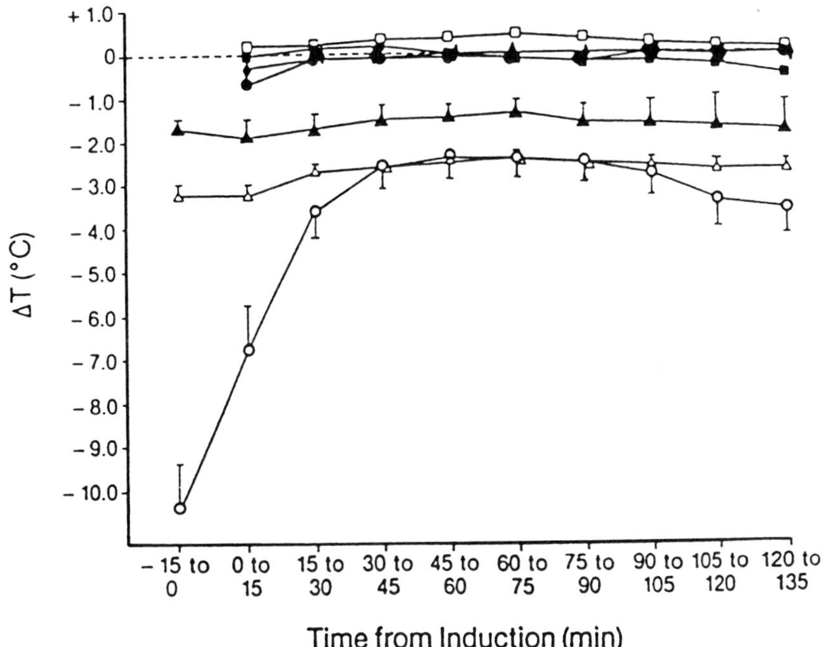


FIG. 9-11. Accuracy of various temperature measurement sites intraoperatively. Accuracy is defined as the difference between tympanic membrane temperature and other temperature measurement sites: □, rectal; ■, bladder; ◆, esophageal; ●, nasopharyngeal; ▲, axillary; △, forehead; ○, great toe. Rectal, bladder, esophageal, and nasopharyngeal temperatures are the most accurate. (From Cork et al[103] with permission.)

Measurement of hemoglobin and hematocrit permits estimation of blood oxygen-carrying capacity and helps guide transfusion therapy. In addition, differences between hematocrit values before and after restoration of intravascular volume with acellular fluids may allow a rough estimate of blood loss.

Serum $Na^+$ rarely changes following trauma and rapid fluid resuscitation. On the other hand, significant and unpredictable changes in serum $K^+$ can occur. Hyperkalemia following trauma is thought to be caused by efflux of $K^+$ from the intracellular space.[238,425] Hypokalemia is more common than hyperkalemia and may result from large intracellular shifts of $K^+$ during maximal adrenal stimulation,[424] since β-2 receptor stimulation activates the ($Na^+$-$K^+$)-ATPase pump and thus moves $K^+$ into the cell.[389,485,506] Shin et al[424] observed $K^+$ levels less than 3.5 mEq/L in massively traumatized patients, which remained low during the entire course of anesthesia even in the presence of acidosis and hypercarbia. A decrease in the serum ionized calcium level during massive transfusion is common, but this reduction is rarely associated with significant hemodynamic alteration. However, when blood transfusion is rapid or citrate clearance is impaired (eg, in hypothermia, renal disease, or hepatic disease), cardiovascular insufficiency may occur.[512] Prolongation of the QT interval on the oscilloscope is a helpful indicator of hypocalcemia with hemodynamic effects during rapid blood and fluid replacement.

Proper control of serum glucose concentration is important in both diabetic and nondiabetic trauma patients, especially those with head injuries. With modern analyzers that use the glucose oxidase enzymatic method, glucose concentrations can be determined accurately in a drop of blood within 30 seconds. Comparable accuracy and efficiency in blood glucose measurement are provided by bedside test strips that use the glucose oxidase reaction.[43] With commercially available portable reflectance meters, the accuracy of determination is further augmented. Of the available paper strips, Dextrostix or Reflotest is designed to be used with a reflectance meter whereas Chemistrip BG or Visidex requires a color chart.[87]

### *Coagulation*

Coagulopathy following acute trauma is a serious complication and has multiple etiologies. Laboratory tests required to differentiate the causes of coagulopathy with reasonable accuracy include complete blood count and differential, prothrombin time (PT), partial thromboplastin time (PTT), platelet count, blood fibrinogen level, and fibrin degradation products (FDP). Blood should be obtained for these tests upon admission to the emergency department since many multiple trauma patients have severe coagulopathy at this stage.[352,386] Serial determination of these parameters is useful intraoperatively but is not practical because of the long time required to obtain results and the unavailability of FDP measurement after hours in many centers. Nevertheless a blood sample should be sent to the laboratory to determine, at least retrospectively, the etiology of any coagulation abnormality.

A convenient method to check clotting status intraoperatively is the "tube test" which involves drawing a plain tube of blood (with no anticoagulant) and observing for coagulation, clot retraction, and clot lysis. Normal blood clots in about 6 to 10 minutes; the clot retracts in 1 hour and starts to lyse after at least 6 hours. If a good clot does not form or does so only after 10 to 20 minutes, clotting factor deficiency is the most likely cause. Failure of clot retraction suggests platelet depletion or dysfunction. Clot lysis earlier than 6 hours indicates fibrinolysis. In severe disseminated intravascular coagulation (DIC) syndrome, clotting factors and platelets are consumed and therefore a clot does not form. This is a well-known phenomenon since it prevents typing and cross-matching of blood.[352]

Thrombelastography is a sophisticated, accurate, and prac-

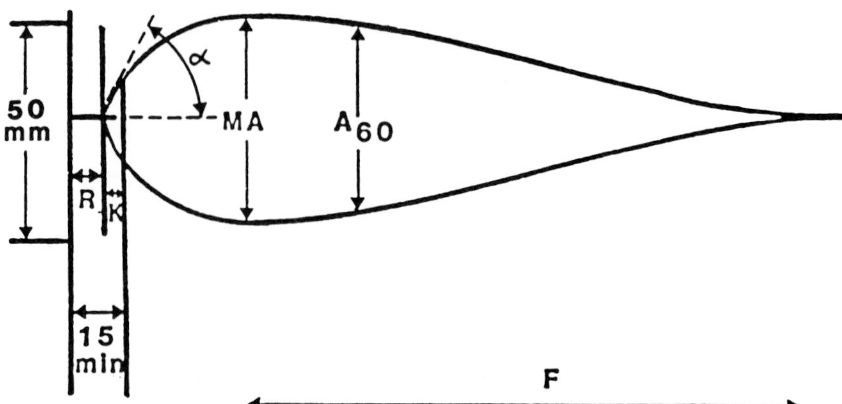


FIG. 9-12. A normal thrombelastogram and its parameters. Parameters are described in Table 9-7.

tical method designed to monitor coagulation. In principle, it is similar to the tube test, but it provides precise quantitation. The thrombelastograph determines the time necessary for initial fibrin formation, rapidity of fibrin deposition, clot consistency, the rate of clot formation, and the times required for clot retraction and clot lysis. The thrombelastograph consists of (1) a cuvette in which the blood (0.35 ml) is deposited; (2) a piston suspended in the cuvette; (3) a pen connected to the piston; and (4) a moving paper for recording. During clot formation, movement of fibrin strands from the wall of the cuvette transmits motion to the piston and the pen which, proportional to these movements, produce the typical thrombelastogram on the recorder. A normal thrombelastogram and the important parameters that serve to determine coagulation abnormalities are shown in Fig 9-12. Table 9-7 gives the definitions and normal values of each of these parameters along with the specific coagulation functions they measure and the coagulation test to which they correspond. Although thrombelastography is useful during liver transplantation,[247,248] open heart surgery,[444] and elective general surgical procedures,[476] its use in trauma patients has not yet gained wide popularity. It may be a useful method of monitoring coagulation in this group of patients as well.

## INDUCTION OF ANESTHESIA

### REGIONAL ANESTHESIA

The selection of regional or general anesthesia for emergency trauma surgery is predicated upon many factors, including (1) the type of injuries; (2) the planned operation; (3) the adequacy of intravascular volume; (4) the presence of coagulation abnormalities; (5) any history of preexisting diseases; and (6) the mental status of the patient.

Regional anesthesia, in the form of peripheral nerve blocks or spinal or epidural anesthesia, is preferred by many anesthesiologists for repair of extremity injuries.[71] Ease of admin-

TABLE 9-7. Features of Each Thrombelastogram Parameter

| PARAMETER | NORMAL VALUE | DEFINITION | SPECIFIC COAGULATION FUNCTION MEASURED | CORRESPONDING COAGULATION TEST |
|---|---|---|---|---|
| *R* | 7 to 14 minutes | Time interval from blood deposition in the cuvette to an amplitude of 1 mm on the thrombelastogram | Time necessary for initial fibrin formation | PTT |
| *K* | 3 to 7 minutes | Time interval between the end of *R* and a point with an amplitude of 20 mm on the thrombelastogram | Rapidity of fibrin buildup and cross-linking | |
| *MA* (maximum amplitude) | 40 to 60 mm | Maximum amplitude of thrombelastogram | Absolute strength of the fibrin clot | Platelet count, platelet function, fibrinogen level, factor VIII and factor XIII activities |
| *O* | 40 to 60° | Slope of the external divergence of the tracing from the *R* value point | Speed of clot formation and fibrin cross-linking | Platelets and fibrinogen |
| $A_{60}$ | 35 to 50 mm | Amplitude of thrombelastogram 60 minutes after maximum amplitude | Beginning of clot lysis | |
| $A_{60}/MA$ | >0.85 | Ratio of $A_{60}$ to *MA* | Whole blood clot lysis index | |
| *F* | >300 minutes | Time from *MA* to return to 0 amplitude | Whole blood clot lysis time | |

istration, possibly decreased intra- and postoperative complications, pleasant patient recovery, and provision of excellent operating conditions are some of the reasons for selecting these techniques.[252] However, this type of anesthesia is not appropriate for the patient with other types of trauma such as cranial, maxillofacial, thoracic, and abdominal injuries for which general anesthesia remains the only choice. Although spinal anesthesia was utilized extensively during World War II[94] and the Vietnam War,[463] the presence of hypovolemia or the possibility of major intraoperative hemorrhage precludes the use of central conduction blockade. In studies by Bonica and coworkers,[62,256] severe hypotension occurred when spinal or epidural anesthesia with sensory levels of T5 were given in the presence of acute blood loss. Additionally, rapid infusion of blood or fluids to restore intravascular volume in an awake patient results in considerable pain at the infusion site when the patient is awake. Coagulation abnormalities are common in the major trauma victim during and after massive transfusion[220] and may be present even before blood and fluid infusion.[352] Coagulation abnormalities are most common in head-injured patients[489] but may also be seen in the presence of injuries producing major tissue destruction or shock.[352] Thus, in order to prevent complications, a coagulation profile must be performed before considering regional anesthesia.

Head injury, alcohol and drug intoxication, metabolic disturbances, or hypoxia in a recently injured patient may produce a spectrum of mental disturbances ranging from coma to agitation. If possible, a clear diagnosis of the etiology of the mental alteration must be established prior to surgery. The airway of the comatose patient must be secured regardless of the type of anesthesia to be administered. Following this, regional anesthesia may be administered if desired. In patients with intact airway reflexes, if other conditions permit, regional anesthesia may be desirable, as it provides the advantage of monitoring mental status during surgery.

## GENERAL ANESTHESIA

The technique used for induction of general anesthesia must allow safe airway management and adequate hemodynamic stability. As described in Chapter 3, the airway can be managed in many ways. However, awake intubation and rapid sequence induction remain the mainstays of airway protection.

The advantages of awake intubation are that the patient retains an intact cough reflex to prevent aspiration and remains breathing until the airway is secured. Sedation with incremental doses of diazepam (2.5 mg), midazolam (1 mg), or droperidol (2.5 mg), and fentanyl (0.05 mg) along with topical anesthesia of the pharynx to the level of the epiglottis produces satisfactory intubating conditions and a high incidence of amnesia.[263] Diazepam and midazolam in doses up to 0.15 and 0.075 mg/kg, respectively, do not appear to produce clinically significant respiratory depression in healthy volunteers; in fact, diazepam may produce enhancement of respiratory drive in some individuals.[20,371] This is not the case when the drug is administered at higher doses,[209,443] to a critically ill or elderly trauma patient, or in combination with other sedatives and opiates. Thus, respiration and oxygenation should be monitored continuously and supplemental $O_2$ given. If the superior laryngeal nerve is blocked, the glottic closure reflex is abolished, but the cough reflex remains intact.[134]

Awake blind intubation can be performed only in the unobstructed, spontaneously breathing patient. It is time consuming, does not fully prevent aspiration, and increases ICP in head-injured patients. Blind intubation techniques should be avoided, if possible, in patients with facial, intraoral, or penetrating airway trauma because of the possibility of entering false passages or carrying foreign bodies into the airway. In these circumstances, intubation is performed under direct vision using a laryngoscope or a flexible fiberoptic bronchoscope.

A rapid sequence induction with cricoid pressure prevents aspiration of blood, secretions, or gastric contents.[156,409] Since the patient is asleep, his cooperation is not needed, and ideal intubating conditions are usually obtained. Disadvantages of this technique include (1) hypotension from the induction dose of hypnotic[35,116]; (2) failure to intubate[35,117]; and (3) hypertension, tachycardia, and resulting impairment of left ventricular performance which cannot be prevented by intravenous lidocaine (1.5 mg/kg) and may be deleterious in patients with cardiovascular or cerebrovascular disease.[90,91] Administration of fentanyl (5 μg/kg) or sufentanil (1 to 2 μg/kg) over a period of 4 to 5 minutes prior to induction, with careful observation of blood pressure and consciousness, has been shown to attenuate but not abolish this stress response.[104,259]

Traditionally, preoxygenation with 100% $O_2$ for a period of 3 to 5 minutes is used to denitrogenate the lung. However, Gold et al[199] showed that only four maximal breaths of 100% $O_2$ suffice to provide arterial oxygenation equal to 5 minutes of preoxygenation in patients with normal lungs. It should be remembered that unconscious and uncooperative patients and those with painful thoracoabdominal injuries may not be able to breathe deeply and thus require a long preoxygenation period. In addition, $Sa_{O_2}$ decreases more rapidly following induction of apnea when preoxygenation is provided with four maximal breaths as compared with oxygen breathing for 3 minutes.[189]

Occasionally, it is necessary to modify the classic rapid sequence induction technique. These modifications are discussed later in this chapter and in Chapters 3 and 11.

## INDUCTION AGENTS

The agent selected for rapid sequence induction should provide rapid loss of consciousness and have minimal undesirable hemodynamic effects. Although anesthetic induction can unmask hypovolemia, causing hypotension in the previously compensated patient, it can also cause hypertension and tachycardia in the normovolemic patient if laryngoscopy and tracheal intubation are performed in light planes of anesthesia. As a general principle, doses of intravenous induction agents must be reduced in the hypovolemic patient to prevent severe cardiovascular depression. This does not result in inadequate anesthesia since the amounts of these drugs required to produce unconsciousness are also decreased with hypovolemia.[7,500] Barbiturates, ketamine, benzodiazepines, and etomidate have all been used for induction. None of these agents appears to be ideal, and since there have been no controlled trials to evaluate their effect in the trauma patient, knowledge in this area is based on an understanding of their pharmacological actions, on clinical experience, and on extrapolation of data from small uncontrolled trauma series or controlled experimental animal work.

### *Barbiturates*

The ultrashort-acting barbiturates (thiopental, methohexital, thiamylal) produce rapid loss of consciousness when given as a bolus and are suitable for use in rapid sequence induction. Maximum depth of anesthesia is produced within 30 to 60 seconds, coinciding with the onset of action of succinylcholine. Thiopental reduces arterial blood pressure by three mechanisms: venous dilatation and peripheral pooling of blood,[141,491] decreased sympathetic tone,[245,431] and myocardial depression.[99] In the normovolemic patient, severe hypotension following thiopental is prevented by compensatory tachycardia[99] and possibly by some vasoconstriction.[161] In the hypovolemic patient, vasoconstriction and tachycardia are already present, and additional compensation may be impossible, resulting in an unacceptable degree of hypotension. Furthermore, rapid injection of thiopental (>175 mg/min), as used in rapid sequence induction, causes greater reduction in blood pressure than slower injection rates (<100 mg/min), making hemodynamic decompensation more likely.[161] Thus, barbiturates must be used cautiously in hypovolemic patients; small repeated doses (25 to 50 mg) should be administered with continuous blood pressure monitoring. Severe hypotension and cardiac arrest occurred when thiopental was given in large doses to hypovolemic soldiers during the Pearl Harbor attack.[215] This, coupled with the general impression that thiopental is dangerous, prompted many clinicians to avoid this drug altogether in acutely hypovolemic patients. More recent studies by Weiskopf et al[500,501] suggest that the cardiovascular depressant effect of thiopental in hypovolemic animals is no more pronounced than that produced by ketamine (Table 9-8). Thus, restoration of blood volume prior to induction of anesthesia, rather than the choice of induction agent, appears to be the key to maintenance of a stable hemodynamic status.

Barbiturates may be selected for their beneficial effects in patients with head and open-eye injuries. Cerebral blood flow decreases in a dose-dependent fashion following thiopental as a result of cerebral vasoconstriction; cerebral oxygen consumption is reduced in parallel with this effect.[417] Thiopental thus decreases ICP in patients with intracranial hypertension and improves cerebral perfusion pressure if systemic arterial pressure is maintained.[418] Thiopental decreases intraocular pressure by several mechanisms: (1) depression of centers in the diencephalon; (2) relaxation of extraocular muscles; and (3) increased aqueous humor outflow[122,331] (see also Chapters 10 and 11).

### *Ketamine*

When administered intravenously, ketamine (2 mg/kg) causes loss of consciousness within 1 minute and is thus a useful agent for rapid sequence induction.[504] In addition, the stimulatory action of ketamine on the cardiovascular system has been a compelling reason for many clinicians to use the

TABLE 9-8 Hemodynamic and Metabolic Changes in Acutely Hemorrhaged (30% of Blood Volume) Swine 5 and 30 Minutes after Minimal Anesthetic Dose (6 mg/kg, intravenously) of Ketamine or Thiopental*

| | 5 MIN AFTER | | 30 MIN AFTER | |
|---|---|---|---|---|
| HEMODYNAMIC AND METABOLIC VARIABLES | *Ketamine % Change from Awake Hemorrhaged Level* | *Thiopental % Change from Awake Hemorrhaged Level* | *Ketamine % Change from Awake Hemorrhaged Level* | *Thiopental % Change from Awake Hemorrhaged Level* |
| Arterial blood pressure (BPa) | −58 | −46 | −26 | −28 |
| Right atrial pressure (RAP) | Negligible decrease | Negligible increase | Negligible decrease | Negligible increase |
| Pulmonary arterial pressure (PAP) | −21 | −5 | −16 | −3 |
| Pulmonary wedge pressure (PWP) | Unchanged | Slight increase | Unchanged | Negligible increase |
| Heart rate (HR) | −30 | −28 | −26 | −26 |
| Stroke volume (SV) | −4 | −6 | +20 | +2.4 |
| Cardiac output ($\dot{Q}_t$) | −35 | −37 | −9 | −18 |
| Systemic vascular resistance (SVR) | −31 | −21 | −20 | −19 |
| Pulmonary vascular resistance (PVR) | +31 | +7 | −12 | +5 |
| Oxygen consumption ($\dot{V}O_2$) | −12 | −13 | +1 | −2 |
| Blood lactate | +94 | +48 | +133 | +49 |
| Renin activity | +322 | +31 | +121 | −34 |
| Epinephrine | +832 | +142 | +300 | −15 |
| Norepinephrine | +216 | +37 | +30 | −58 |

* From Weiskopf et al[501] with permission.

drug during anesthetic induction of acutely traumatized patients.[477] Several clinical reports demonstrated the beneficial hemodynamic effects of this drug for anesthetic induction of hemorrhaging patients, especially when used in combination with pancuronium.[60,88,343] It should be emphasized, however, that in four severely hypovolemic patients described in one of these reports, no beneficial hemodynamic effect of ketamine was noted.[343] More recent studies[282,495] evaluating ketamine induction in critically ill patients demonstrated an overall improvement in hemodynamic and oxygenation parameters following this agent. But these responses were not uniform, and in a small percentage of patients, hypotension, reduced cardiac output, and abnormalities in peripheral oxygen transport occurred. Two severely hypovolemic patients in this series had marked hypotension immediately after ketamine, leading to cardiac arrest in one.[282]

The variability of responses to ketamine among critically ill patients is probably related to the mechanism of its action on the cardiovascular system. The hemodynamic effects of ketamine differ in intact animals and isolated organ preparations. Cardiovascular stimulation in intact animals is caused by the sympathomimetic effects of the drug.[505] In the absence of this effect, ketamine is a myocardial depressant.[128,470] Increased sympathetic activity results from both central and peripheral stimulation of the sympathetic system and presumably a cocaine-like effect, producing elevated plasma catecholamine concentrations.[505] Serum norepinephrine and epinephrine concentrations invariably increase following administration of ketamine. Thus, it is possible that in patients in whom trauma and hemorrhage have produced maximal catecholamine discharge, further liberation of catecholamines by ketamine cannot occur, and myocardial depression with ensuing hemodynamic deterioration develops. Likewise, in catecholamine-depleted patients with long-standing critical illness, the direct myocardial depressant effect of ketamine may be unmasked, and its undesirable hemodynamic action may result. Since the majority of trauma victims are young and healthy prior to the accident, and, with modern resuscitative methods, few victims are severely hypovolemic at the time of anesthetic induction, in most instances ketamine produces few or no adverse hemodynamic effects. In these patients, however, any of the available intravenous anesthetic agents is likely to maintain cardiovascular function if administered in an appropriate dose.

As we mentioned above, results of animal experiments suggest that ketamine in the presence of severe hypovolemia (loss of 30% of blood volume) has at least as much cardiovascular depressant effect as thiopental. In the studies of Weiskopf et al[501,502] both ketamine and thiopental resulted in significant hemodynamic and metabolic derangements (Table 9-8). Interestingly, ketamine, despite being able to elevate serum renin activity, epinephrine, and norepinephrine concentrations far above those produced by thiopental, offered no hemodynamic or metabolic advantage (Table 9-8). In fact, it produced higher blood lactate levels than thiopental, which lasted at least 30 minutes. These experimental findings suggest that in the severely hypovolemic trauma victim, further sympathetic stimulation and serum catecholamine concentration above the level the patient has already produced are not beneficial and may in fact be deleterious.

For obvious ethical reasons, studies in humans similar to those performed by Weiskopf et al[501,502] in animals cannot be performed. In the absence of such data, ketamine or any other intravenous anesthetic agent should be used with certain general principles in mind. First, strong emphasis must be given to correcting the underlying hypovolemia prior to induction. Second, when hypovolemia is severe—as shown by profound hypotension—and uncorrectable, one should avoid administering intravenous anesthetic agents. In most of these patients, intubation can be performed either without anesthetic drugs or with the aid of small doses of narcotic agents (fentanyl, 25 to 50 μg). Third, when hypovolemia is suspected despite vigorous fluid resuscitation and normal arterial blood pressure, doses of intravenous induction agents should be reduced to prevent undesirable hemodynamic consequences. As we suggested earlier, in hemorrhaged animals (30% of blood volume), the anesthetic doses of ketamine and thiopental are 35 to 40% lower than those normally required.[500] In clinical conditions, accurate assessment of the degree of hypovolemia is not possible, and the necessary dose reduction has not been determined. However, empirical reduction of the dose of ketamine in these conditions to 0.5 to 1.0 mg/kg appears to provide adequate anesthesia without reducing arterial blood pressure.

Ketamine may be the agent of choice for inducing anesthesia in the patient with cardiac tamponade[267,505] if the tamponade cannot be relieved under local anesthesia.[448] In some patients, however, there may be a decrease, rather than an increase, in cardiac index and arterial pressure[140] (see also Chapter 15). Another indication for the use of ketamine is the presence of bronchial asthma. Ketamine has been shown to relieve bronchoconstriction and thus is an appropriate agent in the asthmatic patient who requires rapid sequence induction or emergency intubation.[105,231,279]

Ketamine is probably the most extensively used intravenous anesthetic for burn surgery during both early and late phases of the injury. Cardiovascular stimulation and the prolonged postoperative analgesia provided by this agent and the effectiveness of the drug by the intramuscular route are some of the advantages cited by numerous authors. In the acutely burned patient, high doses of ketamine result in prolonged anesthesia, but this may be advantageous since it allows the recovery room nursing staff ample time to position the freshly grafted patient. As in other trauma patients, hypotension and decreased perfusion may follow administration of this drug to burn victims. Tolerance may develop to ketamine following repeated administration, necessitating careful adjustment of its dose.[298]

In trauma victims who do not have significant blood loss or volume depletion due to fluid efflux from the intravascular space, cardiovascular stimulation by ketamine may be undesirable. Hemodynamic changes produced by ketamine include significant increases in heart rate, cardiac index, systemic vascular resistance, and systemic and pulmonary artery pressures, all of which result in significantly increased myocardial oxygen consumption.[505] Although in animals an increase in coronary blood flow commensurate with the increase in myocardial oxygen consumption occurs,[436] these changes may have deleterious effects in patients with hypertension or coronary artery disease. In hypertensive patients a further rise in blood pressure following ketamine might be dangerous, although the drug can be used to induce patients whose hypertension has been controlled. In patients with coronary artery disease, an increase in myocardial oxygen consumption might not be associated with increased blood supply, and ischemia may result. In addition, tachycardia may complicate the course of anesthetic induction in patients with mitral valve disease and atrial fibrillation.

A number of pharmacological agents have been used to block the tachycardia and systemic hypertension produced by ketamine. Pretreatment with intravenous diazepam[240,265,515] (0.1 to 0.2 mg/kg) or droperidol[26] (25 to 50 μg/kg) suppresses ketamine-induced plasma catecholamine increase and resulting hypertension and tachycardia. Intravenous midazolam[504] (0.15 mg/kg) or intravenous thiopental (2 mg/kg) is also effective in preventing this cardiovascular stimulation, and because of relatively similar pharmacokinetic profiles they can be given simultaneously (without mixing) with ketamine. The dose of ketamine should be reduced when these agents are used.

Ketamine is contraindicated in patients with closed-head injury because it increases cerebral blood flow (CBF), cerebral metabolic rate for oxygen ($CMRo_2$), and ICP.[419] These effects appear to be attenuated by prior administration of thiopental,[419] but the reliability of this maneuver remains to be determined. Although earlier studies have demonstrated that ketamine increases intraocular pressure (IOP),[106,510] more recent data show that the drug either has no effect on IOP or causes a slight reduction[14,18,362] (see also Chapter 11).

Metabolic and endocrine responses to ketamine include elevation of serum glucose, adrenocorticotropic hormone (ACTH), and cortisol levels. These responses, however, are transient and unlikely to exacerbate the metabolic and endocrine changes already caused by trauma and surgery.[266]

### *Benzodiazepines*

Benzodiazepines are used either to provide sedation during airway management or regional anesthesia or to produce unconsciousness during rapid sequence induction. Of the three available benzodiazepine derivatives—diazepam, midazolam, and flunitrazepam—only two, diazepam and midazolam, have been used as intravenous anesthetics. Flunitrazepam, although satisfactory as a sedative agent, is not suitable for rapid sequence induction because it fails to produce an acceptable depth of anesthesia within one arm-brain circulation time, leading to great individual variation in drug response.[249] The pharmacological properties of these drugs in healthy individuals are summarized in Table 9-9.

When used for sedation in conjunction with opioid agents in the doses described in Table 9-9, any of these agents provides adequate sedation and allows airway manipulation in the awake state. Wide individual variability in airway reflexes

TABLE 9-9. Characteristics of Diazepam, Midazolam, and Flunitrazepam in Healthy Individuals

| | DIAZEPAM | MIDAZOLAM | FLUNITRAZEPAM |
|---|---|---|---|
| Dose (mg/kg) (sedation in conjunction with narcotic agents for airway management) | 0.05 to 0.15 | 0.05 to 0.1 | 0.005 to 0.015 |
| Dose (mg/kg) (rapid sequence induction) | 0.3 to 0.5 | 0.2 to 0.3 | 0.03 to 0.04 |
| Onset of action (seconds) (after induction dose) | 60 to 120 | 15 to 115 | 40 to 180 (unreliable) |
| Duration (minutes) (after a single dose) | 30 to 45 | 25 to 35 | 15 to 30 (post-operative oversedation) |
| $t_{1/2\alpha}$ (minutes) | 25 to 55 | 6 to 15 | 6 to 30 |
| $t_{1/2\beta}$ (hours) | 20 to 50 | 1.7 to 4 | 23 to 29 |
| $V_D$ (L/kg) | 0.7 to 1.7 | 1.1 to 1.7 | 1.43 to 2.4 |
| Clearance (ml/min/kg) | 0.2 to 0.5 | 6 to 12 | 2.7 to 3.0 |
| Protein binding (%) | 98 | 98 | 95 |
| Hemodynamic effects (induction dose) | Minimal | Decreased SVR<br>Increased venous capacitance | Minimal |
| Respiratory effects | Minimal at doses up to 7 mg<br>Decreased $CO_2$ response | Minimal at doses up to 0.075 mg/kg<br>Decreased $CO_2$ response<br>Occurs faster and lasts longer in patients with COPD than in normals | Decreased $CO_2$ response |

and respiration in response to these drugs, especially in the critically ill trauma patient, dictates careful titration, adequate monitoring, and continuous observation. Occasionally diazepam produces agitation rather than sedation, which becomes more pronounced with increasing doses. Small doses of droperidol (1 to 2.5 mg) are usually quite effective in abolishing this undesirable response. Used in sedative doses, benzodiazepines are unlikely to produce major hemodynamic changes, although careful blood pressure monitoring is essential since hypotension may occur in the acutely traumatized patient.

In anesthetic doses midazolam has a more rapid onset than diazepam.[384,399] However, its onset is slower than that of thiopental or ketamine, ranging from about 30 to 115 seconds with a 0.2 mg/kg dose.[454] Using 0.3 mg/kg, White[504] reported an onset time of between 15 and 60 seconds. Diazepam, 0.5 mg/kg, has been reported to produce unconsciousness within about 60 seconds,[399] but a high incidence of pain and phlebitis at the injection site, especially with such high doses and rapid injection, is an important disadvantage of this drug. In addition, recovery time from diazepam is longer than that from midazolam, since the latter has no active metabolites and is more rapidly excreted.[400] Usually patients are awake and responsive about 45 minutes after an induction dose of midazolam.[504] Results from animal studies suggest that hypovolemia caused by acute hemorrhage reduces anesthetic dose requirement and metabolic clearance and prolongs the elimination half-life of midazolam.[7]

In healthy individuals and in those with stable coronary artery disease, benzodiazepines depress the cardiovascular system less than thiopental.[399] Blood pressure is maintained or decreases slightly after induction with doses of diazepam up to 0.5 mg/kg,[126,399] although larger doses (0.8 mg/kg) may decrease both mean arterial pressure and cardiac output[379] and occasionally produce marked hypotension. Midazolam has comparable benign cardiovascular effects but produces a slightly greater reduction (about 20%) than diazepam in mean arterial blood pressure. This reduction is mainly mediated by a decrease in systemic vascular resistance; the cardiac index is well maintained because of an increase in heart rate.[399]

More detailed evaluation of midazolam's effect on the cardiovascular system has been done in dogs by Gelman and his associates.[192] These authors demonstrated that hypotension produced by midazolam is caused by a decrease in systemic vascular resistance; an increase in venous capacitance causing decreased venous return; and a decrease in myocardial contractility, resulting in diminished cardiac output. These hemodynamic changes are offset by compensatory mechanisms such as increased heart rate; blood mobilization from the spleen and intestine; and increased myocardial contractility, resulting in restoration of cardiac output (Fig 9-13). In the hypovolemic dog, all of these compensatory mechanisms have already been utilized to maintain blood pressure. Thus, administration of midazolam to these dogs would be expected to result in profound hypotension. However, Adams et al[7] found that midazolam produced comparable decreases of blood pressure in normovolemic and hypovolemic dogs (12 versus 23%). The blood pressure was certainly lower in the hypovolemic group, but this was a consequence of hemorrhagic shock rather than of the drug.

If these canine findings can be extrapolated to humans, midazolam appears to be a desirable induction agent for the acutely hemorrhaged patient. Although studies evaluating hemodynamic actions of midazolam in human hemorrhagic shock are not available, indirect observations suggest that this agent is no more advantageous in hypovolemic states than other intravenous anesthetic agents. Lebowitz et al[272] demonstrated that hemodynamic alterations by midazolam were comparable to those of thiopental in critically ill surgical patients without cardiovascular disease. Marty and coworkers[297]

FIG. 9-13. The hemodynamic action of (solid arrows) and the compensatory reaction to (open arrows) midazolam in dogs. Note that venodilatation, diminished myocardial contractility, and reduction in systemic vascular resistance (SVR) following midazolam have the potential of decreasing blood pressure. These effects of midazolam are counteracted by almost immediate blood mobilization from the splanchnic circulation and baroreceptor-mediated increase in heart rate and contractility. (From Reves et al[385] with permission.)

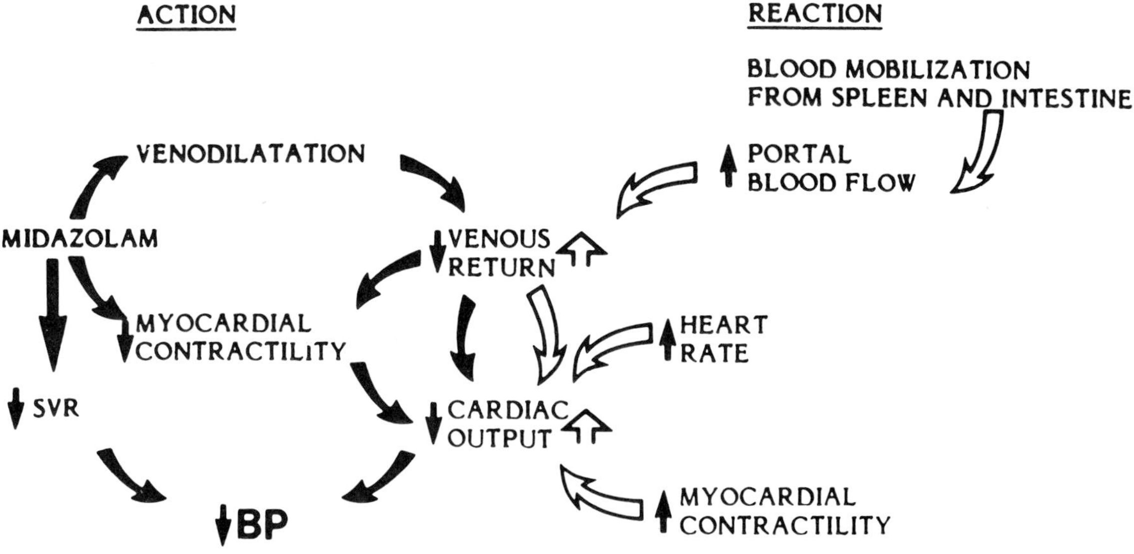

showed that when used for induction of anesthesia, both midazolam and diazepam produce a transient depression of baroreflex function and sustained decrease of sympathetic tone. They caution that "these agents might induce a limited ability to compensate for hemodynamic alterations related to hypovolemia." Finally, Flacke et al,[165] in an elegant study in dogs, demonstrated that the hemodynamic action of diazepam is mediated by the autonomic nervous system. Thus, following trauma and shock, attenuation of central sympathetic response by diazepam and probably by other centrally acting agents such as midazolam and fentanyl might result in significant hemodynamic depression. In view of this, benzodiazepines, like any depressing agent, should be used with caution, in small doses, and with adequate monitoring of cardiovascular function in the hemodynamically compromised trauma patient.

Diazepam decreases CBF and $CMRo_2$ and does not increase ICP in head-injured patients.[109] However, the hypotension induced by diazepam can decrease cerebral perfusion pressure (CPP).[459] Midazolam has similar effects on CBF and $CMRo_2$.[385] In normal men, sleep induced by 0.15 mg/kg midazolam produces 34% reduction in CBF even when a slight rise in $Paco_2$ from 34 to 39 mm Hg occurs. Midazolam, 0.15 to 0.25 mg/kg intravenously, produces little change in ICP in patients with intracranial mass lesions and decreased intracranial compliance; however, the drug does not appear to attenuate the increased ICP response to tracheal intubation. Thus additional measures should be employed to control ICP during anesthetic induction of head-injured patients with midazolam.

Diazepam in doses of up to 10 mg lowers IOP, perhaps by relaxing extraocular muscles,[10,121] although larger doses may cause mydriasis and elevate IOP in patients with acute narrow-angle glaucoma.[134] A significant decrease in IOP has been observed with midazolam,[331] thus it can be used safely during induction of patients with open-eye injuries.

### *Etomidate*

The rapid onset and minimal hemodynamic alteration produced by etomidate are desirable properties for anesthetic induction of the trauma patient. Etomidate produces sleep in one arm-brain circulation time.[201] The minimal dose required to produce anesthesia consistently in 10 seconds is 0.25 mg/kg. In animals, etomidate has been found to have a safety margin four times greater than that of thiopental.[258,383] Pharmacokinetic studies demonstrate very rapid distribution and a large volume of distribution.[482] Etomidate, unlike most other hypnotic agents, has a relatively low degree of serum albumin binding (77%) and high lipid solubility. It is hydrolyzed in the liver with an extraction ratio of 0.5; thus, reductions in hepatic blood flow, as in shock states, or in hepatic metabolism are expected to have only moderate effects on etomidate inactivation.[482] Only 2% of administered etomidate is excreted unchanged in the urine. The metabolites are inert with respect to their sedative activity.[201] Awakening time following administration of this agent is similar to that of thiopental.[229]

The common side effects of etomidate administration are pain on injection, myoclonia, and nausea and vomiting.[176,177,201,225,229,264] Pain is less frequent when larger, more proximal veins are used for injection, and its incidence is also decreased by premedication with intravenous fentanyl (0.1 mg).[176,264] The use of 35% propylene glycol solvent in the formulation of etomidate seems to reduce the incidence of pain on injection.[176,264] Postoperative nausea and vomiting occur in 25 to 50% of patients receiving etomidate for induction of anesthesia.[176] Myoclonic movements occur commonly, although the reported incidence varies between 10 and 70%.[176,177,197,264] They are not associated with epileptiform changes on the electroencephalogram (EEG),[197] and their incidence and severity may also be decreased by fentanyl pretreatment.[176]

A potentially important property of etomidate is its lack of stimulation of detectable histamine release.[132] Stable cardiovascular hemodynamics have been noted with the use of etomidate in healthy patients and in those undergoing coronary artery surgery.[97,114,200,358,458] In the dog hemorrhagic shock model, etomidate was found to be superior to thiopental with respect to hemodynamic stability and survival.[494] From this point of view etomidate appears to be preferable to other intravenous anesthetic agents, with the possible exception of ketamine, in the trauma patient who has hypovolemia, cardiac tamponade, or myocardial injury. However, clinical studies to substantiate this hypothesis are lacking.

One important reason for the relatively uncommon clinical use of etomidate is its inhibitory effect on adrenal steroidogenesis.[487] In the trauma patient, who relies heavily on the metabolic and endocrine stress response, this property of etomidate presents an important disadvantage. Inhibition of adrenal steroidogenesis with etomidate has been described following a single induction dose,[178,486] multiple bolus administration,[149] and continuous infusion.[276,277,486] Patients receiving etomidate show decreased levels of cortisol, diminished cortisol response to ACTH stimulation, and depressed aldosterone levels.[178,486] Recovery of adrenal function occurs usually within 18 to 24 hours, although a longer period of insufficiency has been observed after prolonged sedation with etomidate.[487] Ledingham and Watt[277] reported increased mortality in mechanically ventilated multiple trauma patients receiving continuous infusions of etomidate for sedation. Concomitant use of exogenous steroids may overcome these problems, but data in this realm are scarce and inconclusive.

In summary, etomidate presents some qualities that make it an interesting candidate for use in the acutely traumatized patient. However, the implications of adrenal suppression on postoperative morbidity and mortality in the traumatized patient must be clarified before a strong recommendation for its use can be made.

### *Propofol*

Propofol is a relatively new intravenous anesthetic agent. In a single dose of 2.5 mg/kg, this drug induces anesthesia in an average of 35 seconds, although eyelash reflex disappears approximately 15 seconds later.[120] Some excitatory movements occur during anesthetic induction with this agent, the incidence of which is less than that observed after methohexital or etomidate.[306] Like etomidate, up to 45% of patients may feel pain during injection of propofol into peripheral veins.[255] The drug is distributed and metabolized very quickly;[95] thus, it has a short onset of action, and the recovery of consciousness occurs rapidly.

The hemodynamic effects of an induction dose of propofol are more pronounced than thiopental even in ASA class I or II patients.[306] The cardiovascular effects of propofol have not been tested in acutely traumatized patients, but in ASA class III patients the drug has been shown to decrease arterial blood pressure by up to 40%.[478] Hypotension is caused primarily by decreased systemic vascular resistance,[153] but cardiac output is also reduced if an opioid has been administered before or during induction.[453] In healthy individuals, propofol infusion has little effect on baroreflex response, but the heart rate may remain low despite decreased arterial pressures because of its central sympatholytic and/or vagotonic effects.[119]

Serum cortisol levels fall immediately after injection of propofol.[179,255] This reduction, however, unlike that produced by etomidate, is transient and unlikely to interfere with patient's response to stress.[179]

Hypotension, pain on the injection site, slow abolition of the eyelash reflex, and potential high price will be important drawbacks against choice of this drug in the trauma patient in competition with the currently used intravenous agents.

### *Opioid Agents*

Small doses of opioids, particularly fentanyl, are commonly used prior to injection of intravenous anesthetics to produce sedation as part of the induction sequence. As we mentioned earlier, fentanyl (5 μg/kg) or sufentanil (1 to 2 μg/kg) given over a period of four to five minutes before injection of intravenous anesthetics can attenuate hypertension, tachycardia, and IOP rise in response to rapid sequence induction in normovolemic patients.[89,104,259] Alfentanil (10 μg/kg) also has been shown to prevent pressor and catecholamine responses to laryngoscopy and intubation during anesthetic induction.[113] These drugs should be given with constant monitoring and observation of the patient since they may produce apnea, chest rigidity, hypotension, and seizure-like tonic-clonic movements.[65,318,393]

Opioids are generally not considered anesthetic induction agents for emergency surgery since most available agents do not produce unconsciousness reliably, and they may cause chest or generalized muscle rigidity and have a delayed onset of action and prolonged duration of effect.[21] Alfentanil, however, has a rapid onset of action and a short duration of effect, which have prompted some clinicians to use it for induction, especially when cardiovascular depression is to be avoided.[340,341] Alfentanil has a potency and duration of action approximately one third to one fifth of that of fentanyl. In one series it induced anesthesia faster than midazolam but more slowly than thiopental and etomidate.[341] In healthy patients McDonnell et al[307] demonstrated that a 200 μg/kg dose produced loss of response to voice in 60 seconds. In this study, heart rate and blood pressure were well maintained, although they rose slightly on intubation. Stable heart rates and blood pressure also have been shown during induction with alfentanil in patients with valvular and ischemic heart disease.[340]

Possessing these favorable effects, will alfentanil be a drug of choice for rapid anesthetic induction of the acutely injured patient? In the absence of data and adequate experience with the use of alfentanil for a metabolically hyperactive, possibly hypovolemic, and usually anemic and hypothermic trauma victim, accurate prediction is difficult. There is, however, some evidence to suggest that alfentanil may have drawbacks that counteract its benefits as an induction agent in the acute trauma victim. Silbert et al[429] reported that alfentanil alone at doses of 200 μg/kg could not produce unconsciousness reliably in healthy unpremedicated patients. The addition of intravenous diazepam (0.125 mg/kg) to the induction regimen produced acceptable hypnosis but also resulted in significant hypotension. Significant blood pressure fall also has been reported by Bartkowski and McDonnell[36] with rapid injection of alfentanil (175 μg/kg) alone to patients with cardiovascular disease. Hypotension after alfentanil and other fentanyl derivatives is primarily mediated by decreased brainstem sympathetic output and peripheral vasodilatation.[165] Thus, in the acutely traumatized patient with hyperactive sympathetic tone caused by pain, fear, anxiety, or hypovolemia, rapid administration of alfentanil, especially in conjunction with other hypnotic agents, can deactivate compensatory sympathetic responses and produce significant hypotension.

Anesthetic induction doses of alfentanil often produce generalized muscle rigidity, flexor spasms of arm and jaw, and purposeless movements. Alfentanil-induced muscle rigidity is not associated with increased EEG activity,[44] but muscular hyperactivity in this stage of induction can not only promote gastric fluid regurgitation and thus aspiration, but it can also produce an increase in muscle oxygen consumption as evidenced by decreased arterial oxygen tension and increased base deficit.[44] This increase may be deleterious in the multitrauma patient whose oxygenation may already be compromised. In addition, generalized muscle rigidity increases central venous pressure,[44] resulting in dangerous rises of ICP and IOP in patients with closed-head and/or open-eye injuries. Thus, muscle rigidity and its consequences must be prevented by administering alfentanil simultaneously with a large dose of vecuronium (0.25 mg/kg) or pancuronium (0.20 mg/kg).

### *Muscle Relaxants*

SUCCINYLCHOLINE. Succinylcholine is still the most commonly used muscle relaxant for tracheal intubation during rapid sequence induction. In doses of 1.0 to 1.5 mg/kg, it reliably produces profound muscle relaxation in about 50 to 90 seconds.[37a,86] This dose is deliberately high to achieve rapid onset of paralysis and thus to minimize the risk of regurgitation. Laryngoscopy and tracheal intubation following administration of succinylcholine or any other muscle relaxant should be attempted only when complete neuromuscular blockade is attained, an important point that is commonly overlooked.[86] Monitoring neuromuscular function with a peripheral nerve stimulator will ensure complete blockade and increase safety in emergency situations.

Several side effects of succinylcholine may influence the decision to select it for anesthetic induction of the trauma patient. Succinylcholine may elevate intragastric pressure (IGP) and thus has the potential of increasing the risk of regurgitation. The extent of IGP elevation varies according to the intensity of visible or electromyographically recorded abdominal muscle fasciculation.[312,330] Intragastric pressure after succinylcholine rarely rises above 20 to 30 cm $H_2O$ unless the patient is inadequately anesthetized or paralyzed and coughs or vomits.[312,330] Although the critical IGP value at which regurgitation may occur in unparalyzed man is not known, reflux is seen in human cadavers at an average IGP of 28 cm $H_2O$.[294,295] A similar value has been noted in anesthetized subjects paralyzed with curare if the gastroesophageal angle is normal.[207] Thus, in normal individuals, gastroesophageal reflux solely as a result of succinylcholine-induced fasciculations is unlikely. However, in patients with obesity, hiatus hernia, intra-abdominal pathology, or pregnancy, the lower esophageal sphincter may not function properly, and regurgitation can occur at lower pressures.[344] In addition, use of anticholinergics, opioid analgesics, and intravenous and inhalational agents during induction of anesthesia may promote regurgitation by reducing gastric barrier pressure.[344]

Pretreatment with a subparalyzing dose of nondepolarizing muscle relaxant prevents succinylcholine fasciculations and thus the rise in IGP.[312,330] However, a major controversy surrounds the issue of the need for and appropriateness of this practice in patients with full stomach undergoing emergency surgery. The major objection to "precurarization" is based on the concept that in individuals with normal gastroesophageal junctions succinylcholine-induced IGP increase cannot result in regurgitation because esophageal sphincter tone is increased along with gastric pressure.[434,435] In addition, precurarizing doses of nondepolarizing agents may delay the onset of succinylcholine activity,[118] and pancuronium and gallamine may actually interfere with the competence of the lower esophageal sphincter because of their vagolytic action.[243]

We feel that precurarization of the acute trauma victim adds to the safety of induction because the limited preoperative time often does not allow adequate evaluation of the patient's lower esophageal function. In patients at high risk for regurgitation (eg, hiatus hernia, intra-abdominal pathology), a concomitant rise in gastroesophageal junction tone may not occur. Also, delay in the onset of succinylcholine paralysis by precurarization may be more theoretical than real; it was described in 1971,[118] but since then several investigators have been unable to confirm this finding.[55,100,488] Finally, the use of any nondepolarizing muscle relaxant other than pancuronium or gallamine circumvents the problem of possible decreased esophageal sphincter competence. Precurarization, at least in term pregnant patients, decreases the recovery time from succinylcholine paralysis by approximately 2.5 minutes.[100] Clinically, this may be an advantage when the patient must be awakened because of failed tracheal intubation.

A second side effect of succinylcholine relevant to the trauma patient is increased intracranial and intraocular pressures. In awake or lightly anesthetized patients with compromised intracranial compliance secondary to brain tumors, a bolus dose of succinylcholine (1 to 1.5 mg/kg) produces a rise in ICP of 5 to 10 mm Hg which begins within 1 minute and reaches a peak within 3 minutes after administration of the drug.[315] If untreated, the ICP remains elevated until recovery from paralysis. Whether patients with acute head injury react to succinylcholine in the same way is not known, but we see no reason for them to react differently. The exact mechanism of this phenomenon is unclear, although there is little doubt that fasciculations caused by succinylcholine are responsible for its occurrence.[315,450] It appears that activation of muscle spindle firing by succinylcholine leads to increased afferent neural traffic and cortical electrical activity. This in turn results in augmentation of CBF, cerebral blood volume, and ICP.[268,323] "Defasciculating" doses of nondepolarizing muscle relaxants (metocurine, 0.03 mg/kg; D-tubocurarine, 0.05 mg/kg) given 3 to 5 minutes before anesthetic induction have been shown to prevent succinylcholine-induced ICP increase in both primates and humans[213,450] (Fig 9-14). Thus patients with head injury who require tracheal intubation in the emergency department or the operating room should be pretreated with these agents prior to administration of succinylcholine.

Intraocular pressure elevation following succinylcholine can be damaging, especially in penetrating eye injuries, in which vitreous expulsion can occur. This effect is most prominent when succinylcholine is used in lightly anesthetized patients without pretreatment with nondepolarizing agents. There is much debate about the use of succinylcholine in open-eye injuries. Those who use the drug routinely after pretreatment with a nondepolarizing agent and deep general anesthesia report the absence of further damage to the eye.[280] Others, however, contend that in the light of existing data clearly showing IOP elevation, succinylcholine should not be used at all in open-eye injuries. There is no well controlled, randomized, prospective study available to evaluate the exact role of this drug in open-eye injuries. We feel that there is little need to use succinylcholine in these circumstances since high doses of vecuronium (0.25 mg/kg) allow rapid intubation without adverse effects on IOP. It must be emphasized that laryngoscopy and tracheal intubation or suctioning produce greater increases in ICP and IOP than succinylcholine, if appropriate measures such as opioid pretreatment, deep anes-

FIG. 9-14. Intracranial pressure change (ΔICP) following administration of succinylcholine (Sch) with and without metocurine pretreatment. Asterisks denote statistical significance ($P < .05$). (From Stirt et al[450] with permission.)

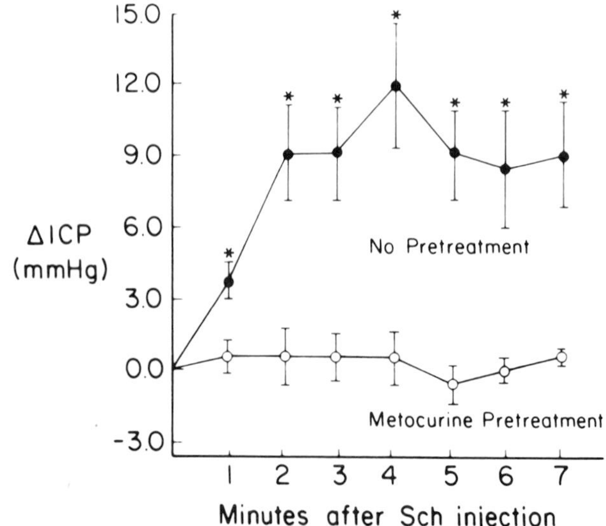

thesia, and lidocaine are not utilized. Further discussion on this subject is offered in Chapter 11.

The third important side effect of succinylcholine is the massive hyperkalemia seen in patients with burns,[299] extensive skeletal muscle injury,[51,304] spinal cord[208] and head trauma,[180,449] and injuries complicated by anoxic encephalopathy.[467] The probable mechanism is increased chemosensitivity of the muscle membrane due to development of receptor sites in extrajunctional areas.[208] This sensitivity develops over a period of a few days to a few weeks. Thus, it is unlikely that succinylcholine given within 24 hours of injury will produce a hyperkalemic response. However, it is prudent to avoid succinylcholine altogether in patients at risk after the first or second posttrauma day. Succinylcholine should also be avoided in patients who present with acute trauma and preexisting neuromuscular diseases, which may produce a hyperkalemic response.[15] A list of these conditions is given in Table 9-10.

Patients with hyperkalemia, such as those with renal failure, probably should not receive succinylcholine. Although only a normal increase (0.5 to 1.0 mEq/L) is seen,[370] it may be sufficient to raise the $K^+$ into the arrhythmogenic range.

The fourth side effect of succinylcholine is contracture or severe muscle spasm that occurs in a variety of conditions. Patients with chronic muscle denervation due to previous trauma, surgery, or malignancy respond to succinylcholine with contracture of the affected muscle which cannot be blocked with precurarizing doses of nondepolarizing muscle relaxants.[27,28] Other conditions resulting in muscle spasm after succinylcholine include myotonia[29] and malignant hyperthermia.[150] Masseter spasm is of concern after succinylcholine because it suggests a possibility that the patient—especially a child—is susceptible to malignant hyperthermia,[391,407] and also may result in difficulties in airway management during the 2- to 3- minute period of its duration. A second dose of succinylcholine or other triggering agent should be avoided in these patients, and if hypercarbia, acidosis, and hyperthermia develop intravenous dantrolene (3 mg/kg) should be administered as soon as possible along with cooling, hemodynamic support and correction of acid-base disturbances. Additional dentrolene of up to 10 mg/kg may be necessary if symptoms persist. It should be emphasized that in children, jaw muscle tone usually increases following a halothane-succinylcholine induction, and this may last at least 45 seconds.[481] This condition appears different from true masseter spasm in which the mouth can barely be opened despite great effort and abolition of evoked muscle twitch in the periphery.[390] Thus, malignant hyperthermia should be suspected in those children in whom increased masticatory muscle tone cannot be easily overcome.[390]

TABLE 9-10. Potassium Response to Succinylcholine in the Presence of Neuromuscular Diseases

| HYPERKALEMIC RESPONSE | NORMAL RESPONSE |
|---|---|
| Hemiplegia | Neurofibromatosis |
| Parkinsonism | Myasthenia gravis |
| Multiple sclerosis | Myasthenic syndrome |
| Encephalitis | Myotonia |
| Ruptured cerebral aneurysm | Myelomeningocele |
| Tetanus | Cerebral palsy |
| Paraplegia | |
| Acute anterior horn disease | |
| Muscular denervation (contracture common) | |
| Duchenne muscular dystrophy | |

Finally, bradycardia and dysrhythmia occur following succinylcholine in children and adults. In children, this may occur after the first dose; in adults a single dose of succinylcholine rarely produces bradycardia or dysrhythmia, although a second dose is frequently followed by this complication. In adults, dysrhythmia (sinus arrest with nodal escape rhythm and nodal rhythm) following a second dose of succinylcholine is more likely when etomidate is used for induction rather than thiopental or midazolam.[2] Pretreatment with nondepolarizing muscle relaxants (D-tubocurarine, 70 μg/kg; pancuronium, 30 μg/kg; or gallamine, 0.3 mg/kg) or with atropine (15 μg/kg) appears to lessen the likelihood of bradycardia in adults.[308] In children, intravenous glycopyrrolate (10 μg/kg) or atropine (20 μg/kg) immediately before anesthetic induction appears to offer reasonable protection.[206]

ALTERNATIVES TO SUCCINYLCHOLINE. Although succinylcholine's rapid onset of action confers advantages in rapid sequence induction, high dose pancuronium (0.20 mg/kg), atracurium (1.5 mg/kg), or vecuronium (0.25 mg/kg) may be substituted if there is any contraindication to its use.[76,278] These muscle relaxants in the doses specified are quite capable of producing rapid paralysis albeit slightly more slowly and less consistently than succinylcholine. Use of a nerve stimulator helps to assess accurately the time appropriate for laryngoscopy and intubation. At these high doses, vecuronium is the best agent since it causes little hemodynamic alteration or prolongation of neuromuscular blockade.[278] Occasionally, however, it produces bradycardia and hypotension, especially when given with large doses of fentanyl or its analogs.[205] Atracurium, because of its histamine-releasing effect, can produce generalized vasodilatation and thus hypotension especially in the hypovolemic trauma victim. Pancuronium is the least desirable agent in normovolemic patients because it produces tachycardia, hypertension, and prolonged paralysis. Thus, except in hypovolemic trauma patients in whom maintenance of elevated heart rate and adequate blood pressure is crucial during anesthetic induction, pancuronium is now seldom used for rapid sequence induction.

Another way of obtaining rapid onset of paralysis with nondepolarizing agents is the use of a subparalytic initial dose followed in a few minutes by the paralyzing dose. The *priming principle,* as this technique was termed by Foldes[171] in 1984, reduces the onset time of paralysis produced by nondepolarizing agents but has several disadvantages. First, onset of neuromuscular blockade is still longer than that produced by succinylcholine. Second, careful adjustment of priming and intubating doses (which are based on body weight) and of the interval between the two is required. For vecuronium, a priming dose of 0.01 mg/kg, a paralyzing dose of 0.1 mg/kg, and a time interval of 4 minutes have been shown to produce 80% twitch depression in 40 to 100 seconds and 100% twitch depression in 60 to 140 seconds.[456] Thus, adequate intubating conditions are achieved within approximately 60 to 90 seconds. In the acutely traumatized patient, preoperative time constraints usually prevent precise determination of body weight, and arbitrarily selected doses may not provide adequate relaxation within a short period of time. Third, a priming dose like precurarization, may produce side effects such as blurred vision, difficulty of swallowing, ptosis, or dyspnea.[442] Although most of these complaints can be alleviated by reassuring the patient, occasionally muscular weakness may result in inadequate airway protection and thus in aspiration of gastric contents.[334] Likewise, uncoordinated movements due to partial paralysis after the priming dose may result in a sudden increase in ICP and IOP, a response that may have deleterious effects in patients with head and open-eye injuries. Fourth, the optimal muscle relaxant, priming and intubating doses, and priming interval have not yet been clearly defined. Varying drugs, doses, and intervals have been used by different investigators with (obviously) varying results.[37a,442,456] We believe that priming should be used only with extreme caution during rapid induction of anesthesia and always with the disadvantages of the technique in mind.

Mivacurium (BW1090) is a short-acting nondepolarizing neuromuscular blocker that is metabolized by human plasma cholinesterase. Preliminary work shows that it provides good intubating conditions within 90 to 120 seconds with doses of 0.20 to 0.25 mg/kg and within 60 seconds at a total dose of 0.3 mg/kg if the drug is given in two divided doses immediately before and after an intravenous anesthetic.[403] Rapid administration of bolus doses of this relaxant exceeding 0.15 mg/kg may be associated with brief hypotension in healthy and, obviously, in hypovolemic patients.[173,451a]

## INTRAOPERATIVE MANAGEMENT

Intraoperative management of the acute trauma victim is a continuum and involves monitoring, diagnosis of unrecognized injuries and newly emerging complications, resuscitation and treatment, and administration of anesthetic and adjunct drugs (Fig 9-15). We have already discussed the various monitoring options available for the anesthesiologist. In this section we will emphasize the remaining aspects of intraoperative management.

### DIAGNOSIS OF UNRECOGNIZED INJURIES AND NEWLY EMERGING COMPLICATIONS

In spite of thorough preoperative evaluation, clinical manifestations of some injuries may not be apparent until surgery. In addition, some trauma-related complications may develop which can only be recognized intraoperatively. Timely diagnosis of these injuries or complications and prompt institution of appropriate therapeutic measures will prevent further physiological deterioration of the trauma victim and at times will be life saving.

Occasionally, external bleeding may not be recognized preoperatively either because it occurs in relatively hidden areas

FIG. 9-15. Schematic representation of specific areas of intraoperative management of acute trauma victim.

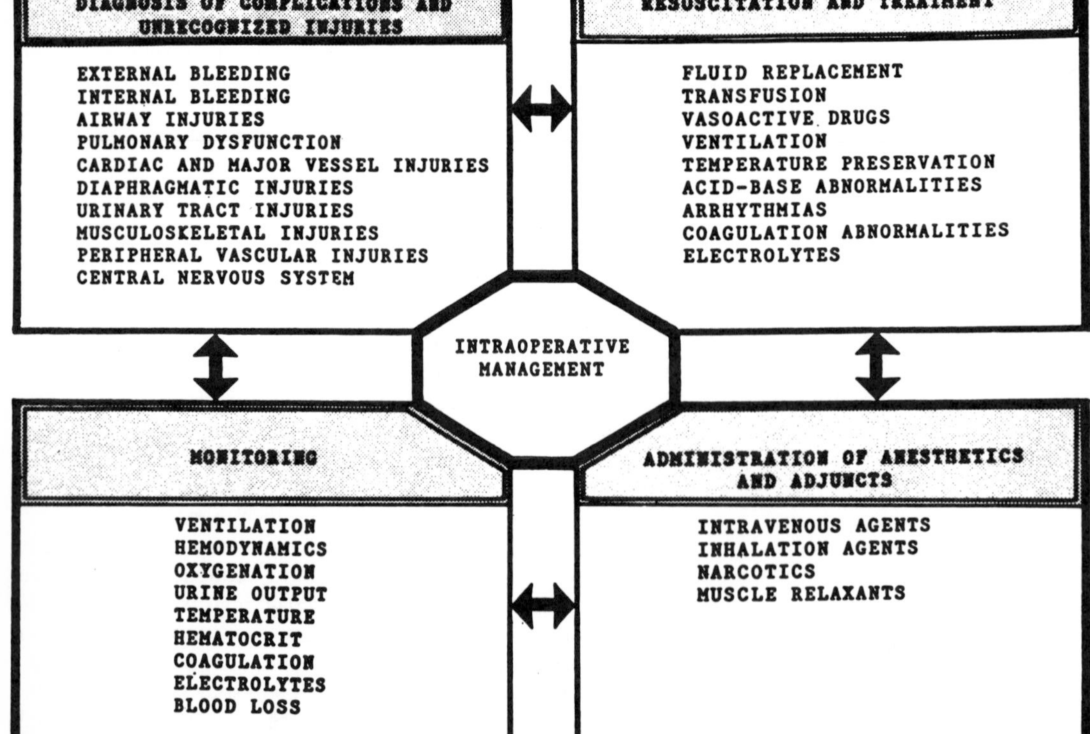

of the body or stops in the emergency department because of hypotension or vascular constriction. Continuing bleeding from the ears, nose, and/or mouth may be recognized only after cleaning blood clots from the face of the trauma victim. Bleeding from the ears and nose should raise the possibility of a basal skull fracture and therefore contraindicate the insertion of gastric or tracheal tubes via the nasal route. The origin of bleeding from the mouth should be identified and treated by an oral surgeon. Patients with pelvic fractures may have associated perineal injuries that may not be recognized preoperatively or even intraoperatively if MAST are not removed, until observation of the floor under the operating table reveals an accumulation of blood dripping from the patient's perineum. Not infrequently, rebleeding from lacerated soft tissues, open wounds at a fracture site, or suddenly from a large lacerated artery occurs; these sites must thus be periodically evaluated. Internal bleeding should be suspected whenever hypotension with decreasing CVP or urine output occurs in the absence of significant surgical or external bleeding. The abdomen, chest, and retroperitoneal space are the common sites of internal hemorrhage since tamponade of bleeding in these areas occurs only after significant blood loss. If a chest tube is already in place, the extent of intrathoracic bleeding can be assessed easily by monitoring drainage. However, when the chest tube is kinked, occluded, or improperly placed, significant blood loss into the pleural space may occur before hypotension ensues. The thigh is another area capable of accommodating a large amount of sequestered blood, but usually blood loss in this area is limited by the tamponading effect of the surrounding muscles. Nevertheless, periodic evaluation for swelling, deformation, and subcutaneous discoloration of limbs may allow diagnosis and surgical treatment of unrecognized fractures simultaneously with the ongoing surgery. The intensity of peripheral pulses may be diminished when injury, thrombosis, or external compression by hematoma occludes the proximal arteries. Periodic evaluation of peripheral pulses may allow rapid diagnosis of this condition. Fluid infusion sites should be checked periodically since catheter dislodgment may result in subcutaneous infiltration of blood or fluid potentially causing compartment syndrome.

Injuries to thoracic organs may become symptomatic during surgery. In some tracheobronchial injuries, airway continuity may not be lost and thus they may go unrecognized preoperatively. If a chest tube is in place, a continuous air leak during positive pressure ventilation and failure of lung reexpansion suggest either airway injury or a diffuse pulmonary parenchymal tear. The neck should be examined a few times, at least during the initial hour of surgery. Progressive swelling, crepitation, and tracheal deviation in this region are all important signs and suggest significant airway or cervical vessel injury. The lung is commonly injured either by the trauma itself or as a result of ventilation and fluid therapy. Pneumothorax is sometimes difficult to diagnose preoperatively either because it is too small or because other injuries make it impossible to obtain a good quality upright chest film. Expansion of a pneumothorax by $N_2O$ and positive pressure ventilation, especially when PEEP is used, results in asymmetrical chest excursion, tympanitic sound on percussion, elevated airway pressure, and, most important, impaired arterial oxygenation. This should be relieved by insertion of a chest tube on that side. If tension pneumothorax occurs, it is accompanied by hypotension and immediate deterioration of patient's condition. This condition should in most instances be treated immediately without waiting for chest X-ray confirmation. A 14-gauge intravenous cannula is inserted anteriorly into the pleural cavity through the second intercostal space, or through the fifth intercostal space at the midaxillary line.

Progressive decline in $Pa_{O_2}$ can also result from lung contusion, aspiration of gastric contents, ARDS, excessive fluid administration, heart failure, and aspiration of blood or secretions. Continuous monitoring of airway pressures, breath sounds, and $Sa_{O_2}$ and measurement of arterial blood gases every 15 to 30 minutes are important for intraoperative recognition of these problems. Air embolization may develop following laceration of a major vein above heart level or after ventilation of a severely lacerated lung with positive pressure.[328] The appearance of air bubbles in a central venous blood sample, nitrogen in the expired air, decreased expiratory $P_{CO_2}$, or elevated pulmonary artery pressures confirms the diagnosis. Occasionally, air may enter the systemic circulation and appear in the arterial blood sample, explaining severe shock or cardiac arrest.

Hypoxemia may also result from fat embolism following fractures of pelvic or long bones. The incidence of this complication has declined recently owing to early operative intervention, but occasionally a multiply injured patient may develop unexplained intraoperative hypoxemia as a result of it. In classic cases, which are rare, accompanying petechiae; snow storm appearance of chest X-ray; pyrexia; and fat globules in the urine, plasma, and retinal vessels help establish the diagnosis.[387] Hyperventilation with ICP monitoring must be instituted as soon as possible, if the surgery must continue and thus the patient cannot be awakened; cerebral embolism with fat globules and severe brain edema may occur in these patients.

A ruptured diaphragm can be missed in the preoperative period.[328] Pneumothorax, because of associated plural injury, occurs frequently in these patients once artificial ventilation is begun. When the diaphragmatic tear is greater than 6 cm, intra-abdominal contents may enter the thoracic cavity and change the quality of the breath sounds. Diaphragmatic rupture must be suspected in the multiple trauma patient when the triad of mediastinal shift, dullness or tympany over the lower thorax, and auscultation of bowel sounds in the chest are present.[333] These physical findings, however, are nonspecific and may be difficult to detect during general anesthesia.

Some cardiac and major vessel injuries may be missed during the preoperative period. Myocardial contusion is thought to accompany up to 75% of major blunt chest injuries.[412] Arrhythmias and cardiac failure may develop in such patients during surgery for an associated injury.[169,440] Electrocardiographic findings in these patients include ST-T segment changes (ST elevation, ST depression, or T wave inversion consistent with ischemia), atrial fibrillation/flutter, bundle branch blocks, and premature ventricular contractions. Elevated CVP in the face of apparent hypovolemia or adequate blood volume in a patient with blunt chest trauma should raise the possibility of cardiac contusion and calls for cardiac output, pulmonary artery pressure, and pulmonary capillary wedge pressure measurements. Other causes of elevated CVP include hypervolemia, cardiac tamponade, acute pulmonary hypertension (pulmonary embolism or contusion), tension pneumothorax, and reduced chest wall compliance caused by muscle rigidity or circular thoracic burns.

Cardiac septal rupture can occur following chest trauma and is associated with systolic murmur, pulmonary vascular congestion, and oxygen step-up found during placement of a pulmonary artery catheter.[513] Depending on the level of the defect, oxygen step-up can be detected at either the atrial or the ventricular level. Cardiac valves may also be disrupted after severe chest trauma. Symptoms following mitral and aortic valve rupture are more severe than those following tricuspid or pulmonic valve injuries and may include manifestations of acute pulmonary edema,[513] mimicking ARDS. Copious secretions and ventilator therapy may make auscultation of heart sounds and thus of a murmur difficult.[329]

Aortic rupture is usually associated with intracranial, abdominal, and musculoskeletal injuries. When bleeding is tamponaded within the adventitia or the surrounding mediastinum, attention may be directed to other injuries, and the ruptured aorta may be missed. Although careful preoperative evaluation of the chest X-ray for upper mediastinal widening, loss of aortic shadow, tracheal or nasogastric tube deviation to the right, and depression of the left main stem bronchus usually indicates this injury,[328] in many cases the diagnosis is missed for hours or days.[513] Intraoperatively, aortic rupture may be suspected if a "pseudocoarctation" syndrome—upper extremity hypertension, lower extremity hypotension, and a systolic murmur over the precordium or left scapula—is present.[513] Unfortunately this syndrome is often absent, and in any case blood pressure is seldom measured from both upper and lower extremities. Thus, once missed preoperatively, aortic rupture may be unrecognized throughout the course of surgery unless additional intraoperative chest X-rays are obtained or sudden complete disruption of the vessel results in severe shock or cardiac arrest.

A urine flow rate in the range of 0.5 to 1.0 mL/kg suggests adequate kidney and other organ perfusion in most instances unless the patient receives diuretics or intravenous radiopaque dye for diagnostic studies. Decreased or absent urine output, however, is not caused only by inadequate kidney perfusion. Urinary tract injuries, kinking, obstruction, and dislocation of a Foley catheter or connecting tubing can all interfere with adequate urine output. The importance of monitoring urine color to diagnose hemoglobinuria and myoglobinuria is discussed in the monitoring section.

Diagnosis of intraoperative development or expansion of intracranial hematomas during surgery for associated injuries is difficult because the signs of these conditions may be masked by the general anesthetic. Intracranial pressure should be measured continuously in head-injured patients, who are operated for associated injuries, by an epidural bolt, subarachnoid or intraventricular catheter, or an intracrebral fiberoptic sensor. When this monitoring is not available, any unexpected change in arterial pressure, bradycardia, dysrhythmia, or change in pupil size should raise the suspicion of increased ICP.[63] Certain extracranial surgical maneuvers can cause increased ICP. Cross-clamping of the thoracic aorta causes an increase in arterial blood pressure and cerebral blood flow.[219] Likewise, sudden lactic acidosis following unclamping of major arteries or deflation of extremity tourniquets can increase ICP.[144] A timely diagnosis of these and the many other possible intraoperative events associated with surgical manipulation requires continuous communication with the surgical team and careful observation of the surgical field.

## RESUSCITATION AND TREATMENT

As we mentioned earlier, ongoing resuscitation together with treatment of developing complications are among the most important tasks of the anesthesiologist who is caring for the multiple trauma victim. The goal is to optimize tissue oxygen transport and utilization by efforts to normalize pulmonary gas exchange, blood volume, blood oxygen-carrying capacity, and cardiac output (see also Chapter 5). Apart from administration of oxygen itself, measures available to optimize these important determinants of tissue oxygenation include ventilation; fluids and blood; inotropes, vasopressors and vasodilators; mechanical aids to optimal cardiac function; maintenance of temperature; and pharmacological agents to treat arrhythmias, acid-base disturbances, and acute exacerbation of preexisting diseases.

### *Ventilation*

Consideration must be given to pulmonary injury, hypovolemia, pericardial tamponade, and closed-head injury during intraoperative ventilation of the trauma patient. Although there are various types of traumatic pulmonary injury—eg, contusion, aspiration pneumonitis, ARDS, and smoke inhalation—the common feature of all is decreased functional residual capacity (FRC) and impaired oxygenation. Occasionally, ordinary anesthesia ventilators may be inadequate because most of them cannot generate sufficient levels of peak inspiratory pressure (PIP) to ventilate these patients. Siemens 900C and 900D (Elk Grove Village, Ill) ventilators can meet this requirement. An Emerson 3MV critical care ventilator (Cambridge, Mass) modified by addition of flow meters, gas blenders, vaporizers, and scavenging system has also been suggested as an alternative[75] (see also chapter 24).

If needed, PEEP is added in small increments (2.5 to 5.0 cm $H_2O$) until optimal arterial oxygenation, as determined by $Pa_{O_2}$, alveolar to arterial $O_2$ difference ($AaD_{O_2}$), $Pa_{O_2}/F_{IO_2}$ ratio, or physiological shunt ($\dot{Q}_{sp}/\dot{Q}_t$), is achieved, as long as blood pressure and cardiac output are maintained within normal ranges.[188,342] Diminution of cardiac output, especially in hypovolemic patients, is a major disadvantage of PEEP. In addition, barotrauma may occur.

High-frequency jet ventilation (HFJV) produces lower peak airway pressures than conventional ventilation.[432] Thus, it can reduce the likelihood of barotrauma and air leak from a lacerated lung. HFJV was also thought to provide more favorable ventilation than conventional intermittent positive pressure ventilation (IPPV), lowering the required levels of PEEP and $F_{IO_2}$. However, based on experience from ICU patients, it is unlikely to provide better $\dot{Q}_{sp}/\dot{Q}_t$ and $Pa_{O_2}$ intraoperatively than conventional ventilation in patients with acute lung injury.[185] Also, the hemodynamic effects of HFJV in normovolemic patients with lung injury are no more favorable than those produced by conventional ventilation if comparable mean airway pressure ($\overline{Paw}$) is used.[185] At $\overline{Paw}$ lower than those used with conventional ventilation, HFJV may improve hemodynamics, but improvement in oxygen delivery is minimal.[185] Further, hemodynamic alterations produced by PEEP are similar whether it is used with conventional ventilation or HFJV.[432] Thus, apart from possibly reducing the likelihood of barotrauma and improving ventilation in patients with lung or tracheobronchial lacerations, HFJV does not appear to offer any advantage intraoperatively over conventional ventilation in normovolemic patients with acute traumatic lung injury. A more recently introduced system, the high-frequency pulse generator (HFPG), may provide improved oxygenation in this group of patients, but clinical experience with this technique is limited.[233]

In hypovolemic patients, mechanical ventilation can compromise both venous return and cardiac output, resulting in marked decrease in blood pressure following each breath. In fact, the difference between the maximal and minimal systolic pressure during the ventilatory cycle has been shown to be the best indicator of hypovolemia in both dogs and humans.[112,361] The decrease in cardiac output and blood pressure is greater with large than with small tidal volumes. Thus, until blood volume is restored, the use of the smallest possible tidal volume at a rate that allows low airway pressures with normal $Paco_2$ may permit improvement in cardiac output, decrease in ventilation-induced cyclic blood pressure changes, and augmentation of mean arterial pressure. It has also been suggested that high frequency ventilation (HFV) may provide a more favorable hemodynamic profile than conventional ventilation in the presence of acute hemorrhage[293] or circulatory shock[185] (Fig 9-16 and Fig 9-17), but the data are inconclusive.

In pericardial tamponade, hemodynamic alterations are essentially the result of right ventricular inflow obstruction.[267] When the chest is closed, spontaneous breathing provides greater cardiac output than positive pressure ventilation, which causes increased intrathoracic pressure and thus reduced venous return and cardiac output.[301,321] PEEP further aggravates the reduction in venous return and cardiac output, especially when used at low respiratory rates (10 to 12 breaths/min)[301,321] (Fig 9-18). It is generally agreed that pericardial tamponade should be evacuated under local anesthesia before general anesthesia is induced.[448] This approach is attractive since it avoids the myocardial depressant effects of anesthetics and the deleterious effects of controlled ventilation. Nevertheless it cannot be used in most cases of traumatic pericardial tamponade since the blood in the pericardial sac is clotted or accumulating rapidly, and patient cooperation is lacking. Some of these patients are anesthetized using a rapid sequence induction technique, thus they will be paralyzed for several minutes after induction during which time spontaneous breathing is not possible, and severe hemodynamic deterioration may occur. Data from animal studies suggest that HFV, by producing lower peak airway pressures than conventional ventilation, might be advantageous in these patients (see Chapter 15).

The necessity for hyperventilation of brain-injured patients frequently raises the question of the effect of mechanical ventilation on cerebral pressure dynamics. Conventional ventilation with PEEP below 30 cm $H_2O$ does not interfere with ICP in closed-head injury patients if the head is elevated 30°.[183] Wide fluctuations in ICP may occur, but mean pressure remains unchanged.[395] Hypotension due to PEEP is more likely than increased ICP and may result in decreased cerebral perfusion pressure both before and after opening of the skull.[183] The fact that ICP fluctuation during the respi-

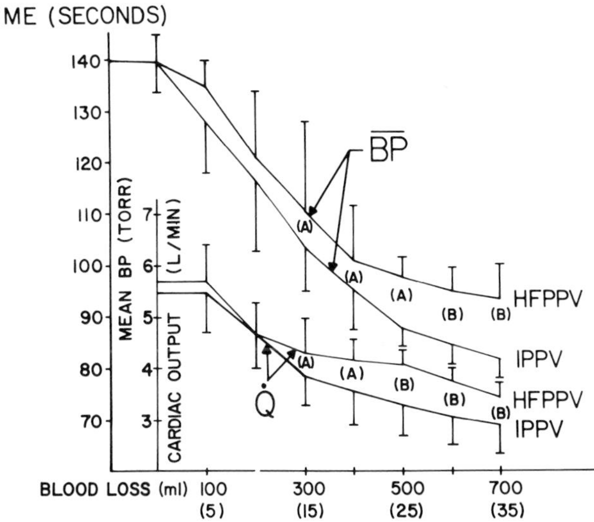


FIG. 9-17. The effect of high frequency positive pressure ventilation (HFPPV) and intermittent positive pressure ventilation (IPPV) on mean arterial blood pressure ($\overline{BP}$) and cardiac output ($\dot{Q}$) during graded hemorrhage in dogs. Figures in parentheses on the abscissa represent percent blood volume removed. Note that both $\overline{BP}$ and $\dot{Q}$ were higher with HFPPV at losses higher than 10% of estimated blood volume. A, $P < .05$; B, $P < .01$. (Courtesy of Dr. Sivam Ramanathan and Lippincott Company. Anesthesiology 1982; 57:A466.)

FIG. 9-16. Arterial blood pressure trace in a hypovolemic dog during high frequency positive pressure ventilation (HFPPV) and intermittent positive pressure ventilation (IPPV). Little change in blood pressure was noted during HFPPV, but IPPV resulted in respirophasic changes in systolic, diastolic, and mean arterial blood pressures. (Courtesy of Dr. Sivam Ramanathan and Lippincott Company. Anesthesiology 1982; 57:A466.)

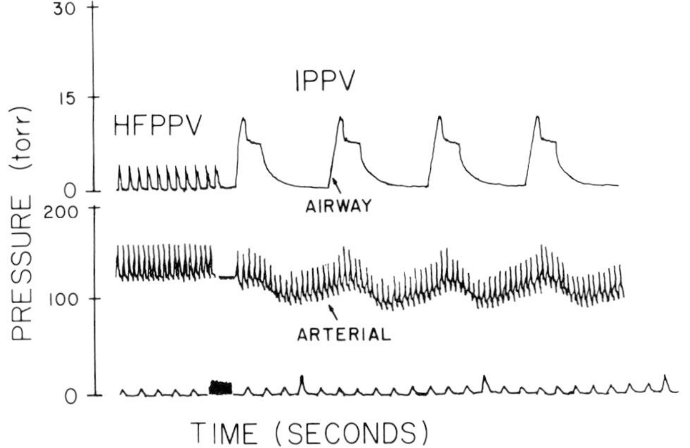

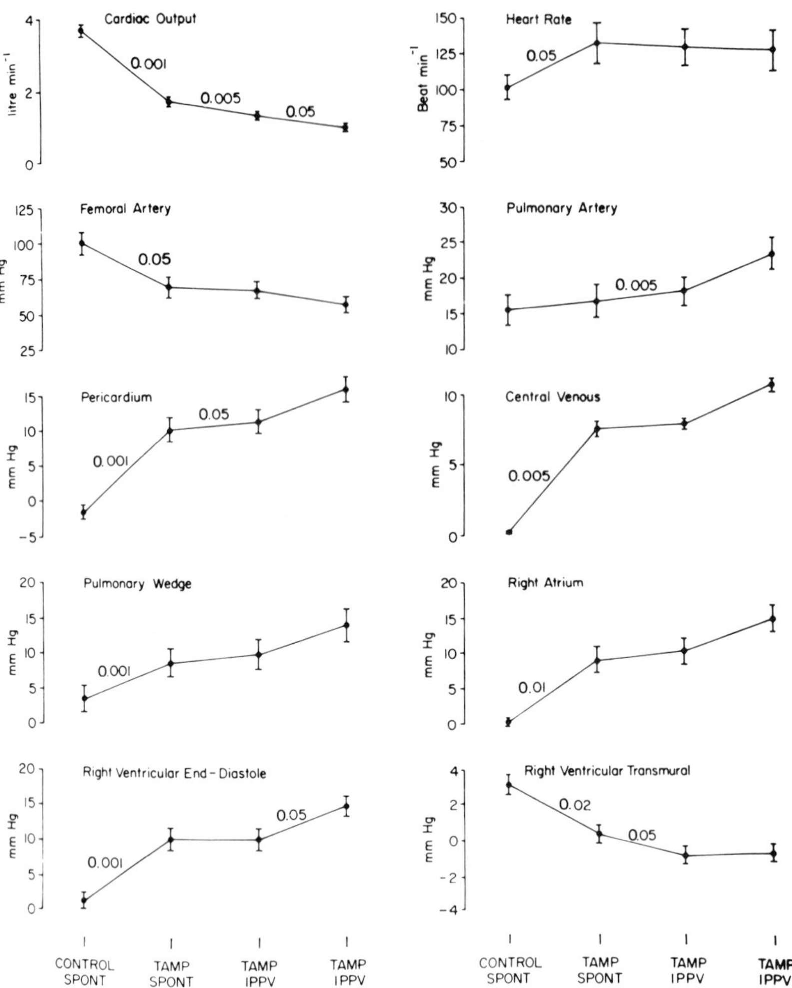


FIG. 9-18. Hemodynamic changes caused by cardiac tamponade (Tamp) in baboons during spontaneous (spont) and intermittent positive pressure ventilation (IPPV) with and without positive end-expiratory pressure (PEEP). Note that cardiac output and transmural right ventricular end-diastolic pressure are significantly greater during spontaneous ventilation than during IPPV with or without PEEP. (From Möller et al[321] with permission.)

ratory cycle is related to changes in intrathoracic pressure has suggested a beneficial effect of HFV, which is associated with smaller changes in intrathoracic pressures, on cerebral hemodynamics. Except for one anecdotal clinical report,[348] studies with HFV have failed to demonstrate any difference in ICP, CBF, and CPP from those observed with conventional ventilation[17,77,469] probably because the mean airway pressure required to produce a given level of ventilation is the same.

The lack of significant ICP increase during mechanical ventilation may be due to the presence of a functional internal jugular valve, the only valve between the brain and the right atrium. Although this valve is competent in most patients, congenital and acquired incompetence has been reported.[135] In these patients, mechanical ventilation is likely to impede venous drainage from the brain and thereby increase ICP. The competence of the internal jugular valve can best be tested by evaluating retrograde jugular blood flow during the cardiac cycle with a noninvasive Doppler flow meter.[135]

### *Fluid Administration*

Much controversy exists about the optimal resuscitation fluid for the severely injured patient. This subject is discussed in Chapter 4 and in an excellent review by Gammage.[190] We use primarily lactated Ringer's solution, which may be supplemented with hydroxyethyl starch (HES). A maximum of 1500 ml of HES is recommended in order to avoid coagulation abnormalities,[216,289] although we are aware that even larger volumes have been shown to cause only minimal hemostatic defects.[421] We have no preset dosage guidelines; patients receive blood and fluids to the following end points: hematocrit between 30 and 35; normal blood pressure, CVP, and urine output; and disappearance of respirophasic changes on the arterial pressure trace.[112,361] When a pulmonary artery catheter is used, we titrate fluid therapy to an adequate cardiac output (4 to 5 L/min), $S\bar{v}O_2$ (75%), and oxygen extraction ratio, calculated as $1 - S\bar{v}O_2$ (0.22 to 0.3).

In two types of trauma—pulmonary contusion and head injury—fluid management is problematic. Overzealous fluid resuscitation may result in pulmonary or cerebral edema. In both conditions intravenous fluids should be administered judiciously, and one must attempt to maintain a relatively "dry state." In patients with pulmonary contusion, arterial blood gases should be observed carefully and, if associated injuries necessitate large amounts of fluid, pulmonary arterial and wedge pressures together with cardiac output and $S\bar{v}O_2$ should be measured to guide fluid and transfusion therapy in accordance with metabolic demand. The type of solution used does not appear critical since both crystalloid and colloid solutions leak in the presence of microvascular injury and increased capillary permeability.[412]

In head injury, similar principles are followed although pulmonary artery catheter monitoring is not required if there is no associated cardiopulmonary dysfunction. Central venous pressure monitoring is usually adequate. In brain-injured patients, the extent and rapidity of ICP changes during resuscitation appear to be influenced by the type of fluid used. Animal studies suggest that isotonic crystalloid solutions produce a greater and more rapid increase in brain water content and ICP (when the head is closed) than colloid or hypertonic salt solutions.[368,373,374,465] (Fig 9-19, upper panel). Thus, albumin, hetastarch, and hypertonic salt solutions are preferred for resuscitation of patients in shock who have concomitant head injuries. Interestingly, however, despite restoration of systemic hemodynamics, CBF and cerebral $O_2$ transport may not be restored to normal with any of the available acellular resuscitation fluids[368,374] (Fig 9-19).

### *Vasoactive Agents and Hemodynamic Support*

Although aggressive fluid infusion is effective in alleviating hypotension in most instances, other means may sometimes be required to support cardiovascular and organ function. Before resorting to such measures, possible causes of intraoperative hypotension and the appropriateness of the contemplated therapy must be considered. Hypotension produced by pneumothorax, cardiac tamponade, surgical occlusion of venous return, and transducer artifact will respond neither to

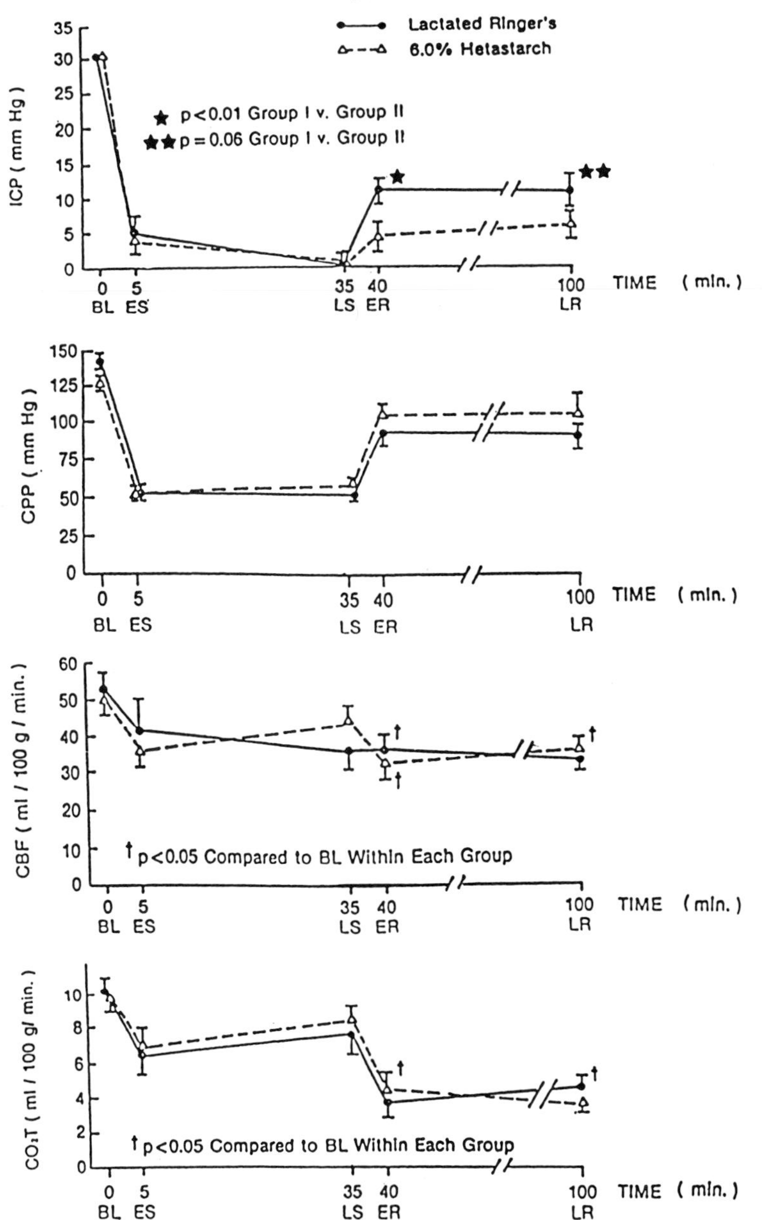


FIG. 9-19. Intracranial pressure (ICP), cerebral perfusion pressure (CPP), cerebral blood flow (CBF), and cerebral oxygen transport ($CO_2T$) in dogs with elevated ICP during hemorrhagic shock and following fluid resuscitation with lactated Ringer's or 6.0% hetastarch. BL, blood loss; ES, early shock; LS, late shock; ER, early resuscitation; LR, late resuscitation. Note that ICP is higher during both early and late resuscitation with lactated Ringer's than with 6.0% hetastarch. There is no difference in CPP, CBF, and $CO_2T$ between dogs resuscitated with lactated Ringer's or 6.0% hetastarch. Note also that despite improvement in systemic hemodynamics, CBF and $CO_2T$ could not be restored to prehemorrhagic shock levels with either solution. (From Poole et al[368] with permission.)

fluids nor to vasopressor therapy, and attempts to treat them in this fashion will result in loss of valuable time and possibly a catastrophic outcome.

Vasopressors should be administered only with vigorous concomitant resuscitation of blood volume. Myocardial failure due to contusion, infarction, valvular disruption, or prolonged hypoxia and peripheral vasodilatation following spinal cord injury are typical indications for intraoperative vasopressor and inotrope therapy in the trauma patient.

In abdominal bleeding with tamponade, hypotension upon opening the abdomen is not uncommon even when patients are resuscitated adequately in the preoperative period. The usual response to such hypotension is to increase the rate of blood and fluid infusion until arterial pressure is restored. Shelly et al[422] showed that in well-resuscitated patients, hypotension is the result of a dramatic decrease in systemic vascular resistance (Fig. 9-20). They suggested the use of vasopressor agents to reduce the amount of blood and fluid infusion required. Thus, in normovolemic abdominal trauma victims, control of hypotension with vasopressor agents may be indicated during laparotomy.

Dopamine or dobutamine infusion at a dose between 4 and 10 μg/kg per minute is started when left ventricular dysfunction is demonstrated by elevated pulmonary artery wedge pressure and depressed cardiac output. Serial ventricular function curves must be constructed to evaluate the effect of therapy and to adjust the dose. Norepinephrine infusion (1 to 4 μg/min) in combination with vasodilators (nitroglycerine or nitroprusside) may be indicated when cardiogenic shock is present. Epinephrine either as a bolus (100 to 200 μg) or as an infusion (1 to 4 μg/min) may be administered for cardiac arrest or severe hypotension.

Hypocalcemia may be present in severe low-flow states, in hypothermia, and during massive transfusion. Serum $Ca^{2+}$ should be monitored under these conditions, but if facilities are not available for rapid $Ca^{2+}$ determination, calcium gluconate (7.5 to 10 mg/kg) or calcium chloride (2.5 to 5 mg/kg) can be administered over a few minutes. Contrary to the old belief that favored calcium chloride in acute states, both calcium gluconate and calcium chloride, given in equivalent doses (approximately 3:1), are equally effective in raising serum $Ca^{2+}$ rapidly.[108] The hemodynamic improvement produced by calcium is brief, but repeated administration should be avoided since refractory ventricular arrhythmias may occur. A list of common vasoactive drugs used in the trauma setting, their mechanism of action, dosage range, and indications is provided in Table 9-11.

Vasodilator agents may be needed for myocardial ischemia or hypertension. Both nitroglycerine and nitroprusside are potent vascular muscle relaxants and can increase CBF. Thus, in the head-injured patient these agents can produce ICP elevation if the skull is not open. Similarly, in patients with

FIG. 9-20. Cardiovascular variables in a patient who developed abdominal tamponade following intra-abdominal bleeding. The shaded area represents the time during which the peritoneal cavity was opened. Vasopressor agents (methoxamine and ephedrine) were administered at 55 minutes. RAP, right atrial pressure; PCW, pulmonary capillary wedge pressure; SVR, systemic vascular resistance; PVR, pulmonary vascular resistance. Hypotension following the release of the tamponade was the result of a decrease in systemic vascular resistance. Following vasopressors, little increase in SVR was noted, but mean arterial pressure increased because of increase in heart rate and cardiac output. (From Shelly et al[422] with permission.)

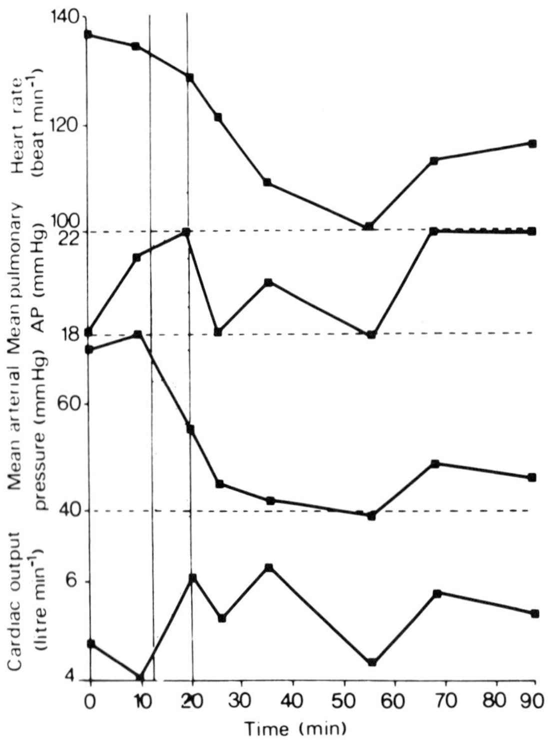


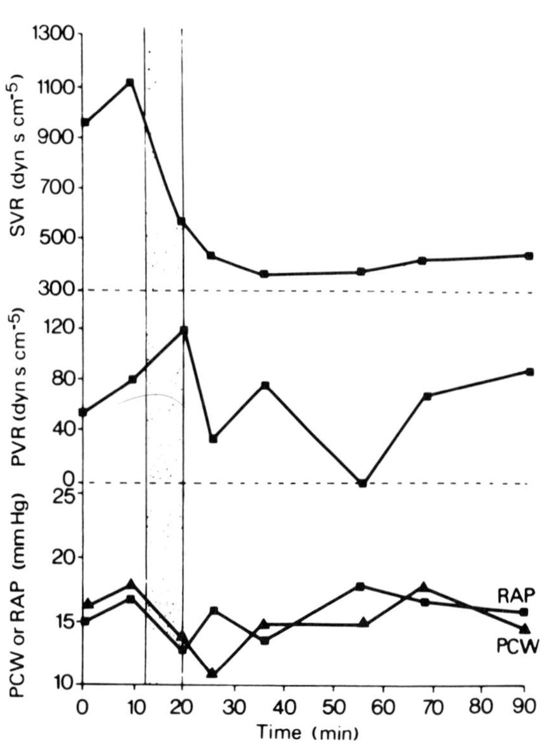

TABLE 9-11. Common Vasoactive Drugs Used Intraoperatively in the Trauma Patient

| DRUGS | MECHANISM OF ACTION | DOSAGE RANGE | INDICATIONS |
|---|---|---|---|
| Epinephrine | Strong $\beta_1$, strong $\beta_2$, moderate $\alpha_1$, moderate $\alpha_2$ | 0.05 to 0.2 μg/kg/min | Severe hypoperfusion<br>Cardiac arrest<br>(0.1- to 0.5-mg bolus) |
| Norepinephrine | Strong $\alpha_1$, strong $\alpha_2$, weak $\beta_1$, no $\beta_2$ | 0.05 to 0.3 μg/kg/min | In Cardiogenic shock with vasodilators (nitroglycerine or nitroprusside) |
| Dopamine | Dopaminergic receptor<br>β receptor<br>β and α receptor<br>α receptor | 1 to 3 μg/kg/min<br>3 to 10 μg/kg/min<br>10 to 20 μg/kg/min<br>>20 μg/kg/min | Low dose, renal vasodilator<br><br>Moderate dose, cardiac inotropy<br>High dose, vasoconstriction |
| Dobutamine | Strong $\beta_1$ | 1 to 5 μg/kg/min<br>5 to 15 μg/kg/min<br>>15 μg/kg/min | Similar to dopamine |
| Calcium gluconate | Direct inotrope | 7.5 to 10 mg/kg | Myocardial depression caused by anesthetics, hypocalcemia, hypothermia |
| Calcium chloride | Direct inotrope | 2.5 to 5 mg/kg | Myocardial depression caused by anesthetics, hypocalcemia, hypothermia |

pulmonary injury they can increase intrapulmonary shunt and aggravate hypoxemia by blunting hypoxic pulmonary vasoconstriction.

Apart from cardiac injuries arrhythmias in the acutely traumatized patient are usually caused by hypoxia, acidosis, hypothermia, or disturbances of serum $Ca^{2+}$ and $K^{+}$. They often disappear once these causes are corrected. However, antiarrhythmic agents may be required to optimize cardiac function until specific therapy takes effect. Tachycardia is the most common rhythm abnormality and is almost always the result of a combination of hypovolemia and pain due to light anesthesia. Adequate replacement of blood volume and increasing the depth of anesthesia (if possible) will slow the heart rate. Tachycardia secondary to left ventricular failure should be treated with intraoperative digitalization and dopamine or dobutamine infusion titrated to optimal pulmonary arterial wedge pressure and cardiac output. Digoxin should be used cautiously in the acute trauma victim since its toxicity may be aggravated by hypokalemia, a frequent occurrence following trauma. The usual dose of digoxin is 0.125 mg, intravenously, twice, with a 20-minute interval between doses. Lidocaine (100 mg, intravenously) followed by continuous infusion at a rate of 2 to 4 mg/min is usually effective in treating ventricular arrhythmias. If lidocaine is ineffective, procainamide up to a total dose of 1000 mg is infused slowly. Bretylium (5 mg/kg, intravenous bolus) over a period of 5 to 10 minutes may be useful in the trauma patient because of its efficacy in controlling ventricular arrhythmias secondary to myocardial ischemia.[226] This dose can be repeated within 30 minutes if the initial dose proves ineffective. Bretylium, however, causes peripheral vasodilatation and hypotension, which may have deleterious consequences in the hypovolemic patient. Ventricular tachycardia is treated with lidocaine (100 mg, intravenously) and DC countershock if lidocaine therapy is ineffective.

For supraventricular arrhythmias, verapamil (0.075 to 0.15 mg/kg, intravenously) is the drug of choice. Hypotension and possibly cardiac arrest may occur if verapamil is given rapidly, especially in anesthetized hypovolemic patients; we administer the drug slowly in 2.5-mg increments. Atrial fibrillation with rapid ventricular rate is treated with digoxin, using a 0.125-mg dose repeated in 20 minutes. Propranolol (0.025 to 0.1 mg/kg, intravenously), given in divided doses, increases the success rate of this treatment.

Complete heart block with hypotension is initially treated with an intravenous infusion of isoproterenol (1 to 1.5 μg/min) and then with a pacemaker once necessary preparations are completed. If a Paceport catheter is already in the pulmonary artery, treatment involves insertion of a pacing wire through the side port and connection to a pacemaker unit; otherwise the pacing wire is introduced into the internal jugular or subclavian vein through a 16-gauge cannula. A recently popularized pacing technique, noninvasive external cardiac pacing, is probably the most appropriate method for intraoperative resuscitation. This device uses two electrodes, of which the larger (posterior) electrode is attached in the left subscapular area, and the anterior electrode is placed on the left lower sternal edge.[155] The device (Ross Research, Marlboro, Mass) can function in both fixed rate and demand mode and unlike older external systems does not produce significant cutaneous nerve stimulation. The approximate pacing current is 80 mA, but the device is capable of delivering currents up to 140 mA.

Not all intraoperative hemodynamic support falls entirely within the domain of the anesthesiologist. Surgeons too have effective measures of improving organ function. Intraoperative thoracotomy with temporary descending aortic occlusion is one of these procedures; it may be required to treat persistent hypotension caused by severe uncontrollable intra-abdominal bleeding.[314] This procedure improves arterial blood pressure effectively and probably increases survival rate following trauma; the survival rate is 30%.[275,314] However, declamping hypotension, myocardial ischemia, coagulation abnormalities, and increased ICP in patients with associated head injury are some of the severe and common complications of this technique. When this procedure is performed, careful monitoring of myocardial ischemia, coagulation, blood pressure, temperature, and ICP (if an intracranial bolt is in place) and instituting appropriate preventive and therapeutic measures against these complications remain the tasks of the anesthesiologist.

Mechanical circulatory assist devices may be required when acute traumatic insult to the heart produces severe myocardial dysfunction refractory to vasoactive agents. Many methods have been designed to provide circulatory support, but intra-aortic balloon counterpulsation is by far the most effective. Reduction of left ventricular work by counterpulsation may benefit patients with myocardial contusion and with traumatic septal and valvular lesions by reducing shunt flow through the interventricular septum[111] and by decreasing mitral regurgitation.

### *Transfusion*

This subject is discussed in detail in Chapter 6. Thus we will deal only with a few salient points.

Although tissue $O_2$ delivery is greater at physiological hematocrit (Hct = 40), satisfactory tissue oxygenation and perfusion are provided at a hematocrit level of 30 if adequate cardiac output is established with aggressive fluid resuscitation[174] (Fig 9-21). Thus, maintenance of Hct between 30 and 35 is our goal during intraoperative transfusion. A period of 30 to 45 minutes is usually required to type and cross-match blood. Extensive use of group O low-titer whole blood by the Armed Forces for at least the past 4 decades[56] suggests that "universal donor" blood can be administered when urgency dictates immediate transfusion. More recently, Schwab et al[406] demonstrated the safety and effectiveness of type O (Rh positive, low titer for males and Rh negative for females) non-cross-matched packed cells in civilian trauma practice. Anti-A and Anti-B titers of the patient whose type is other than O should be determined following universal donor blood if transfusion is to continue with the patient's own type. High titers preclude administration of type-specific blood. If anti-A and anti-B titers cannot be determined, it is wise to continue transfusion with type O blood after 5 units of whole blood or 10 units of packed cells are administered.

Although autotransfusion has been used in some centers, the devices available to process the patient's shed blood require time, effort, and extra attention, reducing the practicality of the technique. However, blood from the chest loses its coagulability, and thus in many emergency departments hemothorax content has been collected into citrate-phosphate-dextrose (CPD)-containing bags and returned to the patient without the use of a cell-washing device.[241] To our knowledge this practice has not been used during intraoperative management of chest trauma victims but may be used in desperate situations. Among artificial blood products perfluorochemicals do not have a place in trauma management, but various stroma-free hemoglobin solutions are likely to be used in the operating room in the future. The recently introduced polymerized pyridoxylated hemoglobin solution (Poly SFH-P) has a hemoglobin concentration of 14 g/dL, a $P_{50}$ of 16 to 20 mm Hg, and colloid oncotic pressure of 20 mm Hg. In animals it can support life at zero hematocrit and improve tissue oxygenation above that provided by red cells alone.[202]

FIG. 9-21. Mean oxygen delivery and oxygen consumption at hematocrits (Hct) 40 and 30 following trauma. Despite a higher oxygen delivery to tissues at hematocrit of 40, oxygen consumption is similar at both hematocrit levels. (From Fortune et al[174] with permission.)

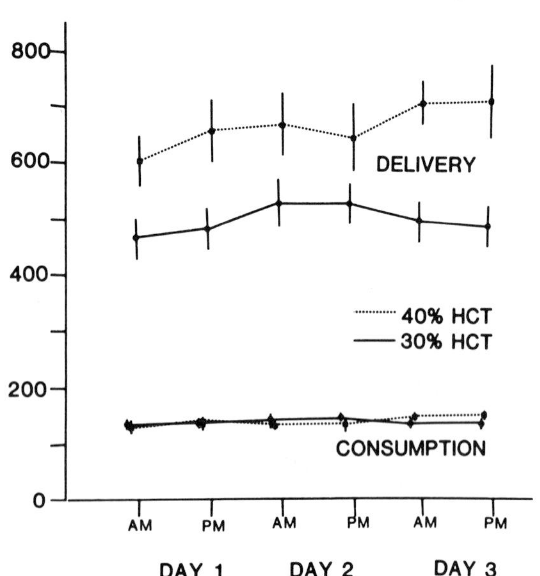


Electrolyte abnormalities ($K^+$ and $Ca^{2+}$) rarely occur during massive transfusion. Hyperkalemia and hypocalcemia are both likely if the rate of transfusion exceeds 30 ml/kg per hour or, for practical purposes, 1 unit of packed red cells every 4 minutes.[1,512] In the hypovolemic patient, hyperkalemia develops because blood is transfused into a contracted intravascular space, and thus the $K^+$ concentration rises rapidly.[451] However, hypokalemia occurs more frequently than hyperkalemia and develops not only from blood transfusion but also as a result of intracellular shift of $K^+$ by trauma-induced sympathetic stimulation.[485] Serum $K^+$ and $Ca^{2+}$ must be measured serially during rapid transfusion.

### *Treatment of Intraoperative Coagulopathy*

Preexisting coagulation abnormalities, DIC, transient dilution of platelets and coagulation factors by resuscitative fluids, and fibrinolysis are common factors producing coagulopathy in the acutely traumatized patient. Hypothermia and diminished tissue perfusion aggravate coagulation abnormalities.[220,480] Thus every effort must be made to maintain normal body temperature and organ perfusion. In the absence of coagulopathy, prophylactic administration of platelets or fresh frozen plasma (FFP) is unwarranted even if coagulation tests (PT, PTT, platelet count, thrombelastogram) indicate platelet or coagulation factor depletion.[69,98,381] In normothermic and well-perfused patients, endogenous release of platelets and coagulation factors prevents dilutional coagulopathy.[381]

If DIC should occur, the treatment is elimination of its causes, which, in the trauma patient, are hemorrhage, hypoperfusion, hypothermia, and tissue damage. As a temporizing measure, however, depleted coagulation components must be replaced with platelet concentrates, FFP, and if necessary, cryoprecipitate. Most hospital blood banks do not store platelets; they should be ordered in advance. Dilutional coagulopathy, is a transient phenomenon,[220] although depleted factors and platelets must be replaced when coagulopathy manifested by generalized bleeding from the surgical wound, intravascular cannula insertion sites, and mucocutaneous membranes is present. Further information on coagulation abnormalities in the trauma patient is provided in Chapters 6 and 7.

### *Prevention and Treatment of Hypothermia*

The preoperative body temperature of the trauma victim is usually low, and there appears to be a direct relation between severity of injury and decrease in body temperature.[246,283,287] The mortality rate following trauma increases with increasing severity of hypothermia both pre- and intraoperatively. In one study, the overall mortality rate was 100% if the core temperature was below 32°C, 69% if below 33°C, and 40% when it was less than 34°C.[246] Also, in patients with similar ISS, the mortality rate of severely hypothermic patients (<32°C) was higher than their moderately or mildly hypothermic counterparts.[246] Exposure to cold, alcohol intoxication, hemorrhage, abnormalities in thermoregulatory mechanisms, inability to shiver, fluid resuscitation, and shock with its resultant decreased metabolism contribute greatly to preoperative hypothermia.[283,287]

The possibility of hypothermia during surgery is also greater in the acute trauma victim than in the elective surgical patient. Intraoperative heat loss increases in patients with spinal cord injuries, burns, large superficial injuries, and ethanol intoxication. Surgical procedures are usually long and involve body cavities—two important factors associated with increased heat loss. Resuscitation with massive amounts of cold fluids and blood products produces further reduction in body temperature. Approximately 67.2 kJ is consumed to warm 1 L of crystalloid solution from ambient to body temperature and 134.4 kJ is required to warm 1 unit of refrigerated blood.[166] The possibility of heat loss following infusion of these agents becomes obvious when it is realized that a drop in body temperature of 1°C requires a loss of only 243.6 kJ.[166,324]

During the intraoperative period, the trauma victim may also be more susceptible to the detrimental effects of hypothermia than elective patients. During elective surgery, because of activation of compensatory cutaneous vasoconstriction, body temperature rarely falls below 34°C;[409a] this level of hypothermia is tolerated well provided ventilation is adequate. It is during the postoperative period that shivering, peripheral vasoconstriction, hypoxemia, delayed drug clearance, increased oxygen consumption, and protein breakdown affect these patients.[85,244] In the major trauma patient, not only is the body temperature more likely to drop below 34°C, but also the impact of hypothermia on already compromised vital functions may be devastating. Reduced cardiac output, cardiac conduction abnormalities, attenuated hypoxic pulmonary vasoconstriction, diminished cerebral and renal blood flow, altered platelet function, and abnormalities of $K^+$ and $Ca^{2+}$ homeostasis, the consequences of hypothermia, further aggravate already poor organ perfusion, oxygenation, blood coagulation, and metabolism.[57,324,480]

Hypothermia increases the solubility of $O_2$ and $CO_2$ in the blood; it thus lowers $Pa{O_2}$ and $Pa{CO_2}$ and raises pH. Since blood gases are measured at 37°C, one may think of correcting the values obtained for the patient's temperature. The correction may be inappropriate for $P{CO_2}$ and pH because several enzyme systems function optimally at "uncorrected" pH values in the physiological range.[378,380] Thus, treatment of acid-base abnormality according to corrected values may interfere with optimal enzyme function. On the other hand, temperature correction for $Pa{O_2}$ is necessary.[322] The drop in $Pa{O_2}$ with hypothermia is dependent upon hemoglobin saturation. $Pa{O_2}$ falls at a rate of 7.5%/°C when saturation is below 90% but only 1.3%/°C when saturation is 100% ($Pa{O_2}$ > 500 mm Hg). In the usual clinical ranges of $O_2$ saturation (90 to 100%), the correction procedure is complex and requires the nomogram described by Andritsch and coworkers.[13]

Hypothermia can be prevented by taking aggressive measures toward heat conservation (Table 9-12). The greatest heat loss takes place in the first hour of anesthesia probably as a result of exposure, prepping, and peripheral vasodilatation during induction. A drop in body temperature of as much as 1.3°C during the first hour of anesthesia has been noted in elective surgical patients. Decreases during the second and third hours were 0.3°C and 0.1°C, respectively.[325] Thus, it is important to institute preventive measures early enough to achieve success.

Data relative to the efficacy of various heat-conserving methods in the trauma patient are lacking. However, information from elective surgery patients suggests that heat loss can be best reduced by maintaining operating room temperature above 21°C.[325] This method, however, cannot eliminate heat loss entirely, and some temperature drop may still occur. Also, at high ambient temperatures (> 22°C) most surgeons will be uncomfortable.

Humidification of inspired gases reduces heat loss by 10 to 15% or 37.8 to 42 kJ/h.[415] As mentioned earlier, a heat loss of 243.6 kJ decreases body temperature 1°C.[166,324] Thus, it is obvious that use of humidification alone will prevent only some of the temperature drop. Inspired gases can be humidified either by heat-moisture exchangers or by electrically heated humidifiers. An absolute humidity of up to 30 mg of $H_2O$/L at 6 L/min of flow can be provided by heat-moisture exchangers.[497] This technique may produce increased inspiratory resistance because of accumulation in the exchanger of moisture, secretions, or blood from the patient's respiratory tract. In our experience, heated humidifiers are more effective than heat-moisture exchangers for the trauma patient. The temperature measured at the proximal end of the endotracheal tube should not exceed 39 to 40°C, and the humidifier should be placed below the patient level to prevent airway burns caused by inadvertent drainage of heated water into the trachea.

TABLE 9-12. Measures to Prevent Heat Loss in the Operating Room

| |
|---|
| *Radiant heat loss* |
| Maintenance of OR temperature above 21°C |
| Draping of the patient immediately after prep |
| *Convective heat loss* |
| Reducing the velocity of high-flow orthopedic air curtains or air conditioners |
| Applying forced-warm air system to the body surface (Bair Hugger) |
| *Conductive heat loss* |
| Warming all sterile prep and irrigating solutions |
| Warming all intravenous infusions |
| *Evaporative heat loss* |
| Drying prepped area quickly |
| Packing moist and exposed tissues |
| Heating and humidifying inspired gases |

Some heat can be conserved by the use of blood warmers if an appropriate warmer is chosen, flow rates are relatively rapid, and the tubing between the warmer and the patient is not long. As we mentioned, a fluid infusion system incorporating a heat exchanger appears to minimize temperature drop in traumatized patients[401] (Fig. 9-7). The value of heating blankets placed between the operating room table and the patient is doubtful at best.[326] This device is generally inadequate because of the relatively small body surface area in contact with the mattress, prevention of adequate heat exchange by vasoconstriction, and the insulating effect of sheets interposed between the patient and the mattress. In addition, the risk of thermal burns has prevented the widespread use of thermal blankets. Reflective blankets (metallized plastic sheeting), on the other hand, may be useful in preserving body heat if more than 60% of the body surface area can be covered.[64] Ordinary clear plastic sheeting has been found equally effective for heat conservation.[324] Delivery of forced-warm air to the body surface (Bair Hugger) is also useful for this purpose.

When used alone, none of the measures described above can decrease heat loss sufficiently to maintain normal body temperature. The combination of heated humidifier and thermal blanket has been shown to be more effective than either humidifier or blanket alone.[466] Joachimsson and coworkers[244] showed that by using all available measures of heat preservation—heated humidifier, thermal blanket, reflective blanket, fluid warmer, and operating room temperature of 21 to 23°C—core temperature could be maintained at preinduction levels during major elective abdominal surgery (Fig. 9-22). Naturally, the rate of heat loss varies from patient to patient. Surgery performed in the abdominal and thoracic cavities of severely injured patients results in the greatest heat loss and warrants the use of multiple heat-preserving measures. In such patients, there may even be a need for invasive rewarming techniques such as cardiopulmonary bypass to resolve this problem.[246] On the other hand, in less severe trauma involving superficial tissues, multiple heat-preserving measures may produce temperature elevation. Of course, body temperature must be monitored at all times in order to adjust it to an optimal level.

Temperature control should continue during the postoperative period. In the recovery room body temperature can be raised by covering the patient with blankets, applying Bair-Hugger, replacing underlying wet sheets with dry ones, and using warmed infusions. A warming blanket placed over rather than underneath the patient is also useful in increasing body temperature. Another warming device is the radiant heater, consisting of three 250-watt infrared lamps directed from the upper thoracic to the suprapubic area. These lamps appear to be very effective in abolishing postoperative shivering.[420] In some institutions, radiant ceiling heaters have also been used intraoperatively to warm severely hypothermic trauma victims.

### *Management of Acid-Base Abnormalities*

Except in head-injured patients, respiratory alkalosis should be avoided by adjustment of alveolar ventilation and measurement of end-tidal $CO_2$ and blood gases. Altered perfusion, hypokalemia, and their consequences occur frequently following severe trauma and may be exacerbated by alkalosis.

In hypovolemic patients, poor tissue perfusion may result in increased production and decreased utilization of lactate, resulting in anion gap acidosis, in which the difference between the concentrations of the cations ($[Na^+] + [K^+]$) and anions ($[Cl^-] + [HCO_3^-]$) is greater than 15 mEq/L.[349] Early metabolic acidosis after trauma is almost always due to accumulation of lactate, although it may rarely be caused by ketoacidosis in alcoholic or diabetic patients.[80] The definitive diagnosis of lactic acidosis is made only by measurement of blood lactate concentration. Normal plasma lactate concentration is 0.5 to 1.5 mmol/L; higher levels, especially above 5 mmol/L, suggest lactic acidosis.[317] Although the proper way to evaluate blood lactate concentration is by measuring the ratio between lactate and pyruvate (lactate/pyruvate > 10 to 15 suggests tissue hypoperfusion),[427] determination of pyruvate in clinical conditions is difficult. Thus, elevated plasma lactate concentrations are generally considered to be sufficient evidence of impaired tissue oxygenation. Blood lactate concentration can be rapidly and inexpensively determined in an operating room laboratory using a recently developed

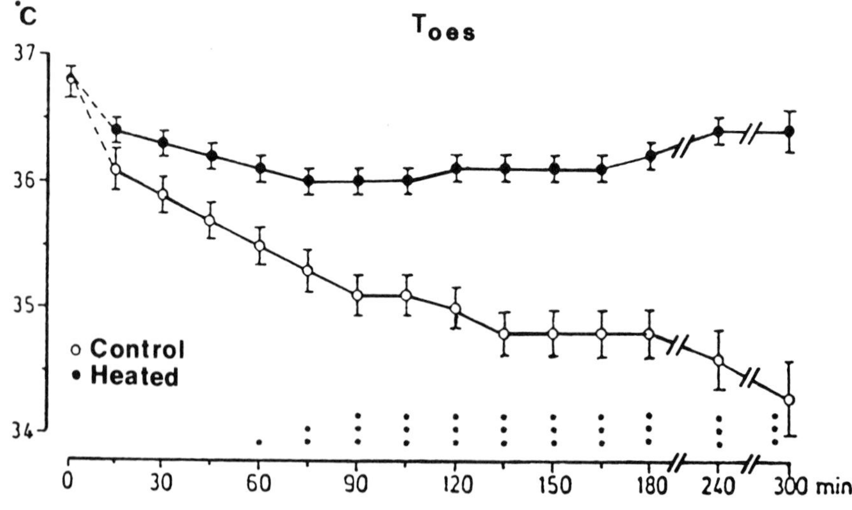


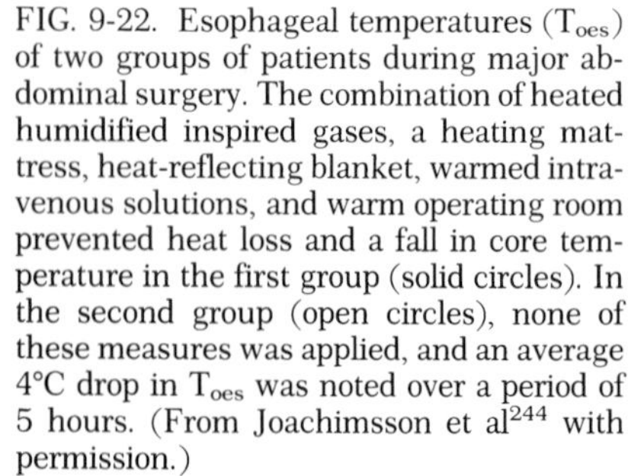
FIG. 9-22. Esophageal temperatures ($T_{oes}$) of two groups of patients during major abdominal surgery. The combination of heated humidified inspired gases, a heating mattress, heat-reflecting blanket, warmed intravenous solutions, and warm operating room prevented heat loss and a fall in core temperature in the first group (solid circles). In the second group (open circles), none of these measures was applied, and an average 4°C drop in $T_{oes}$ was noted over a period of 5 hours. (From Joachimsson et al[244] with permission.)

apparatus (Yellow Springs Instrument Co, Inc, Yellow Springs, Ohio), although most operating room laboratories are not currently equipped with this device. Thus, in most instances, base deficit, computed from measurement of $Pa_{CO_2}$ and pH, is used to determine the severity of acidosis.

The treatment of metabolic acidosis secondary to hypovolemia is restoration of intravascular volume. Once this is accomplished, acidosis will be corrected as lactate production decreases and clearance by the liver increases. There is controversy about the use of sodium bicarbonate in this situation. Until a few years ago, this drug was used routinely in conjunction with volume replacement even in patients with moderate metabolic acidosis secondary to shock. The rationale of such therapy was to "buy time" until intravascular volume was restored and to mitigate against acidosis-induced hemodynamic impairment, arrhythmias, and decreased cardiac responsiveness to endogenous and exogenous catecholamines. More recent data suggest that administration of $NaHCO_3$ in the presence of hypoxic lactic acidosis is associated with pronounced adverse effects: further decrease in cardiac output and blood pressure, decreased tissue oxygenation due to leftward shift of the oxyhemoglobin dissociation curve, precipitation of a hyperosmolar state by the high sodium load, and overshoot alkalosis and its consequences after improvement of tissue perfusion.[49,203] In addition, $NaHCO_3$ does not seem to increase arterial pH and bicarbonate in the presence of tissue hypoxia but rather increases blood lactate to levels above that observed in its absence.[49,203] In view of these findings, alkaline therapy is now rarely used in the treatment of hypoxic or hypovolemic acidosis. However, in severe acidosis ($pH < 7.1$) caused by massive hemorrhage, in which impairment of cardiovascular performance may be partly due to acidosis itself, bicarbonate may be indicated. Whole body base deficit is usually calculated from the formula $0.3 \times BE$ (mEq/L) $\times$ BW (kg) where BE is base excess, and BW is the body weight. Only half of the calculated dose of $NaHCO_3$ is administered, after which the base deficit is reassessed.

Sodium dichloroacetate, a halogenated carboxylic acid that reduces lactate production by stimulating pyruvate dehydrogenase and increasing glycolytic flux, may be a useful alternative to $NaHCO_3$, but its efficacy in acidemic acute trauma victims remains to be determined.[446]

## ADMINISTRATION OF ANESTHETIC AND ADJUNCT DRUGS

In response to trauma, the stressed organism utilizes all available compensatory mechanisms in order to provide adequate blood flow to vital organs and thus sustain life. Preservation of these catecholamine-induced compensatory mechanisms—vasoconstriction, tachycardia, and increased cardiac contractility—is critical during anesthesia. However, the salutary effects of the stress response become deleterious when continued for a prolonged period. Following hypovolemia, prolonged vasoconstriction in non–vital organs results in ischemia, anaerobic metabolism, lactic acidosis, and ultimately death of these tissues and possibly of the patient.[284] Thus, it is not surprising that hemorrhaged animals survive for a shorter period of time when treated with vasoconstrictor agents than their untreated counterparts.[214] Concern about the deleterious effects of vasoconstriction has led investigators to use adrenergic receptor blockers in hypovolemic shock. There are data demonstrating prolonged survival in animals pretreated with these agents.[129] Although we do not advocate the use of $\alpha$ receptor blockade, these experiments indicate the potential for serious complications following prolonged vasoconstriction. Early establishment of adequate intravascular volume during the intraoperative phase, at whatever infusion rate necessary, is the key to prevention of prolonged vasoconstriction. In this way one hopefully can avoid the necessity of administering suboptimal doses of anesthetic agents or use of vasoconstrictors.

Often during the early intraoperative period, the severely traumatized patient can tolerate no more than a "pancuronium/$O_2$" anesthetic, perhaps with small doses of fentanyl. This practice results in awareness of intraoperative events in up to 43% of trauma survivors undergoing surgery for repair of severe injuries.[58] Thus, judicious doses of anesthetic agents should be administered to prevent both sympathetic overactivity and recall, but which anesthetics should be used?

An ideal anesthetic should maintain cardiac output, regional blood flows, and tissue oxygenation at levels similar to those seen in the awake state. Hence, rapid restoration of blood volume would be the only concern of the anesthesiologist managing the patient in traumatic shock. Unfortunately, all anesthetics produce dose-dependent hemodynamic alteration in both normovolemic and hypovolemic patients. Whether these alterations are less with one agent than another in the presence of hypovolemia is not, and probably will not be, known because in clinical conditions, many factors besides the anesthetic agent play roles in the development of hemodynamic changes. Available data from animal studies performed under reasonably controlled conditions are also controversial and inconclusive, providing little help to the clinician (Table 9-13). In this section the characteristics of available anesthesia maintenance agents, as they apply to various types of trauma, will be discussed.

### *Intravenous Agents*

In this group ketamine is the most popular agent and can be administered as a continuous infusion in conjunction with $N_2O$, opioids, and muscle relaxants. The usual infusion rate of ketamine in normovolemic patients is 30 to 50 $\mu$g/kg per minute, but this should be reduced by about 25% after 1 hour to avoid accumulation of ketamine metabolites.[237] In the hypovolemic patient the dose of ketamine should be adjusted according to hemodynamic response.

### *Nitrous Oxide*

Nitrous oxide ($N_2O$) is often used as an adjunct to anesthetics in the healthy patient and is often the sole anesthetic agent in the trauma victim. For many years considered an innocuous drug, recent evidence suggests otherwise. Nitrous oxide is capable of producing myocardial depression and increased systemic vascular resistance from sympathetic stimulation both in normal subjects[146,254] and in patients with coronary artery disease[25,145] (Table 9-14). This effect is also seen when

TABLE 9-13. Results of Studies Comparing Various Anesthetics in Hemorrhaged Animals*

| AUTHOR | SPECIES | ANESTHETICS COMPARED | EXTENT OF HEMORRHAGE | RESULTS |
|---|---|---|---|---|
| Theye et al[462] | Mongrel dog | Cyclopropane (1 MAC)<br>Isoflurane (1 MAC)<br>Halothane (1 MAC) | 10 ml/kg/30 min | Survival times were longer with halothane and isoflurane than with cyclopropane<br><br>Hemodynamic function, $O_2$ uptake, and acid-base balance were better sustained with cyclopropane than with halothane or isoflurane initially when blood loss was mild or moderate, but when blood loss increased these functions were better maintained with halothane or isoflurane than with cyclopropane |
| Longnecker and Sturgill[286] | Sprague-Dawley rats | Halothane (1.25 vol %)<br>Pentobarbital (50 mg/kg)<br>Ketamine (125 mg/kg) | MAP 40 mm Hg during 60-min hemorrhage | Both 24-hour and 7-day posthemorrhage survival rates were higher with ketamine (82%) than with halothane (47%) or pentobarbital (55%)<br><br>Significantly lower incidence of microscopic liver and small intestinal pathology was observed in the ketamine group than in the halothane or pentobarbital group |
| Roberts et al[388] | Mongrel dogs | Halothane (1%) | 10, 20, and 25% of estimated blood volume | No evidence of tissue hypoxia<br><br>MAP, $\dot{Q}_t$, SV, LVEDP decreased, and SVR increased as blood loss increased |
| Horan et al[227,228] | Mongrel dogs | Halothane (1 MAC)<br>Enflurane (1 MAC)<br>Isoflurane (1 MAC) | 20% of estimated blood volume | Cardiovascular function was most depressed with enflurane, least with isoflurane, and halothane was intermediate |
| Weiskopf et al[502] | Mongrel dogs | Halothane (1%)<br>Enflurane (2.5%)<br>Isoflurane (1.6%)<br>Ketamine (5 mg/kg intravenously + 0.25 mg/kg/min infusion) | 10, 20, and 30% of estimated blood volume | With 30% blood loss, arterial blood lactate and base deficit increased in the ketamine group but remained unchanged in the halothane, enflurane, and isoflurane group |
| Idvall[236] | Wistar SPF rats | Ketamine (30 mg/kg intravenously + 1.5 mg/kg/min infusion)<br>Sodium pentobarbital (30 mg/kg intravenously + 6 mg/kg/h infusion) | Moderate (10 ml/kg) | *Moderate bleeding*<br>Ketamine-treated rats had larger $\dot{Q}_t$ and higher BP than unanesthetized rats<br><br>Larger proportion of $\dot{Q}_t$ was distributed to heart, kidneys, skin, and small intestine in the ketamine group |
| | | | Severe (systolic BP 60 mm Hg) | *Severe bleeding*<br>Larger blood loss (36% of blood volume) was necessary to decrease systolic BP to 60 mm Hg in the ketamine group than in the pentobarbital group (23% of blood volume)<br><br>In spite of a larger blood loss, $\dot{Q}_t$ and BP in the ketamine group were higher than those in the barbiturate group 20 min after hemorrhage<br><br>Ketamine maintained higher blood flow to vital organs than barbiturate |
| Longnecker et al[285] | Sprague-Dawley rats | Ketamine (125 mg/kg intramuscularly + 30 mg/kg intramuscular supplements)<br>Enflurane (2.2%) | 2.6 ml/100 g resulting in MAP 30–35 mm Hg for 30 minutes | Tissue hypoxia occurred with enflurane but not with ketamine<br><br>Ketamine, as compared with enflurane, diminished or prevented arteriolar constriction produced by hemorrhage |
| Seyde and Longnecker[411] | Sprague-Dawley rats | Ketamine (125 mg/kg intraperitoneally + 1 mg/kg/min infusion)<br>Halothane (1 MAC)<br>Enflurane (1 MAC)<br>Isoflurane (1 MAC) | 30% of estimated blood volume | $\dot{Q}_t$ and regional blood flows were most like the awake hemorrhaged state under isoflurane anesthesia<br><br>Under ketamine anesthesia, $\dot{Q}_t$ and regional blood flows were closest to the awake state only when the animals were normovolemic |

* The abbreviations used are: MAP, mean arterial pressure; $\dot{Q}_t$, cardiac output; SV, stroke volume; LVEDP,left ventricular and diastolic pressure; SVR, systemic vascular resistance.

$N_2O$ is combined with other anesthetic agents—diazepam, morphine, fentanyl, or halothane.[288,305,438,508]

The effect of $N_2O$ on the hemodynamics of hypovolemic trauma patients is not known. Available data from animal studies suggest that 70% $N_2O$ results in considerable deterioration of cardiovascular compensation for hemorrhage.[499] The sympathetic stimulation caused by $N_2O$ in normovolemic patients does not appear to be beneficial during hypovolemia and may in fact be deleterious, increasing oxygen demand in the face of decreasing supply.[499] In addition, $N_2O$, by reducing $F_{IO_2}$, incurs a risk of hypoxemia. Thus, it may have to be avoided in the presence of pulmonary contusion, aspiration pneumonitis, hypovolemia, or large physiological shunt.

Nitrous oxide must be avoided when pneumothorax or pneumopericardium is present because solubility differences between this agent and nitrogen favor expansion of pleural or pericardial air, which may cause disastrous complications.[142] Although intuitively, one would expect that similar precautions should be taken when subcutaneous or mediastinal emphysema is present, the result of an experimental study in animals showed that use of $N_2O$ did not result in significant volume expansion in these regions.[369]

The use of $N_2O$ may be hazardous in patients with closed-head injury since it dilates cerebral vessels and, in concentrations of 50% or more, causes clinically significant increases in ICP.[327] While this effect can be attenuated by prior administration of diazepam or thiopental,[367] the extent of this action may not be predictable in brain-injured patients.

Nitrous oxide administered in concentrations of 50% or higher for periods longer than 6 hours may reduce the activity of methionine synthase and produce bone marrow dysfunction.[198,355] Megaloblastic anemia, leukopenia, and thrombocytopenia may occur following long exposure to $N_2O$ because of inactivation of vitamin $B_{12}$.[84,198] This effect usually disappears within a few days after discontinuing the agent.[355] Although the clinical significance of this phenomenon has not been elucidated, and overt symptoms do not occur unless $N_2O$ is used longer than 24 hours, in seriously ill trauma patients in whom surgery is prolonged beyond 12 hours, substitution with nitrogen or air may be considered.[84,347]

### *Halogenated Inhalational Agents*

In healthy subjects halothane and enflurane cause a dose-dependent decrease in cardiac output, blood pressure, renal and hepatic blood flows, and an increase in cerebral blood volume.[222] Isoflurane produces little change in cardiac output, but it decreases blood pressure and organ blood flow[222] and also increases cerebral blood volume. There is evidence to suggest that these agents may reduce tissue $O_2$ demand; thus, the balance between supply and demand may not be significantly altered[143] (Table 9-14).

In hypovolemic animals inhalation agents interfere with compensatory cardiovascular mechanisms. Thus, smaller than normal doses produce significant hemodynamic alterations. Studies in hypovolemic animals conducted by Weiskopf and Bogetz[59,499,502] showed that all three agents produced significant decreases in cardiac output, blood pressure, and systemic vascular resistance and increased serum lactate concentrations at lower end-tidal anesthetic concentrations than those usually required in normovolemic patients. However, the lactate increase was small relative to the magnitude of reduction in cardiac output and blood pressure. In equipotent doses, isoflurane appears to produce less profound hemodynamic and metabolic changes than halothane and enflurane.[59,411] Blood flow to vital organs also appears to be better maintained with this agent than with either halothane or enflurane.[411] In its cardiovascular effects, enflurane has a smaller margin of safety between anesthetic and hazardous concentrations than the other inhalation agents.[82] Also, prolonged exposure to enflurane (>9 MAC-hour) results in transient impairment of renal concentrating ability in response to vasopressin.[303] It is probably the least desirable agent in the trauma setting, although all three inhalational agents can be used provided their doses are carefully adjusted according to patient's hemodynamic status. It should be remembered that these effects may be so modified by other factors such as duration of anesthesia, degree of hypovolemia, $P_{CO_2}$, preexisting cardiovascular disease, surgical stress, and other agents that prediction of their effect in a given patient is difficult.[222]

All inhalation agents increase CBF and cerebral blood volume.[464] Although this effect is most pronounced with halothane and least with isoflurane,[136] in animals with cryogenic brain injury, ICP increases to the same extent with both agents even in the presence of hypocapnia.[405] In patients with closed-head injury, elevated ICP coupled with the depressant effects of inhalation anesthetics on mean arterial pressure may decrease cerebral perfusion pressure. Thus, inhalational agents should be avoided in these patients.

### *Narcotic Agents*

Narcotic agents are commonly used during anesthetic maintenance of the trauma patient. Clinically important charac-

TABLE 9-14. Comparative Effects of Nitrous Oxide and the Halogenated Inhalational Agents*

| | NITROUS OXIDE | ISOFLURANE | HALOTHANE | ENFLURANE |
|---|---|---|---|---|
| Myocardial contractility | − | − − | − − − | − − − |
| Systemic vascular resistance | + | − − | − | − |
| Heart rate | No change | + | Slight decrease | Slight decrease |
| Arterial blood pressure | Slight decrease | − − | − − − | − − − |
| Intracranial pressure (in patients with increased ICP at $Pa_{CO_2}$ = 40 mm Hg) | + | + + | + + | + + |
| Total body $O_2$ consumption | Slight decrease | − − | − − | − − |
| Central sympathetic tone | Slight increase | − − | − − | − − |

* −, decrease; +, increase.

teristics of these agents are summarized in Table 9-15. Both morphine and meperidine produce good analgesia but are not suitable for the hypovolemic patient because they release histamine and thus cause hypotension and tachycardia.[167]

Fentanyl, sufentanil, and alfentanil have greater potency with shorter duration of effect and provide greater hemodynamic stability than morphine or meperidine. They have no direct cardiovascular depressant effect and do not cause histamine release.[164,167] The hemodynamic effects of these agents have not been studied in a systematic fashion in patients with hemorrhagic shock, but in a group of patients in septic shock, fentanyl caused little hemodynamic alteration.[447] Nevertheless, these agents can cause hypotension by inhibiting central sympathetic activity, especially in the hypovolemic trauma patient whose apparent hemodynamic stability is maintained by hyperactive sympathetic tone.[165]

The anesthetic doses of fentanyl and its analogs described in Table 9-15 pertain to patients undergoing cardiac surgery. For trauma victims, preset dosage regimens cannot be recommended because the clinical condition of these patients varies widely. The degree of hypovolemia, the intensity of the surgical stimulus, autonomic and somatic responses to surgery, and concomitantly used anesthetics all affect the dosage of these agents. As with other drugs, the doses of fentanyl or its analogs must be reduced in hypovolemic patients. Thus, after adequate fluid resuscitation, incremental doses of fentanyl (50 to 100 μg) or sufentanil (10 to 20 μg) can be administered until the desired effect is obtained. The short duration of action of alfentanil implies frequent injections, which are inconvenient and may result in distraction from other aspects of patient care. For long surgical procedures, alfentanil can be administered by infusion at a rate of approximately 0.5 to 1.5 μg/kg per minute after an initial loading dose of 20 to 75 μg/kg given according to the patient's condition and response. If the patient's hemodynamic status allows, $N_2O$, low doses of an inhalation agent, one of the major tranquilizers (benzodiazepine, midazolam droperidol), and/or a barbiturate can be added. Addition of these agents will hopefully reduce the high incidence of recall reported in trauma patients.[58]

High doses of both fentanyl and sufentanil produce prolonged respiratory and CNS depression. The latter may compromise the ability to assess postoperative CNS function in head-injured patients. Alfentanil offers the advantage of rapid recovery and may be preferable in this group of patients. It is generally believed that narcotics do not alter intracranial pressure dynamics.[163] In two studies from England, however, phenoperidine given as a bolus to patients with traumatic coma produced a decrease in mean arterial pressure without concomitant decrease in ICP.[50,210] These findings suggest a cerebral vasodilatory effect which with decreasing cerebral perfusion pressure, may cause further insult to the brain. Similar findings have also been reported following bolus doses of fentanyl with droperidol in patients and after large doses of sufentanil in animals with intracranial space-occupying lesions.[316] Although the clinical significance of these findings is not yet clear, it is prudent to administer fentanyl or its analogs slowly, after hypocarbia is established and when arterial pressure is near normal.

Agonist-antagonist narcotics given to patients who have received no pure agonist narcotics produce analgesia, sedation, and respiratory depression. In the presence of pure agonist narcotics, these agents act like narcotic antagonists; however, they reverse the respiratory depressant effects of narcotics more than they affect analgesia. Both nalbuphine[269,320] (15-μg/kg increments up to a total dose of 150 μg/kg) and butorphanol[66] (1-mg increments up to a total dose of 3 mg) have been used to antagonize narcotic-induced respiratory depression in the postoperative period. Reversal with nalbuphine, however, is not without side effects; patients may demonstrate sympathetic responses[127] that may lead to pulmonary edema.[53] Plasma epinephrine levels rise following nalbuphine reversal of narcotics.[514]

All agonist-antagonist opiates have a ceiling effect. Thus, the extent of analgesia, somnolence, and respiratory depression reaches a plateau after a certain dose. At this point the analgesia produced by these agents is less intense than that produced by pure agonist narcotics. Thus, unlike pure agonist opiates, these agents usually cannot provide anesthesia on their own and must be used in conjunction with other agents such as potent inhalation agents, barbiturates, or sedatives.[319]

Of the four available agonist-antagonist agents, pentazocine and butorphanol have some hemodynamic depressant

TABLE 9-15. Characteristics of Morphine, Meperidine, Fentanyl, Sufentanil, and Alfentanil

| | MORPHINE | MEPERIDINE | FENTANYL | SUFENTANIL | ALFENTANIL |
|---|---|---|---|---|---|
| Relative potency | 1 | 0.1 | 100 to 200 | 700 to 1200 | 30 to 60 |
| $LD_{50}$ in dogs (mg/kg) | 200 | 700 | 10 | 4 | 59.5 to 87.5 |
| Analgesic dose | 70 to 210 μg/kg | 0.7 to 2.1 mg/kg | 1 to 2 μg/kg | 0.25 μg/kg | 4 to 8 μg/kg |
| Anesthetic dose* | 0.5 to 3 mg/kg | 3 to 10 mg/kg | 50 to 150 μg/kg | 5 to 20 μg/kg | 100 to 300 μg/kg loading dose + 25 to 50 μg/kg/h |
| $MIC_{50}$† | | | 15 ng/mL | | 270 to 400 ng/mL |
| $MIC_{90}$ | | | 25 ng/mL | | |
| $MIC_{95}$ | | | 30 ng/mL | | |
| Cardiovascular stability | +/−‡ | − − | + + + + | + + + + | + + + |
| Histamine release | + + | + + + | − | − | − |
| Respiratory depression | + + | + + | + + + | + + + | + + + |
| Elimination half-life (hours) | 3 | 2.5 | 3.5 | 2.5 | 1.5 |

* Doses used for cardiac surgery. In most trauma patients smaller doses combined with other drugs are sufficient. See text for details of dosage for the trauma patient.

† $MIC_{50,90,95}$, minimum intra-arterial concentration that prevents response to sternotomy incision in 50, 90, and 95% of patients.

‡ −, no; +, yes.

effect, whereas nalbuphine and buprenorphine produce minimal cardiovascular alteration.[319] Nalbuphine is the most commonly used intraoperative agonist-antagonist narcotic because its respiratory depressant effect, unlike that of buprenorphine, is of short duration.

Naloxone antagonizes agonist and agonist-antagonist narcotics. Side effects of this agent include nausea, vomiting, hypertension,[16,457] tachycardia, pulmonary edema,[168] and dysrhythmias[16,309] which, in rare instances, may lead to cardiac arrest.[12] These complications can occur even with naloxone doses as small as 80 μg.[356,375] In narcotic addicts, naloxone produces severe agitation, hypertension, and tachycardia; therefore it should not be given to these patients. Its use in patients with coronary artery disease and in those with limited myocardial reserve may be associated with severe cardiovascular complications although pulmonary edema after naloxone has been described even in healthy teenagers.[375] Naloxone has a short duration of action, and renarcotization may follow a single dose. Continuous infusion of this agent not only prevents renarcotization but also allows titration of the drug and minimizes the risk of sympathetic hyperactivity.

In the trauma setting naloxone is most commonly used for neurological evaluation of head-injured patients following surgery. It is quite possible that naloxone itself can cause an ICP increase in these patients, but we are not aware of any report documenting this point. In any event, naloxone is given as a bolus dose of 1.5 μg/kg, repeated if necessary every 5 minutes until the patient is awake, followed by continuous infusion at a rate of 6 to 12 μg/min.[426] The drip rate is adjusted to maintain a respiratory rate of 12 breaths/min.

Nalmefene is a new analog of naloxone capable of antagonizing opioid-related analgesia and respiratory depression for more than 8 hours.[187] At doses between 0.5 and 2 mg this drug produces a dose-dependent prolongation of opioid antagonism and thus may eliminate the need for naloxone infusion.

### *Muscle Relaxants*

The significant differences among the cardiovascular effects and other properties of different muscle relaxants imply that careful consideration must be given to selecting and using them in the trauma patient. The ganglionic blockade and histamine release caused by D-tubocurarine result in decreased peripheral vascular resistance and hence a decrease in arterial blood pressure. Although ganglionic blockade by D-tubocurarine occurs only with relatively large doses of this drug, histamine release is not dose related.[232,346] Thus, D-tubocurarine must be avoided in the hypovolemic trauma patient. Both pancuronium and gallamine have sympathomimetic effects that are thought to be caused by release of noradrenaline from cardiac adrenergic nerve endings.[74,338] This effect, combined with their well-known vagolytic activity, results in significant tachycardia and at times hypertension. Thus, pancuronium and gallamine are not desirable in normovolemic trauma patients with ischemic heart disease. On the other hand, these agents may not be undesirable in the hypovolemic patient, since they help maintain sympathetic tone and blood pressure during the early resuscitative phase of surgery. It is not known, however, whether a similar degree of rise in blood pressure and heart rate is produced in the hypovolemic, stressed trauma victim as is evoked in the normovolemic patient. Cole and Moreton[96] noted in Vietnam that pancuronium, despite its tendency to raise arterial pressure and heart rate in mildly and moderately wounded soldiers, altered these parameters little following severe trauma.

Metocurine has some histamine-releasing property and, in large doses, can cause hypotension, but its therapeutic index is two to three times that of D-tubocurarine. Its combined use with pancuronium results in augmentation of blockade with smaller doses of each agent and reduction in the incidence and intensity of hemodynamic side effects.[273,274] A pancuronium to metocurine ratio of 1:4 is shown to cause a twofold reduction in expected dosage of each agent.[273] This potentiation, however, does not apply to all combinations of nondepolarizing muscle relaxants, and some pairs of these agents (gallamine plus pancuronium or gallamine plus D-tubocurarine) are simply additive,[493] whereas others (pancuronium plus D-tubocurarine) potentiate each other but to a lesser extent than the pancuronium-metocurine combination.[492,493]

Atracurium's weak histamine-releasing property can produce a transient fall of 15 to 25% in arterial pressure.[37] The dose and rate of injection of atracurium appear to be important in this reaction. Hypotension rarely occurs when the dose is in the range of 0.3 mg/kg[37] and is unlikely if the agent is injected slowly, over about 1 or 2 minutes, even when higher doses (0.6 mg/kg) are given.[408] The effect of this drug on blood pressure in the hypovolemic patient, however, may be more pronounced than normal, since histamine-induced vasodilatation can interfere with compensatory vasoconstriction. Likewise, in the trauma victim on β adrenoreceptor-blocking drugs, atracurium may produce marked hemodynamic depression because epinephrine released from the adrenal glands by histamine cannot act on the cardiovascular system, the direct chronotropic and inotropic effects of histamine are blocked, and the carotid sinus cardioaccelerator reflex is blunted.[402] Vecuronium has little effect on heart rate and hemodynamics since it is devoid of ganglionic blocking, sympathomimetic, and histamine-releasing properties.[160,204,346] Thus, it is the drug of choice in the hypovolemic trauma victim. Cardiovascular actions of the most commonly used muscle relaxants are shown in Table 9-16.

Among drugs under investigation, doxacurium (BWA938U), a long-acting nondepolarizing muscle relaxant, has pharmacological characteristics similar to pancuronium but is devoid of cardiovascular effects and does not cumulate with repeated doses.[262,332] It appears to be an appropriate drug for the trauma patient.

There is wide individual variation in neuromuscular response to nondepolarizing muscle relaxants, probably as a result of pharmacodynamic differences. Nevertheless, an $ED_{50}$ and $ED_{95}$, although with large standard deviations, and an approximate clinical duration for each agent have been established for healthy persons (Table 9-17). Such dose determinations are not available for the acutely injured patient. Several factors associated with trauma may affect the response of these patients to muscle relaxants[242] (Table 9-18) and reduce the accuracy of preset dosage schedules. Adjustment of the maintenance dosage of these agents requires the use of a peripheral nerve stimulator capable of eliciting 2 Hz train-of-four stimuli.

TABLE 9-16. Degree and Mechanism of Cardiovascular Changes Produced

| | GANGLION BLOCKADE | SYMPATHETIC STIMULATION | VAGOLYTIC EFFECT | HISTAMINE RELEASE |
|---|---|---|---|---|
| D-Tubocurarine | + + | − | − | + + + |
| Metocurine | + | − | − | + |
| Gallamine | + | + | + + + | + + |
| Pancuronium | − | + + | + + | − |
| Vecuronium | − | − | − | − |
| Atracurium | − | − | − | + |

* −, none; +, mild; + +, moderate; + + +, marked. (Adapted from Granstad and

What is the effect of massive blood loss on plasma muscle relaxant concentrations? Are incremental doses needed more frequently in this setting? Shanks et al[416] studied the effects on D-tubocurarine pharmacokinetics of massive blood loss involving salvaged autologous blood in patients undergoing surgery for scoliosis. These patients were hemodiluted prior to blood loss, and muscle relaxation was achieved with a bolus of D-tubocurarine, 0.6 mg/kg, and infusion at a rate of 0.18 mg/kg per hour. The results demonstrated that prior fluid loading followed by massive blood loss (up to 4.8 L) did not result in significant reduction in total body D-tubocurarine content. At steady-state concentrations, they estimated that complete central volume loss would result in loss of only 9% of total D-tubocurarine. Trauma patients are usually hypovolemic, but rapid fluid infusion could mimic the conditions of this study in which hemodilution decreased hemoglobin concentrations to as low as 8 g/dL.

One disadvantage of intermediate acting nondepolarizing muscle relaxants is their relatively short duration of action. When vecuronium is used for prolonged trauma surgery, this problem can be circumvented by using a large initial bolus of the drug. The duration of relaxation produced by this agent is linearly dose related, attaining 70 minutes to 10% recovery of single twitch following 0.25 mg/kg.[158] Atracurium cannot be used in this fashion because, as we mentioned above, it produces histamine release and hypotension. An alternative is the use of a continuous infusion.[42,345,354,439] This technique is useful for both atracurium and vecuronium but is more frequently used with the former drug. Approximate infusion regimens are described in Table 9-19 for both agents.

Atracurium is eliminated through several pathways. Hofmann elimination—spontaneous degradation of the drug at normal pH and temperature—together with nonspecific esterase-catalyzed hydrolysis account for 40% of clearance. The remainder of the drug is cleared by hepatic or other nonrenal pathways.[162] The clearance of atracurium by Hofmann elimination and ester hydrolysis, even in the presence of hepatic and renal failure, is an important advantage because the drug can be used for long surgical procedures, such as those performed following trauma, with no accumulation in the body.[139,191] The metabolite of atracurium, laudanosine, accumulates following prolonged use of atracurium but does not reach toxic levels even after infusion of the drug for 2 days.[509]

Blood pH and temperature affect Hofmann elimination. Hypothermia and acidosis, intraoperative events that occur frequently in the trauma patient, reduce the activity of this pathway and thereby prolong the duration of action of atracurium. Hypothermia within the range commonly seen in the trauma patient (33 to 34°C) will prolong its effect by approximately twofold; the duration may be increased by a factor of 5 at 28°C, as observed following cardiopulmonary bypass.[170] Low pH within the range compatible with life probably has less effect than hypothermia on the duration of atracurium paralysis.

Elimination of vecuronium except in large doses, does not depend on normal kidney function (15 to 20% elimination from this route), but abnormal liver function prolongs vecuronium paralysis. Thus, in low perfusion states, decreased liver blood flow may result in prolongation of vecuronium blockade. Also, hypothermia and probably acidosis augment and prolong vecuronium-induced paralysis.[78,184]

TABLE 9-17. Comparative Potency, Clinical Duration, $ED_{50}$, and $ED_{95}$ of Four Commonly Used Nondepolarizing Muscle Relaxants in Healthy Men*

| | POTENCY | CLINICAL DURATION (MINUTES) | $ED_{50}$ (μg/kg) | $ED_{95}$ (μg/kg) |
|---|---|---|---|---|
| D-Tubocurarine | 0.6 | 60 | 270 | 500 |
| Pancuronium | 4.3 | 60 | 35.7 (32 to 40) | 64.4 (58 to 72) |
| Vecuronium | 5.0 | 30 | 30.3 (26 to 36) | 56.2 (49 to 65) |
| Atracurium | 1 | 30 | 147.7 (117 to 187) | 279.3 (235 to 331) |

* Clinical duration is the time from injection to 25% twitch recovery. $ED_{50}$, 50% twitch depression; $ED_{95}$, 95% twitch depression. Numbers in parentheses represent 95% confidence limits. Dosage should be reduced by 20 to 35% when inhalation anesthetics are used. (Adapted from Basta et al[37], Gramstad and Lilleasen[204], and Savarese[402].)

by Moderate Doses of Nondepolarizing Muscle Relaxants*

| HYPOTENSION | HYPERTENSION | BRADYCARDIA | TACHYCARDIA |
|---|---|---|---|
| +++ | − | − | + |
| + | − | − | − |
| − | + | − | +++ |
| − | ++ | − | ++ |
| − | − | − | − |
| + | − | − | −/+ |

Lilleasen[204], Hunter[232], and Norman[346].)

Frequently, muscle relaxants are not reversed following major trauma surgery; hypothermia, thoracoabdominal incisions, the need for hyperventilation following brain injuries, pulmonary complications, hypovolemia, acidosis, and residual anesthetic effect all dictate postoperative ventilation. In less severe cases such as surgery for uncomplicated abdominal stab wounds, open-eye injuries, and severed or fractured limbs, if the body temperature, acid-base balance, oxygenation, and intravascular blood volume are adequate, reversal of muscle relaxants and extubation can be considered. Extubation following inadequate reversal of muscle relaxants in the trauma patient may have severe consequences not only because of resulting respiratory failure but also because of increased risk of aspiration of gastric contents.

## EARLY POSTOPERATIVE CONSIDERATIONS

The conclusion of the surgical procedure is not the end of the trauma patient's resuscitation. The patient must be transported safely, with continued monitoring of heart rate, blood pressure, and $O_2$ saturation. Blood pressure must be stable prior to leaving the operating room, and an esophageal or precordial stethoscope must be kept in place *and used* during transport. The adequacy of the ventilatory system used during transport should be tested in the operating room, especially in patients with severe chest injuries or in those who have developed pulmonary edema or sustained aspiration of blood, secretions, or gastric contents. We ventilate these patients in the operating room with the transport system for about 5 minutes and at the end of this period measure arterial blood gases.

Preparation of the recovery room is important; ample time must be provided to ensure the presence of a ventilator, properly calibrated pressure transducers, and, if necessary, vasoactive drugs. Reevaluation of the following must be performed in the recovery room at frequent intervals: (1) blood pressure; (2) heart rate; (3) temperature; (4) ventilatory function; (5) CNS function; (6) coagulation status; (7) renal function; and (8) neuromuscular block. Lack of surgical stimulation is often accompanied by decreased arterial pressure. Volume requirements may remain quite high from continued bleeding, third-space losses, and chest tube drainage. Heart rate, blood pressure, urine output, and central venous pressure measurements continue to serve as indicators of intra-

TABLE 9-18. Trauma-associated Factors Potentially Affecting the Neuromuscular Response to Nondepolarizing Muscle Relaxants

| FACTORS | POTENTIAL EFFECT |
|---|---|
| Decreased blood volume | Increased response |
| Diminished blood flow to neuromuscular junction | Decreased response |
| Hypothermia | Increased and prolonged response |
| Acute hypokalemia | Increased response |
| Hypocalcemia | Increased response |
| Respiratory acidosis | Increased response |
| Respiratory alkalosis | Decreased response |
| Metabolic acidosis | No change or slight increase |
| Burns (after several days) | Decreased response |
| Changes in plasma proteins and protein binding | Unknown |
| High-dose antibiotics | Increased response |
| Light anesthesia without inhalation anesthetics | Decreased response |

TABLE 9-19. Protocol for Atracurium and Vecuronium Infusion

| ATRACURIUM |
|---|
| Prepare an atracurium solution |
| Average infusion dose is 5 to 7.5 μg/kg per minute. |
| For a 70-kg man undergoing a 3-hour surgical procedure, 7.5 μg × 70 kg × 180 min = 94,500 μg or 94.5 mg of atracurium is needed. |
| Add 100 mg of atracurium to 190 mL of normal saline (200 mL total volume) to create a 0.5 mg/mL infusion solution. |
| Administer an initial loading dose of 0.3 to 0.6 mg/kg atracurium. |
| Monitor neuromuscular function with train-of-four (TOF). |
| When first twitch appears on TOF start infusion at a rate of 9 to 10 μg/kg per minute. |
| Adjust infusion rate to maintain a single twitch on TOF (usual dose is 5 to 9 μg/kg per minute). |
| Discontinue infusion 15 minutes before the end of surgery if muscle relaxant is to be reversed. |
| **VECURONIUM** |
| Follow the same guidelines described above using the following: |
| Average infusion dose of 1 to 2 μg/kg per minute. |
| Vecuronium needed for the patient described above is 25,20 μg or 25 mg. |
| Infusion solution concentration is 0.1 mg/mL (25 mg of vecuronium in 250 mL of saline). |
| Initial loading dose is 0.075 mg/kg. |
| Usual infusion dose is 1 to 2 μg/kg per minute. |

vascular volume. Unless the patient is hemodynamically stable, awake, and alert, continued ventilation is desirable. Hypoxia and hypercarbia are avoided with controlled ventilation and the use of PEEP as needed and tolerated. Intermittent mandatory ventilation (IMV) is used in many hospitals both as a primary ventilatory method when the patient is able to breathe, and for weaning from the ventilator when extubation is planned.[484]

Hypothermia is the rule; Vaughan et al[483] reported a 60% incidence in a normal recovery room population. Certainly a higher incidence of postoperative hypothermia would be expected in trauma patients unless all available means to preserve body temperature are used intraoperatively. Patients often shiver in an attempt to produce heat. Bay et al[38] reported that postoperative shivering can increase oxygen consumption to as much as five times normal levels. This increased need for $O_2$ can strain both respiratory and cardiovascular systems and certainly is undesirable in patients with severe trauma and cardiorespiratory diseases. Hypokalemia has been observed in association with postoperative hypothermia necessitating caution in administration of $NaHCO_3$, insulin, digitalis, or calcium; lethal dysrhythmias may occur in this setting.[57] In addition to the rewarming methods described earlier, intravenous meperidine (25 to 50 mg) abolishes postoperative shivering in the majority of patients within 5 minutes[92] and decreases oxygen consumption, $CO_2$ production, and minute ventilation, although not to normal levels. Significant improvement in arterial pH and bicarbonate levels have been noted following suppression of visible shivering by meperidine.[290] Whether the traumatized patient responds similarly to this drug is not known.

The electrocardiogram should be evaluated for rhythm disturbances, myocardial irritability, and ischemia. Serum electrolytes are determined and corrected if necessary. Urine output is monitored and maintained within adequate limits. Shin et al[423] suggest that determination of creatinine and free water clearances during the first 6 postoperative hours is the most reliable method of predicting the development of posttraumatic renal dysfunction. Creatinine clearance less than 25 ml/min and free water clearance greater than $-15$ ml/h suggest the development of acute renal failure. Decreased urine flow rate is not a good predictor, and the blood urea nitrogen does not rise until at least 24 hours after surgery or trauma. The mental status of the patient should be determined and signs of neurological abnormality carefully evaluated.

When the patient is awake and alert, the temperature is normal, blood pressure and heart rate are stable, arterial blood gases are satisfactory on minimal support, ventilatory criteria for extubation are met, the chest X-ray is free of cardiac and pulmonary abnormalities, and bleeding is controlled, the trachea can be extubated.

## CONCLUSION

The major trauma victim presents to surgery with varying types and severity of injuries, coexisting medical diseases, intoxication, and the resulting physiological disturbances. Frequently, time constraints prevent adequate preanesthetic evaluation, obligating the anesthesiologist to assume a greater responsibility for predicting, recognizing, preventing, and treating potential intraoperative events in these patients than in probably any other population undergoing surgery. Knowledge, experience, vigilance, and adequate intraoperative monitoring are essential ingredients of optimal care. Despite the abundance of literature about the pre- and postoperative care of the acute trauma victim, only a few studies have focused on intraoperative anesthetic care of the injured. Thus, our knowledge in this area remains largely based on clinical experience, some anecdotal reports, and data from animal studies or uninjured patients. Although the urgent need for acquiring information from scientifically oriented clinical studies remains an important fact, certain established basic principles must be adhered to in order to provide safe and rational intraoperative anesthetic care to the acute trauma victim. These principles can be summarized as follows.

1. Anesthetic care of the trauma victim must be individualized, taking into account the nature of the injury and the patient's physiological responses to injury, treatment, and anesthesia.
2. All aspects of care must be prioritized, giving high priority to life-saving or vital organ function-preserving measures and procedures.
3. Acute trauma care requires a team approach; constant coordination and communication among anesthesia, surgery, nursing, radiology, blood bank, and laboratory staff are essential.
4. A fully equipped and prepared operating room must be ready to receive an acute trauma victim at all times.
5. Traumatic shock or altered tissue oxygenation must be recognized and treated in the shortest possible time even when this requires mobilization of all available resources.
6. Appropriate precautions must be taken by all health care workers managing the acute trauma patient to avoid transmission of infectious diseases, especially acquired immunodeficiency syndrome, the incidence of which may be high in this patient population.
7. The condition of the major trauma patient changes rapidly from one moment to the next. It must be evaluated constantly by observation and use of appropriate monitoring techniques during the perioperative period.
8. Rapid administration of blood and fluids may be performed when necessary with appropriate infusion pumps, low-resistance tubing, fluid-warming devices, and large-diameter intravenous cannulas.
9. Selection of monitoring techniques in addition to those routinely used—ECG, arterial blood pressure, body temperature, urine output, inspired $O_2$ concentration, auscultation of breath and heart sounds, end-tidal $CO_2$, and pulse oximetry—must be based on their degree of priority among other diagnostic and therapeutic requirements, the type and severity of injury, any physiological disturbances, and careful estimation of risk and benefit. Direct intra-arterial pressure monitoring should be used in all major trauma victims since it is easy to establish, is not time consuming, provides

valuable information, and is not associated with significant risk.

10. Full stomach, anatomical variations of the airway, hypovolemia, the presence of atherosclerotic coronary and cerebrovascular diseases, and head injury must be given consideration during planning of airway management strategy for the major trauma victim.
11. Ketamine, although considered the anesthetic of choice for induction of anesthesia in the hypovolemic trauma victim, is by no means a substitute for preinduction blood volume restoration. The key to prevention of hypotension or cardiac arrest in the hypovolemic trauma victim is effective restoration of blood volume and administration of intravenous anesthetics at reduced doses and slow rates. In the severely hypovolemic trauma victim, airway management may need to be performed without anesthetics or with small doses of narcotics. A high incidence of recall in survivors following this technique is a small price compared with the potential complications associated with administration of anesthetics. Furthermore, recall may be prevented by administering scopolamine prior to airway intervention.
12. Intraoperative management of the trauma victim involves monitoring, diagnosis of unrecognized injuries or newly emerging complications, resuscitation and treatment, and administration of anesthetic agents. The common goal in each of these tasks is to preserve organ function by optimizing oxygen delivery to and oxygen utilization of tissues. These efforts must be extended into the postoperative period if a successful outcome for the major trauma victim is anticipated.

## REFERENCES


1. Abbott TR. Changes in serum calcium fractions and citrate concentrations during massive blood transfusions and cardiopulmonary bypass. Br J Anaesth 1983;55:753.
2. Abdul-Rasool IH, Sears DH, Katz RL. The effect of a second dose of succinylcholine on cardiac rate and rhythm following induction of anesthesia with etomidate or midazolam. Anesthesiology 1987;67:795.
3. Abraham E, Fink S. Cardiorespiratory and conjunctival oxygen tension monitoring during resuscitation from hemorrhage. Crit Care Med 1986;14:1004.
4. Abraham E, Shapiro M, Podolsky S. Central venous catheterization in the emergency setting. Crit Care Med 1983;11:515.
5. Abraham E, Smith M, Silver L. Continuous monitoring of critically ill patients with transcutaneous oxygen and carbon dioxide and conjunctival oxygen sensors. Ann Emerg Med 1984;13:1021.
6. Accident Facts. Chicago: National Safety Council, 1988:26.
7. Adams P, Gelman S, Reves JG, et al. Midazolam pharmacodynamics and pharmacokinetics during acute hypovolemia. Anesthesiology 1985;63:140.
8. Adams RC, Gray HK. Intravenous anesthesia with pentothal sodium in the case of gunshot wound associated with accompanying severe traumatic shock and loss of blood: report of a case. Anesthesiology 1943;4:70.
9. Aeder MI, Crowe JP, Rhodes RS, et al. Technical limitations in the rapid infusion of intravenous fluids. Ann Emerg Med 1985;14:307.
10. Al-Abrak MH. Diazepam and intraocular pressure. Br J Anaesth 1978;50:866.
11. Aldrete JA, Marron GM, Wright AJ. The first administration of anesthesia in military surgery: on occasion of the Mexican-American War. Anesthesiology 1984;61:585.
12. Andree RA. Sudden death following naloxone administration. Anesth Analg 1980;59:782.
13. Andritsch RF, Muravchick S, Gold MI. Temperature correction of arterial blood gas parameters: a comparative review of methodology. Anesthesiology 1981;55:311.
14. Ausinsch B, Rayborn RZ, Munsen ES, Levy NS. Ketamine and intraocular pressure in children. Anesth Analg 1976;55:773.
15. Azar I. The response of patients with neuromuscular disorders to muscle relaxants: a review. Anesthesiology 1984;61:173.
16. Azar I, Turndorf H. Severe hypertension and multiple atrial premature contractions following naloxone administration. Anesth Analg 1979;58:524.
17. Babinski MF, Albin M, Smith RB. Effects of high frequency ventilation on ICP. Crit Care Med 1981;9:159.
18. Badrinath SK, Vazeery A, McCarthy RJ, Ivankovich AD. The effect of different methods of inducing anesthesia on intraocular pressure. Anesthesiology 1986;65:431.
19. Baele PL, McMichan JC, Marsh HM, et al. Continuous monitoring of mixed venous oxygen saturation in critically ill patients. Anesth Analg 1982;61:513.
20. Bailey PL, Andriano KP, Goldman M, et al. Variability of the respiratory response to diazepam. Anesthesiology 1986;64:460.
21. Bailey PL, Wilbrink J, Zwanikken P, et al. Anesthetic induction with fentanyl. Anesth Analg 1985;64:48.
22. Baker JL, Kelen GD, Sivertson KJ, Quinn TC. Unsuspected human immunodeficiency virus in critically ill emergency patients. JAMA 1987;257:2609.
23. Baker SP, O'Neill B, Haddon W, Long WB. The injury severity score: a method for describing patients with multiple injuries and evaluating emergency care. J Trauma 1974;14:187.
24. Baker SP, O'Neill B, Karpf RS. Introduction to motor vehicle crashes. In: Baker SP, O'Neill B, Karpf RS, eds. Injury Fact Book. Lexington, Mass: Lexington Books, 1984:195.
25. Balasaraswathi K, Kumar P, Rao T, El-Etr A. Left ventricular end-diastolic pressure (LVEDP) as an index for nitrous oxide use during coronary artery surgery. Anesthesiology 1981;55:708.
26. Balfors E, Haggmark S, Nyhman H, et al. Droperidol inhibits effects of intravenous ketamine on central hemodynamics and myocardial oxygen consumption in patients with generalized atherosclerotic disease. Anesth Analg 1983;62:193.
27. Baraka A. Antagonism of succinylcholine-induced contracture of denervated muscles by D-tubocurarine. Anesth Analg 1981;60:605.
28. Baraka A. Suxamethonium-induced muscle contracture following traumatic denervation in man. Br J Anaesth 1978;50:195.
29. Baraka A, Haddad C, Afifi A, Baroody M. Control of succinylcholine-induced myotonia by D-tubocurarine. Anesthesiology 1970;33:669.
30. Barbieri LT, Kaplan JA. Artifactual hypotension secondary to intraoperative transducer failure. Anesth Analg 1983;62:112.
31. Barker SJ, Tremper KK. The effect of carbon monoxide inhalation on pulse oximetry and transcutaneous $Po_2$. Anesthesiology 1987;66:677.
32. Barker SJ, Tremper KK, Gamel DM. A clinical comparison of transcutaneous $Po_2$ and pulse oximetry in the operating room. Anesth Analg 1986;65:805.
33. Barker SJ, Tremper KK, Heitzmann HA, et al. A clinical study of fiberoptic arterial oxygen tension. Crit Care Med 1987;15:403 (abstr).
34. Barker SJ, Tremper KK, Hyatt J, et al. Continuous fiberoptic

arterial oxygen tension measurements in dogs. J Clin Monit 1987;3:48.

35. Barr AM, Thornley BA. Thiopental and suxamethonium crash induction: an assessment of the potential hazards. Anaesthesia 1976;31:23.
36. Bartkowski RR, McDonnell TE. Alfentanil as an anesthetic induction agent: a comparison with thiopental-lidocaine. Anesth Analg 1984;63:330.
37. Basta SJ, Ali HH, Savarese JJ, et al. Clinical pharmacology of atracurium besylate (BW33A): a new nondepolarizing muscle relaxant. Anesth Analg 1982;61:723.

37a. Baumgarten RK, Carter CE, Reynolds WJ, et al. Priming with nondepolarizing relaxants for rapid tracheal intubation: a double-blind evaluation. Can J Anaesth 1988;35:5.

38. Bay J, Nunn JF, Prys-Roberts C. Factors influencing arterial $Po_2$ during recovery from anesthesia. Br J Anaesth 1968;40:398.
39. Bazaral MG, Norfleet EA. Comparison of $CB_5$ and $V_5$ leads for intraoperative electrocardiographic monitoring. Anesth Analg 1981;60:849.
40. Bedford RF. Long-term radial artery cannulation: effects on subsequent vessel function. Crit Care Med 1978;6:64.
41. Bedford RF, Wollman H. Complications of percutaneous radial artery cannulation: an objective prospective study in man. Anesthesiology 1973;38:228.
42. Beemer GH. Continuous infusion of muscle relaxants: why and how. Anaesth Intensive Care 1987;15:83.
43. Belsey R, Morrison JI, Whitlow KJ, et al. Managing bedside glucose testing in the hospital. JAMA 1987;258:1634.
44. Benthuysen JL, Smith NT, Sanford TJ. Physiology of alfentanil-induced rigidity. Anesthesiology 1986;64:440.
45. Benumof JL, Trousdale FR, Alfery DD, Ozaki GT. Large catheter sheath introducers and their side port functional gauge. Anesth Analg 1981;60:216.
46. Benzinger M. Tympanic thermometry in surgery and anesthesia. JAMA 1969;209:1207.
47. Bernstein DP. A new stroke volume equation for thoracic electrical bioimpedance: theory and rationale. Crit Care Med 1986;14:904.
48. Bernstein DP. Continuous real-time monitoring of stroke volume and cardiac output by thoracic electrical bioimpedance. Crit Care Med 1986;14:898.
49. Bersin R, Chatterjee K, Arieff AI. Metabolic and systemic effects of bicarbonate in hypoxic patients with heart failure. Kidney Int 1986;29:180.
50. Bingham RM, Hinds CJ. Influence of bolus doses of phenoperidine on intracranial pressure and systemic arterial pressure in traumatic coma. Br J Anaesth 1987;59:592.
51. Birch AA, Mitchell GD, Playford GA, Lang CA. Changes in serum potassium response to succinylcholine following trauma. JAMA 1960;210:490.
52. Blaisdell FW. General assessment, resuscitation, and exploration of penetrating and blunt abdominal trauma. In: Blaisdell FW, Trunkey DD, eds. Trauma management, vol. 1: abdominal trauma. New York: Thieme-Stratton, 1982:1.
53. Blaise GA, McMichan JC, Nugent M, Hollier LH. Nalbuphine produces side effects while reversing narcotic-induced respiratory depression. Anesth Analg 1986;65:S19.
54. Blitt CD. Invasive intraoperative hemodynamic monitoring. ASA Refresher Courses in Anesthesiology 1984;12:33.
55. Blitt CK, Carlson GL, Rolling GD, et al. A comparative evaluation of pretreatment with nondepolarizing neuromuscular blockers prior to the administration of succinylcholine. Anesthesiology 1981;55:687.
56. Blumberg N, Bove JR. Uncrossmatched blood for emergency transfusion. JAMA 1978;240:2057.
57. Boelhouwer RU, Bruining HA, Ong GL. Correlations of serum potassium fluctuations with body temperature after major surgery. Crit Care Med 1987;15:310.
58. Bogetz MS, Katz JA. Recall of surgery for major trauma. Anesthesiology 1984;61:6.
59. Bogetz MS, Weiskopf RB. Cardiovascular effects of the volatile anesthetics during hypovolemia. Anesthesiology 1984;61:A51.
60. Bond AC, Davies CK. Ketamine and pancuronium for the shocked patient. Anaesthesia 1974;29:59.
61. Bone JR. Regional nerve block anesthesia. Anesthesiology 1945;6:612.
62. Bonica JJ, Kennedy WF, Akamatsu TJ, Gerbershagen HU. Circulatory effects of peridural block, III: effects of acute blood loss. Anesthesiology 1972;36:219.
63. Booij LHDJ. Pitfalls in anaesthesia for multiply injured patients. Injury 1982;14:81.
64. Bourke DL. Intraoperative heat conservation using a reflective blanket. Anesthesiology 1984;60:151.
65. Bowdle TA. Myoclonus following sufentanil without EEG seizure activity. Anesthesiology 1987;67:593.
66. Bowdle TA, Greichen SL, Bjurstrom RL, Schoene RB. Butorphanol improves $CO_2$ response and ventilation after fentanyl anesthesia. Anesth Analg 1987;66:517.
67. Boyd DR. Comprehensive regional trauma and emergency medical service delivery systems: goal of the 1980s. Crit Care Q 1982;5:1.
68. Bratanow N, Polk K, Bland R, et al. Continuous polarographic monitoring of intra-arterial oxygen in the perioperative period. Crit Care Med 1986;13:859.
69. Braunstein AH, Oberman HA. Transfusion of plasma components. Transfusion 1984;24:281.
70. Bready LL, Orr MD, Mote MA. Drug security for emergency surgical procedures. Anesthesiology 1985;63:225.
71. Broadman LM, Mesrobian RB, McGill WA. Regional versus general anesthesia: a survey of anesthesiologist's personal preference. Anesth Analg 1987;66:S20.
72. Brooks DB, Paulus DA, Winkle WE. Infrared heat lamps interfere with pulse oximeters. Anesthesiology 1984;61:630.
73. Brotman S, Browner BD, Cox EF. MAST trousers improperly applied causing a compartment syndrome in lower extremity trauma. J Trauma 1982;22:598.
74. Brown BR, Crout JR. The sympathomimetic effect of gallamine on the heart. J Pharmacol Exp Ther 1970;172:266.
75. Brown DL, Schulz J, Kirby RR. Modification of a critical care ventilator for anesthesia use. Crit Care Med 1987;15:1055.
76. Brown EM, Kristinaprasadi D, Smilen BG. Pancuronium for rapid induction technique for tracheal intubation. Can Anaesth Soc J 1979;26:489.
77. Bunegin L, Smith RB, Sjöstrand UH, et al. Regional organ blood flow during high frequency positive pressure ventilation (HFPPV) and intermittent positive pressure ventilation (IPPV). Anesthesiology 1984;61:416.
78. Buzello W, Schluerman D, Schindler M, Spillner G. Hypothermic cardiopulmonary bypass and neuromuscular blockade by pancuronium and vecuronium. Anesthesiology 1985;62:201.
79. Cahalan MK, Litt L, Botvinick EH, Schiller NB. Advances in noninvasive cardiovascular imaging: implications for the anesthesiologist. Anesthesiology 1987;66:356.
80. Cahill GF, Arky RA, Perlman AJ. Diabetes mellitus. In: Rubenstein E, Federman DD, eds Scientific american medicine: metabolism, section 9. New York: Scientific American Inc, 1987:8.
81. Cales RH, Trunkey DD. Preventable trauma deaths: a review of trauma care systems development. JAMA 1985;254:1059.
82. Calverley RK, Smith NT, Prys-Roberts C. Cardiovascular effects of enflurane anesthesia during controlled ventilation in man. Anesth Analg 1978;57:619.

83. Capan LM, Ramanathan S, Sinha K, Turndorf H. Arterial to end-tidal $CO_2$ gradients during spontaneous breathing, intermittent positive-pressure ventilation and jet ventilation. Crit Care Med 1985;13:810.
84. Caplan RA, Long MC. Prolonged anesthesia: management and sequelae of a two-day general anesthetic. Anesth Analg 1984;63:353.
85. Carli F, Itiaba K. Effect of heat conservation during and after major abdominal surgery on muscle protein breakdown in elderly patients. Br J Anaesth 1986;58:502.
86. Carnie JC, Street MK, Kumar B. Emergency intubation of the trachea facilitated by suxamethonium: observations in obstetric and general surgical patients. Br J Anaesth 1986;58:498.
87. Chang VD, Drucker WR. Management of diabetes mellitus in surgery and trauma. In: Siegel JH, ed. Trauma, emergency surgery and critical care. New York: Churchill Livingstone, 1987:753.
88. Chasapakis G, Kekis N, Sakkalis C, Kolios D. Use of ketamine and pancuronium for anesthesia for patients in hemorhagic shock. Anesth Analg 1973;52:282.
89. Chiu GJ, Stirt JA. Intraocular pressure after "crash" induction with vecuronium or atracurium plus low-dose narcotics. Anesth Analg 1987;66:S28.
90. Chraemmer-Jørgensen B, Høilund-Carlsen PF, Marving J, Christensen V. Lack of effect of intravenous lidocaine on hemodynamic responses to rapid sequence induction of general anesthesia: a double-blind controlled clinical trial. Anesth Analg 1986;65:1037.
91. Chraemmer-Jørgensen B, Høilund-Carlsen PF, Marving J, Christensen V. Left ventricular ejection fraction during anaesthetic induction: comparison of rapid sequence and elective induction. Can Anaesth Soc J 1986;33:754.
92. Claybon LE, Hirsh RA. Meperidine arrests postanesthesia shivering. Anesthesiology 1980;53:S180.
93. Clements FM, deBruijn NP. Perioperative evaluation of regional wall motion by transesophageal two-dimensional echocardiography. Anesth Analg 1987;66:249.
94. Clement FW, Elder CK. Observations on wartime anesthesia. Anesthesiology 1943;4:516.
95. Cockshott ID. Propofol ("Diprivan") pharmacokinetics and metabolism: an overview. Postgrad Med J 1985;61(suppl 3):45.
96. Cole WHJ, Moreton RR. A comparison between pancuronium and tubocurarine administration in injured men. Anesth Analg 1974;53:645.
97. Colvin MP, Savage TM, Newland PE. Cardiorespiratory changes following induction of anaesthesia with etomidate in patients with cardiac disease. Br J Anaesth 1979;51:551.
98. Consenus Conference. Platelet transfusion therapy. JAMA 1987;257:1777.
99. Conway CM, Ellis DB. The haemodynamic effects of short-acting barbiturates: a review. Br J Anaesth 1969;41:534.
100. Cook WP, Schultetus RR, Caton D. A comparison of D-tubocurarine pretreatment and no pretreatment in obstetric patients. Anesth Analg 1987;66:756.
101. Coombs DW, Hooper D, Pageau M. Emergency cimetidine prophylaxis against acid aspiration. Ann Emerg Med 1982; 11:252.
102. Coonan TJ, Hope CE. Cardiorespiratory effects of change of body position. Can Anaesth Soc J 1983;30:424.
103. Cork RC, Vaughan RW, Humphrey LS. Precision and accuracy of intraoperative temperature monitoring. Anesth Analg 1983;62:211.
104. Cork RC, Weiss JL, Hameroff S, Bentley J. Fentanyl preloading for rapid sequence induction of anesthesia. Anesth Analg 1984;63:60.
105. Corssen G, Gutierrez J, Reves JG, Huber FC Jr. Ketamine in the anesthetic management of asthmatic patients. Anesth Analg 1972;51:588.
106. Corssen G, Hoy JE. A new parenteral anesthetic CI 581: its effect on intraocular pressure. J Pediatr Ophthalmol 1967;4:20.
107. Costarino AT, Davis DA, Keon TP. Falsely normal saturation reading with the pulse oximeter. Anesthesiology 1987;67:830.
108. Coté CJ, Drop L, Daniels AL, Hoaglin DC. Calcium chloride versus calcium gluconate: comparison of ionization and cardiovascular effects in children and dogs. Anesthesiology 1987; 66:465.
109. Cotev S, Shalit MN. Effects of diazepam on cerebral blood flow and oxygen uptake after head injury. Anesthesiology 1975; 43:117.
110. Courington FW, Calverley RK. Anesthesia on the western front: the Anglo-American experience of World War I. Anesthesiology 1986;65:642.
111. Cowgill LD, Campbell DN, Clarke DR. Ventricular septal defect due to nonpenetrating chest trauma: use of the intraaortic balloon pump. J Trauma 1987;27:1088.
112. Coyle JP, Teplick RS, Long MC, Davison K. Respiratory variations in systemic arterial pressure as an indicator of volume status. Anesthesiology 1983;59:A53.
113. Crawford DC, Fell D, Achola KJ, Smith G. Effects of alfentanil on the pressor and catecholamine responses to tracheal intubation. Br J Anaesth 1987;59:707.
114. Criado A, Moseda S, Navarro E, et al. Induction of anesthesia with etomidate: hemodynamic study of 36 patients. Br J Anaesth 1980;52:803.
115. Criado A, Reig E, Aruas M, et al. Accidental diagnosis and resuscitation in a case of cardiac tamponade caused by central transvenous catheter. Crit Care Med 1981;9:349.
116. Cromartie RS. Rapid anesthesia induction in combat casualties with full stomachs. Anesth Analg 1976;55:74.
117. Cucchiara R. A simple technique to minimize tracheal aspiration. Anesth Analg 1976;55:816.
118. Cullen DJ. The effect of pretreatment with nondepolarizing muscle relaxants on the neuromuscular blocking action of succinylcholine. Anesthesiology 1971;35:572.
119. Cullen PM, Turtle M, Prys-Roberts C, et al. Effect of propofol anesthesia on baroreflex activity in humans. Anesth Analg 1987;66:1115.
120. Cummings GC, Dixon J, Kay NH, et al. Dose requirements of ICI 35, 868 (propofol, "Diprivan") in a new formulation for induction of anesthesia. Anaesthesia 1984;39:1168.
121. Cunningham AJ, Albert O, Cameron J, Watson AG. The effect of intravenous diazepam on rise of intraocular pressure following succinylcholine. Can Anaesth Soc J 1981;28:591.
122. Cunningham AJ, Barry P. Intraocular pressure physiology and implications for anaesthetic management. Can Anaesth Soc J 1986;33:195.
123. Dammann HG, Müller P, Simon B. Parenteral ranitidine: onset and duration of action. Br J Anaesth 1982;54:1235.
124. Davies JAH, Howells TH. Management of anaesthesia for the full stomach case in the casualty department. Postgrad Med J 1973; (July suppl):58.
125. Davis DA. Anesthesia in the world wars: historical vignettes of modern anesthesia. Philadelphia: FA Davis, 1968:18.
126. Dechène JP, Destrosiers R. Diazepam in pulmonary surgery. Can Anaesth Soc J 1969;16:162.
127. Desmarteau JK, Cassot AL. Acute pulmonary edema resulting from nalbuphine reversal of fentanyl-induced respiratory depression. Anesthesiology 1986;65:237.
128. Diaz FA, Biano JA, Bello A, et al. Effects of ketamine on canine cardiovascular function. Br J Anaesth 1976;48:941.
129. Dietzel W, Massion WH. The prophylactic effect of Innovar in experimental hemorrhagic shock. Anesth Analg 1969;48:968.

130. Dischinger PC, Shanker BS, Kochesfahani D, et al. Automotive collisions involving serious injury or death: an analysis of trends over time (1980–1983) in Maryland. Proceedings of the 29th annual meeting of American Association for Automotive Medicine. 1985:287.
131. Dobb G, Jordan MJ, Williams JG. Cimetidine in the prevention of the pulmonary acid aspiration (Mendelson's) syndrome. Br J Anaesth 1979;51:967.
132. Doenicke A, Lorenz W, Bregl R, et al. Histamine release after intravenous application of short acting hypnotics: a comparison of etomidate, althesin and propanidid. Br J Anaesth 1973;45:1097.
133. Donen N, Twee A, Dashfsky S, Guttormson B. The esophageal obturator airway: an appraisal. Can Anaesth Soc J 1983;30:194.
134. Donlon JV Jr. Anesthesia for eye, ear, nose and throat. In Miller RD, ed. Anesthesia. 2nd. ed. New York: Churchill Livingstone, 1986:1837.
135. Dresser LP, McKinney WM. Anatomic and pathophysiologic studies of the human internal jugular valve. Am J Surg 1987;154:220.
136. Drummond JC, Todd MM, Toutant SM, Shapiro HM. Brain surface protrusion during enflurane, halothane and isoflurane in cats. Anesthesiology 1983;59:288.
137. Dula DJ, Muller HA, Donovan JW. Flow rate variance of commonly used iv infusion techniques. J Trauma 1981;21:480.
138. Duncan GW, Sarnoff SF, Rhode CM. Studies on the effects of posture in shock and injury. Ann Surg 1944;120:24.
138a. Dutky PA, Stevens SL, Maull KI. Factors affecting rapid fluid resuscitation with large-bore introducer catheters. J Trauma 1989;29:856.
139. Eagar BM, Flynn PJ, Hughes R. Infusion of atracurium for long surgical procedures. Br J Anaesth 1984;56:447.
140. Ebert J, Patel K, Gelman S, McElvein RB. The hemodynamic response to ketamine in patients with pericardial tamponade. Anesthesiology 1982;57:A28.
141. Eckstein JW, Hamilton WK, McCammond JM. The effect of thiopental on peripheral venous tone. Anesthesiology 1961;22:525.
142. Eger EI II, Saidman LJ. Hazards of nitrous oxide anesthesia in bowel obstruction and pneumothorax. Anesthesiology 1965;26:61.
143. Eger EI II, Smith NT, Cullen DJ, et al. A comparison of the cardiovascular effects of halothane, fluroxene, ether and cyclopropane in man: a resumé. Anesthesiology 1971;34:25.
144. Eisele JH. New ideas for anesthetic management of trauma. Presented in Anesthesia update. San Diego, Calif: University of California, 1986.
145. Eisele JH, Reitan JA, Massumi RA, et al. Myocardial performance and $N_2O$ analgesia in coronary artery disease. Anesthesiology 1976;44:16.
146. Eisele JH, Smith NT. Cardiovascular effects of 40 percent nitrous oxide in man. Anesth Analg 1972;51:956.
147. Eisenach JC, Nugent M, Miller FA, Mucha P. Echocardiographic evaluation of patients with blunt chest injury: correlation with perioperative hypotension. Anesthesiology 1986;64:364.
148. Elliot GG, Zimmerman GA, Clemmen TP. Complications of pulmonary artery catheterization in the care of critically ill patients. Chest 1979;76:647.
149. Ellis R, Berberich JJ, Ettigi P, et al. Adrenocortical function following multiple anesthesia inductions with etomidate. Anesthesiology 1985;63:571.
150. Ellis FR, Halsall PJ. Suxamethonium spasm: a differential diagnostic conundrum. Br J Anaesth 1984;56:381.
151. Ersoz CJ, Hedden M, Lain L. Prolonged femoral arterial catheterization for intensive care. Anesth Analg 1970;49:160.
152. Eversole WJ, Kleinberg W, Overmann RR, et al. Nervous factors in shock induced muscle trauma in normal dogs. Am J Physiol 1944;140:490.
153. Fahmy NR, Alkhouli HM, Melford I, et al. Hemodynamics, histamine release and plasma catecholamines following induction with Diprivan or thiopental. Anesthesiology 1986; 65:A360.
154. Faist E, Baue AE, Dittmer H, Heberer G. Multiple organ system failure in polytrauma patients. J Trauma 1983;23:775.
155. Falk RH, Zoll PM, Zoll R. Safety and efficacy of cardiac pacing: a preliminary report. N Engl J Med 1983;309:1166.
156. Fanning GL. The efficacy of cricoid pressure in preventing regurgitation of gastric contents. Anesthesiology 1970;32:553.
157. Feigal DW, Blaisdell FW. The estimation of surgical risk. Med Clin North Am 1979;63:1131.
158. Feldman SA. Vecuronium: a variable dose technique. Anaesthesia 1987;42:199.
159. Feliciano DV, Mattox KL, Graham JM, et al. Major complications of percutaneous subclavian vein catheters. Am J Surg 1979;138:869.
160. Ferres CJ, Carson IW, Lyons SM, et al. Haemodynamic effects of vecuronium, pancuronium and atracurium in patients with coronary artery disease. Br J Anaesth 1987;59:305.
161. Fieldman EJ, Ridley RW, Wood EH. Hemodynamic studies during thiopental sodium and nitrous oxide anesthesia in humans. Anesthesiology 1955;16:473.
162. Fisher DM, Canfell PC, Fahey MR, et al. Elimination of atracurium in humans: contribution of Hofmann elimination and ester hydrolysis versus organ-based elimination. Anesthesiology 1986;65:6.
163. Fitch W, Barker J, Jennett WB, McDowall DG. The influence of neuroleptanalgesic drugs on cerebrospinal fluid pressure. Br J Anaesth 1969;41:800.
164. Flacke JW, Bloor BC, Kripke BJ, et al. Comparison of morphine, meperidine, fentanyl, and sufentanil in balanced anesthesia: a double-blind study. Anesth Analg 1985;64:897.
165. Flacke JW, Davis LJ, Flacke WE, et al. Effects of fentanyl and diazepam in dogs deprived of autonomic tone. Anesth Analg 1985;64:1053.
166. Flacke JW, Flacke WE. Inadvertent hypothermia: frequent, insidious, and often serious. Semin Anesth 1983;11:183.
167. Flacke JW, Flacke WE, Bloor BC, et al. Histamine release by four narcotics: a double-blind study in humans. Anesth Analg 1987;66:723.
168. Flacke JW, Flacke WE, Williams GD. Acute pulmonary edema following naloxone reversal of high dose morphine anesthesia. Anesthesiology 1978;47:376.
169. Flancbaum L, Wright J, Siegel JH. Emergency surgery in patients with post-traumatic myocardial contusion. J Trauma 1986;26:795.
170. Flynn PJ, Hughes R, Walton B. Use of atracurium in cardiac surgery involving cardiopulmonary bypass with induced hypothermia. Br J Anaesth 1984;56:967.
171. Foldes F. Rapid tracheal intubation with nondepolarizing neuromuscular blocking drugs: the priming principle. Br J Anaesth 1984;56:663.
172. Foley RW, Harris LS, Pilcher DB. Abdominal injuries in automobile accidents: review of care of fatally injured patients. J Trauma 1977;17:611.
173. Forbes RB, Choi WW, Mehta MP, et al. Cardiovascular effects of BW B1090U during nitrous oxide-oxygen-narcotic anesthesia. Anesthesiology 1987;67:A360.
174. Fortune JB, Feustel PJ, Saifi J. Influence of hematocrit on cardiopulmonary function after acute hemorrhage. J Trauma 1987;27:243.
175. Fowkes FGR, Lunn JN, Farrow SC, et al. Epidemiology in anes-

thesia, III: mortality risk in patients with coexisting physical disease. Br J Anaesth 1982;54:819.
176. Fragen RJ, Caldwell N. Comparison of a new formulation of etomidate with thiopental: side effects and awakening times. Anesthesiology 1979;50:242.
177. Fragen RJ, Caldwell N, Brunner E. Clinical use of etomidate for anesthesia induction: a preliminary report. Anesth Analg 1976;55:730.
178. Fragen RJ, Shanks CA, Molteni A, Avram M. Effects of etomidate on hormonal responses to surgical stress. Anesthesiology 1984;61:652.
179. Fragen RJ, Weiss HW, Molteni A. The effect of propofol on adrenocortical steroidogenesis: a comparative study with etomidate and thiopental. Anesthesiology 1987;66:839.
180. Frankville DD, Drummond JC. Hyperkalemia after succinylcholine administration in a patient with closed-head injury without paresis. Anesthesiology 1987;67:264.
181. Fried SJ, Satiani B, Zeeb P. Normothermic rapid volume replacement for hypovolemic shock: an in vivo and in vitro study utilizing a new technique. J Trauma 1986;26:183.
182. Friedman IM. Alcohol and unnatural deaths in San Francisco youths. Pediatrics 1985;76:191.
183. Frost EA. Effects of positive end-expiratory pressure on intracranial pressure and compliance in brain-injured patients. J Neurosurg 1977;47:195.
184. Funk DI, Crul JF, Van der Pol FM. Effects of changes in acid-base balance on neuromuscular blockade produced by ORG-NC 45. Acta Anaesthesiol Scand 1980;24:119.
185. Fusciardi J, Rouby JJ, Barakat T, et al. Hemodynamic effects of high-frequency jet ventilation in patients with and without circulatory shock. Anesthesiology 1986;65:485.
186. Gaffney FA, Bastian BC, Thal ER, et al. Passive leg raising does not produce a significant or sustained autotransfusion effect. J Trauma 1982;22:190.
187. Gal TJ, Difazio CA. Prolonged antagonism of opioid action with intravenous nalmefene in man. Anesthesiology 1986;64:175.
188. Gallagher TJ, Civetta JM, Kirby RR. Terminology update: optimal PEEP. Crit Care Med 1978;6:223.
189. Gambee AM, Hertzka RE, Fisher DM. Preoxygenation techniques: comparison of three minutes and four breaths. Anesth Analg 1987;66:468.
190. Gammage G. Crystalloid versus colloid: is colloid worth the cost? Int Anesthesiol Clin 1987;25:37.
191. Gargarian MA, Basta SJ, Savarese JJ, et al. The efficacy of atracurium by continuous infusion. Anesthesiology 1984;61:A291.
192. Gelman S, Reves JG, Harris D. Circulatory responses to midazolam anesthesia: emphasis on canine splanchnic circulation. Anesth Analg 1983;62:135.
193. Gerber MJ, Hines RL, Barash PG. Arterial wave-forms and systemic vascular resistance: is there a correlation? Anesthesiology 1987;66:823.
194. Gerner HR, Baker SP, Rutherford RB, et al. Evaluation of the management of vehicular fatalities secondary to abdominal injury. J Trauma 1972;12:425.
195. Gettinger A, DeTraglia MC, Glass DD. In vivo comparison of two mixed venous saturation catheters. Anesthesiology 1987;66:373.
196. Getzen LC, Pollack EW. Short-term femoral vein catheterization: a safe alternative for venous access? Am J Surg 1979;138:875.
197. Ghoneim MM, Yamada T. Etomidate: a clinical and electroencephalographic comparison with thiopental. Anesth Analg 1979;56:479.
198. Gillman MA. Haematological changes caused by nitrous oxide: cause for concern? Br J Anaesth 1987;59:143.
199. Gold MI, Duarte I, Muravchick S. Arterial oxygenation in conscious patients after 5 minutes and after 30 seconds of oxygen breathing. Anesth Analg 1981;60:313.
200. Gooding JM, Corssen G. Effect of etomidate on the cardiovascular system. Anesth Analg 1977;56:717.
201. Gooding JM, Corssen G. Etomidate: an ultrashortacting nonbarbiturate agent for anesthesia induction. Anesth Analg 1976;55:286.
202. Gould SA, Rosen AL, Sehgal LR. Polymerized pyridoxylated hemoglobin: efficacy as an $O_2$ carrier. J Trauma 1986;26:903.
203. Graf H, Leach W, Arieff AI. Evidence for a detrimental effect of bicarbonate therapy in hypoxic lactic acidosis. Science 1985;227:754.
204. Gramstad L, Lilleasen P. Dose-response relation for atracurium, org NC 45 and pancuronium. Br J Anaesth 1982;54:647.
205. Gravlee GP, Ramsey FM, Roy RC, et al. Rapid administration of a narcotic and neuromuscular blocker: a hemodynamic comparison of fentanyl, sufentanil, pancuronium, and vecuronium. Anesth Analg 1988;67:39.
206. Green DW, Bristow ASE, Fisher M. Comparison of I.V. glycopyrrolate and atropine in the prevention of bradycardia and arrhythmias following repeated doses of suxamethonium in children. Br J Anaesth 1984;56:981.
207. Greenan J. The cardio-oesophageal junction. Br J Anaesth 1961;33:432.
208. Gronert GA, Theye RA. Pathophysiology of hyperkalemia induced by succinylcholine. Anesthesiology 1975;43:89.
209. Gross JB, Smith L, Smith TC. Time course of ventilatory response to carbon dioxide after intravenous diazepam. Anesthesiology 1982;57:18.
210. Grummit RM, Goat VA. Intracranial pressure after phenoperidine. Anaesthesia 1984;39:565.
211. Gurman GM, Kriemerman S. Cannulation of big arteries in critically ill patients. Crit Care Med 1985;13:217.
212. Guyton AC. Circulatory shock and physiology of its treatment. In: Guyton AC, ed. Textbook of medical physiology. 6th ed. Philadelphia: WB Saunders, 1981:332.
213. Haigh JD, Nemoto EM, DeWolf AM, Bleyaert AL. Comparison of the effects of succinylcholine and atracurium on intracranial pressure in monkeys with intracranial hypertension. Can Anaesth Soc J 1986;33:421.
214. Hakstian RW, Hampson LG, Gurd FN. Pharmacologic agents in experimental hemorrhagic shock: a controlled comparison of treatment with hydralazine, hydrocortisone, and levarterenol. Arch Surg 1961;83:335.
215. Halford FJ. A critique of intravenous anesthesia in war surgery. Anesthesiology 1943;4:67.
216. Halonen P, Linko K, Myllyla G. A study of haemostasis following the use of high doses of hydroxyethyl starch 120 and dextran in major laparotomies. Acta Anaesthesiol Scand 1987;31:320.
217. Hanowell L, Eisele JH, Downs D. Ambient light affects pulse oximeters. Anesthesiology 1987;67:864.
218. Hansbrough JF, Cain TL, Millikan JS. Placement of 10-gauge catheter by cutdown for rapid fluid replacement. J Trauma 1983;23:231.
219. Hantler CB, Knight PR. Intracranial hypertension following cross-clamping of the thoracic aorta. Anesthesiology 1982;56:146.
220. Hewson JR, Neame PB, Kumar N, et al. Coagulopathy related to dilution and hypotension during massive transfusion. Crit Care Med 1985;13:387.
221. Hiatt JR, Tompkins RK. The importance of nonoperative trauma management in postgraduate surgical education. J Trauma 1987;27:769.
222. Hickey RF, Eger EI II. Circulatory pharmacology of inhaled anesthetics. In: Miller RD, ed. Anesthesia. New York: Churchill Livingstone, 1986:649.

223. Hoar PF, Wilson RM, Mangano DT, et al. Heparin bonding reduces thrombogenicity of pulmonary artery catheters. N Engl J Med 1981;305:993.
224. Hodge D III, Fleisher G. Pediatric catheter flow rates. Am J Emerg Med 1985;3:403.
225. Holdcroft A, Morgan M, Whitwar JG, Lumley J. Effect of dose and premedication on induction complications with etomidate. Br J Anaesth 1976;48:199.
226. Holder DA, Sniderman AD, Frazer G, Fallen EL. Experience with bretylium tosylate by a hospital cardiac arrest team. Circulation 1977;55:541.
227. Horan BF, Prys-Roberts C, Hamilton WK, Roberts JG. Haemodynamic responses to enflurane anaesthesia and hypovolemia in the dog, and their modification by propranolol. Br J Anaesth 1977;49:1189.
228. Horan BF, Prys-Roberts C, Roberts JG, et al. Haemodynamic responses to isoflurane anaesthesia and hypovolemia in the dog, and their modification by propranolol. Br J Anaesth 1977;49:1179.
229. Horrigan R, Moyers J, Johnson B: Etomidate vs. thiopental with and without fentanyl: a comparative study of awakening in man. Anesthesiology 1980;52:362.
230. Horst HM, Obeid FN, Sorensen VJ, Bivins BA. Factors influencing survival of elderly trauma patients. Crit Care Med 1986;14:681.
231. Huber FC, Reves JG, Gutierrez J, Corssen G. Ketamine: its effect on airway resistance in man. South Med J 1972;65:1176.
232. Hunter JM. Adverse effects of neuromuscular blocking drugs. Br J Anaesth 1987;59:46.
233. Hurst JM, Branson RD, DeHaven CB. The role of high-frequency ventilation in post-traumatic respiratory insufficiency. J Trauma 1987;27:236.
234. Hyde MR, Schmidt CA, Jacobson JG, et al. Impalement injuries to the thorax as a result of motor vehicle accidents. Ann Thorac Surg 1987;43:189.
235. Iberti TJ, Paluch TA, Helmer L, et al. The hemodynamic effects of intravenous cimetidine in intensive care unit patients: a double-blind, prospective study. Anesthesiology 1986;64:87.
236. Idvall J. Influence of ketamine anesthesia on cardiac output and tissue perfusion in rats subjected to hemorrhage. Anesthesiology 1981;55:297.
237. Idvall J, Ahlgren I, Aronsen KF, Stenberg P. Ketamine infusions: pharmacokinetics and clinical effects. Br J Anaesth 1979;51:1167.
238. Illner HP, Cunningham JN, Shires GT. Red blood cell sodium content and permeability changes in hemorrhagic shock. Am J Surg 1982;143:349.
239. Iserson KV, Criss E. Combined effect of catheter and tubing size on fluid flow. Am J Emerg Med 1986;4:238.
240. Jackson APF, Dhadphala PR, Callaghan ML, Aberi S. Haemodynamic studies during induction of anaesthesia for open-heart surgery using diazepam and ketamine. Br J Anaesth 1978; 50:375.
241. Jacobs LM, Hsich JW. A clinical review of autotransfusion and its role in trauma. JAMA 1984;251:3283.
242. Jardin F, Farcot JC, Gueret P, et al. Cyclic changes in arterial pulse during respiratory support. Circulation 1983;68:266.
243. Jenkins JG. Pretreatment and "crash" induction. Anesthesiology 1984;61:346.
244. Joachimsson PO, Hedstrand U, Tabow F, Hansson B. Prevention of intraoperative hypothermia during abdominal surgery. Acta Anaesthesiol Scand 1987;31:330.
245. Joyce JT, Roizen MF, Eger EI II. Effect of thiopental induction on sympathetic activity. Anesthesiology 1983;59:19.
246. Jurkovich GJ, Greiser WB, Luterman A, Curreri PW. Hypothermia in trauma victims: an ominous predictor of survival. J Trauma 1987;27:1019.
247. Kang Y, Lewis JH, Navalgund A, et al. Epsilon-aminocaproic acid for treatment of fibrinolysis during liver transplantation. Anesthesiology 1987;66:766.
248. Kang YG, Martin DJ, Marquez J, et al. Intraoperative changes in blood coagulation and thrombelastographic monitoring in liver transplantation. Anesth Analg 1985;64:888.
249. Kanto J, Klotz U. Intravenous benzodiazepines as anaesthetic agents: pharmacokinetics and clinical consequences. Acta Anaesthesiol Scand 1982;26:554.
250. Kaplan JA, King SB. The precordial electrocardiographic lead ($V_5$) in patients who have coronary-artery disease. Anesthesiology 1976;45:570.
251. Kaplan JA, Thys DM. The electrocardiogram and anesthesia. In: Miller RD, ed. Anesthesia. 2nd ed. New York: Churchill Livingstone, 1986:465.
252. Katz J. A survey of anesthetic choice among anesthesiologists. Anesth Analg 1973;52:373.
253. Kaufman RD. Relationship between esophageal temperature gradient and heart and lung sounds heard by esophageal stethoscope. Anesth Analg 1987;66:1046.
254. Kawamura R, Stanley T, English J, et al. Cardiovascular responses to nitrous oxide exposure for two hours in man. Anesth Analg 1980;59:93.
255. Kay NH, Uppington J, Sear JW, Allen MC. Use of emulsion of ICI 35868 (propofol) for the induction and maintenance of anaesthesia. Br J Anaesth 1985;57:736.
256. Kennedy WF, Bonica JJ, Akamatsu TJ, et al. Cardiovascular and respiratory effects of subarachnoid block in the presence of acute blood loss. Anesthesiology 1968;29:29.
257. Kessler MR, Eide T, Humayun B, Poppers PJ. Spurious pulse oximeter desaturation with methylene blue injection. Anesthesiology 1986;65:435.
258. Kissin I, McGee T, Smith LR. The indices of potency for intravenous anesthetics. Can Anaesth Soc J 1981;28:585.
259. Kleinman J, Marlar K, Silva DA, et al. Sufentanil attenuation of the stress response during rapid sequence induction. Anesthesiology 1985;63:A379.
260. Knight RJ. Flow rates through disposable intravenous cannulae. Lancet 1968;2:665.
261. Kondo K, O'Reilly LP, Chiota J. Air embolism associated with an introducer for pulmonary artery catheters. Anesth Analg 1984;63:871.
262. Konstadt S, Thys DM, Reich D, et al. A study of the hemodynamic effects of BW A938U: a new long acting nondepolarizing muscle relaxant. Anesthesiology 1987;167:A369.
263. Kopman AF, Wollman SB, Russ K, Surks SN. Awake endotracheal intubation: review of 267 cases. Anesth Analg 1975; 54:323.
264. Kortilla K, Tammisto T, Aromma U. Comparison of etomidate in combination with fentanyl or diazepam, with thiopentone as an induction agent for general anaesthesia. Br J Anaesth 1979;51:1151.
265. Kumar SM, Kothary SP, Zsigmond EK. Plasma free norepinephrine and epinephrine concentrations following diazepam-ketamine induction in patients undergoing cardiac surgery. Acta Anaesthesiol Scand 1978;22:593.
266. Lacoumenta S, Walsh ES, Waterman AE, et al. Effects of ketamine anaesthesia on the metabolic response to pelvic surgery. Br J Anaesth 1984;56:493.
267. Lake CL. Anesthesia and pericardial disease. Anesth Analg 1983;62:431.
268. Lanier WL, Milde JH, Michenfelder JD. Cerebral stimulation following succinylcholine in dogs. Anesthesiology 1986;64:551.

269. Latasch L, Probst S, Dudziak R. Reversal by nalbuphine of respiratory depression caused by fentanyl. Anesth Analg 1984; 63:814.
270. Leads from the MMWR. Changes in premature mortality: United States, 1984–1985. JAMA 1987;257:1161.
271. Leads from the MMWR. Recommendations for prevention of HIV transmission in health care settings. JAMA 1987;258:1293.
272. Lebowitz PW, Coté ME, Daniels AL, et al. Cardiovascular effects of midazolam and thiopentone for induction of anaesthesia in ill surgical patients. Can Anaesth Soc J 1983;30:19.
273. Lebowitz PW, Ramsey FM, Savarese JJ, Ali HH. Potentiation of neuromuscular blockade in man produced by combinations of pancuronium and metocurine or pancuronium and D-tubocurarine. Anesth Analg 1980;59:604.
274. Lebowitz PW, Ramsey FM, Savarese JJ, et al. Combination of pancuronium and metocurine: neuromuscular and hemodynamic advantages over pancuronium alone. Anesth Analg 1981;60:12.
275. Ledgerwood AM, Kazmers M, Lucas CE. The role of thoracic aortic occlusion for massive hemoperitoneum. J Trauma 1976;16:610.
276. Ledingham I, Finlay WEI, Watt I, McKee JI. Etomidate and adrenocortical function. Lancet 1983;1:1436.
277. Ledingham I, Watt I. Influence of sedation on mortality in critically ill multiple trauma patients. Lancet 1983;1:1270.
278. Lennon RL, Olson RA, Gronert GA. Atracurium or vecuronium for rapid sequence endotracheal intubation. Anesthesiology 1986;64:510.
279. L'Hommedieu CS, Arens JJ. The use of ketamine for the emergency intubation of patients with status asthmaticus. Ann Emerg Med 1987;16:568.
280. Libonati MM, Leahy JJ, Ellison N. The use of succinylcholine in open eye surgery. Anesthesiology 1985;62:637.
281. Lineberger AS, Sprague DH, Battaglini JW. Sinus arrest associated with cimetidine. Anesth Analg 1985;64:554.
282. Lippmann M, Appel PL, Mok MS, Shoemaker WC. Sequential cardiorespiratory patterns of anesthetic induction with ketamine in critically ill patients. Crit Care Med 1983;11:730.
283. Little RA, Stoner HB. Body temperature after accidental injury. Br J Surg 1981;68:221.
284. Longnecker DE. Failure of the peripheral circulation. In: Orkin FK, Cooperman LH, eds. Complications in anesthesiology. Philadelphia: JB Lippincott, 1983:225.
285. Longnecker DE, Ross DC, Silver IA. Anesthetic influence on arteriolar diameters and tissue oxygen tension in hemorrhaged rats. Anesthesiology 1982;57:177.
286. Longnecker DE, Sturgill BC. Influence of anesthetic agent on survival following hemorrhage. Anesthesiology 1976;45:516.
287. Luna GK, Maier RV, Pavlin EG, et al. Incidence and effect of hypothermia in seriously injured patients. J Trauma 1987; 27:1014.
288. Lunn JK, Stanley TH, Eisele J, et al. High dose fentanyl anesthesia for coronary artery surgery: plasma fentanyl concentrations and influence of nitrous oxide on cardiovascular responses. Anesth Analg 1979;58:390.
289. MacIntyre E, Mackie IJ, Ho D, et al. The haemostatic effects of hydroxyethyl starch (HES) used as a volume expander. Intensive Care Med 1985;11:300.
290. MacIntyre PE, Pavlin EG, Dwersteg JF. Effect of meperidine on oxygen consumption, carbon dioxide production, and respiratory gas exchange in postanesthesia shivering. Anesth Analg 1987;66:751.
291. MacKenzie CF, Shin B, Krishnaprasad D, et al. Assessment of cardiac and respiratory function during surgery on patients with acute quadriplegia. J Neurosurg 1985;62:843.
292. Macksood MJ, Setter M. Hydrothorax and hydromediastinum after use of an indwelling percutaneous catheter introducer. Crit Care Med 1983;11:957.
292a. Mangiante EC, Hoots AV, Fabian TC. The precutaneous common femoral vein catheter for volume replacement in critically injured patients. J Trauma 1988;1644.
293. Mankikar D, Ramanathan S, Rock I, Turndorf H. Hemodynamic effects of HFPPV and IPPV during acute hemorrhage. Anesthesiology 1982;57:A466.
294. Marchand P. A study of the forces productive of gastro-oesophageal regurgitation and herniation through the diaphragmatic hiatus. Thorax 1957;12:189.
295. Marchand P. The gastro-oesophageal "sphincter" and mechanism of regurgitation. Br J Surg 1955;42:504.
296. Mark JB, Steinbrook RA, Gugino LD. Continuous noninvasive monitoring of cardiac output with esophageal Doppler ultrasound during cardiac surgery. Anesth Analg 1986;65:1013.
297. Marty J, Gauzit R, Lefeure P, et al. Effects of diazepam and midazolam on baroreflex control of heart rate and on sympathetic activity in humans. Anesth Analg 1986;65:113.
298. Martyn J. Clinical pharmacology and drug therapy in the burned patient. Anesthesiology 1986;65:67.
299. Martyn JAJ, Goldhill DR, Goudsouzian NG. Clinical pharmacology of muscle relaxants in patients with burns. J Clin Pharmacol 1986;26:680.
300. Mateer JR, Thompson BM, Aprahamian C, et al. Rapid fluid resuscitation with central venous catheters. Ann Emerg Med 1983;12:149.
301. Mattila I, Takkunen O, Mattila P, et al. Cardiac tamponade and different modes of artificial ventilation. Acta Anaesthesiol Scand 1984;28:236.
302. Maull KI, Capehart JE, Cardea JA, Haynes BW. Limb loss following military anti-shock trousers (MAST) application. J Trauma 1981;21:60.
303. Mazze RI, Calverley RK, Smith NT. Inorganic fluoride nephrotoxicity: prolonged enflurane and halothane anesthesia in volunteers. Anesthesiology 1977;46:265.
304. Mazze RI, Escue HM, Houston JB. Hyperkalemia and cardiovascular collapse following administration of succinylcholine to the traumatized patient. Anesthesiology 1969;31:540.
305. McCammon RL, Hilgenberg JC, Stoelting RK. Hemodynamic effects of diazepam and diazepam-nitrous oxide in patients with coronary artery disease. Anesth Analg 1980;59:438.
306. McCollum JSC, Dundee JW. Comparison of induction characteristics of four intravenous anaesthetic agents. Anaesthesia 1986;41:995.
307. McDonnell TE, Bartkowski RR, Williams JJ. $ED_{50}$ of alfentanil for induction of anesthesia in unpremedicated young adults. Anesthesiology 1984;60:136.
308. McLeskey CH, McLeod DS, Hough TL, Stallworth JM. Prolonged asystole after succinylcholine administration. Anesthesiology 1978;49:208.
309. Michaelis LL, Hickey PR, Clark TA, Dixon WM. Ventricular irritability associated with the use of naloxone hydrochloride. Ann Thorac Surg 1974;18:608.
310. Mihm FG, Feeley TW, Rodarte A. Monitoring end-tidal carbon dioxide tensions with high frequency jet ventilation in dogs with normal lungs. Crit Care Med 1984;12:180.
311. Mihm F, Halperin B. Noninvasive detection of profound arterial desaturations using pulse oximetry device. Anesthesiology 1985;62:85.
312. Miller RD, Way WL. Inhibition of succinylcholine-induced increased intragastric pressure by nondepolarizing muscle relaxants and lidocaine. Anesthesiology 1971;34:185.
313. Millikan JS, Cain TL, Hansbrough J. Rapid volume replacement

for hypovolemic shock: a comparison of techniques and equipment. J Trauma 1984;24:428.
314. Millikan JS, Moore EE. Outcome of resuscitative thoracotomy and descending aortic occlusion in the operating room. J Trauma 1984;24:388.
315. Minton MD, Grosslight K, Stirt JA, Bedford RF. Increases in intracranial pressure from succinylcholine: prevention by prior nondepolarizing blockade. Anesthesiology 1986;65:165.
316. Misfeldt BB, Jörgensen PB, Spotoft H, Ronde F. The effects of droperidol and fentanyl on intracranial pressure and cerebral perfusion pressure in neurosurgical patients. Br J Anaesth 1976;48:963.
317. Mizock BA. Controversies in lactic acidosis: implications in critically ill patients. JAMA 1987;258:497.
318. Molbegott LP, Flashburg MH, Karasic L, Karlin BL. Probable seizures after sufentanil. Anesth Analg 1987;66:91.
319. Moldenhauer CC, Hug CC Jr. Use of narcotic analgesics as anaesthetics. Clin Anesth 1984;2:107.
320. Moldenhauer CC, Roach GW, Finlayson DC, et al. Nalbuphine antagonism of ventilatory depression following high-dose fentanyl anesthesia. Anesthesiology 1985;62:647.
321. Möller CT, Schoonbee CG, Rosendorff C. Haemodynamics of cardiac tamponade during various modes of ventilation. Br J Anaesth 1979;51:409.
322. Moon RE, Camporesi EM. Arterial $Po_2$ should be corrected for body temperature during hypothermia. Anesthesiology 1987; 67:A20.
323. Mori K, Iwabuchi K, Fujita M. The effects of depolarizing muscle relaxants on the electroencephalogram and the circulation during halothane anesthesia in man. Br J Anaesth 1973;45:604.
324. Morley-Forster PK. Unintentional hypothermia in the operating room. Can Anaesth Soc J 1986;33:516.
325. Morris RH. Operating room temperature and the anesthetized, paralyzed patient. Arch Surg 1971;102:95.
326. Morris RH, Kumar A. The effect of warming blankets on maintenance of body temperature of the anesthetized, paralyzed adult patient. Anesthesiology 1972;36:408.
327. Moss E, McDowell DG. ICP increases with 50% nitrous oxide in oxygen in severe head injuries during controlled ventilation. Br J Anaesth 1979;51:757.
328. Mulder DS, Shennib H, Angood P. Thoracic injuries. In: Maull KI, Cleveland HC, Strauch GO, Wolferth CC, eds. Advances in trauma. Chicago: Year Book Medical Publishers, 1986:193.
329. Munim A, Chodoff P. Traumatic acute mitral regurgitation secondary to blunt chest trauma. Crit Care Med 1983;11:311.
330. Muravchick S, Burkett L, Gold MI. Succinycholine-induced fasciculations and intragastric pressure during induction of anesthesia. Anesthesiology 1981;55:180.
331. Murphy DF. Anesthesia and intraocular pressure. Anesth Analg 1985;64:520.
332. Murray DJ, Mehta MP, Forbes R, et al. Cardiovascular and neuromuscular effects of BWA 938u: comparison with pancuronium. Anesthesiology 1987;67:A317.
333. Murray LB, MacMillan RW, Osler T, Olson JE. Diaphragmatic rupture due to blunt trauma: the case for timely intervention. NY State J Med 1987;87:512.
334. Musich J, Walts LF. Pulmonary aspiration after a priming dose of vecuronium. Anesthesiology 1986;64:517.
335. Nadeau S, Noble WH. Limitations of cardiac output measurements by thermodilution. Can Anaesth Soc J 1986;33:780.
336. Nadeau S, Tousignant M. Use of a urologic set for improved fluid administration rates. Can Anaesth Soc J 1985;32:283.
337. Naguib M, Hassan M, Farag H, et al. Cannulation of the radial and dorsalis pedis arteries. Br J Anaesth 1987;59:482.
338. Nana A, Cardan E, Domokos M. Blood catecholamine changes after pancuronium. Acta Anaesthesiol Scand 1973;17:83.
339. National Center for Health Statistics. Current estimates from the National Health Interview Survey, United States 1982. Vital and Health Statistics, series 10, no. 150. Washington, DC: US Government Printing Office, 1985. US Dept of Health and Human Services publication (PHS) 85-1578.
340. Nauta J, deLange S, Koopman D, et al. Anesthetic induction with alfentanil: a new short-acting narcotic analgesic. Anesth Analg 1982;61:267.
341. Nauta J, Stanley TH, deLange S, et al. Anaesthetic induction with alfentanil: comparison with thiopental, midazolam, and etomidate. Can Anaesth Soc J 1983;30:53.
342. Nelson LD, Civetta JM, Hudson-Civetta J. Titrating positive end-expiratory pressure therapy in patients with early, moderate hypoxemia. Crit Care Med 1987;15:14.
343. Nettles DC, Herrin TJ, Mullen JG. Ketamine induction in poor-risk patients. Anesth Analg 1973;52:59.
344. Nimmo WS. Inhalation of gastric contents. International Anesthesia Research Society Review Course Lectures. 1987:123.
345. Noeldge G, Hinsken H, Buzello W. Comparison between the continuous infusion of vecuronium and the intermittent administration of pancuronium and vecuronium. Br J Anaesth 1984;56:473.
346. Norman J. Neuromuscular blockade. In: Smith G, Aitkenhead AR, eds. Textbook of anaesthesia. Edinburgh: Churchill Livingstone, 1985:166.
347. Nunn JF. Clinical aspects of the interaction between nitrous oxide and vitamin $B_{12}$. Br J Anaesth 1987;59:3.
348. O'Donnell JM, Thompson DR, Layton TR. The effect of high-frequency jet ventilation on intracranial pressure in patients with closed-head injuries. J Trauma 1984;24:73.
349. Oh MA, Carroll HJ. The anion gap. N Engl J Med 1977;297:814.
350. Okamoto K, Komatsu T, Kumar V, et al. Effects of intermittent positive-pressure ventilation on cardiac output measurements by thermodilution. Crit Care Med 1986;14:977.
351. Olsson GL, Hallen B. Pharmacological evacuation of the stomach with metoclopramide. Acta Anaesthesiol Scan 1982;26:417.
352. Ordog GJ, Wasserberger J, Balasubramaniam S. Coagulation abnormalities in traumatic shock. Ann Emerg Med 1985; 14:650.
353. Oreskovich MR, Howard JD, Copass MK, Carrico CJ. Geriatric trauma: injury patterns and outcome. J Trauma 1984;24:566.
354. Ostergaard D, Engbaek J, Ording H, Viby-Mogensen J. A new infusion design for atracurium and vecuronium. Eur J Anaesth 1987;4:87.
355. O'Sullivan H, Jennings F, Ward K, et al. Human bone marrow biochemical function and megaloblastic hematopoiesis after nitrous oxide anesthesia. Anesthesiology 1981;55:645.
356. Partridge BL, Ward CF. Pulmonary edema following low dose naloxone administration. Anesthesiology 1986;65:709.
357. Patel C, Laboy V, Venus B, et al. Acute complications of pulmonary artery catheter insertion in critically ill patients. Crit Care Med 1986;14:195.
358. Patschke D, Bruckner SB, Eberlein HJ, et al. Effects of althesin, etomidate and fentanyl on haemodynamics and myocardial oxygen consumption in man. Can Anaesth Soc J 1977;24:57.
359. Pavlin EG. Anesthesia for the traumatized patient. Can Anaesth Soc J 1983;30:S27.
360. Pender JW, Lundy JS. Anesthesia in war surgery. War Med 1942;2:193.
361. Perel A, Pizov R, Cotev S. Systolic blood pressure variation is a sensitive indicator of hypovolemia in ventilated dogs subjected to graded hemorrhage. Anesthesiology 1987;76:498.
362. Peuler M, Glass DD, Arens JF. Ketamine and intraocular pressure. Anesthesiology 1975;43:575.
363. Phemister DB. Mechanism of surgical shock. JAMA 1945; 127:1109.

364. Philip BK, Philip JH. Avoiding air infusion with pressurized infusion systems: a new hazard (letter). Anesth Analg 1985; 64:377.
365. Philip JH, Philip BK. Pressurized infusion system for fluid resuscitation. Anesth Analg 1984;63:779.
366. Philip BK, Raemer DB, Philip JH. Large-volume fluid resuscitation: prediction of flow capability. Anesthesiology 1982; 57:A107.
367. Phirman JR, Shapiro HM. Modification of nitrous oxide induced intracranial hypertension by prior induction of anesthesia. Anesthesiology 1977;46:150.
368. Poole GV, Prough DS, Johnson JC. Effects of resuscitation from hemorrhagic shock on cerebral hemodynamics in the presence of an intracranial mass. J Trauma 1987;27:18.
369. Poulton TJ, Haldeman LW, Munson ES. Nitrous oxide administration in the presence of subcutaneous emphysema: an experimental model. Can Anaesth Soc J 1982;29:435.
370. Powell R, Miller RD. The effect of repeated doses of succinylcholine on serum potassium in patients with renal failure. Anesth Analg 1975;54:746.
371. Power SJ, Morgan M, Chakrabarti MK. Carbon dioxide response curves following midazolam and diazepam. Br J Anaesth 1983;55:837.
372. Pricolo VE, Burchard KW, Singh AK, et al. Trendelenburg versus PASG application: hemodynamic response in man. J Trauma 1986;26:718.
373. Prough DS, Johnson JC, Poole GV Jr, et al. Effects on intracranial pressure of resuscitation from hemorrhagic shock with hypertonic saline versus lactated Ringer's solution. Crit Care Med 1985;13:407.
374. Prough DS, Johnson JC, Stump DA, et al. Effects of hypertonic saline versus lactated Ringer's solution on cerebral oxygen transport during resuscitation from hemorrhagic shock. J Neurosurg 1986;64:627.
375. Prough DS, Roy R, Bumgarner J, Shannon G. Acute pulmonary edema in healthy teenagers following conservative doses of intravenous naloxone. Anesthesiology 1984;60:485.
376. Puri V, Carlson RW, Bauder JJ, Weil MH. Complications of vascular catheterization in the critically ill. Crit Care Med 1980;8:495.
377. Rafferty TD, Marrero O, Nardi D, et al. Relationship between transcutaneous and arterial carbon dioxide tension in adult patients anesthetized with nitrous oxide-fentanyl and nitrous oxide-enflurane. Anesth Analg 1982;60:504.
378. Rahn H, Reeves RB, Howell BJ. Hydrogen ion regulation, temperature and evolution. Am Rev Respir Dis 1975;112:165.
379. Rao S, Sherbaniuk RW, Prasad K, et al. Cardiopulmonary effects of diazepam. Clin Pharmacol Ther 1972;14:182.
380. Ream AK, Reitz BA, Silverberg G. Temperature correction of $PCO_2$ and pH in estimating acid-base status: an example of the emperor's new clothes? Anesthesiology 1982;56:41.
381. Reed RL, Ciavarella D, Heimbach DM, et al. Prophylactic platelet administration during massive transfusion: a prospective, randomized, double-blind clinical study. Ann Surg 1986;203:40.
382. Rembert FC. State of health at the time of injury. In: Giesecke AH, ed. Anesthesia for the surgery of trauma. Philadelphia: FA Davis, 1976:17.
383. Reves JG. Comparative pharmacology of intravenous anesthetic induction agents. International Anesthesia Research Society review course lectures, 1986:9.
384. Reves JG, Corssen G, Holcomb C. Comparison of two benzodiazepines for anesthesia induction: midazolam and diazepam. Can Anaesth Soc J 1978;25:211.
385. Reves JG, Fragen RJ, Vinik R, Greenblatt DJ. Midazolam: pharmacology and uses. Anesthesiology 1985;62:310.
386. Risberg B, Medegard A, Heideman M, et al. Early activation of humoral proteolytic systems in patients with multiple trauma. Crit Care Med 1986;14:917.
387. Riska EB, Myllynen P. Fat embolism in multiple injuries. J Trauma 1982;22:891.
388. Roberts JG, Foëx P, Clarke TNS, et al. Haemodynamic interactions of high-dose propranolol pretreatment and anesthesia in the dog, III: the effects of haemorrhage during halothane and trichloroethylene anaesthesia. Br J Anaesth 1976;48:411.
389. Rosa RM, Silva P, Young JB, et al. Adrenergic modulation of extrarenal potassium disposal. N Engl J Med 1980;302:431.
390. Rosenberg H. Trismus is not trivial. Anesthesiology 1987; 67:453.
391. Rosenberg H, Fletcher JE. Masseter muscle rigidity and malignant hyperthermia susceptibility. Anesth Analg 1986;65:161.
392. Rosenblatt R, Dennis P, Draper LD. A new method for massive fluid resuscitation in the trauma patient. Anesth Analg 1983;62:613.
393. Rosman EJ, Capan LM, Turndorf H. Another case of probable seizure after sufentanil. Anesth Analg 1987;66:922.
394. Rowe MI, Weinberg G. Transcutaneous oxygen monitoring in shock and resuscitation. J Pediatr Surg 1979;14:773.
395. Rubio JJ, Gilsanz F, Garcia-Sola R, et al. Effects of high-frequency jet ventilation on intracranial pressure and cerebral elastance in dogs. Crit Care Med 1987;15:602.
396. Russell JA, Joel M, Hudson RJ, et al. Prospective evaluation of radial and femoral artery catheterization sites in critically ill adults. Crit Care Med 1983;11:936.
397. Sage DJ, Close A, Boas RA. Reversal of midazolam sedation with anexate ($O 15-1788). Br J Anaesth 1987;59:459.
398. Samra SK. Halothane interference with transcutaneous oxygen monitoring: in vivo and in vitro. Crit Care Med 1983;11:612.
399. Samuelson PN, Reves JG, Kouchoukos NT, et al. Hemodynamic responses to anesthetic induction with midazolam or diazepam in patients with ischemic heart disease. Anesth Analg 1981;60:802.
400. Sarnquist FH, Mathers WD, Blaschke TF. Steady state pharmacokinetics of midazolam maleate. Anesthesiology 1979; 51:S41.
401. Satiani B, Fried SJ, Zeeb P, Falcone RE. Normothermic rapid volume replacement in traumatic hypovolemia: a prospective analysis using a new device. Arch Surg 1987;122:1044.
402. Savarese JJ. Atracurium. International Anesthesia Research Society refresher course lectures, 1986:90.
403. Savarese JJ, Ali HH, Basta SJ, et al. Sixty-second tracheal intubation with BW B1090U after fentanyl-tiopental induction. Anesthesiology 1987;67:A351.
404. Scalfani SJA, Shaftan GW, Mitchell WG, et al. Interventional radiology in trauma victims: analysis of 51 consecutive patients. J Trauma 1982;22:353.
405. Scheller MS, Todd MM, Drummond JC, Zornow MH. The intracranial pressure effects of isoflurane and halothane administered following cryogenic brain injury in rabbits. Anesthesiology 1987;67:507.
406. Schwab CW, Shayne JP, Turner J. Immediate trauma resuscitation with type O uncrossmatched blood: a two-year prospective experience. J Trauma 1986;26:897.
407. Schwartz L, Rockoff MA, Koka BV. Masseter spasm with anesthesia: incidence and implications. Anesthesiology 1984; 61:772.
408. Scott RPF, Savarese JJ, Basta SJ, et al. Atracurium: clinical strategies for preventing histamine release and attenuating the haemodynamic response. Br J Anaesth 1985;57:550.
409. Sellick BA. Cricothyroid pressure to control regurgitation of stomach contents during induction of anesthetic. Lancet 1961;2:404.
409a. Sessler DI, Olofsson CI, Rubinstein EH. The thermoregulatory

threshold in humans during nitrous oxide-fentanyl anesthesia. Anesthesiology 1988;69:357.
410. Severinghaus JW, Naifeh KH. Accuracy of response of six pulse oximeters to profound hypoxia. Anesthesiology 1987;67:551.
411. Seyde WC, Longnecker DE. Anesthetic influences on regional hemodynamics in normal and hemorrhaged rats. Anesthesiology 1984;61:686.
412. Shackford SR. Blunt chest trauma: the intensivist's perspective. J Intensive Care Med 1986;1:125.
413. Shackford SR, Hollingsworth-Fridlund P, Cooper GF, et al. The effect of regionalization upon the quality of trauma care as assessed by concurrent audit before and after institution of a trauma system: a preliminary report. J Trauma 1986;26:812.
414. Shackford SR, MacKersie RC, Hoyt DB, et al. Impact of a trauma system on outcome of severely injured patients. Arch Surg 1987;122:523.
415. Shanks CA. Humidification and loss of body heat during anaesthesia, 1: quantification and correlation in the dog. Br J Anaesth 1974;46:859.
416. Shanks CA, Avram MJ, Ronai AK, Bowsher DJ. The pharmacokinetics of D-tubocurarine with surgery involving salvaged autologous blood. Anesthesiology 1985;62:161.
417. Shapiro HM. Intracranial hypertension: therapeutic and anesthetic considerations. Anesthesiology 1975;43:445.
418. Shapiro HM, Galindo A, Wytei SR, Harris AB. Rapid intraoperative reduction of intracranial pressure with thiopentone. Br J Anaesth 1973;45:1057.
419. Shapiro HM, Wyte SR, Harris AB. Ketamine anesthesia in patients with intracranial pathology. Br J Anaesth 1972; 44:1200.
420. Sharkey A, Lipton JM, Murphy MT, Giesecke AH. Inhibition of postanesthetic shivering with radiant heat. Anesthesiology 1987;66:249.
421. Shatney CH, Deepika K, Militello PR, et al. Efficacy of hetastarch in the resuscitation of patients with multisystem trauma and shock. Arch Surg 1983;118:804.
422. Shelly MP, Robinson AA, Hesford JW, Park GR. Haemodynamic effects following surgical release of increased intraabdominal pressure. Br J Anaesth 1987;59:800.
423. Shin B, MacKenzie CF, Helrich M. Creatinine clearance for early detection of posttraumatic renal dysfunction. Anesthesiology 1986;64:605.
424. Shin B, MacKenzie CF, Helrich M. Hypokalemia in trauma patients. Anesthesiology 1986;65:90.
425. Shires GT, Cunningham JN, Baker CRF, et al. Alterations in cellular membrane function during hemorrhagic shock in primates. Ann Surg 1972;176:288.
426. Shupak RC, Harp JR, Stevenson-Smith W, et al. High-dose fentanyl for neuroanesthesia. Anesthesiology 1983;58:579.
427. Sibbald WR, Calvin JE, Holliday RL, Driedger AA. Concepts in the pharmacologic and nonpharmacologic support of cardiovascular function in critically-ill surgical patients. Surg Clin North Am 1983;63:455.
428. Siegel JH, Dunham CM. Trauma, the disease of the 20th century. In: Siegel JH, ed. Trauma, emergency surgery and critical care. New York: Churchill Livingstone, 1987:1.
429. Silbert BS, Rosow CE, Keegan CR, et al. The effect of diazepam on induction of anesthesia with alfentanil. Anesth Analg 1986;65:71.
430. Simpson ET, Aitchison JM. Percutaneous infraclavicular subclavian vein catheterization in shocked patients: a prospective study in 172 patients. J Trauma 1982;22:781.
431. Skovsted P, Price ML, Price HL. The effects of short acting barbiturates on arterial pressure, preganglionic sympathetic activity and barostatic reflexes. Anesthesiology 1970;33:10.
432. Sladen A. High-frequency jet ventilation in trauma. In: Maull KI, Cleveland HC, Strauch GO, Wolferth CC, eds. Advances in trauma. Chicago: Year Book Medical Publishers, 1986:167.
433. Slogoff S, Keats AS, Arlund C. On the safety of radial artery cannulation. Anesthesiology 1983;59:42.
434. Smith G. Pretreatment with nondepolarizing muscle relaxant does not decrease gastric regurgitation following succinycholine. Anesthesiology 1982;56:408.
435. Smith G, Dalling R, Williams TIR. Gastro-oesophageal pressure gradient changes produced by induction of anaesthesia and suxamethonium. Br J Anaesth 1978;50:1137.
436. Smith G, Thornburn J, Vance JP, Brown DM. The effects of ketamine on the canine coronary circulation. Anaesthaesia 1979;34:555.
437. Smith M, Abraham E. Conjunctival oxygen tension monitoring during hemorrhage. J Trauma 1986;26:217.
438. Smith NT, Eger EI II, Stoelting RK, et al. The cardiovascular and sympathomimetic responses to the addition of nitrous oxide to halothane in man. Anesthesiology 1970;32:410.
439. Sneyd JR. A simple atracurium infusion regimen for intra-abdominal surgery. Br J Anaesth 1986;58:1387.
440. Snow N, Richardson JD, Flint LM. Myocardial contusion: implications for patients with multiple traumatic injuries. Surgery 1982;92:744.
441. Soderstrom CA, Arias JD, Carson SL, et al. Alcohol consumption among vehicular occupants injured in crashes. Alcoholism 1984;8:269.
442. Sosis M, Larijani GE, Marr AT. Priming with atracurium. Anesth Analg 1987;66:329.
443. Spaulding BC, Choi SD, Gross JB, et al. The effect of physostigmine on diazepam-induced ventilatory depression: a double-blind study. Anesthesiology 1984;61:551.
444. Spiess BD, Tuman KJ, McCarthy RJ, Ivankovich AD. Thrombelastography as an indicator of post-cardiopulmonary bypass coagulopathies. J Clin Monit 1987;3:25.
445. Sprung LH. The pulmonary artery catheter: methodology and clinical applications. Baltimore: University Park Press, 1983:73.
446. Stacpoole PW, Harman EM, Curry SH, et al. Treatment of lactic acidosis with dichloroacetate. N Engl J Med 1983;309:390.
447. Stanley TH, Reddy P. Fentanyl-oxygen anesthesia in septic shock. Anesthesiology 1979;51:S100.
448. Stanley TH, Weidauer HE. Anesthesia for the patient with cardiac tamponade. Anesth Analg 1973;52:110.
449. Stevenson PH, Birch AA. Succinylcholine-induced hyperkalemia in a patient with a closed-head injury. Anesthesiology 1979;51:89.
450. Stirt JA, Grosslight KR, Bedford RF, Vollmer D. "Defasciculation" with metocurine prevents succinylcholine-induced increases in intracranial pressure. Anesthesiology 1987;67:50.
451. Stoops CM. Acute hyperkalemia associated with massive blood replacement. Anesth Analg 1983;62:1044.
451a. Stoops CM, Curtis CA, Kovach DA, et al. Hemodynamic effects of mivacurium chloride administered to patients during oxygen-sufentanil anesthesia for coronary artery bypass grafting or valve replacement. Anesth Analg 1989;68:333.
452. Strain JD, Moore EE, Vincent J, et al. Cimetidine for the prophylaxis of potential gastric acid aspiration pneumonitis in trauma patients. J Trauma 1981;21:49.
453. Streisand JB, Nelson P, Bubbers S, et al. The respiratory effects of propofol with and without fentanyl. Anesth Analg 1987;66:S171.
454. Sung YF, Weinstein MS, Hammonds WD, et al. Comparison of midazolam and thiopental for anesthesia induction. Anesthesiology 1982;57:A346.
455. Sutherland GR, Calvin JE, Driedger AA, et al. Anatomic and cardiopulmonary responses to trauma with associated blunt chest injury. J Trauma 1981;21:1.

456. Taboada JA, Rupp SM, Miller RD. Refining the priming principle for vecuronium during rapid-sequence induction of anesthesia. Anesthesiology 1986;64:243.
457. Tanaka GY. Hypertensive reaction to naloxone. JAMA 1974; 228:25.
458. Tarmow J, Hess W, Klein W. Etomidate, althesin and thiopentone as induction agents for coronary artery surgery. Can Anaesth Soc J 1980;27:338.
459. Tateishi A, Maekawa T, Takeshita H, Wakuta K. Diazepam and intracranial pressure. Anesthesiology 1981;54:335.
460. Taylor MB, Whitwam JG. The current status of pulse oximetry: clinical value of continuous noninvasive oxygen saturation monitoring. Anaesthesia 1986;41:943.
461. Thal ER, Bost RO, Anderson RJ. Effects of alcohol and other drugs on traumatized patients. Arch Surg 1985;120:708.
462. Theye RA, Perry LB, Brzica SM. Influence of anesthetic agent on response to hemorrhagic hypotension. Anesthesiology 1974;40:32.
463. Thompson MGE. Anesthesia for battle casualties in Vietnam. JAMA 1967;201:215.
464. Todd MM, Drummond JC, Shapiro HM. Comparative cerebrovascular and metabolic effects of halothane, enflurane and isoflurane. Anesthesiology 1982;57:A332.
465. Todd MM, Tommasino C, Moore S, et al. The effects of acute isovolemic hemodilution on the brain: a comparison of crystalloid and colloid solutions. Anesthesiology 1984;61:A122.
466. Tollofsrud SG, Gunderson Y, Anderson R. Perioperative hypothermia. Acta Anaesthesiol Scand 1984;28:511.
467. Tong TK. Succinylcholine-induced hyperkalemia in near-drowning. Anesthesiology 1987;66:720.
468. Topulos GP, Butler JP. Correction of a recurrent error. Anesthesiology 1985;63:563.
469. Toutant SM, Todd MM, Drummond JC, et al. Cerebral blood flow during high frequency ventilation in cats. Crit Care Med 1983;11:712.
470. Traber DL, Wilson RD, Priano LL. Differentiation of the cardiovascular effects of CI-581. Anesth Analg 1968;47:769.
471. Tremper KK. Transcutaneous $Po_2$ measurement. Can Anaesth Soc J 1984;31:664.
472. Tremper KK, Shoemaker WC. Transcutaneous oxygen monitoring of critically ill patients with and without low flow shock. Crit Care Med 1981;9:706.
473. Tremper KK, Shoemaker WC, Wender D. Monitoring oxygen transcutaneously in critically ill patients. N Engl J Med 1985;312:241.
474. Trunkey DD. Trauma. Sci Am 1983;249:28.
475. Trunkey DD, Sheldon GF, Collins JA. The treatment of shock. In: Zuidema GD, Rutherford RB, Ballinger WF, eds. The management of trauma. 4th ed. Philadelphia: WB Saunders, 1985:105.
476. Tuman KJ, Spiess BD, McCarthy RJ, Ivankovich AD. Effects of progressive blood loss on coagulation as measured by thrombelastography. Anesth Analg 1987;66:856.
477. Tweed WA, Minuck M, Mymin D. Circulatory response to ketamine anesthesia. Anesthesiology 1972;37:613.
478. Ulsamer B, Doenicke A, Laschat M. Propofol im Vergleich zu Etomidat zur Narkoseeinleitung. Anaesthesist 1986;35:535.
479. Vacanti CJ, van Houten RJ, Hill RC. A statistical analysis of the relationship of physical status to postoperative mortality in 68,388 cases. Anesth Analg 1970;49:564.
480. Valeri CR, Feingold H, Cassidy G, et al. Hypothermia-induced reversible platelet dysfunction. Ann Surg 1987;205:175.
481. Van Der Spek AFL, Fang WB, Ashton-Miller JA, et al. The effects of succinylcholine on mouth opening. Anesthesiology 1987;67:459.
482. Van Hamme M, Ghoneim MM, Ambre J. Pharmacokinetics of etomidate, a new intravenous anesthetic. Anesthesiology 1978;49:274.
483. Vaughan MS, Vaughan RW, Cork RC. Postoperative hypothermia in adults: relationship of age, anesthesia, and shivering to rewarming. Anesth Analg 1981;60:746.
484. Venus B, Smith RA, Mathru M. National survey of methods and criteria used for weaning from mechanical ventilation. Crit Care Med 1987;15:530.
485. Vitez T. Potassium and the anesthetist. Can J Anaesth 1987;34:S30.
486. Wagner RL, White PF. Etomidate inhibits adrenocortical function in surgical patients. Anesthesiology 1984;61:647.
487. Wagner RL, White PF, Klein P, et al. Inhibition of adrenal steroidogenesis by the anesthetic etomidate. N Engl J Med 1984;310:1415.
488. Walts LF, Dillon JB. Clinical studies of the interaction between D-tubocurarine and succinylcholine. Anesthesiology 1969;31:39.
488a. Ward CF, Ozaki GT. Pressure-augmented fluid administration: modified system and general results. Crit Care Med 1989;17:70.
489. Wasserberger J, Bundage B, Ordog GL, et al. DIC in head trauma. Ann Emerg Med 1984;13:987.
490. Watson CB, Norfleet EA. Anesthesia for trauma. Crit Care Clin 1986;2:717.
491. Watson WE, Seelye E, Smith AC. The action of thiopentone on the vascular distensibility of the hand. Br J Anaesth 1962;34:19.
492. Waud BE, Waud DR. Interaction among agents that block endplate depolarization competitively. Anesthesiology 1985;63:4.
493. Waud BE, Waud DR. Quantitative examination of the interaction of competitive neuromuscular blocking agents on the indirectly elicited twitch. Anesthesiology 1984;61:420.
494. Wauquier A, Hermans C, Van den Broeck W, et al. Resuscitative drug effects in hypovolemic hypotensive animals, part 1: comparative cardiovascular effects of an infusion of saline, etomidate, thiopental or pentobarbital in hypovolemic dogs. Janssen Research Products, 1981 (unpublished data).
495. Waxman K, Shoemaker WC, Lippmann M. Cardiovascular effects of anesthetic induction with ketamine. Anesth Analg 1980;58:355.
496. Wayne MA, Marvin A. Clinical evaluation of the anti-shock trouser: retrospective analysis of five years experience. Ann Emerg Med 1983;12:342.
497. Weeks DB, Ramsey FM. Laboratory investigation of six artificial noses for use during endotracheal anesthesia. Anesth Analg 1983;62:758.
498. Weiner P, Sznajdler I, Plavnick L, et al. Unusual complications of subclavian vein catheterization. Crit Care Med 1984; 12:538.
499. Weiskopf RB, Bogetz MS. Cardiovascular actions of nitrous oxide or halothane in hypovolemic swine. Anesthesiology 1985;63:509.
500. Weiskopf RB, Bogetz MS. Haemorrhage decreases the anaesthetic requirement for ketamine and thiopentone in the pig. Br J Anaesth 1985;57:1022.
501. Weiskopf RB, Bogetz MS, Roizen MF, Reid IA. Cardiovascular and metabolic sequelae of inducing anesthesia with ketamine or thiopental in hypovolemic swine. Anesthesiology 1984; 60:214.
502. Weiskopf RB, Townsley MI, Riordan KK, et al. Comparison of cardiopulmonary responses to graded hemorrhage during enflurane, halothane, isoflurane and ketamine anesthesia. Anesth Analg 1981;60:481.
503. Wetzel RC, Latson TW. Major errors in thermodilution cardiac output measurement during rapid volume infusion. Anesthesiology 1985;62:684.
504. White PF. Comparative evaluation of intravenous agents for

rapid sequence induction-thiopental, ketamine, and midazolam. Anesthesiology 1982;57:279.
505. White PF, Way WL, Trevor AJ. Ketamine: its pharmacology and therapeutic uses. Anesthesiology 1982;56:119.
506. Williams ME, Rosa RM, Silva P, et al. Impairment of extrarenal potassium disposal by beta adrenergic stimulation. N Engl J Med 1984;311:145.
507. Wong DH, O'Connor D, Tremper KK, et al. Changes in cardiac output after acute blood loss and position change in man. Crit Care Med 1989;17:979.
508. Wong KC, Martin WE, Hornbein TF, et al. The cardiovascular effects of morphine sulfate with oxygen and nitrous oxide in man. Anesthesiology 1973;38:542.
509. Yate PM, Flynn PJ, Arnold RW, et al. Clinical experience and plasma laudanosine concentrations during the infusion of atracurium in the intensive therapy unit. Br J Anaesth 1987;59:211.
510. Yoshikawa K, Murai Y. The effect of ketamine on intraocular pressure in children. Anesth Analg 1971;50:199.
511. Youngberg JA, Miller ED. Evaluation of percutaneous cannulation of the dorsalis pedis artery. Anesthesiology 1976;44:80.
512. Zaloga GP, Chernow B. Hypocalcemia in critical illness. JAMA 1986;256:1924.
513. Zimmerman BL. Uncommon problems in acute trauma. In: Katz J, Benumof J, Kadis LB, eds. Anesthesia and uncommon diseases: pathophysiologic and clinical correlations. Philadelphia: WB Saunders, 1981:635.
514. Zsigmond EK, Durrani Z, Barabas E, et al. Endocrine and hemodynamic effects of antagonism of fentanyl-induced respiratory depression by nalbuphine. Anesth Analg 1987;66:421.
515. Zsigmond EK, Kothary SP, Martinez OA, et al. Diazepam for prevention of the rise in plasma catecholamines caused by ketamine. Clin Pharmacol Ther 1974;15:223.

*Section Two*

# *Specific Injuries*

# Chapter Ten

Sanford M. Miller

# Management of Central Nervous System Injuries

Neurosurgery, one of the newest of recognized medical specialties, is among the oldest of medical therapies. Skulls showing evidence of extensive craniotomy have been found in neolithic burials in Europe[203,208] and pre-Columbian sites in Peru.[260] That these procedures were done at least on occasion for trauma is demonstrated by fracture sites near the craniotomy wound. That patients survived both injury and surgery is shown by evidence of healing around the edges of the skull defect.[208,260] One of the oldest surviving medical documents, the Edwin Smith papyrus (a 1700 BC copy of a treatise probably from 2400 to 2500 BC),[28] describes the symptoms, diagnosis, therapy (if possible), and prognosis of 27 typical cases of head injury and six of spinal trauma. Hippocrates (pre–third century BC)[2] and Galen (second century AD)[3] established treatment criteria—including trephination—for head trauma which remained virtually unchanged for over 2000 years. Anesthesia, asepsis, cerebral localization, and Harvey Cushing improved the outlook for these patients to some degree. Cushing[50] rationalized the indications for surgery in head injuries; his treatment protocol remained standard until recent years, when the development of angiography and computed tomography (CT) scanning made most exploratory surgery unnecessary.[125,248] Laminectomy and cord decompression for spinal injuries was standard therapy through the 17th and 18th centuries, despite many doubts as to its efficacy and a high incidence of wound infection.[119,279] Surgery fell out of favor in the 19th century but was resurrected by Cushing in 1905.[53] Serious questions as to the value of early decompression in spinal injury remain to the present.[297,341,372]

The outlook, however, for most patients with central nervous system injuries remained grim. Cerebral edema, respiratory depression, and infection took a high toll of the brain injured. Those paraplegics who survived their initial insults were doomed to a lingering and uncomfortable downhill course until they succumbed to renal failure and/or infection, generally within 2 years. It was the efforts of a small number of people in the wake of World War II, most notably Sir Ludwig Guttmann in England,[238,336] which stimulated various medical specialists to improve the medical treatment and rehabilitation of patients with spinal cord injuries. Today, most paraplegics can be helped to remarkably well-adjusted and productive lives. Improvement in the nonsurgical therapy of head trauma was largely a product of the 1960s and 1970s, with the use of respiratory support and osmotic diuretics. There is, of course, much room for improvement: mortality from brain injury remains almost 50%,[128] and too many of those who survive are severely disabled.

The population in which central nervous system injuries occur makes any improvement in results of therapy particularly gratifying.[134] The most common causes of this type of trauma are motor vehicle (including bicycle), occupational, and athletic accidents. Thus these patients are generally young (10 to 40 years), male (60 to 80%), and healthy.

Care of the patient with a brain or spinal cord injury involves people—physicians, nurses, and technicians—from many fields of medicine; it is obvious that this discussion must be limited to the areas which primarily involve the anesthesiologist. Those aspects of diagnosis and therapy which are more appropriately the concern of other specialists will be mentioned, if at all, only briefly.

# HEAD INJURIES

## INITIAL EVALUATION AND THERAPY

Intensive care of the head-injured patient must begin as early as possible—in the emergency room if not at the site of the accident—in order to reduce the extension of brain damage that may result from hypoxia and increased intracranial pressure.[32,97,165,256] Several topics will be discussed briefly in this section and described more fully in the discussion of intensive care.

### *Respiration*

Alteration of the ventilatory pattern is a nearly invariable result of brain damage severe enough to produce a marked change in consciousness. Although central neurogenic hyperventilation is most common, some patients exhibit some degree of respiratory depression. Even hyperventilation may be associated with cerebral hypoxia—a result of severe hypocarbic vasoconstriction—which requires supplemental oxygen. Aspiration of regurgitated gastric contents is also a serious risk in the obtunded patient. Thus protection of the airway and maintenance of adequate ventilation are of first concern in anyone with brain injury. *The airway should be cleared and intubation performed at the first suspicion of inadequate respiratory effort or depression of the cough reflex.* There is much less risk in extubating an unnecessarily intubated patient after a couple of hours than in permitting aspiration or prolonged and possibly increasing respiratory depression. When a ventilator is available and arterial blood gases can be monitored, intermittent mandatory ventilation should be instituted, sufficient to maintain $Paco_2$ between 25 and 30 mm Hg.

Another important factor should be considered during intubation: laryngoscopy may produce a marked increase in blood pressure and intracranial pressure (ICP) in any but the most deeply comatose patients. Thiopental in doses of 200 mg or more supplemented, if possible, by lidocaine (1.5 mg/kg, intravenously) will tend to limit or abolish these potentially harmful responses.[21,65,194] Of course, intubation should not be unduly delayed until these drugs are made available. A muscle relaxant (succinylcholine, 1 mg/kg, or vecuronium, 0.25 mg/kg) should be used to facilitate intubation when restlessness or clamping of the jaw makes it difficult. Struggling with an intubation can do more harm than good, since hypercarbia and increased ICP may result. Cricoid pressure should be applied to prevent aspiration of gastric contents during intubation of these patients. Muscle relaxation may have to be continued if restlessness or hyperventilation makes ventilatory control difficult.[32] Immediate cricothyroidotomy or tracheostomy may be required in the presence of maxillofacial or laryngeal injuries. Following intubation, a nasogastric tube should be inserted to empty the stomach.

### *State of Consciousness*

The most striking sign of severe head injury is alteration of consciousness. The Glasgow coma scale (GCS) (Table 10-1) provides an objective evaluation of mental status.[54,258] It should be recorded repeatedly during the early stages of injury—at least every 6 hours, or more frequently if the patient's condition is changing rapidly. Note that one third of the score is based on verbal response. Obviously, allowance must be made for this in patients who are intubated.

TABLE 10-1. Glasgow Coma Scale*

| | |
|---|---|
| Eye opening (E) | |
| Spontaneous | 4 |
| To speech | 3 |
| To pain | 2 |
| Nil | 1 |
| Best motor response (M) | |
| Obeys | 6 |
| Localizes | 5 |
| Withdraws (flexion) | 4 |
| Abnormal flexion | 3 |
| Extensor response | 2 |
| Nil | 1 |
| Verbal response (V) | |
| Oriented | 5 |
| Confused conversation | 4 |
| Inappropriate words | 3 |
| Incomprehensible sounds | 2 |
| Nil | 1 |
| Coma score = E + M + V (ie, 3 to 15) | |

* Adapted from Teasdale and Jennett[258] with permission.

Two factors may affect the initial diagnosis of coma. First, it is well known that a large proportion of serious motor vehicle accidents is associated with alcohol and/or drugs. The effects of these can confuse the evaluation of the injury.[123] Second, hypoxia itself can alter consciousness. Thus, neurologic assessment should not be performed until emergency therapy has been instituted.

### *The Circulatory System*

Hypertension, at times to alarming levels, is very common following head injury, probably as a result of central sympathetic stimulation. It is best not to treat it in the emergency room, pending evaluation of the extent of injury, mass lesions, and ICP.

Hypotension, on the other hand, is a particularly dangerous complication. Cerebral circulation, usually decreased by the initial trauma, may be severely compromised.[182] Decreased blood pressure resulting from brain damage is associated with other terminal signs: marked bradycardia, pupillary dilatation, and agonal respirations.[256] If these are not present, a careful search for a severe associated injury should be instituted immediately: eg, X-rays of the chest, abdomen, and any bones that show indication of fracture; pleural or peritoneal tap.[256] Blood should be obtained for hematocrit, clotting studies, electrolyte determination, typing, and cross-matching. A large-bore peripheral intravenous line should be started, and crystalloids, colloids, and (when available) blood should be given in an effort to restore blood volume. The specific fluids chosen at this time may be less important than the quantity administered.[282] Vasopressors are best avoided since their effects on cerebral circulation, particularly in injured brain, are uncertain.

The possibility of spinal cord injury as a cause of hypotension in these patients should not be overlooked. It is seen in approximately 3% of head-injured patients admitted to the hospital.[202] Spinal shock is usually easily differentiated from hypovolemia. The pulse is normal to slow, the skin is dry and warm, urinary output is usually normal, and peripheral neurologic deficit is present.

If severe secondary injury exists and vital signs cannot be stabilized by volume replacement, immediate surgery is mandatory. It should not be delayed by attempts to refine the evaluation of the patient's condition further. Priorities of surgical treatment in the face of multiple injuries are discussed in Chapter 2. As a rule, brain injuries carry a high priority. When they are associated with other severe injuries, simultaneous surgical intervention must be considered.

### *Intracranial Pressure*

Marshall and Bowers[165] and Becker et al[18] recommend monitoring of ICP in any patient whose coma score following resuscitation is 7 or below. According to Narayan et al,[198] an exception may be made if the patient meets the following criteria: no mass on CT scan, and two of the following three—age under 40, systolic blood pressure above 90, no motor posturing. In this group the incidence of elevated ICP (7%) is virtually the same as the risk of complications from an intraventricular catheter. Several methods of ICP measurement are available.[133,158] A ventricular catheter connected to a standard strain gauge transducer permits withdrawal of cerebrospinal fluid (CSF) to control elevated pressure. However, it may be difficult to insert when hematoma or diffuse brain swelling distorts and/or decreases the size of the ventricle (see Fig 10-2). A subarachnoid bolt is easily inserted under any circumstances, although it may at times give erroneous readings, depending on its placement relative to the site of injury.[276] Epidural bolts have a lower risk of complications but are less accurate than ventricular catheters or subarachnoid bolts and do not permit withdrawal of CSF. Many centers are now monitoring the ICP using an intracerebral fiberoptic sensor which is easy to place and provides accurate information during the first few days after injury (Camino Labs., San Diego, CA). The choice of methods is best left to the judgment and experience of the neurosurgeon.[84] If facilities for monitoring are not available, elevation of ICP should be assumed if the GCS is 7 or below and appropriate therapy undertaken.

Normal ICP pulsates with the heart beat and shows a mean pressure of 10 mm Hg or less. Levels of 10 to 20 mm Hg represent borderline elevation and require appropriate treatment and careful observation. Pressures above 20 mm Hg are considered definitely elevated and, if maintained for more than 1 to 2 hours, should be vigorously treated.[133,165] Pressure fluctuations of varying amplitude and frequency may be noted on the ICP trace. They commonly represent an important sign of intracranial decompensation[84] (see the section on ICP). Management of intracranial hypertension is outlined in Table 10-2.

### *Steroids*

The use of steroids does not seem to be associated with adverse effects. However, they are expensive, and conclusive evidence of a beneficial effect on outcome in head-injured patients is lacking. This issue will be discussed further in the section on critical care.

TABLE 10-2. Management of Intracranial Hypertension*

1. Head elevation 30 degrees and neutral position (no rotation, flexion, or extension)
2. Ventilatory control to $Pa_{CO_2}$ of 25 to 30 mm Hg and $Pa_{O_2}$ of >70 mm Hg. Sedation and muscle relaxation should be used if necessary
3. Blood pressure maintenance: 100 to 160 mm Hg systolic (CPP 70 to 110 mm Hg)
4. Ventricular drainage if possible
5. Evaluation of, and surgery if necessary for, hematoma
6. Avoid hyperthermia
7. Medication, eg, anticonvulsants, diuretics, barbiturates

* Adapted from Marshall and Bowers[165] with permission.

### *Diuretics*

Mannitol is useful both for its osmotic effect in reducing interstitial fluid and its effect in improving regional cerebral blood flow—commonly reduced in adults with head injuries.[29,32,152,199] Since children may show increased, rather than decreased, cerebral blood volume, this agent is probably best avoided in young patients until ICP has been evaluated and other measures taken to reduce it.[33] Rapid infusion of 0.5-1.0 mg/kg over 5 minutes is the usual initial dose.[182] It may be repeated in 4 to 6 hours if necessary.

The use of mannitol has been questioned in the hypotensive multiply injured patient. However, a recent study by Israel et al[122] showed that mannitol lowered ICP while maintaining cerebral perfusion pressure and cardiac indices in a dog model. Thus, mannitol is probably safe if administered in conjunction with other resuscitation measures.

Furosemide has been used in some centers. It seems unreliable by itself in lowering ICP but may be useful in patients with pulmonary edema and resultant decreased $Pa_{O_2}$.[32] It is likely that the combination of mannitol and furosemide may be more effective in reducing ICP and improving cerebral blood flow than either drug used alone.

### *Monitoring and Fluid Replacement*

All head-injured patients in coma will require a large-bore (14 to 16 gauge) peripheral intravenous line, an arterial line, and an indwelling urinary catheter. A nasogastric tube inserted after intubation will prevent gastric dilatation.[256] A central venous or, in the severely injured, pulmonary artery (Swan-Ganz) catheter can aid in assessment of fluid balance. Electrocardiogram (ECG) and temperature should be monitored continuously. Monitoring of intracranial pressure and evoked responses can aid in diagnosis of severity of the injury and in evaluation of response to therapy.

Patients are probably best kept slightly underhydrated in the first 2 days of therapy. 2000 to 2500 mL/day of Ringer's lactate solution is generally adequate in the normal sized adult. Obviously, this volume will have to be increased if diuretics are administered. Volume replacement in excess of daily fluid requirement (eg, hemorrhage, third-space fluid loss) is best provided by colloid solutions (albumin or hetastarch), which may offer the additional benefit of an additive effect on ICP control when used with mannitol or furosemide.[8,9,215] Preliminary data in animals suggest that resuscitation from hemorrhagic shock using hypertonic saline (3.0 to 7.5% solution) may have the benefit of restoring intravascular and interstitial fluid without causing an increase in ICP[105,221] (see also Chapter 4). Further studies will be necessary before hypertonic saline can be recommended in head injury.

A significant number of patients may exhibit hypokalemia in the first hours after head injury. This may be associated with tachycardia and arrhythmias, which will respond promptly to supplementary potassium infusion.[267]

## MECHANISMS AND SURGICAL ASPECTS OF HEAD INJURY

### *Mechanisms*

Two mechanisms, nearly always combined, account for the anatomic derangements seen following head trauma.[248] Concussion-compression results from localized blunt impact. Although the scalp provides some cushioning effect, most of the force is transmitted to the skull, which buckles inward beneath the impacted area. If the compressive force exceeds the elasticity of the skull, it will fracture. Whether or not fracture occurs, the force is transmitted to the cranial contents, resulting in local contusion and diffuse concussion. Acceleration-deceleration injuries result from sudden movement or cessation of movement of the entire head. For instance, in falls or motor vehicle accidents, the rapidly moving head is suddenly brought to a standstill. Large amounts of kinetic energy are transmitted to the cranial contents, and the momentum of the brain causes it to collide with the inner surface of the skull. Shearing forces result from differential acceleration and rebound, and contusion or laceration may occur as the brain is forced against the more irregular contours of the skull or the edges of the dura such as the sphenoid wing or the undersurface of the falx cerebri.[248] As the brain is pulled away from the cranial vault on the side opposite the area of impact, tearing of bridging veins may occur, resulting in subdural hematoma. Rebound of the brain from its initial direction of motion may result in contusion or hematoma in the area opposite the initial injury—contrecoup injury—as the brain once again strikes the inner surface of the skull.

Thus any severe head trauma may result in several types of injury—contusion, laceration, hematoma—over widespread areas of the cranium and its contents. We will restrict our discussion to injuries of relatively immediate surgical importance.

### *Skull Fractures*

Linear skull fractures generally do not require surgery. However, those fractures that cross the paths of the middle meningeal artery or a dural sinus may cause laceration of these vessels and epidural hematoma, which will be discussed below.

Depressed fractures are significant when the depression is greater than the thickness of the skull. Surgical intervention may be necessary if the fracture is compound or if the dura is torn or vessels ruptured.[25,248]

### *Hematomas*

Most surgery in head injury is performed to evacuate hematomas that may occur within the brain substance (intracerebral), beneath the dura (subdural), or between the dura and the skull (epidural).

INTRACEREBRAL HEMATOMAS. Intracerebral hematomas (Fig 10-1) are common, although it is only the recent development of CT scanning which has permitted their true incidence—possibly as high as 23% of severe head injuries—to be recognized. Symptoms are highly variable depending on the size and location of the hematoma. Most importantly, they may, for unknown reasons, occur as late as 10 to 14 days after the initial injury, causing rapid deterioration after a period of improvement.[32] Generally, surgery is not required for small or deep lesions that cause few or no symptoms. These patients are best treated medically with control of ICP. Large surgically accessible hematomas in severely impaired or deteriorating patients are best treated by surgical evacuation.[248]

SUBDURAL HEMATOMAS. Subdural hematomas (Fig 10-2) may be acute (presenting within 24 hours of injury), subacute (presenting between 24 hours and 10 days), or chronic (presenting after 10 days). They are most commonly the result of rupture of arachnoid veins that bridge the space between the brain and the dura. Clinical signs are variable, depending on the size and location of the hematoma and, perhaps most important, the severity of associated injury to the underlying brain. Indeed, much of the relatively poor prognosis associated with acute subdural hematomas may rather result from intracerebral damage.[248] Except for small, asymptomatic he-

FIG. 10-1. Intracerebral hematoma in left temporal lobe. A contrecoup injury secondary to occipital trauma. (Courtesy of Paul R. Cooper, MD.)

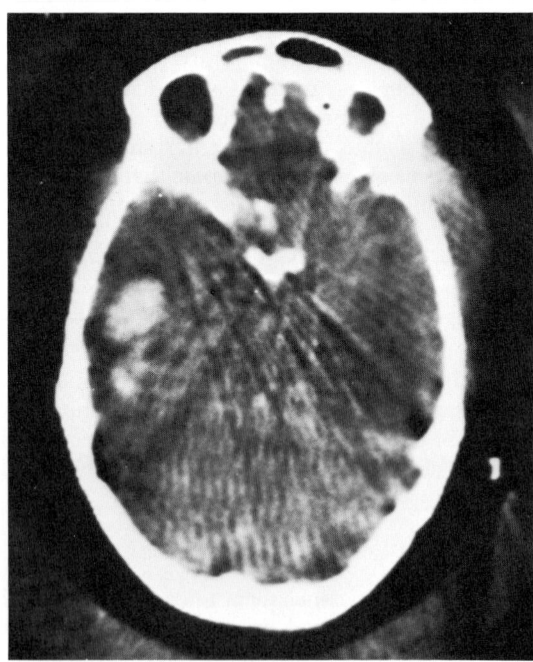

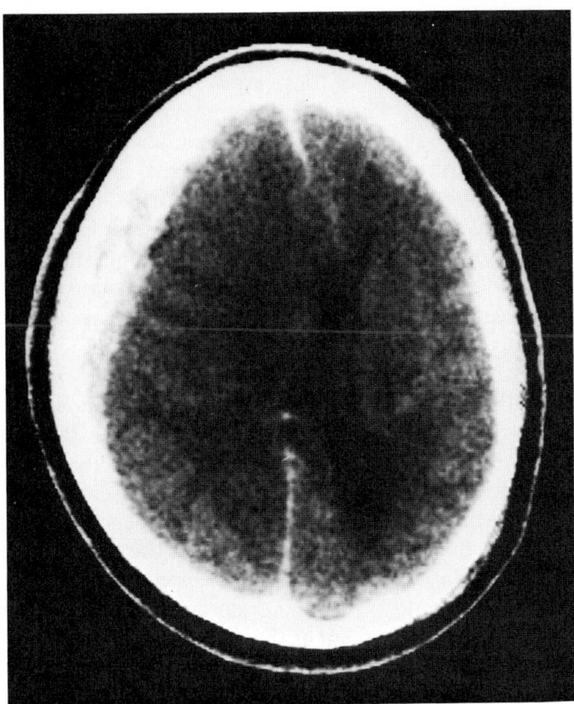

FIG. 10-2. Acute subdural hematoma in left frontal area with severe midline shift and distortion of the ventricles. Note characteristic concave outline. (Courtesy of Paul R. Cooper, MD.)

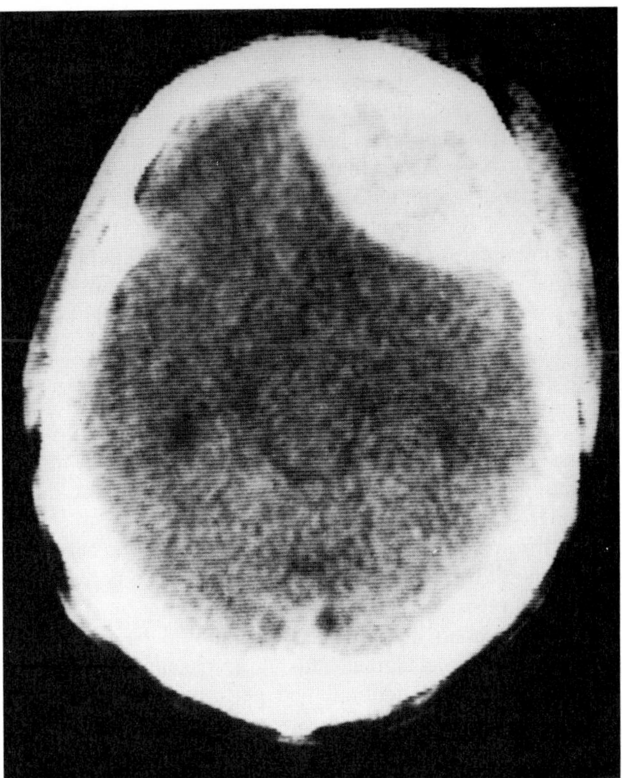

FIG. 10-3. Right frontal epidural hematoma. Note convex outline. (Courtesy of Paul R. Cooper, MD.)

matomas, acute lesions are treated by wide craniotomy and evacuation.[32,248] It should be noted that increased ICP and midline shift may be seen both before *and following* surgery.[32] Intensive medical treatment should thus be continued into the postoperative period.

Subacute—especially those after the first week—and chronic subdural hematomas may be treated by evacuation and continuous drainage through burr holes.[161]

EPIDURAL HEMATOMAS. Epidural hematomas (Fig 10-3) are relatively uncommon, occurring in about 3% of severe head trauma. They result from stripping of the dura from the skull, usually associated with fracture, and laceration of the middle meningeal artery or vein or a dural sinus. Expansion of the hematoma causes further dural separation. The classic clinical course is initial unconsciousness from the primary insult, then neurologic recovery ("lucid interval"), followed over several hours by headache, loss of consciousness, and in untreated patients, by neurologic deterioration and death. However, only a minority of these patients show the classic picture. About one third of patients never regain consciousness, and about one third never lose it. As with other hematomas, treatment is surgical evacuation. If symptoms are progressing rapidly, medical management may help gain time before the patient can reach the operating room.[32]

### Brain Herniation

As a result of supratentorial swelling and/or hematoma, the brain may be forced through the dural folds or the foramen magnum. Four types of herniation are described.[201] Herniation of the medial temporal structures through the tentorial hiatus causes midbrain compression, which results in loss of consciousness, decerebrate rigidity, and dilatation of the ipsilateral pupil from oculomotor nerve compression. Commonly associated with this is herniation of the cingulate gyrus under the falx cerebri (pericallosal herniation), which may be severe enough to compress the anterior cerebral artery and produce weakness of the contralateral lower extremity. Axial herniation of the entire brainstem through the foramen magnum may stretch the arterial supply of the central medulla, resulting in hypertension and bradycardia—the Cushing response[52]—and respiratory irregularities that may culminate in apnea. Herniation of the cerebellar tonsils through the foramen magnum further aggravates medullary symptoms by direct brainstem compression.

Posterior fossa hematomas are rare sequelae of head injury.[183] Although the process of herniation produced by these lesions initially develops rather slowly, abrupt progression may finally occur, producing sudden apnea from axial herniation or bilateral decerebrate rigidity if the cerebellum herniates upward through the tentorial hiatus. In the latter case, the process may be aggravated or precipitated by release of fluid from the lateral ventricles.

Diagnosis of intracranial lesions is made most accurately and expeditiously by the CT scan, which has virtually replaced plain skull films and angiography in those institutions in which a scanner is available.[125,209] Occasionally, in situations in which this facility is lacking, exploratory trephination may be required.[25] CT scans generally require no sedation. Trephination can usually be performed under local anesthesia, although an anesthesiologist should be present to monitor the patient's condition and to evaluate and, if necessary, control the patient's ventilation. General anesthesia should be induced and ventilation controlled via an endotracheal tube for either of these procedures if restlessness or lack of cooperation makes it impossible to keep the patient still without sedation.[47,85] The problems and techniques of general anesthesia in the presence of head injury are described below.

## PREOPERATIVE EVALUATION

The anesthesiologist's first contact with the head-injured patient frequently occurs while he* is being wheeled into the operating suite from the emergency room or X-ray department. History and laboratory studies may be incomplete, and one is thrown back on clinical signs and judgment. Since time is usually of the essence, evaluation should be performed as rapidly as possible.

A presumption of increased ICP should be made if the ICP is not yet available. This is a reasonable conclusion since surgery will generally be performed for intracranial hematoma[32,146] or for shock, which is commonly associated with decreased cerebral perfusion pressure, cerebral hypoxia, and resultant cerebral edema. The patient's state of consciousness, posturing, and pupillary signs may help in ICP evaluation. The lungs should be examined carefully for signs of atelectasis and/or aspiration. Arterial blood gas values and chest X-ray, if available, will aid in diagnosis of pulmonary problems. The course of the patient's blood pressure, intake, output, and hematocrit will aid in assessment of the severity of head or associated injuries and of alterations in blood volume. A history of other medical problems, unless severe, will perhaps complete the clinical picture of the patient but probably will not necessitate change in the anesthetic technique. An ECG and clotting studies can be useful if time is available to perform them since cranial injuries may be associated with abnormalities in cardiac function (dysrhythmias and ST segment changes) and the clotting mechanism.

If anything, only atropine or glycopyrrolate should be given for preoperative medication. Since consciousness and respiration are both critical factors in these patients, any drug that depresses either is strongly contraindicated.

## PERIOPERATIVE MANAGEMENT

Transfer of the patient to the operating table should be done with great care. Unnecessary bouncing can disturb the fragile compensatory mechanisms for hypovolemia and result in a sudden fall in blood pressure—a potential disaster in a patient with cerebral circulatory disturbance. Cervical spine fractures, known or suspected, should be stabilized by a halo brace, cervical traction, or at least by a firm cervical collar before the patient is moved at all.

Decubitus ulcers can start in the operating room as well as anywhere else: pressure points should be padded carefully, and prolonged contact of these areas with cold, wet solutions should be avoided. The patient's temperature should be kept as stable as possible; this can be accomplished by warming the room, warming all intravenous fluids, and/or humidifying the anesthetic gases (which may also provide the additional benefit of aiding in prevention of pulmonary complications).[37]

The following should be inserted in the operating room if not already in place: a large-bore peripheral line (or two if much bleeding is anticipated), an arterial line (radial or femoral), a central venous or pulmonary artery catheter, a nasogastric tube, a temperature probe, and an indwelling urinary catheter. Occasionally, in the most serious situations, corners may have to be cut. There may not be time, for instance, to insert a Swan-Ganz catheter while the patient is rapidly deteriorating from an intracranial hematoma or uncontrolled bleeding. As in any major emergency, the closest communication between the surgeon and the anesthesiologist is required to make such decisions.

Induction of anesthesia and endotracheal intubation carry the same risks at this point as they do in the emergency room. Wide swings in blood pressure, hypoxia or hypercarbia, and bucking on the tube should be avoided. If the patient is not hypotensive, a large (4 to 10 mg/kg) dose of thiopental is given slowly and with careful monitoring of blood pressure.[178,194] Diazepam, up to 20 mg, may be substituted for thiopental in hypotensive patients. An intubating dose of pancuronium (0.08 to 0.1 mg/kg),[156,178] vecuronium (0.1 mg/kg), or atracurium (0.5 mg/kg),[232] and lidocaine (1.0 to 1.5 mg/kg)[22] are given, and the trachea is carefully intubated after hyperventilation. Transient increases in ICP have been reported following the administration of succinylcholine to cats, dogs, and humans, even after high doses of thiopental.[46,148,191,262] Although this effect may be blocked by precurarization,[109,253] we feel that a nondepolarizing muscle relaxant is preferable since ICP and cerebral perfusion pressure (CPP) are not altered by pancuronium, vecuronium, or atracurium.[90,91,232,233,254,270]

We have had no personal experience with etomidate. Its use as an induction agent (1.5 mg/kg) has been reported in a small number of severely head-injured patients.[193,244] Cardiovascular stability was well maintained without an increase in ICP. However, etomidate, even in single doses, suppresses the adrenocortical responses to stress for up to six hours.[79,272] Whether this effect is detrimental is not yet known, but it is probably best not to administer this agent to severely injured patients until its implications are clarified. This problem is discussed more fully in the section on newer therapies.

If surgery is performed within 24 hours of injury, a full stomach should be presumed. In these instances, the doses of nondepolarizing muscle relaxants may be increased to obtain rapid intubating conditions. Pancuronium (0.25 mg/kg), vecuronium (0.25 mg/kg), and atracurium (1.5 mg/kg), intravenously produce relaxation within 60 seconds.[153] During this period the patient should be ventilated while cricoid pressure is applied. Prevention of ICP rise by lowering $Paco_2$ should be given priority over reducing the risk of pulmonary aspiration by cessation of ventilation. Of the three nondepolarizing muscle relaxants, vecuronium has the least potential

* For simplicity, the male gender is used to refer to both sexes. This seems reasonable since the majority of patients with central nervous system injuries are male.

of causing blood pressure and heart rate changes at the high doses recommended.[153,180]

A narcotic technique (generally with fentanyl) is used for maintenance of anesthesia.[77,97,180] Respirations are controlled to maintain $Pa_{CO_2}$ in the 20 to 25 mm Hg range. Used alone, nitrous oxide causes cerebral vasodilatation and increased ICP, even in concentrations as low as 50%.[12,116] This effect is easily blocked by induction agents and hyperventilation and is not generally a problem in the usual course of balanced anesthesia.[12,77] The halogenated agents also dilate the cerebral vasculature and may increase ICP unless $Pa_{CO_2}$ is lowered significantly from preoperative levels, even in spontaneously hyperventilating patients who are hypocarbic before anesthesia.[4,5] Halothane has been shown to increase the extent of secondary brain damage even in the presence of normal ICP,[251] and all of the halogenated anesthetics can increase cerebral edema.[243] These effects may be potentiated by hypotension and decreased cerebral perfusion pressure.[83] It is well known that isoflurane causes only a minimal increase in cerebral blood flow (CBF) in patients (or animals) with normal ICP[68,160,241,263]; however, this advantage over halothane may disappear in the presence of brain injury. In experiments on rabbits, Scheller et al[242] have shown that halothane and isoflurane produce an equal increase in ICP whether $Pa_{CO_2}$ is normal or low, in the presence of a cryogenic lesion. Thus, all halogenated agents should be avoided in the brain-injured patient. Similarly, spontaneous ventilation, sometimes recommended in the older literature,[117] may also be harmful since it is usually inadequate. Although the respiratory pattern may be a useful monitor of brainstem function, our own experience has shown that any problem that affects respiration will also cause changes in cardiac function—bradycardia, premature contractions, arrhythmias, and/or sudden alterations in blood pressure.

Because the patient will have received mannitol preoperatively, he may be somewhat dehydrated when he arrives in the operating room; his hematocrit may not reflect true blood volume status. Blood should be given as it is lost. Packed cells are supplemented with colloid solutions (albumin or hetastarch) or crystalloids as needed. Fluid losses are replaced with Ringer's lactate.[252] We administer sufficient volume to replace urine output, making no provision for third-space shifts or insensible loss, as long as pulmonary artery or central venous and systemic arterial pressures remain stable. The patient's blood volume is thus kept somewhat low. However, any indication of cardiovascular instability should be treated immediately by rapid fluid administration since hypotension in the presence of anesthesia-induced loss of cerebral autoregulation can cause a potentially disastrous reduction of CBF in a patient whose circulation, at least in the injured region of the brain, may already be compromised.

In the recovery room, intubation is maintained with additional doses of narcotic or muscle relaxant as required. Hypertension, a common occurrence after craniotomy, may be controlled with β-blockers or hydralazine. Nitroglycerine and nitroprusside should not be used because they both cause cerebral vasodilatation and may thus increase ICP.[87,106,257] Even if the patient reacts favorably to evacuation of his hematoma, he should remain intubated for several hours postoperatively because rapid brain swelling may occur and negate any decompressive effects of surgery.[151,187] Extubation is performed only when the patient maintains a normal ICP during spontaneous breathing and otherwise meets acceptable extubation criteria. Careful observation should be maintained for several hours after extubation since the patient may still deteriorate at this time if cerebral edema increases.[85]

## INTENSIVE CARE

### *Cerebral Edema, Intracranial Pressure, and Cerebral Blood Flow*

If the brain of an experimental animal is injured, a zone of secondary reaction spreads from the primary region of ischemia and extravasated blood. Within 24 hours, the secondary injury may affect a large part of the involved hemisphere. The exact mechanism of this reaction is not yet known. However, recent experiments suggest a series of interlocked, self-propagating feedback loops (vicious circles) that originate with cell membrane disruption and eventually result in cerebral edema and increased intracranial pressure.[188] The mechanism, basically, is as follows. Hypoxia in the injured area produces reduction of the electron transport chain[219] with uncoupling and release of free radicals and resultant, probably enzyme-induced, breakdown of membrane lipids.[59,66,141] This disruption results in inactivation of important membrane enzymes ($Na^+$,$K^+$-ATPase, cytochrome oxidase, and adenylate cyclase) and loss of the membrane's barrier function and selective permeability. Potassium ion is rapidly released into the extracellular space, displacing the Donnan equilibrium and causing migration of anions, chloride, and water into the surrounding cells. As extracellular potassium concentration ($[K^+]_e$) approaches 10 mEq/L, an active transport mechanism carries additional sodium, calcium, chloride, and water into the cells, which swell rapidly, reducing the extracellular space and further increasing $[K^+]_e$.[14,24,140] Cellular edema thus tends to propagate itself. Swelling of the cells increases the diffusion path for oxygen and carbon dioxide and may also produce some degree of mechanical circulatory impairment. Ischemic hypoxia spreads and causes further cell disruption and edema. In addition, capillary endothelium in the ischemic region also undergoes peroxidative disruption.[16,78,216,217] Intravascular coagulation results. Glial edema and circulatory interference produce further ischemia, cell damage, and edema. Eventually, the edematous zone becomes large enough to increase the ICP, which by reducing CPP and possibly by mechanical circulatory occlusion, further increases the area of damage.[188] The last two stages of this process are shown in Fig 10-4 and Fig 10-5.

Since the primary injury is almost certainly irreversible, the aim of therapy in brain trauma is limitation and, if possible, reversal of the secondary process.[96] Three important principles follow clearly from the above discussion.

1. The earlier that treatment is started, the better the chances of limiting the region of irreversible damage.
2. Maintenance of adequate blood flow and oxygenation in the brain is the prime goal of therapy.
3. Since circulation in the damaged area may be severely compromised, therapeutic measures are largely di-

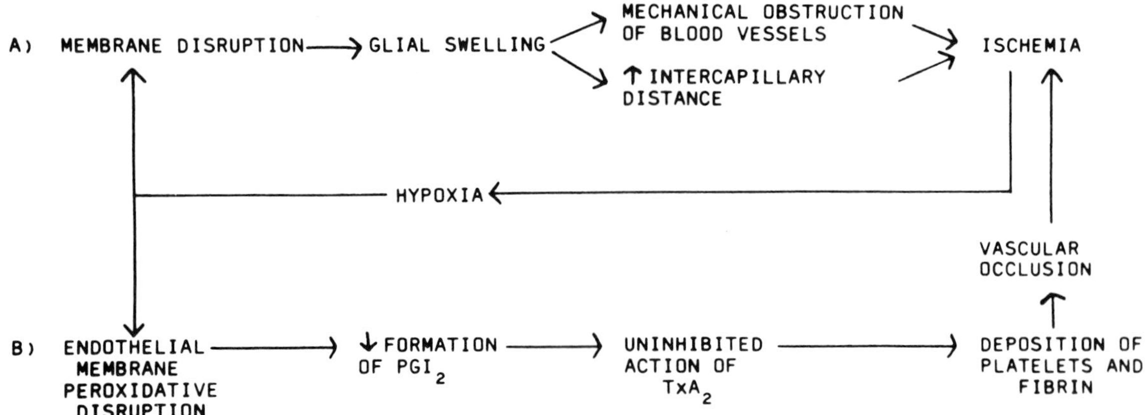


FIG. 10-4. Mechanism of secondary brain injury: tissue hypoxia. Primary brain trauma produces cell membrane disruption by release of free-radicals and resultant peroxidation of membrane lipids. Loss of normal barrier function allows fluid and electrolytes to migrate into the cells, with rapid, severe glial swelling. Increased intercapillary distance and possibly mechanical obstruction of blood vessels cause increasing ischemia and hypoxia. Peroxidative damage to endothelium results in intravascular coagulation and further ischemic hypoxia. ($PGI_2$, prostaglandin $I_2$ (prostacyclin); $T_xA_2$, thromboxane $A_2$). (Adapted from Miller et al[188] with permission.)

rected at normal brain. For instance, osmotic diuretics act by decreasing fluid content and increasing circulation in undamaged regions.[30,199] They have little or no effect (and may actually cause swelling) in the zone of injury.[91,171]

Some understanding of the alterations in ICP and cerebral perfusion caused by brain trauma is necessary to comprehend the bases of intensive care in brain injury. These factors will be discussed before specific therapeutic modes are considered.

FIG. 10-5. Mechanism of secondary brain injury: cerebral edema and raised intracranial pressure. Glial swelling produces increased size of the tissue compartment, ultimately increasing ICP, which, by decreasing CPP and possibly by mechanical vascular occlusion, enlarges the region of damage. The process may be exacerbated by further decrease in CPP resulting from systemic hypotension. ICP, intracranial pressure; CPP, cerebral perfusion pressure; BP, blood pressure. (Adapted from Miller et al[188] with permission.)

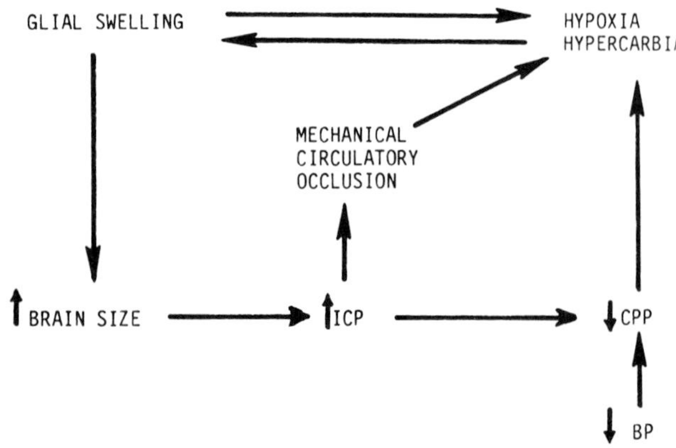


ICP is a function of the interaction of the cranial contents—brain tissue, blood, and CSF—with their rigid container of dura and calvarium. The traditional view of this interaction is basically analogous to a balloon expanding in a rigid box. As one of the components expands another immediately contracts until the limits of compensation are reached. At the point at which the balloon contacts the box walls the pressure increases rapidly and linearly with increase in volume (Fig 10-6).

Recent experimental results show a different picture.[38,163,164] ICP is a smooth logarithmic function of brain volume, up to levels of at least 50 mm Hg (Fig 10-7).[38,163,187] Two mechanisms have been proposed to explain this finding. Chopp et al[38] have found that the elastic resistance of the cerebral vasculature, most probably the veins, is sufficient to cause the observed exponential response. Marmarou and his associates[163,164] and Kosteljanetz,[142] on the other hand, sug-

FIG. 10-6. Idealized volume-pressure relationship. ICP is constant (1–2) until compensation is lost (2–3), at which point pressure rises steeply with increasing volume (3–4). (From Shapiro[246] with permission.)

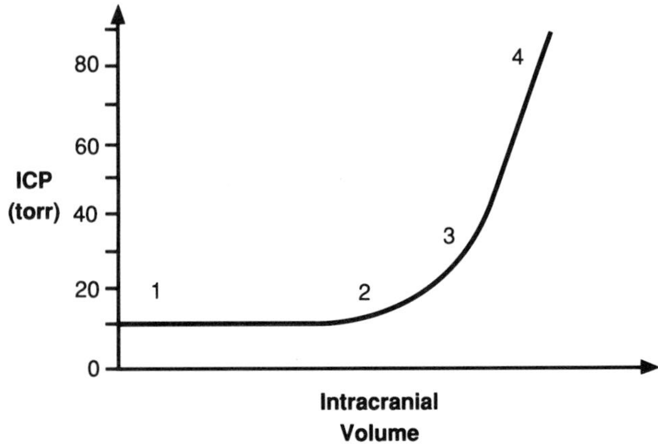

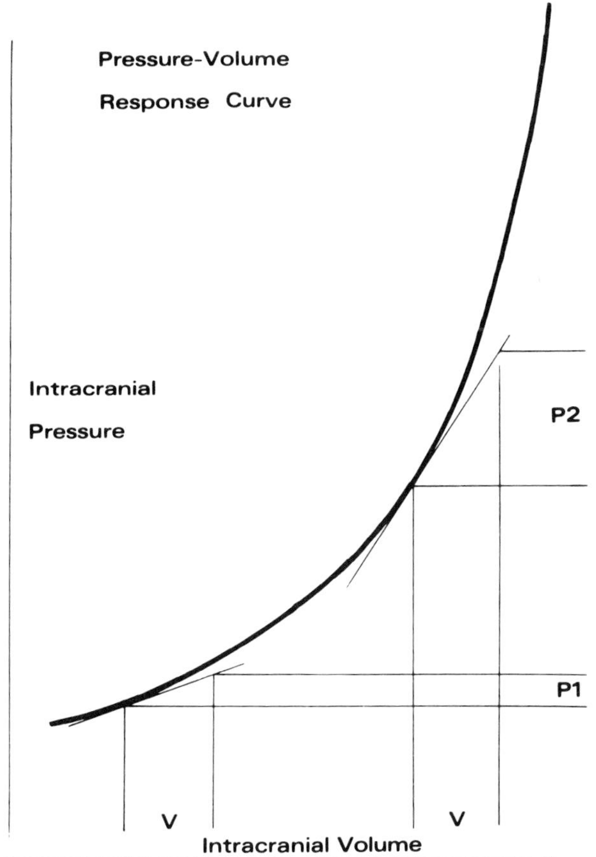


FIG. 10-7. Intracranial volume-pressure curve. As ICP rises, equivalent changes in volume produce increasing pressure response. (From Jones et al[133] with permission.)

gest that alteration of the rate of CSF absorption plays a major role in the response to increasing brain volume. As the tissue compartment expands from brain edema or hematoma, the quantity of CSF decreases in order to maintain constant intracranial volume. However, CSF volume is a function of the equilibrium between its rate of production—virtually constant at any ICP level—and its absorption, which varies logarithmically with changing ICP. As pressure rises, the absorption of CSF increases until equilibrium is reached, generally at a higher pressure level. Of course, these mechanisms are not mutually exclusive; in a recent study Marmarou et al[162] determined that vascular mechanisms accounted for about two thirds whereas CSF parameters were responsible for about one third of the ICP rise in a group of head-injured patients.

The slope of the pressure-volume curve is a function of the compliance (defined as $\Delta V/\Delta P$) of the cranial tissues.[163,187] As they become more stiff, eg, from vasodilatation or edema, compliance decreases, and a small volume increase causes a large increase in pressure. Conversely, if the tissues become more lax, eg, from vasoconstriction or decreasing fluid content, compliance increases, and the curve flattens (Fig 10-8).[187] This effect is seen most clearly during mannitol administration to a patient with increased ICP. As water is absorbed from the tissues, compliance increases, and clinical improvement may occur with little or no ICP change.[186]

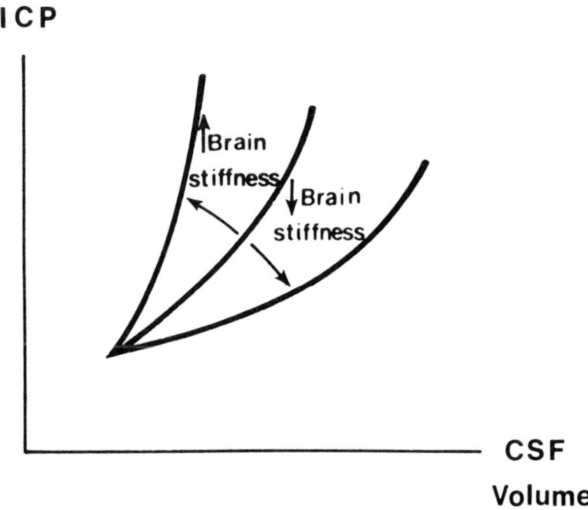


FIG. 10-8. Changing compliance produces a change in the slope of the pressure-volume curve and thus in the magnitude of the volume-pressure response. (Adapted from Miller and Sullivan[187] with permission.)

Of course, the CSF buffer capacity is not unlimited. When it is lost, compliance decreases, and the pressure-volume curve becomes more vertical. Several events may cause this loss of compensation. For instance, rapid expansion of a hematoma may cause brain distortion and herniation into the tentorium or foramen magnum, blocking CSF exit into the spinal subarachnoid space, which provides about one third of the CSF buffer.[163] In this situation, decompensation may occur at relatively low ICP, and a sharp break in the pressure-volume curve will result.

Compliance (or more strictly its reciprocal, elastance, $\Delta P/\Delta V$) is easily measured in the patient with a ventricular catheter or subarachnoid bolt. One mL of fluid is rapidly added to, or to be more safe, withdrawn from, the CSF, and the maximum pressure response is measured. The pressure change is equivalent to the elastance—in Miller's[181] term, the volume-pressure response (VPR). Indeed the entire pressure-volume curve can be estimated from this maneuver by the formula[163,247]

$$\text{PVI} = \frac{\Delta V}{\log_{10} \frac{P_1}{P_2}}$$

where PVI is the pressure-volume index (the volume of fluid required to increase ICP by a factor of 10), and $P_1$ and $P_2$ are, respectively, the higher and lower pressures measured with the volume change. Thus, if V is plotted against the log of the pressure response, a straight line graph is obtained, which will give the VPR to be expected at any level of ICP.[143] PVI is normally 25 mL. It falls soon after brain injury; this may precede and predict the severity of a subsequent rise in ICP.[172] Thus, a reduction to around 20 mL is associated with a normal ICP course; PVI in the range of 15 mL generally indicates manageable ICP elevation, whereas a severely reduced PVI ($\leq$10 mL) is seen in patients who subsequently develop uncontrolled intracranial hypertension. A falling PVI, or equivalently, an increasing VPR (>3 mm Hg/mL at relatively low ICP levels), can also provide an early warning of impending herniation. Decreasing VPR can indicate effectiveness of therapy even before the ICP starts to fall.[152,186]

What is the significance of ICP elevation? Most of the clinical signs attributed to ICP in brain trauma are actually produced by effects on brain or cerebral circulation caused by the same processes that elevate the pressure.[96,187] Increased ICP alone, as in pseudotumor cerebri, is associated only with headache, vomiting, papilledema, and drowsiness even at pressures as high as 90 mm Hg. Brain damage or distortion, as by hematoma, causes the reflex, cardiovascular, and respiratory changes characteristic of brain injury. Ischemia can exacerbate the symptoms produced by brain damage. Nevertheless, the importance of ICP control in the treatment of brain trauma is beyond question. Most therapeutic measures are directed at preventing or reducing elevated ICP, and its level is one of the prime criteria of therapeutic effectiveness. Indeed, there is a strong correlation between ICP level and outcome.[17,170,285] The prognosis of patients with persistent or irreversibly high ICP (>30 mm Hg) is ominous. There is some dispute in the literature as to what pressures should cause concern. According to the generally accepted criteria, normal ICP is 10 mm Hg or less, ICP of 10 to 20 mm Hg is marginally elevated and requires careful observation, and any ICP above 20 mm Hg should be treated urgently.[184,187]

CPP is defined as the difference between mean arterial pressure (MAP) and intracranial pressure (CPP = MAP − ICP). As Fig 10-5 shows, decreasing CPP may be responsible for extension of secondary injury in the presence of cerebral edema.[144] Thus, maintenance of the systemic blood pressure is critically important in treatment of brain injury. CPP should be maintained around 70 to 110 mm Hg to ensure adequate blood supply to the brain.[187] About 20% of patients with increased ICP develop systemic hypertension, the Cushing response.[52,157,239] Although a moderate rise in arterial pressure may help maintain the CPP, an exaggerated effect may be harmful. By increasing filtration pressure in the damaged area, it may increase brain swelling, resulting in further elevation of ICP and extension of ischemia.[71,92,157,245] Management of blood pressure must tread the fine path between maintenance of cerebral perfusion and exacerbation of cerebral edema.

The significance of CBF in brain injury is a more problematic topic. Although there are variations in perfusion among different areas of the brain and between white and gray matter, total CBF normally averages approximately 50 mL/100 g of brain tissue/min. In normal brain, CBF remains constant over a wide range of CPP (40 to 140 mm Hg) as the arterioles constrict with increasing pressure.[187,246] The influence of $CO_2$ is pronounced and virtually linear at $Paco_2$ levels between 20 and 80 mm Hg; a $Paco_2$ increase of 1 mm Hg will increase CBF by approximately 1.0 to 1.5 mL/100 g/min. Arterial oxygen tension has no effect on CBF until hypoxic levels are reached (about 40 mm Hg), below which CBF rises with decreasing $Pao_2$ (see Fig 10-9).[246] This autoregulation is lost, partially or completely, in areas of brain injury, probably because of local increase in lactic acid concentration[16,42,60,121,155,271]. CBF rises or falls with the systemic blood pressure; the vasculature may not respond to

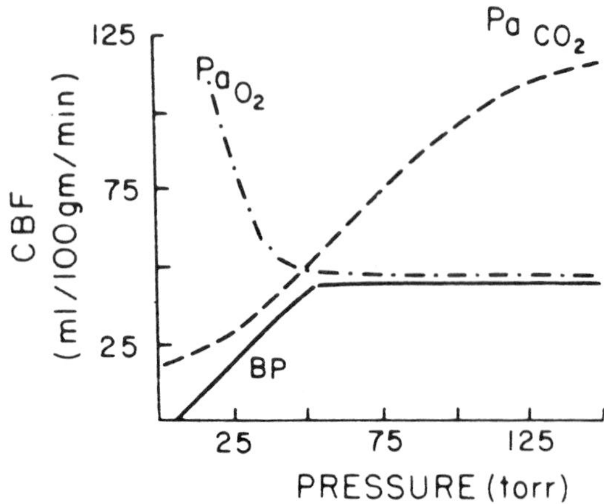


FIG. 10-9. Cerebral blood flow response to changes in $Pao_2$, $Paco_2$, and mean arterial pressure. At MAP above 150 mm Hg, CBF rises with the blood pressure. (From Shapiro[246] with permission.)

blood gas changes. As a result, wide variations in blood flow may be found between injured and normal regions of the brain.[205] Thus, production of vasoconstriction, eg, by decreasing $Paco_2$, in the uninjured region may shunt blood to the damaged area ("inverse steal" phenomenon)[86] unless extensive intravascular coagulation or severe perivascular exudation has occurred, in which case circulation in the area of injury remains low ("no-reflow" phenomenon).[80,182]

Studies have shown no significant correlation between CBF and ICP[73] or between CBF and severity of injury or prognosis.[204] The change in CBF during the course of treatment is significant, however; increasing flow is associated with improvement, whereas decreases indicate a fatal outcome.[147] Obviously, an adequate blood flow (15 mL/100 g of brain/min is regarded as minimal under normal circumstances)[205,255] is required to maintain oxygen supply to the brain. It is likely that considerably higher flows are needed to areas of injury in order to control the accumulation of lactic acid and prevent or limit secondary injury.[16,96]

Since there is one (occasionally incompetent) valve in the internal jugular[67] and no valves in the vertebral veins, cerebral venous blood volume is largely dependent on CVP and head elevation. Thus, increased intrathoracic pressure, as from controlled ventilation, coughing, or straining; hypervolemia; jugular obstruction; or head-down position, can all cause cerebral venodilatation and thereby increase ICP.

### *Respiration and Respiratory Therapy*

Normal respiration in the presence of head trauma generally indicates a mild, unilateral injury in an easily arousable patient. More severe injuries are associated with several types of abnormal ventilatory patterns.[23,82,130] These patterns are generally not reliable indicators of the type or extent of brain damage.[129] However, they are sufficiently varied to justify a brief description.

Central neurogenic hyperventilation is commonly associated with severe cerebral acidosis and/or localized hypoxia,[65,129] pontine damage, and tentorial herniation,[145] although it may (also) be a reflection of the marked increase in metabolism characteristic of brain trauma. It is the most frequent type of abnormal respiration in the head-injured patient. Although hypocapnia is usually mild, occasionally hyperventilation may lower the $Pa_{CO_2}$ so far that severe vasoconstriction may produce cerebral hypoxia.

There are three types of phasic respiration. Some patients exhibit a regular, cyclic variation in respiratory depth (hyperventilation followed by hypoventilation) without apneic periods, called *Cheyne-Stokes variant*. This pattern is generally associated with a rather mild degree of coma.

True Cheyne-Stokes respiration consists of a regular cycle of hyperventilation followed by apnea. It probably results from an exaggerated ventilatory response to increasing $Pa_{CO_2}$, which causes hyperpnea, which in turn lowers the $Pa_{CO_2}$ to the point at which the respiratory drive is abolished until reaccumulation of $CO_2$ again stimulates hyperventilation.[82] Cheyne-Stokes respiration is seen in deep coma and generally indicates a severe injury.

Ataxic ventilation is characterized by inspiratory and expiratory phases that are irregular in both rate and amplitude, with intervening periods of apnea. This pattern is also expressed as gasping or cluster breathing with expiratory pauses. The respiratory rate is usually slow, and minute ventilation is markedly decreased. This is usually an indicator of brainstem damage and is almost always a terminal sign.

Despite these abnormal ventilatory patterns, most patients maintain a relatively normal $Pa_{CO_2}$. However, 85% of victims of severe head injury exhibit an alveolar-arterial $O_2$ gradient of 20 mm Hg or more; occasionally it is severe enough to produce hypoxia.[129] The $O_2$ gradient is probably the result of a ventilation/perfusion ($\dot{V}/\dot{Q}$) mismatch (shunting of air to underperfused alveoli as a result of bronchiolar constriction) and probably also of some degree of interstitial edema. Thus, assisted or controlled ventilation may be necessary in almost any severely head-injured patient. Even in those with severe neurogenic hyperventilation, respiratory control will allow the $Pa_{CO_2}$ to increase and thus raise CBF to more adequate levels. In addition, increased $F_{IO_2}$ permits improved oxygenation of the brain.

Criteria for mechanical ventilation are in some dispute, but the following are reasonable.

1. Respiratory distress, a rate >30/min or <10/min, or an abnormal respiratory pattern
2. Motor posturing or absence of response to pain[174]
3. Abnormal or deteriorating blood gas values
4. Repeated convulsions[174]
5. Signs of aspiration, pneumonitis, or pulmonary edema
6. Increased or increasing ICP
7. Requirement for potent analgesics or sedatives for pain, restlessness, or posturing[174]
8. Concurrent severe pulmonary, cardiac, or upper abdominal injury.

Ventilation is monitored by blood gases and ICP response. A $Pa_{CO_2}$ of 25 to 30 mmHg will usually result in decrease of ICP to normal or near-normal levels.[19,97] $Pa_{CO_2}$ may be lowered, if necessary, to 20 mm Hg, but this should be done only with great care: the extreme vasoconstriction resulting from $Pa_{CO_2}$ below this level may cause inadequate blood flow to the brain and thus cerebral hypoxia. In the normal subject, the cerebrovascular response to hypocarbia is maintained for only about 5 hours.[222] This has raised some question of the value of long-term hyperventilation in the treatment of cerebral edema.[132,269] However, a sustained decrease in CBF seems to occur with prolonged hypocarbia in brain-injured children.[32,114] and probably in brain-injured adults as well.[96] Even after cerebral blood volume (CBV) returns to normal, hypocapnia produces a continuing increase in CSF absorption which may help maintain ICP control.[13] In the adult, continuous ventilatory support not only helps to control the ICP but also prevents hypoxic brain damage resulting from unexpected apnea, respiratory obstruction, or respiratory insufficiency.[19] Mechanical ventilation should be continued until the patient becomes alert enough to follow two-stage commands or until the ICP remains normal for several days—usually a week or less[19]—although in some cases, 2 to 3 weeks of ventilatory support may be necessary.[96] Whether maintenance of hypocarbia is beneficial in adults for this length of time has not been demonstrated conclusively.[269]

Occasionally the patient may resist the ventilator. Chlorpromazine (25 mg, intramuscularly, every 6 hours) or a small dose (1 to 3 mg) of intravenous morphine will usually allow ventilatory assistance or control without unduly masking the neurologic status.[19,165] These agents may not be sufficient in the presence of severe central hyperventilation, and intermittent doses of intravenous muscle relaxants—pancuronium is most usually recommended,[156] vecuronium and atracurium may also be used—may be required. Inability to monitor neurologic signs seems a small price for the benefits obtained from adequate ventilatory control.

Pulmonary physiotherapy, tracheal suctioning, and bronchoscopy are particularly hazardous in the presence of coma. Severe increases of ICP may result from hypercarbia; struggling, or coughing during these maneuvers. The use of sedatives, lidocaine, and/or muscle relaxation with adequate preoxygenation will help limit the patient's reaction to tracheal stimulation. Occasionally, general anesthesia may be required.[65,165,246,278] Controversy exists regarding the optimal route of lidocaine administration to prevent ICP responses to tracheal instrumentation. Although some authors prefer intratracheal instillation,[286] others advise intravenous injection.[113]

### *Diuretics*

The osmotic diuretics exert their beneficial effects primarily on uninjured regions of the brain; blood-brain barrier disruption in the injured region prevents the development of an osmotic gradient.[65,165,246,278] Mannitol is the most commonly used of these agents. Urea is effective in smaller doses, being a smaller molecule, and may be useful in patients who cannot tolerate the volume load required in mannitol therapy.

The standard dose of mannitol is 1.0 to 1.5 g/kg.[55] However, Marshall et al[169] have shown that doses as small as 0.25 g/kg are equally effective, although for a somewhat shorter time, as larger amounts. They demonstrated that a rise in serum osmolarity of 10 mOsm or more is sufficient to lower ICP generally to normal levels. The lower dose permits prolonged use of mannitol to maintain the decrease in ICP. Two dosage schedules are recommended: 0.25 g/kg every 4 hours on a fixed schedule[169] or 20 g as needed, titrated to the patient's ICP.[175] Mannitol has three effects in brain injury: dehydration of the normal brain, as we have already mentioned; increasing CBF and cardiac output, probably by decreasing blood viscosity[30,157,179,196]; and constricting cerebral vessels.[235] It should be noted that the VPR (and the patient's clinical status) may improve before and to a greater degree than the actual fall in ICP.[108,139] Osmotic diuretics are not recommended if serum osmolarity is above 320 mOsm since such a severe increase in osmotic pressure may produce acute renal failure and electrolyte disturbances.[133,182]

Discontinuance of osmotic therapy may be associated with significant ICP "rebound," probably because the serum osmolarity falls below that of the tissues, and water is thus shifted from the vasculature into the brain. This effect is more pronounced if osmolarity is very high.[246] Rebound can probably be moderated by limitation of fluid intake,[118] but this is difficult to recommend in a situation in which hypotension is at least as devastating as a brief elevation of ICP.

In children, head injury may be associated with cerebral hyperemia. Since mannitol may raise CBF and CBV, an increase in ICP may occur, and the patient's condition may deteriorate. Bruce et al[32,33] recommend withholding mannitol therapy until the ICP is known and then using it in the smallest effective doses. Of course, mannitol should not be withheld in children with rapidly progressive deficit and evidence of tentorial herniation since it may be lifesaving in this situation.

The loop diuretics, furosemide and ethacrynic acid, are somewhat controversial. Although they do not reliably lower ICP,[280] they may help reduce the extent of secondary brain injury by decreasing glial swelling.[24,187,265] Indeed, early studies show some evidence of increased survival in patients treated with ethacrynic acid.[287] However, controlled clinical trials have yet to be performed. These agents may aid in preventing hypervolemia and/or pulmonary congestion if given before mannitol therapy.[32,55] They may also potentiate the rate and duration of ICP reduction produced by mannitol.[189,214,228,280] Whether the loop diuretics should be used without mannitol in the therapy of brain injury, however, is a question that remains unanswered.

Occasionally the ICP may become progressively resistant to the effects of diuretics. Worthley et al[283] found that 100 to 250 mL of saline, 5 mmol/mL (29.2%), produced a profound and prolonged decrease in ICP and improved renal function in two patients exhibiting this problem. It appears that these patients had been overtreated with mannitol and were permitted to become hypovolemic. The effect of the saline was thus to increase extracellular fluid volume at the expense of the intracellular compartment. Although it is too early to recommend its routine use, hypertonic saline seems a logical solution in cases similar to these.

### *Steroids*

The controversy surrounding the use of steroids in brain injury has already been mentioned in the discussion of initial therapy. There is no question that usual dose levels of steroids are ineffective.[223] Faupel et al[75] and Gobiet et al[93,94] reported significant reductions in mortality following high dosage schedules of dexamethasone; the former used 100 mg initially and after 6 hours, followed by 4 mg every 6 hours; the latter used 48 mg initially followed by 8 mg every 2 hours during the first and third days and 4 mg every 2 hours on the second and fourth. Miller and Leech[186] demonstrated a sustained decrease in VPR following betamethasone in head-injured patients. Steroid therapy is generally continued for 7 to 8 days. It is possible that like the loop diuretics, steroids reduce the extent of secondary brain injury. Since they are efficient free-radical acceptors, they may prevent membrane disruption by this mechanism.[59] Animal studies show a decreased no-reflow zone following focal ischemia if dexamethasone is administered.[36]

On the other hand, Tornheim and McLaurin[264] could not demonstrate any significant decrease in cerebral edema following dexamethasone in head-injured cats, and Gudeman et al[104] found that high-dose methylprednisolone caused no improvement in ICP, VPR, or survival over low-dose steroids in a clinical study. Similar results were obtained in a group of brain-injured patients with increased ICP given high-dose dexamethasone.[56] The lack of effect on death rate has been confirmed in recent prospective studies by Cooper et al[44] and Braakman et al.[26] It is possible that the doses used in these studies have been too small. Giannotta et al[89] have shown significant improvement in mortality and recovery of speech in patients under 40 years of age receiving very high doses of methylprednisolone (30 mg/kg, two doses 6 hours apart, then 250 mg every 6 hours for six doses, then tapering over 8 days) over those receiving lower doses (ie, doses used in other studies) or placebo. It is also possible that the timing of the first dose is important because circulatory disturbances in the damaged region may prevent the drug from reaching the involved area unless it is given within a short time after injury. The incidence of complications in head-injured patients receiving steroids has been described as decreased,[93] unchanged,[27,167,212] or increased[62,104] by different authors. Although many centers have used high-dose steroid therapy, at least until recently, the questions about its real value in brain injury remain unanswered.[182,192]

### *Anticonvulsants*

Seizure activity in the brain is associated with severe increases in cerebral metabolic rate and resultant vasodilatation. These carry obvious risks of increased ICP, and—if CBF cannot increase adequately—of cerebral hypoxia and acidosis. Note that these effects occur even when motor responses are blocked, as by muscle relaxants or paraplegia. Thus, any patient whose brain injury is severe enough to require intensive care should be treated with prophylactic anticonvulsants.[213] Phenytoin is given in two doses of 250 mg on the first day followed by 100 mg twice a day thereafter. Larger doses may be needed if seizures occur at this dosage level. In patients who are sensitive to phenytoin, phenobarbital may be substituted in doses of 32 mg every 8 hours.[248]

### *General Management (see Table 10-2)*

The patient is kept in semi-Fowler's position, with 20 to 30 degrees of head elevation, in order to decrease jugular venous pressure and cerebral vascular volume by increasing venous drainage.[1,70,210] The head should be maintained in neutral position, by padding if necessary, since rotation, flexion, or extension of the neck may block the jugular veins and increase ICP.[1,120] Temperature is best kept within normal limits. Hyperpyrexia unrelated to infection is seen in about 15% of brain injuries as a result of blood in the ventricles or damage to the hypothalamus or brainstem. It is associated with increased cerebral metabolic requirement and thus represents an additional stress to the injured brain. The usual therapy—ice packs or cold blanket, rectal aspirin, alcohol sponging—should be instituted promptly. Decreasing body temperature might, theoretically, offer the advantage of reducing the cerebral oxygen requirement. However, a therapeutic effect of induced hypothermia has never been demonstrated in cerebral trauma.

As we have already mentioned, blood pressure should be controlled to maintain a CPP of 70 to 110 mm Hg.[236] Hypotension is usually best treated by fluid replacement. This may seem paradoxic in a patient receiving diuretics, but the purpose of mannitol therapy is to dehydrate the brain, not to reduce the blood volume. A normal or somewhat decreased volume of slightly hyperosmolar plasma is the desired therapeutic aim. Thus, fluid losses should be monitored and carefully replaced. Vasopressors should be used cautiously if at all, since their effect on CBF is not well defined. If one is needed, dopamine, with its primarily inotropic action, would seem the best choice.

Hypertension associated with head injury is the result of increased catecholamine production and is thus characterized by increased cardiac output and cardiac work, tachycardia, and normal or somewhat decreased systemic and pulmonary vascular resistance.[41] Sudden increases in blood pressure are usually the result of brain shift or increasing ICP or both. Thus, the initial response to a hypertensive episode should be directed at these factors since reduction of arterial pressure in this situation may severely compromise cerebral perfusion.[182] If ICP is unchanged and no brain shift has occurred, the logical treatment would seem to be β-adrenergic blockade. Indeed propranolol has been shown, in a small group of patients, to bring cardiovascular indices back to, or toward, normal.[231] No ICP change was noted following administration of propranolol in doses as high as 26 mg. The drug is administered at a rate of 1 mg/min until systolic pressure falls below 160 mm Hg, pulse decreases to 55, or pulmonary capillary wedge pressure increases beyond 18 mm Hg. Labetalol, intravenously, in divided doses up to 60 to 100 mg, is effective in reducing blood pressure.[281] Based on our experience, reduction of blood pressure is not associated with ICP elevation in postoperative neurosurgical patients. The drug may be administered as an infusion (1 to 2 mg/min after an initial bolus dose) under close monitoring. Although long considered the antihypertensive agent of choice in head injury, hydralazine may further increase heart rate and cardiac work and has been associated, at least in some patients, with increased ICP.[76,250] Although these results are preliminary, it would seem best to reserve hydralazine (5 to 20 mg) for those cases in which propranolol or labetalol is ineffective. Nitroglycerine and nitroprusside are rapid, potent, and easily controllable agents but are contraindicated in head injury: they cause marked cerebral vasodilatation and may thus increase ICP.[87,107,257]

Intravenous fluids should be supplemented or replaced after 3 or 4 days by oral or tube feeding if there are no gastrointestinal problems (bleeding, diarrhea) to preclude it. If the patient cannot tolerate feedings, total parenteral nutrition (TPN) should be instituted at this time.

Several studies have indicated that parenteral nutrition is associated with better outcome than enteral feeding, possibly because greater amounts of both protein and calories can be administered by this route.[224,229,288] However, a recent controlled prospective study by Young et al[288] showed no significant long-term advantage of TPN over tube feeding, although patients in the former group tended toward a somewhat more rapid neurologic recovery.

Nitrogen balance and respiratory quotient should be monitored carefully during the weeks after injury. Patients with severe cerebral trauma (particularly those with midbrain syndrome) tend to develop a severe hypermetabolic state that lasts about a week, peaking around the third day.[62,63,138] They require a relatively high caloric and protein intake to avoid cachexia, with its attendant possibilities of decubitus ulcers and urinary tract infection.[40,76,108,224,229] Hyperalimentation, however, should be administered cautiously because it may induce hypercarbia.

Hyperglycemia is common after severe head injury.[61,207,220,230] It may result from both the nonspecific response to stress (see Chapter 22) and abnormalities of cerebral metabolism.[230] Although high blood glucose levels seem to correlate with poorer survival, at least in adults,[207,220] it is not known whether these results can be altered by treatment. It may be that neither insulin nor exogenous glucose has any effect at all on outcome.

ICP is monitored until it stabilizes, hopefully at a normal level, for about 24 hours. This usually means maintaining the transducer for 3 to 8 days. If an intraventricular catheter is used, it should probably be removed after 8 days under any circumstances, since the incidence of complications, especially infection, increases with time.[198] However, a recent study in pediatric brain-injured patients suggests that infection risk declines after 6 days, and a single ICP monitoring device may be used as long as necessary, provided surveillance cultures are followed daily.[136]

### *Newer Therapies and Future Possibilities*

Of the newer therapeutic modalities, the barbiturates have been extensively tested clinically. Several studies by Marshall and Shapiro et al[168,171] indicate considerable effectiveness in reducing ICP in patients unresponsive to standard therapy. The value of these agents in the absence of mannitol and hyperventilation is questionable. Sichez et al[249] have reported favorable results from a barbiturate regimen and ventricular drainage, but it is impossible on the basis of their data to make statistical comparisons with other reports.

The therapeutic effect of barbiturates may result from any of several different actions: reduction of ICP by cerebral vasoconstriction (probably the major effect), reduction of cerebral metabolism and oxygen requirement,[137,189] prevention of intravascular coagulation, and reduction of free-radical damage to brain cells.[78,95,188]

Although good results have been reported,[201] serious questions remain about the influence of barbiturates on survival or long-term morbidity.[182,211] In a recent study, Ward et al[274] demonstrated that barbiturate coma offers no benefits and may increase the incidence of complications when used in the absence of intractable intracranial hypertension. In any event, the increased difficulty of care and neurologic evaluation should restrict the use of this therapy to those cases in which a clear indication exists[72,171]: a persistent ICP above 25 mm Hg despite hyperventilation, mannitol, and ventricular drainage. Before barbiturate therapy, mass lesions should be treated surgically, and the patient must be normovolemic (MAP > 70, pulmonary artery diastolic pressure > 8). A Swan-Ganz catheter is necessary in addition to the arterial line and ICP transducer in order to assess both intravascular volume and cardiac output. Rectal temperature should not be allowed to fall below 32°C since severe cardiac arrhythmias, particularly in younger patients, and problems of gas exchange with resultant hypoxia may be caused by the combination of barbiturates and hypothermia.[165,211,227]

Pentobarbital (5 to 10 mg/kg) is administered intravenously as an initial dose and repeated until the ICP falls below 20 mm Hg (preferably below 15 mm Hg) or until serum barbiturate levels are 3 to 5 mg %.[15,165] Levels above 5 mg % seem to offer no increase in therapeutic effect. At these levels, severe burst suppression will be seen on the electroencephalogram (EEG) (it may become isoelectric),[137] deep tendon reflexes may disappear, and the patient usually becomes apneic.[165] The only way to monitor the patient's neurologic status reliably is by evoked potentials and, if these deteriorate, by CT scanning.[68,211]

Barbiturate levels are maintained by infusion at 3 to 5 mg % until ICP remains normal for 24 to 48 hours.[15] The dosage is then tapered gradually over 4 days to avoid the sudden deterioration that may follow abrupt withdrawal.[165] If ICP increases during this period, therapy should be resumed. Blood gases should be followed carefully since decreased pulmonary compliance may require ventilatory adjustment to prevent hypoxia. Hypotension and/or decreased cardiac output is treated by hydration and, if necessary, by dopamine.[133] It is extremely important that CPP be maintained at adequate levels. If ICP cannot be controlled with barbiturate therapy, a fatal outcome is virtually certain.[168,171]

Dimethyl sulfoxide (DMSO) has shown beneficial effects in experimental brain injury[35,58,268] and early clinical trials.[166] It is almost as effective in reducing ICP as pentobarbital[124] without producing alteration of consciousness or hypotension. Like mannitol, the ICP reduction is associated with increased cerebral blood flow.[31] It is not without its own problems, however. DMSO is a very potent diuretic, and unlike mannitol, it can produce significant electrolyte disturbances at therapeutic dose levels. Intravascular hemolysis is regularly seen with higher concentrations, and there may also be some decrease in platelet function. Much more work is obviously needed, both in the laboratory and clinically, if DMSO is to be established in treatment of brain injury.

Etomidate has already been described as an induction agent in the discussion of anesthesia management. It has also been used for long-term management of comatose patients, both as a continuous drip for maintenance of sedation and ICP control and, in bolus doses, to control elevation of ICP and the response to tracheal suctioning.[57,115,218] No attempts have been made to compare its efficacy with that of barbiturates in cases in which ICP could not be controlled by hyperventilation, diuretics, and steroids. By continuous infusion of 0.4 to 1.5 mg/kg/h, etomidate is capable of maintaining adequate sedation and ICP control in most head-injured patients.[57,115,218] Its effects are completely reversed within an hour following cessation of the drip, allowing evaluation of ICP and neurologic status.[115] Bolus doses (0.2 mg/kg) are capable of reducing acute ICP elevations and of preventing the increased ICP caused by chest physiotherapy.[218]

Unfortunately, etomidate is a potent inhibitor of adrenal steroid production and thus blocks the normal physiologic response to stress.[48,272,273] This effect may last for as much as 4 hours after a single dose[79,272] and 4 days after a 20-hour infusion.[273] Although no ill effects have been reported from the brief episodes of adrenal suppression induced by single doses, Ledingham and Watt[150] suggest that long-term use may be associated with increased mortality in multiply injured patients. Their data are retrospective and uncontrolled, and it is possible that concomitant administration of steroids may prevent this effect, if it exists.[273] Nevertheless, it would seem prudent to avoid the use of etomidate in head-injured patients until those questions are answered, unless the benefits derived from its use outweigh the possible hazards.

Propofol is a short-acting, rapidly metabolized intravenous anesthetic agent that has been used in Europe for several years and, has recently been released in the United States. Its use is associated with cardiovascular stability and lack of cumulative effect even after prolonged administration, like etomidate, without significant inhibition of steroidogenesis. It has been administered to a small number of head-injured patients, both for surgical anesthesia[284] and for sedation in the intensive care unit.[74] Arterial blood pressure, ICP, and CPP were well maintained in the latter group of patients throughout a 24-hour infusion (mean dose, 2.88 mg/kg/h). Whether it is capable of reducing an uncontrollable increase in ICP is a question that remains to be answered. If so, it may ultimately prove to be preferable to the barbiturates in this situation.

Several new approaches to medical therapy have been described recently in preliminary studies. CG 3703, a thyrotropin-releasing hormone analog[176]; U-50488H, a κ-opioid receptor agonist[110]; U-74006F, a 21-aminosteroid without corticoid activity[111,293]; and L-644,711, a nondiuretic derivative of the loop diuretics[14], have all been shown to improve survival in head-injured animals. Although clinical evaluation of these or similar drugs is well in the future, it is encouraging to contemplate agents that would be effective without at the same time increasing the difficulty of the patient's care.

An established research technique has been utilized recently in an attempt to refine the management of intracranial hypertension.[10,11,49,240] Catheterization of the jugular bulb with a cannula passed retrograde via the internal jugular vein permits sampling of venous drainage from the brain. A modification of the Fick equation yields

$$\frac{CMRO_2}{CBF} = Cao_2 - Cjvo_2 = AJDo_2$$

where $Cao_2 - Cjvo_2$ is the oxygen content difference between arterial and jugular bulb blood. The left side of the equation represents the relationship between cerebral oxygen demand (cerebral metabolic rate for $O_2$) and oxygen supply (CBF). Normally this ratio is approximately 6. Thus, an increased $AJDo_2$ in a head-injured patient with increased ICP implies that further reduction in CBF, for instance by decreasing $Paco_2$, may lead to cerebral ischemia.[49] The indicated therapy would be to use an agent such as mannitol, which lowers ICP while increasing CBF. On the other hand, a patient with cerebral hyperemia will exhibit a decreased $AJDo_2$ and will probably benefit from hyperventilation since the decrease in $Paco_2$ will bring the CBF into a more normal relation with the $CMRo_2$. The technique may also be helpful in evaluating the effects of antihypertensive medications or barbiturates on the cerebral oxygen supply-demand ratio.

Jugular bulb catheterization may thus offer significant help in the treatment of head-injured patients. There are two limitations to its use.[10] The technique should be restricted to patients who have a diffuse injury, have not suffered a stroke, and do not have a large midline shift or other major focal abnormalities on CT scan. Also, the leftward shift in the hemoglobin dissociation curve caused by alkalosis affects $Cjvo_2$ and may decrease the reliability of $AJDo_2$ measurement in the aggressively hyperventilated patient.[49]

Further experience is needed to determine how often and in which patients management decisions may be altered by knowledge of $AJDo_2$. Questions also remain as to whether there are risks, and if so, what and how great they are, attendant on inserting a catheter into an already unstable cerebral circulation.

Evoked potentials (EPs) also offer the possibility of improvement in evaluation of the comatose patient. The technique involves enhancement of the weak signal produced in the brain by sensory stimulation, and elimination of the "noise" (from the brain's random electric activity, from muscle activity, or from outside electrical interference) that would otherwise mask it. This is accomplished by superimposing a large number of traces, generally 200 to 1000 depending on the sensory modality tested. Fourier transformation increases the signal-to-noise ratio and speeds the analysis, but greater computational capacity is required. The timing (latency) and amplitude of the various waves produced by the stimulus can be analyzed to evaluate both the location and the severity of injury to the brainstem and/or higher centers. Three modalities may be tested: somatosensory (SEP), using the median and/or sural nerves; auditory (AEP), a series of clicks; or visual (VEP), using a flashing light. The short latency waves of the SEP and AEP (<20 msec) indicate brainstem activity and may be analyzed separately (BEP)[99,100] (Fig 10-10).

Thus, EPs are potent indicators of functional capacity over a wide area of the brain, in contrast to, for instance, the CT scan or ICP measurement, which show only anatomic derangement. They have several uses in brain injury. They may provide the only means of neurologic evaluation of the patient receiving muscle relaxants or barbiturates and can demonstrate functional improvement or deterioration in the course of these therapies.[69,200] They indicate the degree and localization of cortical or brainstem impairment in the presence of coma and show which sensory areas are preserved.[99,102,131,225] Most important, EPs are a powerful prognostic tool: recovery

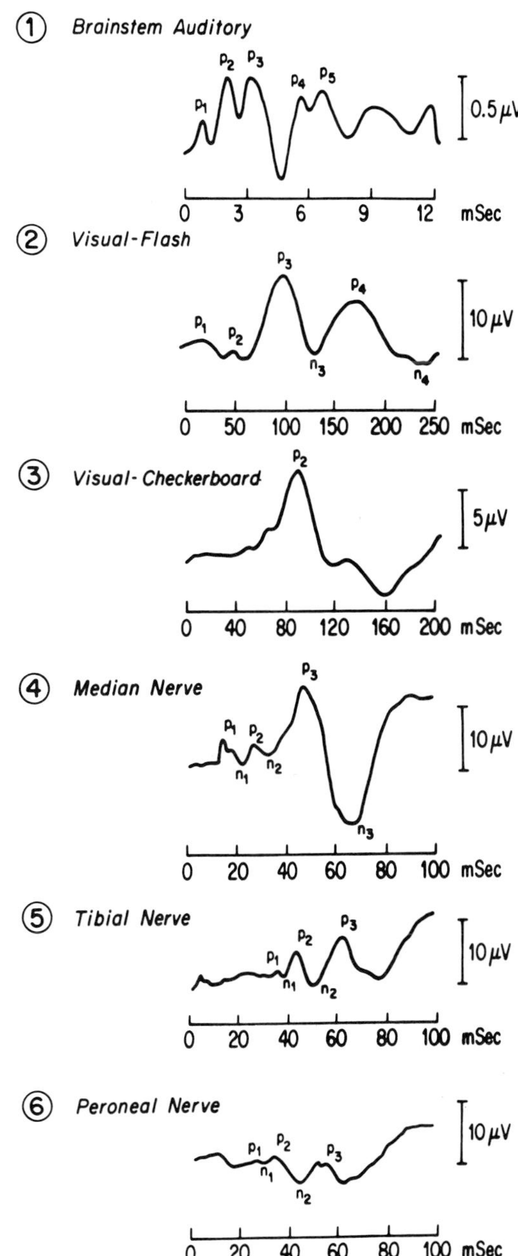


FIG. 10-10. Normal evoked potentials. Different neural pathways produce widely diverse waveforms. (Courtesy of Robert Chabot, PhD, and E. Roy John, PhD.)

is strongly indicated by a moderately altered EP pattern, whereas the patient with marked, diffuse abnormalities will almost certainly have a poor result if he survives[101,197,200,226] (Fig 10-11). Indeed Rappaport et al[226] described a patient in extreme coma who had moderate EP alterations on admission which improved despite persistence of the vegetative state for more than 2 weeks. She recovered completely within 5 months.

Unfortunately, performance of a multimodal EP survey (MEP) is a time-consuming procedure on an instrument that requires a considerable degree of skill to operate and gives results that require considerable training to interpret. Wider

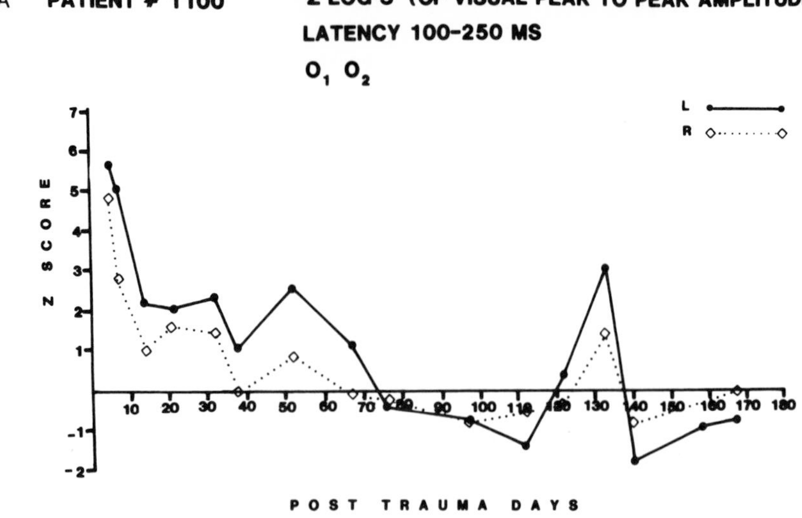


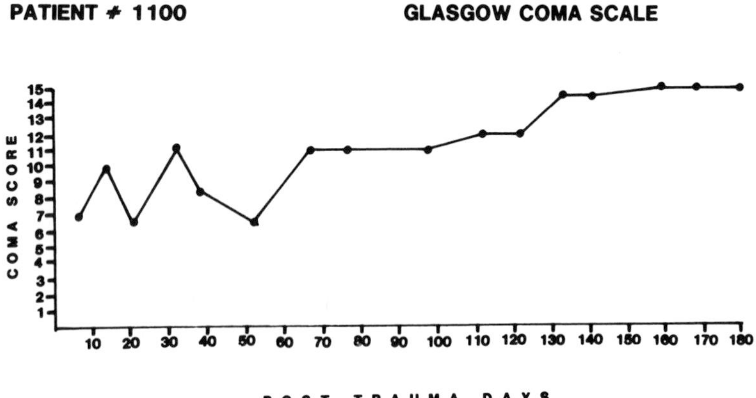


FIG. 10-11. Predictive power of evoked potentials. Variations in latency and amplitude can be analyzed statistically to produce a value, Z, indicating degree of deviation from normal. Since Z is expressed as number of standard deviations from mean normal values, any value beyond ±2 indicates significant derangement. (A) VEPs reached normal values within 2 weeks of injury, although the patient remained comatose for months. This patient eventually recovered with rather severe motor deficits. (B) despite a similar clinical course in the first weeks, this patient's VEPs never approached normal. He remained in a persistent vegetative state and eventually died. (Courtesy of Isabel Alter, PhD, E. Roy John, PhD, and J. Ransohoff, MD.)

use of the technique depends on simplifying both acquisition and interpretation of the data it provides, or alternatively, on an increasing number of people familiar with it. Further experience should also define more precisely the brain regions responsible for the various cortical peaks, particularly those of longer latency, ie, those from association areas. One feels certain that with time EP data will be a most valuable addition to the management of head injury.

## COMPLICATIONS OF SEVERE BRAIN INJURY

The preceding pages have dealt largely with the effects of circulatory and respiratory alterations on the injured brain and conversely with some of the physiologic changes produced by brain damage. It remains to consider the significant pathology that brain injury can induce in other body systems. We can only deal with the most important problems since a complete discussion is beyond the scope of this chapter. The interested reader is referred to Matjasko's excellent review.[173]

### *Pulmonary Complications*

Neurogenic pulmonary edema (NPE) is characterized by the fulminant onset of pulmonary vascular congestion, alveolar hemorrhage, and exudation of protein-rich edema fluid. It is very common in patients who die within an hour of brain injury or hemorrhage,[277] but its incidence decreases with increasing duration of survival. Fortunately, NPE is infrequent, although not unknown, in patients who survive long enough to reach the hospital.

NPE is probably precipitated by the effects of acute brain injury (increased ICP, decreased CPP) on the hypothalamus: massive sympathetic discharge occurs[12,98,195,237] producing a dramatic increase in peripheral vascular resistance and shifting of blood into the pulmonary vasculature. This shift is accompanied by arterial and venous pressure increases in both systemic and pulmonary circulations. Increased pulmonary blood volume and pressure produce structural pulmonary vascular injury and thus alter capillary permeability. Blood and protein-rich fluid can leak from the damaged vessels into the alveoli for a prolonged period, despite the fact that the sympathetic discharge and accompanying cardiovascular changes may cease within minutes.[206,237,261]

Adult respiratory distress syndrome (ARDS) shows a similar clinical and pathologic picture, although its causes may be different. Indeed, it may be difficult to distinguish between them in the head-injured patient. Attempts to differentiate these clinical entities are probably unnecessary since they are

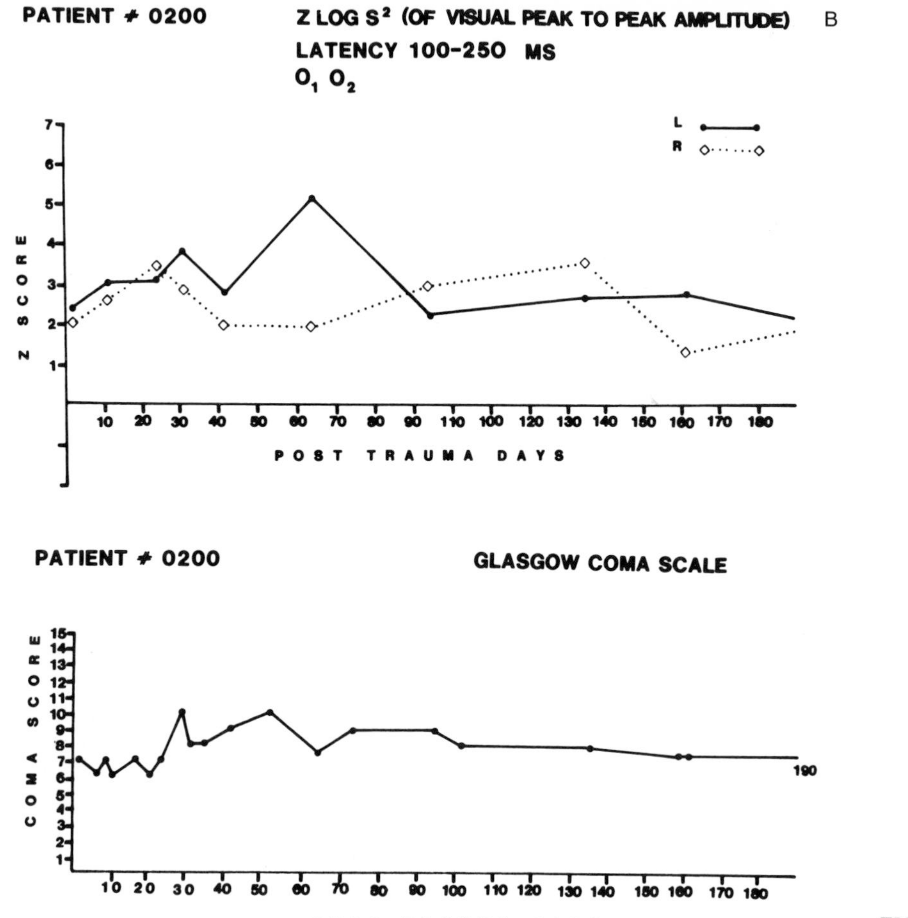


FIG. 10-11. (*Continued*)

treated in the same way. ARDS is the result of pulmonary vascular damage produced by shock, respiratory acidosis, and/or alveolar hypoxia[206] (see Chapter 24). These lead to increased pulmonary vascular resistance and capillary wall disruption. Blood and edema fluid leak into the tissues and alveoli, producing decreased pulmonary compliance, increased intrapulmonary shunt, and increasing hypoxia, which in turn cause further vascular injury. The process may continue until insufficient functional lung remains to maintain life, whatever therapy is used.

Both NPE and ARDS may be prevented by rapid and adequate emergency treatment as already discussed: maintenance of the airway and hyperventilation, control of ICP, and fluid replacement as needed to avoid hypotension.[275] The most vigorous therapy is required for these problems once they occur. In addition to careful fluid replacement (a Swan-Ganz catheter should be used to monitor both pulmonary artery pressures and cardiac output) and ICP control, ventilatory management may be a major problem. $FIO_2$ must be adjusted to maintain adequate $PaO_2$, remembering that a prolonged inspired $O_2$ fraction greater than 0.4 may adversely affect pulmonary gas exchange. The use of positive end-expiratory pressure (PEEP) in head-injured patients is somewhat controversial. Both animal and clinical studies have indicated that usual degrees of PEEP are capable of obstructing jugular venous return, thus increasing CBV and ICP.[6,45,64] However, Frost[81] and Cooper et al[44] have shown that ICP does not increase if the patient is maintained in 30 degree semi-Fowler's position, even at PEEP levels as high as 40 cm $H_2O$. One can conclude, then, that PEEP may be used as required to maintain arterial blood gases but that a 30 degree head-up tilt should be maintained and ICP monitored carefully. It should be recalled that high levels of PEEP are capable of reducing cardiac output[64] and decreasing $O_2$ delivery to the tissues. Adequate hydration is thus critical while PEEP is maintained.

Pulmonary and, rarely, cerebral embolism of fat or venous thrombi is an uncommon cause of pulmonary failure in acute head injury.[173] Embolism is usually seen 24 to 48 hours after trauma and should be considered if pulmonary and/or circulatory deterioration occurs at this time.

### *Cardiac Complications*

The catecholamine release[98] associated with production of NPE also frequently affects the heart. Recent studies[107,177] have shown CPK-MB elevations in almost all the brain-injured patients tested for this enzyme. ECG changes (prolonged QT interval and ST segment depression) were the most common manifestations of cardiac damage. In addition, prolonged sinus tachycardia, sinus arrhythmia, and ventricular tachycardia were seen in this group of patients, two of whom (of the seven in McLeod's study[177]) died—one from lethal cardiac arrhythmias, the other probably from infarction—and two of whom showed evidence of myocardial infarcts but survived.[107]

### Bleeding

Gastrointestinal (GI) bleeding is common following head injury, particularly in comatose patients, nearly 30% of whom show clinical evidence of blood loss from the GI tract.[135] A large proportion of this bleeding is from gastric or esophageal (Cushing's) ulcers classically associated with cerebral pathology.[51] The probable cause of this complication is elevated gastric acidity due to hypothalamic stimulation of vagal activity.[149] Significant hemorrhage or perforation of the stomach or esophagus is thus a common reason for surgery in the postinjury period and should be considered in any patient with abdominal distension, ileus, hypotension, or anemia.[135] The results of a controlled trial of cimetidine (300 mg every 4 hours, intravenously until oral feedings were begun and orally thereafter) have been somewhat equivocal.[112] Although the incidence of GI problems was unchanged, patients receiving cimetidine had a lower incidence of lesions requiring transfusion or surgery. This medication may prove to be a reasonable adjunct to therapy in the head-injured patient.

Clotting disorders, particularly disseminated intravascular coagulation (DIC), are also very common following brain trauma and may represent a significant cause of death from hemorrhage—both intracranial and elsewhere—and intractable cerebral edema.[39,139,190] Associated injuries may also cause DIC, and whether a given case of cerebral hemorrhage has caused or has been caused by DIC may be difficult to determine. Appropriate therapy involves treating the cause, by surgery if necessary, restoring blood volume, and administration of clotting factors such as cryoprecipitate, fresh frozen plasma, and platelets.

### Fluid and Electrolytes

Diabetes insipidus (DI) and inappropriate antidiuretic hormone (ADH) secretion are both reported complications of head trauma.[173] DI is common following basilar skull fractures.[103] Both problems may lead to abnormalities of urine output and electrolyte imbalance. It is important that urine output and serum electrolytes be followed carefully in all severely head-injured patients and that therapy be instituted as soon as problems arise.

## PROGNOSIS AND RESULTS OF THERAPY

The Glasgow outcome scale[127] provides a basis for comparing the results of treatment in different centers and for evaluating new therapeutic measures as they are introduced. There are five categories of results.[127,197]

1. *Good recovery:* complete neurologic recovery or minor deficits that do not prevent the patient from returning to his or her former level of function
2. *Moderately disabled:* deficits present which prevent normal function but allow self-care
3. *Severely disabled:* marked deficits present which prevent self-care
4. *Vegetative:* no evidence of higher mental function
5. *Dead.*

Regardless of the treatment given, several factors are associated with a less favorable prognosis: increasing age, presence of a mass lesion, delay in initial therapy, increased ICP (>40 if mass is present, >20 in diffuse brain swelling), and increasing severity of neurologic abnormalities.[7,34,54,154,170,259] A GCS of less than 5 after 6 hours is almost always associated with a poor outcome, whereas almost all patients with scores greater than 7 at this time make a grade 1 or 2 recovery.[20,88,285] Prognosis is adversely affected in the initial stages of head injury by four avoidable factors: untreated hematoma, hypoxia, hypercarbia, and hypotension.[126,185,234] We have already discussed the vital importance of the earliest possible attention to ventilation and blood volume as a means of minimizing secondary brain injury and avoiding respiratory complications.

Important questions now present themselves. The aggressive management of head injuries requires a large investment of time, equipment, and highly trained personnel. Does this treatment really improve survival?[84] If more patients do survive, what is the quality of their outcome? That is, are we saving them from death only to leave a larger number severely disabled or vegetative—a fate some consider worse than dying? The standard for comparison with newer therapies is the large multinational survey of outcome in 700 cases of brain injury reported by Jennett et al in 1977.[128] Treatment in this study varied widely both within and between the participating institutions: some, but not all patients received hyperventilation, mannitol, and/or steroids. The overall results at 6 months were as follows: dead, 51%; vegetative or severely disabled, 11%; moderate disability, 16%; good recovery, 22%. We may compare these results with those of Miller and his associates[154,164,185] in a group of 158 patients with injuries comparable in severity to those in the earlier study. These patients were treated by a standard protocol of early intubation and ventilation, surgery as required for mass lesions, and continuous monitoring of ICP with aggressive therapy including barbiturates, when necessary, for ICP elevation. They found a 40% mortality, 12% severely disabled or vegetative, and 47% with moderate or no disability. Thus a significant reduction in mortality was achieved with no difference in the incidence of poor results. Other recent studies[17,170,185] also indicate that poor recovery remains around 10% and that any decrease in death rate is associated with an increase in patients making at least an adequate recovery.

A sophisticated statistical analysis of predictive power of the clinical and laboratory data obtainable from head-injured patients has been reported by Narayan et al.[197] They found that although a combination of clinical data (age, GCS, presence of mass lesions, pupillary response, ocular motility, and motor posturing) provided the best single indicator of outcome, the addition of laboratory results could further increase the reliability of predictions based on clinical status. Supplementation of clinical information with MEP results yielded the greatest prognostic power: 89% accuracy with 64% at a 90% confidence level. It should be possible, then, to decide with a high degree of accuracy just which patients are likely to benefit from the prolonged intensive care that may be required to bring them to the best possible neurologic recovery.

## SPINAL CORD INJURIES

The circulation of the spinal cord is more vulnerable to injury than that of the brain. Segmental arteries enter the vertebral canal along the nerve roots and join the longitudinal spinal arteries on the cord surface. The single anterior spinal artery delivers two thirds of the blood supply, and the other third comes from two pairs of posterior spinal arteries (Fig 10-12).[298] There are surface connections between these vessels, but virtually no collateral blood supply exists within the substance of the cord.[298,330] Thus, circulatory disturbance is a prominent aspect of the cord's reaction to injury,[339] a process otherwise similar to, if not identical with, that of the brain (Fig 10-13).[306,310,311,338,355,356] Immediately following blunt trauma or compression, hemorrhages are seen in the central gray matter. Depending on the force applied, a zone of hemorrhage, edema, and necrosis spreads from the central area to involve, in severe injuries, the entire diameter of the cord within 6 to 24 hours.[309,315,355,356] Damage to the gray matter involves only two or three segments at the level of injury. The most significant derangement in spinal cord trauma results from interruption of nerve conduction in the fiber tracts, which isolates the region of the body below the level of injury from cerebral control.

Clinically, there is a generally progressive loss of function during the first 24 hours. As edema subsides or circulation is reestablished, the function in some areas may improve slightly during this period, but in the absence of further injury, the pattern is stable after the first day.[336] The acute stage of spinal cord injury is characterized by loss of nerve function below the injured region: "spinal shock." There is flaccid paralysis of the voluntary muscles, loss of sympathetic tone—and thus hypotension and bradycardia in high thoracic or cervical injuries[348]—and flaccidity of the bladder with urinary retention.

Sympathetic tone returns to some extent in 4 to 7 days. Resting blood pressure returns to, or toward, normal, and there may be a mild hypertensive response (autonomic hyperreflexia) to various stimuli such as pain or bladder distention below the level of the lesion. Reflex activity, of course without higher control, returns after 4 to 6 weeks, and the chronic stage begins. This is characterized by spastic motor paralysis with hyperactive tendon reflexes, occasionally severe autonomic hyperreflexia, and some return of involuntary bladder function. Since the chronic stage is obviously beyond the scope of this chapter, our discussion will be restricted to the management of the patient in spinal shock.

Some terms require definition at this point. *Quadriplegia* or *tetraplegia* is caused by cervical injuries and is characterized by weakness or paralysis of all four extremities. The amount of function remaining in the arms depends, of course, on the level involved, since the brachial plexus originates from the C-5 to T-1 nerve roots. Strictly speaking, *paraplegia* re-

FIG. 10-12. Diagram of spinal cord arterial supply. (From Boyd et al[298] with permission.)

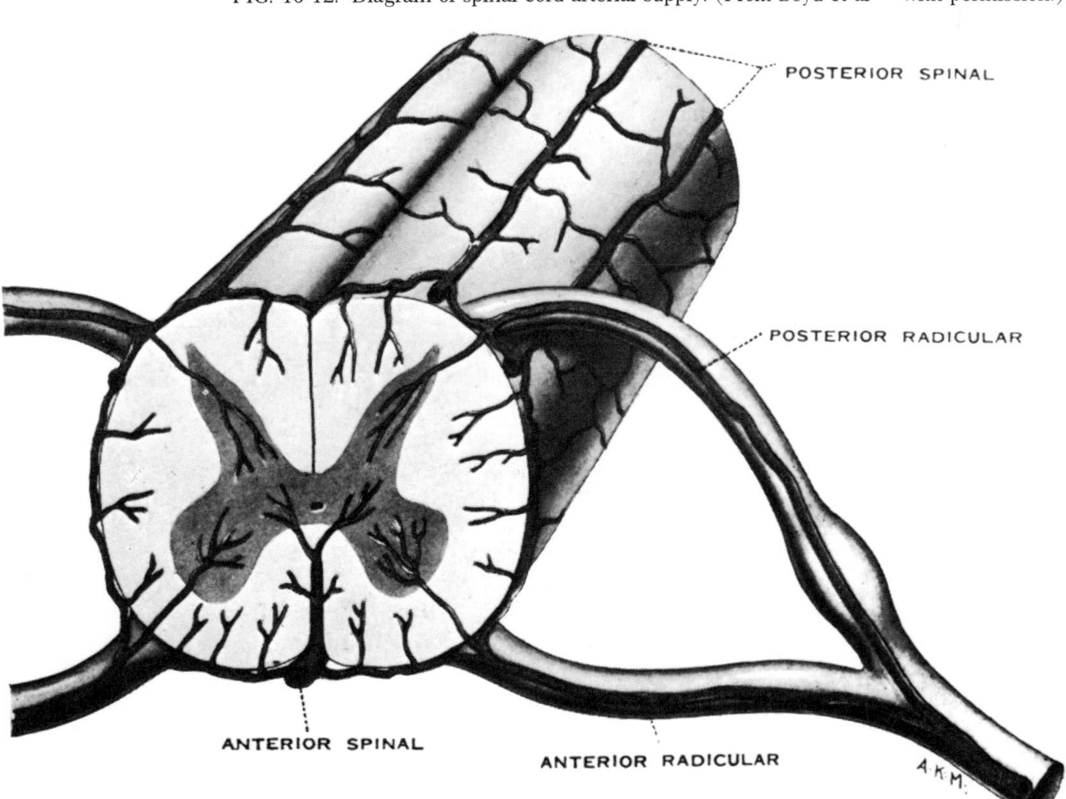

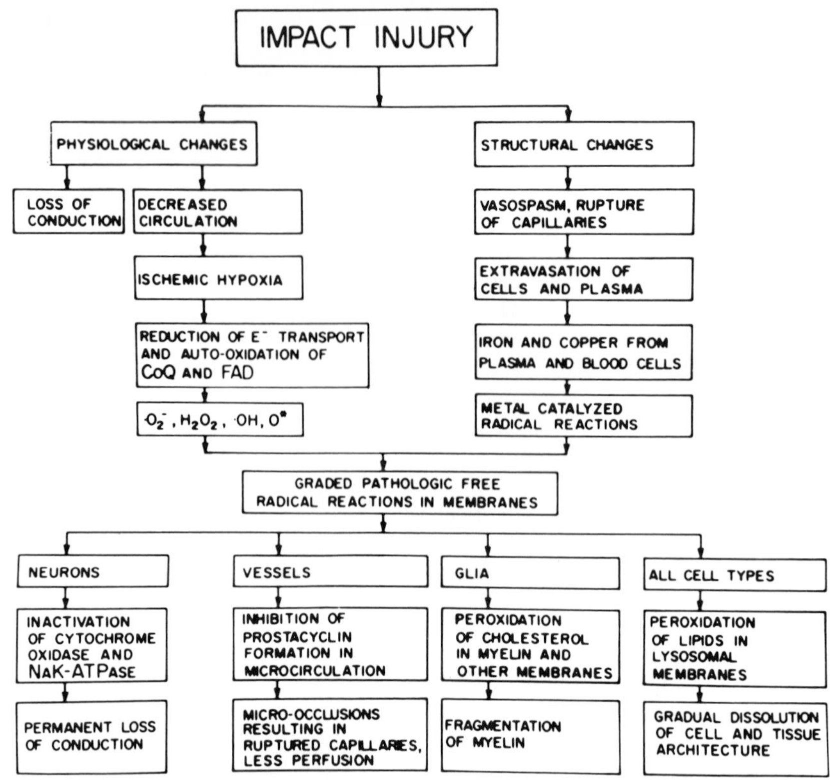


FIG. 10-13. Mechanisms of spinal cord injury. (From Naftchi et al[356] with permission.)

sults from trauma to the thoracic or lumbar spine and thus involves only the lower extremities, although the term is frequently used generically to refer to spinal injury at any level. Lumbar injuries damage the cauda equina and thus produce a peripheral nerve syndrome: flaccid paralysis and bladder atony are permanent, and muscular atrophy, not seen in upper neuron lesions, ultimately results. Total lesions produce complete loss of sensation and motor control below the involved segment; in partial injuries there is some functional sparing, however minimal.

## INITIAL EVALUATION AND TREATMENT

As in brain injury, treatment should be started as soon as possible, preferably at the scene of the accident. This may prevent increased damage to the cord and hopefully limit the secondary injury process.[306,358] Three principles are involved: stabilization of the fracture, maintenance of ventilation, and maintenance of adequate blood pressure.[309,324,333]

At the scene of the accident, the patient is kept in supine position on a flat surface.[359] If a cervical injury may be present, the neck should be fixed in a neutral position by pillows or sandbags. On the patient's admission to the hospital, cervical traction or a halo brace should be applied as soon as possible. Realignment of the spinal canal under X-ray control is the sine qua non of relieving compression and preventing further cord damage.

The phrenic nerve receives fibers mainly from the third and fourth cervical roots, with a smaller contribution from the fifth. Thus, injuries below C-5 are generally associated with adequate ventilation, although the patient's expiratory reserve may be severely diminished (see Table 10-3).[357] Lesions above this level are characterized by ventilatory insufficiency; the patient nearly always requires respiratory support if he is to survive. Even when cord damage is below C-5, ascending cord edema, pulmonary aspiration, or neurogenic pulmonary edema may produce deterioration and necessitate ventilatory support.[305,359,364] Assistance or control of respiration is thus required in patients with obvious signs of respiratory difficulty, history of aspiration or other pulmonary pathology, tachypnea greater than 30 breaths per minute, and/or vital ca-

TABLE 10-3. Expiratory Parameters in Paraplegics During Acute and Chronic Stages*

| | CERVICAL ($n = 6$) | T 1–6 ($n = 5$) | T 7–12 ($n = 9$) | LUMBAR ($n = 3$) |
|---|---|---|---|---|
| FVC 1† | 31.65 | 43.39 | 47.83 | 69.91 |
| 2‡ | 40.78 | 54.81 | 66.69 | 92.23 |
| $FEV_1$ 1† | 37.40 | 56.74 | 44.70 | 58.33 |
| 2‡ | 51.16 | 72.69 | 73.70 | 82.79 |
| $FEV_1$% 1† | 89.30 | 85.20 | 73.10 | 57.00 |
| 2‡ | 90.93 | 92.60 | 83.01 | 64.00 |
| $FEF_{25-75}$ 1† | 89.30 | 85.20 | 73.10 | 57.00 |
| 2‡ | 72.94 | 89.90 | 84.21 | 62.65 |
| PEF 1† | 50 | 58 | 48 | 43 |
| 2‡ | 60 | 54 | 63 | 52 |

* The low values in patients with low thoracic and lumbar levels are probably the result of associated chest injuries. Values are mean percent of predicted in each group (FVC, forced vital capacity; $FEV_1$, forced expiratory volume in 1 second; $FEV_1$%, $FEV_1$/FVC X 100 – timed vital capacity; $FEF_{25-75}$, forced midexpiratory flow; PEF, peak expiratory flow; †, on admission; ‡, after 6 months). (Adapted from Ohry et al[357] with permission.)

pacity less than 500 mL.[329] An arterial line should be inserted in all patients with cervical injuries or in those having thoracic cord damage with associated chest trauma.[367] Any significant adverse change in arterial blood gas values should also be considered an indication for endotracheal intubation.[333]

Intubation may be a major problem in the presence of a cervical fracture since motion of the neck may increase cord compression. It is critically important that hypoxia be corrected by manual ventilation using a mask before the trachea is stimulated by intubation or tracheal suction. Unopposed vagal activity can produce bradycardia and cardiac arrest in hypoxic quadriplegics during airway manipulation.[328,352,353,371] Atropine (0.4 mg, intravenously) will tend to block this reflex somewhat and should be used as a premedicant before tracheal instrumentation is performed.[371]

If possible, intubation should be delayed until the neck is stabilized by tongs or a halo brace. If delay is not possible, an assistant should hold the head firmly in neutral position to prevent further cord damage resulting from movement of the head.[362] The most common type of cervical injury results from flexion of the neck. Thus further flexion, as in the sniffing position, must be avoided, since vertebral dislocation may be increased.[314] Awake nasal intubation, either blind or aided by fiberoptic laryngoscope,[328,353,373] is the method of choice. Sedation may be required to avoid struggling. We generally use small doses of diazepam and fentanyl. The tube is inserted after careful topical anesthesia using 5% cocaine or 4% lidocaine and 0.25 to 0.5% neosynephrine for the nose and 4% lidocaine for the pharynx and trachea. Transtracheal injection should be avoided when a full stomach is suspected. Bilateral superior laryngeal nerve block is recommended by some authors[353] to anesthetize the upper surface of cords and the epiglottis.

In young children or grossly uncooperative (eg, semicomatose) adults or if awake intubation fails, general anesthesia may be required.[314,362] A minimal dose of thiopental is administered to avoid hypotension; lidocaine is given to decrease tracheal reflexes; and pancuronium (0.1 mg/kg), vecuronium (0.1 mg/kg), or atracurium (0.5 mg/kg) is used for muscle relaxation. Succinylcholine is not recommended since (theoretically, at least) muscle fasciculation may exacerbate the cord injury. Because the patient is likely to have gastric dilation, cricoid pressure should be applied in order to prevent regurgitation. This maneuver should be performed with extreme care; too much pressure may further dislocate an unstable fracture.

Airway management after induction of general anesthesia in this group of patients may be associated with the dangers of inability to intubate, airway obstruction, and pulmonary aspiration. The suboptimal position of the head and neck may cause difficulty in directing the tube into the larynx. In addition, patients with extension injuries are commonly fixed in the halo brace with the neck somewhat flexed. In this position, it may be impossible to fit the mask properly to the face between the halo and the chestpiece. The neurosurgeon or orthopedist should be asked to adjust the brace in order to permit airway control. Considering these problems, cricothyroidotomy or tracheostomy may at times be required. This subject is discussed in detail in Chapter 14.

If the quadriplegic patient is permitted to breathe spontaneously, he should be maintained in supine or mild Trendelenburg position so that expiration is facilitated by the pressure of the abdominal contents against the diaphragm.[287] A nasogastric tube should be passed to prevent gastric dilation, and, hopefully, to decrease the risk of regurgitation and aspiration.[287] Decompression of the stomach may also improve ventilatory function. Respiratory problems and their management are discussed in detail in the section on intensive care.

Hypotension is common in patients with high spinal cord injuries because of sympathetic paralysis and vasodilation[266,348] and probably some degree of left ventricular impairment.[351] Although organ blood flow is generally adequate, recent studies have shown that the flow to the cord—especially the damaged area—may be severely decreased.[225,229] Thus, maintenance of the systemic blood pressure may be very important in preventing or at least limiting extension of cord necrosis.[309] Intravenous fluid replacement to a central venous pressure (CVP) or pulmonary capillary wedge pressure (PCWP) of 18 mm Hg seems to be the most efficient means of maintaining cord circulation,[351,359] although too much enthusiasm may result in pulmonary edema.[223] If the patient remains hypotensive despite adequate hydration, atropine, ephedrine, or dopamine will generally restore the blood pressure to normal levels. Naloxone and methylprednisolone may have beneficial effects and will be discussed below.

A central venous line is of great value in management of intravenous fluid replacement. A Swan-Ganz catheter should be inserted for more precise monitoring of hemodynamic status when hypotension is severe or resistant to fluid infusion or if there is evidence of other severe injuries. It may also be useful in diagnosis and management of pulmonary problems.[367] Fluid replacement should be correlated carefully with urine output.[333] A urinary catheter offers the additional benefit of preventing overdistention of the atonic bladder, which may cause urinary tract dysfunction during the chronic stage.[336]

Despite equivocal experimental and clinical results, high dose steroid therapy has been generally accepted for treatment of spinal cord injury.[321,350] However, a large, well-controlled, multicenter clinical study[299] showed that doses of methylprednisolone as high as 1.0 g/day (14.3 mg/kg/day) for 10 days after injury produced no improvement in the degree or extent of paralysis. It now appears that this dose was too low or that the initial dose was given too late to arrest the injury process.[292] This possibility has already been discussed in relation to the use of steroids in brain injury. In experiments with cats Braughler and Hall[300,340] showed that 30 mg/kg of methylprednisolone given within 30 minutes of injury was required to maintain blood flow to an area of cord trauma and that an additional 15 mg/kg dose was needed 2 hours postinjury to avoid neurofilament degeneration. Smaller doses or later administration produced no effect. A followup of the previous multicenter trial[299a] has recently demonstrated a similar beneficial effect in humans. A bolus of methylprednisolone, 30 mg/kg, followed in 1 hour by infusion of 5.4 mg/kg/hr for 23 hours, was associated with improvement in both sensory and motor recovery if (and only if) started within 8 hours of trauma. No increased incidence of wound infection or gastrointestinal bleeding occurred in this group of patients, although they have been seen in other studies.[299,323] If these results are confirmed, they represent the first successful use of medical therapy for spinal cord injury.

There is a possibility that other useful steroids may be found in the future. Anderson et al[293] have noted a beneficial effect of the 21-aminosteroid U-74006F on spinal cord-injured rats. This compound has no corticoid activity but is a potent free-radical acceptor and may exert its effects by preventing cell membrane disruption.

Body temperature should be monitored at all times. Reflex vascular activity, sweating, and shivering are abolished in spinal shock; thus patients with high-level lesions are generally poikilothermic. Hyperthermia is especially hazardous since hypoxia may result from the patient's inability to increase ventilation enough to compensate for increased metabolic demand. Adjustment of room temperature, application of hypo/hyperthermia blankets, and warming or cooling of intravenous fluids can all be useful maneuvers in maintaining normothermia.

Over 25% of patients with spinal cord trauma have secondary injuries.[360,363] Cervical fractures are commonly associated with head trauma of varying severity. Chest and abdominal injuries and rib, pelvic, and long bone fractures are present in a high proportion of patients with thoracic and lumbar spine fractures. A careful and immediate search must be made for these problems because symptoms and signs may be masked by spinal shock. The patient cannot feel pain, abnormal blood gas values may be caused by hemo- or pneumothorax as well as by respiratory depression, and hypotension may indicate internal hemorrhage rather than sympathetic paralysis.

## PERIOPERATIVE CARE

Immediate surgery may be required in thoracic or lumbar fractures to stabilize the spine and/or treat secondary injuries. Fortunately, these patients present few problems for the anesthesiologist. The cardiac sympathetics (T1 to T5) are generally intact and intubation poses no hazard. Although cervical injuries are a much greater anesthetic challenge, surgery can, except in rare instances, be delayed until the hypotensive phase is over.

Important issues in the patient's preoperative evaluation include determination of the level and extent of injury or injuries, stability of the spine, and preexisting medical problems that may affect the anesthetic course. The lungs in particular should be evaluated carefully since aspiration, atelectasis, and pulmonary edema are quite common, especially in association with high thoracic or cervical injuries. A chest X-ray, arterial blood gas determination, and some measure of pulmonary function (at least a vital capacity and inspiratory and expiratory force) are mandatory both to determine preoperative pulmonary status and to provide a baseline for the postoperative period. The blood pressure and its course during the preoperative period should also be noted carefully. The hypotension seen during the first few days following injuries above T-7 has already been described. Some degree of sympathetic hyperreflexia may occur as early as the third day. The patient exhibits wide swings in blood pressure, with hypertensive episodes occurring in response to various kinds of stimulation, especially bladder distention.

Any appropriate premedication may be prescribed for the patient with thoracic or lumbar injury. Depressant drugs should not be used in quadriplegics since respiratory function is already marginal. As we have already discussed, atropine is strongly advisable because it will tend to block the effects of unopposed vagal activity.

If possible, surgery is performed in the patient's bed. Moving anyone with an unstable spine fracture carries a great risk of increasing cord damage. If the cervical fracture is immobilized with a halo brace, transfer is generally not a problem. However, extreme care must be used if the patient is in traction since alteration of the weights may displace the spine.

As in brain injury, careful attention should be paid to padding of pressure points and maintenance of normothermia. Monitoring should be appropriate to the patient's injury and to the procedure performed. An arterial line should be used in all major surgery and in all patients with levels above T-6 since, as we have mentioned, wide and rapid swings in blood pressure may occur. As alluded to earlier, a pulmonary artery catheter may be of great benefit to the quadriplegic for monitoring both fluid replacement and pulmonary status during and after surgery.[367] A urinary catheter will generally be present on arrival in the operating room and may provide a useful monitor of the blood volume.

Induction and maintenance of anesthesia are generally no special problems when the injury is below T-7. Any suitable technique may be used, depending on the patient's general condition and the operation to be performed. Procedures below the sensory level (eg, reduction of lower extremity fractures) may require no anesthesia at all. However, the anesthesiologist should not be lulled into complacency by this: the patient requires the same attention to ventilatory adequacy, blood loss, volume status, temperature, and urinary output as anyone undergoing the same procedure under general anesthesia.

The problems and techniques of intubation in the presence of cervical fractures have been described previously (see also Chapter 14). The principles are the same for those patients who are not intubated before they reach the operating room. A narcotic anesthetic is probably best during the hypotensive phase, whereas an inhalation agent will provide adequate blood pressure control in patients subject to autonomic hyperreflexia.[290,345,371] Enflurane and isoflurane are associated with a lower incidence of cardiac arrhythmias than halothane when serum catecholamine levels increase and are thus agents of choice in normotensive quadriplegics. They should, however, be used with great care in these patients because of their myocardial depressant effect. This, in combination with arteriolar and venous dilatation produced by sympathetic denervation, may produce a precipitous fall in blood pressure, particularly during induction of anesthesia.[345] Loss of sympathetic reflexes may also result in pronounced hypotension during controlled ventilation.[371,373] A prolonged expiratory phase (1:2 or 1:3) should be utilized to minimize the increase in mean airway pressure.[354] Hypotension during anesthesia is usually easily controlled by rapid fluid infusion to a pulmonary capillary wedge pressure or CVP of 18 mm Hg or by vasopressors, preferably dopamine.[351]

Succinylcholine is a major hazard for the paraplegic. In response to denervation, receptor substance proliferates beyond the end plates of voluntary muscle fibers, eventually to invest the entire cell membrane. The muscle becomes "supersensitive" and contracts maximally in response to a concentration of acetylcholine only $10^{-4}$ to $10^{-5}$ that needed to initiate contraction in normal muscle.[294] Potassium ion is released suddenly along the entire length of the fiber rather than gradually as the action potential propagates. This produces a rapid rise in serum $K^+$ levels. Succinylcholine induces an identical response and may be associated with a serum $K^+$ increase of 4 to 10 mEq/L. The extent of this increase is roughly proportional to the amount of paralyzed muscle mass. Within 3 minutes of succinylcholine administration, the serum $K^+$ reaches a peak and may cause irreversible ventricular arrhythmias and cardiac arrest (Fig 10-14, A).[307,335,366] Because of muscle supersensitivity, the severity of this reaction is virtually independent of the dose of succinylcholine administered.[307,366] Although hyperkalemia can be modified somewhat by prior administration of a nondepolarizing muscle relaxant, paralyzing doses are required to eliminate it altogether[335] (Fig 10-14, B). Supersensitivity becomes clinically significant within about a week following denervating injury and lasts for at least 6 months to 2 years even in upper neuron lesions, in which the onset of reflex activity during the chronic phase might be expected to modify the process.[301,342] Thus, although succinylcholine is safe in the first days of paraplegia, it should be avoided completely after the third or fourth day.[342] Pancuronium, vecuronium, and atracurium are safe and effective muscle relaxants for the spinal cord-injured patient.

Careful attention must be paid to maintenance of normothermia in these poikilothermic patients. Proper use of the various methods of temperature control is essential. In prolonged procedures, humidification of inspired gases will not only help maintain the temperature but also may prevent inspissation of pulmonary secretions with possible resultant atelectasis.[37]

Postoperatively, quadriplegics frequently exhibit prolonged respiratory depression. Ventilatory assistance should be maintained until the patient's pulmonary function returns to preoperative levels. This may require from 3 days to a week.

## INTENSIVE CARE

### *Respiration and Respiratory Therapy*

During the early stages of injury, many problems may afflict the paraplegic, and a variety of physicians and other personnel are involved in his care. However, pulmonary complications are the major risks to his life.[305] All spinal cord-injured patients show some degree of respiratory dysfunction, generally in proportion to the level of injury (see Table 10-3).[357] Even in lumbar injuries, flaccidity of the pelvic floor results in significant reduction of ventilatory parameters. The common association of direct pulmonary damage with thoracic spine fractures can complicate ventilatory problems further.[357] In quadriplegia, the degree of respiratory impairment depends critically on the dermatomes involved.[291,327] Injuries below C-5 are associated with normal diaphragmatic function, although the major accessory respiratory muscles, the abdominals and intercostals, are paralyzed. Thus the patient can generally maintain normal tidal volume, but expiratory re-

FIG. 10-14. Serum potassium flux in response to succinylcholine. (A) Comparison of normal, immobilized, paraplegic, and denervated muscle. (B) Inhibition in denervated muscle by pretreatment with nondepolarizing muscle relaxant (gallamine). (From Gronert and Theye[335] with permission.)

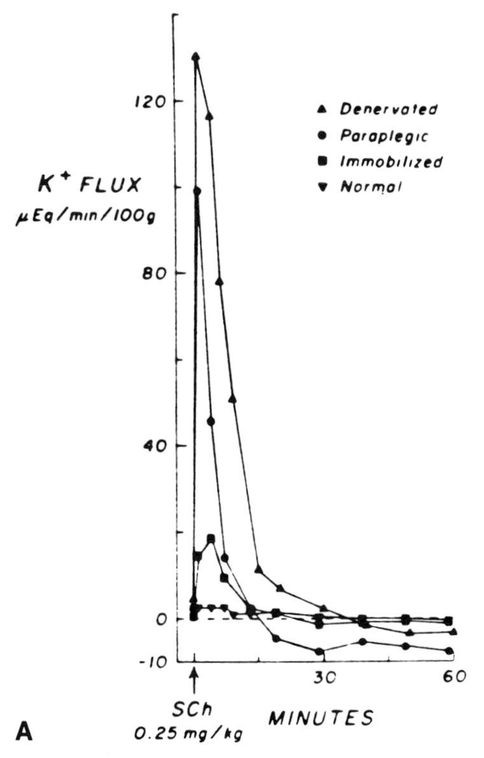


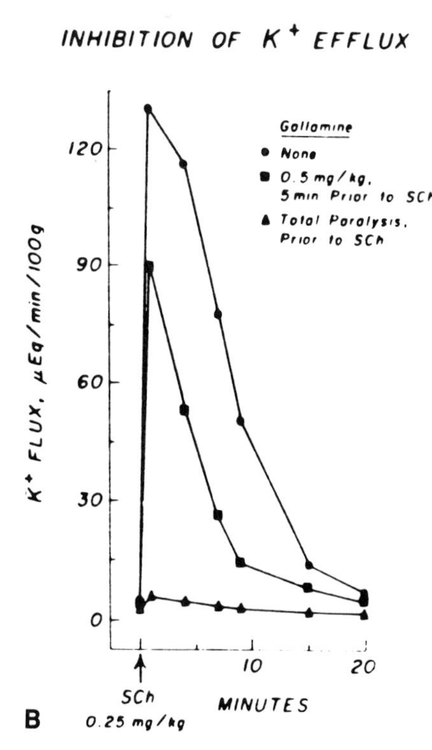

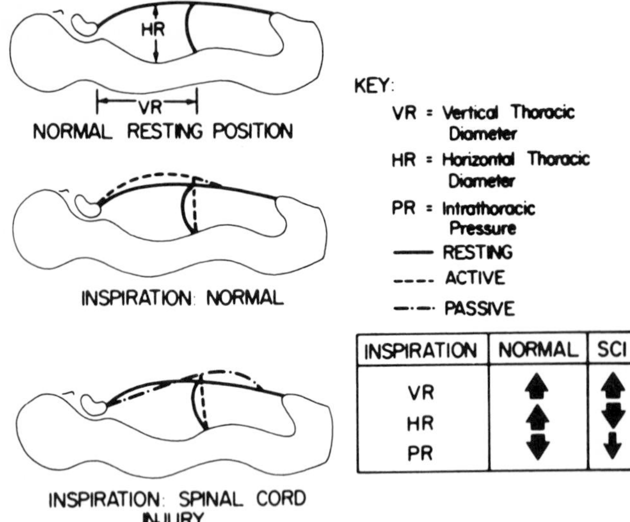


FIG. 10-15. Paradoxic ventilation in the quadriplegic. SCI, spinal cord injury. (From Alvarez et al[291] with permission.)

serve is severely diminished or lost. Some degree of diaphragmatic paralysis is seen with levels of C-4 or C-5 (the major innervation is from C-4). Tidal volume is decreased, and the patient requires ventilatory assistance. With total paralysis of the diaphragm—levels at or above C-3—some form of permanent respiratory support will be necessary. The neck muscles, especially the trapezius and sternocleidomastoids, are preserved in quadriplegia, since they are innervated by cranial nerves. They can provide some degree of inspiratory assistance by elevating the upper part of the thorax.[291,361,370]

Another problem for the quadriplegic is paradoxical respiration (Fig 10-15).[291,370] Loss of the splinting effect of intercostal and abdominal muscle tone causes collapse of the chest wall during descent of the diaphragm and may thus impair tidal volume. Fowler's position should be avoided in the quadriplegic; descent of the abdominal contents is accentuated by loss of abdominal muscle tone, and the diaphragm flattens to the extent that its efficiency of contraction is decreased.[291] Paradoxical collapse of the chest wall further impairs inspiratory volume, and the patient may become hypoxic.[291] Ventilatory parameters tend to improve gradually from the third week to the fifth to sixth month following injury as spasticity improves muscle tone below the level of injury, thus decreasing paradox (Table 10-4). Even patients with C-4 levels can generally maintain normal tidal volumes by the fifth month.[347]

Additional respiratory problems may complicate the picture further.[305,370] Even when ventilation is adequate, quadriplegics commonly exhibit some degree of hypoxia from intrapulmonary shunting during the first week.[347] Pneumonia may result from aspiration and/or retention of secretions. Thirdly, NPE occurs in 50% of quadriplegics, probably as a result of pulmonary capillary damage produced by an explosive sympathetic discharge immediately following injury. The onset of NPE may be delayed for 48 hours or more, until the resumption of sympathetic activity increases venous return to the central circulation.[328] Overinfusion of fluids or blood in an effort to maintain blood pressure may hasten the onset of pulmonary edema or make it worse when it occurs. Thrombophlebitis and pulmonary embolism occur in about 12 to 15% of paraplegics and present a considerably increased risk in a patient whose pulmonary function is already compromised.[317]

Since it is the quadriplegic who suffers the most severe respiratory problems, the following discussion will be directed to the care of this group of patients. It is important to remember that prevention of respiratory failure involves attention to many external factors. Even minor problems in quadriplegics may interfere with the already precarious respiratory reserve.[370]

As discussed earlier, the patient should be maintained in a flat or mild Trendelenburg position if he is breathing spontaneously. The supine position may increase the likelihood of regurgitation and aspiration, particularly if the patient is in traction or halo fixation and cannot turn his head. Thus he should be kept prone or semiprone as much as possible, provided that his tidal volume is not unduly compromised.[370] This is not to imply that his position should not be changed. To the contrary, he should be turned frequently throughout the day—at least every 2 to 3 hours—both to facilitate pulmonary drainage and to avoid decubitus ulcers.[313,359] Adequacy of respiration should be monitored closely, and in the early stages, repeated observation of respiratory rate, vital capacity, tidal volume, inspiratory force, and blood gas values should be performed so that the patient may be intubated at the earliest sign of respiratory depression. Oxygen should be supplemented, if necessary, to maintain a normal $Pa_{O_2}$. Like tracheal

TABLE 10-4. Expiratory Parameters in Quadriplegics*

| | ADMISSION ($n$ = 11) | 3 WEEKS ($n$ = 9) | 5 WEEKS ($n$ = 9) | 3 MONTHS ($n$ = 6) | 5 MONTHS ($n$ = 7) |
|---|---|---|---|---|---|
| FVC | 31.3 ± 6.3 | 36.1 ± 6.3 | 44.9 ± 7.3† | 51.3 ± 7.3† | 57.5 ± 11.5† |
| $FEV_1$ | 27.0 ± 11.5 | 36.1 ± 7.6 | 41.9 ± 6.9† | 47.2 ± 7.9† | 59.1 ± 14.5‡ |
| $FEV_1$% | 84.4 ± 6.1 | 85.3 ± 5.1 | 85.7 ± 4.9 | 86.8 ± 3.4 | 87.5 ± 3.8 |
| $FEF_{25-75}$(L/S) | 1.2 ± 0.43 | 2.0 ± 0.63 | 2.1 ± 0.72† | 2.3 ± 0.77† | 2.4 ± 1.1† |
| Pred (L/S) | 4.4 | 4.4 | 4.4 | 4.2 | 4.3 |

* Significant improvement starts in the fifth week and continues at least into the fifth month. Abbreviations as in Table 3. Pred (L/S), predicted $FEF_{25-75}$. Values are mean ± SD.

† Significantly different from initial measurements ($P < 0.01$).

‡ Significantly different from measurements at 5 weeks ($P < 0.05$). Adapted from Ledsome and Sharp[347] with permission.

intubation, tracheal suctioning is a hazardous procedure in the quadriplegic. Bradycardia and cardiac arrest have been reported as a result of uninhibited vagal reflex activity.[352,353,371] This problem can be prevented by adequate oxygenation—ie, hyperventilation—prior to suctioning and, if this is not sufficient, by atropine.

Chest physiotherapy prevents pulmonary complications and stimulates early recovery of maximal ventilatory function.[291,371] Breathing exercises, diaphragm strengthening, training in use of accessory muscles, and use of assisted cough should start on the first—or first possible—day. An abdominal support can be helpful in maintaining the position of the diaphragm and improving the mechanics of respiration.

Other maneuvers are also helpful in avoiding pulmonary problems.[371] Temperature should be maintained at normal levels. Both hypothermia and hyperthermia are undesirable and can be hazardous. Pulmonary or urinary infections should be treated early and aggressively. If possible, sedation is best avoided or at least minimized. Fluid balance should be monitored carefully by intake/output measurements and daily weight recording in order to decrease the likelihood of pulmonary edema.

Kaufman et al[343] suggest that infections and pulmonary complications may be aggravated by malnutrition. Although caloric expenditure is markedly decreased in spinal injury—to as low as 45% of normal in quadriplegics[308]—there may also be a severe negative nitrogen balance resulting from muscle atrophy. The diet of most patients in the first 2 weeks of hospitalization was found to be inadequate to meet either caloric needs or protein requirements.[308,343] Appropriate attention should be directed at assuring an adequate diet, by tube feeding or intravenous hyperalimentation if necessary, so that the problems of cachexia may be avoided.

Pulmonary embolism, as we have noted above, occurs in about 12 to 15% of paraplegics and carries with it a mortality of 25 to 30%.[317,369] The use of low-dose heparin (5000 U subcutaneously every 12 hours) results in a significant decrease in this risk, virtually without complications. For instance, Epstein et al[318] found no increase in incidence of GI bleeding during this therapy. Thus, prophylactic anticoagulation can be recommended for all paraplegics. Adjusting heparin dose to maintain activated partial thromboplastin time (APTT) at 1½ times normal value seems to result in a lower incidence of thromboembolic complications than the fixed dose schedule.[334] Much higher amounts of heparin—a mean of 13,200 U/dose—are required with this regimen, however, and there may be some increase in hemorrhagic complications. Watson[369] suggests maintenance of heparin for a month, followed by oral warfarin (Coumadin) in doses sufficient to keep prothrombin time between two and three times normal, for 2 months more. The risk of pulmonary embolism is low after the third month. Pulmonary embolism is discussed in detail in Chapter 28.

### Circulatory System

The severe circulatory disturbance caused by cord trauma implies the necessity of maintaining adequate systemic blood pressure and normal or, if possible, increased spinal cord blood flow in order to limit the secondary injury process. Dolan and Tator[312] have shown that increasing blood volume is one of the best ways of accomplishing this end. Unfortunately, as we have discussed in the previous section, this may also seriously increase the risk and severity of pulmonary edema. The effects of various agents on spinal cord blood flow have been investigated in animals. Of the vasopressors, neither dopamine nor isoproterenol significantly increase cord circulation following trauma.[312]

Both thyrotropin-releasing hormone and large doses of naloxone increase systemic blood pressure and spinal cord perfusion in cats.[319,322,326,374] Faden et al[320] demonstrated a marked improvement in functional recovery even if the drug was not administered until 4 hours after injury. More recent studies, however, do not show these effects.[337,368] Although clinical trials of naloxone are in progress, it is too early to evaluate its efficacy in cord-injured patients.[319,325] A recent multicenter clinical trial[299a] has shown that a 5.4 mg/kg bolus followed by 4.0 mg/kg/hr for 23 hours had no beneficial effect. Other dosage schedules, however, were not studied. If it should prove a useful adjunct to therapy, the enormous doses of naloxone which are required may have potentially serious implications for anesthesia. Benthuysen[295] describes great difficulty in maintaining adequate anesthetic depth during laminectomy and stabilization in a paraplegic who had received this drug following injury. The patient was hypertensive, tachycardic, and tachypneic despite administration of 25 μg/kg of fentanyl and 2.7% isoflurane.

### Gastrointestinal Complications

The loss of sympathetic tone associated with acute spinal cord injury predisposes the patient to a number of potentially serious abdominal problems.[304,332] The most common of these is gastric dilatation and ileus, which carry the danger of regurgitation and aspiration if the airway is unprotected. We have already recommended nasogastric intubation following injury. The tube should be left in place until normal gastrointestinal motility returns, usually within 4 to 7 days.[332,370] Intravenous fluids are administered during this period: total parenteral nutrition should be started on the fourth day if gastric atony persists.

Gastrointestinal ulceration, with perforation or bleeding severe enough at times to require surgery, is common following injuries to the cervical or upper thoracic cord.[296,316,332,344,349] Generally seen on the 4th to 20th day following injury, it is probably the result of a combination of gastric hyperacidity from unopposed vagal activity and mucosal ischemia from hypotension. Diagnosis requires a high index of suspicion in the absence of frank hematemesis or melena, since the patient may not feel pain, and the diagnostic signs—fever, tachycardia, abdominal distention—are quite commonly the result of other causes. Anemia and blood in the stools and/or positive X-ray findings will confirm the presence of ulceration or perforation. Unfortunately, neither antacids nor cimetidine seems to provide any prophylaxis against these potentially life-threatening complications.[318,375]

Pancreatitis is another easily missed and occasionally severe complication of acute paraplegia.[302,332] In the absence of abdominal pain, fever may be the only sign. Diagnosis is made on the basis of elevated temperature in the absence of pneumonitis or urinary tract infection, and of course, elevated serum amylase and lipase.

### PROGNOSIS

Unfortunately, neither survival rates nor therapeutic results in paraplegics have been subject to the rigorous statistical analysis that has been accorded to brain injuries. The best available data show that mortality is higher in complete injuries and higher in cervical than in lower-level lesions.[331] Of complete quadriplegics, reported mortality is about 27% within 3 months and 37% in a year; the corresponding data for incomplete cervical lesions are 2 and 17%, respectively.[341] Early deaths are caused most commonly by pulmonary complications or gastrointestinal bleeding.[297] These figures are a composite of results published over an 18-year period (1961 to 1979). More recent results indicate that survival can be markedly improved by aggressive pulmonary therapy.[359]

Other problems are presented by the results of therapeutic trials, surgical or nonsurgical.[324,341,365] There is no standard scale for spinal cord injury corresponding to the Glasgow coma scale. Thus it is impossible to compare patient selection criteria from one study to another, even in the relatively small number of series in which controlled studies have been attempted. It is obvious that some generally accepted scoring system and more controlled studies of relatively large numbers of patients are necessary before effectiveness of various treatments can be statistically evaluated and compared.[303,324]

On the other hand, there is no question that both the duration and quality of life of those patients who survive the acute phase have steadily and significantly improved over the last 40 years.[346] The present long-term outlook for a gratifyingly large number of paraplegics is one of remarkably well-adjusted and productive lives, personally, socially, and vocationally.

## CONCLUSION

Several general principles emerge from the foregoing discussion:

1. Intensive care for the patient with an injury of the central nervous system should ideally start at the scene of the accident. Maintenance of adequate blood pressure and ventilation, stabilization of the spine, and the greatest care in moving and transporting the victim are mandatory to limit secondary reaction and prevent further injury.
2. It is not uncommon for the patient to have multiple injuries, the signs of which may be concealed by coma or sensory paralysis. A scrupulous search for these should be instituted as soon as the cardiovascular and respiratory systems are stabilized.
3. One of the primary concerns in the therapy of severe head injury is control of ICP. All three components of the cranial vault may be treated in order to achieve this end. Thus, head elevation, hypocarbia, and barbiturates reduce CBV; surgery and mannitol can decrease the size of the tissue compartment; and CSF may be withdrawn by ventricular drainage.
4. Most early deaths in spinal cord-injured patients result from pulmonary problems—atelectasis, pneumonitis, and pulmonary edema. Thus, major attention is directed to the respiratory system during the first weeks of treatment, particularly in high thoracic or cervical injuries. One of the oldest maxims in the treatment of spinal injury is "Quads die quietly"—respiratory arrest occurs all too often while the patient is asleep. He must, therefore, be under careful and continuous observation, particularly if he is breathing spontaneously.

Ultimately, prevention must be the answer to reducing the tremendous economic and social costs of central nervous system injuries; thus the major responsibility is societal rather than medical—eg, safer automobiles and workplaces, improved athletic equipment, campaigns to reduce driving after alcohol consumption. Even in the best of all possible worlds, however, accidents will still occur, and it will continue to be our responsibility as physicians to do all in our power to restore the victims to the best possible quality of life.

## REFERENCES

### INTRODUCTION AND BRAIN INJURIES


1. Abbushi W, Kolb E, Herkt G, et al. Klinische und experimentelle Untersuchungen zur Lagerung der Patienten mit Schädel-Hirn-Trauma. Anaesthetist 1979;28:489.
2. Adams F. The genuine works of Hippocrates. New York: W Wood, 1886.
3. Adams F. The seven books of Paulus Aeginita. London: The Syndenham Society, 1846.
4. Adams RW, Cucchiara RF, Gronert GA, et al. Isoflurane and cerebrospinal fluid pressure in neurosurgical patients. Anesthesiology 1981;54:97.
5. Adams RW, Gronert GA, Michenfelder JD. Isoflurane and cerebrospinal fluid pressure in neurosurgery. In Lundberg N, Ponten U, Brock M, eds. Intracranial pressure II. Berlin: Springer-Verlag, 1975:334.
6. Aidinis SJ, Lafferty J, Shapiro HM. Intracranial responses to PEEP. Anesthesiology 1976;45:275.
7. Alberico AM, Ward JD, Choi SC, et al. Outcome after severe head injury. J Neurosurg 1987;67:648.
8. Albright AL, Latchaw RE, Robinson AG. Intracranial and systemic effects of hetastarch in experimental cerebral edema. Crit Care Med 1984;12:496.
9. Albright AL, Latchaw RE, Robinson AG. Intracranial and systemic effects of osmotic and oncotic therapy in experimental cerebral edema. J Neurosurg 1984;60:481.
10. Allen SJ. Management of intracranial hypertension. In: Miner ME, Wager KA, eds. Neurotrauma: treatment, rehabilitation, and related issues. Boston: Butterworth, 1986:41.
11. Allen SJ. Management of intracranial hypertension after head injury. ASA Refresher Course Lectures 1987;15:1.
12. Archer DP, Labrecque P, Tyler JL, et al. Cerebral blood volume is increased in dogs during administration of nitrous oxide or isoflurane. Anesthesiology 1987;67:642.
13. Artru AA. Reduction of cerebrospinal fluid pressure by hypocapnia: changes in cerebral blood volume, cerebrospinal fluid volume, and brain tissue water and electrolytes. J Cereb Blood Flow Metab 1987;7:471.
14. Barron KD, Dentiger MP, Kimelberg HK, et al. Ultrastructural features of a brain injury model in the cat, I: vascular and neuroglial changes and the prevention of astroglial swelling by a fluorenyl(aryloxy)alkanoic acid derivative (L-644,711). Acta Neuropathol 1988;75:295.

15. Bayliff CD, Schwartz ML, Hardy BS. Pharmacokinetics of high dose pentobarbital in severe head trauma. Clin Pharmacol Ther 1985;38:457.
16. Becker DP. The temporal genesis of primary and secondary brain damage in experimental and clinical brain injury. In: Baethmann A, Go KG, Unterberg A, eds. Mechanisms of secondary brain damage. New York: Plenum, 1986:47.
17. Becker DP, Miller JD, Ward JD, et al. The outcome from severe head injury with early diagnosis and intensive management. J Neurosurg 1977;47:491.
18. Becker DP, Miller JD, Young HF, et al. The critical importance of ICP monitoring in head injury. In: Beks JWF, Bosch DA, Brock M, eds. Intracranial pressure III. Berlin: Springer-Verlag, 1976:97.
19. Becker DP, Sullivan HG, Adams WE, et al. Controlled hyperventilation in severe brain injury. In: McLaurin RL, ed. Head injuries. New York: Grune and Stratton, 1975:157.
20. Becker DP, Vries JK, Sakalas R, et al. Early prognosis in head injury based on motor posturing, oculocephalic reflexes, and intracranial pressure. In: McLaurin RL, ed. Head injuries. New York: Grune and Stratton, 1975:27.
21. Bedford RF, Persing JA, Pobreskin L, et al. Lidocaine or thiopental for rapid control of intracranial hypertension? Anesth Analg 1980;59:435.
22. Bedford RF, Winn HR, Tyson G, et al. Lidocaine prevents increased ICP after endotracheal intubation. In: Shulman K, Marmarou A, Miller JD, et al, eds. Intracranial pressure IV. Berlin: Springer-Verlag, 1980:595.
23. Beks, JWF. The effects of increased intracranial pressure on cardiovascular and respiratory function. In: Lundberg N, Ponten U, Brock M, eds. Intracranial pressure II. Berlin: Springer-Verlag, 1975:289.
24. Bourke RS, Kimelberg HK, Daze MA, et al. Studies on the formation of astroglial swelling and its inhibition by clinically useful agents. In: Popp AJ, Bourke RS, Nelson LR, Kimelberg HK, eds. Neural trauma. New York: Raven Press, 1979,95.
25. Braakman R. Emergency craniotomy in severe head injury and the present state of knowledge regarding prognosis. Injury 1983;14:22.
26. Braakman R, Schouten HJA, Blaau-Van Dishoeck M, et al. Megadose steroids in severe head injury. J Neurosurg 1983;58:326.
27. Braun SR, Levin AB, Clark KL. Role of corticosteroids in the development of pneumonia in mechanically ventilated head trauma victims. Crit Care Med 1986;14:198.
28. Breastead JH. The Edwin Smith surgical papyrus. Chicago: University of Chicago Press, 1930.
29. Brown FD, Johns LM, Crockard HA, et al. Response to mannitol following experimental cerebral missile injury. In: Popp AJ, Bourke RS, Nelson LR, Kimelberg HK, eds. Neural trauma. New York: Raven Press, 1979:281.
30. Brown FD, Johns L, Jafar JJ, et al. Detailed monitoring of the effects of mannitol following experimental head injury. J Neurosurg 1979;50:423.
31. Brown FD, Johns LM, Mullan S. Dimethyl sulfoxide in experimental brain injury, with comparison to mannitol. J Neurosurg 1980;53:58.
32. Bruce DA. Management of severe head injury. In: Cottrell JE, Turndorf H, eds. Anesthesia and neurosurgery. 2nd ed. St Louis: CV Mosby, 1986:150.
33. Bruce DA, Schut L, Bruno LA. The role of intracranial pressure monitoring in a pediatric intensive care unit. In: Beks JWF, Bosch DA, Brock M, eds. Intracranial pressure III. Berlin: Springer-Verlag, 1976:323.
34. Bruce DA, Schut L, Bruno LA, et al. Outcome following severe head injuries in children. J Neurosurg 1978;48:679.
35. Camp PE, James HD, Werner R. Acute dimethyl sulfoxide therapy in experimental brain edema, part I: effects on intracranial pressure, blood pressure, central venous pressure, and brain water and electrolyte content. Neurosurgery 1981;9:28.
36. Cerisoli M, Ruggeri F, Amelio GF, et al. Experimental cerebral "no-reflow phenomenon." J Neurosurg Sci 1981;25:7.
37. Chalon J, Ali M, Turndorf H, Fishgrund GK. Humidification of anesthetic gases. Springfield: Charles C Thomas, 1982:19.
38. Chopp M, Portnoy M, Branch C. Hydraulic model of the cerebrovascular bed: an aid to understanding the volume-pressure test. Neurosurgery 1983;13:5.
39. Clark JA, Finelli RE, Netsky MG. Disseminated intravascular coagulation following cranial trauma. J Neurosurg 1980;52:266.
40. Clifton GL, Robertson CS, Grossman RG, et al. The metabolic response to severe head injury. J Neurosurg 1984;60:687.
41. Clifton GL, Robertson CS, Kyper K, et al. Cardiovascular response to severe head injury. J Neurosurg 1983;59:447.
42. Cold GE. Cerebral blood flow in the acute phase after head injury, part 2: correlation to intraventricular pressure (IVP), cerebral perfusion pressure (CPP), $Paco_2$, ventricular fluid lactate, lactate/pyruvate ratio, and pH. Acta Anaesthesiol Scand 1981;25:332.
43. Cooper KR, Boswell PA, Choi SC. Safe use of PEEP in patients with severe head injury. J Neurosurg 1985;63:552.
44. Cooper PR, Moody S, Clark WK, et al. Dexamethasone and severe head injury. J Neurosurg 1979;51:307.
45. Cotev S, Paul WE, Ruiz BC, et al. Positive end-expiratory pressure (PEEP) and cerebrospinal fluid pressure during normal and elevated intracranial pressure in dogs. Intensive Care Med 1981;7:187.
46. Cottrell JF, Hartung J, Giffin JP, et al. Intracranial and hemodynamic changes after succinylcholine administration in cats. Anesth Analg 1983;62:1006.
47. Crockard HA. Early management of head injuries. Br J Hosp Med 1982;27:635.
48. Crozier TA, Beck D, Schlaeger M, et al. Endocrinological changes following etomidate, midazolam, or methohexital for minor surgery. Anesthesiology 1987;66:628.
49. Cruz J, Miner ME. Modulating cerebral oxygen delivery and extraction in acute traumatic coma. In: Miner ME, Wagner KA, eds. Neurotrauma: treatment, rehabilitation, and related issues. Boston: Butterworth, 1986:55.
50. Cushing H. A study of a series of wounds involving the brain and its enveloping structures. Br J Surg 1918;5:558.
51. Cushing H. Peptic ulcers and the interbrain. Surg Gynecol Obstet 1932;55:1.
52. Cushing H. The blood pressure reaction of acute intracranial hypertension, illustrated by cases of intracranial hemorrhage. Am J Med Sci 1903;125:1017.
53. Cushing H. The special field of neurological surgery. Bull J Hopkins Hosp 1905;168:79.
54. Davis RA, Cunningham PS. Prognostic factors in severe head injury. Surg Gynecol Obstet 1984;159:597.
55. De Los Reyes RA, Ausman JI, Diaz FG. Agents for cerebral edema. Clin Neurosurg 1981;28:98.
56. Dearden NM, Gibson JS, MacDowall DG, et al. Effect of high dose dexamethasone on outcome from severe head injury. J Neurosurg 1986;64:81.
57. Dearden NM, McDowall DG. Comparison of etomidate and althesin in the reduction of increased intracranial pressure after head injury. Br J Anaesth 1985;57:361.
58. Del Bigio M, James HE, Camp PE, et al. Acute dimethyl sulfoxide therapy in brain edema, part 3: effect of a 3-hour infusion. Neurosurgery 1982;10:86.
59. Demopoulos HB, Flamm ES, Seligman ML, et al. Membrane perturbations in central nervous system injury: theoretical basis for free radical damage and a review of the experimental data.

In: Popp AJ, Bourke RS, Nelson LR, Kimelberg HK, eds. Neural trauma. New York: Raven Press, 1979:63.
60. DeSalles AAF, Kontos HA, Ward JD, et al. Brain tissue pH in severely head injured patients: a report of three cases. Neurosurgery 1987;20:297.
61. DeSalles AA, Muizelaar JP, Young HF. Hyperglycemia, cerebrospinal fluid lactic acidosis, and cerebral blood flow in severely head-injured patients. Neurosurgery 1987;21:45.
62. Deutschmann CS, Konstantinides FN, Raup S, Cerra FB. Physiological and metabolic response to isolated closed-head injury, part 2: effects of steroids on metabolism, potentiation of protein wasting and abnormalities of substrate utilization. J Neurosurg 1987;66:388.
63. Deutschman CS, Konstantinides FN, Raup S, et al. Physiological and metabolic response to isolated closed head injury, part 1: basal metabolic state, correlations of metabolic and physiological parameters with fasting and stressed controls. J Neurosurg 1986;64:89.
64. Doblar DD, Santiago TV, Kahn AU, et al. The effect of positive end-expiratory pressure ventilation (PEEP) on cerebral blood flow and cerebrospinal fluid pressure in goats. Anesthesiology 1981;55:244.
65. Donegan MF, Bedford RF. Intravenously administered lidocaine prevents intracranial hypertension during endotracheal suctioning. Anesthesiology 1980;52:516.
66. Dorman RV, Dabrowiecki Z, De Medio GE, et al. Effects of cytidine nucleotides on CNS membranes during ischemia. In: Grossman RG, Gildenberg L, eds. Head injury: basic and clinical aspects. New York: Raven Press, 1982:93.
67. Dresser LP, McKinney WM. Anatomic and pathophysiologic studies of the human internal jugular valve. Am J Surg 1987;154:220.
68. Drummond JC, Todd MM, Scheller MS, Shapiro HM. A comparison of the direct cerebral vasodilating potencies of halothane and isoflurane in the New Zealand White rabbit. Anesthesiology 1986;65:462.
69. Drummond JC, Todd MM, U HS. The effect of high dose sodium thiopental on brain stem auditory and median nerve somatosensory evoked responses in humans. Anesthesiology 1985;63:249.
70. Durward QJ, Amacher AL, Del Maestro RF, et al. Cerebral and cardiovascular responses to changes in head elevation in patients with intracranial hypertension. J Neurosurg 1983;59:938.
71. Durward QJ, Del Maestro RF, Amacher AL, et al. The influence of systemic arterial pressure and intracranial pressure on the development of cerebral vasogenic edema. J Neurosurg 1983;59:803.
72. Eisenberg HM, Frankowski RF, Contant CF, et al. High-dose barbiturate control of elevated intracranial pressure in patients with acute head injury. J Neurosurg 1988;69:15.
73. Enevoldsen EM, Jensen FT. The relation between intracranial pressure and regional cerebral blood flow in the acute phase of head injury. In: Beks JWF, Bosch DA, Brock M, eds. Intracranial pressure III. Berlin: Springer-Verlag, 1976:127.
74. Farling PA, Johnston IR, Coppel DL. Propofol infusion for sedation of patients with head injury in intensive care. Anaesthesia 1989;44:222.
75. Faupel G, Reulen HJ, Müller D, et al. Double-blind study on the effects of steroids on severe closed head injury. In: Pappius HW, Feindel W, eds. Dynamics of brain edema. Berlin: Springer-Verlag, 1976:337.
76. Fell D, Benner B, Billings A, et al. Metabolic profiles in patients with acute neurosurgical injuries. Crit Care Med 1984;12:649.
77. Fitch W, Barker J, Jennett WB, et al. The influence of neuroleptanalgesic drugs on cerebrospinal fluid pressure. Br J Anaesth 1969;41:800.
78. Flamm ES, Demopoulos HB, Seligman ML, et al. Barbiturates and free-radicals. In: Popp AJ, Bourke RS, Nelson LR, Kimelberg HK, eds. Neural trauma. New York: Raven Press, 1979:289.
79. Fragen RJ, Shanks CA, Molteni A, et al. Effects of etomidate on hormonal responses to surgical stress. Anesthesiology 1984;61:652.
80. Fraser RAR, Yoshida S, Patterson RH. Focal cerebral ischemia and the "no-reflow" phenomenon. Acta Neurol Scand 1977;50 (Supp 64):5.14.
81. Frost EAM. Effects of positive end-expiratory pressure on intracranial pressure and compliance in brain-injured patients. J Neurosurg 1977;47:195.
82. Frost EAM. Respiratory problems associated with head trauma. Neurosurgery 1977;1:300.
83. Fuchs E, Wüllenweber R. Is there any indication for halothane anesthesia in neurosurgical procedures with increased ICP today? In: Lundberg N, Ponten U, Brock M, eds. Intracranial pressure II. Berlin: Springer-Verlag, 1975:337.
84. Galbraith S. Intracranial pressure monitoring in the management of the head-injured patient. In: Fitch W, Barker J, eds. Head injury and the anaesthetist. Amsterdam: Elsevier, 1985:165.
85. Gelb AW, Manninen PH, Mezon BJ, et al. The anaesthetist and the head-injured patient. Can Anaesth Soc J 1984;31:98.
86. Gennarelli TA, Obrist WD, Langfitt TW, Segawa H. Vascular and metabolic reactivity to changes in $P_{CO_2}$ in head-injured patients. In: Popp AJ, Bourke RS, Nelson LR, Kimelberg HK, eds. Neural trauma. New York: Raven Press, 1979:1.
87. Ghani GA, Sung YF, Weinstein MS, et al. Effects of intravenous nitroglycerin on the intracranial pressure and volume pressure response. J Neurosurg 1983;58:562.
88. Giannotta SL, Weiner JM, Karnaze D. Prognosis and outcome in severe head injury. In Cooper PR, ed. Head injury. Baltimore: Williams and Wilkins, 1987:464.
89. Giannotta SL, Weiss H, Apuzzo MLJ, et al. High dose glucocorticoids in the management of severe head injury. Neurosurgery 1984;15:497.
90. Giffin JP, Cottrell JE, Hartung J, et al. Intracranial pressure, mean arterial pressure and heart rate after rapid paralysis with atracurium in cats. Can Anaesth Soc J 1985;32:618.
91. Giffin JP, Hartung J, Cottrell JE, et al. Effect of vecuronium on intracranial pressure, mean arterial pressure and heart rate in cats. Br J Anaesth 1986;58:441.
92. Go KG. Pathophysiological aspects of brain edema. Cin Neurol Neurosurg 1984;86:77.
93. Gobiet W. The influence of various doses of dexamethasone on intracranial pressure in patients with severe head injury. In: Pappius HM, Feindel W, eds. Dynamics of brain edema. Berlin: Springer-Verlag, 1976:351.
94. Gobiet W, Bock WJ, Liesegang J, et al. Treatment of acute cerebral edema with high dose of dexamethasone. In: Beks JWF, Bosch DA, Brock M, eds. Intracranial pressure III. Berlin: Springer-Verlag, 1976:231.
95. Godin DV, Mitchell MJ, Saunders BA. Studies on the interaction of barbiturates with reactive oxygen radicals: implications regarding barbiturate protection against cerebral ischemia. Can Anaesth Soc J 1982;29:203.
96. Gordon E. Critical care of the patient with head trauma. ASA Annual Refresher Course Lectures 1982;142:1.
97. Gordon E. The management of acute head injuries. In: Gordon E, ed. A basis and practice of neuroanaesthesia. Amesterdam: Exerpta Medica, 1975:249.
98. Graf CJ, Rossi NP. Catecholamine response to intracranial hypertension. J Neurosurg 1978;49:862.
99. Greenberg RP, Becker DP, Miller JD, et al. Evaluation of brain

function in severe human head trauma with multimodality evoked potentials, part 2: localization of brain dysfunction and correlation with posttraumatic neurological conditions. J Neurosurg 1977;47:163.
100. Greenberg RP, Mayer DJ, Becker DP, et al. Evaluation of brain function in severe human head trauma with multimodality evoked potentials, part 1: evoked brain-injury potentials, methods, and analysis. J Neurosurg 1977;47:150.
101. Greenberg RP, Newlon RG, Hyatt MS, et al. Prognostic implications of early multimodality evoked potentials in severely head-injured patients. J Neurosurg 1981;55:227.
102. Greenberg RP, Stablein DM, Becker DP. Noninvasive localization of brain-stem lesions in the cat with multimodality evoked potentials. J Neurosurg 1980;54:740.
103. Griffin JM, Hartley JH, Crow RW, et al. Diabetes insipidus caused by craniofacial trauma. J Trauma 1976;16:979.
104. Gudeman SK, Miller JD, Becker DP. Failure of high dose steroid therapy to influence intracranial pressure in patients with severe head injury. J Neurosurg 1979;51:301.
105. Gunnar W, Jonasson O, Merlotti G, et al. Head injury and hemorrhagic shock: studies of the blood-brain barrier and intracranial pressure after resuscitation with normal saline solution, 3% saline solution and dextran-40. Surgery 1988;103:398.
106. Gupta B, Cottrell JE. Nitroprusside and nitroglycerine induced intracranial pressure changes. In: Shulman K, Marmarou A, Miller JD, et al, eds. Intracranial pressure IV. Berlin: Springer-Verlag, 1980:613.
107. Hackenberry LE, Miner ME, Rea GL, et al. Biochemical evidence of myocardial injury after severe head trauma. Crit Care Med 1982;10:641.
108. Haider W, Lackner F, Schlick W, et al. Metabolic changes in the course of severe acute brain damage. Eur J Intensive Care Med 1975;1:19.
109. Haigh JD, Nemoto EM, DeWolf AM, Bleyaert AL. Comparison of the effects of succinylcholine and atracurium on intracranial pressure in monkeys with intracranial hypertension. Can Anaesth Soc J 1986;33:421.
110. Hall ED, Wolf DL, Althaus JS, von Voightlander PF. Beneficial effects of the kappa-opioid receptor agonist U-50488H in experimental acute brain and spinal cord injury. Brain Res 1987;435:174.
111. Hall ED, Yonkers PA, McCall JM, et al. Effects of the 21-aminosteroid U-74006F on experimental head injury in mice. J Neurosurg 1988;68:456.
112. Halloran LG, Zfass AM, Gayle WE, et al. Prevention of acute gastrointestinal complications after severe head injury: a controlled trial of cimetidine prophylaxis. Am J Surg 1980;139:44.
113. Hamill JF, Bedford RF, Weaver DC, et al. Lidocaine before endotracheal intubation: intravenous or intratracheal? Anesthesiology 1981;55:578.
114. Havill JH. Prolonged hyperventilation and intracranial pressure. Crit Care Med 1984;12:72.
115. Hempelmann G, Dieter K, Volker L, et al. Cerebral protection in neurosurgery, cardiac surgery, and following cardiac arrest. J Cereb Blood Flow Metab 1982;2 (Suppl 1):566.
116. Henriksen HT, Jörgensen PB. The effect of nitrous oxide on intracranial pressure in patients with intracranial disorders. Br J Anaesth 1973;45:486.
117. Hewer AJH. Anaesthesia for neurosurgical emergencies. In: Thornton HL, ed. Emergency anaesthesia. 2nd ed. Baltimore: Williams and Wilkins, 1974:276.
118. Hooshmand H, Dove J, Houff S, et al. Effects of diuretics and steroids on CSF pressure. Arch Neurol 1969;21:499.
119. Horrax G. Neurosurgery: an historical sketch. Springfield: Charles C Thomas, 1952.
120. Hulme A, Cooper R. The effects of head position and jugular vein compression (JVC) on intracranial pressure: a clinical study. In: Beks JWF, Bosch DA, Brock M, eds. Intracranial pressure III. Berlin: Springer-Verlag, 1976:259.
121. Inao S, Marmarou A, Clarke GD, et al. Production and clearance of lactate from brain tissue, cerebrospinal fluid, and serum following experimental brain injury. J Neurosurg 1988;69:736.
122. Israel RS, Marx JA, Moore EE, Lowenstein SR. Hemodynamic effect of mannitol in a canine model of concomitant increased intracranial pressure and hemorrhagic shock. Ann Emerg Med 1988;17:560.
123. Jagger J, Fife D, Vernberg K, Jane JA. Effect of alcohol intoxication on the diagnosis and apparent severity of brain injury. Neurosurgery 1984;15:303.
124. James HE, Camp PE, Harbaugh RD, et al. Comparison of the effects of DMSO and pentobarbitone on experimental brain edema. Acta Neurochir 1982;60:245.
125. Jeffreys RV, Lozada L. The use of the CAT scanner in the management of patients with head injury transferred to the regional neurosurgical unit. Injury 1982;13:370.
126. Jennett B. Avoidable mortality, morbidity and secondary brain damage after recent head injury. In: Baethmann A, Go KG, Unterberg A, eds. Mechanisms of secondary brain damage. New York: Plenum, 1986:319.
127. Jennett B, Bond M. Assessment of outcome after severe brain damage. Lancet 1975;1:480.
128. Jennett B, Teasdale G, Galbraith S, et al. Severe head injuries in three countries. J Neurol Neurosurg Psychiatry 1977;40:291.
129. Jennett S. Pulmonary function in the head-injured patient. In: Fitch W, Barker J, eds. Head injury and the anaesthetist. Amsterdam: Elsevier, 1985:53.
130. Jennett S, North JB. Breathing pattern, response to $CO_2$ and blood gases in cats with experimental increases in intracranial pressure. In: Lundberg N, Ponten U, Brock M, eds. Intracranial pressure II. Berlin: Springer-Verlag, 1975:311.
131. John ER, Alter C, Ransohoff J. Evaluation of coma patients with the brain state analyzer. In: Grossman RG, Gildenberg PL, eds. Head injury: basic and clinical aspects. New York: Raven Press, 1982:259.
132. Jones PW. Hyperventilation in the management of cerebral oedema. Intensive Care Med 1981;7:205.
133. Jones RFC, Dorsch NWC, Silverberg GD, et al. Pathophysiology and management of raised intracranial pressure. Anaesth Intensive Care 1981;9:336.
134. Kalsbeek WD, McLaurin RL, Harris BSH III, et al. The national head and spinal cord injury survey: major findings. J Neurosurg 1980;53:S19.
135. Kamada T, Fusamoto H, Kawano S, et al. Gastrointestinal bleeding following head injury: a clinical study of 433 patients. J Trauma 1977;17:44.
136. Kanter RK, Weiner LB, Patti AM, et al. Infectious complications and duration of intracranial pressure monitoring. Crit Care Med 1985;13:837.
137. Kassell NF, Hitchon PW, Gerk MK, et al. Alterations in cerebral blood flow, oxygen metabolism, and electrical activity produced by high dose sodium thiopental. Neurosurgery 1980; 7:598.
138. Kaufman HH, Bretaudiere JP, Rowlands BJ, et al. General metabolism in head injury. Neurosurgery 1987;20:254.
139. Kaufman HH, Moake JL, Olson JD, et al. Delayed and recurrent intracranial hematomas related to disseminated intravascular clotting and fibrinolysis in head injury. Neurosurgery 1980;7:445.
140. Kimelberg HK, Bourke RS, Steig PE, et al. Swelling of astroglia after injury to the central nervous system: mechanisms and consequences. In: Grossman RG, Gildenberg PL, eds. Head injury. New York: Raven Press, 1982:31.

141. Kontos HA, Povlishok JT. Oxygen radicals in brain injury. Cent Nerv Syst Trauma 1986;3:257.
142. Kosteljanetz M. Acute head injury: pressure-volume relations and cerebrospinal fluid dynamics. Neurosurgery 1986;18:17.
143. Kosteljanetz M. Intracranial pressure: cerebrospinal fluid dynamics and pressure-volume relations. Acta Neurol Scand 1987;75 (Suppl 111):1.
144. Killberg G, Sundbärg G. Reduction of raised intracranial pressure following infusion of mannitol: a review of clinical pressure recordings. In: Beks JWF, Bosch DA, Brock M, eds. Intracranial pressure III. Berlin: Springer-Verlag, 1976:224.
145. Lane DJ, Rout MW, Williamson DH. Mechanism of hyperventilation in acute cerebrovascular accidents. Br Med J 1971;3:9.
146. Langfitt TW. The incidence and importance of intracranial hypertension in head-injured patients. In: Beks JWF, Bosch DA, Brock M, eds. Intracranial pressure III. Berlin: Springer-Verlag, 1976:67.
147. Langfitt W, Obrist WD, Gennarelli TA, et al. Correlation of cerebral blood flow with outcome in head injured patients. Ann Surg 1977;186:411.
148. Lanier WL, Milde JH, Michenfelder JD. Cerebral stimulation following succinylcholine in dogs. Anestheiology 1986;64:551.
149. Larson GM, Koch S, O'Dorisio TM, et al. Gastric response to severe head injury. Am J Surg 1984;147:97.
150. Ledingham I McA, Watt I. Influence of sedation on mortality in critically ill multiple trauma patients. Lancet 1983;1:1270.
151. Leech P, Barker J, Fitch W. Changes in intracranial pressure and systemic arterial pressure during the termination of anaesthesia. In: Lundberg N, Ponten U, Brock M, eds. Intracranial pressure II. Berlin: Springer-Verlag, 1975:342.
152. Leech PJ, Miller JD. The effect of mannitol, steroids and hypocapnia on the intracranial volume/pressure response. In: Lundberg N, Ponten U, Brock M, eds. Intracranial pressure II. Berlin: Springer-Verlag, 1975:361.
153. Lennon RL, Olson RA, Gronert FA. Atracurium or vecuronium for rapid sequence endotracheal intubation. Anesthesiology 1986;64:510.
154. Leuerssen TG, Klauber MR, Marshall LF. Outcome from head injury related to patient's age. J Neurosurg 1988;68:409.
155. Lewelt W, Jenkins LW, Miller JD. Autoregulation of cerebral blood flow after experimental fluid percussion injury of the brain. J Neurosurg 1980;53:500.
156. Lewelt W, Moszynski K, Kozniewska H. Effects of depolarizing, non-depolarizing muscle relaxants and intubation on the ventricular fluid pressure. In: Beks JWF, Bosch DA, Brock M, eds. Intracranial pressure III. Berlin: Springer-Verlag, 1976:215.
157. Long DM, Maxwell RE, Choi KS, et al. Multiple therapeutic approaches in the treatment of brain edema induced by a standard cold lesion. In: Reulen HJ, Schurmann K, eds. Steroids and brain edema. Berlin: Springer-Verlag, 1972:87.
158. Lundberg N. Continuous recording and control of ventricular fluid pressure in neurosurgical practice. Acta Psychiatr Neurol Scand 1960;36 (Suppl 149):1.
159. Lutz HA, Becker DP, Miller JD, Ward JD. Monitoring, management, and the analysis of outcome. In: Grossman RG, Gildenberg DL, eds. Head injury: basic and clinical aspects. New York: Raven Press, 1982:221.
160. Madsden JB, Cold GE, Hansen ES, Bardrum B. The effect of isoflurane on cerebral blood flow and metabolism in humans during craniotomy for small supratentorial cerebral tumors. Anesthesiology 1987;66:332.
161. Markwalder TM. Chronic subdural hematomas: a review. J Neurosurg 1981;54:637.
162. Marmarou A, Maset AL, Ward JD, et al. Contribution of CSF and vascular factors to elevation of ICP in severely head-injured patients. J Neurosurg 1987;66:833.
163. Marmarou A, Shulman K. Pressure-volume relationships: basic aspects. In: McLaurin RL, ed. Head injuries. New York: Grune and Stratton, 1975:233.
164. Marmarou A, Tabaddor K. Intracranial pressure: physiology and pathophysiology. In: Cooper PR, ed. Head injury. 2nd ed. Baltimore: Williams and Wilkins, 1987:159.
165. Marshall LF, Bowers SA. Medical management of intracranial pressure. In: Cooper PR, ed. Head injury. 2nd ed. Baltimore: Williams and Wilkins, 1987:177.
166. Marshall LF, Camp PE, Bowers SA. Dimethyl sulfoxide for the treatment of intracranial hypertension: a preliminary trial. Neurosurgery 1984;14:659.
167. Marshall LF, King J, Langfitt TW. The complications of high dose steroid therapy in neurosurgical patients: a prospective study. Ann Neurol 1977;1:201.
168. Marshall LF, Shapiro HM. Barbiturates for intracranial hypertension: a ten year perspective. In: Schulman K, Marmarou A, Miller JD, et al, eds. Intracranial pressure IV. Berlin: Springer-Verlag, 1980:627.
169. Marshall LF, Smith RW, Rauscher LA, et al. Mannitol dose requirements in brain-injured patients. J Neurosurg 1978;48:169.
170. Marshall LF, Smith RW, Shapiro HM. The outcome with aggressive treatment in severe head injuries, part I: the significance of intracranial pressure monitoring. J Neurosurg 1979;50:20.
171. Marshall LF, Smith RW, Shapiro HM. The outcome with aggressive treatment in severe head injuries, part II: acute and chronic barbiturate administration in the management of head injury. J Neurosurg 1979;50:26.
172. Maset AL, Marmarou A, Ward JD. Pressure-volume index in head injury. J Neurosurg 1987;66:832.
173. Matjasko MJ. Peripheral sequelae of acute head injury. In: Cottrell JJ, Turndorf H, eds. Anesthesia and neurosurgery. 2nd ed. St Louis: CV Mosby, 1986:224.
174. McDowall, DG. Artificial ventilation in the management of the head-injured patient. In: Fitch W, Barker J, eds. Head injury and the anaesthetist. Amsterdam: Elsevier, 1985:149.
175. McGraw CP, Alexander E, Howard G. Effect of dose and dose schedule on the response of intracranial pressure to mannitol. Surg Neurol 1978;10:127.
176. McIntosh TK, Vink R, Faden AI. An analogue of thyrotropin-releasing hormone improves outcome after brain injury: $^{31}P$ NMR studies. Am J Physiol 1988;254:R785.
177. McLeod AA, Neil-Dwyer G, Meyer DHA, et al. Cardiac sequelae of acute head injury. Br Heart J 1982;47:221.
178. McLeskey CH, Cullen BF, Kennedy RD, et al. Control of cerebral perfusion pressure during induction of anesthesia in high-risk neurosurgical patients. Anesth Analg 1974;53:985.
179. Mendelow AD, Teasdale GM, Russell T, et al. Effect of mannitol on cerebral blood flow and cerebral perfusion pressure in human head injury. J Neurosurg 1985;63:43.
180. Messick JM, Newberg LA, Nugent M, et al. Principles of neuroanesthesia for the nonneurosurgical patient with CNS pathophysiology. Anesth Analg 1985;64:143.
181. Miller JD. Clinical aspects of intracranial volume-pressure relationships. In: McLaurin RL, ed. Head injuries. New York: Grune and Stratton, 1975:239.
182. Miller JD. Head injury and brain-ischaemia implications for therapy. Br J Anaesth 1985;57:120.
183. Miller JD. The pathophysiology of head injury. In: Fitch W, Barker J, eds. Head injury and the anaesthetist. Amsterdam: Elsevier, 1985:31.
184. Miller JD, Becker DP, Ward JD, et al. Significance of intracranial hypertension in severe head injury. J Neurosurg 1977;47:503.
185. Miller JD, Butterworth JF, Gudeman SK, et al. Further expe-

rience in the management of severe head injury. J Neurosurg 1981;54:289.

186. Miller JD, Leech P. Effects of mannitol and steroid therapy on intracranial volume-pressure relationships in patients. J Neurosurg 1975;42:274.
187. Miller JD, Sullivan HG. Severe intracranial hypertension. In: Trubuhovich RV, ed. Management of acute intracranial disasters. Int Anesth Clin 1979;17:19.
188. Miller SM, Cottrell JE, Turndorf H, Ransohoff J. Cerebral protection by barbiturates and loop diuretics in acute head trauma: possible modes of action. Bull NY Acad Med 1980;56:305.
189. Millson CH, James HE, Shapiro HM, et al. Intracranial hypertension and brain edema in albino rabbits, Part 3: effect of acute simultaneous diuretic and barbiturate therapy. Acta Neurochirurg 1982;61:271.
190. Miner ME, Kaufman HH, Graham SH, et al. Disseminated intravascular coagulation and fibrinolysis following severe head trauma in children. In: Grossman RG, Gildenberg PL, eds. Head injury: basic and clinical aspects. New York: Raven Press, 1982:251.
191. Minton MD, Grosslight K, Stirt JA, Bedford RF. Increases in intracranial pressure from succinylcholine: prevention by prior nondepolarizing blockade. Anesthesiology 1986;65:165.
192. Molofsky WJ. Steroids and head trauma. Neurosurgery 1984;15:424.
193. Moss E, Powell D, Gibson RM, et al. Effect of etomidate on intracranial pressure and cerebral perfusion pressure. Br J Anaesth 1979;51:347.
194. Moss E, Powell D, Gibson RM, et al. Effects of tracheal intubation on intracranial pressure following induction of anaesthesia with thiopentone or althesin in patients undergoing neurosurgery. Br J Anaesth 1978;50:353.
195. Moss I, Lisbon A, Levine JF, et al. The effects of increased intracranial pressure on respiratory functions. In: Lundberg N, Ponten U, Brock M, eds. Intracranial pressure II. Berlin: Springer-Verlag, 1975:315.
196. Muizelaar JP, Lutz AA, Beck DP. Effect of mannitol on ICP and CBF and correlation with pressure autoregulation in severely head-injured patients. J Neurosurg 1984;61:700.
197. Narayan RK, Greenberg RP, Miller JD, et al. Improved confidence of outcome prediction in severe head injury. J Neurosurg 1981;54:751.
198. Narayan RK, Kishore DRS, Becker DP, et al. Intracranial pressure: to monitor or not to monitor? J Neurosurg 1982;56:650.
199. Nath F, Galbraith S. The effect of mannitol on cerebral white matter water content. J Neurosurg 1986;65:41.
200. Newlon PG, Greenberg RP. Evoked potentials in severe head injury. J Trauma 1984;24:61.
201. Nordby HK, Nesbakken R. The effect of high dose barbiturate decompression after severe head injury. Acta Neurochir 1984;72:157.
202. O'Malley KF, Ross SE. The incidence of injury to the cervical spine in patients with craniocerebral injury. J Trauma 1988;28:1476.
203. Osler W. The evolution of modern medicine. New Haven: Yale University Press, 1921.
204. Overgaard J. Reflections on prognostic determinants in head injury. In: McLaurin RL, ed. Head injuries. New York: Grune and Stratton, 1975:11.
205. Overgaard J. The distribution of regional cerebral blood flow values in traumatic coma. In: Grossman RG, Gildenberg PL, eds. Head injury: basic and clinical aspects. New York: Raven Press, 1982:239.
206. Parham AM, Ducker TB, Redding JS. Lung dysfunction in the presence of central nervous system disease. In: McLaurin RL, ed. Head injuries. New York: Grune and Stratton, 1975:147.
207. Parish RA, Webb KS. Hyperglycemia is not a poor prognostic sign in head-injured children. J Trauma 1988;28:517.
208. Parry TW. Trephination of the living human skull in prehistoric times. Br Med J 1923;1:457.
209. Peyster RG, Hoover ED. CT in head trauma. J Trauma 1982;22:25.
210. Pfenninger E, Kilian J. Die Oberkörper-Hochlagerung bei akutem Schadel-Hirn-Trauma. Anaesthetist 1984;33:115.
211. Piatt JH, Schiff SJ. High dose barbiturate therapy in neurosurgery and intensive care. Neurosurgery 1984;15:427.
212. Pitts LH, Kaktis JV. Effect of megadose steroids on ICP in traumatic coma. In: Shulman K, Marmarou A, Miller JD, et al. Intracranial pressure IV. Berlin: Springer-Verlag, 1980:638.
213. Pitts LH, Martin N. Head injuries. Surg Clin North Am 1982;62:47.
214. Pollay M, Fullenwider C, Roberts PA, et al. Effect of mannitol and furosemide on blood-brain osmotic gradient and intracranial pressure. J Neurosurg 1983;59:945.
215. Poole GV, Prough DS, Johnson JC, et al. Effects of resuscitation from hemorrhagic shock on cerebral hemodynamics in the presence of an intracranial mass. J Trauma 1987;27:18.
216. Povlishock JT, Becker DP, Kontos HA, et al. Neural and vascular alterations in head injury. In: Popp AJ, Bourke RS, Nelson LR, Kimelberg HK, eds. Neural trauma. New York: Raven Press, 1979:79.
217. Povlishock JT, Kontos HA. The pathophysiology of pial and intraparenchymal vascular dysfunction. In: Grossman RG, Gildenberg PL, eds. Head injury: basic and clinical aspects. New York: Raven Press, 1982:15.
218. Prior JGL, Hinds CJ, Williams J, et al. The use of etomidate in the management of severe head injury. Intensive Care Med 1983;9:313.
219. Proctor HJ, Palladino GW, Fillipo D. Failure of autoregulation after closed-head injury: an experimental model. J Trauma 1988;28:347.
220. Prough DS, Coker LH, Lee S, et al. Hyperglycemia and neurologic outcome in patients with closed-head injury. Anesthesiology 1988;69:A584.
221. Prough DS, Johnson JC, Poole GV, et al. Effects on intracranial pressure of resuscitation from hemorrhagic shock with hypertonic saline versus lactated Ringer's solution. Crit Care Med 1985;13:407.
222. Raichle ME, Posner JB, Plum F. Cerebral blood flow during and after hyperventilation. Arch Neurol 1970;23:394.
223. Ransohoff J. The effects of steroids on brain edema in man. In: Reulen HJ, Schurmann K, eds. Steroids and brain edema. Berlin: Springer-Verlag, 1972:211.
224. Rapp RP, Young B, Twyman D, et al. The favorable effect of early parenteral feeding on survival in head-injured patients. J Neurosurg 1983;58:906.
225. Rappaport M, Hall K, Hopkins HK, et al. Evoked potentials and head injury, 1: rating of evoked potential abnormality. Clin Electroencephal 1981;12:154.
226. Rappaport M, Hopkins HK, Hall K, et al. Evoked potential and head injury, 2: clinical applications. Clin Electroencephal 1981;12:167.
227. Rea GL, Rockswold GL. Barbiturate therapy in uncontrolled intracranial hypertension. Neurosurgery 1983;12:401.
228. Roberts PA, Polley M, Engles C, et al. Effect on intracranial pressure of furosemide combined with varying doses and administration rates of mannitol. J Neurosurg 1987; 66:440.
229. Robertson CS, Clifton CL, Grossman RG. Oxygen utilization and cardiovascular function in head-injured patients. Neurosurgery 1984;15:307.
230. Robertson CS, Clifton GL, Grossman RG, et al. Alterations in

cerebral availability of metabolic substrates after severe head injury. J Trauma 1988;28:1523.
231. Robertson CS, Clifton GL, Taylor AA, et al. Treatment of hypertension associated with head injury. J Neurosurg 1983;59:455.
232. Rosa G, Orfei P, Sanfilippo M, et al. The effects of atracurium besylate (Tracrium) on intracranial pressure and cerebral perfusion pressure. Anesth Analg 1986;65:381.
233. Rosa G, Sanfilippo M, Vilardi V, et al. Effects of vecuronium bromide on intracranial pressure and cerebral perfusion pressure. Br J Anaesth 1986;58:437.
234. Rose J, Valtonen S, Jennett B. Avoidable factors contributing to death after head injury. Br Med J 1977;2:615.
235. Rosner MJ, Coley I. Cerebral perfusion pressure: a hemodynamic mechanism of mannitol and the postmannitol hemogram. Neurosurgery 1987;21:147.
236. Rosner MJ, Coley IB. Cerebral perfusion pressure, intracranial pressure, and head elevation. J Neurosurg 1986;65:636.
237. Rosner MJ, Newsome HH, Becker DP. Mechanical brain injury: the sypathoadrenal response. J Neurosurg 1984;61:76.
238. Ross JC, Harris P. Tribute to Sir Ludwig Guttmann. Paraplegia 1980;18:154.
239. Rowan JO, Johnston IH. Blood pressure response to raised CSF pressure. In: Lundberg N, Ponten V, Brock M, eds. Intracranial pressure II. Berlin: Springer-Verlag, 1975:298.
240. Sari A, Matayoshi Y, Yonei A, et al. Cerebral arteriovenous oxygen content difference during barbiturate therapy in patients with acute brain damage. Anesth Analg 1986;65:1196.
241. Scheller MS, Todd MM, Drummond JC. Isoflurane, halothane, and regional cerebral blood flow at various levels of $Pa_{CO_2}$ in rabbits. Anesthesiology 1986;64:598.
242. Scheller MS, Todd MM, Drummond JC, Zornow MH. The intracranial pressure effects of isoflurane and halothane administered following cryogenic brain injury in rabbits. Anesthesiology 1987;67:507.
243. Schettini A. Incompatibility of halogenated anesthetics with brain surgery. In Shulman K, Marmarou A, Miller JD, et al, eds. Intracranial pressure IV. Berlin: Springer-Verlag, 1980: 599.
244. Schulte am Esch J, Themig I, Entzian W. Wirkungen von Etomidat und Thiopental an den Stickoxydulbedingten intrakraniellen Druckansteig. Anaesthetist 1980;29:525.
245. Shalit MN, Cotev S. The Cushing response: a compensatory mechanism or a dangerous phenomenon. In: Lundberg N, Ponten U, Brock M, eds. Intracranial pressure II. Berlin: Springer-Verlag, 1975:307.
246. Shapiro HM. Intracranial hypertension: therapeutic and anesthetic considerations. Anesthesiology 1975;43:445.
247. Shapiro K, Marmarou A. Clinical applications of the pressure-volume index in treatment of pediatric head injuries. J Neurosurg 1982;56:819.
248. Shogan SH, Kindt GW. Injuries of the head and spinal cord. In: Zuidema GD, Rutherford RB, Ballinger WF, eds. The Management of trauma. Philadelphia: WB Saunders, 1985:207.
249. Sichez JP, Melon E, Clergues F, et al. Traumatismes craniocerebraux avec signes precoces de souffrance axiale: traitement par drainage ventriculaire externe et barbituriques. Neurochirurgie 1981;27:205.
250. Skinhøj E, Overgaard J. Effect of dihydralazine on intracranial pressure in patients with severe brain damage. Acta Med Scand 1984;(Suppl 678):83.
251. Smith AL. Barbiturate protection in cerebral hypoxia. Anesthesiology 1977;47:285.
252. Smith DS. Fluid management in neurosurgical anesthesia. ASA Refresher Course Lectures 1983;11:205.
253. Stirt JA, Grosslight KR, Bedford RF, Vollmer D. "Defasciculation" with metocurine prevents succinylcholine-induced increases in intracranial pressure. Anesthesiology 1987;66:50.
254. Stirt JA, Maggio W, Haworth C, et al. Vecuronium: effect on intracranial pressure and hemodynamics in neurosurgical patients. Anesthesiology 1987;67:570.
255. Sundt TM, Jr. Clinical management of severe vasospasm. In: Wishant JP, Sandok BA, eds. Proceedings of the ninth Princeton conference on cerebrovascular diseases. New York: Grune and Stratton, 1975:77.
256. Tabaddor K. Emergency care: initial evaluation. In: Cooper PR, ed. Head injury. Baltimore: Williams and Wilkins, 1982:15.
257. Tabaddor K, Tavares A, Marmarou A, et al. Intracranial pressure and cerebral compliance during hypotension induced by sodium nitroprusside. Acta Neurol Scand 1977;56 (Suppl 64):310.
258. Teasdale G, Jennett B. Assessment of coma and impaired consciousness: a practical scale. Lancet 1974;2:81.
259. Teasdale G, Skene A, Speigelhalter D, et al. Age, severity and outcome of head injury. In: Grossman RG, Gildenberg PL, eds. Head injury: basic and clinical aspects. New York: Raven Press, 1982:213.
260. Tello JC. Prehistoric trephining among the Yamajos of Peru. 18 Session Congress Int des Americanistes 1913;75.
261. Theodore J, Robin ED. Pathogenesis of neurogenic pulmonary oedema. Lancet 1975;2:749.
262. Thiagarajah S, Sophie S, Lear E, et al. Effect of suxamethonium on the ICP of cats with and without thiopentone pretreatment. Br J Anaesth 1988;60:157.
263. Todd MM, Drummond JC. A comparison of the cerebrovascular and metabolic effects of halothane and isoflurane in the cat. Anesthesiology 1984;60:276.
264. Tornheim PA, McLaurin RL. Effect of dexamethasone on cerebral edema from cranial impact in the cat. J Neurosurg 1978;48:220.
265. Tornheim PA, McLaurin RL, Sawaya R. Effect of furosemide on experimental traumatic cerebral edema. Neurosurgery 1979;4:48.
266. Traeger SM, Henning RJ, Dobkin W, et al. Hemodynamic effects of pentobarbital therapy for intracranial hypertension. Crit Care Med 1983;11:697.
267. Trouwborst A, Kooijman J. The alterations of plasma potassium in patients with severe acute head injury. Injury 1984;15:293.
268. Tsuruda J, James HE, Camp PE, et al. Acute dimethyl sulfoxide therapy in experimental brain edema, part 2: effect of dose and concentration on intracranial pressure, blood pressure, and central venous pressure. Neurosurgery 1982;10:355.
269. Turner E, Hilfiker O, Braun U, et al. Metabolic and hemodynamic response to hyperventilation in patients with head injuries. Intensive Care Med 1984;10:127.
270. Unni VKN, Gray WJ, Young HSA. Effects of atracurium on intracranial pressure in man. Anaesthesia 1986;41:1047.
271. Wagner KR, Tornheim P, Eichhold MK. Acute changes in regional cerebral metabolite values following experimental blunt head trauma. J Neurosurg 1985;63:88.
272. Wagner RL, White PF. Etomidate inhibits adrenocortical function in surgical patients. Anesthesiology 1984;61:647.
273. Wagner RL, White PF, Kan PB, et al. Inhibition of adrenal steroidogenesis by the anesthetic etomidate. N Engl J Med 1984;310:1415.
274. Ward JD, Becker DP, Miller JD, et al. Failure of prophylactic barbiturate coma in the treatment of severe head injury. J Neurosurg 1985;62:383.
275. Wauchob TD, Brooks RJ, Harrison KM. Neurogenic pulmonary oedema. Anaesthesia 1984;39:528.
276. Weaver DD, Winn HR, Jane JA. Differential intracranial pressure in patients with unilateral mass lesions. J Neurosurg 1982;56:660.

277. Weisman SU. Edema and congestion of the lungs resulting from intracranial hemorrhage. Surgery 1939;6:722.
278. White PF, Schlobohm RM, Pitts LH, et al. A randomized study of drugs for preventing increases in intracranial pressure during endotracheal suctioning. Anesthesiology 1982;57:242.
279. Wilkins RW. Neurosurgical classics. New York: Johnson Reprint Corp, 1965.
280. Wilkinson HA, Rosenfeld S. Furosemide and mannitol in the treatment of acute experimental intracranial hypertension. Neurosurgery 1983;12:405.
281. Wilson DJ, Wallin JD, Vlachakis ND, et al. Intravenous labetalol in the treatment of severe hypertension and hypertensive emergencies. Am J Med 1983;75:95.
282. Wisner D, Busche F, Sturm J, et al. Traumatic shock and head injury: results of fluid resuscitation on the brain. J Surg Res 1989;46:49.
283. Worthley LIG, Cooper DJ, Jones N. Treatment of resistant intracranial hypertension with hypertonic saline. J Neurosurg 1988;68:478.
284. Wright PJ, Murray RJ. Penetrating cerebral airgun injury. Anaesthesia 1989;44:219.
285. Yano M, Kobayashi S, Otsuka T, et al. Useful ICP monitoring with subarachnoid catheter method in severe head injuries. J Trauma 1988;28:476.
286. Yano M, Nishayama H, Yokota H, et al. Effect of lidocaine on ICP response to endotracheal suctioning. Anesthesiology 1986;64:651.
287. Yen JK, Bourke RS, Popp AJ, et al. Use of ethacrynic acid in the treatment of serious head injury. In: Popp AJ, Bourke RS, Nelson LR, Kimelberg HK, eds. Neural trauma. New York: Raven Press, 1979:329.
288. Young B, Ott L, Twyman D. The effect of nutritional support on outcome from severe head injury. J Neurosurg 1987;67:668.
289. Young B, Rapp RP, Norton JA, et al. Early prediction of outcome in head-injured patients. J Neurosurg 1981;55:300.

## SPINAL CORD INJURIES

290. Alderson JD, Thomas DC. The use of halothane anaesthesia to control automatic hyperreflexia in spinal cord injury patients. Paraplegia 1975;13:183.
291. Alvarez SE, Peterson M, Lunsford BR. Respiratory treatment of the adult patient with spinal cord injury. Phys Ther 1981;61:1737.
292. Anderson DK, Means ED, Waters TR, et al. Microvascular perfusion and metabolism in injured spinal cord after methylprednisolone treatment. J Neurosurg 1982;56:106.
293. Anderson DM, Braughler JM, Hall ED, et al. Effects of treatment with U-74006F on neurological outcome following experimental spinal cord injury. J Neurosurg 1988;69:562.
294. Axelsson J, Thesleff S. A study of supersensitivity in denervated mammalian skeletal muscle. J Physiol 1959;147:178.
295. Benthuysen JL. Naloxone therapy in spinal trauma: anesthetic effects. Anesthesiology 1987;66:238.
296. Berlly HM, Wilmot CB. Acute abdominal emergencies during the first four weeks after spinal cord injury. Arch Phys Med Rehabil 1984;65:687.
297. Bohlmann HH. Acute fractures and dislocations of the cervical spine. J Bone Joint Surg 1979;61A:1119.
298. Boyd JD, LeGros Clark WE, Hamilton WJ, et al. Textbook of human anatomy. London: Macmillan, 1957:725.
299. Bracken MB, Collins WF, Freeman DF, et al. Efficacy of methylprednisolone in acute spinal cord injury. JAMA 1984;251:45.
299a. Bracken MB, Shepard MJ, Collins WF, et al. A randomized controlled trial of methylprednisolone or naloxone in the treatment of acute spinal cord injury. N Engl J Med 1990;332:1405.
300. Braughler JM, Hall ED. Effects of multi-dose methylprednisolone sodium succinate administration on injured cat spinal cord neurofilament degradation and energy metabolism. J Neurosurg 1984;61:290.
301. Brooke MM, Donovan WH, Stolov WC. Paraplegia: succinylcholine-induced hyperkalemia and cardiac arrest. Arch Phys Med Rehabil 1978;59:306.
302. Carey ME, Nance FC, Kirgis HD, et al. Pancreatitis following spinal cord injury. J Neurosurg 1977;47:917.
303. Chahrazi B, Wagner FC, Jr, Collins WF, et al. A scale for evaluation of spinal cord injury. J Neurosurg 1981;54:310.
304. Charney KJ, Juler GL, Comarr EJ. General surgery problems in patients with spinal cord injuries. Arch Surg 1975;110:1083.
305. Cheshire DJE, Coats DA. Respiratory and metabolic management in acute tetraplegia. Paraplegia 1966;4:1.
306. Collins WF. A review and update of experimental and clinical studies of spinal cord injury. Paraplegia 1983;21:204.
307. Cooperman LH. Succinylcholine-induced hyperkalemia in neuromuscular disease. JAMA 1970;213:1867.
308. Cox SAR, Weiss SM, Posuniak EA, et al. Energy expenditure after spinal cord injury: an evaluation of stable rehabilitating patients. J Trauma 1985;25:419.
309. De la Torre JC. Spinal cord injury: review of basic and applied research. Spine 1981;6:315.
310. Demopoulos HB, Flamm ES, Seligman ML, et al. Molecular pathogenesis of spinal cord degeneration after traumatic injury. In: Naftchi NE, ed. Spinal cord injury. New York: SP Medical and Scientific Books, 1982:45.
311. Demopoulos HB, Milvy P, Kakary S, et al. Molecular aspects of membrane structure in brain edema. In: Reulen JJ, Schurman K, eds. Steroids and brain edema. Berlin: Springer-Verlag, 1972:29.
312. Dolan EJ, Tator CH. The effect of blood transfusion, dopamine and gamma hydroxybutyrate on posttraumatic ischemia of the spinal cord. J Neurosurg 1982;56:350.
313. Donovan WH, Dwyer AP. An update on the early management of traumatic paraplegia (nonoperative and operative management). Clin Orthop 1984;189:12.
314. Doolan LA, O'Brien JF. Safe intubation in cervical spine injury. Anaesth Intensive Care 1985;13:319.
315. Ducker TB. Experimental injury of the spinal cord. In: Vinken PJ, Bruyn PW, eds. Handbook of clinical neurology: injuries of the spine and spinal cord, part I. New York: American Elsevier, 1976:9.
316. El Masri W, Cochrane P, Silver JR. Gastrointestinal bleeding in patients with acute spinal injuries. Injury 1982;14:162.
317. El Masri WS, Silver JR. Prophylactic anticoagulant therapy in patients with spinal cord injury. Paraplegia 1981;19:334.
318. Epstein N, Hood DC, Ransohoff J. Gastrointestinal bleeding in patients with spinal cord trauma. J Neurosurg 1981;54:16.
319. Faden, AI. Role of thyrotropin-releasing hormone and opiate receptor antagonists in limiting central nervous system injury. Adv Neurol 1988;47:531.
320. Faden AI, Jacobs TP, Holaday JW. Comparison of early and late naloxone treatment in experimental spinal injury. Neurology 1982;32:677.
321. Faden AI, Jacobs TP, Holaday JW. Thyrotropin-releasing hormone improves neurologic recovery after spinal trauma in cats. N Engl J Med 1981;305:1063.
322. Faden AI, Jacobs TP, Mougey E, et al. Endorphins in experimental spinal injury: therapeutic effect of naloxone. Ann Neurol 1981;10:326.
323. Faden AI, Jacobs TP, Patrick DH, et al. Megadose corticosteroid therapy following experimental traumatic spinal injury. J Neurosurg 1984;60:712.

324. Feuer H. Management of acute spine and spinal cord injuries. Arch Surg 1976;111:638.
325. Flamm ES, Young W, Collins WF, et al. A phase I trial of naloxone treatment in acute spinal cord injury. J Neurosurg 1985;63:390.
326. Flamm ES, Young W, Demopoulos HB, et al. Experimental spinal cord injury: treatment with naloxone. Neurosurgery 1982;10:227.
327. Forner JV. Lung volumes and mechanics of breathing in tetraplegia. Paraplegia 1980;18:258.
328. Fraser A, Edmonds-Seal J. Spinal cord injuries: a review of problems facing the anaesthetist. Anaesthesia 1982;37:1084.
329. Gardner BP, Watt JWH, Krishnan KR. The artificial ventilation of acute spinal cord damaged patients: a retrospective study of forty-four patients. Paraplegia 1986;24:208.
330. Gardner E, Gray DJ, O'Rahilly R. Anatomy: a regional study of human structure. Philadelphia: WB Saunders, 1969:556.
331. Geisler WO, Jousse AT, Wynne-Jones M. Survival in traumatic transverse myelitis. Paraplegia 1977;14:262.
332. Gore RM, Mintzer RA, Calenoff L. Gastrointestinal complications of spinal cord injury. Spine 1981;6:538.
333. Gree BA, Klose KJ. Acute spinal cord injury: emergency room diagnosis, medical and surgical management. In: Green BA, Marshall LF, Gallagher TJ, eds. Intensive care for neurological trauma and disease. New York: Academic Press, 1982:249.
334. Green D, Lee MY, Ito VY, et al. Fixed vs adjusted-dose heparin in the prophylaxis of thromboembolism in spinal cord injury. JAMA 1988;260:1255.
335. Gronert GA, Theye RA. Pathophysiology of hyperkalemia induced by succinylcholine. Anesthesiology 1975;43:89.
336. Guttman L. Spinal cord injuries: comprehensive management and research. 2nd ed. Oxford: Blackwell, 1976.
337. Haghighi SS, Chehrazi B. Effect of naloxone in experimental acute spinal cord injury. Neurosurgery 1987;20:385.
338. Hall ED, Braughler JM. Role of lipid peroxidation in posttraumatic spinal cord degeneration. Cent Nerv Syst Trauma 1986;3:281.
339. Hall ED, Wolf DL. Post-traumatic spinal cord ischemia: relationship to injury severity and physiologic parameters. Cent Nerv Syst Trauma 1987;4:15.
340. Hall ED, Wolf DL, Braughler JM. Effects of a single large dose of methylprednisolone sodium succinate on experimental posttraumatic spinal cord ischemia. J Neurosurg 1984;61:124.
341. Hansebout RR. A comprehensive review of methods of improving cord recovery after acute spinal cord injury. In: Tator CH, ed. Early management of acute spinal cord injury. New York: Raven Press, 1982:181.
342. John DA, Tobey RE, Homer LD, et al. Onset of succinylcholine-induced hyperkalemia following denervation. Anesthesiology 1976;45:294.
343. Kaufman HH, Rowlands BJ, Stein DK, et al. General metabolism in patients with acute paraplegia and quadriplegia. Neurosurgery 1985;16:309.
344. Kiwersky J. Bleeding from the alimentary canal during the management of spinal cord injury patients. Paraplegia 1986;24:92.
345. Lambert DH, Deane RG, Mazuzan JE. Anesthesia and the control of blood pressure in patients with spinal cord injury. Anesth Analg 1982;61:344.
346. Le CT, Price M. Survival from spinal cord injury. J Chron Dis 1982;35:487.
347. Ledsome JR, Sharp JM. Pulmonary function in acute cervical cord injury. Am Rev Respir Dis 1981;124:41.
348. Lehmann KG, Lane JG, Piepmeier JM, Batsford WP. Cardiovascular abnormalities accompanying acute spinal injury in humans. J Am Coll Cardiol 1987;10:46.
349. Leramo OB, Tator CH, Hudson AR. Massive gastroduodenal hemorrhage and perforation in acute spinal cord injury. Surg Neurol 1982;17:186.
350. Lewin MG, Pappius HM, Hansebout RR. Effects of steroids on edema associated with injury of the spinal cord. In: Reulen NJ, Schurmann K, eds. Steroids and brain edema. Berlin: Springer-Verlag, 1972:101.
351. Mackenzie CF, Shin B, Krishnaprasad D, et al. Assessment of cardiac and respiratory function during surgery on patients with acute quadriplegia. J Neurosurg 1985;62:843.
352. Mathias CJ. Bradycardia and cardiac arrest during tracheal suction: mechanisms in tetraplegic patients. Eur J Intensive Care Med 1976;2:147.
353. McKenzie RN. Anesthesia in acute cervical cord injuries. In: Tator CH, ed. Early management of acute spinal cord injury. New York: Raven Press, 1982:219.
354. Morgan BC, Martin WE, Hornbein TF, et al. Hemodynamic effects of intermittent positive pressure respiration. Anesthesiology 1966;27:584.
355. Naftchi NE, Demeny M, Demopoulos H, et al. Effect of pharmacological agents on normalization of molecular and histologic dysfunction following traumatic injury to the spinal cord. In: Naftchi NE, ed. Spinal cord injury. New York: SP Medical and Scientific Books, 1982:29.
356. Naftchi NE, Demeny M, Demopoulos H, et al. The ameliorating effect of pharmacological agents on the traumatically injured spinal cord. In: Parvez H, Parvez S, eds. Advances in experimental medicine: a centenary tribute to Claude Bernard. Amsterdam: Elsevier, 1980:373.
357. Ohry A, Molho M, Rozin R. Alterations of pulmonary function in spinal cord-injured patients. Paraplegia 1975;13:101.
358. Ransohoff J, Benjamin MV, Engler G, et al. Surgical intervention in spinal cord injury. In: Popp AJ, Bourke RS, Nelson LR, Kimelberg HK, eds. Neural trauma. New York: Raven Press, 1979:353.
359. Silver JR. Immediate management of spinal injury. Br J Hosp Med 1983;29:412.
360. Silver JR, Morris WR, Otfinowski JS. Associated injuries in patients with spinal injury. Injury 1980;12:219.
361. Silver JR, Moulton A. The physiological and pathological sequelae of paralysis of the intercostal and abdominal muscles in tetraplegic patients. Paraplegia 1969;7:131.
362. Smith DS. Management of patients with acute and chronic spinal cord injury. ASA Refresher Course Lectures 1983;11:215.
363. Soderstrom CA, McArdle DQ, Ducker TB, et al. The diagnosis of intra-abdominal injury with cervical cord trauma. J Trauma 1983;23:1061.
364. Stewart WB, Wagner FC Jr. Fascicular distribution of spinal cord edema following experimental trauma. In: Popp AJ, Bourke RS, Nelson LR, Kimelberg HK, eds. Neural trauma. New York: Raven Press, 1979:131.
365. Tator CH. Spinal cord cooling and irrigation for treatment of acute cord injury. In: Popp AJ, Bourke RS, Nelson LR, Kimelberg HK, eds. Neural trauma. New York: Raven Press, 1979:363.
366. Tobey RE, Jacobsen DM, Kahlf CT, et al. The serum potassium response to muscle relaxants in neural injury. Anesthesiology 1972;37:332.
367. Troll GF, Dohrmann GJ. Anaesthesia of the spinal cord-injured patient: cardiovascular problems and their management. Paraplegia 1975;13:162.
368. Wallace MC, Tator CH. Failure of naloxone to improve spinal cord blood flow and cardiac output after spinal cord injury. Neurosurgery 1986;18:428.
369. Watson N. Anti-coagulant therapy in the prevention of venous thrombosis and pulmonary embolism in spinal cord injury. Paraplegia 1978–79;16:265.

370. Weber RK. Respiratory management of acute cervical cord injuries. In: Tator CH, ed. Early management of acute spinal cord injury. New York: Raven Press, 1982:213.
371. Welply NC, Mathias CJ, Frankel HL. Circulatory reflexes in tetraplegics during artificial ventilation and general anaesthesia. Paraplegia 1975;13:172.
372. Wilmot CB, Hall KM. Evaluation of the acute management of tetraplegia: conservative versus surgical treatment. Paraplegia 1986;24:148.
373. Yashon D. Spinal injury. New York: Appleton Century-Crofts, 1978:176.
374. Young W, Flamm ES, Demopoulos HB, et al. Effect of naloxone on posttraumatic ischemia in experimental spinal contusion. J Neurosurg 1981;55:209.
375. Zäch GA, Gyr KE, Von Alvensleben E, et al. A double-blind randomized, controlled study to investigate the efficacy of cimetidine given in addition to conventional therapy in the prevention of stress ulceration and haemorrhage in patients with acute spinal cord injury. Digestion 1984;29:214.

# Chapter Eleven

Levon M. Capan
Durgesh Mankikar
William M. Eisenberg

# Anesthetic Management of Ocular Injuries

Among all human sensory modalities, sight is the most dominant; we live in a visual world. The rods and cones in the retinas of the two eyes comprise about 70% of the receptors in the entire body.[137] The approximately 2 million fibers that comprise the optic nerves represent about one third of all afferent nerve fibers projecting information to the central nervous system. So important is the visual system that 6 of the 12 cranial nerves (II, III, IV, V, VI, and VII) are responsible for its innervation. It is natural, therefore, to turn the head toward a disturbance, for instance a loud explosion, in order to judge its direction, type, and magnitude. This may render the face, eyes, and head vulnerable to various types of injuries. However, the orbit houses the eye so effectively that only a relatively small percentage of traumatic insults directed to this area actually cause ocular injury. It is well known that in most individuals the eye cannot be touched by the surface of an open palm applied to the anterior aspect of the orbit. In addition, reflex closure of the eyelids protects the globe from much potential damage.

Ophthalmic injuries, although disfiguring and distressing, are rarely life threatening. Nevertheless, because they may cause blindness, they assume great importance; ocular trauma is the most common cause of unilateral loss of vision throughout the world.[56] Although most patients with ophthalmic injuries do not pose serious problems to the skilled practitioner, slight mismanagement of open-eye injuries can lead to extrusion of intraocular contents and thus, blindness. It is crucial for anesthesiologists, ophthalmologists, and trauma and plastic surgeons to be familiar with the factors that control intraocular volume and tension, and the means by which these parameters can be optimized in the injured eye.

The past 2 decades have seen a remarkable change in ophthalmic surgery.[61] Because of advances in anesthetic techniques and the introduction of operating microscopes and fine surgical instruments and suture materials into clinical practice, operations on the vitreous and retina, which were formerly considered impracticable, can now be performed without difficulty. Anterior and posterior segment ocular reconstruction can be accomplished as a primary or secondary surgical procedure. General anesthesia, by providing a completely immobile eye, by controlling the physiological factors that affect the dynamics of intraocular pressure (IOP), and by eliminating the need for patient cooperation, contributes greatly to the success of this type of reconstructive surgery. General anesthesia, however, may be associated with risks to the eye and/or other systems. Adherence to certain principles will minimize, although not entirely eliminate, these risks.

In this chapter, we intend (1) to review the basic anatomy and physiology of the eye; (2) to highlight the important aspects of ocular injuries as they relate to anesthesiologists; (3) to review briefly the physiology of IOP in the intact and perforated eye; and (4) to discuss the anesthetic management of patients with various types of ocular injuries.

## ANATOMY OF THE EYE

The globe is a slightly asymmetrical sphere consisting of two segments. The smaller anterior segment has a radius of approximately 8 mm, and the posterior segment has a radius of approximately 12 mm. The eyeball is also slightly flattened vertically and has its greatest diameter, approximately 24 mm, in the anterior-posterior axis. The anterior segment, comprising the cornea, aqueous humor, iris, ciliary body, and lens, is divided by the iris into anterior and posterior chambers. The aqueous humor, which has a volume of 0.25 mL in the anterior chamber and 0.06 mL in the posterior chamber, is an optically clear, cell-free, and relatively protein-free fluid with a pH of 7.1 to 7.2 and a specific gravity of 1.003. It has a viscosity of 1.025 to 1.040 relative to water and a low urea and glucose content.[39,132] Aqueous humor is produced in a 6-mm girdle of uveal tissue called the ciliary body. Both clinical and experimental studies indicate that its production is related both to carbonic anhydrase activity and active cation transport, probably mediated by $Na^+$-$K^+$-ATPase.[39,132] Inhibition of either of these enzymes decreases entry of water into the posterior chamber. The flow of aqueous within the eye primarily follows an anterograde path: posterior chamber-pupil-anterior chamber-trabecular meshwork (spaces of Fontana)-Schlemm's canal-aqueous veins-anterior ciliary veins, then into the episcleral vein-orbital venous system to the cavernous sinus-jugular veins and right atrium (Fig 11-1). Thus, obstruction of the intraocular portion of this path and/or elevation of pressure in the venous system interferes with drainage of the aqueous humor and produces an increase in IOP. In an unperforated injured eye, obstruction at the trabecular meshwork may be caused by a collection of blood in the anterior chamber (hyphema) or by anterior displacement of the iris. Delay in treatment of eye injuries may also result in synechiae at various sites in the anterior segment which, by impeding the drainage of aqueous humor, may cause a rise in IOP. Similar events may occur following open-eye injuries when infection or inflammation develops after the perforation is sealed spontaneously or surgically.

The vitreous is a meshwork of collagen fibers occupying the vitreous cavity. Interspersed between and supporting these collagen fibers are hyaluronic acid molecules. Because of the sponge-like ability of the hyaluronic acid, large amounts of water can be retained, allowing the collagen network to expand and fill the veitreous cavity. The normal vitreous has firm adhesions at the vitreous base, an area that straddles the ora serrata, an irregular line at the interior surface of the globe where the neural retina transforms into a visually nonfunctional layer (Fig 11-1). Less firm adhesions occur between the vitreous and the optic disc, macula, along blood vessels, and around areas of chorioretinal scarring. Weaker adhesions exist between the vitreous and the internal limiting membrane of the retina. Thus, detachment of the vitreous either spontaneously or following trauma can cause concomitant retinal damage.

The globe of the eye has three concentric coats: the outer scleral tunic, the middle uvea, and the inner retina.[87] The sclera is collagenous, avascular, and continuous with the dura of the optic nerve posteriorly and the transparent cornea anteriorly. Its compliance is relatively low, thus small increases in intraocular volume may result in sharp elevation of intraocular pressure[196] (Fig 11-2). Contractions of the six external ocular muscles attached to this layer may also result in transient elevation of IOP.

The middle coat consists, from posterior to anterior, of the choroid, ciliary body, and iris. It is a highly vascular structure serving primarily a nutritive function. The ophthalmic artery, a branch of the internal carotid, supplies the uvea via multiple short and two long posterior ciliary arteries that anastomose extensively with the muscular anterior ciliary arteries. There are usually four vortex veins that drain the large network of uveal veins. They emerge through the sclera behind the equator of the globe before forming the orbital veins which empty into the cavernous sinus.[87]

The innermost tunic of the globe is the retina. This delicate 10-cell layer thick transparent structure consisting of neuronal, glial, and vascular tissue varies in thickness from 0.2 to 0.5 mm. Highly specialized, consisting of photoreceptor cells, it is the eye's receptor of visual information. The rod photoreceptors contain the pigment rhodopsin, which functions in dim-light vision. Pigments contained in the cone photoreceptors are responsible for color discrimination and nor-

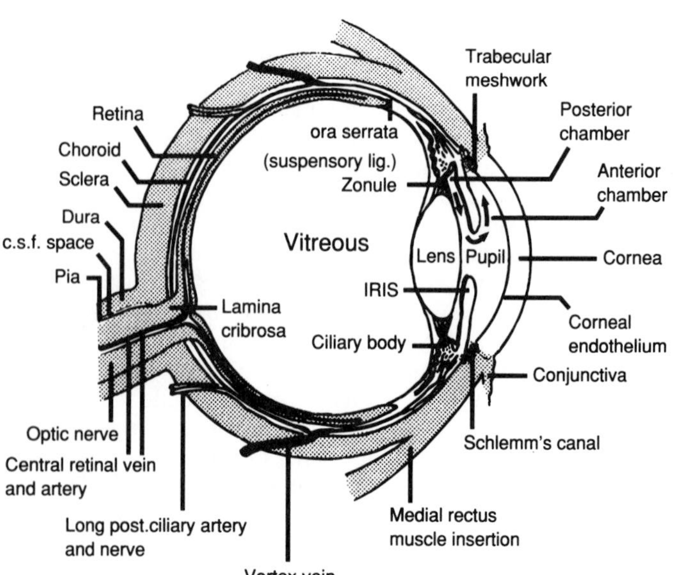


FIG. 11-1. Anatomical organization of the eye.

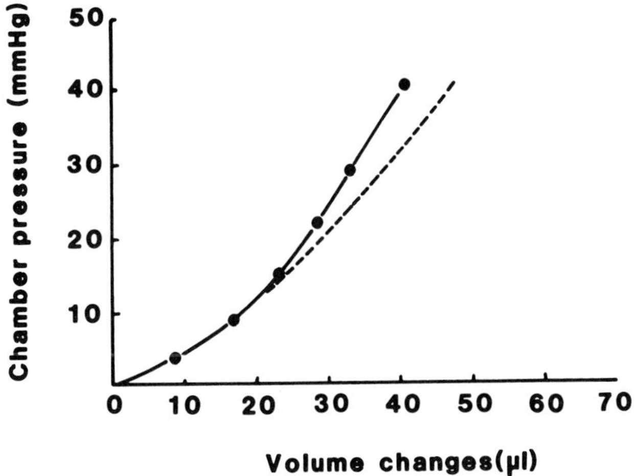


FIG. 11-2. Pressure changes produced by gradual volume increases in the anterior segment of the corneoscleral shell of enucleated human eyes. The solid curve is generated by a computer using the trilinear stress-strain relations of 15 specimens. The broken line is obtained experimentally from 13 specimens using a volume injection technique. (From Woo et al[196] with permission.)

mal daylight vision. The area centralis, the posterior pole of the retina, contains the macula. The macula, a region of retina temporal to the optic nerve head, contains two or more layers of ganglion cells and the highest concentration of cone photoreceptors. The neural retina gradually thins and ends anteriorly at the ora serrata where it is firmly adherent to the choroid. This explains the fact that retinal detachments end at the ora serrata. Although all the elements essential for visual function end at the ora serrata, embryologically the retina continues anteriorly to form the pigmented and nonpigmented cells of the ciliary body and iris.

The retina is supplied by two separate vascular systems. The outer portion of the sensory retina, that closest to the choroid, is supplied by the choroidal circulation, and the inner retina, adjacent to the vitreous body, is supplied by the retinal circulation derived from the central retinal artery, a branch of the ophthalmic artery. The central retinal vessels pierce the dura and arachnoid approximately 12 to 15 mm posterior to the globe and enter the eye in the center of the optic nerve.[87]

## THE SPECTRUM OF OCULAR INJURIES

Every year approximately 100,000 work-related and at least 35,000 to 40,000 sports-related eye injuries occur.[1,187] Assuming that other major causes—falls, assaults, burns, household and vehicular accidents—account for an additional 300,000 cases, approximately 500,000 individuals probably sustain eye injury every year. Fortunately, only a small percentage of these patients have serious ocular damage. Blomdahl and Norell[20] reported a 60.6 per million annual incidence rate for perforating eye injuries in the entire Stockholm population (1.5 million) for the period between 1974 and 1979. If this rate is extrapolated to the United States, approximately 15,000 perforating eye injuries may occur annually. This figure, however, may underestimate the actual number of open eye injuries; a recent population-based report from Maryland has estimated that every year more than 60,000 patients sustain serious ocular injuries requiring hospitalization, and about 20,000 of these patients have open wounds of their eyeball or of the ocular adnexa.[179a] With the growth of the population, it is likely that the number of serious eye injuries (both open and closed) even exceeds these figures which are estimated according to the 1980 census.

Serious eye injuries are more common in men than in women, and the majority of patients are young, their ages ranging between 10 and 40.[20,135,136] A second incidence peak occurs in individuals greater than 70 years of age.[179a] Ocular injuries may be associated with maxillofacial, head, and cervical spine trauma. In one major series, 67% of patients with blunt maxillofacial trauma had associated ocular injuries of which 18% were serious and 3% blinding.[80] Ocular trauma should be suspected when nasal, midfacial, and/or frontal fractures are present; up to 60% of patients with these types of injury may have associated damage of the eye.[80] Ocular injury may be present in 10 to 40% of orbital and periorbital fractures.[62,84,122,146] Associated eye injuries have been reported in up to 8% of head-injured patients.[26]

### TYPES OF EYE INJURIES

Ocular injuries can be divided into two categories: nonpenetrating and pentrating-perforating.

### *Nonpenetrating Eye Injuries*

In this type of injury the ocular coat remains intact but both intra- and extraocular structures may be damaged. In general, forces that give rise to nonpenetrating injuries are either contusive (direct trauma), concussive (indirect or contrecoup trauma), or both.

EYELIDS. Ecchymosis of the eyelids occurs commonly with direct blows to the eye. Although generally considered inconsequential, it may be associated with other more serious orbital or intraocular injuries. More severe eyelid injuries include lacerations, partial avulsions, and complete loss. In cooperative adults surgical treatment of most eyelid injuries can be performed with regional anesthesia and akinesia using infraorbital, supraorbital, or facial nerve blocks. General anesthesia is usually needed in children and in inebriated or uncooperative adults. Retrobulbar block does not produce eyelid anesthesia, but by providing ocular immobility and by allowing conjunctival manipulation it may facilitate surgery. Technical aspects of local or regional anesthesia for the eye will be discussed later in this chapter.

ORBITAL INJURIES. Orbital fractures may result in retrobulbar hemorrhage, subcutaneous emphysema, eyelid anesthesia, and optic nerve avulsion of which the last results in sudden loss of vision. In addition, surgical repair of these fractures may cause ocular damage. Postoperative orbital hematoma, optic nerve damage by fracture manipulation or implant pressure, and excessive pressure on the globe by excessive packing of the maxillary antrum are all eye-threatening complications of surgery in this region.[89] A particularly important injury in this area is the "blowout fracture" which involves the orbital floor, the weakest wall of the orbit.[89] This fracture results from a forceful impact (eg, fist, baseball) to the orbit: a sudden increase in intraorbital pressure fractures the inferior orbital wall. In some instances the inferior rectus and inferior oblique muscles, along with other intraorbital contents, may herniate into the maxillary sinus through the defective orbit (Fig 11-3). Limitation of ocular movements, particularly downward and upward gaze, resulting from this type of injury may result in diplopia.[89]

Occasionally orbital injuries may damage the globe.[62,80,84,89,122,146] Repair of orbital fratures can wait up to 7 to 10 days while periorbital edema is resolving, but associated injuries to the globe usually require urgent intervention. General anesthesia is required for orbital and resultant eye injuries because regional anesthetic techniques rarely produce satisfactory conditions.

EXTRAOCULAR MUSCLES. These injuries are usually caused by a direct blow to the orbit or by projectile-type foreign bodies. Extraocular muscles may be avulsed or entrapped into orbital fractures causing limitation of eye movement. Likewise, hematoma formation within the muscle may interfere with normal motion of the eye.

ANTERIOR SEGMENT. Hyphema, blood in the anterior chamber (Fig 11-4), is usually caused by contusive forces.[32] Trauma from stones, balls, fists, and dashboards frequently produces this type of injury. Severe hyphemas are usually due to iridodialysis, tears in the iris root and anterior portion of the ciliary body. The tear may extend posteriorly and rupture the arterial circle of the ciliary body. Less severe bleeding is usually due to tears in the sphincter or iris stroma (Fig 11-4). Although hyphema is usually caused by a nonpenetrating eye injury, occasionally ocular hypotony may be present, suggesting the presence of a ruptured globe. In children, an interesting finding is the presence of somnolence, which suggests an associated head injury. Although appropriate tests to eliminate the possibility of head injury are mandatory in these patients, usually the results are negative.[42]

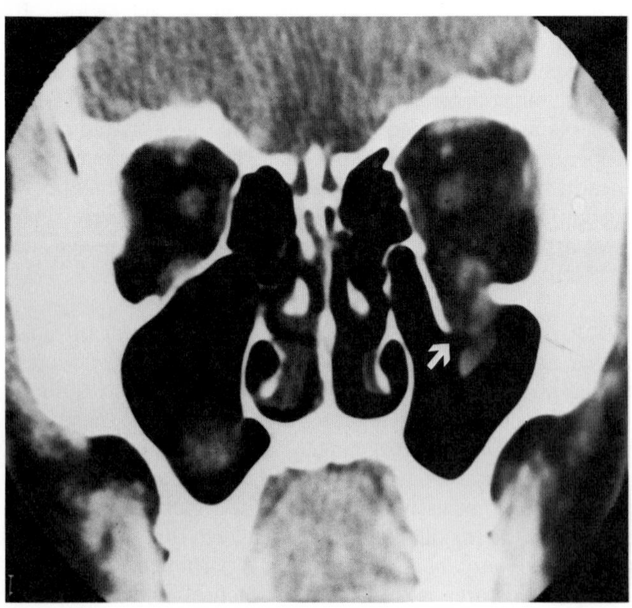

FIG. 11-3. Orbital floor fracture with entrapment of orbital contents (fat, inferior rectus muscle, and inferior oblique muscle) in the maxillary sinus (arrow). The patient had diplopia due to limitation of ocular movement.

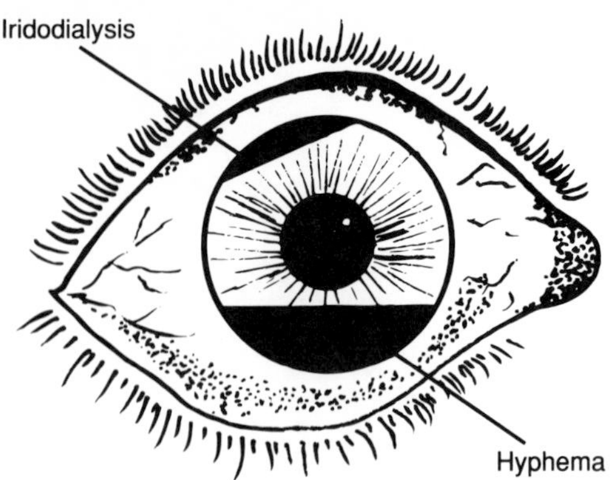


FIG. 11-4. Blood in the anterior chamber (hyphema) obscures distal part of the iris. The lesion seen on the upper portion of the iris is caused by iridodialysis.

The initial management of hyphema is conservative and directed to prevention of rebleeding, which carries a grim prognosis for visual acuity; its incidence in untreated patients varies from 3.5 to 35%.[37,118,178,194] Unfortunately, there are no identifiable risk factors to help predict which patients are likely to rebleed.[28,178] Conservative treatment involves bed rest, bilateral eye patching, and topical mydriatic and cycloplegic agents to dilate the pupil and limit iris movement. $\epsilon$-aminocaproic acid (Amicar), 50 mg/kg, three to four times a day, up to a maximum of 30 g/day, has been suggested by various authors as useful for reducing the likelihood of rebleeding.[37,109,118,139] The side effects of this drug include dizziness, hypotension, syncope, nausea, diarrhea, and cramps, which are more common at higher dose levels.[139] An important complication of hyphema is IOP elevation due to obstruction of the trabecular meshwork and increased volume in the anterior chamber. Thus, IOP should be measured once or twice daily for early recognition of this complication. If the raised IOP fails to respond to conservative medical management, surgery may be indicated.

Surgical intervention is usually indicated for the following conditions: (1) presence of blood staining of the cornea; (2) to prevent the formation of peripheral anterior synechia that results from protracted hyphemas and; (3) prolonged elevation of IOP. Rebleeding appears to be the most important factor producing these complications.[178] Paracentesis, gentle anterior chamber washout, and clot removal can be performed under either local or general anesthesia.[17] Anesethetic management of these patients requires lowering of IOP with anesthetic agents prior to opening the anterior chamber. It is generally believed that surgical intervention adds further risks such as corneal and lenticular injury.

The prognosis of hyphema in patients with sickle cell disease or trait is poor; close monitoring of IOP is required. Early surgical intervention is recommended in these patients, especially when IOP elevation persists.[30,68]

Traumatic narrowing of the anterior angle with resultant

damage to the trabecular meshwork in nonpenetrating injuries with or without hyphemas can result in chronic glaucoma years after the initial injury.

Subluxation or dislocation of the lens may occur if the zonular fibers that hold it in place are damaged. Anterior displacement of the lens, a rare event, comprises both the function of the anterior segment and visual acuity and thus requires early surgical intervention. However, the lens is more commonly dislocated into the posterior segment. In this case, removal is usually not necessary unless significant intraocular inflammation is present. Blunt trauma may also result in cataract formation without subluxation and cause significant loss of vision. If the lens capsule has been ruptured, cataract formation and swelling of the lens due to imbibition of intraocular fluid will develop quickly, resulting in an urgent need for surgical extraction to prevent glaucoma. Occasionally cataracts due to blunt ocular trauma develop slowly over many months. In these cases, elective surgical removal may be required to improve vision. Finally, some apparently nonpenetrating injuries of the globe may be associated with scleral rupture (Fig 11-5). This condition should be suspected whenever the eye is soft compared with the nontraumatized eye. In addition to decreased IOP, signs of a ruptured globe are unequal anterior chamber depth and intraocular, choroidal, and/or subconjunctival hemorrhage.

POSTERIOR SEGMENT. Trauma to the posterior segment of the eye can cause serious visual impairment, but emergency surgery is rarely indicated unless it is associated with an open-eye injury. These injuries are usually treated surgically days or even months after the initial trauma and thus pose little difficulty to the anesthesiologist. Nonpenetrating trauma to the posterior segment may result in the following:

*Retinal Detachment.* Ocular trauma, both nonpenetrating and penetrating-perforating, is the most common cause of retinal detachment in patients below 30 years of age.[10] Dialysis is the most frequent form of retinal tear.[10] Detachment may involve only peripheral areas of the retina and/or the macula. The latter condition is associated with considerable decrease in visual acuity and requires urgent treatment. In patients with nonpenetrating ocular contusions, retinal detachment usually presents from 1 month to many years following ocular trauma. Vitreous hemorrhage and other associated ocular media opacities can add to the delay in diagnosis. Edema and hemorrhage into the retina or the underlying tissues may occur following blunt trauma to the eye and cause decreased vision during the acute stage, especially if they involve the macula. The likelihood of retaining central visual acuity is good in all of these injuries, provided the macula is not involved.

*Vitreous Hemorrhage.* The entry of blood from damaged retinal or choroidal vessels into the vitreous body may result in sudden loss of vision. Occasionally vitreous hemorrhage may be associated with retinal detachment which is difficult to diagnose by ophthalmoscopic examination because blood in the vitreous obscures the view.

Vitreous hemorrhage is treated conservatively during the acute stage since it often resolves spontaneously. Vitrectomy with vitreous suction cutters inserted through the pars plana may be performed when the hemorrhage is associated with retinal detachment or causes decreased visual acuity.

OPTIC NERVE INJURY. Nonpenetrating ocular trauma may cause contusion, laceration, or avulsion of the optic nerve in the narrow bony canal where the nerve leaves the orbit. These injuries result in sudden loss of vision, usually without significant ophthalmoscopic findings. Computed tomography (CT) scanning may be useful in diagnosing optic nerve injury. Conservative treatment with steroid agents may reduce the edema of a contused optic nerve and improve vision. Emer-

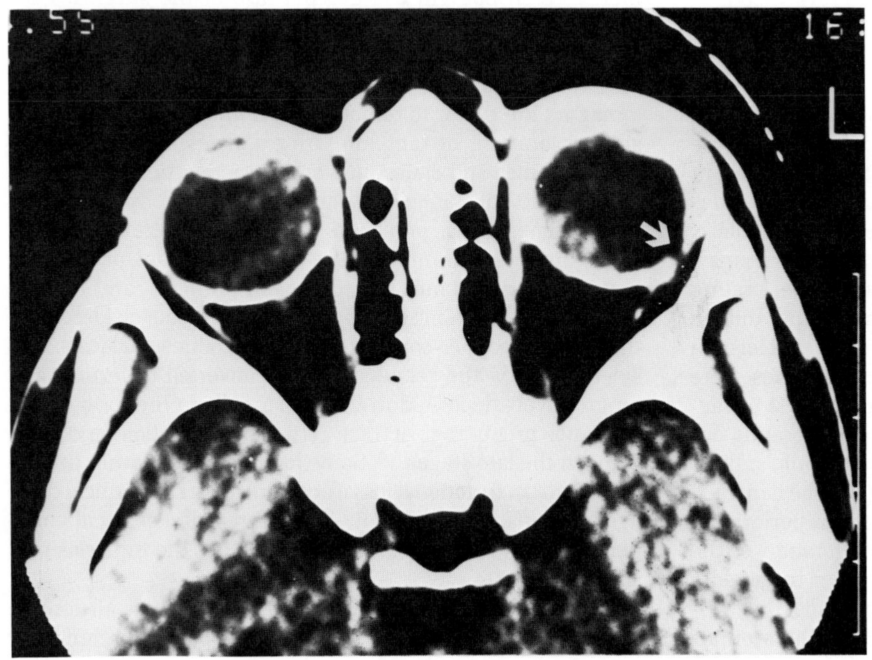


FIG. 11-5. CT scan of a patient with posterior segment perforation of the eye (arrow).

gency surgical treatment may be indicated when the nerve is compressed by orbital structures.

Prolonged pressure on the eyeball by intraorbital contents such as a retrobulbar hemorrhage can result in central retinal artery occlusion. Vision is usually decreased or absent, the IOP is increased, the globe is proptotic, and there is nonperfusion of the central retinal artery. Treatment involves immediate IOP reduction by canthotomy which decompresses the orbit. Pharmacological agents (timolol, acetazolamide, mannitol) are used to help maintain the IOP below the systolic pressure of the central retinal artery.

RUPTURE OF THE CHOROID. Curvilinear tears of the Bruch's membrane (the basal lamina of the retinal pigment epithelium which separates the choroid from the neurosensory retina) -choroid complex may result from blunt (contusion or concussion) injury to the eye. These tears, which are most frequently located temporal and parallel to the disc, may be initially hidden by vitreous or retinal hemorrhage. If the resultant whitish scar involves the macula, visual acuity is usually poor. Contusion to the globe can also cause a hemorrhagic detachment of the choroid from the sclera without rupture of Bruch's membrane. The area of choroidal detachment is seen as a solid dark brown, smooth, elevated mound. Resultant visual acuity depends on its extent and location.

INJURY TO THE OPTIC CHIASM. Contusion injuries of the optic chiasm result in partial blindness. They are usualy produced by falls on the forehead in which hemorrhage, necrosis, or avulsion of the chiasm can occur. In individuals who recover from the initial insult to the brain, bitemporal hemianopsia is seen.

Occasionally, aneurysms or pseudoaneurysms of the carotid artery in the region of the optic chiasm may develop subsequent to trauma. These vascular lesions may produce pressure on the chiasm and cause visual loss. Embolization of these lesions by synthetic particles under fluoroscopic control may reduce the size of the aneurysm and improve vision.

### *Penetrating-Perforating Injuries of the Eye*

This type of injury is characterized by partial (penetrating) or complete (perforating) disruption of the ocular coat. These injuries are treated surgically as soon as possible to prevent infection, extrusion of intraocular contents, and the deleterious effects of foreign bodies on the eye. They are particularly important for the anesthesiologist as their management may, at times, be challenging. As we mentioned above, perforating eye injuries occur in approximately 60 individuals per million population per year.[20] Niiranen[135,136] reports that in Helsinki University Eye Hospital 477 porforating eye injuries were treated between 1970 and 1977, representing 4.7% of admissions. Other eye clinics have reported that perforating eye injuries account for 1.4 to 10% of all ophthalmic admissions.[106,116] Almost any ocular structure that may be damaged by nonpenetrating trauma can also be damaged by perforating insults. The following signs may suggest perforation of the globe[72]: (1) decreased visual acuity; (2) decreased intraocular pressure; (3) change in depth of anterior chamber; (4) displacement or change in shape of the pupil; (5) visible wounds of the cornea or sclera (Fig 11-6); (6) prolapse of ocular tissue (uvea, lens, vitreous, or retina); (7) chemosis (conjunctival edema).

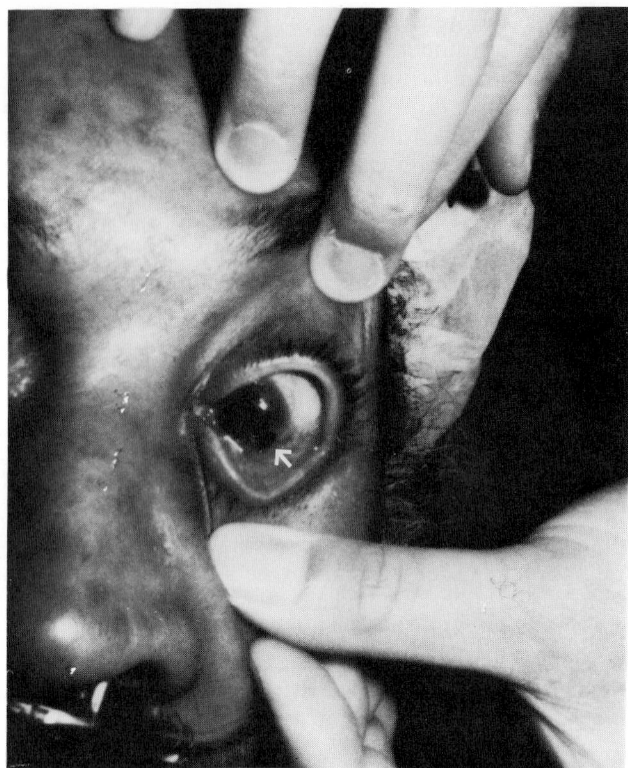

FIG. 11-6. Photograph of a patient who sustained corneoscleral perforation. Note the black puncture site at the inferior limbus (arrow).

During evaluation of perforating injuries the possibility of intraocular foreign bodies should be considered. The physician must be aware not only of the risk of leaving a relatively inert foreign body in the eye but also of the surgical risks involved in its removal. Foreign bodies may be metallic or nonmetallic. Metallic foreign bodies may be magnetic or nonmagnetic. In general, foreign bodies that can be attracted by a magnet are easier to remove than nonmagnetic ones. Gold, silver, platinum, or tantalum are examples of inert metallic foreign bodies and cause little or no reaction in the eye. Inert nonmetallic substances that are also tolerated by the eye include stone, glass, porcelain, carbon, and certain plastics. Lead, zinc, and aluminum are irritants but are usually tolerated. Other irritants are cilia, cloth particles, and organic matter. Iron-containing foreign bodies may cause siderosis of the eye, and copper-containing metals produce chalcosis.[72] In siderosis bulbi the retained iron is converted to ferritin and progressively deposited in the ocular cells in the form of siderosomes producing cataract, retinal degeneration, and glaucoma in the late stages.[176] Some foreign bodies within the eye may result in functional loss by causing both mechanical damage and inflammation. Thus, they represent a surgical emergency and should be removed as soon after the injury as possible.

Diagnosis is made primarily by X-ray, but not all foreign bodies are visible on plain films. A radiopaque foreign body may be intraocular or extraocular. A simple way of determining the location of a radiopaque foreign body by X-ray involves suturing a 12-mm metal ring to the corneal scleral region. Two posteroanterior films (gaze left and gaze right) and two lateral films (gaze up and gaze down) are taken. With the diameter of the metal ring known, a 24-mm circle can be drawn on each of the films outlining the globe. Thus, if the radiopaque material falls within the boundaries of the four circles, it is more likely to be intraocular than extraocular.[72] CT scanning is helpful not only for diagnosing nonradiopaque foreign bodies but also in localizing them within the orbit. Localization requires a CT study in axial and coronal planes with a superimposed grid.[170] However, even with CT scanning, extremely small, multiple, or relatively radiolucent foreign bodies located near the ocular wall may be missed.[180]

Magnet extraction has been used to remove magnetic bodies from the eye.[164] With this method foreign bodies located in either segment can be removed without difficulty. Foreign bodies that cannot be attracted by a magnet or are encapsulated by fibrous tissue or that may cause damage to intraocular structures along the path to the magnet are best removed by vitrectomy instrumentation.[63,148]

In general, penetrating-perforating eye injuries produce more severe ocular damage than nonpenetrating ones. A special category of perforating injuries is the "double-perforating" type that is usually produced by high-velocity foreign bodies, eg, firearm, BB gun, and explosion accidents.[25,171,184] In this form of injury the perforating object produces entry and exit wounds in the eye, causing severe damage to both anterior and posterior segments (Fig 11-7, A and B). Vitrectomy following the initial wound repair has been recommended in the treatment of penetrating injuries to aid in microsurgical intraocular reconstruction of the globe. However, the timing of this procedure is controversial. Some authors recommend vitrectomy within 72 hours of the initial injury[31] whereas others advocate an interval of 4 to 10 days[156] or 15 to 30 days.[76] More recent data fail to show a difference in results between vitrectomies performed within 72 hours of injury and those at longer intervals.[43]

## DIAGNOSIS OF OCULAR INJURIES

Diagnostic principles of ocular injuries do not differ from those applied to other forms of trauma. A brief but pertinent history should be obtained, associated injuries determined, and appropriate eye examinations performed. Ocular history should include key questions about the time, type, and immediate effects of trauma, the state of vision prior to the injury, the degree of visual impairment, and the present complaints. Ophthalmological examination should include tests for visual acuity, ocular movements, diplopia, and pupillary responses to light, along with slitlamp biomicroscopy, fundoscopy, visual field, and gross color testing. Intraocular pressure should be measured in patients with nonpenetrating eye injuries but not in those with open-eye injuries, as the pressure applied to the eye by the tonometer may cause extrusion

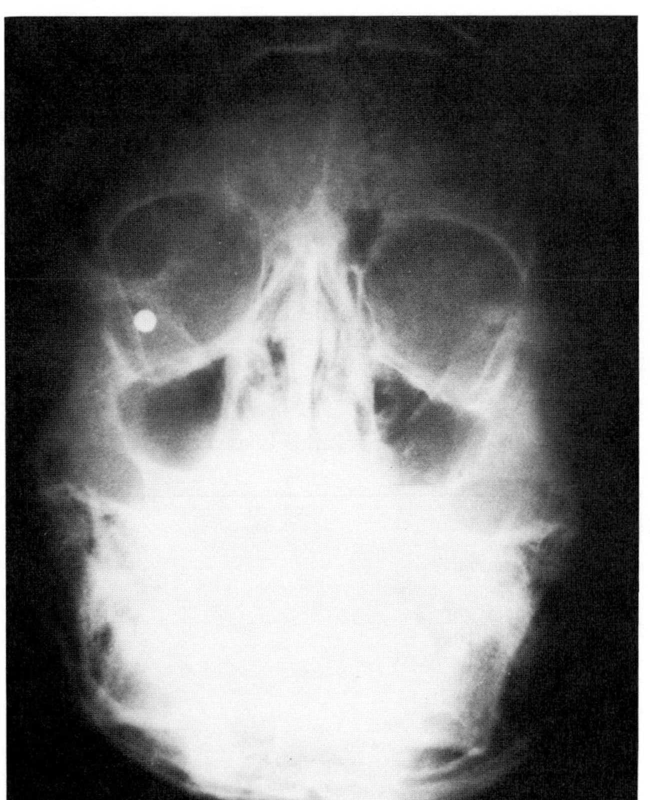


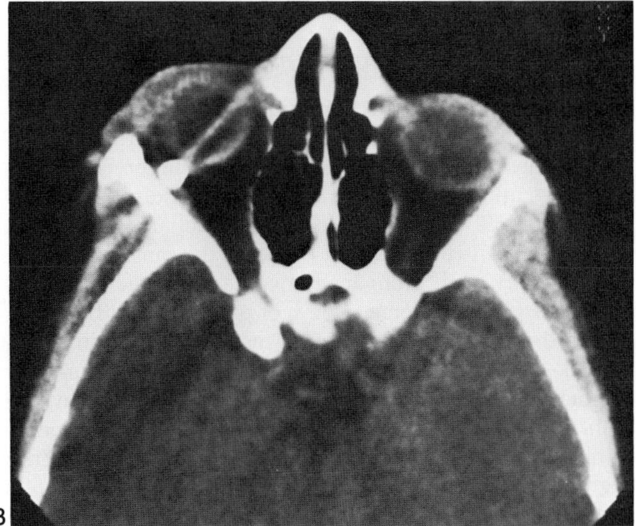


FIG. 11-7. Plain facial X-ray (A) and orbital CT scan (B) of a patient who sustained BB gun injury to the right eye. Note the BB pellet outside the eye suggesting double perforation.

of intraocular contents. Laboratory examinations offer little help; conversely, examination by ultrasound, X-rays, and CT scan may yield important information.

## TREATMENT OF OCULAR INJURIES

Initial treatment of ocular injuries is aimed at preventing further damage to the eye. In this context, administration of analgesic, sedative, and antiemetic agents may help prevent coughing, straining, crying, and vomiting, thus reducing the likelihood of increase in IOP and further damage to the eye. Broad-spectrum antibiotics and tetanus prophylaxis may be given to prevent infectious complications. Finally, placement of an eye shield minimizes further damage to the eye.

Two important goals in treatment of eye injury are preservation of the eyeball and restoration of useful vision. Surgical intervention may be necessary to achieve these goals. The timing of this intervention is dependent upon the patient's concomitant injuries, the type of ocular injury, and the degree of functional impairment. As a general rule, in the polytraumatized patient lifesaving procedures take priority. However, it is important to realize that visual loss results in great disability and that immediate ocular surgical management can often take place without interfering with other resuscitative measures. A perforating eye injury with or without a retained foreign body requires immediate surgical intervention. This urgency is considerably less in most nonperforating injuries unless vision is threatened and conservative therapeutic modalities are ineffective. A closed eye can withstand a brief increase in IOP, but in an open globe even a transient external pressure increase may result in disastrous complications.

## PROGNOSIS OF OCULAR INJURIES

The overall prognosis of ocular injuries improved remarkably from the 1950s to the mid-1970s. In 1959, when Roper-Hall[153] reported the long-term results of surgery for perforating eye injuries at the Birmingham and Midland Eye Hospital, only 45% of patients were able to achieve better than 20/40 vision. In 1976, Eagling,[53,54] from the same institution, and Adhikary et al,[4] from another center, reported a comparably good visual outcome in 62% of patients. Eagling[53] suggested that the improvement was mainly a reflection of improved surgical techniques and better outcome of anterior segment injuries. Indeed, although modern microsurgical techniques have dramatically improved the outlook of penetrating-perforating injuries of the anterior segment, posterior segment involvement continues to carry a guarded prognosis because of the sequelae resulting from these injuries—intraocular fibrous proliferation, traction and rhegmatogenous retinal detachment, and cyclitic membrane formation. Recent reports show little or no improvement in overall outcome in comparison with the findings of Eagling[53,54] and Adhikary et al[4] in 1976. For instance, one correspondence reported that only 54% of patients with penetrating eye injuries regained 20/100 or better vision within 6 months of injury,[152] clearly an outcome no better than that obtained in 1976.

However, considering the heterogeneity of eye injuries, it is inappropriate to compare overall outcome figures of different series. The prognosis of eye injuries is heavily dependent upon certain risk factors. de Juan et al,[44] in a retrospective computer-aided study, demonstrated that the prognosis after a penetrating eye injury was influenced by the location and extent of initial damage and the nature of injury. These authors have found seven risk factors that correlated with final visual outcome (Table 11-1). For example, if visual acuity prior to surgical treatment was better than 5/200, the chance of gaining final vision 5/200 or better would be 97%. Conversely, if the initial acuity was less than 5/200, there was only a 36% chance that the final vision would be 5/200 or better. Likewise the enucleation rate was 2.5% if the initial vision was 5/200 or better but 47% if the initial visual acuity was less than 5/200. Similar relationships were demonstrated between final visual acuity and the remaining risk factors.

Whether the new vitrectomy techniques have improved the outcome of perforating ocular injuries is difficult to determine because, to our knowledge, prospective, patient-stratified studies comparing long-term visual acuity results of conventional and vitrectomy techniques are not available. However, a retrospective case-controlled study indicated that with the probable exception of double perforations and BB gun injuries, vitrectomy does not necessarily improve the prognosis of penetrating eye injuries.[45] The outcome of double-perforating eye injuries, although improved to some extent with vitrec-

TABLE 11-1. Factors Associated with Unfavorable Visual Prognosis (Final Vision <5/200) after Perforating Eye Injuries*

| |
|---|
| Initial vision <5/200 |
| Presence of afferent pupillary defect during initial examination |
| Rupture of the globe by blunt forces |
| Severity of the ocular wound |
| Scleral involvement |
| Extension posteriorly beyond rectus muscle insertion |
| Greater than 10 mm in length |
| Subluxation of lens or loss of lens through the wound into the eye wall |
| Vitreous hemorrhage preventing visualization of the retinal vessels and optic nerve head during ophthalmoscopy |
| Double-perforating injuries and BB gun injuries with intraocular BB pellet |

* From de Juan et al.[44]

TABLE 11-2. Type of Injuries Likely to be Sustained with Blunt Facial Trauma

| |
|---|
| Hyphema |
| Iridodialysis |
| Retinal hemorrhage |
| Macular cyst |
| Corneal/scleral rupture |
| Vitreous hemorrhage |
| Optic nerve abnormality |
| Retinal detachment |
| Dislocated lens |
| Cranial nerve palsy |
| Eye muscle entrapment |
| Enophthalmus |
| Ptosis |

tomy, remains poor; visual success as defined by 5/200 or better vision ranges between 33[151] and 56%.[184]

The prognisis of closed-eye injuries, in terms of visual outcome, is more favorable than that of perforating eye injuries. Although a large percentage of patients (67%) sustaining blunt trauma develop closed-eye injury, a relatively small fraction of these injuries is serious (18%) or blinding (3%).[26] Table 11-2 lists the types of injuries likely to be sustained with blunt facial trauma. The prognosis of optic nerve injury and injury to the central nervous system causing blindness at the time of accident is extremely poor, resulting in permanent blindness in the majority of patients.

## PHYSIOLOGY OF INTRAOCULAR PRESSURE IN THE CLOSED EYE

Normally, the IOP varies between 10 and 24 mm Hg.[41,130] There is little difference between the IOP of the two eyes of an individual, usually less than 5 mm Hg.[87] In animals, the IOP can be measured directly by inserting a hypodermic needle into the anterior chamber and connecting it to a manometer.[100] Because of its invasive nature, this method cannot be used clinically, and the IOP is measured by tonometry.[100] There are three types of tonometers: indentation, applanation, and pneumotonometer. Indentation tonometry (*Schiötz*) measures the depth to which a weighted plunger sinks when applied to the cornea. This method, although still used widely, may give inaccurate results. The applanation tonometer measures the area of corneal flattening under standard pressure with a split-prism doubling device. With pneumotonometry the cornea is flattened by a strong jet of air at a constant and predetermined force. Optical and photocell systems attached to the device measure the difference in the reflection of a beam of light delivered to the cornea. Both the applanation tonometer and pneumotonometer are reliable, but careful technique in applying these tonometers is necessary to avoid artifactual errors.

The following factors have a significant effect on the IOP in the closed eye.

### CHANGES IN THE VOLUME OF INTRAOCULAR CONTENTS

Among the intraocular contents, choroidal blood volume, aqueous humor, and vitreous humor are the three most significant structures capable of volume change.

#### *Choroidal Blood Volume*

The choroid contains arteries and veins. The arterial supply of the choroid is very high and is of the same order of magnitude as hepatic blood flow per unit weight of tissue. This blood flow serves to maintain constant eye temperature in extremes of ambient temperatures and enables the observation of very bright high energy objects by the retina.[18] In monkeys, the rate of circulation through the ciliary processes is 227 gm/min per 100 g of tissue and through the ciliary muscle 163 g/min per 100 g of tissue.[18] The primate retina, iris, ciliary body, and choroid receive 34, 8, 81, and 677 mg/min blood, respectively.[18] Although blood flow to the choroid is high compared with other intraocular structures, oxygen extraction by this layer is not, and venous oxygen content in the anterior uvea is only 4 to 5% less than that of arterial blood.

Like the cerebral circulation, choroidal circulation has its own autoregulation, and the blood volume within the choroid remains constant between mean perfusion pressures of 90 and 130 mm Hg[39,87] (Fig 11-8). However, a sudden increase in arterial blood pressure may increase the thickness of the choroid. This, of course, has a compressive effect on the vitreous which results in a significant increase in IOP.[181] In addition, increased choroidal blood volume may also produce decreased compliance of the ocular coat, facilitating the IOP rise. Usually, this increase is transient because a compensatory increase in aqueous outflow occurs, resulting in renormalization of IOP within a short period of time. Choroidal blood volume, and thus the IOP, begins to decline when the ocular perfusion pressure falls below 90 mm Hg, and at 60 mm Hg choroidal blood volume reaches a minimum[2,39,160] (Fig 11-8). As will be discussed below, compression of the eye by increased choroidal blood volume can lead to prolapse of the vitreous humor and the iris when the eye is open.

The central venous pressure has a greater effect on choroidal blood volume and IOP than the systemic arterial blood pressure.[110] An increase in central venous pressure produces a prompt and proportional increase in IOP.[82,181,190] This increase, is caused not only by elevated choroidal blood volume but also by increased aqueous volume due to impedance of its outflow.

Like the cerebral circulation, choroidal blood volume increases linearly with increased arterial carbon dioxide tension (Fig 11-9). In baboons, choroidal blood flow increases by 3 to 4% for each 7.5 mm Hg increase of $Pa_{CO_2}$ at levels between 34 and 70 mm Hg[192] and is primarily responsible for the linear increase in IOP associated with elevation of $Pa_{CO_2}$[145,157,166,191] (Fig 11-10). Two other factors, increased aqueous humor formation and elevation of central venous pressure, which usually accompany hypercapnia, are less likely to affect the IOP in these circumstances. The formation of aqueous humor from ciliary processes in the posterior chamber is dependent upon the enzyme carbonic anhydrase, the activity of which is influenced by $Pa_{CO_2}$.[145] However, the increase in IOP following elevation of carbon dioxide occurs so rapidly that it is unlikely to be caused by carbonic anhydrase-induced aqueous

FIG. 11-8. The relationship between ocular perfusion pressure and choroidal blood volume. Note the autoregulation between perfusion pressures of 90 and 130 mm Hg. Above these pressures choroidal blood volume increases, and below 90 mm Hg it begins to decline. (From Cunningham and Barry[39] with permission.)

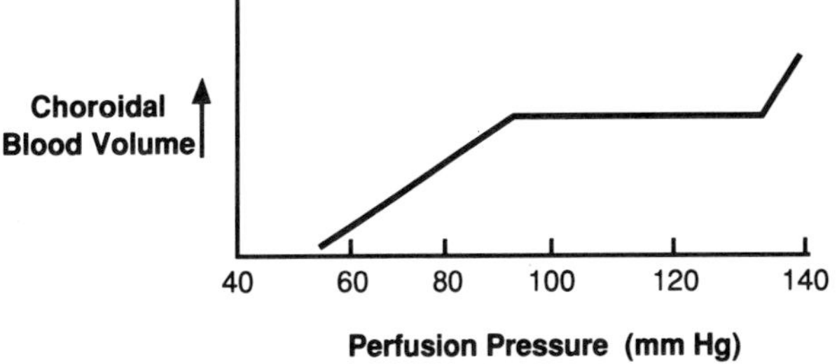

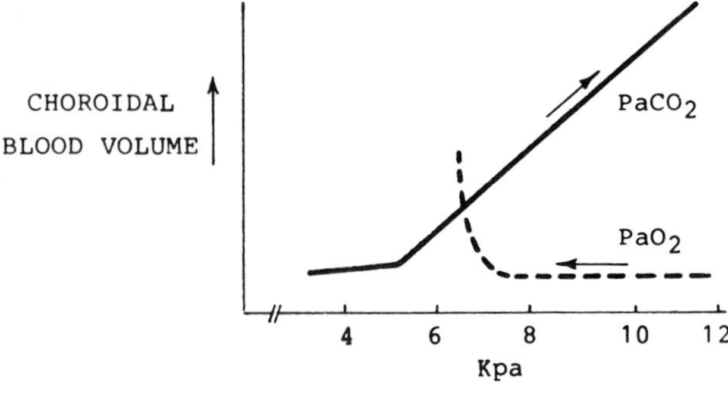


FIG. 11-9. The change in choroidal blood volume as a function of $Pa_{O_2}$ and $Pa_{CO_2}$. Note the linear increase in choroidal blood volume with increase in $Pa_{CO_2}$. Choroidal blood volume remains unaltered at $Pa_{O_2}$ levels down to 7 kPa (50 to 55 mm Hg) below which there is a substantial increase. (From Cunningham and Barry[39] with permission.)

humor formation.[82] Furthermore, administration of acetazolamide prior to hypercapnia cannot prevent IOP elevation.[145] The elevated central venous pressure seen during hypercapnia may contribute to the IOP increase, but the correlation between $Pa_{CO_2}$ and IOP remains unaltered even when central venous pressure is kept constant.[166] It should be noted that although the IOP increases with elevation of $Pa_{CO_2}$, its absolute value usually remains within the normal range (below 25 mm Hg) even at $Pa_{CO_2}$ levels of 76 mm Hg.[166] Lowering $Pa_{CO_2}$ from these high values results in a linear decrease in choroidal blood volume and IOP.[39,166]

FIG. 11-10. Graph showing IOP values as a function of $Pa_{CO_x}$. Note the linear increase in IOP with $Pa_{CO_2}$. Also note that even at $Pa_{CO_2}$ values of 10 kPa (75 mm Hg), IOP did not exceed the upper limit of normal (3 kPa or 22.5 mm Hg). Changes in IOP were not caused by cardiovascular factors because heart rate, arterial blood pressure, and central venous pressure remained unaltered. (From Smith et al[166] with permission.)

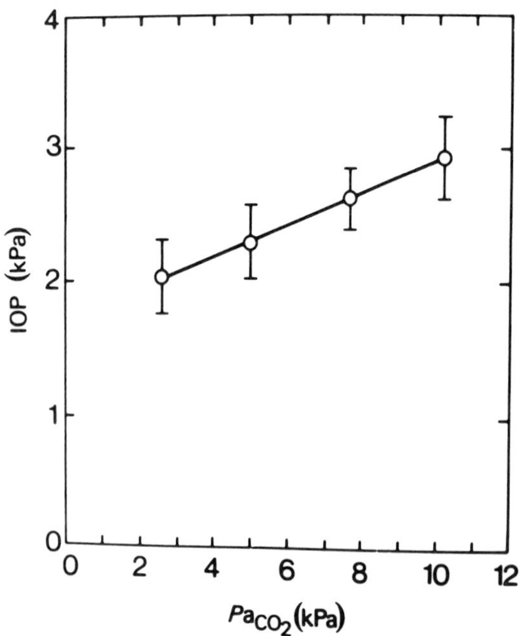


The effects of metabolic acidosis and alkalosis on IOP are opposite those produced by respiratory acid-base disturbances.[39] Intraocular pressure is decreased by metabolic acidosis and increased by alkalosis (Fig 11-11). It is not known whether these changes are caused only by the effects of electrolyte imbalance on choroidal blood flow or if other mechanisms also play a role. The choroidal circulation may be affected by $Pa_{O_2}$.

Hypoxemia produces an increase in choroidal blood volume, whereas hyperoxia causes choroidal vasoconstriction and thus decreased IOP[39] (Fig 11-9). Hypothermia, by causing choroidal vasoconstriction and by decreasing the production of aqueous humor, may also decrease IOP.[39]

### *Changes in Aqueous Humor Volume*

In most physiological conditions, IOP is regulated by the volume of aqueous humor in the anterior segment of the eye. This volume, in turn, is determined by the balance between the rate of production and the drainage from the anterior chamber via the trabecular meshwork (Fontana's spaces) and Schlemm's canal. Aqueous humor is formed at an average rate of 1 to 3 μL (1% of anterior chamber volume) per minute.[39,163] Its volume in the anterior chamber is 0.25 mL, and that in the posterior chamber is 0.05 mL. Production of aqueous humor by the ciliary epithelium in the posterior chamber is an active process. Acetazolamide (Diamox) decreases aqueous humor formation by blocking carbonic anhydrase. After oral administration of acetazolamide (500 mg), IOP decreases by 30 to 40% in about 2 hours.[64] As mentioned above, the aqueous humor drains into Schlemm's canal after crossing the trabecular meshwork (Fontana's spaces) situated in the angle between the cornea and the iris (Fig 11-1). Some aqueous humor (about 10%) diffuses through the sclera into the orbital tissues.[87] The most important factor controlling outflow of aqueous humor is the diameter of Fontana's spaces. These spaces consist of perforated plates arranged in laminar sieves. The eye responds to increased IOP by decreasing the trabecular meshwork resistance to aqueous humor outflow, a phenomenon called *facilitation*. The increased outflow of aqueous produced by this mechanism renormalizes IOP. When IOP is reduced by decreased production of aqueous humor, the term *pseudofacility* is used.

Another important factor controlling aqueous outflow is venous pressure. An increase in venous pressure diminishes the rate of aqueous outflow, increases the volume of aqueous humor in the eye and thus raises the IOP.

Aqueous formation continues over a large range of perfusion pressures but decreases when ocular perfusion is inad-

FIG. 11-11. Relationship between arterial pH and intraocular pressure. (From Cunningham[39] with permission.)

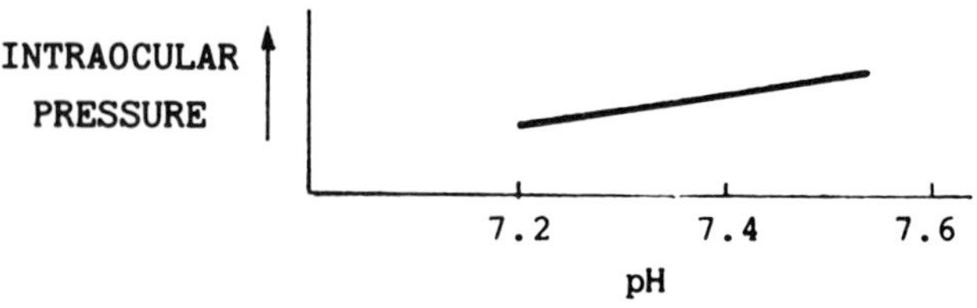

equate.[19] In monkeys, at perfusion pressures below 60 mm Hg, the rate of aqueous flow drops from 2.46 to 0.5 μL/min.[82,130]

### *Changes in Vitreous Humor Volume*

Normally there is little change in the volume of vitreous humor. However, its water content may decrease during dehydration or following administration of diuretic agents. The drug most commonly used to decrease IOP by this mechanism is mannitol, 20%, 1.5 g/kg. The peak effect of this dose of intravenously administered mannitol occurs in 30 to 45 minutes and lasts 5 to 6 hours. Dextran, urea (30% solution), and sorbitol also have been used. Glycerol can be given orally; its onset of action occurs in 10 minutes and the peak effect in 30 minutes. However, this drug should not be given to acutely traumatized patients who will undergo surgery because it increases gastric volume and predisposes the patient to aspiration. Reduction of IOP following these drugs is produced not only by vitreous dehydration; increased plasma oncotic pressure also decreases aqueous humor formation and probably increases its outflow.

## EFFECT OF EXTRAOCULAR PRESSURE ON IOP

Sudden contraction of extraocular muscles and/or eyelid blinking increases IOP by exerting pressure on the globe. The eye may be also compressed by intraorbital contents such as hemorrhage and by external causes such as improper application of a breathing mask or lid retractors or improper positioning of the head during surgery. All of these factors may produce an increase in IOP. However, persistent extraocular pressure results in activation of compensatory mechanisms. Enhancement of aqueous outflow, "aqueous facility," appears to be the most effective IOP-reducing mechanism.[39] Digital pressure on the eye has been used to reduce IOP prior to surgery. The decrease in IOP is greatest during the first minute of this maneuver, but further reduction may occur when the pressure is maintained for 5 minutes or longer.[21,94,95]

## NEURAL REGULATION OF IOP

There is evidence to suggest that centers in the cat diencephalon are responsible for regulating IOP. More than 30 years ago, Von Sallmann and Lowenstein[188] were able to manipulate IOP by selective electrical stimultiaon of these areas. IOP alteration appeared to be mediated by changes in extraocular muscle tone, ocular hemodynamics, and pupillary size. The hypothalamus may also have a role in control of IOP since both increase and decrease in IOP have been noted depending on the stimulated area. It is conceivable that there is a coordinating center in the hypothalamus whose effect is mediated via sympathetic discharge.[39] Central nervous system depressants including opiates and general anesthetics may reduce IOP, at least partly by their effect on these centers.

## EFFECT OF ARTERIAL BLOOD PRESSURE ON IOP

As we discussed above, IOP remains relatively constant during changes in systemic blood pressure over the physiological range. However, there is some evidence to suggest that the change in IOP caused by variations in systemic blood pressure may be dependent upon the initial IOP. The significant correlation demonstrated between IOP and mean arterial pressure in patients with initial IOP less than 11 mm Hg was not present in patients with higher initial pressures.[181]

## EFFECT OF TOPICAL MEDICATIONS ON IOP

Topically applied epinephrine decreases IOP by both α and β receptor stimulation.[130] However, its α effect appears to be predominant. Stimulation of α receptors causes decreased IOP, mydriasis, and increased aqueous outflow facility, whereas β receptor stimulation is associated with decreased IOP without mydriasis or increased outflow facility. It appears that uveal vasoconstriction is the principal mechanism by which epinephrine produces a fall in IOP.[98] Topically applied norepinephrine causes a biphasic response depending on its effect on aqueous outflow resistance. Acetylcholine applied to the eye does not affect IOP, but other parasympathomimetic agents—pilocarpine, physostigmine, and ecothiopate—cause contraction of ciliary muscle and a significant fall in IOP.

## EFFECT OF ANESTHETIC AGENTS ON IOP

All central nervous system depressant agents decrease IOP. Among inhalational anesthetics, the effect of nitrous oxide on IOP has not been specifically determined, but it is believed that a slight increase may occur with this agent.[79] Nitrous oxide may cause a significant increase in IOP when air or sulfur hexafluoride ($SF_6$) is injected into the eye during surgical treatment of retinal detachment.[172] As nitrous oxide is approximately 120 times more soluble and twice as diffusible as $SF_6$, it may enlarge the size of the $SF_6$ bubble and thereby increase pressure.[195] Thus nitrous oxide should be discontinued 10 to 15 minutes prior to injection of $SF_6$ into the eye and avoided for at least 10 days thereafter.[195] Reduction of IOP by halothane, enflurane, and isoflurane[11,51,52,111,150,155] appears to be dose dependent[7,149] and may reach 65% with high inspired concentrations[7] (Table 11-3). However, in most instances IOP falls to 10 to 12 mm Hg during deep general anesthesia.[51,149] Although the mechanism of IOP reduction with these agents is not clear, a combination of factors may be responsible, including relaxation of extraocular muscles, improved aqueous humor outflow, and depression of regulatory centers in the central nervous system.

Among intravenous anesthetic agents, thiopental,[13,46,52,88,97,111,129,159] etomidate,[138] diazepam,[5,38] midazolam,[132] propofol,[129] and droperidol[83,149] reduce IOP by 25 to 50% (Table 11-4). Like the inhalational anesthetics, this effect seems to be caused by depression of the diencephalon, increased aqueous humor facility, and possibly decreased extraocular muscle tone, although a transient elevation of IOP may be noted from myoclonus produced by etomidate.[17a] The effect of ketamine on IOP is controversial. Earlier studies demonstrated a moderate increase of IOP with this agent which was thought to be caused by increased muscle tone, nystagmus, and blepharospasm.[198] However, subsequent research has demonstrated no change or a slight decrease in

TABLE 11-3. Approximate Changes in Intraocular Pressure Caused by Inhalational Agents at Different Inspired Concentrations

| AGENT | INSPIRED CONCENTRATION (%) | CHANGE OF IOP (%) | REFERENCE | COMMENTS |
|---|---|---|---|---|
| Nitrous oxide | | | | Although available data are insufficient, a slight increase in IOP may occur with this agent |
| Halothane | 0.5 to 0.9 (alveolar) | −4 to −20 | 11, 155 | Measurement made in adults and children |
| | 1 | −37 | 7 | Measurements made in adults |
| | 2 | −65 | 7 | Measurements made in adults |
| Enflurane | 1 to 3 | −24 to −40 | 149, 155 | Measurements made in adults |
| Isoflurane | 0.75 to 1.50 (alveolar) | −11 | 11 | Measurements made in children |

IOP with ketamine.[12,13,147] Although narcotic agents cause significant IOP reduction[102,131] (Table 11-5), the nausea and vomiting commonly associated with these agents may result in increased IOP, and thus they are unsuitable for use in awake patients with ophthalmic injuries.

## EFFECT OF ANTICHOLINERGIC AGENTS ON IOP

When applied topically, atropine interferes with the parasympathetic innervation of the iris sphincter and causes pupillary dilatation. In the normal eye the IOP remains unchanged even at extremes of mydriasis. However, in an individual with a shallow anterior chamber caused, for instance, by posttraumatic anterior bulging of the iris, dilatation of the pupil results in obliteration of anterior chamber angle, interference with the drainage of aqueous humor, and elevation of IOP.[132]

When given intramuscularly in usual premedicant doses, the amount of anticholinergic agent that reaches the eye is substantially less than that after topical administration. Mydriatic activity probably occurs only in some patients[102] and appears much later than antisialagogue and cardiac effects.[125] Thus, most patients are anesthetized before mydriasis takes place. Consequently, whether IOP is normal or elevated, atropine, scopolamine, or glycopyrrolate given intramuscularly 45 to 60 minutes prior to surgery causes neither significant mydriasis nor elevation of IOP.[35,102,154,161]

Intravenously administered anticholinergic agents also do not increase IOP in normal eyes. However, their effect on IOP in the glaucomatous eye is not clear. Based on evidence that atropine given by this route produces a greater degree of mydriasis than glycopyrrolate,[70,126] it is prudent to use glycopyrrolate rather than atropine in patients with raised IOP. If atropine is used, concomitant topical administration of miotic agents (1% pilocarpine, one to two drops) may prevent a possible rise of IOP caused by this agent.[3,71]

## EFFECT OF MUSCLE RELAXANTS ON IOP

### *Succinylcholine*

It is well known that succinylcholine increases IOP. This increase occurs within 1 minute of injection, reaches a peak in 2 to 4 minutes, and lasts up to 6 minutes[140] (Fig 11-12). Usually the increase is about 2 to 5 mg Hg, but in some patients elevations as high as 10 mm Hg have been noted.[140] When succinylcholine is given without intravenous or inhalational induction agents, the IOP may rise by 18 mm Hg.[39] Thus, administration of succinylcholine alone to facilitate tracheal intubation in normotensive multiple trauma patients with open-eye injury poses a particular danger to the eye. Not all patients increase IOP following succinylcholine, and in some patients, in fact, the IOP reduction produced by the anesthetic induction agents is well maintained. Usually the pressure increase produced by succinylcholine is independent of the age of the patient, the presence of fasciculation, the change of pupil size, and the route and type of administration—intra-

TABLE 11-4. Change in Intraocular Pressure with Various Intravenous Anesthetic Agents

| DRUG | DOSE | CHANGE IN IOP (%) | REFERENCE | COMMENTS |
|---|---|---|---|---|
| Thiopental | 5 to 7 mg/kg | −35 to −56 | 13, 129, 159 | Measurements made in adults |
| Diazepam | 10 mg | −27 to −46 | 5 | Measurements made in adults |
| Midazolam | 0.2 mg/kg | −30 to −40 | 132 | |
| Etomidate | 0.25 to 0.3 mg/kg | −30 to −53 | 13, 138 | |
| | 20-μg/kg infusion | −61 | 179 | Greater reduction of IOP than that produced by halothane 0.5% and $N_2O$ 60% inspired concentration |
| Propofol | 2.2 mg/kg | −53 | 129 | |
| Innovar | 1 ml/8 kg to 1 ml/20 kg | −12 to −32 | 83, 149 | During EEG determined level I neuroleptanesthesia a slight increase in IOP may occur |
| Ketamine | 1 mg/kg intravenously, pediatric; | ±4 | 12 | Earlier studies showed increase in IOP with ketamine |
| | 2 mg/kg intravenously, adults | −6 | 147 | |

TABLE 11-5. Effect of Commonly Used Opiates on Intraocular Pressure

| OPIATE | DOSE AND ROUTE | CHANGE IN IOP (%) | REFERENCE |
|---|---|---|---|
| Morphine | 10 mg intramuscularly | −19 | 102 |
| Fentanyl | 2.5 μg/kg intravenously | −29 | 131 |
| Alfentanil | 10 μg/kg intravenously | −48 | 131 |

muscular, intravenous bolus, or intravenous infusion.[36] It has been shown that in humans, the increase is greater with small (0.5 mg/kg, intravenously) than with large doses (1.0 mg/kg) of succinylcholine,[88] but no difference has been found between doses of 1.0 and 2.5 mg/kg.[33]

Several factors contribute to the rise in IOP with succinylcholine. Probably most important is the increase in extraocular muscle tension. Extraocular muscles contain two types of fibers: tonic and phasic. Anatomically, tonic fibers are large and irregular with multiple motor nerve endings (*Felderstruktur*) serving to maintain steady binocular vision. The phasic fibers are regular and well defined (*Fibrillenstruktur*) and provide the rapid movements of the eye.[77,193] In cats, response of these fibers to succinylcholine appears to be dose dependent.[55,91] Small doses (10 μg/kg) of succinylcholine produce a transient contracture of phasic muscles without affecting the tonic muscles. With moderate doses of succinylcholine (30 to 75 μg/kg) both tonic and phasic muscles contract, and at very large doses (>100 μg/kg) only tonic muscles are affected. In any case activity of either muscle group is likely to increase IOP, although the rise is probably greater with contraction of tonic muscles. It is conceivable that nondepolarizing agents in pretreatment doses block the stimulating effect of succinylcholine on tonic muscles and diminish the change in IOP. However, section of all extraocular muscles and canthotomy in cats cannot prevent the rise of IOP following succinylcholine.[2,192] Although the rise is smaller in these conditions than with intact extraocular muscles, it may potentially be large enough to cause expulsion of intraocular contents in a perforated eye. The increase in IOP in these conditions is thought to be caused by augmented choroidal blood volume.[2] Another mechanism of IOP increase after succinylcholine is a decrease in aqueous outflow of as much as 21%.[175] Thus, blockade of fasciculations with nondepolarizing muscle relaxants cannot entirely abolish the succinylcholine-induced IOP rise.[120] Techniques described to attenuate the increase in IOP after succinylcholine will be discussed in a later section of this chapter.

FIG. 11-12. Intraocular pressure changes following succinylcholine in intubated and nonintubated patients. Note that the IOP rise caused by succinylcholine is exaggerated by intubation. (From Pandey et al[140] with permission.)

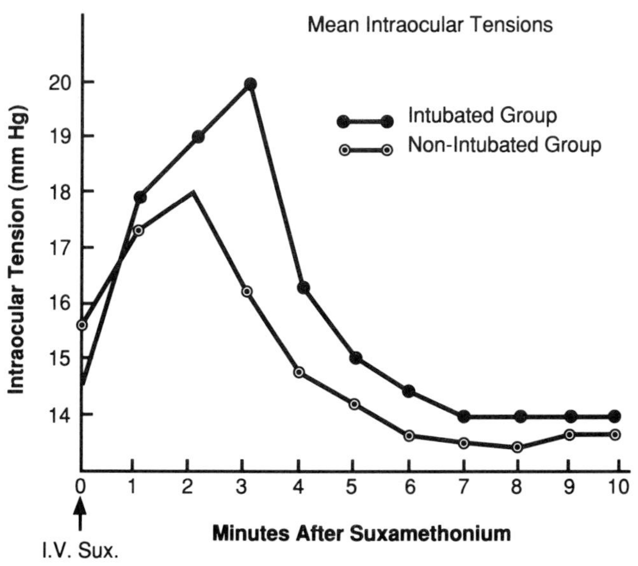


## *Nondepolarizing Muscle Relaxants*

Following administration of nondepolarizing muscle relaxants, IOP either remains unchanged or decreases. The greatest reduction occurs with D-tubocurarine,[6] probably from a combination of factors such as relaxation of extraocular and intraocular muscle tone and autonomic ganglionic blockade producing a decrease in systemic arterial pressure. Pancuronium in paralyzing doses produces little change in IOP if it is administered to deeply anesthetized patients.[6,65] However, in unanesthetized or lightly anesthetized patients this agent can produce significant IOP reduction.[108,168] Following anesthetic induction with thiopental, metocurine alone (0.3 mg/kg) or in combination with pancuronium (metocurine, 0.08 mg/kg, plus pancuronium, 0.02 mg/kg) has been shown to reduce IOP by 30%.[40] Similarly, alcuronium (0.25 mg/kg), when administered with thiopental (5 mg/kg), produces a 40% reduction in IOP within 1 minute of injection.[14] However, this effect of alcuronium could not be detected when measurements were made between 5 and 15 minutes following injection.[65] Fazadinium is a rapidly acting nondepolarizing muscle relaxant which does not increase IOP.[34,75] Although preliminary studies suggest that fazadinium can be a reasonable alternative to succinylcholine during anesthetic induction of perforated eye injuries,[34] the drug is not available in the United States, and the available clinical trials are too limited to be conclusive.

Both atracurium and vecuronium are devoid of any IOP-elevating effect (Fig 11-13). Atracurium has been shown to maintain a stable IOP during maintenance and induction of anesthesia prior to intubation.[99,114,159] In general, similar findings have been demonstrated for vecuronium,[159,165,186] although a more recent report noted an average 23% reduction in IOP 10 minutes after its administration.[86] This reduction was thought to be caused by a decrease in central venous pressure produced by this agent[86] (Fig 11-14).

The combination of nondepolarizing muscle relaxant reversal agents and atropine at the end of surgery does not appear to increase IOP,[102] but detailed studies on this subject are lacking.

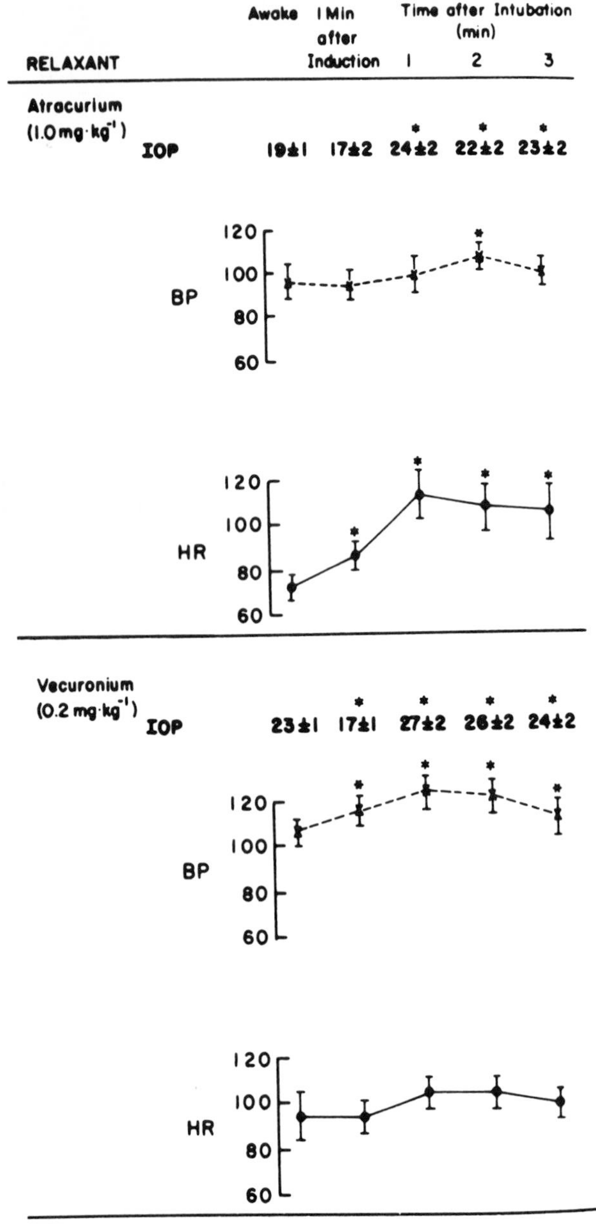


FIG. 11-13. Intraocular pressure (IOP, mm Hg, mean ± SE), mean arterial pressure (BP, mm Hg), and heart rate (HR, beats per minute) changes during each phase of rapid sequence induction with atracurium (1 mg/kg) and vecuronium (0.2 mg/kg). * $P < .05$. Values 1 minute after induction are compared with awake values, and values after intubation are compared with values 1 minute after induction. (From Schneider et al[159] with permission.)

### EFFECT OF LARYNGOSCOPY AND TRACHEAL INTUBATION ON IOP

Laryngoscopy and tracheal intubation are potent stimuli; regardless of the method of anesthetic induction or the type of muscle relaxant used, IOP increases[23,29,50,51,69,99,120,134,140,159,197] (Figs 11-12, 11-13, and 11-15). The methods used to modify laryngoscopy- and intubation-induced sympathetic discharge and IOP elevation will be discussed in a later section of this chapter.

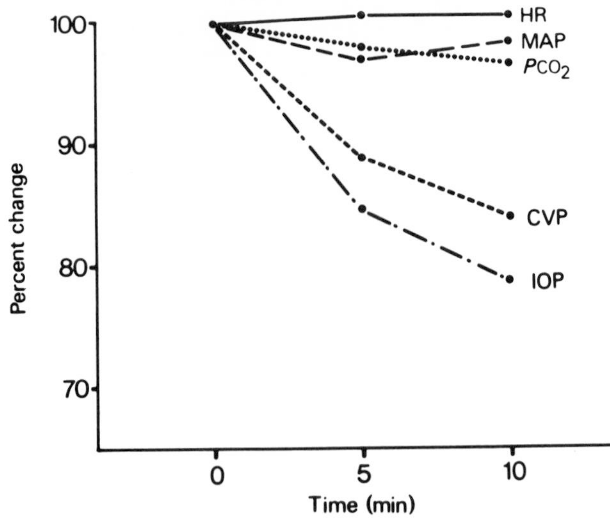


FIG. 11-14. Effect of vecuronium (0.1 mg/kg) administered during anesthetic maintenance on heart rate (HR), mean arterial pressure (MAP), $P_{CO_2}$, central venous pressure (CVP), and intraocular pressure (IOP). Note that a steady decline in IOP follows the reduction of CVP. (From Jantzen et al[86] with permission.)

## PHYSIOLOGY OF INTRAOCULAR PRESSURE IN THE OPEN EYE

In a perforated eye, IOP is approximately equal to the atmospheric pressure. Therefore an episode of extrinsic compression does not cause significant intraocular hypertension but may result in intraocular volume loss or displacement of intraocular contents between the anterior and posterior segments. Indeed, any of the factors that increase the IOP in the

FIG. 11-15. Intraocular pressure changes during rapid sequence induction with atracurium and succinylcholine. The broken line represents the IOP of the atracurium group and the solid line that of the succinylcholine group. A, awake; T, after thiopental; I, after intubation. Note the severe rise in IOP during intubation in both groups. In the group treated with atracurium, IOP remains below awake values. (From Lavery et al[99] with permission.)

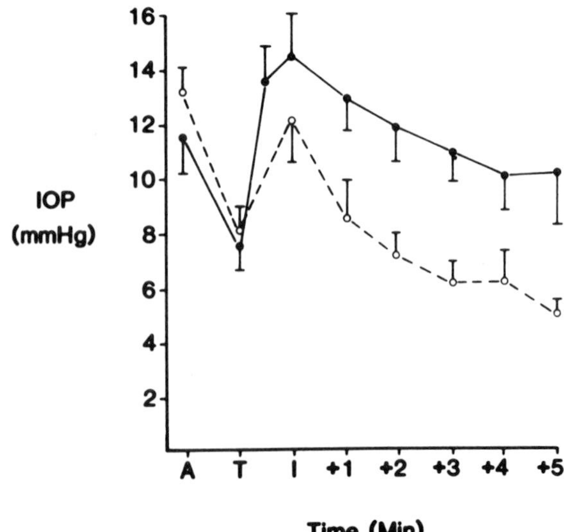

intact eye may produce intraocular volume loss through a surgically or traumatically produced ocular wound even though the pressure in the eye remains atmospheric. Aqueous humor is frequently lost following surgical or accidental opening of an eye to the atmosphere. Small or moderate losses of this fluid at a slow rate, however, usually do not produce significant pressure imbalance, and thus volume does not shift between anterior and posterior segments. However, a sudden loss of fluid through a large wound reduces anterior segment pressure, and may result in forward displacement of iris, lens, and vitreous, and thus in interference with the anatomical and functional integrity of the eye. Loss of virtrous from anteriorly located wounds clearly increases the severity of eye injuries. In addition, two complications may result from sudden foward displacement of the vitreous body: retinal detachment, and intraocular bleeding from disrupted retinal or choroidal blood vessels.

## ANESTHETIC MANAGEMENT OF CLOSED-EYE INJURIES

Generally, two types of patients present for surgery with closed-eye injuries. In the first group the injury is produced by the initial trauma, whereas the second group consists of patients whose perforated globe have been repaired and thus converted to closed-eye injuries. In addition, some patients with intact eyeball but injured periocular tissue may require surgery. Either local (regional) or general anesthesia can be used for surgical treatment of closed-eye injuries. However, general anesthesia is preferred, especially for intraocular procedures, as it renders the eye immobile and does not place excessive demands on the patient's ability to cooperate.

Anesthetic management of closed-eye trauma is easier than that for open-eye injuries. Emergency surgery is rarely required, and there is little possibility that further ocular damage will be produced by anesthesia. A full stomach is not a concern since surgery is performed in most patients at least 1 day after injury. Some patients with closed-eye injury may require surgery to treat traumatic glaucoma. Almost all of these patients are treated with pharmacological agents preoperatively. Some of these drugs may interact with agents used during anesthesia. Echothiopate Iodide (Phospholine Iodide) is a long-acting anticholinersterase agent that reduces IOP by producing miosis. Significant absorption into the systemic circulation occurs following instillation of echothiopate into the conjunctival sac. After several days of treatment, pseudocholinesterase activity may be seriously reduced, and prolonged apnea may result after administration of succinylcholine.[66,141] Timolol, levobunolol and betaxolol, β-adrenergic receptor-blocking agents, are also administered topically to treat glaucoma. Absorption of these drugs from the conjunctiva may result in systemic effects.[158] Thus, they should be used with caution in patients with asthma, congestive heart failure, and heart blocks other than first-degree atrioventricular block. Timolol can also potentiate the cardiovascular effects of inhalational agents and occasionally produce hypotension and bradycardia. Mannitol is used prior to intraocular surgery to reduce IOP. In patients with limited myocardial function, this drug may produce acute circulatory overload and pulmonary edema.

### GENERAL ANESTHESIA

General anesthesia should be smooth during all phases of the anesthetic procedure, especially in patients who require surgery for hyphema, retinal detachment, choroid rupture, or dislocated lens. Sudden changes in IOP in these patients may result in further disruption or displacement of intraocular structures, although we are not aware of any report describing this complication. In patients with high IOP, the ocular incision should be made after inducing hypocapnia ($Paco_2$ = 20 to 30 mm Hg) and a deep level of inhalation anesthesia. Sudden decompression of the eye when the IOP is excessively high may result in prolapse of the iris and vitreous into the anterior chamber or in intraocular bleeding or expulsive hemorrhage. In general, no anesthetic technique is specifically contraindicated in patients with closed-eye injuries.

Frequently, phenylephrine drops (2.5 to 10%) are used topically during the perioperative period to dilate the pupil. Absorption of this drug into the systemic circulation may result in serious hemodynamic and heart rate changes, especially when it is administered during the course of inhalation anesthesia. Administration of the drug 60 to 120 minutes before induction of anesthesia and at the lowest possible concentration (2.5%) may prevent these complications.[183]

### LOCAL (REGIONAL) ANESTHESIA

As we have mentioned above, local or regional anesthesia is an alternative to general anesthesia during surgical management of closed-eye injuries and injuries to the ocular adnexae. However, local anesthesia has its limitations; children and uncooperative adults rarely tolerate surgery awake, and the method may not provide optimal operative conditions in all patients. There are three important requirements for the success of eye surgery under local or regional anesthesia: adequate sedation; complete anesthesia; and immobile eye. Consequently, every effort must be made to achieve these objectives when a regional anesthetic technique is utilized.

#### *Regional Anesthesia for the Repair of Lid Injuries*

The lids are supplied by branches of the trigeminal nerve—the supraorbital, infraorbital, supratrochlear, infratrochlear, and lacrimal nerves[8] (Fig 11-16). Although blocking these nerves individually can produce satisfactory analgesia, infiltration of local anesthetic agents through the lacerated wound edges can be equally effective. When this approach is used, the anesthetic should be injected into the neurovascular plane of the eyelid which lies between the tarsal plate and the orbicularis oculi muscle (Fig 11-17). It is usually necessary to administer either topical anesthesia or retrobulbar block to facilitate manipulation of the conjunctiva during repair of lid lacerations. Local anesthesia for the lids can be provided by injection of a few milliliters of lidocaine (1 to 1.5%) or bupivacaine (0.5%) with or without epinephrine (1/200,000). Topical anesthesia of the cornea or conjunctiva can be provided by two to three drops of tetracaine (1%). Conjunctival and corneal anesthesia produced by this method also allows measurement of the IOP and removal of foreign bodies lodged on the eye surface.

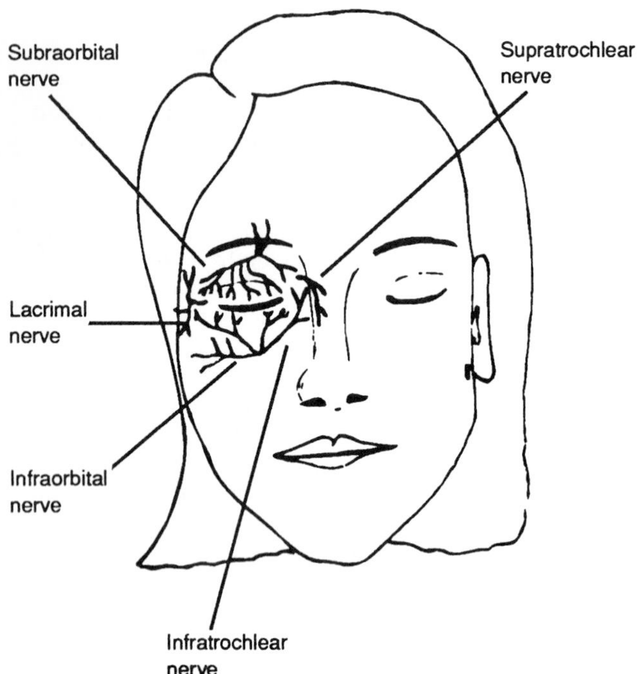


FIG. 11-16. Nerve supply of the eyelids.

## *Regional Anesthesia for Repair of Closed-eye Injuries*

Retrobulbar block has been used for 80 years to provide anesthesia for intraocular surgery. The block has been performed mainly by ophthalmologists and only rarely by anesthesiologists. Thus, it is not surprising that little is published about this subject in the anesthesia literature. In the following discussion, we will summarize only the important aspects of this technique; for more detailed information the reader is referred to three review articles published during the past 15 years.[8,57,58]

FIG. 11-17. Sagittal section of the eyelid showing orbicularis oculi muscle anteriorly, tarsal plate posteriorly, and neurovascular plane in the middle. Satisfactory analgesia can be obtained by injection of local anesthetic agent within the neurovascular plane.

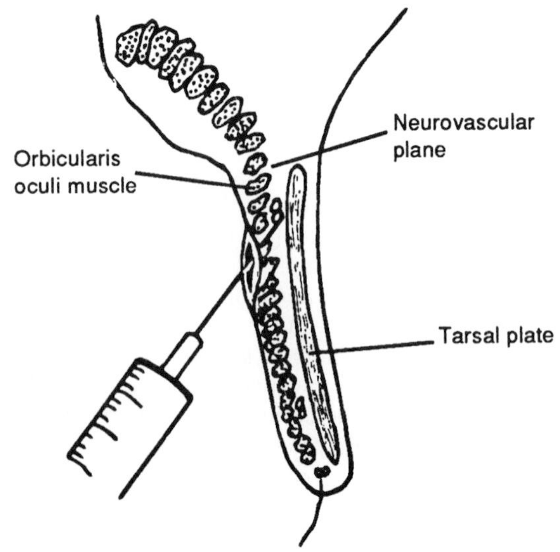


The ciliary ganglion is located behind the eyeball approximately 1 cm from the optic foramen. It lies within the muscle cone of the globe between the optic nerve and the lateral rectus muscle. Sensory nerve fibers arising from intraocular structures enter the ciliary ganglion through the short and long ciliary nerves and then join the ophthalmic branch of the trigeminal nerve (Fig 11-18). Thus, deposition of local anesthetic agents around the ciliary ganglion produces satisfactory anesthesia for surgical procedures performed within the eye.[8]

Retrobulbar block is performed by inserting a 25-gauge 32- to 35-mm-long blunt tip needle through the skin of the lower lid just above the inferior orbital rim slightly medial to its junction with the lateral orbital wall (Fig 11-19). The needle is directed upward and medially toward the apex of the orbit for 3 cm. The needle tip should lie inside the muscle cone, adjacent to the ciliary ganglion. A variety of local anesthetic agents and mixtures has been used (Table 11-6).

It is common to add hyaluronidase (15 to 20 units/mL) and epinephrine (1/200,000) to aid diffusion and rapid onset of anesthesia within the orbit, to delay systemic absorption of the local anesthetic, and to reduce the possibility of retrobulbar hemorrhage. In the conventional method, the patient is asked to maintain an upward and medial gaze to remove the inferior oblique muscle from the path of the needle (Fig 11-19). This position, however, brings the optic nerve, the ophthalmic artery and its branches, the superior orbital vein, and the posterior pole of the globe into close proximity to the tip of the needle. Thus it has been recommended that the globe be positioned either in the neutral position or in a slightly downward and temporal gaze.[144,182] Fig. 11-20 shows the position of the optic nerve in relation to the needle tip at the conventional and modified positions of the eye. In the latter approach, the needle is directed toward the inferior part of the superior orbital fissure instead of the apex, and the needle tip remains lateral to an imaginary sagittal plane passed through the macula. Another modification of the retrobulbar technique is the peribulbar block in which the local anesthetic agent is injected outside the muscle cone, and prolonged orbital pressure is maintained to provide spread to the ciliary ganglion.[58]

Akinesia of the globe requires blocking the motor nerve supply of the extraocular and orbicularis oculi muscles. The motor nerves of the extraocular muscles are located on their inner surfaces. Thus, local anesthetic solution deposited in the retrobulbar space spreads within the muscle cone and blocks these nerves.[8] In most instances, retrobulbar anesthesia also produces orbicularis akinesia,[117] but a separate facial nerve block may be performed to ensure adequate paralysis of the orbicularis muscles and thereby prevent voluntary lid closure. Although the facial nerve can be blocked by several techniques, the methods described by O'Brien and Van Lint are most common. In O'Brien's method, a 25-gauge needle is inserted through the skin slightly below the tragus until the periosteum of the ramus of the mandible is contacted. Then the needle is withdrawn slightly, and 4 to 5 mL of local anetsthetic is injected (Fig 11-21). In Van Lint's method, the peripheral branches of the facial nerve are blocked by injecting local anesthetic solution beneath the facial muscle fi-

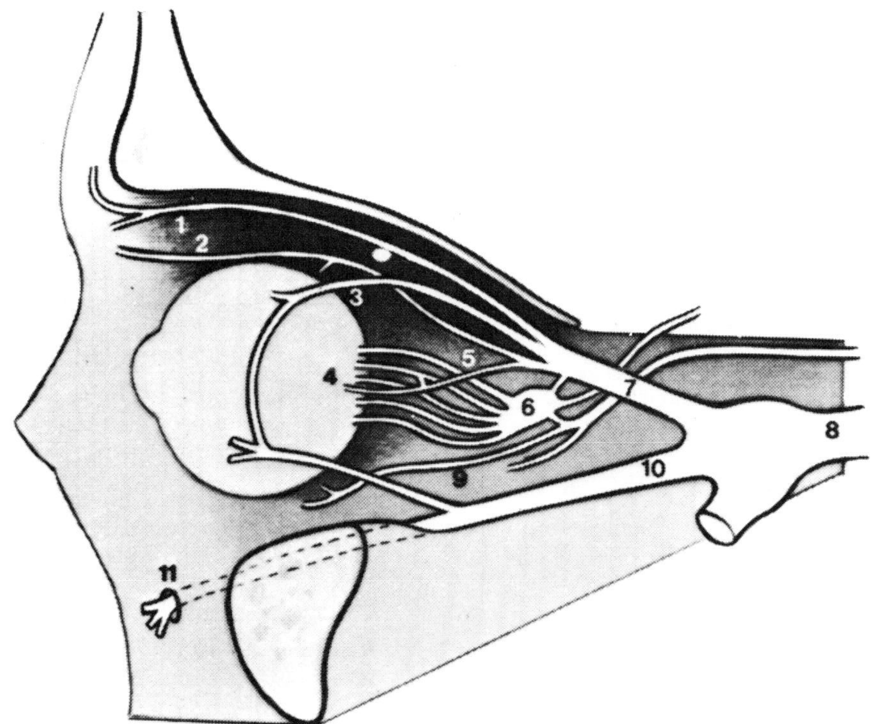


FIG. 11-18. Nerve supply of the globe and the orbit. 1, frontal nerve; 2, infratrochlear nerve; 3, lacrimal nerve; 4, short ciliary nerves; 5, long ciliary nerves; 6, ciliary ganglion; 7, ophthalmic nerve; 8, sensory root of trigeminal nerve; 9, nerve supplying the inferior oblique muscle; 10, maxillary nerve; 11, infraorbital nerve. (From Allen and Elkington[8] with permission.)

bers over the inferior and lateral margins of the orbit (Fig 11-21).

Although complications rarely occur with retrobulbar anesthesia, they can be quite serious and may lead to blindness. The possible complications associated with retrobulbar block, their mechanisms, clinical manifestations, and treatments are shown in Table 11-7. Although the dose of local anesthetic agent injected into the retrobulbar space is small, toxic reactions may occur with intra-arterial injection, possibly due to direct delivery of the drug to the brain by centripetal flow. Brainstem anesthesia may develop due to spread of local anesthetic into the CNS via the optic nerve sheath or the superior orbital fissure.[73] Apnea and loss of consciousness occur frequently with this complication, requiring artificial ventilation.[73] Patients may develop hypertension due to blockade of the vagus depressor nerve, but hypotension may also occur in some patients.[73] Occasionally decreased visual acuity and extraocular muscle palsies may occur in the contralateral eye, probably due to spread of local anesthetic in the CNS. This complication is rare and without permanent sequelae.[9,60] Retrobulbar hemorrhage may interfere with retinal blood flow and thus cause blindness. The eye should be observed care-

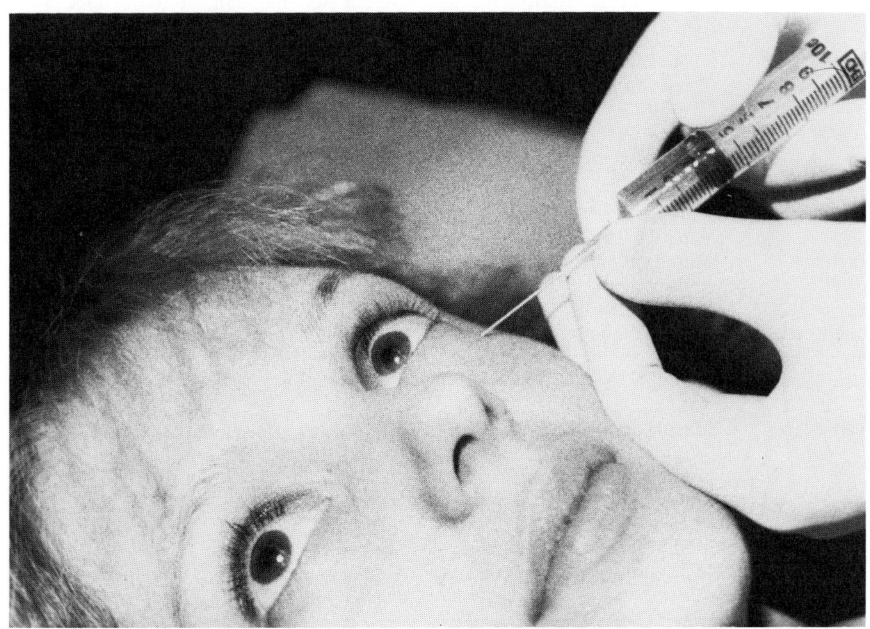

FIG. 11-19. Retrobulbar block. The needle is inserted through the skin immediately above the orbital floor and medial to the lateral wall of the orbit. Note the direction of the needle: posterior, medial, and slightly superior. Classically the patient is asked to look upward and medially. However, recent reports recommend a neutral gaze (see Fig 11–20, A and B).

TABLE 11-6. Concentrations, Volumes, Onset, and Duration of Actions of Local Anesthetic Agents Used for Retrobulbar Block*

| AGENT | CONCENTRATION (%) | VOLUME (ml) | ONSET OF ACTION† (minutes) | DURATION OF ACTION‡ (hours) |
|---|---|---|---|---|
| Lidocaine | 2 | 3 to 5 | 3 to 4 | 3 to 4 |
| Mepivacaine | 2 | 3 to 5 | 3 to 4 | 3 to 4 |
| Bupivacaine | 0.75 | 3 to 5 | 5 to 10§ | 6 to 11 |
| Etidocaine | 1 | 3 to 5 | 3 to 4 | 5 to 9 |

* The volume of local anesthetic described in this table does not include that used for facial nerve block. An additional 5 to 7 mL of local anesthetic solution is used to provide eyelid akinesia with this technique.

† Addition of hyaluronidase (15 to 20 units/mL) reduces the onset time of all local anesthetics.

‡ Addition of epinephrine (1/200,000) prolongs the duration of action of all local anesthetics.

§ Onset of action of bupivacaine may be shortened by mixing it with lidocaine (2%) or mepivacaine (2%).

fully with ophthalmoscopic and tonometric examinations and orbital decompression procedures performed, if necessary, to avoid permanent sequelae.[58] However, retinal vascular occlusion can occur in the absence of retrobulbar hemorrhage due to other causes mentioned in Table 11-7.[173] Thus, ophthalmoscopic examination should be performed following retrobulbar block whenever there is a question about the adequacy of retinal blood flow. Perforation of the globe[58] and injection of local anesthetic agent into the optic nerve sheath[144] can occur during retrobulbar block and require prompt diagnosis and therapeutic intervention (Table 11-7).

## ANESTHETIC MANAGEMENT OF OPEN-EYE INJURIES

Patients with open-eye injuries may present to surgery in a variety of conditions. A small percentage of these patients has other serious associated injuries. These injuries should be given priority; careful evaluation and prompt and efficient treatment should be instituted while ocular injuries are managed conservatively. Anesthesia for surgical management of associated injuries should be planned in such a way that further damage to the injured eye is avoided. Occasionally, immediate surgery may not be indicated for an associated injury,

TABLE 11-7. Possible Complications of Retrobulbar Anesthesia

| COMPLICATION | MECHANISM | CLINICAL MANIFESTATION | TREATMENT |
|---|---|---|---|
| Local anesthetic toxicity | Intravascular injection<br>Direct injection into the CNS via the sheaths of the optic nerve or via the superior orbital fissure (brainstem anesthesia) | Seizures, hypotension, hypertension, bradycardia, respiratory depression, apnea, loss of consciousness | Treatment of seizures, cardiovascular and respiratory support |
| Retrobulbar hemorrhage | Injury to orbital vessels by the needle | Proptosis, increased IOP, bradycardia, dysrhythmia (oculocardiac reflex) | Ophthalmoscopic examination to rule out ischemic damage to the optic nerve and retina<br>Measurement of IOP<br>Excessively high IOP resulting in occlusion of retinal vessels or pallor of optic nerve head requires orbital decompression procedures (eg, lateral cantothomy, release of orbital septum)<br>Anterior chamber paracentesis may be needed to lower IOP in selected patients |
| Retinal vascular occlusion | Retrobulbar hemorrhage<br>Direct trauma to the ophthalmic artery or the optic nerve by the needle<br>Vasoconstriction by epinephrine in the local anesthetic | Decreased or absent vision, observation of occluded retinal vessels during ophthalmoscopy | Decompression of the orbit if retrobulbar hemorrhage present, decompression of optic nerve sheath may be considered if dilated optic nerve sheath is observed on CT |
| Perforation of the globe | Trauma by the needle | Subconjunctival hemorrhage and softening of the eye; symptoms of retinal detachment if retina is perforated | Repair of perforation as soon as possible |
| Injection of local anesthetic into the optic nerve sheath | Trauma by the needle | Sudden transient blindness, optic atrophy; brainstem anesthesia in some cases | In severe cases optic nerve decompression may be considered |

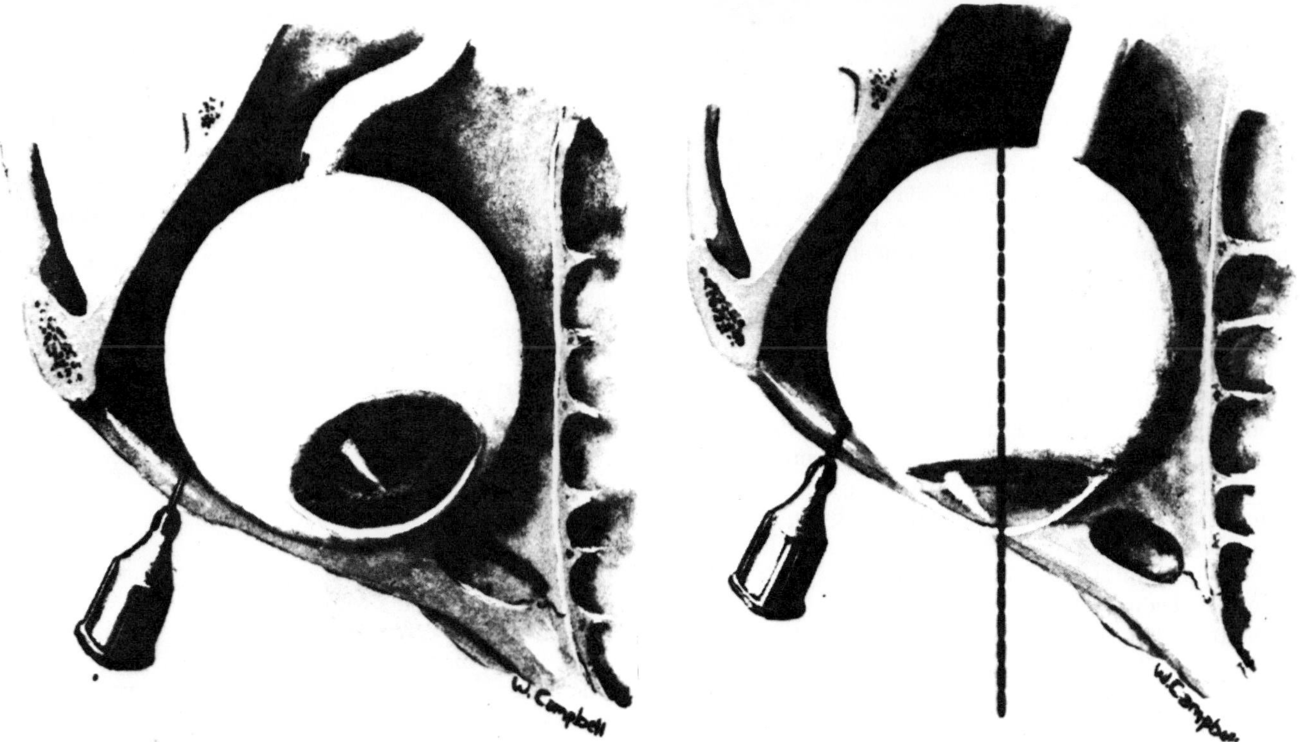

FIG. 11-20. Location of the optic nerve in two different positions of the globe. Left, upward and inward position displaces the optic nerve into the path of the retrobulbar needle. Right, when the eye is in neutral position, the optic nerve remains away from the needle path. (From Pautler et al[144] with permission.)

FIG. 11-21. Facial nerve block to produce eyelid akinesis. In O'Brien's method the needle is inserted slightly below the tragus and the ramus of mandible contacted. Then the needle is withdrawn slightly and 4 to 5 mL of local anesthetic injected. In Van Lint's method the local anesthetic (4 to 5 mL) is injected below the muscle fibers overlying the zygomatic bone at the lateral and inferior margins of the orbit.

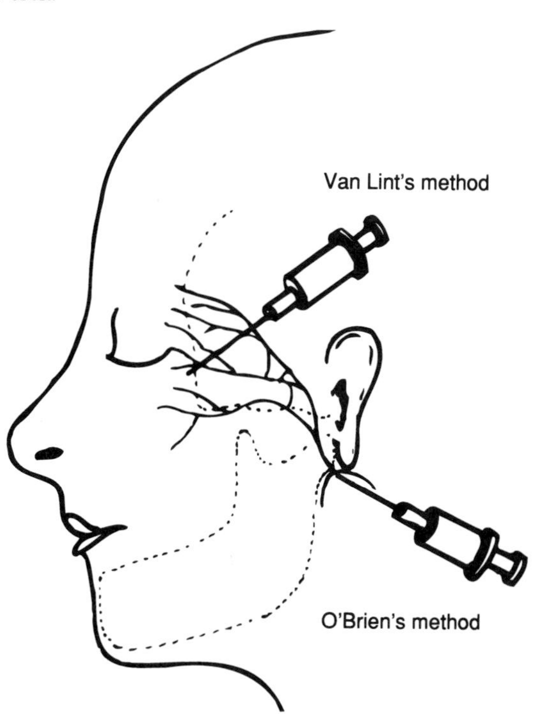


but its presence may create difficulty during anesthetic management of the patient's eye injury; a coexistent cervical spine injury is a characteristic example of this problem.

Usually, however, anesthesia is required for surgical treatment of an isolated eye injury. Most of these patients are young and healthy and have no underlying diseases. Thus, management involves providing smooth anesthetic care to prevent further damage to the eye. However, some elderly patients may present with varying degrees of cardiovascular and pulmonary dysfunction requiring careful perioperative management. Approximately 15 to 20% of open-eye injuries occur in children between the ages of 1 and 9,[20] thus knowledge and skill in pediatric anesthesia are also important.

The importance of careful preanesthetic evaluation with attention to preexisting diseases, prior surgery and anesthesia, current medications, drug allergies, physical examination, and laboratory results cannot be overemphasized. A brief consultation with the ophthalmologist may help in obtaining information about the severity and prognosis of the injury. Although accurate assessment of the damage is not always possible prior to surgery, extreme cases are usually recognized by the ophthalmologist, aiding the anesthesiologist in formulating an anesthetic plan. Special anesthetic techniques may not be necessary if the injured eye is not salvageable.

A common anesthetic problem in acute open-eye injuries is a full stomach. With the exception of protruding or irritant foreign bodies, immediate surgical intervention is not indicated in most instances, and time may be spent preoperatively in evaluation and sedation of the patient. However, waiting more than a few hours for the stomach to empty places the patient at increased risk of ocular infection and extrusion of intraocular contents. Most ocular wounds seal shortly after injury with a thin membrane that prevents the loss of aqueous humor. However, this memebrane cannot withstand sudden ocular hypertension caused by crying, coughing, sneezing, straining, or vomiting which commonly occur in children and in inebriated and/or uncooperative adults. In addition, the conventional period of 8 hours of fasting does not ensure reliable gastric emptying in traumatized patients. Thus, surgery should be performed on open-eye injuries within a few hours of injury and precautions for full stomach taken in all patients. Gastric emptying with a nasogastric tube should not be attempted, since it may evoke coughing and vomiting and result in expulsion of intraocular contents.

Neutralization of gastric acid or emptying the stomach by pharmacological means have received ample attention during the past decade as a prophylactic measure against aspiration pneumonitis. These methods, although effective in most instances, cannot ensure reliable protection. Sodium citrate 0.3 Molar (30 to 40 mL orally), 30 minutes before anesthetic induction, cimetidine (300 mg), or rantidine (150 or 300 mg, by mouth, intramuscularly, or intravenously) 90 minutes before anesthetic induction may provide some protection. Although data are lacking, these drugs do not appear to affect the IOP of a closed eye. Metoclopramide, (10 mg intravenously) 30 minutes before anesthetic induction can accelerate gastric emptying without affecting pH. However, preliminary data demonstrate a tendency of this drug to raise IOP.[142] While further work is needed to substantiate this finding, metoclopramide should be used with caution in open-eye injuries.

Although most intraocular surgical procedures can be performed with a regional anesthetic technique—retrobulbar block for ocular anesthesia and facial nerve block for eyelid akinesis—perforated-eye injuries cannot be repaired by this method. Retrobulbar block is associated with a small but unpredictable incidence of orbital hemorrhage which, by compressing the open eye, may cause extrusion of its contents. Even if there is no retrobulbar bleeding, pressure caused by an intraorbitally deposited local anesthetic agent or by the gentle eye massage used to facilitate spread of the solution may threaten the residual integrity of the eye. Finally, straining by an uncooperative patient during performance of the block or surgery may result in increased venous pressure, choroidal congestion, and thereby expulsion of intraocular contents. Occasionally, topical anesthesia in conjunction with facial nerve block may be used by the ophthalmologist to repair extremely small corneal wounds. However, except for this condition, general anesthesia is the only choice for repair of perforated-eye injuries.

## GENERAL ANESTHESIA

The objectives in anesthetic care of perforated-eye injuries are: (1) overall patient safety; (2) maintenance of decreased extraocular muscle tone; (3) avoidance of elevation in intraocular volume; (4) avoidance of external pressure on the eye; (5) provision of an immobile eye; and (6) minimizing bleeding.

## PREMEDICATION

Premedication should not include drugs likely to increase intraocular volume. Opiates have the potential of causing both ventilatory depression and vomiting, thus increasing choroidal blood volume. A combination of an antisialagogue (atropine, 0.4 mg; scopolamine, 0.6 mg; glycopyrrolate, 0.2 mg) with a benzodiazepine derivative, hydroxyzine (50 to 75 mg) or droperidol (2.5 mg) is usually satisfactory. Scopolamine should be avoided in elderly patients as it may produce agitation. Flunitrazepam (0.02 mg/kg) as a premedicant agent provides adequate sedation and produces a moderate reduction in IOP.[115] Patients who develop blindness of one eye following injury may be extremely agitated and apprehensive. It is therefore important to establish good rapport with them.

## INDUCTION OF ANESTHESIA

Induction represents the most critical period of anesthetic management in patients with open-eye injuries. Anestehetic induction should be smooth with large doses of intravenous anesthetic and muscle relaxant agents. A rapid sequence induction technique is the choice in most patients since the anesthesiologist must assume that the stomach is full. However, this technique is not without hazards[15]: difficulty or failure of intubation or ventilation; muscular responses or movements during cricoid pressure, laryngoscopy and intubation; and cardiovascular responses in the form of tachycardia, hypertension, or hypotension are well-known complications of this technique and may lead to protrusion of intraocular contents and/or aspiration pneumonitis. Nevertheless, these hazards usually can be minimized by careful preoperative evaluation and the use of adqeuate doses of anesthetic induction agents. As described in Chapter 3, the airway should be evaluated thoroughly, and all necessary equipment should be available to overcome difficulties in intubation and ventilation.

During preoxygenation every effort must be made to avoid exerting pressure on the eye by the face mask. Although placement of an eye shield on the damaged side may protect the eye from further injury, allowing the patient to hold the mask on his/her face during preoxygenation may also reduce the risk of mask-induced damage. The patient's head should be elevated 10 to 15° to facilitate venous drainage of the eye.

Any intravenous anesthetic agent can be used as long as the dose is adequate to provide a deep level of anesthesia.[13] Thiopental (5 to 7 mg/kg),[13] etomidate (0.3 mg/kg),[138] and ketamine (2 mg/kg)[13] have all been shown to decrease IOP below awake levels (Table 11-4).

The choice of muscle relaxant for anesthetic induction of open-eye injuries has generated substantial controversy during the last few decades. Shortly after its introduction into clinical practice, succinylcholine was shown to increase IOP.[78] In 1957 expulsion of vitreous during eye surgery was described by Lincoff et al[107] and Dillon et al.[48] During the subsequent 10 years both experimental and clinical research on the subject confirmed the findings of previous investigators that this effect of succinylcholine is caused mainly by contraction of extraocular muscles but also by choroidal congestion.[2,36,55,77,92] Although minimal effects were reported in humans,[105,197] general agreement on the subject led to a search for measures to prevent IOP elevation reliably. Pretreatment with small doses of D-tubocurarine (3 mg),[47,124] gallamine (20 mg),[47,124] pancuronium (1 mg),[96] hexaflurenium (0.4 mg/kg 2 minutes prior to succinylcholine), succinylcholine itself (10 mg),[185] or acetazolamide (500 mg immediately before the anesthetic induction)[27] (Fig 11-22) had been shown to decrease the ocular pressure response to succinylcholine substantially. These findings resulted in frequent use of succinylcholine in conjunction with one or more of these agents until the late 1970s. However, several reports in the second half of the decade showed that neither pretreatment with nondepolarizing agents nor succinylcholine self-taming could reliably prevent the problem.[23,67,120,121] Of the other pretreatment agents, hexaflurenium and acetazolamide gained little popularity because of limited clinical trials.[27,93] During the late 1970s it was shown that pretreatment with diazepam (0.1 mg/kg intravenously) prior to anesthetic induction could attenuate the succinylcholine-induced rise of IOP but without entirely abolishing the response.[5,38] These findings, coupled with the report by Brown et al[24] describing rapid onset of intubating conditions with high-dose pancuronium (0.15 to 0.20 mg/kg), resulted in a significant decline in the use of succinylcholine for anesthetic induction of perforated-eye injuries. In 1985, after a retrospective review of their experience at Wills Eye Hospital in Philadelphia, Libonati et al[106] reported that use of succinylcholine following pretreatment with a nondepolarizing agent and a deep level of general anesthesia was a safe technique for patients with

FIG. 11-22. Graph showing mean IOP changes during induction of anesthesia in patients pretreated with acetazolamide (500 mg intravenously) (broken line) and in patients not treated with this agent (solid line). Although the figure shows almost no change of IOP in acetazolamide-treated patients, in approximately half of the patients some rise in IOP was recorded. A, IOP immediately after injection of acetazolamide and thiopental; B, IOP 2 minutes after administration of thiopental and acetazolamide and immediately before administration of succinylcholine; C, IOP during fasciculations; 1, 2, 3, 4, and 5 represent the time in minutes following intubation. (Redrawn from Carballo[27] with permission.)

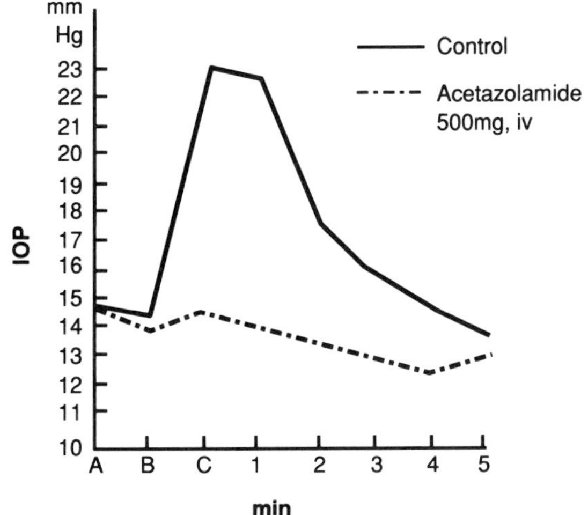


open-eye injuries. None of their 63 patients developed extrusion of intraocular contents. The report was followed by several letters both endorsing[22,49,133] and disparaging[85,152,189] the use of succinylcholine in this setting. The proponents of this technique justify their use of succinylcholine as follows. (1) There has been no published report of eye content extrusion associated with the use of succinylcholine after pretreatment doses of nondepolarizing agents in the presence of deep levels of anesthesia. (2) Tracheal intubation produces a greater degree of IOP rise than succinylcholine. (3) By producing the most rapid intubating conditions, succinylcholine is the safest muscle relaxant overall since it minimizes the possibility of gastric fluid regurgitation and pulmonary aspiration. Those who disagree with the recommendation of Libonati et al[106] contend that (1) there is no randomized prospective study available to justify such a conclusion; and (2) other available techniques provide safe anesthetic induction without jeopardizing the eye. We speculate that the results of future randomized and prospective studies will support the use of succinylcholine as recommended by Libonati et al.[106] Until then, however, the use of succinylcholine should be individualized based on prevailing circumstances.

Nondepolarizing neuromuscular blocking agents provide intubating conditions more slowly than succinylcholine. Thus, these agents are less suitable than succinylcholine for anesthetic induction of patients with perforated-eye injuries. However, several methods have been devised to accelerate the onset of action of these agents even though none achieves the rapidity and reliability of succinylcholine. It has been reported that pancuronium in doses of 0.15 mg/kg produces 90% twitch depression 75 seconds after injection and provides excellent intubating conditions in all patients.[24] Similar twitch depression and intubating conditions could be produced in 60 seconds after a 0.2 or 0.25 mg/kg dose. By using 0.15 mg/kg pancuronium, we have had few patients in whom intubation could not be performed after 75 seconds because of inadequate relaxation. There are several disadvantages associated with high-dose pancuronium. A significant increase in heart rate and blood pressure may occur following its administration, and during tracheal intubation the increase in IOP is the same as that seen after succinylcholine.[103] In addition, large doses of pancuronium may result in prolonged paralysis necessitating postoperative mechanical ventilation. Atracurium and vecuronium, when used in similar large doses, can also provide rapid intubating conditions without causing prolonged paralysis. The recommended dose of vecuronium is 0.25 mg/kg and that of atracurium 1.5 mg/kg.[101] The latter drug, however, may cause generalized flushing and hypotension in some patients due to histamine release.

Some clinicians prefer to inject the usual paralyzing dose of a nondepolarizing muscle relaxant during the preoxygenation period before the intravenous induction agent is given and to wait until muscle weakness develops as manifested by double vision, inability to hold the anesthetic mask, or difficulty in opening the eye.[13,79] At this moment, a large dose of intravenous agent is administered and cricoid pressure applied. After obtaining satisfactory twitch depression (90%) on the neuromuscular function monitor, laryngoscopy is performed and the trachea intubated. An unpleasant sensation of weakness may be felt momentarily by the patient if the injection of induction agent is delayed. Pancuronium (0.08 mg/kg), atracurium (0.6 mg/kg), and vecuronium (0.08 mg/kg) may be adequate to provide satisfactory muscle relaxation within 1 minute after the injection of the anesthetic agent. There is, however, individual variability in response to these muscle relaxants which may result in delay in obtaining adequate intubating conditions. One important point to remember with this technique is that double vision cannot occur in patients whose injured eye is blind or covered with dressings. Thus, reliance on this sign in monocular patients may result in disastrous complications.

The priming principle, which involves administration of subparalytic doses of nondepolarizing agents a few minutes before a large intubating dose, was introduced by Foldes[59] in 1984 as an attempt to shorten the onset of action of nondepolarizing muscle relaxants. This technique may be particularly useful in providing rapid intubating conditions with intermediate-acting muscle relaxants because intubation cannot be achieved in less than 2 minutes even with relatively large doses of vecuronium (0.1 mg/kg) or atracurium (0.5 mg/kg).[123] Thus, shortening the onset time by 1 minute with priming can permit the use of these agents in place of succinylcholine (see also Chapters 3 and 9).

Although preliminary reports demonstrated that by using this technique intubation could be achieved in 60 seconds after injection of the paralyzing dose of vecuronium or atracurium,[119,162] several subsequent reports demonstrated inadequate intubating conditions, unpleasant sensations of weakness, and delayed onset of paralysis.[16,128,169] This was probably due to inadequate knowledge of optimal priming and intubating doses and the interval between them. Tabaoda et al[174] demonstrated that by using a priming dose of 0.01 mg/kg, an intubating dose of 0.1 mg/kg, and a priming interval of 4 minutes, vecuronium could produce rapid and safe intubating conditions. However, there may be individual differences in response among patients depending on age, level of anesthesia, and sensitivity to muscle relaxants.

Laryngoscopy and tracheal intubation cause a greater increase in IOP than succinylcholine, presenting an important threat to the anatomical integrity of a lacerated eye.[23,29,50,51,69,99,120,134,140,159,197] The mechanism of the IOP increase, although unclear, is attributed to an autonomic reflex or an increase in central venous pressure secondary to coughing. However, IOP rises to almost the same level in patients with or without coughing during intubation, suggesting that the autonomic reflex mechanism is more important.[50]

Lidocaine has been used extensively to attenuate the hemodynamic response to intubation. However, conflicting results have been obtained about the effect of this agent on IOP. Smith et al[167] and Murphy et al[134] were unable to demonstrate a beneficial effect of lidocaine (1 to 2 mg/kg) whereas attenuation was noted by others.[50,104,112] These results suggest that lidocaine (1.5 mg/kg) cannot reliably attenuate the intubation-induced rise of IOP. Instillation of lidocaine into the trachea prior to anesthetic induction should be avoided as it may induce coughing. Fentanyl (5 μg/kg) or sufentanil (1 μg/kg) given immediately before rapid sequence induction with intermediate-acting nondepolarizing agents attenuates the rise in IOP caused by intubation.[29] Likewise, large doses of thiopental (7 mg/kg) may be effective in preventing excessive IOP elevation.[13] Thus, deep anesthesia, with a combination of low-dose opiates and relatively large doses of intravenous anesthetic agents, appears to be the most effective method to attenuate the IOP rise during laryngoscopy and intubation.

## MAINTENANCE OF ANESTHESIA

Although not lifesaving, ophthalmic surgery can be life threatening in the presence of multiple trauma, angina, hypertension, congestive heart failure, and various other medical conditions. The risk of surgery being minimal, the main problems are related to the patient's medical condition and the anesthetic management. The choice of anesthetic for maintenance of anesthesia depends on the physical status of the patient and the type of ophthalmic injury. Inhalational anesthetic agents have the advantage of providing smooth anesthesia with ease of control, potentiation of muscle relaxant activity, low incidence of postoperative nausea and vomiting, and adequate control of blood pressure and bronchial tone. The combination of these agents with small doses of narcotic agents provides satisfactory conditions in most instances.

During surgery, "squeezing" of the eyeball by extraocular pressure or choroidal congestion produced by coughing, straining, or bucking should be prevented by deep anesthesia with inhalation anesthetics, narcotics, and muscle relaxants titrated to an appropriate response on the neuromuscular function monitor. Tracheobronchial stimulation in anesthetized patients—movement of the head or tracheobronchial suctioning—should be attempted only after ensuring an adequate level of anesthesia, muscle relaxation, and preferably following slow instillation of lidocaine into the trachea.

Patients with associated lung contusion, aspiration pneumonitis, pulmonary edema, or acute respiratory distress syndrome may have marginal $Pa_{O_2}$, requiring ventilation with pulmonary distending pressures. Intuitively, positive end-expiratory pressure (PEEP), by increasing intrathoracic pressure, should decrease the venous outflow from the eye and present a risk of extrusion of intraocular contents. However, its effect on IOP, to our knowledge, has not been studied in humans. As discussed above, the head-up position (15 to 20°) should be maintained during surgery to facilitate venous drainage.

The oculocardiac reflex, manifested by bradycardia, dysrhythmia, atrioventricular block, or cardiac arrest may occur during manipulation of the eyeball. However, this complication occurs infrequently during repair of eye lacerations because pressure or traction on the eye is avoided. Glycopyrrolate (5 to 7.5 μg/kg intravenously) or atropine (10 to 15 μg/kg intravenously) may decrease the incidence of this reflex in children in a dose-related fashion, but neither drug can prevent bradycardia in every patient.[81,127] In addition, atropine itself may produce arrhythmias if it is given in the presence of halothane anesthesia.[90] Although retrobulbar block is effective in preventing or abolishing the reflex, it should not be utilized in the presence of an open-eye injury because the eye may be compressed by the local anesthetic agent deposited intraorbitally and by the possible development of retrobulbar hematoma following this anesthetic technique. In addition, the reflex can be precipitated by retrobulbar hemorrhage.[177]

Once surgery begins, access to the patient's airway may be difficult. Monitoring of the patient's airway pressure, breath sounds, end-tidal $CO_2$, and oxygen saturation by a pulse oximeter will allow detection of breathing circuit disconnection, airway obstruction, and changes in chest compliance.

## EMERGENCE AND EXTUBATION

During emergence from anesthesia an increase in IOP is likely to occur. Although the adverse consequences of this on the repaired eye are less important than those in an open eye, coughing, straining, or vomiting during this stage may result in intraocular or orbital bleeding, jeopardizing the success of the surgery. Lidocaine (1.5 mg/kg intravenously) may attenuate these responses to emergence and extubation. Shivering after anesthesia may produce a considerable increase of IOP[113] and should be treated with small doses of intravenous narcotics, eg, meperidine (25 mg) and by warming the patient. Patients with a full stomach should be extubated after reasonable return of tracheobronchial reflexes to prevent aspiration of gastric contents.

## EARLY POSTOPERATIVE CARE

During transportation and in the recovery room the patient should be kept in 10 to 20° head-up position to facilitate venous drainage from the eye. Postoperative hypertension may develop in some patients due to pain, anxiety, urinary retention, or other causes. This may contribute to elevation of IOP in the postoperative period; thus it should be treated promptly. Occasionally, mannitol or acetazolamide used before or during surgery may cause intravascular volume depletion which, in the hypovolemic multiple trauma patient, may result in hypotension. Thus, blood pressure and urine output should be measured and appropriate fluids administered when necessary. Nausea and vomiting may occur in some patients; antiemetic agents such as droperidol (2.5 mg) or Compazine (5 to 10 mg) intravenously are usually effective in preventing this complication. Finally, potentially blind patients need the psychological support of all recovery room personnel including the anesthesiologist.

## INDUCTION OF GENERAL ANESTHESIA FOR OPEN-EYE INJURIES IN SPECIAL CONDITIONS

### *Difficult Airway*

In rare instances open-eye injuries may occur in patients in whom the airway may be difficult to manage. As most patients with open-eye injuries also have a full stomach, anesthetic management of these patients may be exceedingly difficult and challenging. The anesthesiologist is faced with the dilemma of conflicting requirements. For the eye injury, tracheal intubation should follow deep anesthesia and paralysis, whereas the presence of a difficult airway may preclude the use of intravenous anesthetic agents and muscle relaxants. An induction method employing spontaneous breathing of inhalation agents, even though it may be satisfactory from the standpoint of the eye injury and airway problems, may be unsafe because of the danger of passive regurgitation and aspiration of gastric contents.

A difficult airway may be caused by preexisting or trauma-induced anatomical abnormalities. Although these problems can be anticipated in most instances, failure to recognize them may lead to disastrous complications during anesthetic induction. Thus, it is important not only to evaluate the airway thoroughly prior to surgery, but also to plan, in advance, management strategies for such difficulties.

OPEN-EYE AND CERVICAL SPINE INJURIES. When an open-eye injury is associated with an acute cervical spine injury, airway management may be necessary as a lifesaving procedure, to provide ventilatory support, and/or as part of anesthetic management for repair of the ocular or other injuries. Tracheostomy or cricothyroidotomy may be required after fixing the head in a neutral position if the airway must be secured immediately in the emergency room. In patients whose breathing is adequate and whose surgery can be delayed for several hours, orotracheal intubation under deep general anesthesia can be performed following reliable immobilization of the cervical spine, preferably with a halo device. However, difficulties may arise in directing the endotracheal tube into the larynx during direct laryngoscopy when the head and neck are stabilized. Thus, some clinicians are reluctant to perform rapid sequence induction in these patients and prefer either tracheostomy or awake intubation with the aid of a fiberoptic laryngoscope. Since awake intubation in a patient with a salvageable open-eye injury is not appropriate, tracheostomy or cricothyroidotomy may be chosen. We base our decision on the result of preoperative airway evaluation: a rapid sequence induction-intubation is used in patients in whom no difficulty of ventilation and intubation is anticipated, but tracheostomy or cricothyroidotomy is performed in the remaining patients. Unfortunately data are scanty in this realm, and decisions are made empirically. It should be noted, however, that even during tracheostomy, coughing evoked by the insertion of the tube may result in extrusion of eye contents. Adequate sedation and intravenous lidocaine (1.5 mg/kg) prior to insertion of the tube may be useful in reducing the risk of this response.

OPEN-EYE AND MAXILLOFACIAL INJURIES. A facial fracture in the presence of an open-eye injury is another condition that should be evaluated carefully before embarking on a rapid sequence induction. Valuable information can be obtained from facial X-rays, CT scans, and consultation with the involved surgeons. In general, facial fractures limited to the upper face do not pose any airway difficulties; thus, rapid sequence induction should not present problems. Midface fractures may result in maxillary instability and intraoral bleeding. In addition, particles of teeth or foreign bodies may be present in the oral cavity or in the larynx and carry the risk of acute airway obstruction following anesthetic induction. Mandibular fractures, particularly those involving the ramus and temporomandibular joint, may cause complete airway obstruction following muscle relaxation. The method of airway management—rapid sequence induction versus cricothyroidotomy or tracheostomy—in patients with facial fractures and open-eye injuries should be decided according to the prevailing circumstances.

OPEN-EYE INJURIES AND PREEXISTING ANATOMICAL ABNORMALITIES. When airway difficulty is anticipated secondary to preexisting anatomical abnormalities such as short neck, small mouth, high-arched palate, receding chin, or protuberant incisor teeth, there are two possibilities: (1) the patient can be ventilated easily by mask but cannot be intubated with direct laryngoscopy; and (2) both ventilation and intubation are difficult. Most patients fall into the first category. In these circumstances it is not unreasonable to induce anesthesia with relatively large doses of thiopental (4 to 7 mg/kg) and a muscle relaxant and then to ventilate by mask with oxygen and inhalational agents while cricoid pressure is applied. When adequate depth of anesthesia and relaxation is obtained, direct laryngoscopy can be performed to visualize the larynx while cricoid compression is maintained by an assistant. If the larynx is visualized, the endotracheal tube can be inserted and its cuff inflated. If direct laryngoscopy and intubation are not possible, a fiberoptic bronchoscope can be inserted orally or nasally through the opening of a face mask designed specifically for this purpose (Patil-Syracuse mask)[143] while ventilation is continued. After insertion of the fiberoptic laryngoscope through the larynx, the endotracheal tube is threaded into the trachea and its cuff inflated. Since the patient is paralyzed and ventilated with an inhalational anesthetic throughout the intubation procedure, coughing or bucking is unlikely to occur, and thus the technique should not pose any danger to the eye. Obviously, when ventilation of the patient proves difficult, this technique cannot be continued; anesthetic gases are turned off and the patient awakened. If difficulty in both ventilation and tracheal intubation in a patient with open-eye injury is anticipated cricothyroidotomy under local anesthesia is the only choice. Fortunately, this situation occurs rarely in practice.

### *Coronary Artery Disease*

Sympathetic response during rapid sequence induction in patients with coronary artery disease may result in myocardial ischemia. The hemodynamic response to laryngoscopy and tracheal intubation may be attenuated by various maneuvers. Ventilation by mask using inhalational agents for 10 to 15 minutes prior to laryngoscopy and intubation while cricoid pressure is applied may blunt the hypertensive and tachycardic response. Alternatively, in normovolemic patients, intravenous administration of $\beta$ receptor-blocking agents such as propranolol or esmolol[74] and/or nitroglycerine before and during anesthetic induction may minimize cardiovascular responses to laryngoscopy and intubation.

### *Bronchospastic Lung Disease*

Patients with a history of bronchospastic lung disease may be induced with thiopental followed by ventilation with a volatile inhalational anesthetic agent prior to intubation. Of course, cricoid pressure should be applied during the 10 to 15-minute period required for a deep level of anesthesia to be achieved.

## CONCLUSION

Trauma to the eye is the most common cause of monocular blindness. It involves young male adults more frequently than their female and elderly counterparts. Emergency surgery is rarely needed for nonpenetrating eye injuries, whereas perforating injuries must be treated surgically as soon as possible to prevent further anatomical and functional deterioration of the eye. During anesthetic management of patients with open-eye injuries, external pressure on the eye and factors that produce choroidal congestion should be avoided.

General anesthesia is preferred for surgery of closed-eye injuries, but these procedures can also be performed with retrobulbar block. The objectives during local (regional) anesthesia are to provide complete anesthesia, an immobile eye, and adequate sedation.

In an open eye, a transient increase in IOP above atmospheric pressure can result in loss of intraocular contents, intraocular bleeding, and retinal detachment. Any one of these complications may severely jeopardize the eye. External pressure can be avoided by careful application of face mask or eyelid retractors, by using an eye shield, by prevention of extraocular muscle contraction, and by avoiding surgical or anesthetic procedures that may result in retrobulbar bleeding. Choroidal congestion can be prevented by avoiding sudden blood pressure increases, hypoxemia, and elevations of central venous pressure and $Pa{CO_2}$. Coughing, straining, vomiting, and crying must be prevented by using adequate sedation and at times, antiemetic drugs.

General anesthesia is the only choice for management of open-eye injuries whereas most closed-eye injuries can be managed with either general or local (regional) anesthesia. Increased intraorbital pressure, the possibility of retrobulbar bleeding, the need for ocular massage, and frequent patient response to needle insertion contraindicates reterobulbar block for repair of open-eye injuries. The key to successful anesthetic management of the open eye is production and maintenance of deep anesthesia by any of the available agents, especially during laryngoscopy and tracheal intubation.

A full stomach is a common accompaniment of open-eye injury; a rapid sequence induction technique is required. During induction succinylcholine without any pretreatment agent (diazepam, nondepolarizing muscle relaxants, or acetazolamide) may cause excessive IOP increase and extrusion of intraocular contents. The available data suggest, although without real proof, that small doses of nondepolarizing agents prior to administration of succinylcholine in deeply anesthetized patients with open-eye injuries may prevent adverse ocular consequences. Although this method can be used with reasonable safety, high doses of nondepolarizing muscle relaxants may also provide intubating conditions within virtually the same time interval as succinylcholine. Since nondepolarizing relaxants do not increase IOP, their use during rapid sequence induction appears safer, at least for the eye, than succinylcholine.

Occasionally the patient with an open-eye injury may have other complicating conditions such as cervical spine injuries, maxillofacial injuries, or preexisting diseases. Safe techniques of anesthetic induction should be provided to such patients.

## REFERENCES


1. Accident Facts. Chicago: National Safety Council, 1986:26.
2. Adams AK, Barnett KC. Anaesthesia and intraocular pressure. Anaesthesia 1966;21:202.
3. Adams AK, Jones RM. Anaesthesia for eye surgery: general considerations. Br J Anaesth 1980;52:663.
4. Adhikary HP, Taylor P, Fitzmaurice DJ. Prognosis of perforating eye injury. Br J Ophthalmol 1976;60:737.
5. Al-Abrak MH. Diazepam and intraocular pressure. Br J Anaesth 1978;50:866.
6. Al-Abrak MH, Samuel JR. Effects of general anaesthesia on the intraocular pressure in man: comparison of tubocurarine and pancuronium in nitrous oxide and oxygen. Br J Ophthalmol 1974;58:806.
7. Al-Abrak MH, Samuel JR. Further observations on the effects of general anaesthesia on intraocular pressure in man: halothane in nitrous oxide and oxygen. Br J Anaesth 1974;46:756.
8. Allen ED, Elkington AR. Local anaesthesia and the eye. Br J Anaesth 1980;52:689.
9. Antoszyk AN, Buckley EG. Contralateral decreased visual acuity and extraocular muscle palsies following retrobulbar anesthesia. Ophthalmology 1986;93:462.
10. Assaf AA. Traumatic retinal detachment. J Trauma 1985; 25:1085.
11. Ausinsch B, Graves SA. Intraocular pressure in children during isoflurane and halothane anesthesia. Anesthesiology 1975; 42:167.
12. Ausinsch B, Rayborn RZ, Munsen ES, Levy NS. Ketamine and intraocular pressure in children. Anesth Analg 1976;55:773.
13. Badrinath SK, Vazeery A, McCarthy RJ, Ivankovich AD. The effect of different methods of inducing anesthesia on intraocular pressure. Anethesiology 1986;65:431.
14. Balamoutsos NG, Tsakona H, Kanakoudes PS, et al. Alcuronium and intraocular pressure. Anesth Analg 1983;62:521.
15. Barr AM, Thornley BA. Thiopentone and suxamethonium crash induction: an assessment of the potential hazards. Anaesthesia 1976;31:23.
16. Baumgarten RK, Reynolds WJ. The priming principle and the open eye-full stomach. Anesthesiology 1985;63:561.
17. Belcher CD III, Brown SVL, Simmons RJ. Anterior chamber washout for traumatic hyphema. Ophthalmic Surg 1985; 16:475.

17a. Berry JM, Merin RG. Etomidate myoclonus and open globe. Anesth Analg 1989;69:256.

18. Bill A. Ocular circulation. In: Moses RA, ed., Adler's physiology of the eye: clinical application. 7th ed. St. Louis: CV Mosby, 1981:191.
19. Bill A. The effect of changes in arterial blood pressure on the rate of aqueous formation in a primate. Ophthalmology 1970; 1:193.
20. Blomdahl S, Norell S. Perforating eye injury in the Stockholm population: an epidemiological study. Acta Ophthalmol 1984; 62:378.
21. Bolling JP, Kurrle RW, O'Day DM. Effect of ocular compression on intraocular pressure. Ophthalmic Surg 1985;16:563.
22. Bourke DL. Open eye injuries. Anesthesiology 1985;63:727.
23. Bowen DJ, McGrand JC, Pamer RJ. Intraocular pressure after pretreatment with pancuronium. Br J Anaesth 1975;48:1201.
24. Brown EM, Krishnaprasad D, Smiler BG. Pancuronium for rapid induction technique for tracheal intubation. Can Anaesth Soc J 1979;26:489.
25. Brown GC, Tasman WS, Benson WE. BB-gun injuries to the eye. Ophthalmic Surg 1985;16:505.
26. Cantore GP, Delfini R, Gambacorta D, Consorti P. Cranio-orbito-facial injuries: technical suggestions. J Trauma 1979;19:370.
27. Carballo AS. Succinylcholine and acetazolamide (Diamox) in anaesthesia for ocular surgery. Can Anaesth Soc J 1965;12:486.
28. Cassel GH, Jeffers JB, Jaeger EA. Wills Eye Hospital traumatic hyphema study. Ophthalmic Surg 1985;16:441.
29. Chiu GJ, Stirt JA. Intraocular pressure after "crash" induction with vecuronium or atracurium plus low-dose narcotics. Anesth Analg 1987;66:S28.
30. Cohen SB, Fletcher ME, Goldberg MF, Jadnock NJ. Diagnosis and management of ocular complications of sickle hemoglobinopathies, V. Ophthalmic Surg 1986;17:369.
31. Coleman DJ. Early vitrectomy in the management of the severely traumatized eye. Am J Ophthalmol 1982;93:543.
32. Collet BI. Traumatic hyphema: a review. Ann Ophthalmol 1982; 14:52.
33. Cook JH. The effect of suxamethonium on intraocular pressure. Anaesthesia 1981;36:359.
34. Couch JA, Eltringham RJ, Magauran DM. The effect of thiopentone and fazadinium on intraocular pressure. Anaesthesia 1979;34:586.
35. Cozanitis DA, Dundee JW, Buchanan TAS, Archer DB. Atropine versus glycopyrrolate: a study of intraocular pressure and pupil size in man. Anaesthesia 1979;34:236.
36. Craythorne NWB, Rottenstein HS, Dripps RD. The effect of succinylcholine on intraocular pressure in adults during general anesthesia. Anesthesiology 1960;21:59.
37. Crouch ER, Frenkel M. Aminocaproic acid in the treatment of traumatic hyphema. Am J Ophthalmol 1976;83:355.
38. Cunningham AJ, Albert O, Cameron J, Watson AG. The effect of intravenous diazepam on rise of intraocular pressure following succinylcholine. Can Anaesth Soc J 1981;28:591.
39. Cunningham AJ, Barry P. Intraocular pressure: physiology and implications for anaesthetic management. Can Anaesth Soc J 1986;33:195.
40. Cunningham AJ, Kelly CP, Farmer J, Watson AG. The effect of metocurine and metocurine-pancuronium combination on intraocular pressure. Can Anesth Soc J 1982;29:617.
41. Davson J. Physiology of the eye. 4th ed. New York: Academic Press, 1980.
42. Deutsch TA, Feller DB. Injuries of the eyes, lids and orbit. In: Zuidema GD, Rutherford RB, Ballinger WF, eds. The management of trauma. 4th ed. Philadelphia: WB Saunders, 1985:243.
43. de Juan E, Sternberg P, Michels RG. Timing of vitrectomy after penetrating ocular injuries. Ophthalmology 1984;91:1072.
44. de Juan E Jr, Sternberg P Jr, Michels RG. Penetrating ocular injuries: types of injuries and visual results. Ophthalmology 1983;90:1318.
45. de Juan E, Sternberg P Jr, Michels RG, Auer C. Evaluation of vitrectomy in penetrating ocular trauma: a case control study. Arch Ophthalmol 1984;102:1160.
46. de Roetth A, Schwartz H. Aqueous humor dynamics in glaucoma: ganglionic blocking agents and thiopental sodium (pentothal) anesthesia on aqueous humor dynamics. Arch Opthalmol 1956;55:755.
47. Dickmann P, Goecke M, Wiemers K. Beeinflussung der intraocularen Drucksteigerung nach Succinylcholin durch depolarisationshemmende Relaxantien. Anaesthesist 1969;18:370.
48. Dillon JB, Sabawala P, Taylor DB, Gunter R. Action of succinylcholine on extraocular muscles and intraocular pressure. Anesthesiology 1957;18:44.
49. Donlon JV. Succinylcholine and open eye injury. Anesthesiology 1986;64:525.
50. Drenger B, Pe'er J, BenEzra D, et al. The effect of intravenous lidocaine on the increase in intraocular pressure induced by tracheal intubation. Anesth Analg 1985;64:1211.
51. Duncalf D. Anesthesia and intraocular pressure. Bull NY Acad Med 1975;51:374.

52. Duncalf D, Foldes FF. Effect of anesthetic drugs and muscle relaxants on intraocular pressure. Int Ophthalmol Clin 1973; 13:21.
53. Eagling EM. Perforating injuries involving the posterior segment. Trans Ophthalmol Soc UK 1975;95:335.
54. Eagling EM. Perforating injuries of the eye. Br J Ophthalmol 1976;60:732.
55. Eakins KE, Katz RL. Response of the medial rectus muscle of the cat to succinylcholine. Nature 1965;207:1398.
56. Editorial: progress in surgical management of ocular trauma. Br J Ophthalmol 1976;60:731.
57. Ellis PP. Retrobulbar injections. Surv Ophthalmol 1974;18:425.
58. Feibel RM. Current concepts in retrobulbar anesthesia. Surv Ophthalmol 1985;30:102.
59. Foldes F. Rapid tracheal induction with nondepolarizing neuromuscular blocking drugs: the priming principle. Br J Anaesth 1984;56:663.
60. Follette JW, LoCascio JA. Bilateral amaurosis following unilateral retrobulbar block. Anesthesiology 1985;63:237.
61. Foulds WS. The changing pattern of eye surgery. Br J Anaesth 1980;52:643.
62. Fradkin AH. Orbital floor fractures and ocular complications. Am J Ophthalmol 1971;67:669.
63. Friberg TR. Long-term visual acuity results after penetrating and perforating ocular injuries. Am J Ophthalmol 1986;101:499.
64. Friedland BR, Mallonee J, Anderson DR. Short term dose response characteristics of acetazolamide in man. Arch Ophthalmol 1977;95:1809.
65. George R, Nursingh A, Downing JW, Welsh NH. Nondepolarizing neuromuscular blockers and the eye: a study of intraocular pressure. Br J Anaesth 1979;51:789.
66. Gesztes T. Prolonged apnoea after suxamethonium injection associated with eye drops containing an anticholinesterase agent: a case report. Br J Anaesth 1966;38:408.
67. Giala MM, Balamoutsos NG, Tsakona EA, et al. Failure of gallamine to inhibit succinylcholine-induced increase in intraocular pressure. Anesthesiology 1979;51:578.
68. Goldberg MF. Sickled erythrocytes, hyphema and secondary glaucoma, I: the diagnosis and treatment of sickled erythrocytes in human hyphemas. Ophthalmic Surg 1979;10:17.
69. Goldsmith E. An evaluation of succinylcholine and gallamine as muscle relaxants in relation to intraocular tension. Anesth Analg 1967;46:557.
70. Greenan J, Prasad J. Comparison of the ocular effects of atropine or glycopyrrolate with two iv induction agents. Br J Anaesth 1985;57:180.
71. Greenstein SH, Abramson DH, Pitts WR. Systemic atropine and glaucoma. Bull NY Acad Med 1984;60:963.
72. Gombos G. Handbook of ophthalmologic emergencies. New York: Medical Examination Publishing Co, 1973.
73. Hamilton RC. Brain stem anesthesia following retrobulbar blockade. Anesthesiology 1985;63:688.
74. Harrison L, Ralley FE, Wynands JE, et al. The role of an ultra short-acting adrenergic blocker (esmolol) in patients undergoing coronary artery bypass surgery. Anesthesiology 1987; 66:413.
75. Hartley JMF, Fidler K. Rapid intubation with fazadinium. Anaesthesia 1977;32:14.
76. Hermsen V. Vitrectomy in severe ocular trauma. Ophthalmologica 1984;189:86.
77. Hess A, Pilar G. Slow fibers in the extraocular muscles of the cat. J Physiol 1963;169:780.
78. Hofman H, Holzer H. Die Wirkung von Musklrelaxantien auf den intraokularen Druck. Klin Monatsbl Augenheilk 1953; 123:1.
79. Holloway KB. Control of the eye during general anaesthesia for intraocular surgery. Br J Anaesth 1980;52:671.
80. Holt JE, Hot GR, Blodgett JM. Ocular injuries sustained during blunt facial trauma. Ophthalmology 1983;90:14.
81. Hunsley JE, Bush GH, Jones CJ. A study of glycopyrrolate and atropine in the suppression of the oculo-cardiac reflex during strabismus surgery in children. Br J Anaesth 1982;54:459.
82. Hvidberg A, Kessing SVV, Fernandes A. Effect of changes in $P_{CO_2}$ and body positions on intraocular pressure during general anesthesia. Acta Ophthalmol 1981;59:465.
83. Ivankovich AD, Lowe HJ. The influence of methoxyflurane and neuroleptanesthesia on intraocular pressure in man. Anesth Analg 1969;48:933.
84. Jabaley ME, Lerman M, Sanders HJ. Ocular injuries in orbital fractures: a review of 119 cases. Plast Reconstr Surg 1975; 56:410.
85. Jantzen J-P, Hackett GH, Earnshaw G. Succinylcholine and open eye injury. Anesthesiology 1986;64:524.
86. Jantzen J-P, Hackett GH, Erdmann K, Earnshaw G. Effect of vecuronium on intraocular pressure. Br J Anaesth 1986;58:433.
87. Jay JL. Functional organization of the human eye. Br J Anaesth 1980;52:649.
88. Joshi C, Bruce DL. Thiopentone and succinylcholine: action on intraocular pressure. Anesth Analg 1975;54:471.
89. Kalisman M, Lachman LJ, Millendorf JB. Management of orbital fractures. Hosp Phys 1984;May:8.
90. Katz RL, Bigger JT. Cardiac arrhythmias during anesthesia and operation. Anesthesiology 1970;33:193.
91. Katz RL, Eakins KE. A comparison of the effects of neuromuscular blocking agents and cholinesterase inhibitors on the tibialis anterior and superior rectus muscles of the cat. J Pharmacol Exp Ther 1966;152:304.
92. Katz RL, Eakins KE. Mode of action of succinylcholine on intraocular pressure. J Pharmacol Exp Ther 1968;162:1.
93. Katz RL, Eakins KE, Lord CO. The effects of hexafluorenium in preventing the increase in intraocular pressure produced by succinylcholine. Anesthesiology 1968;29:70.
94. Kirsch RE. Further studies on the use of digital pressure in cataract surgery. Arch Ophthalmol 1957;58:641.
95. Kirsch RE, Steinman W. Digital pressure, an important safeguard in cataract surgery. Arch Ophthalmol 1955;54:637.
96. Konchigeri HN, Lee YE, Venugopal K. Effect of pancuronium on intraocular pressure changes induced by succinylcholine. Can Anaesth Soc J 1979;26:479.
97. Kornblueth W, Aladjemoff L, Magora F, Gabbay A. Influence of general anesthesia on intraocular pressure in man: the effect of diethyl ether, cyclopropane, vinyl ether and thiopental sodium. Arch Ophthalmol 1959;61:84.
98. Langham ME, Kitazawa Y, Hart RW. Adrenergic responses in the human eye. J Pharmacol Exp Ther 1971;179:47.
99. Lavery GG, McGalliard JN, Mirakhur RK, Shepherd WFI. The effects of atracurium on intraocular pressure during steady state anaesthesia and rapid sequence induction: a comparison with succinylcholine. Can Anaesth Soc J 1986;33:437.
100. Le May M. Aspects of measurement in opthalmology. Br J Anaesth 1980;52:655.
101. Lennon RL, Olson RA, Gronert GA. Atracurium or vecuronium for rapid sequence endotracheal intubation. Anesthesiology 1986;64:510.
102. Leopold IH, Comroe JH. Effect of intramuscular administration of morphine, atropine, scopolamine and neostigmine on the human eye. Arch Ophthalmol 1948;40:285.
103. Lerman J, Kiskis AA. Effects of high-dose pancuronium and endotracheal intubation on intraocular pressure in children. Anesthesiology 1984;61:A434.

104. Lerman J, Kiskis AA. Lidocaine attenuates the intraocular pressure response to rapid intubation in children. Can Anaesth Soc J 1985;32:339.
105. Lewallen WM Jr, Hicks BL. The use of succinylcholine in ocular surgery. Am J Ophthalmol 1960;49:773.
106. Libonati MM, Leahy MJ, Ellison N. The use of succinylcholine in open eye surgery. Anesthesiology 1985;62:637.
107. Lincoff HA, Breinin GM, De Voe AG. The effect of succinylcholine on extraocular muscles. Am J Ophthalmol 1957;43:440.
108. Litwiller RW, Difazio C, Rushia EL. Pancuronium and intraocular pressure. Anesthesiology 1975;42:750.
109. Love DC. Treatment of traumatic hyphema. JAMA 1985; 253:345.
110. Macri FJ. Vascular pressure relationships and the intraocular pressure. Arch Ophthalmol 1961;65:571.
111. Magora F, Collins VJ. The influence of general anesthetic agents on intraocular pressure in man. Arch Ophthalmol 1961;66:806.
112. Mahajan RP, Grover VK, Munjal VP, Singh H. Double-blind comparison of lidocaine, tubocurarine and diazepam pretreatment in modifying intraocular pressure increases. Can Anaesth Soc J 1987;34:41.
113. Mahajan RP, Grover VK, Sharma SL, Singh H. Intraocular pressure changes during muscular hyperactivity after general anesthesia. Anesthesiology 1987;66:419.
114. Maharaj RJ, Humphrey D, Kaplan N, et al. Effects of atracurium on intraocular pressure. Br J Anaesth 1984;56:459.
115. Maillet J, Perier JF, Girard P. Effects of flunitrazepam on intraocular pressure. J Fr Ophtalmol 1982;5:335.
116. Maltzman BA, Pruzon H, Mund ML. A survey of ocular trauma. Surv Ophthalmol 1976;21:285.
117. Martin SR, Baker SS, Muenzler WS. Retrobulbar anesthesia and orbicularis akinesia. Ophthalmic Surg 1986;17:232.
118. McGetrick JJ, Jampol LM, Goldberg MF, et al. Aminocaproic acid decreases secondary hemorrhage after traumatic hyphema. Arch Ophthalmol 1983;101:1031.
119. Mehta MP, Choi WW, Gergis SD, et al. Facilitation of rapid endotracheal intubation with divided doses of nondepolarizing neuromuscular blocking drugs. Anesthesiology 1985;62:392.
120. Meyers EF, Krupin R, Johnson M, Zink H. Failure of nondepolarizing neuromuscular blockers to inhibit succinylcholine-induced increased intraocular pressure. Anesthesiology 1978; 48:149.
121. Meyers EF, Singer P, Otto A. A controlled study of the effect of succinylcholine self-taming on intraocular pressure. Anesthesiology 1980;53:72.
122. Milauskas AT, Feuger GF. Serious ocular complications associated with blowout fractures of the orbit. Am J Ophthalmol 1966;62:670.
123. Miller RD. The priming principle. Anesthesiology 1985;62:381.
124. Miller, RD, Way WL, Hickey RF. Inhibition of succinylcholine-induced increased intraocular pressure by non-depolarizing muscle relaxants. Anesthesiology 1968;29:123.
125. Mirakhur RK. Comparative study of the effects of oral and im atropine and hyoscine in volunteers. Br J Anaesth 1978;50:591.
126. Mirakhur RK, Dundee JW, Jones CJ. Evaluation of the anticholinergic actions of glycopyrronium bromide. Br J Clin Pharmacol 1978;5:77.
127. Mirakhur RK, Jones CJ, Dundee JW, Archer DB. IM or IV atropine or glycopyrrolate for the prevention of oculocardiac reflex in children undergoing squint surgery. Br J Anaesth 1982; 54:1059.
128. Mirakhur RK, Lavery GG, Gibson FM, Clarke SJ. Intubating conditions after vecuronium and atracurium given in divided doses (the priming technique). Acta Anaesthesiol Scand 1986; 30:347.
129. Mirakhur RK, Shepherd WFI. Intraocular pressure changes with propofol ("Diprivan"): comparison with thiopentone. Postgrad Med J 1985;61(Suppl. 3):41.
130. Moses RA. Intraocular pressure. In: Moses RA, Hart WM, Jr, eds. Adler's physiology of the eye: clinical application. 8th ed. St Louis: CV Mosby, 1987;223.
131. Mostafa SM, Lockhart A, Kumar D, Bayoumi M. Comparison of effects of fentanyl and alfentanil on intraocular pressure. Anaesthesia 1986;41:493.
132. Murphy DF. Anesthesia and intraocular pressure. Anesth Analg 1985;64:520.
133. Murphy DF, Davis NJ. Succinylcholine use in emergency eye operations. Can J Anaesth 1987;34:101.
134. Murphy DF, Eustace P, Unwin A, Magner JB. Intravenous lignocaine pretreatment to prevent intraocular pressure rise following suxamethonium and tracheal intubation. Br J Ophthalmol 1986;70:596.
135. Niiranen M. Perforated eye injuries treated at Helsinki University Eye Hospital from 1970 to 1977. Ann Ophthalmol 1981; 13:957.
136. Niiranen M. Perforated eye injuries, thesis. Acta Ophthalmol 1978;135(Suppl):1.
137. Nobach C, Demarest R. The human nervous system: basic principles of neurobiology. 3rd ed. New York: McGraw-Hill Book Co, 1981:388.
138. Oji EO, Holdcroft A. The ocular effects of etomidate. Anaesthesia 1979;34:245.
139. Palmer DJ, Goldberg MF, Frenkel M, et al. A comparison of two dose regimens of epsilon aminocaproic acid in the prevention and management of secondary traumatic hyphemas. Ophthalmology 1986;93:102.
140. Pandey K, Badola RP, Kumar S. Time course of intraocular hypertension produced by suxamethonium. Br J Anaesth 1972; 44:191.
141. Pantuck EJ. Ecothiopate iodide eye drops and prolonged response to suxamethonium. Br J Anaesth 1966;38:406.
142. Parris WCV, Kambam JR, Flanagan JFK, Elliott J. The effects of metoclopramide on intraocular pressure. Anesth Analg 1987; 66:S135.
143. Patil V, Stehling L, Zauder H. Instrumentation and auxiliary equipment. In: Patil V, Stehling L, Zauder H, eds. fiberoptic endoscopy in anesthesia. Yearbook Medical Publishers, Inc., Chicago, 1983, p. 9.
144. Pautler SE, Grizzard WS, Thompson LN, Wing GL. Blindness from retrobulbar injection into the optic nerve. Ophthalmic Surg 1986;17:334.
145. Petounis AD, Chondreli S, Vadaluka-Sekioti A. Effect of hypercapnia and hyperventilation on human intraocular pressure during general anaesthesia following acetazolamide administration. Br J Ophthalmol 1980;64:422.
146. Petro J, Tooze FM, Bales CR, Baker G. Ocular injuries associated with periorbital fractures. J Trauma 1979;19:730.
147. Peuler M, Glass DD, Arens JF. Ketamine and intraocular pressure. Anesthesiology 1975;43:575.
148. Peyman GA, Raichand M, Goldberg MF, Brown S. Vitrectomy in the management of intraocular foreign bodies and their complications. Br J Ophthalmol 1980;64:476.
149. Presbitero JV, Ruiz RS, Riger BM Sr, et al. Intraocular pressure during enflurane and neurolept anesthesia in adult patients undergoing ophthalmic surgery. Anesth Analg 1980;59:50.
150. Radtke N, Waldman J. The influence of enflurane anesthesia on intraocular pressure in youths. Anesth Analg 1975;54:212.
151. Ramsay RC, Cantrill HL, Knobloch WH. Vitrectomy for double penetrating ocular injuries. Am J Ophthalmol 1985;100:586.
152. Rich AL, Witherspoon CD, Morris RE, Feist RM. Use of non-

depolarizing anesthetic agents in penetrating ocular injuries. Anesthesiology 1986;65:108.
153. Roper-Hall MJ. Treatment of ocular injuries. Trans Ophthal Soc UK 1959;79:57.
154. Rosen DA. Anaesthesia in ophthalmology. Can Anaesth Soc J 1962;9:545.
155. Runciman JC, Bowen-Wright RM, Welsh NH, Downing JW. Intraocular pressure changes during halothane and enflurane anaesthesia. Br J Anaesth 1978;50:371.
156. Ryan SJ, Allen AW. Pars plana vitrectomy in ocular trauma. Am J Ophthalmol 1979;88:483.
157. Samuel JR, Beaugie A. Effect of carbon dioxide on the intraocular pressure in man during general anaesthesia. Br J Ophthalmol 1974;58:62.
158. Samuels SI, Maze M. Beta-receptor blockade following the use of eye drops. Anesthesiology 1980;52:369.
159. Schneider HJ, Stirt JA, Finholt DA. Atracurium, vecuronium and intraocular pressure in humans. Anesth Analg 1986;65:877.
160. Schroeder M, Linssen GH. Intraocular pressure and anaesthesia. Anaesthesia 1972;27:165.
161. Schwartz H, de Roeth A, Papper EM. Preanesthetic use of atropine and scopolamine in patients with glaucoma. JAMA 1957; 165:144.
162. Schwarz S, Ilias W, Lackner F, et al. Rapid tracheal intubation with vecuronium: the priming principle. Anesthesiology 1985; 62:388.
163. Sears ML. The aqueous. In: Moses RA, ed. Adler's physiology of the eye: clinical application. St. Louis: CV Mosby, 1981: 204.
164. Shock JP, Adams D. Long-term visual acuity results after penetrating and perforating ocular injuries. Am J Ophthalmol 1985; 100:714.
165. Sia RL, Rashkovsky OM. Org NC 45 and intraocular pressure during anaesthesia. Acta Anaesth Scand 1981;25:219.
166. Smith RB, Aass AA, Nemoto EM. Intraocular and intracranial pressure during respiratory alkalosis and acidosis. Br J Anaesth 1981;53:967.
167. Smith RB, Babinski M, Leano N. The effect of lidocaine on succinylcholine induced increase in intraocular pressure. Can Anaesth Soc J 1979;26:482.
168. Smith RB, Leano N. Intraocular pressure following pancuronium. Can Anaesth Soc J 1973;20:742.
169. Sosis M, Stiner AE, Marr AT. Does the priming principle work? Anesthesiology 1985;63:A340.
170. Spierer A, Tadmor R, Treister G, et al. Diagnosis and localization of intraocular foreign bodies by computed tomography. Ophthalmic Surg 1985;16:571.
171. Sternberg P, de Juan E, Green WR, et al. Ocular BB injuries. Ophthalmology 1984;91:1269.
172. Stinson TW, Donlon JV. Interaction of intraocular $SF_6$ and air with nitrous oxide. Anesthesiology 1979;51:S16.
173. Sullivan KL, Brown GC, Forman AR, et al. Retrobulbar anesthesia and retinal vascular obstruction. Ophthalmology 1983; 90:373.
174. Tabaoda JA, Rupp SM, Miller RD. Refining the priming principle for vecuronium during rapid-sequence induction of anesthesia. Anesthesiology 1986;64:243.
175. Tanifuji Y, Sugahara Y, Mashiko K, et al. Effect of succinylcholine and pancuronium on intraocular pressure and aqueous outflow. Masui Jpn J Anesthesiol 1982;31:600.
176. Tawara A. Transformation and cytotoxicity of iron in siderosis bulbi. Invest Ophthalmol Vis Sci 1986;27:226.
177. Taylor C, Wilson FM, Roesch R, et al. Prevention of oculocardiac reflex in children: comparison of retrobulbar block and intravenous atropine. Anesthesiology 1963;24:646.
178. Thomas MA, Parrish RK, Feuer WJ. Rebleeding after traumatic hyphema. Arch Ophthalmol 1986;104:206.
179. Thomson MF, Brock-Utne JG, Bean P, et al. Anaesthesia and intraocular pressure: a comparison of total intravenous anaesthesia using etomidate with conventional inhalation anaesthesia. Anaesthesia 1982;37:758.
179a. Tielsch JM, Parver L, Shankar B. Time trends in the hospitalized ocular trauma. Arch Ophthalmol 1989;107:519.
180. Topilow HW, Ackerman AL, Zimmerman RD. Limitations of computerized tomography in the localization of intraocular foreign bodies. Ophthalmology 1984;91:1086.
181. Tsamparlakis J, Casey TA, Howell W, Edridge A. Dependence of intraocular pressure on induced hypotension and posture during surgical anesthesia. Trans Ophthalmol Soc UK 1980; 100:521.
182. Unsold R, Stanley JA, DeGroot J. The CT-topography of retrobulbar anesthesia. Graefes Arch Clin Exp Ophthalmol 1981; 217:125.
183. Van Der Spek AFL, Hantler CB. Phenylephrine eye drops and anesthesia. Anesthesiology 1986;64:812.
184. Vatne HO, Syrdalen P. Vitrectomy in double perforating eye injuries. Acta Ophthalmolog (Copenh) 1985;63:552.
185. Verma RS. "Self-taming" of succinylcholine-induced fasciculations and intraocular pressure. Anesthesiology 1979;50:245.
186. Vilardi V, Sanfilippo M, Pelaia P, Gasparetto A. The effect of vecuronium on intraocular pressure during general anesthesia: clinical experiences with Norcuron. Symposium. Geneva Switzerland, April 1983:21.
187. Vinger PF. The incidence of eye injuries in sports. Int Ophthalmol Clin 1981;21:21.
188. Von Sallmann L, Lowenstein O. Responses of intraocular pressure, blood pressure and cutaneous vessels to electrical stimulation in the diencephalon. Am J Ophthalmol 1955;39:11.
189. Weiner MJ, Olk RJ, Meyers EF. Anesthesia for open eye surgery. Anesthesiology 1986;65:109.
190. Williams BI, Peart WS. Effect of posture on intraocular pressure of patients with retinal vein obstruction. Br J Ophthalmol 1978; 62:688.
191. Wilson TM, Le May M, Holloway KB, et al. Experimental and clinical study of factors influencing choroidal blood flow. Trans Ophthalmol Soc UK 1974;94:378.
192. Wilson TM, Strang R, McKenzie ET. The response of the choroidal and cerebral circulations to changing arterial $P_{CO_2}$ and acetazolamide in the baboon. Invest Ophthalmol Vis Sci 1977; 16:576.
193. Wislicki L. Factors affecting intraocular pressure. Proc R Soc Med 1977;70:372.
194. Witteman GJ, Brubaker SJ, Johnson M, Marks RG. The incidence of rebleeding in traumatic hyphema. Ann Ophthalmol 1985;17:525.
195. Wolf GL, Capuano C, Hartung J. Nitrous oxide increases intraocular pressure after intravitreal sulfur hexafluoride injection. Anesthesiology 1983;59:547.
196. Woo SL-Y, Kobayashi AS, Schlegel WA, Lawrence C. Nonlinear material properties of intact cornea and sclera. Exp Eye Res 1972;14:29.
197. Wynands JE, Crowell DE. Intraocular tension in association with succinylcholine and tension in endotracheal intubation: a preliminary report. Can Anaesth Soc J 1960;7:39.
198. Yoshikawa K, Murai Y. The effect of ketamine on intraocular pressure in children. Anesth Analg 1971;50:199.

# Chapter Twelve

Levon M. Capan
Sanford M. Miller
Robert Glickman

# Management of Facial Injuries

Maxillofacial injury has been described in the medical literature since at least 2500 BC.[13] Treating these injuries by wiring the jaws together was first described by Hippocrates around 400 BC.[77] This treatment was apparently forgotten until Guglielmo Salicetti of Italy reintroduced Hippocrates' technique in 1275 AD. Little was written on maxillofacial injuries during the subsequent several centuries. A case report by von Graefe in 1823 describes the introduction of an elastic tube through the nose to prevent suffocation of a coachman who was kicked in the face by a horse,[77] suggesting that the danger of airway obstruction from maxillofacial injury was recognized by this time. In the beginning of the twentieth century Sir Harold Gillies, father of plastic surgery in England, wanted to attach the following statement to the Field Medical Card of soldiers: "If I am looking at Heaven, then I will soon be there!"[77] With this statement he attempted to alert army personnel with facial injuries to the danger of upper airway obstruction in the supine position.

A major advance in the understanding of maxillary fractures was achieved by René LeFort's famous work on cadavers in France in 1901.[57] World War I provided a strong impetus to the establishment of modern surgical and anesthetic techniques. In this era the development of endotracheal anesthesia and the introduction of radiologic diagnosis resulted in a quantum leap in maxillofacial trauma management.[77]

After World War II, efforts were made to establish maxillofacial units utilizing the close cooperation of plastic surgery, oral and maxillofacial surgery, otorhinolaryngology, ophthalmology, and neurosurgery departments. Currently, the treatment of facial trauma falls within the domain of these subspecialities, each of which works independently of the others. Concern about such fragmented care has been raised, and the benefits of an interdisciplinary rather than the existing multidisciplinary system have been emphasized.[20] Progress in maxillofacial injury care during the past two decades has mainly been a result of the following developments: (a) improved diagnosis with computed tomography (CT) scanning; (b) improvements in care of the multiply injured patient; (c) new surgical techniques, such as open jaw reduction and bone grafting; and (d) modern anesthetic, airway management, and monitoring techniques.

The face and head are exposed to all kinds of physical trauma. The gruesome appearance of facial injuries may distract the clinician from less obvious but more critical injuries. This point has been emphasized repeatedly in surgical textbooks, and the reader is advised to focus attention on more important injuries in the absence of life-threatening complications of maxillofacial injury. For the anesthesiologist, however, facial fracture in a patient undergoing emergency surgery presents a formidable challenge and must be put high in the care priority list. This chapter summarizes various aspects of maxillofacial injuries and their management as they pertain to the anesthesiologist.

## INCIDENCE AND ETIOLOGY

It is estimated that three million hospital-treated facial injuries occur in the United States every year, a national incidence rate of 1.4%.[50] More than 90% of these injuries are relatively minor soft tissue lacerations requiring only local infiltration anesthesia in the emergency department for repair.[50] Although large population-based studies are not available, data from Dane County, Wisconsin (population 324,000), suggest that the national incidence of major maxillofacial fractures and lacerations varies between 0.04% and 0.09%,[50] which is roughly comparable to results of population surveys from other countries.[2,72]

The etiology of maxillofacial injuries differs from one locality to the next, depending on socioeconomic characteristics, cultural background, degree of industrialization and urbanization, existing traffic regulations and compliance of motor vehicle drivers with these laws, and the extent of alcohol and drug consumption. A list of the causative factors of these injuries is given in Table 12-1. Before 1970, motor vehicle accidents were the principal cause of maxillofacial fractures; approximately 20 to 50% of these injuries resulted from crashes.[26,50,74,92] Motor vehicle accidents probably remain the predominant cause of this injury for patients treated in private hospitals and in centers located in rural areas, near busy highways, and in developing countries.[1,50,51,54] However, in municipal hospitals and in regions where a mandatory seat belt law is enforced, auto accidents are no longer predominant, and the most common cause of maxillofacial injury is interpersonal violence.[2,14,26,35,54,80a] Among motor vehicles, automobiles are responsible for the majority of maxillofacial injuries, followed by motorcycles, trucks, and other vehicles.[74] In regions where cycling is popular, between 5 and 10% of maxillofacial fractures are caused by bicycle accidents.[59] Sports- and game-related maxillofacial trauma comprises between 2.5 and 28.5% of all facial injuries in published series,[54,60,86] with contact sports, such as football, soccer, and rugby, resulting in the highest incidence.[86] Penetrating weapons are responsible for a relatively small percentage of maxillofacial injuries, although they may produce major facial deformity and tissue loss.

Acute alcohol intoxication is particularly common when the injury is secondary to assault, a motor vehicle accident, or a fall.[64] Some of these patients are also chronic alcoholics. In contrast, patients injured during athletic activities are unlikely to be under the effect of alcohol.[64] Illicit drugs are without doubt contributors to trauma in general, but the extent of their involvement in maxillofacial injury is, to our knowledge, unknown. Sudden unconsciousness resulting from preexisting disease can cause accidents and thus maxillofacial injury. Among these disorders, epileptic seizures and diabetes with hypoglycemia are important contributors. Coronary and cerebrovascular accidents and dysrhythmias are less likely causes of trauma; the victims of maxillofacial injury are usually young (age between 15 and 30) and without significant cardiovascular disease.

TABLE 12-1. Etiological Factors in Maxillofacial Injury

| DIRECT CAUSES | INDIRECT CAUSES |
|---|---|
| Altercation or interpersonal violence | Alcohol intoxication |
| Vehicle accident | Therapeutic or illicit drugs |
| Motorized vehicle | Epileptic seizures |
| Nonmotorized vehicle | Hypoglycemia |
| Pedestrian accident | Coronary and cerebrovascular occlusion |
| Industrial accident | Intracardiac conduction blocks |
| Farm accident | |
| Fall | |
| Sports | |
| Knife, gunshot, shotgun, blast wounds | |
| Thermal trauma | |

## PATHOPHYSIOLOGY OF MAXILLOFACIAL INJURIES

The type and severity of maxillofacial injuries are determined by several factors.

### MECHANISM OF INJURY

In general, maxillofacial injuries are caused by four different types of physical insults: blunt trauma, penetrating trauma, thermal trauma, and explosions. Although there are some similarities among facial injuries produced by each of these mechanisms, distinct differences exist not only in the nature of the resulting facial injury but also of the associated trauma. In blunt trauma the major damage affects the facial skeleton more than the soft tissue. If the injury is caused by an automobile accident, concomitant laceration of soft tissue by a broken windshield is likely. Altercation and sports-related blunt trauma are rarely associated with soft tissue laceration, except for edema and hematoma, which invariably occur. Injuries caused during sport activities are usually simple, and severe facial disruption rarely occurs.[86] Impact interface geometry—the shape and texture of the surfaces by which the face is struck—has an effect on the ultimate type and severity of injury. Car accident victims who strike their face on soft surfaces in the vehicle are less likely to develop severe injuries than those contacting hard surfaces. Likewise, cushioned boxing gloves reduce the likelihood of jaw fractures in boxers,[86] whereas severe injury occurs commonly in altercation victims.

The type and severity of injuries from penetrating trauma depend on the weapon used. Knives usually injure the soft tissue, but intracranial and orbital penetration can also occur.[37] The severity of low-velocity gunshot wounds ranges from mild soft tissue damage without bony involvement to severe facial bone fractures. The tongue and the floor of the mouth are frequently injured; the severity of injury is difficult to predict.[15,21,37] Close-range shotguns, rifles, and high-velocity military missiles produce massive facial destruction and loss of tissue.[31,99] Injuries to the face and jaw from bombs may result in both soft tissue and skeletal destruction, and the resultant edema will rapidly produce upper airway obstruction. Rarely, penetrating injury presents in the form of impalement or Jael's syndrome, so called after the tale of Jael and Sisera.[41,65] Although the appearance of these patients is dramatic and brain and ocular injuries are common, anecdotal reports describe good recovery.[11,41,65,73] Burns produce progressive cutaneous and mucosal edema that may result in airway obstruction within a few hours.

## TOLERANCE OF FACIAL BONES TO IMPACT

The force applied to any part of the body by an impact is traditionally expressed by multiples of $g$, the equivalent of gravitational force. During impact the face is subjected to forces of several $g$. Although women have a lower impact tolerance than men, individual facial bones also differ in fragility.[61] As seen in Fig. 12-1, the nasal bones, the zygoma, the mandibular ramus, and the frontal sinus are less tolerant to impact forces than other facial bones and thus are more apt to break easily. For instance a 30-mph collision can easily result in 80-$g$ forces and thus is sufficient to cause fractures in these bones while sparing others.[56] This fact explains, at least partially, the common occurrence of nasal, zygomatic, and mandibular fractures.

## EXTENT AND DURATION OF FORCE

As expected, the greater the force applied, the greater the severity of a resultant fracture. Similarly, the longer the duration of the impact, the more likely a fracture.[43] Repeated blows to the face also increase the probability of fractures.

## DIRECTION OF THE FORCE

The direction of the force vector usually determines the fracture location. For instance, a force applied to the point of the chin is likely to produce symphyseal and/or bilateral condylar fractures.[54] A lateral blow to the mandibular body produces a direct fracture on the side of the impact and a contralateral fracture of the mandibular angle.[54]

FIG. 12-1. Forces necessary to fracture individual facial bones. (From Luce et al[61] with permission.)

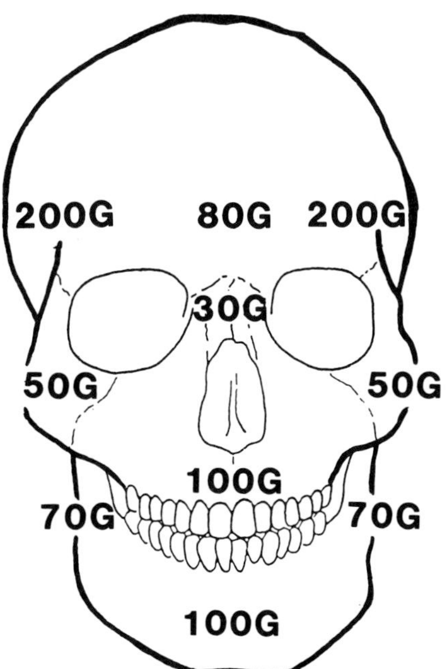


## RESILIENCE OF THE FACIAL BONES AND CUSHIONING EFFECTS OF MUSCLES

Even minor impacts in elderly people with osteoporotic facial bones may produce complicated fractures, whereas young persons may escape a major accident without fractures. Muscles play a significant role in the genesis of jaw fractures, especially of the mandible. They reduce the likelihood of fractures by cushioning the bones if they are relaxed, but strain the bones and may facilitate fractures if they are contracted at the time of the accident.[54]

## FORCE DISPERSION BY FACIAL BONY BUTTRESSES

The facial skeleton is strengthened by structures very much like those used for buildings. The middle third of the face is

FIG. 12-2. (A) Osseous buttresses of the midfacial skeleton. The thin laminar bones are removed. (B) An architectural concept of the bony buttressing of the face. (From Bradley JC et al: Applied surgical anatomy. In: Rowe NL, Killey HC, eds. Maxillofacial injuries. London: Churchill Livingstone, 1985; 19, with permission.)

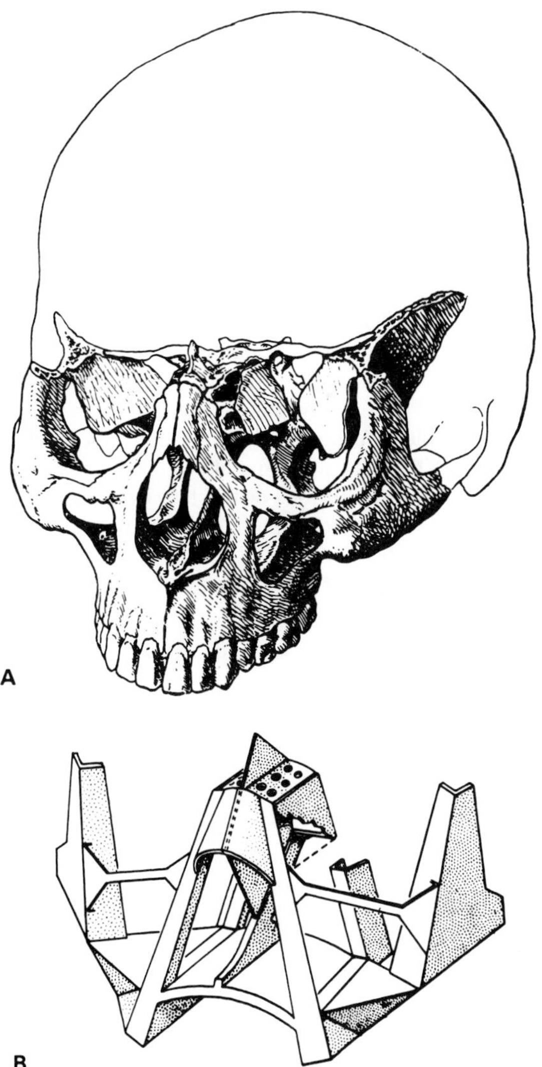

composed of laminar, paper-thin bones reinforced by thick bony buttresses[12] (Fig. 12-2), which are capable of dispersing physiologic or traumatic forces applied at any given point. This distribution of forces prevents, to an extent, fracture of low-resistance facial bones, and, as is discussed below, minimizes energy conduction from the face to the skull or vice versa. The substantial force generated by mastication would probably cause facial and cranial base fractures if such mechanisms did not exist. Likewise, blows to the face or head would cause more severe craniofacial fractures than they actually do.[12] The bony reinforcement of the midfacial skeleton is provided by the following bones: (a) the palate and the floor of the nose, (b) the alveolar process, (c) the lateral and superior rims of the pyriform aperture, (d) the zygomatic complex with its connections to the inferior and lateral orbital margins and the zygomatic arch, (e) the orbital rims, and (f) posteriorly, the pterygoid plates.[12]

A similar mechanism, although architecturally in a different form, exists in the mandible. The strength of this bone, as with all tubular bones, is located in its dense cortical plates. These comprise the buttresses, surrounding the central cancellous bone. The cortex is thicker in the anteroinferior aspect of the mandible and becomes thinner posteriorly at the angle and the condyles.[12]

## TYPES OF INJURY

Most authors divide the face into three anatomic regions. The lower third contains the mandible with its subdivisions: the symphysis, the body, the ramus, the condyle and temporomandibular joint, and the coronoid process. The middle third comprises the maxilla, the nasal bones, the orbits, and the zygomatic bones with their frontal processes. The upper third contains the frontal bone, the frontal sinuses, the frontozygomatic process, and, according to some authors, the nasoethmoid complex. Although this is a convenient classification to review injuries of the maxillofacial skeleton, it does not include soft tissue injuries of the face and does not distinguish central from lateral midfacial fractures. Therefore the following classification is used in this chapter:

1. Soft tissue injuries
2. Mandibular fractures
3. Central midface fractures: LeFort fractures, nasal fractures, nasoethmoidal fractures
4. Lateral midface fractures
5. Upper facial fractures

### SOFT TISSUE INJURIES[84]

Extensive facial avulsion lacerations occurred commonly in car accident victims before 1966 when windshield lamination and bonding were poor. Soft tissue lacerations rarely result in management difficulties and are often repaired in the emergency department under local infiltration or regional anesthesia. Because of the rich vascularity of the face, primary closure, after pressure irrigation and debridement, is possible even in wounds in which treatment has been delayed for as long as 36 hours. Surgical management may be complicated when important structures—branches of the facial nerve, the parotid gland or its duct, or the lacrimal apparatus—are injured. Repair of these injuries often requires a general anesthetic. Hematomas of nasal septal or auricular cartilages require urgent surgery. If not drained rapidly, cartilage necrosis and thus septal or external ear deformity may result.[87]

### MANDIBULAR INJURIES

Because of its prominent position and its morphology the mandible is the third most frequently fractured facial bone after the nose and the zygoma.[87] The severity of fracture varies from a simple nondisplaced or greenstick type to a comminuted type in which the bone is shattered.[54] Mandibular fractures tend to occur in weak areas of the bone: the condyles, the subcondylar area, the angle, or the body in the area of the second bicuspid or the mental foramen. Fractures in the region of the alveolar and coronoid processes occur less frequently[82] (Fig. 12-3A). In elderly edentulous persons with thin cortical bone, the mandible is often broken in the symphyseal and parasymphyseal areas.

There seems to be a relationship between the etiology of the injury and the site of mandibular fracture.[14,74] After automobile accidents the condylar and symphyseal regions are the most common areas injured[74] (Fig. 12-3B). Motorcycle accidents in which the victim's face strikes the pavement result in a larger percentage of alveolar fractures and fewer symphysis fractures than are seen after automobile accidents, although angle, condylar, and body fractures occur with similar frequencies[74] (Fig. 12-3C). The pattern of fracture is different after altercations, most frequently involving the angle, the body, and the condyles[14,74] (Fig. 12-3D).

The U-shape of the mandible permits transmission of impact forces to the contralateral side; thus, more than 50% of mandibular fractures occur in more than one site.[87] Common fracture combinations are of the body and the opposite angle, the body and the opposite subcondylar region, the symphysis and the angle, and the symphysis and both condyles.[87] Thus, a careful search for two or more fracture sites is necessary.[10]

The inferior neurovascular dental bundle, which comprises the inferior alveolar nerve and the inferior dental artery and veins, enters the mandibular canal via the mandibular foramen on the inner surface of the ramus and, after traversing the canal along the mandible, emerges from the mental foramen on the lateral surface of the bone midway between the inferior border and the alveolar crest at the level of the second bicuspid (Fig. 12-4). This bundle is at risk in fractures occurring between the mental foramen and the mandibular foramen. However, the fibrous sheath surrounding the bundle provides considerable support to this structure and explains the low incidence of permanent nerve damage.[12] Lower lip numbness caused by damage to the inferior alveolar nerve or its branches is generally transient, and hemorrhage ceases spontaneously because of the tamponading effect of the bone or retraction of the transected vessels.

Many strong muscles are attached to the mandible and have a tendency to displace fractured bone segments, thereby producing deformities that may affect the selection of surgical and anesthetic management. In addition, displacement of bone fragments may produce encroachment of surrounding

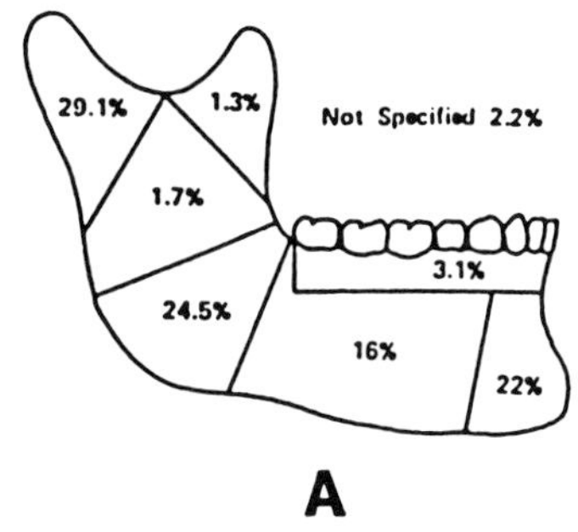


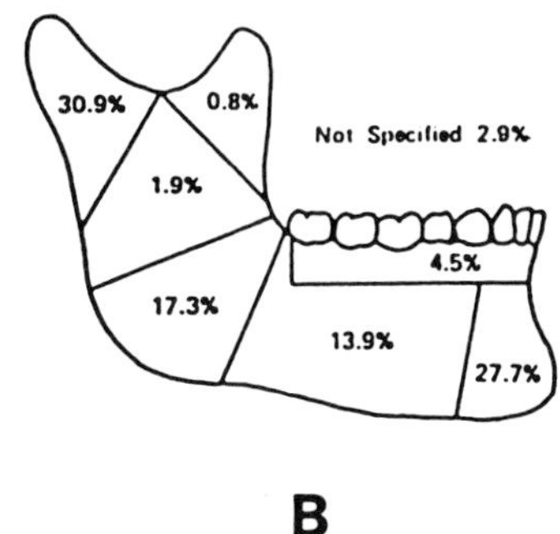


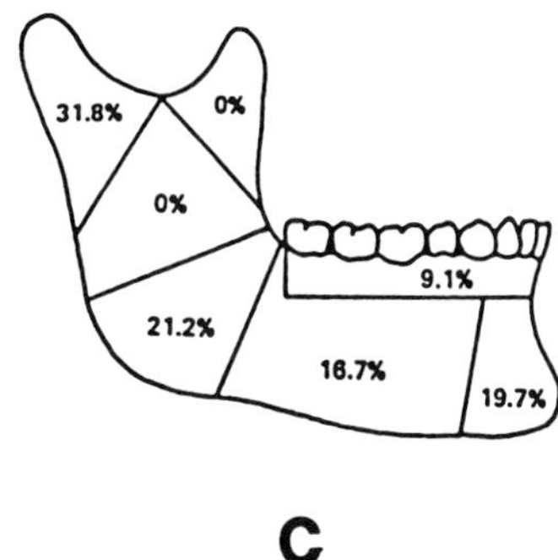


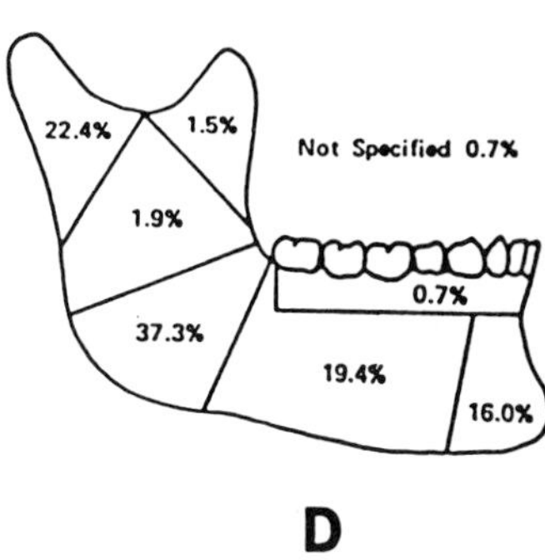


FIG. 12-3. (A) Overall anatomic distribution of mandibular fractures. (B) Anatomic distribution of fractures caused by automobile accidents, (C) motorcycle accidents; and (D) altercations. (From Olson et al[74] with permission.)

soft tissue upon the airway and thus cause airway obstruction. Mandibular muscles are divided into four categories based on their function: (a) elevators, (b) depressor-retractors, (c) retractor, and (d) protrusor[24] (Fig. 12-5).

Of the three elevator muscles, the masseter is the strongest and extends from the medial and lateral surfaces and lower border of the zygomatic arch to the anterior and lateral surfaces and angle of the mandibular ramus (Fig. 12-6). The fan-shaped temporal muscle arises in the temporal fossa, descends medially to the zygomatic arch, and inserts on the coronoid process, the mandibular notch, and the inner surface of the ramus of the mandible. It retracts the mandible in addition to functioning as an elevator (Fig. 12-6). The medial pterygoid muscle originates from the pterygoid fossa of the sphenoid bone and the pyramidal process of the palatine bone and inserts on the inner surface of the ramus and angle of the mandible (Fig. 12-6).

The anterior belly of the digastric, the geniohyoid, and the mylohyoid muscles constitute the depressor-retractor group (Fig. 12-7). Also called the suprahyoid muscles, they originate from the hyoid bone. The digastric and geniohyoid muscles attach to the inferior border of the mentum. The mylohyoid has little effect on movement of the intact mandible because most of its fibers join in the midline at the mylohyoid raphe. Its principal function is to elevate the tongue during swallowing. However, as is discussed later, it exerts considerable force on fractured mandibular segments. The lateral pterygoid muscle, the protrusor muscle of the chin, after originating in two heads from the infratemporal surface of the great wing of the sphenoid bone and the outer surface of the lateral plate of the pterygoid process, inserts into the articular disc of the temporomandibular joint and the anterior surface of the neck of the mandible (Fig. 12-6).

In bilateral parasymphyseal fracture, also called "Andy-Gump" fracture because the retrognathic lower jaw produced by this injury resembles that of a popular comic strip character, the fractured segment of the mandible is pulled downward and backward by the digastric, mylohyoid, and geniohyoid muscles (Fig. 12-8). Such a pull may retract the tongue and intraoral soft tissues into the airway, causing obstruc-

FIG. 12-4. Mandibular foramen, mandibular canal, and mental foramen. The neurovascular bundle travels in the mandibular canal and is prone to injury in body and ramus fractures.

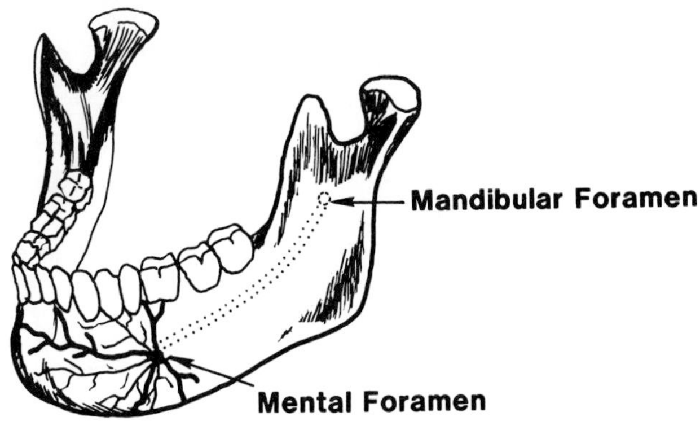

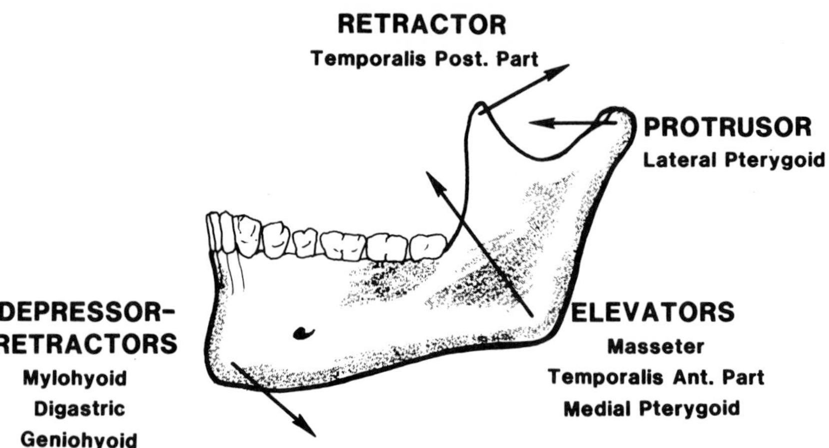


FIG. 12-5. Elevator, depressor-retractor, retractor, and protrusor muscles of the mandible and the direction of fragment displacement produced by them (*arrows*).

tion.[33,54] Fragments of the anterior portion of the mandible can also be displaced medially by the mylohyoid muscles, elevating the tongue and sometimes obstructing the airway.[54] (Fig. 12-9). The posterior fragment of a mandibular fracture anterior to the elevator muscles is usually displaced upward by the masseter and medially by the medial pterygoid muscle, whereas the anterior fragment is pulled downward by the suprahyoid muscles. In condylar and subcondylar fractures, the lateral pterygoid muscle displaces the condyle anteriorly and medially (Fig. 12-10). If the fracture is unilateral the mouth deviates toward the side of injury when opened.[25,87] In bilateral condylar fractures the victim may not be able to open the mouth at all and may present as a gag open bite in which the patient is unable to occlude the anterior portion of the jaw completely.

Muscle pull is not the only factor affecting fragment displacement. The direction of the fracture line is also important. In a mandibular angle or body fracture, the posterior fragment is pulled upward only if the fracture line is directed from posteroinferior to anterosuperior[12,25,54] (Fig. 12-11A). A fracture line in the opposite direction does not permit vertical displacement of the posterior fragment by the elevator muscles because of the locking effect of the anterior fragment and its attached muscles (Fig. 12-11B). Medial displacement of the posterior fragment by the medial pterygoid muscle is also affected by the direction of the fracture line.[12,25,54] If the fracture line extends from posterolateral to anteromedial, there will be no obstacle to movement of the posterior fragment (Fig. 12-11C). In contrast, the large buccal cortical fragment in fractures extending in a posteromedial to anterolateral direction prevents medial displacement (Fig. 12-11D).

Trauma may involve the temporomandibular joint (TMJ). Apart from condylar fractures, two important injuries occur at this site: TMJ dislocation and condylar impaction into the middle cranial fossa. The TMJ is formed by the condyle, the articulating bony socket, the capsule of the joint, the fibrocartilaginous disc, and two synovial pockets above and below the disc[8] (Fig. 12-12). The mouth cannot open unless two separate movements take place within the joint: an initial rotation of the condyle within the capsule and then forward sliding or translation of the condyle.[8] The anterior translation is limited by the bony articular eminence (or tubercle)[8] (Fig.

FIG. 12-6. Bony attachments of lower jaw muscles.

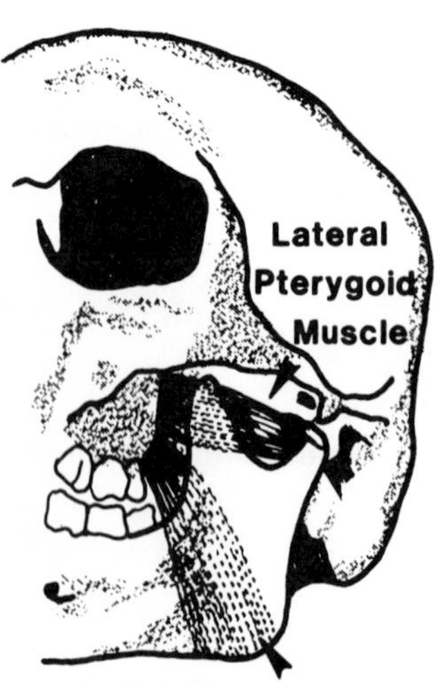


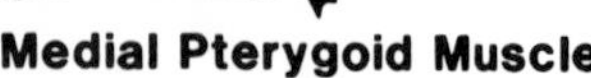


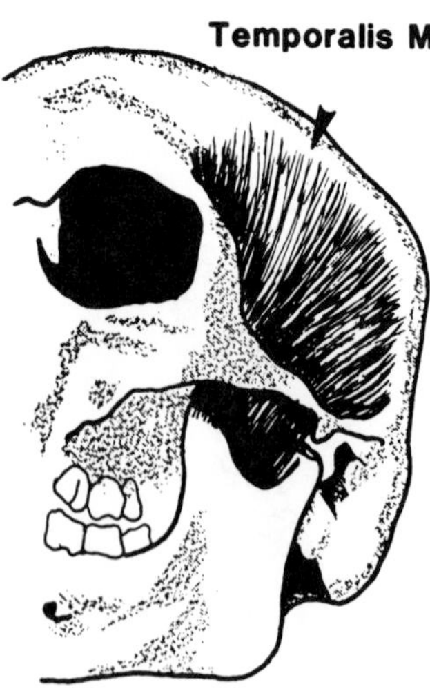


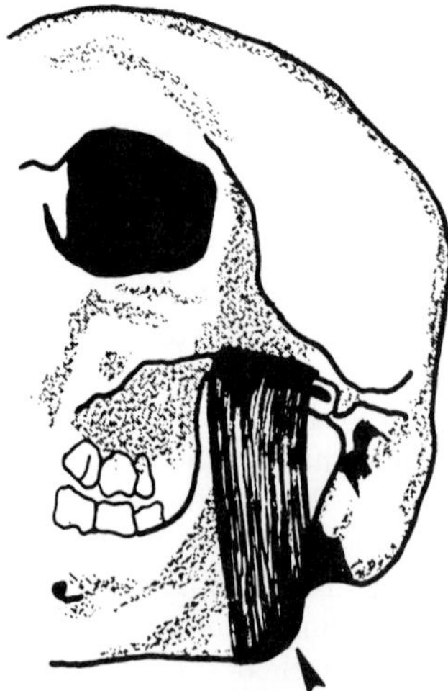

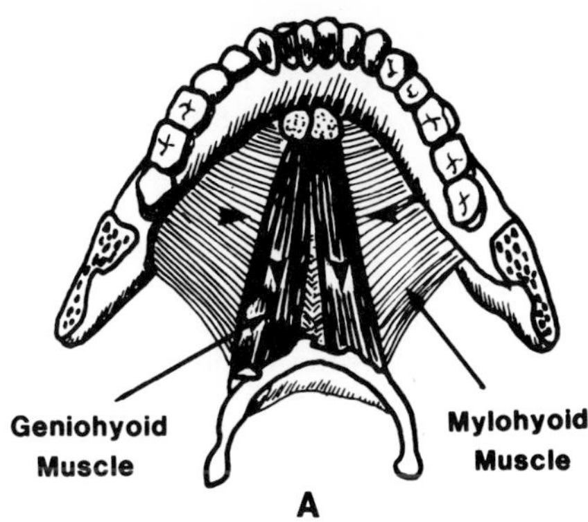


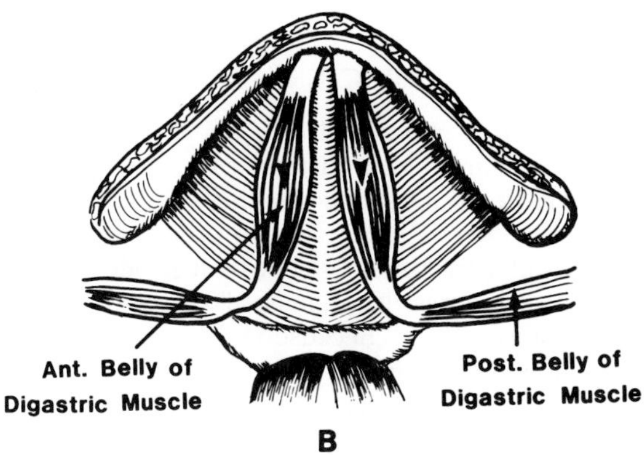


FIG. 12-7. Bony attachments of the depressor-retractor (suprahyoid) muscles. (A) the mandible viewed from the top and (B) from the bottom. Note that the geniohyoid is above and the anterior belly of the digastric is below the mylohyoid muscle. Direction of pull by each muscle is shown with arrowheads.

12-12). The mouth becomes locked in an open position if the condylar head is dislocated anteriorly beyond the articular eminence.[8] If the dislocation is unilateral, the open mouth, in contrast to condylar fractures, deviates away from the involved side.[25,87] Considerable pain and muscle spasm are present in almost all patients. Injection of a few milliliters of local an-

FIG. 12-8. Downward and backward displacement of mandibular fragment in bilateral parasymphyseal fracture. The fragment is pulled by the suprahyoid muscles. Airway obstruction may result.

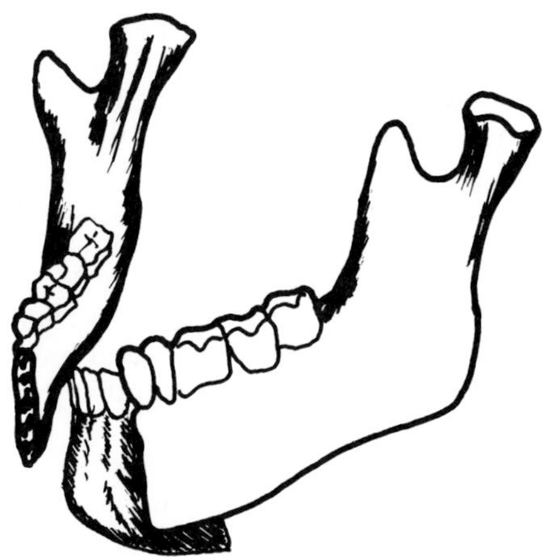

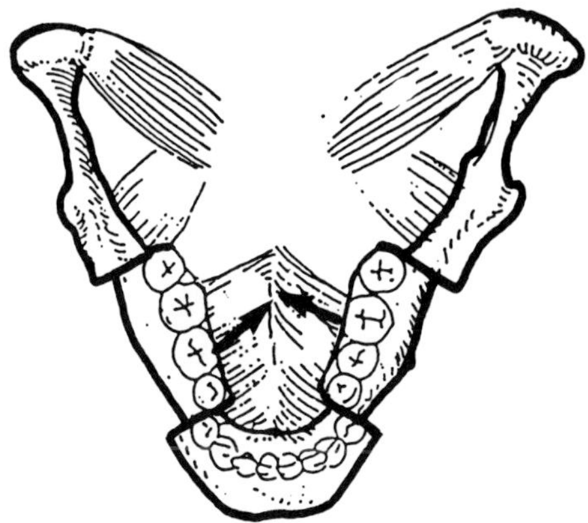

FIG. 12-9. Bilateral double fractures of the mandibular body. The fragments are pulled medially by the mylohyoid muscle. This displacement may push the tongue upward and backward and cause airway obstruction.

esthetic into the connective tissue of the TMJ capsule can result in spontaneous reduction of the dislocation.[25] If this measure is ineffective, manipulation of the mandible for a few minutes by depressing it with the thumbs inserted in the mouth and simultaneous gentle elevation with the fingers from outside the mouth can reduce the dislocation.[25] Intravenous narcotics may be necessary to reduce pain and spasm and facilitate the reduction.

The condyle may become impacted into the cranium through the thin roof of the glenoid fossa when the mandible receives a blow in the mental region with the mouth open.[12,70] This is, however, a rare phenomenon because the elevated margins of the glenoid fossa prevent upward movement of the medial and lateral poles of the condyle.[29] Only a small rounded

FIG. 12-10. Typical anterior and medial displacement of a mandibular condyle fracture. The displacement is caused by the lateral pterygoid muscle. This fracture restricts the patient's ability to open the mouth.

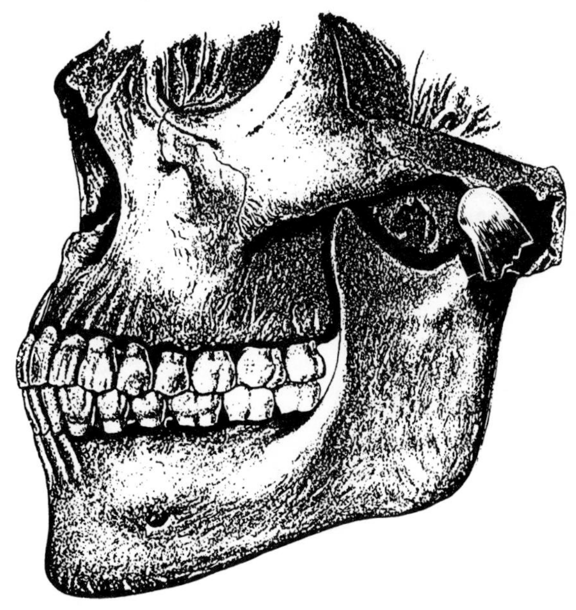

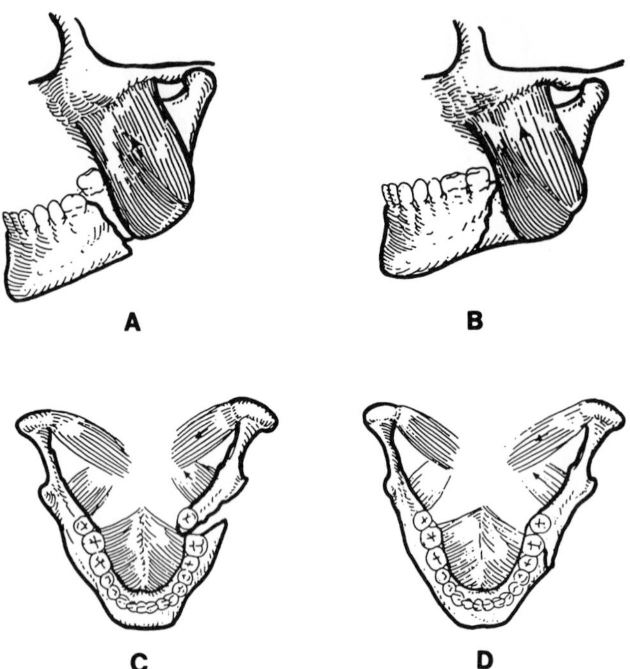


FIG. 12-11. In A and C, the direction of the fracture line is such that the posterior fragment is displaced. In B and D, the movement of the posterior fragment is locked by the anterior fragment because of the favorable direction of the fracture line. (From Kruger GO: Fractures of the jaws. In: Kruger GO, ed. Textbook of maxillofacial and oral surgery. St. Louis: CV Mosby, 1984; 384, 385, with permission.)

FIG. 12-12. The normal temporomandibular joint (TMJ). Arrows on the condyle represent the direction of movements of the condyle during jaw opening.

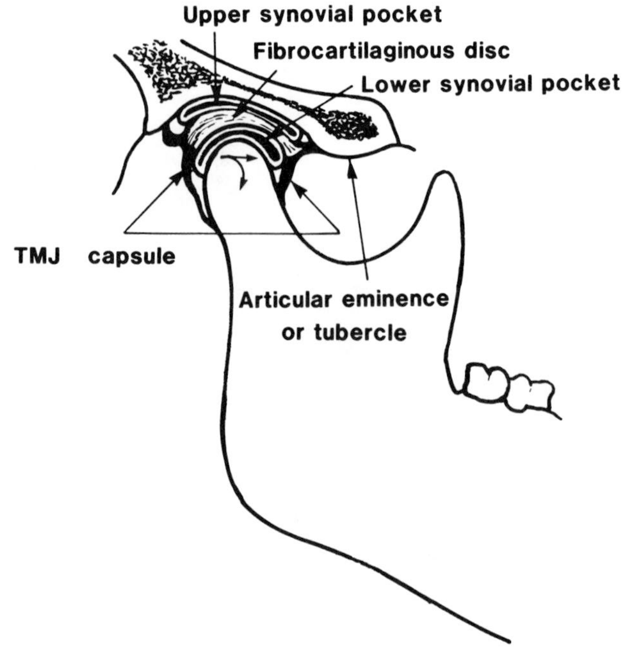


condyle would be likely to reach the center of the fossa and have the potential to penetrate its roof. Fortunately, this configuration is uncommon; only 2.8% of all condyles are rounded.[12] Another reason for the rarity of this type of injury is that the neck of the condyle breaks readily and absorbs most of the impact energy. Thus, the force applied to the cranial base is limited.[12] A potential complication of this type of fracture is severe hemorrhage because of damage to the middle meningeal artery, which runs in proximity to the glenoid fossa.[70] Rarely the condylar head may move posteriorly on the thin tympanic plate, which constitutes part of the posterior nonarticular portion of the glenoid cavity. Although postcondylar soft tissues and the temporomandibular ligament protect this area, fracture and distortion of the bony meatal wall with or without condylar fracture can occur.[12]

## CENTRAL MIDFACE FRACTURES

Unlike mandibular fractures, fragments of the membranous midfacial bones are seldom displaced by muscle pull;[25] the relatively weak muscles attached to these bones cannot exert significant traction. These fractures occur less frequently than mandibular fractures,[25,54] but their incidence, at least in European countries, has remained surprisingly constant over the past 30 years.[49] Because midface fractures involve important adjacent structures, morbidity is high. Both the trauma and secondary infection may involve the nasal cavity, the maxillary antrum, the orbit, and the brain, resulting in major complications. In addition, injuries of cranial nerves, major blood vessels, and the richly vascularized soft tissues are not uncommon.

### *LeFort Fractures*

These fractures were first described by René LeFort[57] in 1901. In an attempt to determine the value of external facial signs and symptoms in predicting the severity of maxillary fractures, he applied forces to the facial skeletons of cadavers. He found little relationship between severity of skeletal injury and external findings, but did notice surprisingly constant fracture lines on the facial skeleton. Based on this observation he divided midfacial fractures into three categories, which are now designated LeFort I, LeFort II, and LeFort III (Fig. 12-13).

In LeFort I or Guerin's fracture, the horizontal fracture line separates the maxillary alveolar process from the rest of the maxilla. The fracture line passes above the nasal floor medially and extends laterally at the same level, involving the maxillary sinuses and the lower third of the septum. It thus mobilizes the palate and the maxillary alveolar process. Posteriorly the fracture line extends to the palatine bones and the lower third of the pterygoid plates (Fig. 12-14). The fracture segment is freely mobile and thus is called "floating jaw." An associated palatal fracture is common and clinically manifested by a line of submucosal ecchymosis. The LeFort I fracture differs from an alveolar fracture in that the latter does not extend to the midline of the palate.

The LeFort II fracture is pyramidal. The fracture begins in the midline at the thick portion of the nasal bone and runs laterally through the lacrimal bones and inferior rim of the

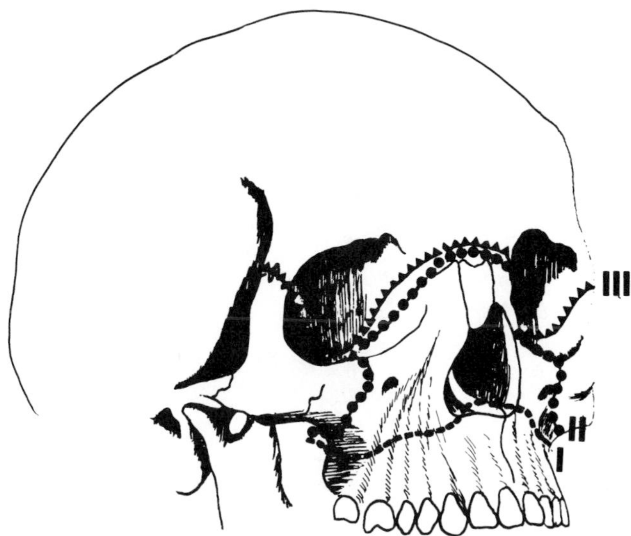


FIG. 12-13. Anterolateral view of fracture lines in LeFort injuries. LeFort I = rectangles; LeFort II = solid circles; LeFort III = solid triangles.

orbit, continuing downward near the zygomaticomaxillary sutures. The fracture line then crosses the lateral wall of the antrum and extends beneath the malar bone (zygoma) toward the pterygomaxillary fossa (Fig. 12-13). Posteriorly the LeFort II fracture involves the upper parts of the pterygoid plates (Fig. 12-14). Significant widening of the inner canthus of the eyes, epicanthal deformity of the bridge of the nose, and damage to ethmoidal cells may be present. Associated basal skull fracture is not uncommon and should be ruled out before embarking on airway manipulation via the nasal route.

The LeFort III fracture is a craniofacial dysjunction in which the entire midfacial skeleton separates from the cranial base. Medially the fracture line originates at the nasofrontal suture and involves the ethmoid bone posteriorly. Laterally it extends through the orbit below the level of the optic foramen to the pterygomaxillary suture and the sphenopalatine fossa; rarely the optic foramen is involved. The fracture then extends laterally and upward, separating the greater wing of the sphenoid bone and the zygoma up to the frontozygomatic suture. Posteriorly, it extends to the sphenopalatine fossa and the uppermost part of the pterygoid plate (Figs. 12-13 and 12-14). The zygomatic arch is fractured at its weakest point in proximity to the zygomaticotemporal suture.

When this fracture is present, the entire midface moves backward and downward parallel to the base of the cranium (Fig. 12-15). The cranial base may be fractured at multiple sites; the cribriform plate is broken in the majority of patients, resulting in rhinorrhea. The posteriorly displaced midface can also impinge upon the oro- and nasopharynx, potentially causing airway obstruction (Fig. 12-15). Craniofacial dysjunction in LeFort III fractures distorts the normal facial configuration; the face is elongated and appears like a dishpan.

In practice, LeFort fractures are rarely bilateral. Usually one side of the face is fractured with one LeFort pattern and the other side with another. A combination of LeFort fractures and nasal, nasomaxillary, nasoethmoidal, or zygomatic fractures is also observed. In more severe injuries, a combination of frontal and maxillary fractures may result in complete separation of the midface and the anterior base of the skull from the main body of the cranium. These injuries are characterized by dysjunction of parts of the frontal bone, the orbital roof, or the sphenoid bone.[22,36,63,67]

FIG. 12-14. Lateral view of the maxillofacial skeleton showing LeFort fracture lines.

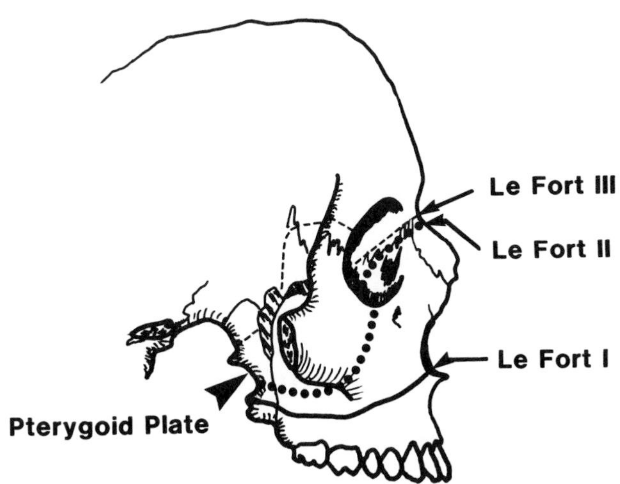


FIG. 12-15. Posteroinferior displacement of entire midface in LeFort III fracture. The dotted line represents the anterior boundary of the maxilla before fracture.

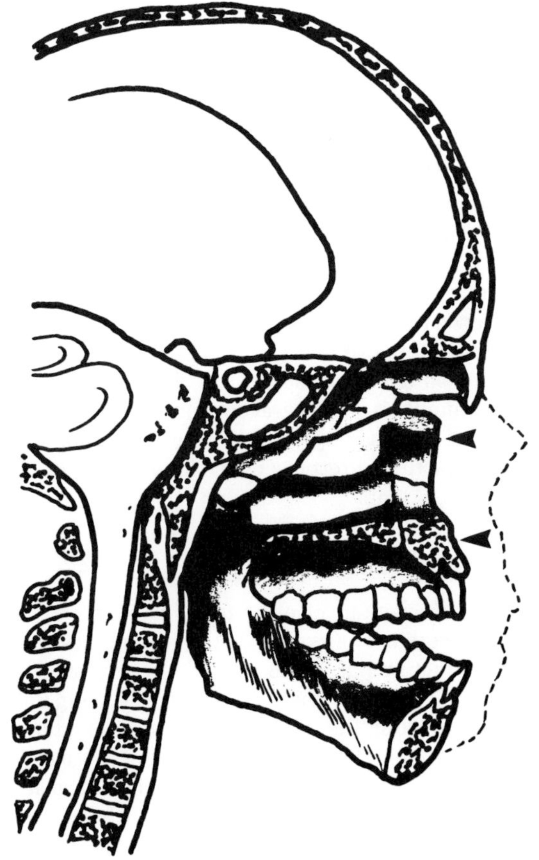

### *Nasal Fractures*

The projection of the nose and the delicate structure of its bones make nasal fractures the most commonly encountered fractures of the face.[10] Nasal fractures may be isolated or combined with maxillary, ethmoidal, and orbital injuries. This fracture is not difficult to recognize; a history of trauma to this region, swelling over the external surface of the nose, and epistaxis strongly suggest the presence of this injury.[62] Radiographic studies add little to the clinical diagnosis. CT scan may be required, however, to differentiate nasal fracture from complex nasoethmoid fractures that require early surgical intervention to prevent infection.[62]

### *Nasoethmoidal Fractures*

Nasoethmoidal fractures differ from nasal fractures in that the cribriform plate of the ethmoid is also broken, potentially resulting in dural fistula and thus infection and pneumocephalus. These injuries are easily missed in the presence of swelling, and clinical findings are often attributed to simple nasal fracture. Ethmoid involvement must be suspected when there are nasal fractures, lacerations of the frontal or nasal region, and bilateral periorbital ecchymosis (spectacle hematoma or racoon eyes). The latter suggests the presence of an anterior cranial base fracture. Nasoethmoid fractures may be associated with orbital, maxillary, frontal, and LeFort fractures. In some of these patients the midface and the cranial base may be separated from the anterior cranial fossa.[22]

Severe ocular injury with initial or subsequent loss of sight may be present in as many as 30% of these patients.[22] Telecanthus, an increase in distance between the medial canthal ligaments, may be observed either immediately after injury or a few days later when the swelling disappears. The canthal ligaments are attached to the inferomedial orbital rim, which is frequently fractured in conjunction with nasoethmoid injuries.[62] Telecanthus suggests the presence of unstable, complex, and severe maxillofacial injury that often requires aggressive management using a combined craniofacial approach.[36] Nasolacrimal duct lacerations occur in about 20% of patients.[22] Carotid-cavernous sinus fistula may develop within a few days to months after injury, resulting in a characteristic pulsating eye.

Nasoethmoid fracture is suspected when epistaxis, depression or comminution of the nasal dorsum, pain and tenderness in the area of the nose, spectacle hematoma, or inferomedial orbital rim fractures are present. Definitive diagnosis is established by CT scan.

## LATERAL MIDFACE FRACTURES

Fractures at this site involve the malar bone, the zygomatic arch, and the orbit. The zygoma is the second most common facial bone fractured after the nose.[10] The masseter muscle is attached to its anteroinferior aspect, and the temporalis fascia is attached along the junction of the facial and temporal surfaces of the frontal process and the superior aspect of the temporal process of this bone. Thus, significant displacement may occur after fractures of the arch or of the zygomaticomaxillary complex. The displaced fragment may impinge on the mandibular coronoid process and produce a limitation of mouth opening (Fig. 12-16), which must be differentiated from trismus secondary to pain and temporalis muscle spasm. The displaced fragment may also intrude upon the lateral wall of the maxilla and produce infraorbital nerve damage.

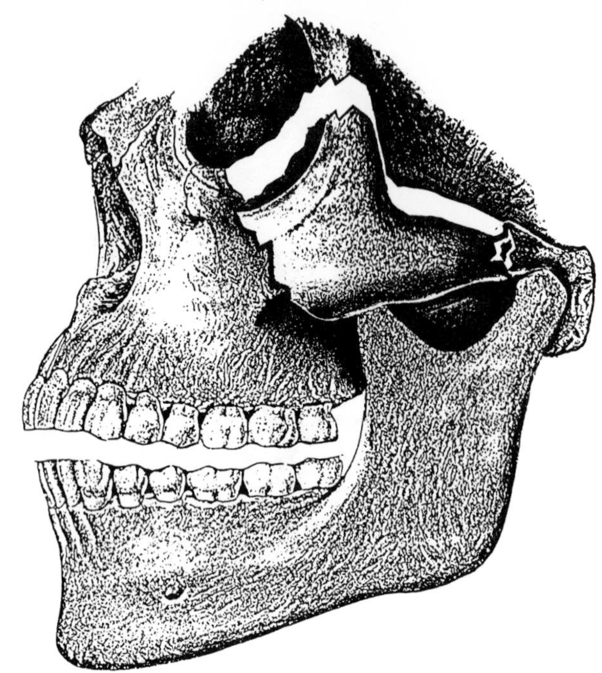

FIG. 12-16. Displaced zygomatic bone impinging on the coronoid process. Mouth opening may be limited because the coronoid process cannot move anteriorly.

Orbital fractures affect eye movement when the external ocular muscles are entrapped by fractured segments. Direct eye injury including optic nerve laceration may occur, requiring careful assessment and timely treatment.

## UPPER FACIAL FRACTURES

These injuries are also termed "frontobasilar fractures" and involve the frontal bone and frontal sinus. Concomitant nasoethmoid, supraorbital, zygomatic, and cranial base fractures are common. Fractures of the frontobasilar region involve the anterior cranial fossa. Thus, frontal lobe contusions, lacerations, cerebrospinal fluid rhinorrhea, pneumocephalus, and periorbital emphysema are common complications of these fractures. Concomitant injury to the skull and the face may sometimes be associated with loss of bone.[36] Significant brain injuries may be easily overlooked because of the silent nature of the frontal lobe and the absence of increased intracranial pressure due to the decompression of cranial contents by mobility of the fracture. In frontal sinus fractures, the nasofrontal ducts may be damaged, resulting in an accumulation of secretions within the sinus and subsequent abscess formation.

# PEDIATRIC FACIAL INJURIES

Facial fractures are infrequent in children, comprising only 1 to 5% of all maxillofacial injuries in major series,[39,76] although in a recent retrospective study 14.5% of maxillofacial injuries occurred in children less than 17 years of age.[38] The frequency of this injury decreases to 1% in children less than 5 years of age.[38] The highly resilient facial bones of children are often able to withstand significant trauma without fracture or, in many instances, with only greenstick fractures. The three-to-one male to female predominance characteristic of adult maxillofacial trauma[98] is not seen in children; in this age group, male predominance is only slight (60% to 40%).[38,40] In the pediatric population the etiology of maxillofacial injury is similar to that of adults except that in children, motor vehicle-pedestrian accidents replace altercations, an important cause of adult maxillofacial trauma.[38] The pediatric maxillofacial injury victim is more prone than adults to have other injuries, especially of the head, extremities, and soft tissues.[38] The large head size and the softness of the long bones explain the high rate of associated injury.

Children tend to sustain mandibular rather than maxillary injuries. Midface fractures do occur in pediatric patients, but are seen mostly in older children at a significantly lower rate than mandibular fractures.[38] The relatively small size of the pediatric maxilla and the lack of pneumatization of the maxillary sinuses appear to be the cause of this predilection. As compared to adults, mandibular fractures in children are more likely to occur at a single site. Unlike adults, pediatric mandibular fractures are generally not displaced by muscle pull because of elasticity of the bone, developing tooth buds, and the high incidence of greenstick fractures.[40] The mandibular condyle is a common site of fracture in children[71] probably because it contains a higher proportion of medullary bone to cortex.[47] These fractures can be overlooked because of physician inexperience and diversion of attention to more obvious injuries, such as lacerations and abrasions.[71] Condylar fracture should be suspected when the child presents with laceration of the chin and mandibular symphysis or body fractures.[71]

In children, facial fractures, especially those close to suture lines, may result in arrest of bone growth. The rapid bone growth of the contralateral side of the face usually results in facial deformity. This complication may also arise from rapid healing and thus malunion if treatment of the fracture is delayed or absent.[25]

Diagnosis of maxillofacial injuries in children is difficult. The apprehension of the child and anxiety of the parent make examination difficult. Complaints, such as pain and malocclusion, are difficult for children to express, especially if they are young. Obtaining the patient's cooperation for X-ray studies is difficult in this age group, and even if they do cooperate, the complex anatomy of the small pediatric mandible, which contains multiple tooth buds, a relatively small amount of cortical bone, and a probable greenstick fracture, makes interpretation difficult. Thus, evaluation with CT scanning is invaluable for both mandibular and maxillary fractures in this age group, whereas in adults this type of evaluation is usually necessary only for middle and upper facial fractures. Sometimes, examination may need to be performed under anesthesia to diagnose these injuries properly.[25]

The treatment principles of maxillofacial injury in pediatric patients differ somewhat from those for adults. Intermaxillary fixation is maintained for a shorter time than in adults; early mobilization of the jaw is the mainstay of treatment because long periods of immobilization may result in ankylosis, especially in condylar and subcondylar fractures.[38] Dentition of many pediatric patients is not appropriate for application of arch bars and interdental wire fixation. Deciduous teeth, mixed dentition, and small permanent teeth make such treatment difficult. Therefore open reduction and internal fixation under general anesthesia shortly after injury are considered by some surgeons the treatment of choice.

## COMPLICATIONS OF MAXILLOFACIAL INJURY

In and of itself, maxillofacial injury is not a devastating condition; however, its complications are. Management of these problems, some of which fall within the realm of the anesthesiologist, requires a clear understanding of their nature.

### AIRWAY OBSTRUCTION

Facial injuries can be responsible for upper and sometimes lower airway impairment that may necessitate immediate intervention. Airway obstruction may develop by several mechanisms. The posteriorly displaced distal fragment of a parasymphyseal mandibular fracture allows the floor of the mouth to fall backward, causing high airway soft tissue obstruction.[33] In bilateral double fractures of the body, the free mandibular segment may be pulled medially by the effect of mylohyoid muscle, pushing the tongue up to the palate and thus obstructing the airway (Fig. 12-9). Similar airway compromise may develop from swelling of the tongue secondary to edema or hematoma[17] (Fig. 12-17). Edema and hematoma may also develop in the pharynx, palate, and floor of the mouth after facial fractures, burns, and penetrating wounds,[16] limiting tongue movement and producing rapid, progressive airway occlusion.[48] The pterygoid plate is the only buttress preventing posterior shift of a midface fracture. If it is broken, the entire midface may move posteriorly, thereby encroaching upon the nasopharynx (Figs. 12-14 and 12-15). In the conscious patient this shift may not result in airway obstruction since mouth breathing is maintained. However, if consciousness is impaired from associated craniocerebral trauma or hemorrhagic shock, the tongue and the epiglottis fall backward against the posterior wall of the pharynx and severe airway obstruction ensues.[9]

Debris, blood clot, tooth fragments, dentures, and foreign bodies in the pharynx may occlude the airway directly or by being aspirated into the tracheobronchial tree.[93] Inhaled loose oral tissue fragments or displaced dental prostheses occasionally lodge in the larynx without causing voice impairment and without producing initial signs of respiratory obstruction.[66] However, when the airway is subsequently manipulated, severe signs of airway obstruction may develop because of displacement of the foreign body or developing edema. Meticulous examination of cervical radiographs for foreign objects is important before attempting intubation.[46] Occasionally, hemoptysis or persistent atelectasis may occur if these foreign bodies are inhaled or pushed into the smaller airways during endotracheal intubation or mechanical ventilation.[52]

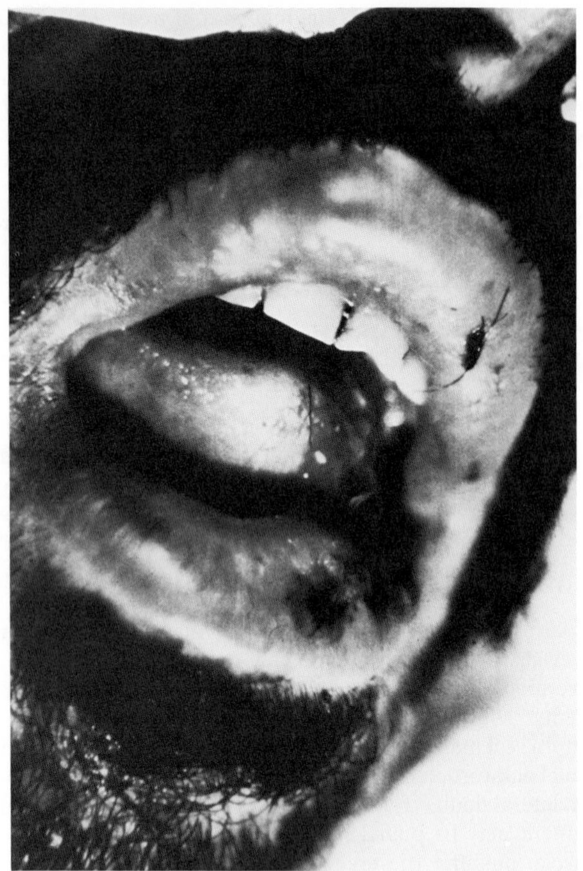

FIG. 12-17. The swollen tongue of a patient who sustained a gunshot wound to the mouth. Swelling on the right (patient's left) side of the tongue is caused by hematoma and associated edema.

Bronchoscopy and sometimes even bronchotomy may be necessary to remove these objects[97] (Fig. 12-18).

Associated head, neck, thoracic, and other injuries complicate the clinical picture. The unconscious patient may have airway problems that vary from simple soft tissue obstruction to significant aspiration with the full-blown asthma-like picture diagnostic of aspiration pneumonitis. Concomitant laryngotracheal injury, if not recognized, may cause progressive dyspnea in unintubated patients in the absence of airway obstruction from the maxillofacial injury. If endotracheal intubation or tracheostomy is performed, respiratory obstruction may develop following extubation or decannulation because of the laryngotracheal pathology.[90] Hemopneumothorax, pneumothorax, or flail chest may confuse the evaluation since each can cause continuing hypoxemia, even in the presence of an established airway.

## HEMORRHAGE

Bleeding from soft tissue lacerations, the mouth, and the nose is a common feature of facial injuries. Significant hemorrhage may result, especially if the temporal or other major branches of the external carotid artery have been injured. In the neck, major vessels, such as the carotid and jugular systems, are susceptible to penetrating injury and shearing wounds. Usually, however, bleeding from lacerations is mild and venous, resulting from muscle and mucosal tears and disruption of emissary veins in the bones. Major hemorrhage from the nose and mouth in closed maxillofacial injuries usually results from lacerations of arteries and veins within the walls of fractured sinuses. Vessels of concern are the anterior and posterior ethmoidal, the internal maxillary, the lingual, and the greater palatine arteries. Nasal, zygomatic, orbital, frontal sinus, nasoethmoid, and anterior cranial fossa fractures are the usual causes of nasal bleeding. However, LeFort and nasoethmoid fractures result in the most profuse hemorrhage. As was mentioned, lacerations of the inferior dental neurovascular bundle may be the cause of bleeding in mandibular body fractures.

Bleeding from facial fractures, although at times serious and life threatening, is usually minor and rarely the cause of severe hypovolemia. Thus in the hypotensive patient with facial injuries, other causes of shock—hemorrhage from other sites, increased intracranial pressure, acute spinal cord injury with bradycardia, and severe alcoholism with nonlethal head injury—must be eliminated. Nevertheless, massive bleeding from facial injuries may sometimes go unnoticed, particularly in patients with impaired consciousness, because the blood is swallowed. In these patients, delay in control of hemorrhage and inadequate intravascular volume restoration may result in a fatal outcome.[69] All patients with acute maxillofacial injury must be assumed to have a full stomach, not only because of recent food intake but also from swallowed blood.

Bleeding from facial lacerations is usually controlled with digital pressure until the lacerated vessel is identified. Blind probing of the wound with surgical clamps should be discouraged; the potential for damage to important facial structures such as the cranial nerves is great with this approach. Bleeding from sinus vessels may be stopped by simple manual repositioning of the bone fragments or by intermaxillary fixation. Anterior packing of the nose with half-inch wide adaptic gauze moistened in a petroleum-jelly-based ointment, such as Bacitracin, often stops mild to moderate bleeding. Combined anterior and posterior nasal packing is necessary to control more profuse epistaxis. Posterior packing can be performed by inserting a 16F or 18F Foley catheter with a 30-mL balloon via the nostril until its tip is seen in the pharynx. The balloon then is filled with air or water and pulled gently against the choana (Fig. 12-19). The catheter should be advanced carefully and the balloon inflated only after the tip is seen in the pharynx since it may enter the cranial vault via a fracture of the cranial base. Alternatively a $4 \times 4$ antibiotic-impregnated gauze pad may be formed into a roll with sutures; this pad is then tied to the tip of a nasally inserted Foley catheter that is withdrawn until the gauze is snugly secured within the posterior pharynx. Anterior packing is then applied as described above.

Although nasal packing is effective for control of bleeding in most patients, a small percentage may not benefit from this technique. Angiography will identify the bleeding site in these patients. If bleeding from an identified vessel is profuse, surgical ligation of its feeding vessel is the treatment of choice. External carotid artery ligation alone is seldom effective because of the rich collateral circulation from the facial, maxillary, and lingual arteries.[69] Ligation of the external carotid artery with clipping of the anterior and posterior ethmoidal arteries along the medial orbital wall is a rapid, safe, and highly successful method of dealing with posterior epistaxis.[42]

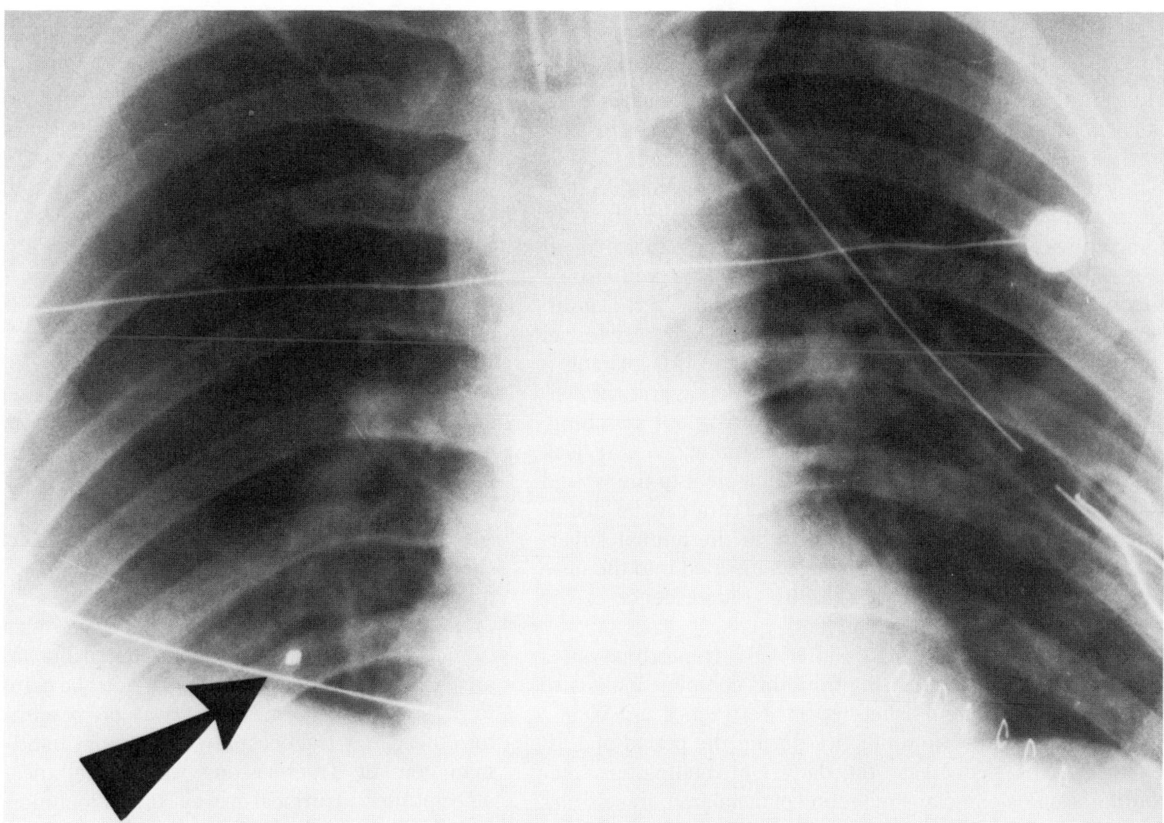

FIG. 12-18. Chest radiogram of a patient demonstrating an aspirated foreign body (*arrow*) in the right lung after a car accident. Removal was not possible with bronchoscopy because of the peripheral location of the aspirated material.

Ligation of the internal maxillary artery within the maxillary sinus is also effective.[69] These procedures can be performed under local anesthesia, but general anesthesia is preferred in most instances. If the rate of hemorrhage is slow, embolization with gelfoam or other substances is the treatment of choice since this procedure does not produce a surgical scar or peripheral nerve damage.[78,81] At Bellevue Hospital, this procedure is performed under local anesthesia with sedation and careful monitoring of hemodynamics and cerebral function. In some of our earlier patients, spillage of the embolizing material into the internal carotid artery resulted in neurologic damage, but this complication has not occurred during the past 5 years.

FIG. 12-19. Control of nasal bleeding with the balloon of a Foley catheter used as a posterior pack and Bacitracin-impregnated gauze as an anterior pack.

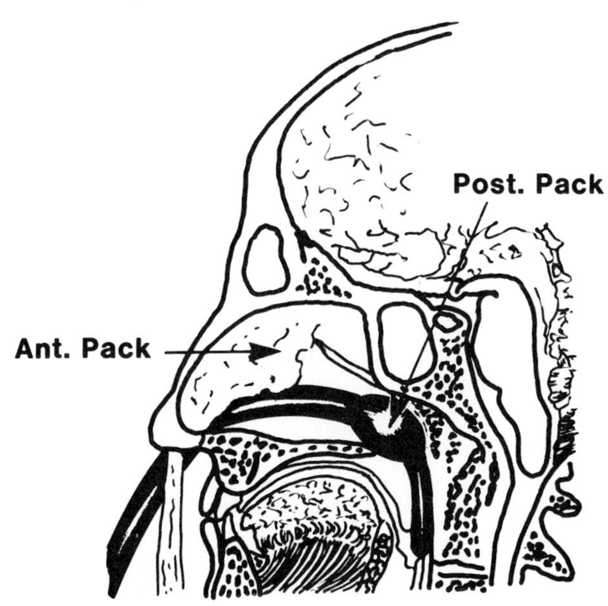


Observation of injured sites for quality of clot information and frequent monitoring of coagulation factors are important since bleeding may be secondary to dilutional coagulopathy or disseminated intravascular coagulation (DIC) caused by release of thromboplastin from concomitantly injured brain or other organs.[79] Treatment involves replacement of coagulation factors.

## CEREBROSPINAL FLUID RHINORRHEA AND OTORRHEA

Cerebrospinal fluid (CSF) rhinorrhea is usually caused by craniofacial injuries in which the base of the cranium is fractured. The cribriform plate is the most common site of bony injury, but damage to other structures in the base of the skull may also cause this complication. It occurs most frequently after maxillary, nasoethmoid, frontal, frontal sinus, and complex frontonaso-orbital fractures. Less frequently CSF presents from the ear. In patients with rhinorrhea or otorrhea, air may enter the cranial vault via the fistula and produce pneumocephalus. Of course, along with air, micro-organisms also gain access to the brain and may cause meningitis, brain abscess, or encephalitis.

In approximately one-third of patients, a CSF leak develops within the first 24 hours of the injury and in more than one-half within 48 hours.[95] In the remaining patients, CSF rhinorrhea develops within 3 months after injury.

It is often difficult to recognize rhinorrhea or otorrhea during the initial stages of maxillofacial trauma when the CSF is mixed with blood and mucus. A commercial paper reagent test designed to identify glucose in normal CSF will also be affected by the glucose in blood. This test, however, can differentiate rhinorrhea from nasal discharge. A simpler test to differentiate CSF from nasal discharge involves placing a handkerchief under the nose for a short period and then allowing the material to dry; CSF will dry without starching, whereas nasal discharge will stiffen the cloth.[16] A CSF leak may also be confused with discharge of tears into the wound after injury to the lacrimal apparatus. Tears can be distinguished by depositing fluorescein dye in the lumbar subarachnoid space and examining pledgets inserted into the nose with a Wood's light after 30 minutes. Fluorescence of the pledgets suggests CSF leakage.[25]

The incidence of meningitis after CSF rhinorrhea varies from 9 to 36%.[95] The mortality from this complication is also variable, ranging in published reports between 1 and 20%.[95] Use of broad-spectrum antibiotics during the period of CSF leakage seems to decrease the danger of meningitis.[25] According to some clinicians reduction of facial fractures during the period of CSF rhinorrhea promotes meningitis. Others believe that positive pressure ventilation by mask facilitates the development of meningeal infection. There is no clear evidence for these suppositions. CSF leakage is often treated conservatively unless large amounts of fluid are draining, drainage is from the cribriform plate and/or posterior ethmoid/sphenoid region, the site of fistula is uncertain or multiple, or the leak is associated with pneumocephalus.[95] Evaluation of the craniofacial region with CT scan is invaluable in assessing these conditions and deciding among therapeutic choices. Surgery involves patching the fistulous tract with a fascia lata graft and patching bony defects with hammered muscle.[95] This procedure is performed by either craniotomy or a transethmoid/sphenoid approach.[95]

## SUBCUTANEOUS EMPHYSEMA AND PNEUMOMEDIASTINUM

These are uncommon complications of facial injury. Air from the maxillary and ethmoid sinuses can communicate with the fascial planes of the neck, and thence with the mediastinum. Air in the mediastinum is a benign complication of facial fractures, but may also be caused by injury to vital organs such as the larynx, trachea, lungs, or esophagus. Appropriate radiographic and endoscopic evaluation of these organs should be performed before pneumomediastinum is labeled a harmless consequence of a facial injury.[18]

## INFECTION

Infection is an important and multifaceted problem in the management of maxillofacial injury. In addition to contamination of the central nervous system by oral micro-organisms, infection in the vicinity of fracture sites, extension into the fascial planes of the face and neck, and even spread to distant sites, such as fractured extremities, can occur.

Fractures of the mandibular angle, body, or parasymphyseal region appear to have a higher infection rate than zygomatic and maxillary fractures, especially if they are compound and involve the teeth.[19] Surprisingly, delay of definitive surgical treatment does not appear to increase the infection rate. Prophylactic use of cephazolin sodium, 1 g intravenously 1 hour before the surgical procedure, and a similar dose 8 hours later has been shown to diminish the incidence of postoperative infections in facial fractures during electively performed definitive surgery.[19]

Extension of infection into the fascial planes of the head and neck a few days after a facial fracture may jeopardize airway continuity. These infections characteristically harbor both aerobic and anaerobic organisms.[83] The patient is treated with 400,000 units of aqueous penicillin G every 4 hours for several days, drainage of the abscess, and further antibiotic therapy depending on the sensitivity of the specific organisms involved. Tracheal intubation to secure the airway for abscess drainage is performed under direct vision using a fiberoptic bronchoscope with the patient sedated but awake. Preoperative CT scan of the face and neck must be carefully evaluated to determine the degree of airway encroachment. Provision for emergency tracheostomy must be at hand during airway management. Tracheostomy under local anesthesia without attempting nonsurgical airway control techniques is indicated if the CT scan reveals a severe airway compromise.

Concern about the possibility of infective endocarditis after elective dental procedures in patients at risk—those with valvular heart disease, prosthetic cardiac valves, etc.—led to the development of an antibiotic prophylaxis protocol by the Committee on Rheumatic Fever and Infective Endocarditis of the American Heart Association (AHA)[88] (Table 12-2). These guidelines are largely aimed at preventing infective endocarditis in electively operated patients and may not necessarily prevent this complication in patients with acute maxillofacial injury whose dentition is damaged before antibiotic administration. Nevertheless, patients at risk should receive such prophylaxis as soon after the injury as possible.

For the last decade, an increasing number of injured patients have been operated concurrently for repair of both facial and orthopedic injuries. The question has been raised whether these patients are at increased risk of orthopedic sepsis due to mouth organisms. Preliminary data suggest that preoperative use of a first-generation cephalosporin eradicates both mouth organisms and *Staphylococcus aureus,* and in these patients, orthopedic sepsis is not likely if only one orthopedic and one oral surgical procedure are performed after the injury. However, in multiply injured patients requiring more than one procedure, certain mouth organisms may be selected by the initial cephalosporin. In these circumstances, throat cultures obtained 24 hours before subsequent surgery will reveal these organisms and permit selection of an appropriate antibiotic.[30]

## MORTALITY

Maxillofacial injuries are seldom life threatening in the absence of associated injuries. In a study from Europe only 84

TABLE 12-2. Recommended Antibiotic Prophylaxis for Infective Endocarditis in Patients Undergoing Oral Surgery

| REGIMEN | DOSAGE |
|---|---|
| Standard regimen (oral route) | Penicillin V, 2.0 g, orally, 1 h before surgery<br>+<br>Penicillin V, 1.0 g, orally, 6 h after the initial dose |
| Standard regimen (parenteral route) | Penicillin G, 2 million units, IV or IM, 30–60 min before surgery<br>+<br>Penicillin G, 1 million units, IV or IM, 6 h after the initial dose |
| Maximal protection regimen | Ampicillin, 1.0 to 2.0 g, IV or IM and Gentamycin, 1.5 mg/kg, IV or IM } 30 min before surgery<br>+<br>Penicillin V, 1.0 g, orally, 6 h after the initial dose<br>or<br>Repeat initial parenteral regimen 8 h later |
| Penicillin allergic regimen (oral route) | Erythromycin, 1.0 g, orally, 1 h before surgery<br>+<br>Erythromycin, 500 mg, 6 h after the initial dose |
| Penicillin allergic regimen (parenteral route) | Vancomycin, 1.0 g, IV slowly over 1 hour, 1 h before surgery |

Adapted from Shulman et al[88].

(2.4%) of 3564 motor vehicle accident victims who died shortly after trauma had maxillofacial injuries.[3] In only 20 of these cases was maxillofacial injury thought to be the definitive cause of fatality.[3] It is suggested that hypoxia, the principal cause of death after maxillofacial trauma, is usually caused by a combination of head injury and massive blood aspiration, rather than airway obstruction from displaced jaw fractures.[3]

## ASSOCIATED INJURIES

Concomitant injury to other regions of the body is a common feature of maxillofacial trauma. These injuries are often more life threatening than the facial injury itself. Overall, associated trauma is present in approximately 50 to 70% of motor vehicle accident victims and 30 to 35% of altercation victims.[3,14,39,61] The number of involved organs and the severity of injury to these organs are also greater after motor vehicle accidents than after altercations.[61] There is a relation between the facial bone fractured and the incidence and severity of associated injuries. When the fracture is limited to facial bones with low impact resistance (nasal bones, zygoma, mandible), both the incidence and severity of concurrent injuries are low. In contrast, the incidence and severity of associated injuries and the mortality rate increase when facial bones with high impact resistance, such as the supraorbital rim and mandibular symphysis, are fractured (Table 12-3).

Head injury frequently occurs with maxillofacial injury, especially after automobile accidents. Its incidence according to published reports varies between 15 and 48%.[14,61,74,92] The risk of serious head injury is higher in upper than in middle or lower facial injuries[56] (Fig. 12-20). Cervical spine injury is reported in 0.2 to 6% of maxillofacial trauma victims.[14,61,74,89,92] Mandibular fractures are usually associated with injuries at the level of the first or second cervical ver-

TABLE 12-3. Relation Between Magnitude of Impact and Incidence and Severity of Associated Injuries in 1,000 Facial Fractures

| | ASSOCIATED INJURIES | | | | | | MORTALITY RATE |
|---|---|---|---|---|---|---|---|
| | *Major (%)* | *Minor (%)* | *Total (%)* | *CNS %* | *Thorax %* | *Abdomen %* | % |
| Low-velocity impact (altercation, minor falls) ($n$ = 359) | 4 | 10 | 14 | 12 | 9.1 | 4 | 0.3 |
| High-velocity impact (MVA, major falls etc.) ($n$ = 661) | 32 | 31 | 63 | 36 | 19.4 | 11.1 | 2.7 |
| A) Fractures of high-impact resistance bones ($n$ = 253) | 50 | 32 | 82 | | | | 5.8 |
| B) Fractures of low-impact resistance bones ($n$ = 408) | 21 | 30 | 51 | | | | 0.7 |

Adapted from Luce et al[61] with permission.

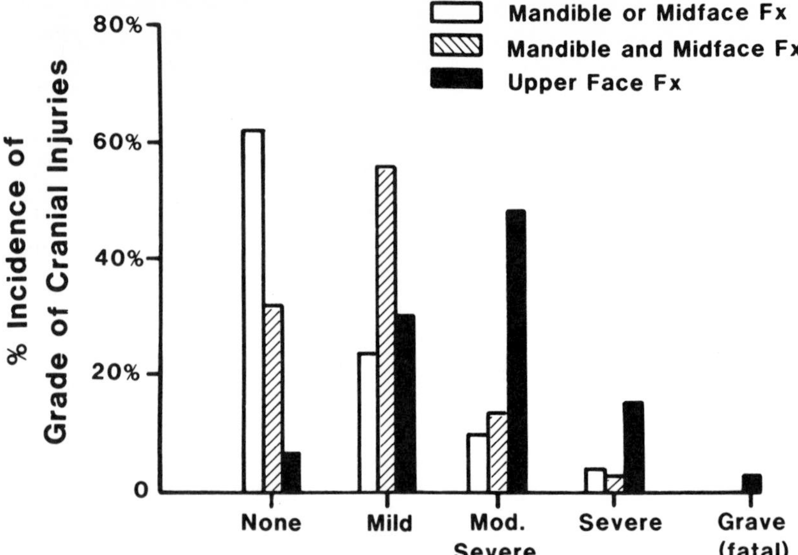


FIG. 12-20. The relationship between lower, middle, and upper facial fractures and severity of head injury. The likelihood of severe head injury increases with upper facial fractures. Lower and middle facial fractures usually are associated with less severe head injury. (From Lee et al[56] with permission.)

tebrae, whereas middle or upper facial trauma is associated with injuries of the lower cervical spine,[58] probably because of differences in direction of the force vectors that accompany trauma to different regions of the facial skeleton.

Since the spinal canal of the upper cervical vertebrae is wide in relation to the spinal cord, neurologic injury is less likely to occur in upper than in lower cervical injuries. The patient with a fracture of the lower face may thus have an associated cervical spine injury without neurologic deficit. Airway management without concern for cervical spine protection in these patients may result in spinal cord damage. It has been suggested that chin laceration, along with other clinical signs and symptoms, should indicate the possibility of cervical spine injury in a patient with maxillofacial injuries.[7,58] However, the most reliable method of ascertaining whether a spine injury is present is radiologic examination. An open mouth view if the patient is able to open the mouth is invaluable for diagnosis of the first and/or second cervical spine fracture-dislocations.

Various cervical structures may be damaged in conjunction with facial injuries after both blunt and penetrating trauma. Associated neck injury is not uncommon in gunshot injuries of the mandible in which the bullet, after shattering the bone, continues its trajectory in the neck.[37,91] In automobile accidents, unrestrained front seat occupants may strike their neck on the steering wheel or dashboard. These patients present with a variety of signs, including shock, airway obstruction, neurologic alterations, cervical hematoma, hemoptysis, and absent peripheral pulses because of carotid or subclavian artery thrombosis. It is not uncommon to ascribe these findings to the maxillofacial injury. Rapid deterioration or death may follow cervical injuries, either shortly after injury or during airway or anesthetic management. This subject is discussed in detail in Chapter 13.

Associated eye injuries occur with a frequency varying from 2.7 to 67% in large series.[39,44,61,74] Fortunately, most of these are minor and do not require specialized anesthetic management. Holt and co-workers[44] found that 67% of 727 patients with blunt maxillofacial trauma sustained ocular injury but that only 18% of these injuries were serious and 3% were blinding. These injuries consisted of hyphema, lens dislocation, intraocular hemorrhage, retinal detachment, optic nerve damage, and rupture of the globe. In rare instances retrobulbar hemorrhage may occur, resulting in severe proptosis that necessitates emergency decompression of the orbit.[75] Sometimes even trivial injuries may cause sudden blindness, probably because of disruption of the optic canal.[4,96]

In many patients with facial fractures, recognition of eye injury may be difficult. Palpebral hematoma and edema often prevent adequate examination. Consultation should be obtained from the ophthalmology department in such patients before administration of an anesthetic. When general anesthesia is required for eye examination, the patient should be considered to have an open globe until proven otherwise.

Thoracoabdominal injuries occur in 5 to 15% of patients presenting to the emergency department with maxillofacial injury.[14,39,61,74,92] Almost any intrathoracic or intraabdominal organ can be injured, but special attention must be given to the search for pneumothorax, hemothorax, aortic trauma, and cardiac contusion; these conditions occur rather frequently, their recognition may be delayed, and they may result in disastrous intraoperative complications if not diagnosed early.

Upper and lower extremity injuries are seen in about 10 to 20% of patients with facial injuries after automobile, motorcycle, and bicycle accidents.[3,39] Hemorrhage from these injuries may be substantial. Injury to extremity vessels and nerves may be detected by clinical tests and angiography.

## MANAGEMENT STRATEGIES

As in any major trauma, hospital management of maxillofacial injuries is a continuum beginning with the patient's arrival in the emergency department and ending when he or she regains full function. The anesthesiologist participates only in certain phases of this care, but it is important to be familiar with the overall management strategy.

After arrival of the patient in the emergency department, an inventory of traumatic injuries is made by rapid primary and secondary surveys. The face is examined to determine the presence of soft tissue and/or skeletal injuries. However, a detailed examination of the face, radiologic evaluation, or definitive therapy is delayed until more emergent problems are addressed. Airway obstruction, pneumothorax, hemothorax, and hemorrhagic shock are the most important problems of this phase and require prompt treatment. All patients with maxillofacial trauma, especially those with neck pain, tenderness, or spasm; chin laceration; and neurologic deficits, must be assumed to have cervical spine injury until X-ray evaluation proves otherwise. If time constraints imposed by the urgency of other conditions preclude such evaluation, the head and neck should be stabilized by spine board, tape, and sandbags or by application of manual axial spine traction before they are manipulated for whatever reason. Appropriate measures should be taken to limit secondary injury in head-injured patients. These include prompt restoration of blood pressure, provision of adequate oxygenation, hyperventilation, and diuretic therapy. Once an adequate airway has been provided, the vascular status has been stabilized, and crucial diagnostic tests have been performed, then attention can be directed to the facial injuries.

The diagnosis of facial injuries is made by physical examination and X-ray evaluation. Physical signs, include contusions, bruises, lacerations, or other evidence of injury to the craniofacial region. Such symptoms as pain or localized tenderness, crepitation from underlying fracture, numbness and paralysis in the distribution of a specific nerve, facial asymmetry and/or deformity, bleeding, visual disturbance, and obstructed respiration are all highly suggestive of serious facial injury. Malocclusion, an abnormal relation of upper and lower jaw dentition, is a very important clinical sign of maxillofacial fracture. It is indicated when the conscious patient states that the bite is abnormal and the teeth of the upper and lower jaw are not meeting each other in the same fashion as they did before the accident. The ability of the patient to open the mouth should be ascertained. Limitation and pain in mouth opening are important keys to the recognition of facial injury. Condylar movement can be detected by introduction of the little finger in the ear canal; absence of condylar movement with opening and closing of the jaw suggests fracture of this part of the mandible.

Definitive diagnosis is made by special X-rays and CT scan. The timing of X-ray evaluation depends on the associated injuries. Patients who are unstable and require immediate operative intervention undergo surgery without obtaining facial X-rays. Likewise, radiographic evaluation of serious associated injuries has a higher priority than that of maxillofacial trauma. In these circumstances, X-ray evaluation of the maxillofacial injury is done when the patient is stabilized; which may at times be days after the accident.

Many X-ray views are available to demonstrate a specific fracture site (Table 12-4). It must be emphasized, however, that some of these techniques require extensive positioning and thus cannot be obtained in the multiply injured patient. For instance, the Panorex view of the mandible that demonstrates the angle, rami, and condyles requires that the patient be upright. Thus, it cannot be obtained in a hemodynamically compromised trauma victim. Likewise, the standard Water's view is obtained with the patient in a prone position. Therefore, a cervical spine X-ray should be obtained to rule out an injury before using this view. Conversely, the availability of a standard Water's view in a given patient, suggests that the spine is intact. In any case these problems of positioning have largely been resolved with the availability of CT scans. In fact, the CT scan has replaced plain facial X-rays in many centers not only because it eliminates these inconveniences but also because of its ability to provide more detailed information. Some centers are also using three-dimensional CT which provides better information than conventional CT scan of maxillofacial fractures.[63a]

TABLE 12-4. Plain Facial X-ray Views to Demonstrate Specific Fractures

| FACIAL X-RAY VIEW | FRACTURE SITE DEMONSTRATED |
|---|---|
| Water's view | Maxilla, zygoma, nose and orbit, sinuses |
| Towne's view | Mandibular rami and condyles, orbital floor |
| Posteroanterior mandible | Mandibular symphysis and body |
| Caldwell posteroanterior | Zygomaticofrontal junction, frontal bone and sinus, orbital roof and medial wall, nasoethmoid region, mandibular rami |
| Lateral skull | Frontal skull, frontal sinus, orbital roof, lateral view of facial bones and zygoma |
| Lateral oblique of the mandible | Mandibular body, angle, rami, condyle, and coronoid process |
| Submentovertex or "jug handle" | Zygomatic arch and nasal bones |
| 180° Panorex | Mandibular angle, rami, and condyles |

The timing of definitive repair of blunt facial injuries is determined by many factors. In some centers maxillofacial injuries are treated immediately after CT scan evaluation of the face if there are no associated injuries or if these injuries do not interfere with hemodynamic stability.[62] Definitive facial reconstruction can also be performed during emergent repair of associated injuries. Most maxillofacial injuries, however, can wait up to 6 days without deleterious effects on the outcome of the repair, provided that soft tissue injuries are treated and intermaxillary fixation is applied. Intermaxillary fixation involves closed reduction of the fracture and fixation of the jaws with wires passing through archbars attached to the upper and lower teeth. In edentulous persons a prosthesis is placed over the gums to provide fixation. These procedures can be done under local anesthesia or regional nerve block in the emergency department without subjecting the patient to the risks of general anesthesia.[25]

Additional surgical treatment is performed electively in patients in whom intermaxillary fixation does not reduce and stabilize the fracture. These procedures vary from closed reduction and fixation of the jaws to internal or external fixation of bone fragments with metal plates, Hoffman apparatus, or bone grafts under general anesthesia. Early internal fixation is favored at present by many surgeons because it provides better function, results in a shorter postoperative recovery and hospital stay, and is not associated with many of the disadvantages of intermaxillary fixation.[53] With this technique, access to the oral cavity for airway control and care of intraoral wounds and rapid return of normal alimentation with full mandibular function are achieved, which are important advantages over intermaxillary fixation.

Postoperatively, attention is directed to prevention of infection, adequate nutrition with liquid formula in patients with intermaxillary fixation, follow-up X-ray studies to ensure optimal fragment alignment, and jaw exercises to prevent ankylosis of the temporomandibular joint.

## AIRWAY AND ANESTHETIC MANAGEMENT

Participation by the anesthesia team in the care of the maxillofacial injury victim may be required during (a) initial management, (b) emergent surgery to repair facial and associated injuries, (c) delayed facial surgery, and (d) management of early postoperative complications.

### INITIAL MANAGEMENT

Airway management is the principal task of the anesthesiologist during this phase. Between 2 and 6% of patients who present to the emergency department with serious maxillofacial injuries require emergency tracheal intubation to relieve airway obstruction, to improve oxygenation, or to initiate hyperventilation for associated head injury.[14,39] Respiratory distress in a patient with acute maxillofacial injury is most commonly caused by airway obstruction, pneumothorax, pulmonary contusion, pulmonary aspiration, or a combination of these factors. Prompt diagnosis of the mechanism of the respiratory distress is mandatory since treatment of each cause is different. In a conscious patient with equivocal breathing difficulty a reliable way to establish the need for immediate airway management is to ask if he or she is getting enough air. In the unconscious patient, evaluation of the airway and auscultation and/or radiographic evaluation of the chest are the only reliable methods. Because cyanosis occurs late in the process of respiratory distress; a change in color should not be a criterion for recognition of airway compromise.

Breathing is characteristically noisy in a patient with partial airway obstruction, although the respiratory efforts of a totally obstructed patient are silent. Intercostal retraction, paradoxical movement of the lower neck and chest, flaring of alae nasi, and stridor are the most important signs of upper airway obstruction. If there is doubt, the examiner should approximate his or her ear to the patient's nose or mouth. If by these maneuvers airway obstruction is confirmed, the next step is to establish its location. Concomitant neck injury may be the cause of airway occlusion. Cervical hematoma, laryngeal deviation, absence of laryngeal protuberance, and subcutaneous emphysema are the usual signs of injury to this region. Likewise, flail chest, sucking chest wound, pneumothorax, and hemothorax are common causes of respiratory distress and should be promptly diagnosed if present.

Many conscious patients with maxillofacial injury breathe more comfortably in a sitting position with the body flexed. In this position, intraoral soft tissue moves forward, relieving airway obstruction. Patients themselves often tend to assume this position; they should be allowed to do so if hemodynamic stability can be maintained.[98]

As was alluded to earlier, airway occlusion from maxillofacial injury is caused by several mechanisms. If it results from simple loss of soft tissue tone, anterior traction on the jaw or tongue or proper placement of an oral or nasal airway usually relieves the problem. A nasal airway is less likely to stimulate gagging if airway reflexes are still present, but should not be used if a nose or cranial base fracture is suspected. If obstruction is caused by a displaced mandibular fracture, anterior traction using a towel clip or wire passed through the mandible will be helpful. Chin lift and jaw thrust may also be effective, but should not be attempted if cervical spine injury has not been ruled out. The mouth should be carefully examined for blood clots, foreign bodies, vomitus, teeth, and dentures. Blood and all vomitus should be removed by suction. It may be necessary to insert fingers in the oral cavity and pharynx to remove blood clots or solid material if the patient is able to open the mouth and is cooperative enough not to bite the fingers of the examiner. Sometimes, airway obstruction is caused by posterior displacement of the entire midface after fracture of the pterygoid plate. Insertion of the fingers into the mouth and palpation of the pterygoid plate immediately posterior and medial to the last upper molar tooth confirm this diagnosis; a characteristic crepitation over this bone is highly suggestive of pterygoid plate fracture. In these instances the palate can be moved anteriorly with the fingers. This maneuver repositions the entire maxilla, thereby relieving the airway obstruction.[25] Oxygen must be administered by face mask or cannula once the airway is cleared.

The maneuvers described are temporary measures. The airway must be secured by more reliable methods to prevent recurrence once the obstruction is initially relieved. Sometimes, chin lift, jaw thrust, anterior traction on the mandible or maxilla, and clearing of debris from the airway may be impossible to perform or insufficient to provide a patent airway, requiring an emergency endotracheal intubation or tracheostomy under emergency conditions. Because of widely varying clinical presentations, no single method of definitive airway control can be recommended for these patients.[23] Nevertheless, certain principles must be followed in order to prevent further complications.

As has been mentioned, the possibility of cervical spine fracture must be kept in mind; if it is not eliminated by appropriate X-ray studies, techniques of cervical spine protection must be utilized. Deeply unconscious patients usually do not experience a significant reaction to laryngoscopy and intubation. On the other hand, conscious patients may be restless, irritable, and uncooperative because of underlying hypoxemia, alcohol intoxication, or respiratory distress. Direct laryngoscopy before intubation may precipitate vomiting and thus loss of airway control and may predispose to aspiration in the sedated patient. It may also increase muscle activity enough to make arterial hypoxemia worse. Moderate sedation with diazepam (5–10 mg) or midazolam (1–3 mg) with or without small doses of fentanyl (0.05–0.1 mg) intravenously usually enables intubation to be done rapidly. These drugs improve the ability to open the mouth in patients who because of pain and jaw muscle spasm cannot do so. Irretrievable steps, such as the use of muscle relaxants or large doses of narcotics, should be avoided before placement of the endotracheal tube, unless the likelihood of easy intubation is high. Apnea may lead to a fatal outcome if the establishment of an artificial airway is time consuming or not possible.

Although it is tempting to try awake nasal intubation, valuable time should not be wasted with this technique. Nasal intubation also carries a great deal of risk in patients with fractures of the cranial base, since there is a possibility of passing the endotracheal tube into the cranium[45] (Fig. 12-21). Thus, in LeFort II and especially LeFort III fractures, nasal intubation is contraindicated. Nasally introduced gastric tubes carry a similar risk.[28,85] It is important not to withdraw a nasogastric tube once it enters the cranial vault. A knot formed during withdrawal of the tube may scrape brain tissue and magnify the injury.[28] Therefore, surgery has been recommended for removal of these tubes.[28] Blind nasal intubation is also precluded by the presence of nasal fractures. The fiberoptic bronchoscope, although recommended for airway control in maxillofacial injuries,[68] may be ineffective during the acute stage of trauma because of poor visualization resulting from excessive blood in the pharynx.

Endotracheal intubation may be performed using a translaryngeal wire or catheter (retrograde intubation) if the patient is able to open the mouth to allow recovery of the wire or catheter from the pharynx.[6] This technique, however, may be unsuccessful because pharyngeal blood precludes visualization and thus recovery of the catheter or wire. Although this problem can be circumvented by continuous pharyngeal suctioning, injection of air through the catheter hub and thus production of air bubbles in the pharyngeal blood may help locate the catheter. The major difficulty during translaryngeal-guided intubation arises during introduction of the endotracheal tube since the tube may become caught on the anterior commissure of the larynx. Manipulation of the wire and thus of the endotracheal tube with the flexible tip of a fiberoptic bronchoscope passed over the wire may alleviate this problem.[55]

FIG. 12-21. Inadvertent introduction of an endotracheal tube into the posterior fossa of the cranium during an attempt at nasotracheal intubation in a patient with severe craniofacial injury. (From Horellou et al[45] with permission.)

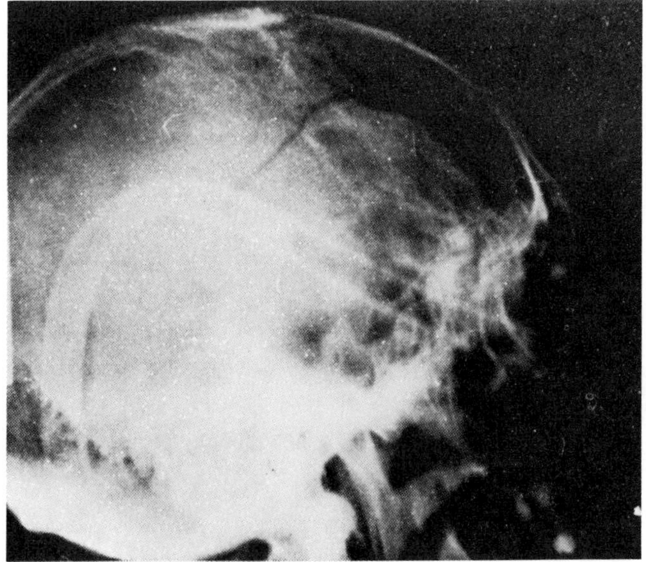

One should always be prepared for emergency cricothyroidotomy since attempts at endotracheal intubation may fail or provoke complete airway obstruction with severe hypoxemia. Cricothyroidotomy is preferred over tracheostomy for emergency airway control because it is easier and faster to perform and does not require extension of the neck, a maneuver that may jeopardize the spinal cord if cervical spine injury is present. This procedure, however, is contraindicated if there is coexisting larygeal injury, particularly cricotracheal separation; the cannula may enter a false passage and produce complete airway obstruction. Cricothyroidotomy is a temporary measure and should be converted to more definitive airway control, such as tracheostomy, once acute hypoxia is relieved. In most instances cricothyroidotomy is performed by the surgeon; the cricothyroid membrane is incised and an 8 mm ID cannula is inserted into the trachea. Alternatively, a 14-gauge intravenous catheter may be inserted percutaneously in the midline and directed caudally through the cricothyroid membrane. Ventilation is accomplished by connecting the catheter to a high-pressure (50 psi) oxygen source or a jet ventilator[94] by means of adapters as described in Chapter 3. Excessive airway pressures may be applied to the lung with this technique if complete outflow obstruction is present.

Conditions in which tracheostomy is required during management of maxillofacial injuries are listed in Table 12-5. In some of these conditions the airway can be controlled initially by endotracheal intubation, allowing tracheostomy to be performed under safe conditions, unless there is unrelievable airway obstruction or associated injuries of the head, spine, or chest.[13] According to published series, emergency surgical airway control is required in 1 to 2.5% of maxillofacial trauma victims.[39,89,98] Tracheostomy is also necessary after intermaxillary fixation if replacement of the orotracheal tube with a nasotracheal tube cannot be accomplished safely.

After the airway is secured and the blood volume restored, patients with maxillofacial injury are transported to the radiology suite for evaluation of their injuries. Continuous monitoring at least of arterial blood pressure and arterial oxygen saturation, along with airway management and other resuscitation equipment and drugs, must be provided during transport and radiologic evaluation.

TABLE 12-5. Indications for Tracheostomy in Maxillofacial Injuries

| |
|---|
| Combined bilateral mandibular fractures and LeFort fractures of the maxilla |
| Extensive lacerations and/or hematoma of the tongue and floor of the mouth |
| Gross posterior displacement of the maxilla with split palate and profuse bleeding from the nasopharynx |
| Gunshot and close-range shotgun injuries of the face |
| Crush-type injuries of the face |
| Extensive facial burns |
| Associated head and cervical spine injuries |

## ANESTHETIC MANAGEMENT OF EMERGENT SURGERY

Repair of maxillofacial injuries is seldom undertaken emergently. However, emergency surgery is frequently performed for associated trauma. Maxillofacial injuries may be concomitantly repaired in stable patients, or intermaxillary fixation may be applied under general anesthesia. Most of these patients arrive in the operating room with an endotracheal or cricothyroidotomy tube in place. The principles of airway management in unintubated patients are described in the previous section. Anesthetic management may be complicated by the presence of pre-existing diseases, acute alcohol intoxication, and recent illicit drug intake. These conditions should be evaluated preoperatively, if possible. Intraoperatively, efforts are directed toward maintenance of normal intravascular volume, oxygenation, temperature, and acid-base status (see Chapter 9). Obstruction of the tracheal tube by blood clots is not uncommon, requiring careful monitoring of peak airway pressure (Fig. 12-22). A progressive decrease in lung compliance may also occur secondary to the development of aspiration pneumonitis pulmonary edema, or atelectasis.

## ANESTHETIC MANAGEMENT OF DELAYED SURGICAL REPAIR

Patients in this group are operated electively and have either recovered or are recovering from their associated injuries. Preoperative evaluation of these patients should assess particularly the presence and extent of concurrent medical problems, history of acute or chronic alcoholism, licit and illicit drug use, associated injuries, and the state of the airway.

Maxillofacial injury may be the result of a fall during a seizure, intracardiac conduction abnormality, transient cerebral ischemia, or a stroke. Similarly, an automobile accident resulting in facial trauma may have been caused by the driver's acute myocardial infarction. Differentiation of these pre-existing conditions from those produced by trauma to the head or heart may at times be difficult. For instance, the accident may be the result of a convulsion that the patient experienced for the first time, yet a seizure in the hospital may be produced by a head injury. Likewise, electrocardiographic changes may reflect a ischemic heart disease or a myocardial contusion acquired during the traumatic event. In any case, accurate diagnosis must be established before surgery.

Acute alcohol intoxication, although very common in the immediate postinjury phase,[64] is rare in hospitalized patients. On the other hand, chronic alcoholism, with its adverse effects on hepatic function, metabolism, and coagulation, is seen frequently in this group of patients. Liver function tests and coagulation profile should be obtained in all patients undergoing delayed facial repair. Zinn et al.[100] demonstrated in a small group of patients that liver function tests are not affected during the first 3 postoperative days in patients with mild alcoholic hepatitis undergoing peripheral surgery. In our institution we delay surgery until liver enzyme levels return to normal. Patients undergoing delayed maxillofacial repair should also be evaluated for alcohol withdrawal symptoms. Tremor, fever, tachycardia, and mental disturbances are suggestive of this syndrome, indicating postponement of surgery and further observation and treatment of the disorder.

A careful history of narcotic abuse should be obtained from all maxillofacial injury victims. Some of these patients may also be abusers of other drugs and alcohol;[33] specific questions should be asked to obtain this information. Cocaine use has increased during the past decade. Patients should be asked whether they abused cocaine within the several hours before coming to the operating room; anesthetics may exacerbate the myocardial ischemia and arrythmias produced by this drug. In a few instances we have found cocaine vials under the tongues of these patients; the mouth should thus be inspected before surgery. Narcotic addicts should receive narcotics perioperatively at doses equivalent to their usual intake.

Although most associated injuries are stabilized at the time of elective maxillofacial repair, clinical, echocardiographic, and radiographic evaluation of chest injuries, such as myocardial and pulmonary contusion, flail chest, and pericardial injury, may be necessary in some patients before surgery. In addition, late complications of trauma, such as sepsis, deep vein thrombosis, and renal failure, should be ruled out.

The airway should be assessed to determine the ease of endotracheal intubation. The patient may not be able to open the mouth or may open it only to a limited extent. Three factors limit mouth opening: intermaxillary fixation, mechanical obstruction, and pain and/or spasm. Intermaxillary wires should be cut before anesthetic induction. However, even when the fixation is released, the patient may be unable to open the mouth because of other factors. Anesthetics and muscle relaxants can relieve muscle spasm or trismus, unless it is long standing and complicated by fibrosis around the joint. On the other hand, they have no effect on mechanical

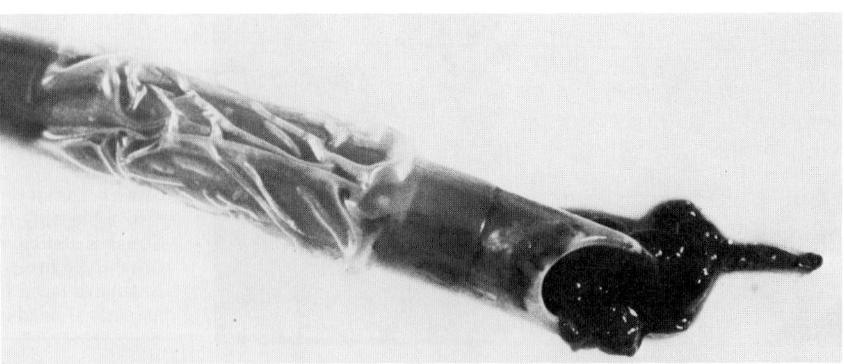

FIG. 12-22. Blood clot obstructing the lumen of an endotracheal tube.

obstruction. The mechanism of limitation can be determined by consulting with the surgeon, by reviewing facial X-rays or CT scan, and by injecting local anesthetic into areas suspected of being the cause of the problem. As was mentioned earlier, two types of fractures cause mechanical limitation of mouth opening: fractures through or near the temporomandibular joint and those involving the zygomatic arch with injury to the temporalis muscle. In the latter condition, the displaced zygomatic bone impinges on the coronoid process of the mandible and prevents its movement. The presence of these fractures can easily be determined by X-rays and consultation with the surgeons. Not infrequently, however, fractures through the temporomandibular joint result only in spasm of surrounding muscles without mechanical obstruction. Incremental doses of diazepam (2.5 mg) or midazolam (1 mg) and fentanyl (0.05 mg) or its analogs can overcome muscle spasm and provide sufficient mouth opening. Alternatively, injection of a few mililiters of lidocaine (1% or 2%) or bupivicaine (0.5%) into the mandibular notch can relieve spasm in these muscles. The degree of soft tissue swelling should also be taken into account when planning the anesthetic.

Patients with minimal or no limitation of jaw movement can be anesthetized with intravenous anesthetics and muscle relaxants and intubated nasally or orally using direct laryngoscopy. Those in whom anatomic variations (short neck, protuberant teeth, retrognathic jaw, etc.), mechanical limitation of jaw opening, or uncertain airway status exist should be managed while awake, preferably with a fiberoptic bronchoscope. The technique of awake sedated endotracheal intubation with topical anesthesia is discussed in Chapter 3. Since the patient does not have a full stomach, the airway can be anesthetized with both superior laryngeal nerve block and transtracheal anesthesia. Nasotracheal intubation is preferred over the oral route because it does not interfere with surgical exposure. Of course, the presence of nasal and cranial base fractures remains a contraindication to nasotracheal intubation. We prefer a regular endotracheal tube to a Rae tube. In the latter, the distance between the nasal curve and the end of the tube is short relative to the distance from the nostril to the larynx; as a result, in some patients, the cuff is positioned between the vocal cords with the potential dangers of cord injury and accidental extubation, especially if a small tube is used.

Any anesthetic can be used for maintenance of anesthesia. We use a combined narcotic-inhalation anesthetic with titrated doses of muscle relaxants guided by a nerve-muscle stimulator. A higher incidence of serious cardiac arrhythmias has been demonstrated with the use of halothane, than with other inhalation anesthetics or fentanyl/droperidol.[27,34] These arrhythmias occur mainly during manipulation of the fractured facial bones. They are often heralded by aberrant conduction and may be prevented by pretreatment with beta-adrenergic blocking agents (practolol, metoprolol, acebutolol).[27] Halothane may also be undesirable when local anesthetic-epinephrine solution is injected into the surgical site to minimize bleeding. The arrhythmogenic serum concentration of epinephrine is three times less in the presence of halothane than it is when enflurane or isoflurane is used.

Although the intraoperative course is usually uneventful, complications occur on rare occasions. The endotracheal tube may be cut during surgery, necessitating its replacement. This may be difficult and unsafe in some instances. A rigid guide wire introduced into the trachea through the partially cut tube acts as a leader and permits "railroading" of an intact tube. Obstruction of the endotracheal tube with secretions and blood occurs, but is less common than during surgery performed in the acute phase of the injury. Endotracheal tube kinking is common. Rarely, air from opened maxillary sinuses may dissect into the fascial planes of the neck and result in subcutaneous, mediastinal, and even pericardial emphysema. This complication is usually recognized postoperatively. Airway obstruction and circulatory embarassment are unlikely unless these spaces are filled with a large amount of air.[80]

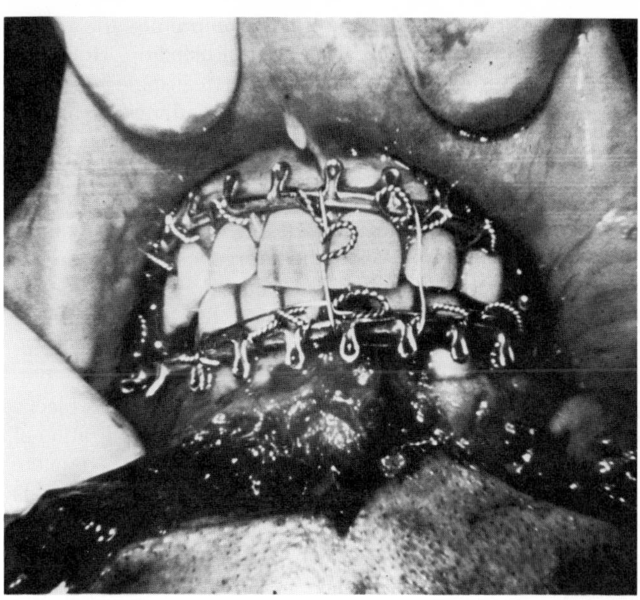

FIG. 12-23. Intermaxillary fixation.

### POSTOPERATIVE PHASE

The endotracheal tube should be left in place at the conclusion of surgery while soft tissue swelling is evaluated, airway reflexes return, and the patient recovers fully from the anesthetic. Dexamethasone, 4–8 mg intravenously, may help diminish soft tissue edema. If intermaxillary fixation is applied, a wire cutter should be taped to the patient's chest for immediate release of the wires in case of airway obstruction with blood clot or vomitus, laryngeal spasm, or soft tissue intrusion on the airway. Only two to four of the wires in the patient's mouth need to be cut (Fig. 12-23). Identification of these wires, however, is difficult for individuals who are not involved in surgical management.[32] Covering these key wires with colored rubber or plastic or leaving them long facilitates emergency jaw release.[5]

## CONCLUSION

Although they may present with impressive deformity, swelling, cuts, and bruises, facial fractures generally do not pose an immediate threat to life unless they compromise the airway or are associated with extensive arterial bleeding. However, associated injuries, particularly of the cervical spine and head, are common and must be suspected before attempting airway management techniques.

Isolated maxillofacial injuries rarely require definitive emergency surgery. Stabilization of fractures, usually by intermaxillary fixation, can be performed under local anesthesia, allowing delay of definitive surgery for up to 6 days without significantly compromising outcome. Regional anesthesia for intermaxillary fixation includes blocks of the inferior alveolar and greater palatine nerves. Supraorbital, nasal, infraorbital, maxillary, and mandibular blocks may also be employed to repair concomitant facial lacerations. These blocks are often supplemented by topical anesthesia or infiltration of the mucosa with local anesthetic agents to ensure complete analgesia during intraoral procedures and, if epinephrine is added, hemostasis.

Emergency surgery for associated injuries or the need for controlled ventilation requires airway management soon after the injury. In these circumstances the face, oral cavity, and neck must be evaluated carefully. No single method of airway control can be uniformly recommended; direct laryngoscopy, translaryngeal-guided intubation, and cricothyroidotomy are the most commonly used techniques when there is no time to evaluate the type and extent of injury. During this stage, irretrievable steps, such as the use of muscle relaxants or large doses of sedative and narcotic agents, should be avoided, and facilities to perform tracheostomy and cricothyroidotomy must be at hand before airway manipulation is attempted. Blind nasal intubation should be avoided in patients with nasal and cranial base fractures since these tubes may enter the cranial vault or periocular fat pad.

Epistaxis is a frequent occurrence after nasal and cranial base fractures. Hemorrhage from these sites is unlikely to cause hypovolemic shock, but in rare instances, serious and insidious bleeding may not be recognized and delay in its control may jeopardize the patient's life. Anterior and posterior nasal packing should be applied if bleeding persists.

Cerebrospinal fluid rhinorrhea is another frequent complication of maxillofacial fractures and may result in central nervous system infection. Nasal intubation is particularly contraindicated in these circumstances.

Postoperatively, if the jaws are wired together, normal laryngeal reflexes are not established, or airway obstruction is anticipated, the endotracheal tube should be left in place until full consciousness returns and periglottic edema subsides. A wire cutter should be available at all times during the postoperative period to prevent catastrophic events caused by endotracheal tube displacement or airway obstruction.

## REFERENCES


1. Abiose BO. Maxillofacial skeleton injuries in the Western States of Nigeria. Br J Oral Maxillofac Surg 1986;24:31.
2. Andersson L, Hultin M, Nordenram A, Ramstrom G. Jaw fractures in the county of Stockholm (1978–1980). (I) General survey. Int J Oral Surg 1984;13:194.
3. Arajarvi K, Lindqvist C, Santavirta S, et al. Maxillofacial trauma in fatally injured victims of motor vehicle accidents. Br J Oral Maxillofac Surg 1986;24:251.
4. Babajews A, Williams JL. Blindness after trauma insufficient to cause bony injury: case report and review. Br J Oral Maxillofac Surg 1986;24:7.
5. Barclay JK. Intermaxillary fixation—a safety measure. Br J Oral Surg 1979;17:77.
6. Barriot P, Riou B. Retrograde technique for tracheal intubation in trauma patients. Crit Care Med 1988;16:712.
7. Bertolami CN, Kaban LB. Chin trauma: a clue to associated mandibular and cervical spine injury. Oral Surg 1982;53:122.
8. Block C, Brechner V. Unusual problems in airway management. Anesth Analg 1971;50:114.
9. Boidin MP. Airway patency in the unconscious patient. Br J Anaesth 1985;57:306.
10. Bowers DG, Lynch JB. Management of facial fractures. South Med J 1977;70:910.
11. Bowsher WG, Smith WP. Severe facial injury by impalement. J Trauma 1984;24:999.
12. Bradley JC, Haskell R, Rowe NL, et al. Applied surgical anatomy. In: Rowe NL, Killey HC, eds. Maxillofacial injuries. London: Churchill Livingstone, 1985:1.
13. Breasted JH. Edwin Smith surgical papyrus. Chicago: University of Chicago Press, 1930.
14. Busuito MJ, Smith DJ, Robson MC. Mandibular fractures in an urban trauma center. J Trauma 1986;26:826.
15. Calhoun KH, Li S, Clark WD, et al. Surgical care of submental gunshot wounds. Arch Otolaryngol Head Neck Surg 1988;114:513.
16. Cawood JI, Thind GS. Supraglottic obstruction. Injury 1983;15:277.
17. Chase CR, Hebert JC, Farnham JE. Post-traumatic upper airway obstruction secondary to a lingual artery hematoma. J Trauma 1987;27:953.
18. Chawla K, Steinbaum S, Alexander LL. Pneumomediastinum occurring in association with facial trauma. NY State J Med 1984;84:9.
19. Chole RA, Yee J. Antibiotic prophylaxis for facial fractures: a prospective, randomized clinical trial. Arch Otolaryngol Head Neck Surg 1987;113:1055.
20. Chuong R, Mulliken JB, Kaban LB, Strome M. Fragmented care of facial fractures. J Trauma 1987;27:477.
21. Cohen MA, Shakenovsky BN, Smith I. Low velocity hand-gun injuries of the maxillofacial region. J Max. fac. Surg. 1986;14:26.
22. Cruse CW, Blevins PK, Luce EA. Naso-ethmoid-orbital fractures. J Trauma 1980;20:551.
23. Davies RM, Scott JG. Anaesthesia for major oral and maxillofacial surgery. Br J Anaesth 1968;40:202.
24. Dingman RO, Natvig P. The mandible. In: Dingman RO, Natvig P, eds. Surgery of facial fractures. Philadelphia: WB Saunders, 1964:133.
25. Edgerton MT, Kenney JG: Emergency care of maxillofacial and otological injuries. In: Zuidema GD, Rutherford RB, Ballinger WF, eds. The management of trauma. 4th ed. Philadelphia: WB Saunders, 1985:275.
26. Eriksson L, Willmar K. Jaw fractures in Malmö 1952–62 and 1975–85. Swed Dent J 1987;11:31.
27. Fergusson NV, Dalgleish JG, Saunders DA. Acebutolol and oral surgery: plasma levels following a single oral dose. Ann Roy Coll Surg Engl 1985;67:124.
28. Fletcher SA, Henderson LT, Miner ME, Jones JM. The successful surgical removal of intracranial nasogastric tubes. J Trauma 1987;27:948.
29. Fonseca GD. Experimental study on fractures of the mandibular condylar process. Int J Oral Surg 1974;89:101.

30. Foster RJ, Collins FJV, Bach AW. Concurrent oral surgery and orthopaedic treatment in the multiple injured patient. Is there an increased incidence of orthopaedic sepsis? J Trauma 1987;27:626.
31. Goodstein WA, Stryker A, Weiner LJ. Primary treatment of shotgun injuries to the face. J Trauma 1979;19:961.
32. Goss AN, Chau KK, Mayne LH. Intermaxillary fixation: how practicable is emergency jaw release? Anaesth Intens Care 1979;7:253.
33. Gotta AW. Maxillofacial trauma: anesthetic considerations. ASA Refresher Courses 1987;15:39.
34. Gotta AW, Sullivan CA, Pelkofski J, et al. Aberrant conduction as a precursor to cardiac arrhythmias during anesthesia for oral surgery. J Oral Surg 1976;34:421.
35. Griffin JM, Nespeca JA. Maxillofacial trauma in the military (an expensive proposition). Milit Med 1986;151:42.
36. Gruss JS. Franto-naso-orbital trauma. Clin Plast Surg 1982;9:577.
37. Gussack GS, Jurkovich GJ. Penetrating facial trauma: a management plan. South Med J 1988;81:297.
38. Gussack GS, Luterman A, Powell RW, et al. Pediatric maxillofacial trauma: unique features in diagnosis and treatment. Laryngoscope 1987;97:925.
39. Gwyn PP, Carraway JH, Horton CE, et al. Facial fractures—associated injuries and complications. Plast Reconstr Surg 1971;47:225.
40. Hall RK. Injuries to the face and jaws in children. Int J Oral Surg 1972;1:65.
41. Harris AMP, Wood RE, Nortje CJ, Grotepass F. Deliberately inflicted, penetrating injuries of the maxillofacial region. (Jael's syndrome). J Cranio-Max-Fac Surg 1988;16:60.
42. Hassard AD, Kirkpatrick DA, Wong FS. Ligation of the external carotid and anterior ethmoidal arteries for severe or unusual epistaxis resulting from facial fractures. Can J Surg 1986;29:447.
43. Hodgson VR. Tolerance of the facial bones to impact. Am J Anat 1967;120:113.
44. Holt JE, Holt R, Blodgett JM. Ocular injuries sustained during blunt facial trauma. Ophthalmology 1983;90:14.
45. Horellou MF, Mathe D, Feiss P. A hazard of naso-tracheal intubation. Anaesthesia 1978;33:73.
46. Jackson CL. Endoscopy for foreign body: report of 178 cases of foreign body in the air and food passages. Ann Otol 1936;45:644.
47. James D. Maxillofacial injuries in children. In: Rowe NL, Williams JL eds. Maxillofacial trauma. Edinburgh: Churchill Livingstone, 1985:538.
48. Javid B. An unusual complication of a mandibular fracture. Compend Contin Educ Dent 1987;8:824.
49. Kahnberg KE, Gothberg KAT. LeFort fractures. (I) A study of frequency, etiology and treatment. Int J Oral Maxillofac Surg 1987;16:154.
50. Karlson TA. The incidence of hospital-treated facial injuries from vehicles. J Trauma 1982;22:303.
51. Karyouti SM. Maxillofacial injuries at Jordan University Hospital. Int J Oral Maxillofac Surg 1987;16:262.
52. Khan RMA. An easily missed foreign body in the respiratory passages. Br J Anaesth 1975;47:628.
53. Klotch DW, Gilliland R. Internal fixation vs. conventional therapy in midface fractures. J Trauma 1987;27:1136.
54. Kruger GO. Fractures of the jaws. In: Kruger GO, ed. Textbook of maxillofacial and oral surgery. St. Louis: CV Mosby, 1984:364.
55. Lechman MJ, Donahoo JS, MacVaugh H. Endotracheal intubation using percutaneous retrograde guidewire insertion followed by antegrade fiberoptic bronchoscopy. Crit Care Med 1986;14:589.
56. Lee KF, Wagner LK, Lee YE, et al. The impact-absorbing effects of facial fractures in closed-head injuries. J Neurosurg 1987;66:542.
57. LeFort R. Etude experimentale sur les fractures de la machoire superiore. Rev Chir 1901;23:208–227, 360–379, 479–507.
58. Lewis VL, Manson PN, Morgan RF, et al. Facial injuries associated with cervical fractures: recognition patterns, and management. J Trauma 1985;25:90.
59. Lindqvist C, Sorsa S, Hyrkas T, Santavirta S. Maxillofacial fractures sustained in bicycle accidents. Int J Oral Maxillofac Surg 1986;15:12.
60. Linn EW, Vrijhoef MMA, deWijn JR, et al. Facial injuries sustained during sports and games. J Maxillofac Surg 1986;14:83.
61. Luce EA, Tubb TD, Moore AM. Review of 1,000 major facial fractures and associated injuries. Plast Reconstr Surg 1979;63:26.
62. Manson PN. Maxillofacial injuries. In: Siegel JH, ed. Trauma, emergency and critical care. New York: Churchill Livingstone, 1987:983.
63. Matras H, Kuderna H. Combined cranio-facial fractures. J Maxillofac Surg 1980;8:52.
63a. Mayer JS, Wainwright DJ, Yeakley JW, et al. The role of three-dimensional computed tomography in the management of maxillofacial trauma. J Trauma 1988;28:1043.
64. McDade AM, McNicol RD, Ward-Booth P, et al. The aetiology of maxillo-facial injuries, with special reference to the abuse of alcohol. Int J Oral Surg 1982;11:152.
65. McKechnie J. A severe craniofacial impalement injury (Jael's syndrome). Br J Oral Maxillofac Surg 1986;24:258.
66. Mehta RM, Pathak PN. A foreign body in the larynx. Br J Anaesth 1973;45:755.
67. Merville L. Multiple dislocations of the facial skeleton. J Max. fac. Surg 1974;2:187.
68. Mulder DS, Wallace DH, Woolhouse FM. The use of the fiberoptic bronchoscope to facilitate endotracheal intubation following head and neck trauma. J Trauma 1975;15:638.
69. Murakami WT, Davidson TM, Marshall LF. Fatal epistaxis in craniofacial trauma. J Trauma 1983;23:57.
70. Musgrove BT. Dislocation of the mandibular condyle into the middle cranial fossa. Br J Oral Maxillofac Surg 1986;24:22.
71. Myall RWT, Sandor GKB, Gregory CEB. Are you overlooking fractures of the mandibular condyle? Pediatrics 1987;79:639.
72. Nair KB, Paul G. Incidence and aetiology of fractures of the facio-maxillary skeleton in Trivandrum: a retrospective study. Br J Oral Maxillofac Surg 1986;24:40.
73. Okumori M, Futamura A, Tsukuura T, et al. Impalement wounds of the head and chest by reinforced steel bars with recovery: an unusual case report. J Trauma 1981;21:240.
74. Olson RA, Fonseca RJ, Zeitter DL, Osbon DB, et al. Fractures of the mandible: a review of 580 cases. J Oral Maxillofac Surg 1982;40:23.
75. Ord RA, Awty MD, Pour S. Bilateral retrobulbar hemorrhage: a short case report. Br J Oral Maxillofac Surg 1986;24:1.
76. Rowe NL. Fractures of the facial skeleton in children. J Oral Surg 1968;26:505.
77. Rowe NL. The history of the treatment of maxillofacial trauma. Ann Roy Coll Surg Engl 1971;49:329.
78. Sakamoto T, Yagi K, Hiraide A, et al. Transcatheter embolization in the treatment of massive bleeding due to maxillofacial injury. J Trauma 1988;28:840.
79. Samman N. Disseminated intravascular coagulation and facial injury. Br J Oral Maxillofac Surg 1984;22:295.
80. Sanford TJ, Shapiro HM, Gallick MN. Pericardial and subcutaneous air after maxillary surgery. Anesth Analg 1987;66:277.
80a. Scherer M, Sullivan WG, Smith DJ, et al. An analysis of 1,423

facial fractures in 788 patients at an urban trauma center. J Trauma 1989;29:388.

81. Schilstra SHA, Marsman JWP. Embolization for traumatic epistaxis. Adjuvant therapy in severe maxillofacial fracture. J Cranio-Max-Fac Surg 1987;15:28.
82. Schrimshaw GC. Malar/orbital/zygomatic fracture causing fracture of underlying coronoid process. J Trauma 1978;18:367.
83. Schroeder DC, Sarha ED, Hendrickson DA, Healey KM. Severe infections of the head and neck resulting from gas forming organisms: report of case. JADA 1987;114:65.
84. Seaton JR. Soft tissue facial injuries related to vehicular accidents. Clin Plast Surg 1975;2:79.
85. Seebacher J, Nozik D, Mathieu A. Inadvertent intracranial introduction of a nasogastric tube, a complication of severe maxillofacial trauma. Anesthesiology 1975;42:100.
86. Seguin P, Beziat JL, Breton P, et al. Sports et traumatologie maxillo-faciale: Aspects etiologiques et cliniques a propos de 46 cas. Mesures de prevention. Rev Stomatol Chir Maxillofac 1986;87:372.
87. Shepherd SM, Lippe MS. Maxillofacial trauma. Evaluation and management by the emergency physician. Emerg Med Clin North Am 1987;5:371.
88. Shulman ST, Amren DP, Bisno AL, et al. Prevention of bacterial endocarditis: a statement for health professionals by the Committee on Rheumatic Fever and Infective Endocarditis of the Council on Cardiovascular Disease in the Young. Circulation 1984;70:1123A.
89. Shultz RC. Facial injuries from automobile accidents: a study of 400 consecutive cases. Plast Reconstr Surg 1967;40:415.
90. Smith AC, Bradley PJ. Progressive dyspnoea following facial injury. Br J Oral Maxillofac Surg 1986;24:28.
91. Stanley RB, Cannalis RF, Colman MF. Gunshot wounds to the mandible with secondary neck injuries. Arch Otolaryngol 1981;107:565.
92. van Hoof RF, Merkx CA, Stekelenburg EC. The different patterns of fractures of the facial skeleton in four European countries. Int J Oral Surg 1977;6:3.
93. Volpe BT, Bradstetter RD. Delayed pneumonia after aspiration of "dashboard" fragment. J Trauma 1985;25:1173.
94. Wagner DJ, Coombs DW, Doyle SC. Percutaneous transtracheal ventilation for emergency dental appliance removal. Anesthesiology 1985;62:664.
95. Westmore GA, Whittam DE. Cerebrospinal fluid rhinorrhoea and its management. Br J Surg 1982;69:489.
96. Wood GD. Blindness following fracture of the zygomatic bone. Br J Oral Maxillofac Surg 1986;24:12.
97. Worsam B. Inhalation of multiple foreign bodies in a motor vehicle accident. Med J Aust 1968; July13:96.
98. Zachariades N, Rapidis AD, Papademetriou J, et al. The significance of tracheostomy in the management of fractures of the facial skeleton. J Max. Fac. Surg 1983;11:180.
99. Zaytoun GM, Shikhani AH, Salman SD. Head and neck war injuries: 10 years experience at the American University of Beirut Medical Center. Laryngoscope 1986;96:899.
100. Zinn SE, Fairley B, Glenn JD. Liver function in patients with mild alcoholic hepatitis, after enflurane, nitrous oxide-narcotic, and spinal anesthesia. Anesth Analg 1985;64:487.

# Chapter Thirteen

Levon M. Capan
Sanford Miller
Herman Turndorf

# Management of Neck Injuries

The neck is tightly packed with vascular, visceral, and neural structures that are prone to injury after trauma to this region, which at times results in life-threatening complications. Fortunately, in the civilian population the neck is injured less frequently than many other regions of the body, largely because of the protection provided by the cervical musculature and adjacent osseous structures—mandible, cervical spine, thoracic cage, and shoulder. Available data from major trauma centers in the United States suggest that only 0.4 to 3.4% of victims of major penetrating trauma sustain significant neck injury.[81,146,222] Except for cervical spine injury, the overall frequency of significant damage to cervical structures after blunt trauma is probably even less than that seen after penetrating trauma.

The mortality rate from civilian penetrating neck trauma is lower (2–6%) than that reported after war injuries (10–15%).[123] This lower rate may be a result of improved management, but one should also bear in mind that the destructive power of military weapons is greater than those generally used by the civilian population.[145] Death after neck trauma is usually caused by airway obstruction, exsanguination, cervical spine injury, or cerebral ischemia due to carotid and occasionally vertebral artery injuries.[110,179]

Considering the abundance of cervical structures likely to be injured and the variety of traumatic mechanisms, it is not surprising that the clinical presentation of neck injuries differs widely from one patient to the next. This variability is reflected in the scarcity of scientifically rigorous, well-controlled, randomized, prospective studies comparing various management techniques. Instead, management principles are based on a large body of retrospective studies and experience from individual patients. Despite the formidable challenges presented not only to the novice but also to the experienced anesthesiologist by many neck injuries, this area of our literature is virtually vacant.

It is customary for surgeons to categorize neck injuries as penetrating or blunt. Although from the anesthesiologist's point of view, there are great similarities between these categories, important differences exist between them, especially in clinical presentation. Thus, in this chapter, injuries caused by penetrating and blunt trauma are discussed separately. Likewise, characteristics of injuries to the airway, food passage, vessels, and neural structures are considered individually for each of the two types of trauma. Cervical spine and cord injuries are discussed in Chapters 10 and 14; therefore they are not elaborated on in this chapter.

## CERVICAL INJURIES CAUSED BY PENETRATING TRAUMA: GENERAL PRINCIPLES

The type of impairment caused by penetrating trauma is to some extent dependent on the region of the neck that is injured. Thus, it is appropriate to review briefly the topographic anatomy of the neck.

### CERVICAL ANATOMY

The classic textbooks on surgical anatomy divide the neck into anterior, lateral, thoracocervical (root of the neck), and posterior regions.[8] The boundaries of the anterior triangle are the midline, the lower border of the mandible, and the anterior border of the sternocleidomastoid muscle. A prominent area in this region is the "laryngeal trapezium," which is bounded superiorly by the hyoid bone, inferiorly by the cricoid cartilage, and laterally by the anterior borders of the sternocleidomastoid.[202] The lateral region of the neck comprises the area under and including the sternocleidomastoid muscle. The posterior triangle is bounded by the middle third of the clavicle inferiorly, the posterior border of the sternocleidomastoid medially, and the anterior border of the trapezius muscle. The thoracocervical region forms a boundary between the neck and the thorax and is occupied by structures that enter and emerge from the thoracic cavity. Wounds in the anterior, lateral, and trapezoid regions compromise the airway more often than those in the posterior region because of their proximity to the larynx, trachea, laryngeal nerves, and the important cervical vessels.[179,202] Penetrating trauma to the thoracocervical region is often associated with severe bleeding because of injury to subclavian, carotid, and/or innominate vessels.[179]

A more recent anatomic classification of penetrating neck injuries is based on division of the neck into three zones according to superficial landmarks[146,172,177] (Fig 13-1). Zone I, also called the root of the neck or the thyrocervical region, is the narrow area below the clavicles.[146,177] According to some authors this area extends from the lower border of the cricoid cartilage to the level of the sternal notch or the medial part of the clavicles.[172] Most of zone I is protected anteriorly by the osseous upper anterior wall of the chest and therefore is injured less often than zone II.[117,138,161,162,191] However, as mentioned above, injuries in this region carry a high risk of mortality because they involve the thoracic structures,[161,162] major vessels, upper mediastinum, lung, trachea, esophagus, and thoracic duct. Zone II is the area between the clavicle or the cricoid cartilage inferiorly and the angle of the mandible superiorly. This area is the most vulnerable to trauma, with resulting injuries of underlying arteries, veins, air and food passages, cervical spine, and thyroid gland. In all series but one,[146] the mortality rate from zone II injuries is low,[117,138,191] probably because most injuries in this region are easy to evaluate and expose surgically. Zone III comprises the area between the angle of the mandible and the base of the skull. Difficulty may arise during repair of the carotid artery in this region because surgical exposure is obscured by the ramus of the mandible.

The platysma muscle has special importance as a landmark in penetrating neck trauma since indications for surgical exploration of the neck wounds are traditionally based on violation of this structure. This muscle lies immediately under the skin, and its thickness, including the skin, does not exceed a few millimeters.

## MECHANISMS OF PENETRATING NECK INJURIES

The majority of penetrating neck injuries in the civilian population are produced by knives or firearms during homicidal

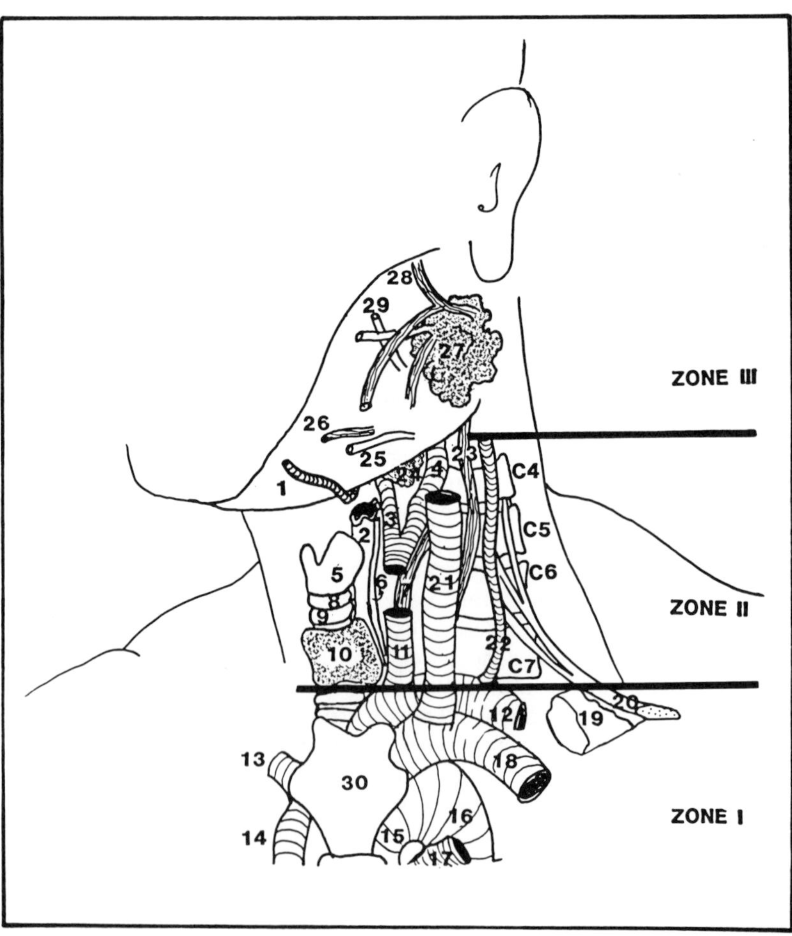


FIG. 13-1. Cervical structures contained in zones I, II and III. (1) facial artery; (2) esophagus; (3) internal carotid artery; (4) external carotid artery; (5) thyroid cartilage; (6) sympathetic trunk; (7) vagus nerve; (8) cricothyroid membrane; (9) cricoid cartilage; (10) thyroid cartilage; (11) common carotid artery; (12) subclavian artery; (13) right innominate vein; (14) superior vena cava; (15) ascending aorta; (16) descending aorta; (17) pulmonary artery; (18) subclavian vein; (19) clavicle; (20) brachial plexus; (21) internal jugular vein; (22) vertebral artery; (23) phrenic nerve; (24) submandibular gland; (25) lingual artery; (26) hypoglossal nerve; (27) parotid gland and duct; (28) facial nerve and its branches; (29) maxillary artery; (30) sternal manubrium. The thoracic duct is not shown in this figure. (Adapted from Ordog[146] with permission.)

or suicidal attempts. Other sharp objects, such as broken bottles, sharp wooden sticks, and a variety of other sharp instruments, are less frequently responsible for producing these injuries. Rarely, penetrating neck injury may be the result of blunt trauma in which the impacting object produces skin and deep tissue penetration. The type, extent, and severity of resulting damage to the cervical structures and thus the morbidity and mortality are, for the most part, dependent on the mechanism of injury.

A brief review of the kinematics of penetrating trauma will help in understanding the mechanisms of various missile injuries. The extent of tissue destruction caused by a damaging object (e.g., bullet) is to some extent related to its kinetic energy. The mass and velocity of the missile determine its energy[90,123,139]:

$$K \text{ (Kinetic energy)} = 0.5 \text{ [M (mass)} \times V^2 \text{ (velocity)]}$$

As this equation shows, the velocity of the object has a more important influence on its destructive power than its mass, and since missiles differ in both velocity and mass, their destructive power varies considerably (Table 13-1). Tissue destruction is a result of transmission of kinetic energy to affected tissue by the missile. The force (F) exerted during passage of the object is determined by the product of its mass (M) and deceleration (X) ($F = MX$). The more tissue mass the missile penetrates, the more rapidly it will slow; the faster the deceleration, the more energy will be transmitted to the surrounding tissue, thereby enhancing the damage. Thus, tissue destruction is proportional to the difference between the kinetic energies of the missile on entry into and exit from the affected region. The affected tissue moves away from the missile path, creating a cavity the size of which will, to some extent, decrease because of return of these structures to or near their original position.[59] Thus, a temporary cavity is produced in the tissue during passage of the missile, and a smaller permanent cavity remains after the missile exits.[59,123] Structures within the permanent cavity are of course damaged, but blood vessels, viscera, or bones at some distance from the projectile path may also be injured by tissue displacement. Injury caused by the latter mechanism is similar to that produced by blunt trauma.[59]

Kinetic energy deposition is not the only factor that determines the extent of tissue disruption. The consistency and flexibility of the impacted tissue also play an important role.[59] Since most tissues in the neck are soft and flexible, they absorb the shock; thus, damage to them is less than would be expected from the same amount of kinetic energy delivered to bone.[123] Also, the greater the frontal area of the missile penetrating the tissue, the greater the amount of tissue contacted. Thus, the missile decelerates quickly, conveying a larger amount of energy to the tissues and increasing destruction. Some missiles expand their frontal area (mushrooming) after leaving the gun and increase tissue destruction. The tumbling of the missile in its path through the tissue and the presentation of its profile at an angle to its path are other factors increasing tissue damage. All nondeforming pointed bullets and some round-nosed bullets yaw 180° in their path through the tissue.[59] Damage to surrounding tissue may also be increased by bouncing, fragmentation, and embolization of bullets within the body.[123]

TABLE 13-1. Velocities of Commonly Used Missiles

| MISSILE TYPE | MISSILE VELOCITY (FEET/SEC) |
|---|---|
| .38 caliber | 800 |
| .45 caliber | 860 |
| .22 caliber | 1100 |
| Shotgun | |
| Birdshot (<.13 caliber) | 1200–1500 |
| Buckshot (>.13 caliber) | 1200–1500 |
| .35 magnum | 1500 |
| 30/30 (deer rifle) | 2200 |
| M-16 | 3200 |

Unfortunately, the pathway of a projectile within the neck is unpredictable.[212] However, if there is more than one penetration, the entrance and exit wounds must be distinguished. Entry wounds are about the same size as the projectile, are rounded, and have a narrow circle of abrasion at their edges. Exit wounds are recognized by a stellate appearance of the skin edges.[123]

A classification system based on the mechanism of injury is suggested by Ordog[145,147] as a predictor of the severity, morbidity, and mortality of penetrating neck injuries. (Table 13-2). According to this classification, severity of injury increases progressively as the weapons change from knives to high-velocity missiles.

## INITIAL EVALUATION AND INTERVENTION

The general condition of the neck injury victim should be evaluated quickly to determine the urgency of intervention. Assessment of airway, ventilatory, circulatory, and central nervous system functions is particularly important. Associated extracervical injuries, although less frequent in penetrating than in blunt trauma, may be present in a significant number of these patients, especially after gunshot and shotgun wounds.[142]

Initial evaluation of any acute trauma patient is done with care priorities in mind. A history of the mechanism of injury; untoward events immediately after the accident or during transport; and changes in neurologic, airway, ventilatory, and hemodynamic status and of the patient's voice quality may be obtained before examination if the patient is stable. However, resuscitation measures must be completed before evaluation of the patient if the airway is obstructed, ventilation is inadequate, and/or hemorrhagic shock is present.

Although a large hematoma with asymmetry of the neck is a reliable indicator of significant vascular injury and airway compression, the absence of visible neck swelling can by no means exclude the possibility of accumulation of blood in deep fascial planes. An expanding neck mass is considered a reliable sign of arterial injury, but occasionally small hematomas located in superficial planes may transmit carotid pulsations and be misinterpreted as a serious injury. Occasionally, early clot formation prevents the development of visible swelling even when important cervical vessels are injured. Some of these patients develop a sudden expanding hematoma some time after injury because of recurrence of bleeding during diagnostic and therapeutic maneuvers. Repeated examination of the neck for swelling and asymmetry is necessary to detect

TABLE 13-2. Severity, Morbidity, and Mortality of Penetrating Neck Injuries Caused by Different Mechanisms

| MECHANISM OF INJURY | PERCENT PATIENTS WITH DAMAGE TO MAJOR CERVICAL STRUCTURES | NUMBER OF MAJOR NECK STRUCTURES INJURED PER PATIENT | MORTALITY RATE (%) | REFERENCES |
|---|---|---|---|---|
| Stab wounds | 20–30 | 2.1 | 0–4.7 | 55, 100, 142, 145, 172, 188 |
| Long-range birdshot shotgun wounds (>12 meters) (type 0) | 0 | 0 | 0 | 145, 147, 148 |
| Long-range birdshot shotgun wounds (>12 meters) (type I) | 0–5 | 0–1 | 0–5 | 145, 147, 148, 189 |
| Low-velocity single bullets | 33–67 | 3.8 | 2.2–12 | 55, 100, 145, 146, 172, 188, 206 |
| Close-range birdshot shotgun wounds (5–12 meters) Type II) | Up to 80 | Multiple | 15–20 | 145, 147, 148 |
| Long-range buckshot wounds | Up to 80 | Multiple | 50 | 145, 148 |
| High-velocity single bullets (rifle) | >90 | Multiple | >50 | 145 |
| Close-range (<5 meters) shotgun (birdshot and buckshot) wounds (type III) | 100 | Multiple | 85–90 | 55, 145, 147, 148, 189 |
| Multiple high-velocity missiles (shrapnel, bomb and mortar fragments) | 100 | Multiple | Up to 90 | 82, 145 |

subtle changes in hematoma size. It is also wise to secure the airway prophylactically under the safest possible conditions if the patient has a hematoma, especially an expanding one.[95]

Respiratory distress after cervical trauma suggests airway obstruction, which may be caused by various mechanisms: aspiration of blood, secretions, or foreign bodies; direct injury to the larynx or trachea; submucosal edema, emphysema, or hematoma; or external compression of the airway by hematoma. Immediate relief of obstruction either by endotracheal intubation or by tracheostomy is of the highest priority. Breath sounds and the adequacy of gas exchange must be evaluated after the airway is established. Pneumothorax may occur following initiation of positive pressure ventilation even when breath sounds are normal before intubation.

Hemorrhage and shock from lacerated cervical vessels require prompt control of bleeding and restoration of blood volume. Bleeding can be controlled by direct pressure on the vessel with a pack or a finger[9] (Fig 13-2). The patient is then transported to the operating room while pressure on the bleeding vessel is maintained. Small wounds may not permit introduction of a finger or gauze to stop bleeding. This problem can be overcome by enlarging the neck wound under local anesthesia, but blind instrumentation should not be used since it may dislodge a clot and allow uncontrollable hemorrhage to occur. Likewise, any intervention that can dislodge a clot by inducing gagging, retching, or vomiting should be deferred. Laryngoscopy, introduction of a nasogastric tube, and scrubbing of the neck should not be attempted in the emergency department if there is no indication for them.

Occasionally a knife or other sharp object is left in the neck. Although radiologic studies allow determination of the depth and location of penetration, it is important to remember that the object may be tamponading a major vessel and should not be removed until the patient is anesthetized and prepared for surgery.

Assessment of distal and proximal carotid and subclavian pulses, bruits, the size and progression of hematomas, and neurologic indicators of hemispheric brain ischemia comprises the physical examination for evaluation of vascular injuries. The physical examination, however, is not always reliable and in at least 20% of instances false-positive or false-negative results are obtained.[120] The reliability of four-vessel cerebral arteriography (carotid and vertebral arteries) exceeds that of physical examination and should be performed in stable patients who are suspected of having cervical vascular injury.[195]

The level of consciousness, motor ability, sensory and cranial nerve functions should be determined and documented.

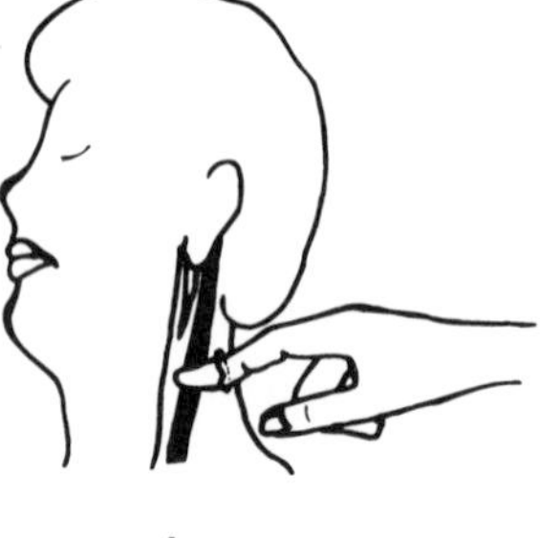


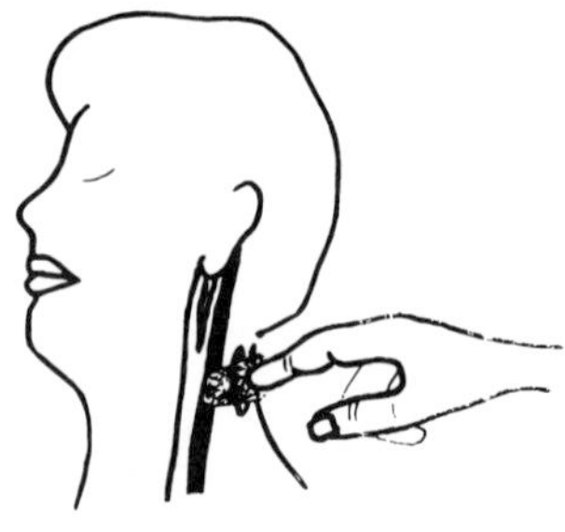


FIG. 13-2. (A) The index finger covered with a sterile glove introduced through the cervical wound tract to apply pressure on the bleeding site. (B) Sterile gauze is introduced through the cervical wound tract to apply pressure on the bleeding site.

TABLE 13-3. Clinical Correlates of Various Cranial Nerve Injuries After Penetrating Neck Trauma

| INJURED NERVE | CLINICAL CORRELATE |
| --- | --- |
| Glossopharyngeal nerve (IX) | Depressed gag reflex |
| Vagus nerve (X) | Hoarseness, breathy voice, weakened cough |
| Recurrent laryngeal nerve | Hoarseness, stridor (bilateral palsy) |
| Superior laryngeal nerve | Hoarseness |
| Accessory nerve (XI) | Impaired shoulder movement |
| Hypoglossal nerve (XII) | Tongue paralysis |

Clinical correlates of cranial nerve injuries seen after penetrating neck trauma are listed in Table 13-3. Brachial plexus injury can be diagnosed by evaluating radial, ulnar, and median nerve function in the upper extremity.

Cervical soft tissue X-rays can detect edema, hematoma, air column obstruction or deviation, and subcutaneous emphysema. In penetrating neck trauma, cervical spine injury is usually the result of gunshot wounds and is uncommon after stab wounds. Cervical spine X-rays should be obtained in all patients with gunshot wounds of the neck to determine not only if the spine is fractured but also the location of the bullet. Although radiologic techniques used for visualization of cervical soft tissues differ from those used for the spine, soft tissues should be examined in available cervical spine X-rays before special soft tissue X-rays are ordered. A chest X-ray must be obtained routinely in all patients with penetrating cervical trauma since many patients have concomitant intrathoracic injuries.

## SURGICAL POLICIES FOR NECK EXPLORATION

Surgical indications for neck exploration after penetrating neck trauma have gone through important modifications in recent years. Familiarity with these policies helps in planning the anesthetic management of these patients.

Undoubtedly, patients with overt signs and symptoms of cervical organ injury (Fig 13-3) and those in whom the missile crosses the midline should undergo surgery as soon as possible.[226a] Surgical indications for patients with minimal clinical signs are controversial and vary considerably from one institution to another. Until the 1970s, all penetrating neck trauma victims whose platysma was violated underwent routine neck exploration. This so-called mandatory exploration policy was based on the observation that patients with stable neck wounds and minimal clinical signs could have injury to major cervical structures and that delay in diagnosis and treatment of these injuries could result in life-threatening complications.[66,93,206,222] This policy is still followed in many institutions.[128] In stable patients, some surgeons who follow this policy prefer to obtain preoperative arteriograms in patients with zone I and zone III injuries to identify additional injuries and to localize the suspected arterial injury.[172,177,226a] These X-rays help in selecting the type of incision and predicting the need for distal and proximal vascular control.[64] In zone II injuries, vascular control is relatively easy, and preoperative arteriography is seldom needed.[181]

The mandatory exploration policy, which is associated with a negative exploration rate of up to 70%,[9,55,66,177] was challenged in the early 1970s by several authors who proposed the policy of selective surgical exploration.[18,188,203] In this ap-

FIG. 13-3. Indications for immediate exploration after penetrating neck trauma.

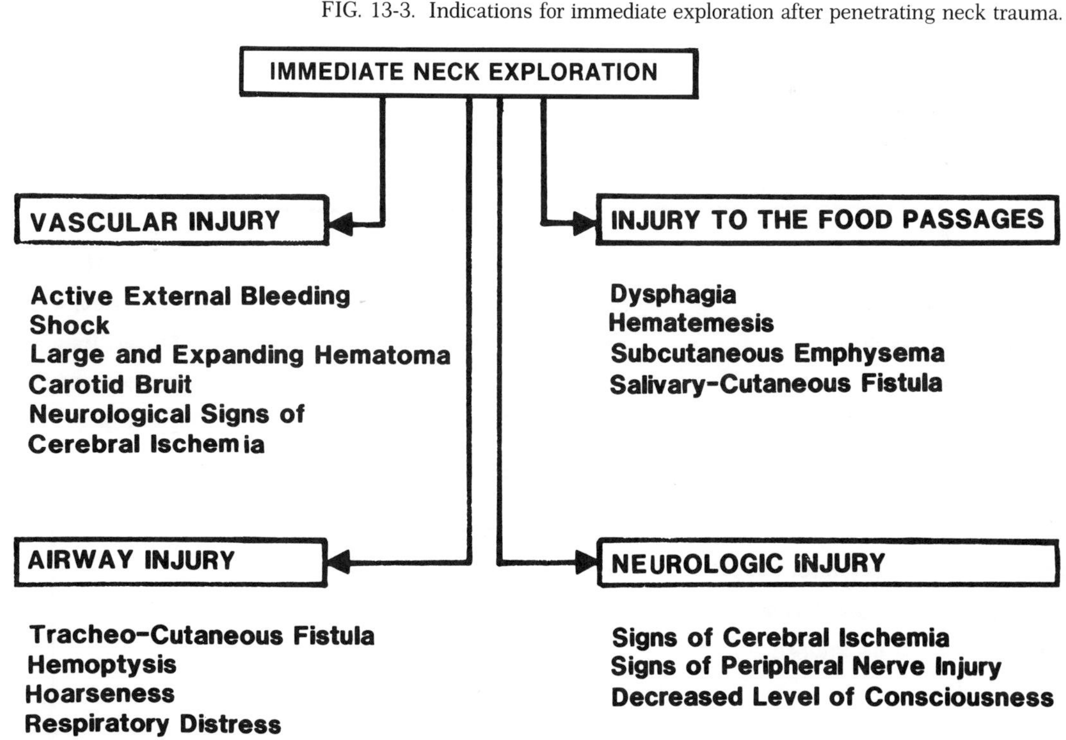

proach, stable patients are observed clinically, and radiologic (angiography and esophagography) and endoscopic (laryngoscopy, bronchoscopy, and esophagoscopy) investigations are performed shortly after admission if vascular, pharyngeal, esophageal, laryngeal, or tracheal injuries are suspected.[142,226a] Patients with positive findings from these diagnostic studies are operated on for repair of their injuries[48,55,161] (Fig 13-4). Many comparative trials have demonstrated no difference in mortality, morbidity, complications, or hospital cost between mandatory and selective approaches.[9,77,138] The selective exploration policy reduces the rate of unnecessary surgery and the small, but in some studies significant, risk of negative exploration.[9,125,172] On the other hand, some injuries may be missed with this approach, as the sensitivity, specificity, and accuracy of radiologic and individual endoscopic examinations are less than 100% and indications for these tests may not be apparent during clinical evaluation.[16]

More recently, selective surgical exploration in combination with mandatory esophagography, angiography, and panendoscopy has been proposed[123,141,221] (Fig 13-5). With this approach major cervical injuries can be identified with an accuracy equal to that provided by surgical exploration.[141] However, the necessity for routine arteriography during observation of stable patients without suggestive findings has lately been questioned.[168a]

Currently, selection of surgical policies is influenced by several factors. Missiles in the vicinity of the pharynx, larynx, trachea, or esophagus are very likely to have damaged these structures.[106] Most surgeons believe that all of these wounds should be explored surgically to prevent complications. Selective surgical exploration requires frequent observation by physician staff and an ability to perform and interpret sophisticated radiologic and endoscopic studies. In centers where such manpower and facilities are not available, mandatory exploration is probably the safest method of managing these patients.[110,123,146] Some authors emphasize the importance of knowing the mechanism of injury in planning surgical treatment of penetrating neck injuries. According to these authors, wounds produced by high-velocity bullets, close-range shotguns, and shrapnel are associated with a high incidence of pathology to major cervical structures, thereby necessitating mandatory exploration.[55,82,145,147,189] Others[16,140] use a selective approach for low (zone I) and high (zone III) cervical injuries and explore all zone II injuries. They claim that surgical exposure in zone I and zone III is difficult, and unlike in zone II, negative exploration in these levels is associated with significant morbidity.

The implications of such widely varying policies on the anesthesia team and on the anesthetic management of these patients are as follows:

- When mandatory exploration is employed for civilian neck injuries, almost all patients admitted to the emergency department with a neck injury deeper than the platysma will need to be anesthetized emergently or urgently. Although appropriate manpower arrangements to meet this requirement must be made, it is also important to realize that between 40 and 70% of these patients have negative findings; thus, the likelihood of experiencing difficulty during anesthetic management will decrease. Nevertheless, careful preoperative evaluation is necessary to identify those patients in whom management difficulties are likely to arise.
- When selective surgical exploration with mandatory radiographic and panendoscopic exploration is employed, almost all admitted patients will require an emergency anesthetic for endoscopic procedures.

FIG. 13-4. Algorithm followed in selective neck exploration policy.

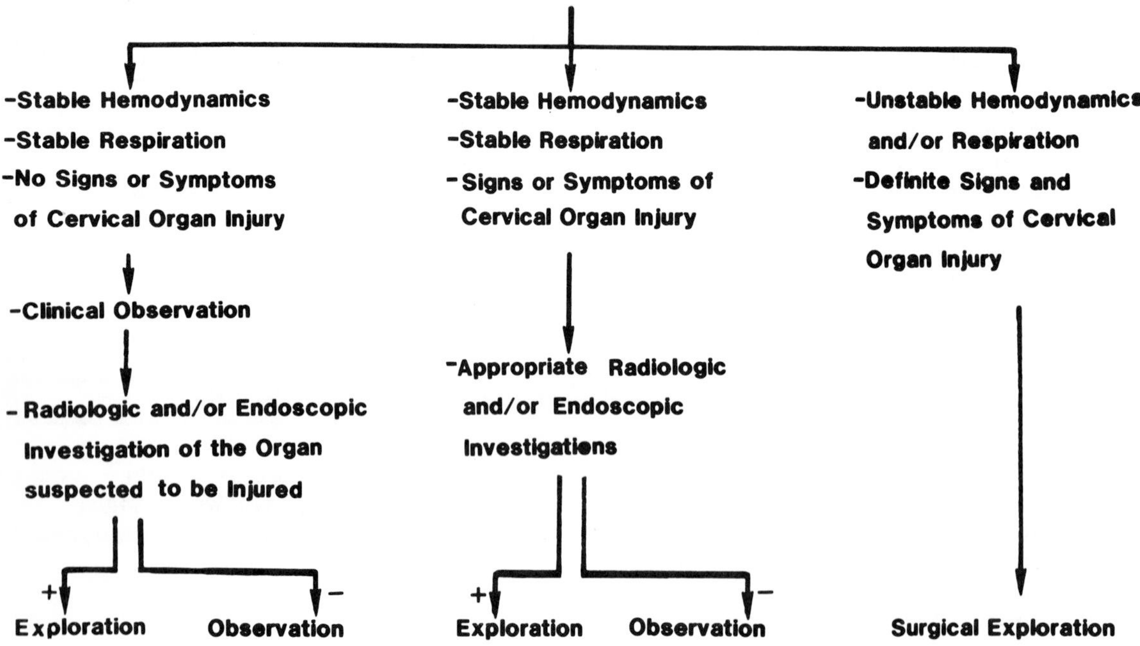

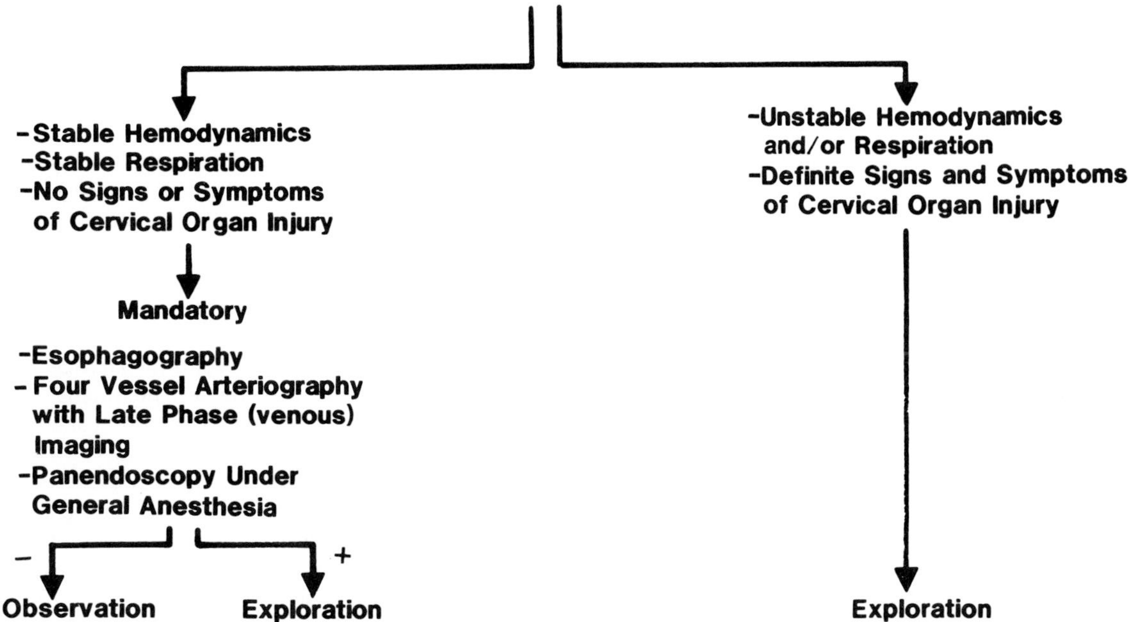


FIG. 13-5. Algorithm followed in modified selective exploration policy.

- When selective surgical exploration without mandatory panendoscopic exploration is employed, the number of patients undergoing general anesthesia will be less than those managed with the two previous approaches, but the likelihood of encountering difficulties during anesthetic management will be increased since the majority of these patients have one or more vital organ injuries. Thus, preoperative evaluation of the victim of penetrating neck trauma with a stable wound and minimal clinical symptoms should include information about the surgical management policy.

## INJURIES OF SPECIFIC NECK STRUCTURES CAUSED BY PENETRATING TRAUMA

### AIRWAY INJURIES

Penetrating injury of the larynx and the cervical trachea is rare compared to injuries to other structures of the neck.[54,96] As seen in Table 13-4, only a relatively small number of penetrating laryngotracheal injuries have been accumulated in published series over the years. The nationwide incidence of these injuries is probably less than that of blunt trauma,[81,202] but they certainly occur more frequently in inner cities where trauma caused by violent crime predominates.[54] The apparent rarity of these injuries is probably due to death from airway obstruction and associated injuries in the prehospital phase and to the protection of the larynx and cervical trachea afforded by the victim's anticipatory lowering of the head to the chest. The majority of these injuries occur as a result of homicidal and suicidal attempts and are produced by stab and gunshot wounds.[202,208] Frequently, multiple wounds are observed on the neck, but more than one airway penetration is rare. Damage to the larynx and trachea varies from tangential injury to complete transection. Often, the entrance wounds and the presenting symptoms are poor predictors of the extent of injury.[202] Associated injuries to adjacent cervical structures are frequent.[54,81,96,97,106,208] Occasionally a fistula may develop between the trachea and adjacent structures, such as the esophagus, carotid artery, superior thyroid artery, or a jugular vein.[208]

TABLE 13-4. Number of Patients with Acute Cervical Airway Injuries Caused by Penetrating Trauma in Published Series

| AUTHOR | PERIOD OF STUDY | NUMBER OF PATIENTS |
|---|---|---|
| Harris and Ainsworth[85] (1965) | 1955–1965 | 4 |
| Harris and Tobin[86] (1970) | 1965–1970 | 6 |
| Le May[106] (1971) | 1967–1968 | 25 |
| Shaia and Cassady[185] (1972) | 1968 | 2 |
| Cohn and Larson[38] (1976) | Not specified | 12 |
| Lambert and McMurry[102] (1976) | 1966–1975 | 13 |
| Trone et al.[217] (1980) | 1965–1978 | 11 |
| Black[17] (1981) | 1977–1978 | 2 |
| Schaefer[180] (1982) | 1965–1978 | 28 |
| Lucente et al.[111] (1985) | 1971–1983 | 18 |
| Angood et al.[7] (1986) | 1974–1984 | 20 |
| Kelly et al.[96] (1985) | 1964–1983 | 78 |
| Gussack et al.[81] (1986) | 1980–1985 | 8 |
| Mathisen and Grillo[118] (1987) | Not specified | 4 |
| Edwards et al.[54] (1987) | 1974–1985 | 14 |
| Stanley et al.[202] (1987) | 1983–1984 | 17 |
| Gussack and Jurkovich[80a] (1988) | 1984–1987 | 12 |
| Schaefer and Close[180a] (1989) | 1978–1988 | 34 |

Penetrating trauma in the laryngeal trapezium often results in laryngotracheal injury.[202] In these so-called cut throat injuries,[52,56] the type of airway compromise is dependent upon the anatomic level of the injury and the structures damaged (Fig 13-6). A penetrating wound above the hyoid bone involves the support muscles of the floor of the mouth, and the base of the tongue tends to fall backward, causing respiratory obstruction. At this level, the oropharynx may also be opened, and severe bleeding may occur from laceration of the facial artery.[56] The superior laryngeal nerve may be severed, resulting in anesthesia of the upper larynx and vocal cords, which can allow aspiration of pharyngeal and gastric contents into the tracheobronchial tree. Wound infection is an important threat after lacerations at this level.

Since the oropharynx lies superficially, penetration at the level of the thyrohyoid membrane results in severe damage, with the epiglottis being extremely vulnerable. A flail epiglottis characteristically produces positional obstruction of the airway. Sitting relieves the obstruction, whereas the supine position allows the epiglottis to fall back and obstruct the larynx.[163] Direct damage to the laryngeal inlet may occur, and laryngeal edema almost invariably takes place a few hours later.

Injuries at the level of the thyroid cartilage are associated with massive bleeding from the thyroid gland, strap muscles, and various neck vessels.[208] The larynx and trachea may be shifted to the contralateral side by the hematoma, causing airway obstruction in extreme situations. Phonation may be affected by damage to the intrinsic laryngeal muscles or recurrent laryngeal nerves. Stridor or partial respiratory obstruction occurs with bilateral recurrent laryngeal nerve injury.

FIG. 13-6. Anatomic levels of open neck injuries and their relation to airway compromises: 1, above the hyoid bone; 2, at the level of the thyrohyoid membrane; 3, at the level of the thyroid cartilage; 4, below the cricothyroid membrane. (From Ellis[56] with permission.)

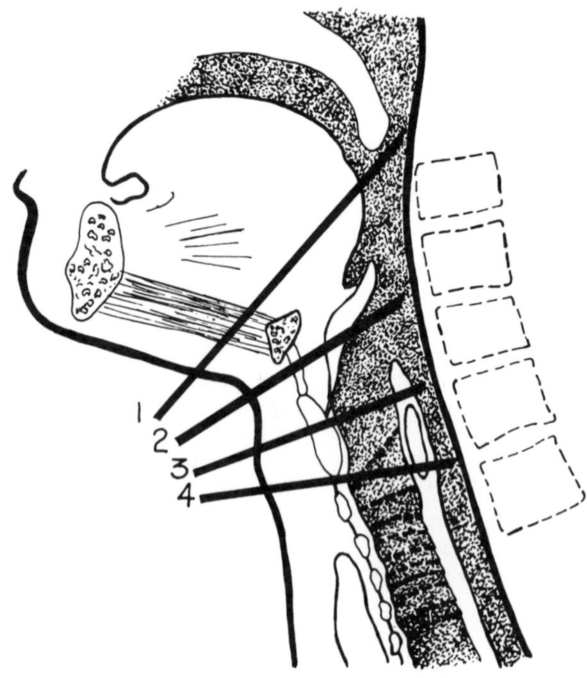


Penetration at or below the cricothyroid membrane carries the risk of partial or total airway obstruction and, if associated with concomitant vessel injury, aspiration of blood into the tracheobronchial tree, resulting in severe hypoxemia.

Depending on the structures damaged, penetrating injuries to cervical sites other than the laryngeal trapezium produce similar effects. Clearly, airway obstruction after penetrating neck trauma occurs by four distinct mechanisms: (a) cervical hematoma causing external pressure and deviation of the larynx or the trachea; (b) aspiration of blood, foreign bodies, or gastric contents into large or small airways; (c) displacement of soft tissue into the upper or lower airway; and (d) bilateral severance of vagus, recurrent laryngeal, superior laryngeal, and/or hypoglossal nerves, producing obstruction either by facilitating aspiration of intraoral contents or by causing abductor paralysis of the vocal cords.

Damage to the laryngeal nerves results in varying and somewhat unpredictable vocal cord positions. The paralyzed vocal cord may be in the midline, or partly, or fully abducted[204] (Fig 13-7). To our knowledge a clear explanation of this variability is not available, and the literature on this subject is controversial, as evidenced by at least nine different hypotheses introduced over the years.[151] Nevertheless, electromyographic studies conducted by Dedo[46] suggest that the behavior of paralyzed vocal cords is best explained by the Wagner-Grossman theory. According to this concept, complete severance of the recurrent laryngeal nerve results in paralysis of all intrinsic laryngeal muscles except the cricothyroid, which is innervated by the external branch of the superior laryngeal nerve. Since the cricothyroid muscle is both adductor and tensor of the vocal cord, complete transection of the recurrent laryngeal nerve results in the involved cord remaining in the paramedian or adducted position. Complete transection of both superior laryngeal and recurrent laryngeal nerves causes the paralyzed vocal cord to be in the intermediate or abducted position. A similar, although very uncommon situation can result from severance of the vagus nerve high in the neck or at the base of the skull.

If the recurrent laryngeal nerve is not completely transected, the position of the vocal cord depends upon the type of nerve fibers damaged. Namiroff and Katz[137] demonstrated that approximately 40% of recurrent laryngeal nerves divide into anterior and posterior branches between 0.6–4 cm from

FIG. 13-7. Possible positions of the vocal cord after recurrent laryngeal nerve injury.

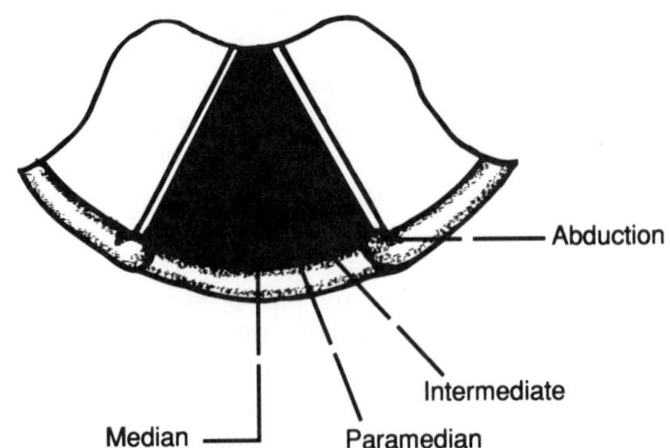

the cricoid cartilage. Gacek et al,[70] using peroxidase tracers, suggested that fibers of the recurrent laryngeal nerve collect into distinct adductor and abductor groups before entering the larynx. Thus, it is possible, although not proven, that damage to an abductor nerve bundle in the presence of an intact external branch of a superior laryngeal nerve can result in a median or paramedian position of the vocal cord, whereas damage to the adductor nerve bundle can produce an intermediate or abducted position.

### *Diagnosis*

Unlike blunt injuries, the timely diagnosis of which requires a high index of suspicion, penetrating injuries to the larynx and the trachea are obvious and dramatic in their presentation.[223,231] A sucking neck wound and progressive hypoxemia are pathognomonic for major laryngotracheal laceration or avulsion.[96,102] Dyspnea and subcutaneous emphysema are present in almost all penetrating laryngotracheal injuries.[54,96] Subcutaneous emphysema, although a frequent sign of airway injury, is not specific as it can be produced by hypopharyngeal or esophageal tears as well. However, when it is secondary to esophageal tears, it is minimal and involves the deep cervical muscles, whereas airway injury usually results in massive subcutaneous and deep neck emphysema.[54] Subcutaneous emphysema caused by airway laceration frequently extends to the mediastinum, pericardium, or even the retroperitoneal space.[58,106] Pneumothorax from associated chest injuries and pleural involvement in zone I injuries or secondary to tracheostomy may accompany airway perforation and be life threatening if not recognized early. Mild to moderate hemoptysis immediately after trauma usually stops if the injury is limited to the larynx or trachea, but continues in the presence of associated vascular injuries.[96] Inhalation of blood elicits frequent coughing spells, compromising patient comfort and oxygenation. Rarely, expectoration of a bullet after a gunshot wound may help establish the diagnosis of airway injury.[208] It is important to remember that sudden airway obstruction may develop in a stable patient after penetrating or blunt trauma; therefore, facilities to establish an emergency airway must be at hand at all times.

In the absence of the signs and symptoms described above, persistent localized pain, that worsens on coughing and swallowing, is highly suggestive of a laryngeal or pharyngeal injury.[106] Local tenderness or evidence of cartilaginous fractures may be present. The trachea may be deviated by a compressing hematoma or avulsion.[106] The voice may be weak with partial tracheal avulsion, or hoarse or even absent when the cords are involved. Dysphonia may not be present, however, as in one series two-thirds of the patients with penetrating laryngotracheal injury had no voice alteration.[106] Very rarely, even these subtle symptoms may be absent initially, and thus penetrating laryngotracheal injury may be missed.

Soft tissue neck X-rays provide ample information and should be obtained in all stable patients.[88] With this technique the larynx can be outlined, the air column and foreign bodies within and in the vicinity of the airway can be demonstrated, and soft tissue edema and retropharyngeal emphysema can be evaluated. In addition these X-rays permit the detection of associated cervical spine injuries. Retropharyngeal emphysema may suggest a pharyngeal or esophageal perforation, in which case contrast swallow studies may be helpful for confirmation of the diagnosis. A negative esophagram, however, cannot reliably rule out esophageal perforation.[97,141,221] A chest X-ray should be obtained in all patients with penetrating neck trauma to detect the presence of pneumothorax, hemothorax, pneumopericardium, and pneumomediastinum.[106]

Indirect laryngoscopy is of limited value in identifying the penetration point, but it is capable of demonstrating edema, hematoma, and blood in the pyriform sinus and vocal cords that suggest indirectly the presence of serious cartilaginous and mucosal injuries.[202] Thus, it may be useful in identifying patients at risk of airway obstruction or further laryngeal damage with endotracheal intubation. Direct laryngoscopy with a fiberoptic bronchoscope is a better method as it permits localization of the penetration point and evaluation of subglottic pathology.[208] Endoscopic examination should be performed in all stable patients before attempting airway intervention.[202,208]

### *Airway Management*

Between 15 and 50% of patients with penetrating laryngotracheal injury have moderate to severe respiratory distress requiring immediate airway management.[54,96,202] Principles of securing the airway are similar to those for blunt laryngotracheal injuries. Primary tracheostomy is recommended by many authors[30,56,106,180a,202] to relieve airway obstruction, although occasionally distorted neck tissues may render rapid location of the trachea difficult. In addition, patients with flail epiglottis cannot be placed in the supine position because the loosely hanging epiglottis, the movement of which becomes gravity dependent, falls backward and causes airway obstruction.[163] Tracheostomy should be performed at least one tracheal ring below the injury to avoid difficulty during surgical repair, infection, and cartilage absorption.[30] At times, airway obstruction may be so severe that the tracheostomy tube may have to be introduced through the neck wound[30,45,106,212,231] even when the wound is above the level of the larynx.[45]

Endotracheal intubation must be performed under direct vision. A blind attempt at intubation carries the risk of introducing the tube into a false passage and producing complete airway obstruction[7,154] (Fig 13-8). Although direct laryngoscopy is sufficient to inspect supraglottic injuries, a fiberoptic bronchoscope should be used to obtain adequate visualization of injuries at or below the glottis.[7,45,154] The cuff of the endotracheal tube should be positioned below the injury to prevent air leak and enlargement of the laceration. Sometimes placing the endotracheal tube in this fashion and keeping it in place for 24 to 48 hours may suffice to allow the injury to heal.[208] In rare instances, the trachea may be transected, and intubation cannot be accomplished. Retrieval of the distal tracheal segment after a cervical incision and introduction of a sterile endotracheal tube is necessary to maintain ventilation.[208]

If an endotracheal tube has been placed under emergency conditions without visualization of the subglottic portion of the airway, it may be necessary to withdraw the tube to slightly above the larynx and to examine the airway with a

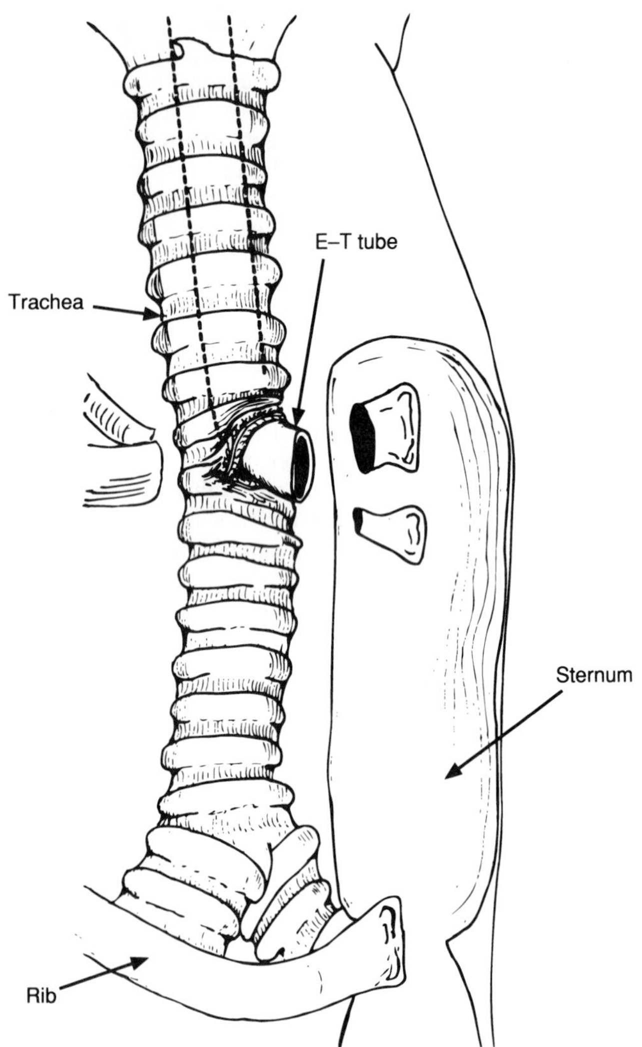


FIG. 13-8. Endotracheal tube entering a false passage at the site of tracheal injury. (From Capan LM, Turndorf HT. Airway management. In Worth M, ed. Principles and practice of trauma care. Baltimore: Williams & Wilkins, 1982; 14, with permission.)

fiberoptic bronchoscope[208] (Fig 13-9). Leakage of air from an injury just below the larynx is usually prevented by positioning the endotracheal tube cuff against the lacerated portion of the trachea; subsequent extubation may be associated with massive air leak, subcutaneous emphysema, and dyspnea.[208]

All airway manipulations should be performed while the patient is awake and breathing spontaneously.[52,56] The use of muscle relaxants and anesthetics should be avoided before the airway is under control. Because the severed larynx or trachea may be held together by the tone of the surrounding muscle, muscle relaxation may result in airway displacement and thus obstruction. The risk of aspiration is also lower in the unsedated awake patient.

Surgical treatment is aimed at restoring and maintaining the airway, providing a functionally acceptable voice, and ensuring that the larynx closes sufficiently to prevent aspiration. Patients with isolated laryngeal hematoma, contusion, pain, dysphonia, or hyoid bone fractures are treated conservatively using voice rest, airway humidification, steroids, and racemic epinephrine. Operative treatment usually involves debridement of damaged mucosa and soft tissue, primary repair of lacerations, and re-establishment of airway continuity if transection has occurred. Laryngoplasty or partial laryngectomy may be necessary for serious laryngeal injuries.[202]

Tracheostomy is performed over an endotracheal tube after initial airway management for laryngeal and high cervical injuries, whereas the trachea is repaired without tracheostomy in low tracheal injuries.[97] A laryngeal stent is used after tracheostomy in some patients after laryngeal injury to prevent endolaryngeal adhesions. Broad-spectrum antibiotics are used for at least 5 to 7 days to prevent infection. Nasogastric tube feeding may be initiated for a similar period after repair of mucosal laceration of the larynx and/or hypopharynx.

Attempts should be made to extubate the trachea soon after surgery to avoid local trauma.[96] After extubation, the airway should be assessed frequently; airway obstruction may develop secondary to laryngeal edema. Postoperative voice rest and airway humidification for a few days are important components of care.[106]

The reported mortality after cervical airway injury is as high as 15%.[96] Death is usually caused by delay in diagnosis and treatment, massive aspiration of blood, missed esophageal injury, associated cervicothoracic vascular injuries, irreversible shock, and injuries to distant organs. Unsuccessful intubation attempts during emergency management may also result in airway obstruction and death.[202] Rarely, tracheal injuries may be missed during surgery performed to repair other cervical structures.

Chronic sequelae of penetrating airway injury include tracheoesophageal fistula, vocal cord paralysis, laryngotracheal stenosis, voice impairment, and recurrent aspiration pneumonitis. Correction of these sequelae may require multiple surgical procedures.

## VASCULAR INJURIES

Cervical vessels are the structures most frequently injured after penetrating neck trauma, resulting in airway obstruction, exsanguination, cerebral ischemia, air embolism, aneurysm, and fistula formation—the most common causes of death following neck injury.[178] Approximately 20–30% of penetrating neck wounds produce significant vascular injuries.[9,37,48,115] All cervical vessels are vulnerable to this type of trauma, but the jugular and subclavian vessels are injured most frequently.[9,16,37,48,146,169]

Injuries to cervical vascular structures vary from tangential lacerations to complete transection. Often, more than one vessel is injured, and damage to multiple sites of the same vessel may be observed. As with vascular injuries of other regions of the body, acute pulsatile hematomas, external bleeding, thrombosis, and fistula formation between the vessel and a hollow viscus—pharynx, trachea, or esophagus—or an artery and vein may occur. Occasionally bullets may lodge in the vascular lumen or embolize to distant sites (Fig 13-10).

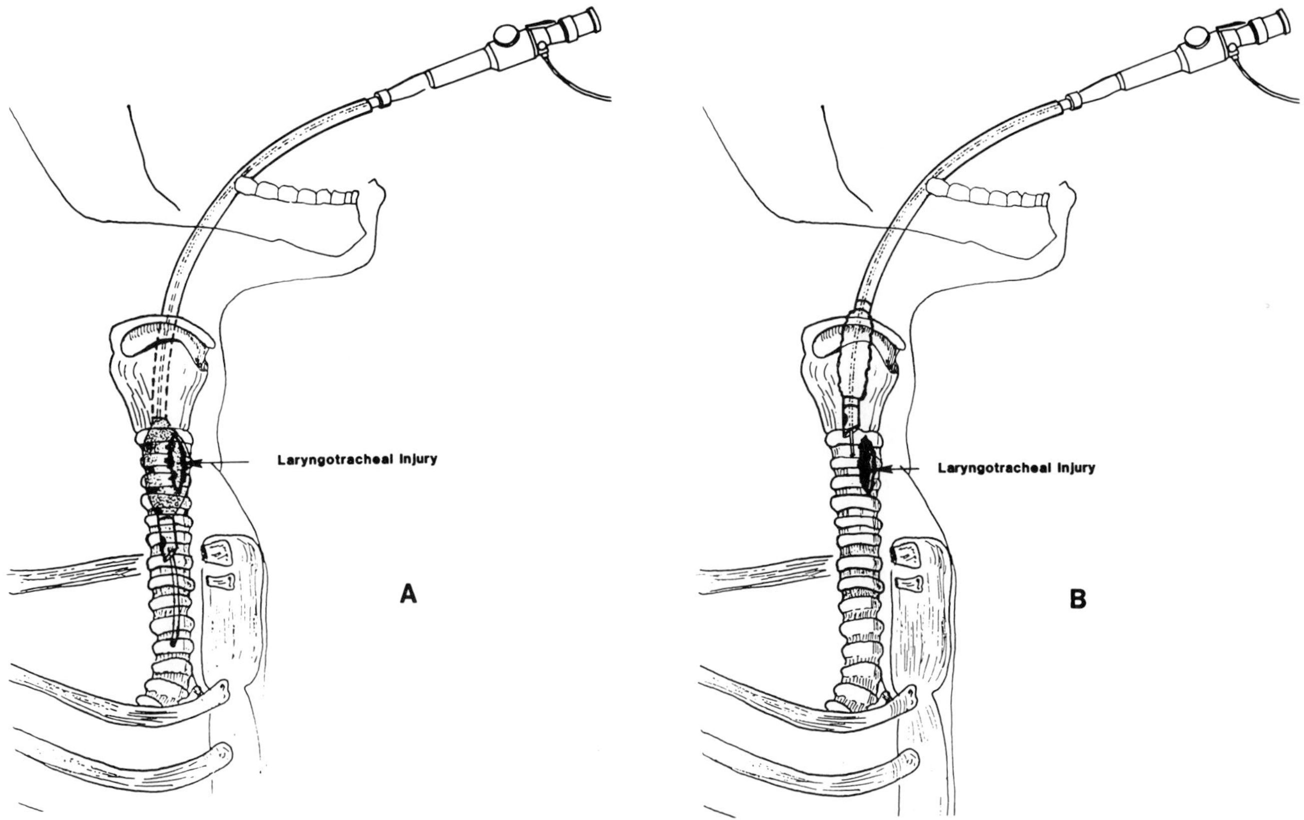


FIG. 13-9. (A) Endotracheal tube cuff positioned against a tracheal laceration. Examination with a fiberoptic bronchoscope shows normal tracheal mucosa. (B) Withdrawal of the endotracheal tube above the larynx allows visualization of tracheal laceration with the fiberoptic bronchoscope.

### *Carotid Artery Injuries*

Among cervical vascular injuries, trauma to the carotid artery is especially important. Penetrating insults are responsible for more than 90% of all reported carotid artery injuries.[196] Most of these patients require an emergency airway management.[128a] The common carotid is injured more frequently than its internal and external branches, probably because of its greater length within the neck.[23,95,175] In addition to the usual complications of vascular trauma, these injuries can also compromise the cerebral blood flow. Neurologic deficits are present in 25–30% of patients because of vessel transection or intraluminal clot formation.[23,64,169,175] Contralateral sensory loss, upper limb paresis, hemiparesis, hemianesthesia, hemiplegia, aphasia, and coma may develop depending on the extent and severity of brain ischemia, infarction, and postischemic cerebral edema.[169] The development and severity of neurologic deficit are determined by several factors: (a) the degree, duration, and site of blood flow reduction; (b) the compensatory capacity of the circle of Willis; (c) the cardiac output and systemic blood pressure; and (d) the magnitude of cerebral edema resulting from the injury.

Ninety percent of the cerebral blood flow, which in normal adults is approximately 800 mL/min, comes from the internal carotids; the remaining 10% is provided by the vertebral arteries. Thus, even partial abrupt occlusion of the common or internal carotid arteries is likely to produce significant reduction in blood flow to the brain if collateral channels are scarce. Neurologic deficit does not occur after isolated external carotid artery injuries.[169] In common carotid artery injuries the extent of neurologic deficit depends on the adequacy of collateral circulation. Since there are extensive connections among the facial vessels, blood may be shunted from the contralateral external carotid circulation to the internal carotid on the injured side and thus perfuse the brain. However, this phenomenon occurs in only half of the healthy population. In the remaining individuals, who do not have a complete circle of Willis, occlusion of the common carotid artery results in reversal of blood flow in the internal carotid artery because resistance through the circle of Willis is greater than that offered by the contralateral external carotid circulation.[170]

Patients with an incomplete circle of Willis also cannot compensate for extracranial internal carotid artery occlusion.[170] The importance of duration of carotid flow cessation is well known to those who utilize cervical plexus block for carotid endarterectomy. The neurologic deficit that follows carotid occlusion in a small percentage of these patients ceases promptly upon rapid release of the vascular clamp, whereas persistent neurologic deficit may follow prolonged occlusion. The critical period of unilateral carotid artery blood flow cessation that is associated with persistent neurologic sequelae

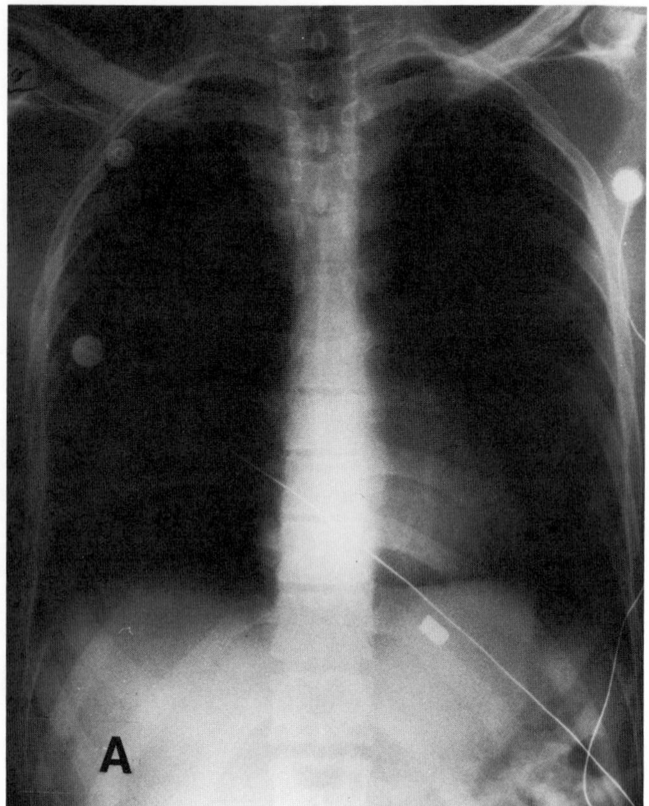


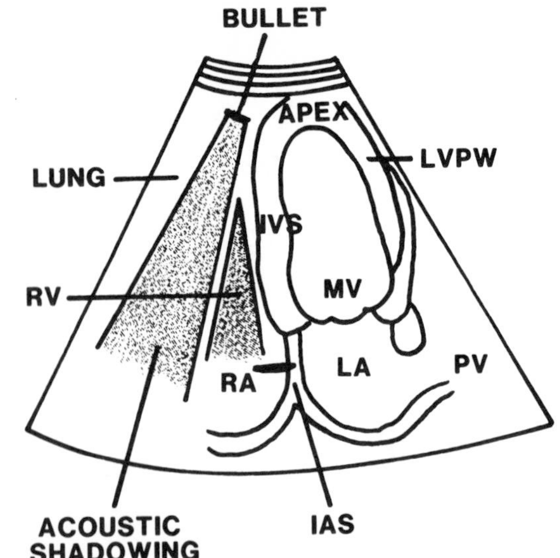


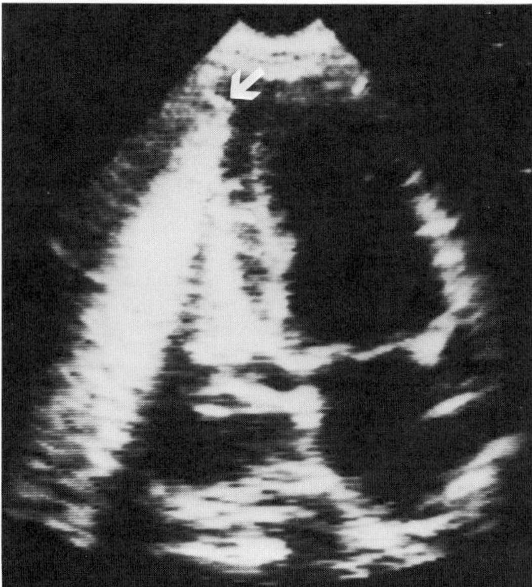


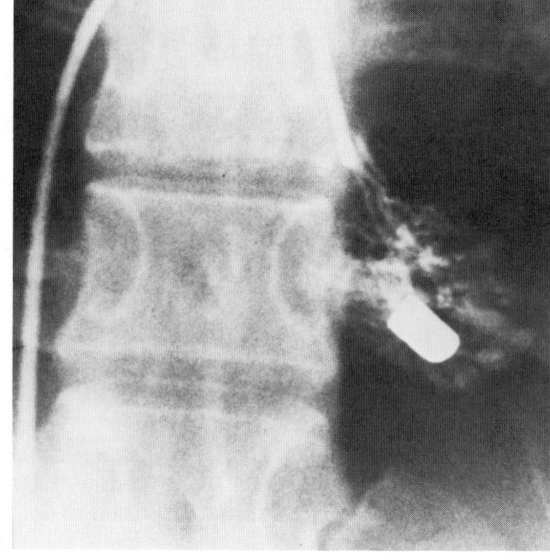


FIG. 13-10. (A) Chest X-ray: (B) 2D echocardiography (apical four-chamber view), and (C), ventriculogram of a patient in whom a bullet, after lacerating the right internal jugular vein, embolized into the right ventricle. Diagnosis was made with 2D echo. Attempts to remove the bullet with cardiac catheterization failed. Ultimately, cardiopulmonary bypass was used to remove it. Note the acoustic shadowing on the 2D-echo produced by the bullet. Abbreviations: RV, right ventricle; LV, left ventricle; IVS, interventricular septum; IAS, interatrial septum; LVPW, left ventricular posterior wall; MV, mitral valve.

in humans is not known. In animals Carter et al[29] demonstrated that complete neurologic recovery was possible when cerebral blood flow (CBF) was reduced to 2 mL/100 g/min for 13 minutes or 5 mL/100 g/min for 33 minutes. More prolonged, although less severe CBF reductions, (8–10 mL/100 g/min for 70 minutes) resulted in fixed neurologic deficit. These findings were similar to those of Marcoux et al[114] who have demonstrated that irreversible histologic damage occurred in the brains of animals whose CBF was reduced to 9–12 mL/100 g/min for 60 minutes. Clinical experience from patients undergoing carotid endarterectomy suggests that reduction of CBF to 8–10 mL/100 g/min, approximately one-fifth of the normal CBF, for 30 minutes does not appear to result in persistent neurologic deficit.[40,73] In acute trauma where such other factors as hypotension, contralateral carotid and vertebral artery insufficiency, and/or poor collateral circulation may also be present, the "critical period" of CBF reduction may be much shorter.

Cardiac output and systemic blood pressure have important effects on CBF after unilateral interruption of the carotid blood flow. Hemorrhage from injured cervical vessels or other associated injuries and cardiac dysfunction caused by coexisting chest trauma or pre-existing diseases may impair cardiac output and systemic blood pressure. Hypotension should be avoided in all phases of care to prevent the exaggeration of cerebral ischemia. Finally, the varying degrees of cerebral edema that follow cerebral ischemia cause an increase in intracranial pressure and thus a decrease in cerebral perfusion.

### *Vertebral Artery Injuries*

Until a few years ago vertebral artery injuries were described infrequently. Rich and Spencer[166] reported an incidence of 0.1% among major vascular injuries encountered in combat and less than 1% in peacetime. During recent years these injuries have been recognized with increasing frequency because of the more common use of four-vessel angiography in patients with penetrating cervical trauma.[78,124,164a] Although in the acute stage vertebral vessel injuries may be manifested by external bleeding and/or hematoma, often these injuries remain occult and are diagnosed only when thrombosis, pseudoaneurysm, or arteriovenous fistula produce neurologic symptoms or an enlarging neck mass.[173] It should be emphasized that a significant number of vertebral artery injuries heal with conservative treatment without neurologic or vascular complications.[78]

Unilateral vertebral artery injuries are usually well tolerated and seldom produce neurologic sequelae if the contralateral vertebral artery is intact and well developed;[78,124] filling of the distal segment of the injured vessel from the opposite side is sufficient to prevent complications. However, injuries of the vertebral artery at or above the level of the first cervical vertebra, the blood supply to the posterior inferior cerebellar artery and thus to the cerebellum and medulla, can produce lateral medullary infarction (Wallenberg's syndrome), which is characterized by fifth, ninth, tenth, and eleventh cranial nerve deficits, ataxia, dysmetria, Horner's syndrome, and loss of pain and temperature sensation on the contralateral side.[78]

### *Subclavian and Other Zone I Vessel Injuries*

Injury to the subclavian artery produces external bleeding, hematoma, shock, pulse deficit, and or bruit.[64] Gangrene of the upper extremity usually does not occur in normal individuals because of extensive anastomoses between the subclavian and other arteries of the neck, shoulder, and chest wall.[178] However, in some instances associated shock and severe arteriosclerosis may set the stage for this complication. If the interruption of the vessel is proximal to the origin of the vertebral artery, then subclavian steal syndrome may occur.[178] Since the brainstem, the inner ear, the upper thorax, and the spinal cord are supplied by the vertebral artery and its branches, patients with subclavian steal syndrome may manifest vertigo, visual disturbances, fainting attacks, and paresis of one or more extremities.[178] These symptoms are often not recognized during initial evaluation and appear only later in the patient's course.

Other vessels that may be injured at the base of the neck are the carotid, innominate, and vertebral arteries and their respective veins. Exsanguinating hemorrhage, a possibility both preoperatively and intraoperatively, is the most prominent risk of zone I injuries. Intraoperative control of bleeding may be difficult and usually requires extension of the classic cervical incision along the anterior border of the sternocleidomastoid muscle toward the anterior chest.[64] An external aortocarotid shunt or even extracorporeal circulation may be necessary to maintain distal blood flow during repair of the innominate artery or combined left common carotid and left subclavian artery injuries.[64,178] The mortality rate of arterial injuries in this region varies between 7 and 30%.[64]

### *Venous Injuries*

Injuries to cervical veins present with bleeding, shock, and hematoma. Venous injuries of the neck pose the danger of air embolism, especially in the hypovolemic patient with airway obstruction. Injury of the internal jugular vein occurs in approximately 11% of patients with penetrating neck wounds.[121] These injuries are usually unilateral and present little difficulty since ligation of the internal jugular vein is associated with little morbidity.[121] Bilateral ligation, however, results in marked facial, lingual, glottic, and cerebral edema and at times death. With time, some reduction of craniocervical swelling can occur, but varying degrees of permanent disfigurement are not uncommon.[121] Thus in bilateral internal jugular vein injuries at least one of the injured vessels should be repaired.[121]

### *Diagnosis*

Diagnosis of vascular injury in the presence of specific physical findings, such as hematoma, external or internal hemorrhage, distal pulse or blood pressure deficit, or bruit, is usually obvious.[98] Unexplained shock in the presence of penetrating neck wound should direct attention to the possibility of a cervical vascular injury, especially in zone I, since it may present with few or no clinical findings.[64] Subclavian artery injuries may be especially difficult to diagnose since overt clinical signs are present only inconsistently.

Neurologic evaluation of these patients should include assessment of mental status, the level of spinal cord injury, cranial and cervicothoracic nerve function, and at times of intracranial pressure, which may be increased because of brain edema after cerebral ischemia. Neurologic deficit in these patients may be caused by regional or global cerebral ischemia and/or direct central or peripheral nervous system injury. Differentiation between these mechanisms permits the appropriate direction of therapeutic efforts.

Chest and soft tissue neck X-rays are invaluable and should be obtained in all patients whose airway and hemodynamic status are stable. In addition to demonstrating soft tissue edema, neck and retropharyngeal hematoma, and widened superior mediastinum, these X-rays may help one recognize narrowing of the airway, pneumothorax, hemothorax, and pulmonary parenchymal changes caused by aspiration of blood, gastric fluid, or foreign bodies. Identification of the site of a bullet or an impaling object, when coupled with information on its entry site, may provide information concerning the missile trajectory and aid in prediction of which structures may be injured.

Arch aortography, which is performed by insertion of a long catheter via the femoral artery, is an important diagnostic test for identification of cervical arterial injuries, especially those located in zone I and zone III[182,195] (Fig 13-11). Venous injuries of the neck can also be demonstrated with late phase films. This test should be performed after the patient's hemodynamic and airway status are stabilized. In addition to confirming the diagnosis of clinically established vascular injury, angiography helps identify the location of injury, providing important advantages both to the surgeon and the anesthesiologist.

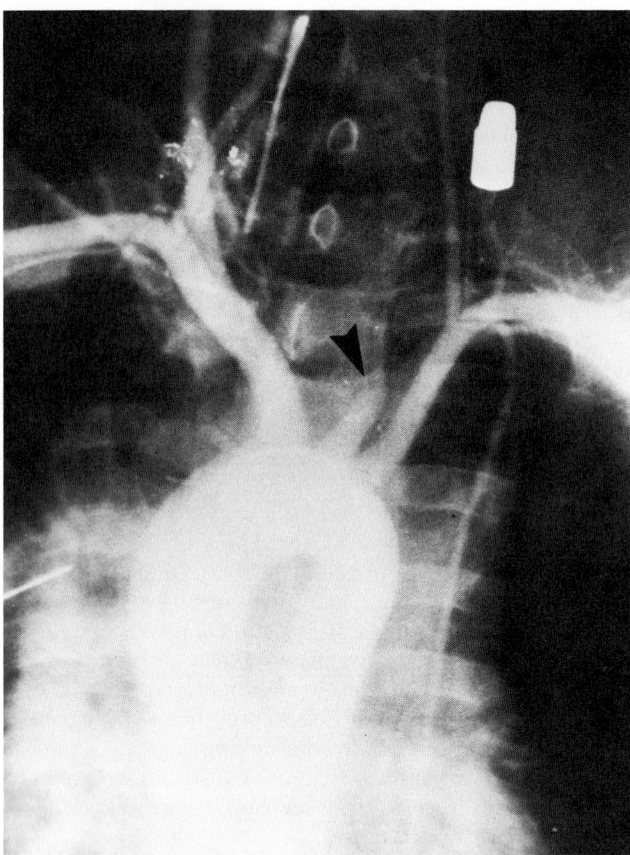

FIG. 13-11. Arch aortogram of a patient who sustained a gunshot wound to the neck. The bullet injured the trachea and then lacerated the left carotid artery. Arrow shows the stump of the left carotid artery. The bullet is lodged in the supraclavicular region.

## *Surgical Considerations*

Of all cervical vascular injuries, those involving the carotid artery present a special challenge to the surgeon and the anesthesiologist. The goal of surgical treatment is to repair all carotid artery injuries in order to provide adequate perfusion to the distal vessels. Repair, depending on the degree of arterial injury, varies from end-to-end vascular anastomosis to interposition of long saphenous vein or Dacron grafts.[169] Distal vessel embolectomy, using a Fogarty catheter, and intraoperative angiography are usually performed to ensure patency of the artery, to confirm the integrity of the reconstructed vessel, and to avoid the severe consequences of inadequate repair. Anticoagulation with heparin (3000–5000 U) into either the central circulation or the repaired vessel is usually initiated if associated injuries, especially head injury, do not contraindicate it. Activated clotting time (ACT) is monitored at frequent intervals. In our institution, if heparin is used, ACT is maintained between 200–250 seconds. Heparin neutralization at the end of the surgery is dependent upon the degree of hemostasis and the ACT value. If used, protamin, 0.5 mg/kg intravenously, is usually sufficient to bring ACT to normal values (80–150 seconds).

In some situations, ligation may be indicated. Ligation or catheter embolization of the external carotid artery or its branches to control bleeding or to close arteriovenous fistulas has been shown to be without significant ischemic complications,[140,169,182,212] although this vessel is repaired by most surgeons whenever possible. Ligation of the common or internal carotid artery is indicated when there is uncontrollable life-threatening hemorrhage or complete occlusion of the vessel with intraluminal thrombus.[212] It has been stated that reestablishment of cerebral blood flow in patients who have already sustained postinjury neurologic deficit may convert an ischemic infarct to a hemorrhagic one,[20,36,213] thereby worsening the outcome. It appears, however, that the outcome of carotid artery repair is affected mainly by the presence of shock and absence of prograde arterial flow; patients with these complications seem to be at a high risk of stroke, although not a hemorrhagic one, after carotid artery repair.[105,213] The extent of prerepair neurologic dysfunction also plays a role. Unless the neurologic deficit is severe and the patient is comatose, the outcome after repair appears to be more favorable than that after ligation.[23,98,105,108,169,178,219] Most surgeons now repair carotid artery injuries in all but comatose patients.[98,105,212,219] However, it is often difficult to determine the degree of neurologic deficit in the acutely traumatized patient. Alcohol and drug intoxication, hypoxia, hypotension, head injury, and some metabolic disturbances may confuse neurologic assessment. Therefore, some surgeons choose to repair internal and common carotid artery injuries in all patients[95,140,169] and to ligate these vessels only in the presence of proven, coexisting, severe associated brain injury or hemorrhagic shock.[169] Interestingly, in one series, carotid artery repair even in comatose patients was not associated with further aggravation of neurologic status, and in fact some improvement was noted.[169]

Internal or external vascular shunts are used in carotid artery repair if the backflow from the distal vessel is scant or the stump pressure is less than 50 mm Hg.[64] In patients with irreparable extensive carotid artery injury and angiographically demonstrated inadequate cerebral collateral circulation, stroke following ligation is unavoidable. Extracranial-intracranial (EC-IC) bypass may be indicated in these patients if the neurologic deficit has been present for only a few hours.[68,74] This procedure involves interposition of an inverted autogenous saphenous vein graft between a branch of the external or common carotid artery and a cortical branch of the middle cerebral artery using a combined cranial and cervical approach. A blood flow of approximately 35 mL/min is delivered to the middle cerebral distribution by this procedure.[74]

In patients who develop postischemic brain edema and coma after carotid artery injury, institution of controlled mechanical ventilation to provide a $PaCO_2$ of 30 mm Hg, administration of mannitol, 0.5 g/kg, and possibly furosemide, 20–40 mg, elevation of the head by 30°, fluid restriction, and intraventricular venting or surgical decompression may be necessary to reduce intracranial hypertension and improve cerebral perfusion.

Embolization techniques have revolutionized the treatment of stable cervical vessel injuries, including those to the vertebral artery.[78] Many patients are now treated by radiologic intervention with embolization of the proximal segment of the injured vessel or of the arteriovenous fistula.[182] In some patients the proximal segment is embolized first to reduce blood loss during subsequent surgery. Selected patients are treated surgically without prior embolization. Almost all therapeutic vertebral artery embolizations in our institution are performed under local anesthesia with sedation while cardiovascular and neurologic functions are monitored continuously. The few neurologic complications that have occurred in a large number of these procedures were related to the embolization of intact vessels adjacent or distal to the vertebral artery. Occasionally when the airway is not secured, cervical hematoma from the injury site or after catheter-induced vascular rupture may result in airway compromise.

### *Anesthetic Management*

As shown in Table 13-5, perioperative anesthetic care of the patients with vascular injury is directed to the following problems.

TABLE 13-5. Perioperative Anesthetic Problems Caused by Cervical Vascular Injuries and Their Management

| PROBLEM | CLINICAL PRESENTATION | MANAGEMENT |
|---|---|---|
| Hemorrhage | a) Active bleeding<br>b) Occult bleeding<br>c) Signs of diminished intravascular volume or shock | a) Control of bleeding<br>b) Clinical and radiologic evaluation to demonstrate occult bleeding<br>c) Restoration of blood volume via lower extremity veins |
| Fistula formation | a) Arteriovenous—murmur<br>b) Vessel to hollow viscera—profuse hemoptysis, hematemesis, or intraoral bleeding | a) Airway protection with a cuffed endotracheal or tracheostomy tube<br>b) Pressure on neck vessels to reduce bleeding |
| Cervical hematoma | a) Tracheal deviation<br>b) Dyspnea<br>c) Stridor | a) Establishment of the airway either by endotracheal intubation or by cricothyroidotomy |
| Air embolism | a) Tachypnea, hypoxemia, hypotension<br>b) Muffled heart sounds (late sign)<br>c) Sudden decrease in end-tidal $CO_2$<br>d) Sudden increase in end-tidal $N_2$ | a) Digital pressure on the lacerated vein or flooding the wound with sterile saline<br>b) Aspiration of air from the right ventricle via a CVP catheter<br>c) Positioning of the patient in left lateral decubitus position<br>d) Respiratory and hemodynamic support<br>e) Closed chest massage |
| Neurologic deficit | a) Spectrum ranging from contralateral sensory loss to coma<br>b) EEG abnormalities | a) Measures to increase cerebral $O_2$ supply<br>b) Measures to decrease cerebral $O_2$ demand |
| Associated injuries | a) Variable depending on the type of injury | a) Correction of physiologic alteration |

HEMORRHAGE. Control of bleeding and restoration of blood volume with fluids and blood products are the hallmarks of management. As described above, bleeding from the wound can be controlled by finger pressure during the initial phase[9,95] (Fig 13-2). Occult bleeding into deep cervical planes and the mediastinum, which is either progressing or initiated by hyperdynamic circulation induced by airway manipulation nor other painful stimuli, cannot be controlled by this method. The surgical team must be ready at all times to intervene when the rate of bleeding to these sites exceeds the maximal fluid infusion rate or when there is airway compromise. In the operating room, the patient should be positioned, prepared, and draped in such a way that access to both sides of the neck, the base of the skull, supraclavicular regions, and both sides of the chest can be gained when necessary. Intravascular volume should be restored before considering the administration of cardiovascular depressant drugs. At least two large-bore venous cannulas must be inserted, taking precautions that the infusion site is not proximal to the suspected venous injury. Since the injured vein is frequently not identified before surgery, it is prudent to insert these lines into lower extremity veins. Persistent or recurring hypotension after infusion of 2,000 mL of lactated Ringer's solution during the initial phase is a fairly reliable indicator of continuing hemorrhage and usually suggests that massive perioperative transfusion will be required. At least ten units of whole blood or packed red blood cells must be available preoperatively, and the need for preparation of additional units must be assessed intraoperatively at frequent intervals. A cell saver, if available, will reduce the amount of bank blood required, and will avoid the need for uncross-matched O-negative blood. Body temperature should be monitored, and such measures as warming of the operating room and intravenous fluids, humidification of the respiratory tract, and use of warming lamps must be considered. Coagulation profile should be monitored either by a tube test or thrombelastogram and appropriate treatment instituted when bleeding diathesis caused by dilution of coagulation factors or DIC occurs. Time constraints often preclude insertion of catheters into the central circulation. Monitoring of the arterial pressure trace for absolute values and waveform changes during ventilation usually suffices to assess intravascular volume. If hypotension and tachycardia preclude transcutaneous insertion of the intra-arterial catheter, a cutdown should be performed. If subclavian artery injury is suspected, the arterial line should be established either in the contralateral radial artery or one of the femoral arteries.

Airway management in severely hypovolemic patients and in those with airway compromise should be done while the patient is awake. If reasonable restoration of blood volume is accomplished during the initial resuscitation phase and if the airway is not compromised, anesthesia can be induced with small doses of opioids, intravenous anesthetics, and a short-acting muscle relaxant to facilitate tracheal intubation, since retching and struggling during airway manipulation of an awake patient may disrupt hemostasis provided by intravascular clot formation.[64] Patients with a difficult airway—anatomic variations, obese individuals with short neck, maxillofacial injuries, etc.—may require a surgical airway. Since some surgeons believe that the risk of infection and thus subsequent disruption of an arterial repair is high after surgery in the presence of a tracheostomy tube, it may be necessary to replace the tracheostomy with an endotracheal tube before surgery. One way to accomplish this in a patient who presents with signs of difficult intubation is as follows. After the patient is anesthetized, the neck is prepped and draped, and the surgeons are scrubbed, judicious doses of opioids and intravenous anesthetics and a paralyzing dose of a muscle relaxant are administered. A 14-gauge intravenous catheter is introduced into the trachea through the tracheostomy site and connected to a Sanders jet ventilator to ensure adequacy of ventilation. While a surgeon holds the catheter in place, the tracheostomy cannula is removed. A long introducer wire then is advanced retrograde through the tracheostomy site, and its tip is recovered from the pharynx. An endotracheal tube is advanced over the wire into the trachea, the cuff is inflated below the tracheostomy site, and the 14-gauge catheter is removed.

Intraoperative anesthetic dosage should be titrated to maintain optimal hemodynamics. A combination of opioids, nitrous oxide, and muscle relaxants is often used, although small doses of potent inhalational agents may be added if the hemodynamic status of the patient permits.

Postoperative management includes observation for bleeding from the operative site, fluid and electrolyte replacement, and assessment and optimization of renal, pulmonary, and cardiovascular functions. Airway obstruction from sudden postoperative bleeding into the neck is managed by opening the wound, evacuating the hematoma, and securing the airway.

FISTULA FORMATION. Rarely, penetrating trauma to the neck results in formation of an arteriovenous fistula or a communication between a vessel and a hollow viscus—pharynx, trachea, or esophagus. An arteriovenous fistula should be suspected when a systolic murmur is auscultated over the neck, although in hypotensive patients the murmur may not be audible. The definitive diagnosis is made by arteriography, which may also indicate the size of the fistula. Patients with vascular to hollow viscus fistula may present with severe hemoptysis, hematemesis, and hypoxemia. Sometimes a blood clot in the fistula tract prevent intravisceral bleeding, but later dislodgement may result in sudden bleeding and aspiration (Fig 13-12). Death due to hemic drowning is not uncommon if the communication is with a large artery; a fatal outcome is less common if the bleeding is from a small artery or a vein. The airway should be secured immediately to prevent further aspiration while pressure is applied to the neck vessels to reduce bleeding. Endotracheal intubation is usually possible, and inflation of the cuff often stops the entry of blood from the pharynx or the opening of the fistula.[226] Tracheostomy or cricothyroidotomy may in some cases be necessary to protect the airway.

CERVICAL HEMATOMA. This complication is a threat to airway patency. In extreme cases patients manifest dyspnea, stridor, cyanosis, and agitation. The trachea may be deviated to the contralateral side. However, airway obstruction may also result from pressure of the hematoma on the veins, which produces mucosal edema within the pharynx, larynx, or trachea.[15,84,149] As expected, tracheal intubation may be diffi-

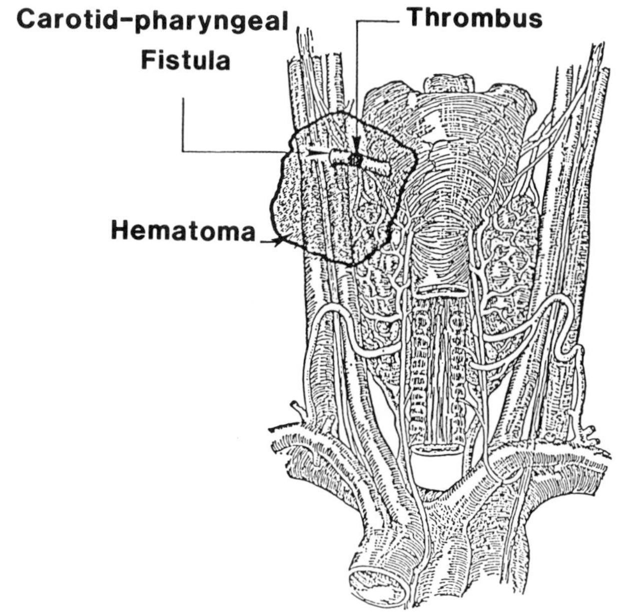


FIG. 13-12. Carotid-pharyngeal fistula surrounded by hematoma. Thrombus within the fistulous tract may dislodge during the early postinjury phase and result in severe intravisceral bleeding.

cult, and preinduction preparation for emergency tracheostomy is mandatory. The airway of these patients should be managed without anesthetics or muscle relaxants since administration of these agents may result in irreversible obstruction. As was mentioned earlier, in many centers early tracheal intubation is carried out prophylactically in order to avoid possible airway compromise by an expanding hematoma.[95]

AIR EMBOLISM. Although intraoperative air embolism is usually recognized as a complication of neurosurgical procedures performed in the sitting position, patients undergoing neck exploration are also at particular risk if a lacerated cervical vein is exposed to the air.[91] The volume and rate of air entry into the venous system are important determinants of the severity of hemodynamic and respiratory abnormalities. As expected, serious physiologic disturbances occur if relatively large volumes of air enter the venous system within a short period of time. In dogs, hemodynamic and respiratory alterations—increased central venous pressure and respiratory rate, decreased systemic arterial pressure, peaked P waves and ST segment depression on the EKG—begin at bolus volumes of 1–1.5 mL/kg.[91] Supraventricular tachycardia occurs at 1.5–2 mL/kg, and fatal ventricular tachycardia ensues at 3–4 mL/kg.[91] It appears that in humans sudden air entry into the venous system in excess of 300 mL is potentially lethal.[91] The deterioration of the patient's condition is caused by obstruction of the right ventricular outflow or the pulmonary arterioles by air bubbles.[91] When nitrous oxide, the solubility of which is 34 times that of nitrogen, is used, the size of the embolus and the potential for adverse consequences increase.

Perhaps of more concern is passage of air into the systemic circulation via a patent foramen ovale or through pulmonary arteriovenous communications. As many as 25% of normal adults have a probe-patent foramen ovale, which may permit right atrial gas under high pressure to enter the arterial side of the circulation. Although the lungs have a remarkable filtering ability,[27] in dogs 0.35 mL/kg/min of air given over a period of 10–20 minutes results in spillover into the arterial system,[89] in which even a small quantity of air may produce fatal complications if it obstructs the coronary or cerebral arteries. In dogs, air volumes of 0.5 mL in the pulmonary vein or of 0.05 mL in the coronary circulation have been shown to be lethal.[89]

The ventilation-perfusion abnormality caused by venous air bubbles in the pulmonary circulation results in an increased alveolar-arterial gradient for both oxygen and carbon dioxide. Increased dead space produces an abrupt decline in end-tidal $CO_2$ tension. Arterial $O_2$ tension may fall to hypoxic levels unless high inspired $O_2$ concentrations are employed. These changes generally resolve within about 30 minutes after venous air entry is halted.[14]

However, in some patients pulmonary microvascular injury caused by air embolism results in increased permeability and pulmonary edema.[34] This self-limiting disorder is characterized by frothy endotracheal secretions, diffuse rales, interstitial and alveolar infiltrates on chest X-ray, and hypoxemia or widened alveolar-arterial $O_2$ gradient in the presence of normal pulmonary artery pressures. The syndrome progresses rapidly; severe hypoxemia may develop, even in the presence of positive end-expiratory pressure ventilation (PEEP). Supportive care alone is usually effective, and marked respiratory improvement occurs within a few hours after cessation of venous air entry.[34]

The immediate circulatory effect of slow venous air entry is an abrupt increase in pulmonary arterial pressure as a result of obstruction of pulmonary vessels with air and probably some fibrin deposits filtered by terminal arteriolar branches.[1,91] A progressive increase in central venous pressure is also noted as the thin-walled right ventricle cannot overcome the increased resistance of the outflow tract or pulmonary arterial obstruction.[1] The decreased left ventricular preload results in diminished cardiac output and systemic arterial pressure, although initially cardiac output and blood pressure may be maintained by a compensatory decrease in systemic vascular resistance and increased heart rate.[1] The combined effects of hypoxemia and hypotension then result in myocardial ischemia that precipitates left ventricular failure. Circulatory effects of bolus air embolism are somewhat different since they include right ventricular failure and a profound decrease in pulmonary and systemic arterial pressures.[1]

These catastrophic effects of air embolism can be prevented only by early detection of venous air entry and elimination of potentially harmful increases in right atrial pressure. Not infrequently, a hissing sound is audible if the volume of air entering the venous system is large enough. The appearance of a classical "mill wheel" murmur has been emphasized by many authors. However, such a change in heart sounds does not occur until other serious physiologic changes are present.[1] Of all the available monitoring techniques, 2D transesophageal echocardiography is probably the most sensitive for detecting air embolism in both venous and arterial systems.[69,76] However, this device is expensive, is not yet generally available in the operating room, and is not safe to use during the acute stage of neck injury if an esophageal injury is not excluded. Precordial Doppler monitor is slightly less sensitive than transesophageal echocardiography.[76] However, it lacks the capability for quantitative measurement of air entry into and dissipation from the lungs. In addition, changes in cardiac rhythm and systemic blood pressure, common intraoperative events in the trauma patient, affect precordial Doppler sounds, reducing its utility in this setting. End-tidal $CO_2$ and, when available, end-tidal nitrogen concentrations should be monitored continuously since a prompt decrease in expired $CO_2$ and an increase in expired nitrogen occurs with clinically significant air embolism.[119] Although end-tidal nitrogen concentration may not rise after small emboli, its increase may precede the change in end-tidal $CO_2$ following significant venous air entry.[119] As pulmonary artery pressure increases immediately after clinically significant venous air embolism, placement of a pulmonary artery catheter in patients undergoing craniotomy in a sitting position has been recommended.[14,116] However, the diagnostic capabilities of a pulmonary artery catheter are not superior to those of end-tidal $CO_2$ or nitrogen monitoring.[119]

Intraoperative treatment of air embolism consists of preventing further air entry, evacuating air already embolized, preventing as much as possible air in the right ventricle from blocking the right ventricular outflow, and correcting the physiologic changes that have resulted.

Immediate measures in a patient whose neck is surgically exposed include head-down positioning and applying pressure over the lacerated veins or, if this is not possible, flooding the surgical field with sterile saline solution. Positive end-expiratory pressure (PEEP) ventilation and use of an antigravity suit, once considered beneficial, have been shown to be ineffective.[215,216] Jugular venous valves located at the thoracic inlet prevent the transmission of PEEP-induced increased right atrial pressure to cervical venous channels.[51] Compression of the internal jugular vein just above the clavicle is effective in preventing further air entry from sites above this level.[215,216]

Evacuation of air from the right atrium is probably the most effective treatment of intraoperative venous air embolism. It must be emphasized, however, that in the setting of severe neck injury the feasibility of placing a right atrial catheter is restricted because of time constraints and technical difficulties. Although the right atrial port of the pulmonary artery catheter has been used for air retrieval,[14,116] its cross-sectional area is only 0.2 $mm^2$ and thus offers high resistance to the aspiration of air.[39] In contrast the Bunegin-Albin multiorifice catheter has a cross-sectional area of 1.8 $mm^2$ and a significantly lower resistance to aspiration.[39] In a comparative study in dogs in which a lethal dose of air was injected via the femoral vein, the amount of air retrieved with the Bunegin-Albin catheter was much greater than that retrieved from the right atrial port of a Swan-Ganz catheter or a single-orifice CVP catheter.[39] (Fig 13-13). It is probably wise to introduce a large multiorifice CVP catheter preoperatively from the side opposite to the injury, if the urgency of surgery permits. The catheter is placed in such a way that its proximal orifice is near the junction of the superior vena cava and the right atrium, and the distal orifice is near the midportion of the right atrium. This placement can be accomplished by advancing a saline-filled catheter connected to an ECG into the superior vena cava until a maximal negative P-wave deflection (without positive component) is seen.

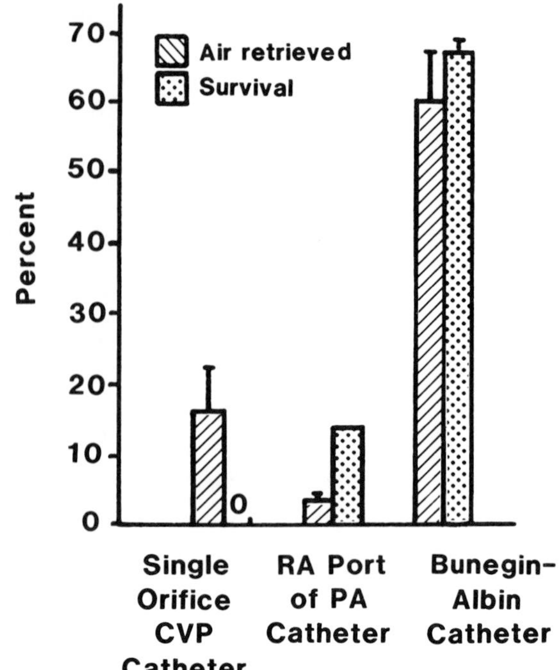


FIG. 13-13. Survival rates and percent air retrieval from the right atrium with three different catheters after a lethal dose (5 mL/kg) of air injection to dogs. (Adapted from Colley and Artru[39] with permission.)

Right ventricular outflow obstruction by air can be alleviated by two maneuvers: placement of the patient in the left lateral decubitus position and closed chest cardiac massage. The purposes of placing the patient in the left lateral decubitus position are to displace the air from the ventricular outflow tract to other sites of the ventricle where it cannot block blood flow and to keep air in the atrium away from the tricuspid valve. The efficacy of this maneuver in improving hemodynamics and survival after venous air embolism has been demonstrated in both animals and humans.[57,91] However, it may be difficult to position patients in the midst of surgery, especially if bleeding is not under control. Likewise, this maneuver is either impossible or fraught with danger if life-threatening arrhythmias, cardiac arrest, or severe hypotension are present.

The purpose of closed chest cardiac massage is to break the large intraventricular air bubble into smaller fragments so that they can enter the pulmonary circulation. The capacity of the pulmonary artery system is larger than that of the right ventricle; thus the air can be accommodated better in this system. This maneuver is easy to perform and can be instituted immediately after the diagnosis is made. In animals external cardiac massage was as effective as placement in the left lateral decubitus position or aspiration of air from the right ventricle, although the resuscitation time was shorter when air was aspirated.[6]

Supportive measures to correct physiologic alterations

caused by venous air embolism include the discontinuation of nitrous oxide, fluid infusion, and administration of inotropes, vasopressors, vasodilators, and antiarrhythmic agents as required. Cardiopulmonary resuscitation should be instituted promptly if cardiac arrest occurs.

NEUROLOGIC DEFICIT. Neurologic injury after carotid artery trauma occurs in three distinct phases: postinjury, intraoperatively during carotid clamping, or after release of the carotid clamp. In all of these phases, neurologic deficit is caused by cerebral ischemia, although the mechanism of ischemia may differ. During the postinjury phase, ischemia is usually caused by clotting of the artery distal to the injury site. During carotid clamping, cerebral injury is secondary to the sudden reduction of blood flow caused by an inadequate collateral circulation. Neurologic deficit after declamping is usually caused by embolism of an atheromatous plaque or blood clot to smaller cerebral vessels. There is little information available about the perioperative management of this complication, and much of it is inferred from experience with carotid endarterectomy. Surprisingly, intraoperative cerebral function monitoring with processed or unprocessed electroencephalography (EEG), a common mode of monitoring in carotid endarterectomy,[19,33,40] has only recently been practiced during repair or ligation of carotid injuries.[63,104] Processed EEG monitors permit even an unexperienced interpreter to recognize cerebral ischemia.[199] Experience with patients undergoing carotid endarterectomy suggests that attenuation of high-frequency activity is the most common EEG change during carotid occlusion; although these changes are often of moderate degree, major changes do occur in a relatively small group (10%) of patients. Postoperative stroke is more likely in patients with major than with minor EEG changes.[19]

Measures designed to protect the brain from the consequences of ischemia may be useful, although very little information is available at this time. Blood pressure must be maintained at normal or slightly elevated levels. In the trauma victim the most important cause of hypotension is hypovolemia; thus vigorous fluid therapy should be instituted. Vasopressor-induced hypertension in normovolemic patients may be beneficial at times since the normal vasoconstrictive response to elevation in systemic pressure is somewhat inhibited in ischemic areas of the brain due to metabolically driven vasodilation. Hence, regional flow to these areas may be augmented selectively. If used, vasopressor agents should be titrated to maintain systolic blood pressure between 130–150 mm Hg. Although intraoperative EEG amplitude and power improve with elevation of systemic blood pressure during carotid endarterectomy, little improvement is noted when the blood pressure exceeds 150 mm Hg.[73,83] In addition, vasopressor infusions are associated with significant complications, including cerebral edema and intracerebral hemorrhage into infarcted tissue. Thus, the routine use of these agents cannot be recommended.

Hypervolemic hemodilution, by increasing capillary blood flow and oxygen delivery, may be beneficial as it has been shown to decrease infarct size and improve CBF and EEG amplitude in patients suffering strokes.[227,228]

Data obtained from patients undergoing carotid endarterectomy suggest that normocapnia should be maintained. However, patients with carotid artery injuries may already have significant brain edema and ICP elevation and thus may benefit from moderate hyperventilation.

Hypothermia, by decreasing cerebral metabolism, can protect the brain against the effects of ischemia. However, the complications of this technique far outweigh its benefits. Cardiac arrhythmias, acidosis, "rewarming shock," and severe coagulopathies are not uncommon. Barbiturates, particularly thiopental and pentobarbital, given before or up to 2 hours after the ischemic insult, have been shown to reduce infarct size and increase survival in experimental animals.[129] Clinical studies using 3–5 mg/kg during carotid endarterectomy, however, showed no clear benefits from this technique.[122,132] In addition, hemodynamic depression may be a significant complication of barbiturate administration to trauma patients. Calcium channel blockers, particularly nimodipine, have been shown to increase blood flow in all areas of the primate cerebral cortex and to lower simultaneously the blood flow threshold for potassium flux and calcium accumulation.[209] The clinical value of these drugs during temporary interruption of blood flow, as in carotid artery injury or clamping, is as yet undefined.

Among inhalational anesthetic agents, isoflurane has a cerebral protective effect similar to that of barbiturates, as demonstrated during carotid artery clamping in carotid endarterectomy.[19,126,130] Critical regional cerebral blood flow (rCBF) is defined as that blood flow below which EEG signs of ischemia occurs. In humans the critical rCBF during isoflurane anesthesia was almost half (< 10 mL/100 g/min) that required during halothane anesthesia (18–20 mL/100 g/min).[126] Thus, it is probably wise to use isoflurane instead of other potent inhalational agents in patients with cerebral ischemia, induced by carotid artery injury, provided that mean arterial blood pressure and cerebral perfusion pressure are kept within the normal range.

It is noteworthy to emphasize that the measures discussed above are primarily effective in ischemic strokes that are caused by carotid artery occlusion. Embolic strokes are probably less responsive to such measures.

ASSOCIATED INJURIES. Outside of the neck, penetrating trauma can produce associated injuries to other organs, but head, maxillofacial, and chest injuries occur most commonly and present additional management difficulties. For instance, neurologic deficit produced by a carotid artery injury may be overlooked in the presence of an associated head injury. Likewise, airway obstruction caused by cervical hematoma may be ascribed to associated maxillofacial injury. These and other possibilities should be considered during the anesthetic and airway management of patients with penetrating vascular injuries of the neck.

## NEUROLOGIC INJURIES

The spinal cord, phrenic nerve, brachial plexus, and autonomic nerves may be injured individually, in combination, or with or without adjacent structures. Approximately one-third of patients with penetrating injury of the cord suffer complete physiologic or, rarely, anatomic transection. The rest develop incomplete lesions resulting in anterior, central, posterior, or

Brown-Séquard syndromes. Neurologic recovery in the patient with a complete lesion is unlikely. Patients with incomplete lesions have a 50% chance of gaining significant neurologic function, although complete recovery is uncommon and a variety of motor, sensory, and autonomic defects persist.[109] Depending on the severity of the cord lesion, varying degrees of airway, hemodynamic, and respiratory management difficulties may arise; these are outlined in Chapters 10 and 14.

One relatively common spinal cord injury is hemisection of the cord, which presents as Brown-Séquard syndrome or some variant of it.[72,155] Ipsilateral areflexic motor paralysis starting just below the level of injury and contralateral sensory and temperature loss from two or three segments below the lesion are the clinical hallmarks of the Brown-Séquard syndrome. The lesion is usually a direct result of penetrating trauma, although vascular compromise, contrecoup injury, and pressure on the spinal cord by foreign bodies or bone fragments may also produce it.[10,109] Consequently, the clinical picture may vary somewhat from that of the classical syndrome, resulting in confusion and delay in reaching the diagnosis.[72] In the acute phase, patients with penetrating spinal cord wounds are treated conservatively with stabilization of the spine, antibiotics to prevent meningitis or epidural abscess, and supportive therapy.[72] However, immediate surgery may be needed to remove foreign bodies or bone fragments impinging on the spinal cord[10] or for associated injuries. Surgery a few days after the initial injury may be required for operative stabilization of the spine or drainage of epidural abscess.

The phrenic nerve may be injured either as a result of trauma or during neck exploration. Frequently patients with unilateral phrenic nerve paralysis and thus a paralyzed hemidiaphragm are asymptomatic.[67] The diagnosis is established by observation of an elevated hemidiaphragm on the chest X-ray (Fig 13-14). Anastomosis of the distal and proximal ends of the nerve may allow return of diaphragmatic function within about a year in some patients.

Bilateral phrenic nerve paralysis results in considerable disturbance of pulmonary function.[67] It is extremely rare after cervical trauma.[174] Postoperative hypoventilation in the presence of complete reversal of neuromuscular blocking agents in an awake patient should suggest this lesion.

Brachial plexus and nerve root injuries present with weakness, paralysis, and sensory disturbances in the affected upper extremity. Anesthetic management of these patients presents no special problems during the immediate postinjury phase. However, a few days after the injury, administration of succinylcholine to these patients may result in contracture of the muscles innervated by the damaged nerve fibers and probably a greater increase of serum $K^+$ than that observed in normal patients.[11] Treatment with small precurarizing doses of nondepolarizing muscle relaxants seems to attenuate this response.[12] A devastating complication of brachial plexus and

FIG. 13-14. Elevated left hemidiaphragm caused by left phrenic nerve transection after a cervical gunshot wound.

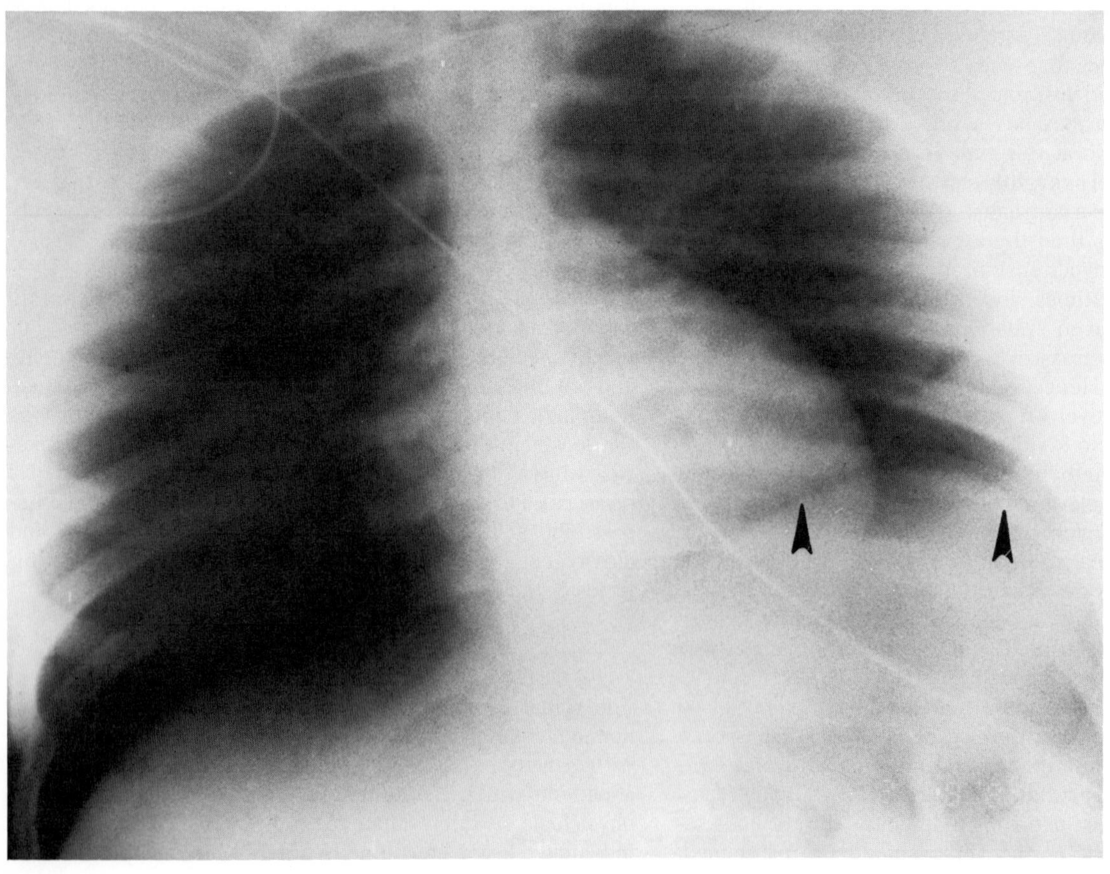

nerve root trauma is the causalgia that becomes obvious a few days after injury, which is manifested by burning pain and sympathetic disturbances over the affected extremity. Treatment involves blocking the sympathetic nerve fibers of the upper extremity as outlined in Chapter 23.

Direct injury to autonomic nerves results in a variety of conditions of interest to anesthesiologists. Injury to the cervical sympathetic chain usually results in Horner's syndrome,[102] but may also cause hypersympathetic dysfunctional states not only in the affected extremities but also on the face and eyes.[211]

Injury to the vagus nerves results in vocal cord paralysis as described previously. In addition, prolongation of the Q-T interval is demonstrated after injury to the right vagus nerve during surgery.[150] This may result in a tachyarrhythmia called "torsades de pointes" or "atypical ventricular arrhythmia," which is characterized by irregular rapid (200–250 beats/min) paroxysms of ventricular activity. Variations in QRS amplitude and polarity occur over 5–20 beats during which the cardiac output is nil and syncope ensues after several seconds. "Torsades de pointes" usually reverts to normal sinus rhythm, but may occasionally degenerate to ventricular fibrillation. Hypokalemia, which is also associated with prolongation of the Q-T interval, is likely to promote the occurrence of prolonged ventricular arrhythmias during such an episode.[150]

Although prolongation of the Q-T interval and "torsades de pointes" have not been described after right-sided neck trauma, they probably occur. Hypokalemia, probably due to increased sympathetic activity from trauma,[190] may be an additional cause of this phenomenon. "Torsades de pointes" can be prevented by administration of β-adrenergic blockers, although the use of these drugs is limited in acute trauma. Treatment of "torsades de pointes" is predicated upon initiation of a rapid ventricular rhythm either pharmacologically (atropine, isoproterenol) or by cardiac pacing, which, by increasing the heart rate, can suppress ventricular extrasystoles. In addition, serum $K^+$ levels should be maintained within the normal range by replacement of this ion and by avoiding ventilatory alkalosis, polyuria, and administration of corticosteroids.[150]

## ESOPHAGEAL INJURIES

Successful management of penetrating injuries of the esophagus depends on early diagnosis and prompt surgical treatment. Both morbidity and mortality are strikingly high if surgical treatment is delayed for longer than 12 hours.[167,186] In appropriately treated patients the overall mortality ranges between 2 and 15%,[75,187,207] although several recent series have reported no mortality after esophageal perforation.[158,221,230]

Recognition of these injuries in the immediate posttrauma period may be difficult and requires a high index of suspicion. The symptoms and clinical findings of esophageal injury are nondiagnostic.[127,221] Often, penetrating trauma injures other cervical structures, diverting the physician's attention from the esophagus. Pain, local tenderness, dysphagia, and odynophagia may all be overlooked during the initial evaluation. Resistance of the neck to passive motion, blood in the nasogastric tube,[187] and moderate subcutaneous emphysema are important but nonspecific signs. Retropharyngeal or prevertebral air on the cervical X-ray indicates the possibility of esophageal or hypopharyngeal perforation (Fig 13-15). Other radiographic signs include retropharyngeal edema, hematoma, and occasionally tracheal deviation. Pneumomediastinum, pneumothorax, and even pneumopericardium may be present, although these findings are more common after thoracic esophageal injury. In gunshot wounds, bullets located in proximity to the esophagus or traversing the midline are likely to have caused esophageal injury.[152]

Neither esophagography nor esophagoscopy alone can rule out esophageal injury with absolute certainty.[97,141,221] A combination of these tests, however, is considered reliable.[221] General anesthesia is required for esophagoscopy since the fiberoptic instrument is unreliable for this purpose[221] and rigid esophagoscopy is quite uncomfortable for the patient.

In most instances, esophageal injuries are accompanied by other trauma to organs.[207] Concomitant airway injuries are common; about 20–25% of victims of tracheobronchial injury also have esophageal injury.[53,60,97]

The most devastating complication of undetected esophageal perforation is infection. Periesophageal inflammation can readily extend to the mediastinum and result in generalized sepsis with multiorgan system failure. Mediastinitis, characterized by mediastinal widening, pleural effusion, and sepsis, develops within 24–48 hours after trauma. Treatment involves prompt drainage, broad-spectrum antibiotic coverage,

FIG. 13-15. Prevertebral air in a patient with perforated hypopharynx after a gunshot wound.

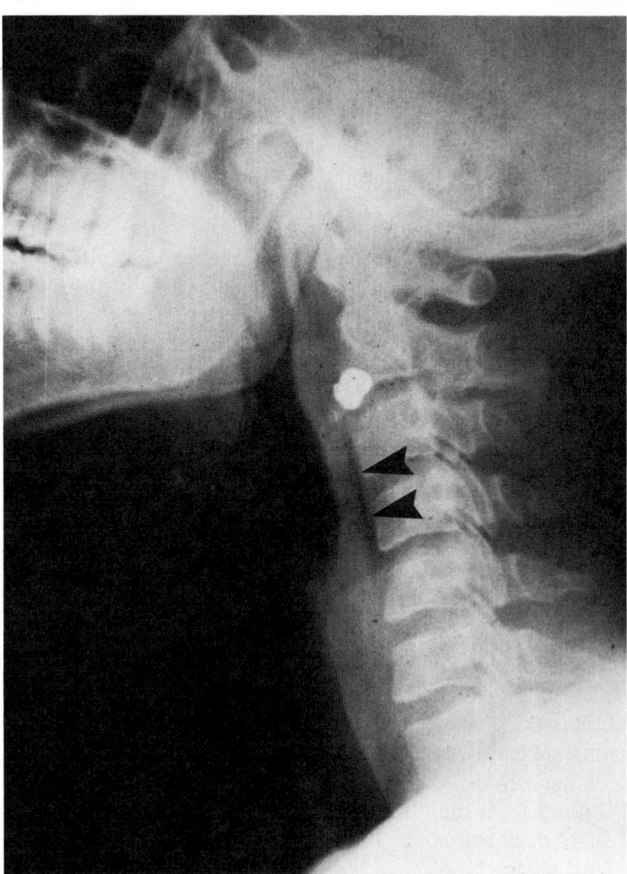

hyperalimentation, and organ support. Tracheoesophageal fistula can develop as a result of trauma or surgery.[74,97] Pulmonary aspiration with severe pneumonitis complicates the clinical course of these patients.

During the acute phase, anesthetic management of isolated penetrating esophageal wounds is the same as that provided to any acute trauma patient. The specific anesthetic technique should depend on the degree of airway difficulty, pulmonary and cardiac dysfunction, hemorrhage, and mental disturbance resulting from associated injuries. When surgery is performed between 12 and 36 hours after the injury, many of these problems have been brought under control and anesthetic difficulties at this time arise from cervical edema and sepsis. Unless, as occurs in rare situations, significant airway distortion from external compression by a paraesophageal collection occurs or the airway mucosa becomes edematous, cervical swelling at this time is usually inconsequential. Sepsis during this stage is also rarely associated with major organ dysfunction. When surgery is delayed longer than 48 hours after injury, most patients develop the full-blown picture of sepsis, especially if appropriate antibiotic treatment has not been used. Perioperative management of these patients should be based on the guidelines provided in Chapters 26 and 27.

Tracheoesophageal fistula usually develops between 6 and 10 days after the injury. Pneumonia caused by aspiration of pharyngeal and gastric contents often results in significant shunting and hypoxemia. Anesthetic management of these patients requires placement of the endotracheal tube cuff at or below the level of the fistulous tract, preferably with guidance of a fiberoptic bronchoscope to prevent further aspiration. Other important measures include adequate tracheobronchial suctioning, titration of PEEP (if necessary), and monitoring of hemodynamic and oxygenation status.

### THORACIC DUCT INJURIES

Penetrating and very rarely blunt trauma to the left side of the root of the neck may injure the thoracic duct. If missed or not ligated during exploration, thoracic duct injuries may result in either chyloma formation in the extrapleural supraclavicular region or in chylothorax if the accumulated lymph in the neck dissects into the pleural cavity.[160,192,210] Fortunately, these complications are rare.

Chyle is a milky-white, slightly alkaline, odorless, bacteriostatic fluid that contains protein and fat at concentrations above serum levels.[210] Thus, its persistent leakage or accumulation in the thoracic cavity results in severe caloric loss. Normally, 1500–2500 mL/day of chyle flows through the thoracic duct. This flow is highly dependent on the level of activity, fat content of the diet, and gastrointestinal function. The flow can be as low as 10 to 15 mL/h in immobilized or starving individuals or in those on gastric suction.[210]

The diagnosis of chylothorax may be difficult if other causes of pleural effusion are superimposed. Nevertheless, a milky-white appearance of the exudate and the demonstration of fat globules, chylomicron bands, and high triglyceride content in the fluid from the chest tube establish the diagnosis.[210] Adequate drainage of the chylothorax fluid and dietary control are two important principles in the management of this problem.[160,210] Dietary control is aimed at maintaining adequate caloric intake as for any critically ill or injured patient and decreasing the flow of chyle. These goals are accomplished by using enteral formulas with a fat content no greater than 1 g/L or a low-fat diet supplemented with medium-chain triglycerides. The fat contained in such formulas tends to select the portal system, rather than the thoracic duct, thereby reducing the flow of chyle.[160] If this regimen is not helpful in reducing chylous leakage, discontinuation of enteral feeding and institution of total parenteral nutrition with adequate caloric and protein intake usually allow spontaneous closure of the fistula.[210]

Ligation of the thoracic duct, although required infrequently, may be indicated in the following situations:[210] (a) excessive chylous drainage, usually more than 1500 mL/day in adults or 100 mL/year of age/day in children; (b) persistent chylous flow despite 2 weeks of conservative treatment; and (c) the development of severe metabolic complications.

In a patient with chylothorax, fluid and electrolyte balance should be assessed and appropriate replacement administered before anesthesia and surgery. The intraoperative responses to anesthetic and adjunct drugs should be monitored carefully since they may be altered because of the depleted serum protein concentration.

## CERVICAL INJURIES CAUSED BY BLUNT TRAUMA

Unlike penetrating trauma in which the cervical wound itself is a major stimulus to suspicion of injuries to various structures, blunt trauma to the neck is often associated with few physical findings even though serious injuries may be present.[7,87,197,200] Therefore, a high index of suspicion must be maintained to avoid the devastating complications of missed injuries. Associated injuries, most notably to the cervical spine, face, head, and chest, are common after blunt neck trauma and frequently complicate treatment.[7,28,135] The management of blunt neck trauma revolves largely around establishment and maintenance of airway patency and integrity of the spine. In addition, injuries to other neck structures, especially the esophagus and carotid arteries, must be recognized and treated in a timely fashion.

### AIRWAY INJURIES

Although the airway is rarely damaged by blunt trauma,[61,81,214] there has been an increase in the frequency of these injuries during the past three decades.[86,134,144,180a] It is, however, likely that with more widespread use of seat belts in automobiles and the declining overall frequency of injury[103] the incidence of blunt laryngotracheal trauma will decrease in the future. In fact, a decline in automobile-related airway trauma has already been reported from one center.[180,180a] Overall only 5–10% of patients who sustain blunt cervical trauma develop airway injury.[81] Thus even in most major trauma centers no more than five such patients are seen annually (Table 13-6).

TABLE 13-6. Number of Patients with Acute Cervical Airway Injuries Caused by Blunt Trauma in Published Series

| AUTHOR | PERIOD OF STUDY | NUMBER OF PATIENTS |
|---|---|---|
| Harris and Ainsworth[85] (1965) | 1955–1965 | 18 |
| Downey et al.[50] (1967) | 1965–1967 | 9 |
| Harris and Tobin[86] (1970) | 1965–1970 | 21 |
| Olson and Miles[144] (1971) | Not specified | 25 |
| Shaia and Cassady[185] (1972) | 1968 | 4 |
| Cohn and Larson[38] (1976) | Not specified | 18 |
| Lambert and McMurry[102] (1976) | 1966–1975 | 10 |
| Trone et al.[217] (1980) | 1965–1978 | 42 |
| Black[17] (1981) | 1977–1978 | 13 |
| Schaefer[180] (1982) | 1965–1978 | 59 |
| Kelly et al.[96] (1985) | 1964–1983 | 2 |
| Angood et al.[7] (1986) | 1974–1984 | 14 |
| Gussack et al.[81] (1986) | 1980–1985 | 4 |
| Mathisen and Grillo[118] (1987) | Not specified | 5 |
| Edwards et al.[54] (1987) | 1974–1985 | 6 |
| Gussack and Jurkovich[80a] (1988) | 1984–1987 | 9 |
| Schaefer and Close[180a] (1989) | 1987–1988 | 34 |

## MECHANISM OF INJURY

The cause is usually a head-on motor vehicle collision in which rapid deceleration causes the extended neck of the unrestrained occupant to strike the dashboard or the steering wheel.[113,223] The victim is often the driver rather than the passenger since the neck is closer to the steering wheel than to the dashboard.[17,138] A similar direct anterior cervical impact can also result during a snowmobile, motorcycle, or all-terrain vehicle accident when an unseen chain, wire, or cable strikes the neck (clothesline injury).[197] Less frequently, laryngeal injury results from a direct blow to the neck during sports or altercations[113] or from strangulation attempts.[201]

In most instances the larynx and trachea are compressed between the impacting object and the vertebral bodies, with resultant ligamentous membrane rupture or fracture of the laryngotracheal cartilages.[136,171] In addition, the glottis closes in anticipation of a blow, converting the trachea to an air-filled rigid tube. A sudden elevation of intraluminal pressure by a compressive force against the chest increases the ligamentous and cartilaginous damage. Cervical hyperextension, by pulling the larynx away from the relatively fixed trachea, facilitates avulsion injury[136,171,183] (Fig 13-16).

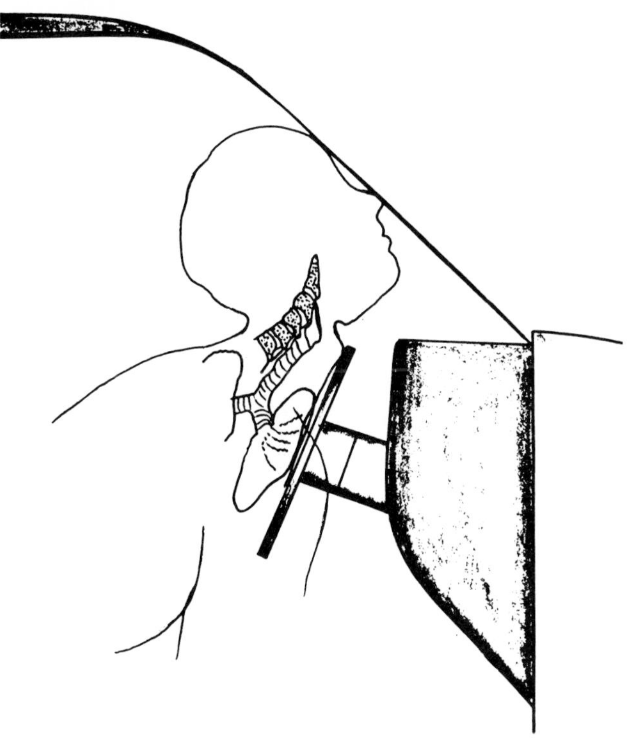

FIG. 13-16. Mechanism of laryngotracheal injury in motor vehicle accidents. Note that (a) the neck is extended, (b) the entire body of the victim moves forward, (c) the chest is compressed against the steering wheel, (d) the neck strikes the steering wheel and (e) the forehead strikes the windshield.

## LARYNGOTRACHEAL PATHOLOGY

The type and extent of laryngotracheal injury are determined by multiple factors: the magnitude and direction of the shearing force, structures affected by the force vector, the position of the cervical spine during impact, the age of the patient, and the consistency of the laryngotracheal cartilage and the soft tissue. Depending on these factors, laryngotracheal contusion, edema, hematoma, laceration, avulsion, and/or fracture and dislocation of the thyroid, cricoid, or tracheal cartilages can occur.[24,135]

The distensible nature of the subglottic and supraglottic submucosa allows rapid accumulation of edema fluid. As the vertical spread of accumulated edema is limited by the conus elasticus, subglottic endolaryngeal swelling tends to be circumferential, thereby increasing the potential for airway obstruction.[200] Sometimes air from the airway or paratracheal tissues also finds its way into the submucosal space and further reduces the luminal diameter of the larynx and or trachea. Air may also cause epiglottic emphysema and further contribute to airway compromise.[176,183] The major portion of submucosal edema and hematoma is formed within about 1 hour after the trauma. Airway obstruction caused by endolaryngeal swelling is unlikely to occur later than 6 hours after injury unless coughing, straining, or speaking increases the quantity of subcutaneous air or reinitiates intramural bleeding.[131] Although fracture can occur in any age group, older persons with calcified cartilages are more susceptible to this type of injury.[113]

Fractures are usually vertical, but horizontal or comminuted fractures also occur[24,159] (Fig 13-17). Both thyroid and cricoid cartilages are composed of hyaline cartilage and are therefore prone to fracture. Cuneiform, corniculate, arytenoid, and epiglottic cartilages are made of fibroelastic tissue, which

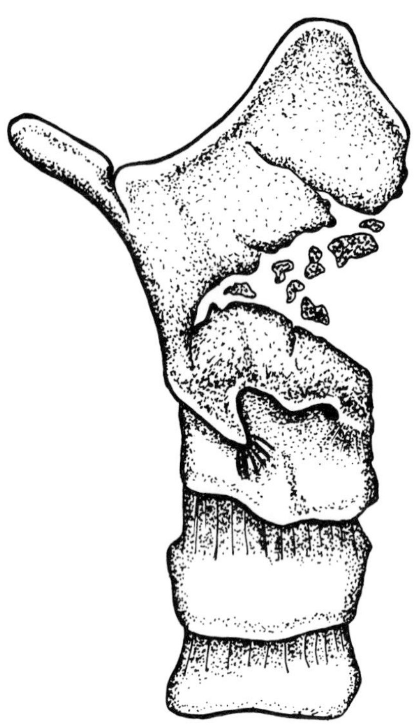

FIG. 13-17. A supraglottic comminuted laryngeal fracture following blunt trauma to the neck. (Adapted from Bryce[24] with permission.)

is more likely to avulse or dislocate than fracture.[31] The arytenoid cartilages are especially liable to dislocate and thus interfere with the function of the thyroarytenoid ligaments (the vocal cords). The hyoid bone, although calcified, is rarely injured because it is protected by the overhanging chin and cushioned by its surrounding muscles.

A system devised by Harris and Ainsworth[85] in 1965 and modified by Potter et al[159] in 1970 may be used to classify the type, location, and severity of injury (Table 13-7). CT scanning allows noninvasive assessment of these injuries based on this classification.[135]

Frequently, soft tissue, supraglottic, glottic, and infraglottic injuries are found in varying combinations in the same patient. The trachea may be lacerated or transected, especially in younger patients in whom intercartilaginous connective membranes are not strong and thus are susceptible to interruption.[4,87,205,214] A common site of transection is the region between the cricoid and the trachea where the connective tissue is relatively weak[4,5,31] (Fig 13-18). Laryngotracheal separation injuries are often accompanied by avulsion of the recurrent laryngeal nerves,[4,5,41,194] causing vocal cord paralysis, usually in adduction.

## ASSOCIATED INJURIES

Cervical spine injury is a very common accompaniment of blunt laryngotracheal injury,[102,144] and must be considered present until proven otherwise.[54,231] The esophagus may be lacerated when it is crushed between the thyroid or cricoid cartilage and the sharp edge of an osteophyte or a fractured fragment of the spine.[164] Tracheoesophageal fistula may develop early after the injury or a few days following corrective surgery. It can be detected radiographically by the presence of an air column in the esophagus.

Closed head injury is a frequent occurrence in this type of trauma[87] and may give the false impression that the airway obstruction is caused by posterior displacement of the tongue and epiglottis in the unconscious patient.[223] Hypoxemia, a frequent finding in laryngotracheal injury, is particularly deleterious in the presence of concomitant head injury as it not only deprives the brain of necessary oxygen and results in further neuronal loss but it also increases cerebral blood flow and thus intracranial pressure.[3,214] Every effort must be made to minimize the hypoxic period. Maxillofacial trauma can occur,[144] but associated mandibular injury is uncommon; the protective effect of the chin prevents damage to the larynx.[17] As in the head-injured patient, airway obstruction caused by neck trauma may be ascribed to concomitant midface injuries. This assumption may lead to performance of an emergency cricothyroidotomy that, as described below, may convert par-

TABLE 13-7. Classification System for Acute Blunt Laryngotracheal Injury

| TYPE OF INJURY | LOCATION OF INJURY | EXTENT OF INJURY |
|---|---|---|
| Soft tissue | Supraglottic, glottic, infraglottic | Superficial mucosal lacerations<br>Hematoma (aryepiglottic folds, arytenoids, vocal cords) |
| Supraglottic | Epiglottis, hypopharynx, aryepiglottic folds, false cords, thyroid cartilage | Epiglottic displacement or avulsion<br>Laceration of false cords<br>Pharyngolaryngeal fistula via false cords<br>Thyroid cartilage fracture<br>Aryepiglottic fold laceration or avulsion |
| Glottic | Thyroid cartilage, vocal cords, arytenoids | Thyroid cartilage fracture<br>Vocal cord laceration<br>Arytenoid avulsion |
| Subglottic | Cricoid ring, trachea | Cricoid cartilage fracture<br>Tracheal cartilage fracture<br>Cricotracheal separation |

(From Potter et al.[159])

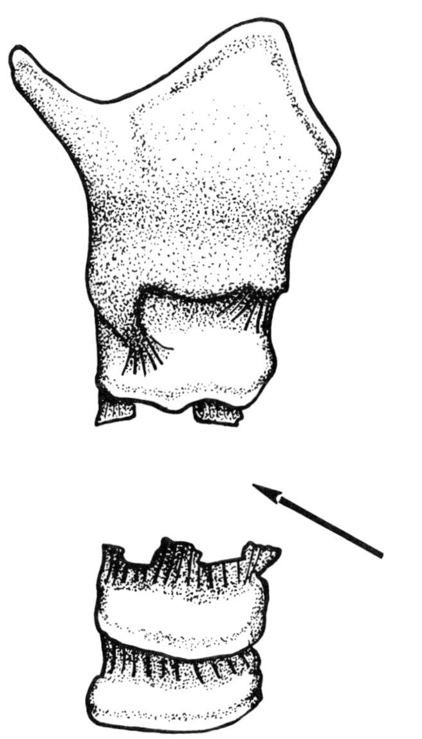

FIG. 13-18. Cricotracheal separation after blunt trauma to the neck. (Adapted from Bryce[24] with permission.)

tial airway obstruction to complete closure. Associated chest injury may produce a wide spectrum of symptoms, diverting suspicion from laryngotracheal injury.[205]

## DIAGNOSTIC CONSIDERATIONS

Early recognition of these injuries is based on a high index of suspicion,[107,223] attention to certain key signs and symptoms,[28,102,135] adequate physical examination,[28] and judicious use of ancillary procedures and radiologic examinations.[135] At times, the absence of symptoms and physical signs results in diagnosis of these injuries during airway management or anesthetic induction when passage of an endotracheal tube becomes difficult or cyanosis develops because of failure to ventilate the lungs.[65,87,193,205,214] However, certain signs and symptoms, although nonspecific, are highly suggestive of laryngeal and tracheal injury.[102,112] Dysphonia is the most common presenting symptom and may vary from mild hoarseness to aphonia depending on the structures involved.[17] The voice may be impaired secondary to cerebral damage and/or injury to laryngeal structures or innervation. Laryngoscopy will usually help differentiate the etiology.[223] A normal appearance of the larynx suggests cerebral damage. A muffled voice suggests injury to the larynx itself, whereas hoarseness is usually caused by injury to laryngeal nerves, laryngeal edema, or hematoma.[50] Vocal impairment cannot be taken as a guide to the severity of injury,[200] but a progressive change in voice quality suggests worsening of the injury and requires prompt intervention.[28] Dyspnea and stridor are frequent symptoms, but may be absent in as many as 30% of patients.[7] Other symptoms include hemoptysis, dysphagia, odynophagia, and cervical pain and tenderness.

Physical examination may reveal cervical ecchymoses, subcutaneous emphysema, or flattening of the anterior neck because of absence of the thyroid cartilage prominence. Gross subcutaneous emphysema is the most common sign of blunt laryngotracheal trauma.[214] Frequently it may dissect into deep tissues, the mediastinum, and the retroperitoneum.[58] Superficial signs usually do not reflect the severity of laryngeal injury; severe laryngeal damage may be present despite minimal soft tissue injury to the anterior aspect of the neck.[28,85,87,99] The mechanisms of symptoms, and signs of blunt laryngotracheal injury are given in Table 13-8.

Definitive diagnosis of suspected laryngotracheal injury is made by radiographic and endoscopic studies. However, performance of these tests during initial management should depend on the patient's condition. Airway obstruction, hemodynamic instability, and life-threatening associated injuries must be treated before these tests are considered. Soft-tissue anteroposterior and lateral neck X-rays are usually helpful in identifying edema and subcutaneous emphysema within the cervical soft tissue and the retropharyngeal space. In addition, one may be able to detect posterior displacement of the epiglottis and distortion of the laryngeal air column.[79] Important signs in lateral cervicofacial X-rays are the position of the hyoid bone in relation to the cervical spine and the mandible and the distance between the mandibular angle and the hyoid cornua. Normally the body of the hyoid bone is located at or below the upper level of the third cervical vertebral body, and the distance between the mandibular angle and the hyoid cornua is more than 2 cm (Fig 13-19). In patients with cricotracheal separation the hyoid bone moves upward and is found above the upper level of the third cervical vertebra on X-ray. Likewise, the distance between the mandibular angle and the hyoid cornua is then less than 2 cm[157,197] (Fig 13-20).

Computed tomography (CT) scanning is an excellent method for diagnosis of laryngeal injuries.[81,135,200] It may detect an unsuspected injury, confirm the diagnosis of a suspected laryngotracheal fracture, and help judge the severity

Table 13-8 Mechanisms of Symptoms, and Signs of Blunt Laryngotracheal Injuries

| SYMPTOMS AND SIGNS | MECHANISMS |
|---|---|
| Subcutaneous emphysema | Cutaneous and mucous membrane lacerations |
| Dysphonia | Edema, hematoma, vocal cord paralysis |
| Dyspnea | Edema, hematoma, displaced cartilage producing airway obstruction |
| Hemoptysis | Laceration of mucous membranes |
| Pain on swallowing | Laceration |
| Loss of laryngeal protuberance | Edema and hematoma or displaced cartilage |
| Atelectasis | Aspiration |
| Pneumothorax | Associated chest injury, mediastinal emphysema, posttracheostomy |

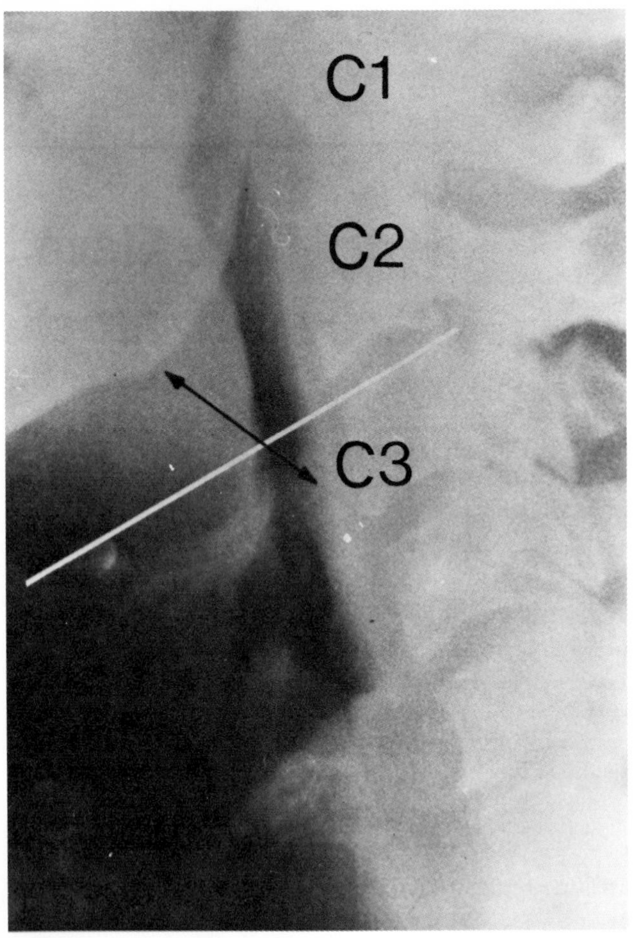


FIG. 13-19. On a normal lateral cervical radiogram the hyoid bone is located at or below the level of the upper surface of the third vertebral body (*white line*), and the distance between the hyoid cornua and the mandibular angle is more than 2 cm (*black line*). Note the continuity of the airway column. (From Polansky et al[157] with permission.)

of fracture preoperatively.[81,180] It can be obtained before or after the airway is secured.

Indirect laryngoscopy gives information about vocal cord mobility, mucosal integrity, endolaryngeal hematoma, arytenoid dislocation, and the degree of distortion of the laryngeal lumen.[144] Unfortunately it is not very useful during initial evaluation of the airway. Associated injuries, hypovolemia, and altered consciousness preclude its use in these patients. Direct laryngoscopy provides important information about the type and the extent of the injury, especially when findings are interpreted in conjunction with those obtained from CT scanning. The conventional laryngoscope blade is not suitable for this purpose as it may lead to acute airway obstruction in awake patients[50,62] and is inadequate for assessment of the cervical trachea. These problems are obviated by using a flexible fiberoptic bronchoscope. Further advantages of this device include minimal cervical spine movement, examination of the naso- or oropharynx,[81] and immediate airway control, if needed, with introduction of an endotracheal tube over the instrument.[7,31,143]

Evaluation of the pharynx, the hypopharynx, and the esophagus is as important as evaluation of the airway. The esophagus is evaluated with a rigid, rather than flexible, esophagoscope and with esophagography.

## MECHANISMS OF AIRWAY OBSTRUCTION

Airway obstruction may develop from several causes.[183] Dislocated arytenoid cartilages may separate from their attachment to the cricoid and move anteromedially to obstruct the larynx. The larynx or trachea may be distorted enough to compromise luminal diameter. Submucosal emphysema, hematoma, and edema may further narrow the tracheal lumen. Partial obstruction of the lumen results in an increase in inspiratory air velocity. Mobilized tissues follow the direction of air flow toward the airway while the subatmospheric pressure in the air stream causes the tissues to move medially, further enhancing the obstruction.[183] In cricotracheal separation injuries, the soft tissue surrounding the trachea usually remains intact, providing airway continuity even though a gap of as much as 8 cm may be present between the separated ends of the airway.[28,87,197,205,214] Paralysis produced by muscle relaxants or weakness from sedatives causes these supporting muscles to lose their tone, resulting in distal fragment displacement and sudden airway occlusion. Severe obstruction may also result from damage to peritracheal tissues caused by the tip of an endotracheal or cricothyroidotomy tube.[87] Total airway closure may also develop spontaneously; some patients arrive in the emergency department with minimal signs, but suddenly develop severe respiratory distress.[28]

Bleeding into the peritracheal tissue may cause a hematoma, which can compress the trachea. Damage to the recurrent laryngeal nerves frequently brings both vocal cords close to the midline, resulting in airway constriction. Interestingly, narrowing of the airway may occur several days or weeks after injury because of nerve entrapment within peritracheal scar tissue.[193] Although damage to the recurrent laryngeal nerves usually results in abductor paralysis, this is not an invariable occurrence, and occasionally airway obstruction may be absent.[159]

Subcutaneous emphysema, although rarely a cause of airway obstruction, is capable of worsening the existing respiratory distress. Struggling or coughing increases the rate of air escape by increasing the intratracheal pressure. Air may enter the mediastinum or the pleural cavities, resulting in early alveolar collapse or even tension pneumothorax.

## AIRWAY MANAGEMENT

The airway should be secured using cervical spine protection measures until the integrity of the spine is assured.[54,102] Injudicious maneuvers, such as forceful neck examination, hypopharyngeal suctioning, changing the patient's position from sitting to supine, and nasogastric tube insertion, should be avoided during the initial stages of trauma as they may precipitate airway obstruction.[87]

The severity of the injury and of the resulting airway compromise determines the type, timing, and extent of airway management. The algorithm provided in Figure 13-21 can be

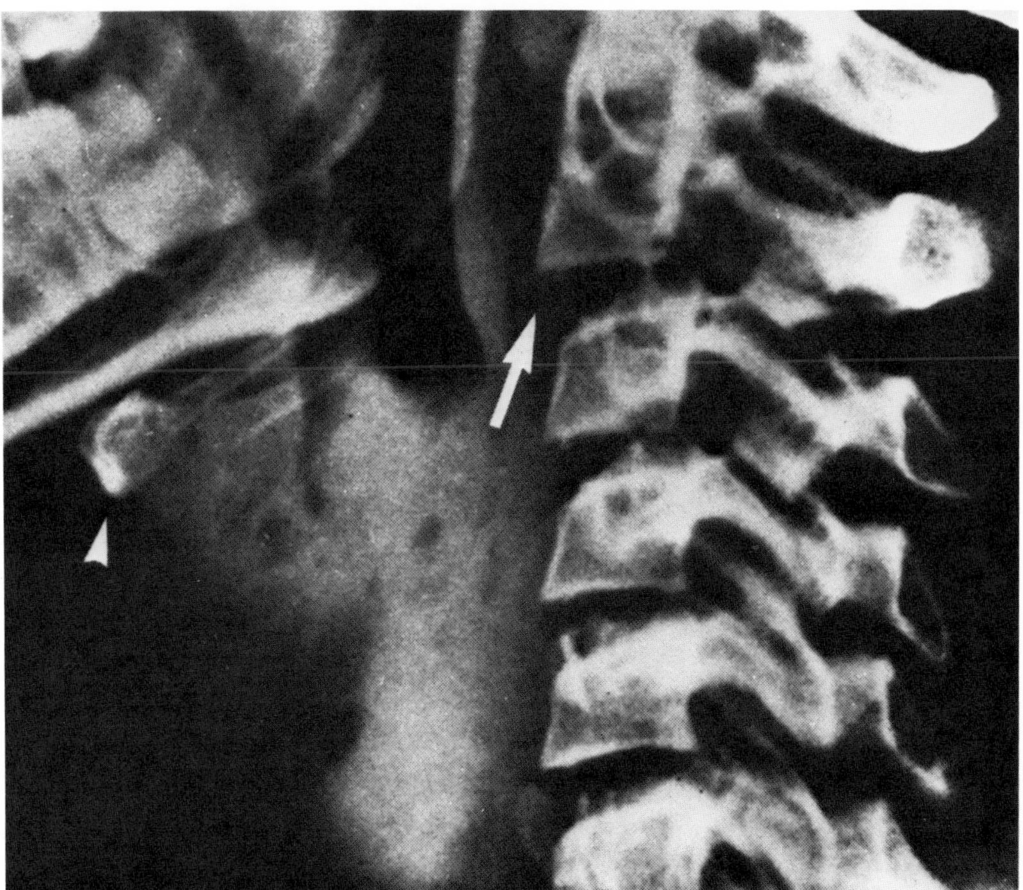

FIG. 13-20. Lateral cervical radiogram of a patient with cricotracheal separation injury. The hyoid bone is elevated above the upper level of the third vertebral body (*arrowhead*). There is no distance between the hyoid cornua and the angle of the mandible. Note the subluxation between C2 and C3 (*arrow*) and the abrupt ending of the airway column at the level of C3. Some retropharyngeal edema and emphysema are also noted. (From Polansky et al[157] with permission.)

used as a guide for decision making. There is little disagreement that immediate tracheostomy rather than endotracheal intubation, should be performed in acutely asphyxiating patients.[28,31,54,85,112,159,198,223] In addition to relieving respiratory obstruction rapidly, tracheostomy reduces intrabronchial pressure and prevents the spread of emphysema into the subcutaneous tissue, mediastinum, and pericardium.[96] Oxygen should be administered by mask during the procedure. Clearly, sedatives or opioids are contraindicated in patients with an obstructed airway. These agents not only eliminate the hypoxic and hypercarbic respiratory drive but also depress the cough reflex and set the stage for aspiration.

Tracheostomy may be extremely difficult in hypoxic and uncooperative individuals, in children, and in those with distorted cervical anatomy or cricotracheal separation. In the latter patients, the distal portion of the trachea retracts into the mediastinum or under the clavicle and may be difficult to find.[28] Delay in identification of the trachea may aggravate hypoxemia, with resulting catastrophic consequences. Unfortunately little can be done to assist the surgeon in these circumstances. It is important to auscultate the lungs and obtain a chest X-ray after tracheostomy since pneumothorax can occur after this procedure.

Initial airway management in the presence of less severe respiratory compromise is somewhat controversial. Many authors advocate immediate tracheostomy without prior endotracheal intubation.[24,86,118,136,143,180,180a,197,217] They prefer this approach because it avoids acute complications induced by attempts at intubation, such as entry into a false passage, damage to injured laryngeal structures, and complete obstruction of a marginally patent airway. Tracheostomy, if elected, should be performed at the lower cervical tracheal rings to prevent tension on and bacterial contamination of the injured region after repair.[231] It should also be performed without extending the neck and with spine protection measures applied if the possibility of cervical spine injury has not yet been eliminated. These constraints give rise to technical difficulties and may be associated with some risks of airway obstruction if prior airway control is not established by endotracheal intubation.[25,112] It must be emphasized that tracheostomy is performed in most patients with laryngeal injuries during definitive surgical repair because the edema after repair and the stent placed to prevent laryngeal stenosis do not permit air movement.

Cricothyroidotomy can provide an adequate airway if the injury is limited to the larynx. However, it aggravates the mu-

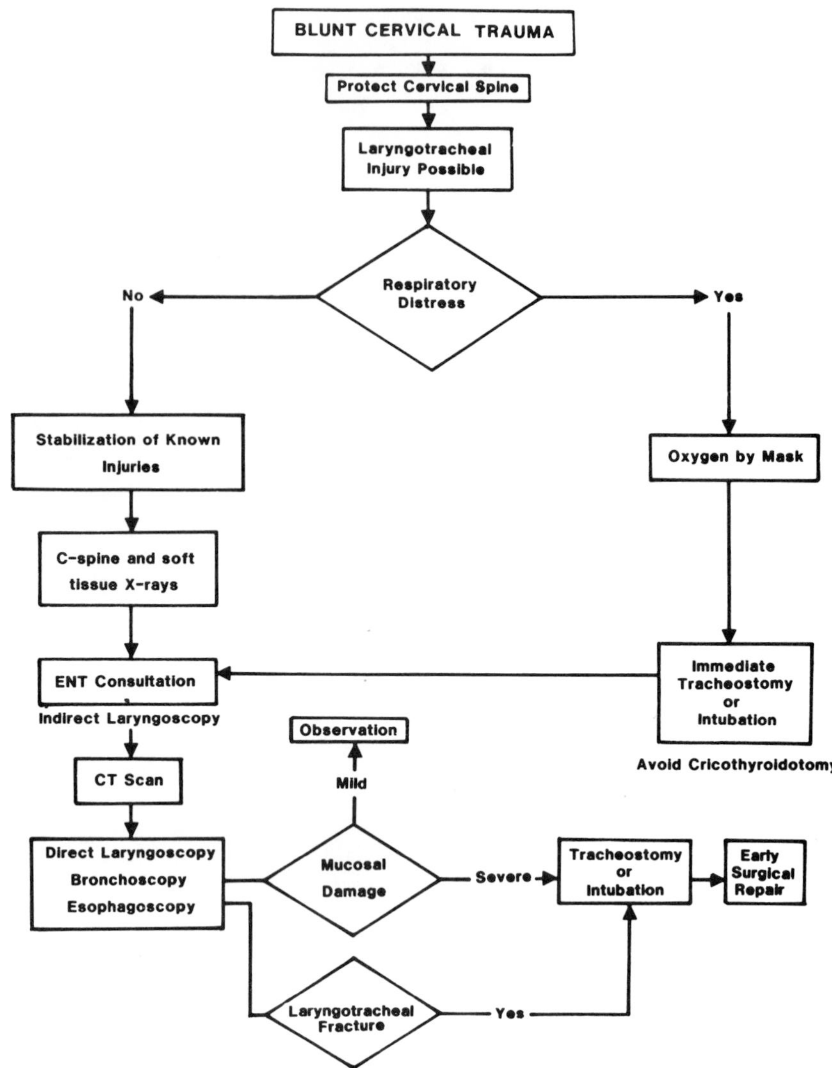


FIG. 13-21. An algorithm for management of laryngotracheal injury caused by blunt trauma.

cosal, ligamentous, and cartilaginous damage already caused by the original trauma. In addition, obliteration of landmarks by edema, subcutaneous emphysema, and cartilage fractures result in technical difficulties. The most important disadvantage of this procedure, however, is the possibility of acute airway obstruction in cricotracheal separation injuries with entry of the cannula into a false passage. Even when the cricothyroidotomy tube remains within the airway, air may escape through a lacerated tracheal wall, preventing adequate ventilation (Fig 13-22). Thus this procedure is contraindicated when blunt laryngotracheal trauma is suspected.[28,81,112]

In practice the laryngotracheal injury is often not recognized during the initial phase of care, and attempts are made to secure the airway with an endotracheal tube using a conventional laryngoscope blade.[87] This procedure is fraught with danger since the tip of the tube may enter a false passage and produce complete airway obstruction and/or extension of damage to glottic and infraglottic structures.[112,197,214,231] Difficulty in advancing the tube and/or appearance of a bulging mass on the anterior surface of the neck suggest entry into a false passage.[44,193]

Many clinicians contend that the airway of patients with blunt laryngotracheal trauma, including those with cricotracheal separation, can be managed safely and rapidly if the procedure is performed under direct vision of the glottis and trachea.[7,41,81,88,96,102,134,214] Use of a conventional laryngoscope is sufficient to prevent damage to supraglottic structures during this procedure, but a fiberoptic bronchoscope should be used to visualize glottic and infraglottic mucosa.[87,205,214] Alternatively, in order to expedite airway control, the larynx can be visualized with a laryngoscope blade, and once the tip of the endotracheal tube is introduced, it is advanced with the aid of a fiberoptic bronchoscope. Blood in the tracheobronchial tree impairs the efficacy of the scope; the suction port of the fiberoptic scope is not large enough to remove massive amounts of blood from the airway. In this situation a rigid pediatric bronchoscope (3.5 mm I.D. and 45 cm length) can be substituted. The endotracheal tube over the rigid bronchoscope is advanced, secured in place, and its cuff inflated once the injured segment is passed. Cervical spine injury must be ruled out before or appropriate protection measures taken during this procedure since the neck must

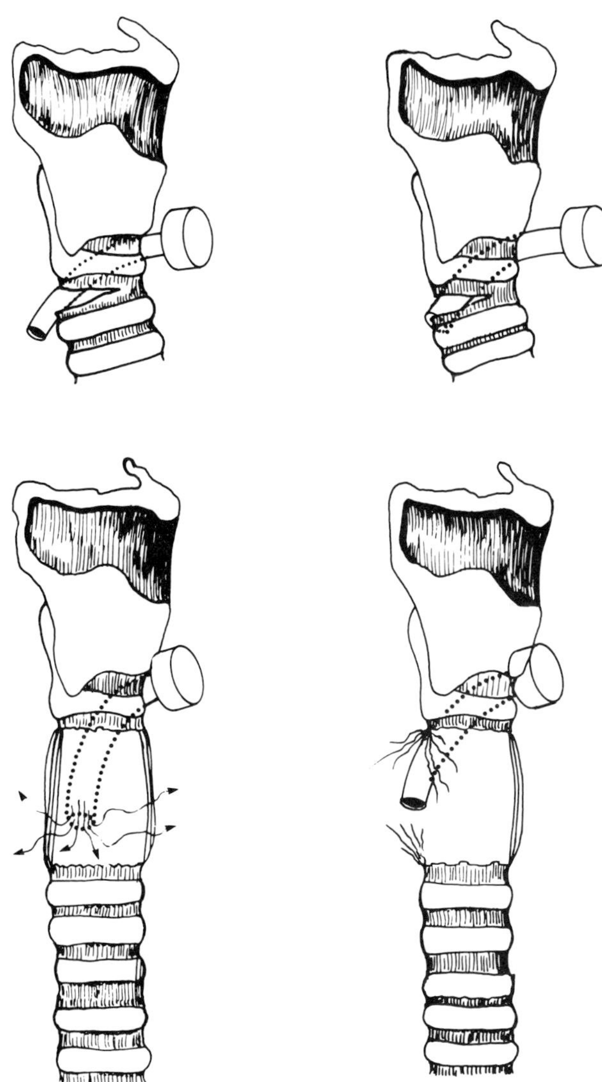

FIG. 13-22. Dangers of cricothyroidotomy in partial (*upper panel*) and complete (*lower part*) cricotracheal separation. The cricothyroidotomy cannula slips through the lacerated tracheal wall (*upper left*) or becomes partially obstructed when its tip is lodged within the lacerated wall (*upper right*). In complete cricotracheal separation the cannula may remain within the tracheal lumen supported by peritracheal tissues (*lower left*), but air leak through these weak tissues prevents adequate ventilation. Peritracheal tissues may be destroyed by the tip or the cuff of the cannula (*lower right*).

be extended during introduction of a rigid bronchoscope. If the injury is severe and the risk of airway obstruction is high, the patient can be ventilated through an adult-sized rigid bronchoscope without an endotracheal tube until the trachea is exposed surgically.[43] The importance of oxygen administration during all of these procedures cannot be overemphasized. In patients with partial airway obstruction but adequate arterial oxygenation, a mixture of helium (50%) and oxygen (50%) may be helpful as it facilitates inspiratory air flow because of its density: one-half to one-third that of air.

In patients without respiratory distress, attention is directed to stabilization of associated injuries and diagnosis of laryngotracheal injury. The need for immediate airway management is uncommon, but the possibility of sudden airway obstruction exists; careful observation and preparedness for emergency airway management are therefore necessary. In these patients, anesthesia and intubation are usually required for panendoscopy, which is performed under elective conditions 24 or more hours after trauma. During this period these patients are treated conservatively using voice rest, bedrest, humidified oxygen, nebulized racemic epinephrine, corticosteroids, and antibiotics.[136,231] During the preanesthetic period indirect laryngoscopy and CT scan findings should be evaluated, and airway patency, hemodynamic status, and associated injuries should be assessed. Since full stomach and airway obstruction are not concerns, anesthetic induction can proceed with the usual intravenous anesthetic and muscle relaxant sequence followed by introduction of a small endotracheal tube. Alternatively, intubation can be performed under fiberoptic bronchoscopic guidance while the patient is awake, sedated, and topically anesthetized or anesthetized and ventilated with a Patil-Syracuse mask.[153]

If anesthesia is required within 12 hours of trauma or shortly after indirect laryngoscopy and CT scan evaluation in a patient without evidence of airway obstruction, either primary tracheostomy or endotracheal intubation can be chosen. If endotracheal intubation is elected, such irreversible steps as administration of intravenous anesthetics or muscle relaxants should not be taken before the airway is secured. These agents may result in severe and uncontrollable airway obstruction by producing a loss of tone in the peritracheal supportive structures or by displacement of the distal segment of the airway in cricotracheal separation injuries. Such complications may even occur with sedative doses of hypnotics and opioids; these drugs should be administered in small doses and repeated only after an adequate time interval and careful assessment of the effect of previous doses. Adequate topical anesthesia of the upper airway is essential before any airway manipulation is attempted. Agitation, straining, and coughing during these maneuvers may result in increased intratracheal pressure, spread of subcutaneous emphysema, and complete airway obstruction.[28]

Children may not tolerate endotracheal intubation under sedation and topical anesthesia. Induction of general anesthesia by mask using inhalational agents and maintenance of spontaneous breathing has been recommended by many clinicians for fasted children or adults.[49,65,183] In our experience this technique is fraught with danger, especially in children who have evidence of partial airway obstruction. Complete airway obstruction ensues secondary to laryngeal spasm and other mechanisms described above.[44] Therefore, tracheostomy under local anesthesia is preferred despite its inherent difficulties. If there is no evidence of airway obstruction and anesthetic induction with inhalational agents is chosen to facilitate endotracheal intubation, the position that allows the most comfortable breathing while awake should be determined, and anesthetic induction performed in this position. Atropine (0.02 mg/kg) or glycopyrrolate (0.01–0.02 mg/kg) should be administered intravenously to prevent laryngeal spasm and bradycardia. Muscle relaxants should probably be avoided since control of ventilation may be impossible if airway obstruction develops. When an adequate level of anesthesia is achieved, an orotracheal tube is placed under direct vision using a pediatric fiberoptic bronchoscope with an external diameter of 2.8 or 3.4 mm. As in adults the procedure should be attempted only in the presence of complete facilities for performing emergency tracheostomy.

The type, extent, and timing of definitive surgical treatment are based on panendoscopy findings and the patient's general condition.[81,86,102] Patients with mild mucosal injuries are treated conservatively as described above.[81] Sometimes tracheostomy is the only surgical treatment required. Occasionally the arytenoid cartilage is relocated endoscopically if the underlying mucosa is not disrupted.[81] Patients with severe mucosal damage or laryngotracheal fractures require surgical exploration, reduction, and internal fixation of cartilaginous fractures; coverage of cartilage surfaces with mucosa; tracheostomy; and placement of a stent in the repaired larynx or trachea.[81] These procedures may be performed immediately after panendoscopy or later. However, it is generally recommended that surgery be performed on hemodynamically stable patients within 24 hours after injury.[24,81,86,102,107,180,217] Cricotracheal separation is repaired immediately after panendoscopy. However, if a primary repair cannot be performed, the distal portion of the trachea is anastomosed to the skin to provide an airway.[118] Most surgeons prefer not to search for the recurrent nerves during the initial procedure; they are difficult to identify and there is a danger of damaging adjacent structures.[194,198] Since the airway has been secured previously, little management difficulty is encountered during definitive repair of laryngotracheal injuries.

## PROGNOSIS

An estimated early mortality rate as high as 30% results from airway obstruction and associated injuries.[134] In surviving patients, laryngotracheal scarring, fibrosis, and contraction result in late complications: breathing difficulties, dysphonia, and recurrent pulmonary aspiration[28,86,107,118,135,193] (Fig 13-23). Granulation tissue and subsequent scar formation are more frequent after blunt than penetrating neck trauma, probably because injury is more extensive.[38,106] Thus, voice and airway impairment after blunt laryngeal trauma are more severe than that produced by penetrating injury.[107] Results of surgical repair from many series are inconsistent and sometimes disappointing.[7,17,38,50,81,85,86,102,107,118,144,180,185,217] Although severity of injury is an important determinant of long-term sequelae,[144,180] delay of diagnosis and treatment for more than 24 hours appears to contribute to the development of late complications.[17,28,31,102,107,118,135,180,223] Additional factors contributing to poor results include multisystem injuries, prolonged systemic hypotension, laryngeal rather than tracheal injury, and a combination of laryngeal and tracheal damage.[7,144,159,180] Although vocal cord mobility after injury suggests that the airway and the voice will be preserved,[107] the airway can be restored and a functional voice is possible even when the cords are paralyzed.[4,118] Infection at the surgical site is an important cause of long-term morbidity; early drainage, interposition of muscle flaps between the trachea and the esophagus (if the esophagus is injured), and broad-spectrum antibiotics have reduced the frequency of this complication.[118,180]

Many patients suffering from blunt laryngotracheal trauma require multiple operative procedures for complications of the injury or of the surgery. In this setting anesthesia is administered most frequently for bronchoscopy, laryngoscopy for assessment of repair and stent removal, endoscopic laser procedures to remove adhesions or a nonfunctioning arytenoid cartilage, repositioning of arytenoids, Teflon injection of the vocal cords, or nerve-muscle pedicle grafts to improve vocal cord function.[4,47,81,118,140,159,184,218] Associated esophageal injuries, especially when initially missed, may also require frequent surgical procedures, such as drainage of a cervical abscess, cervical esophagostomy, gastrostomy, primary repair of the injury or of a tracheoesophageal fistula, and esophageal dilation procedures to treat stenosis.[118,180] All of these procedures require general anesthesia.

## VASCULAR INJURIES

Blunt trauma can injure any vessel in the neck, although these injuries are rare in comparison to those produced by penetrating trauma. Carotid artery injuries are being recog-

FIG. 13-23. Acute and chronic complications of laryngeal injury and their mechanisms.

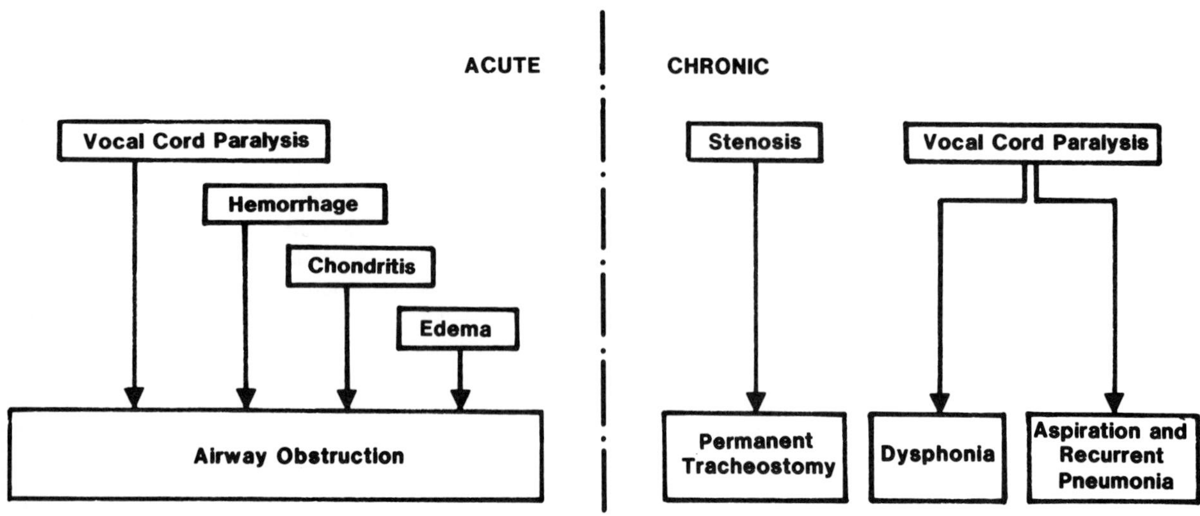

nized with increasing frequency, probably because of greater awareness of their possibility and more liberal use of arteriography in the evaluation of neck trauma. Carotid artery injury following blunt trauma was first reported by Verneuil[220] in 1872, but the first series, comprising 17 cases of this entity, was reported in 1980 by Perry et al.[156] Yamada et al[229] in 1967, Krajewski and Hertzer[101] in 1980, and Kallero et al[94] in 1987 reviewed the subject extensively, but described only a few cases of their own. Information from these reports suggest that only 51 cases of blunt carotid injury were described before 1967,[229] an additional 45 cases between 1967 and 1980,[101] and the total number of reported cases is approximately 200. Protection of the vessel by posterior displacement of the carotid sheath during neck extension explains the rarity of this injury.[197]

Four mechanisms are responsible for blunt carotid artery injury:[42,94,101] (a) direct blow to the artery; (b) sudden hyperextension, contralateral rotation, and lateral flexion of the neck, causing stretching of the artery against the transverse process of the third cervical vertebra or the bony mass of the atlas or axis; (c) intraorally, when the individual falls on a foreign object carried in the mouth; and (d) after basal skull fracture with injury of the intrapetrous portion of the artery. Motor vehicle accidents and falls are the most common causes of blunt carotid trauma,[225] but chiropractic manipulation and direct blows during altercations or such sports as football, rugby, soccer, boxing, or wrestling can also produce this injury.[168]

Although blunt trauma to the neck can lacerate the carotid artery or any other vessel with subsequent bleeding and hematoma formation, the predominant pathology in blunt carotid injuries is either an intimal tear or intramural hemorrhage or scarring.[220,229] Interestingly, in about 25% of patients, no vascular pathology is found.[229] The vascular lumen may be narrowed when an intimal flap is lifted by the stream of blood forming a weblike stenosis or by subintimal dissection with blood. Thrombus may form over the intimal disruption site and progress proximally and distally along the vessel to produce occlusion.[26,101] Perivascular edema or hematoma, hypotension, vasospasm, and increased adhesion of platelets, which are common occurrences after major trauma, increase the tendency to clot formation.[26] A thrombus within the carotid artery may serve as a source of emboli to the cerebral vessels. However, the most frequent source of emboli is an aneurysm, which is formed when there is significant injury to the media.[35,224,225] In severe undiagnosed injuries, pseudoaneurysms may also form, producing a pulsating and sometimes tender mass below the angle of the jaw or in the peritonsillar fossa. Injury and occlusion occur most commonly at or within a few centimeters of the bifurcation, especially in hyperextension-hyperrotation injuries. Less frequently, internal carotid occlusion occurs at the level of the first and second cervical vertebrae.[13] It is important to remember that injury can also occur in the intracranial segment of this artery. Disruption of this vessel's integrity within its cavernous portion results in carotid-cavernous fistula.[225] Carotid artery injuries are almost always unilateral and rarely bilateral.[26,165]

As in cervical airway injuries caused by blunt trauma, the severity of external signs, such as bruising or abrasion of the skin, does not necessarily correlate with the severity of injury to the carotid artery.[13,92,98,229] About 25% of reported cases had either minimal or no visible cutaneous injury. Cervical hematoma, often large, is present in some patients and can shift the trachea to the uninjured side. This finding, however, is not specific to carotid artery injury and may follow laceration of any vessel in the neck (Fig 13-24). Associated mandibular or facial fractures should arouse one's suspicion even though carotid injury is rarely associated with these fractures.

Horner's syndrome, resulting from trauma to the cervical sympathetic chain, is seen in many patients before any other associated neurologic deficit.[92] Some patients may have transient ischemic attacks during the period of thrombus formation before the vessel is totally occluded. They are probably caused by cerebral embolization since the attacks subside once the vessel is completely thrombosed.

The characteristic clinical feature of blunt carotid artery injury is the lucid interval between the time of trauma and the appearance of neurologic symptoms, which range from minor sensory deficits to hemiplegia, dysarthria, decreased consciousness and coma.[26,94,101,156,168,225] The lucid interval varies from less than 1 hour to a few days, but neurologic symptoms usually develop within 24 hours. It is speculated that this interval represents the period necessary for clot propagation to occlude the vessel enough to produce cerebral ischemia. However, neurologic deficit may, as mentioned, also be produced by emboli in the absence of complete carotid occlusion.[101,156]

Diagnosis of carotid artery injuries caused by blunt trauma, unlike those produced by penetrating trauma, is exceedingly difficult. A high index of suspicion is required to recognize these rare injuries, especially when they are associated with more common injuries. In an alert, oriented patient the development of neurologic deficit should raise the possibility of carotid artery injury. This clinical feature is in contrast to that produced by intracranial bleeding in which the patient becomes obtunded by the time focal neurologic signs appear.[101] In the presence of concomitant head injury with decreased consciousness on arrival, the diagnosis is almost impossible, especially when a CT scan shows intracranial hemorrhage. In obtunded patients with focal neurologic signs and a normal CT scan of the head, the possibility of intracranial or extracranial carotid artery injury should be entertained and four-vessel cerebral angiogram, the most definitive diagnostic measure, should be obtained.[101,133,156,225] In fact, angiography is indicated in patients who have sustained blunt cervical trauma even when no neurologic disturbance is apparent.[156] If cerebral angiography cannot be performed, CT of the neck after injection of contrast medium may be useful to establish the diagnosis of carotid artery injury.[94] Digital subtraction angiography may also help deliniate carotid injury, especially pseudoaneurysm formation, during the late phases following trauma.[165]

In many patients blunt carotid injury is diagnosed after the repair of associated injuries. During this phase patients with carotid occlusion complain of head noise or temporal bruit, which can be confirmed by auscultation of the neck. If a carotid-cavernous fistula has developed, an audible bruit, pulsation of the orbit, chemosis, diplopia, visual disturbances, headache, and exophthalmos are observed.[225] Cerebral angiography will confirm the diagnosis in these patients.

Early diagnosis of blunt carotid artery injuries is crucial since little is accomplished by treatment after a cerebral in-

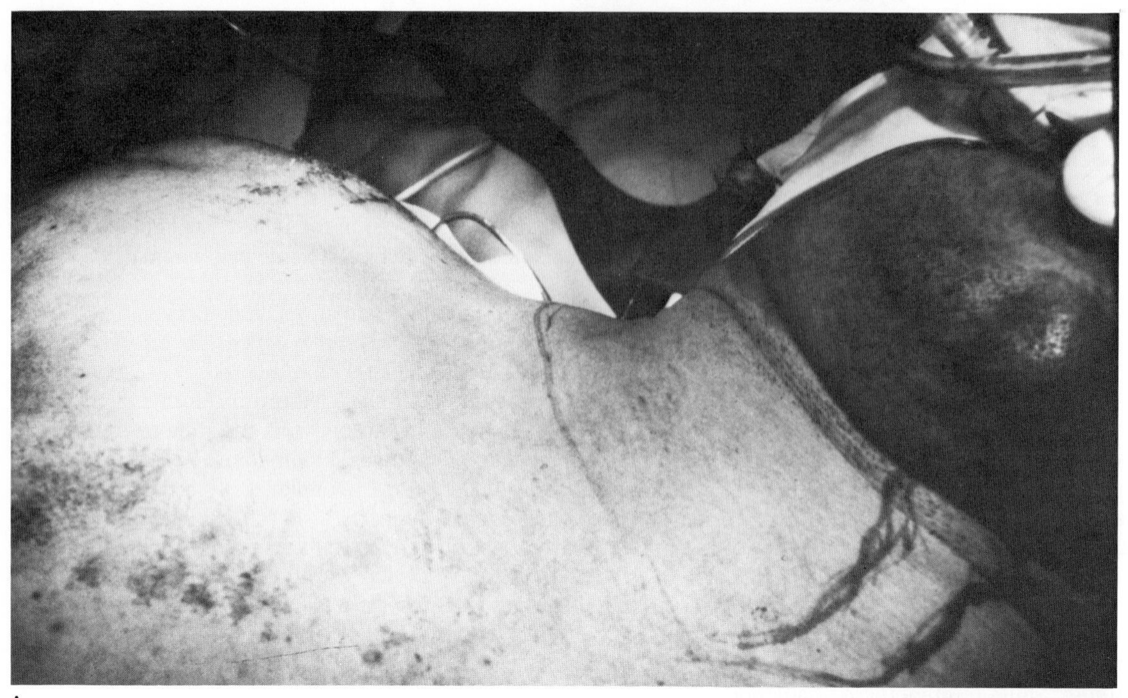

A

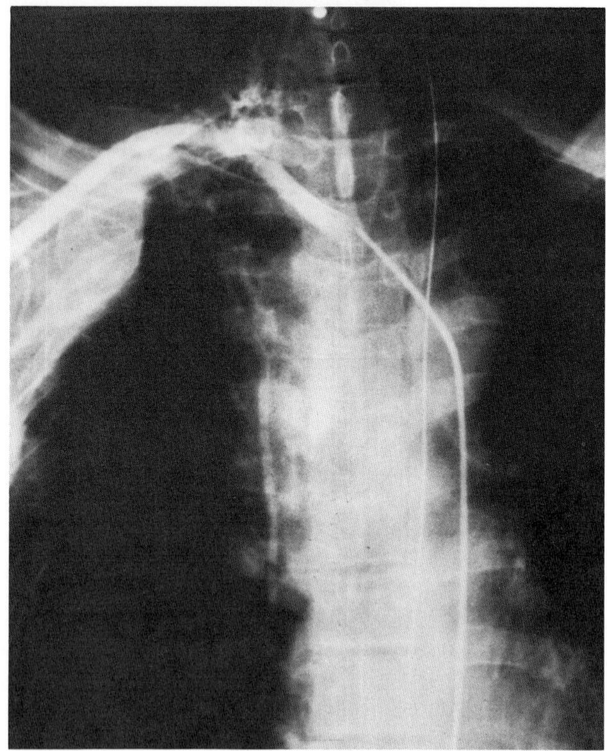

B

FIG. 13-24. A, right-sided neck hematoma shifting the trachea (drawn on the skin) to the left. B, angiographic study of the same patient showing thyrocervical trunk injury. Note the deviation of the air column to the left by the hematoma. This patient sustained a direct blow to to the neck with a lead pipe. Note the absence of skin marks on the neck.

farct has developed. According to Perry et al[156] revascularization is effective in patients with mild neurologic deficits and prograde carotid blood flow, but it accomplishes little in those with complete occlusion, severe neurologic deficits, and altered consciousness. There is, unfortunately, no reliable method to determine the presence of a cerebral infarct. CT scan of the head may be useful, but a negative result does not exclude infarction.[94] Some clinicians consider patients with prolonged (longer than 4–6 hours) severe neurologic symptoms to have a completed infarct and do not recommend revascularization.[42] Welling and coworkers[225] reported that conservative treatment with intravenous heparin for 7 to 10 days followed by oral warfarin for 4 to 6 weeks in patients with relatively new symptoms prevented the development of new deficits.

The treatment of carotid pseudoaneurysms and intracranial carotid-cavernous fistula is also controversial. Pseudoaneurysms can be treated with aneurysmorrhaphy, resection followed by graft interposition, or balloon occlusion of the internal carotid artery above and below the orifice of the aneurysm.[225] Occlusion of the vessel may result in cerebral ischemia after a few hours. Therefore some clinicians (Feliciano D, MD, personal communication) recommend inserting a Fogarty catheter into the internal carotid artery and advancing it to the base of the skull. An EEG is obtained after inflation of the balloon. EEG change with balloon occlusion is an indication for extracranial-intracranial (EC-IC) bypass and subsequent carotid ligation. An alternative is to expose and apply an atraumatic clamp to the carotid artery under local anesthesia and assess neurologic function for 30–60 minutes before ligating the vessel.[35] Graded occlusion of the internal carotid artery with electroencephalographic assessment of cerebral ischemia has also been described.[63] Repair of aneurysms at the base of the skull is technically difficult because the mandible precludes exposure. Although some special surgical approaches can overcome this problem, EC-IC bypass may also be required to supply adequate blood flow to the brain.[68,74] Carotid-cavernous fistula can be treated by embolization or balloon occlusion of the fistula while patency of the internal carotid artery is maintained.[225]

There are no published reports about anesthetic management of blunt cervical vascular injuries. The anesthetic principles discussed for penetrating carotid artery injuries apply to these as well. Tracheal deviation and venous compression with resultant pharyngeal and laryngeal edema may result from hematoma and compromise the airway. Whenever possible, manipulation of the airway should be done under fiberoptic bronchoscopic guidance, with the patient awake. Continuous intraoperative monitoring of brain function using a processed EEG or somatosensory evoked potentials may be helpful.[63,104,199] Arterial pressure should be maintained at normal or slightly elevated levels to provide adequate collateral circulation during carotid clamping.

Among other cervical vessels affected by blunt trauma, subclavian artery injury at the base of the neck may result in bleeding, temporary or rarely permanent upper extremity ischemia, and subclavian steal syndrome.[178] Diagnosis of these rare injuries is difficult since physical examination, noninvasive vascular evaluations, and chest radiograph are frequently normal.[2] A high index of suspicion and liberal use of arteriography are crucial for their recognition. The innominate artery can also be injured in this area, resulting in major bleeding and ischemia of the upper extremity and the brain.[178] The mechanism of injury involves either entrapment of the vessel between the sternum, clavicle, or sternoclavicular joint and the vertebral column or avulsion, with the shearing force generated by displacement of the heart during impact. Deceleration is a relatively rare mechanism of production of these injuries.[178] Clavicular, sternal, or upper rib fractures; shock; mediastinal widening; absence of a radial pulse in one limb; and a blood pressure differential between the upper limbs should arouse suspicion of trauma to the innominate or subclavian arteries. Arch aortography, after control of shock with aggressive fluid infusion, should be performed to establish the diagnosis. As mentioned in the section on penetrating cervical vascular injury, cardiopulmonary bypass may be required for the repair of innominate artery or combined left subclavian-carotid artery injuries to prevent cerebral ischemia. Nonetheless, short periods of innominate artery clamping are tolerated by many patients.

## NEUROLOGIC INJURIES

The brachial plexus is often injured by traction during blunt trauma. Nerve roots may be damaged extradurally or intradurally; the severity of injury may vary from simple stretching to avulsion. Usually the upper roots of the brachial plexus (C5 and C6) are injured extradurally, whereas the lower roots (C7, C8 and T1) are injured intradurally.[22] Motor weakness, pain, and sympathetic dysfunction of the upper extremity are the predominant signs and symptoms of brachial plexus injury. Traction on the cervical sympathetic chain may also occur and result in Horner's syndrome on the affected side. Occasionally cervical sympathetic trauma may result in painless facial and ocular sympathetic hyperactivity, which is termed "Pourfour Du Petit syndrome" after the famous French physician who treated a large number of these patients during the Napoleonic Wars.[211]

Definitive diagnosis of cervical nerve root injuries is made by myelography; obliteration of the dural root sheaths, dilation of the nerve sleeves, pseudomeningocele formation, and extravasation of contrast material are typical radiographic findings.[22,32] Isolated brachial plexus injury is never an emergency, and patients usually present to the anesthesiologist for treatment of pain and reflex sympathetic dystrophy. Sympathetic nerve blocks, as outlined in Chapter 23, may alleviate pain and sympathetic dysfunction to varying degrees. Microsurgical repair is performed in some centers a few weeks after brachial plexus injury. The long duration of these procedures requires special emphasis on proper positioning of the patient, maintenance of normothermia, limitations in the use of enflurane, and appropriate fluid and blood replacement.

## ESOPHAGEAL INJURIES

Esophageal rupture after blunt trauma is uncommon.[75,164] Motor vehicle accidents and falls account for the majority of these injuries.[80,164] The predominant mechanism involves a forceful anterior blow to a hyperextended neck, which crushes the esophagus between the offending object and the cervical vertebra. A sudden intraluminal pressure increase in the esophagus may also play a part. Associated vertebral body fractures may cause esophageal perforation by a sharp edge of fragmented bone. The presence of a large irregular vertebral osteophyte appears to facilitate rupture by acting as a pivot point and/or penetrating the esophagus.[164] In fact many of these patients have either associated cervical spine injury or are elderly. Concomitant laryngotracheal injury in the form of laryngeal fracture, cricotracheal separation, or both may be present, complicating diagnosis and management.[97]

Diagnostic and therapeutic principles of these injuries are the same as those described for penetrating esophageal wounds. Subcutaneous emphysema, dysphagia, odynophagia, and neck tenderness, as well as X-ray findings of gas in cervical soft tissues, retropharyngeal space, or chest, are important signs and symptoms. Cervical spine X-rays should be obtained in all patients to eliminate fractures and dislocations. If air cannot be detected in soft-tissue films, special radiologic techniques should be utilized to enhance detection of small amounts of air.[164] Computed tomography is also useful for this purpose. A combination of esophagrams and rigid esophagoscopy or neck exploration is the definitive method to diagnose this injury. Prompt surgical treatment with primary closure and drainage of paraesophageal spaces is essential for avoiding morbidity and mortality. Fatality in patients with this injury occurs mainly from the sequelae of retropharyngeal abscess and from associated injuries.[164]

The possibility of cervical spine injury should be considered during initial airway management and utmost attention paid to avoid movement of the cervical spine. Other anesthetic considerations are the same as those described in the penetrating esophageal injury section.

## CONCLUSION

The neck is generally protected from trauma by its surrounding muscles and bones. However, once this region is traumatized, injury to cervical structures is very likely. Whether the causative mechanism is penetrating or blunt, injury to one or more of four groups of cervical structures—airway, food passage, vessels, and nerves—may have important acute and chronic consequences, especially when recognition and treatment are delayed. Accurate diagnosis is particularly important for anesthetic and airway management of cervical injuries; the type and severity of injury determine the selection of techniques. The symptoms and signs of all but hypopharyngeal and esophageal injuries are usually obvious after penetrating trauma, and they are thus usually easily recognized. In contrast, diagnosis of these injuries after blunt trauma is notoriously difficult. In this situation, they either present with few ymptoms or signs, or their manifestations are overshadowed by those of more serious injuries. A high index of suspicion should be exercised, and appropriate diagnostic tests should be performed as soon as possible after suspicion is aroused.

Each cervical organ injury presents different management problems, and often more than one structure is injured. Further, concomitant injury to extracervical structures is not uncommon. Thus, each patient presents with an individual group of difficulties for which preset, blanket management recommendations cannot be applied. Instead, it is probably more appropriate to consolidate management principles for each injury and apply them with care priorities in mind. Such an approach requires careful evaluation to predict the injuries that may be present before any intervention is performed. Admittedly some patients with trauma to the cervical region arrive in the emergency department with severe associated injuries and are in need of immediate resuscitation, rather than evaluation. Not infrequently, however, symptoms, signs, and radiographic and endoscopic findings can be coupled with information on the injury mechanism to permit diagnosis of cervical pathology in stable or stabilized patients.

Endotracheal intubation in patients with airway injury or airway compromise should be performed with the aid of a fiberoptic bronchoscope to avoid entry of the tube into a false passage and thus airway obstruction. No irretrievable maneuvers, such as administration of anesthetics and muscle relaxants, should be performed in these patients during initial management. Tracheostomy equipment should be available before any steps are taken to secure the airway. Massive transfusion should be anticipated and preparation for it made in advance in patients with suspected vascular injury. The patient should be prepped and draped in such a way that access to the chest, the contralateral side of the neck, and the base of the skull can be gained at any time during surgery. Brain function may be monitored and brain preservation measures taken if carotid and/or vertebral injuries are present. The possibility of air embolism must be considered and necessary precautions taken whenever possible. The presence of esophageal injury or tracheoesophageal fistula must be suspected and management techniques designed accordingly.

## REFERENCES


1. Adornato DC, Gildenberg PL, Ferrario CM, et al. Pathophysiology of intravenous air embolism in dogs. Anesthesiology 1978;49:120.
2. Aelenock GB, Kazmers A, Graham LM, et al. Nonpenetrating subclavian artery injuries. Arch Surg 1985;120:685.
3. Allen SJ. Management of intracranial pressure after head injury. ASA Refresher Course Lectures 1987;15:1.
4. Alonso WA. Surgical management and complications of acute laryngotracheal disruption. Otolaryngol Clin North Am 1979;12:761.
5. Alonso WA, Pratt LL, Zollinger WK, Ogura JH. Complications of laryngotracheal disruption. Laryngoscope 1974;84:1276.
6. Alvaran SB, Toung TJK, Graff TE, Benson DW. Venous air embolism: comparative merits of external cardiac massage, intracardiac aspiration, and left lateral decubitus position. Anesth Analg 1978;57:166.
7. Angood PB, Attia EL, Brown RA, Mulder DS. Extrinsic civilian trauma to the larynx and cervical trachea—important predictors of long-term morbidity. J Trauma 1986;26:869.
8. Anson BJ, Maddock WG. General considerations; fascia of the neck. In: Anson BJ, Maddock WG, eds. Callander's surgical anatomy. Philadelphia: WB Saunders, 1958:165.
9. Ayuyao AM, Kaledzi YL, Parsa MH, Freeman HP. Penetrating neck wounds. Mandatory versus selective exploration. Ann Surg 1985;202:563.
10. Baghai P, Sheptak PE. Penetrating spinal injury by a glass fragment. Neurosurgery 1982;11:419.
11. Baraka A. Suxamethonium-induced muscle contracture following denervation in man. Br J Anaesth 1978;50:195.
12. Baraka A. Antagonism of succinylcholine induced contracture of denervated muscles by d-tubocurarine. Anesth Analg 1981;60:605.
13. Batzdorf U, Bentson UR, Machleder HI. Blunt trauma to the high cervical carotid artery. Neurosurgery 1979;5:195.
14. Bedford RF. Venous air embolism: a historical perspective. Semin Anesth 1983;2:169.
15. Bexton MDR, Radford R. An unusual cause of respiratory obstruction after thyroidectomy. Anaesthesia 1982;37:596.
16. Bishara RA, Pasch AR, Douglas DD, et al. The necessity of mandatory exploration of penetrating zone II neck injuries. Surgery 1986;100:655.
17. Black RJ. External laryngeal trauma. Med J Aust 1981;1:644.

18. Blass DC, James EC, Reed RJ, et al. Penetrating wounds of the neck and upper thorax. J Trauma 1978;18:2.
19. Blume WT, Ferguson GG, NcNeill DK. Significance of EEG changes at carotid endarterectomy. Stroke 1986;17:891.
20. Bradley EL III. Management of penetrating carotid injuries: an alternative approach. J Trauma 1973;13:248.
21. Brandenburg JH. Management of acute blunt laryngeal injuries. Otolaryngol Clin North Am 1979;12:741.
22. Brophy BP. Supraclavicular traction injuries of the brachial plexus. Aust NZ J Surg 1978;48:528.
23. Brown JM, Graham JM, Feliciano DV, et al. Carotid artery injury. Am J Surg 1982;144:748.
24. Bryce DP. The surgical management of laryngotracheal injury. J Laryngol Otol 1972;86:547.
25. Bryce-Smith R. An anaesthetic technique for tracheostomy. Anaesthesia 1957;12:152.
26. Burrows PE, Tubman DE. Multiple extracranial arterial lesions following closed craniocervical trauma. J Trauma 1981;21:497.
27. Butler BD, Hills BA. The lung as a filter for microbubbles. J Appl Physiol 1979;47:537.
28. Camnitz PS, Shepherd SM, Henderson RA. Acute blunt laryngeal and tracheal trauma. Am J Emerg Med 1987;5:157.
29. Carter LP, Yamagata S, Erspamer R. Time limits of reversible cortical ischemia. Neurosurgery 1983;12:620.
30. Cave-Bigley DJ, Stell PM. Penetrating laryngeal injuries. Injury 1981;13:513.
31. Cavo J, Leonard G, Tzadik A. Laryngeal trauma. In: Maull KI, Cleveland HC, Strauch GO, Wolferth CC, eds. Advances in Trauma. Chicago: Year Book Medical Publishers, 1986:157.
32. Chechick A, Amit Y, Shaked I, et al. Brown-Séquard syndrome associated with brachial plexus injury in neck trauma. J Trauma 1982;22:430.
33. Cho I, Smullens SN, Streletz LJ, Fariello RG. The value of intraoperative EEG monitoring during carotid endarterectomy. Ann Neurol 1986;20:508.
34. Clark MC, Flick MR. Permeability pulmonary edema caused by venous air embolism. Am Rev Respir Dis 1984;129:633.
35. Clarke P. Traumatic aneurysm of the internal carotid artery and rupture of the duodenum following seat belt injury. Injury 1980;12:158.
36. Cohen A, Brief D, Matthewson C Jr. Carotid artery injuries: an analysis of eighty-five cases. Am J Surg 1970;120:210.
37. Cohen ES, Breaux CW, Johnson PN, Leitner CA. Penetrating neck injuries: experience with selective neck exploration. South Med J 1987;80:26.
38. Cohn AM, Larson DL. Laryngeal injury. A critical review. Arch Otolaryngol 1976;102:166.
39. Colley PS, Artru AA. Bunegin-Albin catheter improves air retrieval and resuscitation from lethal venous air embolism in dogs. Anesth Analg 1987;66:991.
40. Collice M, Arena O, Fontana RA, et al. Role of EEG monitoring and cross-clamping duration in carotid endarterectomy. J Neurosurg 1986;65:815.
41. Couraud L, Martigne C, Panconi B. Desinsertion laryngotracheale post-traumatique avec fracture du cartilage cricoide et arrachement des nerfs recurrents. Chirurgie 1980;106:725.
42. Crissey MM, Bernstein EF. Delayed presentation of carotid intimal tear following blunt craniocervical trauma. Surgery 1974;75:543.
43. Dalal FY, Schmidt GB, Bennett EJ, Levitsky S. Fractures of the larynx in children. Can Anaesth Soc J 1974;21:376.
44. Dash HH, Rode GR. Blunt trauma to the cervical portion of the trachea. A case report. Br J Anaesth 1983;55:1271.
45. Davis JR. The fibreoptic laryngoscope in the management of cut throat injuries. Br J Anaesth 1978;50:511.
46. Dedo HH. The paralyzed larynx: an electromyographic study in dogs and humans. Laryngoscope 1970;80:1455.
47. Dedo HH, Rowe LD. Laryngeal reconstruction in acute and chronic injuries. Otolaryngol Clin North Am 1983;16:373.
48. Demetriades D, Stewart M. Penetrating injuries of the neck. Ann Roy Coll Surg Engl 1985;67:71.
49. Donchin Y, Vered IY. Blunt trauma to the trachea. Br J Anaesth 1976;48:1113.
50. Downey WL, Owen RC, Ward PH. Traumatic laryngeal injury: its management and sequelae. South Med J 1967;60:756.
51. Dresser LP, McKinney WM. Anatomic and pathophysiologic studies of the human internal jugular valve. Am J Surg 1987;154:220.
52. Duncan JAT. A case of severely cut throat. Br J Anaesth 1975;47:1327.
53. Ecker RR, Libertini RV, Rea WJ, et al. Injuries of the trachea and bronchi. Ann Thorac Surg 1971;11:269.
54. Edwards WH, Morris JA, DeLozier JB, Adkins RB. Airway injuries. The first priority in trauma. Am Surg 1987;53:192.
55. Elerding SC, Manart FD, Moore EE. A reappraisal of penetrating neck injury management. J Trauma 1980;20:695.
56. Ellis FR. The management of the cut-throat. Anaesthesia 1966;21:253.
57. Ericsson JA, Gottlieb JD, Sweet RB. Closed-chest cardiac massage in the treatment of venous air embolism. N Engl J Med 1964;270:1353.
58. Evans HJR, Citron N. Rupture of the cervical trachea following closed injury of the neck. Injury 1980;12:39.
59. Fackler ML. Wound ballistics. A review of common misconceptions. JAMA 1988;259:2730.
60. Feliciano DV, Bitondo CG, Mattox KL, et al. Combined tracheoesophageal injuries. Am J Surg 1985;150:710.
61. Fitz-Hugh GS, Powell JB. Acute traumatic injuries of the oropharynx, laryngopharynx and cervical trachea in children. Otolaryngol Clin North Am 1970;3:375.
62. Fitz-Hugh GS, Wallenborn WM, McGovern F. Injuries of the larynx and cervical trachea. Ann Otol Rhinol Laryngol 1962;71:419.
63. Fleischer AS, Guthkelch AN. Management of high cervical-intracranial internal carotid artery traumatic aneurysms. J Trauma 1987;27:330.
64. Flint LM, Synder WH, Perry MO, Shires GT. Management of major vascular injuries in the base of the neck. Arch Surg 1973;106:407.
65. Flood LM, Astley B. Anaesthetic management of acute laryngeal trauma. Br J Anaesth 1982;54:1339.
66. Fogelman MJ, Stewart RD. Penetrating wounds of the neck. Am J Surg 1956;91:581.
67. Fraser RG, Peter Pare JA. Diagnosis of diseases of the chest. Philadelphia: WB Saunders, 1979:1872–1878.
68. Fry RE, Fry WJ. Extracranial carotid artery injuries. Surgery 1980;88:581.
69. Furuya H, Suzuki T, Okumura F, et al. Detection of air embolism by transesophageal echocardiography. Anesthesiology 1983;58:124.
70. Gacek RR, Malmgren LT, Lyon MJ. Localization of adductor and abductor motor nerve fibers to the larynx. Ann Otol 1977;86:770.
71. Gelb AW. Anesthetic considerations for carotid endarterectomy. Int Anesthesiol Clin 1984;22:153.
72. Gentleman D, Harrington M. Penetrating injury of the spinal cord. Injury 1984;16:7.
73. Gewertz BL, McCaffrey MT. Intraoperative monitoring during carotid endarterectomy. In: Ravitch MM, ed. Current problems in surgery. Chicago: Year Book Medical Publishers, 1987:481–532.
74. Gewertz BL, Samson DS, Ditmore QM, et al. Management of penetrating injuries of the internal carotid artery at the base of

the skull utilizing extracranial intracranial bypass. J Trauma 1980;20:365.

75. Glatterer MS, Toon RS, Ellestad C, et al. Management of blunt and penetrating external esophageal trauma. J Trauma 1985;25:784.
76. Glenski JA, Cucchiara RF, Michenfelder JD. Transesophageal echocardiography and transcutaneous $O_2$ and $CO_2$ monitoring for detection of venous air embolism. Anesthesiology 1986; 64:541.
77. Golueke PJ, Goldstein AS, Sclafani SJA. Routine versus selective exploration of penetrating neck injuries: a randomized prospective study. J Trauma 1984;24:1010.
78. Golueke P, Sclafani S, Phillips T, et al. Vertebral artery injury—diagnosis and management. J Trauma 1987;27:856.
79. Greene R, Stark P. Trauma of the larynx and trachea. Radiol Clin North Am 1978;16:309.
80. Gulbrandson RN, Gaspard DJ. Steering wheel rupture of the pharyngoesophagus: a solitary injury. J Trauma 1977; 17:74.

80a. Gussack GS, Jurkovich GJ. Treatment dilemmas in laryngotracheal trauma. J Trauma 1988;28:1439.

81. Gussack GS, Jurkovich GJ, Luterman A. Laryngotracheal trauma: a protocol approach to a rare injury. Laryngoscope 1986;96:660.
82. Hadary A, Lernau OZ, Nissan S. Letter to the editor. J Trauma 1986;26:1156.
83. Hansebout RR, Blomquist Jr G, Gloor P, et al. Use of hypertension and electroencephalographic monitoring during carotid endarterectomy. Can J Surg 1981;24:304.
84. Hare RM. Respiratory obstruction after thyroidectomy. Anaesthesia 1982;37:1136.
85. Harris HH, Ainsworth JZ. Immediate management of laryngeal and tracheal injuries. Laryngoscope 1965;75:1103.
86. Harris HH, Tobin HA. Acute injuries of the larynx and trachea in 49 patients. Observations over a 15-year period. Laryngoscope 1970;80:1376.
87. Hermon A, Segal K, Har-El G, et al. Complete cricotracheal separation following blunt trauma to the neck. J Trauma 1987;27:1365.
88. Herrin TJ, Brzustowicz R, Hendrickson M. Anesthetic management of neck trauma. South Med J 1979;72:1102.
89. Hills BA, Butler BD. Air embolism: further basic facts relevant to the placement of central venous catheters and Doppler monitors. Anesthesiology 1983;59:163.
90. Holt CR, Kostohryz G. Wound ballistics of gunshot injuries to the head and neck. Arch Otolaryngol 1983;109:313.
91. Hybels RL. Venous air embolism in head and neck surgery. Laryngoscope 1980;90:946.
92. Jernigan WR, Gardner WC. Carotid artery injuries due to closed cervical trauma. J Trauma 1971;11:429.
93. Jones RF, Terrell JC, Salyer KE. Penetrating wounds of the neck: an analysis of 274 cases. J Trauma 1967;7:128.
94. Kallero BM, Bjorck CG, Bergkvist D. Carotid artery injury caused by blunt cervical trauma: case report. Acta Chir Scand 1987;153:155.
95. Karlin RM, Marks C. Extracranial carotid artery injury. Current surgical management. Am J Surg 1983;146:225.
96. Kelly JP, Webb WR, Moulder PV, et al. Management of airway trauma. I: Tracheobronchial injuries. Ann Thorac Surg 1985; 40:551.
97. Kelly JP, Webb WR, Moulder PV, et al: Management of airway trauma. II: Combined injuries of the trachea and esophagus. Ann Thorac Surg 1987;43:160.
98. Kieffer E, Le Thoai H, Jue-Denis P, et al. Les traumatismes aigus de l'axe carotidien en pratique civile: 15 observations. Chirurgie 1981;107:447.
99. Kirsh MM, Orringer MB, Behrendt DM, Sloan H. Management of tracheobronchial disruption secondary to nonpenetrating trauma. Ann Thorac Surg 1976;22:93.
100. Knightly JJ, Swaninathan AP, Rush BF. Management of penetrating wounds to the neck. Am J Surg 1973;126:575.
101. Krajewski LP, Hertzer NR. Blunt carotid artery trauma. Ann Surg 1980;191:341.
102. Lambert GE, McMurry GT. Laryngotracheal trauma. Recognition and management. JACEP 1976;5:883.
103. Leads from the MMWR. Progress toward achieving the national 1990 objectives for injury prevention and control. JAMA 1988;259:2069.
104. LeBlanc KA, Benzel EC. Trauma to the high cervical carotid artery. J Trauma 1984;24:992.
105. Ledgerwood AM, Mullins RJ, Lucas CE. Primary repair versus ligation for carotid artery injuries. Arch Surg 1980;115:488.
106. Le May SR. Penetrating wounds of the larynx and cervical trachea. Arch Otolaryngol 1971;94:558.
107. Leopold DA. Laryngeal trauma. A historical comparison of treatment methods. Arch Otolaryngol 1983;109:106.
108. Liekwag WG Jr, Greenfield LJ. Management of penetrating carotid arterial injury. Ann Surg 1978;188:587.
109. Lipschitz R. Stab wounds of the spinal cord. In: Vinken PJ, Vruyn GW, eds. Handbook of clinical neurology. Amsterdam: Elsevier/North Holland Publishing Co, 1976:197.
110. Livingstone A. Vascular injuries of the head and neck. Otolaryngol Clin North Am 1983;16:671.
111. Lucente FE, Mitrani M, Sacks SH, et al. Penetrating injuries of the larynx. Ear Nose Throat J 1985;64:406.
112. Mace SE. Blunt laryngotracheal trauma. Ann Emerg Med 1986;15:836.
113. Maran AGD, Stell PM. Acute laryngeal trauma. Lancet 1970;2:1107.
114. Marcoux FW, Morawetz RB, Crowell RM, et al. Differential regional vulnerability in transient focal cerebral ischemia. Stroke 1982;13:339.
115. Markey JC, Hines JL, Nance FC. Penetrating neck wounds: a review of 218 cases. Am Surg 1975;41:77.
116. Marshall WK, Bedford RF. Use of a pulmonary-artery catheter for detection and treatment of venous air embolism: a prospective study in man. Anesthesiology 1980;52:131.
117. Massac E, Siram SM, Leffal LD. Penetrating neck wounds. Am J Surg 1983;145:263.
118. Mathisen DJ, Grillo H. Laryngotracheal trauma. Ann Thorac Surg 1987;43:254.
119. Matjasko J, Petrozza P, Mackenzie CF. Sensitivity of end-tidal nitrogen in venous air embolism detection in dogs. Anesthesiology 1985;63:418.
120. McCormick TM, Burch BH. Routine angiographic evaluation of neck and extremity injuries. J Trauma 1979;19:384.
121. McGovern PJ, Swan KG. Management of bilateral internal jugular venous injuries. Injury 1985;16:259.
122. McMeniman WJ, Fletcher JP, Little JM. Experience with barbiturate therapy for cerebral protection during carotid endarterectomy. Ann Roy Coll Surg Engl 1984;66:361.
123. McSwain NE. Penetrating neck wounds: major advances in the 1980's. In: Maull KI, Cleveland HC, Strauch GO, Wolferth CC, eds. Advances in trauma. Chicago: Year Book Medical Publishers, 1986:135.
124. Meier DE, Brink BE, Fry WJ. Vertebral artery trauma: acute recognition and treatment. Arch Surg 1981;116:236.
125. Merion RB, Harness JK, Ramsburgh SR, Thompson NW. Selective management of penetrating neck trauma. Cost implications. Arch Surg 1981;116:691.
126. Messick JM, Casement B, Sharbrough FW, et al. Correlation of regional cerebral blood flow (rCBF) with EEG changes during isoflurane anesthesia for carotid endarterectomy: critical rCBF. Anesthesiology 1987;66:344.

127. Metzdorff MT, Lowe DK. Operation or observation for penetrating neck wounds? Am J Surg 1984;147:646.
128. Meyer JP, Barrett JA, Schuler JJ, Flanigan P. Mandatory vs selective exploration for penetrating neck trauma. A prospective study. Arch Surg 1987;122:592.
128a. Meyer JP, Walsh J, Barrett J, et al. Analysis of 18 recent cases of penetrating injuries to the common and internal carotid arteries. Am J Surg 1988;156:96.
129. Michenfelder JD, Sundt TM Jr. Cerebral protection by barbiturate anaesthesia: use after middle cerebral artery occlusion in Java monkeys. Arch Neurol 1976;33:345.
130. Michenfelder JD, Sundt TM, Fode N, Sharbrough FW. Isoflurane when compared to enflurane and halothane decreases the frequency of cerebral ischemia during carotid endarterectomy. Anesthesiology 1987;67:336.
131. Miles WK, Olson NR, Rodriguez A. Acute treatment of experimental laryngeal fractures. Ann Otol 1971;80:710.
132. Moffat JA, McDougall MJ, Brunet D, et al. Thiopental bolus during carotid endarterectomy—rational drug therapy? Can Anaesth Soc J 1983;30:615.
133. Morgan MK, Besser M, Johnston I, Chaseling R. Intracranial carotid artery injury in closed head trauma. J Neurosurg 1987;66:192.
134. Mulder DS. Blunt neck injury. In: Hurst JM, ed. Common problems in trauma. Chicago: Year Book Medical Publishers, 1987:135.
135. Myers EM, Iko BO. The management of acute laryngeal trauma. J Trauma 1987;27:448.
136. Nahum AM. Immediate care of acute blunt laryngeal trauma. J Trauma 1969;9:112.
137. Namiroff PM, Katz AD. Extralaryngeal divisions of the recurrent laryngeal nerve. Surgical and clinical significance. Am J Surg 1982;144:466.
138. Narrod JA, Moore EE. Selective management of penetrating neck injuries. Arch Surg 1984;119:574.
139. Newman RK. Penetrating neck trauma. Ear Nose Throat J 1983;62:22.
140. Nolph MB, Richardson JD. Cervical injuries. In: Richardson JD, Polk HC, Flint LM, eds. Trauma, clinical care and pathophysiology. Chicago: Yearbook Medical Publishers, 1987:433.
141. Noyes LD, McSwain NE, Markowitz IP. Panendoscopy with arteriography versus mandatory exploration of penetrating wounds of the neck. Ann Surg 1986;204:21.
142. Obeid FN, Haddad GS, Horst HM, Bivins BA. A critical reappraisal of a mandatory exploration policy for penetrating wounds of the neck. Surg Gynecol Obstet 1985;160:517.
143. Olson NR. Surgical treatment of acute blunt laryngeal injuries. Ann Otol Rhinol Laryngol 1978;87:716.
144. Olson NR, Miles WK. Treatment of acute blunt laryngeal injuries. Ann Otol Rhinol Laryngol 1971;80:704.
145. Ordog GJ. Penetrating neck trauma. J Trauma 1987;27:5.
146. Ordog GJ, Albin D, Wasserberger J, et al. 110 bullet wounds to the neck. J Trauma 1985;25:238.
147. Ordog GJ, Albin D, Wasserberger J, et al. Shotgun "birdshot" wounds to the neck. J Trauma 1987;28:491.
148. Ordog GJ, Wasserberger J, Balasubramaniam S. Shotgun wound ballistics. J Trauma 1988;28:624.
149. O'Sullivan JC, Wells DG, Wells GR. Difficult airway management with neck swelling after carotid endarterectomy. Anaesth Intens Care 1986;14:460.
150. Otteni JC, Pottecher T, Bronner G, et al. Prolongation of the Q-T interval and sudden cardiac arrest following right radical neck dissection. Anesthesiology 1983;59:358.
151. Paparella MM, Shumrick DA. Otolaryngology. Philadelphia: WB Saunders, 1980:2492.
152. Pass LJ, LeNarz LA, Schreiber JT, Estrera AS. Management of esophageal gunshot wounds. Ann Thorac Surg 1987;44:253.
153. Patil VU, Stehling LC, Zauder HL. Instrumentation and auxiliary equipment. In: Patil VU, Stehling LC, Zauder HL, eds. Fiberoptic endoscopy in anesthesia. Chicago: Year Book Medical Publishers, 1983:9.
154. Payne WS, DeRemee RA. Injuries of the trachea and major bronchi. Postgrad Med 1971;49:152.
155. Peacock WJ, Shrosbree RD, Key AG. A review of 450 stab wounds of the spinal cord. South Afr Med J 1977;51:961.
156. Perry MO, Synder WH, Thal ER. Carotid artery injuries caused by blunt trauma. Ann Surg 1980;192:74.
157. Polansky A, Resnick D, Sofferman RA, Davidson TM. Hyoid bone elevation: a sign of tracheal transection. Radiology 1984;150:117.
158. Popovsky J. Perforations of the esophagus from gunshot wounds. J Trauma 1984;24:337.
159. Potter CR, Sessions DG, Ogura JH. Blunt laryngotracheal trauma. Otolaryngology 1978;86:909.
160. Ramzy AI, Rodriguez A, Cowley RA. Pitfalls in the management of traumatic chylothorax. J Trauma 1982;22:513.
161. Rao PM, Bhatti FK, Gaudino J, et al. Penetrating injuries of the neck: criteria for exploration. J Trauma 1983;23:47.
162. Rao PM, Bhatti KF, Ivatury RR, et al. Selective management of penetrating neck wounds. Contemp Surg 1983;23:41.
163. Ray DK. Anaesthesia in a cut-throat injury. Anaesthesia 1962;17:363.
164. Reddin A, Mirvis SE, Diaconis JN. Rupture of the cervical esophagus and trachea associated with cervical spine fracture. J Trauma 1987;27:564.
164a. Reid JDS, Weigelt JA. Forty-three cases of vertebral artery trauma. J Trauma 1988;28:1007.
165. Reyna MT, Cabellon S, Fallon WF. Delayed recognition of carotid artery injury due to blunt trauma. Milit Med 1986;151:450.
166. Rich NM, Spencer FC. Vascular Trauma. Philadelphia: WB Saunders, 1978:260.
167. Richardson JD, Martin LF, Borzotta AP, Polk HC. Unifying concepts in treatment of esophageal leaks. Am J Surg 1985;149:157.
168. Ricotta JJ, Green RM. Trauma to the internal carotid artery following soccer injury. Contemp Surg 1983;23:118.
168a. Rivers SP, Patel Y, Delany HM, Veith FJ. Limited role of arteriography in penetrating neck trauma. J Vasc Surg 1988;8:112.
169. Robbs JV, Human RR, Rajaruthnam P, et al. Neurological deficit and injuries involving the neck arteries. Br J Surg 1983;70:220.
170. Roberts B, Hardesty WH, Holling HE, et al. Studies on extracranial cerebral blood flow. Surgery 1964;56:826.
171. Rogers LF. Injuries peculiar to traffic accidents: seat belt syndrome, laryngeal fracture, hangman's fracture. Texas Med 1974;70:77.
172. Roon AJ, Christensen N. Evaluation and treatment of penetrating cervical injuries. J Trauma 1979;19:391.
173. Roper PR, Guinto FC, Wolma FJ. Posttraumatic vertebral artery aneurysm and arteriovenous fistula: a case report. Surgery 1984;96:556.
174. Rosett R. An unusual cause of postoperative respiratory failure. Anesthesiology 1987;66:695.
175. Rubio PA, Reul GJ, Beall AC, et al. Acute carotid artery injury: 25 years' experience. J Trauma 1974;14:967.
176. Sacco JJ, Halliday DW. Submucosal epiglottic emphysema complicating bronchial rupture. Anesthesiology 1987;66:555.
177. Saletta JD, Lowe RJ, Lim LT, et al. Penetrating trauma of the neck. J Trauma 1976;16:579.
178. Samaan HA. Vascular injuries of the upper thorax and the root of the neck. Br J Surg 1971;58:882.
179. Sankaran S, Walt AJ. Penetrating wounds of the neck: principles and some controversies. Surg Clin North Am 1977;57:139.

180. Schaefer SD. Primary management of laryngeal trauma. Ann Otol Rhinol Laryngol 1982;91:399.
180a. Schaefer SD, Close LG. Acute management of laryngeal trauma. Ann Otol Rhinol Laryngol 1989;98:98.
181. Schenk WG. Neck injuries. In: Moylan JA, ed. Trauma surgery. Philadelphia: JB Lippincott, 1988;429.
182. Sclafani SJA, Panetta T, Goldstein AS, et al. The management of arterial injuries caused by penetration of zone III of the neck. J Trauma 1985;25:871.
183. Seed RF. Traumatic injury to the larynx and trachea. Anaesthesia 1971;26:55.
184. Sessions DG, Ogura JH, Heeneman H. Surgical management of bilateral vocal cord paralysis. Laryngoscope 1976;86:559.
185. Shaia FT, Cassady CL. Laryngeal trauma. Arch Otolaryngol 1972;95:104.
186. Shama DM, Odell J. Penetrating neck trauma with tracheal and esophageal injuries. Br J Surg 1984;71:534.
187. Sheely CH, Mattox KL, Beall AC, DeBakey ME. Penetrating wounds of the cervical esophagus. Am J Surg 1975;130:707.
188. Sheely CH, Mattox KL, Reul GJ, et al. Current concepts in the management of penetrating neck trauma. J Trauma 1975;15:895.
189. Sherman RT, Parrish RA. Management of shotgun injuries: a review of 252 cases. J Trauma 1963;3:76.
190. Shin B, Mackenzie CF, Helrich M. Hypokalemia in trauma patients. Anesthesiology 1986;65:90.
191. Shuck JM, Gregory J, Edwards WS. Selective management of penetrating neck wounds. Ann Emerg Med 1983;12:159.
192. Sinclair D, Woods E, Saibil EA, Taylor GA. "Chyloma": a persistent post-traumatic collection in the left supraclavicular region. J Trauma 1987;27:567.
193. Sirker D, Clark MM. Rupture of the cervical trachea following a road traffic accident: case report. Br J Anaesth 1973;45:909.
194. Snow JB. Diagnosis and therapy for acute laryngeal and tracheal trauma. Otolaryngol Clin North Am 1984;17:101.
195. Snyder WH, Thal ER, Bridges RA, et al. The validity of normal arteriography in penetrating trauma. Arch Surg 1978;113:424.
196. Soderstrom CA, Wasserman DH. Vascular injuries. Emerg Med Clin North Am 1984;2:853.
197. Sofferman RA. Management of laryngotracheal trauma. Am J Surg 1981;141:412.
198. Soothill EF. Closed traumatic rupture of the cervical trachea. Thorax 1960;15:89.
199. Spackman TN, Faust RJ, Cucchiara RF, Sharbrough FW. A comparison of aperiodic analysis of the EEG with standard EEG and cerebral blood flow for detection of ischemia. Anesthesiology 1987;66:229.
200. Stanley RB. Value of computed tomography in the management of acute laryngeal injury. J Trauma 1984;24:359.
201. Stanley RB, Hanson DG. Manual strangulation injuries of the larynx. Arch Otolaryngol 1983;109:344.
202. Stanley RB, Crockett DM, Persky M. Knife wounds into the airspaces of the laryngeal trapezium. J Trauma 28:101, 1988.
203. Stein A, Seaward PD. Penetrating wounds of the neck. J Trauma 1967;7:238.
204. Stevens MH, Stevens CN. Vocal cord paralysis. Ear Nose Throat J 1983;62:519.
205. Storen G, Bugge-Asperheim B, Geiran OR, Dodgson MS. Rupture of the cervical trachea following blunt trauma. J Trauma 1980;20:93.
206. Stromberg BV. Exploration of low-velocity gunshot wounds of the neck. J Trauma 1979;19:381.
207. Symbas PN, Hatcher CR, Vlasis SE. Esophageal gunshot injuries. Ann Surg 1980;191:703.
208. Symbas PN, Hatcher CR, Vlasis SE. Bullet wounds of the trachea. J Cardiovasc Surg 1982;83:235.
209. Symon L. Flow thresholds in brain ischemia, and the effects of drugs. Br J Anaesth 1985;57:34.
210. Teba L, Dedhia HV, Bowen R, Alexander JC. Chylothorax review. Crit Care Med 1985;13:49.
211. Teeple E, Ferrer EB, Ghia JN, Pallares V. Pourfour Du Petit syndrome—Hypersympathetic dysfunctional state following a direct non-penetrating injury to the cervical sympathetic chain and brachial plexus. Anesthesiology 1981;55:591.
212. Thal ER: Injury to the neck. In: Mattox KL, Moore EE, Feliciano DV, eds. Trauma. Appleton and Lange, Norwalk, Conn.: 1988:308.
213. Thal ER, Snyder WH, Hayes R, Perry MO. Management of carotid artery injuries. Surgery 1974;76:955.
214. Thomas RJS. Rupture of the cervical trachea. Med J Aust 1972;1:415.
215. Toung TJK, Ngeow YK, Long DL, et al. Comparison of the effects of positive end-expiratory pressure and jugular venous compression on canine cerebral venous pressure. Anesthesiology 1984;61:169.
216. Toung TJK, Miyabe M, McShane AJ, et al. Effect of PEEP and jugular venous compression on canine cerebral blood flow and oxygen consumption in the head elevated position. Anesthesiology 1988;68:53.
217. Trone TH, Schaefer SD, Carder HM. Blunt and penetrating laryngeal trauma: a 13-year review. Otolaryngol Head Neck Surg 1980;88:257.
218. Tucker HM. Nerve muscle pedicle reinnervation for paralysis of the vocal cord. In: Snow JB, ed. Controversy in otolaryngology. Philadelphia: WB Saunders, 1980:43–50.
219. Unger SW, Tucker WS, Mrdeza MA, et al. Carotid arterial trauma. Surgery 1980;87:477.
220. Verneuil M. Contusions multiples, delire violent, hemiplegie a droite, signes de compression cerebrale. Bull Acad Med (Paris) 1872;1:46.
221. Weigelt JA, Thal ER, Snyder WH, et al. Diagnosis of penetrating cervical esophageal injuries. Am J Surg 1987;154:619.
222. Weil PH, Steichen FM. The treatment of penetrating injuries to the neck. J Trauma 1971;11:590.
223. Weimert TA. Early diagnosis of acute laryngeal injuries. Injury 1980;12:154.
224. Welling RE, Kakkasseril JS, Peschiera J. Pseudoaneurysm of the cervical internal carotid artery secondary to blunt trauma. J Trauma 1985;25:1108.
225. Welling RE, Saul TG, Tew JM, et al. Management of blunt injury to the internal carotid artery. J Trauma 1987;27:1221.
226. Wilson RF, Soullier GW, Wiencek RG. Hemoptysis in trauma. J Trauma 1987;27:1123.
226a. Wood J, Fabian TC, Mangiante EC. Penetrating neck injuries: recommendations for selective management. J Trauma 1989;29:602.
227. Wood JH, Simeone FA, Find EA, et al. Hypervolemic hemodilution in experimental focal cerebral ischemia: elevation of cardiac output, regional cortical blood flow, and ICP after intravascular volume expansion with low molecular weight dextran. J Neurosurg 1983;59:500.
228. Wood JH, Polyjoidia KS, Epstein CM, et al. Quantitative EEG alterations after isovolemic hemodilutional augmentation of cerebral perfusion in stroke patients. Neurology 1984;34:764.
229. Yamada S, Kindt GW, Youmans JR. Carotid artery occlusion due to nonpenetrating injury. J Trauma 1967;7:333.
230. Yap RG, Yap AG, Obeid FN, Horan DP. Traumatic esophageal injuries: 12 year experience at Henry Ford Hospital. J Trauma 1984;24:623.
231. Yarington CT. Trauma involving air and food passages. Otolaryngol Clin North Am 1979;12:321.

# Chapter Fourteen

Richard M. Sommer
R. David Bauer
Thomas J. Errico

# Cervical Spine Injuries

Few diseases or injuries have greater potential for causing death or devastating effects to the quality of life than cervical spine trauma. It usually results from falls, industrial accidents, motor vehicle collisions, gunshot wounds, or athletic activities. The spectrum of disabling conditions that these injuries can cause ranges from minor neck pain to quadriplegia and death.[33] Current diagnostic strategy is directed toward evaluation of both cervical instability and neurologic damage. Management of these patients involves the recognition of injury, immobilization of the spine, restoration of anatomic integrity, and rehabilitation. In addition, recognition and treatment of associated injuries to the head, airway, lungs, and cardiovascular system are important for the care of these patients and improve the probability of survival.

This chapter reviews (a) the acute problems induced by cervical spine instability and spinal cord injury, (b) the physiologic derangements caused by acute and chronic spinal cord damage, and (c) the anesthetic and surgical management strategies followed in these patients. A discussion of spinal cord injury from a different perspective is also offered in Chapter 10.

## EPIDEMIOLOGY

Cervical spine trauma is a disease of industrially developed nations; traffic accidents account for 30–72% of these injuries.[31] A 1981 report estimated that 6,000 automobile passengers die annually in the United States from cervical spine injury.[82] In addition, approximately 500 cases per year of quadriplegia result from automobile accidents. Cervical spine fracture is the most frequent neck injury in severely injured automobile accident victims. It is of note that only 3% of those sustaining severe cervical injury were wearing shoulder-lap belt restraint systems, a fact that confirms reports regarding the effectiveness of these systems in reducing fatal neck injuries.[177]

A California study estimated that the number of acute spinal cord injuries is 53 per million population per year and that the age frequency peaks are 15–35 years and greater than 65 years of age. The risk of quadriparesis was highest for injuries in recreational activities, such as diving.[95,96]

Cervical spine injury statistics are somewhat different in major metropolitan areas. In 1986 at Bellevue Hospital Center in New York City, 36 patients with cervical spine injury were treated by the Department of Neurosurgery. Falls, motor vehicle accidents, gunshot wounds, dives, and crushing trauma were the causes of these injuries (Whitman D, Erickson C, personal communication) (Table 14-1).

With the improvement of medical care it has been recognized that injuries can be exacerbated during transport to and treatment in the hospital. Podolsky and colleagues[127] noted that in traumatized patients 3–25% of spinal cord injuries occur during field stabilization, transit to the hospital, or early in the course of therapy. This finding implies that, in order to prevent additional neurologic disability, care of any severely injured patient must include neck stabilization until cervical fracture is ruled out.

Advances in the treatment and rehabilitation of patients with spinal cord injury have increased their longevity. The increase in the number of patients with these injuries creates a significant financial strain on the economy. The cost of caring for the quadriplegic patient ranges from $35,000 to $75,000 in the first year, and the lifetime cost in the United States for an adult paraplegic averages $750,000.[2,138] These figures do not include lost income from the patient's inability to work.

Since the prognosis for recovery from complete cervical cord lesions is poor, emphasis must be placed first on preventing injury and second on preventing extension of neurologic injury once trauma has occurred. Education, better vehicle design, improved industrial safety, and increased recreational safety are important factors in reducing the incidence and impact of cervical cord injury. The role of the anesthesiologist in preventing the occurrence and extension of cord damage during management of the cervical spine injury victim cannot be overemphasized. His or her skill, knowledge, and judgment in the management of these patients are important ingredients of an optimal prognosis.

## CERVICAL SPINE ANATOMY

The cervical spine consists of seven vertebrae that support and permit motion of the head and neck while protecting the spinal cord. Knowledge of the osseous, ligamentous, and articular anatomy of the region is important for understanding how these functions are accomplished and how trauma to these structures can cause spinal cord injury.[16,81]

### OSSEOUS ANATOMY

The cervical vertebral column consists of five similarly shaped vertebrae, C3–C7, and two highly specialized vertebrae, C1 and C2 (Fig 14-1). The components of a typical vertebra are the body, vertebral arch, and spinous, transverse, and articular processes (Fig 14-2).

The body is the major weight-bearing portion of the vertebra. It is contracted at its waist and enlarged at the superior and inferior ends. Since each vertebra has a diaphysis and two epiphyses it may be considered a miniature long bone.

The vertebral arch protects the spinal cord and consists of two pedicles and two laminae. Each pedicle is attached anteriorly to the vertebral body, whereas the lamina attaches anteriorly to the pedicle and posteriorly in the midline to the contralateral lamina (Fig 14-2). The pedicle is crossed superiorly and inferiorly by spinal nerves that pass through the vertebral notches (Fig 14-3).

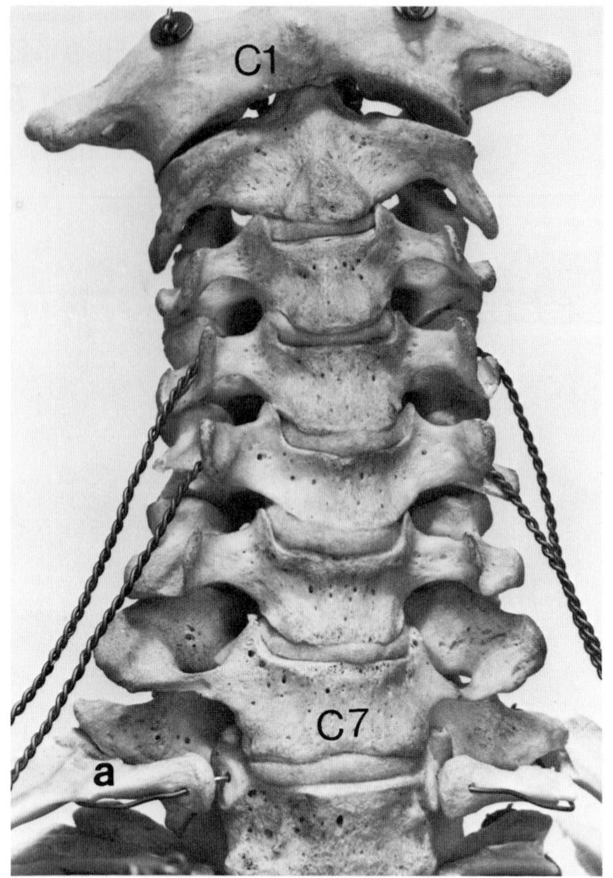


FIG. 14-1. Anterior (a), posterior (b), and lateral (c) views of articulated cervical spine.

The transverse process projects laterally from the junction of the pedicle and lamina and is a muscular insertion site. The cervical transverse process is compound and consists of a posterior, true transverse process and an anterior root or costal process. It terminates in an anterior tubercle with a sulcus for the spinal nerve. Each transverse process has a foramen through which the vertebral artery passes in C1–C6 and the vertebral vein in C7.

The spinous process projects posteriorly from the midline junction site of the lamina. It is directed caudad and is an insertion location for muscles and ligaments. The spinous processes of C2–C6 are bifid, and C7 ends in a large prominence.

The articular processes arise near the junction of the pedicle and lamina. The superior processes arise from the pedicle

TABLE 14-1. Cervical Spinal Cord Injured Patients Treated by The Department of Neurosurgery at Bellevue Hospital in 1986

| SEX | | CAUSE | | NEUROLOGIC INJURY | |
|---|---|---|---|---|---|
| Male | 30 | Falls | 13 | Complete | 20 |
| Female | 6 | Motor vehicle accident | 11 | Incomplete | 16 |
| | | Gunshot wound | 5 | Brown-Séquard syndrome | 3 |
| | | Diving | 6 | Central cord syndrome | 5 |
| | | Crush Injury | 1 | Anterior cord syndrome | 4 |

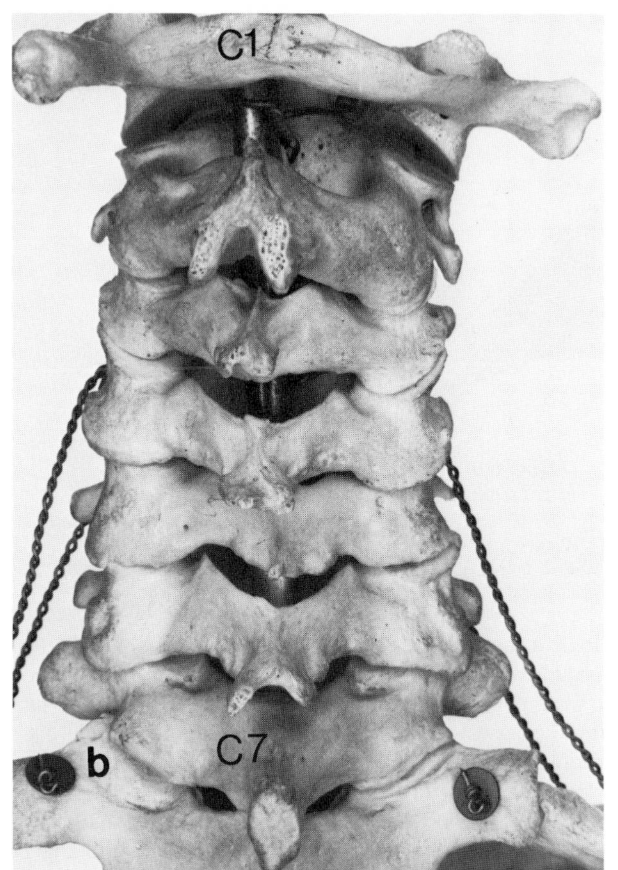


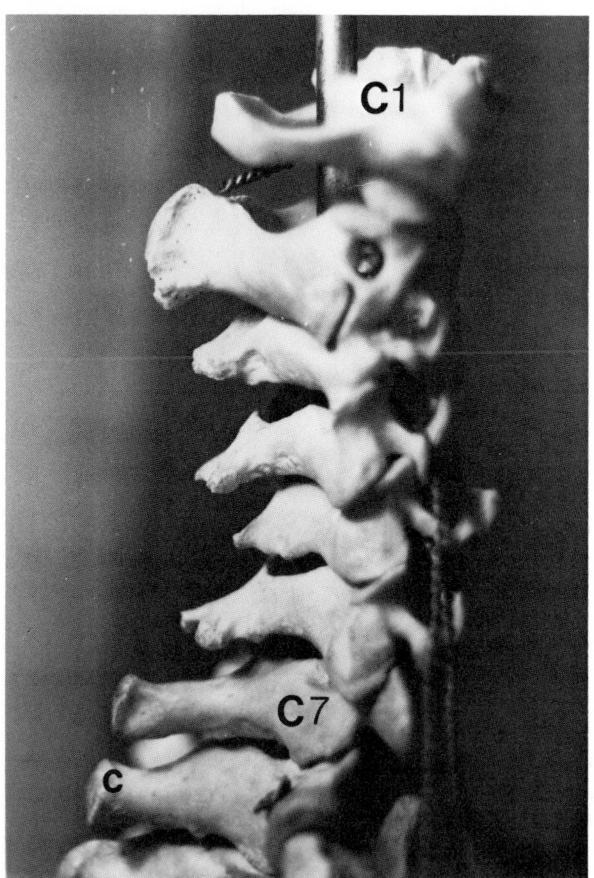


FIG. 14-1. Continued

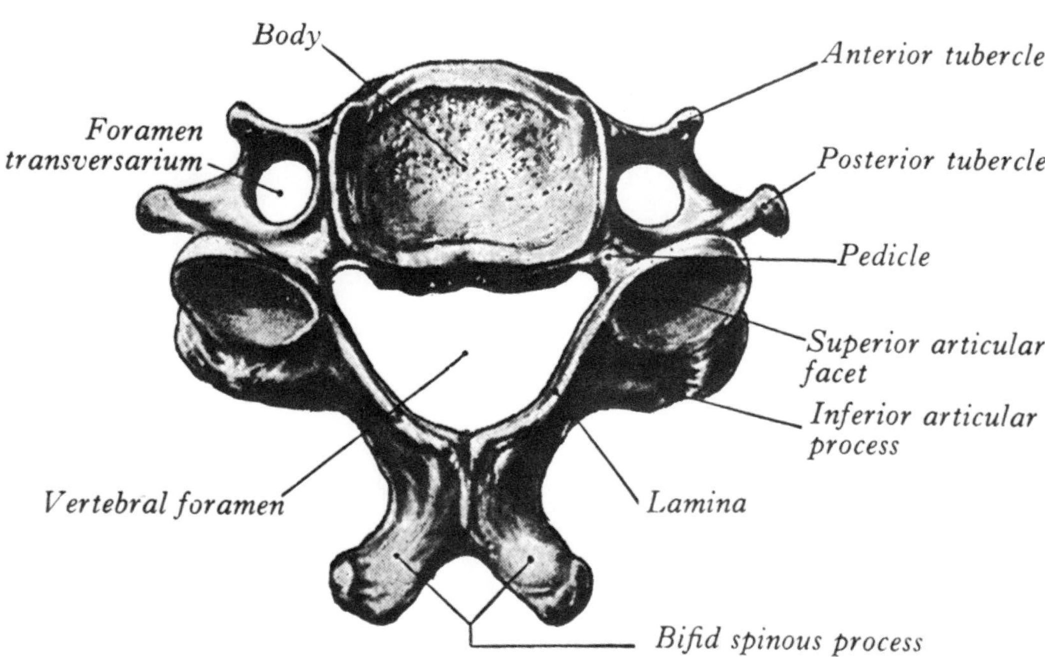

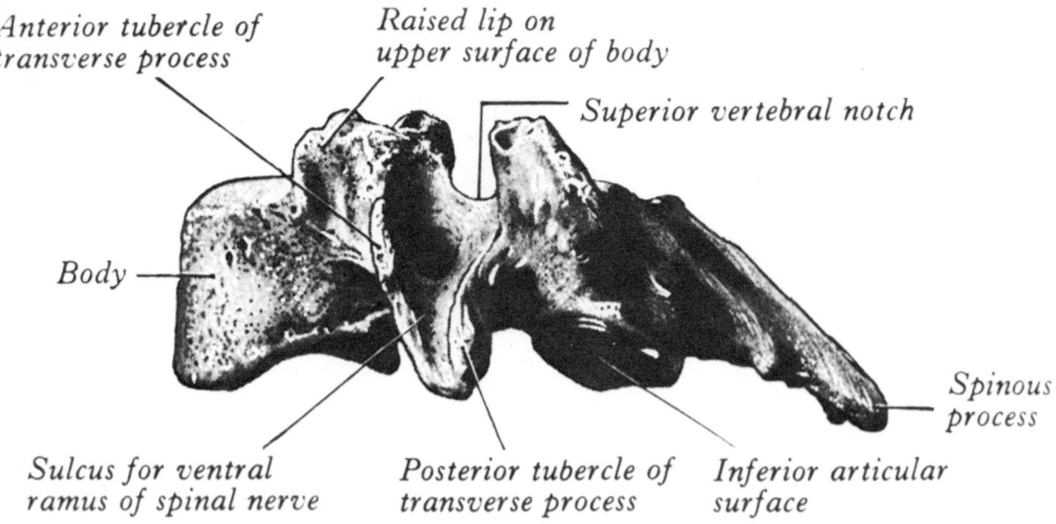


FIG. 14-3. Left lateral view of a lower cervical vertebra. (From Williams PL, Warwick R. Gray's anatomy. 36th ed. New York: Churchill Livingstone, 1980 with permission of the editor and publisher.)

and project posteriorly and superiorly. The inferior processes arise from the lamina and project anteriorly and inferiorly. The pedicles are the posterior contact between the vertebral arches of adjacent vertebrae and prevent forward displacement of the superior vertebra on the inferior one.

Although the functions of C3–C7—providing support to the head and neck and allowing motion of the neck in three planes—are similar, the function and anatomy of C1, the atlas, and C2, the axis, are highly specialized. The atlas is the site of articulation of the head to the neck. It lacks a body and instead consists of an anterior and a posterior arch. There are no articular processes on the atlas. Instead there are paired lateral masses on the superior surface that have foveae for articulation with the occipital condyles of the skull. The lower surface has inferior articular foveae that articulate with the axis. The anterior tubercle of the anterior arch is a muscle insertion site. The posterior part of the anterior tubercle contains a facet, the fovea dentis, for articulation with the dens

FIG. 14-4. Superior view of the atlas. (From Williams PL, Warwick R. Gray's anatomy. 36th ed. New York: Churchill Livingstone, 1980 with permission of the editor and publisher.)

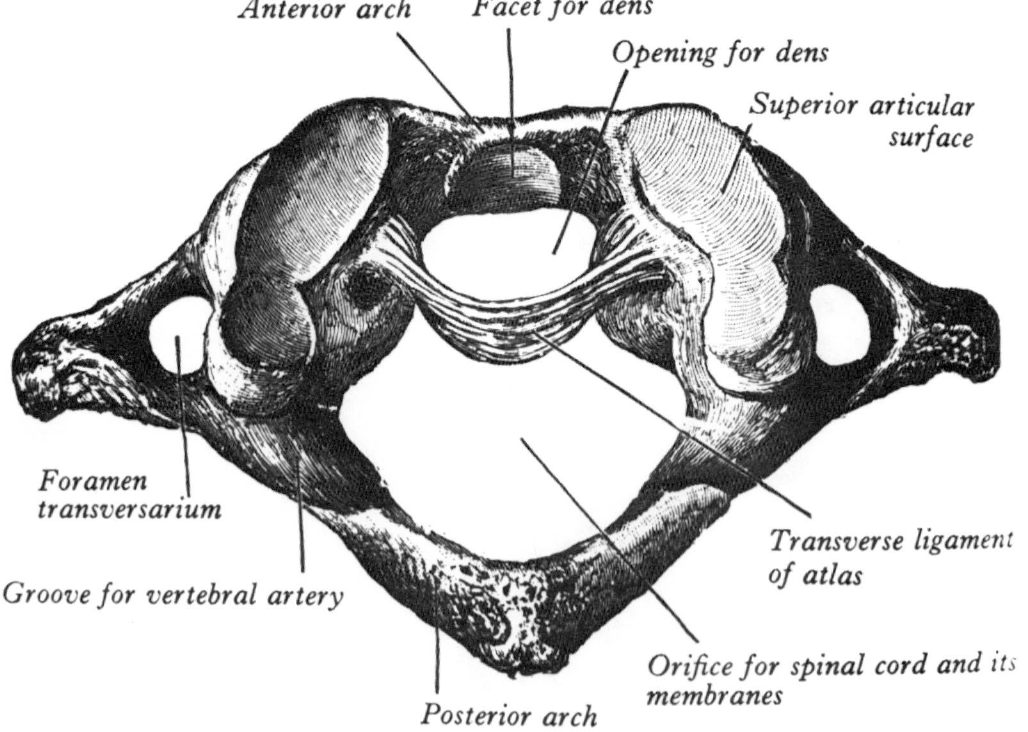

of the axis. The spinous process of the atlas is short and is called the posterior tubercle (Fig 14-4).

The axis, C2, is more similar in appearance to the lower cervical vertebrae than the atlas, but it also contains unique elements. Projecting superiorly from the body of the axis is the dens. The dens or odontoid process is derived embryologically from the body of the atlas. Anterior and posterior articulations and the transverse ligament allow rotation of the atlas on the axis (Figs 14-5 and 14-6). The axis has no superior articular process, but instead has an articular surface that articulates with the inferior articular surface of the atlas. The inferior articular process is similar to those of the remaining cervical vertebrae (Figs 14-4–14-6).

## ARTICULATIONS AND LIGAMENTS

The upper and lower surfaces of the vertebral bodies and the superior and inferior pedicles are the articulation sites of the C2–C7 vertebrae. The joint between the vertebral bodies is a symphysis. It consists of two bony surfaces coated with hyaline cartilage. At the periphery there is a ring-like epiphysis that fuses with the body in early adult life. The cartilage persists and helps enclose the intervertebral disc, which consists of a fibrocartilaginous outer part, the annulus fibrosis, and a fibrogelatinous pulp, the nucleus pulposus, which is virtually incompressible and acts as a shock absorber. The discs are thicker anteriorly than posteriorly and give rise to the anterior convexity or lordosis of the cervical spine. Anterior to the vertebral body, the anterior longitudinal ligament joins adjacent vertebral bodies anteriorly and anterolaterally and limits extension (Figs 14-7 and 14-8). The posterior surfaces of the vertebral bodies are connected by the posterior longitudinal ligament, which tends to check flexion (Fig 14-8). The discs are named for the vertebral body below which they lie. They function to bind adjacent vertebrae together, but allow slight angulation between them. The slight motion that each disc permits between vertebrae enables the substantial mobility of the cervical spine as a whole.

The articular processes are united by synovial joints that consist of a fibrous capsule, synovial membrane, and synovial fluid. They are lined throughout with synovial membrane or articular cartilage. Gliding anterior and posterior motion is permitted at these joints. The articular capsules contribute little to the stability of the cervical spine.

The spine is stabilized posteriorly by the supraspinous ligament, interspinous ligament, and ligamentum flavum (Fig 14-9). The supraspinous ligament runs from the tip of one spinous process to the tip of the next and imparts a high degree of structural integrity to the spinal column. The interspinous ligament is a weak link from the inferior surface of the spinous process to the superior surface of the one below. The ligamenta flava are strong, paired, elastic ligaments that arise from the anterior surface of the lower edge of the superior lamina and attach to the upper part of the posterior

FIG. 14-5. Posterosuperior view of C2. (From Williams PL, Warwick R. Gray's anatomy. 36th ed. New York: Churchill Livingstone, 1980 with permission of the editor and publisher.)

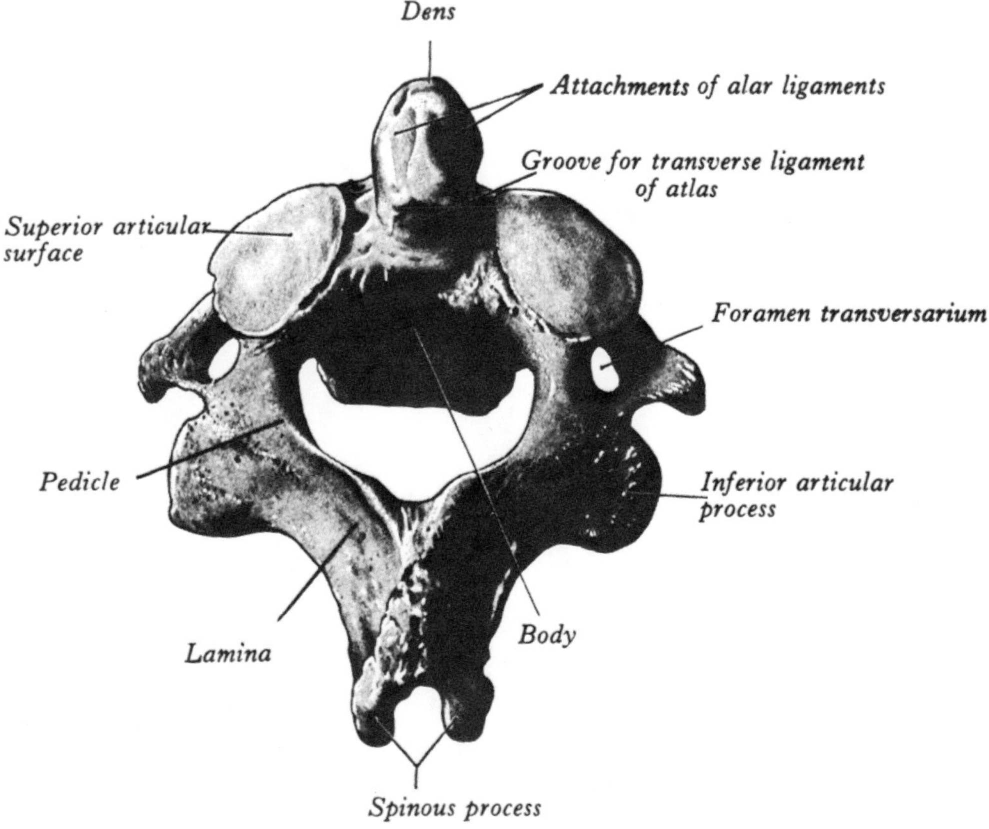

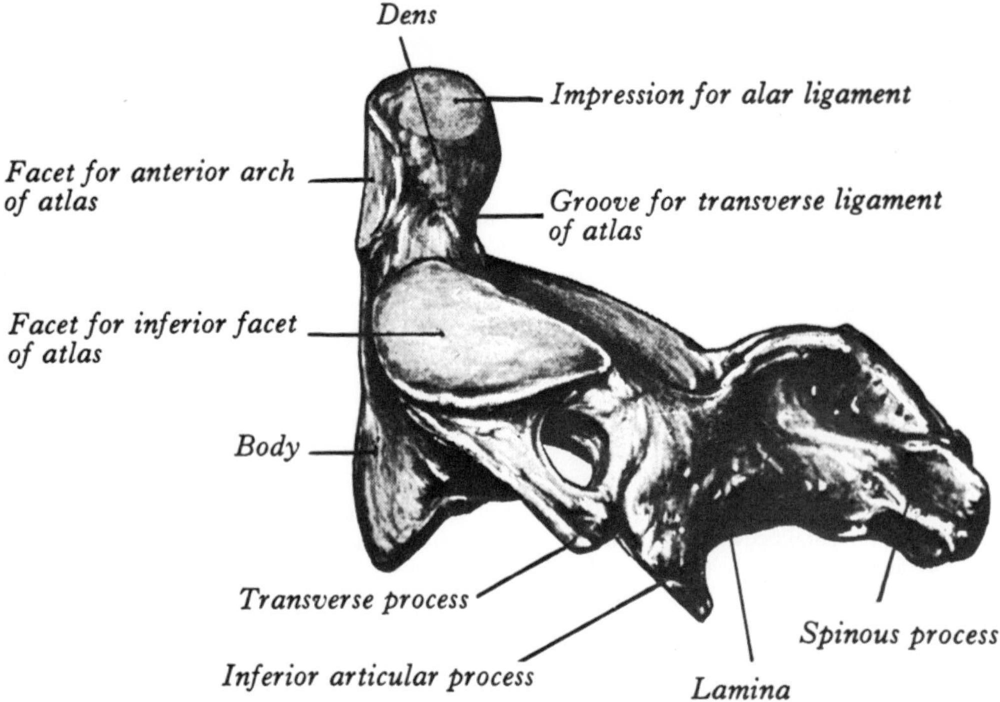


FIG. 14-6. Left lateral aspect of C2. (From Williams PL, Warwick R. Gray's anatomy. 36th ed. New York: Churchill Livingstone, 1980 with permission of the editor and publisher.)

FIG. 14-7. Anterior view of upper cervical spine with ligaments. (From Williams PL, Warwick R. Gray's anatomy. 36th ed. New York: Churchill Livingstone, 1980 with permission of the editor and publisher.)

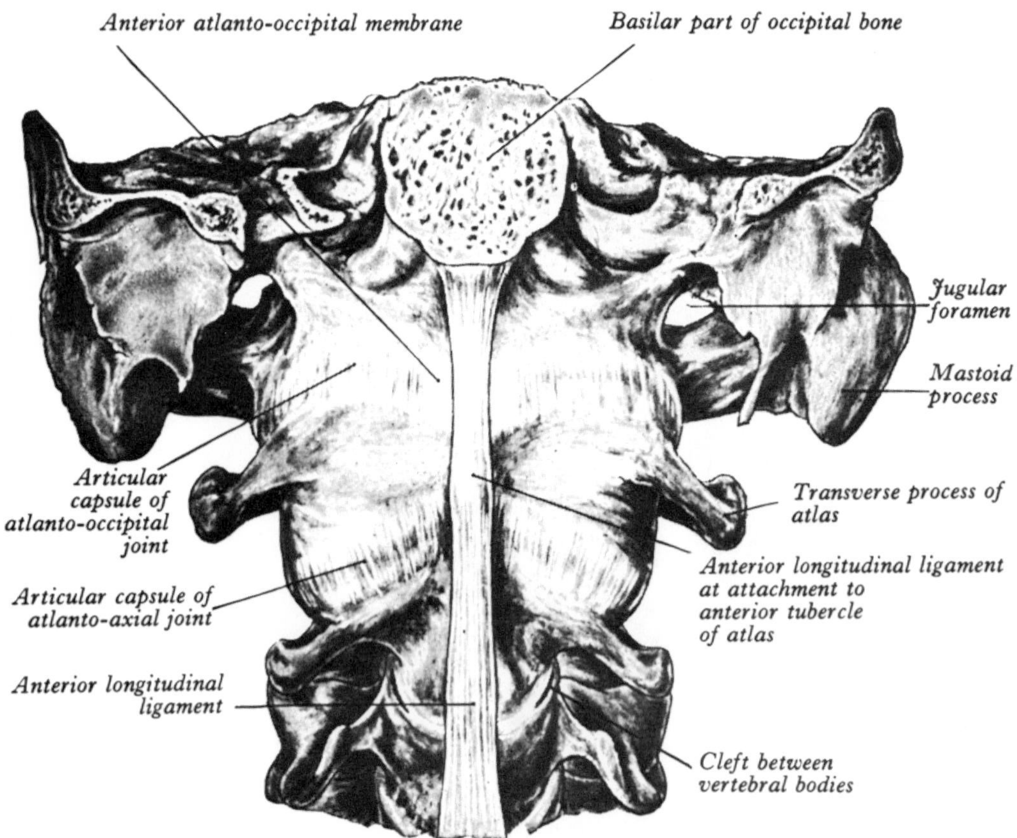

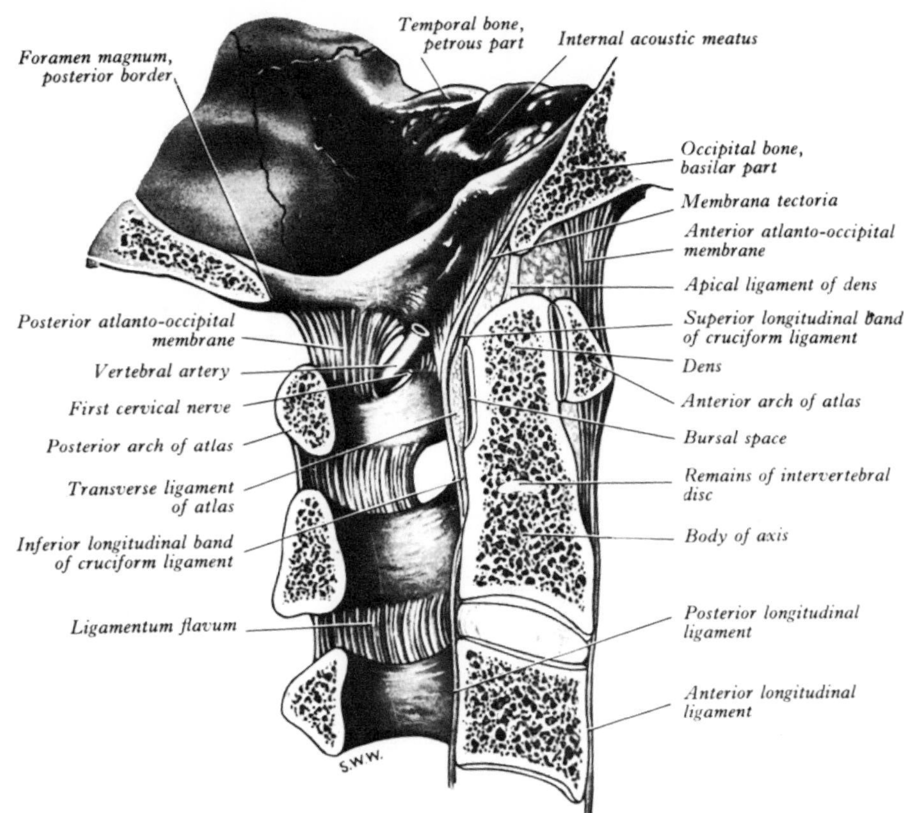


FIG. 14-8. Midsagittal view of cervical spine. (From Williams PL, Warwick R. Gray's anatomy. 36th ed. New York: Churchill Livingstone, 1980 with permission of the editor and publisher.)

surface of the succeeding lamina. Laterally the ligamenta flava approach or blend with the fibrous membranes of the synovial joints, and medially they are separated from each other by a narrow slit. They limit flexion of the cervical spine (Fig 14-9).

Narrow intertransverse ligaments located between succeeding transverse processes add little strength to the spine.

As mentioned earlier, the articulations of the atlas to occiput and axis are specialized. The atlanto-occipital joint is a synovial joint that allows flexion and extension, but no rotation or lateral bending of the head on the atlas. The atlas and axis articulate at three sites to allow rotation of the atlas on the axis and a small amount of flexion and extension. The dens of the axis projects superiorly behind the anterior arch of the atlas and articulates with it through a synovial joint. Laterally, the inferior articular foveae of the atlas articulate with the superior articular surfaces of the axis through synovial joints. The dens is held in place by the cruciform ligament complex, the transverse part of which attaches to the arch of the atlas and is thus called the transverse ligament of the atlas. Synovial cavities between the anterior atlantal arch and the dens and between the dens and the transverse ligament allow rotation. The vertical portion of the cruciform ligament has longitudinal fasciculi, which consist of fibers that attach the body of the axis to the occiput (Fig 14-10).

Other ligaments that stabilize the occiput, C1, and C2 include the apical ligaments, which attach the dens to the occipital bone laterally and restrict rotation (Fig 14-8). The ligamentous attachments of the atlas to the occiput are the anterior and posterior atlanto-occipital membranes, which are superior continuations of the anterior longitudinal ligament and ligamentum flavum, respectively (Fig 14-8). The superior continuation of the posterior longitudinal ligament is the tectorial membrane (Figs 14-8 and 14-10).

## ANATOMY OF THE PEDIATRIC CERVICAL SPINE

The pediatric cervical spine differs from that of the adult because of its cartilaginous nature, ongoing epiphyseal development, and vertebral ossification.[186]

At birth the atlas has three ossification centers: one at the body and one at each of the neural arches. At 3 years the neural arches are closed posteriorly, and by 7 years they are fused to the body of C1 to form a closed ring.

The axis has four centers of ossification: one each for the two neural arches, one for the body, and one for the odontoid process. In young children, the odontoid is attached to the body of C2 by a cartilaginous band, which corresponds to the intervertebral disc. The tip of the dens is also not ossified at birth. By 3 to 6 years of age, ossification of the tip begins, and fusion to the body of C2 takes place.

Os odontoideum occurs when there is complete separation of odontoid from the body of C2. Recent information suggests that it is not a congenital abnormality, but rather a result of

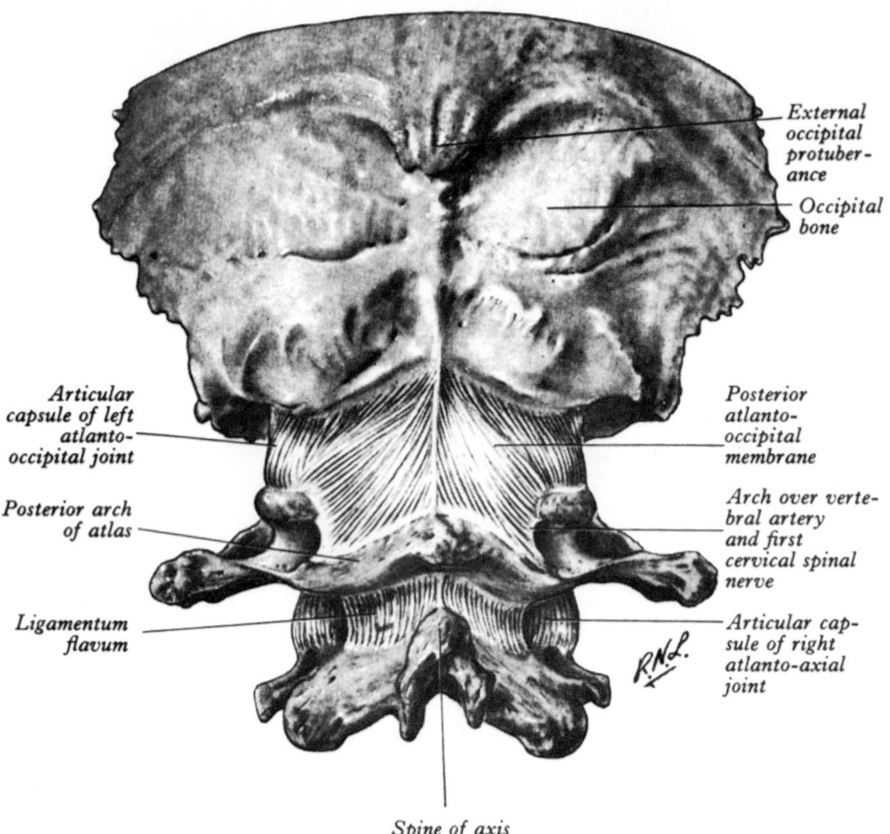


FIG. 14-9. Posterior view of upper cervical spine. (From Williams PL, Warwick R. Gray's anatomy. 36th ed. New York: Churchill Livingstone, 1980 with permission of the editor and publisher.)

a traumatic lesion causing occult odontoid fracture at an early age. Subsequent incomplete healing and bone resorption result in os odontoideum. Clinically significant subluxation of C1–C2 with spinal cord compression can occur in this setting.

The ossification of C3–C7 begins in the two neural arches and the centrum. Complete ossification occurs by 3 to 6 years. Posteriorly, fusion occurs by 2 to 3 years.

As in the adult, the anterior and posterior longitudinal ligaments; the lateral alar, apical dentate, and cruciate ligaments; and the tectorial membrane are critical for providing stability to the cervical spine. The adult elastic properties of these ligaments are not attained until 8 years of age. Thus, abnormal mobility may occur between vertebral bodies with minor trauma.

The angulation of the facet joints in the lower cervical spine changes from 55° to 70° and in the upper cervical spine from 30° to between 60° and 70° by 10 years. Additionally, ossification of the facets does not occur until 7 to 10 years; no significant stability is present until ossification occurs.

## KINEMATICS OF THE CERVICAL SPINE

Kinematics is the branch of mechanics that examines the motion of bodies without consideration of influencing forces.[83] Cervical spine motion is determined by the geometry of the articular surfaces and the mechanical properties of the connecting ligaments. Although the kinematics of this region have been studied in patients and cadaver models, additional investigation and further research are required.

The cervical spine is subject to many types of motion. Movement in the horizontal, vertical, and lateral directions without rotation about an axis is called translation. The cervical spine is also capable of rotatory movements about the vertical axis, lateral bending about the horizontal axis, and anterior flexion and posterior extension around the transverse axis.

The atlanto-occiptal joint has an average range of motion of 13.4° in extension and flexion. Most investigators believe there is no rotation about the vertical axis. The amount of lateral bending possible at the atlanto-occipital joint is controversial; reports range from 7.8° to 40°. The atlantoaxial complex permits 10° of flexion and extension. Up to 47° of rotation about the vertical axis is possible at this joint, accounting for 40 to 50% of the total axial rotation of the neck. This degree of rotation may at times be associated with kinking of the vertebral arteries and the development of vertebrobasilar ischemia and stroke. There is no lateral bending at C1–C2.

Anteroposterior translation greater than 1 mm is abnormal at the occipitoatlantoaxial complex. There can be up to 2 mm

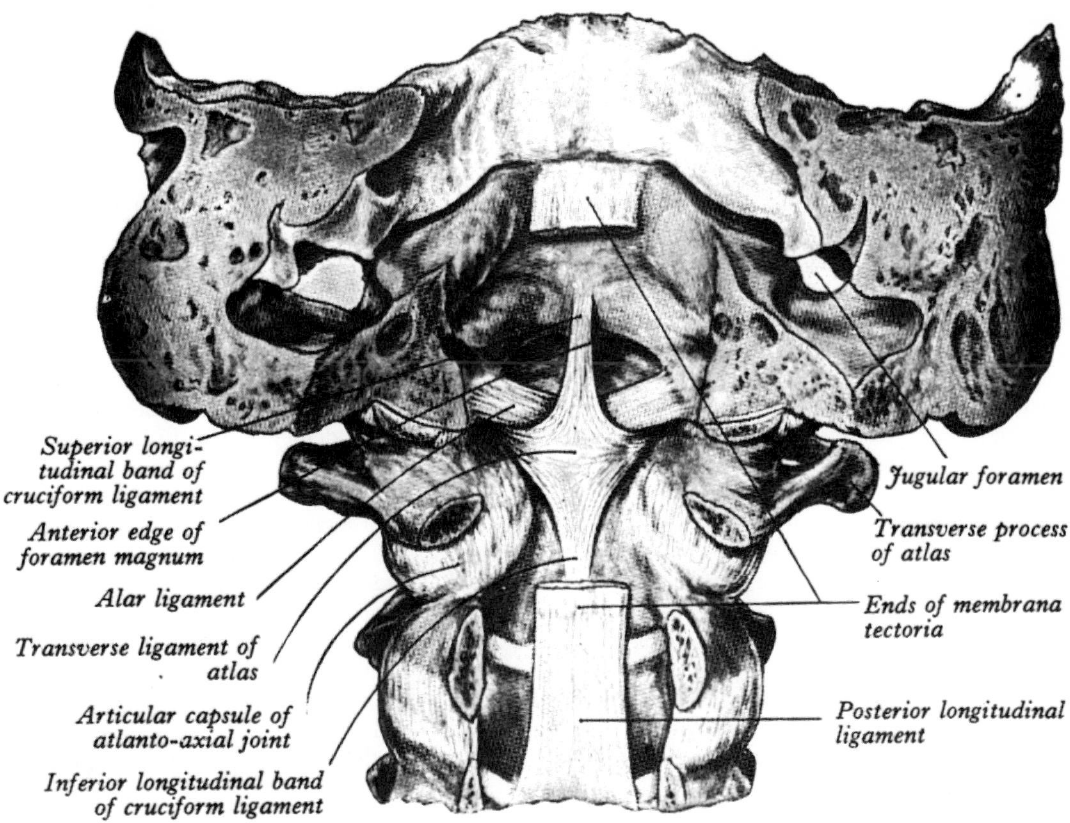


FIG. 14-10. Posterior view of cervical spine with laminae and spinous processes removed. (From Williams PL, Warwick R. Gray's anatomy. 36th ed. New York: Churchill Livingstone, 1980 with permission of the editor and publisher.)

of vertical translation between the occiput and C2, but any additional movement results in rupture of the occipitodentate and alar ligaments. Lateral displacement of C1–C2 greater than 4 mm is abnormal, as is lateral displacement at the atlanto-occipital joint.

Coupling is motion that takes place in one axis while movement is occurring in another axis. It is primarily caused by the geometry of the facet joints. At the C1–C2 joint axial rotation is associated with vertical translation.

The range of motion of the lower cervical spine in the adult decreases with age; the etiology of this decrease is unclear. Pain in the neck and muscles of the upper extremity is also associated with limitation of motion.

The maximum anterior horizontal translation normally observed is 2.7 mm. If one allows for projection magnification in radiographic evaluation, horizontal translation greater than 3.5 mm measured on a lateral film is considered abnormal.

As determined by the stretch test in normal volunteers, vertical translation in the lower cervical spine is normal if less than 1.8 mm of separation exists in the intervertebral interspaces.

Motion of the cervical spine during flexion involves tilting and sliding of the superior vertebra over the inferior. During translation and rotation the joint surface of the inferior vertebra slides upward and forward while the spinous processes separate.

The coupling characteristics of the lower cervical spine are such that during lateral bending the spinous processes rotate to the convexity of the spinal curve. This coupling characteristic helps explain unilateral cervical facet dislocation as a consequence of exaggerated lateral bending. The facet on one side moves too far caudad and the one on the other side moves too far cephalad and consequently is dislocated.

## THE SPINAL CORD AND SPINAL VASCULATURE

The cervical spinal cord is a cylindric extension of the brainstem and occupies two-thirds of the vertebral canal.[188] It is enclosed by the dura, arachnoid, and pia maters, which are separated from each other by the subdural and subarachnoid spaces, respectively. Located at intervals are the paired dorsal and ventral roots of the spinal nerves. They exit from the spinal cord, cross the subarachnoid space, and traverse the dura mater separately. In or near the intervertebral foramina they unite to form the spinal nerves. The ventral spinal roots consist of efferent somatic nerve fibers, whereas the spinal ganglia of the dorsal roots are located proximal to the junction with the ventral root and are formed by afferent sensory nerve fibers.

The spinal cord is suspended by the dentate ligaments.

They are attached to the inner surface of the dura and lateral surface of the cord and thus anchor the cord to the dural surface.

Blood reaches the spinal cord via spinal branches of the vertebral, deep cervical, and anterior and posterior spinal arteries. These vessels contribute to the formation of longitudinal anastomotic channels along the cord. The spinal branches of local arteries give rise to anterior and posterior radicular arteries that approach the spinal cord along the nerve roots (Fig 10-12 in Chapter 10). The anterior arteries are small, whereas the posterior ones supply the dorsal root ganglia. A small number of radicular arteries, four to nine, reach the anterior median sulcus of the spinal cord where they divide into ascending and descending branches.

From the anterior spinal artery, central branches pass into the anterior median fissure and supply the anterior gray column, some of the posterior gray column, the dorsal nuclei, and the adjacent white matter.

The posterior spinal arteries give rise to a pair of longitudinal, frequently anastomosing channels that lie anterior and posterior to the attachments of the dorsal roots. These channels are also supplied by the posterior radicular arteries. The remaining part of the posterior gray column, the posterior white column, and the peripheral parts of the lateral and anterior white columns are supplied by small radially directed vessels from the posterior spinal arteries. Vessels from the pia mater plexus also contribute to the vascular supply of the cord.

The veins of the spinal cord drain into six tortuous, plexiform, longitudinal channels. They are located along the anterior median fissure, the posterior median sulcus, and the sites of attachment of the nerve roots.

## CERVICAL SPINAL CORD INJURIES

### NEUROLOGIC INJURY

The risk of neurologic trauma caused by instability of the cervical spine makes these injuries potentially devastating. Vascular insufficiency resulting from direct pressure on the spinal cord and/or nerve roots is the principal cause of spinal cord injury. Experiments on impact injury have demonstrated that trauma causes mechanical destruction of neuronal elements and/or hemorrhage, decreased vascular perfusion, tissue hypoxia, edema, and necrosis (Fig 10-13, Chapter 10) These changes are time dependent; after injury, partial inhibition of axoplasmic transport is seen in 2 hours, marked block of axoplasmic transport occurs within 4 hours, and complete inhibition of axoplasmic function occurs in 6 hours.[3]

The histology of spinal cord injury has been studied extensively in animals. Seconds after trauma to the cord, flame-shaped hemorrhages appear in the gray matter and in the pia arachnoid. Within 10 minutes hemorrhage spreads to the white matter and begins to affect the microcirculation of the cord.[42] Hemorrhage within the central gray matter spreads to the periphery of the white matter within 4 hours and causes irreversible cystic degeneration and neurolysis. After 24 hours cord necrosis begins and lesions remain unchanged.[113]

It is generally believed that neurons originating and terminating within the central nervous system cannot regenerate after tissue necrosis. Therefore, deficits from spinal cord trauma depend on the initial insult and the success or failure of early resuscitation. Therapeutic modalities aimed at reducing neurologic injury in experimental animals have included selective hypothermia of the spinal cord and the use of hyperosmotic agents, glucocorticoids, hyperbaric oxygen, vasopressors to maintain perfusion, epsilon-aminocaproic acid for membrane stabilization, and dimethyl sulfoxide. Naloxone has been used for spinal cord preservation in the experimental animal with some success. In the human it has been difficult to evaluate these therapeutic techniques primarily because of inability to transport the patient rapidly to a hospital center equipped to do this research. Although steroids have been used, only recently[22a] benefit from their administration has been demonstrated. In humans, spinal cord cooling is technically difficult and therapeutically questionable.[3]

Injury to the vertebral arteries caused by blunt or penetrating trauma to the neck may result in ischemia of the brainstem or spinal cord. The onset may be acute or delayed. The vertebral arteries are prone to injury at their point of entry into the foramen transversarum at C6, in the bony canal from C1–C6, at the atlantoaxial joint due to dislocation, and along their course from the foramen of C1 to their entry into the skull. Indeed, these arteries are subjected to severe stress when the head is rotated in wide arcs, and blood flow is significantly decreased at the extremes of motion. Occlusion of the basilar artery is usually associated with a high mortality rate.[19,68]

Most patients develop incomplete motor and sensory deficits. In incomplete lesions function is preserved more than one level below the injury. Examples of incomplete lesions are those in which sacral sparing is present, distal motor or sensory function exists, or intact somatosensory evoked responses (SSEPs) can be elicited.

A patient who sustains paralysis with no sign of distal sparing may have a complete and irreversible cord lesion. When the period of spinal shock is over, which is heralded by the return of the bulbocavernosus reflex (elicited by pulling on the glans penis, tapping the clitoris, or tugging on an indwelling urinary catheter and obtaining a rectal sphincter response), a definitive diagnosis can be made. If the reflex has returned and complete paralysis continues, there will be no neural recovery.[80,162] The SSEP is absent in patients with complete motor and sensory loss.[72,137] A complete lesion does not necessarily imply a severed spinal cord; the mechanism of this type of neurologic impairement is usually physiologic transection or disruption of cord conduction.

Neurologic injury to the cervical cord may result in complete or partial loss of sympathetic nervous system control. In neurogenic shock peripheral vasodilation occurs because of loss of sympathetic output, resulting in bradycardia, hypotension, and decreased body temperature.[113] Neurogenic shock may also decrease capillary perfusion to the injured spinal cord and thus add secondary damage to the primary injury.

When there is incomplete motor or sensory loss, neurologic examination may reveal a specific pattern of damage. "Cord syndromes" are caused by injury to specific fiber tracts. The damage can be predicted by knowledge of the cross-sectional anatomy of the spinal cord.

*Anterior cord syndromes* are caused by damage to the ventral aspect of the spinal cord and involve mainly the spinothalamic and corticospinal tracts, which carry sensory and motor innervation, respectively. Usually this damage results in immediate partial or complete paralysis with loss of pain and temperature sensation. There is preservation of proprioception, vibration, and deep pressure sensations.[56,178] The primary injury is to the anterior spinal artery, the ventral aspect of the spinal cord, or both. It is the most common spinal cord syndrome and is usually caused by flexion injury of the cervical spine. It may be associated with a retropulsed disc, fracture-dislocation, or vertebral burst fracture. The prognosis for neurologic recovery is guarded. Preservation of the spinothalamic tract with retention of pinprick sensation is a favorable prognostic sign.[113]

*Central cord syndromes* are usually caused by expanding central cord hematomas that compress adjacent pyramidal fibers.[18,80] The syndrome is most commonly seen in older patients, especially those with degenerative spine changes, narrowed spinal canals, and osteophytic ridges, after severe extension injuries.[18,36] The hallmarks of this syndrome are greater motor impairment of the upper than the lower extremities, bladder dysfunction, and varying degrees of sensory loss below the level of the lesion. Fine finger movements are the first affected and last to recover. Lower extremity fibers are protected by their lateral position and recover first. Bladder function also recovers early. A varying degree of recovery is possible, but many patients are left with permanent neurologic deficits.[18,36,178]

The mechanism of *Brown-Séquard Syndrome* is poorly understood, but is probably related to rotation dislocation/subluxation injuries or unilateral pedicle/laminar injuries. There is motor weakness on the side of the lesion and decreased pain and temperature sensation on the contralateral side beginning one or two segments below the level of injury. Significant neurologic recovery often occurs.[36,178]

*Posterior cord syndrome* is marked by the loss of position and vibration sense distal to the lesion, which is caused by involvement of the posterior columns. Rarely seen, it is usually associated with extension injuries.[36,56,178]

## CERVICAL SPINE STABILITY AND SOFT TISSUE, LIGAMENTOUS, AND BONY INJURIES

### SOFT TISSUE INJURIES

Hyperextension or "whiplash" injuries of the neck have received much attention in the literature and in the courts.[78,79] These injuries occur most often during rear-end automobile collisions in which the victim may suffer severe hyperextension of the neck. The head and neck are subjected to acceleration forces of up to 10 *g* (force equal to ten times of that applied by gravity) at impact speeds of only 15 mph.[110] Motion of the head and neck stops only when the back of the head strikes the upper spine. In experimentally produced simple extension strain of the neck, muscle tears were common and produced hemorrhage and spasm. Occasionally, tears of the anterior longitudinal ligament or separation of the disc from the vertebral body was observed.[79,110,122] More severe injuries are noted with hyperextension than with flexion because the potential range of motion is greater. When the neck flexes anteriorly or laterally the head strikes the chest or shoulder. This limitation of motion protects the soft tissues of the neck. Front-end collisions may create posterior soft tissue injury if the flexed head strikes the dashboard or windshield. Tearing of the posterior muscles and ligaments may also occur.[78,79]

The symptoms and signs of soft tissue injury are variable. Often severe pain is experienced immediately after injury, but it may be delayed up to 24 hours. The most prominent immediate finding is muscle tenderness anteriorly and posteriorly. Pain may radiate from the neck to one or both shoulders and down the arms, to the interscapular area, to the chest, and to the occipital region. These patterns of referral are nonneurogenic and can be reproduced by experimental injection of hypertonic saline into the interspinous ligament at any point from C1 to C7.[110] The pain is probably produced by irritation of muscular, ligamentous, joint, and/or intervertebral disc structures.[78,79]

Pain radiating down the arm does not necessarily indicate nerve root compression. Frank disc herniation rarely results from soft tissue injury. However, a frequent postinjury complaint is pain or numbness along the ulnar border of the hand, and objective sensory changes may be present. They are usually caused by scalenus spasm as opposed to true ulnar neuropathy.[79,110]

Cerebral symptoms may be present in the form of confusion, mental dullness, or mild amnesia. Patients may complain of mild headache that is manifested intermittently for months. Blurred vision, tinnitus, and vertigo are common symptoms. Dysphagia is also common and is probably caused by retropharyngeal hematoma or edema.[110] Rarely, hyperextension of the cervical spine in the elderly can cause a large retropharyngeal hematoma, which by displacing the trachea anteriorly may result in signs of acute airway obstruction.[154]

### INSTABILITY OF THE CERVICAL SPINE

Stability of the cervical spine is determined by the integrity of the bones and ligaments. When the integrity of this complex is disrupted abnormal movement may occur that may injure or compress the spinal cord or nerve roots.[84] Instability can thus be functionally defined as weakness of intervertebral bonds that renders them unable to withstand loads tolerated by the normal spine. This weakness implies actual or potential abnormal excursion of one segment on another and therefore actual or potential compromise or irritation of neural elements in the absence of incapacitating deformity or pain from structural changes.[37,56]

The exact determinants of instability are controversial. However, various signs of instability should be sought on plain films.

- "Fanning" of the spinous processes in excess of what is observed at adjacent levels, with or without flexion[151]
- Widening of the intervertebral disc space in excess of that observed at adjacent levels, with or without flexion, extension, or traction[30,151]
- More than 3.5 mm of horizontal displacement of one vertebra relative to its adjacent vertebra, as measured on lateral resting or flexion/extension views[37,180]

- More than 11° of vertebral angulation compared to that of either adjacent vertebra[37,180]
- Disruption of the facet joints, especially with comminuted fractures in and around these joints[37,180]
- Evidence of severe injury, such as multiple fractures at one segment, implying disruption of the anterior or posterior stabilizing complex[37,180]

Atlantal fractures can be either stable or unstable. In all cases the atlantal ring is broken in at least two places. Fractures of the ring in which the transverse ligament is intact are stable, whereas fractures associated with ligament rupture are unstable. Posterior movement of the dens greater than 3 mm behind the anterior ring of the atlas implies significant injury to the transverse ligament.[84]

Fractures of the dens in its middle portion and at the base (types II and III) are unstable since there is associated atlantoaxial instability in all planes of motion. Severe arch fractures of C2, "hangman's fracture," are unstable in flexion at the C2–C3 level.

Despite capsular disruption, unilateral facet dislocations are usually stable unless ligamentous damage is excessive. Dislocations associated with fractures of the facets are usually unstable.[84] Bilateral facet dislocation is a very unstable lesion because most of the ligaments must be destroyed or damaged to allow this type of injury. Fractures through the superior cervical facet with associated extensive ligamentous injury may be very unstable in flexion.[84]

## ATLANTO-OCCIPITAL DISLOCATIONS

Although there are isolated reports of survivors, generally this severe injury is incompatible with life. It is the most common cervical spine injury in fatal motor vehicle accidents.[6,7,27] The mechanism of death seems to be transection of the medulla oblongata or of the spinomedullary junction.[17,46,54]

The mechanism of injury seems to be hyperextension of the head associated with a distraction force to the cranium. The structure primarily responsible for checking these motions is the tectorial membrane; its rupture is required for atlanto-occipital dislocation.[17,46,54] Hyperflexion is prevented by contact between the anterior margin of the foramen magnum and the odontoid.[27]

The diagnosis is made by the demonstration of marked retropharyngeal swelling on the lateral cervical spine film. The anterior portion of the foramen magnum, the basion, normally is directly over the odontoid. The distance between the anterior edge of the foramen magnum and the tip of the posterior arch of the atlas should be the same as the distance from the anterior arch of the atlas and the posterior edge of the foramen magnum. If the ratio of these distances is greater than one, then the head is forward of the spine as the result of atlanto-occipital dislocation.[130] In addition, further injury to the lower cervical spine must be ruled out.

## INJURIES TO THE C1-C2 COMPLEX

Injury to the C1-C2 complex is most commonly caused by force applied to the spine via the base of the skull, and multiple injuries in this region are common.[102,179]

Serious neurologic injury is less common in patients sustaining injury to the upper cervical spine than in those sustaining injury to lower levels. Survivors with these lesions rarely have neurologic sequelae. In part this is due to the relatively small proportion of the canal occupied by the cord in this region[52,102]; the cord and dens each occupy one-third of the available space, and the remaining third is empty. However, when neurologic injury does occur it is frequently fatal. These lesions are commonly found during autopsy of victims of fatal motor vehicle accidents.[6,7]

## FRACTURE OF THE ATLAS

Fractures of the ring of the atlas are most frequently the result of motor vehicle accidents. Other associated cervical spine fractures, especially type I "hangman's fracture" and type II and III odontoid fractures, frequently occur in conjunction with atlantal fractures.[56]

Several major types of C1 ring fracture can be identified. Anterior arch fractures are rare and are usually comminuted and minimally displaced. Posterior arch fractures account for two-thirds of all atlantal fractures and occur at the junction of the posterior arch and lateral mass.[148] They are the result of hyperextension that compresses the posterior arches of the atlas between the occiput and axis pedicles.[58] Lateral mass fractures are uncommon. Fracture lines pass through the articular surface anterior or posterior to the lateral mass on one side of the atlas. Displacement is asymmetric.

Burst fracture of C1 was first described by Jefferson in 1920 and bears his name. The primary force is directed vertically against the skull with downward displacement of the occipital condyles, which drives the lateral masses of C1 apart.[149,150] A classic Jefferson's fracture is a four-part fracture of the ring of C1 with two fractures each in the anterior and posterior arches of C1. Greater force will cause the rupture of the transverse ligament.

Patients present with occipital or neck pain or neck stiffness. Traumatic lesions are always located in the portions of the ring adjacent to the lateral masses and are jagged in appearance. This pattern differs from congenital defects, which are often in the midportion of the arch and are smooth and rounded.[57,150]

Transverse ligament disruption without fracture occurs in the elderly and results from a fall with a blow to the occiput. The average force required to rupture the transverse ligament experimentally is 84 Kg.[58] The same amount of force will also rupture the alar ligaments secondarily. Rupture of the transverse ligament may occur at the midpoint, or it may be associated with an avulsion fracture of the lateral mass on either side of the odontoid. These variants are functionally identical.[58,102] The major diagnostic criterion of this injury is stability on flexion/extension films. The diagnosis of transverse ligament disruption depends on the measurement of the atlantodens interval (ADI) on the lateral radiograph. When the odontoid is intact and shaped normally, the interval on the lateral film between the posterior aspect of the anterior arch of the atlas and the anterior border of the odontoid is the ADI. When the odontoid is deficient, the ADI is measured from a line projected superiorly from the anterior body of the axis and the anterior arch of the atlas. In adults, displacement of 3–5 mm is evidence that the transverse ligament is damaged. If the displacement exceeds 5 mm, the transverse ligament has ruptured and the accessory ligaments are stretched and partially deficient. Displacement greater than 10 mm indicates that all the ligaments have been disrupted.[58] Spasm may make the initial flexion/extension radiographs falsely negative. These patients should be immobilized in a collar, and additional studies should be performed when the spasm subsides.[102]

## ODONTOID FRACTURE

The close interlocking relationship between the atlas and the dens makes them susceptible to common injury. One-third of all fractures of the atlantal ring occur in combination with fractures of the odontoid.[151] Fractures of the odontoid are being reported with increasing frequency, but with decreasing mortality. They may account for 7–14% of cervical spine fractures and occur in conjunction with other cervical spine injuries, skull fractures, mandible fractures, long-bone fractures, and trunk injuries.[115]

The dens is unique in that it is almost completely intraarticular. This anatomic situation has profound effects on the treatment and healing of odontoid fractures. In addition, the atlantoaxial apophyseal joints are horizontal and saddle shaped and add little, if any, anteroposterior stability. A fracture of the dens can therefore create a potentially unstable situation.

An injury to the dens at or above the accessory ligaments leaves the tip fragment floating entirely within synovial cavities.[139,163] The dens is left without periosteal blood supply, and fractures must heal with endosteal new bone formation.

The clinical manifestation of these fractures is usually immediate, with severe high cervical pain and muscle spasm that are aggravated by the slightest motion. Pain may also radiate in the distribution of the greater occipital nerve to the back of the head. Spasm of the neck muscles and severe limitation of motion are the most common physical findings. Neural injury, occurring in 18–25% of cases, may range from high tetraplegia to minimal sensory or motor deficit due to loss of one or several nerve roots.[163]

The diagnosis of odontoid fracture is best made by anteroposterior and lateral tomograms. Since the plane of computed tomography is roughly parallel to the fracture, the fracture may be missed unless sagittal and coronal reconstructions are obtained.[102] These views can sometimes be misleading if the original slices miss the fracture, if the patient has moved, or if there is only minimal displacement.[37]

The differential diagnosis of odontoid fracture must include such anatomic anomalies as os odontoideum. In os odontoideum, the ossicle is smaller than the normal odontoid, usually one-half its size. It is round and is separated from the hypoplastic odontoid by a wide gap. The remnant of the hypoplastic odontoid projects up like a hill above the rest of the ring.[57]

Odontoid fracture results from high-velocity force to the head, but the exact mechanism is unknown. It is probably caused by complex forces, including lateral loading. In about 80% of these fractures, flexion forces the transverse ligament against the posterior aspect of the odontoid and displaces it anteriorly. Extension causes the posterior portion of the anterior ring to impinge on the anterior odontoid with posterior displacement, which is seen in the remaining 20% of fractures.[115]

Classification of odontoid fractures is based upon the level of fracture and is predictive of the likelihood of nonunion[11,139] (Fig 14-11). Type I fractures—avulsion fractures of the tip—are uncommon. The blood supply to the dens is not disturbed, except to the periosteum of the fragment; thus the cervical spine is not rendered unstable. The transverse ligament is intact, and one alar ligament remains attached to the dens. This fracture has a good prognosis.[11]

Type II fractures occur at the junction of the odontoid and the body of C2 and are prone to nonunion.[139,140] The fracture is in the area of the attachment of the accessory ligaments and is the most common type of injury. As a result of ligament damage, excessive motion of the odontoid can occur. The fracture causes a loss of blood supply to the dens. What remains is an area of hard cortical bone with a small surface area. Nonunion is more likely to occur in patients over age 40[11,141] and when the dens is displaced posteriorly.[74]

Type III fractures occur through the body of the axis between the junction of the dens and the axis. These heal well since the fracture occurs through cancellous bone. Although displacement can occur, the injury is usually stable when reduced.[74,151]

Neurologic injury occurs more frequently with posteriorly displaced fractures, as does nonunion. Anteriorly displaced fractures are associated more frequently with other cervical spine injuries, but there are fewer neurologic injuries.[126]

In children, type II fractures are epiphyseal injuries that heal with immobilization alone. In young children, fractures may be caused by a minor fall or other trivial injury, by forceps deliveries, and by major vehicular trauma. The fracture occurs at the junction of the odontoid ossification center (the subdental synchondrosis) with the body. The odontoid fragment almost always angulates anteriorly with respect to the body. Postural reduction should be followed by early rigid immobilization. Stabilization in the extended position should result in union.[8] In these children, an early radiograph is often negative. Persistent symptoms should arouse suspicion, es-

FIG. 14-11. Types of odontoid fractures.

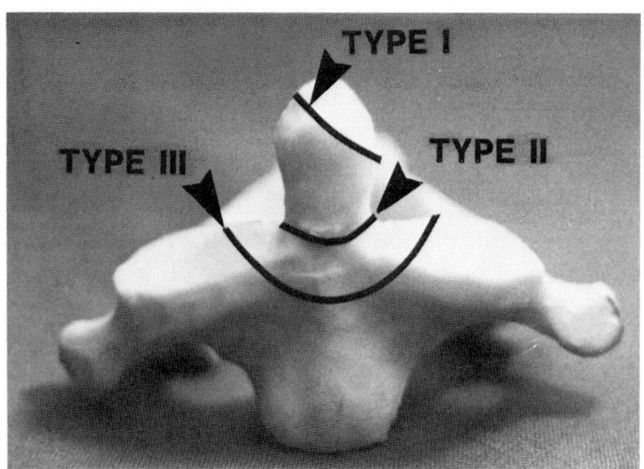

pecially if the child is reluctant to flex or extend the neck. Callus formation can be seen 2 weeks after injury. Operative treatment seems unwarranted in younger children since the rate of union is high.[163] After age 7–10 the synchondrosis fuses, and fractures must be considered identical to their adult counterparts.[150]

### AXIS FRACTURES

Isolated fractures of the body of the axis are uncommon; they are frequently associated with serious facial and thoracic injuries. Neurologic signs are usually transient unless vertebral artery thrombosis occurs.[102]

### TRAUMATIC SPONDYLOLISTHESIS OF THE AXIS

Traumatic spondylolisthesis is characterized by a fracture passing through the neural arch of the axis; it may or may not result in anterior displacement of C2 on C3.[126] The term "hangman's fracture" was given to this lesion because of its similarity to the lesion produced by hanging. Autopsy of prisoners hanged with the knot in the submental position revealed bilateral pedicular axis fractures, and it was postulated that there was complete disruption of the ligaments and disc between C2 and C3. The mechanism of injury was hyperextension with sudden, violent distraction and complete transection of the cord.[62] The dens and the body of the axis were intact.[61]

Today the majority of patients with this lesion are injured in motor vehicle and diving accidents.[62,144] Associated neural injury is relatively uncommon in these patients probably because of the large diameter of the canal at this level, which spares the cord from compression. The absence of distraction forces, which would tear the cranium away, makes this injury different from hanging and makes neurologic injury less probable.[61,62,93] It is the second most common lesion, however, in victims of fatal motor vehicle accidents.[6,7,27]

Diagnosis of this entity is fairly easy. Usually it is clearly evident on the lateral or oblique film. Prevertebral swelling is common and may be associated with more unstable injuries.[126]

Associated head and facial trauma is common in patients with this injury.[61] Head trauma occurs in approximately 70% of patients, and mandibular fractures are more common than maxillary fractures. Frequently there are other upper cervical lesions, such as arch fractures of C1 or C3 and avulsion fractures of C2 and C3.[61] Chest and extremity injuries are also present in over one-thirds of the patients.[126]

The classification of traumatic spondylolisthesis is predicated upon both displacement and angulation of the vertebral bodies on each other.[48,149] Type I fractures are stable and demonstrate no angulation and less than 3 mm displacement. The incidence of neurologic injury is low, but associated cervical spine fractures are common.[101,102] Type II fractures are characterized by significant angulation and translation. Anatomically these are bipedicular fractures in which the anterior longitudinal ligament is shortened but not disrupted. A subset of these fractures, type IIa, is characterized by severe angulation without translation. The anterior disc space is not widened, apparently because of hinging on the anterior longitudinal ligament.[101,102] Type III fractures have severe angulation, displacement, and concomitant unilateral or bilateral facet dislocations.[54,101] This lesion results in separation of the cervicocranium—the skull and first two cervical vertebrae—from the remainder of the cervical spine. The junction between the axis and C3 is a region of high stress, and the neural arch of C2 is the weakest area.[61]

### LOWER CERVICAL FRACTURES AND DISLOCATIONS

Most fractures and dislocations in the lower cervical spine are the result of indirect forces originating in the head or trunk that cause compression or distraction of the neck. Elements of flexion, extension, or rotation may be present. Most injuries are caused by the midair "flight" of the victim in motor vehicle accidents, diving accidents, or head-first falls. Motion of the head is suddenly arrested while the inertia of the rest of the body continues. The resultant force vectors are expended in the spine, and bony or ligamentous injuries result.[163]

A single vector force can cause different injuries in the spine, creating families of injury.[13,75,179] A direct relationship exists between the magnitude of force and severity of injury.[75] There are six common patterns of indirect injury to the lower cervical spine. A comprehensive classification system based upon the mechanism of injury was described by Allen et al.[9] in 1982 (Table 14-2). Each pattern is divided into stages according to the severity of musculoskeletal injury. In all families of injury the injury described in each stage is added to that incurred in the previous stage. The incidence of neurologic damage increases as the stage of the phylogeny goes up.

The families are named according to the dominant force vector leading to failure and also to the presumed attitude of the cervical spine at the time of trauma.[9] "Compressive" indicates that compression accounts for the initial, most conspicuous damage, and "distractive" indicates that tension or shear is the stress producing the most evident structural failure. Ligamentous failure occurs in shear and is inferred from abnormal relationships between vertebrae. Ligaments do not fail in compression. Rotation is not treated as a major injury vector, but rather as a localizing force.

## EARLY PATIENT MANAGEMENT

Treatment of cervical spine trauma begins with the realization that patients with neck, head, facial, and multiple injuries may also have cervical spine instability. All patient care efforts must be directed to prevent the extension of neurologic injury until the stability of the spine can be definitively determined and, if necessary, stabilization achieved.[157] As many as 25% of patients with spinal injuries will develop new or progressive neurologic deficits during initial management, primarily because of the failure to recognize the presence or severity of bony injury.[36,127,133,135] Even when an optimal management strategy is followed, neurologic deterioration after hospitalization may be inevitable in up to 6% of cervical spine injured patients.[107] Management interventions likely to cause such deterioration include early surgery (within 5 days), halo vest application, Stryker frame rotation, skeletal traction application, rotobed rotation, and, of course, airway manipulation.[107]

All phases of care, from the initial evaluation and treatment at the scene to management in the hospital emergency department, should be performed in accordance with the principles of Advanced Trauma Life Support.[10] At the scene, unconscious patients in whom the mode of trauma could have caused spine injury should be treated as if the cervical spine is injured. Alert patients who complain of back or neck pain or tenderness should be treated similarly. Until the cervical spine is immobilized, manual traction must be maintained in order to protect the spine. During transportation and initial hospital management, stabilization is best accomplished with hard collar, sandbags, and tape to a rigid backboard[32,157] (Fig 14-12).

TABLE 14-2. Classificatiion of Lower Cervical Spine Injuries and Characteristics of Each Family of Injury

| CLASSIFICATION | ABBREVIATION | MECHANISM | FREQUENCY | STAGES OF INJURY | PATHOLOGIC FEATURES | REMARKS |
|---|---|---|---|---|---|---|
| Compressive flexion | CF | Compression of vertebral elements while the cervical spine is in flexion | 20% | Stage I (CFS1) | Blunting of the anterior margin of the vertebral body; posterior ligament elements are intact | Compressive force with the spine in flexion at the time of injury creates increasing shear in posterior elements. This links the more severe anterior compression injury with increasing posterior shear and ligamentous failure. |
| | | | | Stage II (CFS2) | Loss of some anterior height and "beaking" of the anterior-inferior vertebral body | |
| | | | | Stage III (CFS3) | Passage of fracture line obliquely from the anterior surface through the subchondral plate without displacement | |
| | | | | Stage IV (CFS4) | Mild (<3 mm) displacement of the inferoposterior margin into the neural canal | |
| | | | | Stage V (CFS5) | Displacement of a vertebral body fragment into the vertebral canal, separation of articular facets, increased distance between spinous processes, and complete failure of the posterior longitudinal ligament | |
| Vertical compression | VC | Neck is in neutral position when force is first applied | 10–15% | Stage I (VCS1) | Fracture through the center of either the inferior or superior endplate of the vertebral body and a cuplike deformity | Posterior portion abuts on or protudes into neural canal. Posterior ligamentous injury can occur if the neck is flexed. Posterior elements may be fractured if the neck is neutral or extended. |
| | | | | Stage II (VCS2) | Fractures through both endplates with minimal displacement | |
| | | | | Stage III (VCS3) | Fragmentation of body with peripheral displacement | |
| Distractive extension | DE | Direction of forces away from the trunk placing the anterior elements under tension | Relatively rare | Stage I (DES1) | Failure of either the anterior ligamentous complex or a transverse fracture of the body; radiographically widening of the disc space | These injuries may be missed on the initial radiographic studies because they are subtle.[9,163] |
| | | | | Stage II (DES2) | Failure of the posterior ligamentous complex allowing displacement of the superior vertebral body posteriorly into the neural canal | |
| Lateral flexion | LF | Direction of compressive injury vector toward the side to which the spine is flexed | Least common | Stage I (LFS1) | Asymmetric, unilateral compression fracture of the vertebral body with a vertebral arch fracture on the ipsilateral side without displacement | |
| | | | | Stage II (LSF2) | Similar to LFS1 with displacement of the arch or separation of the articular processes | |

TABLE 14-2. Classificatiion of Lower Cervical Spine Injuries and Characteristics of Each Family of Injury

| CLASSIFICATION | ABBREVIATION | MECHANISM | FREQUENCY | STAGES OF INJURY | PATHOLOGIC FEATURES | REMARKS |
|---|---|---|---|---|---|---|
| Distractive flexion | DF | Direction of a major force vector away from the trunk with the neck flexed, stressing the posterior elements in tension and producing secondary anterior compression | Most common | Stage I (DFS1) | Failure of the posterior ligamentous complex with facet subluxation in flexion and divergence of the spinous processes at the level of injury; "flexion sprain" | Lateral radiograph is most helpful. Complete loss of contact of facet articulations is seen. Lower facets of superior segment are anterior to the corresponding facets of the lower segments. Oblique views are useful if there is suspicion of this injury since they show disruption of the facet joint.[163] |
| | | | | Stage II (DFS2) | Unilateral facet dislocation | |
| | | | | Stage III (DFS3) | Bilateral facet dislocation: anterior displacement is approximately 50%, with the posterior surface of the superior vertebral articular processes either snugly against the inferior articular processes or in a "perched" position | |
| | | | | Stage IV (DFS4) | Bilateral facet dislocation: vertebral body is displaced anteriorly for its full width, giving the appearance of a "floating" vertebral body | |
| Compressive extension | CE | Major injury vector directed toward the trunk while the head is extended causing compression of posterior elements | 20% | Stage I (CES1) | Unilateral vertebral arch fracture with or without displacement | Ligamentous failure occurs anteriorly between the fractured vertebra and its inferior neighbor and posteriorly with the superior vertebra |
| | | | | Stage II (CES2) | Bilateral laminar fracture without other tissue failure | |
| | | | | Stage III d(CES3) | Same as CES2 with increased severity | |
| | | | | Stage IV (CES4) | Same as CES3 with increased severity | |
| | | | | Stage V (CES5) | Bilateral vertebral arch fractures with full vertebral body displacement anteriorly | |

In the hospital, life-threatening situations are identified and treated during the initial survey and resuscitation phases. Airway, ventilation, and circulation are evaluated and treated as necessary. Hemorrhage is controlled, and neurologic status is assessed. After the initial phase is completed the secondary survey is begun, including a complete neurologic evaluation to determine the presence and extent of injury. Complaints or findings of neck pain or tenderness, weakness, or sensory disturbances of the extremities should alert one to the possibility of spine and/or neurologic injury. If consciousness is altered by head injury, shock, or intoxication, the patient is managed as if these injuries were present.[36] Historical information, which in many cases can be provided by the emergency medical technicians who treated the patient at the scene, is helpful in caring for the patient. Was the patient thrown from a vehicle? Did the patient strike his or her head? Were there signs of paralysis? Has the patient's neurologic status deteriorated? Did the patient lose consciousness?[162] The answers to these questions frequently aid the physician in determining the mechanism and severity of injury and may suggest the possibility of other injuries.

Inspection of the face and head may reveal abrasions, contusions, and lacerations. Anterior head and facial wounds may be indicative of hyperextension injury, whereas posterior wounds may be consistent with flexion injuries.[93]

A thorough neurologic examination should be performed to determine the patient's baseline status and should be repeated at intervals to detect any changes. The level of injury is defined as the lowest spinal cord segment with intact motor and sensory function. Injury at the T1 level results in incomplete loss of function of the intrinsic hand muscles, whereas injury of C8 nerve roots results in paralysis of the interossei and the lumbricals. C7 injury weakens the triceps and limits active elbow extension. C6 injury further weakens the triceps and reduces biceps, brachioradialis, and deltoid function. C5 injury further weakens elbow flexion and paralyzes the deltoid. The diaphragm is innervated from C3–C5, and injuries in this region weaken it to varying degrees. The sensory examination is likewise dermatomal: T1 supplies the undersurface of the proximal arm, C8 the ulnar aspect of the palm and the last two digits, C7 the middle finger and midpalm, C6 the radial digits and the remainder of the palm. C5 supplies the shoulder, whereas the area under the clavicle is supplied by C4. C3 supplies the lower neck and C2 the upper neck.[36] Muscle strength, cutaneous pain sensation, position sensation, and deep tendon reflexes are carefully evaluated and recorded.[173]

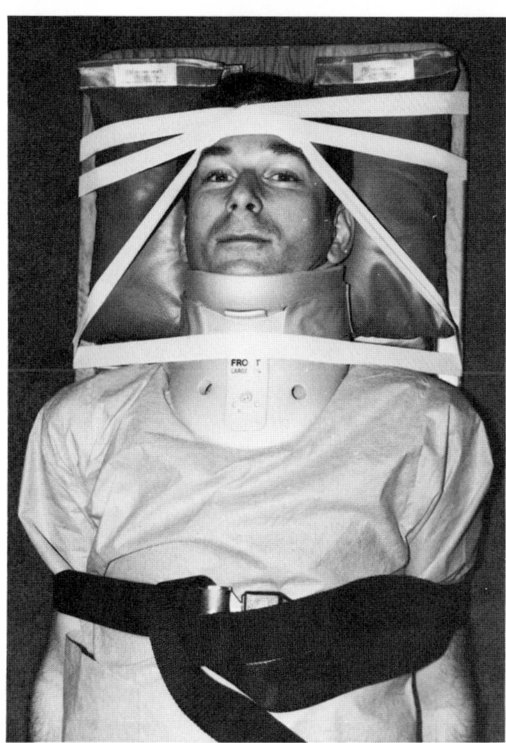

FIG. 14-12. Combination of sandbags on each side of the head, hard collar (Philadelphia collar), and taping of the head and neck to a rigid spine board provides the best cervical immobilization during transport and initial hospital management. The arms and upper torso are immobilized on the spine board by means of restraint belts.

## RADIOGRAPHIC EVALUATION OF CERVICAL SPINE TRAUMA

Radiography is used to determine definitively the presence and extent of damage to the cervical spine. Since it is estimated that up to 50% of patients with these injuries develop neurologic abnormalities, those having radiographic evaluation should be treated as if instability is present until it is conclusively demonstrated that the spine is stable. Therefore, immobilization of the neck should be maintained, and radiographic studies should be initiated on the patient's stretcher. Routine evaluation of the cervical spine consists of anteroposterior, lateral, open mouth, and oblique views.[39]

### ROUTINE STUDIES

A lateral film is usually the first cervical spine radiograph. C7 may not always be visualized with this view because of overlapping shoulder shadows. Since the incidence of isolated C7 injury may be as high as 30%, special techniques should be used when C7 is not demonstrated on the routine lateral view.[39,133] The arms may be pulled inferiorly by an assistant, or a "swimmer's" view may be obtained. Complete analysis of the lateral film includes soft tissue and bone evaluation. Soft tissues often provide significant information about localization of cervical spine trauma. The presence of a prevertebral soft tissue hematoma is closely related to injury to anterior spinal elements. At the level of C3, retropharyngeal width greater than 5 mm is indirect evidence of either hemorrhage or edema. Usually prevertebral hematoma is associated with vertebral fracture, but it may rarely result from avulsion of the anterior longitudinal ligament without fracture of the body. Relatively small hematomas are found with odontoid and compression fractures.[102,125] In children, the prevertebral soft tissue should be one-third the anteroposterior width of the second cervical vertebra. Because crying increases the space, care should be taken when interpreting this sign in children. At the level of C6 the distance from the posterior wall of the trachea to the anteroinferior aspect of C6 should be less than 14 mm in children and 22 mm in adults. However, these measurements are not valid when endotracheal and nasogastric tubes are in place.[39]

On the lateral view, loss of the normal lordotic curve or kyphosis is usually indicative of muscular spasm. However, because it may be a subtle indication of instability after flexion injury, abnormalities in the alignment of the spinous processes should be sought.[78,108] Interpretation of changes in cervical lordosis is highly uncertain, and the chin must be depressed to obtain a meaningful view on the lateral film. Lateral flexion and extension views should be performed on all individuals presenting with loss or reversal of the lordotic curve as their only radiographic abnormality. A full range of motion indicates a normal alignment.[157]

Evaluation of bony anatomy should be made in a routine and organized manner. The tips of the spinous processes form a gentle longitudinal curve, as do the anterior and posterior portions of the vertebral bodies. The fourth curve that is evaluated is the spinolaminar line, the dense white line seen radiographically at the junction of the lamina and spinous process. Interruption of these gentle curves indicates fracture and/or bony displacement. In addition to observing these curves, one should inspect the film for evidence of vertebral fractures, intervertebral angulation in excess of 11°, horizontal displacement in excess of 3.5 mm, widening of the intervertebral disc space, and displacement of the facet joints. Each of these findings may be indicative of spinal instability caused by osseous and/or ligamentous injury[39] (Figs 14-13–14-18). The cervical spine may be injured at more than one level. Thus, each level must be evaluated to identify multiple injuries.[133,146]

The predictive value of a negative lateral cervical spine radiographic study after a careful clinical evaluation is 0.97.[136] In order to raise this value to 1.0 and to avoid missing an unstable injury, open mouth and anteroposterior views of the neck must be obtained.[136]

The open mouth radiograph is required for evaluation of the C1–C2 articulation (Fig 14-19). Fractures of the odontoid are easily identified by this technique. In addition, it evaluates the lateral masses of the atlas and their position relative to C2. Lateral spreading of the masses is indicative of injury. The oblique view is essential for evaluating the facet joints and determining if unilateral fracture or dislocation exists. This view may also confirm the relocation of jumped facets.

When the clinical evaluation indicates that the patient has significant pain without evidence of fracture or dislocation on

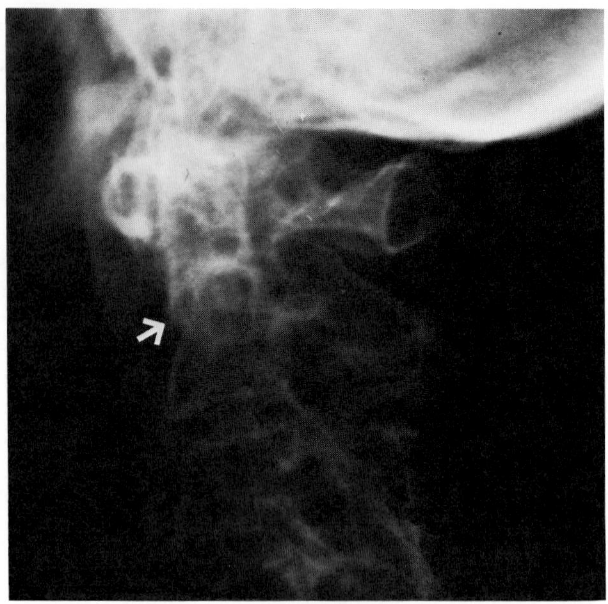

FIG. 14-13. Lateral upper cervical spine film. Arrow shows healed odontoid fracture with residual angulation.

FIG. 14-14. Lateral upper cervical spine film. Odontoid fracture with anterior displacement of C1 on C2 (*arrow*).

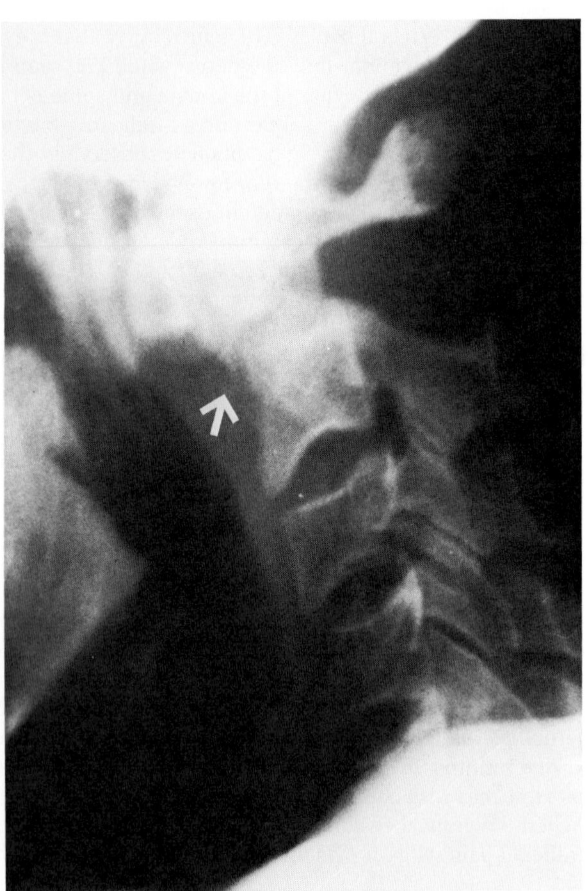

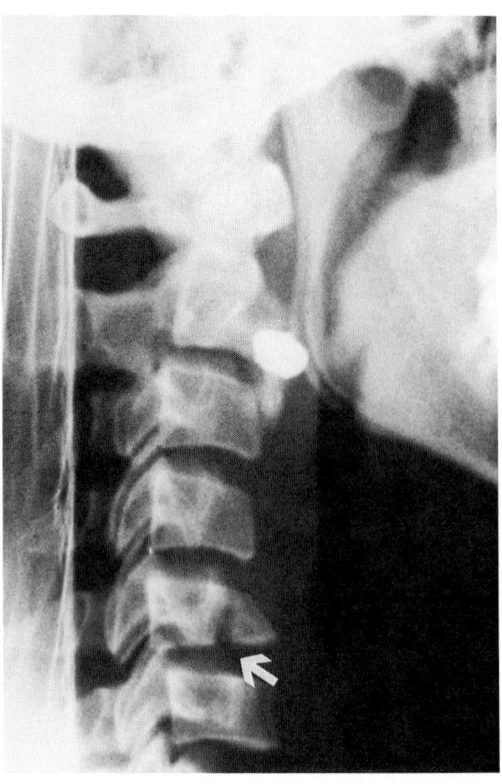

FIG. 14-15. Lateral cervical spine film showing the vertebral bodies of C1–C6. Note the old bullet injury at C2 and recent vertebral body fracture of C5 (*arrow*).

the routine spine series, thin slice and computed tomography (CT) may be helpful in delineating the injury.[39]

SPECIAL STUDIES

*Flexion extension films* may be obtained as part of the initial evaluation. These films may demonstrate displacement that is not visualized on plain films and are used primarily to evaluate instability caused by occult ligamentous injury. Flexion extension views should not be obtained if there is objective evidence of neurologic, bony, or soft tissue injury. For this study the patient should position him- or herself without assistance. Pain and muscle spasm may preclude early use of this technique. As soon as they subside it should be pursued if indicated.[56,157]

*A stress view,* known as the "stretch test," can evaluate the posterior ligaments by placing traction on the skull. Any change in alignment or separation of vertebral bodies is indicative of damage to posterior structures. This evaluation should be obtained only with a physician in attendance. The test is performed while traction is applied to the head, usually by a cloth cervical halter. An initial lateral film is obtained, and then traction is begun with a fairly light weight, usually 15 lb. Traction is increased incrementally, usually 5 or 10 lb at a time, with repeated radiologic and neurologic evaluations. The initial weight and increments are changed depending upon the level of the lesion and the tolerance of the spine. Any change in neurologic status or abnormal separation of anterior or posterior elements constitutes a positive result, and the test is stopped.[9,180,181,183]

*CT and plain tomography* are useful adjuncts. Plain films have been shown to underestimate the presence and severity of spinal fractures at all levels; CT scans are especially useful for lesions that are not visible on plain films. CT allows a thorough evaluation of obscure fractures of posterior elements, as well as providing an accurate display of cross-sectional anatomy at any level[22] (Figs 14-20–14-24).

CT scanning eliminates the need to move a patient with an unstable spine into the lateral position, which is required for tomography. In addition, it displays soft tissue structures accurately and allows visualization of the bony limits of the spinal canal in the axial plane. It is superior to other diagnostic procedures in demonstrating impingement on the neural canal and can be performed more rapidly and with less radiation exposure to the patient.[37,88] Reformatting of CT images can allow heightened awareness of the three-dimensional geometry of fractures, although information can be lost if the patient has moved. Such movement can produce a "pseudofracture" where none actually exists.[37]

Although CT has largely replaced plain tomography, lateral tomography may be useful in many instances, particularly for evaluation of odontoid and anterior atlantal fractures that are parallel to the plane of the CT.[76]

*Myelography* is indicated to visualize optimally the compression of the spinal cord. Lateral C1–C2 puncture and injection of water-soluble nonionic contrast material can be performed with the patient supine. Since this material is completely miscible with CSF, the spinal cord is visualized whether there is blockage or not.

FIG. 14-16. Lateral cervical spine film with fracture and posterior displacement of the vertebral body of C5 into the spinal canal (*arrow*).

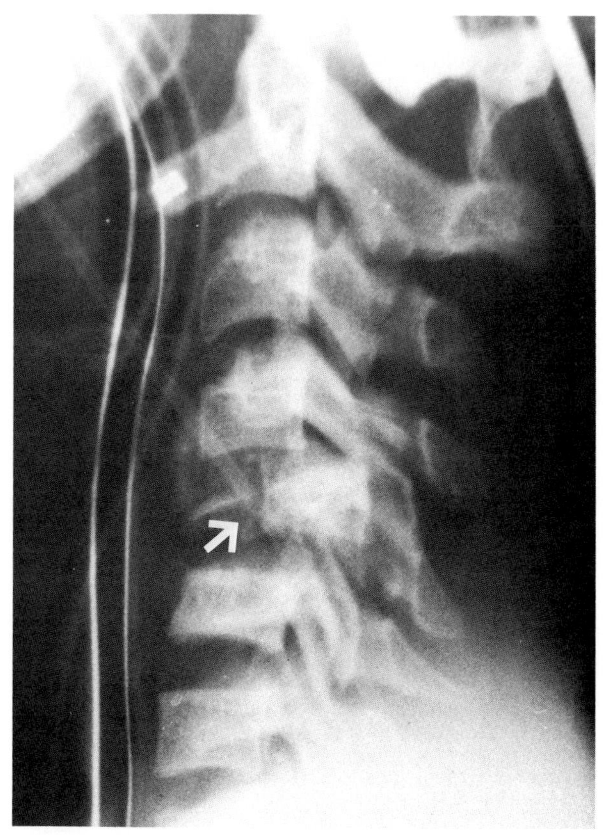

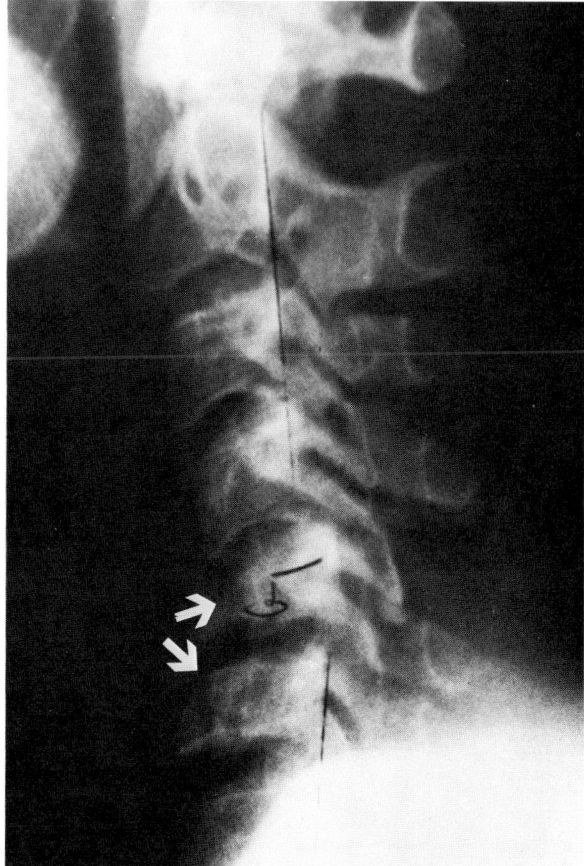

FIG. 14-17. Lateral view of a C5 compression fracture-dislocation and C6 vertebral body fracture (*arrow*). Note interruption of longitudinal black line connecting posterior portion vertebral bodies at C5 level. At C6 level the direction of the line is different from that observed at higher levels.

Plain AP and lateral films are obtained to ascertain the site of bone and spinal cord pathology. This precise localization facilitates targeting of the CT scanner and permits diagnosis of lesions that may be missed if CT or myelography is used separately.[37,69]

*Magnetic resonance imaging* (MRI) has added a powerful tool to the diagnostic armamentarium. The detailed images of bone, muscle, soft tissue, and neural structures that MRI provides may make injury diagnosis easier and more certain. However, the role that this technique will eventually play in spinal trauma is unclear at this time (Fig 14-25).

## DIAGNOSTIC STRATEGY

In the patient with a normal physical examination but an abnormal lateral film, radiographic examination should proceed cautiously. The patient's spine must be stabilized, and static examinations should be performed first. Any bony abnor-

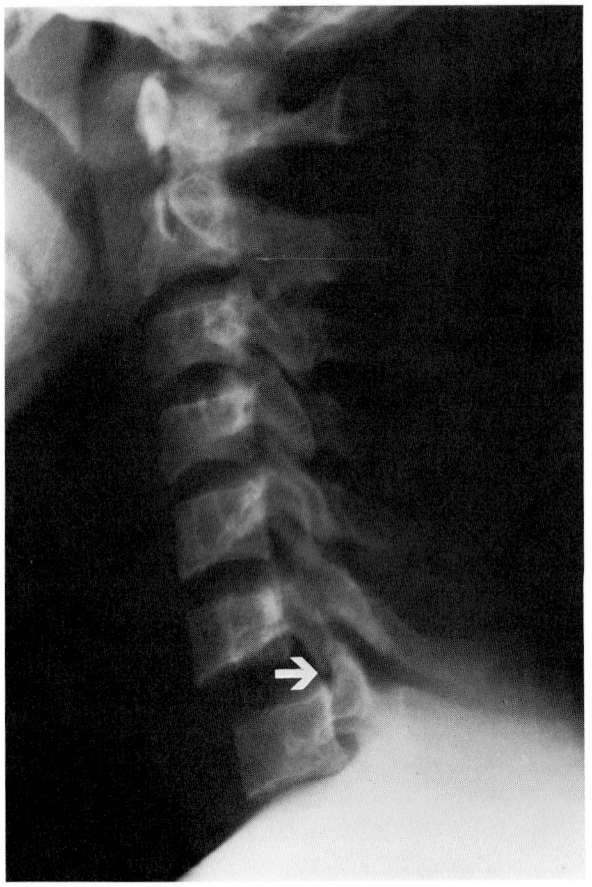

FIG. 14-18. Lateral view of cervical spine with C1–C7 visualized. Note C6–C7 subluxation with locked facets (*arrow*).

mality shown on the initial studies should be further evaluated with CT scan. If there are further indications, a contrast-enhanced CT scan may be obtained.

In patients with neurologic deficits, the sequence and goals of the diagnostic evaluation may be different. In patients with complete lesions, radiologic evaluation should be limited to defining the bony pathology since significant neurologic recovery rarely occurs. A CT myelogram is not indicated. Patients with incomplete lesions should be worked up quickly and aggressively to evaluate and define precisely the presence and location of neurologic compression.

When both the lateral film and the neurologic examination are abnormal in patients with incomplete neurologic injury, the patient should be placed immediately into tongs (the halo device may be applied initially if it is anticipated that it will be part of a patient's definitive care), with traction to maintain overall alignment. Further studies are obtained as indicated,[93] including CT scan and myelography via cisternal puncture.

FIG. 14-19. Open mouth radiogram of cervical spine showing intact odontoid bone and atlantoaxial articulation.

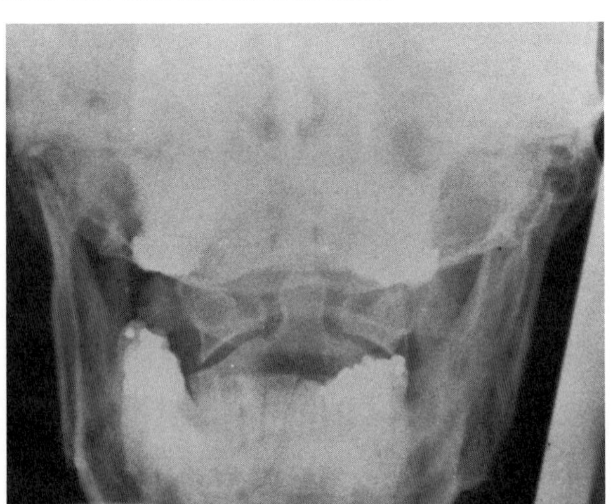

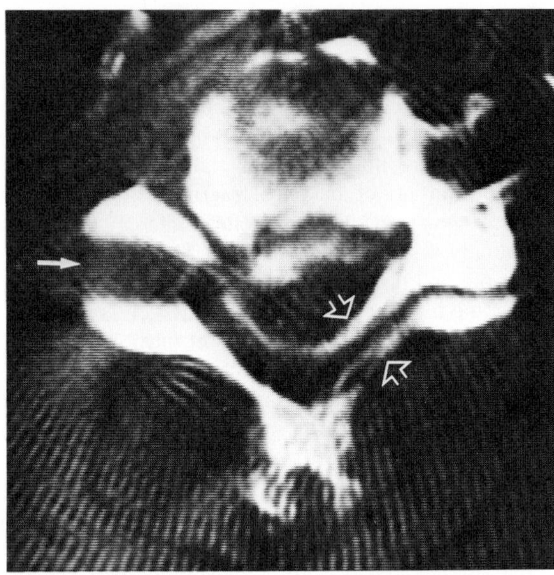

FIG. 14-20. CT scan of lower cervical vertebra demonstrating fractured lamina (*open arrows*) and widened facet joint (*closed arrow*). (Courtesy of Paul Cooper, MD.)

FIG. 14-21. CT scan of lower cervical vertebra demonstrating bilateral laminar fractures (*white arrows*) and vertebral body fracture (*black arrow*). (Courtesy of Paul Cooper, MD.)

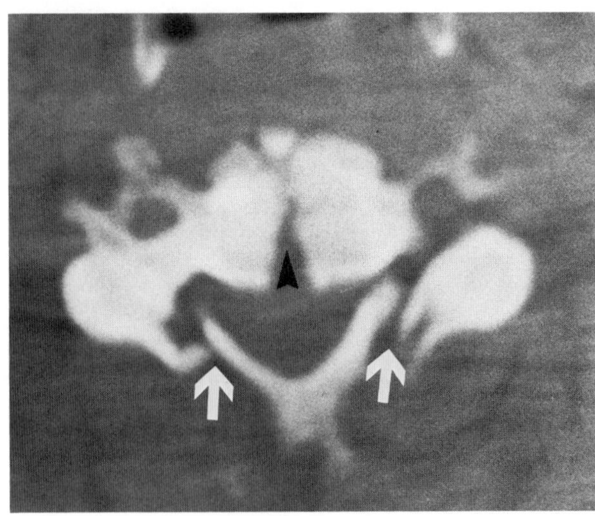

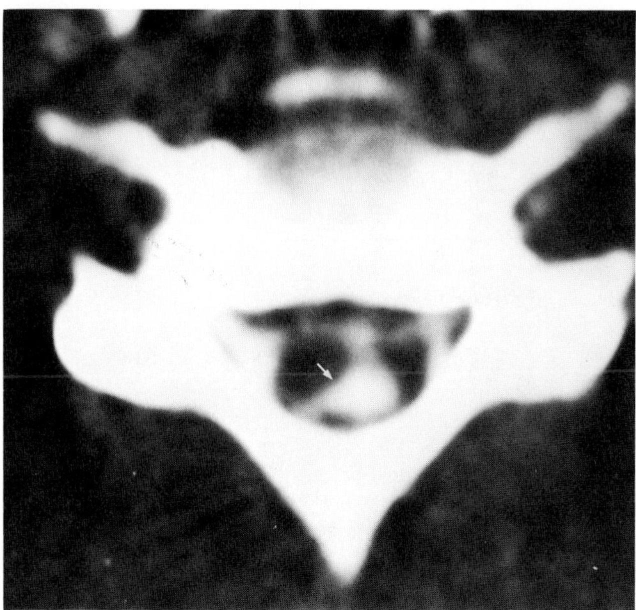

FIG. 14-22. CT scan of lower cervical spine and subarachnoid contrast study. Arrow demonstrates presence of contrast in normal location of spinal cord indicating cord trauma. (Courtesy of Paul Cooper, MD.)

The patient with evidence of head and neck injury, normal plain films, but an abnormal neurologic examination with incomplete neural loss presents a diagnostic problem. Possible diagnoses include osteophytic protrusion into a small canal resulting in contusion of the cord without fracture or subluxation, intervertebral disc herniation that cannot be demonstrated on plain films, or spontaneous reduction of the spinal subluxation that produced the cord injury.[36] CT myelography is obtained in order to visualize the intraspinal pathology.[36,37,93] If these studies are insufficient to determine the mechanism of injury, controlled flexion-extension films may be obtained to rule out subluxation.[36]

### EVALUATION OF PEDIATRIC PATIENTS

Epiphyseal lines can mimic fractures. With few exceptions, the neck has an adult form in children over 8 years of age, and epiphyseal lines are no longer a problem. Before that time, the injured child's neck can be a diagnostic dilemma for all but the most experienced physicians. In general, epiphyseal plates are smooth and regular and can be found in predictable locations accompanied by subchondral sclerotic lines. Fractures are irregular, without sclerosis, and are generally in unpredictable locations.[37]

The child's cervical spine, especially in the upper levels, is much more mobile than the adult spine. Normal ligamentous laxity permits considerable excursion of the atlas, both anteriorly and posteriorly. In flexion, an atlantodens interval of up to 4 mm may be normal. In extension the atlas may appear to sublux cephalad on the dens.[8,76,150]

Pseudosubluxation commonly causes concern, usually at the C2–C3 or C3–C4 levels. It is attributed to a combination of ligamentous laxity, a relatively horizontal orientation of the facet joints, and lesser development of the uncinate processes in younger children. In the fully flexed neck, 3–4 mm of anterior displacement of one body on the subjacent body may be seen. Normally the posterior boundaries of the neural canal, the spinolaminar junction line, are almost straight and can be used to distinguish normal alignment from a pathologic situation.[8,76,150]

Normal anterior wedging of the immature vertebral body can produce the appearance of a compression fracture. Spinous process centers can resemble avulsion fractures.[150] Serious ligamentous disruptions can be detected by an increase in the interspinous distance, loss of parallelism between articular processes, and posterior widening of the disc spaces.[124] Careful attention to these details and matching irregularities on the radiograph with clinical symptoms should prevent over- or undertreatment.

## ANESTHETIC AND PHYSIOLOGIC CONSIDERATIONS

The cervical spine injured patient presents problems that are caused by instability of the cervical spine, spinal cord dysfunction, respiratory compromise, and hemodynamic derangement. With the exception of succinylcholine in sensitive patients, no drug is particularly indicated or contraindicated in the anesthetic management of these patients. Rather, careful attention to the anatomic and physiologic pathology is the requisite for anesthetic care.

### MUSCLE RELAXANTS AND SPINAL CORD INJURY

Cardiac arrest may occur after administration of succinylcholine in patients with extensive muscle damage or denervation, such as that following spinal cord injury, burns, extensive muscle trauma, motor nerve injury, or tetanus.[71] The mechanism involves supersensitivity of the neuromuscular junction to the depolarizing effect of acetylcholine and succinylcholine and the release of large quantities of potassium during muscle contracture.

The increased potassium release is caused by proliferation of motor endplate areas throughout the muscle cell membrane. Normally the acetylcholine receptor is confined only to the neuromuscular junction. In crushed, burned, or denervated muscle acetylcholine receptors proliferate around the injured cell, making the cell more sensitive to both acetylcholine and succinylcholine. Normal depolarization results in a small potassium flux across the muscle cell membrane. When denervated muscle is depolarized the flux of potassium is increased 33–43 times. This potassium enters the circulation, produces acute hyperkalemia, and may cause cardiac asystole. Blockade of the neuromuscular junction with nondepolarizing relaxants reduces the potassium flux until, at doses producing total paralysis, the potassium flux in response to succinylcholine is approximately normal.

Such a response to succinylcholine develops 5–15 days after injury and lasts up to 6 months and possibly longer in patients with upper motor neuron lesions. A very conservative approach to caring for the spinal cord injured patient would

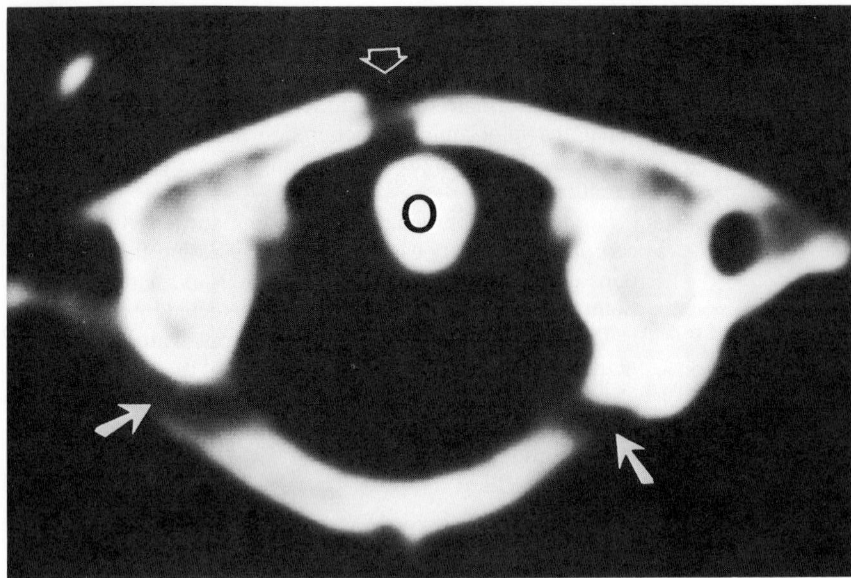


FIG. 14-23. CT scan of the atlas and odontoid process (O) demonstrating fracture of the anterior atlantal ring (*open arrow*) and bilateral fractures of the posterior atlantal ring (*closed arrows*). (Courtesy of Paul Cooper, MD.)

be to avoid succinylcholine entirely in order to be certain that this complication does not occur. Nondepolarizing muscle relaxants present no problem in these patients.

## AIRWAY MANAGEMENT IN CERVICAL SPINE INJURY

The indications for tracheal intubation of patients with cervical spine injury are establishment of an airway for surgery, relief of airway obstruction, treatment of ventilatory failure, provision of a conduit for pulmonary toilet, prevention of aspiration of gastric contents, and the requirement of hyperventilation to reduce or prevent elevated intracranial pressure. The combination of cervical spine instability, a full stomach, unopposed vagal reflexes, hypoxia, hypercarbia, and head, neck, and mouth trauma makes airway management of these patients challenging.

Airway manipulation should be performed in a manner that prevents the extension of neural injury. Even patients with complete injuries should be managed with care since spinal cord compression during airway management may increase edema and cause extension of the injury. It has been demonstrated that airway maneuvers, such as chin lift, jaw thrust,

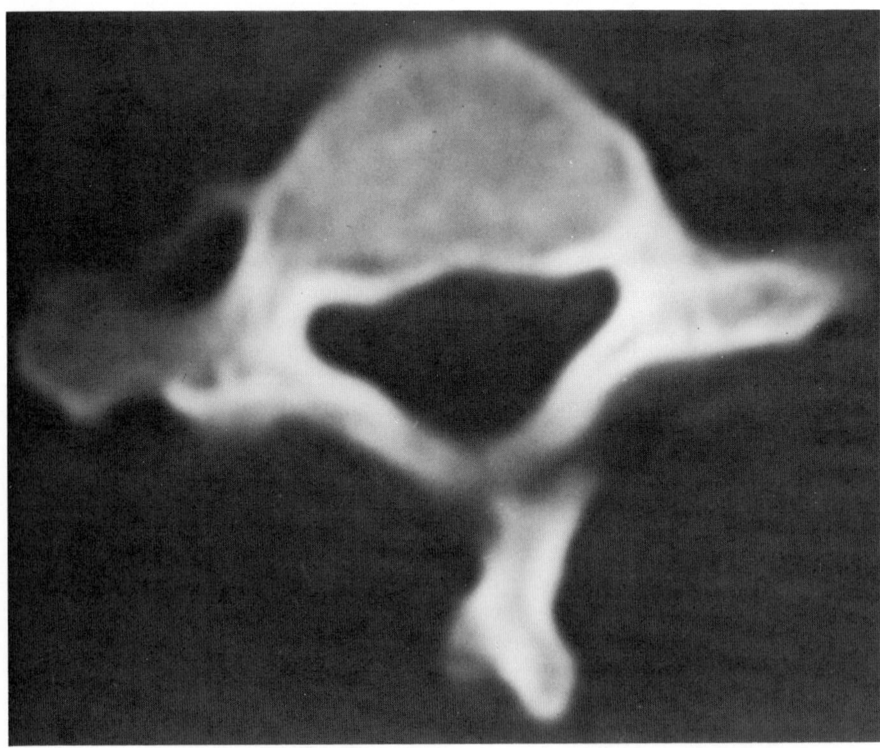

FIG. 14-24. CT scan of the lower cervical spine. Note fractured spinous process. (Courtesy of Paul Cooper, MD.)

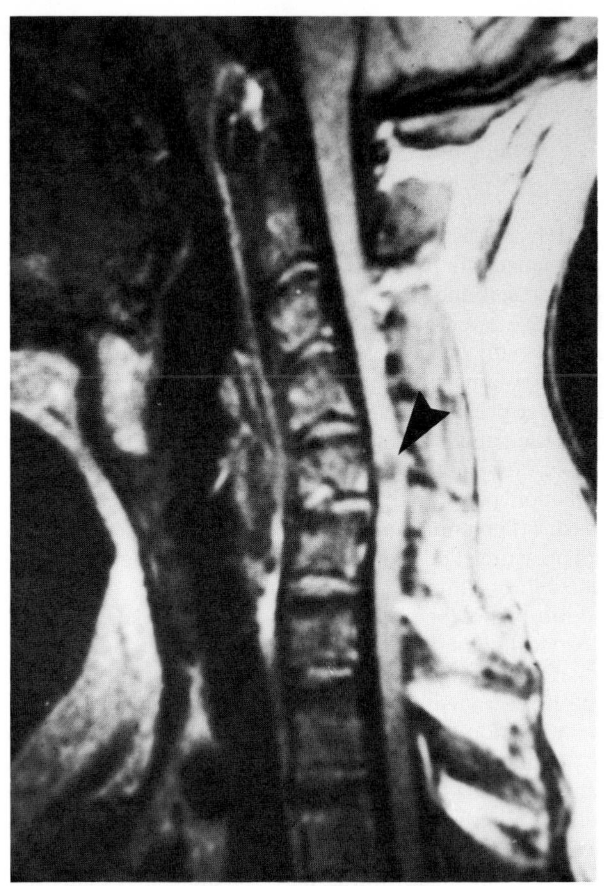

FIG. 14-25. Lateral magnetic resonance image (MRI) of the spine and spinal cord demonstrates severe cord destruction at C5 (*arrow*).

head tilt, oral and nasal airway placement, and orotracheal and nasotracheal intubation, performed without a cervical collar are associated with significant motion of the spine.[12,105] However, placement of soft or Philadelphia collars does not guarantee sufficient limitation of motion. A combination of a Philadelphia collar, sandbags, tape, and spineboard provides the best protection against cervical motion in the absence of cervical traction[63,127] (Fig 14-12). Another technique for stabilizing the neck is to have assistants provide manual traction on the head, neck, and chest during airway manipulation (Fig 14-26). Although this technique is helpful in reducing cervical spine motion during direct laryngoscopy, it may not completely eliminate it and may thereby permit the extension of neural injury.[105]

Acutely injured patients are at risk of aspiration of gastric contents. Likewise, patients who have sustained cervical spine injury several days before airway management may have delayed gastric emptying and may also aspirate.[63,103] Whenever possible, techniques that decrease gastric volume and reduce gastric acidity should be employed before airway manipulation. Metoclopramide,[41,143] sodium bicitrate,[29,60,143] ranitidine,[40,77,114,187] and cimetidine[35,43,60,77,114,166] alone or in combination reduce gastric volume and acidity, but cannot guarantee an empty stomach in all patients. Emptying of stomach contents with nasogastric suction is also valuable, although not foolproof.[103]

Manipulation of the oropharynx, larynx, and trachea during tracheal intubation causes increased vagal tone. If the spinal cord lesion is above the level of the cardioaccelerator nerves (T1–T5), the resulting unopposed vagal activity may cause severe bradycardia. Administering atropine sulfate, 0.4–0.8 mg intravenously, before airway manipulation is useful in preventing bradycardia. Since hypoxemia also contributes to a bradycardic response, one should make certain that the patient is well ventilated and oxygenated before intubation.[45,63]

Some authors suggest that patients with cervical spine instability having elective surgery should be intubated utilizing general anesthesia and muscle relaxation.[45] However, those who promote this technique ignore the fact that direct visualization of the larynx may be difficult in patients who are unable to flex the cervical spine and extend the atlanto-occipital joint, the maneuvers that are normally used to permit visualization of the vocal cords.[47] In addition, lifting the epiglottis or applying pressure to the vallecula during direct laryngoscopy may, if the spine is unstable, cause vertebral movement and extension of neural injury even when traction on the head and neck is maintained.[105]

Direct laryngoscopy may be performed in a sedated and topically anesthetized patient. The advantage that this tech-

FIG. 14-26. Endotracheal intubation of a patient with cervical spine injury using two-man spine protection technique. The first assistant is applying axial traction to the cervical spine while the second is stabilizing the shoulders and the chest.

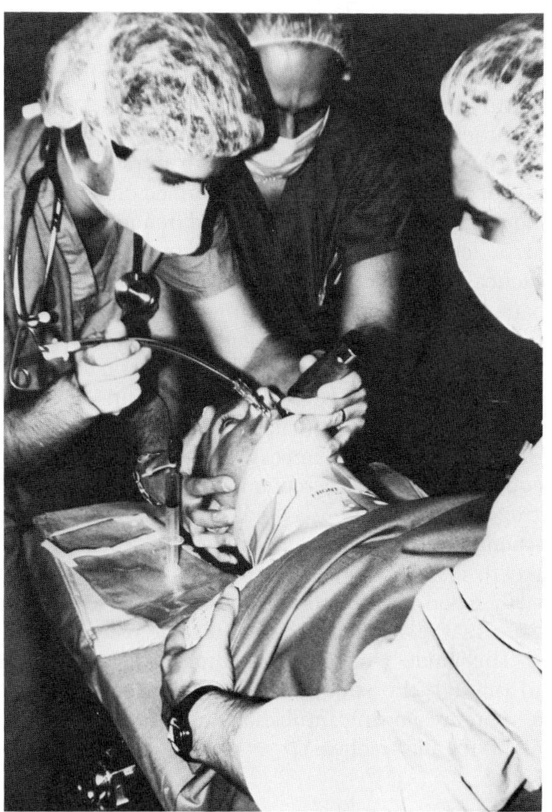

nique offers over general anesthesia is that spontaneous breathing is maintained[158] and visualization of the laryngeal structures need not be as good for intubation to be successful. As one brings the endotracheal tube closer to the larynx the sound of moving air acts as a guide even if the larynx is not visualized. Therefore, the amount of cervical motion required for tracheal intubation would probably be less, and the potential for extension of neural injury would be reduced. Nevertheless, this technique is not as good as one that exerts no pressure on the neck at all.

In elective circumstances, fiberoptic guided tracheal intubation is the technique of choice.[111,116,176] Since the oral and tracheal axes need not be aligned for successful intubation, this technique reduces significantly the risk of extending neural injury. Either the oral or nasal route may be employed; the choice should be guided by the presence or absence of oral, nasal, and/or basilar skull fractures. Intravenous sedatives, topical anesthesia of the airway, and bilateral superior laryngeal nerve blockade increase patient comfort. However, analgesia of the larynx and trachea also increases the risk of aspiration of gastric contents, blood, and secretions by blocking the afferent portions of the laryngeal spasm and cough reflex arcs.[175] Fiberoptic intubation may be performed with the patient sedated and spontaneously breathing or under general anesthesia. If the latter is chosen, the Patil-Syracuse mask should be employed.[123] The sedated technique is easier since the patient ventilates and oxygenates him- or herself, and the anesthesiologist may thus devote more attention to intubation. General anesthesia requires the presence of at least two physicians since one must control the airway and assure ventilation while the other performs the laryngoscopy. Although the fiberoptic technique is the method of choice, one should be aware that it may be difficult to perform if blood or secretions obstruct the view.

A variation of the above technique is to insert a 14-gauge angiocath through the cricothyroid membrane and to jet ventilate the patient through it with oxygen.[87,117,156,161] The patient may then be anesthetized with intravenous agents, and fiberoptic intubation may be performed orally or nasally.

Blind nasal intubation is a useful and frequently successful technique for patients in whom placement of an airway into the trachea with direct laryngoscopy is difficult. However, in the patient with cervical spine injury this technique may prove difficult because the head and neck cannot be manipulated. It is also frequently associated with nasal hemorrhage. Once nasal hemorrhage begins after several unsuccessful intubation attempts, it is difficult to control; under these circumstances it is usually impossible to visualize the larynx subsequently with the fiberoptic instrument.

Retrograde placement of a guide wire through the cricothyroid membrane may be useful to facilitate intubation in patients with cervical spine injury.[91,99,129,169] This technique, especially when used in combination with a fiberoptic bronchoscope, may allow reliable airway management in these patients. The guide wire recovered from the mouth can be passed through the suction port of the fiberoptic bronchoscope, thereby allowing intubation with fiberoptic visualization of larynx and trachea.[134]

In emergent circumstances the patient should be ventilated with a bag, valve, mask, and oxygen. Blind nasal intubation is the technique usually chosen for securing the airway, but it may be difficult to perform if the patient is apneic. Should this technique fail, cricothyrotomy or translaryngeal catheter airway insertion may be the optimal methods to employ.[21,23,152,153,155,156]

Although it is clear that the above techniques are satisfactory for patients in shock or for those in whom intracranial hypertension and an open eye are not considerations, they may cause cerebral herniation and/or extrusion of vitreous in patients with concomitant head and/or eye injuries. Under normal circumstances, if the cervical spine and airway do not present a problem for laryngoscopy and tracheal intubation and if the patient has a normal or high blood pressure, head- or eye-injured patients should have laryngoscopy and tracheal intubation performed after administration of general anesthesia, hyperventilation with oxygen, and maintenance of cricoid pressure. These maneuvers prevent the elevations in intraocular and intracranial pressure caused by laryngoscopy and intubation (see also Chapters 10 and 11). The presence of cervical spine injury complicates this plan, but modifications may permit airway control without risking further injury. If the patient is in shock, airway management can proceed with little regard for associated head or eye injuries since the likelihood of hypertensive and cough response to airway manipulation is small and patient tolerance of general anesthetics is limited by the hypovolemic state. Selected hemodynamically stable patients who have associated head and neck or eye and neck injuries may be managed by establishing the airway with a translaryngeal catheter and jet ventilation with oxygen. General anesthesia can then be induced with thiopental, lidocaine, and muscle relaxant.[20] Muscle relaxant selection should be based upon the need for rapid onset, avoidance of increased intraocular or intracranial pressure, and hemodynamic considerations (see Chapters 9,10,11). Cricoid pressure, which is contraindicated in cervical spine injury, need not be applied if translaryngeal jet ventilation is maintained at a rate of 80–100 breaths/min. Such ventilation prevents aspiration of supraglottic contents.[92] Intubation may then be performed nasally, orally, or through a surgical cricothyrotomy. Although this technique is complex, each element is necessary if the airway must be secured in the face of conflicting demands of cervical instability and head or eye injury.

Establishing the airway in patients with combined neck and certain maxillofacial injuries is also more difficult than usual. If the nasal and oral routes for securing the airway are precluded because of trauma in these areas, a surgical airway is required. Translaryngeal catheter ventilation may be performed as a temporizing measure, but a tracheostomy or cricothyrotomy is ultimately necessary.

In summary, the principles of airway management in patients with cervical spine injury are to immobilize the neck, oxygenate and ventilate before securing the airway, treat with atropine, and prepare for a difficult intubation by having available an assortment of equipment sufficient to deal with any problems that may arise.

## PULMONARY COMPLICATIONS ASSOCIATED WITH CERVICAL SPINE INJURY

### *Ventilatory Insufficiency*

Early mortality from respiratory problems in cervical spine injured patients ranges from 7 to 40%; quadriplegics are at risk of respiratory insufficiency through a variety of mechanisms.[59] The multiply injured patient may be obtunded and have central respiratory depression caused by shock and inadequate brainstem perfusion. Airway obstruction caused by foreign body, hematoma, hemorrhage, soft tissue trauma, facial trauma, or laryngotracheal injury may be present. Rib fractures, hemothorax, and pneumothorax may also contribute to ventilatory failure.[157] Respiratory problems specific to the patient with cervical spine injury result from loss of innervation to the abdominal and intercostal musculature and to the diaphragm. The degree of respiratory insufficiency is determined by the level of spinal cord injury. Spinal cord injury above C4 renders voluntary diaphragmatic respiration impossible. Injuries below this level permit at least some degree of voluntary diaphragmatic control. Very high cervical spinal cord injuries may result in pentaplegia: quadriplegia plus loss of both lower cranial nerve and accessory respiratory muscle functions.[14]

Complete cervical spinal cord injury paralyzes both intercostal and abdominal muscles. These muscles are important to normal ventilation because they stabilize the rib cage and abdominal wall, thereby increasing the efficiency of diaphragmatic contraction. They also permit forced expiration and coughing, which are thus severely compromised or impossible in quadriplegics.[185] Pulmonary function testing of quadriplegic patients without diaphragmatic paralysis or injury has shown a 26% decrease in total lung capacity, 49% decrease in vital capacity, 64% decrease in expiratory reserve volume, and 21% decrease in functional residual volume. Although the forced expiratory volume in 1 second to forced vital capacity ratio is normal, the maximum midexpiratory flow rate is reduced by 40%, and the peak expiratory flow rate is reduced by 53%.[59,109] These derangements increase the risk of pneumonia because of the reduced ability to clear secretions and aspirated material. In addition, small changes in pulmonary compliance are poorly tolerated because of reduced pulmonary reserve. Unilateral diaphragmatic paralysis may be caused by ascending spinal cord swelling, unilateral nerve root injury, or unilateral intramedullary injury that affects the anterior horn cells. Provided the neural elements are not completely destroyed, recovery of diaphragmatic function may be possible.[28]

Arterial $O_2$ and $CO_2$ analysis should be obtained if there is any question of respiratory insufficiency or failure. Even mild levels of hypoxemia and hypercarbia in the cervical spine injured patient should be treated with airway control and mechanical ventilation since compensatory mechanisms are substantially reduced.

In the early postinjury period patients are at risk for further impairment of alveolar ventilation caused by pulmonary edema or pulmonary embolism. Deterioration of the patient's respiratory condition may also be caused by extension of the cone of edema to involve higher spinal segments and to disrupt diaphragmatic activity. In addition, if the cone of edema or hemorrhage extends to the anterolateral portion of the spinal cord at C2 to C4, sleep apnea may occur without any prior change in respiratory findings.[63] Under these circumstances, unless the patient awakens and breathes voluntarily or ventilatory support is provided he or she will die. The greatest risk of sleep apnea is during the first 5 nights after injury.[131]

Alveolar ventilation of the quadriplegic patient is markedly affected by body position. Upright position results in flattening of the diaphragm by gravity and thus a shorter descent of this muscle during inspiration. Ventilation improves in the supine position because the cephalad movement of the diaphragm during expiration allows for a greater descent and lung expansion during the next inspiration[14] (see also Chapter 10).

### *Aspiration of Gastric Contents*

The risk of aspiration of oral secretions, blood, and gastric contents is increased in the unconscious injured patient. In addition, as noted earlier, cervical spinal cord injury reduces pulmonary expiratory reserve and increases the risk of pneumonia if aspiration occurs. Airway control with a cuffed tube reduces this risk and should be established as early as possible.

### *Pulmonary Embolism*

There is a high risk of deep venous thrombosis (DVT) and subsequent pulmonary embolism in patients with traumatic spinal cord injury. A 1965 study of 500 patients reported 66 cases of pulmonary embolus, 15 of which were fatal, within the first 14 days after injury. Deaths due to pulmonary embolism have been reported from 4 to 85 days after spinal cord injury.[51,65] Therefore it has been recommended that quadriplegic patients receive prophylaxis against DVT during the 3 months after their injury. Low-dose heparin, external pneumatic compression, dextran, and graduated compression elastic stockings are effective in DVT prophylaxis.[34] Passive range of motion exercises may also be effective for this purpose. Obese patients and those with previous DVT or pulmonary embolus are at high risk, and anticoagulation should continue, if possible, up to 6 months.[51] Further information on this subject is provided in Chapter 28.

## CARDIOVASCULAR AND CARDIOPULMONARY EFFECTS OF CERVICAL SPINAL CORD INJURY

Hypotension and pulmonary edema are the major early cardiovascular complications of cervical spinal cord injury. Several minutes postinjury, patients demonstrate vasodilation involving all segments of the vascular tree,[112] with resultant hypotension caused by reduced sympathetic output. This condition is termed "spinal shock."

### *Sympathetic Stimulation of Acute Injury*

The immediate response to direct compression of the spinal cord in animals is hypertension and bradycardia.[63,73] Thoracic cord compression yields the greatest pressor response.[5] This effect lasts for 3 to 4 minutes and is mediated by alpha-adrenergic receptors. The subsequent hypotensive phase results from a reduction in alpha-adrenergic activity and can be reversed by an infusion of sympathomimetic agents.[132] In order for the hypertensive response to occur after cervical cord compression, there must be continuity between the cervical and thoracic regions of the cord. Cats with transected spinal cords at T1 had no pressor response to cervical cord compression.[49]

Greenhoot and Mauck[70] showed that the initial response to cervical cord compression in dogs was hypertension and tachycardia followed by sinus pauses, multifocal atrial beats, nodal escape beats, ventricular premature contractions, ventricular tachycardia, and ST and T wave changes. Atropine or section of the vagus nerves abolished bradycardia and arrhythmias, and propranolol abolished the tachycardic response. The conclusion of this study was that the initial effect is one of sympathetic stimulation and reflex parasympathetic activity. In contrast Evans et al.,[53] employing thoracic spinal cord compression in monkeys, demonstrated immediate pressor and bradycardic responses and noted that bradycardia preceded hypertension. The electrocardiogram later showed nodal and premature ventricular beats. Atropine prevented bradycardia, but did not prevent the arrhythmias, which developed 90 seconds after compression. Atropine and propranolol could prevent both brady- and tachyarrhythmias. The authors concluded that the arrhythmias were mediated by both vagal and sympathetic mechanisms; spinal afferent pathways to medullary centers cause the initial bradycardia, whereas efferent sympathetic activity causes hypertension, tachycardia, vasoconstriction, and increased myocardial contractility. Multifocal arrhythmias are caused by simultaneous hyperactivity of both the sympathetic and parasympathetic systems. It should be noted that these arrhythmias may be life threatening; myocardial infarction may occur because of increased cardiac work.[70] Assuming that the hemodynamic response is similar in humans, immediate hypertension caused by spinal cord compression may also produce increased edema and spinal cord hemorrhage and thus extend neuronal damage.

Hypertension is also observed in patients with elevated intracranial pressure. Since these subjects also have pulmonary vascular pressure elevation mediated by alpha-adrenergic stimulation, it is probable that these responses also occur during the hypertensive phase of spinal cord injury.[106,189]

Tibbs et al.[168] demonstrated that cervical spinal cord transection in dogs causes decreased myocardial blood flow because of hypotension and hypoperfusion. Although myocardial ischemia was not demonstrated electrocardiographically in this study, the findings suggest that decreased coronary blood flow after cervical cord transection is caused by decreased mean arterial pressure. Thus, patients with spinal shock who have pre-existent coronary artery disease require careful hemodynamic management.[168]

It has recently been shown that 6 of 22 patients with acute quadriplegia undergoing surgery had left ventricular dysfunction. It was probably a result of quadriplegia, rather than pre-existing ischemic heart disease. Optimal hemodynamic management of these patients involved volume infusion until the pulmonary capillary wedge (PCW) pressure was 18 mm Hg and the use of an inotropic agent (dopamine) if hypotension, acidosis, or low mixed venous $PO_2$ were present.[104]

### *Pulmonary Edema*

Pulmonary edema in spinal cord injured dogs was found to occur at lower central venous pressures than in control animals.[24] In humans, neurogenic pulmonary edema associated with normal pulmonary arterial (PA) and PCW pressures may occur after cervical cord injury.[128,167,189] It has been suggested that the pathophysiology of this phenomenon involves the initial pressor response described above, which causes elevated PA, PCW, and systemic blood pressures. Elevated pulmonary vascular pressures cause immediate hydrostatic pulmonary edema and result in the loss of capillary integrity and the exudation of protein-rich fluid.[100,167,189] Fluid overload may also cause pulmonary edema in spinal cord injury. Early postinjury patients tend to be hypotensive. In order to maintain blood pressure and urine output these patients may receive large quantities of fluid. When spinal shock begins to resolve and intravascular capacity decreases, the blood returned to the heart and lungs increases. If the left ventricle is unable to pump the extra blood returned to it, failure occurs, left atrial and PCW pressures increase, and pulmonary edema develops,[112] which may be potentiated by residual pulmonary capillary damage. The left ventricle is particularly prone to failure since it may sustain injury during the initial hypertensive episode or during the hypotensive, spinal shock phase.[73,104]

### *Spinal Shock*

The period of spinal shock, characterized by hypotension, bradycardia, increased vascular capacitance, flaccid paralysis below the level of injury, areflexia, poikilothermia, and retention of urine and feces, lasts for 3 to 8 weeks after injury.[2] During this period, these patients are especially sensitive to volume loading, drugs, and anesthetics.[170] Hemodynamic management in the intensive care unit and the operating room is best performed if arterial and pulmonary artery catheters are inserted and relevant pressures and indices are evaluated at regular intervals. In addition, measurement of colloid osmotic and oncotic pressures may be helpful in preventing pulmonary edema. Urine output monitoring is mandatory.[2]

Bradycardia is a significant problem in cervical spinal cord injury. The frequency of bradyarrhythmias peaks on day 4 and all arrhythmias resolve by 2 to 6 weeks after injury. The mechanism for bradycardia is presumed to be due to vagal activity in the absence of high thoracic sympathetic output. Administering atropine sulfate 0.4 to 0.8 mg intravenously reduces the risk of this complication as does vagolytic therapy with propanthaline bromide 7.5 to 30 mg orally 4 times daily. External or internal pacemakers may be required for treatment of bradycardia in some cases.[100a,188a]

### *Autonomic Hyperreflexia*

The chronic phase in which spinal reflexes reappear follows the period of spinal shock. This phase is characterized by mass reflexes and autonomic hyperreflexia in a high proportion of patients. Cutaneous, proprioceptive, and visceral stimuli, such as urinary bladder distension, may cause violent muscle spasm and autonomic disturbances.[15]

The symptoms of autonomic hyperreflexia are facial tingling, nasal obstruction, severe headache, shortness of breath, nausea, and blurred vision. The signs are hypertension, bradycardia, arrhythmias, sweating, cutis anserina (goose flesh), cutaneous vasodilation above and pallor below the level of spinal cord injury, and occasionally loss of consciousness and seizures. The precipitous blood pressure increase may lead to retinal, cerebral, or subarachnoid hemorrhage;[145] increased myocardial work; and pulmonary edema.[89] Patients with chronic spinal cord lesions above T6 are at risk for this response; 85% will display it at some time during the course of daily living. Surgery is an especially potent stimulus to autonomic hyperreflexia even in patients who give no previous history of this response.

The neuroanatomic pathway of this syndrome was first described in 1956. Afferent impulses enter the isolated spinal cord and elicit reflex autonomic output over the entire sympathetic outflow below the level of injury, which is not modulated by higher centers as in the neurologically intact subject. This causes vasoconstriction below the level of injury and resultant hypertension, which stimulates baroreceptors and may cause bradycardia via intact vagal pathways to the heart and vasodilation via intact pathways above the injury[89,145] (Fig 14-27).

Therapeutic methods to reduce the hypertension of autonomic hyperreflexia must act below the level of injury. Ganglionic blockers, alpha-adrenergic blockers, catecholamine depleters, direct vasodilators, and general or regional anesthesia have been recommended for prevention or treatment of autonomic hyperreflexia.[97]

Several studies have demonstrated a high incidence of autonomic hyperreflexia when surgery is conducted without anesthesia.[15,98,145] General inhalation anesthesia, when sufficient depth is maintained, has been almost 100% successful in preventing the syndrome.[4,98,145] The use of halothane with spontaneous breathing is associated with more cardiac arrhythmias than the administration of halothane or enflurane with controlled ventilation and normocarbia.[145]

Blockade of afferent pathways by local anesthesia is a technique that can be used to prevent autonomic hyperreflexia. However, for cystoscopic procedures, although topical anesthesia can blunt the response to cystoscope insertion, it cannot block the response to bladder distension.[145] There are isolated reports of the use of epidural anesthesia to block autonomic reflexes,[119,165] but a series of three cases in which epidural anesthesia was used for urologic surgery resulted in two incidents of autonomic hyperreflexia.[25] In contrast, subarachnoid anesthesia is virtually completely successful in preventing the syndrome, and there have been only a few reports of complications associated with its use.[15,25,98,145] Perhaps the

FIG. 14-27. Schematic diagram of the pathophysiology of autonomic hyperreflexia. Dashed line indicates inability of brainstem to communicate neurologically with the lower spinal cord. (Courtesy of Sanford M. Miller, MD.)

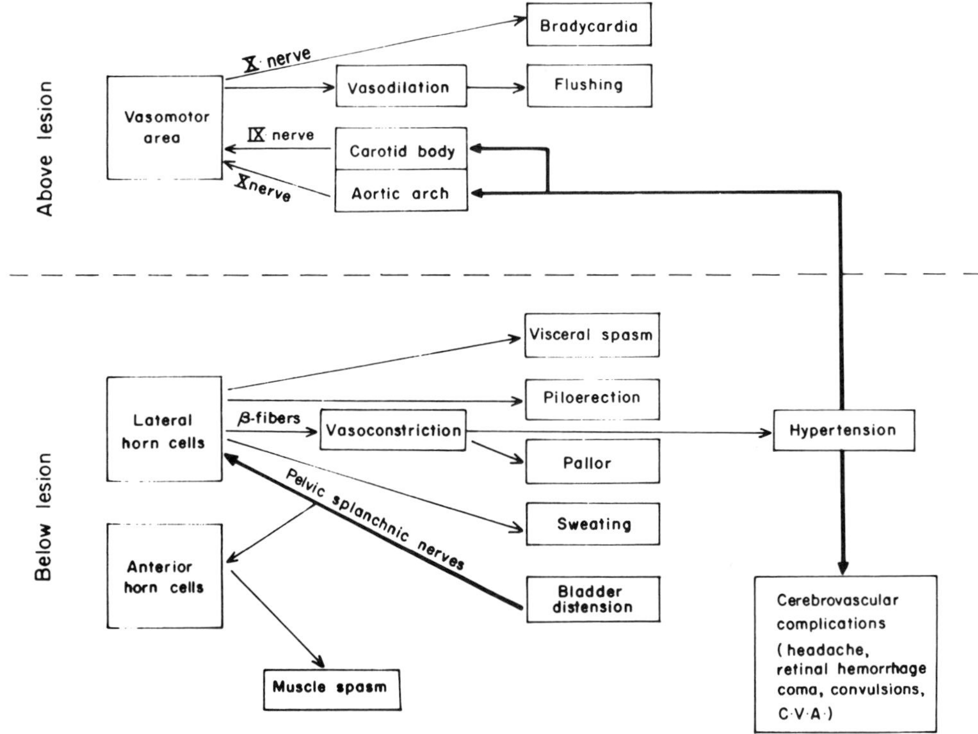

cases in which autonomic hyperreflexia occurred were associated with inadequate block, which could not be detected because of sensory loss due to spinal cord trauma.

## SURGICAL TREATMENT

The specific surgical treatment of patients with cervical spine injury depends upon the exact problem presented by the injury. However, in general, the considerations are neck stability and neurologic disability.

Neurologically intact patients require immediate and long-term neck stabilization to prevent neurologic injury and allow recovery. Those with complete neurologic lesions should receive early stabilization to prevent extension of injury and to permit reduction of edema and any potential recovery. In patients with incomplete injury the primary consideration is identification of any potentially remediable areas of neural compression. Bony fragments, disc material, dislocations, or subluxations that cause neural compression must be identified and corrected in order to provide the best opportunity for recovery. These patients may require traction to correct malalignment or open surgical decompression to remove material impinging on the spinal cord. Finally, even patients with complete neurologic lesions who are diagnosed and treated before the occurrence of permanent damage to the spinal cord may demonstrate remarkable recovery after rapid spinal realignment.[26]

The immediate approach to patient management involves suspicion of spinal injury and radiographic investigation. Those with deteriorating spinal cord or root function need further evaluation with myelography and CT scanning. Instability of the spine is treated immediately with cervical orthoses or traction and later with definitive stabilization. Acute surgical intervention is often necessary when incomplete lesions caused by neural compression are present; decompression and spinal stabilization may improve the chances of neural recovery. Surgery is also indicated when anterior neck injury involving the trachea and esophagus presents a risk of life-threatening airway and septic complications. In this circumstance, the spinal cord is not approached.[113,172] Surgical intervention is not indicated for posterior wounds with complete neurologic deficit.[113]

### ORTHOSES

Cervical orthoses are employed to treat a wide spectrum of clinical problems.[85,86] There are four general categories of support. The soft cervical collar is the least effective appliance in controlling motion in any plane. However, it is comfortable, affords some support, and reminds the patient to restrict neck movement. It is thus useful for treatment of minor muscular spasm. The Philadelphia collar is more massive and slightly more effective than the soft collar in controlling flexion and extension (Fig. 12). However, it does not provide firm control and is very weak in controlling rotation.[127] Poster braces, cervicothoracic braces, and the sterno-occipital-mandibular-immobilizer (SOMI) are more effective in controlling flexion, especially in the upper cervical segments. These orthoses are effective in the treatment of hangman's fractures and in the later stages of odontoid fracture treatment. However, these devices are especially poor at controlling lateral bending and are not indicated for the treatment of unstable fractures.[85,86,90]

The halo, an ambulatory form of skeletal traction, provides rigid fixation of the head and neck. It controls rotation, lateral bending, and sagittal motion, particularly over the upper cervical segments, which are poorly controlled by other braces. Overall, it allows almost no motion between the occiput and the upper thoracic spine. However, there is considerable freedom of motion between adjacent vertebrae, particularly in the saggital plane. It permits flexion of one segment and extension of the next in serpentine fashion.[85,86] For this reason lesions lower in the cervical spine and those with posterior ligamentous damage are unsuitable for treatment in halo.[38,184] Application of the halo device is an invasive procedure, and care must be taken in placement and maintenance of the pins.[66,118]

If a patient wearing a halo vest develops cardiopulmonary arrest and requires external chest compressions, the vest must be opened to expose the chest. Therefore, the necessary wrench should always be available for removing the chest cover (Fig 14-28).

FIG. 14-28. Halo vest applied to a patient with C5-level quadriplegia. Note the wrench taped to his vest to remove the chest cover during a cardiopulmonary resuscitation.

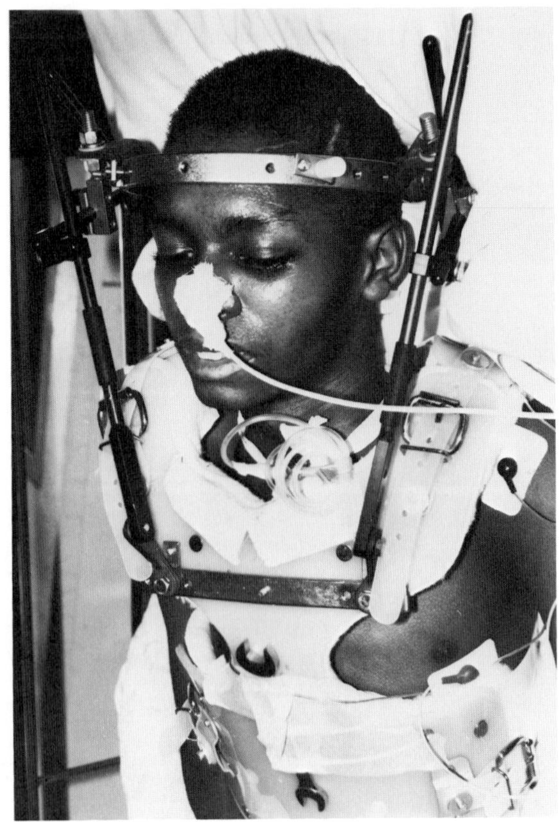

## ACUTE STAGE IMMOBILIZATION

Gardner-Wells tongs are applied easily and quickly in the emergency room. The tongs are applied to the head at its maximum diameter behind the external auditory meatus. Applied early, they can afford added stability in transfers and during radiologic evaluation. Crutchfield tongs are difficult to apply and loosen occasionally.[90]

The halo ring can be applied in the acute phase, allowing both early traction and later definitive care with one invasive procedure. In most cases it is expected that a halo will be used for 3 months or longer. It must be applied with precision and care, usually with a guide. Halo size, pin length, and angulation are all important. There is the potential for a high rate of complications with halo-vest treatment,[66,118] and it probably should not be initiated in the earliest phase of evaluation.[90,184]

## CLOSED REDUCTION

Closed reduction is applicable for many injuries. Spinal traction is applied via a halo device with an initial weight of 15 lb (for lesions below C3), and the weight is increased by increments of 5 lb until reduction is accomplished. Most reductions can be accomplished with less than 40 lb. If large amounts of weight are required, intravenous muscle relaxants should be considered. Reduction must be accompanied by serial neurologic examinations under radiographic control. If additional neurologic deficits occur or an increase in height of one or more intervertebral spaces of more than 5 mm is noted, the attempt at reduction is stopped.[90,94,121]

## OPERATIVE TECHNIQUES

Great controversy exists about the role of surgical intervention in the treatment of cervical spine injuries. Operative treatment is not essential. Many cervical fractures undergo spontaneous fusion ("autofusion") if treated by traction or halo jacket for 8 weeks and intermediate orthosis for additional 8 weeks.[90,184]

The commonly cited indications for surgical fusion are pain reduction, stability, facilitation of nursing care, and avoidance of complications associated with prolonged immobilization,[64,69,90] including recurrent dislocations, osteoporosis, pressure ulcers, thrombophlebitis, and pulmonary embolus, as well as the undesirable psychological changes secondary to prolonged recumbency.[1,121] Fusion may aid the aggressive, overall management of the multiply injured patient.[90] Some authors advocate early surgical intervention to allow for early,

TABLE 14-3. Management of Specific Injuries

| LESION | TREATMENT |
|---|---|
| Soft tissue injuries | Bedrest, neck support, local heat, muscle relaxing medications, neck exercises[50] |
| Atlanto-occipital dislocations | Ventilatory support, gentle traction, halo stabilization, posterior fusion[67,78,110,129] |
| Atlantoaxial injuries | |
| Posterior arch atlas fractures with intact transverse ligament | Cervicothoracic brace for 3–4 months. If nonunion persists then fusion[67,149,171] |
| Posterior arch of atlas with transverse ligament disruption | Upper cervical fusion[54,90] |
| Posterior arch fracture with odontoid fracture | Immobilization until the posterior arch heals,[56] then as per odontoid fracture |
| Transverse ligament disruption | Surgical fusion[58,179] |
| Odontoid fractures | |
| Type I | Collar or brace immobilization[54] |
| Type II | Fusion for all fractures that heal slowly with immobilization[74,90,142,160] |
| Type III | Immobilization with halo traction or skull tongs, then halo brade for 4 months until healed[54,74,90,147] |
| C2 fractures | |
| Nondisplaced, stable | Cervical collar |
| Displaced, unstable | Traction |
| Traumatic spondylolisthesis of the axis | |
| Stable | Halo or Philadelphia collar[58,140,141,147,159] |
| Type I with instability | Traction reduction, then halo vest for 12 weeks[58,159] |
| Type II | Traction, halo vest for 6 weeks[58,159] |
| Type IIa | Halo vest, manual compression[159] |
| Type III | Halo traction, posterior fusion[159] |
| Lower cervical spine fractures and dislocations | |
| Compression flexion | |
| Stable | Halo vest[55,163] |
| Unstable | Halo vest for 3 months; if unstable then fusion[163]; early posterior fusion can also be performed[139] |
| Vertical compression | Halo traction, halo vest for 3 months and posterior fusion if unstable[139,184] |
| Distractive flexion | |
| Unilateral facet dislocation | Traction reduction for 2 weeks and open reduction with fusion if required[139,163] |
| Bilateral facet dislocation | Traction reduction, posterior fusion[121,139,184] |
| Distractive extension | Decompression if needed, immobilization[139] |
| Lateral flexion, unstable | Halo vest, fusion if needed |

halo-free rehabilitation of the patient.[120,163] Aggressive surgical intervention can decrease the duration of hospitalization and reduce the incidence of complications associated with recumbency. It is unclear, however, whether early surgical intervention results in improved neurologic recovery. At least one study showed comparable neurologic improvement in surgically and conservatively treated patient groups.[44]

### *Open Reduction*

This is required when a dislocation is irreducible by closed procedures. In order to effect reduction, the facets are levered into place with a periosteal elevator. A partial excision of the facets may be required if treatment has been delayed. A fusion is required at the same time to restore stability.[1]

### *Decompression*

Routine laminectomy for neural injuries was advocated for many years. However, it has become clear that laminectomy is not indicated and may lead to more neurologic injury and late spinal deformity. Most complete injuries occur instantaneously from impact on the spinal cord at the time of injury. Patients with complete cord lesions do not develop significant neurologic recovery after surgical decompression. Controversy exists about early decompression in an effort to aid root recovery of one or possibly two levels. Return would be of immense value in injuries at C5 or C6 where one level significantly changes the patient's rehabilitative potential.[90,163] However, up to one-third of patients treated conservatively will spontaneously regain one level of root function.[184]

Early reduction is the best and most effective method of decompression in most cases.[1,17] Operative intervention is probably best reserved for incomplete lesions in which neural compression persists after alignment has been restored. Most often an anterior decompression is required to remove bone and/or disc fragment encroaching on the cord.[182]

### *Spinal Fusion*

Spinal fusion continues to be the mainstay of treatment of many cervical injuries. This procedure can be used to create long-term bony stability where ligamentous instability exists. Unlike bony injuries, ligamentous injuries heal poorly because ligamentous tissue is replaced by scar. Under physiologic loads scar stretches; progressive kyphosis or other spinal deformities may result.

It should be understood that, although spinal fusion is performed to provide eventual stability, the degree of immediate stabilization depends upon the surgery performed. The internal fixation should be considered an "internal splint"[69] that allows mobilization of the patient with appropriate external support while bony fusion takes place.

Table 14-3 summarizes the management of specific cervical spine injuries.

## CONCLUSION

Virtually all communication between the brain and the rest of the body passes through the cervical spinal cord. Trauma to the neck, which impinges on the spinal cord, introduces the possibility of devastating or life-threatening injury.

Safe and effective patient management can be assured only if care providers at the accident scene, in transit, and in the hospital stabilize the head and neck until cervical spine injury can be ruled out definitively. In cases where cervical instability is present, external stabilization devices and/or definitive stabilization operations are employed to stabilize the spine and prevent further neurologic injury.

The anesthesiologist deals with problems that are largely determined (a) by the time that has elapsed from injury and (b) by the extent of cord damage. Airway management, which can be difficult because of the necessity of maintaining neck immobilization, may be required for ventilatory failure, treatment of increased intracranial pressure, airway protection, and surgery. Circulatory shock may be present early postinjury in these patients. Those who have recovered from spinal shock are at risk for autonomic hyperreflexia with episodes of hypertension and bradycardia. Management of ventilatory and hemodynamic problems varies from patient to patient. Thus, careful attention to pathophysiologic problems is required; treatment and management proceed from there.

## REFERENCES

1. Aebi M, Mohler J, Zack GA. Indication, surgical technique and results of 100 surgically treated fractures and fracture-dislocations of the cervical spine. Clin Orthop 1986;203:244.
2. Albin MS. Acute cervical spinal injury. Crit Care Clin 1985;1:267.
3. Albin MS, White RJ. Epidemiology, physiopathology, and experimental therapeutics of acute spinal cord injury. Crit Care Clin 1987;3:441.
4. Alderson JD, Thomas DG. The use of halothane anaesthesia to control autonomic hyperreflexia during transurethral surgery in spinal cord injured patients. Paraplegia 1975;13:183.
5. Alexander S, Kerr FWL. Blood pressure responses in acute compression of the spinal cord. J Neurosurg 1964;21:485.
6. Alker GJ, Oh YS, Leslie EV, et al. Postmortem radiology of head and neck injuries in fatal traffic accidents. Radiology 1975;114:611.
7. Alker GJ, Oh YS, Leslie EV. High cervical spine and craniocervical junction injuries in fatal traffic accidents: a radiologic study. Orthop Clin North Am 1978;9:1003.
8. Allen BL, Ferguson RC. Cervical spine trauma in children. In: Bradford D, Hensinger R, eds. The pediatric spine. Thieme, New York: 1985:536.
9. Allen BL, Ferguson RL, Lehman TR, et al. A mechanistic classification of closed, indirect fractures and dislocations of the lower cervical spine. Spine 1982;7:1;27.
10. American College of Surgeons. Advanced Trauma Life Support Course for Physicians, Instructor manual. Chicago: American College of Surgeons, 1984.
11. Anderson LD, D'Alonzo RT. Fractures of the odontoid process of the axis. J Bone Joint Surg 1974;56A:1663.
12. Aprahamian C, Thompson BM, Finger WA, Darin JC. Experimental cervical spine injury model: evaluation of airway management and splinting techniques. Ann Emerg Med 1984;13:584.
13. Babcock JL. Cervical spine injuries: diagnosis and classification. Arch Surg 1976;111:646.

14. Babinski MF. Anesthetic considerations in the patient with acute spinal cord injury. Crit Care Clin 1987;3:619.
15. Barker I, Alderson J, Lydon M, Franks CI. Cardiovascular effects of spinal subarachnoid anesthesia: a study in patients with chronic spinal cord injuries. Anaesthesia 1985;40:533.
16. Basmajian JV. Grant's method of anatomy. 10th ed. Baltimore: Williams & Wilkins, 1980.
17. Bohlman HH. Acute fractures and dislocations of the cervical spine: analysis of three hundred hospitalized patients and a review of the literature. J Bone Joint Surg 1979;61A:1119.
18. Bosch A, Stauffer ES, Nickel VL. Incomplete traumatic paraplegia. JAMA 1971;216:473.
19. Bose B, Northrup BE, Osterholm JL. Delayed vertebrobasilar insufficiency following cervical spine injury. Spine 1985; 10:108.
20. Boucek CD, Gunnerson HB, Tullock WC. Percutaneous transtracheal high-frequency jet ventilation as an aid to fiberoptic intubation. Anesthesiology 1987;67:247.
21. Boyd AD. Tracheostomy and cricothyrotomy. In: Worth M, ed. Principles and practice of trauma care. Baltimore: Williams & Wilkins, 1982:32.
22. Boynton W, Kalb R. Double lumen signs as demonstrated by computer tomography in spine dislocations. Spine 1983;8:910.
22a. Bracken MB, Shepard MJ, Collins WF, et al. A randomized, controlled trial of methylprednisolone or naloxone in the treatment of acute spinal-cord injury. Results of the second national acute spinal cord injury study. N Engl J Med 1990;322:1405.
23. Brantigan CO, Grow JB. Cricothyroidotomy: elective use in respiratory problems requiring tracheostomy. J Thorac Cardiovasc Surg 1976;71:72.
24. Brisman R, Kovach RM, Johnson DO, et al. Pulmonary edema in acute transection of the spinal cord. Surg Gynecol Obstet 1974;139:363.
25. Broecker BH, Hranowsky N, Hackler RH. Low spinal anesthesia for the prevention of autonomic dysreflexia in the spinal cord injured patient. J Urol 1979;122:366.
26. Brunnette DD, Rockswold GL. Neurologic recovery following rapid spinal realignment for complete cervical spinal cord injury. J Trauma 1987;27:445.
27. Bucholz RW, Burkhead WZ. The pathologic anatomy of fatal atlanto-occipital dislocations. J Bone Joint Surg 1979;61A:248.
28. Carter RE. Unilateral diaphragmatic paralysis in spinal cord injured patients. Paraplegia 1980;18:267.
29. Chen CT, Toung TJK, Haupt HM, et al. Evaluation of the efficacy of Alka-Seltzer effervescence in gastric acid neutralization. Anesth Analg 1984;63:325.
30. Cintron E, Gilua L, Murphy W, et al. The widened disc space: a sign of cervical hyperextension injury. Radiology 1981;141:639.
31. Clark K. Injuries to the cervical spine and spinal cord. In: Youmans JR, ed. Neurological surgery. Philadelphia: WB Saunders, 1982:2318.
32. Cline JR, Scheidel E, Bigsby EF. A comparison of methods of cervical immobilization used in patient extrication and transport. J Trauma 1985;25:649.
33. Cloward RB. Acute cervical spine injuries. Clin Symp 1980;32:1.
34. Consensus Conference. Prevention of venous thrombosis and pulmonary embolism. JAMA 1986;256:744.
35. Coombs DW, Hooper D, Pageau M. Emergency cimetidine prophylaxis against acid aspiration. Ann Emerg Med 1982;11:252.
36. Cooper PR. Initial evaluation and management. In: Berczeller PH, Bezkor MH, eds. Medical complications of quadriplegia. Chicago: Year Book Medical Publishers, 1986:1.
37. Cooper PR, Cohen W. Evaluation of cervical spinal cord injuries with metrizamide myelography CT scanning. J Neurosurg 1984;61:281.
38. Cooper PR, Maravilla KR, Sklar FK, et al. Halo immobilization of cervical spine fractures. J Neurosurg 1979;50:603.
39. Dalinka MK, Kessler H, Weiss M. The radiographic evaluation of spinal trauma. Emerg Med Clin North Am 1985;3:475.
40. Dammann HG, Muller P, Simon B. Parenteral ranitidine: onset and duration of action. Br J Anaesth 1982;54:1235.
41. Davies JAH, Howells TH. Management of anesthesia for the full stomach case in the casualty department. J Postgrad Med 1973;(July suppl):58.
42. De La Torre JC. Spinal cord injury: a review of basic and applied research. Spine 1981;6:315.
43. Doble G, Jordan J, Williams JG. Cimetidine in the prevention of the pulmonary acid aspiration (Mendelson's) syndrome. Br J Anaesth 1979;51:967.
44. Donovan WH, Kopaniky D, Stolzmann E, Carter RE. The neurological and skeletal outcome in patients with closed cervical spinal cord injury. J Neurosurg 1987;66:690.
45. Doolan LA, O'Brien JF. Safe intubation in cervical spine injury. Anaesth Intens Care 1985;13:319.
46. Dorr LD, Harvey JP. Traumatic lesions in fatal acute spinal column injuries. Clin Orthop 1981;157:178.
47. Dripps RD, Eckenhoff JE, Vandam LD. Introduction to anesthesia, The principals of safe practice. 6th ed. Philadelphia: WB Saunders, 1982:180–95.
48. Effendi B, Roy D, Cornish B, et al. Fractures of the ring of the axis: a classification based upon the analysis of 131 cases. J Bone Joint Surg 1981;63B:319.
49. Eidelberg EE. Cardiovascular response to experimental spinal cord compression. J Neurosurg 1973;38:326.
50. Eismont FJ, Bohlman HH. Posterior methyl methacrylate fusion for cervical trauma. Spine 1981;6:347.
51. El Masri WS, Silver JR. Prophylactic anticoagulant therapy in patients with spinal cord injury. Paraplegia 1981;19:334.
52. Ersmark H, Löwenhielm P. Factors influencing the outcome of cervical spine injuries. J Trauma 1988;28:407.
53. Evans DE, Kobrine AL, Rizzoli HV. Cardiac arrhythmias accompanying acute compression of the spinal cord. J Neurosurg 1980;52:52.
54. Evarts C. Traumatic occipito-atlantal dislocation: report of a case with survival. J Bone Joint Surg 1970;52A:1653.
55. Fielding JW. Cervical spine surgery: past, present and future potential. Clin Orthop 1985;200:284.
56. Fielding JW, Hawkins RJ. Roentgenographic diagnosis of the injured neck. Instructional course lectures. St. Louis: CV Mosby, 1976.
57. Fielding JW, Hawkins RJ. Atlanto-axial rotatory fixation. J Bone Joint Surg 1979;59A:37.
58. Fielding JW, Hawkins RJ, Sanford RA. Spine fusion for atlanto-axial instability. J Bone Joint Surg 1976;58A:400.
59. Forner JV. Lung volumes and mechanics of breathing in tetraplegics. Paraplegia 1980;18:258.
60. Foulkes E, Jenkins LC. A comparative evaluation of cimetidine and sodium citrate to decrease gastric acidity: effectiveness at the time of induction of anaesthesia. Can Anaesth Soc J 1981;28:29.
61. Francis WR, Fielding JW. Traumatic spondylolisthesis of the axis. Orthop Clin North Am 1978;9:1011.
62. Francis WR, Fielding JW, Hawkins RJ, et al. Traumatic spondylolisthesis of the axis. J Bone Joint Surg 1981;63B:313.
63. Fraser A, Edmonds-Seal J. Spinal cord injuries. Anaesthesia 1982;37:1084.
64. Fried LC. Cervical spinal cord injury during skeletal traction. JAMA 1974;229:181.

65. Frisbie JH, Sasahara AA. Low dose heparin prophylaxis for deep venous thrombosis in acute spinal cord injury patients: a controlled study. Paraplegia 1981;19:343.
66. Garfin SR, Botte MJ, Waters RL, et al. Complications in the use of halo fixation. J Bone Joint Surg 1986;68A:320.
67. Gassman J, Seligson D. The anterior cervical plate. Spine 1983;8:700.
68. Golueke P, Sclafani S, Phillips T, et al. Vertebral artery injury—diagnosis and management. J Trauma 1987;27:856.
69. Green BA, Callahan RA, Klose KJ, et al. Acute spinal cord injury: current concepts. Clin Orthop 1981;154:125.
70. Greenhoot JH, Mauck HP. The effect of cervical cord injury on cardiac rhythm and conduction. Am Heart J 1972;83:659.
71. Gronert GA, Theye RA. Pathophysiology of hyperkalemia induced by succinylcholine. Anesthesiology 1975;43:89.
72. Grundy BL, Friedman W. Electrophysiological evaluation of the patient with acute spinal cord injury. Crit Care Clin 1987; 3:519.
73. Guha A, Tator CH. Acute cardiovascular effects of experimental spinal cord injury. J Trauma 1988;28:481.
74. Hanssen AD, Cabanela ME. Fractures of the dens in adult patients. J Trauma 1987;27:928.
75. Harris JH, Edeiken-Monroe P, Kopaniky DR. A practical classification of acute cervical spine injuries. Orthop Clin North Am 1986;17:15.
76. Harris JH. Radiographic evaluation of spinal trauma. Orthop Clin North Am 1986;17:75.
77. Harris PW, Morison DH, Dunn GL, et al. Intramuscular cimetidine and ranitidine as prophylaxis against gastric acid aspiration syndrome—a randomized double-blind study. Can Anaesth Soc J 1984;31:599.
78. Hohl M. Soft tissue injuries of the neck. Clin Orthop 1975;109:42.
79. Hohl M. Soft tissue injuries of the neck in automobile accidents: factors influencing prognosis. J Bone Joint Surg 1984;56A:1675.
80. Holdsworth F. Fractures, dislocations and fracture-dislocations of the spine: a review paper. J Bone Joint Surg 1970;52A:1534.
81. Hollinshead WH, Rosse C. Textbook of anatomy. Philadelphia: Harper and Row, 1985.
82. Huelke DF, O'Day J, Mendelsohn RA. Cervical injuries suffered in automobile crashes. J Neurosurg 1981;54:316.
83. Jofe MH, White AA, Panjabi MM. Physiology and biomechanics, kinematics. The cervical spine. The Cervical Spine Research Society, Philadelphia: JB Lippincott, 1983:23–35.
84. Johnson RM, Wolf JW Jr. Physiology and biomechanics, stability. In: The Cervical Spine Research Society, ed., The cervical spine. Philadelphia: JB Lippincott, 1983:35–53.
85. Johnson RM, Hart DC, Simmons EF, et al. Cervical orthoses: a study comparing their effectiveness in restricting cervical motion in normal subjects. J Bone Joint Surg 1977;59A:332.
86. Johnson RM, Owens JR, Hart DC, et al. Cervical orthoses: a guide to their selection and use. Clin Orthop 1981;154:34.
87. Jorden RC, Moore EE, Marx JA, Honigman B. A comparison of PTV and endotracheal ventilation in an acute trauma model. J Trauma 1985;25:978.
88. Keene JS, Goletz TH, Lilleas F, et al. Diagnosis of vertebral fractures: a comparison of conventional radiography, conventional tomography and computed axial tomography. J Bone Joint Surg 1982;64A:586.
89. Kiker JD, Woodside JR, Jelinek GE. Neurogenic pulmonary edema associated with autonomic dysreflexia. J Urol 1982;128:1038.
90. King AG. Spinal column trauma. Instructional Course Lectures, vol 35. St. Louis: CV Mosby, 1986.
91. King HK, Wang LF, Khan AK, Woolen DJ. Translaryngeal guided intubation for difficult intubation. Crit Care Med 1987;15:869.
92. Klain M, Keszler H. High-frequency jet ventilation. Surg Clin North Am 1985;65:917.
93. Kornberg M. Upper cervical spine injuries: a review. Contemp Orthop 1986;12:61.
94. Kostiuk JP. Indications for the use of halo immobilization. Clin Orthop 1981;154:46.
95. Kraus JF. A comparison of recent studies on the extent of the head and spinal cord injury problem in the United States. J Neurosurg 1980;53:S35.
96. Kraus JF, Franti CE, Riggins RS, et al. Incidence of traumatic spinal cord lesions. J Chron Dis 1975;28:471.
97. Kurnick NB. Autonomic hyperreflexia and its control in patients with spinal cord lesions. Ann Intern Med 1956;44:678.
98. Lambert DH, Deane RS, Mazuzan JE. Anesthesia and the control of blood pressure in patients with spinal cord injury. Anesth Analg 1982;61:344.
99. Lechman MJ, Donahoo JS, MacVaugh H. Endotracheal intubation using percutaneous retrograde guidewire insertion followed by antegrade fiberoptic bronchoscopy. Crit Care Med 1986;14:589.
100. Lee DS, Kobrine A. Neurogenic pulmonary edema associated with ruptured spinal cord arteriovenous malformation. Neurosurgery 1983;12:691.
100a. Lehmann KG, Lane JG, Piepmeier JM, Batsford WP. Cardiovascular abnormalities accompanying acute spinal cord injury in humans: Incidence, time course and severity. J Am Coll Cardiol 1987;10:46.
101. Levine AM, Edwards CC. The management of traumatic spondylolisthesis of the axis. J Bone Joint Surg 1985;76A:217.
102. Levine AM, Edwards CC. Treatment of injuries in the C1-C2 complex. Orthop Clin North Am 1986;17:31.
103. Luce JM. Medical management of spinal cord injury. Crit Care Med 1985;13:126.
104. MacKenzie CF, Shin B, Krishnaprasad D, et al. Assessment of cardiac and respiratory function during surgery on patients with acute quadriplegia. J Neurosurg 1985;62:843.
105. Majernick TG, Bieniek R, Houston JB, Hughes HG. Cervical spine movement during orotracheal intubation. Ann Emerg Med 1986;15:417.
106. Malik AB. Pulmonary vascular response to increase in intracranial pressure: role of sympathetic mechanisms. J Appl Physiol 1977;42:335.
107. Marshall LF, Knowlton S, Garfin SR, et al. Deterioration following spinal cord injury. A multicenter study. J Neurosurg 1987;66:400.
108. Mazur JM, Stauffer ES. Unrecognized spinal instability associated with "simple" cervical compression fractures. Spine 1983;8:687.
109. McMichan JC, Michel L, Westbrook PR. Pulmonary dysfunction following traumatic quadriplegia. JAMA 1980;243:528.
110. McNab I. Acceleration, extension injuries of the cervical spine. In: Simeone FA, Rothman RH, eds. The spine. Philadelphia: WB Saunders, 1982;647.
111. Messeter KH, Petterson KI. Endotracheal intubation with the fibreoptic bronchoscope. Anaesthesia 1980;35:294.
112. Meyer GA, Berman IR, Doty DB, et al. Hemodynamic responses to acute quadriplegia with or without chest trauma. J Neurosurg 1971;34:168.
113. Meyer PA Jr, Rosen JS, Hamilton BB, et al. Fracture dislocation of the cervical spine: transportation, assessment, and immediate management. In: American Academy of Orthopedic Surgeons, ed. St. Louis: CV Mosby, 1976;171.
114. Morison DH, Dunn GL, Fargas-Babjak AM, et al. A double-blind

comparison of cimetidine and ranitidine as prophylaxis against gastric aspiration syndrome. Anesth Analg 1982;61:988.
115. Mouradian WH, Fietti VG, Cochran GVB. Fractures of the odontoid: a laboratory and clinical study of mechanisms. Orthop Clin North Am 1978;9:985.
116. Mulder JS, Wallace DH, Woolhouse FM. The use of the fiberoptic bronchoscope to facilitate endotracheal intubation following head and neck trauma. J Trauma 1975;15:638.
117. Neff CC, Pfister RC, Sonnenberg EV. Percutaneous transtracheal ventilation: experimental and practical aspects. J Trauma 1983;23:84.
118. Nelson R, Capen D, Garland D, et al. Halo vest stabilization of cervical spine fractures and dislocations. A series review and long term follow-up. Presented at the American Academy of Orthopedic Surgeons Annual Meeting, Atlanta, 1984.
119. Nieder RM, O'Higgins JW, Aldrete JA. Autonomic hyperreflexia in urologic surgery. JAMA 1970;213:876.
120. Norrell H, Wilson CB. Early anterior fusion for injuries of the cervical portion of the spine. JAMA 1970;214:525.
121. O'Brien PJ, Schweigel JF, Thompson WJ. Dislocations of the lower cervical spine. J Trauma 1982;22:710.
122. O'Leary P, Boiardo R. The diagnosis and treatment of injuries of the spine in athletes. In: Nicholas JA, Hershman EB, eds. The lower extermity and spine in sports medicine. St. Louis: CV Mosby, 1986;1171.
123. Patil V, Stehling L, Zauder H, eds. Instrumentation and auxiliary equipment. In: Fiberoptic endoscopy in anesthesia. Chicago: Year Book Medical Publishers, 1983:9.
124. Pennecot GF, Leonard P, Pegrot Des Gauchons S, et al. Ligamentous instability of the cervical spine in children. J Pediatr Orthop 1984;4:339.
125. Penning L. Prevertebral hematoma in cervical spine injury: incidence and etiologic significance. Am J Roentgenol 1981;136:553.
126. Pepin JW, Hawkins RJ. Traumatic spondylolisthesis of the axis: hangman's fracture. Clin Orthop 1981;157:138.
127. Podolsky S, Baraff LJ, Simon RR, et al. Efficacy of cervical spine immobilization methods. J Trauma 1983;23:461.
128. Poe RH, Reisman JL, Rodenhouse TG. Pulmonary edema in cervical spinal cord injury. J Trauma 1978;18:71.
129. Powell WF, Ozdil T. A translaryngeal guide for tracheal intubation. Anesth Analg 1967;46:231.
130. Powers B, Miller MD, Kramer RS, et al. Traumatic anterior atlantooccipital dislocation. Neurosurgery 1979;4:12.
131. Quimby CW, Williams RN, Greifenstein FE. Anesthetic problems of the acute quadriplegic patient. Anesth Analg 1973;52:333.
132. Rawe SE, Perot PL. Pressor response resulting from experimental contusion injury to the spinal cord. J Neurosurg 1979;50:58.
133. Reid DC, Henderson R, Saboe L, Miller JDR. Etiology and clinical course of missed spine fractures. J Trauma 1987;27:980.
134. Riou B, Barriot P, Bodenan P, Viars P. Retrograde tracheal intubation in trauma patients. Anesthesiology 1987;67:A130.
135. Rogers WA. Fractures and dislocations of the cervical spine: an end result study. J Bone Joint Surg 1957;39A:34.
136. Ross SE, Schwab W, David ET, et al. Clearing the cervical spine: initial radiographic evaluation. J Trauma 1987;27:1055.
137. Rowed DW, McLean JAG, Tator CH. Somatosensory evoked potentials in acute spinal cord injury: prognostic value. Surg Neurol 1978;9:203.
138. Roye WP, Dunn EL, Moody JA. Cervical spinal cord injury—a public catastrophe. J Trauma 1987;27:831.
139. Ryan MD, Taylor THK. Odontoid fractures: a rational approach to treatment. J Bone Joint Surg 1982;64B:416.
140. Schatzker J, Rorabek CH, Waddell JW. Fractures of the dens. J Bone Joint Surg 1971;53B:392.
141. Scheiss RJ, deSaussure RL, Robertson JT. Choice of treatment of odontoid fractures. J Neurosurg 1982;51:496.
142. Schlitke LH, Callahan RA. A rational approach to burst fractures of the atlas. Clin Orthop 1981;154:18.
143. Schmidt JF, Jorgensen BC. The effect of metoclopramide on gastric contents after preoperative ingestion of sodium citrate. Anesth Analg 1984;63:841.
144. Schneider RL, Livingston RE, Cave AJE, et al. "Hangman's fracture" of the cervical spine. J Neurosurg 1965;22:141.
145. Schonwald G, Fish KJ, Perkash I. Cardiovascular complications during anesthesia in chronic spinal cord injured patients. Anesthesiology 1981;55:550.
146. Shear P, Hugenholtz H, Richard MT, et al. Multiple noncontiguous fractures of the cervical spine. J Trauma 1988;28:655.
147. Sherk HH. Fractures of the atlas and odontoid process. Orthop Clin North Am 1978;9:973.
148. Sherk HH, Nicholson JT. Fractures of the atlas. J Bone Joint Surg 1970;52A:1017.
149. Sherk HH, Snyder B. Posterior fusions of the upper cervical spine: indications, techniques and prognosis. Orthop Clin North Am 1978;9:1091.
150. Sherk HH, Schut L, Lane JM. Fractures and dislocations of the cervical spine in children. Orthop Clin North Am 1976;7:563.
151. Shields CC, Stauffer ES. Late instability in cervical spine fractures secondary to laminectomy. Clin Orthop 1976;119:144.
152. Simon RR, Brenner BE. Emergency cricothyroidotomy in the patient with massive neck swelling: part 1: anatomical aspects. Crit Care Med 1983;11:114.
153. Simon RR, Brenner BE, Rosen MA. Emergency cricothyroidotomy in the patient with massive neck swelling: part 2: clinical aspects. Crit Care Med 1983;11:119.
154. Smith JP, Morrissey P, Hemmick RS, et al. Retropharyngeal hematomas. J Trauma 1988;28:553.
155. Smith RB. Transtracheal ventilation during anesthesia. Anesth Analg 1974;53:225.
156. Smith RB, Myers EN, Sherman H. Transtracheal ventilation in pediatric patients. Br J Anaesth 1974;46:313.
157. Soderstrom CA, Brumback RJ. Early care of the patient with cervical spine injury. Orthop Clin North Am 1986;17:3.
158. Sosis M, Possanza C. Anaesthesia for the patient with an unstable neck. Anaesth Intens Care 1986;14:328.
159. Southwick WO. Current concepts review: management of fractures of the dens (odontoid process). J Bone Joint Surg 1980;62A:482.
160. Spence KF, Dedser D, Sell HW. Bursting atlantal fractures associated with rupture of the transverse ligament. J Bone Joint Surg 1970;52A:543.
161. Spoerel WE, Narayan PS, Singh NP. Transtracheal ventilation. Br J Anaesth 1971;43:932.
162. Stauffer ES. Fractures and dislocations of the spine—part I: the cervical spine. In: Rockwood CA, Green DP, eds. Fractures in adults. 2nd ed. Philadelphia: JB Lippincott, 1984:932.
163. Stauffer ES. Management of spine fractures C3-C7. Orthop Clin North Am 1986;17:45.
164. Stauffer ES, Kelly EG. Fracture dislocations of the cervical spine; instability and recurrent deformity following treatment by anterior interbody fusion. J Bone Joint Surg 1977;59A:45.
165. Stirt JA, Marco A, Conklin KA. Obstetric anesthesia for a quadriplegic patient with autonomic hyperreflexia. Anesthesiology 1979;51:560.

166. Strain JD, Moore EE, Markovchick VJ, Van Duzer-Moore S. Cimetidine for the prophylaxis of potential gastric acid aspiration pneumonitis in trauma patients. J Trauma 1981;21:49.
167. Theodore J, Robin E. Speculations on neurogenic pulmonary edema. Am Rev Respir Dis 1976;113:405.
168. Tibbs PA, Young B, Todd EP, McAllister RG, Hubbard S. Studies of experimental spinal cord transection—part IV: effects of cervical spinal cord transection on myocardial blood flow in anesthetized dogs. J Neurosurg 1980;52:197.
169. Tobias R. Increased success with retrograde guide for endotracheal intubation. Anesth Analg 1983;62:366.
170. Troll GF, Dohrmann GJ. Anesthesia of the spinal cord injured patients: cardiovascular problems and their management. Paraplegia 1975;13:162.
171. van der Bout AH, Dommisse GF. Traumatic atlantooccipital dislocation. Spine 1986;11:174.
172. Wagner FC, Cheharzi B. Spinal cord injury: indications for operative intervention. Surg Clin North Am 1980;60:1048.
173. Wagner FC, Cheharzi B. Neurologic evaluation of cervical spine injuries. Spine 1984;9:507.
174. Walls RM. Orotracheal intubation and potential cervical spine injury. Ann Emerg Med 1987;16:373.
175. Walts LF. Anesthesia of the larynx in a patient with a full stomach. JAMA 1965;192:705.
176. Wang JF, Reves JG, Gutierrez FA. Awake fiberoptic laryngoscopic tracheal intubation for anterior cervical spinal fusion in patient with cervical cord trauma. Int Surg 1979;64:69.
177. Watson N. Road traffic accidents, spinal injuries and seat belts. Paraplegia 1983;21:63.
178. Weir DC. Roentgenographic signs of cervical injury. Clin Orthop 1975;109:11.
179. White AA III, Panjabi MM. Clinical biomechanics of the spine. Philadelphia: JB Lippincott, 1978.
180. White AA III, Johnson RM, Panjabi MM, et al. Biomechanical analysis of clinical stability in the cervical spine. Clin Orthop 1975;109:85.
181. White AA III, Panjabi MM, Saha S, et al. Biomechanics of the axially loaded cervical spine; development of clinical test for ruptured ligaments. J Bone Joint Surg 1975;57A:582.
182. White AA III, Southwick WO, Panjabi MM. Clinical stability in the lower cervical spine: a review of past and current concepts. Spine 1976;1:15.
183. White AA III, Panjabi MM, Posner I, et al. Spinal stability: evaluation and treatment. In: American Academy of Orthopedic Surgeons, eds. Instructional Course Lectures. St. Louis: CV Mosby, 1983.
184. Whitehill R, Richman J, Glasser JA. Failure of immobilization of the cervical spine by the halo vest. A report of five cases. J Bone Joint Surg 1986;68A:326.
185. Whitelaw WA. The respiratory pump. In: Guenter CA, Welch MH, eds. Pulmonary Medicine, 2nd ed. Philadelphia: JB Lippincott Co, 1982:51–55.
186. Wilberger JE Jr. Spinal cord injuries in children. Mount Kisco, NY: Futura Publishing, 1986.
187. Williams JG. $H_2$ receptor antagonists and anaesthesia. Can Anaesth Soc J 1983;30:264.
188. Williams PL, Warwick R. Gray's anatomy. 36th ed. New York: Churchill Livingstone, 1980.
188a. Winslow EBJ, Lesch M, Talano JV, Meyer PR Jr. Spinal cord injuries associated with cardiopulmonary complications. Spine 1986;11:809.
189. Wray NP, Nicotra MB. Pathogenesis of neurogenic pulmonary edema. Am Rev Respir Dis 1978;118:783.

A portion of this chapter was previously published by Drs. Bauer and Errico in: Bauer RD, Errico TJ, Waugh TR, Cohen W. Evaluation and diagnosis of cervical spine injuries: a review of the literature. Cent Nerv Sys Trauma 1987;4:71. It is used with permission of the publisher.

# Chapter Fifteen John Jackson

# Management of Thoracoabdominal Injuries

Patients with thoracoabdominal injuries pose unique and complex challenges to the clinical anesthesiologist. Hemorrhagic shock, cardiac dysfunction, and impending respiratory failure may all be encountered in a single patient whose life-threatening injuries require immediate surgery. Successful anesthetic management may hinge on one's ability to define problems accurately and to reconcile quickly seemingly conflicting pathophysiologic constraints. At times doing so requires extremely imaginative exercises in applied pharmacology; just as frequently it requires a timely stroke of good luck in terms of what physiologic insults the patient can withstand temporarily.

This chapter discusses some of the clinical and physiologic data that are crucial to the anesthetic management of these patients. A digression about monitoring is warranted at this point. The following sections are at times rather detailed in their discussion of hemodynamic data. This information represents that fund of knowledge that the astute and experienced clinician would utilize in managing a patient whose rapidly deteriorating clinical status might preclude sophisticated monitoring. The goal of any monitoring tool is to obtain maximal knowledge at minimal cost to the patient. In the setting of cardiothoracic, vascular, or severe abdominal trauma, the most critical cost may be the delay in getting the patient to the operating room.

## BLUNT CHEST TRAUMA

Nonpenetrating injuries to the chest wall may be easily overlooked during emergency department evaluation of a patient with multiple trauma. However, signs of blunt thoracic injury should alert the anesthesiologist to the possibility of an underlying pulmonary or myocardial contusion and its attendant complications. Statistically, hypoxia, exsanguination, and associated extrathoracic injuries are the three most common causes of death from blunt chest trauma, which is the leading fatal thoracic disorder in persons under the age of 45.[244]

The particularly treacherous nature of blunt thoracic trauma can be appreciated in terms of basic physical principles. The kinetic energy imparted to the chest wall by an object is determined by the difference between the object's impacting and residual velocities. Blunt injuries result in maximal energy transmission to the thorax since the residual velocity of the impacting object is zero.[80] This energy can cause one or more of the following categories of intrathoracic injuries: (a) rib fractures with or without flail chest, (b) parenchymal injury, ie, pulmonary contusion/laceration, (c) hemothorax/pneumothorax, (d) tracheobronchial disruption, and (e) diaphragmatic rupture. In addition, cardiac and great vessel injuries may occur and are discussed later in this chapter.

### RIB FRACTURES

Rib fractures are a common feature of major thoracic trauma. The incidence of serious complications increases with the number of ribs fractured. This increase is undoubtedly a reflection of the greater traumatic forces associated with multiple rib fractures, and fatal cardiorespiratory complications occur in 5 to 7% of these patients.[172,244] Multiple rib fractures most commonly involve the seventh through tenth ribs and thus are often associated with hepatic or splenic lacerations. Acute gastric dilation commonly accompanies left-sided fractures and may increase the likelihood of acid aspiration.

Early studies suggested a statistical association between fractures of the upper five ribs and more serious internal injuries.[177] First rib fractures in particular were said to herald a high incidence of multiple internal injuries and/or the occurrence of subclavian artery trauma.[168,207,241] However, more recent data indicate that upper rib fractures are not necessarily associated with either a higher incidence or greater severity of concurrent internal injuries.[121] In particular, the simple presence of a first rib fracture does not by itself constitute an indication for subclavian arteriography. The first rib, because of its low cervical location and broad flat anatomy, probably requires a particularly intense, but localized blow to sustain a fracture. Thus, associated injuries of the chest, abdomen, and heart may not be especially frequent, although an association may exist between first rib fractures and severe maxillofacial or neurologic injuries.[114,167]

Even in the absence of underlying cardiopulmonary trauma, rib fractures may contribute to serious pulmonary complications. The associated pain and reflex muscle splinting can exacerbate alveolar hypoventilation, resulting in retention of secretions and atelectasis. The key to preventing this sequence of events is adequate analgesia. Systemic narcotics are physiologically unattractive for this purpose because of the attendant respiratory depression. The use of intercostal nerve block is a better approach to the management of rib fractures; improvement in vital capacity has been documented in patients after thoracotomy.[57,150] The only serious disadvantage is the high blood level of local anesthetic that may result from intercostal blocks.[195,230] Comparable analgesia of longer duration and with less potential for systemic toxicity may be achieved with continuous thoracic epidural analgesia.[46]

## FLAIL CHEST AND PULMONARY CONTUSION

The term "flail chest" refers to the paradoxical inspiratory retraction and expiratory expansion of an unstable chest wall segment that commonly occur as a result of sequential segmental rib fractures. The involved ribs are often fractured in at least two locations, resulting in a chest wall or sternal segment that moves independently of the remaining thorax during respiration. The greater the number of adjacent rib fractures, the greater the likelihood of a flail segment. However, visible flailing is also dependent on the compliance of the underlying lung. Decreased lung compliance results in an increase of the atmospheric-to-intrapleural pressure gradient during spontaneous breathing, which in turn promotes the paradoxical movement of the flail segment. Flail injuries of the posterior chest wall are less common, probably because of the protection afforded by the paraspinous muscles. However, the clinician should specifically examine this area for evidence of multiple segmental rib fractures since the heavy musculature may also obscure the movement of an obviously flail segment. Reported mortality rates for patients with flail chest injuries have ranged from 10 to 50%.[175,192] The continued high mortality is most closely associated with intrathoracic or extrathoracic hemorrhage and lethal head trauma. Fatalities are rare in patients with isolated flail chest injury.

Historically, gas exchange abnormalities accompanying a flail chest were attributed to the presumed hypoventilation produced by the inspiratory retraction of the flail segment.[48] The concept of "Pendelluft" arose from Brauer's early work on thoracoplasty.[22] He noted that decostalized chest wall segments exhibited inspiratory retraction and expiratory expansion. This pendulum-like motion was incorrectly attributed to the intrapulmonary exchange of respiratory gases between the normal lung and the underlying flail segment. Although intuitively appealing, the Pendelluft phenomenon has not been confirmed by laboratory or clinical investigations.[130,191] In fact, minute ventilation and oxygen uptake may be slightly greater on the side of the flail segment (Fig 15-1).[48]

The hypoxemia and respiratory failure that accompany flail chest injuries are predominantly a reflection of underlying pulmonary contusion.[27] Chest wall instability, except in severe cases, probably plays a less important role.[38] Although Pendelluft does not contribute to hypoventilation, pain from rib fractures may elicit chest wall splinting and result in regional hypoventilation of perfused alveoli. This $\dot{V}/\dot{Q}$ mismatch is the principal cause of hypoxemia in victims of pulmonary contusion. In the approach to the acutely injured patient, it is particularly important to realize that the onset of hypoxemia and the appearance of pulmonary X-ray abnormalities may be delayed for 4 hours or longer after the traumatic episode. The hypoxemia is also likely to be progressive; further deterioration of arterial oxygen tension should be expected over the first 24 hours.[53,72,100,245]

As alluded to earlier, the pathophysiologic basis of the hypoxemia in pulmonary contusion is a mismatch between pulmonary ventilation and perfusion.[91,156] The energy imparted to the chest at the moment of impact precipitously increases intra-alveolar pressure, resulting in rupture of the alveolar-capillary interface. Pathologically, this rupture produces intra-alveolar hemorrhage and edema in the absence of parenchymal laceration. The exact pathogenesis is unknown, but most

FIG. 15-1. Minute ventilation and $O_2$ uptake may actually be greater on the side of the flail segment. (From Duff et al[48] with permission.)

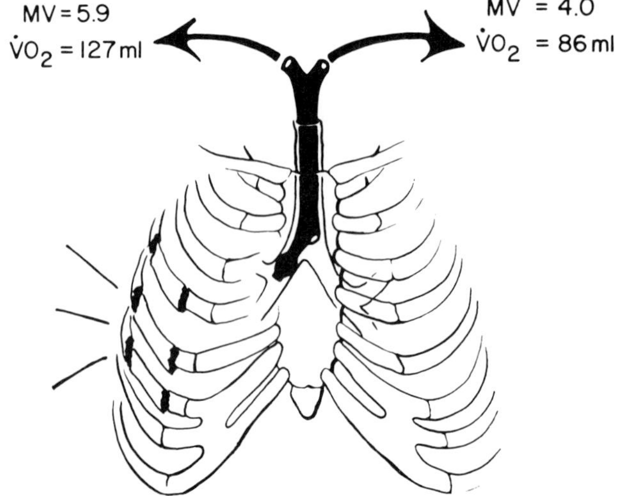

experimental data support a mechanism analogous to blast trauma. In blast trauma, a high pressure wave compresses the thorax, resulting in a compression injury that is then exacerbated and/or extended by the shearing forces of the subsequent rapid intrathoracic pressure reversal, which produces a decompressive injury.[114]

In laboratory models, the severity of such injuries is influenced by the thickness and compliance of the overlying chest wall.[114,249] Thus, obesity may be protective for the patient sustaining an isolated pulmonary contusion. Paradoxically, an injury to the highly elastic thoracic cage of the younger individual may result in a minimally damaged chest wall accompanied by a severe underlying pulmonary contusion, whereas the same forces applied to the brittle thorax of a more elderly person might result in multiple rib fractures but perhaps a less severe parenchymal insult. In this regard it should be noted that patients with pulmonary contusion and concomitant flail chest are more likely to require intubation, but do not have a higher mortality than those having an intact thorax.[103]

Unfortunately, there is evidence that aggressive fluid resuscitation, which is often necessary for the massively traumatized patient, may exacerbate the congestive atelectasis of the contused lung. In addition, for reasons that are not entirely clear, profound edema may develop concurrently in the normal lung. In animal models of pulmonary contusion, there is a decrease in pulmonary blood flow to the contused lung that is associated with increased pulmonary vascular resistance in vessels supplying the contused region. A concurrent decrease in resistance of the precapillary vessels in the noncontused area allows for deleterious, "luxury" perfusion of the normal lung. In the setting of concurrent rapid transfusion, the relaxation of precapillary pulmonary arterioles allows for the transmission of high flow and high pressures directly to the unprotected pulmonary capillaries in previously normal areas of the lung.[73] An as yet unproven hypothesis is that vasoactive mediators enhancing pulmonary capillary permeability may exacerbate the process.

Therapy for flail chest injuries has evolved with greater understanding of its pathophysiology. When the Pendelluft concept held sway, sandbagging and external traction devices were used to stabilize the flail segment and thus, it was hoped, to minimize wasted ventilation. When increasing experience was gained with mechanical rspirators, the use of prolonged (3–4 weeks) controlled mechanical ventilation was proposed as a form of "internal pneumatic stabilization."[7] Controlled hyperventilation prevented the paradoxical retractions of spontaneous inspiratory efforts until the flail segment healed. Trinkle and others have demonstrated the safety and efficacy of a more selective use of ventilatory therapy in patients with flail chest injuries.[10,179,198,199,228] Morbidity, mortality, and hospital cost may be significantly reduced by restricting mechanical ventilation to patients meeting standard criteria for ventilatory failure (hypoxia, tachypnea) and alterations in lung mechanics (low tidal volume and low vital capacity).[26] More recently, a randomized controlled trial of ventilatory and nonventilatory management has shown a shortened therapeutic course for nonventilated (mask CPAP) patients.[16a] In this study, epidurally administered narcotics were an integral part of the nonventilatory management, and these patients also had a significantly reduced incidence of pulmonary infections.

Therapy for the underlying pulmonary contusion is largely supportive, but early effective analgesia and aggressive pulmonary toilet are essential. The anesthesiologist frequently encounters these patients when they require surgery for life-threatening extrathoracic injuries. A common therapeutic dilemma is that of a patient in hemorrhagic shock with a severely contused lung. The possibility of an associated increase in pulmonary capillary permeability creates the potential for excerbating intra-alveolar edema by aggressively replenishing the known depletion in intravascular volume. Given these conflicting choices, fluid administration in these patients should be guided by pulmonary artery catheterization as soon as possible. However, prolonged hypovolemic shock with the potential for irreversible ischemic injury to the kidney and other organs would seem to be the greater risk, given the relatively treatable nature of the lung injury.[166]

Optimal fluid management of these patients remains an area of controversy, with theoretical advantages being claimed for both crystalloid and colloid resuscitation regimens. There are data suggesting that the interstitial leak of pulmonary fluid may be prevented or minimized by maintaining the colloid osmotic pressure; experimentally, the use of colloid volume expanders has been associated with less gain in overall weight and water content of the injured lung.[228] Other animal models of pulmonary contusion also support a strategy of minimizing crystalloids, adequate volume resuscitation with colloid, and forced diuresis.[33,47,227] In contrast, clinical studies have demonstrated the efficacy of crystalloid-based regimes,[17] but to date no randomized trials have been conducted.[218]

Patients progressing to respiratory failure (tachypnea, hypoxia, hypercarbia) require ventilatory assistance, but the specific modality chosen should depend on the clinical situation. Possible ventilatory modalities include continuous positive airway pressure (CPAP) via a well-fitting face mask, controlled ventilation with titrated doses of positive end-expiratory pressure (PEEP), low-rate intermittent mandatory ventilation (IMV) with PEEP,[42] and a combination of IMV with PEEP and high-frequency ventilation. Administration of an expiratory distending pressure is the key element in all these ventilatory maneuvers (see also Chapter 24). As it does with other causes of adult respiratory distress syndrome, PEEP usually improves oxygenation by increasing the compromised FRC, especially in cases of bilateral contusions. In patients with severe but localized contusions, PEEP may exacerbate the contusion by producing gas trapping in alveoli adjacent to the damaged pulmonary capillaries.[156] Failure to respond to mechanical ventilation with PEEP is commonly caused by bacterial pneumonias. These patients may be particularly vulnerable to infections since there is evidence that hypovolemia and crystalloid resuscitation depress the contused lung's ability to clear bacteria.[178]

Adequate pain relief using systemically or spinally administered narcotics, intercostal nerve blocks, or epidural analgesia with local anesthetics may improve ventilatory mechanics,[128a] assist in clearance of airway secretions, and facilitate chest physiotherapy. In addition, as alluded to earlier, they may play a key role in the success of the nonventilatory management of the patient with a flail chest.

More controversial measures include large doses of corticosteroids (methylprednisolone, 30 mg/kg). They may have theoretical advantages in the treatment of the contused lung,[213] but their clinical use has been largely restricted to a low-risk group of patients who are not expected to require mechanical ventilation.[65] A consensus seems to exist that the attendant risk of immunosuppression does not warrant their routine use in patients at high risk for colonization and opportunistic infection.[33] Again there are few controlled studies documenting the clinical efficacy of steroids, and they may needlessly threaten a critically ill population with a variety of undesirable side effects.

There are only a few absolute restrictions in the anesthetic management of these patients. Because of the potential for delayed hypoxemia, a high inspired oxygen concentration should be used even if the initial arterial oxygen tension is acceptable. Since hypovolemia may preclude the use of inhalation agents, a narcotic-oxygen technique is often the most suitable approach. Moribund patients are best served by a relaxant-oxygen-ventilator anesthetic so that all available hands and minds can be marshalled to the resuscitative effort. However, it should be remembered that neurologically intact survivors may recollect unpleasant intraoperative events when low-dose anesthetic agents are used.[16] At the other extreme is the hemodynamically stable patient with a pulmonary contusion who requires a peripheral orthopedic or plastic procedure. In these instances, an inhalation agent might be advantageous with a view to relatively early extubation. In patients with localized pulmonary contusion it is important to realize that these agents may have the potential to inhibit hypoxic pulmonary vasoconstriction and thus increase intrapulmonary shunt.

## TRAUMATIC PNEUMOTHORAX

Both blunt and penetrating thoracic injuries may result in traumatic pneumothorax, but pneumothorax can occur without apparent rib injuries. The most common cause is lung puncture produced by the penetration of displaced rib fractures. Subcutaneous emphysema is the most sensitive clinical sign; however, its specificity is low and its presence is not an indication for chest tube insertion. Massive subcutaneous emphysema in the absence of pneumothorax may be seen in patients sustaining lung injury who have chronic pleural adhesions from pre-existing pleural disease.[166]

The detrimental cardiovascular effects of tension pneumothorax are believed to be due to the mechanical compression of the heart and great vessels. However, experimental preparations do not support mechanical obstruction to venous return as a pathophysiologic mechanism.[90,190] Unilateral tension caused by free air within the pleural space transmits incompletely to the mediastinum or contralateral pleural space, causing only slight changes in the superior vena cava, carotid artery, and pulmonary artery pressures.[90] In awake animals with intrapleural pressure as high as 25 cm $H_2O$, cardiac output remains unchanged because of a compensatory increase in heart rate. Instead it is likely that lung collapse causes intrapulmonary shunting and that the resultant hypoxemia is the primary pathophysiologic derangement.[90] In anesthetized patients, compensatory tachycardia may not occur, which may exacerbate the resultant cardiovascular deterioration. With bilateral tension pneumothoraces, both hypoxemia and compression of the great vessels may contribute to hypotension and/or cardiac arrest.

Pneumothorax ranks second to rib fracture as the most common injury in patients with chest trauma,[222] and in one large series it was noted in 40% of patients.[47] A chest X-ray should be obtained in all traumatized patients to rule out the possibility of pneumothorax or other chest injuries. Although it is preferable to obtain an upright film to facilitate the detection of a pneumothorax, this position may be impossible or contraindicated in patients who are experiencing severe hemorrhage or in those with suspected cervical spine or severe head injury. It is therefore important to realize that the supine chest radiograph can detect most pneumothoraces large enough to require immediate thoracosotomy.[222] Intrapleural free air in supine patients tends to move to the highest portion of the chest, which corresponds to the cardiophrenic or anteromedial and subpulmonic spaces.[221] However, although an experienced radiologist may be able to recognize the radiolucency of free air in this area, particularly on a lateral radiograph, other physicians may easily miss this finding. Moreover, small pneumothoraces may easily go undetected even when the chest X-rays are obtained in the upright position. Computed tomography of the chest has been shown to be more sensitive than chest X-ray for the detection of occult pneumothoraces (Fig 15-2).[223] In one series of 15 head-injured patients, CT enabled detection of 11 pneumothoraces that were missed on plain chest radiograms.[223] If available, a CT study should be considered in patients undergoing general anesthesia or mechanical ventilation after blunt thoracoabdominal injuries.

Even small pneumothoraces of traumatic origin should be treated with thoracostomy tube drainage and suction.[98] Expectant therapy is particularly inappropriate for the patient who may require intubation and positive pressure ventilation during surgery for extrathoracic injuries. Preoperatively it is important to ascertain that the thoracostomy tube is placed accurately and that effective re-expansion of the lung has occurred. Failure to aspirate air during the initial thoracentesis of a patient with subcutaneous emphysema may occur when the needle is not long enough to enter the pleural space. This is a frequent mistake in the young heavily muscled patient who is commonly encountered in the trauma setting. Rarely, a ruptured esophagus or major bronchus may not communicate with the pleural space and yet result in massive subcutaneous emphysema.[166]

Intraoperative hemodynamic collapse may occur in the patient whose pneumothorax is unrecognized preoperatively. In these patients, expansion of intrapleural air frequently creates a tension pneumothorax after intubation and positive pressure ventilation. When nitrous oxide is used, its potential for expanding closed air-containing spaces may also exacerbate the problem. Thorough preoperative evaluation and intraoperative vigilance should avoid this emergency. Precipitous hypoxemia, hypotension, absent breath sounds, tracheal devia-

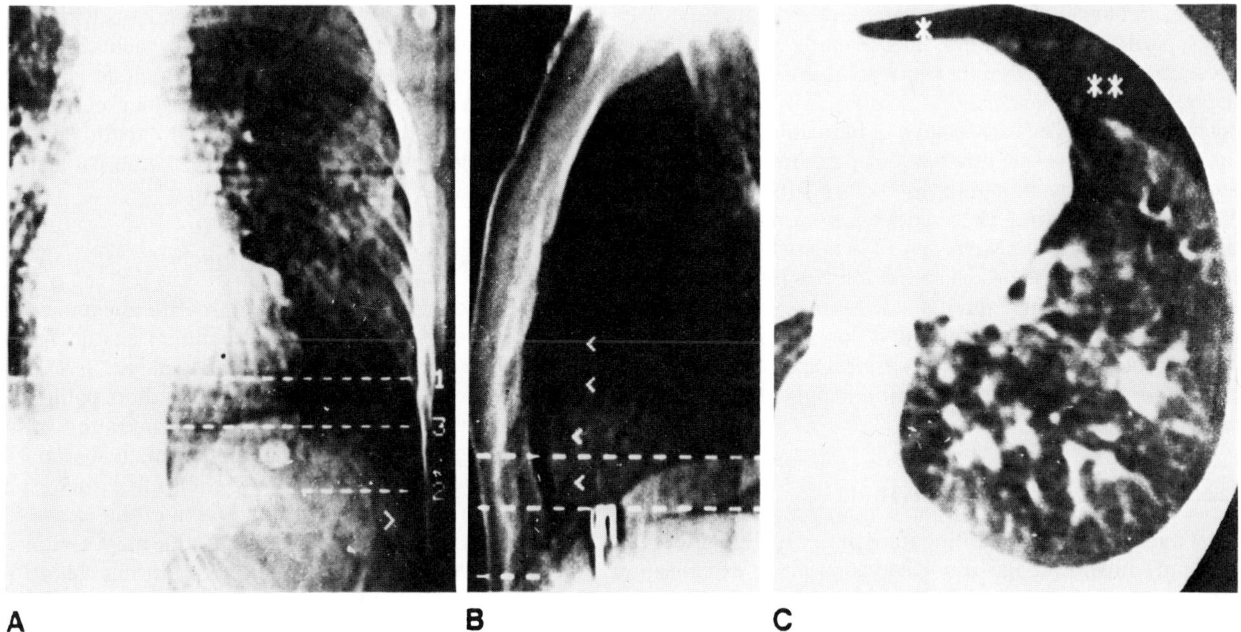


FIG. 15-2. (A) Scout view of supine chest CT scan. Note the small pneumothorax at the left costophrenic angle (*arrowhead*). Broken lines numbered 1, 3, and 2 indicate the locations of axial scans obtained. (B) Scout view of supine lateral chest CT scan. Note the small pneumothorax at the costophrenic angle (*arrowheads*). (C) Axial CT scan obtained from line 2 of A, demonstrating the pneumothorax at cardiophrenic angle (*) and anteromedial plural space (**). (From Tocino et al[223] with permission.)

tion, and increased airway pressure may all be present in the classical presentation. This is a life-threatening emergency that requires immediate thoracostomy or evacuation of the pleural space with a large-bore needle.

## TRAUMATIC HEMOTHORAX

Hemothorax may occur with both penetrating and nonpenetrating thoracic trauma and is usually caused by blood emanating from cardiac, great vessel, pulmonary parenchymal, or chest wall injury.[216] Most of these patients are initially managed with tube thoracostomy. This procedure allows for continual quantification of the blood loss, and with an appropriate drainage system, the recovered blood can be reinfused after filtration. Patients with massive hemothoraces who remain hypotensive despite aggressive transfusion may require an emergency room thoracotomy. These patients require only intubation, ventilation with 100% oxygen, and a muscle relaxant. The surgical objective is to relieve any cardiac tamponade or to control arterial bleeding or aortic dissection by applying a proximal occlusion clamp. The best results are seen in patients with penetrating injuries.[8]

## DIAPHRAGMATIC RUPTURE

Traumatic rupture of the diaphragm is a relatively uncommon injury, seen in 2–3% of patients with blunt chest trauma. However, a delay in diagnosis continues to contribute to morbidity and mortality.[56] Associated injuries occur in virtually all cases and are the major determinants of persistently high mortality rates, which range between 15 and 20%.[12,56] Rupture of the left hemidiaphragm accounts for 70 to 75% of these injuries,[12] presumably because of the shielding effect of the underlying mass of the liver on the right. It is important to remember that the gastric herniation and distention accompanying left-sided injuries may place these patients at increased risk for acid aspiration.

Diagnostic clues on plain radiographs include elevation of the affected hemidiaphragm, intrathoracic displacement of abdominal organs with loss of the normal overlying diaphragmatic contour, and the obviously errant course of a nasogastric tube.[9,165] However, diagnosis by plain film may be difficult or misleading when the X-ray is obtained in an upright position and when the patient is mechanically ventilated (with or without PEEP). Under these conditions, the displaced abdominal organs may be pushed back into their normal location, thus obscuring the diaphragmatic disruption. Conversely, radiographs obtained at end-expiration with the patient in the Trendelenburg position may facilitate the diagnosis. In selected cases, computed tomography may be useful, but the abnormalities to be sought are the same as those seen on the plain film; that is, interruption of diaphragmatic contour and/or displacement of fat or bowel loops posterior or lateral to the disrupted diaphragmatic margin.[222] However, the diagnosis of most diaphragmatic ruptures which occur as a result of blunt abdominal trauma, is often made only at the time of laparotomy. In this regard it should be noted that, although peritoneal lavage alone (see section on abdominal trauma) is unreliable in detecting diaphragmatic rupture,[184] the diagnosis may be made definitively by demonstrating the egress of peritoneal lavage fluid through a functioning thoracostomy tube.[31]

Although intrathoracic herniation of the abdominal viscera

may be an obvious finding at laparotomy, diaphragmatic ruptures, particularly small ones, may be easily overlooked in the presence of life-threatening thoracic injuries.[235] Intraoperatively, the anesthesiologist may notice a change in pulmonary compliance if there is any degree of herniation of the abdominal viscera. However, this particular finding may easily be attributed to surgical manipulation of the lung. Postoperative difficulties in weaning these patients from mechanical ventilation should arouse suspicion of a missed diaphragmatic hernia. Thoracic and/or abdominal injuries may rarely result in an intrapericardial diaphragmatic hernia. Small pericardial herniations may easily be missed at the time of thoracotomy, and laparotomy is the preferred surgical approach since it allows for inspection of both the injured and contralateral side of the diaphragm.[233]

## PENETRATING TRAUMA OF THE LUNG

Most patients with penetrating lung injury require only thoracostomy tube drainage and observation for re-expansion of the lung and resolution of the hemothorax. Actual parenchymal damage is rarely significant enough to require lobectomy or pneumonectomy.[98] However, patients sustaining these injuries may be encountered during emergency department resuscitation or when they require surgery for nonpulmonary injuries. The anesthesiologist must be aware that these patients are at risk of systemic air embolism during mechanical ventilation as a result of traumatic bronchovenous fistulas.[139] Peak airway pressures as high as 100 cm $H_2O$ may be required during resuscitative thoracotomy in patients with penetrating lung trauma.[86] These increased intrabronchial pressures have been shown to contribute to the transmission of air through traumatic bronchial-to-pulmonary venous communications. When such injuries are produced in experimental animals, air emboli are frequently observed in the coronary arteries (Fig 15-3).[86]

## TRACHEOBRONCHIAL INJURIES

Injuries to the tracheobronchial tree are uncommon sequelae of thoracic trauma, but their recognition is critical to the planning of appropriate anesthetic management. Serious concomitant injuries occur in less than half of these patients, usually as a result of direct trauma from penetrating missles. Although reports have documented traumatic disruptions at almost every level of the tracheobronchial tree, the vast majority of these injuries occur within 2.5 cm of the carina.[116]

Sudden forceful compression is the most common insult causing tracheobronchial injuries during blunt thoracic trauma.[116] This anteroposterior compression combined with simultaneous lateral expansion of the lungs can result in severe traction on the pericarinal portion of the trachea. Another possible mechanism for these injuries is an acute increase in intrabronchial pressure resulting from reflex glottic closure at the moment of impact. A third possibility is shearing forces at points of fixation of the intrathoracic airways caused by rapid deceleration, accounting for the preponderance of disruptions near the carina.

FIG. 15-3. Air emboli in the coronary arteries of a dog subjected to penetrating lung injury. (From Graham et al [86] with permission.)

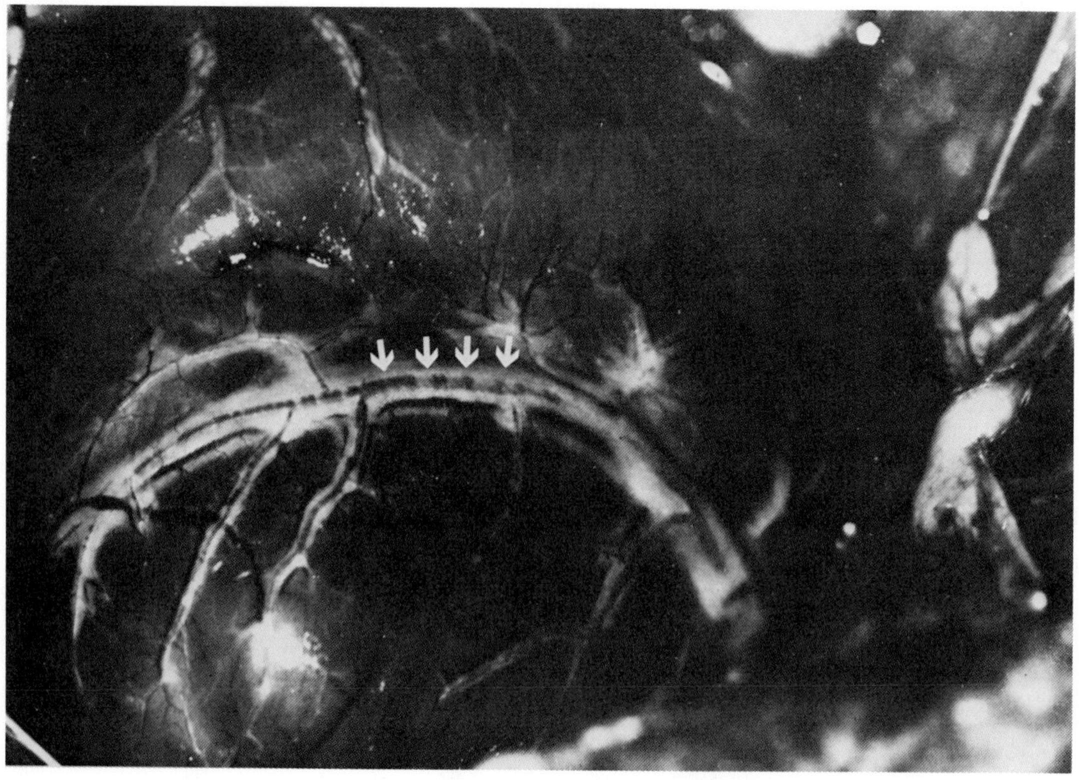

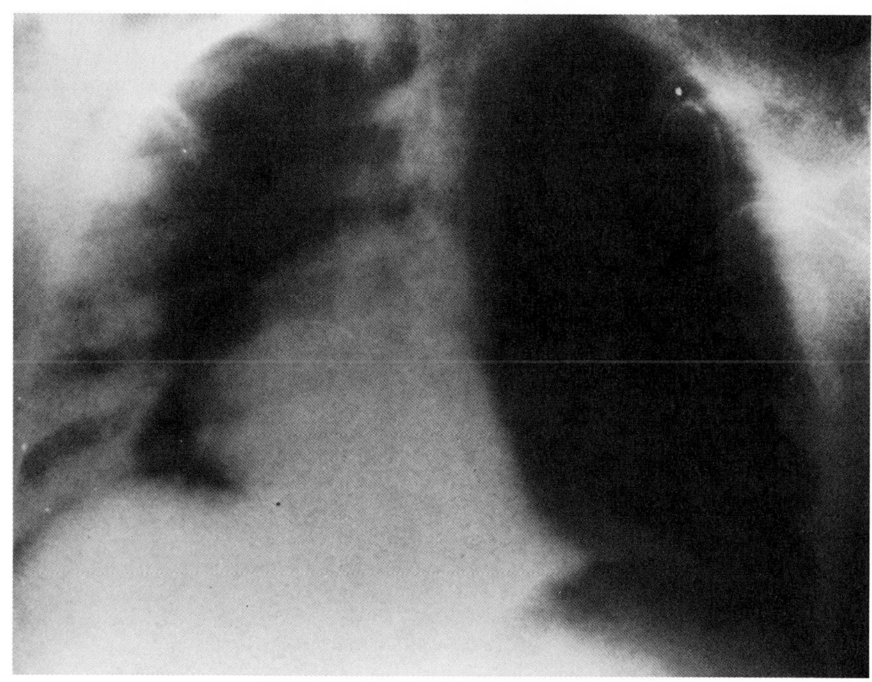

FIG. 15-4. Chest roentgenogram after transection of left mainstem bronchus. Note apex of the left lung at the level of carina. (From Mills et al.[146] with permission.)

Dyspnea, cough, painful hemoptysis, and subcutaneous emphysema are the most common clinical findings in patients with tracheobronchial disruption.[87] However, a surprising number of patients (10%) are nearly asymptomatic, accounting for the frequent delays in diagnosis. Two distinct clinical patterns have been described, depending on whether the site of disruption communicates freely with the mediastinal pleura.[114] When there is free communication, pneumothorax obviously results, and tube thoracostomy and suction characteristically fail to re-expand the affected lung. In the absence of communication with the pleural space, there is little or no pneumothorax, but if present, it resolves appropriately with placement of a chest tube.

In addition to pneumothorax and pneumomediastinum, indicative radiographic findings include subcutaneous and deep cervical emphysema. With complete transection of a mainstem bronchus, the superior margin of the affected lung characteristically drops below the level of the transection. This occurs because the lung is deprived of its normal bronchial tethering in the thoracic cage (Figs 15-4 and 15-5).[146] This radiographic finding is relatively specific. In otherwise uncomplicated pneumothorax, the superior border of the col-

FIG. 15-5. Schematic representations of tracheobronchial disruptions. A, with communication into the pleural space; apex of ipsilateral lung at level of carina. B, no communication with pleural space, therefore no pneumothorax; mediastinal air may be the only radiographic abnormality. (From Mills et al[146] with permission.)

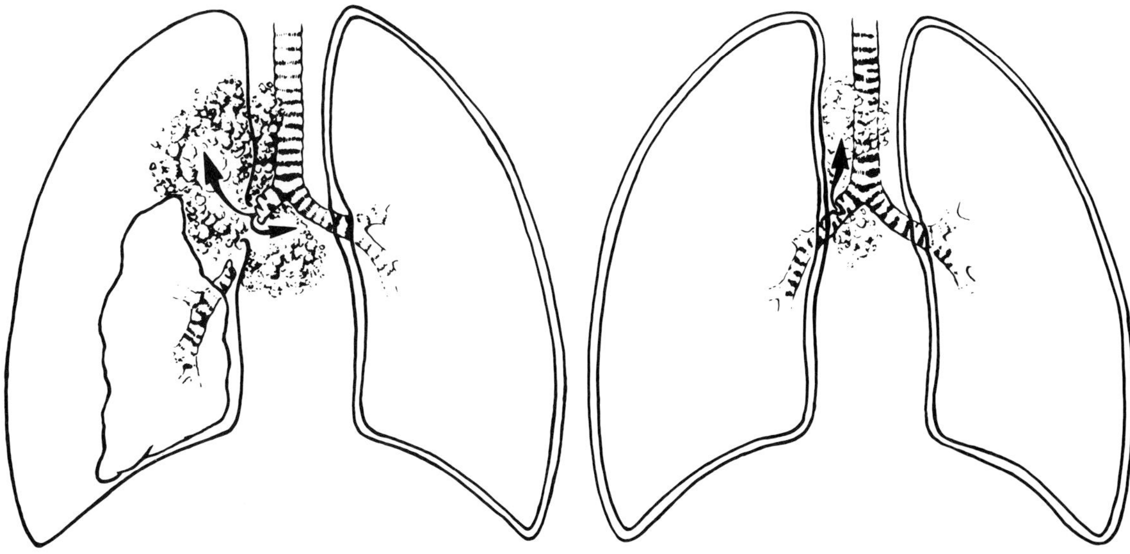

lapsed lung is above the level of the ipsilateral distal bronchus. There are few suggestive physical findings other than subcutaneous emphysema and the occasionally noted Hamman's sign, a crunching sound synchronous with the heart beat. It is produced by air within the mediastinum and may be confused with a pericardial or pleural friction rub.

Blind endotracheal intubation without endoscopic visualization of the tracheobronchial tree is unwise in the presence of tracheal disruption. It is unlikely to be successful because of posterior displacement of the distal trachea, and it may produce further trauma. In addition, acute airway obstruction may develop when the endotracheal tube enters a false passage and occludes the tracheal lumen. Patients with complete high tracheal separations usually require direct control of the airway via a transverse cervical incision. The most common site of these "clothesline" or steering wheel injuries is between the cricoid cartilage and the second tracheal ring.[99] The repair is usually by end-to-end anastomosis performed after a surgically guided oral intubation of the distal tracheal segment and removal of the initial surgically established airway.

There are several acceptable ways of managing the airway when the disruption and the distal segment can be visualized clearly. Under direct vision, a double-lumen tube (or a long cuffed endotracheal tube) can be inserted distal to the tracheal tear or, in the case of bronchial disruption, into the contralateral bronchus. Alternatively, one can visualize directly the area of disruption with a fiberoptic bronchoscope and then use the instrument as a stent over which an endotracheal tube can be passed into the distal tracheal segment. This approach is equally acceptable for bronchial disruption, although it is preferrable to intubate the uninjured bronchus selectively for ventilation during bronchial repairs. Techniques employing high-frequency jet ventilation using uncuffed catheters in the contralateral bronchus have also been described.[169] Regardless of the method chosen, a variety of sterile, long endotracheal tubes should be available for insertion into the distal airway at the time of surgery.

## CARDIAC TRAUMA

Trauma to the heart, with an estimated yearly incidence of 900,000 cases, may be the most common unsuspected fatal visceral injury in accident victims.[164] The reported incidence of cardiac injury in trauma patients varies from 6 to 76%.[153,162] Thus, its true incidence is in fact unknown, yet it is probably a seriously underdiagnosed complication in multiple trauma victims. This underdiagnosis is particularly regrettable since the nature and severity of the cardiac injury may have important implications for the anesthetic management of those patients whose noncardiac injuries necessitate urgent surgical intervention.

Since cardiac trauma is underdiagnosed, the anesthesiologist should suspect it in any patient with blunt or penetrating injury to the chest or upper abdomen. However, this generalized suspicion should be enhanced by an ability to recognize the subtle clinical and hemodynamic findings characteristic of the most common cardiac injuries. For example, cardiac tamponade is a final common pathway for many traumatic injuries of the heart, and familiarity with its frequently atypical presentation in the trauma patient may facilitate the diagnosis of a variety of far more esoteric cardiac lesions. Therefore, this section begins with a detailed analysis of the clinical findings and pathophysiology of cardiac tamponade, with emphasis on features peculiar to its presentation in the multiple trauma patient.

### CARDIAC TAMPONADE

In patients with penetrating cardiac trauma, the two most common causes of immediate death are exsanguinating hemorrhage and cardiac tamponade.[215] Both of these conditions may also be seen in the majority of survivors.[215] In multiple trauma patients, blood loss from other thoracic or nonthoracic injuries may exacerbate the overall volume deficit. Since aggressive expansion of intravascular volume may produce clinical improvement in patients suffering from either hypovolemic shock or cardiac tamponade, the anesthesiologist must remain strongly suspicious of the latter diagnosis in victims of thoracic trauma with complicating hypovolemia.

#### *Clinical Features and Pathophysiology*

To a certain extent the nature of the cardiovascular or extrathoracic injury determines the clinical presentation and makes the diagnosis of tamponade difficult. Beck's triad of cervical venous distention, hypotension, and muffled heart sounds is seen in less than 50% of cases of traumatic tamponade.[243,246] Agitation, combativeness, and cool vasoconstricted extremities are seen in patients with tamponade, but these are also quite common nonspecific findings in patients with hypovolemic shock. Concurrent drug or ethanol intoxication that has contributed to the traumatic injury may also obscure the neurologic picture of cerebral hypoperfusion resulting from cardiac tamponade. Paradoxical inspiratory distention of the neck veins (Kussmaul's sign) is characteristic of cardiac tamponade. However, it may be extremely difficult to demonstrate this relatively subtle physical finding in the acutely traumatized patient.

Given this frequently ambiguous clinical picture, the diagnosis of cardiac tamponade is often made on the basis of hemodynamic data. A paradoxical pulse, although not specific for cardiac tamponade, is a classical physical sign that is often noted in patients with this condition. Pulsus paradoxus refers to a greater than 10 mm Hg inspiratory decline in the systolic arterial pressure. This phenomenon is simply an exaggeration of the normal 3–6 mm Hg respirophasic variation. Total paradox or complete disappearance of the peripheral pulse during inspiration may be seen with very severe tamponade.[35] It is important to emphasize the lack of specificity of this finding. For example, it has been observed in patients with uncomplicated hypovolemia from a variety of causes. Conversely, its absence does not exclude the presence of tamponade. A concurrent atrial septal defect, severe left ventricular failure, or aortic regurgitation are all possible associated lesions that may preclude a paradoxical pulse.

Although the factors generating the paradoxical pulse are complex, they exert their hemodynamic effects through two fundamental synergistic mechanisms.[138] The first involves the normal respirophasic fluctuation of left ventricular afterload. Transmural aortic pressure increases with the inspiratory reduction of intrathoracic pressure (Fig 15-6).[182,183] As a result, during inspiration the left ventricle must contract against an increased impedance to achieve the same arterial pressure generated during expiration. Such acute elevations in afterload decrease the left ventricular ejection fraction. Also, it has been shown that preload-independent indices of contractile performance, such as the end-systolic volume index, are exquisitely sensitive to afterload (Fig 15-7).[25] Thus, the overall decrease in stroke volume may be exacerbated by simultaneously compromised diastolic filling and the resultant reduction in stroke volume mediated by the Starling phenomenon.[101,239] This is an excellent example of a situation where blood pressure cannot be equated with ventricular afterload. With reduction in the intrapleural pressure, transmural aortic pressure (left ventricular afterload) rises, and this increase in afterload mediates the reduction in blood pressure.

Underfilling of the left ventricle is the second basic mechanism causing the pulsus paradoxus of cardiac tamponade. It occurs because of leftward displacement of the interventricular septum during inspiration. Normally, the inspiratory reduction in intrathoracic pressure enhances the pressure gradient from the systemic veins to the right heart, and right ventricular volume is accomodated without significant septal shift because of right ventricular free wall expansion. Accumulation of pericardial fluid can severely restrict this expansion, causing septal encroachment on the left ventricle and a resultant decrease in its diastolic size.[88,193,197] Thus, cardiac tamponade accentuates the normal phenomenon of ventricular interaction whereby filling or distention of one ventricle alters the compliance properties of the other.[13,189] The increase in pericardial volume increases intrapericardial pressure and acutely shifts the left ventricular pressure-volume curve up and to the left.[174] Therefore, given this reduction in chamber compliance, left ventricular pressures in the normal or even elevated range may be consistent with significant reductions in ventricular size.

The contribution of ventricular interaction and septal shift to the production of paradoxical pulse varies directly with the degree of venous distention.[138] Therefore, in most cases of cardiac tamponade, high venous pressures should greatly enhance right ventricular filling as intrathoracic pressure declines during inspiration.[74] However, patients with traumatic tamponade and hypovolemia may present without an elevated central venous pressure. Hypovolemia also significantly lowers the slope of the pericardial pressure-volume curve, creating the potential for severe tamponade with only modestly elevated right atrial pressure (Fig 15-8).[4,200] In the absence of an exaggerated gradient for inspiratory venous return, significant right ventricular distention may not occur, and the paradoxical pulse may be absent. Therefore, in acute traumatic tamponade, concurrent hemorrhagic shock may preclude the development of the elevated central venous pressure and paradoxical pulse that are the classical hemodynamic findings of tamponade in medical patients. Although aggressive fluid resuscitation will undoubtedly benefit the hypovolemic trauma victim with acute tamponade,[41] the initially favorable clinical response may lead to a further delay in diagnosis and therapy of the underlying cardiac problem.

Equalization of elevated intrapericardial and ventricular filling pressures is a common pathophysiologic finding in patients with cardiac tamponade. Intrapericardial pressure (IPP) is determined by the total intrapericardial volume and the compliance properties of the pericardium.[174] Since the pericardium is an intrathoracic structure, the IPP normally approximates intrapleural pressure. During quiet respiration it

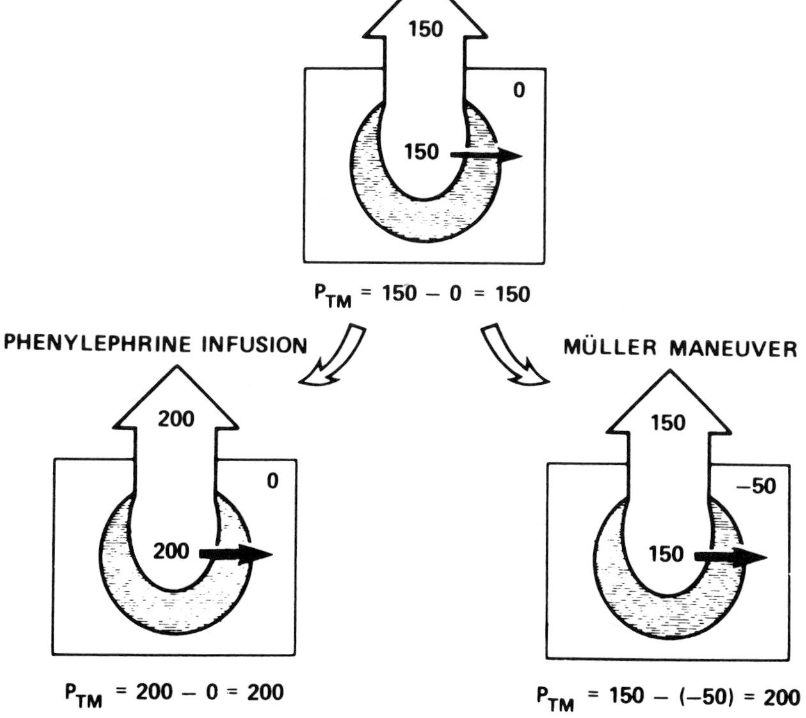


FIG. 15-6. Pharmacologic and respirophasic interventions may both produce equal changes in transmural aortic pressure. The square box represents the thorax. $P_{TM}$, transmural aortic pressure. (From Bude et al[25] with permission.)

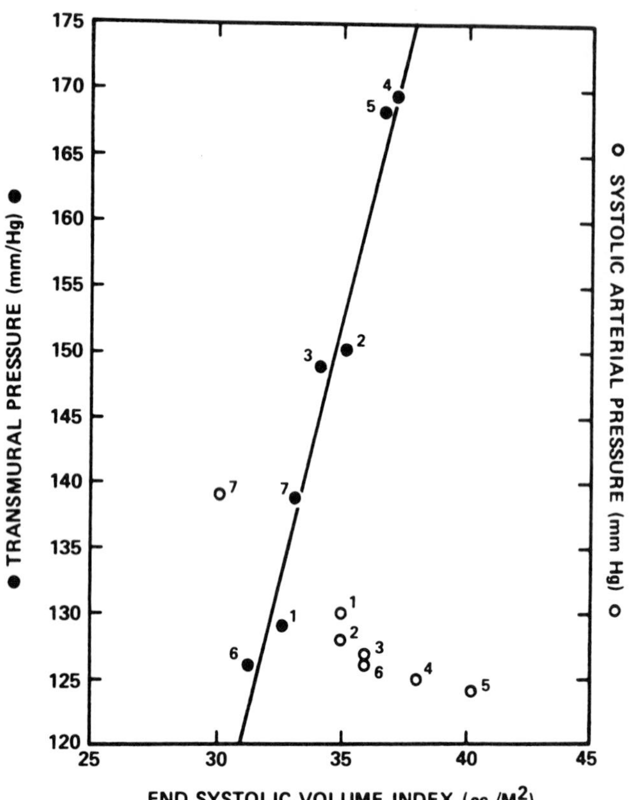


FIG. 15-7. The end-systolic volume index, an afterload-sensitive index of contractility, varies directly with transmural aortic pressure. The graph is constructed from one patient during various phases of two individually performed Müller maneuvers. Open circles denote systolic arterial pressure, whereas solid circles the transmural pressure. The numbers denote the following: 1 = control values; 2 = early strain and 3 = late strain phases of the −30 cm $H_2O$ Müller maneuver; 4 = early strain; 5 = late strain; 6 = early recovery, and 7 = late recovery phases of the −60 cm $H_2O$ Müller maneuver. (From Buda et al[25] with permission.)

FIG. 15-8. Hypovolemia decreases the slope of the pericardial pressure-volume curve. (From Shabetai et al[200] with permission.)

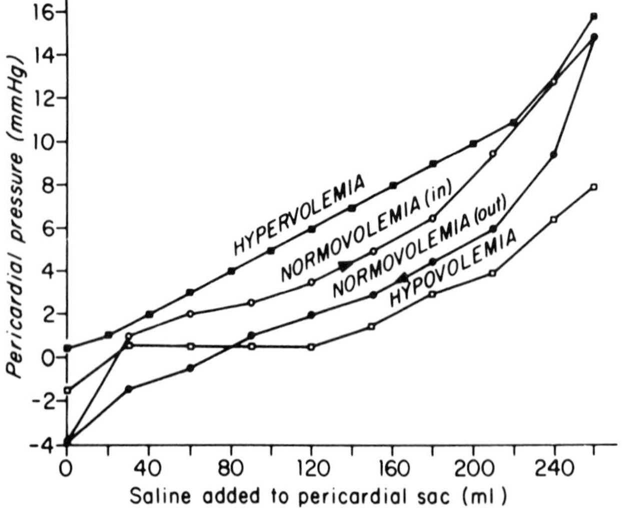


may be slightly subatmospheric, and it is usually several mm Hg lower than ventricular diastolic pressure.[200] When intrapericardial fluid accumulates, assuming that intracardiac volumes remain constant, the total intrapericardial volume increases. The IPP inevitably rises and eventually equilibrates with the systemic venous pressure. A compensatory increase in the latter is the only means of maintaining a constant intracardiac volume. Thus, in compensated cardiac tamponade, intrapericardial, systemic venous, and right ventricular end-diastolic pressures are identical.[173] Ultimately, these pressures rise together to the level of the left ventricular diastolic pressure, although the latter may remain significantly higher in patients with pre-existing left ventricular dysfunction. However, in patients with uncomplicated tamponade, objective indices of myocardial contractility are usually normal, and decreases in left ventricular stroke volume are entirely a reflection of diastolic underfilling.

With the reduction in stroke volume, cardiac output may become rate dependent. Sympathetically mediated tachycardia and vasoconstriction are observed in most patients with tamponade.[200] Less commonly, pericardial distention may elicit vagally mediated depressor reflexes,[69,71] and profound bradycardia has been described in severely hypotensive patients as a preterminal event.[70]

Patients with cardiac tamponade are also at risk for myocardial ischemia. Coronary blood flow is directly compromised by systemic hypotension, whereas the accompanying compensatory tachycardia results in a rate-related reduction of the overall time for diastolic coronary perfusion. The other deleterious effect of tachycardia is that it maintains the level of myocardial oxygen demand that would otherwise decline because of the reduced left ventricular stroke work.[118,157] It has been shown experimentally that the first measurable decrease in systolic pressure results in a reduction in coronary blood flow on the order of 40%. With the onset of significant hypotension, coronary blood flow is only one-third of normal, and the percentage of cardiac output delivered to the coronary vascular bed is 20% of that achieved at comparable degrees of hypotension caused by hemorrhagic shock.[237] The fact that tamponade-induced hypotension often occurs in the setting of high ventricular filling pressures dictates that the pressure gradient for subendocardial perfusion is preferentially compromised.[64,237] At the same time, the increased intrapericardial pressure may impede systolic coronary flow by causing extravascular compression of epicardial vessels.[102] Nevertheless, recent data from experimental work in dogs suggest that, even with severe tamponade which produces coronary blood flow reduction, myocardial ischemia and thus decreased contractility are unlikely to occur because of a proportional decrease in myocardial work due to decreased systemic blood pressure, stroke volume, and biventricular stroke work indices.[104,105]

## *Diagnosis*

As alluded to earlier, cardiac tamponade often proves to be an extremely elusive diagnosis in the trauma patient. Since it may occur in association with a variety of cardiothoracic or abdominal injuries, the clinical features of these entities often overshadow even the more classic signs of acute tamponade.

Therefore the anesthesiologist should be familiar with the ancillary diagnostic findings of this readily treatable emergency.

There are no radiographic findings specific for cardiac tamponade. Acute hemopericardium caused by cardiac laceration results only infrequently in pericardial distention sufficient to produce cardiomegaly on a chest roentgenogram.[127] A widened mediastinum may be seen in cases associated with aortic dissection.

A variety of electrocardiographic abnormalities may be seen in patients with cardiac tamponade. Elevation of the ST segments occurs with many pericardial disorders, although with accumulation of significant pericardial blood the QRS voltage also may be diminished. Electrical alternans (phasic alteration of R wave amplitude) is a more specific indication of cardiac tamponade, but may also be seen in the patient with tension pneumothorax. Total electrical alternans (phasic alterations of both the P and R wave amplitudes) is a rare but perhaps pathognomonic sign of cardiac tamponade.[28]

Echocardiography is extremely useful in diagnosis and preoperative assessment of the patient with suspected tamponade. However, its performance should never delay potentially lifesaving pericardiocentesis/pericardiotomy in the moribund patient with clinical and hemodynamic findings compatible with the diagnosis. In addition to defining the size of the effusion the experienced echocardiographer may provide other physiologic data of use to the anesthesiologist in planning intraoperative management. For example, demonstration of right ventricular diastolic collapse is a valuable sign of impending tamponade and may be associated with a significant reduction in cardiac output before any decrease in systemic blood pressure occurs.[122] The sensitivity of right ventricular diastolic collapse as a marker of cardiac tamponade has been found to be 92%. The specificity and predictive value of the test are 100%, and its accuracy is 94%.[202] These findings suggest that echocardiagraphic demonstration of right ventricular collapse may be a more reliable sign than pulsus paradoxus. It should be remembered that patients with hypertrophic ventricles or those with high intraventricular pressures (tricuspid regurgitation) may not develop this sign, even with a considerable amount of pericardial blood or fluid. Because of its greater compliance, collapse of the right atrium may occur even earlier than right ventricular collapse during the course of cardiac tamponade.

### *Anesthetic Management*

The concept of "primum non nocere" is particularly relevant to the anesthetic management of the patient with cardiac tamponade. The minimal goals of providing both patient comfort and optimal surgical conditions may be achieved only at the price of critical derangement in the pathophysiologic mechanisms that are maintaining circulatory stability. Success requires adequate monitoring and the judicious use of fluids, anesthetics, and vasoactive drugs.

What constitutes adequate monitoring is often determined by the presence or absence of associated cardiac injuries. Certainly any patient with traumatic tamponade should have continuous electrocardiographic and direct intra-arterial pressure monitoring. Since any pericardiotomy carries with it the risk of precipitous blood loss, a central venous or pulmonary artery catheter is helpful in assessing accurately the expected shifts in intravascular volume. A previously healthy patient with tamponade caused by a suspected epicardial laceration may be adequately managed with a central venous line alone. In such patients myocardial contractility should be normal, and there is a low probability of significantly disparate ventricular function. Patients with severe cardiac, pulmonary, or multiple extrathoracic injuries pose an entirely different set of risks. Acute valvular dysfunction, pulmonary contusion, and concurrent hemorrhage from extrathoracic injuries may impose complex physiologic insults on the cardiovascular system. Pulmonary arterial catheterization in these instances may yield indispensable information for reconciling the frequently conflicting treatment priorities in these patients.

Since left ventricular volume is reduced in cardiac tamponade, some hemodynamic improvement can usually be achieved with restoration of intravascular volume. In an animal model of acute tamponade, volume expansion alone increased cardiac output and specifically improved both renal and cerebral perfusion.[144] It is interesting that one of the early reports on the salutary effects of volume administration in patients with cardiac tamponade dealt with victims of thoracic trauma.[41] More recent experimental work in normovolemic dogs with acute cardiac tamponade showed little benefit from volume resuscitation.[105] Likewise, the efficacy of volume expansion in patients with chronic effusion has been questioned.[112] However, filling pressures in these patients are characteristically quite high, except in those with severe dehydration.[4] Maximizing cardiac output and perfusion pressure may require markedly elevated filling pressures, especially if the effusion is quite large or if ventricular compliance is poor as a result of septal encroachment. Therefore, in patients with acute tamponade, it may be necessary intentionally to elevate the wedge pressure above the normal range in order to achieve an end-diastolic volume that in turn maximizes stroke volume.

Since tachycardia is a key compensatory mechanism for maintaining cardiac output in patients with tamponade, every effort should be made to support the heart rate intraoperatively. Atropine can be useful if pericardial distention, laryngoscopy, or surgical manipulation elicit vagally mediated reflexes.

Vasodilators are rarely beneficial in stabilizing the patient with traumatic tamponade. In other low cardiac output states these agents maximize forward flow by reducing systemic impedance to left ventricular ejection.[34] Vasodilators are thus theoretically attractive in cardiac tamponade, which is characterized by reduced stroke volume and high systemic vascular resistance. However, in animal models of acute tamponade, only hydralazine significantly increases cardiac output in the absence of concurrent volume administration.[144] The exact mechanism of hydralazine's beneficial effect is unclear. In addition to decreasing impedance to ejection it may elicit direct and reflex increases in myocardial contractility.[113] This drug may also aggravate an imbalance between myocardial oxygen demand and supply. Although hydralazine increases total coronary blood flow, it preferentially dilates epicardial vessels and may produce hypoperfusion of the subendocardium.[77] Balanced (venous and arteriolar) vasodilators increase cardiac output in animals with tamponade, but only with concurrent augmentation of intravascular volume.[144] The vasodilator-volume combination is ineffective in patients with chronic tamponade,[112] and vasodilators alone predictably precipitate catastrophic hypotension in hypovolemic trauma patients.

Inotropic support is unlikely to improve cardiac function significantly in the patient with acute tamponade. Cardiac tamponade may properly be viewed as a derangement in loading conditions on a ventricle, the intrinsic contractile performance of which is normal or perhaps supranormal as a result of maximal catecholamine stimulation. The only exception is the possible development of ischemic contractile dysfunction, the severity of which could potentially be exacerbated by positive inotropic agents. There are animal data supporting the efficacy of isoproterenol in the setting of acute tamponade; however, the increases in stroke volume achieved in clinical studies are small.[59,226] More importantly, there is little to suggest that any of these drugs enhance vital organ perfusion.[133]

Most patients with traumatic tamponade should be brought to the operating room for pericardial decompression. However, pericardiocentesis or surgical drainage should be performed immediately in the emergency department if severe shock or cardiac arrest occurs. Hemodynamically unstable patients should receive a high inspired oxygen concentration and aggressive fluid resuscitation while the surgeons prepare and drape. The removal of even a small amount of fluid or blood via pericardiocentesis or a subxyphoid incision performed under local anesthesia can improve cardiac performance dramatically.[132] Most of the increase in stroke volume and cardiac output occurs with the initial fluid evacuation because patients with large, acutely developing effusions are operating on an extremely steep portion of the pericardial pressure-volume curve (Fig 15-9).[97,133,173] With relief of extramural compression, both right and left ventricular end-diastolic volumes rise, allowing immediate increases in stroke volume mediated by the Starling mechanism. General anesthesia can then be induced with fewer pathophysiologic constraints. Ketamine (1 mg/kg) may be preferable to more vasodilating intravenous agents. However, ketamine depresses myocardial contractility[231] and may precipitate hemodynamic deterioration when used in the presence of hypovolemia and maximal sympathetic outflow.[238] Every effort should be made to minimize intraoperative increases in intrathoracic pressure since they will impede venous return further and exacerbate underfilling of the cardiac chambers.[149]

Airway pressure rise during positive pressure ventilation, especially with the use of PEEP, may aggravate hemodynamic abnormalities produced by cardiac tamponade. There is evidence from dog studies that high frequency jet ventilation (rate 60–120 breaths/min) may prove beneficial, since it is associated with lower peak airway pressure, and thus results in higher cardiac output than conventional mechanical ventilation.[85a]

## MYOCARDIAL CONTUSION

Myocardial contusion is the most common injury resulting from nonpenetrating trauma to the heart.[78] It is diagnosed in about 20% of patients sustaining severe blunt chest trauma, but its true incidence in this population may be as high as 55%.[106,211] Underdiagnosis remains a serious problem because the cardiac lesion may be clinically silent or its symp-

FIG. 15-9. Hemodynamic effects of decompression of acute cardiac tamponade with serial 50-ml withdrawals of pericardial fluid in three patients. The greatest hemodynamic changes occur with the initial aspirations of small volumes of fluid while right atrial and pericardial pressures remain in equilibrium. Little improvement in atrial pressure and to some extent in brachial artery pressure is noted after the fall of pericardial pressure below that of atrial pressure. EXP = expiration; INSP = inspiration. (From Reddy et al[173] with permission.)

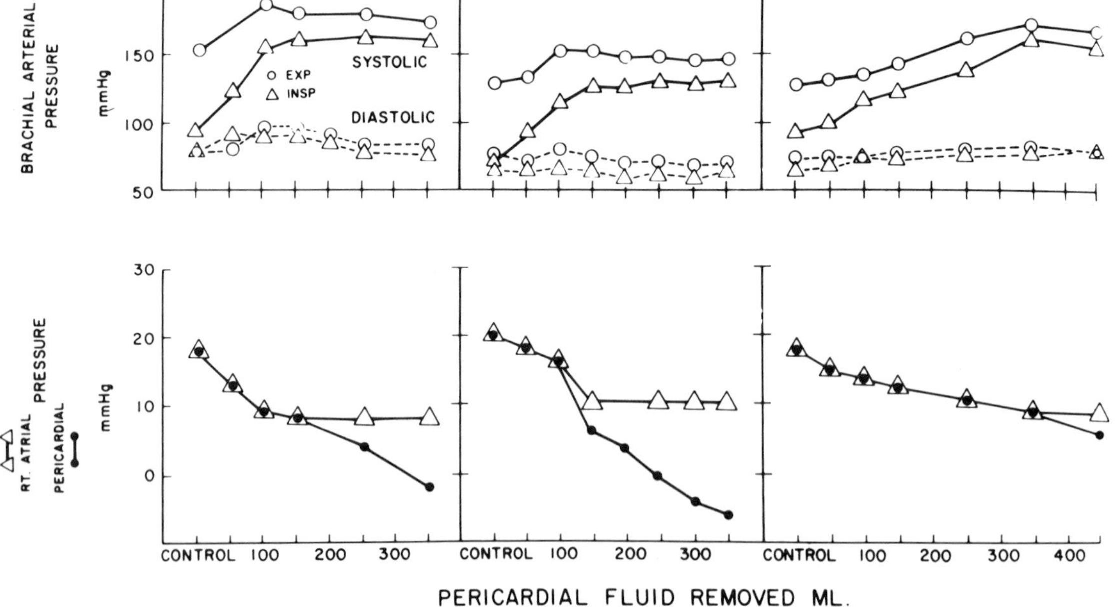

toms attributed to more obvious chest wall injuries. In addition, commonly employed diagnostic tests usually reveal only nonspecific abnormalities.[171]

Patients sustaining a myocardial contusion characteristically report symptoms compatible with an acute myocardial infarction.[124] Most patients can readily differentiate this squeezing, angina-like discomfort from the pain of their concomitant chest wall injuries. However, unlike angina pectoris, the pain of a myocardial contusion is characteristically unresponsive to nitrates.[124] Myocardial contusion may be associated with ventricular septal rupture, valve disruption, coronary artery lacerations, or myocardial wall rupture. In these instances overt clinical signs and symptoms permit easy and early diagnosis of the injury. When myocardial contusion is not associated with other cardiac injuries or is asymptomatic, diagnosis may be extremely difficult. Intraoperative use of myocardial depressant agents and/or large compartmental fluid shifts may result in significant reduction of myocardial contractility and hypotension.

Abnormal electrocardiograms are extremely common in these patients, but changes other than nonspecific ST segment and T wave abnormalities are seen in less than 50%.[210] The changes are very variable in both time of onset and duration. Nonspecific changes may persist for as long as a month after the traumatic episode.[124] Persistent ST segment elevation may reflect pericardial injury, inflammation, or the development of a ventricular aneurysm. Dysrhythmias are the most common complications of traumatic cardiac injury. Premature ventricular contractions are most frequent, but varying degrees of heart block, intraventricular conduction delay, and the entire spectrum of supraventricular dysrhythmias have all been described. Ventricular tachycardia degenerating to fibrillation may be a frequent cause of sudden death in these patients. In animal models, the more malignant dysrhythmias are seen with more severe impact injuries.[35,120]

Many trauma centers routinely utilize creatine kinase (CK) isoenzyme analysis as an adjunct to the diagnosis of myocardial contusion, but its value as a diagnostic test is presently uncertain. One problem is the possibility of falsely elevated MB fractions when the total CK exceeds 20,000 units, a not infrequent finding in victims of severe traumatic injury. Published criteria for the diagnosis in this setting are that the total CK-MB should exceed 50 U/L, and that the CK-MB be ≥5% of the total CK.[51a] Using these criteria, Healey et al[92a] found a strong correlation between an increased CK-MB and the subsequent occurrence of cardiac complications. In addition, the best diagnostic sensitivity and specificity was achieved with the concurrent presence of CK-MB positivity and ECG changes. However, other workers have found no correlation between CK-MB elevation and clinicaly significant myocardial contusions.[111]

Given the equivocal data provided by these routine diagnostic tests, referral institutions have utilized more sophisticated and invasive measures to diagnose cardiac contusions. Pyrophosphate scintigraphy is useful in diagnosing myocardial infarctions, but has been found to be too insensitive to detect traumatic cardiac injury.[21] A very practical constraint is that chest wall hemorrhage and muscle necrosis may interfere with the detection of muscle necrosis in the underlying right ventricle. Radionuclide angiography has shown focal myocardial wall motion defects in 68% of patients with blunt chest trauma.[210] Although such techniques are rarely available in the emergency setting, these results demonstrate that myocardial contusion may be a frequently missed clinical diagnosis. Two-dimensional echocardiography is a valuable noninvasive diagnostic aid. Very specific abnormalities are seen in patients with contusions. A clinical study has shown that patients with myocardial contusions and abnormal echocardiograms have an increased incidence of perioperative hypotension.[50] In addition, such other lesions as mural thrombi, valvular disruption, and effusions can be demonstrated.[145,160] Two-dimensional echocardiography combined with serial ECG and CPK-MB determinations probably provides the best combination for diagnosing myocardial contusion.[219]

Whatever the value of these more sophisticated tests in delineating the presence of myocardial contusion, it must be acknowledged that there is also controversy as to the clinical importance of this injury. As in many other areas in the trauma literature it is often critically important to consider findings in the light of the patient population under study. Young patients, who are likely to be free of preexisting coronary or myocardial disease, may be at particulaly low risk for clinically significant morbidity from a myocardial contusion. Thus, Beresky et al,[14] in a population almost exclusively of young trauma victims, found that the "diagnosis" of myocardial contusion was of no importance as a predictor of subsequent cardiac morbidity. They accordingly urged restraint in the widespread use of expensive monitoring and extensive diagnostic tests. However, it may be that clinicians are simply better informed as to the prevalence of this problem, and as a result, they are routinely employing the type of intensive monitoring and aggressive therapies which together are resulting in a decline in patient morbidity. For example, a variety of studies[55,62,66,94a] have demonstrated that the patient with a myocardial contusion is not at increased risk for general anesthesia. However, it should be reiterated that as in patients with myocardial infarction, it may be that the skill and increased awareness of clinicians has played an important role in producing these improved outcome statistics.

Although there are clinical similarities between myocardial infarction and contusion, the pathophysiology of the traumatic injury is significantly different. Experimental data suggest that, at least acutely, coronary blood flow increases to both contused and noncontused areas of the myocardium.[232] However, spasm in the coronary microvasculature may ultimately impede this augmented perfusion through the large coronary vessels and result in accentuation of interstitial hemorrhage and edema.[2]

The right ventricle (RV) is particularly vulnerable to contusion probably because of its proximity to the anterior chest wall. Its presentation may be unfamiliar to the clinician accustomed to dealing with the left ventricular pathology that predominates in nontraumatic cardiovascular disease. Radionuclide angiography has documented the preponderance of right ventricular injury in victims of blunt chest trauma.[210] In addition it has been shown that the contused RV usually maintains a relatively normal level of systolic performance (RV stroke-work index), albeit at a higher preload (RV end-diastolic index).[212] This ability of the RV to function as a highly compliant, volume-responsive pump may, however, be compromised in patients who go on to develop respiratory failure and secondary pulmonary hypertension. Elevations in PVR may precipitate failure of this thin-walled chamber designed for low-resistance work and may unmask intrinsic contractile dysfunction resulting from the initial contusion injury.

As in patients with cardiac tamponade, ventricular interaction may elicit a hemodynamic profile consistent with biventricular failure. When an elevated PVR decreases the ejection fraction of the afterload-sensitive right ventricle (Fig 15-10,) the resultant fall in transpulmonary blood flow directly reduces the filling of the preload-dependent left ventricle (Fig 15-11). Left ventricular (LV) diastolic filling may also be physically compromised by the septal encroachment produced by right ventricular distention.[23] Although this further decreases LV preload and stroke volume, the LV filling pressure may remain relatively constant or increase because of the accompanying deterioration in compliance. These pathophysiologic considerations are summarized in Figure 15-12.

The potential pitfall in intraoperative management is to misinterpret the rising LV filling pressure and decline in cardiac output as indicative of primary left ventricular failure. Proceeding on this assumption could lead to unnecessary inotropic support and disastrously inappropriate fluid restriction in the face of overwhelming clinical evidence of hypovolemia. Although there is no ideal therapy for pulmonary hypertension and right heart failure, a combination of vasodilators and appropriate replenishment of intravascular volume is probably the best approach. Nitroprusside or nitroglycerin can be used; the latter may be clinically safer since hypotension from arteriolar dilation is less likely. The decrease in pulmonary artery pressure is often less than dramatic, but venodilation may allow treatment of hypovolemia without exacerbating right ventricular distention.

FIG. 15-10. The negative curvilinear relationship between right ventricular ejection fraction and pulmonary vascular resistance in patients with RV contusions. (From Sutherland et al[210] with permission.)

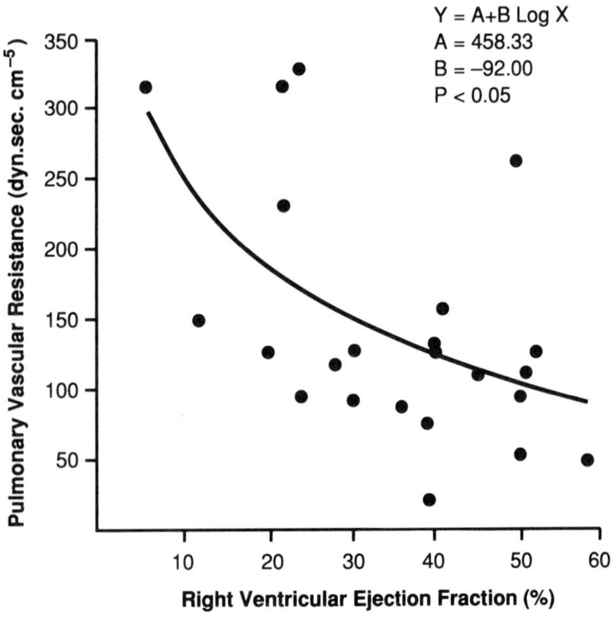


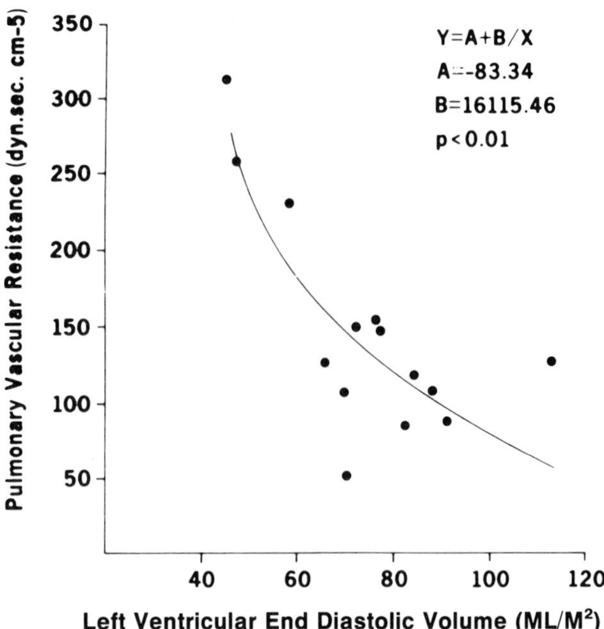


FIG. 15-11. The negative curvilinear relationship between LV end-diastolic volume index and PVR in patients with isolated RV contusions. Pulmonary hypertension decreases LV preload. (From Sutherland GR et al[210] with permission.)

If myocardial contusion is diagnosed preoperatively, a careful assessment of the risks and benefits of performing immediate surgery must be considered. With the exception of true emergencies, all surgery should probably be delayed for 2 to 3 days until myocardial function improves.[224] However, concurrent extracardiac injuries often necessitate immediate surgery, and there are good data to indicate that these procedures may be performed at relatively low cardiac risk.[14,55,62,203]

Although appropriate analogies may be made between traumatic myocardial necrosis and that accompanying acute myocardial infarction, there are important differences as well.[35] The most obvious difference, and that with perhaps the most favorable implications for anesthetic management, is that these injuries occur most frequently in patients under the age of 40.[55] Thus, it is statistically unlikely that the traumatically injured myocardium is concurrently afflicted with diffuse coronary artery disease. In addition, the nature of the injury is such that myocardial damage is usually localized, and the likelihood of global ventricular dysfunction is correspondingly reduced.[35] For example, studies employing electrocardiographic-gated ventriculography have documented a low incidence of global ventricular dysfunction in patients meeting standard enzymatic and electrocardiographic criteria of myocardial contusion. However, as alluded to earlier, it may also be that these standard criteria are too broad and are delineating a large patient population that is at relatively low perioperative risk.[14,111,204] It is likely that sophisticated noninvasive studies (2D-echo, radionuclide ventriculography, thallium scanning) will assume an increasing role in the risk stratification of this large group of patients.[55,66,204,236]

With these considerations in mind, it is inappropriate to

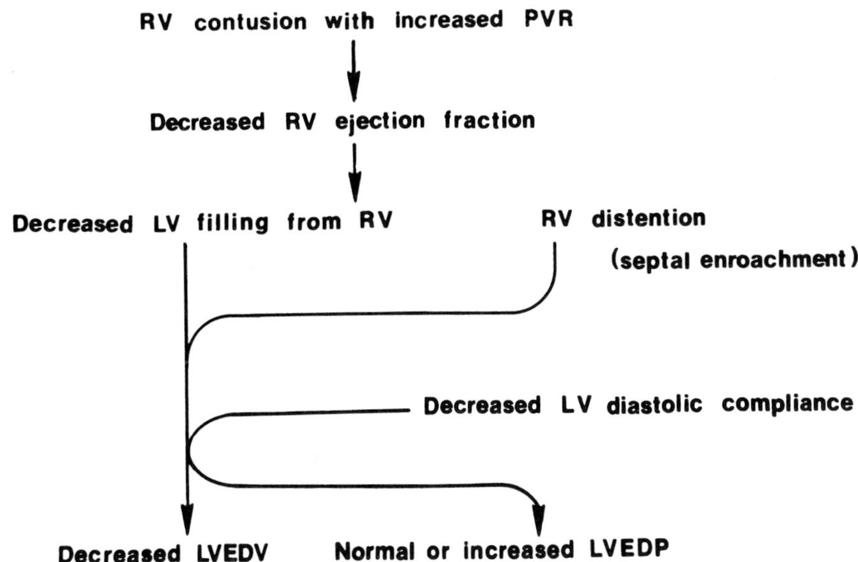


FIG. 15-12. Mechanism of interrelated right (RV) and left ventricular (LV) dysfunction during myocardial contusion and cardiac tamponade.

generalize about indications for invasive monitoring in these patients. However, pulmonary arterial catheterization should be routinely utilized in that small group of patients in whom ventricular dysfunction either is strongly suspected on clinical grounds or established on the basis of a sophisticated noninvasive examination, eg, 2D-echocardiography, radionuclide ventriculography, etc. For example, preoperative echocardiographic abnormalities have been shown to be predictive of perioperative hypotension.[50] In a probably larger group of patients, the catastrophic nature of extracardiac injuries (eg, large intravascular losses in a patient with a severe pulmonary contusion) may be an overwhelming indication for similarly aggressive monitoring. However, it is equally clear that, unlike an acute myocardial infarction, a diagnosis of myocardial contusion per se is insufficient grounds for invasive monitoring in the patient requiring emergency surgery.

There are few proscriptions on anesthetic technique, although known pulmonary vasoconstrictors are contraindicated. Practically, the goals of management are correction of hypoxemia and avoidance/treatment of hypercarbia and acidosis. Patients with suspected pulmonary contusions should always receive a high inspired oxygen concentration because of the possibility of delayed hypoxemia. The clinician who chooses to add nitrous oxide to the inspired gas mixture must be wary of this agent's potential for aggravating pulmonary hypertension in certain settings.[119] When postoperative ventilation is planned, it may be preferable to adopt a high-dose narcotic-oxygen/air-relaxant technique.

## CORONARY ARTERY INJURY

Coronary artery occlusion is a rare complication of blunt cardiac trauma.[162] Injury to the coronary arteries was distinctly uncommon in Parmley's autopsy series of 546 cases of nonpenetrating cardiac trauma.[162] He reported only nine cases of coronary artery rupture and a tenth involving an intimal tear. However, a number of clinical reports have documented that blunt chest trauma may indeed result in coronary artery occlusion.[206,234] In these cases myocardial infarctions evolved after the traumatic injury in patients without pre-existing coronary atherosclerosis.

Several mechanisms may be involved in the pathogenesis of myocardial infarction after blunt chest trauma. In perhaps the simplest scenario, the forces accompanying an episode of blunt trauma could dislodge a previously adherent intramural plaque, resulting in intraluminal obstruction of the involved coronary artery.[181] Patients with pre-existing atherosclerotic heart disease also may be at increased risk for infarction because of trauma-induced hemorrhage into a plaque, which is known to be richly vascularized with fragile, thin-walled capillaries.[152] A third possible mechanism of ischemic injury is trauma-induced coronary vasospasm. Although spasm also occurs in normal vessels, angiographically visualized spasm often occurs at a site of atherosclerotic narrowing.[95] Other etiologies of traumatic infarction include coronary thrombosis due to vascular trauma, direct transection of the coronary arteries, coronary embolization, and dissecting aneurysm.[234]

In the absence of other major cardiovascular injuries, the anesthetic requirements of these patients approximate those of a patient with "natural" coronary artery disease. A variety of anesthetic techniques are consistent with the hemodynamic goals of avoiding tachycardia and extremes of blood pressure. In the young trauma victim with good ventricular function, a deep, combined narcotic-inhalation anesthetic is ideal since intraoperative sympathetic reflexes are reliably blunted, while myocardial contractility and oxygen consumption are appropriately depressed. There is admittedly no ideal induction technique for the patient with ischemic heart disease and a full stomach. A variety of intravenous, "rapid-sequence" techniques are acceptable, including narcotic and/or etomidate inductions combined with either succinycholine or a rapid acting, non-depolarizing relaxant. In the setting of severe skeletal muscle injury the non-depolarizing relaxants may be preferable, despite their slower onset, because of the possibility of succinylcholine-induced hyperkalemia. Although the hypovolemic patient may already be tachycardic, the potential for exacerbation of this problem with pancuronium should be avoided. Rapid-sequence narcotic inductions probably should be performed with fentanyl rather than sufentanil, as inductions with the latter, in conjunction with nonsympathomimetic relaxants, have resulted in profound bradycardia, heart block and sinus arrest.

All patients with suspected coronary arterial trauma should have continuous intraoperative display of a modified V5 lead along with the capability to display each of the six standard limb leads. Ischemic changes occur most frequently in anterolateral leads since the left anterior descending coronary artery is the vessel most often involved in traumatic injury.[234] Transient, recurrent ST segment elevation is particularly suggestive of coronary spasm; empiric therapy with sublingual nifedipine may be worthwhile in these patients.

Total occlusion of the left anterior descending coronary artery by whatever mechanism may precipitate congestive heart failure secondary to extensive anteroseptal myocardial infarction. Patients may also develop potentially resectable left ventricular aneurysms. Restoration of intravascular volume losses must be guided by the pulmonary capillary wedge pressure since acute ischemia usually decreases left ventricular compliance. Measurement of cardiac output is also desirable because optimal contractile performance may be achieved only over a rather narrow range of filling pressures. Immediate revascularization may be considered, but diagnostic angiography is rarely feasible in these patients who frequently have other life-threatening injuries.

When emergency surgery is required, preoperative insertion of an intra-aortic balloon pump should be considered, especially if inotropic agents have failed to maintain adequate arterial blood pressure. Experimental data demonstrate a relationship between mean arterial pressure and coronary blood flow to noncontused areas of myocardium.[232] Preservation of the intact portion of the myocardium may be essential for survival of patients with extensive infarctions. Intra-aortic counterpulsation decreases myocardial work while simultaneously augmenting left ventricular ejection and coronary perfusion. The hemodynamic improvement, although rarely immediate, is often dramatic over the course of a few hours. Filling pressures and metabolic acidosis characteristically decline while cardiac output, blood pressure, and urine output increase. Inotropes can be weaned gradually, and their withdrawal often decreases ventricular irritability.

Patients with an acutely ischemic and dysfunctional myocardium require aggressive monitoring for optimal titration of anesthetic and vasoactive drugs. A depressed myocardium does not necessarily contraindicate the use of anesthetic agents that may further depress contractile function. For example, control of ventricular afterload by utilizing any of the vasodilating inhalation agents may offset potentially deleterious myocardial depression.[185] On the other hand, an oxygen-relaxant-narcotic technique (note the order) produces the smallest physiologic effect and has the additional benefit of simplicity. This may be a particularly important factor in cases in which fluid resuscitation, hemodynamic monitoring, and adjustment of inotropic agents and intra-aortic balloon timing may occupy the majority of the anesthesiologist's time. The narcotic component of the anesthetic must be titrated against its hemodynamic effects. The use of arbitrary, predetermined doses of narcotics is inappropriate for a hypovolemic patient in cardiogenic shock.

## CARDIAC RUPTURE

Rupture of the heart is a common cause of immediate death in victims of both blunt and penetrating thoracic trauma. In nonpenetrating injuries, decelerative forces imparted to the blood within the cardiac chambers may result in significant wall stress and precipitate myocardial rupture.[124] This is a probable mechanism of cardiac rupture from blunt chest trauma sustained in automobile accidents. As might be expected, the thin-walled atria are the structures most frequently involved.[35] Blunt chest trauma also may result in indirectly penetrating cardiac injuries. In these cases, sudden acceleration or deceleration may impale the heart against a fractured rib or sternal fragment, which may be the only external sign of thoracic injury.

Directly penetrating injuries are the more frequent cause of cardiac perforations. In most series, right ventricular perforations predominate, although a comparable incidence of left ventricular injuries has been described.[215] However, because of the higher immediate mortality associated with ventricular trauma, patients with atrial perforations are more frequently encountered in the operating room.

The clinical presentation of cardiac rupture or perforation is determined by the status of the pericardium.[35] With an open pericardial wound, blood extravasating from the heart drains freely into the pleural space, producing a hemothorax. Occasionally, clotted blood or the adjacent lung may occlude the pericardial tear.[35] In these cases cardiac tamponade eventually develops, although as described earlier, the hemodynamic picture may be equivocal in the presence of hypovolemia.

Ventricular septal rupture may also result from blunt or penetrating trauma. Most traumatic perforations occur near the apical portion of the septum.[35] These patients usually present in congestive heart failure. Differentiation from acute valvular insufficiency or severe myocardial contusion may be difficult. A harsh holosystolic murmur is usually audible along the left sternal border, but it may be absent or very soft in the presence of shock or severe hypovolemia. Pulsed-Doppler echocardiography may suggest valvular rupture, a variety of intracardiac arteriovenous fistulas, or a simple ventricular septal defect.[54,125,135] The latter diagnosis may be made or confirmed at the time of pulmonary arterial catheterization by obtaining blood gas values of right atrial, right ventricular, and pulmonary arterial samples. An acute septal perforation results in an oxygen saturation stepup at the level of the right ventricle or pulmonary artery.

There are few specific anesthetic problems posed by the patient with myocardial rupture or perforation. The management of the patient with complicating tamponade has been described earlier. Operative management of atrial and ventricular disruptions is fairly straightforward. Most surgeons perform a median sternotomy because it allows exposure of all the mediastinal structures except the esophagus. Atrial injuries are oversewn while ventricular lesions are closed with pledgeted sutures. Cardiopulmonary bypass is rarely required.

Although traumatic ventricular septal defects may close

spontaneously, most of them require surgical closure. Repair is usually done through the left ventricle, utilizing cardiopulmonary bypass. Vasodilators, such as nitroprusside, often produce some degree of clinical and hemodynamic improvement. These agents augment forward flow by decreasing the systemic impedance to ejection. Peak left ventricular systolic pressure declines, and the transseptal pressure gradient favoring left to right shunting is correspondingly reduced. However, vasodilators are contraindicated in severely hypovolemic patients.

## VALVULAR INJURIES

Rupture of the cardiac valves is a rare and often unsuspected cause of cardiac failure in victims of thoracic trauma. Unfortunately, acute dyspnea is often attributed to more obvious concurrent injuries, such as pulmonary contusion, flail chest, or pneumothorax. The clinical diagnosis may be further obscured by hypovolemia or pericardial effusion, both of which may decrease the intensity of the diagnostic murmurs.

The aortic valve is most frequently involved, followed in order by the mitral and tricuspid valves.[124] Damage to the pulmonic valve is extremely rare and is usually the result of penetrating trauma.[124] Penetrating wounds of the heart may disrupt any of the valves, but they usually occur in the context of complex cardiac injuries and rarely as isolated lesions.

The exact mechanisms producing valvular disruption with blunt chest trauma are unknown. Sudden, forceful chest wall compression may acutely increase intra-aortic or intraventricular pressure to a level sufficient to destroy valvular tissue. Although most patients have normal underlying anatomy, preexisting valvular disease may increase the possibility of traumatic rupture. The forces associated with blunt trauma also have been reported to precipitate rupture or dysfunction of bioprosthetic valves.[20,136,176,188]

The hemodynamic effect of valvular insufficiency depends on the volume of regurgitant flow and the compliance properties of the recipient chamber.[35] Chronic valvular insufficiency causes eccentric dilation of the recipient chamber and a resultant increase in its compliance.[187] Thus, large regurgitant volumes are accommodated with relatively small increases in pressure. In contrast, after acute valvular disruption, comparable regurgitant volumes precipitously increase pressure in a recipient chamber, the size and compliance of which are normal.

In acute aortic insufficiency, retrograde flow increases ventricular diastolic volume, but its ultimate magnitude is limited by the precipitously rising left ventricular diastolic pressure. Its rate of rise may be sufficiently rapid to cause premature closure of the mitral valve, ie, before atrial systole.[131] This limit on the end-diastolic volume curtails potential increases in the stroke volume mediated by the Starling mechanism. In addition, a reflex sympathetic response produces tachycardia and vasoconstriction.

Moderate tachycardia increases net forward flow in acute aortic insufficiency by preferentially decreasing the diastolic time available for retrograde flow.[60,107] Although the total regurgitant volume decreases, there is no significant reduction in the transmitral filling volume. A lower systemic vascular resistance will beneficially reduce the pressure gradient favoring regurgitation. Anesthetic and relaxant drugs should be chosen with these hemodynamic principles in mind. One approach is to use a narcotic-oxygen-relaxant technique and control detrimental increases in systemic resistance with a vasodilator, such as nitroprusside. This method also minimizes myocardial depression. Isoflurane may be useful in patients with less critical hemodynamic compromise. Peripheral vasodilation may partly counteract its mild myocardial depressant effect.[201]

These patients obviously require continuous intra-arterial pressure monitoring, and in most cases pulmonary arterial catheterization is advisable. A pulmonary artery catheter with pacing capability is ideal since bradycardia can precipitate catastrophic left ventricular distention. It is important to remember that the wedge pressure may underestimate the left ventricular end-diastolic pressure (LVEDP) if the precipitously rising LVEDP closes the mitral valve prematurely.[131] The wedge or left atrial pressure can then no longer reflect the LVEDP, which continues to rise as regurgitation continues across the incompetent aortic valve.

Inotropes may be necessary in patients with massive regurgitation, but they are contraindicated when associated aortic dissection is present. Increased contractility may exacerbate shear forces on the already disrupted aortic wall. Patients who cannot be stabilized on inotropes and vasodilators require emergency valve replacement. Balloon counterpulsation is contraindicated because it will augment the diastolic pressure gradient, favoring regurgitation.

Rupture of the mitral valve acutely elevates left atrial and pulmonary capillary pressure as a left atrium of normal size and compliance suddenly receives the systolic regurgitant jet from the high pressure left ventricle. Fulminant pulmonary edema usually develops and is much more common than in patients with acute aortic insufficiency. The characteristic harsh holosystolic murmur that radiates to the apex is easily differentiated from the blowing diastolic murmur of aortic insufficiency.

The determinants of mitral regurgitant volume are the size of the regurgitant orifice and the magnitude of the ventriculoatrial pressure gradient.[84] It is important to realize that the mitral valve area may fluctuate in size when the entire valve and its annulus are not rigidly calcified.[18] Furthermore, changes in orifice area will alter the regurgitant volume to as great a degree as changes in the systolic ventricular pressure gradient.[18] This follows from the mathematical relationship describing regurgitant volume (RV).

$$RV \propto ROA \times PG$$

where ROA = regurgitant orifice area and PG = ventriculoatrial pressure gradient.[84]

The anesthetic management of patients with acute mitral regurgitation closely parallels that for patients with acute aortic incompetence. Mild tachycardia, by decreasing diastolic filling time, decreases ventricular size and regurgitant area. Vasodilators decrease the impedance to forward ejection and thus lower the ventriculoatrial pressure gradient.[83] Agents such as nitroprusside that also dilate the venous system, may decrease ventricular size, as well as the pressure gradient.[32]

Rupture of the tricuspid valve is rare, and the diagnosis can be easily overlooked since symptoms and clinical findings may be unimpressive in the absence of pulmonary hypertension.[35] The right atrium and vena cava are highly compliant structures; therefore even large regurgitant volumes may only elevate the CVP minimally. Concurrent hypovolemia may effectively unload the right atrium and obscure the diagnosis further. The phenomenon of silent tricuspid regurgitation is well known to clinicians who frequently encounter intravenous drug abusers with tricuspid endocarditis. These individuals may even tolerate total excision of the valve as long as their pulmonary artery pressures are normal. When clinical and hemodynamic data are unimpressive, echocardiography may provide essential diagnostic information. Demonstration of right ventricular volume overload in the absence of a left-to-right shunt should raise the possibility of tricuspid incompetence, and integrity of the valve itself may be assessed with pulsed-Doppler echocardiography.[148]

Initially trivial tricuspid regurgitation may become hemodynamically significant if the patient develops acute respiratory failure and pulmonary hypertension. These present an acute afterload stress for the right ventricle, a thin-walled chamber designed only for low-pressure work. Regurgitation through a minimally damaged tricuspid valve may increase as the right ventricle contracts against this elevated resistance. Retrograde ejection into the low-pressure right atrium beneficially reduces right ventricular wall tension at the price of a decrease in forward stroke volume. The decrease in transpulmonary blood flow underloads the left ventricle; as a result, cardiac output and left-sided filling pressures decline. Unfortunately these data may be misinterpreted as reflecting hypovolemia in a setting where aggressive transfusion can only worsen right ventricular distention.

Therapy should be directed to the underlying respiratory failure and pulmonary hypertension. The latter may be at least partially responsive to vasodilators. Repair or replacement of the tricuspid valve is rarely necessary since right ventricular output usually improves dramatically with resolution of pulmonary hypertension.

## TRAUMATIC INJURIES OF THE AORTA AND GREAT VESSELS

During blunt chest trauma, abrupt deceleration of the thorax applies a shearing force to the aortic wall, which is greatest at the origin of the subclavian artery and, in the ascending aorta, at the level of the coronary arteries.[147] Traumatic disruption of the aorta is immediately fatal in approximately 85% of cases.[35] A minority survive because of containment and tamponade of the hemorrhage by adjacent mediastinal structures. Often the adventitia remains intact and prevents exsanguination. Sudden aortic rupture may develop in these patients some time later.

Penetrating chest trauma may also involve the great vessels. Depending on whether the vessels are injured at an intrapericardial or extrapericardial location, the clinical presentation is usually one of acute tamponade or massive hemothorax.[35] These patients usually sustain one or more penetrating cardiac injuries as well, but severe hypovolemia may account for the frequently atypical hemodynamic findings.

Clinical findings of aortic rupture include a diagnostic triad that is seen in more than 50% of cases[35]: increased arterial pressure and pulse amplitude in the upper extremities, decreased pressure and pulse amplitude in the lower extremities, and a widened superior mediastinum on the chest radiograph. Other clinical and radiographic findings are shown in Table 15-1. Of the radiographic signs, the combined presence of widened right paraspinal interface, broadened paratracheal stripe, displacement of the nasogastric tube to the right, and opacified pulmonary window may facilitate recognition of this injury.[94] An active search for these clinical and radiographic findings is important during evaluation since as many as one-third of patients with aortic rupture have minimal or no external signs of chest trauma.[63,115]

Although the particular constellation described constitutes the classical presentation, clinical studies have documented that initial complaints and physical findings are poor indicators of the presence or absence of aortic rupture.[208] In addition, ancillary studies, which often prove crucial in making the diagnosis, are also subject to several limitations. For example, anteroposterior (AP) chest radiographs usually demonstrate a widened mediastinum in patients with acute aortic injuries. However, this sign is not a universal finding, and when present it is more frequently caused by conditions other than aortic rupture.[61,89,94] A contributing practical constraint is that chest radiographs of trauma victims are often obtained in the supine position, which may cause a normal mediastinum to appear widened.[194] Although there are distinguishing characteristics[82] of such "pseudo-widening" on a supine AP view, these fine radiologic points may be overlooked easily in the emergency department setting. Another practical and critical point is the importance of obtaining serial chest radiographs in the patient with suspected aortic rupture. One clinical study has reported that initial chest films were normal in 28% of patients who were subsequently proved to have aortic rupture; these patients went on to exhibit abnormalities on plain films in 6 to 36 hours after presentation.[205]

Computed tomography (CT) is assuming growing importance in the radiologic diagnosis of thoracic vascular trauma, but its use should obviously be restricted to hemodynamically stable patients with equivocal radiographic findings. Compared to plain radiographs, CT should provide superior defi-

TABLE 15-1. Common Clinical and Radiographic Features of Aortic Rupture

| CLINICAL | RADIOGRAPHIC |
|---|---|
| Increased arterial pressure and pulse amplitude of upper extremities | Widened mediastinum |
| Decreased arterial pressure and pulse amplitude of lower extremities | Unsharp aortic contours |
| Retrosternal or interscapular pain | Widened paraspinal interfaces |
| Hoarseness | Opacified pulmonary window |
| Systolic flow murmur over the precordium or medial to the left scapula | Broadened paratracheal stripe |
| Neurologic deficits in the lower extremities | Displacement of the left mainstem bronchus |
| | Rightward deviation of the esophagus |
| | Sternal and/or upper rib fractures |
| | Left hemothorax |

be superior at demonstrating any congenital abnormalities of the mediastinum [persistent left superior vena cava (SVC), right aortic arch, etc.] that may produce a radiographic appearance of mediastinal widening.[222] However, despite optimistic reports of earlier studies,[93] computed tomography has proved to be vulnerable to both false-positive and false-negative results in the diagnosis of aortic trauma; thus, current opinion discourages its use.[58,82] Aortography remains the definitive diagnostic procedure, and it should probably be performed whenever aortic injury is suspected (Figs 15-13A and 15-13B),[61,82,140] even though the yield of positive aortography in acute trauma victims with widened mediastinum is only 17%.[81]

After confirming the diagnosis by aortography, surgical repair should be accomplished as soon as possible. There is currently no consensus as to the best operative technique for repairing traumatic disruption of the descending aorta. Ischemia of the abdominal viscera and spinal cord may occur during the period of proximal aortic clamping; the reported incidence of paraplegia in survivors ranges from 1.0 to 11.7%.[147] Prophylactic measures for preserving spinal cord viability include the use of partial cardiopulmonary bypass, heparin-coated shunts, partial left heart bypass, cerebrospinal fluid drainage, and systemic hypothermia; none is of proven benefit.[39,43,109] Crawford and others have reported comparable results without bypass or shunting.[5,39] The "clamp and sew" approach places a premium on the aortic occlusion time and thus may not be suitable for all surgeons. However, the technique is a particularly appealing one in the trauma victim since associated injuries may pose strong contraindications to systemic anticoagulation.

The presumed mechanism of paraplegia in these patients is ischemia of the cord from mechanical interruption of its blood supply during the period of aortic cross-clamping. Monitoring of somatosensory evoked cortical potentials (SEP) may be useful in heralding spinal cord ischemia.[40] However, ischemia occurring only at the anterior portion of the cord may not be detected by this method. Loss of motor function with preservation of SEPs during aortic cross-clamping has been described.[217] More reliable clinical monitoring of spinal cord function may be achieved by recording electrical signals from the spinal cord evoked by an electrode placed on the scalp over the motor cortex.[123] However, this method may induce epileptiform activity in seizure-prone patients. Thus, further studies are needed to determine its accuracy and safety. It is also possible that spinal cord damage is mediated by deleterious increases in intracranial[92] and intraspinal[155] pressures associated with occlusion of the thoracic aorta. This possibility is intriguing because this process could potentially be exacerbated by vasodilators. Since vasodilator treatment may be crucial to preservation of cardiac performance during the period of proximal aortic clamping, further developments in this area should be followed closely.

The kidney is the abdominal organ at greatest risk for ischemic injury during the period of aortic occlusion. Experimentally, clamping of the thoracic aorta is associated with decreased renal blood flow, glomerular filtration rate, and urine output[180]; further reduction (3–5%) in renal blood flow occurs with concomitant administration of vasodilators.[79] In a retrospective clinical study of patients sustaining injuries of the thoracic aorta, subsequent renal dysfunction occurred in 27% of cases and was found to be unrelated to patient age, severity of injury, initial blood pressure, or interval between injury and thoracotomy.[209] Cross-clamping of the aorta was the only factor adversely affecting renal outcome, although interestingly enough, no relationship was found between renal failure and total cross-clamp time. However, at least in this retrospective study, preserving distal perfusion (use of shunts, partial bypass, etc.) was associated with a lower incidence of postoperative renal dysfunction. It is probably also reasonable to suggest the use of mannitol and/or low-dose dopamine as part of a strategy for renal protection similar to that commonly used in abdominal aortic aneurysm surgery.

In addition to the electrocardiogram, intraoperative hemodynamic monitoring should include a *right* radial arterial line and a lower extremity arterial line for monitoring of distal aortic pressure. In all but the most emergent cases, pulmonary arterial catheterization is also desirable because proximal aortic occlusion imposes a severe afterload stress on the left ventricle. Other specifics of intraoperative management vary depending on the operative technique favored by the surgeon.

During simple proximal aortic clamping, the left ventricle experiences a precipitous increase in afterload; the pulmonary capillary wedge pressure often increases in parallel with the proximal arterial (ie, right radial) pressure, necessitating intervention with vasodilators. These agents also allow appropriate transfusion during the period of proximal occlusion without fear of aggravating ventricular distention. Declamping hypotension can be minimized by raising the wedge pressure slightly just before releasing the clamp while tapering the vasodilators concurrently. At least three large-bore indwelling venous catheters are recommended when the surgeon employs this technique. Blood loss may be quite large after release of the aortic clamp.

Partial cardiopulmonary bypass, utilizing a femoral vein to femoral artery circuit, is another operative method for aortic injuries. With this technique distal aortic perfusion is assured, although this is of unproven benefit with reasonably short clamping times.[39] In addition, the perfusionist's regulation of venous drainage to the heart provides control over left ventricular preload. The degree of mechanical drainage varies with pump flow; maintaining a relatively constant flow rate in the extracorporeal circuit immeasurably simplifies accurate titration of the vasodilators used to control proximal aortic and cardiac filling pressures. The femoral arterial cannula may also be used for transfusion after release of the aortic clamp; this is a comforting safety net in the event of torrential hemorrhage from any of the vascular anastomoses. The major disadvantages of partial bypass are the usual risks of extracorporeal circulation—air, particulate emboli, disconnection, etc.—and the requirement for systemic heparinization, which may increase the operative blood loss and transfusion requirement. Any resultant dilutional thrombocytopenia may be aggravated by functional platelet defects from pump-related trauma. The incidence of paraplegia is unaltered by the use of femoral-femoral bypass.

Certain features of anesthetic management are constant regardless of the surgical technique. A double-lumen endobronchial tube is desirable for several reasons.[44] The ability to collapse the left lung facilitates surgical exposure. Equally

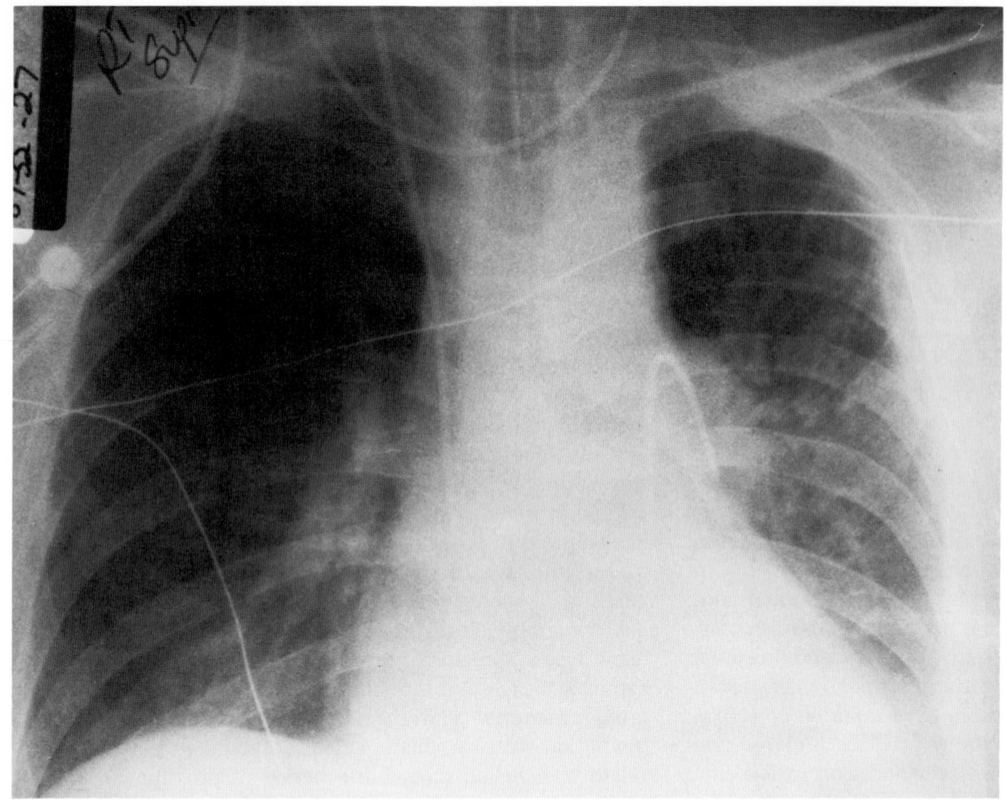

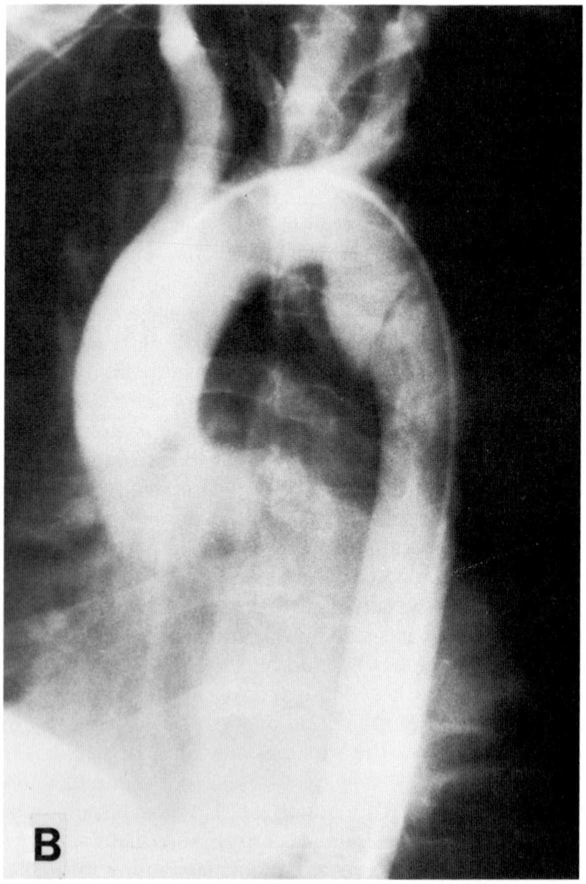

FIG. 15-13. Supine chest X-ray (A) and aortogram (B) of a patient who was involved in a motor vehicle accident and developed lower extremity fractures. Widened mediastinum on the chest X-ray was initially attributed to the supine position of the patient. Thirty-six hours after admission, a pulmonary angiogram was performed to rule out pulmonary embolism as a cause of his persistent hypoxemia. In the late phase of this study the enlarged appearance of the aorta prompted the performance of an aortogram, which demonstrated an intimal and medial tear of the descending aorta (B). Immediate repair of the vessel with 14 minutes of aortic clamp time resulted in no neurologic deficit.

important, however, is the ability to isolate the dependent right lung from the parenchymal hemorrhage that inevitably occurs in the left lung as a result of surgical retraction. This can be a particularly serious problem in patients who are heparinized for femoral-femoral bypass. These severely hypovolemic patients are good candidates for myocardial depression or vasodilation and the consequent hypotension associated with inhalation anesthetics. A fentanyl-oxygen-relaxant technique is probably the best approach, with vasodilators used as necessary to decrease vascular resistance during the period of aortic clamping.

Trauma is confined to the ascending aorta in less than 10% of patients. These patients usually present with cardiac tamponade, and there may be concurrent involvement of the coronary arteries and/or aortic valve. Repair of these lesions requires complete cardiopulmonary bypass with cardioplegia for myocardial preservation.

Survival after traumatic avulsion of the arch vessels is extremely rare, but successful repairs have been reported. Most surgeons utilize total cardiopulmonary bypass to induce profound hypothermia. The arch repair then is completed during a period of total circulatory arrest.[49,52] At the present time, pharmacologic approaches to protect the brain during circulatory arrest are of unproven benefit. Although barbiturates reduce cerebral metabolism, the effect is not additive to that conferred by hypothermia alone.[6,142,143]

## ABDOMINAL TRAUMA

Victims of abdominal trauma are at risk of two major life-threatening sequelae: exsanguinating hemorrhage and chemical or bacterial peritonitis.[3] Although dramatic strides have been made in reducing morbidity and mortality from these causes, the major remaining challenge is to reduce the diagnostic delays that often occur in these patients because of a high frequency of concurrent, life-threatening extra-abdominal injuries.

### OCCULT ABDOMINAL TRAUMA

In an effort to decrease patient morbidity and minimize unnecessary operations, surgeons have become more conservative in their use of exploratory laparotomy. Although this has undoubtedly contributed to some missed diagnoses, at least one study of operative findings in an unselected group of patients would seem to support this approach. Laparotomies were negative in 25% of patients with blunt abdominal trauma.[96] However, the anesthesiologist should always consider the possibility of occult abdominal hemorrhage when clinical signs of hypovolemia complicate the course of procedures associated with modest measurable blood loss.

#### *Peritoneal Lavage*

Very often the decision not to explore the abdominal trauma victim is made on the basis of a negative peritoneal lavage. This test was introduced by Root in 1965[186] and is deservedly popular given its low incidence of complications and high accuracy in detecting intra-abdominal hemorrhage. Over the years, practical aspects of the test have become relatively standardized, with the threshold for surgical exploration being 50,000 red blood cells/mL fluid.[36,186] The incidence of false-positive lavages is negligible,[158] which usually translates into a less than 2% rate of completely negative abdominal exploration.[163] A low rate of negative exploration is consistent with good clinical practice since peritoneal lavage is not an infallible diagnostic technique and false-negative results are known to occur frequently in a variety of specific clinical situations. For example, a ruptured diaphragm may allow intraperitoneal blood to drain into the thorax, and the diaphragm itself may produce a tamponading effect on bleeding abdominal viscera.[68] Isolated injury of retroperitoneal structures should not be associated with positive results, but false-positive results may occur because of migration of red blood cells into the peritoneum or insertion of the lavage tube into the retroperitoneal space. Finally, peritoneal lavage has been shown to be particularly unreliable in patients with gunshot wounds of the lower chest and abdomen.[220] In this population the false-negative rate may be as high as 25%.[37]

#### *Injuries to the "Thoracic Abdomen" and Retroperitoneum*

In the search for occult abdominal injury, particular attention should be directed to two clinically and radiographically silent areas, the thoracic abdomen and the retroperitoneal space.[68] Patients with penetrating wounds of the lower chest have a high incidence of associated intra-abdominal injuries; conversely thoracic injuries occur in only one-fourth of patients with penetrating upper abdominal wounds.[67] The latter finding may be surprising to the clinician accustomed to thinking of the diaphragm's low position on chest roentgenograms. However, during a Valsalva maneuver, as commonly occurs immediately before injury, the diaphragm may reach as high as the third rib anteriorly,[98] preventing associated intrathoracic injuries in many patients with upper abdominal trauma. Studies have documented a high incidence of diaphragmatic injury in patients with stab and gunshot wounds to the abdomen.[151] Thus, a significant number of patients with intra-abdominal hemorrhage may be at risk of a false-negative peritoneal lavage by virtue of their concurrent diaphragmatic injury. Therefore, a more liberal approach toward abdominal exploration may be warranted in this group of patients.

If a laparotomy is undertaken in a patient with a penetrating chest wound, placement of an ipsilateral chest tube is warranted, even in the absence of known intrathoracic injury.[98] Prophylactic chest tubes protect against the possibility of tension pneumothorax induced by positive pressure ventilation or by air traversing the diaphragmatic rent during laparotomy. It is important to remember that only about 25% of patients with ruptured diaphragm have classical clinical findings (see the section on diaphragmatic rupture).

### ABDOMINAL INJURIES ASSOCIATED WITH THORACIC VASCULAR TRAUMA

Patients with injuries of the thoracic vasculature are an important subgroup of thoracic trauma victims who may be particularly at risk of a missed diagnosis of serious abdominal trauma. The seemingly catastrophic nature of the thoracic vascular injury may divert attention from even the most obvious clinical signs of abdominal injury. Such concurrent injuries are not at all uncommon, being reported in almost half of the victims of blunt thoracic aortic transections.[19] Active intra-abdominal bleeding occurs quite frequently in these patients and is the most common cause of persistent or recurrent hypotension. The most common sources of intra-abdominal hemorrhage are the spleen, liver, and mesentery.[19] These diagnoses must be considered if the thoracotomy fails to reveal an obvious bleeding source. However, patients who are known to have sustained thoracoabdominal injuries and who survive the acute traumatic episode may still be candidates for immediate exploratory laparotomy, even if angiography has documented a thoracic aortic transection. Several reports in the surgical literature support the safety of a brief delay of thoracic aortic repair, if the clinical picture and positive peritoneal lavage mandate abdominal exploration.[1,19] Free rupture of the aortic hematoma is rare in the hospital setting, and patients who are hypotensive on this basis are unlikely to be saved by emergency repair.

## PERICARDIAL INJURY IN ABDOMINAL TRAUMA VICTIMS

Conversely, it is also important to entertain the diagnosis of common life-threatening thoracic injuries in patients with abdominal trauma. In particular, the possibility of pericardial injury or rupture should always be considered seriously. Figure 15-14 illustrates that even large pericardial wounds may produce nonspecific changes on the electrocardiogram. Smaller pericardial defects are more common and may be less likely to decompress freely, creating the possibility of tamponade or cardiac herniation. Pericardial injury is an important diagnosis to consider when a patient deteriorates unexpectedly during the course of a seemingly negative laparotomy. The only clue may be the finding of inexplicably high intravascular filling pressures. Transabdominal decompressive pericardiectomy may be lifesaving in these instances.[76]

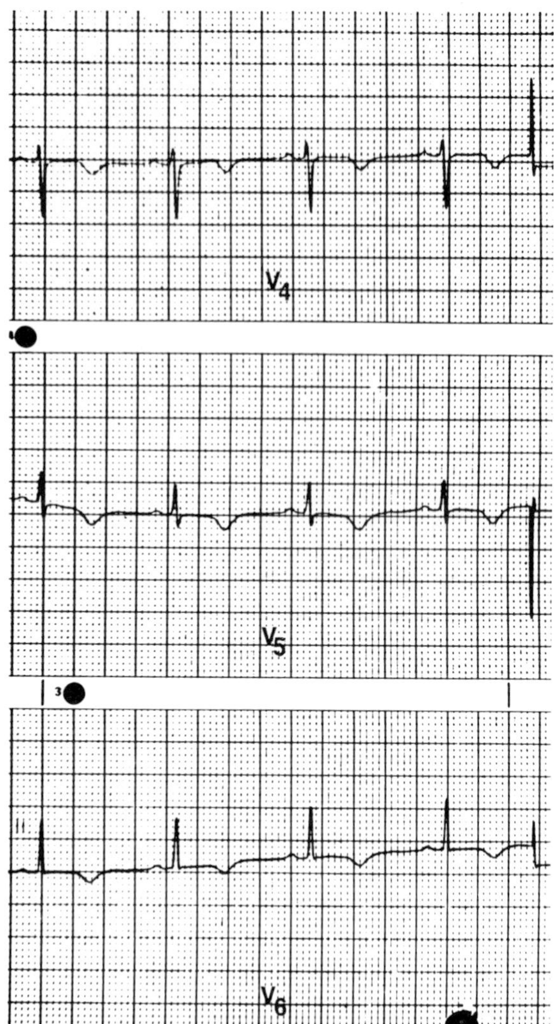


FIG. 15-14. ECG changes in a patient with severe orthopedic and abdominal trauma. Note that the presence of only nonspecific ST-T wave changes makes the diagnosis of pericardial injury difficult. Massive disruption of the pericardium was discovered at the time of thoracotomy for pleural decortiation. Luckily, the very severity of the pericardial defect made cardiac herniation unlikely in this case.

## RETROPERITONEAL INJURIES

The retroperitoneal space is a truly hidden area of the abdomen in that it is not sampled by peritoneal lavage. Fortunately, the location of the pancreaticoduodenal complex in the mid-upper abdomen is relatively well protected, and serious injuries are infrequent.[170] However, diagnostic delays often contribute significantly to immediate morbidity and mortality. Hyperamylasemia has been reported to occur in 48 to 91% of patients after blunt pancreatic trauma, but serum amylase may also be normal after injuries producing severe pancreatic destruction.[3] Perforation of the gastrointestinal tract may also result in hyperamylasemia, and a particular association with retroperitoneal duodenal injuries has been described.[15] The pancreas is most often injured by anteroposterior crushing forces that impale the organ against the spinal column; those patients usually complain of steady upper abdominal and back pain. Intraoperatively there is always the potential for immediate and torrential blood loss, particularly if there is associated trauma to the adjacent portal venous system.[19]

## ABDOMINAL VASCULAR INJURIES

Isolated abdominal vascular trauma is associated with a mortality rate of 30 to 60%; these injuries are responsible for the majority of deaths after blunt or penetrating trauma to the abdomen.[108] Although retroperitoneal or visceral tamponade may obscure the diagnosis occasionally, the presentation is usually quite dramatic, with most patients arriving in profound shock. Major vascular trauma should be suspected in any severely hypotensive patient after an episode of abdominal trauma. Hemorrhage is the most common cause of death in these patients; at least two large-bore intravenous catheters are required to replenish intravascular volume. Saphenous vein "cutdowns" or other lower extremity cannulas are unacceptable as the primary intravenous lines because clamping of the inferior vena cava may be necessary during repair of vena caval or iliac vein injuries. Trauma to the inferior vena cava has been reported in almost 50% of cases of major abdominal vascular trauma and reported mortality rates range from 35 to 53%.[134]

Anesthetic considerations are similar to those described for patients with hemorrhagic losses from thoracic vascular trauma. Profound hypovolemia and systemic hypotension preclude the use of the vasodilating inhalation agents. Truly moribund patients should be intubated awake, paralyzed, and ventilated with 100% oxygen. A narcotic-oxygen-relaxant technique is appropriate for conscious but hypotensive patients. Ketamine (1–2 mg/kg) is a popular induction agent because of its sympathomimetic properties. However, it is a direct myocardial depressant, and experimental preparations have demonstrated that this effect may predominate in the presence of severe hypovolemia.[238]

## INJURIES TO THE ABDOMINAL VISCERA

There are few anesthetic implications of injuries confined to the solid organs of the abdomen. However, intraoperative resuscitation of these patients, particularly those with hepatic trauma, can be extremely challenging. Exsanguination remains the most common cause of immediate death after injury to the parenchymal organs (liver and spleen), although the frequency of death from hemorrhage has been markedly reduced over the past decade.[170] Despite this progress, mismanagement of abdominal injuries accounts for the majority of preventable deaths after multiple trauma.

### *Splenic Trauma*

The spleen is the most commonly injured organ in blunt abdominal trauma and is also frequently involved in penetrating wounds of the left lower chest and upper abdomen.[225] An important clinical feature of splenic trauma is the frequency of serious associated intra-abdominal injuries, which occur in 36.5% and 94%, respectively, of patients sustaining splenic damage from blunt and penetrating trauma.[225]

Diagnostic peritoneal lavage is extremely accurate in determining the presence of splenic and associated intra-abdominal injury. Routine splenectomy for ruptured spleen is undergoing reappraisal because of increasing data that link splenectomy, done at any age and for any reason, with a high incidence of subsequent overwhelming bacterial infection.[11,196] However, some studies have demonstrated that nonoperative management of splenic rupture in adults may be associated with significant morbidity because of surgical delay.[129] Repairing the spleen (splenorrhaphy) during laparotomy is another approach that has become highly popular in recent years.

### *Hepatic Trauma*

The liver is the second most commonly injured intra-abdominal organ; liver lacerations are the most common abdominal injuries that result in death.[29,51] Overall mortality from hepatic trauma has dropped dramatically from the 60% level reported during World War I to the 10 to 20% level characteristic of most current civilian series. Exsanguinating hemorrhage remains the leading cause of operative death.[51] Associated injuries occur in 85 to 90% of victims of hepatic trauma, and overall mortality is directly proportional to the number of other organs involved.[29] It must be emphasized that the vast majority of liver injuries (85 to 90%) heal spontaneously and require only surgical drainage.[170] The minority of complex injuries pose inordinate surgical and resuscitative challenges.

Although the diagnosis of hepatic trauma is often made only at the time of laparotomy, preoperative findings that may suggest its presence include right lower rib fractures, elevated right hemidiaphragm, and right pleural effusion or pneumothorax.[154] Computed tomography may also be useful in the diagnosis of limited parenchymal lacerations and intrahepatic hematoma.[141] The latter are frequently found to exhibit no active bleeding at the time of exploration; thus, serial tomographic studies may be useful in nonoperative management of a select group of clinically stable patients.[229]

Patients with suspected serious hepatic injuries should be prepared and draped from the sternal notch to the upper thighs before inducing anesthesia. If the hepatic veins and retrohepatic vena cava are damaged, control of the intrapericardial vena cava may be necessary. In these instances, extension of the abdominal incision as a median sternotomy may be unavoidable.[51,170] These patients are best managed with a narcotic-oxygen-relaxant technique. Intermittent periods of hepatic ischemia may be an unavoidable part of the surgical repair. In this milieu, it would seem unwise to challenge further the hepatic microsomes with any of the halogenated agents. Moreover, myocardial depression and vasodilation are unnecessary handicaps during a procedure that may repeatedly provoke episodes of hemorrhagic hypotension.

The principles of surgical repair of complex liver injuries include adequate hemostasis by control of individual vessels, conservative debridement of necrotic tissue, and drainage of the hematoma.[159] The inevitably massive transfusion often results in the development of clinically significant coagulopathy, necessitating aggressive resuscitation with blood components (see Chapters 6 and 7).[51] Hypothermia and acidosis are preventable aggravators of any coagulopathy. Acidosis directly inhibits ADP-dependent platelet aggregation and also retards the interaction of the other coagulation factors. Hypothermia slows the coagulation process and induces platelet sequestration. Routine measures should include warming of all infused and irrigating fluids. An extremely efficient but often overlooked measure is heated humidification of the inspired anesthetic gases. Raising the ambient temperature is also unquestionably desirable, but some compromise with the surgeon's comfort must be accepted to maintain operative efficiency. If sufficient coagulopathy does occur, it is often the better part of valor to pack the liver parenchyma temporarily and make a brief retreat to the intensive care unit. Doing so allows for further resuscitation with blood components and correction of residual hypothermia and acidosis and has not been shown to be associated with an increased incidence of infection.[30,214]

Patients with actively bleeding hepatic injuries represent truly inordinate surgical challenges. Blind attempts at controlling bleeding from the hepatic parenchyma may only extend areas of vascular trauma and thereby perpetuate the hemorrhage. In these cases, isolation of the hepatic vascular bed may be lifesaving. The surgeon may employ any of a number of specific techniques, but all of these involve hepatic inflow occlusion, ie, clamping the hepatic artery, portal vein, and common bile duct (Pringle maneuver) (Fig 15-15).[170] Hemodynamic changes associated with portal triad clamping alone include an increase in mean arterial pressure (21%) and systemic vascular resistance (48%) and decreased pulmonary capillary wedge pressure (10%) and cardiac index (17%).[45] Hemorrhage that persists despite packing and the Pringle maneuver may indicate injury to the hepatic vein or retrohepatic vena cava, which will necessitate control of the infrahepatic and suprahepatic vena cava. Usually the incision is extended to a median sternotomy, and a vascular tourniquet is applied to the IVC within the pericardium. A decrease in venous return of 60% or more may be anticipated with IVC occlusion, which usually results in immediate hemodynamic deterioration in these patients who are often already severely hypovolemic.[117]

FIG. 15-15. The Pringle maneuver and placement of an atrial-caval shunt divert blood flow away from the retrohepatic inferior vena cava. (From Anderson CB, Ballinger WF. In Zuidema GD, Rutherford RB, Ballinger WF, eds. The management of trauma. 4th ed. Philadelphia: WB Saunders, 1985, with permission.)

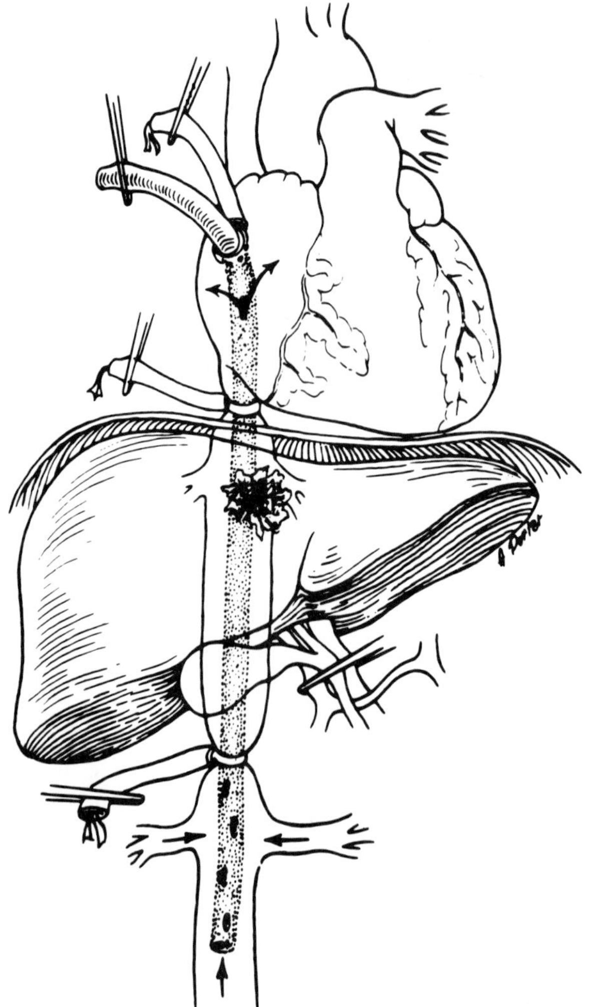

Simultaneous clamping of the abdominal aorta has been recommended as an expedient although certainly unphysiologic means of maintaining perfusion pressure until caval integrity is established.[117] Although technically more difficult, the use of an atrial-caval shunt may represent a more physiologic approach.[247] A 36F chest tube or an endotracheal tube is inserted through the right atrial appendage and into the inferior cava, with the tip at the level of the renal veins. Two tourniquets are applied, one at the level of the intrapericardial inferior vena cava and the other around the suprarenal vena cava. When an endotracheal tube is used, its cuff is inflated and positioned above the renal veins. In combination with the Pringle maneuver, this diverts all blood supplying the juxtahepatic inferior vena cava (Fig 15-15).[3] Atrial placement of the shunt achieves a bloodless field and allows for rapid transfusion through the exposed cannula.[117]

MAS TROUSERS

Military antishock trousers (MAST) are an adjunctive resuscitative device that the anesthesiologist may encounter during acute management of the patient with abdominal injuries. It was originally theorized that inflating the trousers to a pressure above venous pressure produced internal autotransfusion by shunting blood from the lower extremities toward the heart.[24] However, more recent studies suggest that they increase blood pressure primarily by increasing ventricular afterload and that the external counterpressure may directly compromise perfusion to organs within the confines of the trousers.[75,242] The applied force also may be responsible for a demonstrated 14% decrease in vital capacity, which could be seriously detrimental to patients with pre-existing respiratory compromise.[137]

External counterpressure of only 20 to 30 mm Hg theoretically controls hemorrhage from arterial vessels by external tamponade and by promoting clot formation. Thus, excessive pressures are unnecessary and may exacerbate hypoperfusion of intra-abdominal organs. It is critical that the leg segments be inflated before the abdominal segment. Otherwise, the abdominal segment may act as a venous tourniquet on the lower extremities.[19] This effect is also produced by using the abdominal segment alone. Therefore, when deflating the trousers, the abdominal segment should be deflated first, followed by deflation of the two leg segments. There are several case reports of compartment syndromes resulting from such incorrect inflation-deflation sequences.[24,240] MAS trousers should not be deflated until a pump to reinflate the device is available; uncontrollable bleeding or hypotension may result if this simple safety device is omitted. It is obvious that improper use of these devices is fraught with serious complications, and several of the purported benefits are in considerable dispute at this time. Their in-the-field use should clearly be restricted to highly trained personnel (see also Chapters 4 and 9).

## CONCLUSION

The victim of thoracic and/or abdominal trauma is often an eminently salvagable individual who has sustained a potentially fatal cardiopulmonary insult. One key to success in the anesthetic management of these patients is the ability to recognize quickly common life-threatening problems that may present in clinically atypical fashion, eg, "hypovolemic tamponade." Accurate definition of the patient's problems must then be followed by a triage process whereby therapeutic compromises are accepted with respect to relatively treatable problems in an effort to avoid potentially irreversible complications in other areas. Thus, transient exacerbation of a patient's pulmonary contusion may be accepted as the price for warding off ischemic renal failure. However, this process is further complicated by the specter of a missed diagnosis that inevitably haunts the clinician who cares for these patients. These injuries, by the nature of the organs involved (heart, lungs, great vessels, etc), are characteristically "impressive," requiring intense concentration for an optimal therapeutic result. The inevitable danger is an inordinate narrowing of the clinical focus such that even classic findings of serious concurrent injuries may be overlooked entirely.

## REFERENCES


1. Akins CW, Buckley MJ, Daggett W, et al. Acute traumatic disruption of the thoracic aorta: a ten-year experience. Ann Thorac Surg 1981;31:305.
2. Allen RP, Liedtke AJ. The role of coronary artery injury and perfusion in the development of cardiac contusion secondary to non-penetrating chest trauma. J Trauma 1979;19:153.
3. Anderson CB, Ballinger WF. Abdominal injuries. In: Zuidema GD, Rutherford RB, Ballinger WF, eds. The management of trauma. Philadelphia: WB Saunders, 1985:449.
4. Antman EM, Cargill V, Grossman W. Low-pressure cardiac tamponade. Ann Intern Med 1979;91:403.
5. Antunes MJ. Acute traumatic rupture of the aorta: repair by simple aortic cross-clamping. Ann Thorac Surg 1987;44:257.
6. Astrup J, Skovsted P, Gjerris F, et al. Increase in extracellular potassium in the brain during circulatory arrest: effects of hypothermia, lidocaine, and thiopental. Anesthesiology 1981;55:256.
7. Avery EE, Morch ET, Benson DW. Critically crushed chests. J Thorac Cardiovasc Surg 1956;32:291.
8. Baker CC, Thomas AN, Trunkey DD. The role of emergency room thoracotomy in trauma. J Trauma 1980;20:848.
9. Ball T, McCrory R, Smith JO, et al. Traumatic diaphragmatic hernia: errors in diagnosis. AJR 1982;138:633.
10. Barone JE, Pizzi WF, Nealon TF, Richman H. Indications for intubation in blunt chest trauma. J Trauma 1986;26:334.
11. Barrett J, Sheaff C, Abuabara S, Jonasson O. Splenic preservation in adults after blunt and penetrating trauma. Am J Surg 1983;145:313.
12. Beal SL, McKennan M. Blunt diaphragm rupture. A morbid injury. Arch Surg 1988;123:828.
13. Bemis CE, Serur JR, Borkenhagen D, et al. Influence of right ventricular filling pressure on left ventricular pressure and dimensions. Circ Res 1974;34:498.
14. Beresky R, Klingler R, Peake J. Myocardial contusion: when does it have clinical significance. J Trauma 1988;28:64.
15. Berne CF, Donovan AJ, Hagen WE. Combined duodenal pancreatic trauma. The role of end-to-side gastrojejunostomy. Arch Surg 1968;96:712.
16. Bogetz MS, Katz JA. Recall of surgery for major trauma. Anesthesiology 1984;61:6.

16a. Bolliger CT, Van Eeden SF. Treatment of multiple rib fractures: Randomized controlled trial comparing ventilatory and nonventilatory management. Chest 1990;97:943.

17. Bongard FS, Lewis FR. Crystalloid resuscitation of patients with pulmonary contusion. Am J Surg 1984;148:145.
18. Borkenhagen DM, Serur JR, Gorlin R, et al. The effect of left ventricular load and contractility on mitral regurgitant orifice size and flow in the dog. Circulation 1977;56:106.
19. Borman KR, Aurbakken CM, Weigelt JA. Treatment priorities in combined blunt abdominal and aortic trauma. Am J Surg 1982;144:728.
20. Brady PW, Deal CW. An unusual cause of mitral incompetence: post-traumatic paraprosthetic mitral incompetence. J Trauma 1988;28:259.
21. Brantigan CO, Burdick D, Hopeman R, et al. Evaluation of technetium scanning for myocardial contusion. J Trauma 1978;18:460.
22. Brauer L. Erfarhrugen und Uberlegungen zur Lungenkollapstherapie. Beitr Klin Tuberk 1909;12:49.
23. Brinker JA, Weiss JL, Lappe DL, et al. Leftward septal displacement during right ventricular loading in man. Circulation 1980;61:626.
24. Brotman S, Browner BD, Cox EF. MAS trousers improperly applied causing a compartment syndrome in lower-extremity trauma. J Trauma 1982;22:598.
25. Bude AJ, Pinsky MR, Ingels NB, et al. Effect of intrathoracic pressure on left ventricular performance. N Engl J Med 1979;301:453.
26. Bugge-Asperheim B, Svennevig JL, Birkeland S. Hemodynamic and metabolic consequences of lung contusion following blunt chest trauma. Scand J Thorac Cardiovasc Surg 1980;14:295.
27. Burns D, Stool EW. Blunt chest trauma. In: Bordow RA, Stool EW, Moser KM, eds. Manual of clinical problems in pulmonary medicine. Boston: Little, Brown and Co, 1980.
28. Callaham ML. Pericardiocentesis in traumatic and nontraumatic cardiac tamponade. Ann Emerg Med 1984;13:924.
29. Carmona RH, Lim RC, Clark GC. Morbidity and mortality in hepatic trauma. Am J Surg 1982;144:88.
30. Carmona RH, Peck DZ, Lim RC. The role of packing and planned reoperation in severe hepatic trauma. J Trauma 1984;24:779.
31. Carter JW. Diaphragmatic trauma in southern Saskatchewan—an 11 year review. J Trauma 1987;27:987.
32. Chatterjee K, Parmley WW, Swan HJC, et al. Beneficial effects of vasodilator agents in severe mitral regurgitation due to dysfunction of subvalvular apparatus. Circulation 1973;48:684.
33. Clemmer TP, Fairfax WR. Critical care management of chest injury. Crit Care Clin 1986;2:759.
34. Cohn JN, Franciosa JA. Vasodilator therapy of cardiac failure. N Engl J Med 1977;297:27.
35. Cohn PF, Braunwald E. Traumatic heart disease. In: Braunwald E, ed. Heart disease: a textbook of cardiovascular medicine. Philadelphia: WB Saunders, 1988:1535.
36. Cox EF, Dunham CM. A safe technique for diagnostic peritoneal lavage. J Trauma 1983;23:152.
37. Cox EF, Siegel JH. Blunt trauma to the abdomen. In: Siegel J, ed. Trauma, emergency surgery and critical care. New York: Churchill Livingston, 1987:883.
38. Craven KD, Oppenheimer L, Wood LDH. Effects of contusion and flail chest on pulmonary perfusion and oxygen exchange. J Appl Physiol 1979;47:729.
39. Crawford ES, Walker HSJ, Saleh SA, Normann NA. Graft replacement of aneurysm in descending aorta: results without bypass or shunting. Surgery 1981;89:73.
40. Coles JG, Wilson GJ, Sima AF, et al. Intraoperative detection of spinal cord ischemia using somatosensory cortical evoked po-

tentials during thoracic aortic occlusion. Ann Thorac Surg 1982;34:299.
41. Cooper FW Jr, Stead EA Jr, Warren JV. The beneficial effect of intravenous infusions in acute pericardial tamponade. Ann Surg 1944;120:822.
42. Cullen P, Modell JH, Kirby RR, et al. Treatment of flail chest. Use of intermittent mandatory ventilation and positive end-expiratory pressure. Arch Surg 1975;110:1099.
43. Cunningham JN, Laschinger JC, Merkin HA, et al. Measurement of spinal cord ischemia during operations upon the thoracic aorta. Ann Surg 1982;196:285.
44. Das BB, Fenstermacher JM, Keats AS. Endobronchial anesthesia for resection of aneurysms of the descending aorta. Anesthesiology 1970;32:152.
45. Delva E, Camus Y, Paugam C, et al. Hemodynamic effects of portal triad clamping in humans. Anesth Analg 1987;66:864.
46. Dittman M, Ferstl A, Wolff G. Epidural analgesia for the treatment of multiple rib fractures. Eur J Intens Care Med 1975;1:71.
47. Dougall AM, Paul ME, Finlay RJ, et al. Chest trauma—current morbidity and mortality. J Trauma 1977;17:547.
48. Duff JH, Goldstein M, McLean APH, et al. Flail chest: a clinical review and physiological study. J Trauma 1968;8:63.
49. Dumanian AV, Hoehsema TD, Sautschi DR, et al. Profound hypothermia and circulatory arrest in the surgical treatment of traumatic aneurysm of the thoracic aorta. J Thorac Cardiovasc Surg 1970;59:541.
50. Eisenach JC, Nugent M, Miller FA Jr, Mucha P. Echocardiographic evaluation of patients with blunt chest injury: correlation with perioperative hypotension. Anesthesiology 1986;64:364.
51. Elerding SC, Aragon GE, Moore EE. Fatal hepatic hemorrhage after trauma. Am J Surg 1979;138:883.
51a. ElAllaf M, Chapelle J, ElAllaf D, et al. Differentiating muscle damage from myocardial injury by means of the serum creatine kinase (CK) isoenzyme MB mass measurement total CK activity ratio. Clin Chem 1987;32:291.
52. Ergin MA, O'Connor J, Guinto R, Griepp RB. Experience with profound hypothermia and circulatory arrest in the treatment of aneurysms of the aortic arch. J Thorac Cardiovasc Surg 1982;84:649.
53. Erikson DR, Shinozaki T, Beckman E, Davis JH. Relationship of arterial blood gases and pulmonary radiographs to the degree of pulmonary damage in experimental pulmonary contusion. J Trauma 1971;11:689.
54. Eskilsson J. Tricuspid insufficiency caused by nonpenetrating chest trauma: report of two cases diagnosed by Doppler cardiography. Acta Med Scand 1985;218:347.
55. Fabian TC, Mangiante EC, Patterson CR, et al. Myocardial contusion in blunt trauma: clinical characteristics, means of diagnosis, and implications for patient management. J Trauma 1988;28:50.
56. Fallazadeh H, Mays ET. Disruption of the diaphragm by blunt trauma: new dimensions of diagnosis. Am J Surg 1975;41:337.
57. Faust RJ, Nauss LA. Post-thoracotomy intercostal block: comparison of its effects on pulmonary function with those of intramuscular meperidine. Anesth Analg 1976;55:542.
58. Federle MP, Brant-Zawadski J. Computed tomography in the evaluation of trauma. (2nd ed.) Baltimore: Williams & Wilkins, 1986.
59. Finnegan RE, Schroll M, Robinson S, Harrison DC. Action of pharmacological agents in experimental cardiac tamponade. Am Heart J 1971;81:220.
60. Firth BG, Dehmer GJ, Nicod P, et al. Effect of increasing heart rate in patients with aortic regurgitation. Am J Cardiol 1982;49:1860.
61. Fishbone G, Robbins DI, Osborn DJ, et al. Trauma to the thoracic aorta and great vessels. Radiol Clin North Am 1973;11:543.
62. Flancbaum L, Wright J, Siegel JH. Emergency surgery in patients with post-traumatic myocardial contusion. J Trauma 1986;26:795.
63. Fleming AW, Green DC. Traumatic aneurysms of the thoracic aorta. Report of 43 patients. Ann Thorac Surg 1974;18:91.
64. Frank MJ, Nadimi M, Lesniak LJ, et al. Effects of cardiac tamponade on myocardial performance, blood flow and metabolism. Am J Physiol 1971;220:179.
65. Franz JL, Richardson JD, Grover FL, et al. Effects of methylprednisolone sodium succinate on experimental pulmonary contusion. J Thorac Cardiovasc Surg 1974;68:842.
66. Frazee RC, Mucha P, Farnell MB, Miller FA. Objective evaluation of blunt cardiac trauma. J Trauma 1986;26:510.
67. Freeark R. Penetrating wounds of the abdomen. N Engl J Med 1974;291:185.
68. Freeark R. The abdomen in the patient with multiple injuries. Can J Surg 1982;25:178.
69. Friedman HS, Lajam F, Zaman Q, et al. Effect of autonomic blockade on the hemodynamic findings in acute cardiac tamponade. Am J Physiol 1967;212:549.
70. Friedman HS, Gomes JA, Tardio AR, Haft JI. The electrocardiographic features of acute cardiac tamponade. Circulation 1974;50:260.
71. Friedman HS, Lajam F, Gomes JA, et al. Demonstration of a depressor reflex in acute cardiac tamponade. J Thorac Cardiovasc Surg 1977;73:278.
72. Fulton RL, Peter ET. The progressive nature of pulmonary contusion. Surgery 1970;67:499.
73. Fulton RL, Peter ET. Physiologic effects of fluid therapy after pulmonary contusion. Am J Surg 1973;126:773.
74. Gabe IT, Mason DT, Gault JH, et al. Effect of respiration on venous return and stroke volume in cardiac tamponade. Br Heart J 1970;32:592.
75. Gaffney FA, Thal ER. Hemodynamic effects of medical antishock trousers (MAST) garment. J Trauma 1981;21:931.
76. Garrison RN, Richardson JD, Frey DE. Diagnostic transdiaphragmatic pericardiotomy in thoracoabdominal trauma. J Trauma 1982;22:147.
77. Gascho JA, Martins JB, Marcus ML, Kerber RE. Effects of volume expansion and vasodilators in acute pericardial tamponade. Am J Physiol 1981;232:449.
78. Gay W. Blunt trauma to the heart and great vessels. Surgery 1982;91:507.
79. Gelman S, Reeves JC, Fowler K, et al. Regional blood flow during cross-clamping of the thoracic aorta and infusion of sodium nitroprusside. J Thorac Cardiovasc Surg 1983;85:287.
80. Gerblich AA, Kleinerman J. Editorial—blunt chest trauma and the lung. Am Rev Respir Dis 1977;115:369.
81. Gerlock AAJ, Muhletaler CA, Coulam CM, et al. Traumatic aortic aneurysm. Validity of esophageal tube displacement sign. AJR 1980;135:713.
82. Godwin JD, Tolentino CS. Thoracic cardiovascular trauma. J Thorac Imag 1987;2:32.
83. Goodman DJ, Rosen RM, Holloway EL, et al. Effect of nitroprusside on left ventricular dynamics in mitral regurgitation. Circulation 1974;50:1025.
84. Gorlin R, Dexter L. Hydraulic formula for the calculation of the cross-sectional area of the mitral valve during regurgitation. Am Heart J 1952;43:188.
85. Goto K, Goto H, Benson KT, et al. Efficacy of high frequency ventilation in cardiac tamponade. Anesth Analg 1990;70:375.
86. Graham JM, Beall AC, Mattox KL, Vaughn GD. Systemic air embolism following penetrating trauma to the lung. Chest 1979;72:449.

87. Grover FL, Ellestad C, Arom KV, et al. Diagnosis and management of major tracheobronchial injuries. Ann Thorac Surg 1979;28:384.
88. Guberman BA, Fowler NO, Engel PJ, et al. Cardiac tamponade in medical patients. Circulation 1981;64:633.
89. Gundry SR, Williams S, Burney RE, et al. Indications for aortography. Radiography after blunt chest trauma: a reassessment of the radiographic findings associated with traumatic rupture of the aorta. Invest Radiol 1983;18:230.
90. Gustman P, Yerger L, Wanner A. Immediate cardiovascular effects of tension pneumothorax. Am Rev Respir Dis 1983;127:171.
91. Hankins JR, Gonzalez MH, Hanashiro PK, et al. The treatment of major chest trauma in a research facility. Am Rev Respir Dis 1971;103:492.
92. Hantler CB, Knight PR. Intracranial hypertension following cross-clamping of thoracic aorta. Anesthesiology 1982;56:146.
92a. Healey MA, Brown R, Fleiszer D. Blunt cardiac injury: Is this diagnosis necessary? J Trauma 1990;30:137.
93. Heiberg E, Wolverson MK, Sundaram M, et al. CT in aortic trauma. AJR 1983;140:1119.
94. Heystraten FM, Rosenbusch G, Kingma LM, et al. Chest radiography in acute rupture of the thoracic aorta. Acta Radiol 1988;29:411.
94a. Hiatt JR, Yeatman LA, Child JS. The value of echocardiography in blunt chest trauma. J Trauma 1988;28:914.
95. Hillis LD, Braunwald E. Coronary artery spasm. N Engl J Med 1978;299:695.
96. Hockerstedt K, Airo I, Karaharju E, Sundin A. Abdominal trauma and laparotomy in 158 patients. Acta Chir Scand 1982;148:9.
97. Holt JP. The normal pericardium. Am J Cardiol 1970;26:455.
98. Hood RM. Trauma to the chest. In: Sabiston DC, Spencer FC, eds. Surgery of the chest. Philadelphia: WB Saunders, 1990:383.
99. Hood RM. Injury to the trachea and major bronchi. In: Hood RM, Boyd AD, Culliford AT, eds. Thoracic trauma. Philadelphia: WB Saunders, 1989;245.
100. Hopkinson BR, Border JR, Schenk WD. Experimental closed chest trauma. J Thorac Cardiovasc Surg 1968;55:580.
100a. Lehmann KG, Lane JG, Piepmeier JM, et al. Cardiovascular abnormalities accompanying acute spinal cord injury in humans: Incidence, time course and severity. J Am Coll Cardiol 1987;10:46.
101. Imperial ES, Levy MN, Zieske H Jr. Outflow resistance as an independent determinant of cardiac performance. Circ Res 1961;9:1148.
102. Jarmakani JMM, McHale PA, Greenfield JC. The effect of cardiac tamponade on coronary hemodynamics in the awake dog. Cardiovasc Res 1975;9:112.
103. Johnson JA, Cogbill TH, Winga ER. Determinants of outcome after pulmonary contusion. J Trauma 1986;26:695.
104. Johnston WE, Vinter-Johansen T, Klopfenstein HS, et al. Effect of cardiac tamponade on left ventricular contractility. Anesthesiology 1988;69:A45.
105. Johnston WE, Vinter-Johansen T, McGiver AC, et al. Efficacy of intravascular volume resuscitation in dogs with acute cardiac tamponade. Ann Thorac Surg 1988;45:667.
106. Jones JW, Hewitt RL, Drapanas T. Cardiac contusion: a capricious syndrome. Ann Surg 1975;181:567.
107. Judge TP, Kennedy JW, Kennett LJ, et al. Quantitative hemodynamic effects of heart rate in aortic regurgitation. Circulation 1971;19:355.
108. Kashuk JL, Moore EE, Millikan JS, Moore JB. Major abdominal vascular trauma—a unified approach. J Trauma 1982;22:672.
109. Katz NM, Blackstone EH, Kirklin JW, Karp RB. Incremental risk factors for spinal cord injury following operations for acute traumatic aortic dissection. J Thorac Cardiovasc Surg 1981;81:669.
110. Keeling MM, Gray LA, Brink MA, et al. Intraoperative autotransfusion: experience in 725 consecutive cases. Ann Surg 1983;197:536.
111. Keller KD, Shatney CH. Creatine phosphokinase-MB assays in patients with suspected myocardial contusion: diagnostic test or test of diagnosis. J Trauma 1988;28:58.
112. Kerber RE, Gascho JA, Litchfield R, et al. Hemodynamic effects of volume expansion and nitroprusside compared with pericardiocentesis in patients with acute cardiac tamponade. N Engl J Med 1982;307:929.
113. Khatri I, Vemura N, Notargioromo A, Freis ED. Direct and reflex cardiostimulating effects of hydralazine. Am J Cardiol 1977;40:38.
114. Kirsh MM. Acute thoracic injuries. In: Siegel J, ed. Trauma, emergency surgery and critical care. New York: Churchill-Livingstone, 1987:863.
115. Kirsh MM, Behrendt DM, Arringer MB, et al. The treatment of acute traumatic rupture of the aorta: A ten year experience. Ann Surg 1976;184:308.
116. Kirsh MM, Orringer MB, Behrendt DB, Sloan H. Management of tracheobronchial disruption secondary to non-penetrating trauma. Ann Thorac Surg 1976;22:93.
117. Kudsk KA, Sheldon GF, Lim RC. Atrial-caval shunting after trauma. J Trauma 1982;22:81.
118. Lake CI. Anesthesia and pericardial disease. Anesth Analg 1983;62:431.
119. Lappas DG. Left ventricle performance and pulmonary circulation following addition of nitrous oxide to morphine during coronary artery surgery. Anesthesiology 1975;43:61.
120. Law VK, Viano DC, Doty DB. Experimental cardiac trauma—ballistics of a captive bolt pistol. J Trauma 1982;21:39.
121. Lazrove S, Harley DP, Grinnell VS, et al. Should all patients with first rib fractures undergo arteriography? J Thorac Cardiovasc Surg 1982;83:532.
122. Leimgruber PP, Klopfenstein HS, Wann LS, Brooks HL. The hemodynamic derangement associated with right ventricular diastolic collapse in cardiac tamponade: an experimental echocardiographic study. Circulation 1983;68:612.
123. Levy WJ, York DH, McCaffrey M. Motor evoked potentials from transcranial stimulation of the motor cortex in humans. Neurosurgery 1984;15:287.
124. Liedtke AJ, DeMuth WE. Nonpenetrating cardiac injuries: a collective review. Am Heart J 1973;86:687.
125. Lindenbaum G, Larrieu AJ, Goldberg SE, et al. Diagnosis and management of traumatic ventricular septal defect. J Trauma 1987;27:1289.
126. Lindsey D, Nivin TR, Finley PR. Transient elevation of serum activity of MB-isoenzyme of creatine phosphokinase in drivers involved in automobile accidents. Chest 1978;74:15.
127. Lorell BH, Braunwald E. Pericardial disease. In: Braunwald E, ed. Heart disease: a textbook of cardiovascular medicine. Philadelphia: WB Saunders, 1988:1484.
128. Ludwig RM, Wangenstein SL. Aortic bleeding and effect of external counterpressure. Surg Gynecol Obstet 1968;127:253.
128a. Mackersie RC, Shackford DR, Hoyt DB, Karagianes TG. Continuous epidural fentanyl analgesia: Ventilatory function, improvement with routine use in therapy of blunt chest trauma. J Trauma 1987;27:1207.
129. Mahon PA, Sutton JE. Nonoperative management of adult splenic injury due to blunt trauma: a warning. Am J Surg 1985;149:716.
130. Maloney JV, Schmutzer KJ, Raschke E. Paradoxical respiration and "Pendelluft." J Thorac Cardiovasc Surg 1961;41:291.

131. Mann T, McLaurin LP, Grossman W, et al. Assessing the hemodynamic severity of acute aortic regurgitation due to infective endocarditis. N Engl J Med 1975;293:108.
132. Manyari DE, Kostuk WF, Purves P. Effect of pericardiocentesis on right and left ventricular function and volumes in pericardial effusion. Am J Cardiol 1983;52:159.
133. Martins JB, Manuel W, Marcus ML, Kerber RE. Comparative effects of catecholamines in cardiac tamponade: experimental and clinical studies. Am J Cardiol 1980;46:59.
134. Mattox KL. Abdominal venous injuries. Surgery 1982;91:497.
135. Mattox KL, Limacher MC, Feliciano DV, et al. Cardiac evaluation following heart injury. J Trauma 1985;25:758.
136. Mazzucco A, Rizzoli G, Faggian G, et al. Acute mitral regurgitation after blunt chest trauma. Arch Intern Med 1983;143:2326.
137. McCabe JB, Seidel DR, Jagger JA. Antishock-trouser inflation and pulmonary vital capacity. Ann Emerg Med 1983;12:290.
138. McGregor M. Pulsus paradoxus. N Engl J Med 1979;301:480.
139. Meier GH, Wood WJ, Symbas PN. Systemic air embolization from penetrating lung injury. Ann Thorac Surg 1979;27:161.
140. Merrill WH, Lee RB, Hammon JW, et al. Surgical treatment of acute traumatic tear of the aorta. Ann Surg 1988;207:699.
141. Meyer AA, Crass RA, Lim RC, et al. Selective nonoperative management of blunt liver injury using computed tomography. Arch Surg 1985;120:550.
142. Michenfelder JD. The interdependency of cerebral functional and metabolic effects following massive doses of thiopental in the dog. Anesthesiology 1974;41:231.
143. Michenfelder JD. Hypothermia plus barbiturates: apples plus oranges? Anesthesiology 1978;49:157.
144. Millard RW, Fowler NO, Gabel M. Hemodynamic and regional blood flow distribution responses to dextran, hydralazine, isoproterenol and amrinone during experimental cardiac tamponade. J Am Coll Cardiol 1983;1:1461.
145. Miller FA, Seward JB, Gersh BJ. Two dimensional echocardiographic findings in cardiac trauma. Am J Cardiol 1982;50:1022.
146. Mills SA, Johnston FR, Hudspeth AS, et al. Clinical spectrum of blunt tracheobronchial disruption illustrated by seven cases. J Thorac Cardiovasc Surg 1982;84:49.
147. Mitchell RL, Enright LP. The surgical management of acute and chronic injuries of the thoracic aorta. Surg Gynecol Obstet 1983;157:1.
148. Miyatake K, Okamoto M, Kinoshita N, et al. Evaluation of tricuspid regurgitation by pulsed Doppler and two-dimensional echocardiography. Circulation 1982;66:111.
149. Moller CT, Schoonbee CG, Rosendorf C. Haemodynamics of cardiac tamponade during various modes of ventilation. Br J Anaesth 1979;51:409.
150. Moore DC. Intercostal nerve block for postoperative somatic pain following surgery of thorax and upper abdomen. Br J Anaesth 1975;47:284.
151. Moore JB, Moore EE, Thompson JS. Abdominal injuries associated with penetrating trauma in the lower chest. Am J Surg 1980;140:724.
152. Moritz AR. Trauma, stress and coronary thrombosis. JAMA 1954;156:1306.
153. Moritz AR, Atkins JP. Cardiac contusion: an experimental and pathologic study. Arch Pathol 1938;25:445.
154. Novick TL, Moylan JA. Hepatic trauma. In: Moylan JA, ed. Trauma surgery. Philadelphia: JB Lippincott 1988:197.
155. Nugent M, Kaye MP, McGoon DC. Effects of nitroprusside on aortic and intraspinal pressures during thoracic aortic cross-clamping. Anesthesiology 1984;61:A68.
156. Oppenheimer L, Craven KD, Forkert L, Wood LDH. Pathophysiology of pulmonary contusion in dogs. J Appl Physiol 1979;47:718.
157. O'Rourke RA, Fischer DP, Escobar EE, et al. Effect of acute pericardial tamponade on coronary blood flow. Am J Physiol 1967;212:549.
158. Pachter HL, Hofstetter SR. Open and percutaneous paracentesis and lavage for abdominal trauma. A randomized prospective study. Arch Surg 1981;116:318.
159. Pachter HL, Spencer FC, Hofstetter SR, Coppa GF. Experience with finger fracture technique to achieve intrahepatic hemostasis in 75 patients with severe injuries of the liver. Ann Surg 1983;197:771.
160. Pandian NG, Skorton DJ, Doty DB, Kerber RE. Immediate diagnosis of acute myocardial contusion by two-dimensional echocardiography: studies in a canine model of blunt chest trauma. J Am Coll Cardiol 1983;2:488.
161. Parham AM, Yarbrough DR, Redding JS. Flail chest syndrome and pulmonary contusion. Arch Surg 1978;113:900.
162. Parmley LF, Manion WC, Mattingly TW. Nonpenetrating traumatic injury of the heart. Circulation 1958;18:371.
163. Parvin S, Smith DE, Asher WM, et al. Effectiveness of peritoneal lavage in blunt abdominal trauma. Ann Surg 1975;181:255.
164. Patterson JE, Hetzl A. Vital statistics in the United States 1978. Washington: US Department of Health, Education and Welfare, Public Health Service, 1978:1–6.
165. Perlman SJ, Rogers LF, Mintzer RA, et al. Abnormal course of nasogastric tube in traumatic rupture of left hemidiaphragm. AJR 1984;142:85.
166. Peters RM. Chest trauma. In: Moser KM, Spragg RG, eds. Respiratory emergencies. St. Louis, CV Mosby, 1982:132.
167. Philips EH, Rogers WF, Gaspar MR. First rib fracture: incidence of vascular injury and indications for angiography. Surgery 1981;89:42.
168. Pierce GE, Maxwell JA, Boggan MD. Special hazards of first rib fractures. J Trauma 1975;15:264.
169. Pizov R, Shir Y, Eimerl D, et al. One-lung high frequency ventilation in the management of traumatic tear of bronchus in a child. Crit Care Med 1987;15:1160.
170. Polk HC, Flint LM. Intra-abdominal injuries in polytrauma. World J Surg 1983;7:56.
171. Potkin RT, Werner JA, Trobaugh JB, et al. Evaluation of noninvasive tests of cardiac damage in suspected cardiac contusion. Circulation 1982;66:627.
172. Rappoṙt RL, Allen RB, Curry GJ. The fractured rib—a significant injury. Arch Surg 1955;71:7.
173. Reddy PS, Curtiss EI, O'Toole JD, Shaver JA. Cardiac tamponade: hemodynamic observations in man. Circulation 1978;58:265.
174. Refsum H, Junemann M, Lipton MJ, et al. Ventricular diastolic pressure-volume relations and the pericardium. Circulation 1981;64:997.
175. Rehlihan M, Litwin MS. Morbidity and mortality associated with flail chest injury. A review of 85 cases. J Trauma 1973; 13:663.
176. Reinfeld HB, Agatston AS, Robinson MJ, Hildner FJ. Bioprosthetic mitral valve dysfunction following blunt chest trauma. Am Heart J 1986;111:800.
177. Richardson JD, McElvein RB, Trinkle JK. First rib fracture: a hallmark of severe trauma. Ann Surg 1975;181:251.
178. Richardson JD, Woods D, Johanson WG, Trinkle JK. Lung bacterial clearance following pulmonary contusion. Surgery 1979;86:730.
179. Richardson JD, Adams L, Flint LM. Selective management of flail chest and pulmonary contusion. Ann Surg 1982;196:481.
180. Roberts AJ, Nora JD, Hughes WA, et al. Cardiac and renal re-

sponse to cross-clamping of the descending thoracic aorta. J Thorac Cardiovasc Surg 1983;86:732.
181. Roberts WC, Maron BJ. Sudden death while playing professional football. Am Heart J 1981;102:1061.
182. Robotham JL, Lixfeld W, Holland L, et al. Effects of respiration on cardiac performance. J Appl Physiol 1978;44:703.
183. Robotham JL, Rabson JL, Bromberger-Barnea B, et al. The effects of increasing negativity of pleural pressure on the left heart in a closed chest right heart bypass preparation. Circulation 1978;57 and 58(suppl):II-107.
184. Rodriguez-Morales G, Rodriguez A, Shatney CH. Acute rupture of the diaphragm in blunt trauma. Analysis of 60 patients. J Trauma 1986;26:438.
185. Roizen MF, Hamilton WK, Sohn YJ. Treatment of stress-induced increases in pulmonary capillary wedge pressure using volatile anesthetics. Anesthesiology 1981;55:446.
186. Root HD, Hauser CW, McKinley CR, et al. Diagnostic peritoneal lavage. Surgery 1965;57:633.
187. Ross J Jr, Sonnenblick EH, Taylor RR, et al. Diastolic geometry and sarcomere length in the chronically dilated canine left ventricle. Circ Res 1971;28:49.
188. Rumisek JD, Robonowitz M, Virmani R, et al. Bioprosthetic heart valve rupture associated with trauma. J Trauma 1986;26:276.
188a. Winslow EBJ, Lesch M, Talano JV, et al. Spinal cord injuries associated with cardiopulmonary complications. Spine 1986;11:809.
189. Ruskin J, Bache RJ, Rembert JC, et al. Pressure-flow studies in man: effect of respiration on left ventricular stroke volume. Circulation 1973;48:79.
190. Rutherford RB, Hurt HH, Brickman RD, et al. The pathophysiology of progressive tension pneumothorax. J Trauma 1968;8:212.
191. Sarnoff J, Gaensler EA, Maloney JV. Electrophrenic respiration. The effectiveness of contralateral ventilation during activity of one phrenic nerve. J Thorac Cardiovasc Surg 1950;19:929.
192. Schall MA, Fischer RP, Perry JF. The unchanged mortality of flail chest injuries. J Trauma 1979;19:492.
193. Schiller NB, Botvinick EH. Right ventricular compression as a sign of cardiac tamponade. Circulation 1977;56:774.
194. Schwab CW, Lawson RB, Lind JF, et al. Aortic injury: comparison of supine and upright portable chest films to evaluate the widened mediastinum. Ann Emerg Med 1984;13:896.
195. Scott DB, Jebson PJR, Braid DP, et al. Factors affecting plasma levels of lignocaine and prilocaine. Br J Anaesth 1972;44:1040.
196. Sekikawa T, Shatney CH. Septic sequelae after splenectomy for trauma in adults. Am J Surg 1983;145:667.
197. Settle HP, Adolph RJ, Fowler NO, et al. Echocardiographic study of cardiac tamponade. Circulation 1977;56:951.
198. Shackford SR, Smith DE, Sairns CK, et al. The management of flail chest. A comparison of ventilatory and nonventilatory treatment. Am J Surg 1976;132:759.
199. Shackford SR, Virgilio RW, Peters RM. Selective use of ventilator therapy in flail chest injury. J Thorac Cardiovasc Surg 1981;81:194.
200. Shabetai R, Fowler NO, Guntheroth WG. The hemodynamics of cardiac tamponade and constrictive pericarditis. Am J Cardiol 1970;26:480.
201. Shimosato S, Carter JG, Kemmatsu O, et al. Cardiovascular effects of prolonged administration of isoflurane in normocarbic human volunteers. Acta Anaesthesiol Scand 1982;26:27.
202. Singh S, Wann LS, Schuchard GH. Right ventricular and right atrial collapse in patients with cardiac tamponade—a combined echocardiographic and hemodynamic study. Circulation 1984;70:966.
203. Snow N, Richardson JD, Flint LM. Myocardial contusion: implications for patients with multiple trauma injuries. Surgery 1982;92:744.
204. Soliman MH, Waxman K. Value of a conventional approach to the diagnosis of traumatic cardiac contusion after chest injury. Crit Care Med 1987;15:218.
205. Stark P. Traumatic rupture of the thoracic aorta: a review. CRC Crit Rev Diagn Imaging 1984;31:229.
206. Stern T, Wolf RY, Reichart B, et al. Coronary artery occlusion resulting from blunt trauma. JAMA 1974;230:1308.
207. Sturm JT, Strate RG, Mowlem A, et al. Blunt trauma to the subclavian artery. Surg Gynecol Obstet 1974;138:915.
208. Sturm JT, Perry JF, Olson FR, et al. Significance of symptoms and signs in patients with traumatic aortic rupture. Ann Emerg Med 1984;13:876.
209. Sturm JT, Billiar TR, Luxenberg MG, Perry JF. Risk factors for the development of renal failure following the surgical treatment of traumatic aortic rupture. Ann Thorac Surg 1987;43:425.
210. Sutherland GR, Calvin JE, Driedger AA, et al. Anatomic and cardiopulmonary responses to trauma with associated blunt chest injury. J Trauma 1981;21:1.
211. Sutherland GR, Driedger AA, Holliday RL, et al. Frequency of myocardial injury after blunt chest trauma as evaluated by radionuclide angiography. Am J Cardiol 1983;52:1099.
212. Sutherland GR, Cheung HW, Holliday RL, et al. Hemodynamic adaptation to acute myocardial contusion complicating blunt chest injury. Am J Cardiol 1986;57:291.
213. Svennevig JL, Bugge-Aspesheim B, Bjorgo S, et al. Methylprednisolone in the treatment of lung contusion following blunt chest trauma. Scand J Thorac Cardiovasc Surg 1980;14:301.
214. Svoboda JA, Peter ET, Dang CV, et al. Severe liver trauma in the face of coagulopathy: a case for temporary packing and early reexploration. Am J Surg 1982;144:717.
215. Symbas PN. Cardiac trauma. Am Heart J 1976;92:387.
216. Symbas PN. Acute traumatic hemothorax. Ann Thorac Surg 1978;26:195.
217. Takaki O, Okumura F. Application and limitation of somatosensory evoked potential monitoring during thoracic aortic aneurysm surgery: a case report. Anesthesiology 1985;63:700.
218. Taylor GA, Miller HA, Shulman HS, et al. Symposium on Trauma 1. Controversies in the management of pulmonary contusion. Can J Surg 1982;25:167.
219. Tenzer ML. The spectrum of myocardial contusion: a review. J Trauma 1985;25:620.
220. Thal ER, May RA, Beesinger D. Peritoneal lavage: its unreliability in gunshot wounds of the lower chest and abdomen. Arch Surg 1980;115:430.
221. Tocino IM, Miller MH, Fairfax WR. Distribution of pneumothorax in the supine and semirecumbent critically ill adult. AJR 1985;144:901.
222. Tocino IM, Miller MH. Computed tomography in blunt chest trauma. J Thorac Imaging 1987;2:45.
223. Tocino IM, Miller MH, Frederick PR, et al. CT detection of occult pneumothorax in head trauma. AJR 1984;143:987.
224. Torres-Mirabal, Gruenberg JC, Talbert JG, Brown RS. Ventricular function in myocardial contusion. Crit Care Med 1982;10:19.
225. Traub AC, Perry JF. Injuries associated with splenic trauma. J Trauma 1981;21:840.
226. Triester B, Gianelly RE, Cohn KE, Harrison DC. The circulatory effects of isoproterenol, acetylstrophanthidin, and volume loading in acute pericardial tamponade. Cardiovasc Res 1967;3:299.
227. Trinkle JK, Furman RW, Hinshaw M, et al. Pulmonary contusion—pathogenesis and effect of various resuscitative measures. Ann Thorac Surg 1973;16:568.

228. Trinkle JK, Richardson JD, Franz JL, et al. Management of flail chest without mechanical ventilation. Ann Thorac Surg 1975;19:355.
229. Trunkey DD, Shires GT, McClelland RN. Management of liver trauma in 811 consecutive patients. Ann Surg 1974;179:722.
230. Tucker GT, Moore DC, Bridenbaugh PO, et al. Systemic absorption of mepivacaine in commonly used regional block procedures. Anesthesiology 1972;37:277.
231. Urthaler F, Walker AA, James TN. Comparison of the inotropic action of morphine and ketamine studied in canine cardiac muscle. J Thorac Cardiovasc Surg 1976;72:142.
232. Utley JR, Doty DB, Collins JC, et al. Cardiac output, coronary flow, ventricular fibrillation and survival following varying degrees of myocardial contusion. J Surg Res 1976;20:539.
233. Van Loenhout RMM, Shiphorst TJMJ, Wittens CHA, Pinckaers JA. Traumatic intrapericardial diaphragmatic hernia. J Trauma 1986;26:271.
234. Vlay SC, Blumenthal DS, Shoback D, et al. Delayed acute myocardial infarction after blunt chest trauma in a young woman. Am Heart J 1980;100:907.
235. Ward RE, Flynn TC, Clark WP. Diaphragmatic disruption secondary to blunt abdominal trauma. J Trauma 1981;21:335.
236. Waxman K, Soliman MB, Braunstein P, et al. Diagnosis of traumatic cardiac contusion. Arch Surg 1986;121:689.
237. Wechsler AS, Auerbach BJ, Graham TC, Sabiston DC. Distribution of intramyocardial blood flow during pericardial tamponade: correlation with microscopic anatomy and intrinsic myocardial contractility. J Thorac Cardiovasc Surg 1974;68:847.
238. Weiskopf RB, Bogetz MS, Roizen MF, Reid IA. Cardiovascular and metabolic sequelae of inducing anesthesia with ketamine or thiopental in hypovolemic swine. Anesthesiology 1984;60:214.
239. Wilken DEL, Charlier AA, Hoffman JIE, et al. Effects of alterations in aortic impedance on the performance of the ventricles. Circ Res 1964;14:283.
240. Williams TM, Knopp R, Ellyson JH. Compartment syndrome after anti-shock trouser use without lower-extremity trauma. J Trauma 1982;22:595.
241. Wilson JM, Thomas AN, Goodman PC, Lewis FR. Severe chest trauma -morbidity—implication of first and second rib fracture in 120 patients. Arch Surg 1978;113:846.
242. Wilson RF. Science and shock. A clinical perspective. Ann Emerg Med 1985;14:714.
243. Wilson RF, Bassett JS. Penetrating wounds of the pericardium or its contents. JAMA 1966;195:513.
244. Wilson RF, Murray C, Antonenko DR. Nonpenetrating thoracic injuries. Surg Clin North Am 1977;57:17.
245. Wise AJ, Topuzlu C, Mills EL, Page HG. The importance of serial blood gas determinations in blunt chest trauma. J Thorac Cardiovasc Surg 1968;56:520.
246. Yao ST, Vanecko RM, Printen K, et al. Penetrating wounds of the heart: a review of 80 cases. Ann Surg 1968;168:67.
247. Yellin AE, Chaffee CB, Donovan AJ. Vascular isolation in the treatment of juxtahepatic venous injuries. Arch Surg 1980;102:566.
248. Young GP, Purcell TB. Emergency autotransfusion. Ann Emerg Med 1983;12:180.
249. Zuckerman S. Experimental study of blunt injuries of the lung. Lancet 1940;2:219.

Chapter Sixteen

Katie P. Patel
Levon M. Capan

Gilbert J. Grant
Sanford M. Miller

# Musculoskeletal Injuries

Management of musculoskeletal injuries comprises the major workload of most trauma centers. In 1957 Braunstein,[18] reviewing the findings of 1,000 automobile accidents in which at least one person was injured, noted that musculoskeletal injuries as a whole were the most common type of trauma; indeed lower extremity injuries alone were second in frequency only to head trauma. A Swedish study showed that 85% of men in the population sustained at least one injury in the course of a lifetime. Twenty-nine percent of the injuries were to the upper extremities and another 29% to the lower extremities, although only 16–20% of these required inpatient care.[26] A fracture incidence of 43% to 85% has been documented after motorcycle accidents and other types of blunt trauma.[129] Penetrating trauma, although capable of producing severe musculoskeletal damage, is generally less likely to cause this type of injury than blunt trauma.

## PRESENTATION AND MANAGEMENT

Presentation and management of musculoskeletal injuries vary widely according to their anatomic location, mechanism, type and severity, and association with other injuries.

### ANATOMIC LOCATION

Upper extremity fractures, although not uncommon in the multiply traumatized patient, generally produce little hemodynamic alteration and may be overlooked or neglected temporarily until life-threatening injuries are brought under control. In contrast, fractures or dislocations of the spine, pelvis, or lower extremities frequently present with major hemorrhage, neurologic deficit, and adjacent vascular compromise, necessitating rapid treatment. In and of themselves, fractures of the chest wall, including the ribs, clavicle, sternum, and scapula, usually pose no threat to life, but they are generally associated with serious intrathoracic injuries that require careful and expeditious management.

### MECHANISM OF INJURY

Musculoskeletal injuries are produced by various mechanisms that, to some extent, determine their location, type, and severity. For instance, a recent survey demonstrated that the incidence of multiple skeletal injury after motor vehicle accidents was higher than in victims suffering falls or assaults.[129] It is not surprising that motor vehicle-pedestrian impact often produces devastating musculoskeletal injuries; the forces generated by this type of accident exceed 100,000 foot-pounds as compared to domestic or sporting injuries in which the force is generally in the range of 100–500 foot-pounds.[24] Passive, low-velocity, crushing trauma—for instance, when a vehicle overturns and rolls over the victim's body—generally produces less severe damage than a deceleration injury in which the person's body is actively thrown and then comes to an abrupt stop against a solid object, eg: a street or a windshield. In deceleration injury a moment of explosive force shatters bones, ruptures ligaments, and produces a wide displacement of bone fragments. Such severe musculoskeletal injury is not only difficult to repair but may also be associated with injuries to adjacent neural and vascular elements.

Injuries produced by simple falls usually involve isolated bones and, unless the patient is elderly, cause little morbidity or anesthetic difficulty. In contrast, falls from a high altitude can produce severe musculoskeletal and associated injuries, the severity of which is affected by six variables[47,240]: (1) the orientation of the body at impact; (2) the area over which the force is distributed; (3) the magnitude of the force, which increases with altitude; (4) the material impacted; (5) the duration of impact; and (6) the age and physical condition of the patient. Landing on the feet results in a high load per unit area, increasing the likelihood of lower extremity fractures. The material impacted and the duration of impact are interrelated. Elastic surfaces cause increased impact duration and less morbidity.

In general, penetrating musculoskeletal injuries are less severe than those seen after blunt trauma. Further, stab and bullet wounds are generally less severe than close-range shotgun injuries that, by producing severe and multiple skeletal injuries, may result in limb loss in up to 14% of victims.[233] Appropriate attention to the mechanism of injury during the preoperative evaluation may assist the physician in predicting the type and severity of injury and associated intraoperative complications.

## TYPE AND SEVERITY OF INJURIES

In general, musculoskeletal injuries are divided into two categories: closed and open. Closed injuries, if they do not involve the lower extremity long bones, the pelvis, or the spine and are not associated with vascular and neurologic injuries, rarely result in anesthetic difficulties. Hemorrhage, fat embolism syndrome, atelectasis, pneumonia, and thromboembolism are common complications of spine and lower extremity fractures.

Open or compound fractures usually result from high-energy impact and are classified into three categories (Table 16-1).[78,204] The rate and severity of fracture-related complications, such as infection, delay in union or non-union, and amputation, increase as severity increases from type I to type III. Although little information exists about the correlation of this classification with non-fracture-related complications (pulmonary problems, generalized sepsis), it is reasonable to assume that the more severe the injury, the more frequent and severe the systemic complications.

TABLE 16-1. Classifications of Open Musculoskeletal Injuries

|  |  |
|---|---|
| Type I: | Circumscribed lesion of the skin produced by a spike of bone piercing the skin from within |
| Type II: | Trauma-induced open fracture with contusion of the surrounding skin and damage to the underlying musculature |
| Type III: | Type II injury complicated by injury to vessels, nerves, and entire muscle groups resulting in functional deficits |
| Type IIIA: | Adequate soft tissue coverage of a fractured bone despite extensive soft tissue laceration or flaps, or high-energy trauma regardless of the size of the wound |
| Type IIIB: | Extensive soft tissue loss with periosteal stripping and bone exposure |
| Type IIIC: | Open fracture associated with arterial injury requiring repair |

(Adapted from Rittman et al[204] and Gustilo et al[78]).

## ASSOCIATION WITH OTHER INJURIES

In addition to damaging the musculoskeletal system, penetrating trauma, high-energy impact, and crush injuries produce concomitant injuries to both local and distant structures. Locally, the most commonly injured structures are the vessels and nerves. Concomitant orthopedic and vascular trauma is infrequent but often serious; the incidence in the lower extremity varies between 0.1%[188] and 3%.[96] A variety of vascular injuries may occur: thrombosis, intimal flap, transection, pseudoaneurysm, and arteriovenous fistula. Arteries, veins, or both may be injured, but the adverse consequences of arterial or combined injuries, which are produced by limb ischemia, are much more devastating than those of venous injuries. Some fracture-dislocations are notorious for injuring specific vessels. For instance, axillary artery disruption from an anterior dislocation of the shoulder,[8] subclavian artery injury from high upper extremity trauma,[252] axillary artery injury from humeral fracture,[100] brachial artery injury from posterior dislocation of the elbow,[89] and popliteal artery injury from posterior dislocation of the knee or from tibiofemoral fracture[258] occur rather frequently. In general, acute arterial interruption is tolerated better in the upper extremity than in the lower, probably because of the extensive upper extremity collateral circulation and a greater tendency to atherosclerosis in lower extremity vessels. The most important considerations in preventing amputation of the involved extremity after vascular injury are prompt recognition and repair. In addition to obvious bleeding from the wound, pulselessness, pallor, pain, paresthesias, and paralysis, often described in textbooks as the "five Ps" of arterial injury, are the presenting signs of this type of trauma. A distal pulse, however, may be present in a significant number of these patients, especially in those with upper extremity injuries, because of incomplete side-wall lacerations and the rich collateral circulation.[64] Formal arteriograms provide adequate evaluation, but may delay surgical repair as much as 2 to 3 hours. Therefore, some surgeons prefer to obtain percutaneous arteriography in the emergency department or the operating room and proceed with surgery expeditiously, even though the information obtained with this technique is clearly inferior to that obtained in the radiology suite.[55] The administration of contrast media during the initial evaluation or after completion of vascular repair is not without danger. Intravascular contrast media produce peripheral vasodilation that may be associated with severe hypotension in the hypovolemic trauma victim.[68] In addition acute renal failure may develop when potentially nephrotoxic contrast media are administered to a hypovolemic patient; adequate hydration before injection is necessary to avoid this complication.

Earlier reports suggested that fixation of skeletal injuries, with open internal stabilization or external fixators, should be given precedence to prevent distortion of the repaired vessels during later skeletal manipulation. The more recent trend is to repair the vessels first in order to avoid prolonged ischemia distal to the injury.[6]

When segmental arterial resection is performed, heparin is administered systemically to maintain a slightly elevated activated clotting time (200–225 sec)[144] or locally using 50 units/mL solution via a Fogarty catheter passed into the vessel.[55] Compartment syndrome caused by swelling of ischemic skeletal muscle develops frequently; fasciotomy involving all compartments of the limb is performed to avoid limb loss from this complication. In most instances, compartment syndrome produces obvious swelling of the extremity and pain. In equivocal cases direct measurement of compartment pressure may be necessary. A pressure above 40 mm Hg in a normotensive patient (lower if the patient is hypotensive) is an indication for fasciotomy.[192]

Controversy exists about the repair of venous injuries. Rich et al.[198] recommend the repair of injured veins, whereas others contend that ligation is preferable in upper extremity venous injuries or in hemodynamically unstable patients with lower extremity injuries.[84,212] Many surgeons believe that major injuries of lower extremity veins (common femoral, superficial femoral, or popliteal) should be repaired even though thrombosis occurs in most of these vessels within a few days.[145]

Spinal cord injury, complete or incomplete, is the most important concern in spine trauma. These injuries are discussed in Chapters 10 and 14. Peripheral nerves may also be damaged in extremity trauma. For instance, sciatic nerve injury is not uncommon after posterior dislocation of the hip. Peripheral nerve injury is a serious threat to limb function; its presence in severe open fractures is often an indication for amputation. Functional, sensory, and motor loss should be evaluated before any operative intervention. Primary nerve repair is seldom required during emergency surgery of salvageable extremities, but identification and marking of the ends of damaged nerves during this phase may facilitate the definitive surgery that is performed later.

Associated distant injuries are common after blunt trauma and less frequent after penetrating musculoskeletal trauma. When they are life threatening, these injuries require primary attention. If the patient is unconscious, musculoskeletal injuries may be missed easily during the initial evaluation. In one study, injuries of the spine, pelvis, femur, or tibiofibular complex occurred in 31% of obtunded head trauma victims, underscoring the importance of routine radiologic evaluation of these patients.[129]

Several classification systems attempt to grade the severity of injury and predict the viability of a limb after trauma.[74,96,266] The first of these systems was proposed by Gregory and co-workers[74] in 1985 based on a retrospective review of a small number of traumatized patients. They devised an index for the "mangled extremity syndrome," which was defined as significant injury to three of four major structures (integument, nerve, vessel, and bone) in the same extremity. The scoring system is based on the severity of injury to each of the limb structures and on overall injury severity, the lag time between injury and surgery, age of patient, and the presence of pre-existing disease and shock. A score of 20 is the demarcating point between a functionally retrievable and a probably nonviable extremity. In all patients with scores of less than 20, limb salvage was achieved, whereas amputation was unavoidable if the score was above 20. This or a similar classification system may aid in deciding between extremity repair and amputation.

## CHANGING CONCEPTS IN MANAGEMENT STRATEGIES

Until a few years ago treatment of musculoskeletal injuries in the multiple trauma victim was given a low priority. After lifesaving procedures—management of the obstructed airway, ventilation, and volume replacement—operations on life-threatening injuries of the thorax, abdomen, and cranium were performed immediately while fractures were treated initially with splinting or traction, although debridement and closure of open fractures were always carried out soon after trauma. Definitive fixation was often delayed for several days until the patient was in an adequate hemodynamic and metabolic condition. Currently, although cranial and thoracoabdominal surgery still have a high priority, most centers do not delay surgical fixation of fractures in the multiply injured patient. According to findings from Europe[273] and those of Border's group in the United States,[113,228] early operative stabilization of fractures results in improved nursing care, early patient mobilization, and improved respiratory function with decreased likelihood of ventilatory failure. Data from others have confirmed that multiply injured patients receiving immediate fixation of long bone and pelvic fractures had less postoperative pulmonary dysfunction, fewer infectious complications, and a decreased need for intensive care than those in whom delayed stabilization was selected. (Table 16-2).[70,101,127] There is evidence to suggest that the effectiveness of early stabilization in reducing pulmonary morbidity and sepsis increases with increasing injury severity.[101] It is important to realize, however, that the policy of completing sur-

TABLE 16-2. Pulmonary and Septic Complications after Early and Late Stabilization

| PARAMETER | IMMEDIATE FRACTURE FIXATION | TRACTION 10 DAYS | TRACTION 30 DAYS |
|---|---|---|---|
| Ventilator days | 3.4 ± 2.6 | 9.7 ± 8.8 | 21 ± 14 |
| ICU Days | 7.5 ± 3.8 | 15 ± 12 | 27 ± 16 |
| Febrile days (>101°F) | 3.8 ± 4 | 8.8 ± 7 | 13 ± 11 |
| Positive blood cultures (per patient) | 0.05 | 0.50 | 3.7 |

(Adapted from Seibel et al.[228])

gical skeletal fixation "on the night of injury" applies to stable trauma patients. When hemodynamic instability, compromised oxygenation, abnormal acid-base status, or clotting defect are present, delay of orthopedic surgery remains the safest approach.[228] The prolonged surgical repair required for severe extremity injuries often taxes the patient's limited physiologic reserves and may result in an unacceptably high risk of acute and chronic morbidity or mortality.

How does early fracture stabilization reduce pulmonary and septic complications? Several mechanisms have been postulated: (a) decreased fat embolization, (b) improved matching of ventilation and perfusion, (c) decreased pain from motion of the fracture, and (d) absence of fracture hematoma. Skeletal traction does not prevent the movement of bone fragments. Thus, intravasation of fat particles and embolization, especially to the lungs, are likely with this type of treatment. With rigid internal or external fixation of bone fragments, the frequency of fat embolization appears to decrease.[203] The early ability to sit and ambulate after rigid bone fixation allows the chest to assume a vertical position and thus to benefit maximally from chest physiotherapy. Atelectasis and ventilation/perfusion mismatch are therefore less likely to occur with this approach than when the patient is maintained in an enforced supine position. Ambulation is also facilitated by the decrease in pain from movement of the fracture site. The last factor, the absence of hematoma and necrotic tissue around the fracture site after early fracture stabilization, is most effective in reducing pulmonary and septic complications. Necrotic tissue at the fracture site in patients on traction stimulates phagocytosis. The presence of an increased number of activated leukocytes and platelets within a periosseous hematoma facilitates the occurrence of embolization to the lung and the release of such substances as complement split products, fibrin split products, prostaglandins, and leukotrienes that can precipitate sepsis, pulmonary edema, or acute respiratory distress syndrome.[228]

The clinical picture, treatment goals, and anesthetic management of skeletal injuries, although quite similar in principle, vary in detail from one type of fracture to another. Regional anesthesia has gained wide popularity among clinicians for emergency limb trauma during the past decade. However, not all types of musculoskeletal injuries are amenable to this technique. Certainly, ongoing hemorrhage and resulting hypovolemia contraindicate the use of regional anesthetic techniques, especially those that result in significant central sympathetic blockade. Because the scope of this chapter precludes discussion of all types of musculoskeletal injuries, its focus is on the following three subjects that are of interest to anesthesiologists: (1) hip fracture, (2) pelvic injuries, and (3) fat embolism.

## THE FRACTURED HIP

Hip fractures comprise the largest group of serious fractures in the elderly. Approximately 85% of hip fractures occur in persons over 65 years of age, and the remaining 15% are relatively equally distributed among younger age groups.[250] In the elderly group, women, because of their tendency to osteoporosis, are two to three times more likely to suffer the injury than men.[119] Likewise, whites are more likely to have this fracture than blacks.[119] A fall at home is the principal cause of injury in the elderly,[250] whereas in the younger age group, vehicular, sports, and industrial accidents and falls from a high altitude are the main causes of hip fractures or fracture dislocations.[46,165] In 1985, about 247,000 hip fractures occurred among persons over age 45 in the United States,[165] an incidence of about 0.1% for the entire population but 1.9–2.5% for individuals older than 55 years. Comparison of these figures with that of 200,000 hip fractures annually in the United States estimated by Lewinnek et al.[119] in 1980 suggests that the incidence is increasing steadily. Indeed, an age-specific comparative survey from England demonstrated an almost threefold increase in the incidence of hip fracture between 1958 and 1983.[16] This trend is likely to continue because of the increasing number of elderly persons in the population. Thus, the frequency of hip fractures can be expected to double or triple by the end of the first quarter of the next century unless effective preventive measures are applied.

The cost of hip fractures in the United States was $7.3 billion in 1983,[91] which represents a significant impact on our health care economy. This cost is expected to rise continuously. However, more important than the economic aspect is the effect of this injury on the lifestyle of the patient and family. Hip fracture in an elderly person may signal the end of his or her independent life and the beginning of institutionalization. The death rate from hip fracture and its surgical treatment (between 2.7 and 30% depending on the study) is also significant and actually exceeds that of many diseases involving more vital organs or requiring more complex surgical procedures. For instance, in our institution the overall mortality from coronary artery bypass surgery is less than 1% and that of open heart surgery in general is about 6%, well below the rates reported in many studies for hip fractures.

Several problems must be addressed in the anesthetic management of the hip fracture victim. In the young individual who sustains the fracture during a major accident, the immediate problems of associated severe injuries must be dealt with along with management of the hip trauma. Many of these multiple trauma victims are hospitalized for a prolonged period during which they receive repeated anesthetics for a wide variety of surgical procedures, only one of which may be for repair of the hip fracture. Postinjury sepsis, multiple organ failure, and severe physiologic derangements are common in this group of patients and require careful management. The elderly patient with a hip fracture is also likely to have chronic and/or acute medical problems that were either caused by the injury or responsible for it. An elderly patient sustaining a hip fracture after a fall resulting from a Stokes-Adams attack is a perfect example of the latter situation. Thus, utmost concern for concurrent pathophysiologic derangement and a thorough review of the patient's medical history, including any drug intake, are essential components of care.

### TYPES OF HIP INJURIES

#### *Dislocations and Fracture-Dislocations of the Hip*

These rare injuries result from an indirect force.[200] The hip joint is most commonly dislocated posteriorly in automobile accidents in which the flexed hip is pushed backward when the knee strikes the dashboard while the body is moving forward.[200] Anterior dislocation is less frequent and results from a force to the abducted femur. It can occur after falls or skiing accidents.[200] Characteristically the hip remains abducted and externally rotated. The sciatic and peroneal nerves may be injured, resulting in an inability to dorsiflex the foot. Associated pelvic and femoral fractures are common; radiographs should include the entire pelvis and the femur. The patient with dislocation or fracture-dislocation of the hip presents with severe pain. Immediate closed reduction under general anesthesia is mandatory in order to prevent aseptic necrosis of the femoral head. Reduction requires considerable force and may sometimes be unsuccessful. Computed tomography (CT) evaluation of the joint after an attempt at closed reduction may indicate the necessity for open reduction. Rarely, the femoral head may dislocate centrally and cause acetabular fracture. The presence of this injury suggests severe impact and almost always serious injuries to other systems.

### *Fractures of the Proximal Femur*

Four distinct fracture sites are distinguished on the proximal femur: subcapital, transcervical, intertrochanteric, and subtrochanteric (Fig 16-1). Subcapital and transcervical fractures are within the hip joint and are referred to as femoral neck or intracapsular fractures. Intertrochanteric and subtrochanteric fractures are outside the joint and are referred to as extracapsular fractures. Some differences exist between intracapsular and extracapsular fractures regarding the patient's age, mechanism of fracture, mortality rate, healing, the incidence of aseptic necrosis, and hemorrhage around the fracture site.[126] Intracapsular fractures are more likely to occur in a younger age group (60–70 years old); extracapsular fractures are more frequent in older patients (70–90 years old). Intracapsular fractures often occur before the fall, as a result of twisting of the foot or the leg, whereas in extracapsular fractures the fall usually precedes the fracture. This temporal relationship may be important for the anesthesiologist; the occurrence of the fracture before the fall decreases the likelihood of serious coexisting cardio- or cerebrovascular disease. Healing of intracapsular fractures is slower than that of extracapsular fractures. Aseptic necrosis is also more likely with intracapsular than with extracapsular fractures. However, the mortality rate after intracapsular fracture is lower than that after extracapsular fractures. Bleeding into the periosseous soft tissue from injured vessels around the proximal femur is usually less in intracapsular (about 800 mL) than in extracapsular (about 1200 mL) fractures.[126]

Subtrochanteric fractures, although not uncommon in the elderly, tend to occur in the younger age group, usually as a result of high-energy trauma. Thus, the comparisons described above are not relevant to these or any other fractures of the proximal femur in young individuals.

Surgical treatment of hip fractures varies according to their site. Intracapsular fractures are first reduced, and then multiple screws are driven through the longitudinal axis of the femoral neck into the cortical bone of the femoral head (Fig 16-2). If there is little chance of successful reduction and firm fixation, a common occurrence in the elderly patient, then primary replacement of the femoral head with a one-piece Austin-Moore prosthesis (Fig 16-3) or a two-piece biopolar prosthesis is the usual procedure. In the rare patient with a femoral neck fracture superimposed on significant underlying degenerative arthritis of the hip, primary total hip replacement may be required.

The surgical goal in extracapsular intertrochanteric or subtrochanteric fractures is similar: reduction and stabilization of the fracture followed by mobilization of the patient. After positioning the patient on a fracture table, the injured extremity is reduced and stabilized with a two-piece prosthesis consisting of a heavy lag-screw that is placed through the femoral neck into the femoral head and an attached side plate that is fixed to the femoral shaft with multiple screws (Fig 16-4) This system provides strong and reliable fixation.

PATIENT CHARACTERISTICS

The multiple trauma victim with an associated hip injury is often young and healthy, and apart from the acute metabolic, endocrine, and hemodynamic consequences of trauma, the likelihood of pre-existing physiologic derangement is small. The elderly patient with an isolated hip fracture, on the other hand, often presents with a variety of medical conditions. Often these pre-existing diseases are well controlled with appropriate medication, but frequently the physiologic derangement resulting from compensated or uncompensated organ dysfunction increases the risk of morbidity and mortality after anesthesia and surgery,[95,133,146] especially emergency procedures.[166,251,269] The physiologic derangement seen in these patients are the result of three factors: the natural effects of aging, pre-existing diseases, and the injury itself.

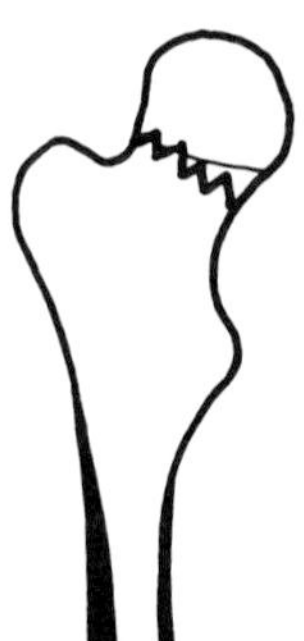


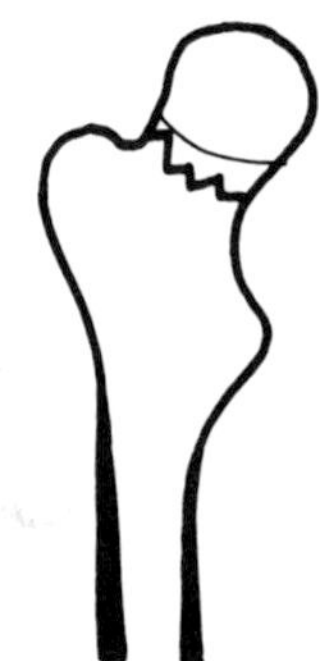


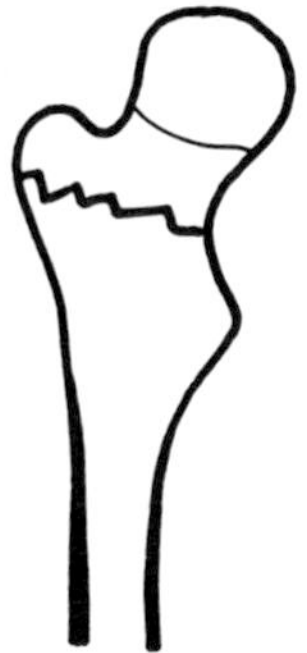


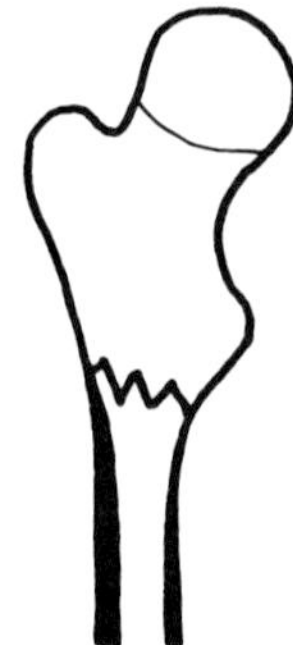


FIG. 16-1. Four common sites of hip fracture.

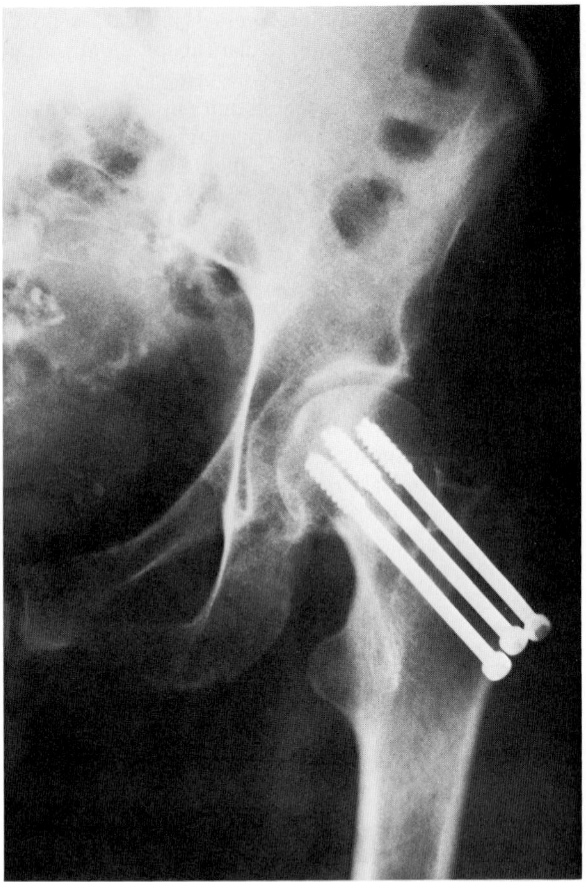

FIG. 16-2. Multiple stabilizing screws inserted into the femoral head after reduction of a intracapsular fracture.

## *Physiologic Changes in the Elderly*

Although the extent of decline in physiologic function with advancing age varies from one individual to another and thus chronologic and biologic age do not necessarily correlate, a gradual decrease in organ function occurs after age 30. In most individuals this decline is small until age 50 or 60 and does not interfere with their response to stress. However, after the sixth decade of life, the decreased reserve capacity becomes obvious during times of stress, such as anesthesia, trauma, and surgery. Ultimately, basal function diminishes to a critical level, threatening the individual's existence even in the absence of stress (Fig 16-5).[53]

BASAL METABOLIC RATE. The basal metabolic rate declines about 1% per year after age 30. Thus not only is the degradation of anesthetic and adjunct drugs slower in elderly patients than their younger counterparts but also intraoperative and postoperative hypothermia is more common and prolonged. Perioperative hypothermia in these patients is largely a result of decreased heat production and altered thermoregulation caused by general anesthesia.[141] It is not uncommon for elderly patients to develop moderate hypothermia even under spinal anesthesia. Some shivering does occur in the elderly to prevent the decline in body temperature, but the associated increase in oxygen consumption may be inadequately compensated for by the limited pulmonary and myocardial reserve, and myocardial ischemia, hypoxemia, increased systemic vascular resistance, and at times anaerobic metabolism and lactic acidosis may result.[141]

RESPIRATORY FUNCTION. The efficacy of protective airway reflexes decreases in elderly persons,[186] increasing the likelihood of perioperative aspiration of pharyngeal secretions or foreign bodies. Large doses of sedative and narcotic agents may interfere further with the function of these already compromised airway reflexes. Thus, the assessment of airway reactivity, avoidance of heavy sedation, and protection of the lungs with an endotracheal tube until the return of adequate airway reflexes after surgery are important care considerations in the elderly.[186] Degeneration of musculoskeletal structures with aging not only limits the movements of the cervical spine and temporomandibular joint and renders airway management of the elderly individual with intact teeth difficult but it also interferes with lung expansion and causes decreased lung volumes. Kyphosis and chest wall rigidity caused by these degenerative changes, coupled with reduced muscle mass and strength of the diaphragm and other respiratory muscles, reduce total lung volume, maximum breathing capacity, and vital capacity (Fig 16-6)[187,259] Aging also brings about parenchymal changes in the lung: alveolar ducts dilate, many interalveolar septa disappear, and the elastic recoil of

FIG. 16-3. Austin-Moore prosthesis replacing the femoral head and neck of a patient with intracapsular hip fracture.

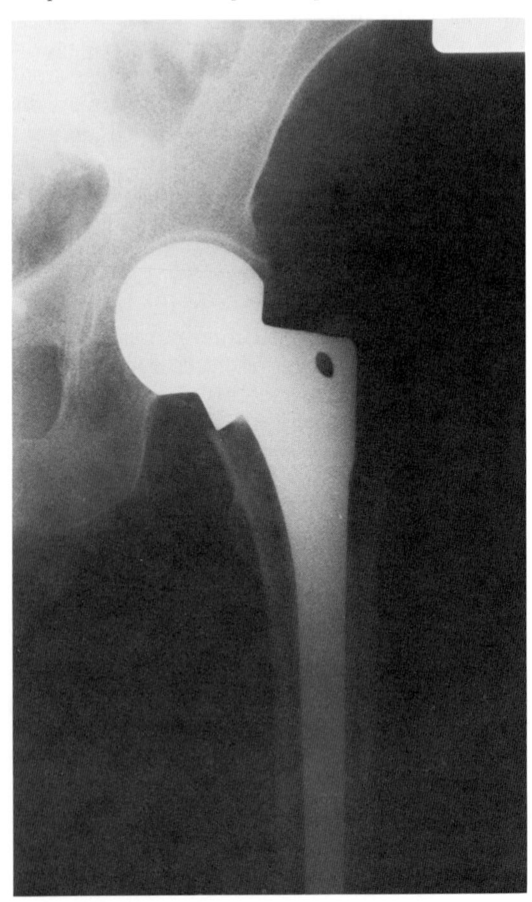

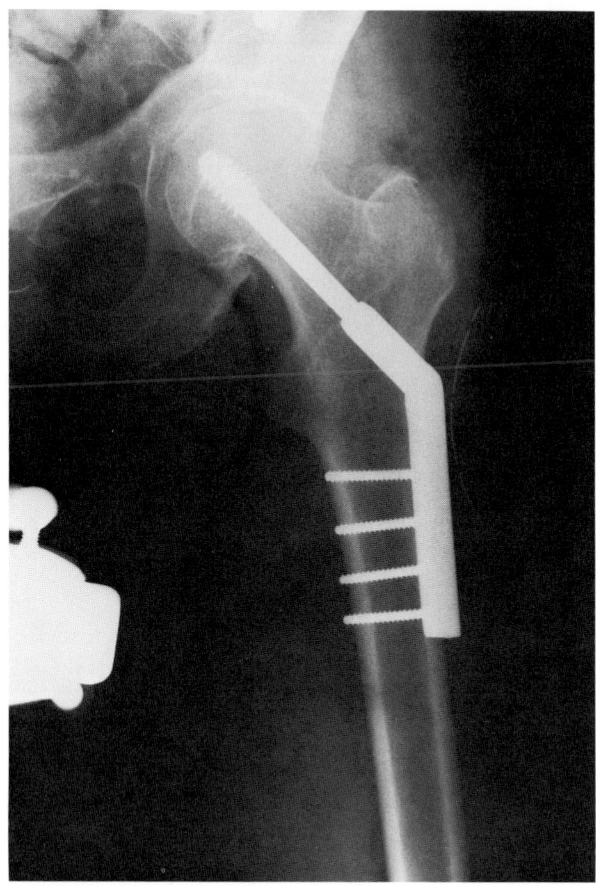

FIG. 16-4. Fracture stabilization system for extracapsular fractures consisting of a heavy lag-screw and an attached side plate.

the lung decreases.[259] All of these morphologic changes reduce the stability of the pulmonary framework that maintains the patency of terminal bronchioles during expiration.[187] The small airways begin to collapse earlier in expiration, increasing the "closing volume" and the "closing capacity" of the lung. Thus, the fraction of tidal ventilation that occurs below

FIG. 16-5. The rate of decline in various physiologic measurements with age. (Adapted from Evans[53] with permission.)

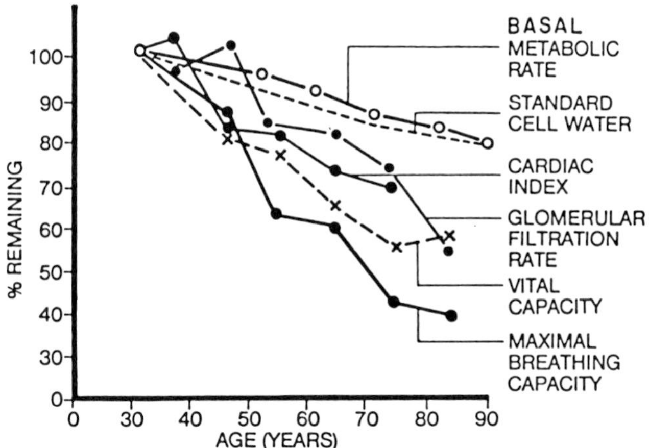


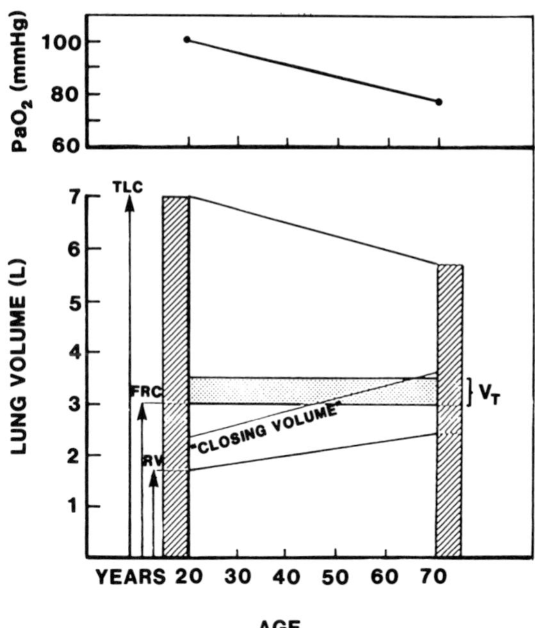


FIG. 16-6. Physiologic changes in $PaO_2$ (*upper panel*) and various lung volumes with age. (Adapted from Pontoppidan et al[187] with permission.)

closing volume increases, predisposing the patient to air trapping, exacerbated ventilation/perfusion ($\dot{V}/\dot{Q}$) abnormalities, and hypoxemia. The $PaO_2$ of the elderly individual with no acute pulmonary changes can be predicted from the following formula described by Raine and Bishop[190]:

$$PaO_2\ (\text{mmHg}) = 103.7 - (0.24 \times \text{age})$$

The $PaO_2$ reduction that normally occurs with a change of body position from upright to supine is also exaggerated in elderly patients for the reasons described above.[261]

The normal respiratory response to hypoxia and hypercarbia is also diminished in the elderly.[112] Further blunting of this response by opioids and inhalational anesthetics leaves the elderly patient unprotected during perioperative hypoxemic periods. Supplemental oxygen must be provided to these patients for at least 24 hours postoperatively.

CARDIOVASCULAR FUNCTION. Age-related cardiovascular changes are summarized in Table 16-3. Basically, cardiac reserve is diminished because of impaired pump function and loss of elasticity of the vascular tree. Myocardial fibrosis, calcification of the endocardium and cardiac valves, narrowing of the coronary and other vital organ vessels, and hypertrophy of the left ventricle all contribute to the diminished reserve and inability of the elderly individual to compensate for the stress of injury, surgery, and anesthesia. These changes are also responsible for the frequent development of hypertension and ischemic heart disease in the elderly.

RENAL AND HEPATIC FUNCTION Both renal and hepatic functions are decreased in the elderly even when the clinical examination and routine laboratory tests are normal. The de-

TABLE 16-3. Age-Related Cardiovascular Changes and their Anesthetic Consequences

| CARDIOVASCULAR PARAMETER | CHANGE | MECHANISM | CONSEQUENCE DURING ANESTHESIA |
|---|---|---|---|
| Resting heart rate | Decrease | Decreased sinoatrial node activity<br>Decreased catecholamine content and adrenergic receptors | Increased incidence of ventricular dysrhythmias |
| Ability to increase heart rate | Decrease | Decreased sinoatrial node activity<br>Decreased catecholamine content and adrenergic receptors<br>Diminished baroreceptor response | Decreased response to vagolytic agents<br>Decreased ability of the heart to compensate for the myocardial depressant effects of anesthetics<br>Decreased ability of the heart to compensate for intravascular volume depletion |
| Stroke volume (at rest and during stress) | Decrease | Myocardial fiber atrophy<br>Increased amount of connective tissue replacing heart muscle<br>Diminished response to circulating catecholamines | Decreased responsiveness to stress<br>Increased $O_2$ extraction by peripheral tissues during stress<br>Delayed onset of intravenously administered anesthetic agents<br>Faster onset of inhalational agents |
| Cardiac index (at rest and during stress) | Decrease | As described for stroke volume | As described for stroke volume |
| Peripheral vascular resistance | Increase | Decreased arterial distensibility due to replacement of elastic tissue with fibrous connective tissue | Decreased cardiac output<br>Contracted blood volume<br>Hypertension |
| Organ blood flow | Decrease | Arteriosclerosis<br>Decreased distensibility of vessels | Decreased ability to compensate for increased demand and/or decreased supply, such as hypotension. |

cline in renal function results from a reduced glomerular filtration rate (1.5% for every year after age 30) and impaired tubular function.[92,215] Glomerular filtration decreases because of decreased cardiac output and internal aging of the glomeruli, which is manifested histologically by glomerular fibrosis and capillary degeneration. The ability of the kidney to excrete anesthetics, muscle relaxants, other metabolized drugs, and normal body waste products is decreased.

As the muscle mass of the geriatric patient is decreased, creatinine production is less than that of young patients. Thus, normal serum creatinine levels do not rule out the presence of limited renal excretory function.[141] Creatinine clearance is a far more reliable index of renal function in the elderly and may be as low as 33% of normal values by age 70.[215] In contrast, an elevated serum creatinine level in a patient in this age group suggests serious renal dysfunction.

The best indicator of altered hepatic function in the elderly is the bromosulfophthalein (BSP) retention test.[248] This test is considered abnormal if more than 10% of BSP is retained in the serum 30 minutes after injection. Based on this test, a gradual decline in hepatic function has been observed in patients over age 50.[248]

With decreasing hepatic function, the capacity of the liver to conjugate lipid-soluble drugs is impaired. Thus, many drugs that rely on hepatic conjugation for clearance are retained, with a resultant prolonged increase in concentration and a reduced dose requirement in the elderly. Thiopental dosage, for instance, is decreased in patients of age 60 and above.[29,141] Likewise, as compared with young adults, a fivefold increase in the plasma concentration of propranolol, which is eliminated almost entirely on the first pass through the liver, may be seen in aged patients without evidence of hepatic, renal, or cardiac disease.[141] Diazepam elimination is also prolonged in the elderly because of altered hepatic biodegradation.[141]

Advanced age may also have some effects on serum protein levels and drug binding to these proteins. Not only are serum proteins decreased in the elderly but also the affinity of some drugs to proteins is less. Thus, slightly more free drug is available in the serum, increasing its clinical effects. The effects of thiopental, etomidate, and temazepam are augmented by this mechanism, whereas midazolam, lidocaine, propranolol, and meperidine binding is unaltered in the elderly.[274]

It is clear from the above discussion that close attention to drug dosing is extremely important in the elderly if toxicity and prolongation of effects are to be avoided.

CENTRAL NERVOUS SYSTEM (CNS) FUNCTION. Aging brings about changes in cognitive, sensory, motor, and autonomic functions.[141] Cerebral perfusion pressure and oxygen consumption are decreased. It is also possible that cerebral autoregulation is altered in the elderly, exposing them to the risk of cerebral ischemia during hypotension. Varying degrees of dementia are not uncommon in the elderly and may be due to decreased cerebral blood flow or localized areas of cerebral infarction.

### *Pre-Existing Diseases*

In addition to the age-dependent decline in organ function, an increased prevalence of disease contributes to the increased perioperative morbidity and mortality of elderly persons with hip fracture. A detailed survey revealed pathologic findings in 92% of 204 female geriatric hip fracture victims. Cardiovascular diseases were present in 78%, mental abnormalities in 39%, pulmonary diseases in 14%, endocrinopathies in 12%, and neurologic disturbances in 10% of these patients.[82] Obviously many patients suffered from more than one disease, a situation confirmed by other surveys of the geriatric population.[270] A list of commonly encountered pathologic conditions in patients with hip fracture is shown in Table 16-4. Since many of these patients have been under medical care for their diseases before injury, they commonly present with a history of drug therapy, often with multiple medications. In the series described above 87% of female patients were receiving drug therapy before hip fracture.[82] Digitalis preparations, β-blockers, calcium channel blockers, and antihypertensives are the most commonly used medications. Such polypharmacy may increase the risk of perioperative drug interactions. Also noteworthy is the frequent observation that alcohol, sedative, and psychotropic drugs are used in excess by some elderly hip fracture victims.[193,249] Review of these disease states and concurrent drug therapy is beyond the scope of this chapter. The reader is referred to Chapter 8 and several other excellent reviews on this subject.[83,207,242]

### *Physiologic and Pathologic Disturbances Produced by the Injury*

The $PaO_2$ reduction seen in elderly patients with hip fracture is in excess of the degree of age-related change predicted by the standard formula of Raine and Bishop.[131,190,220] It is generally considered that this profound decrease in $PaO_2$ is related to the fracture and its consequences. The mechanism of this phenomenon has not been clearly defined. It may be related to atelectasis and pneumonia resulting from prolonged perioperative supine positioning. However, hypoxemia has been noted in patients with no radiologic evidence of pulmonary pathology and in those seen shortly after injury.[220] Posttraumatic microthromboembolism without clinical and radiologic signs is another possibility, but there is little evidence to prove this hypothesis. Pulmonary fat emboli can be found in 80–90% of long bone fractures, especially after prolonged immobilization, although clinically apparent fat embolism syndrome occurs only in approximately 1% of these patients.[231,232] In fact, an increase in $V_D/V_T$ ratio lasting 1 to 5 days after injury has been demonstrated in up to 89% of patients.[131] It is possible that platelets activated by this mechanism may aggregate in the blood and subsequently accumulate in the pulmonary vascular bed. However, treatment of patients with hip fracture with the platelet aggregation inhibitor aprotinin failed to elevate the $PaO_2$ despite increasing blood platelet counts.[220] It seems likely that the excess reduction in $PaO_2$ is caused by a combination of the injury-related factors described above.

TABLE 16-4. Commonly Encountered Pre-Existing Pathologic Conditions in Elderly Patients with Hip Fracture

| SYSTEM | PATHOLOGIC CONDITION |
|---|---|
| Cardiovascular | Hypertension |
| | Congestive heart failure |
| | Atrial fibrillation |
| | Various intracardiac conduction blocks |
| | Sick sinus syndrome |
| | Ventricular extrasystole |
| | Angina |
| | History of myocardial infarction |
| | Valvular lesions |
| | Intermittent claudication |
| | Status postcoronary artery bypass surgery |
| Respiratory | Reactive airway disease |
| | Emphysema |
| | Pneumonia |
| Neurologic | Cerebral vascular accident |
| | Dementia |
| | Parkinson's disease |
| | Epilepsy |
| Endocrine | Diabetes |
| | Thyroid disease |
| Others | Deafness |
| | Meniere's syndrome |
| | Glaucoma |
| | Cataract |
| | Osteoarthritis |
| | Poor self-care |

Based on our own experience and reports from other institutions.

Patients with hip fracture may also develop deep vein thrombosis (DVT) and occasionally pulmonary embolism. As described by Virchow in 1856 three major factors are thought to contribute to DVT—venous stasis, changes in blood constituents, and damage to the vessel wall. Immobilization after hip fracture results in venous stasis. Plasma fibrinogen, factor VIII, and the platelet count increase 12–24 hours after injury and produce a hypercoagulable state.[90] Damage to vessel walls can occur during the traumatic event. To our knowledge, this damage has not been shown in patients with hip fracture, but considerable distortion of the femoral vein has been demonstrated with manipulation of the leg during total hip replacement.[241] Unfortunately, clinical signs and routine coagulation tests are of little value as early indicators of DVT. On the other hand measurement of blood factor VIII-related antigen (F VIII:Ag) and factor VIII procoagulant activity (F VIII:C) has been shown to be a useful indicator of hypercoagulability and intravascular coagulation.[213] Disproportionate increases occur in both F VIII:Ag and F VIII:C activities in patients developing DVT.[163] In addition, the F VIII:Ag/F VIII:C ratio increases in the presence of DVT.[213] Measurement of these factors may make early diagnosis of DVT possible in hip fracture patients in the future. Further information on DVT and pulmonary embolism is offered later in this chapter and in Chapter 28.

## THE TIMING OF SURGERY FOR HIP FRACTURE

Deciding when a hip fracture should be repaired is often difficult and is a subject of major controversy. Three views emerge from numerous reports in the literature. According to the old view, hip fracture is an emergency, and surgery should be performed urgently.[137] Lowell[126] stated,

> The patient is usually in his best state of health the moment before injury and a fractured hip is a surgical emergency. The pain and immobilization in the interval between fracture and fixation only increase the severity of associated medical conditions and slide the patient along a continuing path of deterioration.

He recommended, however, that such medical problems as cardiorespiratory disease, anemia, and diabetes should be brought under control before surgery is done within 12–24 hours of injury. There is evidence that a delay in reduction and internal fixation of femoral neck fractures increases the incidence of delayed union and avascular necrosis of the femoral head.[20] According to the second view, emergency surgery is not indicated and may increase morbidity and mortality following hip fracture repair.[3,108,124,275] The protagonists of this view suggest adequate general preparation to optimize the patient's status.

A more modern concept, which represents the third view on the issue, is to perform surgery immediately after adequate optimization of coexisting medical complications. Certain conditions, such as hyperglycemia, atrial fibrillation with rapid ventricular rate, and bronchospasm, are easy to recognize and treat. Evaluation of other diseases, such as myocardial ischemia, may require extensive tests that may not be possible in an acutely injured patient. The approach described by Schultz et al.[225] permits both evaluation and treatment of underlying hemodynamic, respiratory, and metabolic derangements in patients with hip fracture. Their protocol is shown in Figure 16-7. After an admission workup, the patient is transferred to a special care unit where a pulmonary artery catheter is introduced to obtain physiologic measurements including ventricular function curves. If medical problems are found during this period, appropriate therapy is instituted and a repeat profile obtained to ensure adequate optimization. Surgery is performed as soon as the underlying abnormalities are corrected. The physiologic surveillance of the patient is continued throughout the postoperative period. By using this approach, Schultz et al.[225] modified the widespread notion of orthopedic surgeons that patients should undergo surgery within 24 hours after the fracture. They stated that the "appropriate time for surgery should be accurately determined and chosen on the basis of optimal physiologic balance." The mortality rate in their monitored group was 2.9% as opposed to 29% in the unmonitored group, despite a mean interval of 3.7 days between admission and operation.

## CHOICE OF ANESTHESIA

Spinal and epidural anesthesia are the two most commonly used techniques for hip fracture repair because they reduce surgical blood loss,[41] decrease the likelihood of DVT and pulmonary embolism[44] and attenuate the stress response to trauma and surgery.[42] Decreased blood loss is brought about by sympathetic blockade-induced lower extremity vascular changes that include diminished blood flow in small vessels and decreased venous pressure.[149] Since, during meticulous surgery, most bleeding is from small vessels, the decrease in blood flow to these vessels produced by epidural or spinal anesthesia results in a decreased blood loss. A few studies have demonstrated a reduction in surgical blood loss during general anesthesia with induced hypotension. However, generalized vascular changes in the elderly, who are the most likely group of patients to present for hip surgery, may preclude the use of a hypotensive technique, or render it unsafe.

The trauma- and surgery-induced coagulation response is also altered by epidural and spinal anesthesia.[43,147] A summary of these changes is provided in Table 16-5. Surgery induces an intraoperative hypocoagulable state and postoperative hypercoagulability. Enhanced fibrinolysis and decreased factor VIII activity are mainly responsible for the intraoperative changes.[147] Decreased platelet, antithrombin III, and fibrinogen levels result from hemodilution, rather than from active mechanisms.[43] Hypocoagulability during surgery is likely to prevent clot formation. In contrast, venous thrombosis may occur during the postoperative or postinjury phase because of the presence of hypercoagulation. Epidural or spinal anesthesia extending into the postoperative phase reduces the likelihood of venous thrombosis by the following mechanisms:[148] (a) increasing lower extremity blood flow; (b) counteracting the effects of factors inhibiting fibrinolysis; (c) reducing factor VIII activity; and (d) possibly decreasing platelet aggregation, which may be a direct effect of the local anesthetic, rather than a result of anesthetic technique.[36] General anesthesia does not prevent postoperative deep vein thrombosis.

The suppression of the general stress response to lower ex-

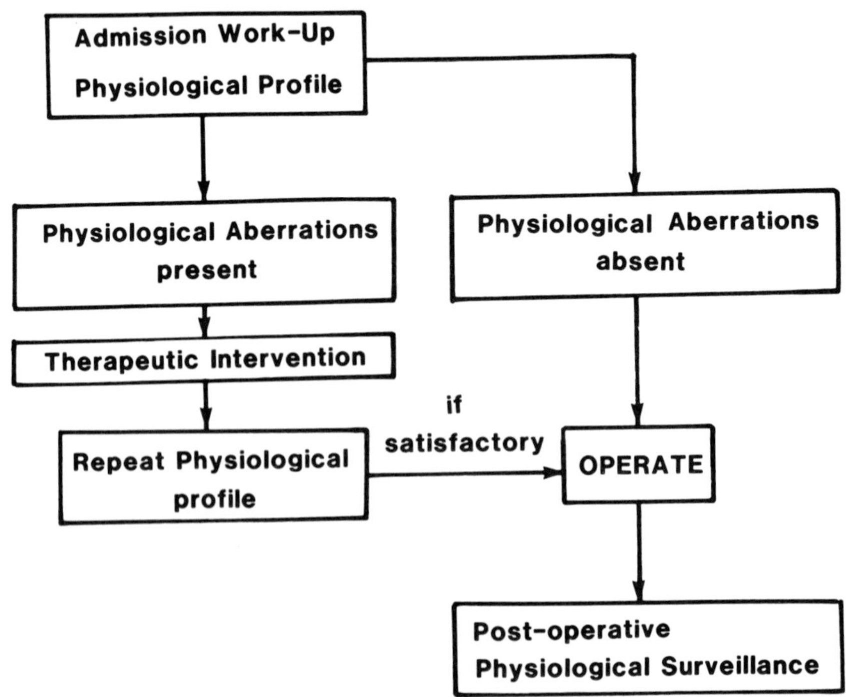


FIG. 16-7. Management algorithm for hip fracture proposed by Schultz et al. (Adapted from Schultz et al[225] with permission.)

TABLE 16-5. Intraoperative and Postoperative Changes of Hemostasis

| INTRAOPERATIVE (HYPOCOAGULABLE) | POSTOPERATIVE (HYPERCOAGULABLE) |
|---|---|
| Increased fibrinolysis | Decreased fibrinolysis |
| Decreased factor VIII activity | Increased factor VIII activity |
| Decreased platelet activity | Increased platelet activity |
| Decreased antithrombin III | Increased antithrombin III |
| Decreased fibrinogen | Increased fibrinogen |

tremity trauma or surgery by limb denervation was first demonstrated by Egdahl[52] in 1959. Recently, Davis et al.[42] were able to demonstrate that a low, predominantly unilateral spinal anesthesia is sufficient to suppress the neuroendocrine response to elective hip surgery. Whether blocking of the neuroendocrine and hemodynamic response to surgery is beneficial has, to our knowledge, not yet been clearly determined. In any case such suppression does not occur with general anesthesia unless extremely large doses of narcotic or inhalation agents are administered.

Some authors also claim that regional anesthesia is more effective than general anesthesia in reducing postoperative confusion and maintaining mental function in the elderly.[30] Postoperative confusion occurred in 44% of elderly patients with femoral neck fractures in one series.[14] In contrast to the general belief, the rate of this complication did not appear to be reduced by regional anesthesia. Instead, it correlated closely with a history of pre-existing mental depression and with the use of drugs with anticholinergic effects. Many psychotropic agents commonly used by the geriatric population contain anticholinergics and thus contribute to postoperative mental dysfunction. An important cause of postoperative confusion is the hypoxemia that, as previously mentioned, is common in this group of patients.[14]

Despite the advantages of regional anesthesia described above, postoperative mortality is affected little by the choice of anesthetic technique. Between 1977 and 1984, seven prospective randomized trials compared the mortality rate of hip fracture surgery under general and regional anesthesia (Table 16-6). In only one of these trials could a significant reduction in both short- and long-term mortality with regional anesthesia be demonstrated,[140] whereas another showed reduction only in short-term mortality.[139] In the remaining five studies neither short- nor long-term mortality was significantly reduced, although there was a tendency to a lower death rate when regional anesthesia was employed.[37,41,138,265,267] Unfortunately each of these trials contained a relatively small number of patients, reducing the significance of their results. More recently, two prospective trials, each comparing postoperative mortality of more than 500 elderly hip fracture victims after spinal and general anesthesia concluded that the type of anesthesia had no effect on short- or long-term mortality of these patients. (Table 16-7).[45,257] In the light of available information, these results can be interpreted in the following ways:

- Physiologic derangements caused by the hip fracture or its surgical repair are so great that they cannot be counteracted effectively by the relatively minor beneficial effects of regional anesthesia.
- The beneficial effects of regional anesthesia are offset by known (hypotension, stress of being awake during surgery, medication with sedatives and narcotics, etc.) or unknown side effects of the technique.
- Death in these patients is determined by the presence of pre-existing conditions and the development of postoperative complications, and regional anesthesia has little effect in improving either of these factors.

In fact, in the two large trials mentioned above, a clear linkage was demonstrated between hip fracture mortality and the pre-existing condition of the patient and/or postoperative complications. (Table 16-8).[45,257]

Although a useful criterion to demonstrate the efficacy of a therapeutic method, mortality may be too crude and insensitive an index to show differences between therapeutic modalities. Thus, future work that selects more sensitive indices may be able to show differences between regional and general anesthesia for hip fracture surgery.

TABLE 16-6. Mortality Rates from Hip Fracture Repair with General and Regional Anesthesia in Seven Prospective Trials Conducted Between 1977 and 1984

| AUTHORS | TYPE OF REGIONAL ANESTHESIA | MEAN AGE (YR) | MORTALITY GA (%) | MORTALITY REGIONAL ANESTHESIA (%) | STATISTICAL SIGNIFICANCE (*p*) |
|---|---|---|---|---|---|
| Couderc et al.[37] (1977) | Epidural | 86 | 24 | 14 | NS |
| McLaren et al.[140] (1978) | Spinal | 76 | 28 | 7 | <0.005 |
| McKenzie et al.[138] (1980) | Spinal | 75 | 15 | 10 | NS |
| White & Chappell[265] (1980) | Spinal or psoas block | 80 | 0 | 0 (spinal)<br>7 (psoas) | NS |
| Davis and Larenson[41] (1981) | Spinal | 80 | 13 | 4.5 | NS |
| Wickstrom et al.[267] (1982) | Epidural | 81 | 6.5 | 6 | NS |
| McKenzie et al.[139] (1984) | Spinal | 74 | 16 (2 wk mortality) | 4 (2 wk mortality) | <0.05 |
| McKenzie et al.[139] (1984) | Spinal | 74 | 18 (2 mo mortality) | 17 (2 mo mortality) | NS |

GA = general anesthesia.

TABLE 16-7. Short- and Long-Term Results of Two Prospective Studies Comparing Mortality Rates of Hip Fracture Surgery with General and Spinal Anesthesia

| AUTHORS | TOTAL NUMBER OF PATIENTS | MEAN AGE (YR) | SHORT-TERM MORTALITY[a] SPINAL (%) | SHORT-TERM MORTALITY[a] GENERAL (%) | LONG-TERM MORTALITY[b] GENERAL (%) | LONG-TERM MORTALITY[b] SPINAL (%) |
|---|---|---|---|---|---|---|
| Valentin et al.[257] (1986) | 578 | 79 | 6 | 8 | 32 | 28 |
| Davis et al.[45] (1987) | 538 | 79.5 | 6.6 | 5.9 | 20.4 | 20.4 |

[a] Cumulated mortality 28 and 30 days after surgery in Valentin et al. and Davis et al. study, respectively.
[b] Cumulated mortality 2 years and 1 year after surgery in Valentin et al. and Davis et al. study, respectively.

## INTRAOPERATIVE ANESTHETIC CARE

The objectives of intraoperative management of the elderly hip fracture victim are careful titration of anesthetic and adjunct drugs, provision of adequate sensory analgesia and motor paralysis, prolonged postoperative pain relief, prevention of pulmonary aspiration, avoidance of major hemodynamic respiratory and metabolic disturbances, and preservation of body temperature. These objectives can be realized regardless of the anesthetic method employed. Recently, there has been a trend among clinicians toward combining regional and general anesthetic techniques, which allows maintenance of a plane of general anesthesia that is often just deep enough to enable the patient to tolerate an endotracheal tube. Preliminary data suggest but do not prove an overall reduction of morbidity with this technique.[196,276]

### *General Anesthesia*

Generally, longer elimination half-lives, lower volume of distribution, and decreased clearance of drugs increase the effects and duration of anesthetic agents in the elderly. For instance, the dose of thiopental should be reduced by 30 to 40%[29] because the decreased initial distribution volume results in higher plasma concentrations than are seen in young persons.[93] Diazepam's duration of action is also greatly prolonged in the elderly. The elimination half-life of fentanyl is increased by 350%, necessitating prolongation of the dose interval.[222] Age does not seem to affect alfentanil pharmacodynamics,[116] but does slow its elimination.[227] Thus, reduced doses of intravenous anesthetics and opioids are sufficient in elderly patients.

TABLE 16-8. Factors Correlating with Mortality after Hip Fracture Surgery

| FACTORS INCREASING SHORT-TERM[a] MORTALITY | FACTORS INCREASING LONG-TERM[b] MORTALITY |
|---|---|
| Preoperative | |
| Coronary artery disease | Coronary artery disease |
| Congestive heart failure | Congestive heart failure |
| Arrhythmias | Arrhythmias |
| ASA status III and IV | Dementia |
| Age above 85 | Age above 85 |
| Male sex | Surgical delay (>24 h) |
| Trochanteric fracture | Male sex |
| | ASA status III and IV |
| Postoperative | |
| Cerebrovascular accident | Cerebrovascular accident |
| Pneumonia | Pneumonia |
| Acute renal failure | Acute renal failure |

[a] Short-term refers to 1 month postoperative mortality.
[b] Long-term refers to 1 to 2 years postoperative mortality.
(From Valentin et al[257] and Davis et al[45] with permission.)

Muscle relaxation is often necessary to permit manipulation of the fractured limb. Intermediate-acting nondepolarizing muscle relaxants (atracurium or vecuronium) are preferred since they are less likely to produce residual postoperative paralysis in the elderly.[33] Nevertheless, a nerve stimulator must be used regardless of the type of muscle relaxant employed.

A faster rate of alveolar partial pressure rise, coupled with a lower blood-gas partition coefficient of inhalational agents in the elderly, results in a more rapid induction than in young persons.[118] Consequently, the hemodynamic effects of these agents are abrupt in the elderly. Among the three potent inhalational agents, isoflurane is probably the best choice for the aged as it is metabolized the least, does not sensitize the heart to catecholamines, enables rapid emergence from anesthesia, produces good muscle relaxation, maintains the cardiac output reasonably well, and probably has the least effect on the cerebral circulation. Coronary artery steal and thus regional myocardial ischemia[23] are possibilities with this agent, but the importance of this phenomenon in humans is unclear.

Glycopyrrolate is probably the best choice for reversal of neuromuscular blocking agents in the elderly as it is associated with a low incidence of tachycardia.

A disadvantage of general anesthesia is that it provides little postoperative pain relief. Thus, other analgesic techniques as described in Chapter 23 are required.

### *Regional Anesthesia*

Excellent sensory and motor blockade for manipulation and surgery in the lower extremity is obtained with spinal, epidural, or lumbosacral plexus anesthesia. To administer these blocks, we usually place the patient in the lateral decubitus position with the injured side uppermost. For spinal anesthesia either 1% tetracaine or 0.75% bupivacaine is administered. The dose of these anesthetics should be adjusted carefully to avoid high levels of blockade and therefore hypotension. The usual doses of hyperbaric tetracaine and bupivacaine for hip surgery are 8–10 mg and 10–12 mg, respectively. If a hyperbaric solution is used, the patient should be placed in the supine position immediately after injection of the anesthetic to allow spread of the agent to the injured side. Alternatively, hypobaric tetracaine can be used to provide anesthesia only of the nondependent (fractured) hip, although the patient must be maintained in the lateral position for a longer period of time. The usual hypobaric concentration of 0.1% tetracaine is generally inadequate to provide satisfactory motor blockade; 0.15% tetracaine produces adequate muscle relaxation.[104] If the operation is performed in the lateral decubitus position, as for insertion of an Austin-Moore prosthesis, hypobaric spinal anesthesia may be associated with patient discomfort because of pressure-induced pain in the unanesthetized dependent hip. In these circumstances, after adjusting the level of anesthesia in the nondependent part of the body, hyperbaric anesthetic solution can be administered through the same needle to provide anesthesia to the dependent side.

Winnie[271] noted that hypotension occurred most commonly when the patient was transferred from the gurney to the fracture table after spinal anesthesia. Fluid loading before administration of the anesthetic is thus very important in order to maintain hemodynamic stability.

Technical difficulties may arise during spinal puncture in up to 10% of elderly patients, probably because of perivertebral calcification.[45] In our experience, epidural anesthesia is easier and more successful than spinal anesthesia in these patients. It permits a more accurate adjustment of the anesthetic level by intermittent injection of the agent through an indwelling catheter. Hypotension also occurs more gradually during epidural anesthesia than during spinal anesthesia, allowing time for treatment with fluids. The occasionally seen delayed or incomplete blockade of the $L_5$-$S_1$ segment with this technique can be prevented by using a high concentration of local anesthetic (lidocaine 2% or bupivacaine 0.75%).

Mixing epidurally or intrathecally administered local anesthetics with morphine or opioid agents may provide prolonged postoperative analgesia. Morphine, 0.2–0.4 mg, can be added to subarachnoid tetracaine or bupivacaine solution without any adverse effects on the quality of anesthesia.[105] Higher doses of morphine (1 mg) result in an unacceptably high incidence of side effects, such as respiratory depression, nausea, vomiting, and pruritus.[40] The recommended dose of morphine that may be added to epidurally administered lidocaine or bupivacaine is 4 mg.[234] Fentanyl, 200 μg, added to epidural bupivacaine solution has been shown to have several beneficial effects: shorter time of local anesthetic spread, greater duration of analgesic block, better sedation during operation, and reduction of shivering episodes.[216] However, this mixture may be associated with several disadvantages: reduction of motor blockade, incomplete sacral blockade, occasional itching and bladder dysfunction after surgery, and delayed intestinal transit.[216]

Meperidine, the only narcotic with local anesthetic effects, can produce surgical anesthesia and prolonged postoperative analgesia (24–36 h) if injected into the subarachnoid space at a dose between 0.5 and 1.0 mg/kg.[54] The moderate hypotension that follows administration of 1.0 mg/kg appears to be caused by reduced systemic vascular resistance.[38] Subarachnoid meperidine provides some motor block[38,54] and is associated with delayed respiratory depression similar to that seen with morphine, especially if parenteral narcotics are administered. All patients who are given spinal narcotics, especially morphine, should be observed closely for at least 12–18 hours after the last injection.

The lumbosacral plexus can be blocked by depositing 30–35 mL of 1.5% lidocaine or 0.5% bupivacaine in the psoas compartment as described by Chayen et al.[28] and Winnie et al.[272] The plexus is sandwiched between the quadratus lumborum muscle anteriorly and the psoas muscle posteriorly. The patient is placed in the lateral decubitus position with the injured side uppermost. A line is drawn between the iliac crests to locate the L4-L5 interspace. The block needle is introduced at the level of the posterior superior iliac spine 5 cm lateral to the lumbar spinous process (Fig 16-8). A 15-cm 20-gauge block needle connected to a nerve stimulator is advanced perpendicularly to the patient's back until a twitch of the quadriceps muscle is elicited with a current of 0.5–0.7 mA. Alternatively, the psoas compartment can be located by the loss of resistance technique. To obtain satisfactory anesthesia in the hip region,[9,169] the sciatic nerve must also be blocked by using 10–15 mL of local anesthetic solution. In experienced hands the success rate of psoas block is 90%.[28]

FIG. 16-8. Surface landmarks to determine the injection point (⊗) of psoas compartment block. The vertical dashed line connects the iliac crests and helps in locating the L4-L5 interspace. The injection point is at the level of the posterior superior iliac spine approximately 5 cm lateral to the lumbar spinous process. If the psoas compartment cannot be located with this approach, the needle entry point is moved cephalad toward the vertical dashed line for about 1–3 cm. (From Chayen et al[28] with permission.)

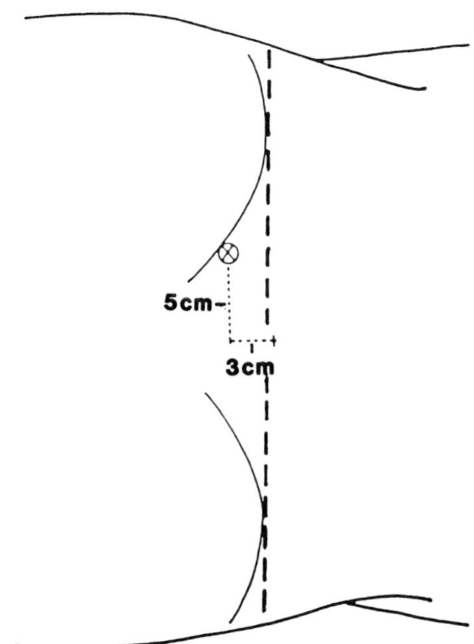

### *Prevention of Pulmonary Aspiration*

As mentioned earlier, pharyngeal, laryngeal, and airway reflexes are depressed in many elderly persons.[186] Intraoperatively administered sedatives and narcotics may depress these reflexes further and result in pulmonary aspiration in patients with a full stomach. General anesthesia with an endotracheal tube to protect the airway is the safest choice when depressed airway reflexes are suspected.

### *Minimizing Hemodynamic, Respiratory, and Metabolic Disturbances*

The patient with hip fracture may have an intravascular fluid deficit of up to 1200–1500 mL[126,242] because of hematoma around the fracture site and poor oral intake after injury. Preoperative evaluation and restoration of intravascular volume with fluids and blood will minimize intraoperative hypotension. Adequate oxygen transport to vital organs must be maintained. In young trauma victims there is little difference in oxygen consumption when the hematocrit is between 30 and 40, even though oxygen delivery is greater at a hematocrit of 40.[60] This lack of difference may not apply to the elderly trauma victim who cannot increase cardiac output during hemodilution or stress.[210] Thus, it is wise to maintain the hematocrit between 35 and 40 in these patients during the perioperative period. All efforts must be made to avoid tachycardia, hypertension, and hypotension during the perioperative period in order to prevent ischemia and possibly infarction of the heart or brain. In addition to routine intraoperative monitoring, an arterial line and a central venous pressure line (pulmonary artery catheter, if necessary) must be inserted as an aid to hemodynamic management. Because of a high incidence of ischemic heart disease, all elderly patients with hip fracture must be monitored with electrocardiogram leads II and $V_5$. Blood gas levels must be measured frequently to assess oxygenation and acid-base status.

Occasionally the entire hip may require replacement. In these instances, the use of polymethyl methacrylate cement to secure the acetabular and femoral prostheses may result in a fall in arterial pressure and hypoxemia. Hypotension is more common after insertion of the cement into the femoral shaft than into the acetabulum. The cement is supplied as the liquid monomer; powdered methylmethacrylate polymer is used to induce polymerization of the monomer. The two are mixed together before application. The liquid monomer is highly toxic and is responsible for the hemodynamic changes: peripheral vasodilation, increased cardiac output, tachycardia, and hypotension. Thus, the cement should be used when it is as stiff as possible in order to minimize the residual concentration of the monomer.

Embolism of air introduced into the femoral shaft during reaming of the femur is another mechanism of hypotension.[4,123] The air can easily escape into open venous channels upon insertion of the cement, which may produce an intramedullary pressure as high as 1900 mm Hg.[123] Reaming of the femur itself contributes greatly to the increase in intramedullary pressure and causes a decline in systemic and pulmonary artery pressure with an associated reduction in left ventricular $dP/dt_{max}$.[195] This hemodynamic change is thought to be mediated by a neurally transmitted reflex.[195] Venting of the femoral shaft should theoretically reduce the pressure in the medullary cavity, but has been shown to have little effect.[123] Therefore, arterial blood pressure should be monitored closely during reaming of the femur and application of cement. Intravascular volume must be replaced adequately before cement application to limit hypotension. Measures to detect embolism—transesophageal echocardiography, precordial Doppler, end-tidal $CO_2$, and end-tidal nitrogen—must be at hand. Hypoxemia after insertion of the prosthesis may last up to 30 minutes. It is probably caused by pulmonary embolism of crushed medullary fat during insertion of the femoral prosthesis.[106] Methylmethacrylate is a fat solvent and may predispose to fat embolism by increasing absorption of fat from the femoral marrow.[123] However, hypoxemia, as was mentioned, occurs frequently in the elderly even without the application of cement.[131,220] Supplemental oxygen must be administered for at least 24 hours postoperatively whether the patient received spinal or general anesthesia, and arterial oxygen saturation should be checked frequently.

### *Body Temperature Preservation*

Diminished heat-generating ability in the elderly dictates the preservation of body temperature by warming the operating room, surgical prep solutions, and intravenous fluids. The use of heated humidifiers or heat-moisture exchangers may be necessary. Shivering must be prevented or treated as it increases oxygen consumption by as much as 400%.[128]

In hypothermic patients, assessment of blood gases requires the application of a correction factor for $PaO_2$ but not for $PaCO_2$ and pH. The treatment of pH on the basis of temperature-corrected values may result in suboptimal enzyme function.[155,194]

## POSTOPERATIVE COMPLICATIONS

Pneumonia, myocardial infarction, congestive heart failure, cerebrovascular accident, arrhythmias, acute renal failure, bleeding gastric ulcer, deep vein thrombosis, and pulmonary embolism are the major complications of hip fracture and are associated with high mortality. Management of these complications is discussed separately in other chapters of this book.

Deep venous thrombosis (DVT) occurs in about 25–30% of patients with hip fracture.[151] Various prophylactic regimens, including subcutaneous heparin (5000 units every 8 to 12 hours daily), dextran infusion (500 mL), aspirin (3–6 tbl/day), combined heparin-dihydroergotamine, warfarin, and cyclic compression of the calf veins with a Venodyne® unit have been used.[61,219] Heparin prophylaxis has been somewhat disappointing in preventing thromboembolic complications after orthopedic trauma. Data compiled from eight randomized prospective trials of subcutaneous heparin prophylaxis are shown in Table 16-9.[35] As can be seen, the incidence of DVT with heparin prophylaxis is almost half of that without heparin.

TABLE 16-9. Effect of Subcutaneous Heparin in Preventing Thromboembolic Complications After Orthopedic Trauma[a]

| GROUPS | TOTAL NUMBER | NUMBER OF PATIENTS WITH | | | |
|---|---|---|---|---|---|
| | | DVT | NONFATAL PE | FATAL PE | BLEEDING COMPLICATIONS |
| Heparin prophylaxis | 321 | 82 | 4 | 5 | 4 |
| No heparin prophylaxis | 303 | 148 | 0 | 7 | 6 |

[a] Data from eight randomized trials.
Abbreviations: DVT = deep vein thrombosis; PE = pulmonary embolism.
(Adapted from Collins et al[35] with permission.)

However, the incidence of fatal and nonfatal pulmonary embolism remains unaffected by heparin prophylaxis.

## MANAGEMENT OF PELVIC INJURIES

Pelvic fractures represent a significant cause of mortality and disabling morbidity because of their association with major organ system trauma and their proximity to major blood vessels and nerves and to the genitourinary and gastrointestinal tracts. Early mortality is caused by intractable external hemorrhage from compound fractures or from expanding or ruptured retroperitoneal hematomas, whereas late mortality is often secondary to pelvic or generalized sepsis and multiorgan failure following soft tissue injuries and prolonged low-flow states. Neurologic injuries causing peripheral neuropathy, lower extremity motor dysfunction, and chronic pain[174,175,263]; genitourinary injuries resulting in incontinence and impotence; and pelvic injuries leading to diminished weight-bearing capacity account for most chronic morbidity and disability.

Trauma victims who have sustained pelvic fracture present with a wide spectrum of injury severity. Much of this variability is attributable to the type of pelvic fracture and to other organ system trauma.[99] In general, however, patients can be classified into one of three major categories. Exsanguinating hemorrhage occurs from external bleeding in open fractures or from retroperitoneal hematoma in closed fractures in about 0.5–1% of patients.[154,221] These patients almost always arrive in the hospital with either severe hypotension or cardiac arrest and rarely respond to any resuscitative measures. Approximately 75% of pelvic fracture victims are hemodynamically stable and have a relatively uncomplicated course, requiring initial emergency department evaluation, admission to the orthopedic surgery service, and pain relief. Later in the course of their hospitalization some of these patients may require urgent[69] or elective[260] surgery for repair of bony and ligamentous pelvic disruptions. The remaining 25% of patients with pelvic fracture are in the intermediate group, usually presenting in a critical condition with varying degrees of overall injury severity, hemorrhage, and hemodynamic instability. Associated extrapelvic injuries involving the head, neck, face, thorax, abdomen, and long bones are often significant factors affecting outcome in this group of patients.[99,159,255]

### CLASSIFICATION OF PELVIC FRACTURES

In order to assess the type and severity of pelvic fractures and to aid in formulating a management plan, surgeons have devised various classification systems.[50,62,159,164,179,256] Although from the standpoint of anesthetic management there is little necessity for knowing the details of these systems, some knowledge of their bases is helpful in assessing injury severity and in making a rough prediction of complications, morbidity, and mortality.

#### *Mechanism of Injury*

Pelvic fractures result from three well-defined forces on the pelvic girdle: anteroposterior compression, lateral compression, and vertical shear.[229] Although pelvic fracture is seldom the result of a unidirectional force since significant stresses frequently act in other directions, the dominant distorting force is usually in one direction. Anteroposterior compression forces on the pelvic ring push the anterior pelvic component (symphysis and rami) backward, producing a lateral strain on the relatively weak anterior ligaments of the sacroiliac joints. The posterior sacroiliac ligaments are strong and are usually not affected. Therefore, they act like the spine of a book, promoting tearing and separation of the anterior ligaments by laterally directed stress. This separation is then reflected to the anterior pelvic components, resulting in separation of the symphysis pubis and thus giving the pelvis the appearance of an open book (open book fracture) (Fig. 16-9). Anteroposterior forces can also cause fractures of the pubic rami. These fractures usually result from motor vehicle accidents or entrapment of the victim between two objects.

Lateral forces cause ramus fractures and separation of the symphysis pubis but not without involvement of the posterior pelvic components. With lateral displacement of the anterior pelvic components, the posterior pelvis is forced medially, and fracture of the anterior portion of the sacrum may occur. Lateral forces acting on the femur produce a different pattern, sually resulting in fracture of the acetabulum. Motor vehicle-pedestrian accidents and falls from an altitude onto the victim's side are the usual causes of these injuries.

Vertical shear forces produce the most devastating pelvic injuries since they are almost always associated with substantial bleeding. Fracture dislocation in the vicinity of the

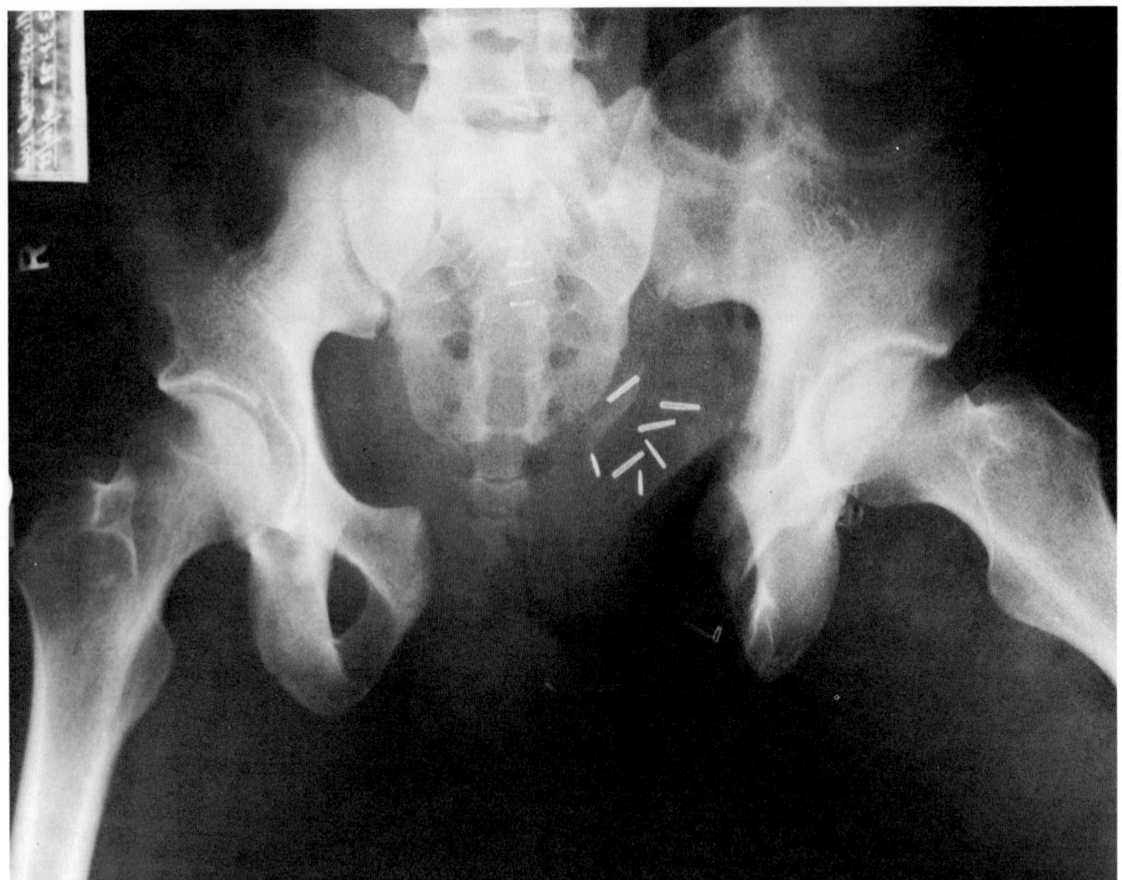

FIG. 16-9. Anteroposterior pelvic X-ray of a motorcycle accident victim. Note the symphyseal dysjunction giving the pelvis the appearance of an open book.

sacroiliac joint allows migration of the entire hemipelvis superiorly, and hemorrhage results from vessels that are lacerated or transected by the fracture fragments. Falls from an altitude onto the legs or the ischial spine generally produce this type of injury.

### *Fracture location*

The fracture may involve the pelvic ring or the wing of the ilium. Pelvic ring fractures may produce serious structural distortion, hemorrhage, and damage to the abdominopelvic organs. Iliac wing fractures, although painful, can generally be ignored unless they also involve the acetabulum or sacroiliac joint. Fractures that primarily involve the posterior portion of the pelvic ring are more commonly associated with concomitant organ and vessel injuries, massive hemorrhage, and late complications and thus have a higher mortality rate than pure anterior pelvic fractures.[67]

### *Stability of the Fracture*

Movement of bone fragments in unstable fractures is a constant threat to adjacent soft tissue, organs, and vessels. Instability of the pelvis is largely diagnosed by direct palpation and by applying pressure to the anterior iliac spines; movement of the fracture during this manipulation defines the unstable pelvis. Cryer and coworkers[39] also consider the pelvis unstable if there is symphysis pubis diastasis or if the gap between bone fragments is greater than 0.5 cm on anteroposterior pelvic X-ray. Morbidity and mortality are considerably less in stable than in unstable injuries.

### *Open, Closed, and Comminuted Fractures*

A major difference in morbidity and mortality exists between open and closed pelvic fractures. Open fractures, in which the fracture site communicates with the air via lacerations in the perineum, buttocks, or vagina, have an increased rate of hemorrhagic and infectious complications (Fig 16-10).[199] Comminuted fractures cause a greater degree of pelvic instability and hemorrhage and produce more morbidity and mortality than noncomminuted fractures. Thus, an unstable, open, comminuted posterior pelvic ring fracture accompanied by a vertical shear injury to the sacroiliac joint with cephalad displacement of the hemipelvis would be at an extremely high risk for major hemorrhage, associated injuries, and infection.[59,67]

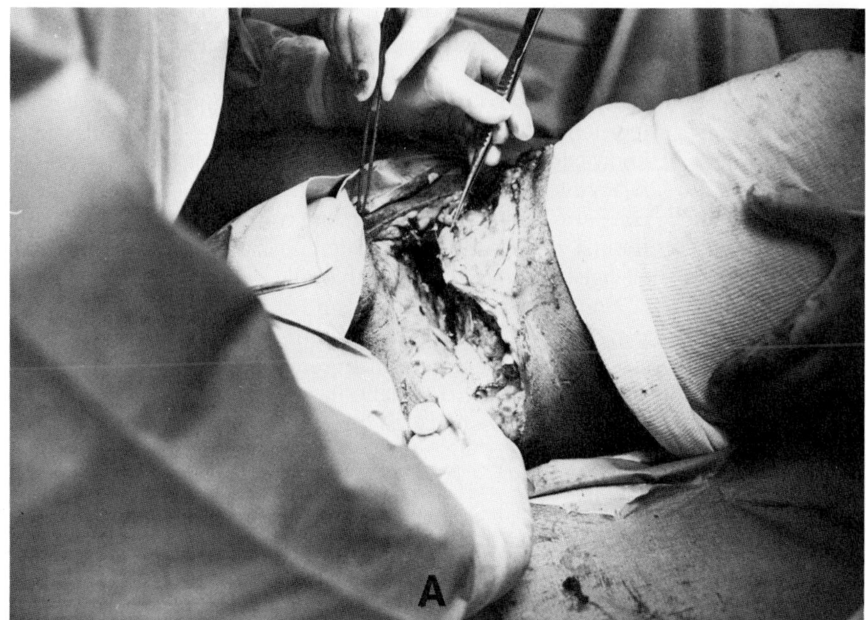


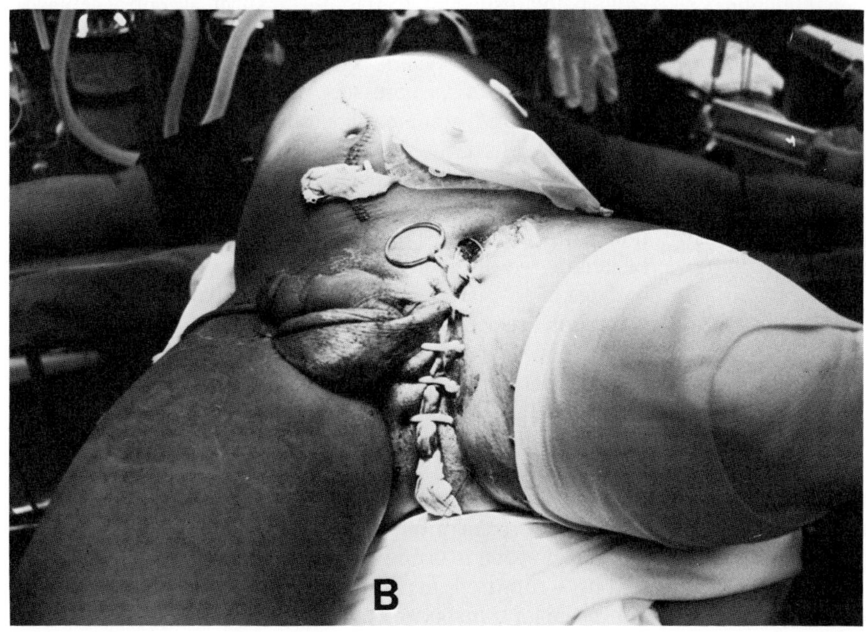


FIG. 16-10. (A) Open pelvic fracture with severe perineal injury involving the rectum after a motorcycle accident. (B) The same patient after laparotomy, debridement and closure of the wound, and colostomy. Note also the amputated left leg.

## DIAGNOSIS

Identification of pelvic fracture in the trauma patient is based on information about the mechanism of injury, physical examination, and diagnostic tests. Pelvic fracture should be strongly suspected if the injury is caused by a motor vehicle accident, crushing impact, fall from a height, or penetrating trauma (gunshot, shotgun, stab, or impalement),[161,230] which cause, respectively, 60%, 30%, 5%, and 5% of these injuries.[110] The presence of suprapubic pain; significant low back pain, or extremity shortening, weakness, and/or diminished sensation should suggest pelvic fracture.[255] These complaints can easily be overlooked or ignored by the evaluating physician in the presence of more prominent symptoms and signs of hemorrhage and associated injuries.

Physical examination may reveal swelling in the suprapubic and groin areas, point tenderness of the pubis and/or iliac spines, and swelling and ecchymosis of the medial thigh, genitalia, and lumbosacral area.[229] Swelling and ecchymosis, which result from dissection of sequestered pelvic blood through the fascial planes, develop gradually and may be absent if prehospital transport time is less than 30 minutes. Lacerations of the buttock, groin, and perineum may be seen and are likely to be indicators of open (compound) fractures.[229] Bleeding from the urethral meatus, vagina, or anal orifice is a common sign of pelvic fracture and is associated with genitourinary or rectal injury. Evidence of pelvic instability should be sought by applying anteroposterior and lateral pressures to the anterior iliac spines.[229] A positive finding should alert one to the possibility of fracture of the posterior pelvic elements and the attendant risk of bleeding.[67] Rectal examination is of crucial importance; it not only permits assessment of rectal sphincter tone, which if flaccid indicates the presence of nerve injury, but also provides information about injury to the genitourinary tract, the second most frequent direct complication of pelvic fracture.[255] The presence of blood and/or bone fragments in the rectum is a strong sign of intestinal perforation. A free-floating, superiorly displaced, or edematous prostate gland indicates an injury to the membranous portion of the urethra, the most common genitourinary complication of pelvic fractures in men. In women, urethral injury is less frequent, probably because the urethra is short and the urogenital diaphragm is less well developed.[255]

Definitive diagnosis of pelvic fractures is made by X-ray. An anteroposterior pelvic X-ray must be obtained routinely in all major blunt trauma victims at the same time as chest and cervical spine films to avoid delay in recognition of pelvic injuries.[160] Although adequate visualization of pelvic fractures can be achieved only with at least two additional oblique X-rays,[255] the difficulties and dangers of positioning the patient during initial evaluation and resuscitation make anything more than this single anteroposterior view impractical and hazardous. If further information is needed, computed tomography (CT) scanning of the pelvis is obtained as it provides the most accurate identification of bony injuries[22,51] without requiring alteration of the patient's position. In most instances, transporting the patient to the radiology suite does not present an additional inconvenience since CT scanning is usually necessary to evaluate injuries of other regions of the body.

## MANAGEMENT STRATEGY

The severe acute physiologic derangements seen in 30–40% of pelvic fracture victims require active early resuscitation efforts. In the emergency department they should be performed according to the American College of Surgeons Advanced Life Support guidelines (see Chapter 2). Depending on the staffing structure of the trauma center, a member of the anesthesia department might be assigned to the emergency department and participate actively in the resuscitation of the patient, or he or she may be available for emergency consultation when complex airway management problems arise during the resuscitation phase. Under any circumstances, it is appropriate to establish an institutional policy of informing the anesthesiology department as soon as the ambulance personnel notify the emergency department that the victim is en route to the hospital. Doing so enables the anesthesia team to make final preparations not only in the operating room but also in the angiography suite to which many pelvic trauma patients are transported directly from the emergency department.

At the conclusion of initial evaluation and resuscitation, the duration of which varies between 5 and 30 minutes, the hemodynamic condition of the patient falls into one of the three possible categories: (a) normotensive and stable, (b) severely hypotensive (systolic BP < 60 mm Hg, exsanguinating), or (c) mild to moderately hypotensive (systolic BP 80–100 mm Hg) but stable with ongoing fluid resuscitation. The overall management plan of each of these conditions differs substantially and is controversial in some instances, but most centers follow the algorithm shown in Figure 16-11. Adequate knowledge of the management strategy will enhance the efficacy of the anesthesiologist. Of course, the importance of constant communication among various specialties of the trauma team cannot be overemphasized, and the anesthesiologist is no exception to this rule.

Normal systolic blood pressure and hemodynamic stability can be achieved in nearly two-thirds of pelvic fracture patients who arrive in shock. In this group detailed evaluation of associated injuries, especially those involving the thorax and abdomen, is possible with use of diagnostic peritoneal lavage, additional X-ray studies, and while CT scanning of the pelvic fracture is addressed. Depending on the result of these evaluations, a decision is made whether the patient will be transported to the operating room, the angiography suite, or directly to the intensive care unit.

In exsanguinating patients, management options are restricted. These patients are rushed to the operating room, while being resuscitated en route, for surgical control of bleeding. Anesthetic management of these patients involves ventilation with oxygen, aggressive volume replacement, administration of vasopressors, treatment of acid-base abnormalities, and other cardiopulmonary resuscitation measures as required.

The management protocol for patients whose systolic blood pressure can be maintained between 80–100 mm Hg with fluid resuscitation is somewhat controversial; however, all clinicians agree on giving priority to the treatment of any associated life-threatening injuries. Abdominal injuries are most commonly associated with pelvic fractures and require early recognition. Thus, the management strategy is guided by diagnostic peritoneal lavage (DPL) performed shortly after the initial evaluation and resuscitation. As is discussed later, this diagnostic method is associated with some pitfalls in the presence of pelvic fractures, but gross blood from the peritoneal cavity is an indication for abdominal exploration to control hemorrhage from intraperitoneal organs. The pelvic retroperitoneal space is examined during exploratory laparotomy; finding a ruptured, expanding, or pulsating hematoma is an indication for transporting the patient to the angiography suite for embolization. If the DPL is negative, the decision to perform diagnostic angiography is based on the rate of bleeding; a transfusion requirement greater than 4 units within the first 24 hours or 6 units in less than 48 hours is, according to some authors, an indication for this test and for embolization if it reveals arterial bleeding.[69,159] Similarly, angiography is performed in any patient with a documented pelvic fracture in whom other specific sites of hemorrhage cannot be demonstrated once 4 units of blood have been given during the initial hours after trauma. Efforts to control pelvic bleeding in the operating room and/or the angiography suite usually last longer than 3 to 4 hours. After angiography and possibly embolization of the bleeding artery, management objectives are directed to continuation of resuscitation as necessary and management of newly discovered or previously ignored associated injuries and of the pelvic fracture.

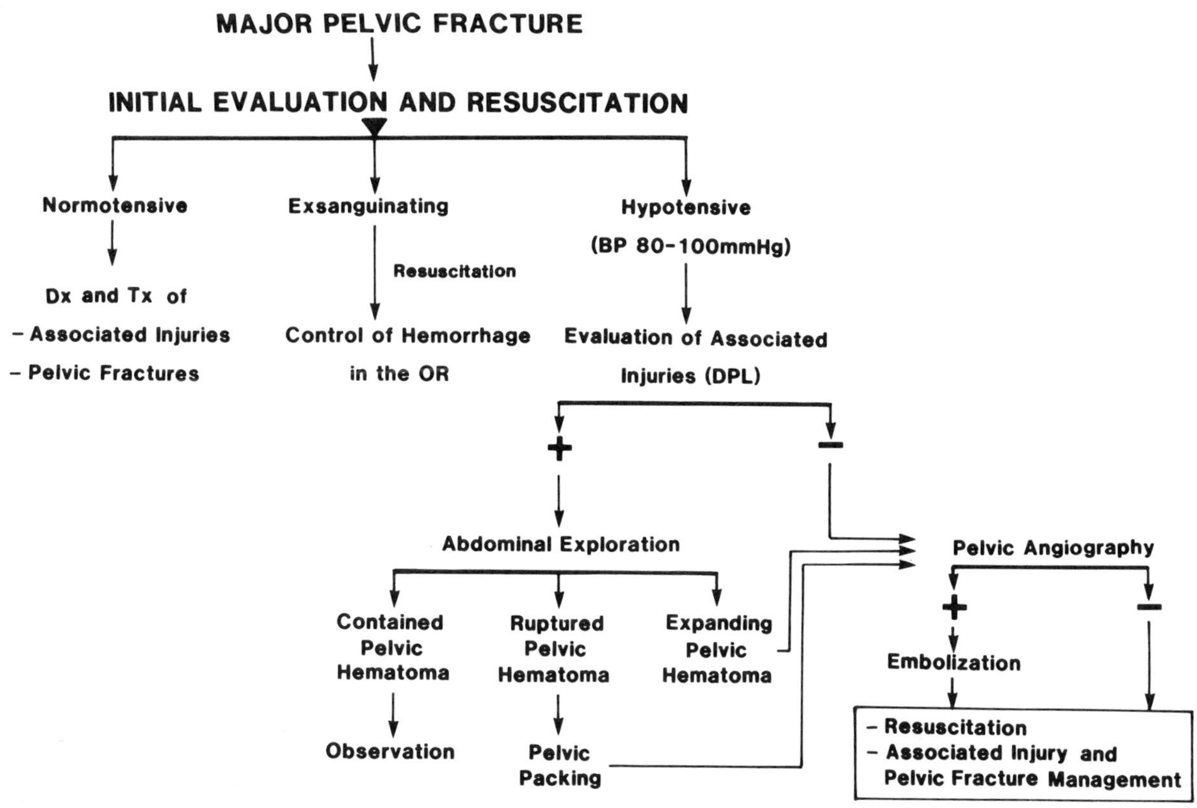


FIG. 16-11. The algorithm followed in most centers for initial evaluation and treatment of major pelvic fractures.

## COMPLICATIONS OF PELVIC FRACTURES AND THEIR MANAGEMENT

### *Hemorrhage*

As mentioned, hemorrhage is the most frequent acute complication and the foremost concern in the initial management of major pelvic fractures. As can be seen in any pelvic angiogram, a close relationship exists between the bony pelvis and the rich pelvic vasculature (Fig 16-12). Brotman and coworkers[19] have described the arterial network of the pelvis as four interconnected collateral loops: posteromedian, anteromedian and two laterals. The segmental vertebral plexus and the lumbar, medial sacral, posterior division of the internal iliac, iliolumbar, lateral sacral, and superior gluteal arteries form the posteromedian loop (Fig 16-13). Some of these vessels traverse the posterior wall of the bony pelvis, whereas others pass through the sacral foraminae, explaining the frequent occurrence of arterial damage associated with fracture or dislocation of the sacroiliac joint, sacrum, or ilium. The anteromedian vascular loop is formed by branches of the anterior division of the internal iliac artery that interconnect with the gonadal, superior epigastric, and superior rectal arteries and with tributaries of the external iliac and femoral vessels.[19] This loop supplies blood to the pubis, ischium, perineum, and pelvic viscera and is injured in pubic fractures and symphysis pubis separation. The lateral loop is formed by collaterals between the femoral and internal iliac arteries.

Veins accompanying these arteries are also at great risk of

FIG. 16-12. A normal pelvic angiogram showing the close relationship between the pelvic skeleton and the arterial network. (Courtesy of Richard Lefleur, MD.)

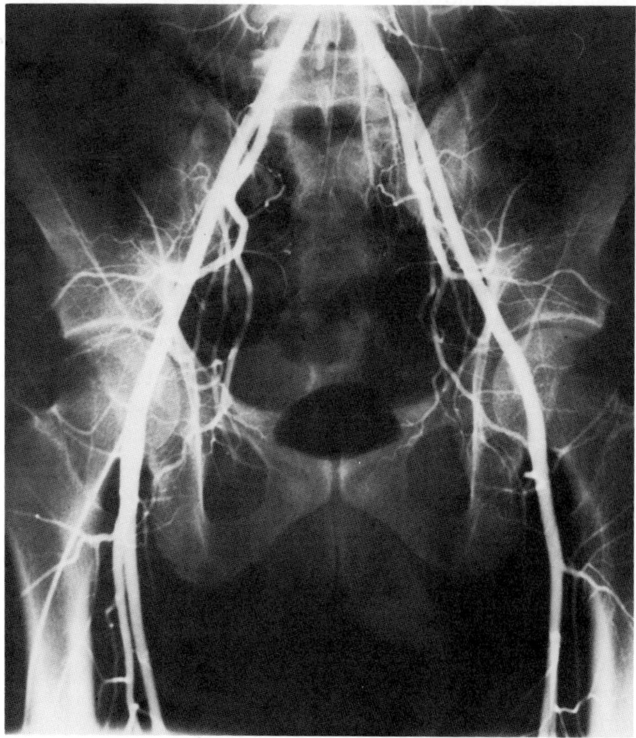

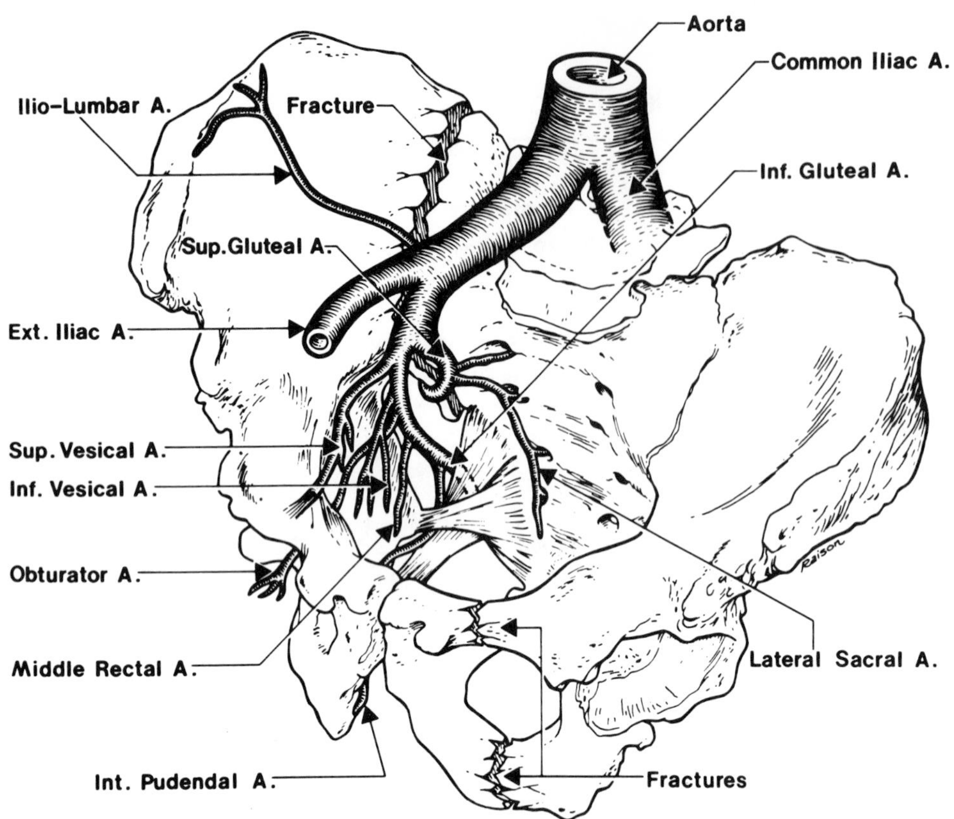


FIG. 16-13. The relationship between pelvic skeleton and most posteromedian loop arteries. (From Brotman et al[19] with permission.)

being injured directly in pelvic fractures. In addition, the link between the superior rectal vein and the valveless portal venous system contributes to the abundance of bleeding from the pelvic veins, since pelvic venous injury can result in reversal of portal flow away from the liver and toward the pelvis.[19]

This rich interconnection of vessels explains why occlusion of a single trunk, such as the hypogastric (internal iliac) artery, does little to decrease hemorrhage after pelvic trauma.[59,229] In addition, single-vessel injury is rare; pelvic fractures are usually associated with multiple injuries to small arteries and veins,[98] although in only 6–18% of patients is hemorrhage primarily from the arterial system.[39,66]

The pelvis has been described as a vascular sink because it represents a distensible reservoir for blood flowing antegrade from the aorta and retrograde from the portal circulation.[19] The retroperitoneal space can accommodate several liters of blood before any appreciable tamponade occurs.[229] Nevertheless the main factor limiting the extent of hemorrhage from pelvic fractures is the tamponading effect of the pelvic tissues. As high pressures are capable of overcoming this effect, bleeding from pelvic arteries is more severe than that from pelvic veins. In open pelvic fractures, however, both arterial and venous systems may bleed profusely because of the lack of any resistance to outflow.[199]

Many attempts have been made to predict the extent of hemorrhage that might be expected after specific pelvic injuries. However, none of the systems, which classify pelvic fractures according to location, number, and stability of fractured components of the pelvic ring, can identify with high reliability the specific victims who are likely to exsanguinate. The most recent of these classification schemes, proposed by Cryer et al,[39] divides pelvic fractures into two categories: stable and unstable. By their definition stable fractures include those in which displacement of the fractured segment is less than 0.5 cm. Open book fractures, which involve disruption of the pubic symphysis, are not included in this category even though they may be stable. Unstable fractures include open book fractures and all fractures with greater than 0.5 cm displacement on an anteroposterior pelvic radiogram. Based on this classification, one can be 90% confident that 50–69% of patients with unstable fractures will require 4 or more units and 30–49% more than 10 units of blood during the ensuing 48 hours.

Recognition that hemorrhage is occurring is not difficult. Hypotension, acute reduction of the hematocrit, increased heart rate, and, if available, a decrease in central venous pressure in the face of vigorous administration of fluids and blood are all important signs of this condition and can indicate the diagnosis even to those who do not deal with pelvic fractures on a regular basis. Difficulty arises, however, in differentiating the site of bleeding in the multiple trauma victim—whether it is from the pelvic fractures or from associated injuries and whether it is arterial or venous. These distinctions are important because measures required to control the hemorrhage vary according to the site of bleeding.

The most common extrapelvic sources of hemorrhage include long bone fractures and intrathoracic and abdominal injuries. Diagnosis of long bone fractures and intrathoracic injuries is relatively straightforward, requiring only physical examination and skeletal and chest X-rays. Diagnostic peritoneal lavage (DPL) is the initial test of choice for diagnosis of intra-abdominal hemorrhage. Ideally, after examination of the urethral meatus and rectum, a Foley catheter and a nasogastric tube should first be inserted to decrease the likelihood of injury to the stomach and bladder. A supraumbilical cutdown with direct visualization of the peritoneum, instead of the usual infraumbilical approach, avoids perforation of a bulging retroperitoneal hematoma and diminishes the likelihood of a false-positive lavage.[99]

DPL will yield one of three results: (1) gross blood; (2) grossly negative lavage with negative microscopic fluid analysis, which is a good indicator of the absence of significant intra-abdominal pathology[66]; and (3) negative peritoneal lavage with positive microscopic analysis. Gross blood aspirated from the peritoneal cavity is an indication for immediate laparotomy and takes precedence over the management of pelvic hemorrhage. Positive lavage fluid analysis (RBC > 100,000/mm$^3$, WBC > 500/mm$^3$) also indicates bleeding from intraperitoneal organs. There is, however, a significant incidence of negative laparotomy in patients with pelvic fracture who have a positive DPL. The incidence of false-positive results in the presence of pelvic fractures may be as high as 28%.[97,171] This high incidence is attributed to the migration of blood from the retroperitoneum into the peritoneal cavity,[199] rupture of the hematoma, or perforation of the retroperitoneal hematoma by the trochar. Mortality from unnecessary laparotomy in these patients is high because of uncontrollable bleeding; it reached 30% in one study.[97] For this reason, some authors have suggested abdominal CT scans and/or abdominal and pelvic angiography as an adjunct to DPL before deciding on laparotomy.[66]

Differentiation between arterial and venous bleeding in pelvic fractures is best made by angiography via one of the femoral arteries or, if both are injured, via an axillary artery (Fig 16-14). Although the pelvic veins are injured more frequently than the arteries, venography is not performed since interpretation of this study is exceedingly difficult. Nevertheless, late phase angiography may sometimes show a site of venous bleeding.

MANAGEMENT OF BLEEDING. As in any acutely bleeding patient, the measures employed to optimize the condition of the hemorrhaging pelvic trauma victim can be divided into two major categories: adequate replacement of blood loss and control of bleeding.

Replacement of blood loss requires effective fluid resuscitation with at least two large-bore catheters, while keeping in mind that lower extremity intravenous access is contraindicated and that warmed fluids should be employed to minimize hypothermia and its complications. Techniques of rapid warmed fluid infusion are discussed in Chapter 9. The importance of blood bank support in hemodynamically unstable patients, whether they are managed in the emergency de-

FIG. 16-14. (A) Pelvic angiogram showing extravasation of radiopaque dye from injured superior gluteal artery (*arrow*). (B) Selective angiogram obtained from the same patient demonstrating better visualization of the lesion (*arrow*). (Courtesy of Richard Lefleur, MD.)

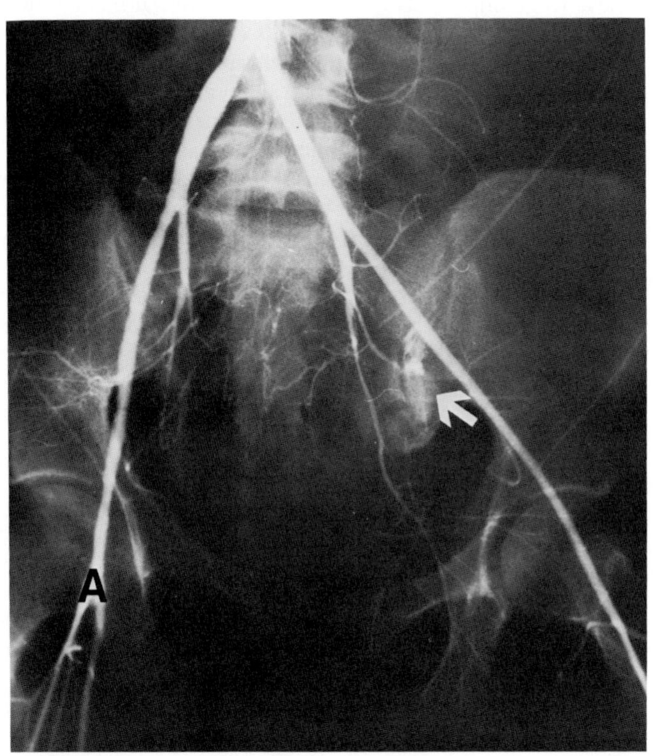


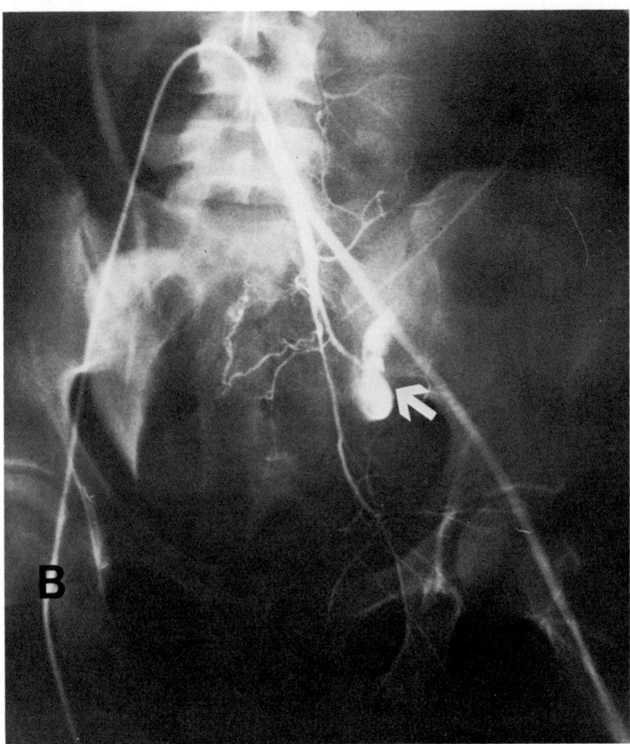

partment, the operating room, or the angiography suite, cannot be overemphasized. Several series describe an average blood requirement of as much as 16 units in the hemodynamically unstable patient.[59,159,171,230] A detailed discussion of massive blood transfusion is offered in Chapter 6.

Various measures are available to control bleeding. None of these is under the direct control of the anesthesiologist, but their use, indications, and complications are intimately related to overall patient care. External bleeding from bone or soft tissues in open pelvic fractures can be controlled with direct suture, ligation of the vessel, or packing of the wound in the emergency department until more definitive measures can be taken in the operating room. In traumatic hemipelvectomy, the transected vessels may contract and bleeding may cease; however, an increase in blood pressure caused by painful manipulations may result in sudden exsanguination. These patients should be taken to the operating room immediately; the pelvic vessels should be ligated under controlled conditions, followed by completion of the hemipelvectomy and wide debridement.[122,152,205]

A contained pelvic hematoma encountered during laparotomy should not be explored.[39,88,256] Release of a retroperitoneal tamponade may result in torrential bleeding from multiple sites with no possibility of achieving surgical control before the patient exsanguinates. If the hematoma is found to be ruptured when the abdomen is opened or rupture occurs during surgery, several options are available. Cross-clamping of the aorta below the origin of the renal arteries decreases the rate of bleeding. As mentioned, ligation of the hypogastric artery has little effect on pelvic hemorrhage. Likewise, balloon catheterization of the hypogastric vessels via infrarenal aortotomy has met with limited success. Packing of the pelvis with laparotomy pads or sterile towels can stop the bleeding effectively and allow repair of any other abdominal injuries.[160] After this repair is completed, the patient may be transferred to the angiography suite for embolization. In a preliminary report, intraoperative embolization of the severely bleeding vessel, using a slurry of autologous blood clot (30 mL) combined with microfibrillar collagen, thrombin, and calcium, stopped the hemorrhage.[221] Although the complications of operative embolization may exceed those of the angiographic approach, its risks may be acceptable in exsanguinating patients.

Control of bleeding from pelvic fractures has been greatly improved during the last decade by the use of three measures: pneumatic antishock trousers (PASG or MAST), orthopedic external fixators, and, as has already been discussed, angiographic embolization techniques. PASG, according to some authors, should be applied to all hemodynamically unstable patients with pelvic fractures in the prehospital phase, especially if transport time exceeds 10 minutes.[159,160] An advantage of this device, in addition to reduction of blood loss and thus improvement of hemodynamics, is provision of some degree of realignment of the fractured fragments. If PASG is not applied in the prehospital phase, its application during the initial evaluation period after a brief examination of the pelvis, external genitalia, rectum, and lower extremities may result in dramatic reduction in venous, but not arterial, blood loss and improvement in hemodynamics.[48,159,160] Thus, it may serve as a diagnostic tool to identify major arterial bleeding and to determine the need for angiography if failure to achieve hemodynamic stability within 2 hours of application occurs.[59] The recommended inflation pressure of the garment is 30–40 mm Hg; at this pressure the device can be left in place for as long as 24 to 48 hours.[48,160] It should be emphasized, however, that some authors feel that this device is associated with serious disadvantages in the hospital as it prevents observation of and ready access to the patient's abdomen, groin, and perineum and causes difficulty in performing selective angiography.[59,164] Deflation of the garment in the operating room or the angiography suite may result in sudden hypotension. It should thus be deflated one segment at a time. In open pelvic fractures or in those with associated lacerations of the thigh, buttocks, or perineum, deflation of the device may be followed by profuse bleeding; the floor must be checked periodically to detect it. Application of the garment may also produce an increase in intracranial pressure, which may be deleterious if the patient has also sustained a closed head injury. Cephalad displacement of intra-abdominal organs may compromise the patient's ventilation; endotracheal intubation and controlled ventilation should be given serious consideration after application of PASG. Finally, skin and muscle necrosis may result from PASG if inflation pressures greater than 30–40 mm Hg are used and protective padding between the skin and the garment is not employed.

Application of external fixation has gained wide popularity in the past 5 years (Fig 16-15). These devices limit pelvic hemorrhage by several mechanisms. They reduce the volume of the pelvic retroperitoneal space by approximating the displaced fracture fragments. Thus, the volume at which bleeding is tamponaded is reduced. Since, in the majority of patients, bleeding is mainly from small vessels on the edges of the fractured bones, patient movement promotes additional bleeding. External fixators reduce this effect by stabilizing these fragments.[253] The advantages of external fixation over PASG are manifold. First, it permits easy access to the lower part of the body, facilitating the performance of peritoneal tap, urethrography, cystography, and femoral angiography. Second, it enables early mobilization of the patient. Third, it does not effect ventilation and intracranial pressure. External fixators are easy to use; they can be applied in the emergency department under local anesthesia in about 10 minutes. The most important disadvantage of external fixators is that they are somewhat inadequate in stabilizing posterior pelvic fractures, allowing bleeding to continue from these sites. Recent advances in pelvic fracture management have demonstrated that early (within 12–36 hours of trauma) open reduction and internal fixation of pelvic fractures is possible and provides better results than external fixators.[69] Of course, this method cannot be used for initial management of hemorrhage, but it may be useful in situations where bleeding persists for several hours.

Transcutaneous angiographic embolization of bleeding arteries has revolutionized pelvic fracture management. Since this technique is effective in controlling only arterial bleeding, proper diagnosis is necessary using both clinical and angiographic measures. The most commonly used embolization materials are Gelfoam and stainless steel coil.[171] Gelfoam permits recanalization of the occluded vessel within 7 to 8 weeks after treatment, allowing restoration of blood supply to the

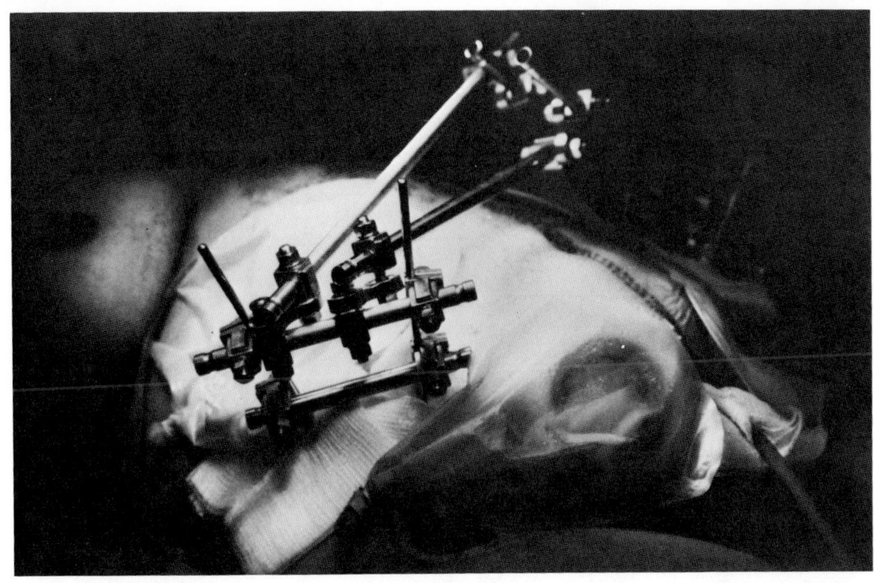

FIG. 16-15. External pelvic fixation device applied to a woman who sustained abdominal and pelvic injuries following motor vehicle-pedestrian accident. The fixator shown on one side of the patient connects in the midline with a similar part of a stabilizing frame from the contralateral pelvis.

pelvic organs.[160] Thrombogenic stainless steel coils, by leaving the vascular lumen patent, have reduced the complications associated with embolization of nonbleeding vessels.[171] Since severe hemodynamic changes occur during embolization, a level of anesthetic care similar to that used in the operating room is essential.[171] The success rate of embolotherapy in management of hemorrhage from pelvic fracture is between 85–95%.[160]

## ASSOCIATED INJURIES

Injuries associated with pelvic fractures can be divided into two categories: pelvic and extrapelvic. Extrapelvic organ injuries are not directly related to the pelvic trauma, but are discussed briefly in this section.

### *Pelvic Organ Injuries*

As has already been mentioned, the frequency of genitourinary complications is second only to that of hemorrhage. The posterior membranous and supramembranous urethra and the urinary bladder are at great risk of injury in pelvic fractures. The incidence of posterior urethral injury in association with pelvic fractures is 58%, of bladder injury alone is 32%, and of combined urethral and bladder injury is 10%.[31] The high incidence of urethral damage results from the immobility of this structure in the pelvis. The vulnerability of the bladder increases when it is full at the time of trauma; thus inebriated patients are more likely to sustain bladder injury than sober victims. Genitourinary injuries occur more frequently after pubic arch fractures than after isolated iliac, acetabular, or sacral fractures, although displacement of the urinary tract by pelvic hematoma occurs with both anterior and posterior pelvic injuries.[31] More than 75% of bladder ruptures are extraperitoneal, and the extravasated urine, which can easily become infected if not recognized, contaminates the pelvic hematoma, resulting in sepsis. Nevertheless, mortality and morbidity after extraperitoneal ruptures are lower than after intraperitoneal ruptures, especially if diagnosis of the latter is delayed.[31] Severe pelvic injuries result in separation of the membranous and supramembranous portions of the urethra. A concomitant injury to the periprostatic venous plexus in these circumstances results in a large hematoma that displaces the prostate gland cephalad and posteriorly.

Placement of a Foley catheter, which is essential during the initial management of major trauma, requires great caution in a patient with pelvic fracture. Such physical signs as an elevated, edematous, or nonpalpable prostate; perineal, scrotal, or penile discoloration and swelling; or blood from the urethral meatus suggest urethral injury and preclude catheterization. Attempts to pass a urinary catheter in these circumstances may further damage the urethra, introduce infection, and possibly increase the rate of impotence and incontinence.[31] However, physical signs alone are not sufficient to diagnose urethral injury. In one retrospective study 57% of men who sustained urethral injury after pelvic fractures had no suggestive physical signs.[125] It takes some time after the injury for perineal discoloration and swelling to occur and for blood to appear in the urethra. Thus, men examined within 1 hour of injury, which is usually the case in urban trauma centers, may not yet have developed these signs. Therefore, it is prudent to perform a retrograde urethrogram routinely in all patients with pelvic fracture before insertion of a Foley catheter during initial management.[31,125]

The classic sign of extraperitoneal bladder rupture is similar to that of pelvic hematoma: a diffuse prominence in the suprapubic area with minimal restriction of abdominal wall mobility. Patients with intraperitoneal rupture show abdominal rigidity and decreased mobility of the abdominal wall. The definitive diagnosis is made by a finding of extravasation of contrast media on a cystogram (Fig 16-16). The initial surgical treatment of both bladder and urethral injuries is suprapubic cystostomy, which should be performed as soon as the resuscitation is completed.[31]

Other organs that may be damaged by sharp fragments of the pelvis include the intestines, pelvic organs, and neural

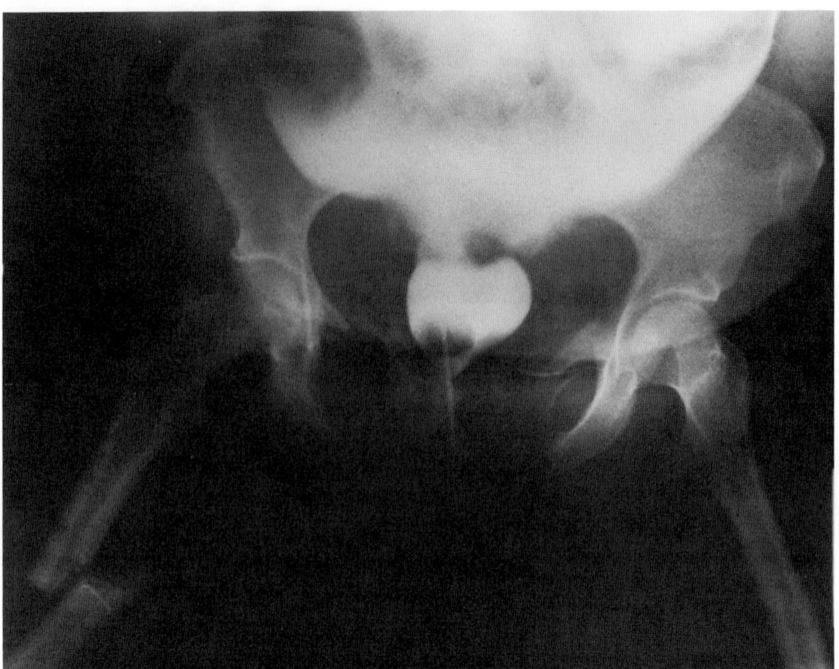

FIG. 16-16. Cystogram showing diffuse leakage of contrast material into the peritoneal cavity in a patient with intraperitoneal bladder rupture. Note the spread of contrast material between radiolucent intestinal loops. In extraperitoneal ruptures the contrast material spreads only to the perivesicular regions. Note also the displaced right femoral shaft fracture.

structures. Intestinal injury can occur anywhere between the jejunum and the anus; however, the rectum and sigmoid colon are the most common sites of injury. Severe sepsis within a few days of trauma is inevitable if the intestinal injury is missed. A diverting colostomy during the initial surgery followed by generous saline irrigation of the distal intestinal segment decreases the likelihood of sepsis, but still leaves a significant percentage of patients at risk. Infection of the soft tissues surrounding the pelvis by aerobic and/or anaerobic organisms occurs frequently, and the patient generally requires multiple operating room visits for debridement.

Gynecologic injuries are infrequent. However, the enlarged pregnant uterus is at significant risk of injury in pelvic fractures. Laceration or rupture of the uterus during the third trimester frequently results in major bleeding, placental disruption, and fetal demise. These injuries may be fatal to the mother as well if recognition and treatment are delayed. Anesthetic management of the injured pregnant patient is discussed in Chapter 19.

Among neural structures, lumbosacral plexus injury may cause serious neurologic abnormalities of the lower extremity and pelvic organs.[174,175] Even in the absence of clinically apparent neurologic signs, injury to the lumbosacral plexus is demonstrated by electromyographic abnormalities in up to 64% of patients with sacral fracture and sacroiliac joint separation.[263]

### *Extrapelvic Injuries*

Pelvic fractures rarely occur as isolated injuries; they are usually associated with other life-threatening extrapelvic trauma involving the head, thoracoabdominal organs, diaphragm, and/or long bones. The signs and symptoms of both pelvic fractures and other injuries may be masked by concomitant head injury, necessitating routine DPL and CT scan evaluation. Associated diaphragmatic rupture is not uncommon and may complicate anesthetic induction by rendering the gastroesophageal junction incompetent and by increasing intrapulmonary shunt because of compression of the lungs by abdominal organs.

## SEPSIS

Contamination of open wounds in the pelvic region or of a pelvic hematoma causes sepsis. The incidence of sepsis is especially high in open fractures in which communication between the pelvic space and external environment results in infection of a pelvic hematoma. Aggressive measures, such as a diverting colostomy in patients with perineal wounds whether or not intestinal injury is present, multiple debridements, frequent dressing changes, and administration of appropriate antibiotics, appear to decrease the incidence and severity of this complication.[199] In rare life-threatening infections such heroic measures as hemipelvectomy may be necessary.[199]

## RESPIRATORY DISTRESS

Respiratory distress occurs rather frequently after major pelvic fractures. During the initial phase of trauma, aspiration pneumonitis, lung contusion, overtransfusion, head injury, and airway obstruction from associated maxillofacial injuries may all be responsible for deteriorating respiratory function. Two additional mechanisms unique to pelvic fractures may also play an important role in the development of respiratory distress. In severe fractures the cephalad spread of a retroperitoneal hematoma displaces the diaphragm, producing a significant decrease in lung volume, atelectasis, and ventilation-perfusion abnormalities. In addition, application of PASG results in cephalad displacement of intra-abdominal contents and compression of the diaphragm, again compromising ventilation.

Many patients arrive in the emergency department in respiratory distress and require immediate airway management. Pulmonary function in those who are not in respiratory distress must be observed carefully since this complication may develop within a short period. In an intubated patient with pelvic fracture, continuously rising airway pressure, declining hematocrit, and hypoxemia should alert the clinician to the possibility of an expanding retroperitoneal hematoma. It is also prudent to intubate the trachea prophylactically and initiate mechanical ventilation if PASG is applied. Sudden respiratory distress a few days after pelvic fracture is likely to be caused by fat- or thromboembolism.

## COAGULATION ABNORMALITIES

As in most multiple trauma patients, coagulation abnormalities occur frequently after major pelvic fractures. Figure 16-17 summarizes the mechanism of coagulopathy in massive trauma and shock.[173] Hypothermia, acidosis, pre-existing liver dysfunction, and tissue hypoxia from hemorrhagic shock are all responsible for the development of this complication. In some patients, especially those with brain or liver trauma, coagulopathy occurs immediately after the injury as a result of massive tissue thromboplastin release.[170] Disseminated intravascular coagulation (DIC) in these circumstances produces further deterioration of oxygenation, thereby aggravating the coagulation dysfunction.

All available resources must be utilized to treat hypothermia. Heat lamps, covering the patient's body with plastic sheets, elevating the room temperature, warming all intravenous fluids, irrigating the stomach with warm saline (if gastrointestinal perforation is ruled out), and heating and humidifying inspired gases will increase or at least maintain the temperature. Of course, shock and acidosis should be treated aggressively by administration of fluids and bank blood, control of bleeding, and at times by use of vasoactive agents. Periodic evaluation of the coagulation profile by observing the degree of oozing from the surgical field and by measuring platelet counts, PT, PTT, fibrinogen (normal, greater than 200 mg/dL) and fibrin split products (normal, less than 10 mg/mL) permits the assessment of the patient's response to therapeutic measures. Alternatively a tube test can be performed to determine clotting function (see Chapter 9). Factor replacement using platelet concentrates and fresh-frozen plasma should be considered if oozing continues.

## ACUTE RENAL FAILURE

With aggressive fluid resuscitation and monitoring, the incidence of this complication has declined during the past two decades. Nevertheless it still occurs in patients with severe bleeding and prolonged shock. Detailed information on this subject is provided in Chapter 25.

## MORTALITY

The majority of studies published before 1970 reported a mortality rate from pelvic fractures between 9 and 50%.[58,87,179] Improvement in trauma care and use of therapeutic embolization and external fixation of fractures during the past two decades have reduced this rate, but even with these advanced methods, overall mortality from this injury remains high, varying in most reports between 5 and 15%.[48,159,256,277] Many factors affect the mortality rate. Mucha and Farnell[159] noted that 42% of patients who presented to the emergency department in shock died, whereas mortality was only 3.4% in those who were hemodynamically stable on admission to the hospital. The mortality rate is high, reaching 40–50%, in open pelvic fractures,[185,214] although more recently Richardson et al.,[199] using an aggressive management protocol, were able to reduce the mortality from these fractures to 5.5%. Mortality is also high in unstable fractures of the posterior pelvic elements, ranging between 12 and 39% in recent reports.[67,79,159,164,230] Age appears to affect the death rate. Dove and co-workers[48] found that 64% of patients who died were over the age of 60, and no patient over the age of 70 survived. In summary, despite significant improvements in management of pelvic fractures during recent years, elderly patients; those with open, unstable, and posterior pelvic fractures; and

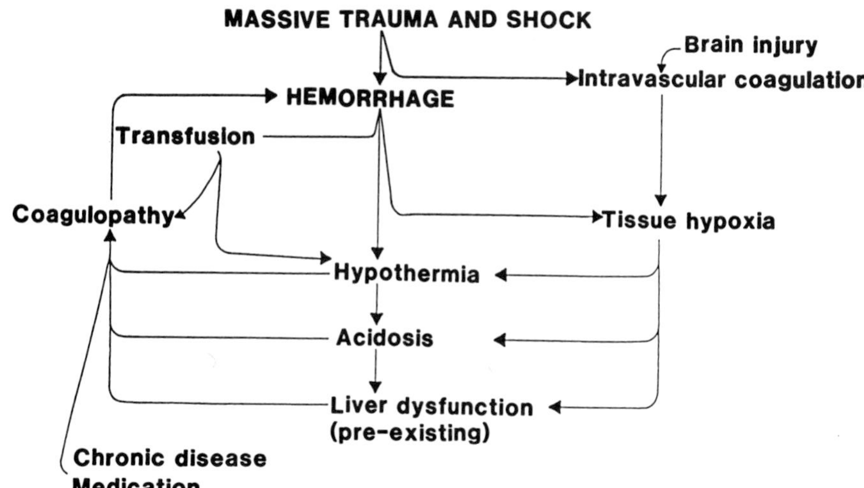


FIG. 16-17. Interacting mechanisms of coagulation abnormalities in multiple trauma victims. (From Patt et al[173] with permission.)

those presenting with exsanguination or hemodynamic instability die at a high rate. It must be emphasized, however, that in many instances death is not directly from the pelvic injury, but rather from associated vital organ trauma. Mucha and Farnell[159] noted that in only 12% of all deaths was pelvic fracture the direct cause. Further improvements in management of these injuries may bring about a better survival rate.

## FAT EMBOLISM

The pathologic and clinical manifestations of fat embolism were first described in the 19th century by Zenker, Wagner, and von Bergman.[150,180,183] Since that time extensive work has been done and numerous reviews[72,157,182,183,206,232,271,268] have been written on the subject; however, many aspects of fat embolism remain poorly understood, and disagreement on its etiology, pathophysiology, diagnosis, and treatment persists. Although fat embolism has been associated with many nontraumatic disorders,[106,235] it is most common after skeletal injury.[201] Thus, an awareness and thorough understanding of this entity are necessary when dealing with trauma patients. This section provides an overview of the topic as it applies to the management of the trauma patient with musculoskeletal injuries.

### INCIDENCE

The incidence of fat embolism is difficult to determine because no uniformly accepted set of diagnostic criteria exist. Fat can be identified in the lungs of as many as 95% of musculoskeletal trauma victims at autopsy,[181] but not all of these patients display the clinical syndrome. Some authors have emphasized the frequent occurence of posttraumatic subclinical fat embolism characterized by the presence of laboratory abnormalities but no clinical symptoms.[136,201] These patients appear to be a subset of the larger group defined by postmortem examination. More than half of the 118 patients with fractures in one prospective series exhibited laboratory abnormalities, although only two demonstrated clinical signs.[201] These two patients appear to represent the more severe end of the spectrum: the clinical fat embolism syndrome. It is clear, then, that laboratory and autopsy findings are of little significance since they seldom correlate with identifiable clinical abnormalities.

The lack of universally accepted diagnostic criteria coupled with the frequent existence of various concomitant injuries and pathologic processes in these patients has made it very difficult to standardize patient populations for study. Undoubtedly, this is one reason for the varying incidences reported in the literature. Although several series determined the incidence of clinical fat embolism in patients with major musculoskeletal injury to be 0.25–1.2%,[181] others have concluded that the figure is as high as 19–29%.[77,121,202] In fact, as Gossling and associates[71] surmise, it may be nearly impossible to collect accurate data on the incidence of fat embolism syndrome since it probably often coexists with other causes of posttraumatic respiratory insufficiency.

Many authors agree that the fat embolism syndrome is most likely to occur in patients with multiple long bone and pelvic fractures, especially those involving the middle and proximal part of the femoral shaft.[32,49] The syndrome seems to have an age predilection. Young men and elderly patients with fractures are important populations at risk.[150]

### PATHOPHYSIOLOGY

Although over the years many authors have attempted to explain the clinical and pathologic findings associated with fat embolism, the pathophysiologic basis of this complication remains controversial. When one examines the plethora of existing hypotheses, two main theories emerge. One, first proposed by Gauss[63] in 1924, suggests that the consequences of fat embolism are a result of physical obstruction of the pulmonary vasculature with embolized fat. The second theory maintains that chemical changes, both in the blood and in the lungs, are of major importance, a position originally enunciated by Lehman and Moore in 1927.[115]

Central to the mechanical theory of fat embolism is the concept that marrow fat gains access to the venous circulation after injury. It is postulated that increased pressure in the marrow cavity resulting from trauma, motion of bone fragments, and/or intramedullary nailing procedures forces the marrow into venous sinusoids from which the fat travels to the lungs and occludes pulmonary capillaries. There is much clinical and experimental evidence to support this hypothesis. Experience from Vietnam demonstrated a lower incidence of hypoxemia—a feature of the fat embolism syndrome—in those casualties whose open fractures resulted in decompression of the medullary cavity of the bone than in those who suffered closed compressive injuries.[34] In rabbits the application of slight uniform pressure with an elastic bandage to a fracture site has been shown to increase intravasation of marrow by raising intramedullary pressure.[86] Another clinical study demonstrated fat in the venous drainage from fractured extremities.[2] In this study, the size and number of fat globules were larger in those patients who developed the clinical fat embolism syndrome. Animal studies have confirmed the presence of fat in the circulation within seconds of injury,[156] and it has been shown that fat found in the lungs originated from bone marrow.[86,109,156,218,237] Obstruction of the lung vessels by fat can lead to cor pulmonale when the compensatory capabilities of the pulmonary vasculature are exceeded. Such mechanical obstruction of lung vessels was demonstrated in rabbits by Peltier,[177] who also showed that neutral fat, not free fatty acids, was responsible for the obstruction. More recently Hagley[81] has drawn attention to the clinical counterpart of this laboratory observation by describing acute cor pulmonale within a few hours of injury in patients with fulminant fat embolism syndrome.

Sometimes fat gains access to the systemic circulation. Embolization to the brain, kidney, and myocardium in the fulminant syndrome may be a result of increased right atrial and ventricular pressures, which result in passage of fat globules through a probe-patent foramen ovale, although convincing evidence that these particles cannot traverse the pulmonary capillaries is lacking.[56] Of course, in the presence of a cardiac septal defect, embolized fat can enter the systemic circulation even in the absence of increased pulmonary vascular resistance.

Lequire and colleagues[117] also believed that the fat embolism syndrome results from simple mechanical obstruction of the lungs by fat. They postulated, however, that the fat that embolizes to the pulmonary vasculature originates from both traumatized fat depots and the coalescence of blood lipids as a result of physicochemical alterations associated with trauma. By invoking both mechanical and chemical means, Lequire's group bridged the two main theories. Peltier[177] also incorporated both mechanisms in his theory of the biphasic pathology of fat embolism. In elegant animal studies he demonstrated that the initial phase of the process is obstructive in nature, and the second phase, which appears after a short (hours) delay, is due to the chemically toxic effects of fat in the lungs. Currently this is the most widely accepted view among clinicians.

The chemical theory, originally proposed by Lehman and Moore,[115] states that lipids that are normally present in the blood coalesce into larger molecules as a result of trauma. More recently, much of the thrust of the chemical theory of fat embolism has focused on the toxic properties of free fatty acids (FFA). In fact free fatty acids are directly toxic to the lungs, causing interstitial hemorrhage, edema, and chemical pneumonitis secondary to destruction of capillary endothelium.[177,180,183] This inflammatory effect of fatty acids in the lung has been confirmed,[172] and some authors have found a correlation between free fatty acid levels and hypoxemia in clinical studies.[168,201]

There is, however, controversy about the origin of the fatty acids. Peltier[177,180,181,183] has proposed that they are liberated in the lungs as a result of the action of increased pulmonary lipase on neutral embolic fat. Others have postulated that the offending fatty acids originate in the periphery. It is well known that the FFA level increases regularly in response to elevated catecholamine levels,[135] and increased levels have been noted after both trauma and surgery.[135,142,168,262] However, there is little current evidence to suggest that FFA derived from peripheral adipose tissue is important in the development of fat embolism syndrome.[223] Mays[135] speculates that FFA levels may be further elevated if liver function is compromised since the liver has an important role in clearing FFA from the circulation. If this is true, coexisting shock, by reducing liver blood flow, should exacerbate the level and toxic effects of FFA. One would also expect greater derangement of pulmonary function to occur with ongoing fat embolism during surgery since hepatic blood flow is decreased by both general and spinal anesthesia.[65]

Some argue that isolated elevation of the peripheral FFA level may not be of paramount importance. Rather, they maintain that the proportion of FFA binding to albumin in the blood may be the main determinant of toxicity. Bergentz[12] suggested that stress-induced fatty acids produced outside the lungs do not result in pulmonary toxicity because their destructive effects are neutralized by albumin binding. In an interesting retrospective analysis, Moylan and co-workers[158] noted that trauma patients who developed fat embolism syndrome had serum albumin levels lower than the asymptomatic group; they suggested that clinical symptoms develop when serum albumin is decreased, for instance, in the catabolic multisystem trauma patient. However, not all investigators subscribe to this notion.

A host of other mechanisms have been proposed for the pathophysiology of fat embolism. Coagulation abnormalities have been implicated by some authors. It has been suggested that fat, which is thromboplastic, triggers disseminated intravascular coagulation (DIC).[217] Several authors have also described fibrinolytic system failure after trauma.[13,107,191,197] Platelet counts are lower in patients with fat embolism syndrome than in patients with similar trauma but without the syndrome.[197] In a prospective study, McCarthy et al.[136] found that the extent of thrombocytopenia was inversely proportional to the lung dysfunction determined by the alveolar-arterial oxygen difference. However, other investigators have not noted DIC in patients with fat embolism.[25]

Clearly, it has not yet been firmly elucidated whether the pathophysiologic changes seen in fat embolism syndrome are caused by neutral fat, free fatty acids, other factors, or a combination of these. In view of its unclear etiology and pathophysiology, Bradford and colleagues[17] have suggested that the fat embolism syndrome be referred to as "posttraumatic respiratory insufficiency." Use of this name for the syndrome makes good sense as it clearly identifies the end result of the pathophysiologic process.

## CLINICAL PRESENTATION AND DIAGNOSIS

Through the years there has been debate about the diagnostic criteria that define the fat embolism syndrome. Thus, a thorough knowledge of the signs and symptoms of the syndrome and a high index of suspicion are needed if the diagnosis is to be made in a timely fashion.

A symptom-free latent period of about 12–48 hours after trauma usually precedes the clinical manifestations of fat embolism.[77,177] Peltier,[180] however, has emphasized that many patients have no latent period and further states that, if careful attention is given to making the diagnosis, a latent period will rarely be seen. This view has been substantiated by others who reported that signs of fat embolism occurred within 12 hours in one-third of their patients.[247] Hagley[80,81] has more recently described the existence of a fulminant form of fat embolism syndrome that presents as acute cor pulmonale, respiratory failure, and/or embolic neurologic phenomena within a few hours of injury.

A characteristic feature of fat embolism syndrome is a petechial rash, usually on the upper portion of the body, including the axillae, upper arms and shoulders, chest, neck, and conjunctivae.[12,176,180,268] Rarely, the rash appears on the abdomen or thighs.[180] There is still a debate about how the petechiae develop, but they probably result from occlusion of dermal capillaries by fat and increased capillary fragility.[268] If there is a pathognomonic sign of fat embolism, it is this rash, and its presence has been said to establish the diagnosis.[176] Several series have reported petechiae in 53–95% of patients with diagnosed fat embolism syndrome.[76,77,153,176,202] The rash usually appears between 12 and 96 hours after injury,[176] but may be evanescent, sometimes lasting for only a few hours.[72,180] One wonders whether, by more careful observation, this sign can be detected more frequently than is usually reported. In any event, the presence of a petechial rash in the characteristic anatomic distribution in a patient with a history of trauma should alert the clinician to the possibility of fat embolism syndrome. Unfortunately, petechiae do not appear early enough in the process to permit institution of possible pharmacologic prophylaxis.[224]

Other physical findings seen in the fat embolism syndrome include tachypnea, dyspnea, rales, and cyanosis.[180] Clinically, the respiratory impairment resembles that seen in adult respiratory distress syndrome (ARDS). Nonspecific findings of fever and tachycardia have been noted. Allardyce et al.[2] state that a fever of 38.6°C and a pulse rate of 110/min should arouse suspicion. In another series, fever was present in all patients who developed fat embolism syndrome[76]; however, Pazell and Peltier[176] found that fever was not helpful in diagnosing the syndrome.

Central nervous system (CNS) signs are not uncommon in the syndrome and, in at least one retrospective series, were the most common findings.[247] In another series, a change in level of consciousness was noted in 86% of patients.[176] Although focal deficits have been noted, CNS signs are usually nonspecific and nonlateralizing and range from impaired consciousness to decerebrate rigidity and convulsions. In unanesthetized patients a change in consciousness is frequently the first sign of fat embolism syndrome.[162] Progression from initial restlessness and anxiety to confusion and coma occurs in many patients.[94] CNS signs in most cases are probably caused by cerebral hypoxia resulting from pulmonary fat embolism, although embolization of cerebral vessels with fat occurs occasionally.[77] Cerebral edema caused by a combination of hypoxemia, embolic ischemia, and toxic FFA-induced cerebrovascular disruption contributes to the neurologic deterioration.[143] Any change in CNS status in a trauma patient should alert the physician to the possibility of fat embolism, although obviously such other diagnoses as subdural or epidural hematoma, alcohol intoxication and withdrawal, or drug overdose must also be entertained. Generally, the onset of coma in patients with intracranial hematoma occurs earlier than 12 hours after injury and often is preceded by headache, nausea, and vomiting if unconsciousness was not present immediately after trauma. Coma associated with fat embolism generally begins more than 12 hours after injury and is often preceded by restlessness and delirium.[268]

A rare clinical scenario, which is pertinent to the anesthesiologist, is lack of recovery from anesthesia. In patients unsuspected of having intraoperative fat embolism syndrome this lack of recovery may be attributed to the prolonged effects of anesthetics and opioids. Occasionally the patient may become agitated a few hours after anesthesia without recovery of consciousness. This may easily result in the administration of sedative and opioid agents and a further delay in recognition of cerebral involvement. Although sedation of these patients after neurologic examination is indicated, evaluation of the brain with CT scan should be performed early in the postoperative period. If intraoperative fat embolism syndrome, as evidenced by hemodynamic and metabolic abnormalities, petechiae, and other signs and symptoms, is suspected, termination of surgery and anesthesia as quickly as possible and evaluation of neurologic function should be considered.

Acute renal failure and coronary ischemia from fat embolism to renal and coronary vessels, although possible, occur rarely.[206] The kidney appears to have a great ability to clear embolized fat. In addition, shock, which is often associated with this syndrome, results in renal vasoconstriction, decreasing the quantity of fat globules distributed to this organ. Death, sometimes sudden, from embolization of fat globules into coronary vessels can occur not only because of acute myocardial failure but also dysrhythmias secondary to involvement of the cardiac conduction system.[226]

Retinal signs may be present in the form of fluffy white exudates caused by occlusion of retinal vessels with fat.[180] In one retrospective series, retinal signs were detected by fundoscopic examination in 46% of patients.[247] Conjunctival petechial hemorrhages often occur concomitantly with the previously described petechial rash over the upper portion of the body.

In view of the difficulty of diagnosing the fat embolism syndrome, it is not surprising that many laboratory tests have been suggested, one of the more useful being measurement of the arterial blood gases. Hypoxemia, which is common after lower extremity fractures,[136] has been attributed to subclinical fat embolism and considered to be an early indicator of the clinical syndrome in patients at risk. However, it is often inapparent in fat embolism: developing before signs of respiratory distress,[10,11,34] it can be detected only if blood gases are measured. Riseborough and Herndon[201] noted an abnormally low $PaO_2$ in patients with severe fractures compared to a group whose fractures were less severe. In a prospective study of 50 consecutive patients with uncomplicated extremity fractures, McCarthy et al.[136] found that, although 74% of patients exhibited $PaO_2 < 80$ mm Hg on room air, no patients developed clinical fat embolism. Thus, the mere presence of hypoxemia at this level does not seem to confirm the diagnosis of fat embolism syndrome, although it may indicate subclinical fat embolism. Tachakra and Sevitt's[245] prospective data support this reasoning, as an arterial $PO_2 < 80$ mm Hg was discovered in 32 (64%) of 50 uncomplicated fracture patients, although only 4 developed the fat embolism syndrome.

On the other hand, many authors have discovered a substantial degree of hypoxemia in patients with fat embolism syndrome; a large majority exhibit room air $PaO_2$ values well below 60 mm Hg.[11,76,77,153] This finding has led Lindeque et al.[121] to consider isolated hypoxemia with $PaO_2 < 60$ mm Hg in room air as a diagnostic criterion for fat embolism syndrome in patients with fractures. Arterial hypoxemia in these patients has been attributed to ventilation-perfusion inequality and intrapulmonary shunting.[10,11] Although hypoxemia is present in nearly all cases of fat embolism syndrome, there have been reports of patients with the syndrome and a normal $PaO_2$,[2] so that the absence of hypoxemia cannot rule out the diagnosis when it is supported by other signs and symptoms. Initial $PaCO_2$ elevation occurs in some patients, but is not characteristic of this syndrome; rather, some degree of respiratory alkalosis, secondary to tachypnea and hyperventilation, is usual.[76,153] Later, as respiratory failure progresses, $PaCO_2$ rises.[136]

The chest roentgenogram has been used as a diagnostic aid in some cases of fat embolism syndrome. The characteristic appearance is evenly distributed fleck-like pulmonary shadows, increased pulmonary markings, and dilation of the right side of the heart.[150] The fleck-like shadows give the roentgenogram a "snowstorm" appearance.[94] Some authors have emphasized the presence of bilateral patchy infiltrates, primarily in perihilar and basilar areas, which could be confused with pulmonary edema except for the absence of vascular congestion or pleural effusion.[73,132] The ECG may be useful if it shows patterns of acute cor pulmonale or myocardial ischemia,[180] but in the absence of extensive pulmonary involvement it is usually normal.

Much has been written about the role of serum lipase determination in fat embolism. Although increased serum lipase levels have been demonstrated in trauma patients,[176,184] the significance of this finding has been questioned.[27] In one study, for example, serum lipase was found to be elevated in patients without fat embolism syndrome, but was normal in patients with the syndrome, prompting Ross[211] to conclude that the serum lipase level is not only without value but may be misleading.

Many have attempted to measure fat in the blood for use as a marker of the syndrome, but the amount of circulating fat does not correlate with the severity of the clinical picture.[77] The normal variation in serum lipid levels makes interpretation of test results difficult.[180] A clinical report noted a postfracture alteration in lipoprotein electrophoretic patterns that persisted longer in patients who went on to develop the fat embolism syndrome than in those who did not.[254] The cryostat technique of identifying fat globules in sections of rapidly frozen clotted blood, originally described by Hauman, was found to be a sensitive test for diagnosing clinical and subclinical fat embolism in one prospective series.[27] One group has measured activated complement (C5a) and found it to be sensitive but not specific for predicting the occurrence of the syndrome.[224]

A myriad of other laboratory tests have been used in an attempt to establish the diagnosis of the syndrome. Some have claimed that detection of fat in the urine after staining with Sudan or o-red-oil is indicative of a significant degree of fat embolism.[180] However, this is certainly not a reliable finding: lipuria could not be demonstrated in a single instance in a group of patients with established fat embolism syndrome.[224] Fat globules in tracheal aspirates have been said to be diagnostic of the syndrome, but others have not found sputum examination helpful since fat is normally present in sputum.[180] Sampling of blood from the pulmonary artery catheter after inflation of its balloon probably yields a high concentration of fat globules and permits quantitative analysis, but the diagnostic significance of this approach is not certain at this time.

A decrease in hematocrit occurs within 24–48 hours after fat embolism[201] and is attributed to intra-alveolar hemorrhage.[177] Rokkanen et al.[208] showed that two-thirds of patients with fat embolism syndrome had hemoglobin levels < 10 gm/dL, whereas only 25% of a control group of trauma patients had such low values. However, the use of hemoglobin determinations to predict the development of or to diagnose fat embolism syndrome in trauma patients has not been widely reported. Alterations in coagulation tests and thrombocytopenia, which occur frequently after fat embolism, have been investigated as a possible tool in aiding the diagnosis of fat embolism, but Allardyce et al.[2] failed to demonstrate any consistent differences in coagulation parameters or platelet counts in fracture patients with or without the clinical syndrome.

Efforts aimed at standardizing diagnostic criteria for fat embolism have not been lacking. In the last decade, Gurd and Wilson[77] defined precise criteria on which to base the diagnosis of fat embolism. According to these authors a positive diagnosis required the presence of at least one of three major clinical features (respiratory insufficiency, cerebral involvement, or petechial rash), four of five minor clinical features (pyrexia, tachycardia, retinal changes, jaundice, or renal changes), and fat macroglobulemia. In another series the fat embolism syndrome was diagnosed if a young patient with fractures had any combination of pyrexia, tachypnea, tachycardia, or CNS involvement along with a $PaO_2$ less than 50 mm Hg.[162] A scoring system was designed by Alho and associates[1] to establish the diagnosis: one point each was given for a "snowstorm" chest roentgenogram, skin petechiae, ocular petechiae, mental disturbances, axillary temperature > 38°C, a decrease in hemoglobin > 2.5 g% per day in the absence of hemorrhage, or platelet count < 120,000/μL. A $PaO_2$ < 60 mm Hg was given two points. Scores were tabulated daily, and the cumulative score over 5 days was used to make the diagnosis. More recently, Schonfeld and colleagues[224] described a fat embolism index score in which signs and symptoms were assigned point values as follows: petechiae (5), diffuse alveolar infiltrates (4), $PaO_2$ below 70 mm Hg (3), confusion (1), fever 38°C or greater (1), pulse 120/min or greater (1), and respiratory rate 30/min or greater (1). In the study, scores were ascertained during the first 3 days of hospitalization and considered to be diagnostic for fat embolism syndrome if they reached a level of 5 or more. Recently Lindeque and colleagues[121] proposed the simple set of diagnostic criteria shown in Table 16-10. They claim that these sensitive criteria not only permit instant diagnosis of fat embolism syndrome but also obviate the problem of underdiagnosis. By using this set of criteria Lindeque et al.[121] reported that the incidence of fat embolism syndrome, which by using Gurd and Wilson's[77] criteria would be 13%, was actually 29%.

These efforts to standardize diagnostic criteria, although sporadic, are encouraging. Since the signs and symptoms of fat embolism are often nonspecific, diagnosis of the syndrome is difficult. With the exception perhaps of petechiae, there are no pathognomonic signs. Also, it is clear that there is no specific laboratory test for the syndrome.

## TREATMENT

Since the pathophysiology of fat embolism syndrome has not yet been defined clearly, it is not surprising that proposed

TABLE 16-10. Clinical Criteria Proposed by Lindeque et al.[121] for Diagnosis of Fat Embolism Syndrome after Long Bone Fracture(s)[a]

| |
|---|
| $PaO_2$ <60 mm Hg in room air |
| $PaCO_2$ >55 mm Hg or pHa <7.3 |
| Spontaneous respiratory rate >35 breath/min (even after adequate sedation) |
| Clinical signs of increased work of breathing (dyspnea, accessory muscle use) and tachycardia |

[a] The presence of at least one of these findings in a patient with long bone fracture(s) establishes the diagnosis of fat embolism syndrome.

treatment regimens vary widely. Prevention and supportive therapy are the primary management aims.

Through the years, many authors have emphasized the importance of maintaining intravascular volume in fat embolism syndrome, a view supported by abundant clinical and laboratory evidence.[21,85] The severity of the syndrome is directly related to the degree and duration of associated shock. In a retrospective series patients who had systolic blood pressure < 100 mm Hg and tachycardia > 120 beats/min had a mortality rate twice that of those with normal blood pressure and pulse rate, underscoring the importance of prevention or prompt treatment of hypovolemia.[176] Shock, by producing pulmonary damage on its own, can intensify the lung injury caused by fat embolism syndrome. More importantly it causes a severe decrease in cardiac preload that, in the face of increased pulmonary vascular resistance from fat embolism, can bring cardiac output to a halt.[180] Aggressive fluid resuscitation must be initiated early to restore intravascular volume, improve preload, and establish optimal cardiac output. Appropriate monitoring should be used to avoid fluid overload since the margin of safety of fluid resuscitation is diminished in the presence of pulmonary hypertension. Central venous pressure monitoring is usually sufficient, but measurement of pulmonary artery and pulmonary artery wedge pressures, and cardiac output must be considered in the fulminant syndrome. Albumin has been recommended for volume resuscitation along with balanced electrolyte solution, since it not only restores blood volume but also binds fatty acids, reducing their potential for lung damage.[120,168]

Acute right heart failure caused by elevated pulmonary vascular resistance is a major threat to life in the fat embolism syndrome. Death from acute cor pulmonale as a result of fat embolism was described as early as 1921,[180] and its existence has been documented in more recent case reports.[80] Therapy of acute cor pulmonale in fat embolism includes an inotrope, fluids, and a pulmonary vasodilator, such as isoproterenol.[81]

The lung is the primary target organ in fat embolism, necessitating the use of aggressive ventilatory therapy. Harman and Ragaz[85] witnessed a dramatic decline in mortality with administration of oxygen in their animal model of fat embolism. Since that report the importance of early oxygen therapy and close monitoring of arterial blood gases has been emphasized.[71,162,183] Mechanical ventilation preferably with positive end-expiratory pressure (PEEP) must be instituted whenever simple oxygen administration is insufficient to maintain adequate arterial oxygenation or when ventilation is inadequate.[71,162] High-frequency jet ventilation, although it permits monitoring of cerebral function by reducing the requirement for sedatives and analgesics, probably offers little advantage over conventional ventilation in terms of oxygenation.[114,239] Diuretics may be required to treat pulmonary edema caused by the pulmonary hypertensive effect of fat embolism.[189]

High-dose corticosteroid treatment was introduced into clinical practice in an effort to limit the FFA-induced inflammatory reaction in the lung. Initial favorable results with the use of these agents in three patients by Ashbaugh and Petty[5] in 1966 were followed by numerous reports suggesting the prophylactic administration of steroids to patients at risk for this syndrome.[57,102,111,209,238,243,264] These recommendations have been confirmed by the results of three separate prospective randomized double-blind trials.[1,121,224] Methylprednisolone was the agent used in all three studies, and the initial intravenous doses of the drug ranged between 7.5 mg/kg and 30 mg/kg. A similar dose was repeated during the course of the syndrome, but the number of doses and the interval between them varied widely in each study. High-dose prophylactic corticosteroid treatment was effective in preventing development of the syndrome in all three trials. In two studies $PaO_2$ in corticosteroid-treated patients was higher than in untreated patients.[1,121] A reduction in serum FFA levels was noted in at least one.[121] Some patients in all trials, however, developed fat embolism syndrome despite high-dose corticosteroids. Also, it appears that the use of corticosteroids is not critical in the treatment of the established syndrome since, in one of these trials, seven of nine patients who did not receive the drug and developed the syndrome recovered.[224] Recent prospective randomized multicenter trials that tested the effect of high-dose corticosteroids in ARDS could not demonstrate any beneficial effect from these agents.[15] Although ARDS was produced by a wide variety of mechanisms and in general the pulmonary insult caused by fractures and FFA is probably less severe than that induced by such other mechanisms as sepsis and aspiration pneumonitis, in most instances the pulmonary consequences of fat embolism syndrome are indistinguishable from ARDS. Thus it is possible that forthcoming rigorously controlled multicenter studies directed to this subset of ARDS may also demonstrate little benefit from these agents. Presently, however, it appears that high-dose corticosteroids, if given early in the course of the fat embolism syndrome, offer some advantages in preventing decreased $PaO_2$ and in reducing pulmonary morbidity from this complication.

Another factor in the etiology of fat embolism is the time of operative fixation of the fracture.[244] In a prospective study, Riska and Myllynen[202] observed a decreased incidence of fat embolism syndrome in fracture patients treated with early internal fixation compared to a control group treated nonoperatively. This difference may have been due to reduction of local tissue pressure around the fracture brought about by opening and draining the fracture hematoma. This hypothesis is supported by a dog study that demonstrated less fat release from the femur during reaming of an open versus a closed fracture.[130] A retrospective review by the same group[246] also revealed that fat embolism syndrome did not develop in patients treated with immediate intramedullary nailing as compared to those treated with delayed fixation. Proponents of early fracture stabilization emphasize that earlier patient mobilization decreases the likelihood of development of pulmonary complications attendant on prolonged bedrest.[130] In addition this approach prevents recurrent fat embolization produced by movement of fracture fragments during management with skeletal traction.[245] It should be emphasized, however, that intramedullary reaming of long bones with various currently available rods is also associated with significant fat embolization. Thus, not only should this procedure be performed gently, but if careful monitoring of hemodynamics and oxygenation reveals serious alterations, other surgical alternatives, such as external fixation, should be considered.

Use of a tourniquet has been proposed as a prophylactic

measure in averting fat embolization. Its use on the involved limb appears to be logical in that egress of fat into the systemic circulation is prevented at least until the tourniquet is released. Peltier[178] has in fact advocated the use of a tourniquet in all procedures involving bone trauma. An opposing view was expressed by Hagley,[80] who reported a case of massive fat and thromboembolism resulting in the death of a patient with leg fractures after tourniquet release during surgery.

Successful cardiac and pulmonary fat embolectomy has been described,[167] although admittedly this procedure constitutes heroic therapy and requires acute diagnostic acumen.

The prognosis in patients with cerebral manifestations of fat embolism is poor. However, with continuous intracranial pressure (ICP) measurement, periodic CT evaluation of the head, and institution of measures that optimize cranial pressure dynamics and cerebral perfusion, one may hope to reduce brain edema and thus improve the outcome.[143] These measures include maintenance of hypocapnia ($PaCO_2$, 23–30 mm Hg), administration of diuretics (mannitol and furosemide) and high-dose corticosteroids, elevation of the head, and prevention of straining and coughing. Seizure prophylaxis and treatment should also be instituted. A discussion of ICP control and management of convulsions is offered in Chapter 10.

The most common cause of death in fat embolism syndrome is pulmonary failure, and as has been mentioned, since the syndrome may coexist with other posttraumatic pulmonary problems, it is practically impossible to collect accurate statistics on the mortality of the fat embolism syndrome itself.[71] In the series of Burgher and co-workers[25] of 36 cases of fat embolism syndrome, mortality was 33%. Guenter and Braun[76] reported no deaths in a retrospective series of 54 patients with fat embolism syndrome who were treated primarily with supportive oxygen and respiratory care. These results contrast with the overall mortality rates of 12–35% reported in the literature. However, it appears that despite the unavailability of specific therapy, improvement in supportive treatment has reduced the high mortality rate described in the older literature.

## REFERENCES


1. Alho A, Saikku K, Eerola P, et al. Corticosteroids in patients with a high risk of fat embolism syndrome. Surg Gynecol Obstet 1978;147:358.
2. Allardyce DB, Meek RN, Woodruff B, et al. Increasing our knowledge of the pathogenesis of fat embolism: a prospective study of 43 patients with fractured femoral shafts. J Trauma 1974;14:955.
3. Allen HL, Metcalf DW. Fractured hip. A study of anesthesia in the aged. Anesth Analg 1965;44:408.
4. Anderson KH. Air aspirated from the venous system during total hip replacement. Anaesthesia 1983;38:1175.
5. Ashbaugh DG, Petty TL. The use of corticosteroids in the treatment of respiratory failure associated with massive fat embolism. Surg Gynecol Obstet 1966;123:493.
6. Ashworth EM, Dalsing MC, Glöver JL, Reilly MK. Lower extremity vascular trauma: a comprehensive, aggressive approach. J Trauma 1988;28:329.
7. Bach BR Jr, Wyman ET Jr. Financial charges of hospitalized motorcyclists at Massachusetts General Hospital. J Trauma 1986;26:343.
8. Baratta JB, Lim V, Mastromonaco E, Edillon EL. Axillary artery disruption secondary to anterior dislocation of the shoulder. J Trauma 1983;23:1009.
9. Barrett JB, Mostarlic O. Psoas compartment block. Anaesthesia 1986;41:1057.
10. Benoit PR, Hampson LG, Burgess JH. Respiratory gas exchange following fractures: the role of fat embolism as a cause of hypoxemia. Surg Forum 1969;20:214.
11. Benoit PR, Hampson LG, Burgess JH. Value of arterial hypoxemia in the diagnosis of pulmonary fat embolism. Ann Surg 1972;175:128.
12. Bergentz SE. Fat embolism. Prog Surg 1968;6:85.
13. Bergentz SE, Nilsson IM. Effect of trauma on coagulation and fibrinolysis in dogs. Acta Chir Scand 1961;122:21.
14. Berggren D, Gustafson Y, Erikisson B, et al. Postoperative confusion after anesthesia in elderly patients with femoral neck injuries. Anesth Analg 1987;66:497.
15. Bernard GR, Luce JM, Sprung CL, et al. High-dose corticosteroids in patients with the adult respiratory distress syndrome. N Engl J Med 1987;317:1565.
16. Boyce WJ, Vessey MP. Rising incidence of fracture of the proximal femur. Lancet 1985;1:150.
17. Bradford DS, Foster RR, Nossel HL. Coagulation alterations, hypoxemia and fat embolism in fracture patients. J Trauma 1970;10:307.
18. Braunstein PW. Medical aspects of automotive crash injury research. JAMA 1957;163:249.
19. Brotman S, Soderstrom CA, Oster-Granite M, Cisternino S, et al. Management of severe bleeding in fractures of the pelvis. Surg Gynecol Obstet 1981;153:823.
20. Brown JT, Abrami G. Transcervical femoral fracture. A review of 195 patients treated by sliding nail-plate fixation. J Bone Joint Surg 1964;46B:648.
21. Bruecke P, Burke JF, Lam KW, et al. The pathophysiology of pulmonary fat embolism. J Thorac Cardiovasc Surg 1971;61:949.
22. Buckley SL, Burkus JK. Computerized axial tomography of pelvic ring fractures. J Trauma 1987;27:496.
23. Buffington CW, Romson JL, Levine A, et al. Isoflurane induces coronary steal in a canine model of chronic coronary occlusion. Anesthesiology 1987;66:280.
24. Burgess AR, Poka A, Brumback RJ, et al. Pedestrian tibial injuries. J Trauma 1987;27:596.
25. Burgher LW, Dines DE, Linscheid RL, Didier EP. Fat embolism and the adult respiratory distress syndrome. Anesth Analg 1974;53:664.
26. Carlsson GS, Svardsudd AK, Carlsson S, et al. A study of injuries during life in three male populations. J Trauma 1986;26:364.
27. Chan KM, Tham KT, Chow YN, Leung PC. Post-traumatic fat embolism—its clinical and subclinical presentations. J Trauma 1984;24:45.
28. Chayen D, Nathan H, Chayen M. The psoas compartment block. Anesthesiology 1976;45:95.
29. Christensen JH, Andreasen F. Individual variation in response to thiopental. Acta Anaesthesiol Scand 1978;22:303.
30. Chung F, Meier R, Lautenschlager E, et al. General or spinal anesthesia: which is better in the elderly? Anesthesiology 1987;67:422.
31. Clark SS, Prudencio RF. Lower urinary tract injuries associated with pelvic fractures. Diagnosis and management. Surg Clin North Am 1972;52:183.
32. Cobb CA Jr, Hillnaj JW. Fat embolism. In: American Academy of Orthopedic Surgeons, eds. Instructional course lectures. Chicago: American Academy of Orthopedic Surgeons, 1961:122.
33. Coleman SA, Boyce WJ, Cosh PH, McKenzie PJ. Outcome after general anesthesia for repair of fractured neck of femur. A ran-

domized trial of spontaneous v. controlled ventilation. Br J Anaesth 1988;60:43.
34. Collins JA, Gordon WC Jr, Hudson TL, et al. Inapparent hypoxemia in casualties with wounded limbs. Pulmonary fat embolism? Ann Surg 1968;167:511.
35. Collins R, Scrimgeour A, Yusuf S, Peto R. Reduction in fatal pulmonary embolism and venous thrombosis by perioperative administration of subcutaneous heparin. N Engl J Med 1988;318:1162.
36. Cooke ED, Bowcock SA, Loyd MJ, Pilcher MF. Intravenous lignocaine in prevention of deep venous thrombosis after elective hip surgery. Lancet 1977;2:798.
37. Couderc E, Mange F, Duvaldestin P, Desmonts JM. Resultats comparatifs de l'anesthesie generale et peridurale chez le grand viellard dans la chirurgie de la hauche. Anesth Analg Reanim 1977;34:987.
38. Cozian A, Pinaud M, Lepage JY, et al. Effects of meperidine spinal anesthesia on hemodynamics, plasma catecholamines, angiotensin I, aldosterone, and histamine concentrations in elderly men. Anesthesiology 1986;64:815.
39. Cryer HM, Miller FB, Evers BM, et al. Pelvic fracture classification: correlation with hemorrhage. J Trauma 1988;28:973.
40. Cunningham AJ, McKenna JA, Skene DS. Single injection spinal anaesthesia with amethocaine and morphine for transurethral prostatectomy. Br J Anaesth 1983;55:423.
41. Davis FM, Laurenson VG. Spinal anaesthesia or general anaesthesia for emergency hip surgery in elderly patients. Anaesth Intens Care 1981;9:352.
42. Davis FM, Laurenson VG, Lewis J, et al. Metabolic response to total hip arthroplasty under hypobaric subarachnoid or general anaesthesia. Br J Anaesth 1987;59:725.
43. Davis FM, McDermott E, Hickton C, et al. Influence of spinal and general anaesthesia on haemostasis during total hip arthroplasty. Br J Anaesth 1987;59:561.
44. Davis FM, Quince M. Deep vein thrombosis and anaesthetic technique in emergency hip surgery. Br Med J 1980;281:1528.
45. Davis FM, Woolner DF, Frampton C, et al. Prospective, multicenter trial of mortality following general or spinal anaesthesia for hip fracture surgery in the elderly. Br J Anaesth 1987;59:1080.
46. Dedrick DK, Mackenzie JR, Burney RE. Complications of femoral neck fracture in young adults. J Trauma 1986;26:932.
47. DeHaven H. Mechanical analysis of survival in falls from heights of fifty to one hundred fifty feet. War Med 1942;2:586.
48. Dove AF, Poon WS, Weston PAM. Haemorrhage from pelvic fractures: dangers and treatment. Injury 1982;13:375.
49. Duis HJT, Nijsten MWN, Klasen HJ, Binnendijk B. Fat embolism in patients with an isolated fracture of the femoral shaft. J Trauma 1988;28:383.
50. Dunn AW, Morris HD. Fractures and dislocations of the pelvis. J Bone Joint Surg 1968;50A:1639.
51. Dunn EL, Berry PH, Connally JD. Computed tomography of the pelvis in patients with multiple injuries. J Trauma 1983;23:378.
52. Egdahl RH. Pituitary-adrenal response following trauma to the isolated leg. Surgery 1959;46:9.
53. Evans TI. The physiological basis of geriatric general anaesthesia. Anaesth Intens Care 1973;1:319.
54. Famewo CE, Naguib M. Spinal anaesthesia with meperidine as the sole agent. Can Anaesth Soc J 1985;32:533.
55. Feliciano DV, Herskowitz K, O'Gorman RB, et al. Management of vascular injuries in the lower extremities. J Trauma 1988;28:319.
56. Findlay JM, DeMajo W. Cerebral fat embolism. Can Med Assoc J 1984;131:755.
57. Fischer JE, Turner RH, Herndon JH, Riseborough EJ. Massive steroid therapy in severe fat embolism. Surg Gynecol Obstet 1971;132:667.
58. Fleming WH, Bowen JC III. Control of hemorrhage in pelvic crush injuries. J Trauma 1973;13:567.
59. Flint LM, Brown A, Richardson JD, Polk HC. Definitive control of bleeding from severe pelvic fractures. Ann Surg 1979;189:709.
60. Fortune JB, Feustel PJ, Saifi J, et al. Influence of hematocrit on cardiopulmonary function after acute hemorrhage. J Trauma 1987;27:816.
61. Fredin HO, Rosberg B, Arborelius M, Jr, Nylander G. On thromboembolism after total hip replacement in epidural analgesia; a controlled study of dextran 70 and low-dose heparin combined with dihydroergotamine. Br J Surg 1984;71:58.
62. Froman C, Stein A. Complicating crushing injuries of the pelvis. J Bone Joint Surg 1967;49B:24.
63. Gauss H. The pathology of fat embolism. Arch Surg 1924;9:593.
64. Gelberman RH, Menon J, Fronek A. The peripheral pulse following arterial injury. J Trauma 1980;20:948.
65. Gelman SI. Disturbances in hepatic blood flow during anesthesia and surgery. Arch Surg 1976;111:881.
66. Gilliland MG, Ward RE, Flynn TC, et al. Peritoneal lavage and angiography in the management of patients with pelvic fractures. Am J Surg 1982;144:744.
67. Gilliland MD, Ward RE, Barton RM, et al. Factors affecting mortality in pelvic fractures. J Trauma 1982;22:691.
68. Goldberg M. Systemic reactions to intravascular contrast media. Anesthesiology 1984;60:46.
69. Goldstein A, Phillips T, Sclafani SJA, et al. Early open reduction and internal fixation of the disrupted pelvic ring. J Trauma 1986;26:325.
70. Goris RJA, Gimbrere JSF, van Niekerk JLM, et al. Early osteosynthesis and prophylactic mechanical ventilation in the multitrauma patient. J Trauma 1982;22:895.
71. Gossling HR, Ellison LH, DeGraff AC. Fat embolism. The role of respiratory failure and its treatment. J Bone Joint Surg 1974;56A:1327.
72. Gossling HR, Pellegrini VD Jr. Fat embolism syndrome. A review of the pathophysiology and physiological basis of treatment. Clin Orthop 1982;165:68.
73. Greenberg HB. Roentgenographic signs of posttraumatic fat embolism. JAMA 1968;204:540.
74. Gregory RJ, Gould RJ, Peclet M, et al. The mangled extremity syndrome (MES): a severity grading system for multisystem injury of the extremity. J Trauma 1985;25:1147.
75. Grieco JG, Perry JF. Retroperitoneal hematoma following trauma: its clinical importance. J Trauma 1980;20:733.
76. Guenter CA, Braun TE. Fat embolism syndrome—changing prognosis. Chest 1981;79:143.
77. Gurd AR, Wilson RI. The fat embolism syndrome. J Bone Joint Surg 1974;56B:408.
78. Gustilo RB, Mendoza RM, Williams DN. Problems in the management of type III (severe) open fractures: a new classification of type III open fractures. J Trauma 1984;24:742.
79. Gylling SF, Ward RE, Holcroft JW, et al. Immediate external fixation of unstable pelvic fractures. Am J Surg 1985;150:721.
80. Hagley SR. Fulminant fat embolism syndrome—case reports. Anaesth Intens Care 1983;11:167.
81. Hagley SR. The fulminant fat embolism syndrome. Anaesth Intens Care 1983;11:162.
82. Haljamäe H, Stefansson T, Wickström I. Preanesthetic evaluation of the female geriatric patient with hip fracture. Acta Anesth Scand 1982;26:393.
83. Halsey MJ. Drug interactions in anaesthesia. Br J Anaesth 1987;59:112.

84. Hardin WD, Adinolfi MF, O'Connell RC, Kerstein MD. Management of traumatic peripheral vein injuries. Primary repair or vein ligation. Am J Surg 1982;144:235.
85. Harman JW, Ragaz FJ. The pathogenesis of experimental fat embolism. Am J Pathol 1950;26:551.
86. Hausberger FX, Whitenack SH. Effect of pressure on intravasation of fat from the bone marrow cavity. Surg Gynecol Obstet 1972;134:931.
87. Hawkins L, Pomerantz M, Eiseman B. Laparotomy at the time of pelvic fracture. J Trauma 1970;10:619.
88. Henao F, Aldrete JS. Retroperitoneal hematomas of traumatic origin. Surg Gynecol Obstet 1985;161:106.
89. Hennig K, Franke D. Posterior displacement of brachial artery following closed elbow dislocation. J Trauma 1980;20:96.
90. Hirsh J. Hypercoagulability. Semin Hematol 1977;14:409.
91. Holbrook TL, Grazier K, Kelsey JL, Stauffer RN. The frequency of occurrence, impact and cost of selected musculoskeletal conditions in the United States. Chicago: American Academy of Orthopedic Surgeons, 1984.
92. Hollenberg NK, Adams DF, Solomon HS, et al. Senescence and the renal vasculature in normal man. Circ Res 1974;34:309.
93. Homer TD, Stanski DR. The effect of increasing age on thiopental disposition and anesthetic requirement. Anesthesiology 1985;62:714.
94. Horne RH, Horne JH. Fat embolization prophylaxis. Arch Intern Med 1974;133:288.
95. Hospital Mortality, PAS Hospital U.S. 1974–1975. Ann Arbor, MI: Commission on Professional and Hospital Activities, 1977.
96. Howe HR, Poole GV, Hansen KJ, et al. Salvage of lower extremities following combined orthopedic and vascular trauma. Am Surg 1987;53:205.
97. Hubbard SG, Bivins BA, Sachatello CR, Griffin WO. Diagnostic errors with peritoneal lavage in patients with pelvic fractures. Arch Surg 1979;114:844.
98. Huittinen V, Slatis P. Postmortem angiography and dissection of the hypogastric artery in pelvic fractures. Surgery 1973;73:454.
99. Hurst JM. Initial management of pelvic fractures. In: Hurst JM, ed. Common problems in trauma. Chicago: Year Book Medical Publishers, 1987:237.
100. Jensen BV, Jacobsen J, Andreasen H. Late appearance of arterial injury caused by fracture of the neck of the humerus. J Trauma 1987;27:1368.
101. Johnson KD, Cadambi A, Seibert GB. Incidence of adult respiratory distress syndrome in patients with multiple musculoskeletal injuries: effect of early operative stabilization of fractures. J Trauma 1985;25:375.
102. Kallenbach J, Lewis M, Zaltzman M, et al. Low-dose corticosteroid prophylaxis against fat embolism. J Trauma 1987;27:1173.
103. Kallos T. Impaired arterial oxygenation associated with use of bone cement in the femoral shaft. Anesthesiology 1975;42:210.
104. Kallos T, Smith TC. Continuous spinal anesthesia with hypobaric tetracaine for hip surgery in lateral decubitus. Anesth Analg 1972;51:766.
105. Kalso E. Effects of intrathecal morphine injected with bupivacaine on pain after orthopaedic surgery. Br J Anaesth 1983;55:415.
106. Katz DA, Ben-Ezra J, Factor SM, et al. Fatal pulmonary and cerebral fat embolism in systemic lupus erythematosus. JAMA 1983;250:2666.
107. Keith RG, Mahoney LJ, Garvey MB. Disseminated intravascular coagulation: an important feature of the fat embolism syndrome. Can Med Assoc J 1971;105:74.
108. Kenzora JE, McCarthy RE, Lowell JD, Sledge CB. Hip fracture mortality. Relation to age, treatment, preoperative illness, time of surgery, and complications. Clin Orthop 1984;186:45.
109. Kerstell J. Pathogenesis of posttraumatic fat embolism. Am J Surg 1971;121:712.
110. Kinzl L, Burri C, Coldewey J. Fractures of the pelvis and associated intrapelvic injuries. Injury 1982;14:63.
111. Kreis WR, Lindenauer SM, Dent TL. Corticosteroids in experimental fat embolism. J Surg Res 1973;14:238.
112. Kronenberg RS, Drage CW. Attenuation of the ventilatory and heart rate responses to hypoxia and hypercapnia with aging in normal men. J Clin Invest 1973;52:1812.
113. LaDuca JN, Bone LL, Seibel RW, Border JR. Primary open reduction and internal fixation of open fractures. J Trauma 1980;20:580.
114. Lee A, Simpson D. High frequency jet ventilation in fat embolism syndrome. Anaesthesia 1986;41:1124.
115. Lehman EP, Moore RM. Fat embolism: including experimental production without trauma. Arch Surg 1927;14:621.
116. Lemmens HJM, Buurm AGL, Bovill JG, Hennis PJ. Pharmacodynamics of alfentanil as a supplement to nitrous oxide anaesthesia in the elderly patient. Br J Anaesth 1988;61:173.
117. Lequire VS, Shapiro JL, Lequire CB, et al. A study of the pathogenesis of fat embolism based on human necropsy material and animal experiments. Am J Pathol 1959;35:999.
118. Lerman J, Gregory GA, Willis MM, et al. Age and solubility of volatile anesthetics in blood. Anesthesiology 1984;61:139.
119. Lewinnek GE, Kelsey J, White AA, et al. The significance and a comparative analysis of the epidemiology of hip fracture. Clin Orthop 1980;152:35.
120. Liljedahl SO, Westermark L. Aetiology and treatment of fat embolism. Report of five cases. Acta Anesthesiol Scand 1967;11:177.
121. Lindeque BGP, Schoeman HS, Dommisse GF, et al. Fat embolism and the fat embolism syndrome. A double-blind therapeutic study. J Bone Joint Surg 1987;69B:128.
122. Lipkowitz G, Phillips T, Coren C, et al. Hemipelvectomy, a lifesaving operation in severe open pelvic injury in childhood. J Trauma 1985;25:823.
123. Loach A. Anesthesia for surgery of the lower limb. In: Loach A, ed. Anaesthesia for orthopaedic patients. London: Edward Arnold Publishing, 1983:46.
124. Lorhan PH, Shelby EA. Factors influencing mortality in hip fractures. Anesth Analg 1964;43:539.
125. Lowe MA, Mason JT, Luna GK, et al. Risk factors for urethral injuries in men with traumatic pelvic fractures. J Urology 1988;140:506.
126. Lowell JD. Fractures of the hip. N Engl J Med 1966;274:1418.
127. Lozman J, Deno C, Feustel PJ, et al. Pulmonary and cardiovascular consequences of immediate fixation or conservative management of long bone fractures. Arch Surg 1986;121:992.
128. Macintyre PE, Pavlin EG, Dwersteg JF. Effect of meperidine on oxygen consumption, carbon-dioxide production, and respiratory gas exchange in postanesthesia shivering. Anesth Analg 1987;66:751.
129. Mackersie RC, Shackford SR, Garfin SR, Hoyt DB. Major skeletal injuries in the obtunded blunt trauma patient: a case for routine radiologic survey. J Trauma 1988;28:1450.
130. Manning JB, Bach AW, Herman CM, Carrico CJ. Fat release after femur nailing in the dog. J Trauma 1983;23:322.
131. Martin VC. Hypoxaemia in elderly patients suffering from fractured neck of femur. Anaesthesia 1977;32:852.
132. Maruyama Y, Little JB. Roentgen manifestations of traumatic pulmonary fat embolism. Radiology 1962;79:945.
133. Marx GF, Mateo CV, Orkin LR. Computer analysis of postanesthetic deaths. Anesthesiology 1973;39:54.

134. Matzch T, Karlsson B. Moped and motorcycle accidents—similarities and discrepancies. J Trauma 1986;26:538.
135. Mays ET. The effect of surgical stress on plasma free fatty acids. J Surg Res 1970;10:315.
136. McCarthy B, Mammen E, LeBlanc LP, Wilson RF. Subclinical fat embolism: a prospective study of 50 patients with extremity fractures. J Trauma 1973;13:9.
137. McGoey PF, Evans J. Fractures of the hip: immediate versus delayed treatment. Can Med Assoc J 1960;83:260.
138. McKenzie PJ, Wishart HY, Dewar KMS, et al. Comparison of the effects of spinal anesthesia and general anesthesia on postoperative oxygenation and perioperative mortality. Br J Anaesth 1980;52:49.
139. McKenzie PJ, Wishart HY, Smith G. Long-term outcome after repair of fractured neck of femur. Br J Anaesth 1984;56:581.
140. McLaren AD, Stockwell MC, Reid VC. Anaesthetic techniques for surgical correction of fractured neck of femur. Anaesthesia 1978;33:10.
141. McLeskey CH. Anesthesia for the geriatric patient. Adv Anesth 1985;2:32.
142. McNamara JJ, Molot M, Dunn R, et al. Lipid metabolism after trauma. Role in the pathogenesis of fat embolism. J Thorac Cardiovasc Surg 1972;63:968.
143. Meeke RI, Fitzpatrick GJ, Phelan DM. Cerebral oedema and the fat embolism syndrome. Intens Care Med 1987;13:291.
144. Menzoian JO, LoGerfo FW, Doyle JE. Management of vascular injuries to the leg. Am J Surg 1982;144:231.
145. Meyer J, Walsh J, Schuler J, et al. The early fate of venous repair after civilian vascular trauma. A clinical, hemodynamic and venographic assessment. Ann Surg 1987;206:458.
146. Mircea N, Constantinescu C, Jianu E, et al. Risk of pulmonary complications in surgical patients. Resuscitation 1982;10:33.
147. Modig J, Borg T, Bagge L, Saldeen T. Role of extradural and of general anaesthesia in fibrinolysis and coagulation after total hip replacement. Br J Anaesth 1983;55:625.
148. Modig J, Borg T, Karlström G, et al. Thromboembolism after total hip replacement: role of epidural and general anesthesia. Anesth Analg 1983;62:174.
149. Modig J, Malmberg P, Karlström G. Effect of epidural versus general anaesthesia on calf blood flow. Acta Anaesthesiol Scand 1980;24:305.
150. Mokkhavesa S, Shim SS, Patterson FP. Fat embolism: clinical and experimental studies with emphasis on therapeutic aspects. J Trauma 1969;9:39.
151. Montrey JS, Kistner RL, Kong AY, et al. Thromboembolism following hip fracture. J Trauma 1985;25:534.
152. Moore WM, Brown J, Haynes JL, Viamontes L. Traumatic hemipelvectomy. J Trauma 1987;27:570.
153. Moore P, James O, Saltos N. Fat embolism syndrome: incidence, significance and early features. Aust NZ J Surg 1981;51:546.
154. Moreno C, Moore EE, Rosenberger A, et al. Hemorrhage associated with pelvic fracture: a multispeciality challenge. J Trauma 1986;26:987.
155. Morley-Forster PK. Unintentional hypothermia in the operating room. Can Anaesth Soc J 1986;33:516.
156. Morton KS, Kendall MJ. Fat embolism: its production and source of fat. Can J Surg 1965;8:214.
157. Moylan JA, Evenson MA. Diagnosis and treatment of fat embolism. Annu Rev Med 1977;28:85.
158. Moylan JA, Birnbaum M, Katz A, Everson MA. Fat emboli syndrome. J Trauma 1976;16:341.
159. Mucha P Jr, Farnell MB. Analysis of pelvic fracture management. J Trauma 1984;24:379.
160. Mucha P Jr, Welch TJ. Hemorrhage in major pelvic fractures. Surg Clin North Am 1988;68:757.
161. Murr PC, Moore EE, Lipscomb R, Johnston RM. Abdominal trauma associated with pelvic fracture. Trauma 1980;20:919.
162. Murray DG, Racz GB. Fat-embolism syndrome (respiratory insufficiency syndrome). J Bone Joint Surg 1974;56A:1338.
163. Myllynen P, Kammonen M, Rokkanen P. The blood F VIII: Ag/F VIII:C ratio as an early indicator of deep venous thrombosis during post-traumatic immobilization. J Trauma 1987; 27:287.
164. Naam NH, Brown WH, Hurd R, et al. Major pelvic fractures. Arch Surg 1983;118:610.
165. National Center for Health Statistics: Advance data from vital and health statistics: 1985 summary: national hospital discharge survey. Hyattsville, MD: Public Health Service. 1986 (U.S. Public Health Service Publ. No (PHS) 86-1250.)
166. Nehme AE. Groin hernias in elderly patients. Am J Surg 1983;146:257.
167. Nelson CS. Cardiac and pulmoanry fat embolectomy. Thorax 1974;29:134.
168. Nixon JR, Brock-Utne JG. Free fatty acid and arterial oxygen changes following major injury. A correlation between hypoxia and increased free fatty acid levels. J Trauma 1978;18:23.
169. Odoom JA, Zuunmond WWA, Sih IL, et al. Plasma bupivacaine concentrations following psoas compartment block. Anaesthesia 1986;41:155.
170. Ordog GJ, Wasserberger J, Balasubramaniam S. Coagulation abnormalities in traumatic shock. Ann Emerg Med 1985;14:650.
171. Panetta T, Sclafani SJA, Goldstein AS, et al. Percutaneous transcatheter embolization for massive bleeding from pelvic fractures. J Trauma 1985;25:1021.
172. Parker FB Jr, Wax SD, Kusajima K, Webb WR. Hemodynamic and pathological findings in experimental fat embolism. Arch Surg 1974;108:70.
173. Patt A, McCroskey BL, Moore EE. Hypothermia-induced coagulopathies in trauma. Surg Clin North Am 1988;68:775.
174. Patterson FP, Morton KS. Neurologic complications of fractures and dislocations of the pelvis. Surg Gynecol Obstet 1961;112:702.
175. Patterson FP, Morton KS. Neurological complications of fractures and dislocations of the pelvis. J Trauma 1972;12:1013.
176. Pazell JA, Peltier LF. Experience with sixty-three patients with fat embolism. Surg Gynecol Obstet 1972;135:77.
177. Peltier LF. Fat embolism. III. The toxic properties of neutral fat and free fatty acids. Surgery 1956;40:665.
178. Peltier LF. Fat embolism: the prophylactic value of a tourniquet. J Bone Joint Surg 1956;38A:835.
179. Peltier L. Complications associated with fracture of the pelvis. J Bone Joint Surg 1965;47A:1060.
180. Peltier LF. The diagnosis of fat embolism. Surg Gynecol Obstet 1965;121:371.
181. Peltier LF. Fat embolism. A current concept. Clin Orthop 1969;66:241.
182. Peltier LF. Fat embolism: an appraisal of the problem. Clin Orthop 1984;187:3.
183. Peltier LF. Fat embolism, a perspective. Clin Orthop 1988;232:263.
184. Peltier LF, Adler F, Lai SP. Fat embolism: the significance of an elevated serum lipase after trauma to bone. Am J Surg 1960;99:821.
185. Perry JF. Pelvic open fractures. Clin Orthop 1980;151:41.
186. Pontoppidan H, Beecher HK. Progressive loss of protective reflexes in the airway with the advance of age. JAMA 1960;174:2209.
187. Pontoppidan H, Geffins B, Lowenstein A. Acute respiratory failure in the adult. N Engl J Med 1972;287:690.

188. Porter MF. Arterial injuries in an accident unit. Br J Surg 1967;54:100.
189. Price GFW, Goodwin NM. Hypoxaemia and leucopaenia after fractures. Injury 1980;12:115.
190. Raine JM, Bishop JM. A-a difference in $O_2$ tension and physiological dead space in normal man. J Appl Physiol 1963;18:284.
191. Rammer L, Saldeen T. Inhibition of fibrinolysis in posttraumatic death. Thromb Diat 1970;24:68.
192. Ransom KJ, Shatney CH, Soderstrom CA, Cowley RA. Management of arterial injuries in blunt trauma of the extremity. Surg Gynecol Obstet 1981;153:241.
193. Ray WA, Griffin MR, Schaffner W, et al. Psychotropic drug use and the risk of hip fracture. N Engl J Med 1987;316:363.
194. Ream AK, Reitz BA, Silverberg G. Temperature correction of $pCO_2$ and pH in estimating acid-base status. Anesthesiology 1982;56:41.
195. Reikeras O. Cardiovascular reactions to intramedullary reaming of long bones in dogs. Acta Anaesth Scand 1987;31:48.
196. Reiz S, Balfors E, Sorensen MB, et al. Coronary hemodynamic effects of general anesthesia and surgery. Modification by epidural analgesia in patients with ischemic heart disease. Reg Anesth 1982;7:S8.
197. Rennie AM, Ogston D, Cooke RJ, Douglas AS. The fibrinolytic system after trauma and in patients with fat embolism. J Bone Joint Surg 1974;56B:421.
198. Rich NM, Jarstfer BS, Geer TM. Popliteal artery repair failure. Causes and possible prevention. J Cardiovasc Surg 1974;15:340.
199. Richardson JD, Harty J, Amin M, Flint LM. Open pelvic fractures. J Trauma 1982;22:533.
200. Riegstad A. Traumatic dislocation of the hip. J Trauma 1980;20:603.
201. Riseborough EJ, Herndon JH. Alterations in pulmonary function, coagulation and fat metabolism in patients with fractures of the lower limbs. Clin Orthop 1976;115:248.
202. Riska EB, Myllynen P. Fat embolism in patients with multiple injuries. J Trauma 1982;22:891.
203. Riska E, Von Bonsdorff H, Hakkinen S. Primary operative fixation of long bone fractures in patients with multiple injuries. J Trauma 1977;17:111.
204. Rittman WW, Schibli M, Matter P, et al. Open fractures: long term results in 200 consecutive cases. Clin Orthop 1979;138:132.
205. Rodriguez-Morales G, Phillips T, Conn AK, Cox EF. Traumatic hemipelvectomy: report of two survivors and review. J Trauma 1983;23:615.
206. Roger JA, Stirt JA. fat embolism syndrome. Semin Anesth 1987;6:176.
207. Roizen MF. Anesthetic implications of concurrent diseases. In Miller RD, ed. Anesthesia. 2nd ed. New York: Churchill Livingstone, 1986;255–359.
208. Rokkanen P, Lahdensuu M, Kataja J, Julkenen H. The syndrome of fat embolism: analysis of thirty consecutive cases compared with trauma patients with similar injuries. J Trauma 1970;10:299.
209. Rokkanen P, Alho A, Avikainen V, Karaharju E, et al. The efficacy of corticosteroids in severe trauma. Surg Gynecol Obstet 1974;138:69.
210. Rosberg B, Wulff K. Hemodynamics following normovolemic hemodilution in elderly patients. Acta Anaesth Scand 1981;25:402.
211. Ross APJ. The value of serum lipase estimations in fat embolism syndrome. Surgery 1969;65:271.
212. Ross SE, Ransom KJ, Shatney CH. The management of venous injuries in blunt extremity trauma. J Trauma 1985;25:150.
213. Rossi EC, Green D, Rosen JS, et al. Sequential change in factor VIII and platelets preceding deep vein thrombosis in patients with spinal cord injury. Br J Haematol 1980;45:143.
214. Rothenberger DA, Fischer RP, Strate RG, et al. The mortality associated with pelvic fractures. Surgery 1978;84:356.
215. Rowe JW, Andres R, Tobin JD, et al. The effect of age on creatinine clearances in man—a cross-sectional and longitudinal study. J Gerontol 1976;31:155.
216. Rucci FS, Cardamone M, Migliori P. Fentanyl and bupivacaine mixtures for extradural blockade. Br J Anaesth 1985;57:275.
217. Saldeen T. Intravascular coagulation in the lungs in experimental fat embolism. Acta Chir Scand 1969;135:653.
218. Saldeen T. Fat embolism and signs of intravascular coagulation in posttraumatic autopsy material. J Trauma 1970;10:273.
219. Salzman EW, Harris WH, DeSanctis RW. Anticoagulation for prevention of thromboembolism following fractures of the hip. N Engl J Med 1966;275:122.
220. Sari A, Miyauchi Y, Yamashita SH, et al. The magnitude of hypoxemia in elderly patients with fractures of the femoral neck. Anesth Analg 1986;65:892.
221. Saueracker AJ, McCroskey BL, Moore EE, Moore FA. Intraoperative hypogastric artery embolization for life-threatening pelvic hemorrhage: a preliminary report. J Trauma 1987; 27:1127.
222. Schmucher DL. Alterations in drug disposition. In: Stephen CR, Assaf RAE, eds. Geriatric anesthesia. London: Butterworth Publishing, 1986;155–188.
223. Schnaid E, Lamprey JM, Viljoen MJ, et al. The early biochemical and hormonal profile of patients with long bone fractures at risk of fat embolism syndrome. J Trauma 1987;27:309.
224. Schonfeld SA, Polysongsang Y, Dilisio R, et al. Fat embolism prophylaxis with corticosteriods: a prospective study in high-risk patients. Ann Intern Med 1983;99:438.
225. Schultz RJ, Whitfield GF, LaMura JJ, et al. The role of physiologic monitoring in patients with fractures of the hip. J Trauma 1985;25:309.
226. Schwartz DA, Finkelstein SD, Lumb GD. Fat embolism to the cardiac conduction system associated with sudden death. Hum Pathol 1988;19:116.
227. Scott JC, Stanski DR. Decreased fentanyl and alfentanil dose requirements with age. A simultaneous pharmacokinetic and pharmacodynamic evaluation. J Pharmacol Exp Ther 1987; 240:159.
228. Seibel R, LaDuca J, Hassett JM, et al. Blunt multiple trauma (ISS 36), femur traction, and the pulmonary failure-septic state. Ann Surg 1985;202:283.
229. Seibel RW, Border JR, Flint LM. Pelvic trauma. In: Richardson JD, Polk HC, Flint LM, eds. Clinical care and pathophysiology. Chicago: Year Book Medical Publishers, 1987:421.
230. Semba RT, Yasukawa K, Gustilo RB. Critical analysis of results of 53 Malgaigne fractures of the pelvis. J Trauma 1983; 23:535.
231. Sevitt S. The significance of fat embolism. Br J Hosp Med 1973;9:784.
232. Sevitt S. The significance and pathology of fat embolism. Annu Clin Res 1977;9:173.
233. Shah PM, Ivatury RR, Babu SC, et al. Is limb loss avoidable in civilian vascular injuries? Am J Surg 1987;154:202.
234. Shapiro LA, Hoffman S, Jedeikin R, Kaplan R. Single-injection epidural anesthesia with bupivacaine and morphine for prostatectomy. Anesth Analg 1981;60:818.
235. Shapiro MP, Hayes JA. Fat embolism in sickle cell disease. Report of a case with brief review of the literature. Arch Intern Med 1984;144:181.
236. Sheikh MA. Respiratory changes after fractures and surgical skeletal injury. Injury 1982;13:489.

237. Sherr S, Gertner SB. Production and recovery of pulmonary fat emboli in dogs. Exp Mol Pathol 1974;21:63.
238. Shier MR, Wilson RF, James RE, et al. Fat embolism prophylaxis: a study of four treatment modalities. J Trauma 1977;17:621.
239. Sjöstrand U. High frequency positive pressure ventilation: a review. Crit Care Med 1980;8:345.
240. Snyder RG. Human tolerance to extreme impacts in free fall. Aerospace Med 1963;34:695.
241. Stamatakis JD, Kakkar VV, Sagar S, et al. Femoral vein thrombosis and total hip replacement. Br Med J 1977;2:223.
242. Stehling LC. Anesthetic considerations for the patient with a fractured hip. In: Zauder HL, ed. Anesthesia for orthopaedic surgery, Philadelphia: FA Davis, 1980:29–66.
243. Stoltenberg JJ, Gustilo RB. The use of methylprednisolone and hypertonic glucose in the prophylaxis of fat embolism syndrome. Clin Orthop 1979;143:211.
244. Svenningsen S, Nesse O, Finsen V, et al. Prevention of fat embolism syndrome in patients with femoral fractures. Immediate or delayed operative fixation? Ann Chir Gynecol 1987;76:163.
245. Tachakra SS, Sevitt S. Hypoxaemia after fractures. J Bone Joint Surg 1975;57B:197.
246. Talucci RC, Manning J, Lampard S, et al. Early intramedullary nailing of femoral shaft fractures: a cause of fat embolism syndrome. Am J Surg 1983;146:107.
247. Thomas JE, Ayyar DR. Systemic fat embolism: a diagnostic profile in 24 patients. Arch Neurol 1972;26:517.
248. Thompson EN, Williams R. Effect of age on liver function with particular reference to bromosulphalein excretion. Gut 1965;6:266.
249. Thompson TL II, Moran MG, Nies AS. Psychotropic drug use in the elderly (Part 1). N Engl J Med 1983;308:134.
250. Tideiksaar R. Falls in the elderly. Bull NY Acad Med 1988;64:145.
251. Tingwald GR, Cooperman M. Inguinal and femoral hernia repair in geriatric patients. Surg Gynecol Obstet 1982;154:704.
252. Tomazsek DE. Combined subclavian artery and brachial plexus injuries from blunt upper-extremity trauma. J Trauma 1984;24:161.
253. Trafton PG, Herndon JH. External fixators in fracture management. In: Maull KI, Cleveland HC, Strauch GO, Wolferth CC, eds. advances in trauma. Chicago: Year Book Medical Publishers, 1986:257–260.
254. Treiman N, Waisbrod V, Waisbrod H. Lipoprotein electrophoresis in fat embolism: a Preliminary report. Injury 1981;13:108.
255. Trunkey DD. Pelvic injuries. In: Najarian JS, Delaney JP, eds. Trauma and critical care surgery. Chicago: Year Book Medical Publishers, 1987:147.
256. Trunkey DD, Chapman MW, Lim RC, Dunphy JE. Management of pelvic fractures in blunt trauma injury. J Trauma 1974;14:912.
257. Valentin N, Lomholt B, Jensen JS, et al. Spinal or general anaesthesia for surgery of the fractured hip. Br J Anaesth 1986;58:284.
258. Wagner WH, Calkins ER, Weaver FA, et al. Blunt popliteal artery trauma: one hundred consecutive injuries. J Vascular Surg 1988;7:736.
259. Wahba WM. Influence of aging on lung function—clinical significance of changes from age 20. Anesth Analg 1983;62:764.
260. Ward EF, Tomasin J, Vander Griend RA. Open reduction and internal fixation of vertical shear pelvic fractures. J Trauma 1987;27:291.
261. Ward RJ, Tolas AG, Benveniste RJ, et al. Effect of posture on normal arterial blood gas tensions in the aged. Geriatrics 1966;21:139.
262. Warner WA. Release of free fatty acids following trauma. J Trauma 1969;9:692.
263. Weiss EB. Subtle neurological injuries in pelvic fractures. J Trauma 1984;24:983.
264. Wertzberger JJ, Peltier LF. Fat embolism: the effect of corticosteroids on experimental fat embolism in the rat. Surgery 1968;64:143.
265. White JWC, Chappell WA. Anaesthesia for surgical correction of fractured femoral neck. A comparison of three techniques. Anaesthesia 1980;35:1107.
266. Whitman GR, McCroskey BL, Moore EE, et al. Traumatic popliteal and trifurcation vascular injuries: determinants of functional limb salvage. Am J Surg 1987;154:681.
267. Wickström I, Holmberg I, Steffansson T. Survival of female geriatric patients after hip fracture surgery. A comparison of 5 anaesthetic methods. Acta Anaesthesiol Scand 1982;26:607.
268. Wilkins KE. Fat embolism. In: Zauder HL, ed. Anaesthesia for orthopedic surgery. Philadelphia: FA Davis, 1980:147.
269. Williams JS, Hale HW. The advisability of inguinal herniorrhaphy in the elderly. Surg Gynecol Obstet 1966;122:100.
270. Wilson LA, Lawson IR, Braws W. Multiple disorders in the elderly: a clinical and statistical study. Lancet 1962;2:841.
271. Winnie AP. Spinal anesthesia for hip pinning given with the patient supine. JAMA 1969;207:1663.
272. Winnie AP, Ramamurthy S, Durrani Z, Radonjic R. Plexus blocks for lower extremity surgery. New answers to old problems. Anesth Rev 1974;1:11.
273. Wolff G, Dittmann M, Ruedi T, et al. Koordination von Chirurgie und Intensivmedizin zur Vermeidung der posttraumatischen respiratorische Insuffizienz. Unfallheilkunde 1978;81:425.
274. Wood M. Plasma drug binding: implications for anesthesiolgists. Anesth Analg 1986;65:786.
275. Wyant GM, Cockings EC. A study in geriatric anesthesia—fractured neck of the femur. Can Anaesth Soc J 1963;10:567.
276. Yaeger MP, Glass DD, Neff RK, Brinck-Johnsen T. Epidural anesthesia and analgesia in high-risk surgical patients. Anesthesiology 1987;66:729.
277. Zannis VJ, Wood MD. Laparotomy for pelvic fracture. Am J Surg 1980;140:841.

# Chapter Seventeen

*Katie P. Patel*
*Levon M. Capan*
*Gilbert J. Grant*
*Sanford M. Miller*

# *Management Principles for Microvascular Surgery*

A revolution in reconstructive surgery commenced in 1960 with the introduction of the operating microscope, microsurgery instruments, and microsutures into clinical practice. This technology permitted anastomosis of disrupted vessels as small as 1 mm or less in diameter and reattachment of small injured nerves, resulting in both esthetic and functional restoration of limbs or other parts of the body. In the United States the first replantation was performed by Malt and McKhann[53] in 1962 on a 12-year-old boy who had sustained an above-elbow amputation. This was followed by replantation of amputated digits by Kleinert and Kasdan[46] in 1963. Since then microsurgery has become an important subspecialty, saving many traumatically amputated parts of the body. Experience gained in this specialty over the years has resulted not only in improvement and innovation of techniques but also in development of realistic indications for surgery. The overuse that occurred during the early years of microsurgery has been replaced by improved patient and procedure selection.

Despite major advances in surgical techniques, optimal perioperative anesthetic management remains undefined. Several reviews describing anesthetic management for this type of surgery during the past decade are based on experience of individual centers, rather than on scientifically rigorous data.[8,15,36,51,74] Consequently, a wide variety of anesthetic techniques and agents has been advocated. This review summarizes the current understanding of perioperative anesthetic care of traumatized patients undergoing various microvascular procedures. The information presented in this chapter is based on our clinical experience supported by available data in the anesthetic and surgical literature.

## GENERAL CONSIDERATIONS

Microsurgery in the trauma victim is performed for the following purposes:

- To restore a completely amputated part (replantation)
- To restore the circulation of an incompletely severed part (revascularization)
- To reconstruct skin, muscle, and bone (free flap transfer)
- To repair nerve injuries

Although the number of centers with the capacity to perform these procedures has increased during the past few years, most trauma victims are still transferred to institutions specializing in this type of surgery. Thus, some anesthesiologists are rarely involved in the care of these patients, whereas for others administration of anesthesia for a microsurgical procedure has become an almost daily routine. At Bellevue Hospital Center approximately 30 limb replantations, 40 revascularizations, and 100 free flap transfers are performed every year (Table 17-1). Survival rates of replanted, revascularized, and transferred tissues has reached 80%, 95%, and 99%, respectively. These procedures are time consuming. The average time required for replantation of the first amputated digit is approximately 4 hours; each subsequent digit takes

TABLE 17-1. Replantations, Revascularizations, and Free Flap Transfers Performed at Bellevue Hospital Center, New York, 1985–1987*

| PROCEDURE | 1985 | 1986 | 1987 |
|---|---|---|---|
| Replantations | | | |
| Number of procedures | 21 | 32 | 29 |
| Mean age | 33 yr | 34 yr | 33 yr |
| Age range | 3–65 yr | 6.5–83 yr | 3.5–69 yr |
| Mean length of procedure | 9.5 h | 7.5 h | 7.5 h |
| Number of reoperations** | 9 (7) | 5 (3) | 3 (2) |
| Graft survival rate | 66.6% | 81.2% | 75.8% |
| Revascularizations | | | |
| Number of procedures | 34 | 31 | 40 |
| Mean age | 34 yr | 33 yr | 32 yr |
| Age range | 11–75 yr | 12–73 yr | 16 mo–63 yr |
| Mean length of procedure | 7.5 h | 7.5 h | 6 h |
| Number of reoperations** | 4 (3) | 5 (1) | 0 (0) |
| Graft survival rate | 91.1% | 93.5% | 95% |
| Free flaps† | | | |
| Number of procedures | 85 | 109 | 97 |
| Mean age | 39 yr | 37 yr | 38 yr |
| Age range | 14–69 yr | 12–63 yr | 16–72 yr |
| Mean length of procedure | 10 h | 8.5 h | 7 h |
| Number of reoperations | 12 | 18 | 11 |
| Graft survival rate | 99% | 90.8% | 98.9% |

* Courtesy of William Shaw, MD.

** Numbers in parentheses represent the number of reoperations which failed to improve graft survival.

† Includes trauma and nontrauma cases.

about 2 to 3 hours. Free flap transfers take an even longer time, ranging between 7 and 20 hours depending on the type of the flap, the skill and experience of the surgical team, and the type and severity of intraoperative complications. Reoperation to repair an occluded anastomosis, to relieve venous obstruction, and to control bleeding is relatively frequent and is required in approximately 10–20% of patients.

## REPLANTATION

The goal in replantation of an amputated part is re-establishment not only of morphologic continuity but also of function. Thus, the success of surgery is based on the survival as well as the degree of recovery of sensation and mobility of the replanted part. The repair of damaged nerves, tendons, bones, joints, and soft tissues is as important as that of vessels. Not all amputated limbs are replantable; careful patient selection based on well-established clinical criteria and the individual assessment of each patient is as important a determinant of tissue survival and function as the technical skills of the operating team.[47,62] Many factors influence the decision to embark on the replantation of an amputated limb.[34] A warm ischemic period of the amputated part exceeding 4 hours reduces the probability of replant survival, whereas a delay of 12 hours is a definite contraindication for replantation.[27,47] Placing the part in a dry plastic bag and surrounding it with another bag containing an ice and water mixture (4°C) increases the permissible ischemia time of digits to 24 or more hours and of the forearm to 12 hours.[8,62] Nevertheless, a period of cold ischemia exceeding 10 hours seems to decrease the functional recovery rate of replanted digits.[96]

A large muscle mass in the amputated part reduces the endurance time and the survival rate of the replant.[98] Additional factors, such as surgical dissection and use of a tourniquet, become critical in exacerbating the ischemia and increasing the chances of muscle necrosis and infection with both aerobic and anaerobic organisms.[56] Furthermore in these patients the risk of acidosis, hyperkalemia, and renal failure increases, whereas the possibility of regaining useful limb function is small.[56] Thus, the indications for reattachment of major limbs are more restricted than those for digits. In order to increase the likelihood of replant survival, amputated major parts are perfused with physiologic solutions or the patient's own blood via temporary shunts during the preparation phase. The wrist, however, does not contain a large muscle mass and responds favorably to replantation. Unfavorable results (insensate foot) obtained after lower extremity replants and the progressive improvement in design of lower extremity prostheses have reduced the enthusiasm for reattachment procedures in this area, except for limbs that have sustained a very brief period of ischemia.

The type of injury is another determinant of successful replantation. Sharp guillotine amputations are more amenable to replantation than severe avulsion and crush injuries or those with severe contamination.[47] Anatomic considerations play an important role in patient selection; thumb and multiple finger injuries are definite indications for urgent replantation, even in the presence of severe crush or avulsion damage since they provide the major portion of hand function. Obviously, valuable time should not be wasted on limb reattachment if severe life-threatening associated injuries are present.[27,47] However, with adequate preservation of the amputated limb, replantation is usually possible after the high-priority procedures are done.[98] Pre-existing medical problems have also been cited as absolute contraindications for replantation surgery.[27,47] However, with recent improvements in intraoperative monitoring and anesthetic management, the decision to operate must be based on an assessment of anesthetic and surgical risk for each patient. Anastomosis may be difficult if the vessel quality is affected by atherosclerosis, diabetes, or hypertension. The decision to perform replantation is thus also influenced by the patient's age. The small diameter of structures in the amputated parts may preclude repair in small children, although replant survival in children less than 16 years old was similar to that of adults in one study,[39] and, unlike adults, gratifying results were obtained in another after proximal upper limb replantation in children.[99]

## REVASCULARIZATION

As mentioned earlier, the term "revascularization" implies restoration of circulation to parts that are incompletely amputated, even if the tissues in continuity are minimal. Consequently, care considerations for replantation apply also to revascularization. Often the extent of tissue damage cannot be assessed preoperatively because of pain caused by examination of the limb. Thus, the decision to amputate or revascularize the injured extremity is often made after the patient is anesthetized.

## FREE FLAP TRANSFER

Unlike replantation, which is performed as an emergency, reconstruction with free flap transfer is usually performed urgently or electively. In the trauma patient this procedure is most commonly used to cover open wounds of the extremities. High-energy impact injuries frequently produce large losses of extremity tissue, including skin, fat, muscle, or even bone. After initial debridement, cleansing, and external fixation, these wounds must be covered with muscle and skin to prevent sepsis, osteomyelitis, and pain and to accelerate wound healing.[32] This can be done safely within the first week after injury if the open area remains dressed and moist. In the presence of bone loss, non-union is also a major threat. Substantial soft tissue loss that leaves only tendons and bone precludes coverage with split-thickness skin grafts and necessitates reconstruction with flaps, which in some instances must also contain bone.[37,38,59,66,86] Survival of these large flaps is not possible unless an adequate blood supply is provided. Thus, a unit of tissue with its principal artery and vein must be raised and implanted in the injured area by anastomosing its vessels to those of the recipient site.

Blood supply to the skin is provided by two types of arteries[78]: musculocutaneous and direct cutaneous arteries. Musculocutaneous arteries are the end branches of muscle perforators. These vessels rise obliquely within the subcutaneous fatty layer and reach the subdermal-dermal layer, forming an extensive network[16] (Fig 17-1A). Direct cutaneous arteries are located between the anterior muscle fascia and the deep subcutaneous fascia. Characteristically these vessels run parallel to the muscle fascia and the skin and are accompanied by a pair of veins called venae comitantes (Fig. 17-1B). Muscular blood supply is provided by segmental arteries that generally run parallel to the muscle along its undersurface[17] (Figs 17-1A and 17-1B). Segmental arteries form the pedicle of the flap. Thus, a viable skin flap includes the skin, the subcutaneous tissue, and the direct cutaneous artery (Fig 17-1B). Likewise a viable free myocutaneous flap can be raised by isolating the skin, the subcutaneous tissue, and the muscle with its pedicle (Figs 17-1A and 17-1B). Dissection should be parallel to the included artery in order to avoid damage to the vessel or the pedicle. A number of donor sites may be used, including some containing bone or even visceral organs. These donor sites have already been mapped and their nutrient arteries specified (Table 17-2). Recent understanding of anatomy has also enabled plastic surgeons to describe angiosomes in various regions of the body.[86] These units, consisting of skin and subcutaneous tissue, are supplied by multiple vessels and can be implanted with high reliability. Although the angiosome concept is currently used for rotation flaps, it is likewise used to define free flap territory.

After being raised, the flap is transferred to the recipient site and its pedicle anastomosed with appropriate vessels. The recipient site vessels are usually identified anatomically, but in severely distorted wounds, doppler studies or preoperative angiography may be necessary.

## REPAIR OF NERVE INJURIES

Whether associated with vessel damage or otherwise, the quality of nerve repair is critical to the achievement of adequate function. Crush injuries, proximal lesions, a delay of

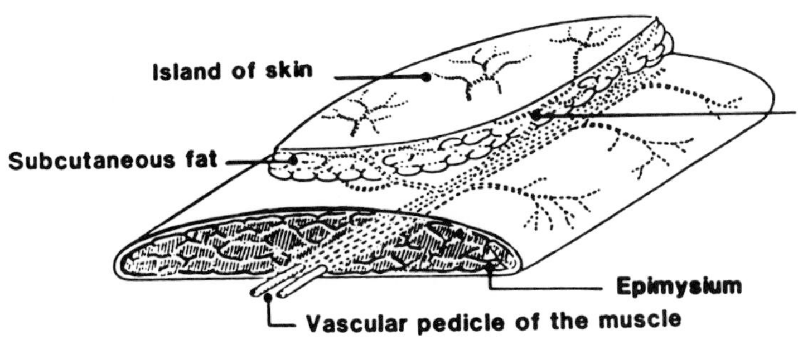


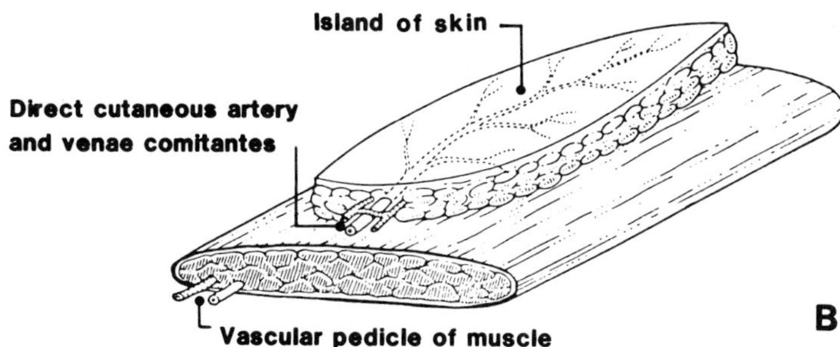


FIG. 17-1. The blood supply to the skin from musculocutaneous perforators (A) and direct cutaneous arteries (B). Note that the vascular pedicle of the muscle and the direct cutaneous artery and vena comitantes run parallel to the skin and muscle. (From Cormack GC, Lamberty BGH. The arterial anatomy of skin flaps. London: Churchill Livingstone, 1986; 65, 77, with permission.)

TABLE 17-2. Commonly Raised Flaps and Their Arteriovenous Supply

| FLAP DONOR SITE | ARTERIOVENOUS SUPPLY |
|---|---|
| Skin flaps | |
| Scalp | Superficial temporal |
| Scalp | Occipital |
| Deltopectoral | Internal mammary perforator |
| Myocutaneous flaps | |
| Latissimus dorsi | Thoracodorsal |
| Rectus femoris | Lateral femoral circumflex |
| Tensor fascia lata | Lateral femoral circumflex |
| Groin | Superficial circumflex iliac |
| Vascularized bone flaps | |
| Rib | Posterior cutaneous |
| Iliac crest | Deep circumflex iliac |
| Fibula | Peroneal |
| Osterocutaneous flaps | |
| Fibula and overlying skin | Peroneal |
| Iliac crest and overlying skin | Deep circumflex iliac |
| Specialized parts | |
| Great toe | Dorsalis pedis |

more than 48 hours, and a large gap between nerve ends affect nerve regeneration adversely and thus reduce the likelihood of successful repair.

Differentiation of motor and sensory elements is important for nerve regeneration. Various methods, such as electrical stimulation[30] or measurement of acetylcholinesterase content in the axons, have been used for this purpose. The authors believe that evoked potential monitoring may be a useful tool to distinguish between motor and sensory funiculi and assist the surgeon in the correct apposition of the nerves. Recovery of function after repair is a slow process, lasting up to 2 years. Although results of repair are assessed by both subjective and objective analysis of motor and sensory function, the patient's own assessment of his or her function provides the best means of evaluating nerve regeneration.

## PATHOPHYSIOLOGIC CONSIDERATIONS

Whether the surgery involves replantation of an amputated part, revascularization, or transfer of a flap, a wide variety of pathophysiologic events at the microvascular level determines the patency of anastomosed vessels and thereby the survival of implanted tissue. Although some of these factors have been recognized since the birth of microvascular surgery, other important factors have been appreciated only recently.

Essentially, the patency of the vessel is affected by interrelated extraluminal and intraluminal factors. During microvascular surgery these factors may reduce blood flow to the graft by constricting its vessel(s) and/or by promoting platelet aggregation with subsequent clot formation.

### EXTRALUMINAL FACTORS

These factors result from changes in the vessel wall and extravascular tissue. The blood vessels between 1 and 4 mm internal diameter that are used for microvascular anastomosis have a considerable amount of smooth muscle in their walls.[51] These muscles normally respond to sympathetic stimuli, which obviously cannot affect the denervated vessel wall. However, vascular spasm can still occur with surgical manipulation, cold, and reflex activity, despite the maximal dilation induced by accumulation of metabolites around the vessel during surgery.[45] Sympathetic control of vessels proximal and distal to the denervated area remains intact and adds its effects to the physical and chemical influences exerted on the vessel wall. Another factor that may affect vascular diameter is pressure in the tissue bed. It may increase because of edema, prolonged ischemia, or inadequate venous outflow and exert sufficient external pressure to constrict or even obstruct the vessel.[70]

Blood flow to the graft is governed by the laws of Laplace and Hagan-Poiseuille.[15,51,77] Laplace's law states that the intraluminal pressure required to keep the vessel open is greater in a constricted than in a dilated vessel:

$$P = 2T/R$$

where P is the intraluminal pressure, T the vascular wall tension, and R the radius of the vessel wall. The greater the pressures exerted on the vessel wall by autonomous vessel tone and extravascular tissue pressure, the greater the intraluminal pressure required to keep the vessel open. Thus the critical closing pressure, which by definition is the external pressure required to obstruct the vessel totally, decreases when the vessel is already constricted.[11]

The Hagan-Poiseuille law states that flow through a vessel is proportional to the driving pressure (pressure difference over the length of the vessel) and the fourth power of the radius:

$$\text{Flow} = \frac{\Delta P \pi r^4}{8 \eta L}$$

where $\Delta P$ is driving pressure, $\eta$ is blood viscosity, r is vessel radius, and L is vessel length.

Thus, in a dilated vessel the substantially increased blood flow allows reduction in the driving pressure needed to maintain adequate circulation. In contrast, a constricted vessel requires disproportionately high driving pressures to maintain vascular patency.

Viewed from these perspectives, it becomes obvious that the first requisite to ensure adequate flow to the graft is to maintain maximal dilation in the anastomosed vessel.

### INTRALUMINAL FACTORS

As already discussed, blood flow is proportional to the driving pressure, the magnitude of which is largely determined by systemic blood pressure. Adequate blood pressure varies from one patient to another, depending on history of preoperative hypertension, age, intravascular blood volume, and the extent of atherosclerosis. Nevertheless in a young individual with minimal atherosclerosis a systolic blood pressure of no less than 100 mm Hg provides satisfactory perfusion.[51] Allowing the systemic blood pressure to fall below this level results not only in a decline in perfusion pressure but may also cause stimulation of the renin-angiotensin and vasopressin systems with resulting vasoconstriction.[51] The vasoconstrictive effect of these reflexes in the skin and muscle, however, may be overridden by low pressure receptors stimulated by a full vascular compartment.[51] Thus, the second and third requisites to ensure adequate blood flow to the graft are provision of adequate perfusion pressure and adequate intravascular volume.

As can be seen from the Hagan-Poiseuille equation, blood viscosity also plays an important role in determining blood flow through the graft. Generally the higher the viscosity, the lower the blood flow. The effect of viscosity in the microcirculation, however, is more complex than that described by the Hagan-Poiseuille equation. A gradual decrease in intravascular pressure occurs as blood flows through the vasculature (Fig 17-2). Thus at the arteriolar level blood pressure is approximately 40 mm Hg, whereas in the venules it is 20 mm Hg.[70] The flow rate at the arteriolar level, although lower than that in the aorta, is increased relative to the diameter of the vessel. For a non-Newtonian fluid, such as blood, an increase in relative velocity produces an increase in shear rate (pressure-generated flow) and decreased viscosity.[51] In fact, the normal blood viscosity in the arterioles and capillaries is lower than that in the large arteries and approaches that of the plasma.[51] This reduction in viscosity results from alignment of the erythrocytes in the arteriolar lumen with their surfaces parallel to each other (Fig 17-3). The space between the edges of the erythrocytes and the vessel wall is occupied by plasma. Such regularity in red cell alignment is a direct result of the relative increase in velocity of arteriolar blood flow and the high elasticity of erythrocytes.

When the shear rate decreases or the red cells lose their elasticity (as in acidosis or sickling), this streamlining of the erythrocytes disappears and capillary blood viscosity increases, resulting in a reduction of blood flow. This decrease in shear rate results from decreased arterial blood pressure and increased venous resistance caused either by active vasoconstriction or by an excessive increase in whole blood viscosity. Normally the enlargement in vessel caliber during the transit of blood from the capillaries into the venules results in a sudden fall in flow rate. If such a decrease in venular shear rate reaches a critical value below which erythrocytes lose their axial streamlining (Fig 17-3), the viscosity of the blood within the venule increases. This effect, coupled with collisions of the erythrocytes with the vessel walls, results in increased resistance to capillary outflow and a concomitant reduction of blood flow at this level as well. Thus, a progressive decrease in flow in both the capillaries and venules reaches a point where red cells tend to aggregate and occlude the lumen of the vessel.

FIG. 17-2. The mean pressure in various segments of the vascular system.

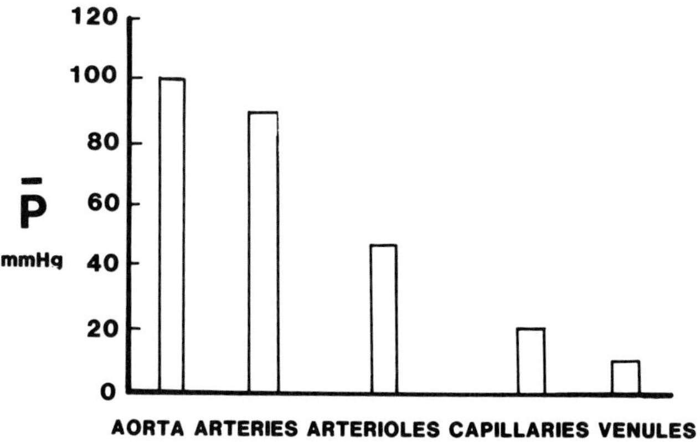


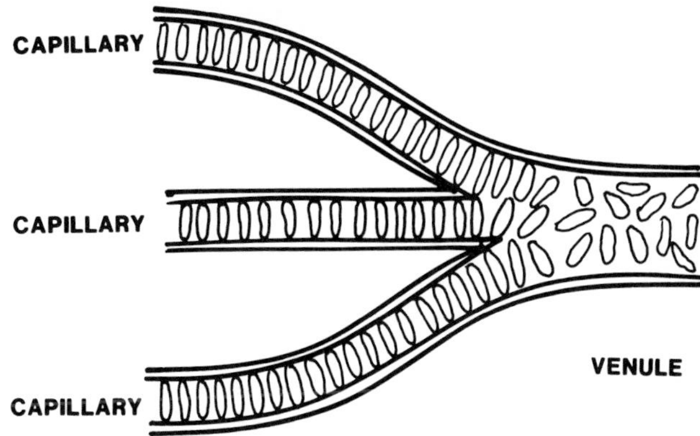


FIG. 17-3. The relative increase in velocity in the capillaries results in streamlining of the erythrocytes with reduction of viscosity. In the venules the blood velocity is lower than in the capillaries. Erythrocytes tend to lose their streamlining with a resultant increase in blood viscosity.

Several other factors influence the viscosity of blood: high hematocrit, increased plasma concentrations of fibrinogen and macroglobulins, and infusion of fluids with high molecular weight, eg, dextran. Of these, hematocrit is of prime importance; lowering the hematocrit is usually sufficient to improve blood flow even when the plasma contains an elevated concentration of high molecular weight substances. One important reason why the overall viscosity of blood decreases and its flow in the microcirculation improves with infusion of dextran or albumin is the hemodilution caused by these high molecular weight agents. Thus, the fourth requisite to provide adequate blood flow to the graft is to maintain a low blood viscosity, which can be achieved mainly by keeping the hematocrit at relatively low levels, usually at 30.

Probably the most important intraluminal factor that jeopardizes graft flow is thrombotic occlusion of the anastomosed vessel. Perioperative microvascular thrombosis occurs in 10 to 20% of cases and is more common after replantation of digits than following free flap transfer. Occult intimal damage from the injury appears to be the reason for this high rate of thrombosis.[82] The major event that initiates microvascular thrombosis after significant injury to the vascular endothelium is adherence of platelets to the exposed collagen and subendothelial structures. Formation of an enzyme-substrate complex between galactosyl residues in the collagen and glucosyl-transferase on the platelet membrane appears to be the mechanism of platelet adhesion to the vascular wall.[13] Simultaneously, increased platelet aggregation at the damaged vascular site takes place (primary aggregation).

After the reversible primary aggregation, an irreversible secondary aggregation occurs in which secretory granules within the platelets release calcium, serotonin, adenosine triphosphate (ATP), adenosine diphosphate (ADP), collagenase, elastase, and platelet factors (release-I reaction). Thromboxane $A_2$ ($TxA_2$), formed by the metabolism of membrane-bound arachidonic acid, plays an important role in the release-I reaction. A release-II reaction also takes place during the secondary aggregation phase in which cathepsin, acid hydrolase, and fibrinogen released from the α granules stimulate platelet aggregation. This reaction is stimulated by thrombin and high levels of collagen. Of all the substances released, ADP has the greatest effect in enhancing secondary platelet aggregation, thereby rapidly increasing the size of the thrombus. The clot formed up to this point contains primarily platelets and therefore is termed "white clot." In the microvasculature the "white clot" is sufficient to cause occlusion. As thrombosis progresses, fibrin and erythrocytes build up via the extrinsic coagulation pathway to produce a completely developed clot.[13]

Recent data have pointed out the importance of arachidonic acid metabolites in microvascular clot formation.[13] Both the vascular endothelium and the outer layer of the platelets contain a large amount of arachidonic acid, which is converted to prostaglandins $G_2$ ($PGG_2$) and $H_2$ ($PGH_2$) via the cyclo-oxygenase pathway after the injury. There is, however, a substantial difference in the metabolism of $PGG_2$ and $PGH_2$ in the platelets and the vascular wall (Fig 17-4). In the platelet, $PGG_2$ is converted to $TxA_2$ and $TxB_2$ by the enzyme, thromboxane synthetase. These end products, especially $TxA_2$, are potent stimulants of platelet aggregation and cause vasoconstriction. A completely different set of biochemical events takes place in the vascular wall where $PGH_2$ and $PGG_2$ are converted by the enzyme, prostacyclin synthetase, to prostacyclin ($PGI_2$), a potent vasodilator and a powerful inhibitor of platelet aggregation. Thus, the balance between intraluminal thromboxane ($TxA_2$ and $TxB_2$) and prostacyclin ($PGI_2$) activity is an important determinant of clot formation. As discussed later, this balance can be manipulated, at least theoretically, in favor of the prostacyclin pathway with clinically available pharmacologic agents. $PGI_2$ and $TxA_2$ produce their effects on platelet aggregation via the adenine nucleotide mechanism. $PGI_2$ stimulates adenyl cyclase, whereas $TxA_2$ inhibits it. Adenyl cyclase is necessary for production of intracellular 3′5′cyclic AMP, which inhibits platelet aggregation. Thus, the fifth requisite to maintain vascular patency and therefore adequate blood flow to the graft is to prevent adhesion and aggregation of platelets to the vascular wall and to each other, respectively, by both mechanical and pharmacologic means.

## MEASURES TO OPTIMIZE GRAFT BLOOD FLOW

Basically these measures can be divided into two categories: (a) those involving the surgical technique and (b) those unrelated to the surgical technique.

### MEASURES INVOLVING THE SURGICAL TECHNIQUE

In most instances in which the patient's metabolic and hemodynamic status is maintained optimally, blood flow and thus the survival of the graft are primarily determined by the appropriateness of patient selection and the surgical technique employed.[31] Although an extensive discussion on microsurgical techniques is beyond our expertise and the scope of this review, a few basic principles deserve to be mentioned.

Before anastomosis the vessel should be examined under the highest magnification to rule out damage, intimal tears, intraluminal clot, or fibrin deposition. Only normal vessels

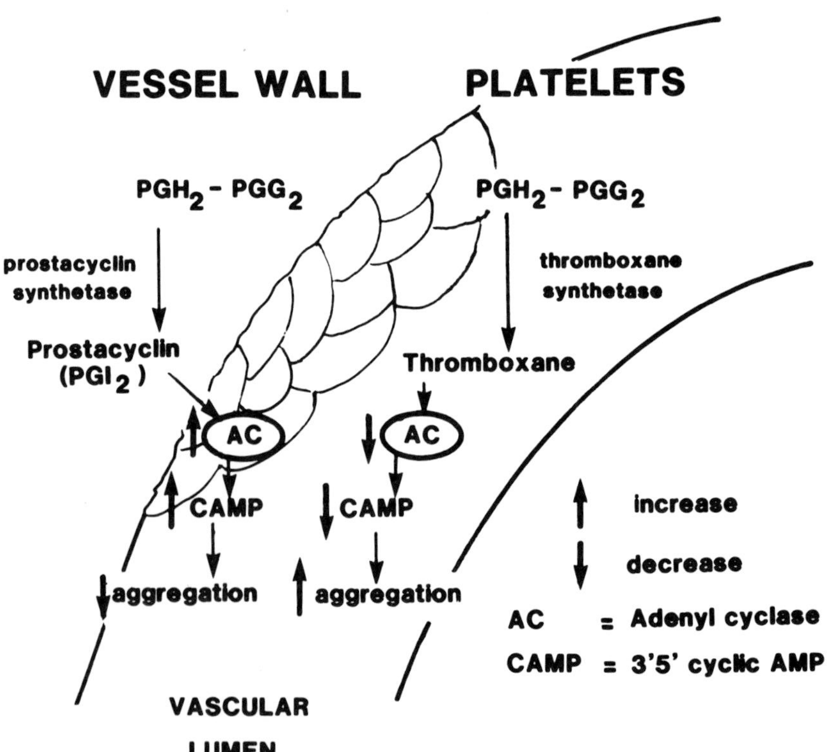


FIG. 17-4. Arachidonic acid metabolism in the vessel wall and platelets and the effect of metabolites on platelet aggregation.

with good pulsatile flow should be anastomosed. If the vessel is damaged, adequate debridement should be performed and blood clots removed. The largest possible vessel supplying the graft must be selected for anastomosis. Whenever possible end-to-side, rather than end-to-end, anastomosis into larger vessels is preferred since vasospasm is less likely to occur with this method. Excessive longitudinal tension on the anastomosed vessel promotes vasospasm, especially on the venous side. If this situation is likely, interposition of free vein graft(s) may be necessary. Kinking or twisting of the vessel should also be avoided by appropriate adjustment of the length of the vascular graft. If the anastomosed vessel constricts, it should be dilated by using undiluted topical lidocaine (4%), bupivacaine (0.5%), papaverine, or verapamil. If spasm persists despite these measures, mechanical dilation of the vessel with a vessel dilator or a jeweler's forceps may be effective. The graft tissue must be kept warm by using warm saline, heat lamps, or both. After the anastomosis is completed the patency of the vessel must be checked for both antegrade and retrograde flow.[14] Occlusion of the anastomosis immediately after its completion usually results from poor technique; it should be taken down and redone. Before wound closure adequate hemostasis must be achieved; perivascular hematoma is an important cause of vessel occlusion. Likewise, fasciotomy may be necessary to decompress swollen muscle compartments, which may bring about vessel occlusion. During closure of the wound the revascularized region should be monitored constantly to avoid compression of the vascular pedicle.

At the conclusion of surgery, dressings should be applied loosely to prevent compression of the anastomosed vessels. Postoperative factors that may result in venous obstruction and tissue edema must be treated. The grafted region should be elevated to promote venous drainage and decrease swelling. Medicinal leeches have been applied on the graft tissue to reduce venous congestion (Fig 17-5). In addition leeches secrete a powerful anticoagulant, hirudin, which has the potential of reducing thrombotic complications.[5] If these measures are ineffective in abolishing venous stasis, reoperation may be required.

## MEASURES UNRELATED TO THE SURGICAL TECHNIQUE

### *Hemodynamic Management*

Of the five basic requisites described in the previous section to ensure adequate blood flow to the graft, four can be attained by providing optimal total body circulation. The meaning of "optimal total body circulation" in the context of microvascular surgery differs slightly from the usual definition. MacDonald[51] and Jakubowski et al.[40] suggest that a slightly hyperdynamic circulation is required to provide optimal graft

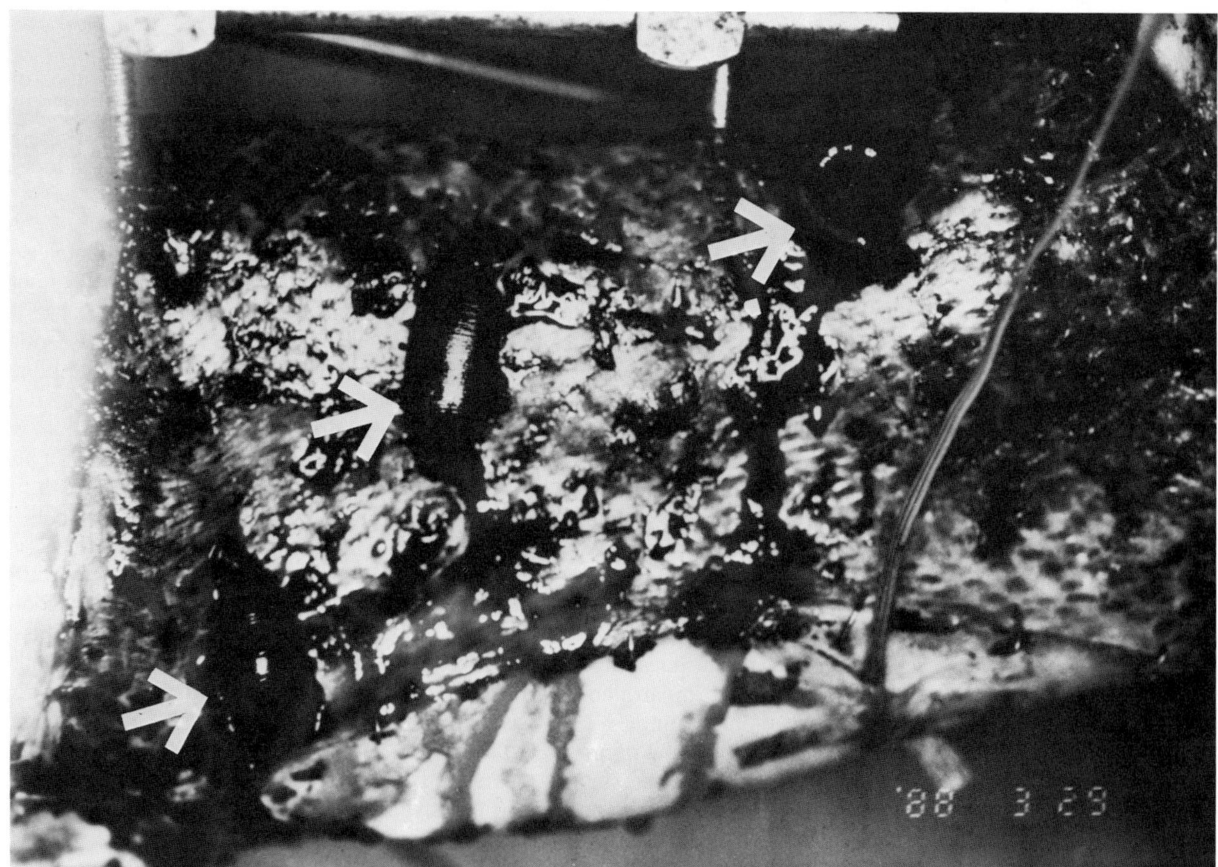


FIG. 17-5. Medicinal leeches (*arrows*) applied on a free flap to reduce venous congestion.

flow. They recommend raising cardiac filling pressures deliberately to 2–3 mm Hg above the patient's normal value with fluid infusion to achieve increased cardiac output and simultaneous skin and muscle vasodilation. Since low blood viscosity is crucial for the adequacy of microcirculation, they suggest that the volume of infused acellular fluids should exceed that of transfused blood by several-fold so that a hypervolemic hemodilution with a hematocrit value between 30 and 35 is maintained. Most clinicians agree with these guidelines,[15] even though there are few data to prove the superiority of a hyperdynamic circulation over normal hemodynamics. Of course, these management principles should be applied only after ensuring adequate cardiac reserve since the adequacy of peripheral oxygen transport in hypervolemic hemodilution depends on the ability of the heart to increase its stroke volume.

Often the extent of blood loss during surgery is difficult to quantitate because more blood is lost in the surgical drapes than on sponges or in the suction container. In emergency replant surgery, a significant amount of blood may have been lost preoperatively without a significant change in systemic blood pressure, yet sudden hemodynamic depression may occur after induction of anesthesia. Major blood loss invariably occurs if the limbs are severed at proximal sites, such as the forearm, arm, or leg. In reconstructive free flap transfers, continuous capillary and venous bleeding occurs during preparation of the donor and recipient site, amounting usually to 1000–1500 mL. Deliberate hypotension during this phase may reduce blood loss, but blood pressure should be restored before microvascular anastomoses are performed. Serial measurements of blood pressure, pulse, hematocrit, and urine output must be performed to determine the adequacy of blood volume and hemodynamics.

Although the suggestion has been made that the monitoring of urine output coupled with noninvasive measurement of blood pressure is satisfactory,[51] we prefer to monitor blood pressure in these patients with an indwelling arterial catheter. The urine output must be maintained at a minimum of 1 mL/kg/h to ensure satisfactory perfusion. If a central venous line is inserted, we aim to maintain the pressure at 1 or 2 mm Hg above the patient's control value. In the majority of patients, however, we titrate our infusions according to the changes in amplitude of the arterial pressure trace with respiration since the sensitivity of this method is equal to or even exceeds that of central venous pressure (CVP).[69] Using this method, fluids are infused generously until the difference in amplitude of the arterial trace during controlled inspiration and expiration is minimal or disappears. Pulmonary artery catheterization is seldom necessary; we do use it, however, during the infrequently performed major limb replantations in which blood loss may exceed 4000–5000 mL.

Controversy continues about the choice of infusion fluids. Used alone, crystalloids theoretically have the disadvantage of disappearing rapidly from the intravascular compartment and thus being less effective than colloids in maintaining volume expansion and hemodilution.[40,51] In addition, the tissue edema produced by these solutions may jeopardize the survival of the flap.[40] None of these suppositions, however, is based on objective determinations. Thus, we continue to use mainly isotonic crystalloid solutions for fluid replacement. In many centers, dextran 40 is administered routinely. This is done not only to take advantage of its colloid osmotic effect, which by drawing water into the intravascular compartment increases plasma volume, improves blood flow, produces hemodilution, and causes passive capillary dilation, but also to reduce the likelihood of thrombosis, since this agent by increasing the negative charge on platelets decreases their adhesiveness to foreign substances. The recommended dosage is 500 mL administered over a period of 1 hour starting shortly after anesthetic induction. Thereafter, the patient receives 500 mL every 12–24 hours for 5 or 6 days postoperatively. The peak effect of dextran 40 occurs approximately 4 hours after infusion and lasts at least 12 hours. Recently, we have been administering this agent as a 25 mL/h infusion after a 500-mL loading dose to provide sustained action. Possible complications of dextran 40 include circulatory overload, hemorrhage due to coagulation abnormality, anaphylactic reaction (incidence 0.003–0.038%), and renal damage.

### *Prevention of Thrombosis*

As has been discussed, proper surgical technique is the most effective means of prevention of thrombosis at the site of anastomosis. However, additional pharmacologic measures may contribute to prevention of clot formation. As evidenced by their waxing and waning clinical use during the past 30 years, the efficacy and reliability of some of these agents have not been well established. Nevertheless in clinical conditions where doubt exists about the success of surgical repair, these measures are often utilized.

HEPARIN. The anticoagulant effect of heparin is mainly derived from accelerated antithrombin activity, which inhibits thrombin activation.[29,62,75] In addition heparin reduces platelet adhesiveness by blocking the thrombin-induced release-II reaction[20] and inhibits the conversion of fibrinogen to fibrin.[75] However, thrombosis in microvascular surgery is mediated primarily by adhesion and aggregation of platelets, the extent of which is predominantly determined by the amount of ADP release and the balance between $PGI_2$ and $TxA_2$.[13] The thrombin-induced release-II reaction is thus not essential for platelet aggregation.[52] In addition, heparin, by inhibiting adenyl cyclase, decreases platelet cyclic AMP content and thus neutralizes the antiaggregatory effect of $PGI_2$.[13] It would seem logical then to expect that heparin should have little value in prevention of microvascular thrombosis and, in fact, may be deleterious through its neutralizing effect on $PGI_2$. Indeed, Ketchum[43] has shown that the patency rate of vessels repaired with concomitant heparin treatment was no different from those repaired without heparin administration. Recently, however, Greenberg et al.[29] showed that in rabbits continuous intravenous heparin infusion (500 units bolus followed by 45 μl/h for 3 days after microvascular anastomosis) increased the vascular patency rate from 19 to 69%. Puckett,[71] in a separate experimental study, also found that locally applied heparin was effective in protecting the anastomosis. Currently, heparin prophylaxis is used in only a few centers because of its doubtful effect on thrombosis prevention and its potential bleeding complications. If, however, the results obtained from these animal studies can be reproduced in humans, heparin may gain in popularity.

ASPIRIN AND INDOMETHACIN. Aspirin blocks the enzyme cyclo-oxygenase, thus inhibiting the formation of $PGG_2$ and $PGH_2$. Its blocking effect on platelet and endothelial cell cyclo-oxygenase is dose related; platelet cyclo-oxygenase is blocked with lower aspirin levels than endothelial cell cyclo-oxygenase.[10] Thus, the balance between $PGI_2$ and $TxA_2$ can be shifted in favor of the former by using low-dose aspirin. Currently in most institutions aspirin, 3 mg/kg/day, is given daily for 3 to 4 weeks postoperatively until the anastomosis is completely re-endothelialized. In our institution, 325 mg of aspirin is administered rectally before surgery and continued orally at this dose daily for a few days.

Indomethacin acts on phospholipase $A_2$, an enzyme necessary for the production of arachidonic acid. Thus, indomethacin results in a reduction of both $PGI_2$ and $TxA_2$, as well as primary degradation products of arachidonic acid. In microvascular surgery this agent is seldom used.

DEXTRAN. The use of this agent in microvascular surgery has been discussed in the previous section.

EXPERIMENTAL ANTITHROMBOTIC AGENTS. Pluronic F68, a synthetic polyglycol that is administered parenterally, reduces the adhesiveness of platelets in experimental anastomoses; it has not been used clinically.[44] Topical application of magnesium sulfate has been used in an attempt to reduce microvascular thrombosis experimentally without any appreciable benefit.[23] Activation of the fibrinolytic system may be impaired after prolonged ischemia of the amputated parts. Fibrinolytic agents such as streptokinase may be useful in these circumstances. In one study streptokinase, in an initial bolus of 100,000 U followed by 5,000 U daily, was used in six patients with distal hand ischemia. Reperfusion of the hand was established in four patients.[41] Further work is necessary to determine the efficacy of these agents in microvascular surgery.

### *Measures to Enhance Vasodilation or Prevent Vasospasm*

Surgical measures to prevent or treat intraoperative vasospasm have already been discussed. Additional measures that are known to produce vasodilation may improve blood flow to the graft and prevent vascular spasm.

SYMPATHETIC BLOCKADE. Although sympathetic blockade has no effect on the denervated vessels of the amputated part or of the raised free flap, it may increase the flow of blood to and from the graft by producing vasodilation in the recipient site.[70,74] There is some evidence to substantiate this supposition. For instance, surgical sympathectomy and epidural anesthesia have been shown to increase graft flow during reconstructive vascular surgery, such as aortoiliac or femoropopliteal bypass.[18,88] In radial forearm flaps, combined cervical and brachial plexus block with bupivacaine 0.375% caused a 50% increase in blood flow to the flap.[45] Likewise, in anecdotal reports epidural bupivacaine was shown to reestablish blood flow to a lower extremity microvascular free flap,[93] whereas block of the brachial plexus increased the arterial flow to replanted fingers by 102 to 786%.[7,60] It may be critical to administer these blocks in young patients (age < 25 years) whose vessels tend to constrict, especially after surgical manipulation.

In spite of these findings, however, available data are not sufficient to prove that sympathetic blockade improves graft survival. Epidural blockade, by producing hypotension, may cause an overall reduction of blood flow to the graft.[91] In one instance decreased perfusion of the graft was noted despite a steady blood pressure.[91] It is possible that, in some patients, vasodilation in adjacent normal tissues produced by sympathetic blockade may result in a "steal" phenomenon, decreasing blood flow to the graft.

Sympathetic blockade can be provided by several methods. Continuous epidural anesthesia using intermittent doses of 0.25–0.5% bupivacaine (5 mL/h) or 1.5% lidocaine (5 mL/h) or infusion of these local anesthetics (0.1 mL/min) after an initial loading dose of 15–20 mL provides satisfactory sympathetic blockade of the lower extremity.[18,74,93] For the upper extremity, brachial plexus block using axillary, supraclavicular, interscalene, subclavian perivascular,[94] or the modified axillary approach described by Ang et al.[2] can be administered. All of these techniques are amenable to placement of a catheter adjacent to the plexus,[2,21,33,49,54,56,76,79] and thus continuous sympathetic blockade may be maintained with doses of local anesthetics similar to those used for epidural anesthesia. Adrenaline (1:100,000–1:200,000) added to the local anesthetic increases the cardiac output and thus blood flow to the fingers, yet local vasoconstriction produced by this agent during axillary brachial plexus block prevents an increase in circulation to the arm.[19,60] In addition to producing vasodilation in the involved extremity, these blocks have the advantages of reducing the stress response if they are used during surgery, allowing administration of lower doses of general anesthetic, and providing effective postoperative analgesia.[74]

Satisfactory upper extremity sympathetic blockade can also be obtained with stellate ganglion block using 0.25–0.5% bupivacaine or 1% lidocaine (5–10 mL). Although continuous stellate ganglion block by injection of local anesthetics through a catheter is possible, this block is usually performed intermittently when there is doubt about the patency of graft vessels in the postoperative period. Radial, ulnar, and median nerve blocks at the wrist also provide good sympathetic blockade after digital surgery and reduce the likelihood of the "steal" phenomenon that may accompany proximal plexus blocks.[70] The ulnar and median nerves are anesthetized through catheters inserted surgically or percutaneously adjacent to the nerves,[70] whereas the radial nerve is blocked by semicircumferential subcutaneous injection of the lateral aspect of the wrist. Intravenous regional block (IVRB) using low-concentration local anesthetics (lidocaine 0.5%, prilocaine 0.5%, or bupivacaine 0.25%) also provides effective sympathetic blockade of the extremities, but this effect often disappears with removal of the tourniquet 1 or 2 hours after injection of the local anesthetic agent. The use of guanethidine (15–30 mg) or reserpine (2.5 mg) in 30–50 mL isotonic saline or local anesthetic solution during IVRB may provide prolonged sympathetic blockade lasting up to 7 days.[26,35]

Selective α-adrenergic blockade by systemic administration of phentolamine, phenoxybenzamine, chlorpromazine, or thymoxamine has been employed both experimentally and clinically to improve blood flow to the graft,[1,25,74] but all of these agents have the potential of producing profound hypotension and tachycardia, which limits their clinical usefulness. In addition, these agents do not protect against the direct vascular smooth muscle contraction that results from surgical manipulation. The β-adrenergic agonist isoxuprine has also been used successfully for this purpose,[24] but this drug too has systemic side effects, such as tachycardia, hypotension, and tremor.

GANGLIONIC BLOCKERS AND DIRECT VASODILATORS. Trimethaphan, a ganglionic blocking agent, can also produce vasodilation, but does not protect against vasospasm. Nitroglycerine, hydralazine, and sodium nitroprusside are direct vascular smooth muscle relaxants and have the potential of preventing or treating vasospasm. Nitroglycerine tends to have a greater effect on the venous than on the arterial side. Thus, its beneficial effect in microvascular surgery, in which the primary focus is on dilating the arterioles and increasing the inflow to the graft, is limited. However, recent data describe an important property of nitroglycerine: reduced platelet deposition on the injured arterial wall.[48] Hydralazine is a longer-acting agent, and therefore, its vasodilator effect is difficult to control. In addition this drug often produces reflex tachycardia, treatment of which requires a β-adrenergic blocking agent with the risk of vasoconstriction. Sodium nitroprusside is probably the most logical choice among all vasodilators; its short duration of action allows it to be controlled easily. Nitroprusside is capable of preventing or treating vasospasm and, if used properly, can relax vascular smooth muscle without producing profound hypotension. The drug is administered via a central venous line and is titrated to a systolic blood pressure around 100 mm Hg. Using this method in patients undergoing free flap transfer, Aps and co-workers[3] reported a significant reduction in intraoperative vasospasm during microvascular surgery.

MAINTENANCE OF TEMPERATURE. Vasodilation caused by ischemia and denervation in an amputated part or a raised flap is more than counteracted by a concomitant local decrease in temperature.[4,45] Warming the amputated part with irrigation solution or heating lamps improves blood flow[45] by reducing the effects of hypothermia: vasoconstriction, hemoconcentration, increased red cell aggregation, and increased whole blood and plasma viscosity.[51] If the overall temperature of the body is also low, further reduction in graft blood flow occurs because of increased vasomotor tone in the innervated skin, which is mediated by direct stimulation of cutaneous vessels by cold and indirectly through the vasomotor centers that are in turn stimulated by perfusion of cold blood. Sympathetic input to innervated vessels is probably negligible during anesthesia, but gains importance during the recovery period. Thus, temperature preservation during microsurgery is vital in order to maintain blood flow to the graft and should be achieved with two objectives in mind: adequate body temperature and adequate graft temperature. Hypothermia during general anesthesia is caused by impaired heat production and heat conservation. The degree of impairment in heat production varies from one individual to the other and is maximal in the elderly and in infants.

Little can be done to increase heat production during anesthesia, but several measures can and should be employed to conserve heat. In an anesthetized patient heat is lost by four different mechanisms: evaporation, radiation, conduction, and convection. Of these, evaporation and radiation are the main sources of heat loss. Measures to reduce evaporative heat loss include the delivery of warm and humidified gases to the patient by incorporating heated humidifiers or heat-moisture exchangers in the anesthesia circuit. Administration of the anesthetic in a closed or semiclosed circuit is also effective, because with low fresh gas inflow the effectiveness of the exothermic and moisture-producing reaction between $CO_2$ and soda lime is augmented. In order to overcome radiative heat loss, as much of the patient's surface area as possible should be covered with plastic sheeting. Often more than one anatomic region is operated upon during microsurgery; thus, the effective block of radiant heat loss may not be possible. Heat loss by conduction can be minimized by warming all fluids administered to the patient. Convective heat loss results from the movement of cold air across exposed body areas. Thus, it can be minimized by warming the operating room to between 21°C and 24°C and by covering as much of the patient as possible with protective blankets or plastic sheeting. More detailed information on general temperature preservation is provided in Chapter 9.

Graft temperature can best be preserved by exposing the graft to appropriate heating lamps.[45] The duration of exposure and the distance between the lamp and the graft must be adjusted carefully to prevent burn injury. Solutions used for wound irrigation must also be warm to prevent heat loss.[45] The graft should not be wrapped in wet packs during dissection as this technique promotes heat loss.

Recent data suggest that postoperative shivering is primarily a result of decreased cortical inhibition of spinal reflex hyperactivity.[81] However, maintenance of body temperature may minimize shivering and help avoid vasoconstriction in the grafted tissue. If postoperative shivering occurs, treatment with intravenous meperidine, 15–25 mg, along with measures to warm the patient rapidly, will minimize the duration of vasoconstriction.

A temperature elevation of 1°C or 2°C toward the end of a 10- to 12-hour general anesthetic for replantation or free flap transfer is not uncommon.[12,15,74] The exact cause of this effect is not clear. Sepsis has been suggested as a cause, although evidence for its occurrence is lacking. Closure of surgical wounds while heat-conserving measures are functional may also result in pyrexia. The most likely cause, however, is the endocrine-metabolic response to surgery, which is frequently manifested by hyperthermia 12–24hours after an operation. In fact, a correlation between steroid output and temperature rise in patients undergoing prolonged surgery under general anesthesia has been described by Cochrane,[15] who observed that patients receiving regional anesthesia had lower serum cortisol levels and less elevation of temperature than those who received general anesthesia. The increase in body temperature usually continues in the recovery room. Treatment includes discontinuing heat-preserving measures, cooling the patient, and using antipyretics, such as aspirin suppositories.

MAINTENANCE OF NORMOCARBIA. Hypocapnia should be avoided as it increases peripheral vascular resistance and decreases the cardiac output, jeopardizing the blood flow to the graft.[51] In contrast, hypercapnia may increase bleeding and result in cardiac dysrhythmias, although it produces vasodilation. Thus, normocapnia must be maintained throughout the surgical procedure to provide adequate blood flow to the graft.

PREVENTION OF PAIN AND AGITATION. Both pain and anxiety cause an increase in vasomotor tone; thus, adequate pain control and prevention of anxiety and agitation during emergence from anesthesia are important. Extending regional anesthesia into the postoperative period will provide excellent analgesia and decrease the likelihood of agitation. For lower extremity procedures, epidural anesthesia provides good analgesia, but may also cause hypotension. Epidural narcotics, although devoid of vasodilator effect, provide adequate postoperative pain relief without the risk of hypotension.

POSTOPERATIVE SMOKING. One cigarette yields 0.4–1.6 mg of nicotine, which stimulates the autonomic nervous system to release catecholamines. Vasoconstriction, blood pressure elevation, and tachycardia resulting from cigarette smoking may jeopardize graft flow. Each cigarette also causes a 42% decrease in distal blood flow velocity and, at times, vasospasm. Rao et al.[73] demonstrated in rabbits that spasm induced by cigarette smoke was dose dependent and decayed over a period of 10 minutes. It is important not only that the patient refrain from smoking but also that visitors not be allowed to smoke in the patient's room.

## MONITORING OF GRAFT PERFUSION

The first requirement for preventing loss of revascularized tissue is early detection of perfusion failure during the postoperative period.[31] Perfusion failure requiring early surgery occurs in approximately 6–15% of free tissue transfers.[31,50] Only 70–75% of replanted digits are viable, some only after urgent re-exploration and anastomotic repair. The techniques employed to monitor graft perfusion and their advantages have been summarized by Sanders[77] (Table 17-3). Monitoring of graft temperature is sufficient to detect perfusion failure in finger replants.[77] On the other hand, temperature monitoring is not satisfactory in determining the adequacy of most free flaps because heat from the surrounding well-vascularized tissues may affect the temperature of a nonviable graft.[77] Differential temperature monitoring, which involves measuring the gradient between the graft and the surrounding normal tissue, may have predictive value, but only 24 or more hours after flap insertion, which is sometimes too late.[42] Although a consensus has not been reached about the most satisfactory monitoring technique, transcutaneous oxygen, laser Doppler, ultrasound Doppler, tissue pH monitoring, and photoplethysmography appear to be promising techniques.[42,77]

## ANESTHETIC CONSIDERATIONS

### PREOPERATIVE ASSESSMENT

Preoperative evaluation of patients undergoing free flap transfer is usually similar to that required for any electively operated patient, but a few additional areas must be assessed carefully. Typically, open wounds with significant tissue loss are only debrided and fractures are externally fixed during the immediate postinjury phase; free flap coverage of the wound is delayed until the patient's overall condition and associated injuries are stabilized. The presence of consequences of multiple trauma, such as associated head, maxillofacial, or thoracoabdominal injuries; postinjury sepsis; fat- or thromboembolism; and single- or multiorgan failure must be sought for and their effects on hemodynamics, oxygenation, acid-base status, and blood chemistry assessed carefully. Depending on their severity, any of these conditions may result in a complicated intra- and postoperative course, resulting at times in death. Thus, there is little justification to administer an anesthetic for free flap surgery in these situations. In addition, based on animal studies, septic foci, even though remote from the site of microvascular surgery, may promote clot formation within the anastomosed vessel[61] and thus often preclude this type of surgery.

Occasionally if the patient's oxygenation and hemodynamic condition permit, free flap transfer is performed during the emergency procedure. A common example of this is the transfer of skin from the sole of an amputated foot to the stump. The firmness of sole skin provides excellent coverage in this region and allows uncomplicated application of a leg prosthesis. Preoperative evaluation and intraoperative management of these patients are similar to that of trauma victims undergoing emergency replantation or revascularization procedures.

Preoperative evaluation and optimization for emergency replantation or revascularization usually begin before the patient's arrival in the emergency department. Telephone communication with the referring medical facility, usually by the plastic surgeon, may prevent many perioperative complications. Since, in most patients with partially or completely amputated limbs, major hemorrhage often occurs before the patient reaches medical care, optimal fluid resuscitation must take place in the referring hospital before the patient is transferred. It is also essential that major associated injuries be evaluated in the referring institution and that the replantation center be informed about them. Good communication with the referring facility clarifies these aspects of the patient's condition and care, augmenting the efficacy of patient management in the referring center and permitting appropriate arrangements with the departments which will be involved in management.

In the emergency department, if not precluded by hemorrhage or associated injuries, a brief interview with the patient about past medical history, medications, drug allergies, and

TABLE 17-3. Microvascular Monitoring Techniques

| METHOD | DESCRIPTION | ADVANTAGES | DISADVANTAGES | COMMENTS |
|---|---|---|---|---|
| Temperature | Measures the surface or deep temperature (depending on probe used) | Inexpensive and simple to use; baseline values for survival well established in digital replantation; noninvasive and continuous | Good only for end-organ systems (replanted parts); flaps may remain warm due to environmental factors, but be nonviable | Very adequate and most widely used for monitoring of replants |
| Doppler ultrasound probe | Measures blood flow in larger caliber vessels | Readily available and can determine direction of flow; can distinguish arterial from venous flow | Does not give quantitative value or measure capillary flow, may read adjacent vessels and give a false-negative reading; of limited use with deeply buried anastomoses | Occasionally useful for intermittent check of flow, but difficult to adapt for continuous monitoring; hard to position probe over pedicle consistently |
| Pulsed Doppler cuff | Measures blood flow directly through small vessels by implanted cuff | Continuous with instantaneous response; waveform analysis possible; inexpensive; quantitative | Invasive; infection, vascular thrombosis, or anastomosis disruption possible; requries removal | May be useful for buried flaps |
| Laser Doppler | Measures movement of red cells in the capillary network by Doppler shift of laser light | Continuous & noninvasive; detects either arterial or venous obstruction; probes to monitor buried transfers are available; can monitor all types of tissue transfers | Expensive; requires calibration to establish baseline (intraoperatively); no absolute flow value is obtained; clotted blood and exudate interfere with recording; measures only 1–2 mm in depth | Either this method, PPG, or pH measurement will probably be most commonly used in the future |
| Transcutaneous $O_2$ | Measures tissue $PO_2$ diffusing through the skin | Continuous; baseline easily established; can test flow by having patient inhale $O_2$; rapid response time for loss of arterial inflow | Useful on skin only and requires heating the tissue to obtain local hyperemia; cannot monitor deep flaps; halothane and $N_2O$ interfere with $TcO_2$ measurements; probe is large | Probe must be fixed to the skin; requires frequent calibration; effects of venous occlusion not known |
| Photoplethysmography (PPG) | Uses reflected light to measure minute changes in tissue volume associated with pulsatile blood | Noninvasive; waveform can predict venous obstruction | Requires experience to interpret waveform; no definite zero level | Useful with replants, skin, and muscle flaps |
| Tissue pH | Measures pH of tissue | Continuous; possibly more sensitive in evaluating survival of distal or marginal flap tissue | Slower detection than laser Doppler; requires inserted probe (invasive); normal values vary widely | May not indicate loss of perfusion for 3 hours or more |
| Fluroscein | Measures fluroscein in the tissue following intravenous injections | Relatively inexpensive and useful for skin flaps; minimally invassive; will detect problems earlier than clinical evaluation only, and can detect venous obstruction by fluorscein buildup | Venous obstruction may lead to fluroscein buildup in the tissue; requires repeated injections; not yet adapted for continuous monitoring | Useful for replants and skin flaps but not for deep flaps, muscle, etc; must compare to control area for baseline |
| Radioisotope scanning or clearance | Measures flow of radioactive substance "into" (scanning) or "out of" (clearance) the tissue | Helpful in deeply placed osseous flaps, eg, free fibular transfer | Not continuous and cannot be repeated frequently due to radiation hazard and accumulation | Limited usefulness |
| Hydrogen washout | Measures hydrogen concentration in the revascularized part after inhalation of hydrogen gas | Sensitive; repeated measurements possible | Requires special gas mixtures and electrodes; not continuous | |

(From Sanders[77] with permission.)

previous anesthetic experiences is obtained, and information about the anesthetic procedure and immediate postanesthetic period is provided. Although hypovolemia requiring active fluid resuscitation is rarely, if ever, associated with finger or hand injuries, it is often present during the preanesthetic period in arm and lower extremity injuries. Blood loss in these patients is often controlled by a pneumatic tourniquet, the pressure of which must be checked periodically. Pain and anxiety, which are present in almost all patients, can be controlled with small titrated intravenous doses of narcotics (morphine sulfate, 3–4 mg; fentanyl, 0.05–0.1 mg) and benzodiazepines (diazepam, 2.5 mg; midazolam, 1–3 mg). Using doses of these drugs sufficient to lead to depression of mental status and airway reflexes must be avoided. Hematocrit is the only laboratory test that is obtained for all patients; however, other tests, including electrolytes, blood gases, chest radiogram, and electrocardiogram, are obtained if the patient's age, medical history, physical findings, and extent of injury make them necessary.

## INTRAOPERATIVE CONSIDERATIONS

Unlike many patients having free flap transfer, almost all patients undergoing replantation procedures have a full stomach; measures to prevent aspiration, such as the use of rapid sequence induction for general anesthesia and avoidance of excessive sedation during regional anesthesia, are important. The choice between general and regional anesthesia for microvascular surgery is more of an institutional than an objective decision since there are no data available to show the superiority of one approach over the other. Although regional anesthesia offers some advantages, such as a stress-free operation and prolonged sensory, motor, and sympathetic block extending into the postoperative phase, few patients can remain immobile comfortably on an operating table for many hours unless supplementary sedation or light general anesthesia is also administered. In free flap transfers the donor and recipient sites may be widely separated, and regional anesthesia alone may not be feasible. Therefore, general anesthesia, alone or in combination with regional anesthesia, is administered in most centers.

### *General Anesthesia*

Low blood-gas solubility, minimal metabolism, and a peripheral vasodilatory effect with relatively small reduction in cardiac output make isoflurane the anesthetic agent of choice for microvascular surgery.[8,15] Enflurane, on the other hand, is associated with fluoride release, which may have a toxic effect on the renal-collecting tubules, resulting in vasopressin-resistant high-output renal failure if the anesthetic is administered longer than 9 MAC hours.[58] Data about the comparative effects of isoflurane and regional anesthesia on skin and muscle vasodilation are not available, but evaluation of these techniques individually suggests that the vasodilation caused by isoflurane is comparable with that produced by regional anesthesia.[7,19,22] Thus, isoflurane combined with nitrous oxide, supplemental doses of opioids, and muscle relaxants provides adequate graft perfusion and blunting of autonomic responses. Its high cost compared to other potent inhalational agents, which is probably the only disadvantage of this agent, can be minimized by using it in a low-flow anesthetic circuit. Doing so is also beneficial from the standpoint of heat conservation.

The blood-gas solubility coefficient of isoflurane is 1.4, which is close to those of halothane (2.3) and enflurane (1.9), anesthetics with intermediate blood-gas solubility. Partial recovery (75% of end-tidal concentration) from these anesthetics is affected little by prolonged exposure, but complete recovery (10% of end-tidal concentration) is disproportionately prolonged.[55,83] For instance, the partial recovery time from halothane is 4 minutes after 10 minutes of anesthesia and 6 minutes after 10 hours of administration. In contrast, complete recovery after 10 minutes of halothane anesthesia is 30 minutes, extending to 9 hours after a 10-hour administration.[55] Thus, delayed emergence is likely to occur after prolonged anesthesia with these agents. Postoperative agitation is another important disadvantage of potent inhalational anesthetics administered without adjunct drugs.[12] Agitation, coughing, bucking, and retching during emergence must be avoided since they increase catecholamine secretion and may result in spasm of the anastomosed vessel. Since the presence of a full stomach in most of these patients dictates extubation of the trachea after the return of airway reflexes, the anesthetic technique should be modified in such a way that recovery is rapid, smooth, and yet without the danger of pulmonary aspiration. Maintaining the inspired isoflurane concentration deliberately low throughout the procedure by supplementation with opioid agents and/or regional anesthesia shortens the complete recovery time and provides a smooth emergence. In addition, we discontinue isoflurane approximately 1 hour before the end of surgery to decrease recovery time further. Opioids are given whether or not supplemental regional anesthesia is administered to prevent coughing and bucking on the endotracheal tube and to provide postoperative analgesia in the absence of regional anesthesia.

Concern has been raised about the reaction of nitrous oxide after prolonged administration with vitamin $B_{12}$, a bound coenzyme of methionine synthase, which converts its centrally located cobalt from the monovalent (Cob (I) alamin) to the bivalent form (Cob (II) alamin). In this form methionine synthase, which is essential for methylation of homocystein to methionine and $N^5$-methyl tetrahydrofolate to tetrahydrofolate, cannot function.[63] Methionine synthase is a key link between two important cycles that are essential for the synthesis of S-adenyl-methionine (SAM), an important intermediary metabolite in methylation reactions, and of folic acid. Thus, inactivation of methionine synthase by nitrous oxide can bring these two cycles to a halt, reducing tissue methionine concentrations and trapping folate; this results in functional folate deficiency with impairment of folate-dependent reactions. Clinically, these disorders may be manifested as bone marrow depression, including megaloblastic anemia, leukopenia, and thrombocytopenia, and neurologic dysfunction consistent with spinal cord degeneration within a few weeks of exposure to nitrous oxide.[63] However, despite the potentially serious biochemical effects of nitrous oxide, its widespread use in routine anesthesia practice rarely produces detectable adverse clinical sequelae. It is now well established that administration of this agent for up to 24 hours to healthy surgical patients causes little overt harm, even though megaloblastic bone marrow changes do occur in most patients.[63] Cellular changes are not seen in the blood of patients without pre-existing bone marrow dysfunction because mature granulocyte stores are usually adequate to prevent pancytopenia for about 3 days. In critically ill surgical patients and in those with pre-existing subclinical $B_{12}$ deficiency, such as strict vegetarians, nitrous oxide toxicity may be apparent after a shorter period of administration.[63] It appears then that administration of nitrous oxide to healthy patients undergoing microvascular procedures of up to 24 hours is safe. After this period, it is prudent to substitute air for this agent. It may also be prudent to use air instead of nitrous oxide after a shorter period of exposure in severely injured patients since megaloblastic bone marrow changes have been shown even after brief administration of nitrous oxide to these patients.[64]

Diffusion of nitrous oxide into the endotracheal tube cuff can result in a rise of intracuff pressure to well above mucosal capillary pressure within a few hours. In order to prevent tracheal mucosal damage, intracuff pressure must be checked periodically and excess air removed. Alternatively, the cuff may be filled with anesthetic gases or water.

### *Regional Anesthesia*

As was mentioned before, the prolonged duration of microvascular surgery limits the usefulness of regional anesthesia as the sole anesthetic technique. However, in many institutions including ours, it is employed in conjunction with general anesthesia for reasons already discussed. Since the duration of most microvascular procedures exceeds that of available local anesthetics and extending analgesia into the postoperative period is desirable, placement of an indwelling catheter at the block site for injection of top-up doses is a necessity. Such catheter techniques are available for both upper and lower extremity blocks.

UPPER EXTREMITY BLOCKS. Anesthesia of the upper extremity is readily achieved by blockade of the brachial plexus using one of the three classic approaches: interscalene, subclavian perivascular, and axillary.[72,94] The supraclavicular approach is now rarely used because it is associated with a high incidence of pneumothorax. Winnie[94] emphasizes that the brachial plexus and the major vessels of the upper extremity are enveloped in a continuous sheath of fascia that extends from the cervical vertebrae to the distal axilla. He points out the analogy between epidural anesthesia and the perivascular approach to the brachial plexus. In both techniques, local anesthetic solution deposited into a distinct space surrounds the nerves to produce anesthesia, and thus the larger the volume of local anesthetic, the greater the extent of the block.

The axillary technique is chosen most commonly for surgical procedures of the distal forearm and hand because it is technically the easiest to perform. This approach is not associated with the complications sometimes seen with the subclavian perivascular and interscalene techniques: subarachnoid injection, vertebral artery injection, pneumothorax, phrenic nerve block, and stellate ganglion block. The main disadvantage of this approach, however, is its frequent failure to block the musculocutaneous nerve which exits from the neurovascular bundle before the sheath enters the axilla. Failure to anesthetize this nerve results in preservation of motor function to the forearm flexors and in retention of lateral forearm sensation. To sensure blockade of the musculocutaneous nerve, a large volume (40 mL) of local anesthetic should be injected in order to achieve sufficient proximal spread within the sheath. If necessary, the nerve can be blocked by injection of 5–7 mL of local anesthetic into the coracobrachialis muscle just superior to the axillary artery. The sensory component of the nerve can also be blocked separately by injection of local anesthetic at the level of the epicondyles in the groove between the biceps and brachioradialis muscles. In this manner, an incomplete axillary nerve also leaves the investing sheath of the brachial plexus at a high level, and thus insufficient proximal spread of the local anesthetic may result in sparing of some upper arm sensation. Again, this situation can usually be avoided if a sufficient volume of local anesthetic is used.

Nerves that are within the sheath in the axilla may also remain unblocked despite deposition of the local anesthetic into the perivascular space; the radial nerve remains unanesthetized most frequently. In a study on cadavers Thompson and Rorie[89] demonstrated that each component of the brachial plexus is separately packaged in a sheath that originates as a septum from the main brachial sheath. Thus, they speculated that the local anesthetic solution could not penetrate through some of the septa to block the nerve within it. Based on these findings, some clinicians suggested blockade of each nerve separately within the perivascular sheath. More recent data by Partridge et al.[67] showed that the axillary sheath is made up of numerous thin layers of velamentous fascia with no free space between the layers, suggesting that the injected solution can easily find its way to the nerves without being hampered by these septa. Thus, Winnie's[94] original concept of depositing the local anesthetic within the fascial sheath without the necessity of blocking individual nerves has been confirmed once more. Clinical support for this concept also comes from the fact that complete anesthesia may be achieved whatever the specific technique employed to block the brachial plexus by the axillary approach; success rates are similar with transarterial fixation, perivascular, nerve stimulator, and paresthesia techniques.[28,90,97] Why then do some nerves remain unblocked? A satisfactory explanation has yet to be given for this phenomenon, but it appears that injection within the tense neurovascular bundle produced by 90° abduction of the arm favors distribution of the local anesthetic anteriorly and medially within the sheath, reducing its access to the radial nerve.[80,92] Injection while the patient's arm is positioned at the side may overcome this problem, but this can be done only if a catheter is in placed.

The subclavian perivascular approach is useful for surgical procedures between the midportion of the arm and the midportion of the forearm, including the elbow. In this technique, onset of anesthesia is slower than with the axillary approach. However, as the brachial plexus is most compact at this level, incomplete anesthesia occurs less frequently. Complications of this block include pneumothorax; intravascular injection; and block of the stellate ganglion, vagus, and recurrent laryngeal nerves.

The interscalene approach is generally used for manipulations of the shoulder and surgery on the shoulder and upper arm. However, it provides good anesthesia even for surgical procedures performed on the hand. In this technique, anesthesia is relatively rapid in onset and is usually complete within 10 minutes. However, because of the arrangement of the roots of the brachial plexus at this level, anesthesia in the distribution of the ulnar nerve may be slow to develop. In addition to subarachnoid and vertebral artery injections, complications of this block are the same as those seen with the subclavian perivascular approach. However, it is unlikely that pneumothorax will result from a carefully performed interscalene block.

Whichever approach to the brachial plexus is chosen, a separate block of the intercostobrachial and medial brachial cutaneous nerves is necessary if tourniquet pain is to be averted. These nerves are not part of the brachial plexus and must be blocked independently to permit painless use of the tourniquet for prolonged periods. This is readily accomplished by infiltrating 3–5 mL of anesthetic subcutaneously over the axillary sheath.

The choice of technique in limb trauma patients is influenced by several considerations, including the site of surgery, specific anatomic findings, ease of performance, and familiarity with the technique. For example, despite the fact that an axillary approach would be well suited for surgery on the hand, a superficial skin infection or lymphadenopathy of the axilla dictates a supraclavicular or interscalene approach. Another important factor is the patient's ability or desire to cooperate in positioning. Severe pain may limit the manipulations necessary to achieve the proper exposure necessary to perform an axillary block. Similarly, an intoxicated patient may not be cooperative enough to permit performance of the block. In both of these situations, interscalene or subclavian perivascular techniques, which require a minimal amount of positioning, may be the best choice.

Coexisting disorders may also influence the selection of one approach over another. For example, in a patient with pneumothorax contralateral to an arm injury, one may not wish to risk the development of bilateral pneumothorax. In this situation, the axillary approach to the brachial plexus, which is associated with negligible risk, might be the best choice if it would provide adequate surgical anesthesia. Similarly, in an asthmatic patient it would be preferable not to use a technique that might block the stellate ganglion and precipitate an asthmatic attack.

Indwelling catheter placement providing continuous anesthesia for operations on the upper extremity and postoperative pain relief, is possible with each of these techniques. Various catheter placement techniques have been described by several authors.[21,33,49,54,57,76,79] The technique we generally use at our institution has been described by Ang et al.[2] and does not require elicitation of paresthesias or the use of a nerve stimulator (Fig 17-6). The arm is externally rotated, abducted to approximately 70°, and extended at the elbow. The axillary neurovascular bundle is then palpated as a cord lying against the humerus between the biceps and triceps muscles approximately 4 cm below the humeral insertion of the pectoralis muscle. After location of the neurovascular bundle, the overlying skin is aseptically cleansed and draped. A skin wheal is raised using a small amount of local anesthetic just medial to the neurovascular bundle, and a small skin puncture is made in the center of the wheal in order to facilitate the unhindered passage of the plexiflex needle (Burron Medical). This needle has a bevel of 45° so that a change in resistance can be appreciated easily during insertion through the fascia. The plexiflex needle, over which a plastic cannula is fitted, is then attached to a syringe filled with 5 mL of sterile normal saline. The syringe-needle unit is then advanced slowly through the skin incision at an angle of 30 to 40° parallel and just medial to the neurovascular bundle. As the unit is advanced, constant pressure is maintained on the barrel of the syringe. When the perivascular sheath is punctured, a "pop" will be appreciated, as will loss of resistance to injection. The 18-gauge cannula is then threaded off the plexiflex needle into the axillary sheath. A thin-walled polyamide catheter is advanced through the cannula while the arm is adducted to facilitate its passage. Resistance to passage of the catheter is encountered at 12–15 cm, at which time the cannula is removed. The catheter is then sutured in place and covered with a sterile dressing.

The latency of onset, which may be as long as 30 minutes, is an important disadvantage of brachial plexus block. Various local anesthetics and their combinations have been used to shorten the onset time, but it is important to emphasize that pain in patients with upper extremity injuries decreases the latency of onset of analgesia and of paralysis by approximately 35 to 40%.[65] Pain-induced high-frequency nerve impulses are thought to be the mechanism of this short latency. The latency of the block is shortest with 3% 2-chloroprocaine (35–40 mL). Sensory and motor blockade with this agent begins within about 5 minutes; complete block occurs in 10 minutes. Carbonation of local anesthetics has also been shown to reduce the onset time of brachial plexus block. Interestingly, however, recent work has shown that, although in both interscalene and subclavian perivascular approaches the onset time of carbonated lidocaine was decreased by 40% compared to lidocaine hydrochloride,[84,85] alkalinization of bupivacaine without added epinephrine did not confer any clinical advantage over the standard formulation of the drug in subclavian perivascular blockade.[6]

LOWER EXTREMITY BLOCKS. Continuous epidural anesthesia is the regional anesthetic technique of choice for lower extremity microvascular surgery because unlike the upper extremity, anesthesia of the entire lower extremity with a single plexus block is not possible. Hypovolemia from hemorrhage is a frequent complication of lower extremity amputations, limiting the feasibility of epidural anesthesia for replantation procedures. On the other hand, this technique may be useful in elective free flap transfers. A combination of a three-in-one block, which involves depositing 20–25 mL of local anesthetic into the femoral sheath to anesthetize the femoral, obturator, and lateral cutaneous nerves,[95] and a sciatic nerve block can

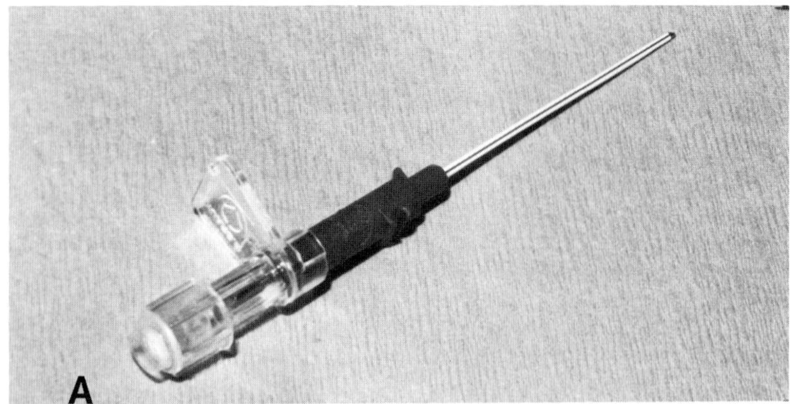

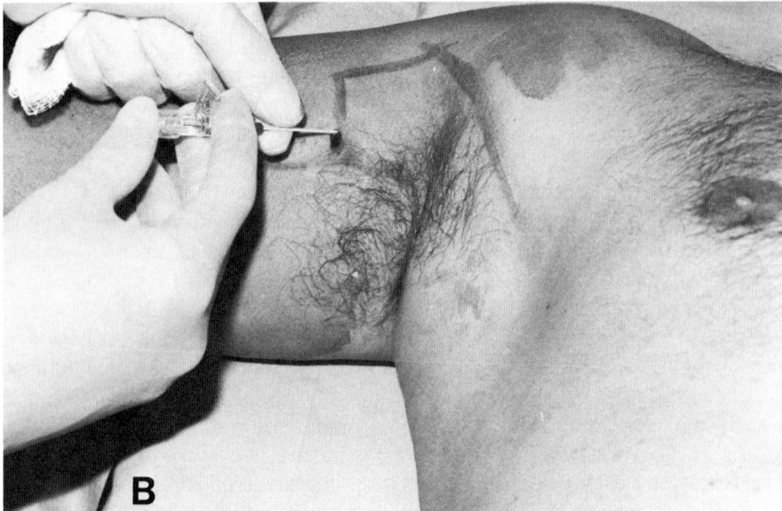

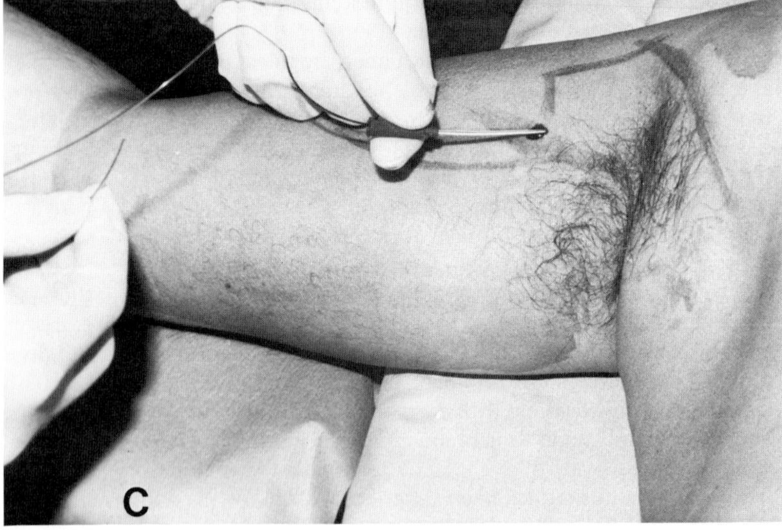

FIG. 17-6. The technique of continuous brachial plexus block via axillary approach. (A) The plexiflex needle-cannula assembly (supplied by Burron Medical). (B) The entry site of the plexiflex needle-cannula assembly in the groove between the biceps and triceps muscles 4 cm below the humeral insertion of the pectoralis muscle. (C) After puncture of the fascia, the needle is withdrawn while the cannula is advanced. A polyamide catheter is advanced through the cannula until resistance is encountered at 12–15 cm. (D) The cannula is withdrawn, and the polyamide catheter is left in place.

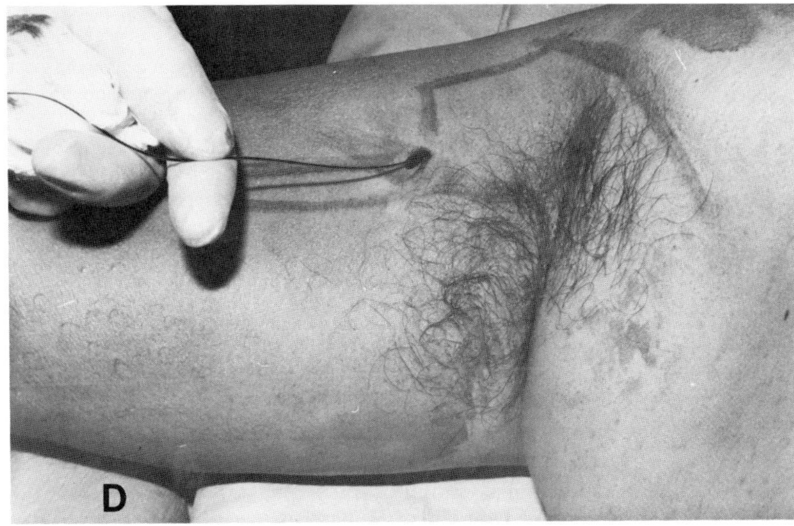


FIG. 17-6. Continued.

produce complete surgical anesthesia of the lower extremity. This technique requires proper positioning of the painful limb, and is not widely accepted.

## PERIOPERATIVE COMPLICATIONS

Reference has already been made to the frequent occurrence of hypothermia and to its prevention and correction. Pressure necrosis and peripheral neuropathy are two important preventable complications of prolonged microvascular surgery. With properly placed protective padding and constant observation of the patient, such complications should occur rarely. However, each position presents specific problems. In the supine position occipital alopecia results from prolonged resting of the head on a firm pillow or doughnut, especially if the lengthy anesthesia is also associated with blood loss and hypotension.[68] The use of a soft, contoured pillow and intermittent repositioning of the head prevent this complication. Fortunately, regrowth of hair invariably occurs between 6 months and 1 year. Decubitus ulcers are not uncommon and can be prevented by covering the operating table with sheepskin or preferably with a 4-inch thick eggcrate-type foam mattress. Peripheral neuropathy, especially of the brachial plexus and ulnar nerve, occurs in the supine position if the arm is abducted more than 90°, if the elbows are not padded adequately, or when there has been prolonged contact with metal surfaces.

The lateral decubitus position, which is used for harvesting of latissimus dorsi and serratus anterior muscle flaps, may give rise to axillary neurovascular compression; a soft towel roll placed in the dependent axilla prevents this complication. In this position cervical and brachial nerves may be stretched if the head is not maintained in a neutral position. The dependent malar eminence and eye may be damaged; a soft foam pad under the cheek and careful taping of the eye can prevent these problems. Abduction of the nondependent arm to facilitate harvesting may result in a brachial plexus stretch injury manifested postoperatively by numbness and weakness of the arm. Intraoperative positional changes may result in unrecognized pressure points; frequent observation of patient position will prevent this problem.

As has been mentioned, intraoperative and postoperative graft failure is generally a result of poor surgical technique. However, occasionally simple interventions by the anesthetic team may improve graft perfusion. For instance elevation of blood pressure with fluids[51] or administration of a stellate ganglion block or a top-up dose of a local anesthetic via the epidural or brachial plexus catheter[93] may result in improvement of the color of the graft.

The rate of thromboembolism, although it might be expected to be high after prolonged immobilization, is low probably because most patients are young and healthy and are ambulatory within a few days after surgery.

## POSTOPERATIVE CONSIDERATIONS

Prevention of pain and agitation is the principal care consideration during the postoperative period. Epidural narcotics provide excellent postoperative analgesia without the risk of hypotension associated with local anesthetics. Detailed information about epidural narcotics is provided in Chapter 23. Perfusion failure of the graft is most likely to occur during the first 48 hours after surgery; after this period graft circulation is unlikely to fail. Thus, the color, capillary filling, and temperature of the graft must be monitored continuously during this period.[31] Perfusion failure may be due to arterial or venous compromise or both. Differentiation between arterial and venous perfusion failure is important since the indication for repeat surgery is to some extent dependent on the mechanism. Arterial occlusion dictates immediate surgery, whereas venous occlusion may sometimes be alleviated by applying medicinal leeches[5] or by allowing the graft to ooze until new venous channels are established. A mild to moderate degree of oozing from the graft site is not uncommon, especially in composite grafts containing bone and muscle. The extent of bleeding must be monitored carefully to regulate fluid and blood transfusion and to determine the need for and timing of surgery.

## REFERENCES


1. Aarts HF. Regional intravascular sympathetic blockade for better results in flap surgery: an experimental study of free-flaps, island flaps and pedicle flaps in the rabbit ear. Plast Reconstr Surg 1980;66:690.
2. Ang ET, Lassale B, Goldfarb G. Continuous axillary brachial plexus block—a clinical and anatomical study. Anesth Analg 1984;63:680.
3. Aps C, Cox R, Mayou B, Sengupta T. The role of anaesthetic management in changing peripheral blood flow in patients undergoing free flap transfer. Ann Roy Coll Surg Engl 1985;67:175.
4. Awwad AM, White RJ, Webster MHC, Vance JP. The effect of temperature on blood flow in island and free skin flaps: an experimental study. Br J Plast Surg 1983;36:373.
5. Batchelor AGG, Davison P, Sully L. The salvage of congested skin flaps by the application of leeches. Br J Plast Surg 1984;37:358.
6. Bedder MD, Kozody R, Craig DB. Comparison of bupivacaine and alkalinized bupivacaine in brachial plexus anesthesia. Anesth Analg 1988;67:48.
7. Berger A, Tizian C, Zenz M. Continuous plexus blockade for improved circulation in microvascular surgery. Ann Plast Surg 1985;14:16.
8. Bird TM, Strunin L. Anaesthetic considerations for microsurgical repair of limbs. Can Anaesth Soc J 1984;31:51.
9. Bloch EC. Hyperthermia resulting from tourniquet application in children. Ann Roy Coll Surg Engl 1986;68:193.
10. Burch JW, Stanford N, Majerus PW. Inhibition of platelet prostaglandin synthetase by oral aspirin. J Clin Invest 1978;61:314.
11. Burton AC, Yamada S. Relation between blood pressure and flow in the human forearm. J Appl Physiol 1951;4:329.
12. Caplan RA, Long MC. Prolonged anesthesia—management and sequelae of a two-day general anesthetic. Anesth Analg 1984;63:353.
13. Chang WHJ, Petry JJ. Platelets, prostaglandins, and patency in microvascular surgery. J Microsurg 1980;2:27.
14. Chow SP, Huang CD, Chan CW. Microvascular anastomosis of arteries under tension. Br J Plast Surg 1982;35:82.
15. Cochrane DF. Anaesthesia for microvascular surgery. Clinical Anesthesiology 1987;1:747.
16. Cormack GC, Lamberty BGH. The direct cutaneous system of vessels. In: Cormack GC, Lamberty BGH, eds. The arterial anatomy of skin flaps. London: Churchill Livingstone, 1986:65.
17. Cormack GC, Lamberty BGH. The principles of the musculocutaneous system. In: Cormack GC, Lamberty BGH, eds. The arterial anatomy of skin flaps. London: Churchill Livingstone, 1986:77.
18. Cousins MJ, Wright JC. Graft, muscle, skin blood flow after epidural block in vascular procedures. Surg Gynecol Obstet 1971;133:59.
19. Cross GD, Porter JM. Blood flow in the upper limb during brachial plexus anaesthesia. Anaesthesia 1988;43:323.
20. Danese CA, Haimov M. Inhibition of experimental arterial thrombosis in dogs with platelet deaggregating agents. Surgery 1971;70:927.
21. DeKrey JA, Schroeder CF, Buechel DR. Continuous brachial plexus block. Anesthesiology 1969;30:332.
22. Dolan WM, Stevens WC, Eger EI II, et al. Cardiovascular and respiratory effects of isoflurane-nitrous oxide anaesthesia. Can Anaesth Soc J 1974;21:557.
23. Engrav LH, Benjamin CI, Crandall H, Perry JF. Experimental effects of heparin or magnesium sulfate on the patency of microvascular anastomoses. Plast Reconstr Surg 1975;55:618.
24. Finseth F. Clinical salvage of three skin flaps by treatment with a vasodilator drug. Plast Reconstr Surg 1979;63:304.
25. Finseth F, Adelberg MG. Prevention of skin flap necrosis by a course of treatment with vasodilator drugs. Plast Reconstr Surg 1978;61:738.
26. Glynn CJ, Basedow RW, Walsh JA. Pain relief following postganglionic sympathetic blockade with I.V. guanethidine. Br J Anaesth 1981;53:1297.
27. Gold AH, Lee GW. Upper extremity replantation: current concept and patient selection. J Trauma 1981;20:551.
28. Goldberg ME, Gregg C, Larijani GE, et al. A comparison of three methods of axillary approach to brachial plexus blockade for upper extremity surgery. Anesthesiology 1987;66:814.
29. Greenberg BM, Mathias M, May JW Jr: Therapeutic value of intravenous heparin in microvascular surgery: an experimental vascular thrombosis study. J Plast Reconstr Surg 1988;82:463.
30. Hakstian RW. Funicular orientation by direct stimulation. An aid to peripheral nerve repair. J Bone Joint Surg 1968;50A:1178.
31. Harashina T. Analysis of 200 free flaps. Br J Plast Surg 1988;41:33.
32. Harris GD, Nagle DJ, Lewis VL, Bauer BS. Accelerating recovery after trauma with free flaps. J Trauma 1987;27:849.
33. Hempel V, van Finck M, Baumgartner E. A longitudinal supraclavicular approach to the brachial plexus for the insertion of plastic cannulas. Anesth Analg 1981;60:352.
34. Hing DN, Buncke HJ, Alpert BS, Gordon L. Indications for replanting amputated parts. Hosp Phys 1986;2:13.
35. Holland AJC, Davies KH, Wallace DH. Sympathetic blockade of isolated limbs by intravenous guanethidine. Can Anaesth Soc J 1977;24:597.
36. Hynynen M, Eklund P, Rosenberg PH. Anaesthesia for patients undergoing prolonged reconstructive and microvascular plastic surgery. Scand J Plast Reconstr Surg 1982;16:201.
37. Iwaya T, Haric K, Yamada A. Microvascular free flaps for the treatment of avulsion injuries of the feet in children. J Trauma 1982;212:15.
38. Jackson IT, Scheker L. Muscle and myocutaneous flaps on the lower limb. Injury 1981;13:324.
39. Jaeger SH, Tsai TM, Kleinert HE. Upper extremity replantation in children. Orthop Clin North Am 1981;12:897.
40. Jakubowski M, Lamont A, Murray WB, DeWit SL. Anaesthesia for microsurgery. S Afr Med J 1985;67:581.
41. Jelalian C, Mehrhof A, Cohen IK, et al. Streptokinase in the treatment of acute arterial occlusion of the hand. J Hand Surg 1985;10A:534.
42. Jones BM. Predicting the fate of free tissue transfers. Ann Roy Coll Surg Engl 1985;67:63.
43. Ketchum LD. Pharmacological alterations in the clotting mechanism: use in microvascular surgery. J Hand Surg 1978;3:407.
44. Ketchum LD, Wennen WW, Masters FW, Robinson DW. Experimental use of pluronic F68 in microvascular surgery. Plast Reconstr Surg 1974;53:288.
45. Khashaba AA, McGregor IA. Haemodynamics of the radial forearm flap. Br J Plast Surg 1986;39:441.
46. Kleinert HE, Kasdan ML. Salvage of devascularized upper extremities, including studies on small vessel anastomosis. Clin Orthop 1963;29:29.
47. Kleinert HE, Jablon M, Tsai TM. An overview of replantation and results of 347 replants in 245 patients. J Trauma 1980;20:390.
48. Lam JYT, Chesebro JH, Fuster V. Platelets, vasoconstriction, and nitroglycerine during arterial wall injury. A new antithrombotic role for an old drug. Circulation 1988;78:712.
49. Lee VC, Abram SE. Continuous brachial plexus anesthesia. Axillary sheath cannulation using a spinal needle-intravenous catheter combination. Regional Anesth 1987;12:139.
50. Lineweaver WC, Buncke HJ. Complications of free flap transfer. Hand Clin 1986;2:347.
51. MacDonald DJF. Anaesthesia for microvascular surgery. A physiologic approach. Br J Anaesth 1985;57:904.
52. MacFarlane DE, Walsh PN, Mills DCB, et al. The role of thrombin

in ADP-induced platelet aggregation and release: a critical evaluation. Br J Haematol 1975;30:457.

53. Malt RA, McKhann CF. Replantation of severed arms. JAMA 1964;189:716.
54. Manriquez RG, Pallares V. Continuous brachial plexus block for prolonged sympathectomy and control of pain. Anesth Analg 1978;57:128.
55. Mapleson WW. Quantitative prediction of anesthetic concentrations. In: Papper EM, Kitz RJ, eds. Uptake and distribution of anesthetic agents. New York: McGraw-Hill, 1963:104–109.
56. Matsuda M, Kato N, Hosoi M. The problem in replantation of limbs amputated through the upper arm region. J Trauma 1981;21:403.
57. Matsuda M, Kato N, Hosoi M. Continuous brachial plexus block for replantation in the upper extremity. The Hand 1982; 14:129.
58. Mazze RJ, Calverley RK, Smith NT. Inorganic fluoride nephrotoxicity: prolonged enflurane and halothane anesthesia in volunteers. Anesthesiology 1977;46:265.
59. McConnell CM, Hyland WT, Neale HW. Microvascular free groin flap soft-tissue coverage of the extremities. J Trauma 1980; 20:593.
60. McGregor AD, Jones WK, Perlman D. Blood flow in the arm under brachial plexus anaesthesia. J Hand Surg 1985;10B:21.
61. McLean NR, Ellis H. Does remote sepsis influence the potency of microvascular anastomoses? Br J Plast Surg 1988;41:395.
62. Murphy RC, Robson MC. Microvascular surgery in trauma. In: Kerstein MD, ed. Management of vascular trauma. Baltimore: University Park Press, 1985:148–173.
63. Nunn JF. Clinical aspects of the interaction between nitrous oxide and vitamin $B_12$. Br J Anaesth 1987;59:3.
64. Nunn JF, Chanarin I, Tanner AG, Owen ERTC. Megaloblastic bone marrow changes after repeated nitrous oxide anaesthesia. Br J Anaesth 1986;58:1469.
65. Okasha AS, EL-attar AM, Soliman HL. Enhanced brachial plexus blockade. Effect of pain and muscular exercises on the efficiency of brachial plexus blockade. Anaesthesia 1988;43:327.
66. Olson RM, Wood MB, Irons GB. Microvascular free-flap coverage of mechanical injuries to the upper extremity. Am J Surg 1982;144:593.
67. Partridge BL, Katz J, Benirschke K. Functional anatomy of the brachial plexus sheath: implications for anesthesia. Anesthesiology 1987;66:743.
68. Patel KD, Henschel EO. Postoperative alopecia. Anesth Analg 1980;59:311.
69. Perel A, Pizov R, Cotev S. Systolic blood pressure variation is a sensitive indicator of hypovolemia in ventilated dogs subjected to graded hemorrhage. Anesthesiology 1987;67:498.
70. Phelps DB, Rutherford RB, Boswick JA. Control of vasospasm following trauma and microvascular surgery. J Hand Surg 1979;4:109.
71. Puckett CL. Therapeutic value of intravenous heparin in microvascular surgery: an experimental vascular thrombosis study. Plast Reconstr Surg 1988;82:471.
72. Raggi RP. Balanced regional anesthesia for hand surgery. Orthop Clin North Am 1986;17:473.
73. Rao VK, Morrison WA, O'Brien B McC. Effect of nicotine on blood flow and patency of experimental microvascular anastomosis. Ann Plast Surg 1983;11:206.
74. Robins DW. The anaesthetic management of patients undergoing free flap transfer. Br J Plast Surg 1983;36:231.
75. Rosenberg RD. Actions and interactions of antithrombin and heparin. N Engl J Med 1975;292:146.
76. Sada T, Kobayashi T, Murakami S. Continuous axillary brachial plexus block. Can Anaesth Soc J 1983;30:201.
77. Sanders WE. Principles of microvascular surgery. In: Green DP, ed. Operative hand surgery vol 2. New York: Churchill Livingstone, 1988:1049–1103.
78. Sasaki GH. Vascular anatomy and physiology of the skin and muscle flaps. Applications in reconstructive surgery. In: Habal MB, Morain WD, Lewin ML, Parsons RW, Woods JE, eds. Advances in plastic and reconstructive surgery. vol 2. Chicago: Year Book Medical Publishers, 1986:227.
79. Selander D. Catheter technique in axillary plexus block. Presentation of a new technique. Acta Anaesth Scand 1977;21:324.
80. Selander D. Axillary plexus block: paresthetic or perivascular. Anesthesiology 1987;66:726.
81. Sessler DI, Israel D, Pozos RS, et al. Spontaneous post-anesthetic tremor does not resemble thermoregulatory shivering. Anesthesiology 1988;68:843.
82. Speat TH, Gaynor E, Stemerman MB. Thrombosis, atherosclerosis, and endothelium. Am Heart J 1974;87:661.
83. Stoelting RK, Eger EI II. The effects of ventilation and anesthetic solubility on recovery from anesthesia. Anesthesiology 1969;30:290.
84. Sukhani R. Winnie AP. Clinical pharmacokinetics of carbonated local anesthetics. I: subclavian perivascular brachial block model. Anesth Analg 1987;66:739.
85. Sukhani R, Winnie AP. Clinical pharmacokinetics of carbonated local anesthetics. II: interscalene brachial block model. Anesth Analg 1987;66:1245.
86. Takami H, Takahashi S, Ando M. Microvascular free musculocutancous flaps for the treatment of avulsion injuries of the lower leg. J Trauma 1983;23:473.
87. Taylor GI, Palmer JH. The vascular territories (angiosomes) of the body: experimental study and clinical applications. Br J Plast Surg 1987;40:113.
88. Terry HJ, Allan JS, Taylor GW. The effect of adding lumbar sympathectomy to reconstructive arterial surgery in the lower limb. Br J Surg 1970;57:51.
89. Thompson GE, Rorie DK. Functional anatomy of the brachial plexus sheaths. Anesthesiology 1983;59:117.
90. Tuominen MK, Pitkanen MT, Numminen MK, Rosenberg PH. Quality of axillary brachial plexus block. Comparison of success rate using perivascular and nerve stimulator techniques. Anaesthesia 1987;42:20.
91. Van Twisk R, Gielen MJM, Pavlov PW, Robinson PH. Is additional epidural sympathetic block in microvascular surgery contraindicated? A preliminary report. Br J Plast Surg 1988;41:37.
92. Vester-Andersen T, Broby-Johansen U, Bro-Rasmussen F. Perivascular axillary block. VI: the distribution of gelatine solution injected into the axillary neurovascular sheath of cadavers. Acta Anaesthesiol Scand 1986;30:18.
93. Weber S, Bennett CR, Jones NF. Improvement in blood flow during lower extremity microsurgical free tissue transfer associated with epidural anesthesia. Anesth Analg 1988;67:703.
94. Winnie AP. Perivascular techniques of brachial plexus block. In: Winnie AP, Hakansson L, eds. Plexus anesthesia. Perivascular techniques of brachial plexus block. WB Philadelphia: WB Saunders, 1983:117.
95. Winnie AP, Ramamurthy S, Durrani Z. The inguinal perivascular technique of lumbar plexus anesthesia. Anesth Analg 1973;52:989.
96. Yoshimura M, Nomura S. Critical determinants in restoring function of reattached digits. Ann Acad Med 1982;11:218.
97. Youssef MS, Desgrand DA. Comparison of two methods of axillary brachial plexus anaesthesia. Br J Anaesth 1988;60:841.
98. Zhong-Wei C, Meyer VE, Kleinert HE, Beasley RW. Present indications and contraindications for replantation as reflected by long-term functional results. Orthop Clin North Am 1981;12:849.
99. Zuker RM, Stevenson JH. Proximal upper limb replantation in children. J Trauma 1988;28:544.

# Chapter Eighteen

Robert Pascucci
James Walsh

# Evaluation and Management of the Injured Child

Accidental injuries and deaths are all too common in childhood. In the United States, 19 million children each year (three in every ten) are injured severely enough to seek medical care or to restrict their usual activity.[108,159,173] Although most of these injuries are minor and without serious morbidity, accidents remain the leading cause of death in children and young adults (Table 18-1). There are approximately 22,000 deaths per year due to trauma in children under the age of 19, and for each death, there are another 40 to 50 nonlethal injuries requiring hospital admission.[117] These admissions constitute a significant portion of total hospital days in the pediatric age group.[90] Whether or not treatment involves surgery, anesthesiologists are becoming increasingly involved in management of the injured child.

When childhood trauma is analyzed from the perspective of epidemiology, it becomes apparent that the child sustains different injuries at different levels of growth and development[108,159,181] (Table 18-2). For example, the crawling infant, the physically clumsy preschooler, and the adolescent display different behaviors; these differences in behavior patterns make each group susceptible to different agents of injury. The infant explores with the mouth and therefore is susceptible to choking or poisoning; the preschooler is more likely to grab and to slip or fall, thereby sustaining a burn or a head injury. The adolescent is often involved in motor vehicle, diving, or gunshot injuries.[201] As the child grows older, personality factors, such as sex (males more at risk), general level of activity, temperament, and attentiveness, gain in influence.[28,179] It is also interesting to note that children who have sustained three or more separate injuries between birth and 5 years of age are at increased risk of being injured in the next 5 years of their life.[29]

The environment of the child also influences the incidence and type of injury. Most childhood accidents occur in environments where children spend most of their day: home and school.[196] Parents play an important role, with their level of attentiveness, preoccupations, and state of health influencing the safety of the child.[179] Child abuse is also a growing problem; approximately one million children are abused in the United States every year, and it is estimated that between 2,000 and 5,000 children die annually as a result of this type of trauma.[148] Death is often a result of major head and abdominal injuries in these young (age between 0 and 6) children.[55,148] As the child grows into adolescence and young adulthood, family influence is reduced in proportion, and the peer group and other entities gain in influence. Although death rates for other age groups have fallen over the past 20 years, those for adolescents and young adults have risen, with motor vehicle accidents, drowning, and homicide accounting for much of the increase.[17] Substance abuse (alcohol and other drugs) is frequently involved in adolescent injuries, and such substances are often present in patients brought to the operating room for trauma surgery (Walsh JW, Bruce DL, unpublished data).

The quality of care delivered at the site of injury may influence outcome greatly, especially when the child is hypoxic or hypovolemic; several authors have called for more intensive training of emergency personnel in pediatric airway management and resuscitation.[132,213] From the trauma scene, the injured child is usually brought to the community hospital

TABLE 18-1. Major Causes of Death in Pediatric Patients, 1980*

| | LESS THAN 1 YEAR | 1–4 YEARS | 5–14 YEARS |
|---|---|---|---|
| All causes | 1,288.3 | 63.9 | 30.6 |
| Malignant neoplasms | 3.2 | 4.5 | 4.3 |
| Major cardiovascular diseases | 27.8 | 3.2 | 1.3 |
| Respiratory diseases | 32.7 | 2.8 | 0.8 |
| Congenital abnormalities | 260.9 | 8.0 | 1.6 |
| Accidents | 33.0 | 25.9 | 15.0 |
| Homicide | 5.9 | 2.5 | 1.2 |
| All other | 924.8 | 17.9 | 6.4 |

* Data from National Center for Health Statistics. Rates per 100,000 population in specified age group.

emergency department for treatment.[212] Management may continue there, or with a growing trend toward regionalization of health care, transfer of the seriously injured child to a pediatric trauma center may be considered.[178,189,248] The American Pediatric Surgical Association has proposed the establishment of a two-tier system of care, with the regional "optimal" pediatric trauma center serving as a resource center for all hospitals in its catchment area.[211] Because the total volume of pediatric trauma cases is small (approximately 25% of adult volume), each pediatric trauma center would need to serve a relatively large area to maintain a critical number of patients and a high level of expertise. Several such centers have been established, and there is evidence that the specialized care provided by them has resulted in a greater salvage rate among children who sustain major trauma.[119]

The anesthesiologist may be called upon for assistance in a number of ways in pediatric trauma management. Initial resuscitation in the emergency department frequently involves the anesthesiologist. Subsequent surgery, if necessary, and postoperative care in the postanesthesia recovery room or the intensive care unit require the expertise of the anesthesiologist as well. Should transfer to another institution be required, the anesthesiologist may be part of the team providing safe transport.[251]

This chapter first considers the role of the anesthesiologist in providing initial life support to the pediatric trauma victim. A more thorough assessment of the injured child, with emphasis on particular concerns during the perioperative period, is then presented. Possible techniques of anesthetic management of both major and minor injury are considered. The provision of critical care for the injured child, together with appropriate care for several typical childhood injuries, is then discussed, and the chapter concludes with brief comments on prognosis and prevention.

## EMERGENCY RESUSCITATION AND STABILIZATION

Coronary artery disease is rare in children, and the young, healthy heart is able to withstand a great deal more insult than that of the adult. It is unlikely that a primary myocardial lesion or dysrhythmia is responsible for a child's cardiac arrest. More commonly, the arrest results from respiratory compromise with hypoxemia, severe loss of intravascular volume, and/or massively increased intracranial pressure. Rapid correction of these abnormalities is critical; once gas exchange is normalized and circulating volume restored, cardiac stabilization is usually accomplished easily.

### AIRWAY MANAGEMENT

An adequate airway must be established at once. In most children, simple positioning is the key to successful correction of airway obstruction. Although the urgency to restore the airway in children with suspected cervical spine injury is the same as in those without such injury, special care must be exercised to avoid undue flexion or extension of the neck when cervical injury may be present. Splinting or sandbag-

TABLE 18-2. Injury Deaths, United States, 1980*

| INJURY TYPE | LESS THAN 1 YEAR | 1–4 YEARS | 5–14 YEARS | 15–19 YEARS | TOTAL |
|---|---|---|---|---|---|
| Motor vehicle | | | | | |
| Occupant | 218 | 493 | 1122 | 7246 | 9079 |
| Pedestrian | 13 | 435 | 1005 | 757 | 2210 |
| Motorcycle | 1 | 8 | 120 | 788 | 917 |
| Pedal cycle | 0 | 16 | 387 | 159 | 562 |
| Other | 20 | 264 | 285 | 480 | 1049 |
| Total | 252 | 1216 | 2919 | 9430 | 13,817 |
| Bicycle | 0 | 4 | 25 | 10 | 39 |
| Burn | 177 | 735 | 535 | 348 | 1795 |
| Drowning | 91 | 693 | 795 | 1012 | 2591 |
| Choking/suffocation | 439 | 214 | 205 | 131 | 989 |
| Foreign body | 1 | 4 | 2 | 2 | 9 |
| Poison | 22 | 83 | 52 | 293 | 450 |
| Falls | 44 | 111 | 89 | 209 | 453 |
| Other | 140 | 253 | 602 | 824 | 1819 |
| TOTAL | 1166 | 3313 | 5224 | 12,259 | 21,962 |

* Data from National Center for Health Statistics.

ging of the neck early in the course of resuscitation may prevent an inadvertent increase in pressure on the cervical cord. If there is no suspicion of such injury, the neck should be flexed gently and the head extended to achieve the "sniffing" position. A folded towel placed under the occiput is helpful; in infants, this measure is often not necessary because of the relatively large head and protuberant occiput. The trachea of the infant or child lacks the firm cartilaginous support of the adult, and extreme hyperextension may collapse, rather than improve, the airway.

Anterior displacement of the jaw and tongue relieves soft tissue obstruction of the airway. A straight anterior thrust of the jaw by displacement of the mandible seems to work best. Continuous, gentle positive pressure may then "splint" the airway open. Airway adjuncts may prove useful. A properly sized oral airway encircles the tongue comfortably without inducing gagging. Awake patients may be managed better with a nasopharyngeal airway, although there is significant risk of nasal bleeding as the device is passed through the enlarged adenoid bed typical of childhood.

As the airway is being restored, other necessary equipment is assembled. Oxygen is administered as soon as it can be made available; even if significant airway obstruction remains, hypoxemia can often be corrected by increasing the $F_{IO_2}$. In general, triangularly shaped masks, such as the "Trimar" or the "Rendell-Baker-Soucek," fit children somewhat better than more oval designs and may offer the added advantage of less dead space. Most children are easily ventilated with a self-refilling type of resuscitator eg, the "Ambu-bag".

If adequate ventilation cannot be achieved, the possibility of airway obstruction by a foreign body must be entertained. Various authors have recommended back blows, chest thrusts,[111] abdominal thrusts,[126] or a combination of maneuvers[16,52,90,186] as initial treatment for removing a foreign body from the airway. The National Conference on CPR recommends back blows and chest thrusts, which act as an artificial cough, for patients younger than 1 year of age. When circumstances allow, the back blows should be administered four times rapidly, between the shoulder blades, while the child is held with the head lower than the trunk (Fig 18-1). Chest thrusts, applied in the same location as cardiac compression (ie, one finger-breadth below the midsternum for infants and the lower sternum for older children), or abdominal thrusts are then applied, the foreign body removed, and ventilation re-evaluated (Fig 18-2). When such injuries as cervical spine fracture are present or suspected and the patient cannot be moved, subxiphoid abdominal thrusts should be performed. In patients older than 1 year, the Heimlich maneuver (applied six to ten times in rapid succession) is recommended as the initial treatment of foreign body in the airway.[195] It should be remembered that complications (eg, organ laceration) from both the chest thrust[126] and abdominal thrust[171] have been reported in pediatric patients and that abdominal thrusts may be more dangerous in children younger than 8 years of age.[16]

If the child is unconscious, removal of foreign material in the upper airway may be attempted initially with a gentle finger sweep of the posterior pharynx (avoiding trauma to the airway) or preferably with an instrument under direct vision. Material that has entered the trachea or bronchus may require bronchoscopic removal. However, a foreign body that has lodged in or beyond a mainstem bronchus in a child is rarely responsible for life-threatening airway obstruction. Removal of such an object can usually wait until it can be performed in the controlled environment of the operating room.

Blunt or penetrating trauma to the larynx and upper airway can impede ventilation by disrupting the tracheobronchial tree.[66,70,235] Such cases may require emergency surgical intervention (tracheotomy or cricothyroidotomy) or insertion of a rigid ventilating bronchoscope into the trachea under direct

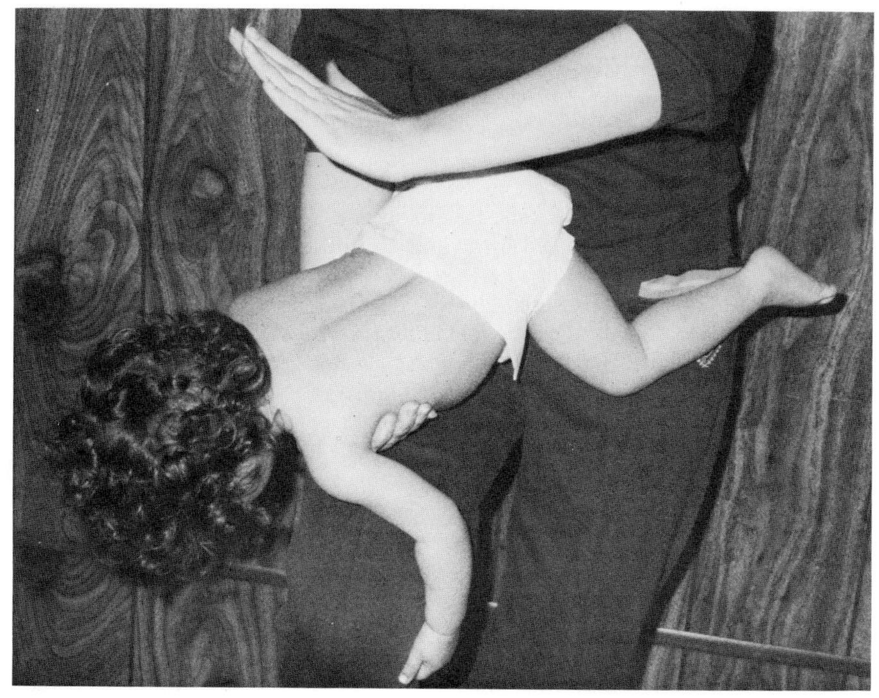

FIG. 18-1. Airway foreign body—back blow.

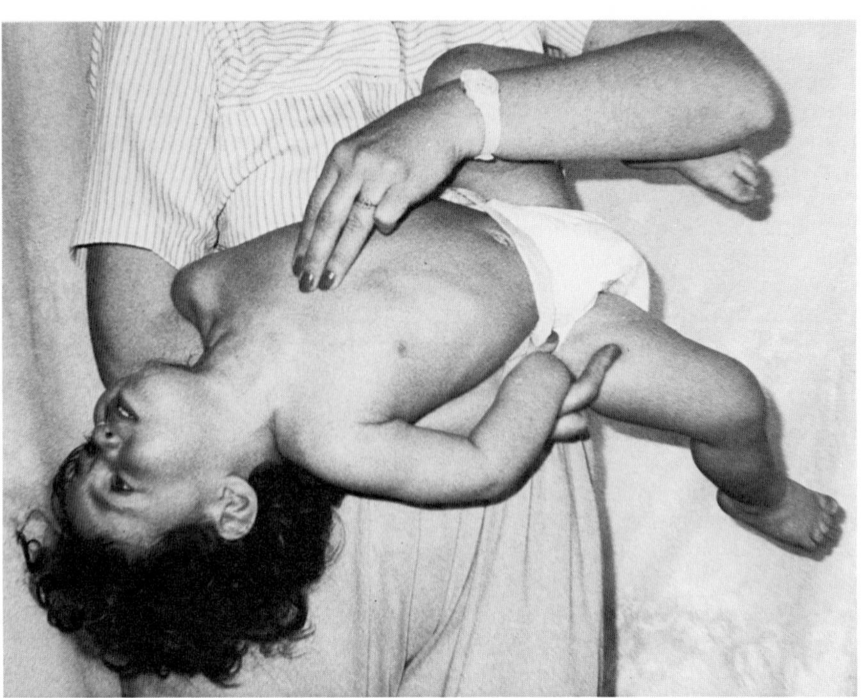

FIG. 18-2. Airway foreign body—chest thrust.

vision. If an endotracheal tube is placed by direct laryngoscopy, the possibility of its entering a false passage must be assessed immediately before high inflating pressures are delivered.[43]

Blood, secretions, loose teeth, soft tissue distortion, and edema compromise the airway frequently. In such cases it may be appropriate to proceed directly to laryngoscopy and intubation or, in more severe situations, to cricothyroidotomy or tracheotomy. Surgical cricothyroidotomy in children younger than 8 years of age is not desirable as it is associated with a high incidence of laryngeal injury. Many authors now recommend needle cricothyroidotomy in these relatively small children[173] (Fig 18-3). With the head in a slightly extended position (neutral position if a cervical spine fracture has not been excluded), the cricothyroid membrane is identified, and a large plastic intravenous catheter (with needle stylet) angled 45° caudally is inserted through the skin and membrane into the trachea. The needle is removed as the catheter is advanced; air should be aspirated freely. A jet ventilator, intermittent high-flow oxygen, or a ventilating bag is attached with a 3.0 mm endotracheal tube adaptor. With these techniques, normoxia can usually be re-established, improving the patient's condition and allowing time for more definitive measures.[63,195]

## ENDOTRACHEAL INTUBATION

Endotracheal intubation provides a secure airway, minimizing the risks of gastric distension and regurgitation and allowing better regulation of $F_{IO_2}$, airway pressures, and ventilatory pattern. However, intubation should not be the first priority; ventilation and oxygenation come first. Unsuccessful endotracheal intubation without prior oxygenation may compromise resuscitation efforts.

The larynx of the infant and child is positioned at a slightly higher level than that of the adult, corresponding to vertebral levels C3-C4, rather than C5-C6.[138] The epiglottis is shorter and more U-shaped as well, particularly in the neonate.[138] Because of these characteristics, laryngeal exposure and intubation are more easily accomplished with a straight laryngoscope blade (eg, Miller or Wis-Hipple) than a curved one.

The narrowest point of the adult upper airway is the glottis; in the child from birth to approximately 10 years of age, however, the subglottic region is narrowest.[138] A cuff is thus not required to seal this area in the child. Trauma to the subglottic region by an endotracheal tube that fits too snugly must be avoided, as severe long-term consequences may result.[177] The appropriate endotracheal tube is one that achieves a good seal and thus lessens the likelihood of aspiration but that still allows slight leakage of gas around it.[142] Typical endotracheal tube sizes are given in Table 18-3. The proper size of an endotracheal tube for children at or above 2 years of age may be estimated by adding 16 to the child's age (in years) and then dividing by 4. A more rapid, but rough estimate of proper tube size is to choose one the same size as the child's fifth finger[113] or one that approximates the size of the child's nostril. Once intubation has been accomplished, careful positioning and secure taping are essential to ensure good ventilation of both lungs; a shift of only a centimeter may be significant in a small child. The length of the airway from the child's teeth to the midtrachea may be estimated using one of three equations described by Morgan and Steward[189]: airway length = 14.5 + (Age − 3) × 0.6 for ages 3–14 years, height (cm)/10 + 5 cm for all ages, or 12 + weight(kg)/5 for all ages.

Blind nasotracheal intubation is somewhat more difficult in the child than in the adult, but it may be successful and is quite useful in the patient with cervical spine injury. It should

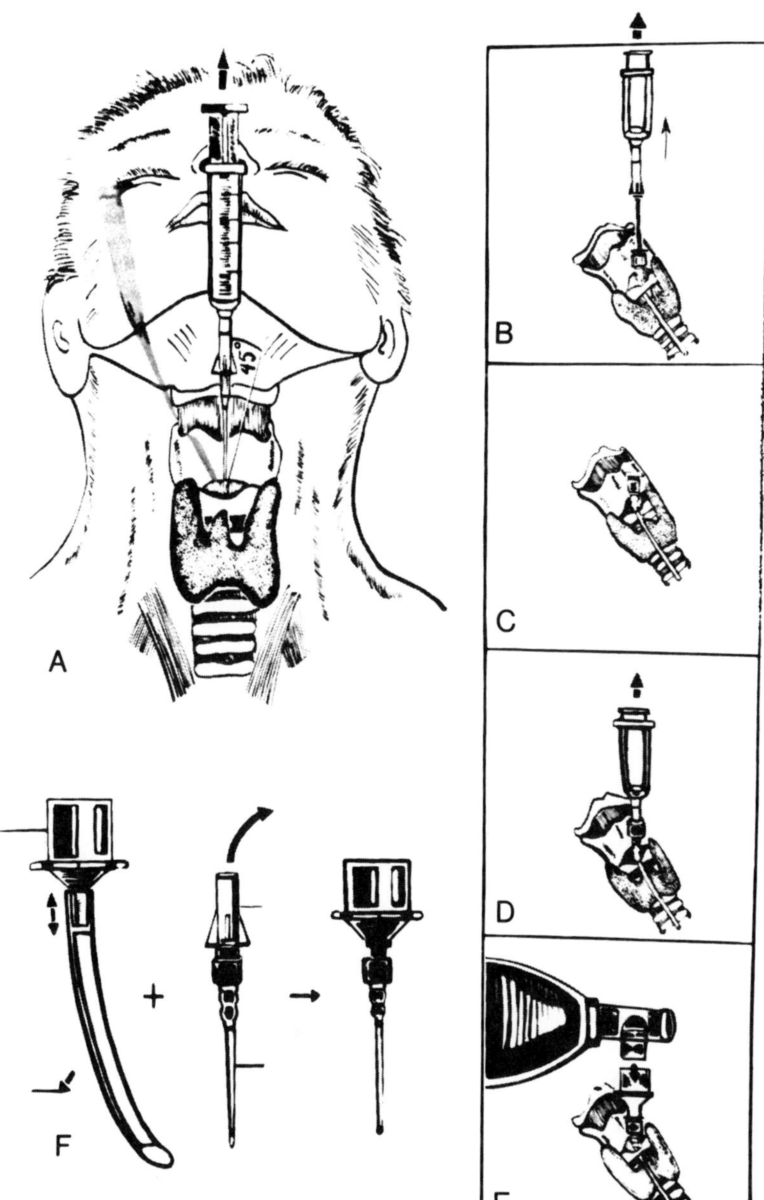


FIG. 18-3. Emergency ventilation with cannula through cricothyoid membrane. (From Mayer TA: Emergency management of pediatric trauma. Philadelphia: WB Saunders Co., 1985, with permission.)

be performed only with extreme care in children younger than 10 years of age since severe pharyngeal bleeding may result from trauma to the adenoids. This technique should not be used if there is a suspicion of basal skull fracture (intracranial placement)[234] and may be hazardous in the presence of a pharyngeal tear (false passage). Basal skull fractures are commonly manifested by cerebrospinal fluid rhinorrhea, Battle's sign, raccoon eyes, and/or bleeding from the ears.[245]

Fiberoptic endoscopy and intubation, with a pediatric fiberscope in the hands of the experienced clinician, are invaluable, although the size of the instrument used in most centers may preclude its use in patients requiring endotracheal tubes smaller than 4.0- to 4.5-mm.[202] For the past several years a fiberoptic scope with an external diameter of 2.7 mm (Olympus PF, Type 27M), allowing intubation with a 3.0-mm endotracheal tube, has been available.[149] Wire-guide

TABLE 18-3. Endotracheal Tube and Laryngoscope Blade Sizes for Children

| AGE | TUBE SIZE* | LARYNGOSCOPE BLADE |
|---|---|---|
| Premature newborn | 2.5 mm ID | Miller 0 |
| Term newborn | 3.0 mm ID | Miller 0 or 1 |
| 6 months | 3.5 mm ID | Miller 1 |
| 1 year | 4.0 mm ID | Miller 1, Wis-Hipple 1.5 |
| 18 months | 4.5 mm ID | Miller 1, Wis-Hipple 1.5 |
| 2 years and above | $\frac{16 + \text{age (yr)}}{4}$ | Miller 2<br>Wis-Hipple 1.5<br>Macintosh 2 |

Uncuffed tube <10 years old or <6 mm ID; cuffed tube >10 years old or >6 mm ID. Typical endotracheal tube sizes for age; tubes 0.5 mm ID larger and smaller should also be available.

techniques, both anterograde and retrograde, have been successful in some patients who would otherwise have required tracheostomy.[254] Intubation in the patient with cervical spine injury may require repeated attempts with more than one of these techniques[127,139]; it is essential to have extra personnel at the bedside whose sole responsibility is to stabilize the head and neck, maintaining gentle but firm axial traction during manipulation. Whenever possible, intubation in these patients should be delayed, to be performed after external stabilization of the neck.

## VENTILATION

Once the airway is established, ventilation must be coordinated with chest compressions during CPR, the standard recommendation being one breath for each five compressions. (Table 18-4).

Although sophisticated monitoring methods may be utilized if available, the most reliable indicators of adequate ventilation in emergencies are symmetric breath sounds, adequate chest wall movement, and clinical improvement. Chest wall and pulmonary compliance vary from moment to moment during resuscitation, particularly in the presence of chest or abdominal trauma. Thus, such measurements as airway pressures may not consistently reflect tidal volume. Undue resistance to ventilation or newly occurring asymmetric breath sounds may suggest a developing pneumothorax that requires prompt attention. Bleeding in the airway may result in clotting and occlusion of the endotracheal tube; therefore, frequent irrigation and suctioning are essential.

Additional guidance may be obtained from arterial blood gas analysis, end-tidal $CO_2$ measurement, and noninvasive oximetry. Arterial blood gases guide oxygen administration and correction of acidosis. End-tidal $CO_2$ monitoring tracks the adequacy of both ventilation and pulmonary perfusion and may thus serve as an indicator of the overall effectiveness of resuscitation. A pulse oximeter allows beat-to-beat assessment of arterial oxygen saturation, with less susceptibility to some of the factors that affect transcutaneous $PO_2$ and $PCO_2$ measurement, eg, poor skin perfusion in a hypovolemic patient.[69]

## HEMODYNAMIC MANAGEMENT

### *Re-Establishment of Circulation*

External chest compression provides subnormal but adequate circulatory support; it should be employed not only after complete cardiac arrest but also at any time that spontaneous cardiac output seems inadequate. The rate and technique should vary with the child's age, with younger children requiring a faster rate and less effort to accomplish chest compression (Table 18-4). The carotid pulse is difficult to palpate in children, and palpation of the brachial or femoral pulses may serve as a guide to the adequacy of the effort. If external compression fails to provide adequate circulation, especially if there is evidence to suggest intrathoracic trauma, the chest should be opened without delay and internal cardiac compression applied, gently squeezing the heart between the palms of the hands. It should be remembered that, although elevation of the legs may be helpful, use of the head-down (Trendelenburg) position has no place in the management of shock.[54]

TABLE 18-4. Values for CPR in Pediatric Patients

| | INFANT | CHILD | ADOLESCENT |
|---|---|---|---|
| Chest compressions per minute | 120 | 100 | 80 |
| Chest compressions—depth (inches) | ½–1 | 1–1½ | 1½–2 |
| Breaths per minute | 24 | 20 | 16 |

### *Venous Access*

The techniques and landmarks for venous cannulation are identical in children and adults. The internal and external jugular veins, the axillary vein, and the femoral vein can usually be cannulated percutaneously, even in small infants. The internal jugular vein can be cannulated by using either the low approach, inserting the needle slightly above the clavicular notch,[214] or the traditional high approach. Coté et al.[58] found a greater success rate and lower incidence of morbidity with the high cervical approach. The subclavian vein is relatively difficult to reach. Many authors discourage its use in children younger than 6 to 7 years of age because of a high rate of complications, especially pneumothorax.[7,173] The saphenous and brachiocephalic systems may be entered percutaneously or by surgical cutdown. Care should be taken to establish intravenous lines of sufficient caliber to allow rapid fluid resuscitation. Intravenous lines should be positioned in such a way that they will be secure and accessible intraoperatively, and there should be reasonable certainty that venous continuity between the insertion site and the heart is and will remain intact. Children with severe intra-abdominal or retroperitoneal hemorrhage may have inferior vena cava injury, precluding placement of intravenous lines in the lower extremity. It is often wise to establish two or more access points on opposite sides of the diaphragm. Intravenous lines placed before the child arrived in the hospital should be untaped and reinspected.

Although access to the central circulation may provide a more direct route to the heart, it is not essential. It is more beneficial to establish a reliable intravenous line peripherally than to waste precious time in repeated attempts at central line placement. Central venous pressure measurements add little to the initial management of pediatric trauma patients and can wait until the patient is more stable.

If venous access is delayed unavoidably, certain resuscitation drugs—for instance, atropine, epinephrine, and lidocaine—may be administered intratracheally.[264] The usual doses are diluted to a volume of several milliliters with sterile water and injected into the endotracheal tube; a few large breaths will distribute the drug across the pulmonary bed, with subsequent rapid absorption and direct return to the heart.

Intraosseous fluid administration has received renewed attention as a technique for emergency vascular access.[123,222]

A large-bore needle (eg, an 18-gauge spinal needle) is placed into the intramedullary space of a large bone, such as the tibia, femur, or iliac crest. Fluids and drugs, including plasma, saline, lactated Ringer's solution, sodium bicarbonate, and catecholamines, can be infused into the marrow cavity from which they enter the nutrient and emissary veins of the bone. Infusions can be maintained by gravity or pressure pump; in infants, rates as high as 100 mL/h are usually well tolerated. Complications of intraosseous infusions are surprisingly infrequent and include osteomyelitis or other infections, growth plate injuries, and leakage of fluid around the puncture site.

### *Intravascular Volume*

Resuscitation will be unsuccessful if hypovolemia remains uncorrected. It is our impression that the child subjected to an ongoing loss of intravascular volume responds somewhat differently than the adult under similar circumstances. The adult, as blood loss continues, becomes progressively tachycardic and hypotensive; hypotension may be used as an indicator of the need for volume replacement. The child also becomes tachycardic; blood pressure however; is much better preserved than in the adult owing to the child's highly responsive sympathetic nervous system and ability to constrict the blood vessels. A child can be drastically hypovolemic and still sustain a relatively normal blood pressure; when the volume loss finally exceeds the limits of this compensation (greater than 25–30% of the blood volume) the subsequent fall in blood pressure is catastrophic, and loss of cardiac output with subsequent cardiac arrest may occur within minutes. It is inappropriate then to assume that the child is doing well and is not hypovolemic simply because the blood pressure is adequate. Volume replacement must be initiated early, guided by the history, evidence of poor perfusion, tachycardia, and response to fluid challenge.

External blood loss can usually be controlled simply by applying pressure to the wound. Care must be taken if the wound overlies a fracture site, especially in the skull. An assessment must be made for unrecognized internal bleeding.

Volume resuscitation should begin with isotonic crystalloid solutions, such as Ringer's lactate or 0.9% sodium chloride,[121] initially 15–20 mL/kg, approximating 25% of the estimated blood volume. If the child fails to respond, the fluid challenge may be repeated three to four times. If the patient's condition improves transiently only to deteriorate, there may be ongoing blood loss, or the infused crystalloid solution may be redistributing out of the intravascular space.[121] A patient who requires several fluid challenges to correct perfusion probably needs blood replacement to maintain intravascular volume and oxygen-carrying capacity. Type 0-negative or, if available, cross-matched packed red cells should be given in aliquots of 5–15 mL/kg. Colloid solutions may be used if blood is not available or if crystalloid administration exceeds 30–40 mL/kg.

It is preferable to administer volume aliquots by direct syringe infusion. This technique allows immediate correction of the volume deficit, permits the clinician to judge the child's response to the added volume, and may also improve the accuracy of record keeping. A satisfactory response to restoration of intravascular volume will be manifested by success of resuscitation, slowing of the heart rate, improved perfusion, and correction of metabolic acidosis.

Use of MAST (military antishock trousers) has been recommended by some as adjunct treatment in the child who does not respond promptly to volume administration. MAST is a three-compartment pneumatic device that compresses the legs and lower abdomen. It can fit patients as small as 18 kg (40 lb).[186] MAST improves blood pressure by increasing systemic vascular resistance and by transferring blood from the lower extremities to the central circulation. This device therefore is contraindicated in the presence of pulmonary edema. MAST is also used to stop retroperitoneal pelvic bleeding in children.[92] Because of abdominal compression, pediatric patients may experience respiratory compromise with MAST. As the patient's condition improves, MAST should be released one compartment at a time, and after each step the hemodynamic status of the patient should be observed. Additionally, arterial blood gases should be monitored at frequent intervals since acidic metabolic products from tissues under the MAST may be released during deflation. Although there is much information on the use of MAST in adults (Chapters 4 and 9), little data have been published on its pediatric use.

In moribund patients in whom volume loss is suspected and hemodynamic stability cannot be achieved, thoracotomy and supradiaphragmatic aortic clamping may be indicated.[226] Failure to respond to these measures is an ominous sign[18] and suggests the presence of inferior vena cava injury.

The process of volume resuscitation is complicated in the patient with head injury and raised intracranial pressure. Crystalloids may expand the brain's interstitial space, causing an increase in intracranial pressure and a decrease in cerebral perfusion pressure.[93] This does not mean, however, that hypovolemia should be left untreated or undertreated as adequate cardiac output and cerebral oxygenation are crucial for brain preservation. In these situations there must be frequent communication between the neurosurgeon or neurologist and those directing the resuscitation effort. Resuscitation with hypertonic saline may offer the advantage of restoring intravascular volume without raising the intracranial pressure, but its clinical use in pediatric trauma patients remains to be investigated.[210] Colloid solutions should be administered to patients with severe brain injuries if excessive volumes of crystalloid solutions are required for resuscitation.

## RESUSCITATION DRUGS

The drugs used in pediatric resuscitation are similar to those used in adults; doses are noted in Table 18-5.[131] Epinephrine is clearly the most useful of all resuscitation drugs. Although the drug has both alpha- and beta-adrenergic stimulating effects, there is much evidence to suggest that the alpha (vasoconstrictive) effect is the one of greatest importance in restoring cerebral and coronary perfusion. Epinephrine should be one of the first drugs given for cardiac arrest; specific indications include asystole, bradyarrythmias, fine ventricular fibrillation, and (as an infusion) for pressor support following resuscitation.

The use of other resuscitation drugs is, as in adults, controversial. It seems justified to continue to include glucose, calcium, and bicarbonate among the list of such drugs for

TABLE 18-5. Pediatric Resuscitation Drugs*

| DRUG | DOSE | COMMENTS |
|---|---|---|
| Atropine | 0.02 mg/kg | Indications: Bradycardia.<br>Cautions: Administer full dose; partial doses may paradoxically slow rate by central vagal stimulation |
| Epinephrine | 10 μg/kg (0.1 cc/kg of 1/10,000 solution) | Indications: Asystole, to stimulate cardiac activity; to convert fine ventricular fibrillation to a coarse fibrillation before electroshock; to increase vascular tone and perfusion pressure |
| $NaHCO_3$ (sodium bicarbonate) | 1–2 mEq/kg (initial) 0.5–1 mEq/kg (repeat) | Indications: Metabolic acidosis<br>Cautions: Avoid excessive administration; dilute 1:1 with sterile water for infants, infuse slowly; repeat doses guided by measurements of arterial gases and pH |
| Calcium chloride<br>Calcium gluconate | 10–30 mg/kg<br>30–90 mg/kg | Indications: Hypocalcemia; hyperkalemia; hypermagnesemia; Ca-channel blocker overdose<br>Cautions: May aggravate digoxin toxicity; extravasation may yield tissue necrosis; rapid administration may produce bradycardia; ??toxic effects intracellularly |
| Lidocaine | 1 mg/kg (bolus)<br>15–50 μg/kg/min (infusion) | Indications: Ventricular tachycardia or ectopy<br>Cautions: Metabolism slowed in congestive failure; avoid in high degrees of AV block; rapid administration may cause seizures; infusion rarely needed in children |
| Bretylium | 5 mg/kg (initial) 10 mg/kg (repeat) to cumulative maximum of 30 mg/kg | Indications: Ventricular tachycardia or fibrillation<br>Cautions: Nausea, vomiting in the awake patient if given too fast |
| Dextrose | 0.5–1.0 g/kg (2–4 cc/kg of 25% solution) | Indications: Hypoglycemia (documented or suspected)<br>Cautions: Hypertonic solution—administer slowly; do not overtreat |
| Naloxone | 10 μg/kg; repeat as needed | Indications: Suspected narcotic overdose<br>Cautions: If effective, watch for renarcotization as the drug wears off |

* All drugs are intended for intravenous administration; atropine, lidocaine, and epinephrine may be diluted with sterile water and given intratracheally. The intracardiac route is hazardous and should be avoided if possible.

pediatric resuscitation, however, as the circumstances of an arrest in an infant or child may suggest a special need for these agents. Special attention to the evaluation and treatment of hypoglycemia in infants and small children[205] and to hypocalcemia during rapid infusion of citrated blood products is required.

The usual response to trauma is hyperglycemia, which may cause a hyperosmolar state, diuresis, and hypovolemia. Administration of exogenous glucose to prevent glycolysis may further aggravate both hyperglycemia and hypovolemia. Blood glucose should be monitored throughout the perioperative period with glucose administered only as indicated.[256]

Serum ionized calcium ($Ca^{++}$) levels are usually maintained within normal limits in children if the rate of blood transfusion is less than 30 mL/kg/h.[2] However, in the presence of hypothermia and hemodynamic instability, which are commonly seen in the injured pediatric patient, reduction of $Ca^{++}$ may occur at slower transfusion rates.[2] If hypocalcemia does occur, calcium chloride (10%) or calcium gluconate (10%) can be used with equal efficacy to raise serum ionized calcium levels quickly.[63] If calcium gluconate is used, the dose should be three times that of calcium chloride, as the gluconate salt contains one-third the amount of elemental calcium as the chloride.

Sodium bicarbonate should be diluted with sterile water before use and administered slowly to infants and small children to avoid rapid osmolar shifts.[136] It is important to note that convincing evidence for a beneficial effect of sodium bicarbonate is lacking, despite its long history of recommended use. In addition, $CO_2$ liberated from its metabolism can readily diffuse into cells and increase acidosis further at this site. Therefore, its use should probably be restricted to patients with severe extracellular acidosis ($pH < 7.1$). In these patients a transient increase in arterial pH may contribute to recovery of spontaneous cardiac activity.

## TEMPERATURE PRESERVATION

Restoration and preservation of normal body temperature are essential in children as the cold infant will remain acidotic and poorly perfused. The child readily loses heat on exposure to the external environment and during the rapid administration of unwarmed fluids or cold blood. Also, heat production is decreased during the initial phase of severe trauma.[65] This period is termed the "ebb" phase, which is normally followed by an increase in heat production in the "flow phase." In severe trauma, the transition to the flow phase may be delayed, resulting in prolonged hypothermia. A warm room, radiant heaters, warming blankets, and heating and humidification of inspired gases help maintain the patient's temperature. Shaver et al.[244] demonstrated preservation of core and epicardial temperature in dogs resuscitated from hypovolemic shock with Ringer's lactate given at 37°C. The patient's esophageal or rectal temperature should be monitored with a thermometer capable of measuring a wide range of temperatures. Severe hypothermia (temperature less than 32°C) may occur and should be corrected aggressively. Aggressive attempts at pharmacologic or electrical therapy to improve cardiac function will be unsuccessful until rewarming is accomplished.

### DEFIBRILLATION

Defibrillation can usually be accomplished with external DC electroshock at 2–4 J/kg.[116] Persistent ventricular ectopy after successful defibrillation is unusual in children. Once myocardial perfusion is restored and hypoxemia and hypothermia are corrected, cardiac rhythm is generally well maintained, and continuous infusion of antiarrhythmics is not necessary.

## ASSESSMENT OF THE INJURED CHILD

The initial assessment of the injured child is most important since it is the basis of the provisional diagnosis and the institution of a specific therapeutic plan. The assessment process is a dynamic one. All currently available information must be considered, and the working diagnosis and plan must be updated continuously by new information and by the child's response to therapy.[121]

### HISTORY

The importance of obtaining an adequate history cannot be overemphasized. Information about the mechanism of the current injury will suggest areas needing special attention in the physical examination. Pertinent details of the child's past health, pre-existing disease, and prior anesthetic experiences should be sought. A few moments spent inquiring about medications and allergies may be invaluable to later management; these may have been overlooked by previous historians. One should inquire about the extent of the child's injuries, degree of physiologic disturbance, and the planned medical and surgical treatment. The child's course since entry into the hospital, especially with regard to response to therapy, must be reviewed. Finally, a brief discussion with the child's parents about the proposed anesthetic and surgical procedures and risks is appropriate.

### INITIAL EVALUATION

A complete physical examination is necessary in all patients who have sustained more than minor injury. The physician must perform this evaluation systematically, assessing the need for rapid intervention in vital areas, while ensuring that no area of the examination is neglected.[76,121] Often, examination, diagnosis, and therapy must proceed simultaneously since they are interdependent.

Blunt, rather than penetrating, trauma is most commonly seen in children, and multisystem involvement is not unusual. Often the trauma has been one-sided, as in a vehicle-pedestrian accident. In such cases, external wounds are commonly accompanied by injuries to underlying tissues on the same side.[170] A rapid appraisal of the child "from across the room," even before detailed examination is begun, may offer clues to the extent of injury and the areas likely to be involved.

Airway, breathing, and circulation are of first priority in evaluation. If the airway is compromised in any way or if the patient's level of consciousness is depressed sufficiently to blunt normal protective reflexes, then endotracheal intubation is indicated. It may be performed in the emergency department using anesthetics as needed. In most instances, the patient should be assumed to have a full stomach and managed accordingly. If the circumstances of the trauma suggest cervical spine injury, careful stabilization of the head and neck with gentle axial traction during intubation is necessary.

Patients who may have increased intracranial pressure (ICP), even if they do not appear comatose, should have appropriate anesthetic precautions taken to prevent further ICP elevation during intubation. These include hyperventilation by mask before laryngoscopy and pretreatment with an ultrashort-acting barbiturate (eg, thiopental, 2–4 mg/kg); lidocaine, 1.5 mg/kg IV; and/or muscle relaxation.[72,270,276] Care should be taken to avoid depressing cardiovascular performance. It is better to err on the side of early intubation than to have serious airway difficulties develop a few hours later, which require emergency intubation under less controlled circumstances.

If the need for airway control is not acute, possible difficulties in intubation may be planned for preoperatively. The presence of certain congenital abnormalities, such as cystic hygromas, hemifacial microsomia, Pierre-Robin syndrome, or the Hunter/Hurler group of disorders, may be considered "red flag" warnings of potentially difficult airway and intubation.

Adequacy of oxygenation and ventilation should be ensured. Physical examination of the chest may reveal such abnormalities as assymetry of breath sounds, tracheal deviation, or displacement of the cardiac apex, which may indicate injury within the mediastinum or pleural cavities. Open chest wounds, hemothorax, pneumothorax, and flail chest require correction or stabilization; depending on the lesion, placement of chest tubes and positive-pressure ventilation may be necessary. If increased ICP is suspected, modest hyperventilation should be begun in the emergency department.

Cardiac performance, blood pressure, and peripheral perfusion are evaluated next. Cardiac tamponade is rare in children, but should not be overlooked; muffled heart sounds, dyspnea, a weak thready pulse, and distended neck veins suggest the diagnosis. Hypotension is more commonly caused by hypovolemia and is manifest by tachycardia, peripheral vasoconstriction, and generally normal or increased systemic blood pressure. Recurrent deterioration of vital signs after an initial improvement with rapid fluid infusion suggests continuing blood loss. Although possible, it is unlikely that in older children hypovolemic shock will result purely from closed head or even closed extremity injury; in these patients other causes of intravascular volume loss should be sought.[14] Closed head injury, however, can be the cause of hemorrhagic shock in young children with open cranial sutures.

### NEUROLOGIC STATUS

A brief neurologic examination that evaluates the level of consciousness and notes any focal findings is essential. Anesthetic techniques may require modification in order to reduce intracranial pressure. Focal deficits suggest a mass lesion in the brain or spinal cord that may require immediate attention; in addition, documentation of pre-existing deficits for comparison with postoperative findings may be invaluable. A smaller proportion of pediatric head trauma victims require surgical intervention as compared to adults (6% versus 30%).[261] It should be remembered that a large percentage of children with head injuries show evidence of disseminated intravascular coagulation (DIC)[185] and may show ECG abnormalities as well, eg, prolonged qTc.[219] Neurovascular compromise of an extremity may require immediate therapy and will influence the anesthetist's choice of sites for arterial and venous access.

### ABDOMEN AND PERIPHERAL AREAS

Abdominal distension resulting from acute gastric dilation is extremely common in injured children, and placement of a nasogastric or orogastric tube will assist the abdominal examination, ease ventilation, and lessen the risk of regurgitation and aspiration of gastric contents. Although significant loss of blood into the peritoneal cavity may result from injury to solid intra-abdominal organs, current pediatric surgical practice favors a nonoperative approach in pediatric blunt abdominal trauma, with diagnostic peritoneal lavage, careful observation, and CT scan evaluation, unless significant hemodynamic instability is present.[224,226,259] During the observation period, particularly in battered children and after motor vehicle accidents, the possibility of hollow viscus perforation should be considered and appropriate diagnostic maneuvers and periodic examinations performed.[148,169] Associated injuries are common (55%) after blunt abdominal trauma and require an aggressive radiographic imaging protocol.[226]

Physical examination of other areas is completed as circumstances allow. The anesthesiologist may not require as detailed an assessment of more peripheral areas, but the general plan of treatment for the child should be known so that appropriate anesthetic management for further diagnostic and therapeutic procedures may be anticipated.

### LABORATORY

Studies of particular interest to the anesthesiologist include radiographs of the chest and cervical spine; blood count and coagulation tests; measurement of serum electrolytes, glucose, and ionized calcium; and arterial blood gases. Unless there is evidence to the contrary, it should be assumed that laboratory values were normal before the injury. Blood should be dispatched to the blood bank for typing, cross-match, and preparation of adequate quantities of blood and blood components. More sophisticated radiologic examinations, including angiography, nuclear isotope scans, and CT scans of the head and body, may be helpful to both surgeon and anesthesiologist. It is mandatory, however, that these procedures be performed expeditiously and efficiently, although only after some degree of stability has been achieved. In many cases, it is appropriate for the child to be accompanied to the diagnostic area by the anesthesiologist, who will provide monitoring and life support during the procedure. Continued close supervision of the patient in transport from the emergency department to the operating room or intensive care area is essential to anticipate and prevent decompensation enroute.

## ANESTHETIC CONSIDERATIONS FOR MINOR SURGERY

One of the most important contributions that the anesthesiologist can make to the child's care is as a calm, warm, and caring individual who will devote his or her entire attention to the patient during the frightful perioperative period.[143] The child who is able to understand will respond positively to a simple explanation of what is wrong, what is being done to remedy the problem, and what the proposed future course of therapy will be. Painful but necessary examinations or procedures must not be omitted in order to be kind to the child. However, the patient should be warned about painful procedures, and their necessity should be explained as simply as possible. The anesthesiologist should try, as preparations for anesthesia and surgery are being made, to maintain close physical contact with the child, speaking in a calm, reassuring, but firm voice and explaining events as they are happening. Hypnotic techniques, such as monotony of voice and distraction and displacement of the child's concentration, are helpful. Most children respond better to direct, simple adult conversation than to obviously strained and artificially sweet "baby talk."

The diagnosis and treatment of minor trauma may, in the frightened child with a painful injury, require sedation, anesthesia, and analgesia. In many cases, infiltration with a local anesthetic agent, moderate doses of analgesic agents, and physical restraint are sufficient. Administration of fentanyl slowly, 2–3 μg/kg IV, was shown to provide satisfactory analgesia and sedation for repair of minor facial injuries in a study of 2,000 pediatric patients. Only three apneic apisodes occurred in this series, and all were treated successfully with naloxone.[27] Heavy sedation with combinations of narcotics, barbiturates, and other tranquilizers should not be used because of extended duration of action and the danger of aspiration pneumonitis. Some centers are equipped to allow inhalation of *low* concentrations of nitrous oxide (typically 50% $N_2O$, balance $O_2$) during painful procedures. Such an option should only be offered under the guidance of strict protocols previously approved by the department of anesthesia. One trained staff member should be assigned to monitor the patient's condition closely during the procedure. If the child remains uncooperative during simple measures or if the extent of surgery or of physical and psychological trauma is particularly great, more complete anesthetic management may be required.

The request of emergency personnel that the anesthesiologist be available to give "a little anesthesia" is fraught with hazard.[260] Although minor cases may allow the relatively elective scheduling of surgery, it must be remembered that gastric emptying time is delayed even after a minor injury and that the patient must be managed with appropriate protection against aspiration of gastric contents. Preparation for such management must be made even if a fasting period has ensued and even if a regional technique is planned, as the need to convert from an unsatisfactory regional anesthetic to a general anesthetic occurs frequently in children.

The incidence of gastric content aspiration in children during anesthesia is higher than that in adults.[199] The relatively small stomach, air swallowing with crying, strenuous diaphragmatic breathing, and encroachment of abdominal organs on the stomach (especially in infants) may result in a significant increase in intragastric pressure, forcing gastric contents into the esophagus.[229] In addition, upper airway obstruction, for instance from laryngeal spasm, is more common in children than in adults during anesthesia, and the resulting increase in the pleuroperitoneal pressure gradient may promote regurgitation of gastric contents.[229] The risk of pneumonitis after aspiration of gastric contents also appears to be greater in children than in adults, even in the absence of trauma and recent food ingestion. Several studies have demonstrated lower pH and relatively larger gastric fluid volume in fasting children than in adults.[60,162,230]

If time permits, preoperative prophylactic measures should be employed to reduce the risk of aspiration pneumonitis. These include mechanical emptying of the stomach and esophagus, neutralization of gastric acidity with antacids or $H_2$-receptor blocking agents, acceleration of anterograde gastric emptying, and augmentation of gastric barrier pressure by pharmacologic means. However, none of these measures is capable of entirely preventing regurgitation, vomiting, aspiration, or pneumonitis. Therefore, all possible protective measures must be employed during anesthesia to prevent these complications. A detailed discussion of anesthetic management of the full stomach is given in Chapter 3, and the specific areas pertinent to the pediatric patient are offered in the section on anesthesia for major trauma in this chapter.

Evacuation of the stomach by means of a nasogastric tube reduces the volume of gastric contents. However, total emptying of the stomach by this method cannot be ensured, even in the absence of particulate matter in the stomach.[4] In addition, introduction of a nasogastric tube in the awake, uncooperative child may be difficult. If a nasogastric tube is already in place, it should not be removed during the anesthetic induction. Although the competence of the gastroesophageal sphincter is altered by the nasogastric tube, cricoid pressure will occlude the esophagus without blocking the tube. The patent nasogastric tube then may act as a "blow-off" valve and prevent a rise in intragastric pressure.[227,231] Although antacid agents are effective in reducing gastric acidity, they frequently increase gastric fluid volume and may promote regurgitation and pulmonary aspiration. Cimetidine, 7.5 mg/kg orally, given to electively operated children 1 to 3 hours before surgery can reduce gastric fluid volume and increase its pH above 2.5.[101] In the traumatized child in whom gastric emptying is delayed, the value of this drug may be reduced. Metoclopramide stimulates anterograde emptying of gastric contents, coordinates gastroduodenal peristalsis, and increases gastric barrier pressure. One study has shown that this drug could be of value in decreasing the risk of aspiration in the injured child undergoing surgery.[198] However, additional data are needed before routine use of metoclopramide can be recommended for aspiration prophylaxis in the injured child.

Premedication may be helpful in some instances and is permissible if there is no serious compromise of airway or consciousness. Atropine or glycopyrrolate decreases secretions if given intramuscularly 30–45 minutes before surgery; their effect on heart rate is achieved better by intravenous administration immediately before induction.[23,265] In addition, glycopyrrolate, 0.01 mg/kg, or atropine, 0.02 mg/kg IV, given immediately before anesthetic induction prevents the bradycardia or dysrhythmia caused by repeated succinylcholine administration or laryngoscopy.[109] Pain should be relieved with narcotics once the diagnosis of injury and the management strategy are established. Sedation and amnesia may be achieved with intravenous diazepam or other sedatives, but these agents must be administered with caution since both respiratory depression and hypotension may occur in hypovolemic children.

## REGIONAL ANESTHESIA FOR MINOR TRAUMA

Regional anesthetic techniques may be used in cooperative, hemodynamically stable injured children.[249] Uncomplicated procedures on the fingers may best be performed under digital block, which may be performed by the surgeon or anesthesiologist; solutions without epinephrine should be used. Intravenous regional anesthesia (Bier blocks) and brachial plexus blocks are quite effective for minor upper extremity surgery. In all regional techniques, an adequate concentration and volume of agent (Tables 18-6 and 18-7) should be used and sufficient time allowed for the development of a good block; testing of the block before anesthesia has set in will undermine the child's confidence in the technique. In many instances regional anesthesia is administered in conjunction with general anesthesia to minimize the total dosage of intravenous and inhalation agents, to shorten the recovery period, to provide postoperative analgesia, and to maintain vasodilation during replantation surgery. A detailed description of regional anesthetic techniques for children is beyond the scope of this chapter; the reader is referred to two recent publications on this subject.[67,277]

Intravenous regional anesthesia using 0.5% lidocaine is appropriate for the repair of tendon lacerations, closed fractures, and other distal injuries of the upper extremity.[44,85] The technique is the same as that used in adults. The volume of drug injected should be sufficient to perfuse the venous distribution of the arm. The total volume required is 10–15 mL for ages 1–4, 15–20 mL for ages 5–7, and 20–30 mL for ages 8–12.

Brachial plexus block is suitable for suturing of extensive lacerations or reduction of fractures of the arm and forearm. The axillary approach is recommended for children; the axillary artery is easily palpated, and entry of the needle tip into

TABLE 18-6. Suggested Maximum Doses of Local Anesthetics for Regional Blocks in Children*

| DRUG | TYPE OF BLOCK | MAXIMUM DOSE | CONCENTRATION (%) |
|---|---|---|---|
| Lidocaine | IV regional | 3–5 mg/kg | 0.5 |
| | Peripheral nerve block | 7–10 mg/kg without epinephrine** | 1 |
| | Caudal-epidural | 7–10 mg/kg without epinephrine** | 1.0–2.0 |
| | Spinal | 1–2.5 mg/kg | 2.0–5.0 |
| Bupivacaine | Peripheral nerve block | 3–5 mg/kg* | 0.5 |
| | Caudal-epidural | 3–5 mg/kg* | 0.5 |
| | Spinal | 0.3–0.4 mg/kg | 0.75 |
| Tetracaine | Peripheral nerve block | 2 mg/kg | 0.2 |
| | Caudal-epidural | 2 mg/kg | 0.2 |
| | Spinal | 0.2–0.5 mg/kg | 0.5 |

* Available data on regional anesthetic drugs in children are sparse; this information should be regarded only as a guideline.

** The dose may be increased by 25–30% with addition of epinephrine 1:200,000.

the perivascular sheath is accompanied by a definite "pop," aiding injection of local anesthetic solution in the vicinity of the plexus. With the use of insulated needles and nerve stimulators capable of delivering electrical currents as low as 0.3–0.5 mA, the plexus can be located and appropriate local anesthetic injected. Although this technique may be performed with uninsulated needles as well,[188] the nerve can be located more precisely with insulated needles.[15,88] Children may be more frightened by the supraclavicular and interscalene approaches to the plexus, and the risk of complications and ineffective block in a struggling, uncooperative child is high. However, it has been suggested that these disadvantages may be minimized by use of the recently described parascalene approach.[67] Lidocaine, 1%, usually with epinephrine, 5 μg/mL, is the recommended drug because of its rapid onset and minimal toxicity, although some physicians prefer to use bupivacaine, 0.25–0.5%. The recommended volume of agent is 0.5 mL/kg. Thus, the total volume of injected local anesthetic is 3 mL for the neonates, 6–9 mL for ages 1–3, 9–12 mL for ages 4–6, and 15–30 mL for ages 7–15.[249]

Although experience is limited, intercostal nerve block may be used in children to provide analgesia after chest trauma.[249] Two technical points should be kept in mind when performing blocks in children. First, the needles should not be inserted any deeper than 1 to 2 mm under the rib because the pleura is in close proximity to the skin. Second, the block should not be attempted medially to the angle of the rib because there are no intercostal muscles in this region. The total dose of bupivacaine 0.25–0.5 % used is 2–3 mg/kg. Rothstein and colleagues[225] reported that absorption of bupivacaine-epinephrine solution from the intercostal space is more rapid in small children than is usually observed in adults, probably as a result of the relatively greater cardiac output in children. Since they observed blood concentrations occasionally greater than 3 μg/mL when a dose of 4 mg/kg was administered, they recommend that doses greater than 3 mg/kg should not be used.

TABLE 18-7. Suggested Volumes of Local Anesthetic Solutions for Various Regional Blocks in Children

| TYPE OF BLOCK | VOLUME |
|---|---|
| IV regional (Bier) | 0.5–1.0 mL/kg |
| Brachial plexus | 0.5 mL/kg |
| Lumbar epidural | 0.5–0.75 mL per spinal segment |
| Caudal (sacral segments only) | 3 mL minimum volume, plus 1 mL for each age >3 years |

Peripheral nerve block for lower extremity surgery is used less frequently, probably because both the sciatic and femoral nerves must be blocked, necessitating multiple needle punctures. However, isolated femoral nerve block may relieve quadriceps muscle spasm and thus provide analgesia in patients with femoral shaft fractures awaiting surgery.[25]

In hemodynamically stable patients undergoing lower extremity procedures, spinal anesthesia or lumbar or caudal epidural anesthesia may be employed. Spinal anesthesia may be administered even to children younger than 1 year of age.[1] The lumbar puncture should be performed below the third lumbar vertebra because the spinal cord terminates at this level in infants. Lidocaine 5% in dextrose in a dose of 1.5–2.5 mg/kg provides satisfactory analgesia to T4–T6.[182] Abajian et al.[1] used tetracaine (1%) 0.22–0.32 mg/kg in high-risk infants without significant complications. Yaster and Maxwell[277] suggest the use of 0.5–0.6 mg/kg tetracaine in an equal volume of dextrose 10%. Subarachnoid bupivacaine 0.75%, 0.3–0.4 mg/kg, may also provide satisfactory analgesia.[30] Epidural anesthesia is used less frequently. The distance from the skin to the lumbar epidural space increases from 1.5 cm in children 1 year of age to 2.5 cm in those 10 years of age.[249] The dose of lidocaine (1–2%) with 1/200,000 epinephrine is 6–8 mg/kg.[182] A similar dose is used for caudal epidural block.[257]

Pediatric patients who have received a regional anesthetic commonly require sedation, which may depress respiration and obtund tracheobronchial reflexes. In the traumatized child with recent food ingestion, these effects may set the stage for pulmonary aspiration of gastric contents. Induction of general anesthesia using a rapid sequence technique should be considered in those children who require excessive doses of sedative and narcotic agents.

Whenever regional anesthesia is employed, the anesthesiologist must be prepared to treat the complications of local anesthetic toxicity. Appropriate agents should be at hand for emergent management of seizures and cardiovascular collapse, and drugs and equipment necessary for rapid sequence induction and intubation must be prepared in advance.

Obviously any minor surgical procedure can be performed under general anesthesia, which is discussed in the next section.

## ANESTHETIC CONSIDERATIONS FOR MAJOR SURGERY

It should be emphasized that transport of the seriously injured patient to the operating room is a period of particular risk. It is wise for the anesthesiologist to supervise this transfer personally, if possible. Intravenous lines, endotracheal and nasogastric tubes, and other catheters must be secured, and the child, if conscious, must be supervised to ensure that he or she does not disturb them. In addition, assessment and modification of therapy can continue, and time may be spent in comforting the patient.

Major emergency surgery in the child usually requires general anesthesia.[253,256] Spinal or peridural anesthesia, although reasonable in elective or minor surgery, is unwise in the trauma patient with uncertain blood volume and increased vascular tone.

### PREMEDICATION

Children with acute head injury and/or multiple system trauma should not receive premedication. In awake, responsive patients premedication may be given after stabilization of the circulation. Anticholinergic agents may be given early or immediately before anesthetic induction to decrease pharyngeal secretions. The intravenous route is preferred since absorption of intramuscularly injected drugs may be poor. Morphine sulfate (0.05–0.1 mg/kg) or fentanyl (0.002–0.004 mg/kg) IV, usually provides satisfactory analgesia within a few minutes after injection. Sedative drugs are rarely needed if adequate rapport has been established between the physician and the child. Agitation in a traumatized child or adult may be due to hypoxia, which should be ruled out before giving sedatives or narcotics. Benzodiazepines or barbiturates may be used in small doses; the latter may be less desirable because of the risk of hypotension in the hypovolemic patient. Barbiturates may also have a paradoxical stimulant and antianalgesic effect in some children.[252] Droperidol has sedative, antisialogogue, and antiemetic effects. However, it causes restlessness, anxiety, and motor disturbances in some patients. In addition, hypotension may occur in hypovolemic children because of its alpha-receptor blocking effect.

### INDUCTION OF ANESTHESIA

#### *Airway Management*

All trauma patients arriving in the operating room within 24 hours after injury should be considered to have a full stomach. Thus, a rapid sequence induction and intubation technique should be chosen to manage the airway. In children, bradycardia is easily produced during intubation because of direct vagal stimulation by instrumentation of the airway and the parasympathomimetic effects of succinylcholine. Thus, unlike adults, children should be given atropine or glycopyrrolate intravenously immediately before induction if these drugs have not been administered earlier.[109] Head-up tilt, a usual position for the rapid sequence induction technique, is presumed to prevent gastric regurgitation into the pharynx. However, the hydrostatic pressure exerted by this position, especially in a small child with a short esophagus may not counteract the pressure generated in the stomach (Fig 18-4). Therefore, this position appears to be of little value in pediatric patients.[229]

Children have a relatively smaller functional residual capacity (FRC) and a larger oxygen consumption than adults, resulting in the possibility of hypoxemia during an extended laryngoscopy. Monitoring of arterial oxygen saturation with pulse oximetry is extremely valuable during this period. If rapid intubation cannot be accomplished, the patient should be ventilated by mask, additional medication given as needed, and another attempt at laryngoscopy and intubation made; cricoid pressure must be maintained throughout.

When the airway is compromised by trauma or a congenital anomaly, a difficult intubation may be anticipated. In these instances, rapid sequence induction may not be safe. Alternatives include awake intubation using blind nasal, oral, or fiberoptic methods.[95] As mentioned earlier, a fiberoptic bronchoscope with an external diameter of 2.7 mm (Olympus PF, Type 27m), allowing intubation of the trachea with an endotracheal tube as small as 3.0 mm ID, has become available.[146] A slightly larger device with an outside diameter of 3.5 mm accommodates an endotracheal tube of 4.5 mm ID or greater. Retrograde intubation by passing a guide wire or epidural catheter through the cricothyroid membrane and recovering it from the mouth is another alternative in the awake patient. However, intubation by this technique may be impossible if the child cannot or will not open the mouth.[34,254] Awake tracheal intubation may be difficult or impossible in a frightened, struggling child, but it is usually quite successful in reasonably cooperative or obtunded children. Tracheostomy or cricothyroidotomy may be necessary when a secure airway cannot be established with the above techniques. During this procedure the child should be given oxygen by face mask and monitored carefully.

#### *Induction Agents*

Whenever possible, administration of anesthetics to hypovolemic children should be avoided. Rapid administration of blood and fluids before anesthesia restores the intravascular volume in the majority of patients. If correction of hypovolemia without the immediate surgical control of hemorrhage

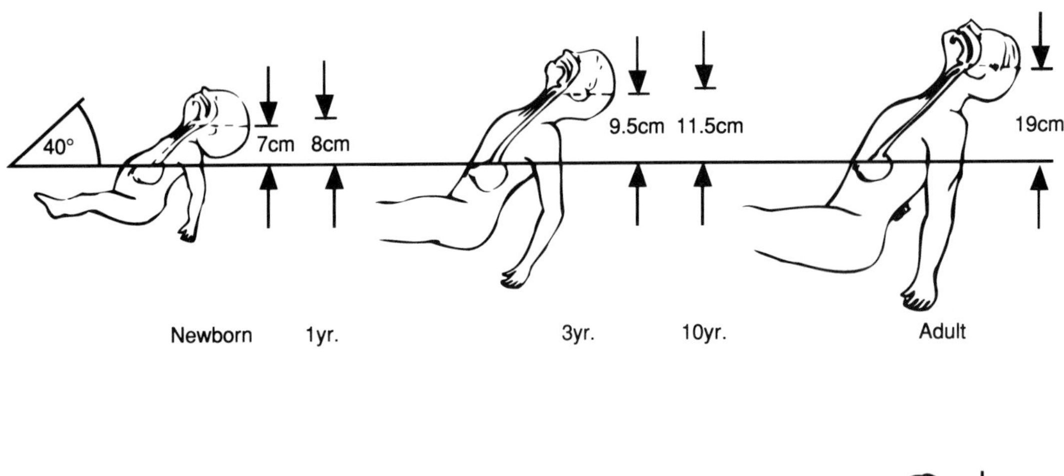


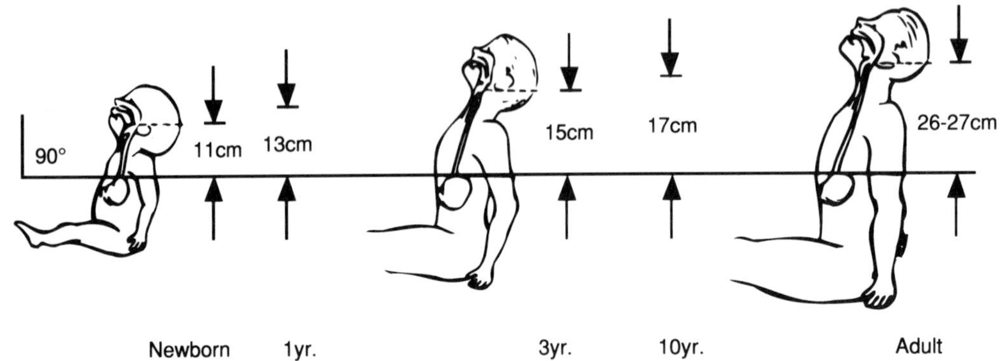


FIG. 18-4. The hydrostatic pressure exerted by the length of esophagus in 40° and 90° head-up tilt at various ages. Note that in children head-up tilt affords little protection against movement of gastric contents into the pharynx. (From Salem et al[229] with permission.)

is not possible, the anesthetic agent(s) and technique(s) with the least potential to perturb the compensatory responses to hemorrhage must be chosen. However, it should be remembered that all anesthetic agents may cause significant hemodynamic derangements; they cannot be viewed as substitutes for the maintenance of circulating blood volume.

The requirement for intravenous anesthetics is reduced after trauma and hemorrhage because (a) the distribution volume for the drug is decreased; (b) dilutional hypoproteinemia occurs so that less drug is bound to proteins and more free drug is available,[274] and (c) during hemorrhage the blood flow to myocardium and brain is well maintained; thus, these organs probably receive a greater fraction of the administered drug in hypovolemic patients than in those in the normovolemic state.[208,267]

Ketamine causes sympathetic stimulation, and studies in hemorrhaged rats have demonstrated the maintenance of venous tone[130] and tissue oxygenation[134,157] and more favorable survival rates compared to other anesthetics.[156] This drug has been advocated for use in adults with hemorrhagic shock.[33,47,197] More recently, however, Seyde and Longnecker[236] demonstrated a significant reduction in cardiac output and regional blood flow in hemorrhaged rats anesthetized with ketamine. Weiskopf et al.,[269] in a well-controlled study, failed to document any advantage of ketamine over thiopental as an induction agent in hemorrhaging swine. These authors found that ketamine, in spite of increasing plasma epinephrine and norepinephrine concentrations and renin activity above already elevated levels, depressed mean systemic blood pressure, heart rate, cardiac output, and systemic vascular resistance. Plasma lactate levels increased and remained elevated 30 minutes after administration of ketamine. In hemorrhaged cats, Wong and Jenkins[273] found that ketamine raised the systemic arterial pressure without necessarily improving perfusion. Although it is difficult to extrapolate these animal data to traumatized children, it appears that the purported benefits of ketamine are minimal in moderately or severely hypovolemic patients. In mild hypovolemia, however, ketamine may be preferable, as it maintains systemic blood pressure. In normovolemic children the dose of ketamine is inversely related to age. Infants require doses four times higher than children 5 to 6 years of age.[154] However, the sleep dose of this drug is 35–40% less in hypovolemic than in normovolemic animals.[267] The dose should thus be adjusted according to the child's age and intravascular volume. The usual intravenous dose of ketamine in normovolemic, unpremedicated children is 2–6 mg/kg (Table 18-8). Ketamine has been shown to increase intracranial pressure in patients with space-occupying lesions; thus it should be avoided in children with closed-head injuries.[243,276] However, intraocular pressure does not seem to increase with this drug; therefore it can be used safely in children with open-eye injuries.[9] It should be remembered that ketamine does not preserve laryngeal reflexes,[35,259] and its use during anesthetic

TABLE 18-8. Doses of Anesthetic Agents used for Uncompromised Children during General Anesthesia

| DRUG | DOSE | COMMENTS |
|---|---|---|
| Thiopental | 2–8 mg/kg | Rapid induction; protection against increase in ICP; avoid in hypotension/hypovolemia |
| Methohexital | 2–3 mg/kg | Same as above; may induce seizures in susceptible patients |
| Ketamine | 2–6 mg/kg | Neuroleptic; maintains blood pressure and systemic vascular resistance |
| Diazepam | 0.1–0.3 mg/kg | Amnesia, sedative; generally safe, but can cause respiratory and cardiac depression in the seriously ill |
| Midazolam | 0.05–0.3 mg/kg | Same as diazepam; ??induction agent |
| Fentanyl | 2–4 μg/kg | Rapid onset, short duration of action; no histamine release; larger doses acceptable, but carry the risk of prolonged respiratory depression |
| Morphine | 0.1–0.2 mg/kg | Longer duration of action; some histamine release |
| Succinylcholine | 1–4 mg/kg | Rapid action; bradycardia common in children |
| Pancuronium | 0.08–0.15 mg/kg | Protective of heart rate and blood pressure |
| D-tubocurarine | 0.6 mg/kg | Potent histamine releaser |
| Metocurine | 0.4 mg/kg | Minimal cardiovascular effect |
| Atracurium | 0.4 mg/kg | Slight histamine release |
| Vecuronium | 0.08–0.10 mg/kg | No cardiovascular effects |

induction should be accompanied by full stomach precautions. Ketamine may produce emergence reactions in children, although the frequency of this complication is less than that seen in adults.[271] Diazepam (0.15–0.3 mg/kg IV) or other available benzodiazepines appear to attenuate these reactions.[271]

Thiopental may be used as an induction agent in normovolemic traumatized children. There is a wide variation in the pediatric response to intravenous thiopental. In pediatric patients with a full stomach, a rapid and smooth anesthetic induction is important since coughing, bucking, or retching in response to laryngoscopy may promote regurgitation and vomiting, thereby increasing the risk of aspiration. Coté and coworkers[59] recommended that normovolemic unpremedicated children (5–15 years) should receive approximately 5–6 mg/kg of intravenous thiopental to ensure a smooth anesthetic induction. This dose of thiopental in children whose intravascular volume is depleted may result in disastrous complications. The anesthetic requirement for thiopental is decreased by 25–35% in hypovolemic animals.[267]

In normovolemic adults thiopental acts as a direct myocardial depressant.[68] It has little effect on resistance vessels, but significant dilation occurs in capacitance vessels.[78] Thus, the net hemodynamic effect is a dose-dependent decrease in arterial blood pressure, stroke volume, and cardiac output.[49,56] In hypovolemic patients thiopental may produce severe hypotension and even cardiac arrest. In 1941 Halford,[118] based on his experiences at Pearl Harbor, described the use of thiopental in hemorrhagic shock as an "ideal method of euthanasia." Likewise, Beecher[20] stated that "avoiding the use of thiopental in shock can reduce the early mortality rate in war surgery." The results of experimental studies also suggest that thiopental given in minimal anesthetic doses to hypovolemic animals causes severe hemodynamic derangement.[269] Similar cardiovascular effects should be expected with other ultrashort-acting barbiturates. These effects are due at least partly to the reduction in sympathetic activity and alteration of baroreflex control by these agents.[38,45,137]

Benzodiazepines are used infrequently in children as intravenous induction agents. In normovolemic adults these drugs exhibit minimal cardiovascular depressant effects. Both diazepam and midazolam cause a transient depression of the baroreflex response and a sustained decrease of sympathetic tone, although the baroreflex depression is less pronounced than that caused by the inhalational agents.[164] In sympathectomized dogs, diazepam does not produce untoward hemodynamic effects, which suggests that the cardiovascular effects of this drug are indirect in nature.[86] Thus, hypovolemic trauma victims with increased sympathetic tone may be more vulnerable to diazepam than normovolemic patients. Although the hemodynamic effects of midazolam (0.15–0.3 mg/kg) are similar to those of thiopental (3–4 mg/kg),[147,217] midazolam is less reliable in inducing anesthesia in children.[232] It decreases systemic blood pressure by decreasing systemic vascular resistance, venous return, and cardiac contractility and output to a greater extent than diazepam.[217] In acutely hypovolemic dogs, the hypotensive effect of midazolam is potentiated.[3] Etomidate is seldom used in trauma victims because it interferes with the patient's response to stress unless it is administered in conjunction with steroids (see Chapter 9).

In severely hypovolemic patients who require immediate surgery, administration of even small amounts of intravenous anesthetics may result in cardiac arrest. In these instances the authors prefer to administer small doses of fentanyl (0.5–2 μg/kg) followed by a rapidly acting muscle relaxant for intubation. The possibility of patient awareness of intraoperative events with this technique may be a small price to pay for the prevention of more disastrous complications.

### *Muscle Relaxants*

The muscle relaxant used in severely injured children during rapid anesthetic induction should have the following characteristics: (a) rapid onset of action, (b) minimal hemodynamic effect, (c) lack of effect on intracranial or intraocular pressures, and (d) no histamine-releasing properties. Vecuronium has all of these characteristics, although this is not to say that other muscle relaxants should not be used in the presence of trauma. For instance, in the absence of certain injuries and disease states (ie, open-eye injury, burns, skeletal muscle disorders, etc.), succinylcholine is considered the drug of choice. Pancuronium may be advantageous in children whose cardiac output is heart-rate dependent.

Succinylcholine given IV, 2 mg/kg, results in paralysis within 20–30 seconds in 95% of infants and neonates.[100] The neuromuscular blocking effect of this drug in older children is more pronounced, and smaller doses (1–1.5 mg/kg) may suffice to produce adequate paralysis. In the severely hypovolemic patient whose muscle blood flow is decreased, larger doses may be needed; however, this is probably more of a theoretical than a practical consideration. Succinylcholine (4 mg/kg) administered intramuscularly also produces adequate relaxation, but its onset is prolonged (mean, 3.5 minutes).[152] This time may be prolonged further in children in whom significant blood volume depletion and compensatory reduction of muscle blood flow diminish absorption of the drug. Thus, whenever possible, the intravenous route should be used.

Most children under the age of 5 do not fasciculate vigorously after succinylcholine; thus, pretreatment with a nondepolarizing muscle relaxant is not needed.[228] In older children these drugs may be administered at approximately one–tenth of the intubating dose listed in Table 8 to prevent fasciculations. Fentanyl, 0.002 mg/kg, or alfentanil 0.05 mg/kg IV, given 2 minutes before succinylcholine, has been shown to be more effective in preventing fasciculations in children than the nondepolarizing muscle relaxants.[150,151] Succinylcholine causes vagal stimulation; bradycardia or dysrhythmia may occur, especially after repeated doses. As mentioned earlier, premedication with atropine (0.02 mg/kg) or glycopyrrolate (0.01 mg/kg) IV, before anesthetic induction is effective in preventing this complication.[109] In unpremedicated patients this response to succinylcholine is usually transient, but should be treated promptly with atropine after rapid evaluation of the patient's airway and oxygenation. Succinylcholine increases intraocular and intracranial pressures; thus it should not be used in children with open-eye or head injuries. These subjects are discussed in detail in Chapters 10 and 11. Succinylcholine may cause massive life-threatening hyperkalemia in burn patients and in those with congenital myotonias, extensive muscle damage, and spinal cord injuries.

Succinylcholine is a potent triggering agent for malignant hyperthermia, which is manifested clinically by increasing body temperature, elevation of end-tidal $CO_2$, metabolic acidosis, tachycardia, hypotension, and oliguria. When malignant hyperthermia (MH) occurs in a trauma patient, one may not have the option of discontinuing the anesthetic and postponing surgery. In these instances, anesthesia should be continued with agents having the least potential to trigger the syndrome, and treatment of the crisis should be carried out during surgery and in the postoperative period. Ketamine, nitrous oxide, narcotics, barbiturates, benzodiazepines, and nondepolarizing muscle relaxants are considered relatively safe. The rubber breathing circuit, if one is being used, should be replaced, as the release of previously absorbed inhalational agents may trigger MH.[160] Dantrolene, 2–3 mg/kg IV, should be administered and incremental doses up to a total of 10 mg/kg given as indicated. Treatment of acidosis with bicarbonate, of hyperthermia with surface cooling and gastric and bladder irrigation, and treatment of hemodynamic instability with fluids and vasoactive agents should be considered.

MH is a rare event, occurring in 1 anesthetized child in 15,000. More frequently, isolated masseter spasm occurs in response to succinylcholine during anesthetic induction, especially when the drug is administered in conjunction with halothane. Although earlier reports suggested that many of these patients show succeptibility to MH on subsequent muscle testing and recommended postponement of elective surgery,[87,220,221,240] more recent data from Van Der Spek and coworkers[263] demonstrate that isolated masseter spasm occurs rather routinely in deeply anesthetized children and does not seem to be associated with a high incidence of a hypermetabolic state or hyperthermia. Thus, many authors now believe that even elective surgery can proceed with nontriggering agents while monitoring end-expired $CO_2$, venous and/or arterial blood gases, blood pressure, pulse, and muscle tone.[24,114] Should a hypermetabolic state develop, the treatment protocol described for MH is instituted.

Atracurium provides effective neuromuscular blockade. Its $ED_{95}$ for train of four twitch depression in normal children is between 170–280 μg/kg.[99] Intubating conditions can be produced in 2 minutes by giving 2.5–3 times this dose (0.3–0.6 mg/kg) as a bolus.[99] In adults and probably in children, a larger dose (1.5 mg/kg) reduces this time to 1 minute.[149] Atracurium is metabolized rapidly by ester hydrolysis and Hoffman elimination, and complete recovery usually occurs within 50–70 minutes.[102] The breakdown products of clinical doses are not likely to have neuromuscular, cardiovascular, or central nervous system effects, even in anephric patients.[46,79,135] Hypotension caused by histamine release may occur after rapid injection of more than 0.4 mg/kg of atracurium. Although the incidence and intensity of this response in pediatric patients appear to be less than that seen in adults and that produced by d-tubocurarine, in hypovolemic traumatized children this effect of atracurium may be deleterious. In trauma victims with uncertain blood volume, atracurium, if used, should be administered slowly to minimize its untoward cardiovascular effects.[241] Onset of neuromuscular blockade after atracurium injection is considerably longer than that observed after succinylcholine. This represents a disadvantage during rapid sequence induction, because the $PaO_2$ in pediatric patients declines at a faster rate than that of adults during apnea. Priming patients with small doses of atracurium 2 to 3 minutes before administration of the drug has been proposed as a method of reducing the onset time in adults.[94,193] This method, however, should not be used in traumatized patients, because the initial dose may result in significant weakness, during which time regurgitation and aspiration may occur. We prefer to ventilate patients by mask while applying cricoid pressure until full paralysis occurs after a single bolus.

Vecuronium is a monoquaternary homologue of pancuronium.[184] The potency of this drug is essentially the same in infants, children, adolescents, and adults.[81,103] The onset of action of vecuronium in infants is slightly shorter than that in children or adolescents.[81] A bolus dose of 70–80 μg/kg produces intubating conditions within 2 minutes.[81,103] In adults higher doses (0.25 mg/kg), produce intubating conditions within 60 seconds.[149] This decrease in onset time with high doses is also likely in pediatric patients. The duration of action of this drug is approximately 40–60 minutes; infants have a slightly longer recovery time than children. The hemodynamic effects of vecuronium differ from those of d-tubocurarine and pancuronium. No serious changes in systemic or regional hemodynamics have been noted with vecuronium.[81,103,233] Although the cardiovascular effects of vecuronium have not been studied in hemorrhaging or hypovolemic trauma victims, our limited clinical experience suggests remarkable safety. Vecuronium does not increase intraocular or intracranial pressure.

In children, intubating conditions can be obtained by 0.08 mg/kg pancuronium, 0.34 mg/kg metocurine, 0.6 mg/kg d-tubocurarine, or 3.4 mg/kg gallamine.[104] As in adults, d-tubocurarine (dTC) causes hypotension in children by releasing histamine[191] and by producing partial ganglionic blockade. The extent of histamine release is proportional to the dose administered. The large dose of dTC required for intubation of a traumatized child results in significant hypotension, especially if the patient is hypovolemic. Infants may require higher initial doses of dTC (on a body weight basis) than older children because they have a larger extracellular volume. Likewise the drug is cleared more slowly in neonates and infants than in children or adolescents, probably because of decreased glomerular filtration rate.[82,172] Metocurine is a derivative of dTC with less potential for causing histamine release.[155] In clinical doses (0.34 mg/kg) metocurine does not produce hypotension. However, in large doses, it may decrease blood pressure. In addition, 3.5–4 minutes are required to obtain intubating conditions after administration of metocurine, making it a poor choice for rapid sequence induction.

Pancuronium and gallamine cause tachycardia and mild hypertension, primarily by a vagolytic effect. Although pancuronium is the most widely used relaxant, either agent can be used in the hypovolemic trauma patient. In pediatric patients, intubating conditions with pancuronium (0.08 mg/kg) can be obtained within a shorter time after administration of the drug (1–3 minutes) than in adults.[26,155] However, this period is longer than the onset of action of succinylcholine. The administration of pancuronium in divided doses does not shorten this time in pediatric patients and may be associated with the risk of pulmonary aspiration.[26] In adults, doses of 0.2–0.25 mg/kg provide intubating conditions within 1 minute.[39] Doses of this magnitude probably provide similar results in children. It should be remembered that the volume of distribution of drugs in hypovolemic trauma victims is decreased, and fluid resuscitation results in dilutional hypoproteinemia, thereby increasing the unbound fraction of pancuronium. Thus, the neuromuscular effect of pancuronium is likely to be potentiated and its onset shortened in these children. Mivacurium, 0.2 mg/kg, abolishes the twitch response in children in about 2 minutes without adverse cardiovascular effects.[106] It is likely that at higher doses this drug can provide satisfactory intubating conditions in a shorter period of time and be a reasonable alternative to succinylcholine for rapid sequence induction.

## MAINTENANCE OF ANESTHESIA

The same agents employed in adult trauma surgery may be used in children. Patients who are volume repleted may be managed with inhalation anesthetics. As a generalization, patients who are in shock or markedly hypovolemic tolerate all anesthetics poorly. These patients may be best managed with a carefully titrated oxygen-narcotic-muscle relaxant technique, although the incidence of recall of surgery with this method is high.[31]

Morphine and meperidine should be avoided in hypovolemic patients since they produce histamine release with resulting hypotension because of increased venous capacitance and arterial vasodilation. In children, fentanyl, 2–10 μg/kg, provides good analgesia and does not cause this hemodynamic instability. The injection of large doses (25–50 μg/kg) of fentanyl is hemodynamically well tolerated by infants and neonates.[51,129] Because the volume of distribution for fentanyl is larger in neonates than in adults,[141] a given dose should produce lower plasma fentanyl concentrations in neonates. In hypovolemic trauma victims the volume of distribution for fentanyl decreases. Thus, higher plasma fentanyl concentrations and hypotension may ensue if the dose is not reduced. A prolonged elimination half-life and an increased sensitivity of the brain to fentanyl result in long-lasting ventilatory depression after relatively large doses of this drug in neonates.[141] However, the characteristic redistribution of fentanyl from the brain to the pharmacodynamically inert tissues may somewhat decrease this period of respiratory depression.[51] Sufentanil is five times more potent than fentanyl and has a shorter duration of action. Although this drug has not been studied in hypovolemic children, its hemodynamic effects appear to be similar to those of fentanyl.[128]

The presence of undue tachycardia in children, even if the systemic blood pressure is normal, usually indicates hypovolemia with compensatory vasoconstriction. Administration of the usual clinical doses of an inhalation anesthetic to such a child will rapidly produce marked hypotension and, at times, cardiac arrest. In addition, the uptake of inhaled anesthetics and consequent effects on the organ systems are unpredictable in the patient with deficient blood volume or cardiac function. Alveolar concentration of anesthetic agents tends to rise rapidly if pulmonary blood flow is decreased, and a higher concentration of the agent is delivered to the brain and heart since perfusion to these organs is usually maintained in shock. Excessive depth of anesthesia and myocardial depression may thus be achieved without warning.

Nitrous oxide in healthy normovolemic patients causes a mild sympathetic stimulation that offsets its myocardial depressant effect, resulting in only minimal hemodynamic changes.[266] However, its cardiovascular effects vary depending on several factors, including background sympathetic activity, condition of the patient, and the primary anesthetic agent.[22] The cardiovascular effects of nitrous oxide in hypovolemic children are not known. However, data from one animal study suggest that it produces cardiovascular depression similar to that caused by equipotent doses of halothane.[266] Both halothane (0.25 MAC) and nitrous oxide (70%) in this study caused significant deterioration in compensatory mechanisms for hemorrhage and an increase in blood lactate level. When hypovolemic shock and cardiac and pulmonary compromise are not present, nitrous oxide may be used in concentrations as high as 70%. Careful monitoring of hemodynamic and oxygenation variables and adjustment of nitrous oxide concentration are necessary in severely traumatized children.

In healthy, normovolemic children, both halothane and enflurane cause dose-dependent depression of ventricular function.[10,11] At inspired halothane concentrations of 2%, the systolic blood pressure, pulse rate, and cardiac output decrease by 10–25%. The systemic vascular resistance remains relatively constant. In contrast, isoflurane (end-tidal concentration, 2.2%) produces little alteration in cardiac output, but decreases systemic vascular resistance.[272] The preload remains relatively constant during both halothane and isoflurane anesthesia. Newborns and infants seem to show similar but exaggerated hemodynamic responses to these agents.[36,238] All potent inhalational anesthetics depress baroreceptor reflexes in a dose-dependent fashion.[73,144] There are no data about the hemodynamic effects of inhalational agents in hypovolemic pediatric patients. However, clinical impression suggests that these agents interfere with all of the compensatory mechanisms that occur in response to hemorrhagic shock. The blunted baroreflex responses and sympathetic activity result in both resistance and capacitance vessel dilation, decreased venous return, decreased cardiac output, and impaired tissue oxygenation in hypovolemic patients.

The alterations in microcirculatory blood flow that occur in response to shock seem to be modified by inhalational agents. However, it is not clearly known whether these effects are beneficial or deleterious. Experimental studies by Theye et al.,[8,262] comparing the influence of cyclopropane, halothane, and isoflurane on survival and the hemodynamic, metabolic, and sympathoadrenal responses to hemorrhagic shock demonstrated a less deleterious effect with halothane and isoflurane than with cyclopropane. These results were consistent with the hypothesis that anesthetics associated with decreased sympathetic activity provide better tissue perfusion than those producing increased sympathetic effect. In contrast to this finding, Longnecker and Sturgill[156] demonstrated a better survival rate with ketamine than with halothane. In two subsequent experimental studies, the improvement in outcome after ketamine was shown to be due to improved microcirculatory blood flow and tissue oxygenation.[34,157] However, recent experimental data suggest that inhalational anesthetics, particularly isoflurane, provide better tissue oxygenation than ketamine.[236,268]

The above experimental findings may not apply strictly to the clinical situation. In the traumatized patient, in addition to bleeding, there is significant alteration in metabolic and endocrine function. In addition, injured patients receive more than one anesthetic or adjunct drug, the cardiovascular effects of which may be unpredictable. Finally, other factors, such as positive-pressure ventilation, increased intra-abdominal pressure from peritoneal blood or MAST trousers, pneumothorax, hemothorax, or hemopericardium, may modify the patient's response to inhalational or intravenous agents. The effect of the unlimited permutations of these factors on hemodynamics in a given child is difficult to predict, and anesthetic management should be based on the patient's overall clinical condition.

## VENTILATION

Ventilation should be controlled in most patients to ensure adequate gas exchange. An adult ventilator may be used in children weighing 10 kg or more; pediatric bellows are available for use in smaller children. Manual ventilation may be desirable if wide changes in pulmonary compliance are anticipated, such as may occur in abdominal and thoracic trauma. An adult anesthesia circuit can be used in patients who weigh less than 10 kg, provided that ventilation is controlled. However, most anesthesiologists choose a T-piece system, such as the Mapleson circuit. Care must be taken to ensure that a fresh gas inflow adequate to prevent rebreathing is provided; a flow of two and one-half to three times the expected minute ventilation is appropriate.[122] In head-injured children in whom hyperventilation and hypocapnia are desired, an increase in fresh gas inflow proportionate to the required increase in minute ventilation is necessary.

## MONITORING

All children should be monitored with at least a precordial stethoscope, ECG, blood pressure cuff, and temperature probe. The width of the blood pressure cuff should be one-half to two-thirds the length of the child's upper arm. If measurement of blood pressure by auscultation is difficult, a commercially available Doppler device that detects blood flow may be used. Respiratory monitoring should include measurement of airway pressures, arterial blood gases, $F_{IO_2}$, and end-tidal $CO_2$, as indicated by the clinical condition. End-tidal $CO_2$ measurement, which is mandatory in many states, may be useful in detecting such intraoperative events as circuit disconnection or leak, accidental extubation, endobronchial intubation, and malignant hyperthermia.[62] The transcutaneous oxygen ($P_{tc}O_2$) monitor usually provides accurate determination of $PaO_2$ in children and can provide on-line assessment of trends in tissue oxygen delivery. Thus, it is useful in the operating room as an early indicator of shock. Some models may be affected by the use of halothane. Pulse oximetry devices measure arterial oxygen saturation and for the most part do not depend on adequate skin perfusion, which may be compromised in trauma patients.[69] In hemodynamically unstable patients, however, accurate assessment of oxygen delivery to the tissues may not be possible with the use of pulse oximetry.[13] A detailed discussion of this subject may be found in Chapter 5.

Invasive monitoring is used in more seriously injured children. An indwelling urinary catheter, if not contraindicated by urethral trauma, is most helpful; a urine output of 0.5–1.0 mL/kg/h should be maintained. An arterial line can usually be placed percutaneously, even in small children. Recommended sites include the radial, dorsalis pedis, and posterior tibial arteries. We avoid the brachial artery, which may have a limited collateral circulation, and the temporal artery, where even very small amounts of retrograde flow (as with flushing) may enter the cerebral circulation.[75] In children, a good sense of volume status and cardiovascular performance may be obtained from the heart rate and the arterial trace alone. With hypovolemia, the entire arterial waveform shows an exaggerated oscillation with positive-pressure ventilation, and the dicrotic notch, which normally appears in the middle third of the pressure downstroke, is close to the diastolic pressure line.[89] An arterial pressure trace in a child that does not show a brisk upstroke usually indicates compromise of myocardial contractility.

Measurement of the central venous pressure (CVP), although useful, is generally not a first priority and may be accomplished after initial stabilization is completed. CVP catheters are most easily placed through the external and internal jugular veins and the femoral vein, using the Seldinger technique. The subclavian vein is a good choice for those experienced in its use; catheter placement from the brachiocephalic system is reasonable, but often not successful in small children. Once CVP measurement is established, it is best used to monitor trends rather than absolute values, allowing titration of volume infusions to effect.

More sophisticated monitoring of the cardiovascular system may be obtained with the placement of a thermodilution pulmonary artery catheter. Both 5F and 7F sizes are available, and some thought must be given to catheter length to ensure that the final position of the proximal (CVP) port will be in the right atrium or thoracic vena cava. Normal values for pulmonary capillary wedge pressure, cardiac index, and systemic and pulmonary vascular resistances in children above 6–8 weeks of age are the same as those of adults.[218]

## HEMOTHERAPY

Adequate intravascular volume and circulating red cell mass should be maintained with infusions of isotonic crystalloid, colloid, red cells, or whole blood as needed. Whole blood, as fresh as can be made available, is appropriate for rapid replacement of blood loss, especially in very young children in whom replacement of individual components of a relatively small intravascular volume may be technically difficult. Component therapy is better suited to treatment of specific deficiencies in the more stable patient, as well as to overall conservation of resources. A hematocrit of 25–30% is adequate in most instances; a higher value is preferable in newborns. Packed red blood cells can be used to correct normovolemic anemia in any pediatric patient; a useful rule of thumb is that 1 mL of packed cells per kilogram of body weight will raise the hematocrit approximately 1%. For example, in order to raise the hematocrit from 25 to 30% in a 12-kg child, approximately 60 mL of packed red cells will be required. Simple protein losses can be replaced with 5% albumin.

Replacement of clotting factors and platelets should be considered as blood losses approach one blood volume (Table 18–9). After replacement of one blood volume, most children will have platelet counts equal to 50% or greater of the initial level.[61] Platelets may be administered when the platelet count has fallen to less than 100,000 $mm^{-3}$ and continued blood loss is anticipated, or when clinical signs of coagulopathy occur during massive transfusion. One unit of platelets per

TABLE 18-9. Normal Blood Volumes and Replacements

NORMAL BLOOD VOLUMES

85 mL/kg—newborn
80 mL/kg—infant
75 mL/kg—child
70 mL/kg—adult

COMPONENT THERAPY

| *Loss* | *Replacement Product* |
|---|---|
| Whole blood (rapid losses) | Whole blood |
| Red cells (normovolemia) | Packed red cells |
| Coagulation factors (prolonged PT or PTT) | Fresh-frozen plasma |
| Platelet (decreased number or function) | Platelets (0.1 unit/kg raises count by 25,000/$mm^3$) |

10 kg of body weight (0.1 units/kg) will raise the platelet count by approximately 25,000 $mm^{-3}$. A higher dose (0.3 units/kg) may be preferable for the initial treatment of clinically apparent coagulopathy.[61]

The plasma present in red cell packs, along with the child's ongoing ability to replace clotting factors, should prevent coagulopathy due to factor deficiency during massive transfusion until several blood volumes have been replaced.[89] Should factor replacement become necessary, fresh-frozen plasma, 15 mL/kg, will provide adequate levels for coagulation.[133] In all cases of intraoperative coagulopathy, causes other than platelet or factor deficiency (eg, DIC or transfusion reaction) should also be considered and appropriate diagnostic and therapeutic modalities employed (see Chapters 6 and 7).

The rapid administration of blood products, especially red cells that have been subjected to lengthy storage, can result in acute hyperkalemia.[255] However, hypokalemia is a more common occurrence after transfusion (see Chapter 6). Occasionally, one may see evidence of chelation of circulating calcium ions by the citrate anticoagulant. As stated earlier, serum $Ca^{++}$ levels are usually maintained if the transfusion rate is less than 30 mL/kg/h.[2] However, calcium should be administered if the systolic blood pressure falls acutely with transfusion, or if ECG evidence of hypocalcemia (prolonged QT interval) develops. If measurements of ionized calcium are unavailable, calcium, either as the chloride (50–100 mg) or the gluconate (150–300 mg), may be administered empirically for each 100 mL of citrated blood product transfused.

Although there is some evidence that hetastarch may offer some advantages in fluid resuscitation,[124] the use of plasma expanders (dextran, hetastarch) has not been well studied in children. Fluosol-DA, a perfluorochemical, is capable of loading and unloading oxygen when the recipient breathes supplemental oxygen. However, data from adults suggest that Fluosol-DA does not increase arterial oxygen content appreciably and is ineffective in severely anemic patients.[107] In addition, this agent caused severe anaphylactic reactions in some patients, resulting in discontinuation of its trials in the United States. Stroma-free hemoglobin may be beneficial in severe hemorrhage, but it is not available at this time (see Chapter 6).

## TEMPERATURE PRESERVATION

Children easily become hypothermic in the operating room. Traumatic shock enhances hypothermia further. Heating the room, to as much as 85° F for infants, before the child's arrival decreases temperature loss. Care must be taken to warm intravenous solutions and to attempt to minimize heat loss by use of a heating blanket, radiant heat source, warmed irrigation solutions, and an airway heater/humidifier. The patient's skin should be dried promptly after prepping or washing. Clear plastic drapes, closely adherent to the patient and preferably including the head, minimize heat losses through the skin and allow continuous assessment of the patient's color and perfusion.

## MAINTENANCE OF BLOOD GLUCOSE

Small children have only moderate liver glycogen stores, and these can be depleted rapidly during the stress of injury. Although children respond initially to stress with hyperglycemia, hypoglycemia may develop despite high levels of circulating catecholamines. Serum glucose levels should be monitored and hypoglycemia treated as necessary with moderate increases in glucose administration. Except in head-injured children in whom excess serum glucose may be associated with poor outcome, the "maintenance" IV solution may include some glucose and some salt; a typical solution is 5% dextrose and 0.33% saline. If rapid volume infusion is needed, however, this should be accomplished with an isotonic solution, such as normal saline or Ringer's lactate.

## EMERGENCE

At the conclusion of anesthesia, the decision to remove the endotracheal tube should depend on the patient's (a) circulatory and respiratory status, (b) body temperature, (c) state of consciousness and tracheobronchial reflexes, (d) recovery from muscle paralysis, and (e) the type and extent of trauma and surgery. Before extubation, blood pressure, pulse rate, and cardiac rhythm should be within acceptable limits, and tidal volume, respiratory rate, and vital capacity should be adequate. End-tidal $CO_2$ and arterial blood gas measurement with the patient breathing spontaneously will help determine the adequacy of ventilation. Hypothermia, a frequent finding in traumatized children, decreases $O_2$ availability to the tissues (see Chapter 5). In addition, in the presence of residual anesthetic agents, hypothermia may depress normal ventilatory responses to hypercapnia and hypoxia in the recovery room.[74,194,216] Thus, postoperative mechanical ventilation at high inspired $O_2$ concentrations should be provided until the body temperature is raised to 35–36° C. Patients undergoing surgery for acute trauma should be extubated only after they recover their tracheobronchial reflexes. This simple measure will reduce the incidence of aspiration of gastric contents during the postoperative period.

In children, removal of the endotracheal tube while the patient is in a light plane of anesthesia may activate protective airway reflexes and result in laryngospasm and breath-holding. This is a relatively common problem in pediatric patients and can be prevented by observing the expiratory air flow. The child who can generate a rapid expiratory flow is unlikely to develop laryngospasm after extubation. The treatment of laryngospasm includes forceful displacement of the mandible anteriorly; this distracts the hyoid bone and epiglottic cartilage and provides a glottic opening. By opening the child's mouth and upper airway, this maneuver allows administration of oxygen by positive pressure, which will help open the laryngeal inlet. In some instances, the administration of small doses of succinylcholine may be necessary to abolish the spasm. However, succinylcholine in a hypoxic child may cause serious arrhythmias; thus, proper ECG monitoring is essential.

Adequate recovery from muscle relaxants must be ensured with a neuromuscular monitor. When satisfactory communication between child and anesthesiologist is possible, such clinical signs as sustained head lift and measurement of forced vital capacity may help determine the adequacy of reversal. In infants, evaluation of these signs is obviously not possible. Preoperative assessment of neuromuscular function (posture, vigor, muscle tone, respiration, etc.) provides a baseline for comparison with the child's condition at the end of surgery. Contrary to older belief, the anticholinesterase dose required for infants is not greater than that for adults.[98] In fact, Fisher et al.[83] demonstrated that the infant's requirement for neostigmine is about 0.025 mg/kg, which is approximately half of the adult dose. The time course of onset and duration of action of neostigmine are similar in infants, children, and adults. The infant dose of edrophonium (1 mg/kg) is, on the other hand, the same as that required by adults.[84,180] Edrophonium has a more rapid onset of action (2.3 ± 0.5 minutes) than neostigmine (7.4 ± 2.2 minutes).[84,180] The changes in heart rate and systolic blood pressure that may be produced by these drugs can be minimized by administration of atropine (0.01 mg/kg) 30 seconds before giving the reversal agent.[84]

Finally, the type and extent of trauma and surgery should be taken into account before removing the endotracheal tube. Pulmonary complications—atelectasis, embolism, aspiration of blood or gastric contents, etc.—may occur during the traumatic event. These complications should be recognized during the perioperative period and plans made for ventilatory therapy after surgery. Pulmonary complications are common in patients requiring large amounts of blood and fluids. Prolonged shock after the injury may be associated with respiratory distress syndrome, which also requires postoperative ventilation. Patients with head injuries may not regain consciousness immediately after surgery and therefore should be kept intubated to prevent pulmonary aspiration. These patients may also require postoperative hyperventilation to control intracranial pressure.

If extubation is contemplated, the anesthesiologist should ensure that the stomach is emptied. Supplemental oxygen should be given by face mask during the postanesthetic recovery period since many children develop unacceptably low $PaO_2$ levels when they breathe room air during this time.[192]

Postoperative pain relief can be provided by intravenous morphine 50–100 μg/kg, meperidine, 100–300 μg/kg, or methadone, 100–200 μg/kg.[153] If the clinical setting allows, fentanyl may be administered as a continuous infusion of 1–2 μg/kg/hr. For older, cooperative children, patient controlled analgesia (PCA) may be a good choice. Administration of epidural narcotics has been shown to provide excellent and safe postoperative analgesia in children 3 to 13 years of age.[243] The recommended dose of morphine is 1 mg for ages 3–7 years, 1.5 mg for 7–10 years, and 2 mg for 10–13 years. The total volume injected should not exceed 5 mL. Similar doses are given subsequently when the child complains of pain. Rapid and effective analgesia can also be obtained with epidural sufentanil (0.75 μg/kg), but the duration of analgesia with this agent is relatively short (3 hours).[21] Children receiving epidural narcotics should be kept in a unit where frequent measurement of respiratory rate, tidal volume, and arterial blood gases is possible. Parents should be allowed to visit as soon as possible, even if only for a brief period of time, for the child's and their own comfort.

## CRITICAL CARE OF THE INJURED CHILD

Perioperative care for the injured child is best provided in a multidisciplinary setting in which the staff members have significant experience in pediatric critical care.[53,64,140,211] Ongoing input from physicians of different specialties, nursing personnel, respiratory and physical therapists, nutritionists, and others will assist the child's recovery and minimize complications. Coordination of this care remains the responsibility of the primary physician.

It is common practice to approach the care of seriously ill children in a system-oriented fashion. This section reviews briefly the special aspects of the systems approach to the child. Detailed discussions of each system are offered in other chapters.

### CARDIOVASCULAR AND RESPIRATORY SYSTEMS

Optimal cardiovascular performance can be assured by manipulating the factors contributing to cardiac output—heart rate and stroke volume. Children tolerate tachycardia well, and in younger children with small, fairly noncompliant ventricles, cardiac output is essentially rate dependent. If an increase in output is needed, raising the heart rate to 120–160 beats/min is a reasonable first step. Stroke volume is augmented initially with volume infusion; central venous and pulmonary capillary wedge pressures may be deliberately raised to the 10–15 mm Hg range. It is not unusual to administer large fluid volumes to relatively small children in the course of this treatment, as large third-space losses and capillary leaks are common. If intravascular volume has been maximized and cardiac output is still poor or if there is particular concern about minimizing fluid administration, as in patients with cerebral edema or ARDS, vasopressor agents are added. Dopamine remains the most popular agent in our practice, partly because of its beneficial effects on renal and splanchnic perfusion at low doses. Other agents may be used as needed (Table 18-10). In an occasional child, vasodilating agents, such as nitroprusside, nitroglycerin, and hydralazine, improve cardiac performance. Our goal is to maintain adequate tissue perfusion, and the absence of metabolic acidosis is a reasonable marker of this in the child.

Some form of respiratory assistance is required for most children in the intensive care unit. The provision of increased $F_{IO_2}$ by mask or mist tent may be all that is necessary. Intubated children may be managed with CPAP alone or with mechanical ventilation and PEEP. Generally, it is advisable to provide some form of continuous distending airway pressure. Resistance to gas flow through small endotracheal tubes can be minimized by trimming tube length and by careful attention to humidification and suctioning to loosen and remove secretions. Chest physiotherapy is very helpful in children both to prevent atelectasis and re-expand collapsed segments of the lung.[112] Particular attention should be given to choosing a proper endotracheal tube in infants and children.

TABLE 18-10. Medications Commonly Used in Pediatric Critical Care*

| DRUG | DOSE | COMMENTS |
|---|---|---|
| Dopamine | 2–5 μg/kg/min | Renal-splanchnic effect |
| | 5–10 μg/kg/min | Some beta-sympathomimetic action |
| | 10–20 μg/kg/min | Alpha-effects begin |
| | | Indications: Low-output state; impaired renal or splanchnic perfusion |
| | | Cautions: Tachydysrhythmias; excessive vasoconstriction |
| Isoproterenol | 0.05–2.00 μg/kg/min | Indications: Bradycardia; refractory status asthmaticus |
| | | Cautions: Vasodilator; may lower blood pressure; may precipitate tachyarrhythmias; increases myocardial oxygen requirement and may aggravate myocardial ischemia |
| Dobutamine | 5–15 μg/kg/min | Indications: Low-output state |
| | | Cautions: Tachycardia and dysrhythmias |
| Epinephrine | 0.05–1.00 μg/kg/min | Indications: Refractory low-output state |
| | | Cautions: Higher doses may cause intense vasoconstriction |
| Nitroprusside | 0.5–10.0 μg/kg/min | Indications: Low-output state with myocardial failure; hypertension |
| | | Cautions: Easily produces hypotension; toxic metabolites if use is prolonged |

* Medications are best administered by a continuous-infusion pump capable of accurate delivery at low flow rates.

Uncuffed tubes do not seal the airway completely, and may allow pharyngeal contents to enter the trachea, especially in the presence of an audible leak. In one study the incidence of aspiration in endotracheally intubated children was 16%; more than half of these patients developed changes on chest X-ray.[97] On the other hand, very large tubes may result in postextubation croup.[142]

Ventilators used in pediatric practice are of two types. A volume-preset ventilator is appropriate for most children weighing 10 kg or more; we favor relatively large tidal volumes (10–15 mL/kg) and low rates to minimize alveolar collapse. Infants and smaller children may be better managed with a time-cycled, pressure-limited ventilator, which allows more rapid rates and fine tuning of the inspiratory time; we find that the use of a prolonged inspiratory time or even an inverse I:E ratio improves oxygenation in some particularly ill children. At high rates, gas trapping and inadvertent PEEP occur with most neonatal ventilators.[247] This results in delivery of a tidal volume less than the preset value. Similar decreases in tidal volume can be observed when airway resistance is increased.[247] All ventilators should be capable of providing intermittent mandatory ventilation; the continuous-flow technique may offer less resistance than solenoid-controlled mechanisms in small children.

## FLUIDS-METABOLISM-NUTRITION

Many formulas exist for calculation of fluid requirements. One simple method for estimating "maintenance" rates of fluid administration is outlined in Table 18-11. It should be remembered that this estimation assumes normal temperature, adequate urine output, and no unusual fluid gains or losses; the actual clinical situation may be quite different. Careful monitoring of serum electrolytes, glucose, calcium, phosphate, BUN, and creatinine will guide fluid and metabolic management. The syndrome of excessive ADH secretion is common in children, particularly in the surgical population, and must be diagnosed promptly and treated with fluid restriction. In the early postoperative or posttrauma period, oliguria may be caused by prerenal azotemia, renal failure, or inappropriate ADH secretion. Differential diagnosis can be made by evaluation of urinary and serum findings (Table 18-12). Hypoglycemia and hypocalcemia are frequently seen, particularly in smaller children.

Nutritional support is critical in facilitating recovery from severe trauma. Assessment of nutritional status and early institution of enteral or parenteral feeding benefit most children. Caloric requirements are relatively greater in children than adults because of the need for growth; recovery from serious illness or trauma, with accelerated metabolism and repair of tissues, increases these requirements further[246] (see Chapter 22).

TABLE 18-11. Fluid and Electrolyte Requirements

| BODY WEIGHT | WATER REQUIREMENT | ELECTROLYTES |
|---|---|---|
| 0–10 kg | 4 mL/kg/h | $Na^+$—2–3 mEq/kg/day |
| 10–20 kg | 40 mL plus 2 mL/kg/h for each kg over 10 | $K^+$—1–2 mEq/kg/day |
| >20 kg | 60 mL plus 1 mL/kg/h for each kg over 20 | $Cl^-$—2–3 mEq/kg/day |

## BLOOD AND COAGULATION FACTORS

An adequate circulating red cell mass must be maintained to ensure tissue oxygen delivery. We attempt to maintain a minimum hematocrit of 25–30% or, if there is significant compromise of pulmonary function, 35–40%. The white cell count is followed for evidence of infection, although it is often elevated simply by stress and trauma. Coagulation factors may require supplementation by infusion of fresh-frozen plasma. If fibrin split products are found in the serum, disseminated intravascular coagulation may be present; the coagulopathy is also treated with fresh-frozen plasma, but the primary cause must be sought and treated as well. Dilutional thrombocytopenia is occasionally seen, and platelet transfusion to maintain the platelet count above 50,000/mm$^3$ is appropriate. Transfusion therapy must be used when needed, but careful consideration should be given to the associated risks of disease transmission and adverse reactions (see also Chapters 6 and 7).

## INFECTION

Culture and sensitivity testing is performed as clinically indicated and antibiotic therapy adjusted by these results. The Gram stain is often helpful in sorting out the presence and cause of bacterial infection. Prophylactic use of antibiotics in the immediate perioperative period is felt to be beneficial by many physicians, but it is important that they be employed for only a limited time and then discontinued. Nonbacterial infections in the otherwise healthy child recovering from trauma are unusual, but may occur and contribute to clinical illness (see also chapters 26 and 27).

## GASTROINTESTINAL SYSTEM

Stress ulcers are not uncommon in children. In adults the use of prophylactic antacids and/or $H_2$-receptor antagonists seems to be warranted.[110] In adults, antacids, 30 mL/hr, seem to be more effective than cimetidine, 300 mg IV every 6 hours, in raising gastric pH and reducing the incidence of bleeding.[209] Goudsouzian et al.[101] found that children require larger doses (7.5 mg/kg) of cimetidine than adults. In pediatric patients with burn injury, Martyn[165] demonstrated that oral antacids, 15–30 mL every 3 hours, and/or cimetidine, IV 7.2 mg/kg every 6 hours, did not effectively control increased gastric acidity and bleeding, although antacids were superior to cimetidine in controlling gastric pH. The decreased efficacy of cimetidine in pediatric burn patients may be due to its rapid clearance by the kidney or other organs. More recent data suggest that ranitidine given intravenously in doses of 1.5 mg/kg every 6 hours provides effective prophylaxis against acute gastric mucosal damage in 80% of critically ill children.[158] Orally administered ranitidine was ineffective in this study

TABLE 18-12. Differential Diagnosis of Prerenal Azotemia, Renal Failure, and Inappropriate ADH Secretion in the Postoperative or Posttrauma Period

| | PRERENAL AZOTEMIA | RENAL FAILURE | INAPPROPRIATE ADH |
|---|---|---|---|
| | Urinary Examination | | |
| Urine volume | Decreased | Decreased | Decreased |
| RBC, protein cast, and tubular cells | Absent | Present | Absent |
| Urine/plasma ratio | | | |
| Osmolarity | >1.5/1 | <1.1/1 | >1.5/1 |
| Urea | >10/1 | <10/1 | >10/1 |
| Creatinine | >10–20/1 | <10/1 | >10/1 |
| Sodium | <20 mEq/L | >20 mEq/L | >20–25 mEq/L |
| FENa | <1% | >2–3% | >2–3% |
| | Serum Examination | | |
| BUN | Normal or increased | Increased | Normal or decreased |
| Creatinine | Normal or increased | Increased | Normal or decreased |
| Sodium | Normal | Normal, increased, or decreased | Decreased |
| Potassium | Normal or increased | Increased | Normal |
| Calcium | Normal | Decreased | Normal |
| Phosphate | Normal | Increased | Normal |

FENa = fraction of total filtered Na+ that is excreted in the urine.

probably because of defective absorption from gastrointestinal mucosa.[158] Gastric pH should be monitored during prophylactic therapy and maintained above 4.0.

## RENAL FUNCTION

A urine output of 0.5–1.0 mL/kg/h is a reasonable minimum. Oliguria may be due to prerenal, renal, or postrenal factors, and a differential diagnosis must be made as shown in Table 18-12 (see also Chapter 25). Acute tubular necrosis in the postresuscitative period is managed with fluid adjustment, diuretics, and dialysis as necessary. Peritoneal dialysis is quite effective in children, and hemodialysis is rarely needed.[77]

The presence of hematuria suggests renal trauma, which should be evaluated by intravenous pyelography. Simple contusion is often the source of the bleeding. Management should include generous fluid administration to encourage good urine flow; some physicians add mannitol to this regimen.

## CUTANEOUS AND MUSCULOSKELETAL SYSTEM

Injuries to the extremities may be managed simply with immobilization or may require multiple surgical procedures and microvascular anastomoses. The nursing staff caring for these patients in the intensive care unit must regularly assess perfusion of all tissues and alert the responsible physician if there is neural or vascular compromise. The anesthesiologist may suggest and provide sympathetic blockade of an extremity to improve graft perfusion.

Loss of the protective function of the skin is occasionally a problem, particularly in the burned patient. Pediatric burn victims often receive a significant amount of care from anesthesiologists during resuscitation, debridement, and reconstructive or plastic surgical procedures. Management of these patients can be extremely demanding and requires a thorough knowledge of the pathophysiologic processes involved. Presented here is a brief description of some anesthetic considerations for pediatric burn patients; for a more detailed discussion of the burn patient, the reader is referred to Chapter 20.

Thermal injuries represent a major source of morbidity and mortality in the pediatric population, accounting for several thousand childhood deaths each year in the United States.[120] Scald injuries are most frequent among toddlers, and flame burns are the commonest cause of injury in children between 4 and 12 years of age. Other common agents are electricity and chemicals. Many of these injuries are the result of child abuse.[167]

Initial resuscitation focuses on the respiratory and cardiovascular systems. The face, oral, and nasal areas and the upper airway are injured frequently. Early intubation should be performed in patients who are beginning or can be expected to develop airway edema, as the child with a relatively small airway is very susceptible to obstruction from the injury. Inhalation of steam or pulmonary irritants can result in parenchymal injury. Carbon monoxide, which may be inhaled during a fire, combines with hemoglobin and produces decreased oxygen-carrying capacity. It is important to remember that commercially available pulse oximeters cannot distinguish between oxyhemoglobin and carboxyhemoglobin[12] and that standard blood gas machines measure oxygen tension only in plasma. These monitors thus cannot evaluate blood oxygen content.

The plasma volume becomes depleted rapidly in burn patients due to losses through the burned tissue and to the increased permeability of vascular structures to proteins and electrolytes.

Fluid and drug administration in the burn patient is influenced by the amount of body surface area involved in the injury. The "rule of nines" is useful in estimating the percent of body surface area burned in an adult. In children, however, the proportions differ according to age, with the head representing more and the legs less of total body surface area. Available charts allow for calculation of burn area in the injured child (Fig 18-5).

In large burns (more than 30% of the body surface area), fluid resuscitation may require more than 4 mL/kg/% burn. There are several formulas available (see Chapter 20) to serve as guidelines for fluid administration. The pediatric patient, with different proportions of body surface area, water turnover, and body water distribution to weight at different ages, requires frequent observation and modification of therapy to maintain homeostasis. Pediatric patients with burns over 50% or more of their body surface area may have fluid requirements well in excess of those predicted by standard formulas.[120,200] One suggested fluid regimen is given in Table 18-13. Monitoring of urine output, CVP, arterial pressure, and pulmonary artery pressures may be required for management.

A large portion of thermally injured children develop hypertension during the acute phase of their injury.[206] The magnitude of this complication may be such as to cause seizures and encephalopathy. Burned and resuscitated children typically develop increases in heart rate, cardiac index, blood and urine catecholamines, and activity of the renin-angiotensin-aldosterone system. These children also demonstrate increases in intravascular volume and vasoconstrictor activity.[207] Treatment with analgesics (eg, morphine, 0.1–0.2 mg/kg), diuretics (furosemide, 1 mg/kg), or vasodilators (hydralazine, 0.2–0.3 mg/kg) may be required during this period to

FIG. 18-5. This chart of body areas, together with the table showing the percentage of surface area of head and legs at various ages, can be used to estimate the surface area burned in a child. (Reproduced by permission from Solomon JR: Crit Care Clin 1985; 1:161.)

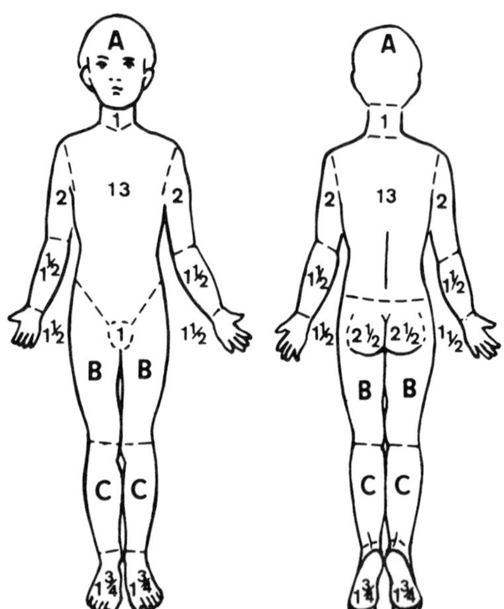


**PERCENTAGE OF SURFACE AREA OF HEAD AND LEGS AT VARIOUS AGES.**

| AREA IN DIAGRAM | AGE IN YEARS 0 | 1 | 5 | 10 | 15 |
|---|---|---|---|---|---|
| A = ½ of head | 9½ | 8½ | 6½ | 5½ | 4½ |
| B = ½ of one thigh | 2¾ | 3¼ | 4 | 4¼ | 4½ |
| C = ½ of one lower leg | 2½ | 2½ | 2¾ | 3 | 3¼ |

TABLE 18-13. Fluid Therapy in Burns (First 24 hours)

Normal Requirements

3–10 kg: 100 mL/kg
10–20 kg: 1,000 mL + 50 mL/kg for each kg over 10 kg
>20 kg: 1,500 mL + 20 mL/kg for each kg over 20 kg

given as ⅕–¼ normal saline in 5% dextrose administered in equal amount each 8 hours ______ mL

PLUS Burn Requirements

3 mL/kg/1% BSA (2 mL/kg/1% BSA if less severe) given as: ______ mL
Colloid
¼ ______ ⅓ ______ ½ ______ ______ mL
(BSA 20% +), (BSA 35% +), (BSA 50% +)
Remainder as Ringer's lactate in 5% dextrose (20–40 mmol/L sodium bicarbonate added in severe burns ______ mL

Half volume of burn requirements (colloid + Ringer's lactate) administered in first 8 hours and remainder over the subsequent 16 hours.

Reproduced with permission from Solomon JR: Crit Care Clin 1985, 1:163.
BSA = burn surface area.

prevent complications of hypertension. With convalescence, the vasoconstrictor activity resolves, although the hypervolemic state may persist throughout the hospital stay.

The markedly elevated metabolic rate that occurs in burned children is associated with changes in nutritional requirements, tissue catabolism, and alterations in renal and hepatic functions. These factors, combined with fluid, electrolyte, membrane, and target organ changes, result in derangements of pharmacokinetics and pharmacodynamics.[166] Massive hyperkalemia can occur with succinylcholine adminstration in burn patients[145]; although the patient may be safe for the first 5–7 days after injury, many authors recommend avoiding depolarizing relaxants entirely until at least 1 year postburn. Burn patients show resistance to nondepolarizing muscle relaxants, which peaks approximately 2 weeks after injury and then gradually disappears.[168] There are often changes in requirements for narcotics, sedatives, and other drugs.[57,166]

Burn victims, especially children, require multiple anesthetics for wound debridement and dressing changes. Many of these hypermetabolic children have had multiple halothane anesthetics; there has been no evidence of halothane hepatitis.[115,166] Ketamine is also commonly used with success. Low-dose (1.5–2 mg/kg IM) ketamine produces amnesia and analgesia with rapid recovery.[250] High-dose (5–6 mg/kg IM) ketamine results in satisfactory operative conditions, but is associated with prolonged postoperative recovery.[70] Tolerance to ketamine may develop after repeated doses; therefore, the dose should be titrated to effect.[271] More important than particular anesthetic agents is attention to particular problems, such as temperature and fluid management, which require creative and thoughtful solutions. Placement of the blood pressure cuff, ECG leads, and venous cannulas may be difficult because of pain or surgical requirements. All manipulations should be made as aseptically as possible as these children are extremely susceptible to infection. A smooth emergence is desirable, especially after placement of a fresh skin graft.

Although few anesthesiologists practice in a major burn center, all should be familiar with the basic management of the burned patient. Aggressive treatment of the airway and fluid status must begin immediately, often in the general or community hospital, before transfer to the specialized institution.

## CENTRAL NERVOUS SYSTEM

Frequent neurologic examinations should be performed on the child with head injury, documenting the global level of consciousness, pupillary responses, and presence of any focal signs.[203] Progressive deterioration in any of these signs should prompt immediate clinical reassessment and suspicion of increased intracranial pressure (ICP), which results from an acute increase in the volume of the intracranial contents within the closed cranial vault. Emergency reduction of ICP can usually be obtained with hyperventilation and acute dehydration using furosemide and/or mannitol. Since most brain-injured children exhibit cerebral hyperemia (see below), mannitol, which may increase cerebral blood volume and flow, should be given only if hyperventilation fails to improve the patient's condition or if rapid neurologic deterioration occurs. Otherwise, its use is recommended only after ICP monitoring is established (see Chapter 10).

The clinician must then establish the etiology of the ICP increase. An emergency CT scan will define the presence of a surgically treatable lesion, such as a subdural or epidural hematoma. If present, immediate decompression is required. It is much more likely, however, that a specific focal lesion is not present, as most children with increased ICP after closed head trauma have scattered punctate hemorrhages or diffuse cerebral edema.[41,42] The incidence of traumatic intracranial mass lesions in children is lower than that of adults.[41,176,183] However, nearly 50% of children who sustain head injury develop acute cerebral hyperemia shortly after trauma, which produces a significant increase in ICP.[42] This so-called secondary injury should be treated promptly. Secondary brain injury may also occur if hypovolemia, hypoxia, hypercarbia, hypotension, or increased ICP is allowed to continue.

Electrocardiographic abnormalities, including prolonged qTc, U waves, notched T waves, and ventricular arrhythmias, are common (75%) in head-injured infants and children.[219] Thus, careful monitoring of the ECG is required.

The appearance of clinical signs of increased ICP, a slow deterioration of global level of consciousness to a Glasgow coma scale of 6 or less (Table 18-14), or the need for therapies that preclude repeated neurologic examinations (eg, anesthesia and surgery, paralysis) are all indications for direct monitoring of ICP. When direct monitoring has been established, an attempt is made to maintain the ICP at less than 15 mm Hg, with a cerebral perfusion pressure of 50 mm Hg or greater. A number of agents and techniques are of use in this effort:

TABLE 18-14. Glasgow Coma Scale*

| | | | |
|---|---|---|---|
| Eyes | Open | Spontaneously | 4 |
| | | To verbal command | 3 |
| | | To pain | 2 |
| | No response | | 1 |
| Best motor response | To verbal command | Obeys | 6 |
| | To painful stimulus | Localizes pain | 5 |
| | | Flexion—withdrawal | 4 |
| | | Flexion—abnormal (decorticate rigidity) | 3 |
| | | Extension (decerebrate rigidity) | 2 |
| | | No response | 1 |
| Best verbal response | | Oriented and converses | 5 |
| | | Disoriented and converses | 4 |
| | | Inappropriate words | 3 |
| | | Incomprehensible sounds | 2 |
| | | No response | 1 |
| TOTAL | | | 3–15 |

* The Glasgow Coma Scale assists in documenting the patient's global level of consciousness. The verbal responses may be difficult to assess in the young child or in the intubated patient; a best approximation must be made.

- cardiovascular support, to ensure adequate cerebral perfusion
- oxygenation, to maintain $PaO_2$ greater than 100 mm Hg
- hyperventilation, with $PaCO_2$ initially 28–32 mm Hg; acute elevations of ICP can be treated with further lowering of the $PaCO_2$
- dehydration, using furosemide or mannitol at first and then fluid restriction to half maintenance to maintain serum osmolarity at 300–310 mosm/L
- 30° head-up tilt with the head midline, to maximize jugular venous drainage
- seizure control, using prophylactic diphenylhydantoin (loading dose of 10 mg/kg, followed by 5 mg/kg per day, attempting to maintain a serum level of 10–15 mg/L) or another drug to prevent seizures with the associated increase in cerebral metabolic rate and blood flow
- temperature control, to maintain normothermia and avoid the increased blood flow associated with fever
- sedation and pain control, using narcotics and/or low doses of diazepam; although these may cloud the neurologic examination, they are essential to interrupt painful stimuli that might cause abrupt increases in ICP
- paralysis, which controls ICP by preventing coughing and bucking and by relaxing abdominal muscle tone, thus promoting venous drainage

If ICP elevation is refractory to the above measures, a continuous infusion of barbiturate may be begun.[163,215,237] We use pentobarbital at an 8–16 mg/kg loading dose, followed by a 1 mg/kg/h maintenance infusion to achieve a serum level of approximately 20 mg/L; higher levels may be used, but carry a greater risk of cardiovascular depression. If ICP is still uncontrolled, hypothermia to 32°C, as a last effort, may be added (see Chapter 10).

If successful, therapy is maintained for at least 72 hours or for 24 hours after the latest dangerous ICP elevation and then is withdrawn gradually in a sequence inverse to the above. It is often a great effort to treat these children, but that effort is frequently rewarded with good results.[5] Children with increased ICP after head trauma have an excellent prognosis for return to normal life, provided that the pressure can be controlled, secondary brain injury does not occur, DIC does not supervene, and brainstem auditory evoked potentials remain intact.[40,41,96,161,185] However, the combination of head injury and multiple trauma is shown to be associated with a 2.5 times higher incidence of death or vegetative state than either injury alone.[175]

Other forms of brain injury are also seen. Near-drowning accounts for many admissions to pediatric intensive care units throughout the country. Although ischemic injury to many organs is seen in near-drowning, injury to the brain and the lungs dominates our attention in caring for these children. The prognosis is reasonably good for children who have not had prolonged submersion, do not have increased ICP, and are not in cardiac arrest on hospital admission.[186] It appears that neither hypothermia nor barbiturate coma improves the outcome or increases the number of neurologically intact children after hypoxic or ischemic cerebral injury. In fact, hypothermia seems to increase the incidence of septicemia in near-drowning victims.[32]

Hypothermia complicates near-drowning and other injuries. Children cool rapidly because of their large surface area and limited reserves for heat production. Attempts at resuscitation of the severely hypothermic child must include active core rewarming, as spontaneous cardiac activity may not return until the body temperature is above 34–35°C; resuscitation efforts, even if prolonged, should not be abandoned until warming has been accomplished. Detailed discussion on near-drowning is offered in Chapter 21.

### PSYCHOSOCIAL ASPECTS

The child and family must be supported through the illness. Feelings of guilt are common, not only in the parents but particularly on the part of siblings. Young children do not understand the true causes of illness or injury and often feel as if it were their fault that their brother or sister was hurt. Parents and siblings should be encouraged to visit the child in the intensive care unit; if possible, professional psychological counseling should be provided to assist them through the crisis.

## CONCLUSION

Trauma in the child is not, in absolute numbers, as frequent as trauma in the adult, yet it accounts for significant morbidity and mortality in an otherwise healthy population.

Head injury, either alone or in combination with multiple other injuries, is seen in a large number of cases.[223] Mayer et al.[174] reported that up to 75% of children with multiple trauma had head injury. As noted above, management of diffuse cerebral edema is the most significant aspect of care for these children. The prognosis is, fortunately, reasonably good.[40,161,204]

Blunt trauma predominates in the child; injury is related to falls or motor vehicle accidents. Diffuse thoracic and abdominal damage is common, but the diagnosis of the problem is often more difficult because of the child's inability to give an exact history and because of the lack of external signs to localize the injury.

The complications that arise during the course of treatment are not very different from those seen in adults. Shock, sepsis, ARDS, renal failure, nutritional depletion, and the like all occur in the seriously ill child and are managed in much the same way as in the adult.

The prognosis for recovery from severe injury in the child is good. The overall health and vigor of the tissues do much to improve the outlook for these young patients. Similarly, the cost-benefit ratio for intensive care is better in children than in adults. The healthy child sustaining a major injury may require many months of intensive care and rehabilitation, but has a reasonable chance of complete recovery and can become a contributing, productive member of society. The physician assisting in the treatment of these children then receives the satisfaction of seeing rewarding and successful outcomes.

Much needs to be done. Research into the mechanisms of injury and of the common complications thereof is continuing, and participation of the anesthesiologist in such areas as the patterns of lung injury and repair is welcomed. It cannot be overemphasized that, particularly in pediatrics, prevention is better than cure. Perhaps the most direct beneficial effect each of us can have on the problem of pediatric trauma is to educate ourselves and our own friends in home and vehicular safety; simply fastening our seat belts and placing our children in approved car seats will do more for us and, by example, for our associates than patching up the pieces with the best pediatric critical care.

## REFERENCES


1. Abajian JC, Mellish P, Browne AF, et al. Spinal anesthesia for surgery in the high-risk infant. Anesth Analg 1984;63:359.
2. Abbott TR. Changes in serum calcium fractions and citrate concentrations during massive blood transfusions and cardiopulmonary bypass. Br J Anaesth 1983;55:753.
3. Adams P, Gelman S, Reves JG, et al. Midazolam pharmcodynamics and pharmacokinetics during acute hypovolemia. Anesthesiology 1985;63:140.
4. Adelhoj B, Petring OU, Hagelsten JO. Inaccuracy of preanesthetic gastric intubation for emptying liquid stomach contents. Acta Anaesth Scand 1986;30:41.
5. Alberico AM, Ward JD, Choi SC, Marmarou A, Young HF. Outcome after severe head injury. J Neurosurg 1987;67:648.
6. Allen TH, Steven IM. Prolonged nasotracheal intubation in infants and children. Br J Anaesth 1972;44:835.
7. American Heart Association. Textbook of advanced life support (abridged). Dallas: American Heart Association, 1983:263.
8. Arbon DH, Theye RA. Lactic acidemia during hemorrhagic hypotension and cyclopropane anesthesia. Anesthesiology 1972;37:634.
9. Ausinsch B, Rayburn RL, Munson ES, et al. Ketamine and intraocular pressure in children. Anesth Analg 1976;55:773.

10. Barash PG, Glanz S, Katz JD, et al. Ventricular function in children during halothane anesthesia: an echocardiographic evaluation. Anesthesiology 1978;49:79.
11. Barash PG, Katz JD, Firestone S, et al. Cardiovascular performance in children during induction: an echocardiographic comparison of enflurane and halothane. Anesthesiology 1979;51:S315.
12. Barker SJ, Tremper KK. The effect of carbon monoxide inhalation on pulse oximetry and transcutaneous $PO_2$. Anesthesiology 1987;66:677.
13. Barker SJ, Tremper KK, Gamel DM. A clinical comparison of transcutaneous $PO_2$ and pulse oximetry in the operating room. Anesth Analg 1986;65:805.
14. Barlow B, Niemirska M, Gandhi R, Shelton M. Response to injury in children with closed femur fractures. J Trauma 1987;27:429.
15. Bashein G, Haschke RH, Ready B. Electrical nerve location: numerical and electrophoretic comparison of insulated vs. uninsulated needles. Anesth Analg 1984;63:919.
16. Basic life support for infants and children. Standards and guidelines for cardiopulmonary resuscitation (CPR) and emergency cardiac care (ECC). JAMA 1980;244:453.
17. Bass JL, Gallagher SS, Metha KA. Injuries to adolescents and young adults. Pediatr Clin North Am 1985;32:31.
18. Beaver BL, Colombani PM, Buck JR, et al. Efficacy of emergency room thoracotomy in pediatric trauma. J Pediatr Surg 1987;22:19.
19. Bedford RF, Persing JA, Pobereskin LH, et al. Lidocaine or thiopental for rapid control of intracranial hypertension. Anesth Analg 1980;59:435.
20. Beecher HK. Resuscitation and anesthesia for wounded men. Springfield, IL: Charles C Thomas, 1949.
21. Benlabed M, Ecoffey C, Levron J-C, et al. Analgesia and ventilatory response to $CO_2$ following epidural sufentanil in children. Anesthesiology 1987;67:948.
22. Bennett GM, Loeser EA, Kawamura R, et al. Cardiovascular responses to nitrous oxide during enflurane and oxygen anesthesia. Anesthesiology 1977;46:227.
23. Berghem L, Bergman U, Schildt B, et al. Plasma atropine concentrations determined by radioimmunoassay after single-dose IV and IM administration. Br J Anaesth 1980;52:597.
24. Berry FA. Succinylcholine and trismus. Anesthesiology 1989;70:161.
25. Berry FR. Analgesia in patients with fractured shaft of femur. Anaesthesia 1977;32:576.
26. Bevan JC, Donati F, Bevan DR. Attempted acceleration of the onset of action of pancuronium. Effects of divided doses in infants and children. Br J Anaesth 1985;57:1204.
27. Billmire DA, Neale HW, Gregory RO. Use of IV fentanyl in the outpatient treatment of pediatric facial trauma. J Trauma 1985;25:1079.
28. Bijur PE, Golding J, Haslum M, Kurzon M. Behavioral predictors of injury in school-age children. Am J Dis Child 1988;142:1307.
29. Bijur PE, Golding J, Haslum M. Persistence of occurrence of injury: can injuries of preschool children predict injuries of school-aged children. Pediatrics 1988;82:707.
30. Blaise GA. Spinal anaesthesia for minor paediatric surgery. Can Anaesth Soc J 1986;33:227.
31. Bogetz MS, Katz JA. Recall of surgery for major trauma. Anesthesiology 1984;61:6.
32. Bohn DJ, Biggar WD, Smith CR, et al. Influence of hypothermia, barbiturate therapy, and intracranial pressure monitoring on morbidity and mortality after near-drowning. Crit Care Med 1986;14:529.
33. Bond AC, Davies CK. Ketamine and pancuronium for the shocked patient. Anaesthesia 1974;29:59.
34. Borland LM, Swan DM, Leff S. Difficult pediatric endotracheal intubation: a new approach to the retrograde technique. Anesthesiology 1981;55:577.
35. Bosomworth PP. Ketamine symposium—comment by moderator. Anesth Analg 1971;50:471.
36. Boudreaux JP, Schieber RA, Cook DR. Hemodynamic effects of halothane in the newborn piglet. Anesth Analg 1984;63:731.
37. Brandom BW, Rudd GD, Cook DR. Clinical pharmacology of atracurium in pediatric patients. Br. J Anaesth 1983;55: 117S.
38. Bristow JD, Prys-Roberts C, Pickering A, et al. Effects of anesthesia on baroreflex control of heart rate in man. Anesthesiology 1969;31:422.
39. Brown EM, Krishnaprasad D, Smiler BG. Pancuronium for rapid induction technique for tracheal intubation. Can Anaesth Soc J 1979;26:489.
40. Bruce DA, Schut L, Bruno LA, et al. Outcome following severe head injuries in children. J Neurosurg 1978;48:679.
41. Bruce DA, Raphaely RC, Goldberg AI, et al. Pathophysiology, treatment and outcome following severe head injury in children. Child's Brain 1979;5:174.
42. Bruce DA, Alavi A, Bilaniuk L, et al. Diffuse cerebral swelling following head injuries in children: the syndrome of "malignant brain edema". J Neurosurg 1981;54:170.
43. Capan LM, Turndorf H. Airway management. In: Worth MH, ed. Principles and practice of trauma care. Baltimore: Williams & Wilkins, 1982:2.
44. Carrell ED, Eyring EJ. Intravenous regional anesthesia for childhood fractures. J Trauma 1971;11:301.
45. Carter JA, Clarke TNS, Prys-Roberts C, et al. Restoration of baroreflex control of heart rate during recovery from anesthesia. Br J Anaesth 1986;58:415.
46. Chapple DJ, Clark JS. Pharmacological action of breakdown products of atracurium and related substances. Br J Anaesth 1983;55:11S.
47. Chasapakis G, Kekis N, Sakkalis C, et al. Use of ketamine and pancuronium for anesthesia for patients in hemorrhagic shock. Anesth Analg 1973;52:282.
48. Chernow B, Holbrook P, D'Angona DS, et al. Epinephrine absorption after intratracheal administration. Anesth Analg 1984;63:829.
49. Christensen JH, Andreasen F, Kristoffersen MB. Comparison of the anesthetic and haemodynamic effects of chlormethiazole and thiopentone. Br J Anaesth 1983;55:391.
50. Clergue F, Desmonts JM, Duvaldestin P, et al. Depression of respiratory drive by diazepam as premedication. Br J Anaesth 1981;53:1059.
51. Collins C, Koren G, Crean P, et al. Fentanyl pharmacokinetics and hemodynamic effects in preterm infants during ligation of patent ductus arteriosus. Anesth Analg 1985;64:1078.
52. Committee on Accidents and Poison Prevention, American Academy of Pediatrics: First aid for the choking child. Pediatrics 1981;67:744.
53. Conn AW. Intensive care for the injured child. In: Surgical staff of the Hospital for Sick Children, Toronto, eds. Care for the injured child. Baltimore: Williams & Wilkins, 1975:36.
54. Coonan TJ, Hope CE. Cardio-respiratory effect of change in body position. Can Anaesth Soc J 1983;30:424.
55. Cooper A, Floyd T, Barlow B, et al. Major blunt abdominal trauma due to child abuse. J Trauma 1988;28:1483.
56. Conway CM, Ellis DB. The hemodynamic effects of short acting barbiturates. Br J Anaesth 1969;41:534.
57. Coté CJ, Petkav AJ. Thiopental requirements may be increased

in children reanesthetized at least one year after recovery from extensive thermal injury. Anesth Analg 1985;64:1156.
58. Coté CJ, Jobes DR, Schwartz AJ, et al. Two approaches to cannulation of a child's internal jugular vein. Anesthesiology 1979;50:371.
59. Coté CJ, Goudsouzian NG, Liu LMP, et al. The dose response of intravenous thiopental for the induction of general anesthesia in unpremedicated children. Anesthesiology 1981;55:703.
60. Coté CJ, Goudsouzian NG, Liu LMP, et al. Assessment of risk factors related to the acid aspiration syndrome in pediatric patients—gastric pH and residual volume. Anesthesiology 1982;56:70.
61. Coté CJ, Liu LMP, Szyfelbein SK, et al. Changes in serial platelet counts following massive blood transfusion in pediatric patients. Anesthesiology 1985;62:197.
62. Coté CJ, Szyfelbein SK, Goudsouzian NG, et al. Intraoperative events diagnosed by expired carbon dioxide monitoring in children. Can Anaesth Soc J 1986;33:315.
63. Coté CJ, Eavey RD, Todres ID, Jones DE. Cricothyroid membrane puncture: oxygenation and ventilation in a dog model using an intravenous catheter. Crit Care Med 1988;16:615.
64. Crone RK. Pediatric intensive care. In: ASA Refresher Courses in Anesthesiology. vol 9. Philadelphia: JB Lippincott, 1981:21.
65. Cuthbertson DP, Fell GS, Rahimi AG, et al. Environmental temperature and metabolic response to injury. Protein, mineral and energy metabolism. Adv Exp Biol Med 1973;33:409.
66. Dalal FY, Schmidt GB, Bennett EJ, et al. Fractures of the larynx in children. Can Anaesth Soc J 1974;21:376.
67. Dalens B, Vanneuville G, Tanguy A. A new parascalene approach to the brachial plexus in children: comparison with the supraclavicular approach. Anesth Analg 1987;66:1264.
68. Dauchot PJ, Rasmussen JP, Nicholson DH, et al. On-line systolic time intervals during anesthesia in patients with and without heart disease. Anesthesiology 1976;44:472.
69. Deckardt R, Steward DJ. Noninvasive arterial hemoglobin oxygen saturation versus transcutaneous oxygen tension monitoring in the preterm infant. Crit Care Med 1984;12:935.
70. Demling RH, Ellerbee S, Jarrett F. Ketamine anesthesia for tangential excision of burn eschar: a burn unit procedure. J Trauma 1978;18:267.
71. Donchin Y, Vered IY. Blunt trauma to the trachea. Br J Anaesth 1976;48:1113.
72. Donegan MF, Bedford RF. Intravenously administered lidocaine prevents intracranial hypertension during endotracheal suctioning. Anesthesiology 1980;52:516.
73. Duke PC, Trosky S. The effect of halothane with nitrous oxide on baroreflex control of heart rate in man. Can Anaesth Soc J 1980;27:531.
74. Edelist G. The effect of hypothermia on the respiratory response to carbon dioxide. Can Anaesth Soc J 1970;17:551.
75. Edmonds JF, Barker GA, Conn AW. Current concepts in cardiovascular monitoring in children. Crit Care Med 1980;8:548.
76. Eichelberger MR, Randolph JG. Pediatric trauma: an algcrithm for diagnosis and therapy. J Trauma 1983;23:91.
77. Ellis D, Gartner JC, Galvis AG. Acute renal failure in infants and children: diagnosis, complications, and treatment. Crit Care Med 1981;9:607.
78. Etsten B, Li TH: Hemodynamic changes during thiopental anesthesia in humans: cardiac output, stroke volume, total peripheral resistance, and intrathoracic volume. J Clin Invest 1955;34:500.
79. Fahey MR, Rupp SM, Fisher DM, et al. The pharmacokinetics and pharmacodynamics of atracurium in patients with and without renal failure. Anesthesiology 1984;61:699.
80. Fifield GC. Multiple trauma in children. Postgrad Med 1984;75:111.
81. Fisher DM, Miller RD. Neuromuscular effects of vecuronium (ORG NC 45) in infants and children during $N_2O$, halothane anesthesia. Anesthesiology 1983;58:519.
82. Fisher DM, O'Keefe C, Stanski DR, et al. Pharmacokinetics and pharmacodynamics of d-tubocurarine in infants, children and adults. Anesthesiology 1982;57:203.
83. Fisher DM, Cronnelly R, Miller RD, et al. The neuromuscular pharmacology of neostigmine in infants and children. Anesthesiology 1983;59:220.
84. Fisher DM, Cronnelly R, Sharma M, et al. Clinical pharmacology of edrophonium in infants and children. Anesthesiology 1984;61:428.
85. Fitzgerald B. Intravenous regional anesthesia in children. Br J Anaesth 1976;48:485.
86. Flacke JW, Davis J, Flacke WE, et al. Effects of fentanyl and diazepam in dogs deprived of autonomic tone. Anesth Analg 1985;64:1053.
87. Flewellen EH, Nelson TE. Halothane-succinylcholine induced masseter spasm: indicative of malignant hyperthermia susceptibility? Anesth Analg 1984;63:693.
88. Ford DJ, Pither C, Raj PP. Comparison of insulated and uninsulated needles for locating peripheral nerves with a peripheral nerve stimulator. Anesth Analg 1984;63:925.
89. Furman EB: Massive transfusions in Children. Semin Anesth 1984;3:127.
90. Gallagher SS, Guyer B, Kotelchuck M, et al. A strategy for the reduction of childhood injuries in Massachusetts: SCIPP. N Engl J Med 1982;307:1015.
91. Gann DS. Emergency management of the obstructed airway. JAMA 1980;243:1141.
92. Garcia V, Eichelberger M, Ziegler M, et al. Use of military antishock trouser in a child. J Pediatr Surg 1981;16:544.
93. Geeverghese KP. Basic considerations. Int Anesth Clin 1977;15:1.
94. Gergis SD, Sokoll MD, Mehta M, et al. Intubation conditions after atracurium and suxamethonium. Br J Anaesth 1983;55:83S.
95. Giesecke AH Jr. Anesthesia for trauma surgery. In: Miller RD, ed. Anesthesia. New York: Churchill Livingstone, 1986:1819.
96. Goitein KJ, Amit Y, Fainmesser P, et al. Diagnostic and prognostic value of auditory nerve brainstem evoked responses in comatose children. Crit Care Med 1983;11:91.
97. Goitein KJ, Rein AJ-JT, Gornstein A. Incidence of aspiration in endotracheally intubated infants and children. Crit Care Med 1984;12:19.
98. Goudsouzian NG. Muscle relaxants in infants and children. Can Anaesth Soc J 1985;32:S27.
99. Goudsouzian NG. Atracurium in infants and children. Br J Anaesth 1986;58:23S.
100. Goudsouzian NG, Gionfriddo M. Muscle relaxants and children. Semin Anesth 1984;3:50.
101. Goudsouzian NG, Coté CJ, Liu LMP, et al. The dose response effects of oral cimetidine on gastric pH and volume in children. Anesthesiology 1981;55:533.
102. Goudsouzian NG, Liu LMP, Coté CJ, et al. Safety and efficacy of atracurium in adolescents and children anesthetized with halothane. Anesthesiology 1983;59:459.
103. Goudsouzian NG, Martyn JJA, Liu LMP, et al. Safety and efficacy of vecuronium in adolescents and children. Anesth Analg 1983;62:1083.
104. Goudsouzian NG, Martyn JJA, Liu LMP, et al. The dose response effect of long-acting nondepolarizing neuromuscular blocking agents in children. Can Anaesth Soc J 1984;31:246.
105. Goudsouzian NG, Liu LMP, Gionfriddo M, et al. Neuromuscular effects of atracurium in infants and children. Anesthesiology 1985;62:75.

106. Goudsouzian NG, Alifimoff JK, Eberly C, et al. Neuromuscular and cardiovascular effects of mivacurium in children. Anesthesiology 1989;70:237.
107. Gould SA, Rosen AL, Sehgal LR, et al. Fluosol-DA as a red-cell substitute in acute anemia. N Engl J Med 1986;314:1653.
108. Gratz IR. Accidental injury in childhood: a literature review on pediatric trauma. J Trauma 1979;19:551.
109. Green DW, Bristow ASE, Fisher M. Comparison of IV glycopyrrolate and atropine in the prevention of bradycardia and arrhythmias following repeated doses of suxamethonium in children. Br J Anaesth 1984;56:981.
110. Greene WL, Bollinger RR. Cimetidine for stress-ulcer prophylaxis. Crit Care Med 1984;12:571.
111. Greensher J, Mofenson HC. Emergency treatment of the choking child. Pediatrics 1982;70:110.
112. Gregory GA. Respiratory care of the child. Crit Care Med 1980;8:582.
113. Gregory GA. Induction of anesthesia. In: Gregory GA, ed. Pediatric anesthesia. New York: Churchill-Livingston, 1983:437.
114. Gronert GA. Management of patients in whom trismus occurs following succinylcholine. Anesthesiology 1988;68:653.
115. Gronert GA, Schaner PJ, Gunther RC. Multiple halothane anesthesia in burn patients. JAMA 1968;205:878.
116. Gutgesell HP, Tacker WA, Geddes LA, et al. Energy dose for ventricular defibrillation in children. Pediatrics 1976;58:898.
117. Guyer B, Gallagher SS. An approach to the epidemiology of childhood injuries. Pediatr Clin North Am 1985;32:5.
118. Halford FJ. A critique of intravenous anesthesia in war surgery. Anesthesiology 1943;4:67.
119. Haller JA, Shorter N, Miller D, et al. Organization and function of a regional pediatric trauma center: does a system of management improve outcome? J Trauma 1983;23:691.
120. Harmel RP, Vane DW, King DR. Burn care in children: special considerations. Clin Plast Surg 1986;13:95.
121. Harris BH, Eichelberger MR, Haller JA, et al. Trauma in children: a symposium. Contemp Surg 1983;22:123.
122. Harrison GA. Ayre's T-piece: a review of its modifications. Br J Anaesth 1964;36:115.
123. Harte FA, Chalmers PC, Walsh RF, et al. Intraosseous fluid administration: a parenteral alternative in pediatric resuscitation. Anesth Analg 1987;66:687.
124. Haupt MT, Rackow EC. Colloid osmotic pressure and fluid resuscitation with hetastarch, albumin, and saline solutions. Crit Care Med 1982;10:159.
125. Heimlich HJ. A life-saving maneuver to prevent food choking. JAMA 1975;243:398.
126. Heimlich HJ. First aid for choking children: back blows and chest thrusts cause complications and death. Pediatrics 1982;70:120.
127. Hemmer D, Lee TS, Wright BD. Intubation of a child with cervical spine injury with aid of a fiberoptic bronchoscope. Anaesth Intens Care 1982;10:163.
128. Hickey PR, Hansen DD. Fentanyl and sufentanil-oxygen-pancuronium anesthesia for cardiac surgery in infants. Anesth Analg 1984;63:117.
129. Hickey PR, Hansen DD, Wessel DL, et al. Pulmonary and systemic hemodynamic responses to fentanyl in infants. Anesth Analg 1985;64:483.
130. Hoka S, Takeshita A, Yamamato K, et al. The effects of ketamine on venous capacitance in rats. Anesthesiology 1985; 62:145.
131. Holbrook PR, Mickell J, Pollack MM, et al. Cardiovascular resuscitation drugs for children. Crit Care Med 1980;8:588.
132. Holmes MJ, Reyes HM. A critical review of urban pediatric trauma. J Trauma 1984;24:253.
133. Hurvitz CH. Hematologic considerations in the surgical patient. In: Gans SL, ed. Surgical pediatrics—nonoperative care. New York: Grune and Stratton, 1980:183.
134. Idvall J. Influence of ketamine anesthesia on cardiac output and tissue perfusion in rats subjected to hemorrhage. Anesthesiology 1981;55:297.
135. Ingram MD, Sclabassi RJ, Cook DR, et al. Cardiovascular and electroencephalographic effects of laudonosine in "nephrectomized" cats. Br J Anaesth 1986;58:145S.
136. James LS. Emergencies in the delivery room. In: Fanaroff AA, Martin RJ, eds. Neonatal-perinatal medicine. St. Louis: CV Mosby, 1983:185.
137. Joyce JT, Roizen MF, Eger EI II. Effect of thiopental induction on sympathetic activity. Anesthesiology 1983;59:19.
138. Kaplan RF, Graves SA. Anatomic and physiologic differences of neonates, infants and children. Semin Anesth 1984;3:1.
139. Kapp JP. Endotracheal intubation in patients with fractures of the cervical spine. J Neurosurg 1975;42:731.
140. Keene AR, Cullen DJ. Therapeutic intervention scoring system: update 1983. Crit Care Med 1983;11:1.
141. Koehntop DE, Rodman JH, Brundage DM, et al. Pharmacokinetics of fentanyl in neonates. Anesth Analg 1986;65:227.
142. Koka BV, Jeon IS, Andre JM, et al. Postintubation croup in children. Anesth Analg 1977;56:501.
143. Korsch BM. The child and the operating room. Anesthesiology 1975;43:251.
144. Kotrly KJ, Ebert TJ, Vucins EJ, et al. Effects of fentanyl-diazepam-nitrous oxide anaesthesia on arterial baroreflex control of heart rate in man. Br J Anaesth 1986;58:406.
145. Krishna G, Haselby KA, Rao CC, et al. The pediatric patient. In: Stoelting RK, Dierdorf SF, eds. Anesthesia and co-existing diseases. New York: Churchill Livingstone, 1983:741.
146. Laravuso RF, Perloff WH. Difficult pediatric intubation. Anesthesiology 1986;64:668.
147. Lebowitz PW, Cote ME, Daniels AL, et al. Cardiovascular effects of midazolam and thiopentone for induction of anaesthesia in ill surgical patients. Can Anaesth Soc J 1983;30:19.
148. Ledbetter DJ, Hatch EI, Feldman KW, et al. Diagnostic and surgical implications of child abuse. Arch Surg 1988;123:1101.
149. Lennon RL, Olson RA, Gronert GA. Atracurium or vecuronium for rapid sequence endotracheal intubation. Anesthesiology 1986;64:510.
150. Lindgren L, Saarnivaara L. Effect of competitive myoneural blockade and fentanyl on muscle fasciculations caused by suxamethonium in children. Br J Anaesth 1983;55:747.
151. Lindgren L, Saarnivaara L. Increase in intragastric pressure during suxamethonium-induced muscle fasciculations in children: inhibition by alfentanil. Br J Anaesth 1988;60:176.
152. Liu LMP, De Cook TH, Goudsouzian NG, et al. Dose-response to intramuscular succinylcholine in children. Anesthesiology 1981;55:599.
153. Lockhart CH. Maintenance of general anesthesia. In: Gregory GA, ed. Pediatric anesthesia. New York: Churchill Livingstone, 1983:463.
154. Lockhart CH, Nelson WL. The relationship of ketamine requirement to age in pediatric patients. Anesthesiology 1974;40:507.
155. Loftness SL, Lockhart CH. Pitfalls in the use of anesthetic agents in children. Int Anesth Clin 1985;23:201.
156. Longnecker DE, Sturgill BC. Influence of anesthetic agent on survival following hemorrhage. Anesthesiology 1976;45:516.
157. Longnecker DE, Ross DC, Silver IA. Anesthetic influence on arteriolar diameters and tissue oxygen tension in hemorrhaged rats. Anesthesiology 1982;57:177.
158. Lopez-Herce J, Velasco LA, Codoceo R, et al. Ranitidine prophylaxis in acute gastric mucosal damage in critically ill pediatric patients. Crit Care Med 1988;16:591.

159. Lovejoy FH, Chaffee-Bahamon C. The physician's role in accident prevention. Pediatr Rev 1982;4:53.
160. Lowe HJ, Titel JH, Hagler KJ. Absorption of anesthetics by conductive rubber in breathing circuits. Anesthesiology 1971;34:283.
161. Mahoney WJ, D'Souza BJ, Haller JA, et al. Long term outcome of children with head trauma and prolonged coma. Pediatrics 1983;71:756.
162. Manchikanti L, Colliver JA, Marrero TC, et al. Assessment of age-related acid aspiration risk factors in pediatric, adult, and geriatric patients. Anesth Analg 1985;64:11.
163. Marshall LF, Smith RW, Shapiro HM. The outcome with aggressive treatment in severe head injuries: Part II. Acute and chronic barbiturate administration in the management of head injury. J Neurosurg 1979;50:26.
164. Marty J, Gauzit R, Lefevre P, et al. Effects of diazepam and midazolam on baroreflex control of heart rate and on sympathetic activity in humans. Anesth Analg 1986;65:113.
165. Martyn JAJ. Cimetidine and/or antacid for the control of gastric acidity in pediatric burn patients. Crit Care Med 1985;13:1.
166. Martyn JAJ. Clinical pharmacology and drug therapy in the burned patient. Anesthesiology 1986;65:67.
167. Martyn JAJ, Szyfelbein SK. Pathophysiology and management of burn trauma in children. Semin Anesth 1984;3:75.
168. Martyn JAJ, Liu LMP, Szyfelbein SK, et al. The neuromuscular effects of pancuronium in burned children. Anesthesiology 1983;59:561.
169. Mason Cobb L, Vinocur CD, Wagner CW, et al. Intestinal perforation due to blunt trauma in children in an era of increased nonoperative treatment. J Trauma 1986;26:461.
170. Matlak ME. Abdominal injuries. In: Mayer TA, ed. Emergency management of pediatric trauma. Philadelphia: WB Saunders, 1985:328.
171. Matlak ME. Foreign bodies. In: Mayer TA, ed. Emergency management of pediatric trauma. Philadelphia: WB Saunders, 1985:490.
172. Matteo RS, Lieberman IG, Salanitre E, et al. Distribution, elimination, and action of d-tubocurarine in neonates, infants, children and adults. Anesth Analg 1984;63:799.
173. Mayer TA. Initial evaluation and management of the injured child. In: Mayer TA. ed. Emergency management of pediatric trauma. Philadelphia: WB Saunders, 1985:1.
174. Mayer T, Matlak ME, Johnson DG, et al. The modified injury severity scale in pediatric multiple trauma patients. J Pediatr Surg 1980;15:719.
175. Mayer T, Walker ML, Matlak ME. Causes of morbidity and mortality in severe pediatric trauma. JAMA 1981;245:719.
176. Mayer T, Walker MC, Shasha I, et al. Effect of multiple trauma on outcome of pediatric patients with neurologic injuries. Child's Brain 1981;8:189.
177. Maze A, Bloch E. Stridor in pediatric patients. Anesthesiology 1979;50:132.
178. McCoy C, Bell MJ. Preventable traumatic deaths in children. J Pediatr Surg 1983;18:505.
179. McCue Horwitz S, Morgenstern H, DiPietro L, Morrison CL. Determinants of pediatric injuries. Am J Dis Child 1988;142:605.
180. Meakin G, Sweet PT, Bevan JC, et al. Neostigmine and edrophonium as antagonists of pancuronium in infants and children. Anesthesiology 1983;59:316.
181. Meller JL, Shermeta DW. Falls in urban children. Am J Dis Child 1987;141:1271.
182. Melman E, Penuelas J, Marrufo J, et al. Regional anesthesia in children. Anesth Analg 1975;54:387.
183. Miller JD, Butterworth JF, Gudeman SK, et al. Further experience in the management of severe head injury. J Neurosurg 1981;54:289.
184. Miller RD, Rupp SM, Fisher DM, et al. Clinical pharmacology of vecuronium and atracurium. Anesthesiology 1984;61:444.
185. Miner ME, Graham SH, Gildenberg PL, et al. Disseminated intravascular coagulation, fibrinolytic syndrome following head injury in children—frequency and prognostic implications. Pediatrics 1982;100:687.
186. Modell JH. Treatment of near-drowning: Is there a role for H.Y.P.E.R. therapy? Crit Care Med 1986;14:593.
187. Mofenson HC, Greensher J. Management of the choking child. Pediatr Clin North Am 1985;32:183.
188. Montgomery SJ, Raj PP, Nettles D, et al. The use of the nerve stimulator with standard unsheathed needles in nerve blockade. Anesth Analg 1973;52:827.
189. Morgan GAR, Steward DJ. Linear airway dimensions in children including those with cleft palate. Can Anaesth Soc J 1982;29:1.
190. Morse TS. The child with multiple injuries. Emerg Med Clin North Am 1983;1:175.
191. Moss J, Rosow CE, Savarese JJ, et al. Role of histamine in the hypotensive action of d-tubocurarine in humans. Anesthesiology 1981;55:19.
192. Motoyama EK, Glazener CH. Hypoxemia after general anesthesia in children. Anesth Analg 1986;65:267.
193. Nagashima H, Nguyen HD, Lee S, et al. Facilitation of rapid endotracheal intubation and atracurium. Anesthesiology 1984;61:A289.
194. Nashat FS, Neil E. The effect of hypothermia on baroreceptor and chemoreceptor reflexes. J Physiol (Lond) 1955;127:59P.
195. National Conference on Cardiopulmonary Resuscitation and Emergency Cardiac Care: Pediatric basic life support. JAMA 1986;255:2954.
196. National Safety Council. Accident facts 1983 edition. Chicago: National Safety Council, 1983.
197. Nettles DC, Herrin TJ, Mullen JG. Ketamine induction in poor risk patients. Anesth Analg 1973;52:59.
198. Olsson GL, Hallen B. Pharmacological evacuation of the stomach with metoclopramide. Acta Anaesth Scand 1982;26:417.
199. Olsson GL, Hallen B, Hambraeus-Jonzon K. Aspiration during anesthesia: a computer-aided study of 185,358 anaesthetics. Acta Anaesth Scand 1986;30:84.
200. O'Neill JA. Fluid resuscitation in the burned child—a reappraisal. J Pediatr Surg 1982;17:604.
201. Ordog GJ, Prakash A, Wasserberger J, Balasubramaniam S. Pediatric gunshot wounds. J Trauma 1987;27:1272.
202. Ovassapian A, Dykes MHM. Difficult pediatric intubation—an indication for the fiberoptic bronchoscope. Anesthesiology 1982;56:412.
203. Pascucci RC. Head trauma in the child. Intens Care Med 1988;14:185.
204. Pfenninger J, Kaiser G, Lutschig J, Sutter M. Treatment and outcome of the severely head injured child. Intens Care Med 1983;9:13.
205. Pildeo RS, Lilien LD. Carbohydrate metabolism in the fetus and neonate. In: Fanaroff AA, Martin RJ, eds. Neonatal-perinatal medicine. St. Louis: CV Mosby, 1983:845.
206. Popp MB, Freidberg DL, MacMillan BG. Clinical characteristics of hypertension in burned children. Ann Surg 1980;191:473.
207. Popp MB, Silberstein EB, Srivastrava LS, et al. A pathophysiologic study of the hypertension associated with burn injury in children. Ann Surg 1981;193:817.
208. Price HL. A dynamic concept of the distribution of thiopental in the human body. Anesthesiology 1960;21:40.
209. Priebe HJ, Skillman JJ, Bushnell LS, et al. Antacid versus cimetidine in preventing acute gastrointestinal bleeding. A ran-

domized trial in 75 critically ill patients. N Engl J Med 1980;302:426.

210. Prough DS, Johnson C, Poole GV, et al. Effects on intracranial pressure of resuscitation from hemorrhagic shock with hypertonic saline versus lactated Ringer's solution. Crit Care Med 1985;13:407.
211. Ramenofsky ML, Morse TS. Standards of care for the critically injured pediatric patient. J Trauma 1982;22:921.
212. Ramenofsky ML, Luterman A, Curreri PW, et al. EMS for pediatricians: optimum treatment or unnecessary delay? J Pediatr Surg 1983;18:498.
213. Ramenofsky ML, Luterman A, Quindlen E, et al. Maximum survival in pediatric trauma: the ideal system. J Trauma 1984;24:818.
214. Rao TL, Wong AY, Salem MR. A new approach to percutaneous catheterization of the internal jugular vein. Anesthesiology 1977;46:362.
215. Rea GL, Rockwold GL. Barbiturate therapy in uncontrolled intracranial hypertension. Neurosurgery 1983;12:401.
216. Regan MJ, Eger EI II. Ventilatory responses to hypercapnia and hypoxia at normothermia and moderate hypothermia during constant-depth halothane anesthesia. Anesthesiology 1966;27:624.
217. Reves JG, Fragen RJ, Vinik R, et al. Midazolam: pharmacology and uses. Anesthesiology 1985;62:310.
218. Robinson S. Anesthesia for congenital heart disease. In: Gregory GA, ed. Pediatric anesthesia. New York: Churchill Livingstone, 1983:607.
219. Rogers MC, Zakka KG, Nugent SK, et al. Electrocardiographic abnormalities in infants and children with neurologic injury. Crit Care Med 1980;8:213.
220. Rosenberg H, Fletcher JE. Masseter muscle rigidity and malignant hyperthermia susceptibility. Anesth Analg 1986;65:161.
221. Rosenberg H, Reed S, Heiman T. Masseter spasm, rhabdomyolysis and malignant hyperpyrexia. Anesthesiology 1980;53:S248.
222. Rosetti VA, Thompson BM, et al. Intraosseous infusion: an alternative route of pediatric intravascular access. Ann Emerg Med 1985;14:885.
223. Rosman NP, Oppenheimer EY, O'Connor JF. Emergency management of pediatric head injuries. Emerg Med Clin North Am 1983;1:141.
224. Rothenberg S, Moore EE, Marx JA, et al. Selective management of blunt abdominal trauma in children—the triage role of peritoneal lavage. J Trauma 1987;27:1101.
225. Rothstein P, Arthur GR, Feldman HS, et al. Bupivacaine for nerve blocks in children: blood concentrations and pharmacokinetics. Anesth Analg 1986;65:625.
226. Ryckman FC, Noseworthy J. Multisystem trauma. Surg Clin North Am 1985;65:1287.
227. Salem MR, Wong AY, Fizzotti GF. Efficacy of cricoid pressure in preventing aspiration of gastric contents in paediatric patients. Br J Anaesth 1972;44:401.
228. Salem MR, Wong AY, Lin YH. The effect of suxamethonium on the intragastric pressure in infants and children. Br J Anaesth 1972;44:166.
229. Salem MR, Wong AY, Collins VJ. The pediatric patient with a full stomach. Anesthesiology 1973;39:435.
230. Salem MR, Wong AY, Mani M, et al. Premedicant drugs and gastric juice pH and volume in pediatric patients. Anesthesiology 1976;44:216.
231. Salem MR, Joseph NJ, Heyman HJ, et al. Cricoid compression is effective in obliterating the esophageal lumen in the presence of a nasogastric tube. Anesthesiology 1985;63:443.
232. Salonen M, Kanto J, Iisalo E, Himberg JJ. Midazolam as an induction agent in children: a pharmacokinetic and clinical study. Anesth Analg 1987;66:625.
233. Saxena PR, Dhasmana KM, Prakash O. A comparison of systemic and regional hemodynamic effects of d-tubocurarine, pancuronium and vecuronium. Anesthesiology 1983;59:102.
234. Seebacher J, Nozik D, Matheiu A. Inadvertent intracranial introduction of a nasogastric tube, a complication of severe maxillofacial trauma. Anesthesiology 1975;42:100.
235. Seed RF. Trauma injury to the larnyx and trachea. Anaesthesia 1971;26:55.
236. Seyde WC, Longnecker DE. Anesthetic influences on regional hemodynamics in normal and hemorrhaged rats. Anesthesiology 1984;61:686.
237. Schable DH, Cupit GC, Swedlow DB, et al. High-dose pentobarbital pharmacokinetics in hypothermic brain-injured children. J Pediatrics 1982;100:655.
238. Schieber RA, Namnoum A, Sugden A, et al. Hemodynamic effects of isoflurane in the newborn piglet: comparison with halothane. Anesth Analg 1986;65:633.
239. Schulte-Steinberg O. Neural blockade for pediatric surgery. In: Neural blockade in clinical anesthesia and management of pain. Philadelphia: JB Lippincott, 1980;521.
240. Schwartz L, Rockoff MA, Koka BV. Masseter spasm with anesthesia: incidence and implications. Anesthesiology 1984; 61:772.
241. Scott RPF, Savarese JJ, Basta SJ, et al. Atracurium: clinical strategies for preventing histamine release and attenuating haemodynamic response. Br J Anaesth 1985;57:550.
242. Shapiro HM, Wyte SR, Harris AB. Ketamine anesthesia in patients with intracranial pathology. Br J Anaesth 1972;44:1200.
243. Shapiro LA, Jedeikin RJ, Shalev D, et al. Epidural morphine analgesia in children. Anesthesiology 1984;61:210.
244. Shaver J, Camarata G, Taleisnik A, et al. Changes in epicardial and core temperatures during resuscitation of hemorrhagic shock. J Trauma 1984;24:957.
245. Shogan SH, Kindt GW. Injuries of the head and spinal cord In: Zuidema GD, Rutherford RB, Ballinger WF, eds. The management of trauma. 4th ed. Philadelphia WB Saunders, 1985:169.
246. Siegler RL. Nutritional support. In: Mayer TA, et al. management of pediatric trauma. Philadelphia: WB Saunders, 1985:125.
247. Simbruner G. Inadvertent PEEP in mechanical ventilation of the newborn infant. J Pediatr 1986;108:589.
248. Simon JE, Smookler S, Guy B. A regionalized approach to pediatric critical care. Pediatr Clin North Am 1981;28:677.
249. Singler RC. Pediatric regional anesthesia. In: Gregory GA, ed. Pediatric anesthesia. New York: Churchill Livingstone, 1983:481.
250. Slogoff S, Allen GW, Wessels JV, et al. Clinical experience with subanesthetic ketamine. Anesth Analg 1974;53:356.
251. Smith DF, Hackel A. Selection criteria for pediatric critical transport teams. Crit Care Med 1983;11:1.
252. Steward DJ. Psychological preparation and premedication in pediatric anesthesia. In: Gregory GA, ed. Pediatric anesthesia. New York: Churchill Livingstone, 1983:423.
253. Steward DJ, Creighton RE. Anesthetic management of the injured child. In: Surgical Staff, The Hospital for Sick Children, Toronto, eds. Care of the injured child. Baltimore: Williams & Wilkins, 1975:26.
254. Stiles CM. A flexible fiberoptic bronchoscope for endotracheal intubation in infants. Anesth Analg 1974;52:1017.
255. Stoops CM. Acute hyperkalemia associated with massive blood replacement. Anesth Analg 1983;62:1044.
256. Striker TW. Anesthesia for trauma in the pediatric patient. In:

Gregory GA, ed. Pediatric anesthesia. New York: Churchill Livingstone, 1983:899.
257. Takasaki M, Dohi S, Kawabata Y, et al. Dosage of lidocaine for caudal anesthesia in infants and children. Anesthesiology 1977;47:527.
258. Taylor GA, Fallat ME, Potter BM, Eichelberger MR. The role of computed tomography in blunt abdominal trauma in children. J Trauma 1988;28:1660.
259. Taylor PA, Towey RM. Depression of laryngeal reflexes during ketamine anesthesia. Br Med J 1971;2:688.
260. Templeton JJ, Broennle AM. Emergency department anesthetic management. In: Fleisher G, Ludwig S, eds. Textbook of pediatric emergency medicine. Baltimore: Williams & Wilkins, 1983:43.
261. Templeton JM, O'Neill JA. Pediatric trauma. Emerg Med Clin North Am 1984;2:899.
262. Theye RA, Perry LB, Brzica SM. Influence of anesthetic agent on response to hemorrhagic hypotension. Anesthesiology 1974;40:32.
263. Van Der Spek AFL, Fang WB, Ashton-Miller JA, et al. Increased masticatory muscle stiffness during limb muscle flaccidity associated with succinylcholine administration. Anesthesiology 1988;69:11.
264. Ware JT. Endotracheal drug therapy. Am J Emerg Med 1983;1:72.
265. Warren P, Radford P, Manford MLM. Glycopyrrolate in children. Br J Anaesth 1981;53:1273.
266. Weiskopf RB, Bogetz MS. Cardiovascular actions of nitrous oxide or halothane in hypovolemic swine. Anesthesiology 1985;63:509.
267. Weiskopf RB, Bogetz MS. Haemorrhage decreases the anesthetic requirement for ketamine and thiopentone in the pig. Br J Anaesth 1985;57:1022.
268. Weiskopf RB, Townsley MI, Riordan KK, et al. Comparison of cardiopulmonary responses to graded hemorrhage during enflurane, halothane, isoflurane and ketamine anesthesia. Anesth Analg 1981;60:481.
269. Weiskopf RB, Bogetz MS, Roizen MF, et al. Cardiovascular and metabolic sequellae of inducing anesthesia with ketamine or thiopental in hypovolemic swine. Anesthesiology 1984;60:214.
270. White PF, Schlobohm RM, Pitts LH, et al. A randomized study of drugs for preventing increases in intracranial pressure during endotracheal suctioning. Anesthesiology 1982;57:242.
271. White PF, Way WL, Trevor AJ. Ketamine—its pharmacology and therapeutic uses. Anesthesiology 1982;56:119.
272. Wolf WJ, Neal MB, Peterson MD. The hemodynamic and cardiovascular effects of isoflurane and halothane anesthesia in children. Anesthesiology 1986;64:328.
273. Wong DHW, Jenkins LC. The cardiovascular effects of ketamine in hypotensive states. Can Anaesth Soc J 1975;22:339.
274. Wood M. Plasma drug binding: implications for anesthesiologists. Anesth Analg 1986;65:786.
275. Wyte SR, Shapiro HM, Turner P, et al. Ketamine-induced intracranial hypertension. Anesthesiology 1972;36:174.
276. Yano M, Nishiyama H, Yokota H, et al. Effect of lidocaine on ICP response to endotracheal suctioning. Anesthesiology 1986;64:651.
277. Yaster M, Maxwell LG. Pediatric regional anesthesia. Anesthesiology 1989;70:324.

# Chapter Nineteen

*Sivam Ramanathan*
*Robert M. Porges*

# *Anesthetic Care of the Injured Pregnant Patient*

Trauma has recently become the most frequent cause of maternal death in this country.[178] Although maternal mortality due to other causes, such as infection, hemorrhage, and thromboembolism, has declined over the years, the number of maternal deaths due to suicide, homicide, and motor vehicle accidents has risen steadily (Fig 19-1). Accidental injuries occur in 6–7% of all pregnant patients,[14,55,122,147,155] and in some instances serious injuries threaten both maternal and fetal welfare. Trauma kills more women under age 35 than any other cause.[55] In addition, trauma in pregnancy is becoming increasingly common because socioeconomic factors force more and more pregnant women to work until late in pregnancy.[14]

During the early 1970s, basic deficiencies existed in the ability of the U.S. health care system to render optimal care to injured pregnant patients. The intervening years have seen great improvement not only in the subspecialty disciplines but also in equipment required for management of both high-risk pregnancy and trauma.[121] Management of trauma is unique during pregnancy not only because two lives are at stake but also because the signs, symptoms, patterns, and severity of injury may be altered by pregnancy.[56,91,122] For instance, certain pathologic conditions of pregnancy, such as eclamptic convulsions, may mimic head trauma. Traumatic placental abruption or laceration may cause extensive disseminated intravascular coagulation (DIC).[46,122] A team approach involving obstetricians, trauma surgeons, perinatologists, anesthesiologists, and nursing staff is vital to a satisfactory fetomaternal outcome.[107,121] An obstetrician should always be consulted to follow the course of pregnancy, even when the injury does not involve the reproductive organs.

This chapter is presented in two sections. The first section deals with obstetric and surgical approaches to the injured pregnant patient. The second section, which is divided into two parts, deals with anesthetic evaluation and management.

## OBSTETRIC AND SURGICAL CONSIDERATIONS

If women are pregnant two to three times during a span of 30 years, then the likelihood of pregnancy in any woman between 15 and 45 years of age seen in an emergency department is 6.5 to 7%. Pregnant women may be more prone to accidental trauma because of a shift in the body's center of gravity.[10] Motor vehicle accidents are the major cause of trauma to pregnant women. Falls, burns, firearm injuries, stab wounds, poisoning, or electrocution[8,10,14,46,54,55,71,91,97,101,147,155,178,194] also occur, although less frequently (Table 19-1). Head injury is the commonest cause of death in victims of automobile accidents. The victim with multiple injuries will probably lose the fetus as a result of placental separation, hypovolemic shock, or both. This is particularly true after blunt abdominal trauma sustained in an automobile accident. In a series of 103 cases of blunt abdominal trauma, maternal mortality reached 80% when hypovolemic shock developed.[122] The incidence of pelvic fractures in severely injured automobile accident victims

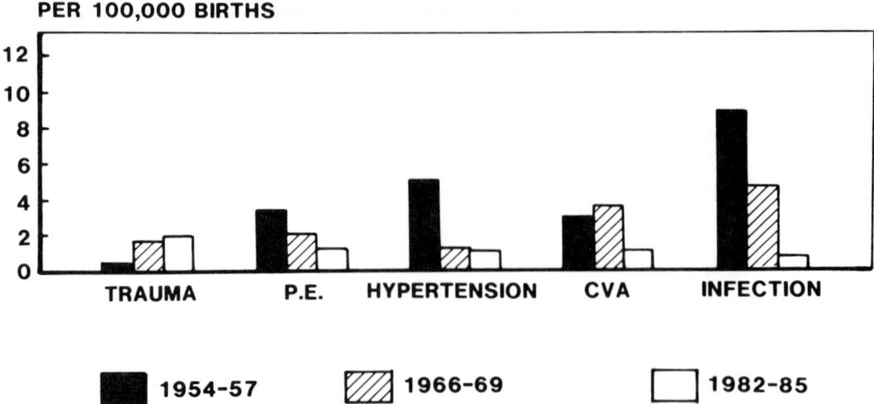


FIG. 19-1. Changing trends in maternal mortality in Massachusetts. Note that trauma has become the leading cause of maternal death. Abbreviations: PE = pulmonary embolism; CVA = cerebro-vascular accident. (From Sachs et al[178] with permission.)

is high, and the majority of pregnant patients with pelvic fractures also sustain placental separation. Fetal loss is generally proportional to the severity of maternal injury.[64a] The most common cause of fetal death is maternal death, followed by placental separation.[54]

Health care professionals should exercise a high degree of suspicion that any injured woman of reproductive age may be pregnant. The date of the last menstrual period (LMP), when available, is helpful. If the data of the LMP is not available or the pregnancy is in the early stages, the diagnosis becomes difficult. Radioimmune assay of the β-subchain of chorionic gonadotropin can be used to diagnose pregnancy before the first missed period. The salient features in the history include previous pregnancies, presence of medical complications, and previous surgery.[91] In the event of life-threatening injuries, all possible diagnostic techniques should be used, without regard to the potential harmful fetal effects of radiation or diagnostic drugs. On the other hand, the abdomen should be protected with lead shields when other parts of the body are being X-rayed.[55] This is especially necessary in women who are not overtly pregnant because fetal tissues are most vulnerable to radiation during early gestation. The number of films taken of the abdomen and pelvis and the dose of radiation should be recorded. This subject is discussed in more detail in the section on diagnostic irradiation in this chapter.

TABLE 19-1. Types of Trauma in Pregnant Women

| TYPE | COMMENTS |
|---|---|
| Automobile | Head injury (traumatic coma) |
| | Rupture of intra- and extrathoracic blood vessels |
| | Rupture of spleen, liver, bowel, uterus |
| | Placental separation |
| | Rib and pelvic fractures |
| | Fetal injuries |
| | Blunt trauma |
| Falls | Multiple fractures |
| | Head injury |
| | Rupture of spleen |
| | Blunt trauma |
| Firearms | Fetal injury |
| | Uterine injury |
| | Abdominal injury |
| | Occasionally self-inflicted |
| Stab wounds | Uterine injury |
| | Fetal injury |
| | Visceral injury |
| Poisoning | Snake bites |
| | Suicide |
| | Accidental ingestion |
| Burns | CO poisoning |
| Suicide | Ante- or postpartum depression |
| Electrocution | Lightning |
| | Burns |
| | Fetal cardiac asystole |
| | Maternal cardiac asystole |

Sources of data: Jeikkenen et al,[104] Aderet et al,[8] Albright et al,[10] Baker,[14] Civil et al,[46] Crosby,[55,56] Edner et al,[71] Haycock H,[91] Neufeld et al,[147] Patterson,[155] Sachs et al,[178] and Sorenson et al.[194]

The initial care of the trauma patient must include assessment of the airway, circulating fluid volume, and fetal welfare. Endotracheal intubation may be needed to establish the airway. During the stabilization period in the emergency department, two intravenous lines must be started: one in the upper and the other in the lower extremity.[91] Using either extremity alone may result in inadequate volume infusion if the subclavian vein or inferior vena cava is injured. In addition, the inferior vena cava may be obstructed by the gravid uterus; thus, lifesaving medications injected into a lower extremity vein during cardiopulmonary resuscitation may not gain rapid access to the central circulation. When the patient is in shock, Ringer's lactate (RL) must be used to restore circulating volume until blood becomes available.[91] *Technical Bulletin 64*, published by the American College of Obstetricians and Gynecologists, recommends the use of tetanus toxoid for women who have not previously been immunized. Tetanus immunoglobulin does not affect the fetus adversely.[37] When using medical antishock trousers (MAST) the abdominal compartment must not be inflated.

## IMMEDIATE MANAGEMENT OF TRAUMA

The algorithm in Fig 19-2 provides guidelines for managing a traumatized pregnant patient. If the mother's condition is stable, the status of the fetus or the extent of the uterine injury will dictate further management. When a viable fetus shows signs of distress despite resuscitative measures, cesarean delivery must be performed immediately. When a premature fetus sustains trauma in utero, a cesarean section (CS) may

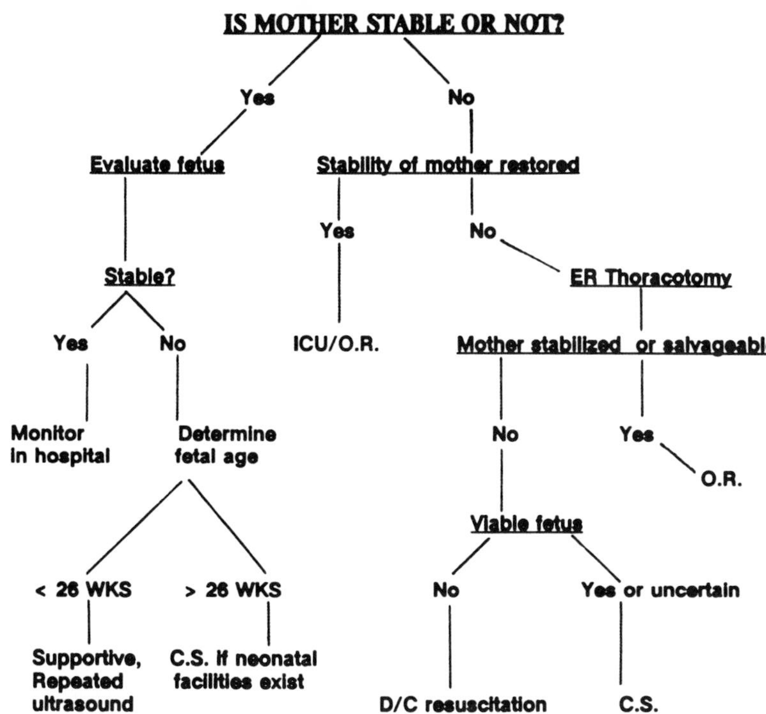


FIG. 19-2. Algorithm for management of trauma and delivery in pregnant patients. Abbreviations: ER = emergency room; CS = cesarean section; D/C = discontinue. (Adapted from Neufeld et al.[147])

be performed to allow repair of neonatal injuries. Unfortunately, the advantages of urgent neonatal surgery are hard to evaluate because of the inability to gauge the severity of fetal injury at the time of first maternal evaluation. Consequently, the benefits of an emergency CS should be weighed carefully against the severity of fetal trauma and the gestational age of the fetus.

A nonviable fetus in distress should be treated conservatively in utero by optimizing maternal oxygenation and circulation.[147] A fetus that shows no signs of distress should be monitored with external ultrasound. Since premature labor is always a threat in these patients, an external tocotransducer must be used to detect the onset of contractions. Should premature labor ensue, β-mimetic therapy may be instituted.

When confronted with a gravely injured mother carrying a viable gestation, the physician must attempt primary repair of all maternal wounds even at the expense of a distressed fetus. The best chances for fetal survival are afforded by restoring normal maternal physiology without delay. Performing cesarean section at the time of surgery for trauma will unnecessarily prolong the operation and increase blood loss. Even when the postoperative condition is critical, the mother who delivers vaginally within 24 hours will tolerate the stress of vaginal delivery better than the stress of prolonged surgery in the immediate posttrauma period.[147] Vaginal delivery in the early postoperative period has not been shown to be deleterious for the mother or the fetus. However, if the maternal condition is stable and if her viable fetus shows signs of distress, cesarean section should be performed. Other reasons for cesarean section include uterine rupture and situations in which the uterus mechanically limits maternal repair. Fetal death is not an indication for cesarean section. Finally, if the mother is not deemed salvageable, a viable fetus should be removed by casarean section in the emergency department.

Active vaginal bleeding demands prompt investigation. It may be due to a heavy menstrual period, expulsion of the products of conception, or trauma to the uterus or the lower birth canal. A pelvic examination should be performed at the earliest opportunity. If the examination discloses a closed cervix and a normal-sized uterus, vaginal bleeding is most likely due to a heavy menstrual period. However, this finding alone does not rule out the possibility of abortion. The approximate amount of vaginal hemorrhage, the passage of any products of conception, and the original size of the uterus should be recorded accurately. Any tissue passed from the vagina should be submitted for pathologic verification, without which the diagnosis of pregnancy cannot be upheld. Despite increased pelvic vascularity, pregnant women are not more likely to sustain injuries to their lower birth canals than nonpregnant subjects. Vaginal lacerations, which may be the source of significant bleeding, may be easily repaired without endangering a pregnancy.

Lower abdominal distension may result from pregnancy or other causes. A distended bladder should be ruled out by catheterization. Monitoring of urinary output is also useful in managing hypovolemic shock. Hematuria may be a sign of pelvic fracture and/or a ruptured uterus. X-ray studies of the pelvis should be performed to detect displaced pelvic bone fragments that may damage the fetus. A nasogastric tube should also be inserted at the earliest opportunity.[121]

A seriously injured woman usually passes through a radiology facility for X-ray studies of her skull, chest, abdomen, and pelvis. This may be the appropriate time for rapid pelvic ultrasonography.[64a] In a matter of minutes, a pregnancy as early as 6 to 8 weeks may be diagnosed by this method. To detect early pregnancies, patients are normally instructed to drink large volumes of water to fill the urinary bladder. The full bladder provides a better sonic window for visualizing the uterus. When a Foley catheter is present in an injured patient, the bladder may be filled rapidly by clamping the catheter for one-half to 1 hour while increasing the rate of intravenous hydration. In urgent situations, the bladder may be filled with normal saline. When the uterus is large enough to be palpated above the pubic symphysis, there is less need for a full bladder.

The usefulness of ultrasonography as a diagnostic tool can hardly be overstated, especially in a patient unable to give a history.[64a] Ultrasound provides an immediate means of (a) establishing the presence of pregnancy, (b) determining whether the fetus is alive or dead, (c) assessing the gestational age, (d) quantitating fetal breathing movements, which are reliable indices of fetal well-being,[78] (e) diagnosing placental abruption,[86] and (f) diagnosing fetal injuries. Edner et al.[71] reported a case in which a bullet that perforated the uterus of the mother also entered the skull of the fetus, inflicting a superficial injury. An ultrasound examination showed the bullet in the fetal skull and also revealed the absence of injury to the fetal brain.

The next logical step in patient evaluation is to determine the presence or absence of major uterine injury. The pregnant uterus is prone to injury because of its size. Absence of vaginal bleeding, lack of amniotic fluid leak (as shown by nitrazine test paper), and presence of a normal fetal heart rate point against major trauma to the uterus and its contents. A perforated uterine wall is almost invariably associated with pain and hemodynamic instability.[55] Surgeons often perform a minilaparotomy to explore the peritoneal cavity for evidence of bleeding or ruptured viscus. The presence of an enlarged uterus may interfere with abdominal exploration, especially in the second trimester. Needle paracentesis may also be less accurate and more dangerous in the second trimester.[121] Rothenberger and colleagues[176] have suggested open peritoneal lavage via a catheter inserted through a supraumbilical incision. Aspiration of 10 mL of blood is considered a positive test. When aspiration is negative, the peritoneal cavity is lavaged with 1000 mL of Ringer's lactate. If the lavage fluid contains an RBC count of 100,000 cells/mm$^3$, WBC count of 500 cells/mm$^3$, or an amylase concentration of 175 U/dL or if the lavage fluid escapes through the Foley catheter or a chest tube, the test is considered positive. By a combination of open lavage, minilaparotomy, and ultrasonography, one should be able to diagnose uterine injury with reasonable accuracy. However, a uterine tear may occasionally be situated between the leaves of the broad ligament, resulting in retroperitoneal hemorrhage that is undetectable by routine diagnostic tests.

Surgical treatment of a ruptured uterus depends on the nature of the rupture. A very small tear of the uterine wall without damage to the amniotic sac may be treated by simple repair. Larger uterine rents result in extrusion of the fetus and placenta into the abdomen. In this case, after removal of the fetus and placenta, the decision must be made whether the uterus should be preserved. Often, the patient's plans for future childbearing will not be known, which may dictate a conservative approach. However, preserving the uterus should not be undertaken at the expense of adequate hemostasis. Uterine rupture at the placental implantation site invariably results in abruption of the placenta and therefore necessitates termination of pregnancy. Bleeding from the torn wall of the gravid uterus may be profuse. The diagnosis of uterine rupture may not be apparent on initial inspection when the classical signs of visceral perforation are absent. On rare occasions, after complete extrusion of its contents, the wall of the uterus may contract sufficiently to control bleeding temporarily from myometrial and placental vessels. Thus, these patients should be followed carefully for at least 48 hours.

Separation, laceration, or abruption of the placenta may result from direct trauma to the uterus.[46] A blunt impact over the placental implantation site may result in formation of a hematoma between the uterine wall and the placenta, leading to complete placental separation. This process is associated not only with immediate fetal death but also with substantial maternal effects. Bleeding from the site of abruption into the uterine wall may cause hypovolemic shock and further damage to the myometrium (Couvelaire uterus). Since the damaged myometrium contracts ineffectively around the blood vessels, the patient may continue to bleed. Placental abruption may also lead to DIC,[147,174] which may predispose to further bleeding. Blunt trauma to the abdomen may also result in injury of the fetal skull and long bones, which is recognizable on X-ray or ultrasound examination. A fetus may be killed by violent external impact, even in the absence of direct injury to the placenta or uterus.[147]

Ordinarily, the timing and mode of delivery of patients with placental abruption depend upon the condition of the fetus and mother. If the fetal heart rate shows no signs of distress and the pregnancy is sufficiently mature, one may allow vaginal delivery to occur, provided that proper facilities for fetal monitoring are available. If the fetus is dead after complete abruption, one may choose to permit vaginal delivery if the patient's condition is stable. However, a primigravida with a very tightly closed cervix may require laparotomy and cesarean section regardless of fetal condition when uterine size increases rapidly. Generally, vaginal delivery is preferable when there are no signs of intra-abdominal bleeding and the fetus is dead.

Although trauma is implicated in many instances of abruption, one must remember the nontraumatic causes. Wide fluctuations of blood pressure, compression of the inferior vena cava by the gravid uterus, uterine anomalies, adenomyosis, sudden decompression of the uterus, and leiomyomas may predispose to abruption. A seriously injured pregnant patient who is unresponsive and lying supine is especially vulnerable to this complication. Certain crush injuries of the lower extremities may also alter intravascular pressures, enhancing placental separation.

Trauma may contribute to the onset of spontaneous labor. Rupture of the membranes usually results in onset of labor within 24 to 48 hours.[147] The more advanced the pregnancy, the greater will be the time lag. If spontaneous labor occurs before the 34th week, one may attempt to inhibit uterine contractions with ritodrine, a beta-sympathomimetic agent.[16] Ritodrine may cause maternal hypertension, cardiac tachyarrhythmias, hyperlactacidemia,[168] hypokalemia, and hyperglycemia.[21,112,162] Subcutaneous or intravenous injection of 0.25 mg of terbutaline may also be used for this purpose.[162]

During the course of treatment of major trauma in the third trimester, one should not overlook the possibility of pre-eclampsia. This complication may have begun before the traumatic event. Accurate diagnosis of pre-eclampsia may be difficult in view of the wide fluctuations of blood pressure, diminished urinary output, and aberrant reflexes caused by the injury. In addition, head injury in a traumatized patient may mimic eclamptic convulsions. Although one must search actively for intracranial bleeding in a trauma victim presenting with convulsions, the possibility of eclampsia should never be overlooked. A computed tomography scan may be useful in differentiating eclampsia from intracranial hematoma. Painful stimuli may induce seizure in eclamptic patients and therefore should be kept to a minimum.

Pregnant women are prone to a variety of other injuries. Urinary tract injuries occur more frequently in pregnant women because the bladder becomes an abdominal organ early in the second trimester. In view of the proximity of the bladder to the lower uterine segment, hematuria may signify trauma to the uterus, as well as to the bladder. Pregnancy increases the risk of spontaneous aortic dissection because of hyperdynamic circulation and increased blood volume, which may also increase the risk of traumatic aortic dissection.[147] Increased intra-abdominal pressure may increase the risk of diaphragmatic herniation. The spleen and liver may be more prone to rupture, especially in women with pre-eclampsia.[147]

## BURNS

Four percent of all women of childbearing age dying of burns are pregnant.[192] Assessing the adequacy of intravenous fluid therapy is difficult in pregnant patients because of pregnancy-induced changes in blood volume and vascular permeability. This difficulty is compounded further by fluid shifts and serum electrolyte abnormalities caused by the burn itself. Respiratory tract burns may result in maternal and fetal hypoxia. Increased maternal carbon monoxide (CO) levels can produce significant CO levels in fetal blood since fetal hemoglobin has a higher affinity for CO than maternal hemoglobin.[192] Secondary infection of burned areas is likely to produce fetal septicemia and death; therefore, judicious antimicrobial therapy must be instituted. Although burns involving less than 40% of the body surface are associated with a maternal mortality less than 3%, burns over 60% are fatal to more than 80% of women.[134] Fetal mortality ranges from 17 to 27% in burns involving 40% of maternal body surface area and exceeds 50% when the burned area covers more than half of the body surface.[134] Severe burns and accompanying sepsis are associated with high maternal blood levels of arachidonic acid (prostaglandin precursors), which may cause premature labor.[192] Uterine activity should therefore be monitored by external transducers. Tocolytic therapy with ritodrine may be instituted if the patient's condition is stable. If the burn involves less than 30% of body surface area, attempts should be made to treat the mother adequately while using tocolytic therapy to supress premature labor.[134] When thermal injury involves greater than 30% of the body surface, obstetric intervention should be considered within the first 24 hours if the gestational age exceeds 26 weeks.[134,192]

## DIAGNOSTIC IRRADIATION

The diagnostic irradiation that is vital to the care of a traumatized patient may be teratogenic.[73,143] The most frequent abnormalities that may result from irradiation are mental retardation, microphthalmos, pigmentary degeneration of the retina, genital and skeletal malformations, and cataracts. A radiation dose as small as 5–15 rads is known to cause fetal death in early murine pregnancy. Most human organogenesis is complete at 16 weeks of gestation. However, the central nervous system (CNS) may be damaged even after 16 weeks. Neuroblasts are found in the human from about 16 days postconception until about 2 weeks after birth. They can be destroyed by a 25-rad exposure. A woman who was exposed to intense irradiation from an atomic bomb explosion in late pregnancy is known to have delivered a spastic child.

Most human data are collected from patients after exposure to therapeutic rather than diagnostic radiation. Studies in mice show that when the radiation dose does not exceed 10 rads, the anomaly rate is not distinguishable from background. At 20 rads, the incidence of malformations is definitely increased. Diagnostic X-ray studies in which the pregnant uterus is not in the direct path of the beam do not expose the fetus to appreciable irradiation if appropriate beam columnation and pelvic shielding are used.[64a] When studies that may expose the uterus to direct irradiation—X-rays of the pelvis, hips, lumbar spine, sacrum, and abdomen—are required, the number of views and exposures must be limited. Intravenous pyelogram, cystogram, and pelvic angiography may also occasionally be needed. During angiography, fluoroscopy must be kept to a minimum. The use of video playback equipment may allow more viewing time and thus minimize exposure to as little as 2 rads per examination. The possible exception is angiography for pelvic hemorrhage, in which the dose may exceed 5 rads. In view of the seriousness of this condition, the study must be performed and the patient be informed of the possible risk to the fetus. Contrast media used for angiography do not affect the fetus adversely.[147]

When computed tomography (CT) is needed, a dosimeter can be placed directly on the maternal abdomen to measure the skin dose. During CT exposures, the dose is approximately 3 rads to any volume of tissue that is irradiated directly. During the scan the patient should be moved in such a way that there is no overlap of adjacent slices. Some recommend small gaps between tissue slices during exposure. Myelograms may be avoided by the use of a CT scan. A small dose of intrathecal metrizimide may be used to provide contrast. Whatever the study, an accurate record of all X-ray doses must be kept for future reference.

The National Council on Radiation Protection (NCRP-Report #39) has published guidelines for the maximum permissible dose (MPD) for pregnant patients. The fetal MPD is 0.5 rem. The MPD for adult workers is 5 rem per year. Radiation from protons, neutrons, or alpha particles is more damaging than the same dosage from gamma rays or X-rays.

## CARDIOPULMONARY RESUSCITATION

A traumatized pregnant patient may require cardiopulmonary resuscitation (CPR) in the emergency department or in the operating room. CPR of a pregnant woman is unique not only because two lives are at stake but also because pregnancy itself influences management decisions since (a) cardiorespiratory physiology changes, (b) the supine position may introduce problems, (c) the fetus faces severe hypoxic complications, (d) a perimortem cesarean section may be needed to save the mother and/or the fetus, and (e) the neonate may require resuscitation.[122]

### Cardiorespiratory Physiology

Maternal cardiac output, blood volume, alveolar ventilation, and oxygen consumption increase during pregnancy. During apnea the pregnant patient's $PaO_2$ decreases rapidly. From early in the second trimester, the classic signs of hypovolemia, such as vasoconstriction and clammy skin, may be absent, necessitating central venous pressure (CVP) monitoring to manage hypovolemic arrest. Decreased functional residual capacity (FRC), the presence of enlarged breasts, congestion of the tracheal mucous membranes, and narrowing of the glottis may interfere with airway management and external cardiac massage (ECM). The placenta changes maternal circulation to a high flow-low resistance circuit sensitive to perfusion pressure. So long as blood $PO_2$ and pH remain within normal limits, the placenta offers only limited resistance to blood flow.[122] However, should these values decrease, placental vascular resistance increases.[122] The evidence for an increased flow requirement comes from fetal heart tracings obtained during open-heart surgery. Higher than conventional flow rates and perfusion pressures are required to maintain a normal fetal heart pattern during cardiopulmonary bypass.[119,162]

### Supine Position

The gravid uterus compresses both the aorta and the inferior vena cava (IVC). Aortocaval compression intensifies fetal acidosis. During CPR, the uterus should be shifted to the left by wedging a sandbag under the right hip. Animal experimentation has shown that the difficulty of CPR is increased by IVC compression.[108] Since the aorta may be compressed by the gravid uterus, an absent femoral pulse should not be taken as indicative of inefficient ECM.

### Fetal Hazard

Even a brief interruption in uterine blood flow affects the fetal condition. Whereas prolonged maternal cardiac arrest results in fetal death, inadequate oxygenation during resuscitation may result in neurologic sequelae or physical abnormalities in the growing fetus. Excessive administration of vasopressor agents during CPR can cause uteroplacental vasoconstriction.[122] The sensitivity of the alpha receptors in the uteroplacental circulation is augmented during maternal acidosis. The only method of assessing the adequacy of fetal oxygenation during CPR is to monitor the fetal heart rate (FHR). Carotid pulse and end-tidal $CO_2$ monitoring may be used to assess the adequacy of maternal vital organ perfusion during CPR. An end-tidal $CO_2$ of 1.5 to 1.8% usually signifies effective external cardiac compression.[83]

### Emergency Cesarean Section

When CPR does not generate a carotid pulse or adequate end-tidal $CO_2$ or when it fails to maintain an adequate fetal heart rate, a CS must be performed immediately. Delivering the baby offers the following advantages. It improves maternal cardiac filling, thereby improving the possibility of successful CPR; ECM is performed more effectively after the baby is born; it gives the fetus a chance of survival in case maternal CPR fails; and it diminishes fetal exposure to drugs administered during CPR. The longer the delay between the onset of arrest and delivery, the less are the chances of fetal and maternal survival. If, however, ECM appears to be effective, it may be continued for 8–10 minutes. If a spontaneous pulse is not restored within this time, emergency CS must be performed. Should the CS fail to revive the mother, open chest massage (OCM) is indicated.[122] OCM is particularly useful in patients who have sustained hypovolemic cardiac arrest from trauma, placenta previa, placental abruption, ruptured uterus, pericardial tamponade, or tension pneumothorax.[122]

When the gestation is less than 24 weeks, emergency CS is usually not performed because the fetus is too small to survive and the delivery is unlikely to have any significant impact on maternal cardiovascular dynamics.[122] However, in gestations greater than 25 weeks, emergency CS is likely to affect maternal and/or fetal survival favorably. Guidelines for managing patients with gestation between 26–32 weeks differ from those for managing patients with gestation more than 32 weeks. In the former group, one must seriously consider OCM before performing emergency CS. Should OCM prove successful, delivery may be delayed so that fetal viability improves. Even a slight prolongation of intrauterine life is likely to improve the chances of fetal survival, especially when the gestation is less than 28 weeks. If, however, OCM proves to be ineffective, the fetus must be delivered forthwith.[122] An algorithm for CPR management in pregnant patients is presented in Fig 19-3.

### CPR Procedure

Since the actual technique of CPR in pregnant patients is similar to that in nonpregnant patients, only those aspects that differ are discussed in this section. Chest thump and external cardiac compression are done in the usual manner.[122] Tracheal intubation is preferred to other means of airway management because of the increased risk of aspiration during pregnancy. An endotracheal tube no larger than 7.0 or 7.5 mm should be used. The endotracheal tube can also be used for tracheal instillation of epinephrine (1–2 mg in 10 mL normal saline) when an intravenous line is not available.[127] Epinephrine must be used regardless of its effects on uteroplacental blood flow because of its beneficial actions on maternal circulation.[40] An external Doppler device or a real-time echo instrument must be used to monitor the FHR.

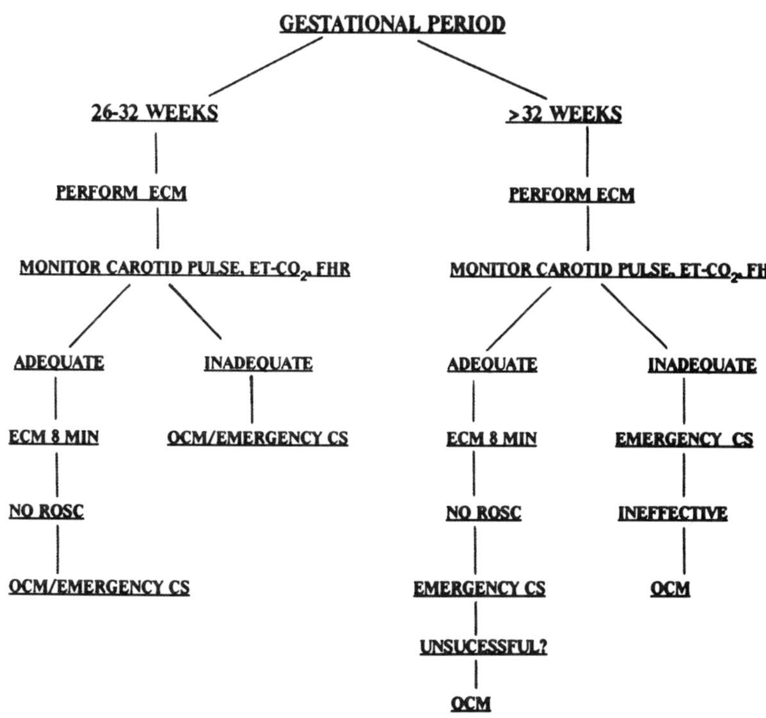


FIG. 19-3. Algorithm for management of cardiopulmonary resuscitation in pregnant patients. Abbreviations: ECM = external cardiac massage; OCM = open cardiac massage; ET-$CO_2$ = end-tidal $CO_2$; ROSC = return of spontaneous circulation; FHR = fetal heart rate; CS = cesarean section. (Adapted from Lee et al.[122])

In pregnancy, the $PaCO_2$ is normally 32–34 mm Hg, a fact to be remembered when ventilation parameters are evaluated. Excessive hyperventilation will diminish uteroplacental blood flow. To prevent acidosis-induced vasoconstriction, an arterial pH of 7.3 or less should be corrected.[122] The need for sodium bicarbonate administration must be assessed by frequent arterial blood gas measurements. Excessive sodium bicarbonate must be avoided since metabolic alkalosis will compromise fetal oxygenation further by causing a leftward shift of the oxyhemoglobin dissociation curve. External DC cardioversion has been safely done in pregnant patients without electrical hazard to the fetus. However, the FHR must be monitored closely immediately after application of the shock or after administration of beta-blockers, vasoactive agents, or calcium channel blocking agents.

Recently, it has been proposed that the mechanism by which external cardiac compression produces blood flow to the brain is related to increased intrathoracic pressure.[177] Animal experiments have shown that maneuvers that increase intrathoracic pressure deliver higher carotid flow to the brain than conventional ECM.[23,177] These maneuvers include simultaneous chest compression and ventilation (SCV-CPR), the use of abdominal binders during ECM, and abdominal counterpulsation. Of these, abdominal binding and counterpulsation are not practical in patients with advanced gestation. The use of these newer methods of CPR has not been investigated in pregnant women, and therefore, they should be attempted only when all other methods of reviving the mother have failed. Occasionally the fetus may sustain cardiac arrest in utero. If the diagnosis of fetal asystole is made in time, external massage of the fetal heart may be performed by digital pressure through the maternal abdomen until arrangements can be made for delivery.[149]

## PERIMORTEM CESAREAN SECTION

Since time immemorial, perimortem cesarean sections have been performed to save the fetus. Numa Pompilus of Rome (715 BC) decreed that the fetus must be removed from a dead woman before she was buried. Julius Caesar himself was said to have been extricated from his dead mother; hence derived the name of the procedure. Katz et al.[110] reviewed 188 cases of perimortem deliveries in the years between 1879 and 1985. A fetus delivered within 5 minutes of maternal death has the best chance of survival. The longer the delay between maternal death and delivery, the smaller is the likelihood of fetal survival and normal neurologic outcome. Koppe et al.[115] reviewed the outcomes of 54 infants who were born severely asphyxiated. They found that normal neurologic outcome is possible in infants in whom 15–30 minutes were required to restore spontaneous respiration after delivery. This indicates the resistance of the fetal brain to hypoxic damage and the enormous resilience that the neonatal brain possesses. After 30 minutes, the outlook for survival, as well as normal neurologic outcome, becomes dismal. Consequently, in the event of maternal demise after the 28th week of gestation, a perimortem cesarean section should be performed at the earliest opportunity.[55,110,121] Although some consultation with family members is desirable, the absence of consultation should not deter the performance of the procedure.

## ANESTHETIC CONSIDERATIONS

In an attempt to keep pace with the demands of the growing fetus, every physiologic system of the mother undergoes significant changes.[56] The fetus is totally dependent on the mother for its oxygen supply. However, maintaining adequate maternal $PaO_2$ alone will not guarantee adequate fetal oxygenation. Meticulous attention should thus be paid to maintenance of an adequate uteroplacental blood flow. Proper anesthetic management of a pregnant woman requires a thorough understanding of the physiologic demands of pregnancy, the mechanisms of transplacental respiratory gas transfer, optimization of fetal oxygenation, and the potential harmful effects of the commonly used anesthetic and nonanesthetic agents. In this section changes in maternal physiology and the way they relate to anesthetic management are reviewed.

### CHANGES IN MATERNAL PHYSIOLOGY

#### *Cardiovascular System*

The changes in the cardiovascular system are important to the anesthesiologist.[32,33,132,133,204] The heart is displaced upward and shifted to the left and anteriorly. The cardiac size may be increased due both to hypertrophy and dilation, resulting in left axis deviation and nonspecific ST-segment changes on the ECG. Other ECG changes may include Q waves in leads III and AVF. Echocardiography reveals increased left ventricular end-diastolic volume. Premature atrial and ventricular contractions occur more frequently in pregnant than in nonpregnant patients. Both heart rate and stroke volume increase from early in the first trimester and reach a peak at 28–32 weeks (Fig 19–4). Two types of functional murmurs may be heard: a pulmonary midsystolic murmur and a supraclavicular systolic murmur produced by blood flow in the brachiocephalic trunks.[120]

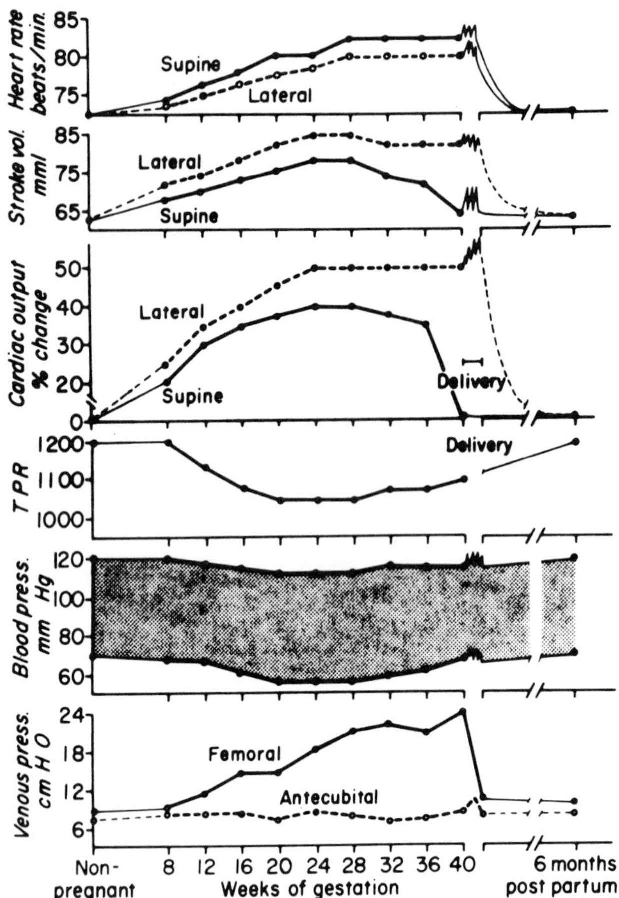


FIG. 19-4. Heart rate, cardiac output, total peripheral resistance (TPR), blood pressure, and venous pressure changes in pregnancy. Note that cardiac output is lower and heart rate is higher in lateral than in supine position because of compression of the inferior vena cava in the supine position by the gravid uterus. Fluctuation in hemodynamic parameters during labor is due to labor pains. (From Bonica[33] with permission.)

#### *Blood Volume Changes*

Plasma volume and red and white blood cell (RBC and WBC) volumes increase from the middle of the first trimester and peak during the early third trimester.[32–34,126,132,133] The increase in plasma volume is greater than that in RBC mass, which results in physiologic anemia (Fig 19-5). The specific gravities of whole blood and plasma are reduced, and blood viscosity declines approximately 12%. Despite the increase in blood volume, there is no evidence of circulatory overload. Central venous pressure (CVP) remains unaltered. In a healthy gravida, the CVP will rise from 8 to only 10 cm $H_2O$ after infusion of 1 L of crystalloid solution in 20 minutes. The increased blood volume not only facilitates transplacental gas exchange but also enables the parturient to tolerate the substantial blood loss that she is likely to incur during delivery. Hemodilution and augmented renal function decrease the serum concentrations of blood urea nitrogen (BUN), creatinine, and glucose.[126] There is a net gain of sodium, potassium, calcium, and water in pregnancy.[17,60,130] Both intra- and extracellular water compartments increase in size, with a slightly greater increase in the intracellular compartment.[130]

The increase in plasma volume accounts for only 20–25% of the increase in extracellular fluid (ECF); the remainder is due to an increase in the interstitial fluid compartment. The gain in water and electrolytes in different body compartments is shown in Table 19-2.

#### *Aortocaval Compression*

After 20 to 24 weeks of gestation, the gravid uterus may compress both the inferior vena cava and the aorta (Fig 19-6). Inferior vena caval compression occurs in over 90% of term pregnant patients and may reduce venous return to the heart and thereby the maternal cardiac output.[111] The vertebral venous plexus, which drains into the azygous vein, provides collateral circulation when the inferior vena cava is obstructed.[33] The lower aorta and its branches may be compressed and shifted to the left,[4] decreasing uteroplacental blood flow. The renal blood flow is also reduced, affecting the glomerular filtration rate.

The supine position thus causes profound changes in maternal hemodynamics (Fig 19-7). Cardiac output, systemic

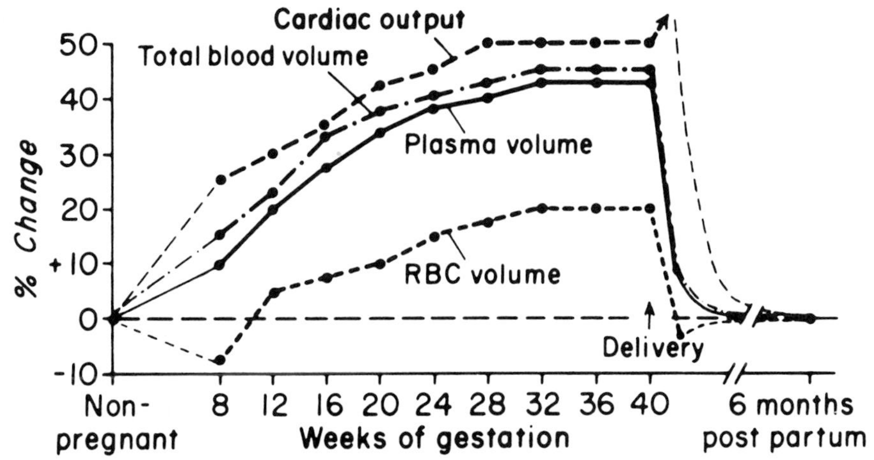


FIG. 19-5. Cardiac output, plasma volume, and RBC volume changes in pregnancy. Note that in early pregnancy, the RBC volume tends to decrease before it starts increasing and that the increase in plasma volume is greater than the increase in RBC, resulting in physiologic anemia. (From Bonica[33] with permission.)

blood pressure, and pulmonary blood volume decrease in this position.[65,183] The patient compensates by increasing her peripheral vascular resistance (vasoconstriction) and/or her heart rate. This compensatory mechanism is capable of maintaining systemic pressure in 70% of patients. In the rest, arterial pressure decreases and the patient may faint, especially when collaterals are not well developed. When sympathetic tone is reduced by regional block, a more profound and precipitous reduction in cardiac output occurs because of reduced compensatory vasoconstriction. Bienarz et al.[27] showed that, although brachial and femoral artery pressures are equal in the supine normotensive patient, the femoral systolic pressure falls 20 mm Hg below the brachial pressure in the presence of hypotension, signifying increased aortic compression.

ANESTHETIC IMPLICATIONS. The increase in blood volume, together with the presence of peripheral vasodilation, makes the detection of hypovolemia difficult in traumatized pregnant patients in the second and third trimesters. Classical signs of hypovolemia, such as peripheral venous constriction and cold and clammy skin, may not be present in pregnant patients until volume loss is severe.[91] Positional hypotension may mimic hypovolemia. The normal increase in the maternal heart rate may introduce errors in assessing the adequacy of the circulating volume. ECG changes resulting from pregnancy may be confused with those produced by myocardial contusion.[91] Physiologic anemia may be confused with that produced by hemorrhage in a patient who has sustained trauma. When doubt exists about the circulating fluid volume, a CVP catheter must be used.

The following precautions should be taken to minimize aortocaval compression. Patients should be prophylactically hydrated with crystalloid solutions before regional or general anesthesia is administered, a noncompressible sandbag should be wedged under the right hip to displace the uterus 15° to the left during anesthesia; and femoral arterial pressure may be used as a guideline to assess the degree of aortic compression.[70]

TABLE 19-2. Fluid and Electrolyte Gain in Pregnancy

| TISSUE OR FLUIDS | GRAM | WATER (L) | Na+ (mmol) | K+ (mmol) |
|---|---|---|---|---|
| Fetus | 3400 | 2.0 | 290 | 155 |
| Placenta | 650 | 0.3 | 60 | 40 |
| Uterus | 800 | 1.2 | 100 | 5 |
| Breasts | 405 | 0.4 | 30 | 40 |
| Plasma volume | 250 | 1.25 | 150 | 60 |
| Interstitial fluid | 1680 | 1.68 | 240 | 10 |
| Maternal fat | 3345 | — | — | — |
| Totals (approximate) | 12,500 | 7.53 | 950 | 360 |

### *Respiratory System*

The nasopharynx, the larynx, the trachea, and the bronchi may appear reddened and swollen because of capillary engorgement. The glottic opening may be narrower than in nonpregnant subjects. The vertical dimension of the chest decreases while anteroposterior and transverse diameters increase due to rib flaring.[32,33,132,133] Because of increased pulmonary blood volume, lung markings are increased, simulating mild congestive heart failure. Tidal volume, respiratory rate, minute ventilation, and alveolar ventilation increase starting early in pregnancy (Fig 19-8, Table 19-3), whereas dead space remains unchanged. Residual volume, expiratory reserve volume, and functional residual capacity (FRC) decrease consistently. Closing capacity (CC) and closing volume remain unaltered.[15,52] However, the difference between FRC and CC is reduced, which may predispose to ventilation-perfusion abnormalities. At an $F_{IO_2}$ of 1, the mean $PaO_2$ of a term pregnant patient is 60–70 mm Hg lower than that of a nonpregnant female.[164]

Because of increased alveolar ventilation, the $PaCO_2$ falls to 33–35 mm Hg by the third month of pregnancy and remains at that level until delivery.[33] Arterial pH increases slightly. Plasma $HCO_3^-$ and base excess decrease as a result of increased renal bicarbonate excretion to compensate for the respiratory alkalosis.

ANESTHETIC IMPLICATIONS. Because of diminished FRC, $O_2$ stores in the lungs are decreased. In the presence of increased total body oxygen consumption ($\dot{V}O_2$), decreased $O_2$ stores imply that the rate and magnitude of decrease in $PaO_2$ in an apneic pregnant patient are greater than in nonpregnant

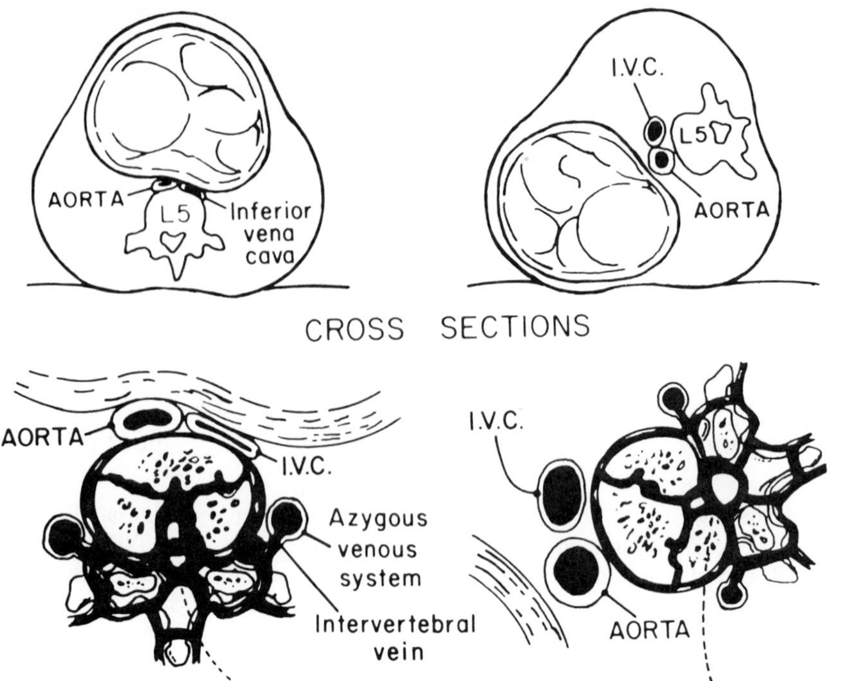


FIG. 19-6. Compression of the aorta and inferior vena cava (IVC) by the gravid uterus. Note that both blood vessels are compressed against the 5th lumbar vertebra, the vertebral venous plexus is distended in the supine position because it provides collateral circulation, and the plexus is less distended in the lateral position because the IVC compression is relieved. (From Bonica[33] with permission.)

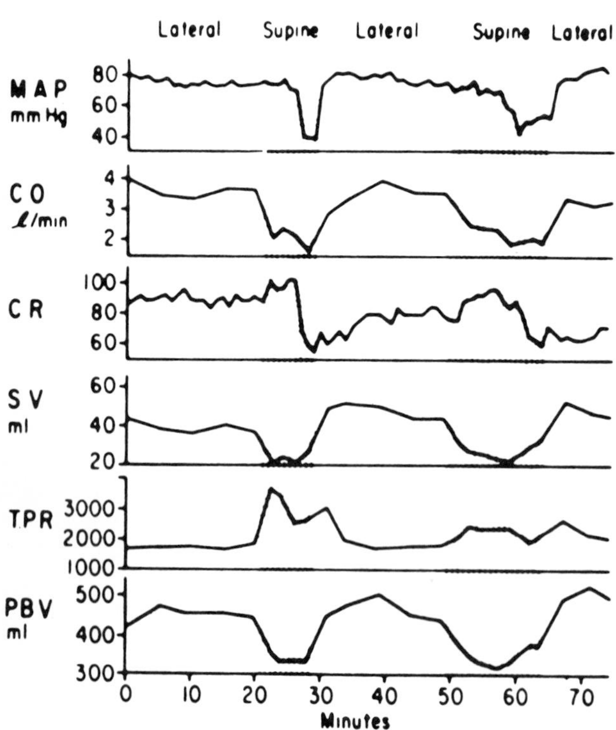


FIG. 19-7. Hemodynamic effects of supine position in late pregnancy. The compensatory increase in CR and TPR maintained MAP for a short period of time, following which the patient developed a marked hypotension. Abbreviations: MAP = mean arterial pressure; CO = cardiac output; CR = cardiac rate; SV = stroke volume; TPR = total peripheral resistance; PBV = pulmonary blood volume. Note the reduction in MAP, CO, SV, and PBV in supine position. (Adapted from Scott[183] with permission.)

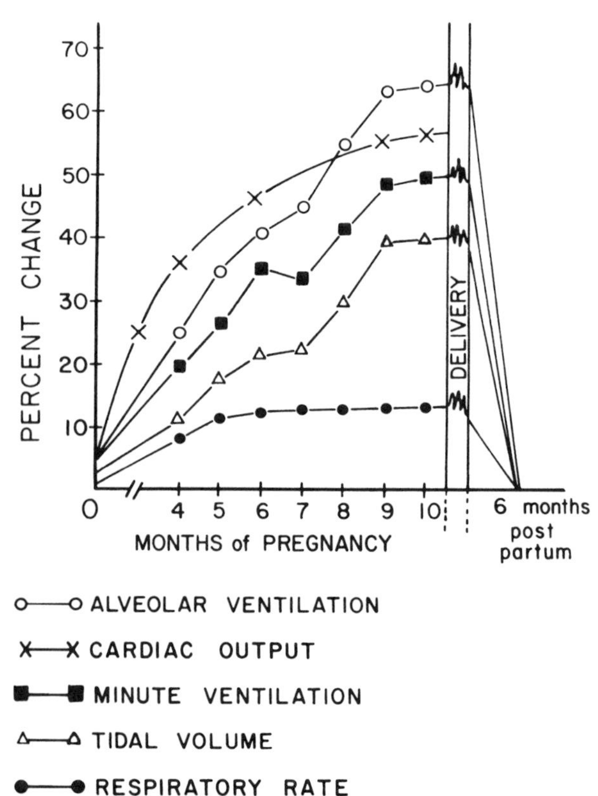


FIG. 19-8. Pregnancy-induced changes in some respiratory parameters. Note that changes begin to occur very early in pregnancy and that the increase in minute ventilation is mainly due to increased tidal volume. (From Bonica[32] with permission.)

TABLE 19-3. Summary of Pregnancy-Induced Changes in Lung Function Measurements

| MEASUREMENT | CHANGE | % CHANGE OVER NONPREGNANT |
|---|---|---|
| Minute ventilation | Increased | 50 |
| Dead space | No change | 0 |
| Alveolar ventilation | Increased | 70 |
| Respiratory rate | Increased | 40 |
| Tidal volume | Increased | 40 |
| Airway resistance | Decreased | 36 |
| Lung compliance | No change | 0 |
| Chest wall compliance | Decreased | 45 |
| Expiratory reserve volume | Decreased | 20 |
| Residual volume | Decreased | 20 |
| Functional residual capacity | Decreased | 20 |
| Closing volume and closing capacity | No change | 0 |

patients.[133] Pregnant patients should inhale 100% oxygen to denitrogenate the lungs for at least 5 minutes before induction of general anesthesia. This will minimize the risk of hypoxia during endotracheal intubation. Maternal exposure to increased $F_{IO_2}$ for a few hours will not produce harmful fetal effects, such as premature closure of the ductus arteriosus.[104] Although the increased cardiac output of the pregnant patient would normally slow the uptake of inhalation agents, this effect is counteracted by diminished FRC and increased alveolar ventilation, with the net result that anesthetic uptake is more rapid.[133]

Because of capillary engorgement, nasal intubation may be hazardous and must be resorted to only when absolutely essential. Proper precautions, such as pretreating the nasal mucosa with phenylephrine or cocaine, should be taken before attempting nasal intubation.[100] The hypocarbia of pregnancy must be remembered when adjusting respiratory parameters.

### *Gastrointestinal System*

The stomach and intestines are progressively displaced cephalad by the enlarging uterus. In addition, the stomach may be divided into antral and fundal pouches, preventing proper mixture of antacids within the stomach.[9,93] Intragastric pressure rises during pregnancy, with further elevation occurring in lithotomy and Trendelenburg positions.[195] Lind et al.[125] noted that, although the pressure gradient between stomach and esophagus was normal in pregnant patients without heartburn, it was significantly lower in patients with heartburn because of the decreased competence of the gastroesophageal sphincter.[125] This alteration in pressure gradient predisposes to esophageal reflux. Although the total quantity of both basal and histamine-stimulated acid output decreases in midpregnancy, it increases to greater than nonpregnant levels toward term.[145]

Wald[208] showed that, during the third trimester, the gastrointestinal transit time is prolonged, probably as a result of increased progesterone levels. During labor, there is further prolongation of gastric emptying time. Davison et al.[61] noted that pregnant patients with heartburn have prolonged gastric emptying time compared to controls. Other factors contribute to the prolongation of gastric emptying time in hospitalized trauma victims: pain and anxiety, sedatives and analgesics, and abdominal injury.

ANESTHETIC IMPLICATIONS. The above-mentioned factors put the traumatized pregnant patient at increased risk of pulmonary aspiration of gastric contents. The most reliable way of preventing aspiration (if a general anesthetic is required) is a rapid sequence induction followed by endotracheal intubation while cricoid pressure is applied to occlude the esophagus. Inhalational anesthesia administered through a face mask without endotracheal intubation definitely carries the risk of aspiration of gastric contents after the 20th week of pregnancy. Before this time, the pregnant patient may not be at increased risk if she has fasted for at least 10 hours.[215] It is generally accepted that a gastric fluid pH of 2.5 or less and a gastric fluid volume of 25 mL or more increase the risk of acid aspiration syndrome in hospitalized patients.[131] Several studies have shown that judged by these criteria 60–90% of all surgical patients are at risk.[50,131,171,180,206,210]

Prophylactic use of antacids or $H_2$-blockers, such as cimetidine or ranitidine, is effective in elevating gastric fluid pH and decreasing the volume of gastric fluid.[50,68,79,128] The currently recommended oral antacid is sodium citrate.[206] Fifteen to 30 mL of 0.3 M sodium citrate administered 30 minutes before induction of anesthesia is effective in elevating gastric fluid pH.[206] Water-soluble antacids are preferred to particulate preparations containing magnesium hydroxide or aluminum hydroxide because pulmonary aspiration of particulate antacid is associated with severe pneumonitis. Cimetidine should be used with caution in patients with bronchial asthma because it may precipitate bronchospasm due to the unopposed action of $H_1$-receptors in the bronchial wall.[146] Parenteral administration of cimetidine may also precipitate cardiac arrhythmias or cardiac arrest by its action on myocardial $H_2$-receptors.[28,48,184] A single dose of cimetidine is known to reduce propranolol metabolism.[75] Cimetidine is also known to prolong postoperative somnolence.[118] Another $H_2$-blocker, ranitidine, is believed to lack enzyme-inducing properties. A 50-mg injection of ranitidine will maintain a high gastric fluid pH and a low gastric fluid volume for 6–8 hours.[58] An oral dose of 150 mg offers protection for 10–12 hours. The drug has received only limited trial in pregnant patients.[36]

Cimetidine crosses the placental barrier and attains significant levels in fetal blood.[92] Caution must be exercised in using this drug in early pregnancy because its fetal effects are not completely known. Metoclopramide, a dopamine antagonist that accelerates gastric emptying and increases lower esophageal sphincter tone, may be beneficial in reducing the risk of aspiration.[215] The drug crosses the placenta and has undergone only a limited clinical trial.[39] Its fetal effects are unknown at this time; therefore it is best avoided in early pregnancy. In addition, the use of intravenous metroclopramide may cause systemic hypotension, especially in hypovolemic patients.[154] Belladonna agents, such as atropine and glycopyrrolate, affect gastric fluid pH negligibly.[199]

It should be emphasized that none of these agents is totally reliable in lowering gastric volume or increasing the pH of the gastric contents. Rapid sequence induction is still required for any nonelective general anesthetic.

Practical guidelines for prevention of aspiration pneumonitis are summarized in Table 19-4.

### Blood Coagulation

Blood is hypercoagulable in pregnancy. The serum fibrinogen concentration increases from 300 mg/dL to over 480 mg/dL.[35] A progressive rise in serum fibrin degradation products is also seen in the third trimester (Friedman S, Ramathan S, unpublished data).[133] Platelet count remains unchanged, but concentrations of factor VII, VIII, IX, and X are increased.[133,174] Concentrations of factor XI and XIII decrease. Prothrombin time, partial thromboplastin time, bleeding time, and clotting time remain within normal limits.

Maximum amplitude and r and k times of the thrombelastogram remain within normal limits. Although the plasminogen level itself remains unchanged,[216] the activity of plasminogen activator is decreased and that of plasminogen inhibitor is increased, resulting in delayed fibrinolysis.[35,133] Pregnancy-induced changes in coagulation factors are summarized in Table 19-5.[174]

ANESTHETIC IMPLICATIONS. Placental laceration or abruption produced by abdominal trauma may lead to DIC and/or hypofibrinogenemia. When evaluating these conditions the clinician must remember the elevated fibrinogen level in pregnancy.[46,122] A fibrinogen concentration of 300 mg%, although normal for a nonpregnant patient, may signify coagulopathy in a pregnant patient.

Thromboembolic complications are more frequent in pregnancy.[35] Precautions to minimize deep vein thrombosis (DVT) must be instituted without delay.

### Renal Function and Sodium and Water Balance

The renal pelvis and calices dilate together with the ureters because of increased progesterone.[17,24,60,133] This effect begins early in pregnancy and may persist as late as 12 weeks after delivery. The glomerular filtration rate (GFR) and renal plasma flow (RPF) increase 60% and 30%, respectively, with the result that BUN and creatinine decrease.[24]

The increase in GFR and RPF cause increased natriuresis in pregnancy. Increased concentrations of progesterone, arginine-vasopressin (AVP), melanocyte-stimulating hormone (MSH), and prostaglandins produce further natriuresis. Thus, approximately 20,000–30,000 mmol/24 h of sodium may be filtered through the kidneys in a pregnant woman. If all the filtered sodium were to be excreted in the urine, the pregnant subject would develop circulatory collapse rapidly. Sodium must therefore be reabsorbed by the renal tubules. Indeed, the pregnant patient retains a net of 4–6 mmol/day of sodium, which is stored in both fetal and maternal compartments. This increase in renal tubular sodium reabsorption is perhaps the single most important change in renal function during pregnancy.[17,60] It is caused by elevated levels of aldosterone, deoxycorticosterone acetate, prostaglandins, and estrogens and increased activity of the renin-angiotensin system. The factors that cause increased sodium filtration or reabsorption are shown in Table 19-6.

TABLE 19-4. Prevention of Aspiration

| |
|---|
| Use regional anesthesia whenever possible |
| Use endotracheal anesthesia—rapid sequence induction with cricoid pressure. Do not use mask anesthesia. |
| If time permits, use two-dose cimetidine regimen: 300 mg PO hs the previous night and 300 mg IM 1 hour before induction, in late pregnancy. |
| For urgent surgery, use sodium citrate 15–30 mL PO one-half hour before surgery. Use sodium citrate in early pregnancy. |
| Use caution during extubation. Wait for full recovery of laryngeal reflexes before extubation. |

TABLE 19-5. Coagulation Changes in Pregnancy

| | |
|---|---|
| Fibrinogen | 4.0–6.5 g/L |
| Factor II | 100–125% |
| Factor V | 100–150% |
| Factor VII | 150–250% |
| Factor VIII | 200–500% |
| Factor IX | 100–150% |
| Factor X | 150–250% |
| Factor XI | 50–100% |
| Factor XII | 100–200% |
| Factor XIII | 35–75% |
| Antithrombin III | 75–100% |
| Antifactor Xa | 75–100% |
| Plasminogen activator | Decreased |
| Plasminogen inhibitor | Increased |

### Water Balance in Pregnancy

Plasma osmolarity (P-osm) decreases 8–10 mosm/L in pregnancy.[17,60] Only a small fraction of this reduction is due to reduced blood urea levels. A reduction in P-osm of this magnitude induces diuresis in nonpregnant subjects. The fact that polyuria does not occur in pregnant subjects makes it likely that the osmotic thresholds for both thirst and vasopressin release are set at levels 10 mosm lower than in nonpregnant subjects. Ability to excrete a fluid load is also impaired in pregnancy.

### Body Fluids and Intravenous Therapy

Given a liter of water to drink, the pregnant patient will reduce her osmolarity 10 mosm/L just like a nonpregnant patient,

TABLE 19-6. Factors Affecting Sodium Balance in Pregnancy

| FACTORS INCREASING Na+ FILTRATION | FACTORS INCREASING Na+ REABSORPTION |
|---|---|
| Renal plasma flow | Na-K ATPase |
| Glomerular filtration | Deoxycorticosterone |
| Progesterone | Prostaglandin (vasodilation) |
| Prostaglandin | Renin-angiotensin system |
| Arginine-vasopressin | Increased ureteral pressure |
| | Supine-upright posture |
| | Prolactin, estrogen |

but this value will return to the usual level of 280 mosm/L within 2 hours.[60] The excess water is eliminated by increased diuresis in the first trimester. However, during the last trimester, the volume of urine produced in response to hydration is reduced.[126] Yet, the osmolarity still returns to the prehydration level. It is believed that the excess water migrates into the extravascular compartment, thereafter to be excreted perhaps more slowly by the kidneys.

The hemodilution of pregnancy affects the concentration of many substances. Serum total protein and albumin concentrations and plasma oncotic pressure (POP) decrease.[165] Intravenous infusion of 1.5 to 2 L of crystalloid solution reduces plasma oncotic pressure (POP). Concomitant administration of at least 50 g of albumin is necessary to prevent this fall.[165] However, acute reduction of POP is not usually associated with serious pulmonary complications.[165]

Mathru et al.[135] reported that prior colloid infusion minimized systemic hypotension from spinal anesthesia in pregnant patients. However, we were unable to demonstrate any fetal or maternal advantages of colloid prehydration before epidural anesthesia.[165] Thus 1 to 1.2 L of crystalloid infusion seems safe and efficient for minimizing regional-anesthesia-induced hypotension. One must exercise caution when using nonelectrolyte solutions (dextrose 5 or 10% in water) in pregnant subjects because of the risk of both maternal and fetal hyponatremia, hyperglycemia, and hyperlactacidemia.[126]

Ringer's lactate (RL) solution is used extensively for hydration and has been found to be safe. Despite the lactate content (28 mmol/L), RL infusion does not cause increased lactate levels in the mother or the fetus. Plasmalyte A solution, which contains acetate instead of lactate, is associated with increased fetal lactate levels,[167] probably caused by inhibition of placental glycolysis by acetate ions.[214] Plasmalyte A solution should therefore be used with caution in pregnant patients. Rapid infusion of normal saline solution may decrease maternal arterial blood pH and should perhaps be avoided.[167] Body temperature is also affected by rapid fluid infusion; infusion of 1 L of crystalloid solution at room temperature may decrease the patient's body temperature by 0.5° C or more.[173]

Maternal hypoglycemia is associated not only with decreased fetal breathing movements (FBM) and EEG activity[30] but is also implicated in teratogenesis.[90] Assessment of FBM is becoming an important tool in evaluating fetal well-being.[78] Infusion of glucose has been shown to improve both FBM and fetal EEG activity.[169] The rate of administration of glucose should be regulated to maintain maternal serum glucose between 80 and 120 mg/dL. Maternal hyperglycemia (> 120 mg/dL) is associated with increased fetal lactate[114] and umbilical vein insulin levels, which may cause neonatal hypoglycemia.[129,138] When glucose administration is desired, the rate of administration should not exceed 25 g/h.[138] At lower rates, the placenta seems able to metabolize glucose through the aerobic glycolytic pathway.[138] Increased anaerobic lactate production does not occur, and the risk of neonatal hypoglycemia is minimal.[138,167] Thus, prophylactic hydration can be attained with RL solution containing no more than 20 g of glucose before induction of regional anesthesia.

In pregnant patients, even a short period of starvation leads to ketosis more rapidly than in nonpregnant subjects. Conversely, eating a meal is associated with a more rapid and pronounced rise in the blood concentrations of insulin and nutrients. The accelerated development of starved and fed states enables the mother to ensure an adequate fuel supply to the fetus (Fig 19-9).[65,81] Prolonged fasting must therefore be avoided in pregnant patients awaiting surgery. If oral food intake is not feasible, appropriate intravenous fluid therapy must be prescribed. The urine must be checked often for the presence of ketones.

ANESTHETIC IMPLICATIONS. A fluid challenge is often given to differentiate between prerenal and renal causes of oliguria. Since the urinary response to a fluid load may be delayed in pregnancy, sufficient time must be allowed before instituting further therapy. Dehydration, starvation, and ketosis result quickly in undesirable fetal and maternal effects. Overt maternal hypo- and hyperglycemia are deleterious to the fetus. Since the tubular reabsorptive capacity for glucose decreases and glycosuria may occur at normal serum glucose levels, one must exercise caution in using urine glucose levels as an index for insulin therapy in pregnant diabetics. It is interesting to note that administration of glucose in quantities of as little as 5 g may abolish ketosis in pregnant subjects.

### *Endocrine System*

During pregnancy, the anterior lobe of the pituitary gland undergoes hypertrophy and secretes more ACTH and TSH. Although the posterior lobe does not enlarge, its secretory activity is also increased. The plasma concentrations of free and bound plasma cortisol, androgen, and aldosterone increase without clinical evidence of hypercorticism.[133] Pregnancy also causes increased levels of thyroxin-binding globulin. In order to maintain a euthyroid state, the thyroid gland becomes hypertrophic. Radio-iodine uptake is markedly elevated, and there may be slight thyroid enlargement.[133] The basal metabolic rate also increases by at least 15%. Human chorionic somatomammotropin (hCS, human placental lactogen), which is biologically and immunologically similar to growth hormone,[94] is the major peptide hormone synthesized by the

FIG. 19-9. Accelerated fed state (*light area*) and fasted state (*dark area*) in nonpregnant and pregnant subjects. Arrows indicate meals. Note the rapid development of the fed state after eating and the starved state after brief starvation in the pregnant subjects. (From Frienkel[81] with permission.)

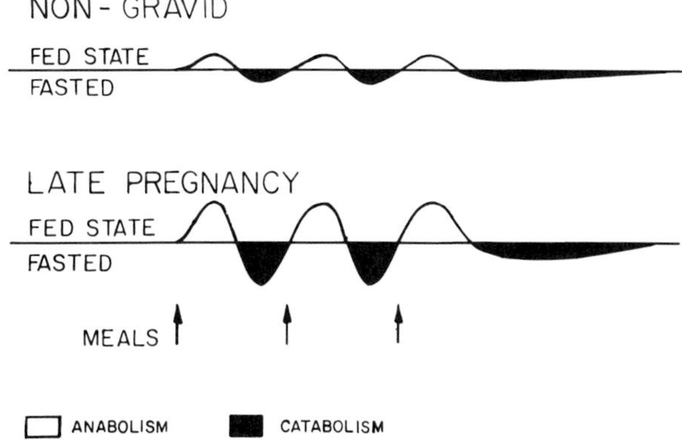

placenta. hCS has multiple biologic activities, including hyperglycemia and lipolysis. Because of the increased anti-insulin activity of pregnancy caused by increased lactogen and placental insulinase, pancreatic beta cell activity increases.[133] For other hormonal changes, see the section on renal function in this chapter.

### *Serum Cholinesterase Activity*

Pregnancy causes a reduction in serum cholinesterase activity starting soon after the 10th week of gestation (Fig 19-10).[172,187] It remains suppressed throughout pregnancy and reaches its lowest level on the third postpartum day. Despite this reduction, dibucaine, fluoride, and chloride levels remain within normal limits.[156,172] Although anecdotal reports have described prolonged apnea after succinylcholine in pregnant patients, the majority of these patients respond normally to succinylcholine.[29]

ANESTHETIC IMPLICATIONS. Since rapid intubation of the trachea is essential in pregnant patients, a full paralyzing dose of succinylcholine should be used. A reduction in the dosage of succinylcholine in view of the decreased enzyme level may result in unsatisfactory intubating conditions and may predispose to aspiration of gastric contents. Prolonged use of muscle relaxants in pregnant patients may result in paralysis and subsequent contracture of the fetal limb muscles.[162] This complication may occur when an injured pregnant patient in the third trimester requires prolonged curarization to facilitate mechanical ventilation.

### *Placental Physiology*

Respiratory gas exchange, which follows the laws of simple diffusion, takes place between the mother and the fetus in the intervillous space.[139] Gas exchange in the placenta is mainly flow limited because the transfer efficiency depends on the oxygen-transport capacity of the fetal circulation and not on the diffusion gradient between maternal and fetal circulation.[139] Fetal hemoglobin has a higher affinity for oxygen than that of the mother. Thus, for a given $PO_2$, the fetal oxygen saturation is greater than that of the mother. The $P_{50}$ levels of fetal and maternal hemoglobin are 20 and 27 mm Hg, respectively.[139] The leftward shift of the fetal oxyhemoglobin dissociation curve is partly due to diminished content of 2–3 diphosphoglyceraldehyde (2–3 DPG).

FIG. 19-10. Serum cholinesterase values in pregnant and nonpregnant patients. (Adapted from Schnider and Webster.[188])

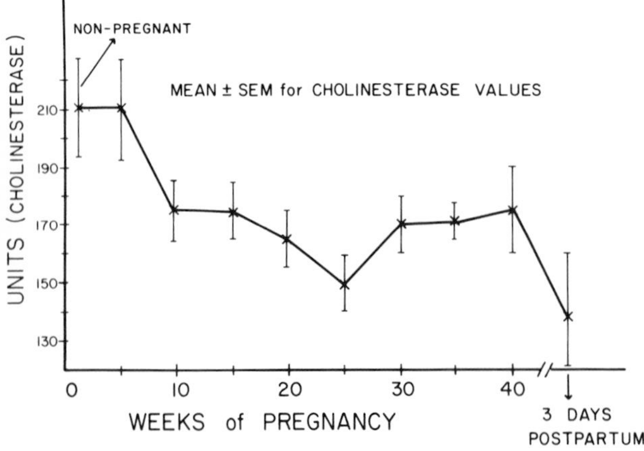


In the placenta, oxygen diffuses from the intervillous space into the fetal circulation, and $CO_2$ diffuses in the reverse direction (Fig 19-11). When the mother breathes room air, the oxygen diffusion gradient between the maternal artery and the fetal umbilical artery (UA) is 80 mm Hg. The diffusion gradient for $CO_2$ is approximately 22 mm Hg.[161] Umbilical artery blood contains more $H^+$ than maternal blood because of the higher $P_{CO_2}$ and not because of metabolic acidosis.[161] The transfer of $CO_2$ from UA blood into the intervillous space not only decreases maternal blood pH but increases UA blood pH as well. The maternal oxyhemoglobin dissociation curve thus shifts to the right while the fetal curve shifts to the left. Therefore, transplacental oxygen transfer is regulated by a change in the oxygen affinity of maternal and fetal hemoglobin due to altered $H^+$ concentrations on both sides (double Bohr effect). In order to achieve the same degree of efficiency without the Bohr effect, the diffusion gradient and/or the uteroplacental blood flow would have to increase considerably.[139]

$CO_2$ transfer is regulated by the diffusion gradient and the Haldane effect. Although $CO_2$ diffuses readily across biologic membranes, a continuous supply of free $CO_2$ must be available at the placenta for diffusion. Because the fetal blood carbonic anhydrase content is low, the rate of $CO_2$ formation from $H_2CO_3$ may not be sufficiently rapid.[139] In order to maintain ionic equilibrium within the RBC, when $HCO_3^-$ enters the cell, $Cl^-$ diffuses out (Fig. 19-11). This ensures continuous $HCO_3^-$ entry into the cell for further processing. Because the fetal hemoglobin has now gained $H^+$ due to increased oxygenation, $CO_2$ is driven out of amino acids, thus further augmenting the diffusion gradient across the placenta. On the maternal side, the deoxygenated alkaline blood now more readily accepts the incoming $CO_2$. The $HCO_3^-$ leaves the maternal RBC in exchange for $Cl^-$ entering the cell from the maternal plasma. Thus, the transfer of $CO_2$ from the fetus to the mother is facilitated by the double Haldane effect.[139,151]

ANESTHETIC IMPLICATIONS. There are some simple steps one can take to optimize gas exchange across the placenta.

- Both respiratory and metabolic alkalosis should be avoided in the mother. Alkalosis shifts the maternal oxyhemoglobin dissociation curve to the left and impairs the release of oxygen from hemoglobin. Levinson et al.[124] showed that mechanical hyperventilation of the mother impaired fetal oxygenation. Although hyperventilation also caused a reduction in uterine blood flow, respiratory alkalosis was a more important factor in producing fetal hypoxia. Similarly, metabolic alkalosis induced by $NaHCO_3$ may also impair fetal oxygenation.[160]
- Aortocaval compression should always be avoided.
- Enriching maternal inspired air with oxygen improves fetal oxygen stores and acid-base status. (Fig 19-12).[164] During prolonged surgery, maternal arterial pH and blood gas tensions should be measured frequently and maintained at optimal levels.

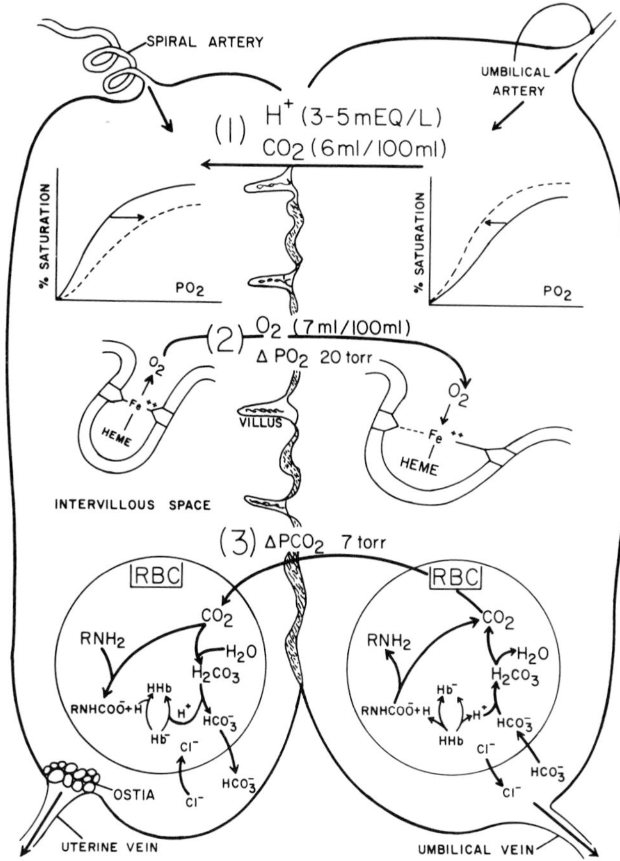


FIG. 19-11. Schematic representation of the double Bohr and double Haldane effect in augmenting transplacental gas transfer. $H^+$ and $CO_2$ leave the fetal circulation and enter the maternal circulation. The fetal oxyhemoglobin dissociation curve shifts to the left, and the maternal oxyhemoglobin curve shifts to the right. Oxygen diffuses from the maternal intervillous space into the fetal RBC. Because of the Haldane effect, fetal hemoglobin releases $CO_2$ from carbamino compounds ($RNHCO_2$). Continuous supply of $HCO_3^-$ is ensured by extracellular chloride (Cl) migration. Maternal hemoglobin readily accepts the incoming $CO_2$ due to the reverse Haldane effect. $RNH_2$ = n-terminal histidine amino acids. (From Ramanathan[162] with permission.)

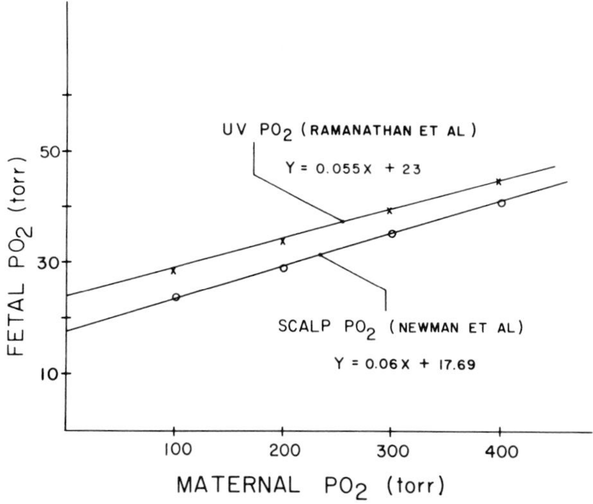


FIG. 19-12. Relationship between maternal $PaO_2$ and fetal umbilical vein (UV) and scalp $PO_2$. (From Ramanathan et al[164] with permission.)

- Maternal stress causes a significant increase in catecholamine levels, impairing uterine blood flow and fetal oxygenation.[189] Maternal pain must therefore be avoided by the judicious use of sedatives or analgesics. A combination of meperidine and promethazine has been found to be safe.[156,190]
- Prolonged hyperthermia may also increase maternal catecholamine levels and interfere with fetal oxygenation.[186]
- Systemic hypotension from any cause is associated with reduced uteroplacental blood flow and should be corrected at the earliest opportunity. Maternal hypovolemia should be corrected by crystalloid infusion or blood transfusion when indicated. The incidence and severity of systemic hypotension due to spinal or epidural anesthesia may be minimized by prophylactic infusion of 1500 to 2000 mL of RL. If hypotension occurs despite this measure, ephedrine should be administered intravenously in 5-mg increments until the systolic pressure reaches at least 100 mm Hg. Should ephedrine prove ineffective, a small dose of phenylephrine (100-μg bolus) may be tried. In an adequately hydrated patient, this dose of phenylephrine is unlikely to produce any harmful fetal effects.[163] However, the routine use of pure alpha-receptor agonists is not advisable for treatment of maternal hypotension because they may reduce uterine blood flow significantly.[159]

## TERATOLOGY

Ever since the thalidomide tragedy, the teratogenic effects of maternally administered drugs have been the focus of numerous studies. A pregnant trauma victim may be exposed to several drugs during her stay in the hospital, and if surgery is required, she may also be exposed to anesthetics and diagnostic irradiation. Although many studies with impressive results have been done on animals, only a limited number of human studies are available on the subject at present. Extrapolation of the findings of animal experiments to human situations is difficult because high doses of the drugs are used in animals, there may be species differences in metabolic pathways of and fetal susceptibility to exogenous teratogens, and drugs that are not teratogenic to animals may be teratogenic to humans or vice versa. The classic example is streptomycin, which does not produce ototoxicity in animal fetuses, but is known to do so in humans. Conversely, salicylates and corticosteroids are teratogenic to animal fetuses, but may not be teratogenic in humans. Nevertheless, the use of animal fetuses to study teratogenesis is a common requirement before drugs are released for public use. Animal experiments may draw attention to a problem that may otherwise go unnoticed. Diphenylhydantoin was shown to be a teratogen in animals long before human data were available. The same is true of diethylstilbestrol.

Genetic make-up, maternal age, nutritional status, and coincidental diseases may influence the teratogenic potential of a drug.[45] There is a high incidence of alcohol and/or other drug abuse among trauma victims. Both alcohol and abusable drugs, such as narcotics and diazepam, are implicated in teratogenesis.

Since 1978 the Swedish catalogue of registered pharmaceutical specialties (FASS) has presented information on pregnancy and breast-feeding. All drugs are assigned to one of the following pregnancy categories: A, $B_1$, $B_2$, $B_3$, C, and D. The letters refer to information based on human data and the figures to animal data. Pregnancy risks are classified into categories A to D. Drugs are classified into groups I to IV with respect to their potential for being secreted into the breast milk.

### *Pregnancy Risks*

*Category A*: These drugs have been used by a large number of women and are not associated with any increase in fetal malformation or disturbances in the reproductive process.

*Category B*: These drugs have been used only by a limited number of patients. They are not known to be associated with any harmful effects.

*Category C*: These drugs have either caused or have been suspected of causing disturbances in the reproductive process, without being directly teratogenic to the fetus.

*Category D*: These drugs are known to have caused fetal malformation.

The drugs in category A include local anesthetics, cardiac glycosides, and theophylline. Category B is subdivided into three subgroups: $B_1$, $B_2$, and $B_3$

- *Group $B_1$*: Reproduction studies in animals have not indicated any harmful effects.
- *Group $B_2$*: Reproduction-toxicology studies are incomplete.
- *Group $B_3$*: Reproduction-toxicology studies have shown an increased incidence of fetal damage or other deleterious effects on the reproductive process.[22]

### *Breast-Feeding Risks*

*Group I*: These drugs do not enter the breast milk.

*Group II*: These drugs enter the breast milk, but are not likely to affect the neonate in therapeutic dose ranges.

*Group III*: These drugs enter the breast milk in quantities that may affect the infant even when therapeutic doses are employed.

*Group IV*: There is no information as to whether or not these drugs enter the breast milk.

In clinical practice, drugs are often prescribed in combination. For instance, trimethoprim (Category $B_3$) and ergotamine (Category C) are prescribed together for migraine. The combination is usually assigned to the more harmful category, in this instance category C. The intended therapeutic use of the drug also may modify the assignment of category. For instance, phenobarbital is assigned to category D when used in combination with other drugs for the treatment of epilepsy, but is placed in category A when used for sedation. Assignment of pregnancy and breast-feeding risks for some commonly used drugs is shown in Table 19-7.[22]

TABLE 19-7. Pregnancy and Breast-Feeding Risks*

| TYPE OF DRUG | PREGNANCY | BREAST MILK |
|---|---|---|
| Analgesics | | |
| Codeine, dextropropoxyphene | A | II |
| Methadone, morphine, meperidine | C | II |
| Fentanyl | C | IV |
| Anesthetics | | |
| Enflurane | A | IV |
| Halothane, ketamine, thiopental | A | II |
| Methotexital | $B_2$ | II |
| Propanidid | $B_1$ | IV |
| Bupivacaine, lidocaine | A | II |
| Etidocaine | $B_1$ | IV |
| Antiaddiction | | |
| Disulfiram | $B_1$ | IV |
| Nalaxone | $B_1$ | IV |
| Antiasthmatic | | |
| Theophylline | A | II |
| Anticonvulsants | | |
| Phenytoin, valproic acid | D | II |
| Antihistamines | | |
| Brompheniramine, chlorpheniramine | A | II |
| Antiemetics | | |
| Diphenhydramine, cyclizine | A | II |
| Antibiotics | | |
| Aminoglycosides | D | IV |
| Cephalosporin | A | II |
| Penicillins | A | II |
| Sulfonamide | C | II |
| Tetracycline | $B_3$ | II |
| Para-amino salicylic acid | A | IV |
| Ethambutol | A | II |
| Rifampin | C | II |
| Acyclovir | $B_1$ | IV |
| Chloramphenicol | C | III |
| Erythromycin | $B_2$ | II |
| Metronidazole | $B_2$ | II |
| Trimethoprim | $B_3$ | II |
| Antimalarials | | |
| Chloroquine | D | II |
| Hydroxychloroquine | D | IV |
| Antitussives, expectorants | | |
| Opium derivatives | A | IV |
| Acetylcysteine (Mucomyst) | $B_2$ | IV |
| Iodides | C | III |
| Caffeine | A | IV |
| Autonomics | | |
| Dobutamine, norepinephrine | $B_2$ | IV |
| Dopamine | $B_3$ | — |
| Ephedrine (epinephrine) | A | IV |
| Pseudoephedrine | $B_2$ | III |
| Terbutaline | A | II |
| Isoproterenol | A | IV |
| Anticholinergics | | |
| Atropine | A | III |
| Glycopyrrolate | $B_2$ | IV |
| Scopolamine | $B_1$ | I |
| Cardiovascular | | |
| Disopyramide, procainamide | $B_2$ | IV |
| Quinidine | D | II |
| Beta-adrenoreceptor blocker | | |
| All preparations | C | II |
| Vasodilators | | |
| Isosorbide | $B_1$ | IV |
| Verapamil | A | IV |
| Nicotinic acid | $B_2$ | IV |
| Nifedipine | $B_2$ | IV |
| Nitroglycerine | $B_2$ | IV |
| Hydralazine, reserpine | A | II |

TABLE 19-7. Pregnancy and Breast-Feeding Risks (*continued*)

| TYPE OF DRUG | PREGNANCY | BREAST MILK |
|---|---|---|
| Antihypertensives | | |
| Clonidine, prazosin | $B_2$ | IV |
| Diazoxide | C | IV |
| Trimethaphan | C | IV |
| Alpha-methyldopa | A | III |
| Diuretics | | |
| Bendroflumethiazide | C | IV |
| Chlorothiazide | C | III |
| Furosemide | C | I |
| Spironolactone | A | III |
| Anticoagulants | | |
| Heparin | $B_2$ | I |
| Dicumarol | C | III |
| Warfarin | D | II |
| Streptokinase | C | IV |
| Protamine | $B_2$ | IV |
| Corticosteroids | | |
| Beclomethasone | $B_3$ | IV |
| Antithyroid drugs | | |
| Carbimazole, Propylthiouracil | C | II |
| Hypnotics, sedatives | | |
| Phenobarbital (anticonvulsant) | D | III |
| Benzodiazepines | C | III |
| Hydroxyzine | A | IV |
| Meprobomate | $B_3$ | III |
| Chlorpromazine | A | II |
| Antipsychotics | | |
| Amitriptyline | A | III |
| Imipramine | C | II |
| Lithium | D | II |
| Oxytocics | | |
| Methyl ergometrine | C | II |
| Oxytocin | A | IV |

* (From Berland et al.[22])

For the sake of convenience, Hutchings[96] has subdivided the prenatal period into three periods: (1) the predifferentiation period, (2) the period of the embryo, (3) the period of the fetus. A drug that is teratogenic in one period may not produce abnormalities in the other two.[96]

The predifferentiation period extends from the fertilization of the oocyte to its implantation in the endometrium. This period lasts 6 days in rats and humans. Except for some reports of altered behavior caused by phenothiazine exposure in this period,[212] most workers agree that the fetus is least vulnerable to teratogenicity during this period.[96]

The period of the embryo extends from early germ layer differentiation to the completion of major organ formation; that is, from the sixth day to the eighth week of gestation in humans.[96,156] The embryo is maximally susceptible to teratogens during this time. The agent may damage the actively proliferating cells, resulting in a structurally defective embryo. With increasing gestational age in this period, the fetus becomes more resistant to teratogenic drug effects.

The period of the fetus extends from the eighth week to delivery. The fetal brain grows very rapidly during this period. In humans, myelination of the nervous system takes place from the seventh month of intrauterine life to the first few months of extrauterine life.[7] Fetus and neonate, although refractory to gross structural damage, remain vulnerable to more subtle brain defects, particularly in actively proliferating areas. This may produce brain dysfunction in infancy or early childhood.

The teratogenic process can therefore be generally divided into two major categories: morphologic teratogenicity, which involves gross structural alteration of an organ, and behavioral teratogenicity, which involves subtle brain dysfunction, such as learning disability.[96] Behavioral teratogenesis may occur with or without gross CNS structural abnormality. Two other factors may also play a role in teratogenicity in fetuses born of trauma victims: the stress of the trauma and of hospital confinement may be associated with an increased incidence of congenital malformations and mental retardation,[6,85,201] and hypoglycemia is associated with defective ossification of the axial skeleton and defective morphogenesis of the embryonic neural tube.[90] Improper intravenous fluid therapy in a trauma victim may result in hypoglycemia. Frequent blood sugar determinations are therefore necessary in traumatized pregnant patients receiving prolonged parenteral fluid therapy.

It is beyond the scope of this discussion to describe exhaustively the effects of all teratogens. This section discusses the teratogenic effects of the most commonly used drugs and anesthetics.

### *Morphologic Teratogens*

ANTICOAGULANTS. Oral anticoagulants, such as warfarin, are contraindicated in pregnancy. Exposure during the first trimester is associated with fetal nasal hypoplasia and chondrodysplasia punctata.[89] Exposure during the second and third trimester may result in optic atrophy, microcephaly, mental retardation, and other CNS abnormalities (Warfarin embryopathy). If anticoagulants are required during pregnancy, heparin is preferred to oral anticoagulants.[20,96]

LITHIUM. This drug is implicated in congenital malformations (Ebstein's anomaly).[22]

DIETHYLSTILBESTROL. Intrauterine exposure to this drug causes malformations of the genitourinary tract and sometimes adenocarcinoma of the vagina in later life.

TRANQUILIZERS. Diazepam taken in early pregnancy is associated with oral clefts.[179,182] There may be a small risk of congenital heart disease with the use of meprobomate and chlordiazepoxide.[140]

PHENOTHIAZINES. Despite a suspicion that antenatal exposure to phenothiazines may be associated with cardiovascular malformations, these drugs are considered to be generally safe.[190] Hydroxyzine may be used safely in a pregnant patient.

SALICYLATES. Intrauterine exposure to aspirin causes neural tube defects, ophthalmic malformation, and eventration in the rat. Neonatal platelet dysfunction has been reported in humans.[96] Acetaminophen may be used as a safe analgesic and antipyretic in pregnant patients.[150]

ANTICONVULSANTS. Children born to epileptic women have a malformation rate two to three times higher than controls.[19,31] The defects include oral clefts and cardiac anomalies. Fetal dilantin syndrome is the name given to a combination of severe facial anomalies and mental retardation. Both barbiturates and dilantin are also implicated in a fetal coagulopathy resembling vitamin K deficiency.

NARCOTICS. Methadone produces CNS and skeletal abnormalities in laboratory animals.[96] Morphine causes reduced fetal brain size with reduced amounts of DNA, RNA, and total protein content in the brain.[197] Cranioschisis and exencephaly are also reported with morphine use. Heroin is also implicated in CNS malformations. Pretreatment of the mother with a narcotic antagonist, such as nalorphine or naloxone, blocks the teratogenic effects of both single and multiple doses of the narcotic.[84]

ANESTHETICS. All available data on the teratogenicity of anesthetics are based on animal experimentation. There are no reliable well-controlled prospective studies available from human beings. $N_2O$ is associated with increased fetal resorption, reduced fetal size, and skeletal abnormalities;[207] because of its action on methionine synthase, it may also interfere with folate metabolism by affecting vitamin $B_{12}$.[20,43] However, recent studies in humans show that the incidence of teratogenicity is not increased after administration of $N_2O$ in early pregnancy for procedures lasting less than 6 hours.[11,53,136] Chronic exposure to trace anesthetics in the operating room is implicated in an increased incidence of miscarriage and congenital abnormalities.[47,196]

Using a microbial assay system, Baden et al.[13] noted that fluoroxene was more mutagenic than other halogenated ether anesthetics. Mice exposed to 0.4 MAC per day had an increased incidence of pregnancy resorption, fetal death, and decreased birth weight. Acute exposure to halothane (0.8% for 12 hours) was associated with increased fetal skeletal abnormalities in rats.[18] A more recent report suggests that halothane, isoflurane, and enflurane are not associated with increased teratogenicity.[137] Thus, based on the evidence available to us, we cannot say with certainty that a short exposure to an inhalational anesthetic is associated with any significant fetal teratogenic effect. Enflurane and halothane are in pregnancy category A (Table 19-7).[22] Local anesthetics, including lidocaine, are devoid of teratogenic potential.[82] High inspired concentrations of halothane have been shown to be associated with metabolic disturbances in the rat brain suggestive of cerebral hypoxia. Low to moderate inspired concentrations (0.4%) were not associated with any significant change in the metabolic status of the brain.[205] Pentobarbital administered in high doses to the mother (200 mg/kg) has been shown to protect the fetal rat brain against hypoxia.[205]

### *Behavioral Teratology*

FETAL ALCOHOL SYNDROME. Infants born to chronic alcoholic women exhibit prenatal and postnatal growth retardation and craniofacial anomalies. During the neonatal period, tremulousness, hyperactivity, and irritability are seen, suggesting a withdrawal state that may persist for months. Hyperactivity in the preschool-aged child with evidence of mental retardation has also been noted.[202]

FETAL HYDANTOIN SYNDROME. This syndrome is associated with low IQ scores and mild to moderate mental retardation.

FETAL TRIMETHADIONE SYNDROME. This syndrome is characterized by facial anomalies, developmental delay, and speech difficulty.[96]

AMPHETAMINE. An estimated 570,000 American women of childbearing age use amphetamine-containing diet pills. Amphetamines cause an elevation in the catecholamine content of the fetal brain. The offspring may show increased nondirected locomotion.[96]

BARBITURATES. Infants born from mothers on chronic barbiturate treatment may exhibit a withdrawal syndrome characterized by overactivity, restlessness, disturbed sleep, excessive crying, diarrhea, and vomiting.[63] High doses of barbiturates administered to the mother may cause decreased neonatal response to environmental stimuli.

OPIATES. Approximately 34,000 women of childbearing age, including 10,000 to 12,000 in a methadone maintenance program, are among the 150,000 opiate-dependent persons in the New York metropolitan area. Passively addicted neonates show signs of acute narcotic withdrawal (hyperreflexia, tremors, and irritability). Infants may not become symptomatic for 2–4 weeks after birth because of fetal storage and prolonged metabolic clearance of narcotic agents. Neonates exposed to narcotics in utero (morphine, methadone, heroin) experience less quiet sleep and more active rapid eye movement (REM) sleep. Morphine exposure may be associated with neonatal tolerance to the drug.[218] In early childhood, they demonstrate poor intellectual and cognitive abilities. Heroin exposure is linked with uncontrollable temper and impulsiveness in early childhood. After prenatal exposure to methadone, the compound persists in the brain and liver of the offspring at least until 20 days of age. This suggests that the hyperactivity, increased lability state, and sleep disturbance may be due to the slow clearance of methadone. In summary, both clinical and animal studies suggest that prenatal exposure to opiates produces biphasic effects, the acute phase consisting of an abstinence syndrome with increased CNS arousal followed by such changes in behavior as hyperactivity, disturbed sleep, and increased lability state. Tables 19-7 and 19-8 summarize the teratologic potential of some of the morphologic and behavioral teratogens. For more information on drug effects, see the section on drug abuse in this chapter.

ANESTHETICS. Only limited human data are available on this subject. The fetal brain is more sensitive to inhalational agents than the adult brain.[87] Intrauterine exposure to halothane and enflurane for short periods has been shown to impair learning in mice.[41] These learning defects were found to be present even in the second generation. Intrauterine exposure to halothane also increases murine postnatal autotolerance to the anesthetic. In addition, halothane exposure reduces brain weight of the offspring.[42]

Subtle neurobehavioral testing of early neonates has shown

TABLE 19-8. Teratogenicity of Some Commonly Used Drugs*

| AGENT | MORPHOLOGIC TERATOLOGY | BEHAVIORAL TERATOLOGY |
|---|---|---|
| Anticoagulants | Optic atrophy<br>Microcephaly | Mental retardation |
| Diazepam (humans) | Oral clefts | |
| Phenothiazines (humans) | ? Congenital heart disease | |
| Salicylates | Neonatal platelet dysfunctions, neural tube defects, eye defects | |
| Dilantin (humans) | Facial anomalies; neonatal vitamin K deficiency | Mental retardation |
| Narcotics | Cranial anomalies, reduced DNA, RNA in the brain | Hyperactivity, insomnia, motor incoordination, neonatal withdrawal, neonatal tolerance |
| Anesthetics: Subacute exposure to trace anesthetics ($N_2O$, halothane) (humans) | Fetal loss, ? congenital anomalies | |
| Acute exposure | Skeletal abnormalities, fetal resorption | Learning difficulties, deranged neurobehavior in the first 24 hours |
| Barbiturates (humans) | Fetal vitamin K deficiency | Withdrawal symptoms, decreased reactivity |
| Alcohol (humans) | Craniofacial and limb defects | Withdrawal syndrome, hyperactivity in neonatal life and preschool period, low IQ |
| Amphetamine | Altered brain catecholamine levels | Hyperactivity, impaired locomotion |
| Phencyclidine | Cranial anomaly | Hyperactivity |
| Antenatal stress (humans) | | Mental retardation, defective motor development |
| Hypoglycemia (humans) | Skeletal abnormalities | |
| Diabetes with acetonuria (humans) | Neural tube defects | Low IQ |
| Antibiotics | | |
| Aminoglycosides (humans) | Cranial nerve, renal abnormalities | None known |
| Cephalosporins | None known | None known |
| Erythromycin | None known | None known |
| Metronidazole | None known | None known |
| Penicillin | None known | None known |
| Sulfonamides | Hemolytic anemia, thrombocytopenia | None known |
| Tetracyclines | Impaired bone growth, stained teeth | None known |

* Teratogenic effect reported in human beings is indicated as (humans). The remaining teratogenic possibilities are based on animal studies.

that intrauterine exposure to general anesthetics,[57] local anesthetics, or analgesics may impair the behavior of the infant. However, one may conclude based on currently available data that CNS depressants have a more pronounced effect on neonatal neurobehavior than local anesthetic agents, especially in the first 24 hours of fetal life.[3] In a prospective study of 570 infants whose mothers received anesthesia, no significant differences were found in the developmental status of the children at 4 years of age, regardless of the type of obstetric analgesia or anesthesia.[57]

### *Anesthetic Implications*

A traumatized pregnant patient may receive many potentially teratogenic drugs and therapeutic irradiation. Whenever possible, the anesthesiologist should use standard medications when anesthetizing pregnant patients. A brief exposure to general anesthetic drugs is unlikely to result in fetal abnormalities. Caution must be exercised in using antibiotics during surgery. For more teratogenic implications of anesthetics, refer to the section on anesthesia guidelines in this chapter.

## DRUG ABUSE IN PREGNANCY

Trauma and drug abuse often go hand in hand. Drug abuse during pregnancy is associated with serious maternal and fetal complications. Unfortunately, the number of young women who abuse drugs, both narcotic and nonnarcotic, is on the increase.[148] Table 19-9 lists drugs that may be abused by

TABLE 19-9. Commonly Abused Drugs in Pregnancy

| DRUG | ABSTINENCE SYNDROME: Mother | ABSTINENCE SYNDROME: Fetus | TERATOGENICITY: Morphologic | TERATOGENICITY: Behavioral |
|---|---|---|---|---|
| Ethyl alcohol | Yes | Yes | Facial anomalies<br>IUGR, FAS | Learning disability; delayed milestones |
| Narcotics | Yes | Yes | IUGR, reduced brain weight | Learning disability |
| Barbiturates | Yes | Yes | None reported | — |
| Benzodiazepines | Yes | Yes | Cleft palate | — |
| Cocaine | Yes | — | Genitourinary | ? |
| Amphetamines | ?Yes | — | — | — |
| Marihuana | Yes | ? | Like FAS | ? |
| LSD | Yes | No data | No data | No data |
| Phencyclidine | Yes | — | ? | No data |

Abbreviations: FAS = fetal alcohol syndrome; LSD = lysergic acid diethlamide; IUGR = intrauterine growth retardation. The character — signifies none reported and ? signifies that possibility is suspected.

the pregnant patient, and Table 19-10 gives a summary of maternal and perinatal problems in drug abusers.

In a general hospital in New York City 6–10% of women admitted to the labor ward test positive for cocaine in their urine. A recent bulletin from the Drug Abuse Warning Network of the National Association on Perinatal Addiction Research and Education indicates that 10% of all newborns in this country have been exposed to an illegal drug in utero. A vast majority of addicts do not seek antenatal medical care and usually go to a hospital only when unforeseen accidents happen.

Pregnant trauma victims who have abused drugs present many problems to the anesthesiologist. Specific problems have been described under each drug category. Other problems may include treatment of acute overdose, recognition and treatment of withdrawal, poor general condition of the patient, multisystem involvement, perioperative cardiovascular and hemodynamic problems, prolonged recovery from anesthesia, withdrawal symptoms in the neonate, and poor neonatal condition.

TABLE 19-10. Maternal and Neonatal Outcome in Drug Abusers

| PROBLEMS | % ABUSERS | % CONTROLS |
|---|---|---|
| Maternal problems | | |
| Meconium-stained amniotic fluid | 21.2 | 13.8 |
| Maternal anemia | 13.2 | 8.2 |
| Premature membrane rupture | 12.2 | 7.8 |
| Antenatal hemorrhage | 3.0 | 1.2 |
| Multiple birth | 3.4 | 1.2 |
| Neonatal condition at birth | | |
| Birth weight (2–2.5 kg) | 21 | 7.0 |
| Birth weight (2.5 kg or heavier) | 69 | 89.0 |
| Prematurity (<38 weeks) | 18.5 | 9.8 |
| Apgar <6 (5 min) | 7 | 3.2 |
| Postnatal problems | | |
| Jaundice | 12.7 | 8.2 |
| Aspiration pneumonia | 9.2 | 1.8 |
| Transient tachypnea | 6.6 | 2.5 |
| Hyaline membrane disease | 3.6 | 1.5 |
| Congenital malformations | 2.4 | 0.5 |

(From Ostrea and Chavez.[153])

### *Alcohol*

This is the substance most commonly abused by pregnant patients. Regardless of the gestational period, alcohol causes adverse fetal effects.[116,141,175] These are seen only when the mother drinks heavily (5 or more drinks on a single occasion or 45 drinks per month; 1 drink = 15 mL of alcohol). A small risk does, however, exist in moderate drinkers (less than 45 drinks per month but never 5 or more drinks on a single occasion). Occasional alcohol consumption does not seem to be associated with serious fetal sequelae.[116,141,175] Increased blood alcohol levels impair metabolism of vital nutrients and interfere with nucleic acid turnover in the fetal brain.

Problem drinkers frequently abuse a variety of other substances, including narcotics. Chronic use of alcohol increases cross-tolerance to other depressant drugs as a result of either pharmacodynamic tolerance or increased metabolism through enzyme induction.[98]

The alcohol withdrawal syndrome is characterized by tremulousness, hyperreflexia, hallucinations, tremulous delirium, and tonic-clonic seizures. Respiratory alkalosis (with or without reduced serum $Mg^{++}$ levels) is implicated in the genesis of delirium tremens.

Chronic alcohol use also causes multiple organ damage and nutritional insufficiencies: fatty necrosis of the liver, cerebral atrophy, polyneuropathy, Wernicke's encephalopathy, skeletal myopathy, and cardiomyopathy.[157] Cardiomyopathy may be associated with decreased cardiac output and increased vasoconstriction. In addition, alcoholics may suffer from dehydration and hypokalemia due to vomiting caused by gastritis and/or poor fluid intake.[157]

Heavy drinking is associated with the fetal alcohol syndrome[116,157] (see the section on teratology). In addition, neonates may develop a withdrawal syndrome that may be delayed for 24 hours. The symptoms of neonatal withdrawal include excessive crying, irritability, and seizures. The condition may be treated with phenobarbital, 3–5 mg/kg.[76]

ANESTHETIC IMPLICATIONS. If the patient is in delirium tremens due to alcohol withdrawal, prompt treatment is necessary to prevent circulatory collapse. Hyperthermia may occur if the delirium is not treated promptly. Hyperthermia increases maternal catecholamine levels and thus may interfere with placental circulation. Fluid-electrolyte imbalance (hypokalemia and hypomagnesemia) and hypoglycemia must be corrected. Caution must be exercised in administering large amounts of glucose because of the possible development of encephalopathy due to thiamine depletion.[157] Lidocaine may be used for treating cardiac arrhythmias. Diazepam in small amounts may be used to control the delirium.

All patients who have abused alcohol must have their liver function evaluated. Severe liver disease is associated with resistance to the action of d-tubocurarine due to increased binding of the drug by $\gamma$-globulin.[67] In patients with hepatic cirrhosis the onset of action of pancuronium may be delayed and its total duration of action prolonged because of the increased volume of distribution of the drug.[69] Similarly, the action of vecuronium may be prolonged in patients with liver disease. Whenever a nondepolarizing relaxant is used, a neuromuscular monitor must be employed. Unless cirrhosis is so advanced as to decrease the concentration of pseudocholinesterase, the action of succinylcholine is not affected significantly.

Patients who have abused alcohol demonstrate resistance to the action of CNS depressant drugs, such as thiopental and inhalational agents.[104] The dose of thiopental must be individualized, and the drug must be titrated to obtain the desired response. Administration of excessive doses of thiopental may be hazardous because of diminished protein binding, the possibility of cardiomyopathy,[38] and increased fetal CNS depression. Similarly, the use of excessive concentrations of volatile agents may lead to cardiovascular depression. Small amounts of narcotics may be tried when higher than usual concentrations of volatile agents are needed to produce adequate anesthesia.

The use of regional block obviates some of the problems associated with general anesthesia. However, circulating fluid volume must be optimized to avoid the consequences of sympathetic denervation. Polyneuropathy is not a contraindication to regional anesthesia, but any existing neurologic impairment must be documented before this technique is used to avoid future litigation.[38] Regional anesthesia may be hazardous in the presence of coagulopathy caused by advanced liver disease. Two additional factors may predispose to local anesthetic toxicity: decreased protein binding (hypoalbuminemia) and delayed metabolism of amide agents. Even at moderate doses, toxic side effects may be seen.[38,51] Lidocaine is preferable to bupivacaine because it is less cardiotoxic. 2-Chloroprocaine, which is an ester, may be ideal under these circumstances. Ester hydrolysis is usually so efficient that, in all but those with advanced liver disease, a normal rate of metabolism may be expected. Precautions with reference to the use of 2-chloroprocaine are outlined under anesthesia guidelines in this chapter.

The use of spinal anesthesia may circumvent the problem of local anesthetic toxicity. However, the rapid hypotension produced by this technique dictates meticulous attention to prophylactic intravenous hydration and proper patient positioning to avoid aortocaval compression. Spinal opiates may be used for postoperative pain relief.

Caution is necessary in inserting nasogastric tubes because of the possible occurrence of esophageal varices. Patients who are acutely intoxicated are at increased risk of gastric aspiration. They usually require smaller anesthetic doses. Since serum ammonia levels are high in stored blood, the use of fresh blood transfusion is recommended.

### *Narcotics*

Maternal narcotic addiction affects both the mother and her fetus, and the abuse of such narcotics as heroin is on the increase. Street heroin also contains quinine, talc, or starch, which contribute further to morbidity in the abuser. The heroin addict frequently abuses other legal and illegal drugs and alcohol.

Maternal problems in a drug addict include the abstinence syndrome and multiple organ dysfunction. When the drug in question is a $\mu$-receptor agonist, withdrawal symptoms appear within 8–12 hours after the last dose.[98] Typically, they include anxiety, restlessness, lacrimation, tremors, hot and cold flushes, tachycardia, tachypnea, and muscle spasms. Cardiovascular collapse may result from dehydration, starvation, and disorders of acid-base balance. The withdrawal of methadone takes 24–48 hours to produce symptoms, which are usually less intense. The meperidine abstinence syndrome appears within 2–4 hours and reaches a peak within 24 hours.[98]

Patients who have received a high dose of methadone for maintenance may experience withdrawal even when the dose is reduced gradually. Withdrawal also follows discontinuation of semisynthetic opioid drugs, such as pentazocine, nalbuphine, butorphanol, and buprenorphine.[99] As a rule, symptoms associated with the semisynthetic drugs are less severe than those seen with heroin withdrawal. The semisynthetic opioids have different actions on the various opioid receptors. Generally speaking, those that antagonize the $\mu$-receptor—for instance, pentazocine, nalbuphine, and butorphanol—may produce the withdrawal symptoms in addicts.[99] Epidural administration of butorphanol may also precipitate withdrawal symptoms.[211] Buprenorphine, which has a partial agonistic action on the $\mu$- receptor, may suppress symptoms caused by morphine withdrawal when given in small doses, but in high doses may precipitate withdrawal. Naloxone and naltrexone are potent antagonists of the $\mu$- receptor and therefore must not be used in opioid-dependent patients.[99]

A thorough preanesthetic evaluation of all systems must be made. Persons who have been previously detoxified may be receiving methadone or 1-$\alpha$-actylmethadol (LAAM), which has a longer duration of action than methadone.[157] Clonidine ($\alpha_2$-agonist) has been used to control withdrawal symptoms associated with sympathetic nervous system hyperactivity. Abrupt discontinuation of clonidine may cause such symptoms as anxiety, hypertension, and tachycardia. Therapy with beta-blockers and/or sodium nitroprusside may be necessary to control clonidine withdrawal symptoms.[157] Clonidine overdose may cause sedation and hypotension.

Infants born of heroin users have a lower birth weight compared to those born of mothers on a supervised methadone program.[198] The incidence of fetal distress is highest in polydrug users. Meconium aspiration and premature delivery are other causes of fetal morbidity. Maternal withdrawal may lead to fetal withdrawal in utero, resulting in increased fetal oxygen consumption. Maternal withdrawal may also be responsible for initiating uterine contractions, which may further interfere with fetal oxygenation.[153] Human studies have not shown an increased incidence of congenital malformations in methadone users; however, animal studies have implicated this drug in causing impaired intellectual function.[96] Methadone administration may also interfere with the ability of the fetus to increase respiratory motions when the mother is given 5% $CO_2$ to inhale, thus demonstrating its profound effect on the fetal CNS.[170] Heroin has been shown to produce congenital cranial anomalies in fetuses exposed to the drug in utero.[96]

Heroin, methadone, and other opioids cause a neonatal withdrawal syndrome characterized by irritability, fever, vomiting, shrill cry, and diarrhea.[198] The symptoms must be recognized and treated promptly to avoid neonatal death. The treatment usually consists of administration of paregoric (camphorated tincture of opium).[76] Phenobarbital may be given if multiple drug exposure is suspected. Diazepam is the least efficacious drug for the treatment of neonatal abstinence syndrome.

ANESTHETIC IMPLICATIONS. Since venipuncture may be a problem in intravenous drug abusers, internal jugular or subclavian vein cannulation may be needed. Patients must be given their maintenance methadone dose. If narcotics are required for analgesia, meperidine and/or methadone may be used. In general, oral, epidural, and intrathecal narcotics produce lower plasma levels than IV or IM injections and therefore cause less euphoria. Thus, development of readdiction is less likely with these routes. Narcotics that antagonize $\mu$-receptor activity must not be used lest they precipitate withdrawal.[218]

If general anesthesia is required, thiopental may be used for induction. Anesthesia is preferentially maintained with inhalation agents. The use of narcotics is not recommended intraoperatively. Isoflurane may be preferable to halothane since it undergoes very little hepatic metabolism. Postoperative pain relief may be provided by epidural injection of local anesthetic or morphine, both of which diminish the total narcotic requirement. Patients who are acutely intoxicated must have their airway protected with an endotracheal tube. Hypotension should be treated with vasopressors and intravenous fluid administration. Incremental doses of naloxone may be necessary to counteract respiratory depression in severe cases.

### *Barbiturates*

Tolerance develops more slowly to barbiturates than it does to opioids. An addict may ingest up to 2 g of barbiturate without showing signs of intoxication.[98] Even in those who frequently abuse the drug, the lethal dose does not increase at the same rate at which tolerance develops,[98] with the result that a barbiturate abuser has little safety margin. Barbiturates may be abused solely for their effects on the CNS, to suppress withdrawal from alcohol, or to supplement the effects of impure street heroin. A barbiturate abuser may concomitantly abuse benzodiazepines and other sedative drugs.

The manifestations of chronic barbiturism include (a) slow thinking, (b) untidy personal habits, (c) emotional instability, and (d) neurologic signs (cerebellar incoordination, nystagmus, and dysarthria). Barbiturate withdrawal is more life threatening than narcotic withdrawal. Symptoms start within 24–72 hours after the last barbiturate dose[157] and include tremors, nervousness, grand mal seizures, and psychosis. The EEG usually shows spike-dome activity, which may or may not be associated with seizures.[157] The patient is remarkably sensitive to photic stimulation. Severe hallucinations may also occur. Although such problems as endocarditis or hepatitis are not usually seen in barbiturate abusers, there are other concerns. Barbiturates are potent enzyme inducers; they modify the action of several drugs, such as anticoagulants, and may accelerate the metabolism of many anesthetics. Cross-tolerance to other CNS depressants may develop. The neonate usually shows signs of withdrawal, which respond to phenobarbital administration. Chronic use of barbiturates (except when used for treating epilepsy) is not associated with teratogenicity. Regional anesthesia, whenever possible, is preferable to general anesthesia in chronic barbiturate abusers.

Acute intoxication is managed with tracheal intubation and positive-pressure ventilation. Measurements of barbiturate blood levels may be helpful. A blood level of 2 mg/dL in a comatose patient is usually due to secobarbital or pentobarbital poisoning, whereas a level of 11–12 mg/dL is suggestive of barbital or phenobarbital intake.[157] Barbiturates cause diminished cardiac output, peripheral vasodilation, and systemic hypotension. The following measures should be taken to correct hypotension: nursing the patient on her side to avoid aortocaval compression, optimizing circulating fluid volume, and administering ephedrine in intermittent injections or continuous infusion. The fetal heart rate must be monitored continuously. Forced diuresis and alkali administration are recommended to accelerate the rate of elimination of the drug.[157] Occasionally, hemodialysis or peritoneal dialysis may be required.

### *Benzodiazepines*

Diazepam may be abused by pregnant women. The abstinence syndrome resembles that produced by barbiturate withdrawal. Neonates are also prone to develop withdrawal, which responds to benzodiazepine administration. As stated before, the use of diazepam in the first trimester is associated with cleft palate in the neonate; it may also produce decreased muscle tone and altered temperature regulation.

### *Cocaine*

Five million Americans use cocaine regularly,[44] among whom are some pregnant women. Cocaine may be inhaled or self-administered parenterally. Cocaine addicts may suffer from persecutory delusions. Its use rapidly leads to physical dependence. Sudden discontinuation of the drug does not cause observable changes in behavior; however, patients do complain of a craving for the drug, hyperphagia, and depression.[113] Occasionally a withdrawal syndrome may develop, consisting of delirium and sleeplessness. However, there is no need for slow withdrawal of the drug. The mood changes that often follow cocaine withdrawal may be treated with tricyclic antidepressants.

Cocaine prevents catecholamine reuptake at sympathetic synapses. It produces hypertension, tachycardia, and placental vasoconstriction and abruption. It also causes premature uterine contractions, which may result in premature labor or spontaneous abortion. Cocaine crosses the placenta and stimulates the fetus with the result that fetal body movement increases in the third trimester.[44] The infant's neurobehavior is also affected at birth.[44] In addition, problems due to intravenous use of impure drug may develop. Lung damage is known to occur in those who smoke coca paste.[157] The nasal septum may become ulcerated in those who use it nasally.

Acute cocaine intoxication causes excitement, convulsions, tachyarrhythmias, hypermetabolic state, acidosis, and circulatory collapse. Convulsions may be controlled with diazepam and tachyarrhythmias with beta-blockers.[103] General anesthesia may be hazardous in a cocaine abuser because of a possible elevation in circulating catecholamine levels. Hypertension, tachycardia, and cardiac arrhythmias, especially in the presence of such sensitizing agents as halothane, may occur. In addition, the acute use of cocaine is associated with increased anesthetic requirements.[200] Thus, regional anesthesia is preferable whenever possible. When general anesthesia is required, a balanced technique may be used.

### *Central Nervous System Stimulants*

AMPHETAMINES. Amphetamine and its d-isomer dextroamphetamine are powerful CNS stimulants. The toxic syndrome caused by amphetamine is usually indistinguishable from that caused by cocaine.[98] Amphetamine, like cocaine, blocks the reuptake of norepinephrine; the effects of both drugs are believed to be mediated through dopaminergic sites in the CNS.[98] Tolerance develops rapidly to the euphorigenic effects of amphetamines but not to its toxic effects, thus increasing the possibility of toxic psychosis.[98] Prolonged use of amphetamines may result in microvascular damage and depletion of dopamine from the caudate nucleus.[72] Withdrawal symptoms resemble those produced by cocaine.[98]

Acute amphetamine toxicity is characterized by hypertension, tachycardia, irritability, sweating, hyperpyrexia, and convulsions.[98] Diazepam or chlorpromazine is recommended to control these symptoms. Acidification of the urine enhances excretion of the drug.[98]

Acute administration of amphetamine has been shown to increase MAC in animals in a dose-dependent manner. Chronic administration may, however, reduce MAC because of catecholamine depletion in the brain.[105] The use of general anesthetic agents that sensitize the myocardium to circulating catecholamines may be hazardous because of the increased likelihood of cardiac arrhythmias. Cardiac arrest has been reported during induction of general anesthesia with thiopental in an amphetamine abuser.[181] Such sympathetic stimulants as ketamine are also better avoided. Pulmonary edema occurred in one patient during general anesthesia with halothane.[193] It is interesting to note that pulmonary edema is also a frequent complication of tocolytic therapy with the sympathomimetic agent ritodrine. Because epidural anesthesia diminishes the intensity of sympathetic activity, it is the preferred technique whenever possible. Chronic amphetamine use suppresses appetite and causes ketosis and dehydration.[98] Therefore, circulating fluid volume must be expanded adequately before epidural blockade. Ketonuria must be corrected by judicious administration of glucose. To treat systemic hypotension caused by regional anesthesia, a direct acting vasopressor, such as phenylephrine, may be needed, especially when ephedrine fails to restore blood pressure.

CANNABINOIDS (MARIHUANA). The effects of marihuana are attributed to 1–9 tetrahydrocannabinol (THC). A moderate dose produces euphoria followed by sleepiness. Higher doses produce hallucinations and delusions.[98] Tachycardia and postural hypotension occur in some cases. THC increases the circulating blood volume and decreases sweating.[98] Smoking marihuana causes bronchitis and an asthma-like syndrome.[98] Tolerance usually develops, and sudden withdrawal may result in nervousness, irritability, and insomnia.

Marihuana use is not uncommon among pregnant women.[12,80] Chronic use is associated with premature or precipitate labor, an increased incidence of fetal distress, and possibly of intrauterine growth retardation. The babies may have altered response to photic stimulation, altered neurobehavior, and a peculiar high-pitched cry (cri de chat).[80] A teratogenic effect resembling fetal alcohol syndrome is also described.[80]

PSYCHEDELICS. Lysergic acid diethylamide (LSD) produces hallucinations that may last for hours. Its central effects are believed to be mediated by the effects of the drug on the tryptaminergic raphe neurons of the midbrain.[98] Occasionally the individual may experience terrifying hallucinations, which are often referred to as a "bad trip." Subsequent bad trips may be experienced without being provoked by the drug.[5] This is called the "flashback" syndrome; it may be exacerbated by phenothiazine exposure, psychic trauma, or alcohol. The syndrome has also been reported in the postoperative period.[102] LSD and related compounds possess in vitro anticholinesterase activity. Thus, there exists a theoretical possibility that the duration of ester drugs, such as succinylcholine, may be prolonged in chronic LSD users.[102]

Phencyclidines (angel dust) may also be abused by pregnant patients. The drug may be smoked, ingested, or administered intravenously.[157] Users may exhibit catatonic muscular rigidity, sweating, and a neurodissociative state. Phencyclidine prevents reuptake of dopamine, 5-OH-tryptamine, and norepinephrine by synaptosomes.[98] The phencyclidine receptor may be related to the $\sigma$- opioid receptor.[98] Abrupt withdrawal results in feelings of fear and facial twitching. Infants born of mothers who use the drug often manifest neurobehavioral changes.[98] Phencyclidine overdose may result in coma, convulsions, respiratory depression, hyperthermia, hypertension, and possible intracranial hemorrhage.[157] Acidification of urine hastens the renal excretion of the drug. Phenothiazines must not be used for the treatment of acute psychosis associated with phencyclidine use because they may potentiate the anticholinergic effect of the agent.[157]

## OPERATING ROOM MANAGEMENT

This section explores how best to plan an anesthetic approach based on the mechanisms by which pregnancy influences management of the trauma victim and the effects of intrauterine drug exposure on the fetus. Both obstetric and nonobstretic surgical interventions may have to be made simultaneously on rare occasions. For instance, abdominal trauma in a term pregnant patient may be managed by laparotomy not only to treat injury to abdominal organs but also to deliver the baby when the uterus is involved extensively.

If conditions permit, the pregnant patient should be adequately prepared before surgery. Fluid, electrolyte, and major blood volume deficits should be corrected by transfusion and acellular fluids. Fresh blood is preferable to stored blood because it contains a greater concentration of 2–3 DPG.[95] Diminished 2–3 DPG content may impair oxygen release by maternal hemoglobin in the intervillous space. Ringer's lactate (RL) should be infused when crystalloids are required. Maternal blood glucose concentration should be maintained between 80 and 120 mg/dL, although glucose administration rate should not exceed 25 g/h. In severely hypovolemic subjects, central venous pressure monitoring is required for proper fluid replacement. The pitfalls of assessing circulatory fluid volume in pregnant patients have been previously discussed. An indwelling arterial cannula is also indicated during surgery for major trauma.

When placental abruption is suspected, coagulation tests are necessary. Every attempt should be made to correct any clotting abnormalities before surgical intervention. If coagulation deficits are suspected, platelets, cryoprecipitate, and fresh-frozen plasma must be prepared before surgery. The use of heparin is not recommended in managing obstetric DIC. Since fetal oxygen delivery depends on maternal hemoglobin concentration, adequate red cell replacement is vital in pregnant patients.

Pain and anxiety should be relieved in the preoperative period to minimize the stress response, which reduces uterine blood flow. A combination of meperidine and phenothiazine is safe to use, provided the patient is hemodynamically stable. Barbiturates may be useful for sedation.[156] Atropine may also be used safely for premedication.

An attempt must be made to raise the pH of the gastric contents. Because teratogenic studies are not available, cimetidine or ranitidine should be used with great caution during the fetal organogenesis period. Sodium citrate, 15–30 mL PO, may be used in patients in the first trimester. In the second trimester, cimetidine or ranitidine may be prescribed orally if sufficient time is available. In urgent situations, sodium citrate can be used regardless of the gestational period. If a belladonna preparation is desired, glycopyrrolate, which undergoes only limited placental transfer, may be preferable to atropine.[144]

From the late second trimester, pregnant patients should not be left supine because of the possibility of aortocaval compression. A history of lightheadedness or faintness may help diagnose susceptibility to supine hypotension. Epidural or spinal anesthesia may produce severe hypotension if the patient is supine. Similarly, acute vasodilation caused by thiopental induction may also cause systemic hypotension. Therefore, the uterus must always be displaced to the left during surgery by a noncompressible sandbag wedged under the right hip.

Whenever possible, conduction anesthesia should be used in the pregnant patient. Doing so avoids the multiple agents required for general anesthesia. Prophylactic intravenous hydration with 1.0 to 1.2 L of crystalloid solution will minimize systemic hypotension due to spinal or epidural anesthesia. Blood pressure should be determined frequently after the block, and if systolic pressure falls below 100 mmHg, ephedrine should be injected in 5-mg increments to restore normotension.[59] If ephedrine is ineffective, 100-μg increments of phenylephrine may be administered. In well-hydrated patients, neither ephedrine nor phenylephrine is associated with adverse fetal effects.[161–163,166]

The fetus cannot effectively metabolize local anesthetics, such as mepivacaine, that require ring-hydroxylation. These agents should therefore not be used in pregnant patients. The serum elimination half-life of mepivacaine is more than 9 hours in the neonate. Amide local anesthetics, such as lidocaine and bupivacaine, that depend on N-dealkylation for metabolism are safer. The fetus and newborn, like the adult, convert lidocaine by dealkylation to monoethylglycine xylidide (MEGX), before further hydrolysis.[77] It takes twice as long for the fetus to metabolize lidocaine as it does for the mother. The fetus dealkylates bupivacaine to pipecole xylidine (PPX).[64]

For elimination of local anesthetics, the fetus depends not only on its own metabolic pathways, which are quite similar to those of the adult, but on placental clearance as well. This speaks for the need for the maintenance of adequate uteroplacental flow at all times. Because of rapid placental clearance, the serum concentration of lidocaine required for producing fetal CNS toxicity is 2.5 times greater than that required in the newborn.[77] A hypoxic fetus initiates circulatory adaptations to maximize blood supply to the brain, which include hepatic vasoconstriction. This decreases fetal ability to metabolize local anesthetics. Reduced blood pH and decreased protein binding increase the proportion of ionized to non-ionized fractions in the fetal circulation, which predisposes to increased CNS toxicity.[158]

Although earlier reports claimed that the use of lidocaine was associated with decreased neonatal neurobehavior scores, subsequent studies have not shown this effect.[1–3] The authors have used lidocaine with epinephrine for regional anesthesia in all stages of gestation in the past 14 years and have not seen any serious maternal, fetal, or neonatal side effects.

Epinephrine added to the local anesthetic mixture does not decrease uterine blood flow if maternal systemic perfusion pressure is maintained.[106] Large clinical series that used epinephrine-containing local anesthetic agents in pregnant patients have also not reported any adverse fetal outcome.[88] Bupivacaine has also been used extensively in obstetric regional anesthesia. Because 0.75% bupivacaine has been implicated in fatal maternal cardiac arrhythmias, one should use only 0.5% bupivacaine for regional anesthesia. Bupivacaine is more cardiotoxic than lidocaine and produces cardiac toxicity at subconvulsant anesthetic concentrations.[62] Chloroprocaine is hydrolyzed rapidly by plasma cholinesterase, and therefore its fetal uptake is negligible. Although it was popular until a few years ago, several reports of permanent paraplegia resulting from accidental subarachnoid injection have appeared in the literature.[142] The neurotoxicity of 2-chloroprocaine is believed to be due to the antioxidant, sodium bisulfite.[209] Although 2-chloroprocaine is presently being marketed using ethylene diamine tetra-acetic acid as the antioxidant, insufficient data exist about its safety. One should therefore exercise extreme caution in using chloroprocaine for epidural anesthesia in injured patients who may have sustained occult spinal injuries. Lidocaine, bupivacaine, and tetracaine are safe for spinal anesthesia.

Pregnancy causes a 15% reduction in dose requirement for both spinal and epidural anesthesia.[133] The rate of spread of both spinal and epidural anesthesia is increased in pregnant patients. The increased spread of epidural anesthesia has been demonstrated even in early pregnancy.[74,133] The onset of spinal anesthesia is faster and the duration of sympathetic, sensory, and motor block is longer in pregnant than in nonpregnant patients. Thus, hypotension may develop very rapidly in a pregnant patient. During surgery under regional anesthesia, intravenous sedation may be required to minimize anxiety and stress. Meperidine may be used if supplementation of regional anesthesia is needed.

Severe maternal hypovolemia is likely to result in fetal hypoxia due to reduced uteroplacental blood flow. The hypoxic fetus increases its cerebral blood flow to maximize oxygen supply to the brain. Reduced fetal cardiac output, increased fetal blood pressure, and bradycardia are often present. Animal experiments have shown that administration of general anesthesia to the mother abolishes the hypertensive and bradycardic response to hypoxia in the fetus without improving its oxygenation.[203,216] However, the fetal cardiac output may not change even at a 1.5% inspired concentration of halothane. Every attempt must therefore be made to improve maternal circulation as quickly as possible. It is interesting to note that the maternal administration of naloxone intensifies the fetal bradycardic response to hypoxia.[117]

Before induction of general anesthesia, the lungs should be denitrogenated for 5 minutes to avoid maternal and fetal hypoxemia. Rapid sequence thiopental-succinylcholine induction and intubation with cricoid pressure should be done in all injured pregnant patients regardless of gestational age. It is advisable to use agents that have a history of safe use. If the patient is hypotensive, ketamine (1 mg/kg) may be used intravenously for induction. Caution must be exercised in using higher doses of ketamine because it has been shown to increase intrauterine pressure. This effect is, however, not seen in the third trimester.[152] Anesthesia can be maintained using $N_2O$ supplemented with meperidine; d-tubocurarine or pancuronium may be used for muscle relaxation. The pros and cons of using $N_2O$ in pregnancy have been discussed previously.

Some anesthesiologists prefer to use inhalational agents because they relax the myometrium and may prevent premature labor. Despite a 27% reduction in fetal blood pressure, halothane anesthesia is associated with normal fetal regional blood flow, cardiac output, heart rate, and acid-base status.[25] Isoflurane, however, decreases fetal cardiac output and causes progressive fetal acidosis in animal experiments.[26] Isoflurane must therefore be used with caution in traumatized pregnant patients. Fetal MAC is less than adult MAC for halothane.[87] Glycopyrrolate and neostigmine may be used for reversal of the muscle relaxant at the end of the surgical procedure.

Except for a few retrospective studies, there are no well-controlled prospective studies regarding fetal outcome after maternal surgery.[66,123,188,191] Pelvic surgery (appendectomy) and Shirodkar procedures carry a higher fetal mortality and a higher incidence of premature labor.[191] No anesthetic technique or agent appears to be superior to another with respect to the incidence of premature labor, abortion, perinatal mortality, or teratogenic effects.[64a,185,188] Duncan et al[66] reported a higher risk of abortion with general than with regional anesthesia in mothers undergoing surgery during the first or second trimester of their pregnancy. However, many authors believe that the nature of the surgery rather than the type of anesthetic determines pregnancy outcome.[49]

Maternal $PaCO_2$ should be measured frequently and maintained between 33 and 36 mm Hg during long surgical procedures. Maternal acid-base status should also be maintained within normal limits to optimize gas exchange across the placenta. Excessive hyperventilation should be avoided. Similarly, maternal hypothermia and hyperthermia may affect fetal temperature and oxygenation.[186] Whenever possible, the fetal heart rate should be monitored continuously during surgery.[109] Maternal hypoxemia during surgery causes loss of baseline variability of the fetal heart tracing.[109] Tocolysis may be used if the patient develops premature labor. Postoperative pain relief may be provided with epidural or intrathecal narcotics.

## CONCLUSION

Successful management of an injured pregnant patient involves physicians from many disciplines. Pregnancy must always be suspected in any trauma victim of childbearing age. The type and extent of trauma must be assessed quickly. Hemodynamic status must be stabilized at the earliest opportunity. Because the fetus is precariously dependent on its mother for its oxygen needs, an uninterrupted supply of oxygenated blood must be provided to the fetus at all times. The importance of maintaining adequate uteroplacental blood flow cannot be overemphasized. The short- and long-term fetal effects of many medications administered to the mother are also cause for concern. A working knowledge of how pregnancy modifies normal physiology will aid in tailoring anesthetic administration to suit the need of the traumatized pregnant patient. A systematic approach must be planned for managing trauma victims who have abused drugs. A perimortem cesarean section may be needed to salvage the fetus when the mother succumbs to her injuries. The number of working women is steadily on the increase; thus more and more women are being exposed to the risk of minor and major trauma. Therefore, we are likely to be seeing more injured pregnant patients in the future.

## REFERENCES


1. Abboud TK, Kim KC, Noueihed R, et al. Epidural bupivacaine, chloroprocaine or lidocaine for cesarean section; maternal and neonatal effects. Anesth Analg 1983;62:914.
2. Abboud TK, Raya J, Sadri S, et al. Fetal and maternal cardiovascular effects of atropine and glycopyrrolate. Anesth Analg 1983;62:426.
3. Abboud TK, Sarkis F, Blikian A, et al. Lack of adverse neonatal neurobehavioral effects of lidocaine. Anesth Analg 1983;62:473.
4. Abitbol MM. Aortic compression by pregnant uterus. NY State J Med 1976;76:1470.
5. Abraham HD. Visual phenomenology of the LSD flash. Arch Gen Psychiatry 1983;40:884.
6. Abramson JH, Singh AR, Mbambo V. Antenatal stress and the baby's development. Arch Dis Child 1961;36:42.
7. Adamson SK, Joelsson I. The effect of pharmacologic agents upon the fetus and the newborn. Am J Obstet Gynecol 1966;96:437.
8. Aderet NB, Cohen I, Abramowicz JS. Traumatic coma during pregnancy with persistent vegetative state; case report. Br J Obstet Gyneacol 1984;91:939.
9. Albright GA, Joyce TH, Ferguson JE, et al. Physiology of Pregnancy. In: Albright GA, Ferguson JE, Joyce TH, Stevenson DK, eds. Anesthesia in obstetrics. Maternal, fetal and neonatal aspects. Boston: Butterworths, 1986:41.
10. Albright J, Sprague B, El-Khoury G, et al. Fractures and Pregnancy. In: Buschbaum HJ, ed. Trauma in pregnancy. Philadelphia: WB Saunders, 1979:142.
11. Aldridge LM, Tunstall ME. Nitrous oxide and the fetus. A review and the results of a retrospective study of 175 cases of anaesthesia for insertion of shirodkar suture. Br J Anaesth 1986;58:1348.
12. Alpert J, Day N, Dooling E, et al. Maternal alcohol consumption and newborn assessment. Neurobehav Toxicol Teratol 1981;3:195.
13. Baden JM, Kelley M, Wharton RS, et al. Mutagenicity of halogenated ether anesthetics. Anesthesiology 1977;46:346.
14. Baker DP. Trauma in the pregnant patient. Surg Clin North Am 1982;62:275.
15. Baldwin GB, Moorthi DS, Whelton JA, et al. New lung functions and pregnancy. Am J Obstet Gynecol 1977;127:235.
16. Barden TP, Peter JB, Merkatz IR. Ritodrine hydrochloride: a betamimetic agent for use in preterm labor. Obstet Gynecol 1980;56:1.
17. Barron WM, Lindheimer MD. Renal sodium and water handling in pregnancy. In: Wynn RM, ed. Obstetrics and gynecology manual. Vol 13. 1984:36.
18. Basford AB, Fink BR. The teratogenicity of halothane in the rat. Anesthesiology 1968;29:1167.
19. Beeley L. Adverse effects of drugs in the first trimester of pregnancy. Clin Obstet Gynecol 1981;8:261.
20. Beeley L. Adverse effects of drugs in later pregnancy. Clin Obstet Gynecol 1981;8:275.
21. Benedetti TJ. Life-threatening complications of betamimetic therapy for preterm labor inhibition. Clin Perinatol 1986;13:843.
22. Bergland F, Flodh H, Lundborg P, et al. Drug use during pregnancy and breast-feeding: a classification system for drug information. Acta Obstet Gynecol Scand 1984;126(suppl):5.
23. Berkowitz ID, Rogers MC. The physiology of cerebral blood flow during cardiopulmonary resuscitation. 1988;35:S23.
24. Berman LB. The pregnant kidney. JAMA 1974;230:111.
25. Biehl DR, Tweed A, Cote J, et al. Effect of halothane on cardiac output and regional blood flow in the fetal lamb in utero. Anesth Analg 1983;62:489.
26. Biehl DR, Yarnell R, Wade IG, et al. The uptake of isoflurane by the fetal lamb in utero: effect on regional blood flow. Can Anaesth Soc J 1983;30:581.
27. Bienarz J, Maqueda E, Caldeyro-Barcia R. Compression of the aorta by the uterus in late human pregnancy. Am J Obstet Gynecol 1966;95:781.
28. Black JW, Duncan AM, Durant CJ, et al. Definition and antagonism of histamine $H_2$-receptors. Nature 1972;385:390.
29. Blitt CD, Petty WC, Alberternst EE. Correlation of plasma cholinesterase activity and duration of action of succinylcholine during pregnancy. Anesth Analg 1977;56:78.
30. Bocking A, Adamson L, Cousin A. Effects of intravenous glucose injections on human fetal breathing movements and gross fetal body movements at 38 to 40 weeks of gestational age. Am J Obstet Gynecol 1982;142:606.
31. Bodendorfer TW. Fetal effects of anticonvulsant drugs. Drug Intell Clin Pharm 1978;12:14.
32. Bonica JJ, ed. Principles and practice of obstetric analgesia and anesthesia. vol 1. Philadelphia: FA Davis, 1966.
33. Bonica JJ. Obstetric analgesia and anesthesia. 2nd ed. Amsterdam: World Federation of Societies of Anesthesiologists, 1980:1.
34. Bonica JJ. Maternal physiologic and psychologic alterations during pregnancy and labor. In: Cosmi EV, ed. Obstetric anesthesia and perinatology. New York: Appleton-Century-Crofts, 1981:19.
35. Brakman P. The fibrinolytic system in human blood during pregnancy. Am J Obstet Gynecol 1966;94:14.
36. Brater D, Peters M, Eshelman F, et al. Clinical comparison of cimetidine and ranitidine. Clin Pharmacol Ther 1982;32:484.
37. Briggs GG, Freeman RK, Yaffe SJ. Drugs in pregnancy and lactation. Baltimore: Williams & Wilkins, 1986.
38. Bruce DL. Alcoholism and anesthesia. Anesth Analg 1983;62:84.
39. Bylsma-Howell M, Riggs KW, McMorland GH. Placental transport of metoclopramide. Assessment of maternal and neonatal effects. Can Anaesth Soc J 1983;30:487.
40. Caplan RA, Ward RJ, Posner K, Cheney FW. Unexpected cardiac arrest during spinal anesthesia, a closed claims analysis of predisposing factors. Anesthesiology 1988;68:5.
41. Chalon J, Tang CK, Ramanathan S, et al. Exposure to halothane and enflurane affects learning function of murine progeny. Anesth Analg 1981;60:794.
42. Chalon J, Hillman D, Gross S, et al. Intrauterine exposure to halothane increases murine postnatal autotolerance to halothane and reduces brain weight. Anesth Analg 1983;62:565.
43. Chanarin I, Deacon R, Lumb M, et al. Vitamin $B_{12}$ regulates folate metabolism by the supply of formate. Lancet 1980;2:505.
44. Chasnoff IJ, Burns WJ, Schnoll SH, Burns KA. Cocaine use in pregnancy. N Engl J Med 1985;336:666.
45. Churchill WA, Berendes HW, Nemore J. Neuropsychological deficits in children of diabetic mothers. A report from the collaborative study of cerebral palsy. Am J Obstet Gynecol 1969;105:257.
46. Civil ID, Talucci RC, Schwab CW. Placental laceration and fetal death as a result of blunt abdominal trauma. J Trauma 1988;28:708.

47. Cohen EN, Belleville JW, Brown BW. Anesthesia, pregnancy and miscarriage. A study of operating room nurses and anesthetists. Anesthesiology 1979;35:343.
48. Cohen J, Whectman AP, Dvagie HJ, et al. Life-threatening arrhythmias and intravenous cimetidine. Br Med J 1979;2:768.
49. Cohen SE. Risk of abortion following general anesthesia for surgery during pregnancy: anesthetic or surgical procedure. Anesthesiology 1986;65:706.
50. Coombs DW, Hooper D, Colton T. Preanesthetic cimetidine alteration of gastric fluid volume and pH. Anesth Analg 1979;58:183.
51. Covino BG, Vassallo HG. Local anesthetics: Mechanism of action and clinical use. New York: Grune and Stratton, 1976.
52. Craig DB, Toole MA. Airway closure in pregnancy. Can Anaesth Soc J 1975;22:665.
53. Crawford JS, Lewis M. Nitrous oxide in early human pregnancy. Anaesthesia 1986;41:900.
54. Crosby WM. Automobile injuries and blunt abdominal trauma. In: Buschbaum HJ, ed. Trauma in pregnancy. Philadelphia: WB Saunders, 1979:101.
55. Crosby WM. Traumatic injuries during pregnancy. Clin Obstet Gynecol 1983;26:902.
56. Cruikshank DP. Anatomic and physiologic alterations of pregnancy that modify the response to trauma. In: Buschbaum HJ, ed. Trauma in pregnancy. Philadelphia: WB Saunders, 1979: 21.
57. Dailey PA, Baysinger CL, Levinson G, et al. Neurobehavioral testing of the newborn infant. Clin Perinatol 1982;9:191.
58. Dammann HG, Muller P, Simon B. Parenteral ranitidine: onset and duration of action. Br J Anaesth 1982;54:1235.
59. Datta S, Alper MH, Ostheimer GW, et al. Method of ephedrine administration for hypotension and nausea during spinal anesthesia for cesarean section. Anesthesiology 1983;58:184.
60. Davison JM. Renal hemodynamics and volume homeostasis in pregnancy. Scand J Clin Lab Invest 1984;169(suppl):15.
61. Davison JS, Davison MC, Hay DM. Gastric emptying time in late pregnancy and labour. J Obstet Gynecol Br Comm 1970;77:37.
62. De Jong RH, Ronfield RA, De Rosa RA. Cardiovascular effects of convulsant and supraconvulsant doses of amide local anesthetics. Anesth Analg 1982;61:3.
63. Desmond MM, Schwanekke RP, Wilson GS. Maternal barbiturate utilization and neonatal withdrawal symptomatology. J Pediatrics 1972;80:190.
64. Di Fazio CA. Metabolism of local anesthetics in the fetus, newborn and the adult. Br J Anaesth 1979;51:295.
64a. Drost TF, Rosemurgy AS, Sherman HF, et al. Major trauma in pregnant women: maternal/fetal outcome. J Trauma 1990;30:574.
65. Justins DM. Anesthesia for Obstetrics. In: Churchhill-Davidson HC, ed. A Practice of anaesthesia. Chicago: Year Book Medical Publishers, 1984:1069.
66. Duncan PG, Pope WDB, Cohen MM. Fetal risk of anesthesia and surgery during pregnancy. Anesthesiology 1986;64:790.
67. Dundee JW, Gray TC. Resistance to d-tubocurarine chloride in the presence of liver damage. Lancet 1957;2:16.
68. Dundee JW, Moore J, Johnston JR, et al. Cimetidine and obstetric anesthesia. Lancet 1981;2:252.
69. Duvaldestin P, Agoston S, Henzel D, et al. Pancuronium; pharmacokinetics in patients with liver cirrhosis. Br J Anaesth 1978;50:1131.
70. Eckstein KL, Marx GF. Aortocaval compression and uterine displacement. Anesthesiology 1974;40:92.
71. Edner U, Erasmie U, Gentz J, et al. Intrauterine cranial gunshot wound in a 32-week fetus. J Trauma 1988;28:1605.
72. Ellinwood EH Jr. Amphetamines/anorectics. In:Handbook of drug abuse. National Institute on Drug Abuse. Washington DC: US Government Printing Office, 1979:221.
73. Elliot G, Rao T. Pregnancy and radiographic examination. In: Haycock CE, ed. Trauma and pregnancy. Littleton, MA: PSG Publishing, 1985:67.
74. Fagraeus L, Urban BJ, Bromage PR, et al. Spread of epidural anesthesia in early pregnancy. Anesthesiology 1983;58:184.
75. Feely J, Wilkinson GR, Alastair A, et al. Reduction of liver blood flow and propranalol metabolism. N Engl J Med 1981;304:692.
76. Finnegan LP, Michael H, Leifer B, Desai S. An evaluation of neonatal abstinence modalities. Natl Inst Drug Abuse Res Monogr Ser 1983;49:282.
77. Finster M, Pedersen H. Placental transfer and fetal uptake of drugs. Br J Anaesth 1979;51:255.
78. Fishburne JI. Fetal monitoring in high risk pregnancy. In: James FM, Wheeler AS, eds, Obstetric anaesthesia: The complicated patient. Philadelphia: FA Davis, 1982:1.
79. Foulkes E, Jenkins LC. A comparative evaluation of cimetidine and sodium citrate to decrease gastric acidity. Effectiveness at the time of induction of anesthesia. Can Anaesth Soc J 1981;28:29.
80. Fried P. Marihuana use by pregnant women and effects of offspring: an update. Neurobehav Toxicol Teratol 1983;3:195.
81. Frienkel N. Of pregnancy and progeny. Diabetes 1980;29:1023.
82. Fujinaga M, Mazze RI. Reproductive and teratogenic effects of lidocaine in Sprague-Dawley rats. Anesthesiology 1986;65:626.
83. Garnett AR, Ornato JP, Gonzalez ER, et al. The clinical value of end-tidal carbon dioxide monitoring during cardiopulmonary resuscitation. JAMA 1987;257:512.
84. Geber W, Schramm LC. Congenital malformations of the central nervous system produced by narcotic analgesics in the hamster. Am J Obstet Gynecol 1975;123:705.
85. Goodman AS, Yakovac WC. The enhancement of salicylate teratogenicity by maternal immobilization in the rat. J Pharmacol Exp Therap 1963;142:351.
86. Grannum PA. Ultrasound examination of the placenta. Clin Obstet Gynecol 1983;10:459.
87. Gregory GA, Wade JG, Biehl DR, et al. Fetal anesthetic requirement (MAC) for halothane. Anesth Analg 1983;62:9.
88. Gunther RE, Belleville JW. Obstetrical caudal anesthesia: II. A randomized study comparing 1% mepivacaine with 1% mepivacaine plus epinephrine. Anesthesiology 1972;37:288.
89. Hall J, Pauli RM, Wilson KM. Maternal and fetal sequelae of anticoagulation during pregnancy. Am J Med 1980;68:122.
90. Hannah RS, Moore KL. Effects of fasting and insulin on skeletal development in rats. Teratology 1971;4:135.
91. Haycock CE. Emergency care of the pregnant traumatized patient. Emerg Med Clin North Am 1984;2:843.
92. Hodgkinson R, Glassenberg R, Joyce TH. Comparison of cimetidine (Tagamet®) for safety and effectiveness in reducing gastric acidity before elective cesarean section. Anesthesiology 1983;59:86.
93. Holdsworth JD. Mixing of antacids with stomach contents. Anaesthesia 1980;35:641.
94. Hollingsworth DR. Alterations of maternal metabolism in normal and diabetic pregnancies. Differences in insulin-dependent, non-insulin dependent, and gestational diabetes. Am J Obstet Gynecol 1983;146:417.
95. Hunt TM, Semple MJ. Blood transfusion. In: Churchill-Davidson HC, ed. A Practice of Anaesthesia. Chicago: Year Book Medical Publishers, 1984:587.
96. Hutchings DE. Behavioral teratology: a new frontier in neurobehavioral research. In: Johnson EM, Kochhar DM, eds. Teratogenesis and reproductive toxicology. Handbook of experimental pharmacology. New York: Springer-Verlag, 1983:207.
97. Jackson FC. Accidental injury, the problem and the initiative.

In: Buschbaum HJ, ed. Trauma in pregnancy. Philadelphia: WB Saunders, 1979:1.

98. Jaffe JH. Drug addiction and drug abuse. In: Gilman AG, Goodman LS, Rall TW, Murad F, eds, the Pharmacologic basis of therapeutics. New York: MacMillan Publishing, 1985:532.
99. Jaffe JH, Martin WR. Opioid analgesics and antagonists. In: Gilman AG, Goodman LS, Rall TW, Murad F, eds. The pharmacologic basis of therapeutics. New York: MacMillan Publishing, 1985:491.
100. James FM III, Wheeler AS, Dewan DM. Obstetric anesthesia: the complicated patient. Philadelphia: FA Davis, 1988.
101. Jeikkinen JE, Rinne RI, Alahuhta SM, et al. Life support for 10 weeks with successful fetal outcome after fatal maternal brain damage. Br Med J 1985;290:1237.
102. Jenkins LC. Anesthetic problems due to drug abuse and dependence. Canad Anaesth Soc J 1972;19:461.
103. Johnsson S, O'Meara M, Young JB. Acute cocaine poisoning. Importance of treating seizures and acidosis. Am J Med 1983;75:1061.
104. Johnston RE, Kulp RA, Smith TC. Effects of acute and chronic ethanol administration on isoflurane requirement in mice. Anesth Analg 1975;54:277.
105. Johnston RR, Way WL, Miller RD. Alteration of anesthetic requirement by amphetamine. Anesthesiology 1972;36:357.
106. Jouppila R, Jouppila P, Kuikka J, et al. Placental blood flow during cesarean section under lumbar extradural analgesia. Br J Anaesth 1978;50:275.
107. Kammerer WS. Nonobstetric surgery in pregnancy. Med Clin North Am 1987;71:551.
108. Kasten GW, Martin TS. Resuscitation from bupivacaine induced cardiovascular toxicity during partial inferior vena cava occlusion. Anesth Analg 1986;65:341.
109. Katz JD, Hook R, Barash PG. Fetal heart rate monitoring in pregnant patients undergoing surgery. Am J Obstet Gynecol 1976;125:267.
110. Katz VL, Dotters DJ, Droegmueller W. Perimortem cesarean delivery. Obstet Gynecol 1986;68:571.
111. Kerr MG, Scott DB, Samuel E. Studies of the inferior vena cava in late pregnancy. Br Med J 1964;1:532.
112. Kirkpatrick C, Quenon M, Desir D. Blood anions and electrolytes during ritodrine infusion during preterm labor. Am J Obstet Gynecol 1980;138:523.
113. Kleber HD, Gawin FH. Cocaine abuse: a review of current and experimental treatments. Natl Inst Drug Abuse Res Monogr Ser 1984:112.
114. Knepp NB, Shelly WC, Kumar S, et al. Effects on newborn of hydration with glucose in patients undergoing cesarean section with regional anesthesia. Lancet 1980;1:645.
115. Koppe JG, Kleiverda G. Severe asphyxia and outcome of survivors. Resuscitation 1984;12:193.
116. Kruse J: Alcohol use during pregnancy. AFP 1984;29:199.
117. Lagamma EF, Irskowitz J, Rudolf AM. Effects of naloxone on fetal circulatory responses to hypoxemia. Am J Obstet Gynecol 1983;143:933.
118. Lam AM, Parkin JA. Cimetidine and prolonged post-operative somnolence. Can Anaesth Soc J 1981;28:450.
119. Lamp MP, Manners JM. Fetal heart monitoring during open heart surgery. Br J Obstet Gynaecol 1981;88:669.
120. Lang RM, Borrow KM. Pregnancy and heart disease. Clin Perinatol 1985;12:551.
121. Lavin JP, Polsky SS. Abdominal trauma during pregnancy. Clin Perinatol 1983;10:423.
122. Lee RV, Rogers BD, White LM, Harvey RC. Cardiopulmonary resuscitation of pregnant women. Am J Med 1986;81:311.
123. Levine W, Diamond B. Surgical procedures during pregnancy. Am J Obstet Gynecol 1961;81:1046.
124. Levinson G, Shnider SM, de Lorimer AA. Uterine blood flow and fetal acid-base changes after bicarbonate administration to the pregnant ewe. Anesthesiology 1974;40:340.
125. Lind JF, Smith AM, Coopland AT, et al. Heartburn in pregnancy—a manometric study. Can Med Assoc J 1968;98:571.
126. Lind T. Fluid balance during labor: a review. J Roy Soc Med 1983;76:870.
127. Lindsay SL, Hanson GC. Cardiac arrest in near term pregnancy. Anaesthesia 1987;42:1074.
128. Longstreth GF, Go VLW, Malagelda JR. Cimetidine suppression of nocturnal gastric secretion in active duodenal ulcer. N Engl J Med 1981;304:692.
129. Lucas A, Adrian TE, Aynsley-Greene A, et al. Iatrogenic hyperinsulinism at birth. Lancet 1980;1:144.
130. MacGillivray I. Pre-eclampsia: the hypertensive disease of pregnancy. London: WB Saunders, 1983:116.
131. Manchikanti L, Kraus JW, Edds SP. Cimetidine and related drugs in anesthesia. Anesth Analg 1982;61:595.
132. Marx GF, Orkin LR. Physiology of obstetrics anesthesia. Springfield, IL: Charles C Thomas, 1969:96.
133. Marx GF, Bassell GM. Physiologic considerations of the mother. In: Marx GF, Bassell GM, eds. Obstetric analgesia and anesthesia. New York: Elsevier, 1980:21.
134. Mathews RN. Obstetric implications of burns in pregnancy. Br J Obstet Gynaecol 1982;89:603.
135. Mathru M, Rao TLK, Kartha RK, et al. Intravenous albumin administration for prevention of spinal hypotension during cesarean section. Anesth Analg 1980;59:655.
136. Mazze RI. Nitrous oxide during pregnancy; editorial. Anaesthesia 1986;41:897.
137. Mazze RI, Wilson AI, Rice SA, et al. Effects of isoflurane on reproduction and fetal development in mice. Anesth Analg 1984;63:249.
138. Mendiola J, Graylack LJ, Scanlon JW. Effects of intrapartum glucose infusion on the normal fetus and newborn. Anesth Analg 1982;61:32.
139. Metcalfe J, Bartels H, Moll W. Gas exchange in the pregnant uterus. Am J Obstet Gynecol 1967;47:782.
140. Milcovich L, van den Berge BJ. Effects of perinatal meprobomate and chlordiazepoxide on human embryonic and fetal development. N Engl J Med 1974;291:1268.
141. Mills JL, Gzaubard BI, Harley EE, et al. Maternal alcohol consumption and birth weight. JAMA 1984;252:1875.
142. Moore DC, Spierdig K, van Kleef JD. Chlorprocaine neurotoxity: four additional cases. Anesth Analg 1982;61:15.
143. Mossman KL. Medical radiodiagnosis and pregnancy: evaluation of options when pregnancy status is uncertain. Health Physics 1985;48:297.
144. Murad SHN, Conklin KA, Tabsh KMA, et al. Atropine and glycopyrrolate: hemodynamic effects and placental transfer in the pregnant ewe. Anesth Analg 1981;60:710.
145. Murray FA, Erskine JP, Fielding J. Gastric secretion in pregnancy. J Obstet Gynecol Brit Emp 1957;64:373.
146. Nathan RA, Segall N, Glover GC, et al. The effects of $H_1$ and $H_2$ antihistamines on histamine inhalation challenges in asthmatic patients. Am Rev Respir Dis 1979;120:1251.
147. Neufeld JDG, Moore EE, Marx JA, Rosen P. Trauma in pregnancy. Emerg Med Clin North Am 1987;5:623.
148. Nibyl JR. Drug use in pregnancy. Philadelphia: Lea and Febiger, 1988:193.
149. Nicolaides KH, Rodeck CH. In utero resuscitation after cardiac arrest in a fetus. Br Med J 1984;288:900.
150. Niederhoff H, Zahradnaik HP. Analgesics during pregnancy. Am J Med 1984;83:117.
151. Nunn JF. Applied respiratory physiology. 2nd ed. Boston: Butterworths, 1977:340.

152. Oats JN, Vasey DP, Waldron BA. Effects of ketamine on the pregnant uterus. Br J Anaesth 1979;51:1163.
153. Ostrea EM, Chavez CJ. Perinatal problems (excluding neonatal withdrawal) in maternal addiction: a study of 830 cases. J Pediatr 1979;94:292.
154. Park GR. Hypotension following metoclopramide administration during hypotensive anaesthesia for intracranial aneurysm. Br J Anaesth 1978;50:1268.
155. Patterson RM. Trauma in pregnancy. Clin Obstet Gynecol 1984;27:32.
156. Pedersen H, Finster M. Anesthetic risk in the pregnant surgical patient. Anesthesiology 1979;51:439.
157. Petersdorf RG et al. Opiates and synthetic analgesics. Commonly abused drugs. Alcohol. Sedatives, stimulants and psychotropic drugs. In: Petersdorf RG, Adams RD, Braunwald E, Isselbacher KJ, Martin JB, Wislon JD, eds. Harrison's principles of internal medicine. New York: McGraw-Hill, 1983:1278–1301.
158. Ralston DH, Shnider SM. The fetal and neonatal effects of regional anesthesia in obstetrics. Anesthesiology 1978;48:34.
159. Ralston DH, Shnider SM, de Lorimer AA. Effects of equipotent ephedrine, metaraminol, mephentermine and methoxamine on uterine blood flow in the pregnant ewe. Anesthesiology 1974;40:354.
160. Ralston DH, Shnider SM, de Lorimer AA. Uterine blood flow and fetal acid-base changes after bicarbonate administration to the pregnant ewe. Anesthesiology 1974;40:348.
161. Ramanathan S. The biochemical profile of a well-oxygenated human fetus. Anesthesiology 1984;61:A85.
162. Ramanathan S. Obstetric anesthesia. Phildelphia: Lea and Febiger, 1988.
163. Ramanathan S, Grant GJ. Vasopressor therapy for hypotension due to epidural anesthesia for cesarean section. Acta Anaesthesiol Scand 1988;32:559.
164. Ramanathan S, Gandhi S, Arismendy J, et al. Oxygen transfer from mother to fetus during cesarean section under epidural anesthesia. Anesth Analg 1982;61:576.
165. Ramanathan S, Masih AK, Rock I, et al. Maternal and fetal effects of hydration with crystalloids or colloids before epidural anesthesia. Anesth Analg 1983;62:673.
166. Ramanathan S, Friedman S, Moss P, et al. Phenylephrine for treatment of maternal hypotension due to epidural anesthesia. Anesth Analg 1984;63:262.
167. Ramanathan S, Masih AK, Ashok U, et al. Concentrations of lactate and pyruvate in maternal and neonatal blood with different intravenous fluids used for prehydration before epidural anesthesia. Anesth Analg 1984;63:69.
168. Richards SR, Chang FE, Stempel LE. Hyperlactacidemia associated with acute ritodrine infusion. Am J Obstet Gynecol 1983;146:1.
169. Richardson B, Hohimer AR, Muegler P, et al. Effects of glucose concentration on fetal breathing movements and electrocortical activity in fetal lambs. Am J Obstet Gynecol 1982;142:678.
170. Richardson BS, O'Grady JP, Olsen GD. Fetal breathing movements and the response to carbon dioxide in patients on methadone maintenance. Am J Obstet Gynecol 1984;150:400.
171. Roberts RB, Shirley MA. Reducing the risk of acid aspiration during cesarean section. Anesth Analg 1974;53:859.
172. Robertson GS. Serum cholinesterase deficiency. II: pregnancy. Br J Anaesth 1966;38:361.
173. Rock I, Ramanathan S, Gandhi S, et al. Serum chemistry and oncotic pressure changes due to hydration before epidural anesthesia. Anesthesiology 1982;57:A394.
174. Romero R. The management of acquired hemostatic failure in pregnancy. In: Berkowitz RL, ed. Critical care of the obstetrical patient. London: Churchill Livingstone, 1983:219.
175. Rosett HL, Weiner L. Alcohol and pregnancy: a clinical perspective. Annu Rev Med 1985;36:73.
176. Rothenberger D, Quattlebaum F, Zebol J, et al. Diagnostic peritoneal lavage for blunt trauma in pregnant women. Am J Obstet Gynecol 1977;129:497.
177. Rudikoff MT, Maughan WL, Effron M, et al. Mechanisms of blood flow during cardiopulmonary resuscitation. Circulation 1980;61:345.
178. Sachs BP, Brown DAJ, Driscoli SJ, et al. Maternal mortality in Massachusetts: trends and prevention. N Engl J Med 1987;316:667.
179. Safra MJ, Oakley GP. Association between cleft lip with or without cleft palate and prenatal exposure to diazepam. Lancet 1975;2:478.
180. Salmenpera M, Kortilla K, Kalima T. Reduction of the risk of acid pulmonary aspiration in anesthetized patients after cimetidine premedication. Acta Anaesth Scand 1980;24:25.
181. Samuels SI, Maze A, Albright G. Cardiac arrest during cesarean section in a chronic amphetamine abuser. Anesth Analg 1979;58:528.
182. Saxen I, Saxen L. Association between maternal intake of diazepam and oral clefts. Lancet 1975;2:498.
183. Scott DB. Inferior vena caval occlusion in late pregnancy and its importance in anesthesia. Br J Anaesth 1968;40:120.
184. Shaw RG, Mashford ML, Desmond PV. Cardiac arrest after intravenous injection of cimetidine. Med J Aust 1980;2:629.
185. Shelley WC. Anesthetic considerations for nonobstetric surgery. Clin Perinatol 1982;9:135.
186. Shelley WC, Gutsche BB. Anesthesia for the febrile parturient. In: James FM, Wheeler AS, eds. Obstetric anesthesia: the Complicated patient. Philadelphia: FA Davis, 1982:297.
187. Shnider SM. Serum cholinesterase activity during pregnancy, labor and the puerperium. Anesthesiology 1966;26:335.
188. Shnider SM, Webster GM. Maternal and fetal hazards of surgery during pregnancy. Am J Obstet Gynecol 1965;92:891.
189. Shnider SM, Wright RC, Levinson G, et al. Uterine blood flow and plasma norepinephrine—changes during maternal stress in the pregnant ewe. Anesthesiology 1979;50:524.
190. Slone D, Siskind V, Heinonen OP, et al. Antenatal exposure to phenothiazines in relation to congenital malformations, perinatal mortality rate, birth weight and intelligence quotient score. Am J Obstet Gynecol 1977;128:486.
191. Smith BE. Fetal prognosis after anesthesia during gestation. Anesth Analg 1963;42:521.
192. Smith BK, Rayburn W, Feller I. Burns and pregnancy. Clin Perinatol 1983;10:383.
193. Smith DS, Gutsche BB. Amphetamine abuse and obstetrical anesthesia (letter). Anesth Analg 1980;59:710.
194. Sorensen VJ, Bivins BA, Obeid FN, Horst HM. Trauma in pregnancy. Henry Ford Hosp Med J 1986;34:101.
195. Spence AA, Moir DD, Finlay WEI. Observations on intragastric pressure. Anaesthesia 1967;22:249.
196. Spence AA, Cohen EN, Brown BW, et al. Occupational hazards for the operating room-based physician. JAMA 1977;238:955.
197. Steele WJ, Johanesson T. Effects of prenatally-administered morphine on brain development and resultant tolerance to analgesic effect of morphine in offspring of morphine treated rats. Acta Pharmacol Toxicol 1975;36:243.
198. Stimmel B, Goldberg J, Reisman A, et al. Fetal outcome in narcotic dependent women. Am J Drug Alcohol Abuse 1982–83;9:383.
199. Stoelting RK. Responses to atropine, glycopyrrolate and Riopan on gastric fluid pH and volume in adult patients. Anesthesiology 1978;48:367.
200. Stoelting RK, Craesser CW, Martz RC. Effects of cocaine ad-

ministration on halothane MAC in dogs. Anesthesiology 1975;54:422.

201. Stott DH. Physical and mental handicaps following a disturbed pregnancy. Lancet 1957;1:1006.
202. Streissguth AP, Herman CS, Smith DW. Intelligence behaviour and dysmorphogenesis in fetal alcohol syndrome: a report on 20 patients. J Pediatrics 1978;92:363.
203. Swartz J, Cummings M, Pucci W, et al. The effects of general anesthesia on the asphyxiated fetal lamb in utero. Can Anaesth Soc J 1985;32:577.
204. Ueland K, Metcalfe J. Circulatory changes in pregnancy. Clin Obstet Gynecol 1975;18:41.
205. Vannucci RC, Wolf JW. Oxidative metabolism in the fetal rat brain during maternal anesthesia. Anesthesiology 1978;48:238.
206. Viegas OJ, Ravindran RS, Shumacker CA. Gastric fluid pH in patients receiving sodium citrate. Anesth Analg 1981;60:521.
207. Vieira E. Effect of the chronic administration of nitrous oxide 0.5% to gravid rats. Br J Anaesth 1979;51:283.
208. Wald A. Effects of pregnancy on gastrointestinal tract. Dig Dis Sci 1982;27:1015.
209. Wang BC, Hillman DE, Spielholz NI, et al. Chronic neurological deficits and nesacaine CE—an effect of the anesthetic 2-chloroprocaine or the antioxidant, sodium bisulfite? Anesth Analg 1984;63:445.
210. Watson DW. Effects of glycopyrrolate and cimetidine on gastric volume and acidity in patients awaiting surgery. Br J Anaesth 1978;50:1247.
211. Weintraub SJ, Naulty S. Acute abstinence syndrome after epidural injection of butorphanol. Anesth Analg 1985;64: 452.
212. Werhoff J, Havlena J. Postnatal behavioral effects of tranquilizers administered to the gravid rat. Exp Neurol 1962;6: 263.
213. Wharton RS, Mazze RI, Baden JM, et al. Fertility, reproduction and postnatal survival in mice chronically exposed to halothane Anesthesiology 1978;48:167.
214. Williamson JR. Glycolytic control mechanisms. Inhibition of glycolysis by acetate and pyruvate in the isolated perfused rat heart. J Biol Chem 1965;240:2308.
215. Wyner J, Cohen SE. Gastric volume in early pregnancy. Anesthesiology 1982;57:209.
216. Yarnell R, Biehl DR, Tweed WA, et al. The effects of halothane anesthesia on the asphyxiated fetal lamb in utero. Can Anaesth Soc J 1983;30:474.
217. Ygge J. Change in blood coagulation and fibrinolysis during the puerperium. Am J Obstet Gynecol 1969;104:2.
218. Zimmerberg B, Charap AD, Glick SD. Behavioral effects of in utero administration of morphine. Nature 1974;257:376.

# Chapter Twenty

Gary W. Welch

# Care of the Patient with Thermal Injury

Each year more than 2 million people suffer thermal injury in the United States.[1] Of those so injured, 90,000 require hospital treatment. Approximately 20,000 have injuries severe enough to require admission to a specialized care center. Demling quotes a probability of anyone's being burned during his or her lifetime of almost 1.5%.[43] Although the majority of injuries occur in individuals 17 to 44 years of age and in men between the ages of 17 and 30, almost one-third of those incurring a major injury are under 17 and one-fifth are over the age of 45.[93] As a result of improved education, prevention, and therapy, the mortality from thermal injury has declined to 2.0–2.7 per 100,000 population during the past several years.[1,5] This represents a 31% decrease in the death rate and a 24% decrease in the total number of deaths from burns in 1987 as compared to 1977.[1] Approximately 5,000 persons died from burns and fires in 1987.[1]

In 1985, the $LA_{50}$ at the Shriners Burn Institute Cincinnati Unit was slightly above 80%, nearly 2.5 times that of 1940.[5] $LA_{50}$ is defined as percent body surface area burn that results in death in 50% of persons. Decreased mortality from burn injury also has been reported by other major centers in the nation.[109,158] One must remember, however, that mortality can differ in different burn units; at least two studies have correlated decreased mortality with rapid closure of the burn wound.[158,179] Yet, patients over the age of 60 with major thermal injury continue to have a poor prognosis. Anous and Heimbach[8] suggest that Baux's formula, which states that percent mortality in thermal injury is equal to the sum of the patient's age and percent burn, is still valid for elderly patients.

The skin is one of the larger organs of the body and, in the average adult, weighs approximately 2.5 kg. Loss of significant amounts of skin presents the individual with a life-threatening situation because of metabolic stress, loss of body heat and fluid, and immunosuppression. Fractures of major bones or peritonitis produce an increase in the metabolic rate of 30 to 50%. Burns, however, have a very profound effect on oxygen consumption; a 50% body surface burn produces a 70% increase in metabolic rate (Fig 20-1).[175] This increase has been correlated with increased catecholamine secretion, but other hormones may also play a role. A major goal of burn therapy therefore is to ameliorate or eliminate these potentially life-threatening conditions.

## BURN CLASSIFICATION

Classically, burn wounds are classified as first, second, or third degree according to depth. First-degree burns correspond to a profound sunburn and are characterized by pain and erythema. Second-degree burns are characterized by involvement of the dermis and vesicle formation accompanied by pain. A third-degree burn is defined as total destruction of the skin and extension of injury into the subcutaneous fat. This results in a very tough, leathery eschar that is insensitive to pain because of coagulation of nerve endings. Preservation of the epithelial elements allows regeneration to occur after first- and second-degree burns; thus the wound will heal gradually. Although healing occurs, patients with large superficial burns have initial fluid requirements as great as those with third-degree injury. Inadequate resuscitation may actually re-

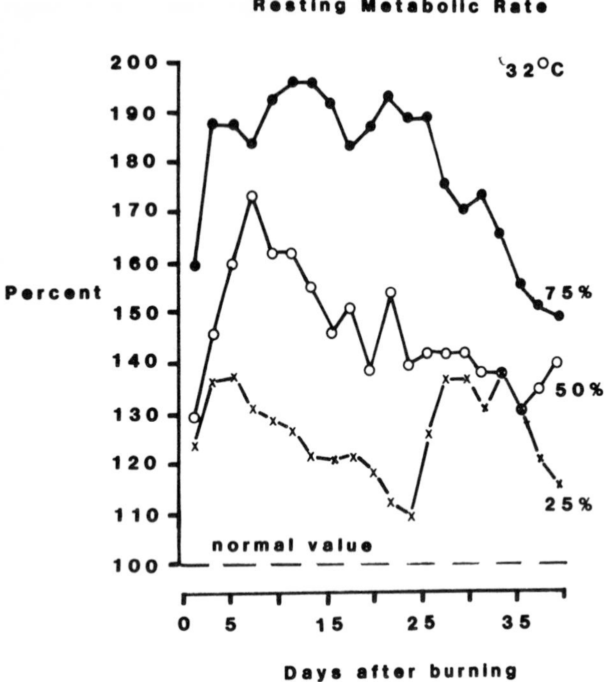


FIG. 20-1. Percent elevation of resting metabolic rate after burns covering 25, 50, and 75% of total body surface area. All patients were treated at an ambient temperature of 32°C. (Reproduced with permission from Davies JWL: J Roy Soc Med 1982;75(suppl 1):20.)

sult in conversion of a second- to a third-degree burn. Until the wound heals, infection is a constant threat. Third-degree burns can heal only by contracture and scarring, and after extensive injury, a persistent granulating bed remains.

A newer classification divides burn wounds into partial and full thickness and further subdivides partial-thickness wounds into superficial and deep burns (Fig 20-2). This division of burn wounds by depth has prognostic importance and also provides an estimate of the requirements for subsequent grafting. Patients with significant partial-thickness injury require aggressive resuscitation and wound protection as healing progresses. Patients with full-thickness injury additionally require multiple operative procedures to provide timely coverage of the burned area.

## IMMEDIATE CARE

Initial treatment of the burn patient is very similar to other forms of trauma therapy. Airway and ventilatory status must be evaluated. If the injury occurred in an enclosed area or as a result of steam and there is evidence of burns of the face, singed nasal hairs, or burns of the uvula, oropharynx, or upper airway, airway obstruction may occur precipitously. It is possible to assess upper airway obstruction by monitoring the inspiratory limb of the flow-volume loop. Doing so requires a cooperative patient and rather sophisticated equipment; hence, some clinicians have recommended prophylactic intubation, rather than waiting for evidence of obstruction to occur.[166] Once edema begins to develop, airway management can be very difficult and sometimes impossible. As discussed later, a surgical approach to the airway during this phase should be considered only in those patients who have developed acute complete or near-complete obstruction and in whom rapid oro- or nasotracheal intubation is impossible; tracheostomy is associated with a higher rate of complications than nonsurgical airway management in burn patients.[51,83,120] In the absence of the above signs and symptoms, the patient initially is usually able to maintain adequate ventilation and oxygenation. Supplemental oxygen should be administered in any case to counteract potential carboxyhemoglobinemia. Assessment of the airway should require only a short time. Simultaneously, venous access should be obtained for administration of fluids and drugs.

With any burn injury larger than 30% of the total body surface area (TBSA), a generalized increase in capillary permeability may develop as a result of direct thermal injury and secondary processes.[7] These secondary changes may be the result of vasoactive substances, such as leukotrienes, prostaglandins, and oxygen radicals released from burned tissue.[44] Attempts to alter permeability changes by using specific antagonists have, however, been unsuccessful.[43]

Increased capillary permeability to plasma proteins and

FIG. 20-2. Partial-thickness thermal injury leaves the hair follicles and sebaceous glands intact, and hence reepithelialization will occur. Full-thickness burns destroy these skin appendages and extend into the subcutaneous fat. (Reproduced with permission from Welch GW: Curr Rev Clin Anesth 1983;4:50.)

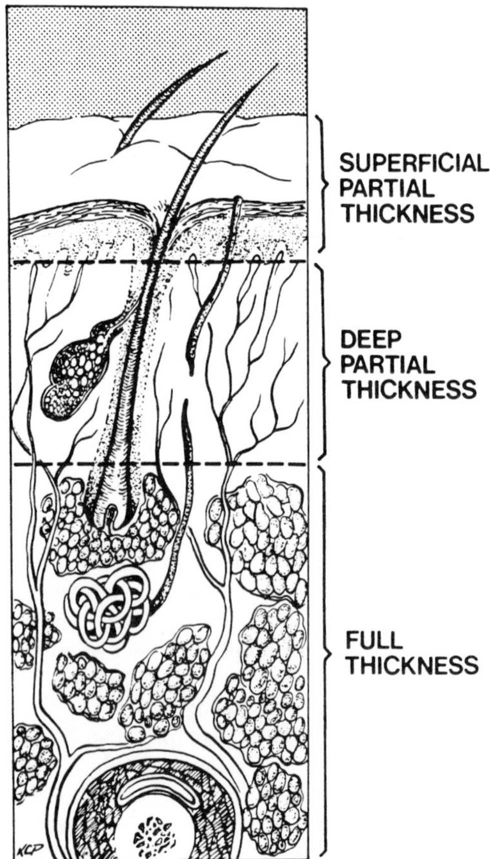

fluid results primarily from severe impairment of microvascular integrity. In animals, large endothelial cell gaps have been demonstrated that permit the passage of large protein molecules. These persist for several days.[44] Other factors that promote fluid shift into the extravascular space are hypoproteinemia, loosening of the interstitial matrix, impairment of vascular basement membrane, increased osmotic pressure in burned tissue, and a generalized decrease in cellular transmembrane potential from a normal value of −90 mV to −70 to −80 mV.[44] Fluid loss from the vascular bed results in significant hypovolemia; major thermal injury thus requires large volumes of fluid, and large-bore intravenous catheters should be used. Peripheral veins may be difficult to locate; the internal jugular or subclavian veins may be used even if it is necessary to place the catheter through eschar. A Swan-Ganz catheter introducer allows large volumes of fluid to be administered rapidly; it can be used subsequently for placement of a pulmonary artery catheter, which allows one to follow physiologic profiles and aids in guiding therapy. An increased risk of endocarditis has been reported in burn patients after pulmonary artery catheterization, however.[52] There is also evidence of damage to the tricuspid and pulmonary valves,[16] which may then serve as a nidus for thrombus formation and the development of endocarditis. Strict aseptic technique in placement and exacting care of the insertion site should minimize these problems.

A Foley catheter should also be placed in order to measure urine output on an hourly basis and to demonstrate hemoglobin or myoglobin in the urine. Low urine output during the initial phases of burn resuscitation is nearly always secondary to inadequate fluid replacement. Conversely, urine flow between 0.5–1.0 mL/kg/min suggests adequate kidney perfusion if the patient is not hyperglycemic and has not received hypertonic saline solution.

To the inexperienced clinician, a patient with major thermal injury can be a shocking experience. Although the patient may not be in pain, there is a tendency to provide analgesics. If these are necessary during the early phase of evaluation and resuscitation, small repeated doses (1–2 mg) of intravenous morphine should be administered. Intramuscular narcotics are not absorbed during this period. Repeated intramuscular doses accumulate and are subsequently absorbed as peripheral perfusion returns to normal, resulting in overnarcotization and possible respiratory arrest.[99]

## FLUID RESUSCITATION

The previously mentioned capillary leak results in intravascular volume depletion as fluid translocates into the interstitial space. As a result, hematocrit increases and cardiac output decreases. With burns involving more than 20% of the TBSA, profound hypovolemia results. Children are more susceptible to this condition than adults and may develop hypovolemia with burns of as little as 10–20% of the TBSA.[109] Volume replacement therefore is the cornerstone of initial therapy.[44]

With improvement in understanding of the pathophysiology of burns and with the development of burn centers, the majority of patients with thermal injuries receive adequate volume replacement. The major problem facing the burn patient at present is edema formation in both burned and nonburned tissues resulting from aggressive fluid resuscitation. Progression of upper airway edema after large cutaneous burns with or without smoke inhalation is greatly facilitated by rapid fluid infusion.[67] Pulmonary edema is uncommon even after administration of large volumes of fluid unless an inhalation injury is present.[44] However, chest wall edema may occur, and by reducing chest wall compliance, it can result in increased work of breathing and at times in respiratory insufficiency.[44] Edema formation may also increase the tissue pressure in the burned area, resulting in the reduction of blood flow. This reduction, together with decreased tissue oxygen tension, may produce necrosis of damaged but viable cells, thereby increasing the extent of injury and risk of infection.

Thus, volume replacement in burn injury has two objectives: adequate restoration of blood volume and minimizing of edema formation in both damaged and intact tissues. These objectives are of particular importance in modern burn treatment, which, as is discussed in the next section, involves early burn wound excision. In this setting both hypovolemia and/or excessive tissue edema increase operative risk. In addition, it has been demonstrated that fluid retention in excess of 4500 mL/m$^2$ TBSA/48 h (corrected for fluid loss from the burn wound) is an accurate predictor of mortality after a burn.[22]

The time course of edema formation differs in injured and uninjured tissues because different mechanisms are involved. In the injured region the magnitude of edema is determined by the volume of blood flow through the microcirculation. Since the blood flow to these tissues is decreased immediately after injury, significant edema does not occur until fluid resuscitation is initiated. After this period, gradual tissue swelling occurs and reaches a maximum within 8–12 hours if hypovolemia is corrected. Burns involving a large proportion of the body surface produce severe hypovolemia, which takes a longer time to correct. In this situation tissue swelling is delayed by the hypovolemia, and maximum edema formation usually occurs 18–24 hours after injury. In uninjured tissue, swelling results primarily from decreased plasma oncotic pressure produced by hypoproteinemia and the previously mentioned capillary leak. Since plasma protein concentration reaches its minimum 8–12 hours after injury, maximum edema formation in the intact tissues develops within this time.[44]

Intravenous therapies using crystalloid and colloid in varying proportions have been developed based on weight and percent of body surface injured (Fig 20-3). The Evans formula requires 1 mL/kg/% burn of a salt-containing solution and 1 mL/kg/% burn of a colloid solution, such as blood or plasma, to initiate fluid therapy. In addition, 2,000 mL of 5% dextrose solution is given for insensible losses.[54] The Brooke modification of the Evans formula calls for 0.5 mL/kg/% burn of a colloid solution and 1.5 mL/kg/% burn of crystalloid solution. The Parkland formula utilizes Ringer's lactate at a rate of 4 mL/kg/% burn; as in the modified Brooke formula, colloid-containing solutions are not administered during the first 24 hours (Table 20-1). Because of the generalized increase in capillary permeability, it was felt that any albumin given to the patient in the first 24 hours would be lost to the interstitial space, and therefore it would be of greater benefit to give only crystalloids. All of these formulas require that half the calculated volume be given in the first 8 hours, half the re-

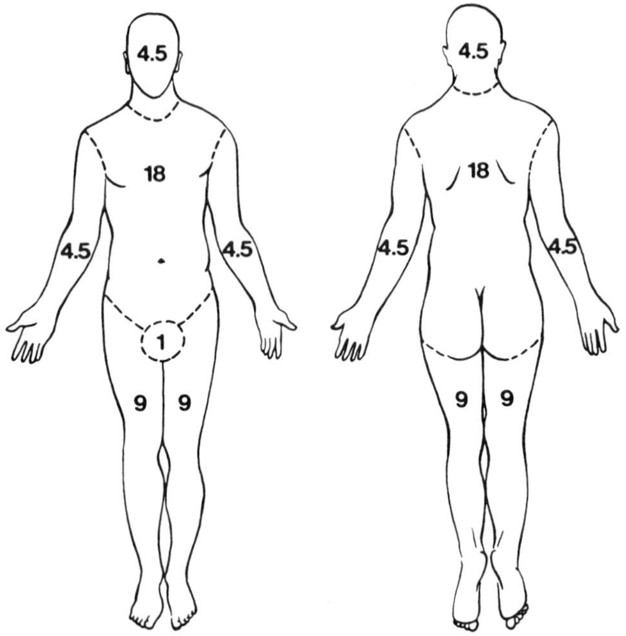


FIG. 20-3. Total body surface burn can be determined by the "rule of nines." (Reproduced with permission from Welch GW: Curr Rev Clin Anesth 1983;4:50.)

TABLE 20-1. Formulas to Guide Initial Fluid Resuscitation after Burn Injury

Evans formula*
  1.0 mL crystalloid/kg/% burn/24 h
  1.0 mL colloid/kg/% burn/24 h
  2,000 mL 5% dextrose in water/24 h
Brooke formula*
  1.5 mL crystalloid/kg/% burn/24 h
  0.5 mL colloid/kg/% burn/24 h
  2,000 mL 5% dextrose in water/24 h
Modified Brooke formula*
  2.0 mL Ringer's lactate/kg/% burn/24 h
Parkland formula*
  4.0 mL crystalloid/kg/% burn/24 h
Hypertonic lactated saline**
  Volume adjusted to promote a urine flow of 30 mL/h with a solution containing 300 mEq/L sodium, 200 mEq/L lactate, and 100 mEq/L chloride. Usually this amounts to 2 mL/kg/% burn/24 h
Dextran-crystalloid-protein***
  Dextran 40 or dextran 70 ≥ 2 mL/kg/h to maintain plasma dextran levels at or in excess of 2 g/dL and crystalloid as needed (1.0 mL/kg/% burn/8 h) during the first 8 hours after injury. This is followed by plasma protein 0.5–1.0 mL/kg/% burn/16 h with necessary additional crystalloid infusion.

* 50% of calculated volume is given during the first 8 hours, 25% of calculated volume is given during the second 8 hours, and 25% of callculated volume is given during the third 8 hours.

** Hypertonic saline is usually administered during the first 8 hours. Elevation of serum $Na^+$ concentration above 160 mEq/L dictates replacement of hypertonic solution with isotonic saline.

*** Used in patients admitted in shock to restore adquate volume and perfusion rapidly.

mainder in the next 8 hours, and the remaining fluid be given over the last 8 hours of resuscitation.

It should be emphasized that these and the more recently developed regimens shown in Table 1 are designed only to guide fluid administration. Rigid adherence to these formulas without appropriate monitoring of tissue perfusion, fluid retention, and edema formation frequently results in suboptimal therapy. For example, in small children who require more fluid than adults for burns of relatively similar size, the use of the Parkland formula gives a resuscitative fluid volume that is even less than their basal requirements.[108] Some protocols, such as the Parkland formula, do not account for evaporative or other water losses. These losses should be replaced using 5% dextrose solution. Evaporative water loss is calculated as follows:

$$\text{Evaporative water loss (mL/h)} = (25 + \%\ \text{TBSA burned}) \times \text{TBSA}$$

In a 70-kg patient with a 50% burn this loss is about 125 mL/h.

In an effort to reduce the volume of fluid administered and diminish edema, a formula has been developed that uses hypertonic lactated saline solution[44] containing 300 mEq/L of sodium, 200 mEq/L lactate, and 100 mEq chloride administered at a rate sufficient to maintain urine output at 30 mL/h. (Table 20-1). In the adult patients studied, the average volume infused was 1.8 mL/kg/% burn/24 h. The majority of this volume is given during the first 8 hours after the injury. Resuscitation is then continued by isotonic crystalloid and colloid solutions. Although the volume administered is reduced compared to the other formulas, the sodium load is increased by this regimen. It is important to realize that the topical antibiotic used in many of these patients, 0.5% silver nitrate, removes sodium from the serum; therefore the net sodium load is less than that delivered. Caldwell and Bowser[21] compared a hypertonic lactated Ringer's solution to Ringer's lactate as a resuscitation fluid for severely burned children. They were able to demonstrate a reduced water load in those patients receiving the hypertonic fluid. By 48 hours, sodium balance was equal in both groups as a result of greater sodium excretion in the group receiving the hypertonic solution. Similar studies with hypertonic saline in patients over the age of 60 showed hemodynamic stability and good urine flow in spite of a reduced cardiac index.[17] Jelenko and his group modified the hypertonic saline formula by adding albumin to the infusion.[80] This technique reduced both the amount of fluid administered and the time needed to resuscitate the patient. If serum sodium reached 160 mEq/L or serum osmolality exceeded 340 mosm/L water, Ringer's lactate alone was administered.

There is little information about the use of hetastarch for early fluid resuscitation of burn victims. The large size of this molecule leads to a long vascular retention time, making it an appropriate fluid for burn resuscitation. However, coagulation abnormalities may result from large doses of hetastarch infusion, mediated mainly by its dilutional effect on coagulant proteins. There is some evidence that hetastarch, like albumin, may displace coagulant proteins from the intravascular to the interstitial space, but the significance of this phenomenon in producing coagulation abnormalities has not yet been determined.[92] A new hydroxyethylstarch, pentastarch, which is less hydroxylated than hetastarch and thus has a shorter vascular retention, has been used by Waxman et al.[172] to resuscitate burn patients after the first day of injury. In this trial 500 mL of 10% pentastarch was as effective as 5% albumin in improving hemodynamics and oxygen transport. These findings suggest that pentastarch may also be useful during the first 24 hours of resuscitation of burn patients. They also demonstrate that inadequate cardiac function after burn injury is usually caused by hypovolemia, rather than by burn-induced myocardial depression,[172] a concept that is supported by others as well.[114]

Dextran-40 and dextran-70 have adequate volume effects and thus have been used during initial resuscitation of burns of greater than 50% of TBSA. A plasma dextran concentration of 2 g/dL or more is necessary to obtain adequate colloid osmotic and volume-retaining effects from this agent. This can be achieved by infusion rates of 2 mL/kg/h.[44] As with hetastarch, coagulation abnormalities are likely with dextran if large volumes are administered. Therefore, this agent is administered during the first 8 hours of burn injury to obtain rapid restoration of intravascular volume; it is then replaced with albumin solution, 0.5–1.0 mL/kg/% burn, for the next 16 hours. Crystalloids are administered as needed with both colloid solutions.[44]

Occasionally, patients undergoing resuscitation have fluid requirements far in excess of predicted volumes. The prognosis for such patients is poor. The postulated mechanism is release of toxins from the burn wound that affect cellular function.[12,139] In an attempt to remove such toxins, Warden et al.[170] have performed plasma exchange with moderate success in patients with refractory burn shock. Whether the beneficial effect of this therapy is due to removal of toxins or to the administration of colloid has not yet been determined.

Data comparing two groups of patients, however, one of which received crystalloid alone and the other a combination of crystalloid and albumin, showed improved cardiovascular function in those patients receiving colloid during resuscitation.[49] Additional studies have also supported early administration of colloid to animals with thermal injury.[23] Although some controversy still exists regarding the use of colloid early in resuscitation of burn patients, the author prefers solutions that contain 12.5 g of albumin for every liter of crystalloid administered.

## ESCHAROTOMY

The accumulation of interstitial fluid that follows major thermal injury, in combination with the constrictive eschar produced by a third-degree burn, may cause compression of neurovascular bundles, resulting in ischemia of the extremities and development of progressive neurologic deficit. During the initial period of resuscitation, one should evaluate the patient frequently to determine whether such compression is developing. This can be done using a Doppler flow probe to monitor the pulses in the deep palmar arch and the posterior tibial arteries. If there is evidence of neurovascular compromise, escharotomies should be performed. Incisions are made through the eschar to allow swelling to occur. Since this procedure is done through a third-degree burn, it is painless and relatively bloodless and can be performed without anesthetics.

## TOPICAL ANTIBIOTICS

After resuscitation, the major threat to the patient is infection of the burn wound. Multiple therapies have been tried, including a salve that, among other ingredients, contained moss from the skull of a person who had been hanged.[128]

The development of mafenide acetate as a topical antibiotic by the U.S. Army Institute for Surgical Research was clearly a breakthrough. It is used as a cream, usually applied to the wound twice a day. Mafenide acetate has a broad spectrum of antibacterial activity. It is a carbonic anhydrase inhibitor and therefore causes some diuresis. It is also painful when applied to a partial-thickness burn.

Silver sulfadiazine was developed in the early 1970s. It is used in much the same way as mafenide acetate. Although it is not painful on application, it may produce transient leukopenia and tissue deposits of silver after application.[167]

Silver nitrate in a concentration of 0.5% is applied with gauze dressings. The major complication of silver nitrate therapy is hyponatremia. Additionally, anything coming in contact with the solution will be stained black.

Betadine has also been used as a topical antibiotic, but is associated with metabolic acidosis and elevated serum iodine levels (Table 20-2).

## EXCISION

Excision of the burn wound to fascia and closure of the remaining area with skin grafts within the first few days after injury is a common practice in many centers. Among the claimed advantages of this technique are reduction in endotoxin and inflammatory mediator release, decrease in systemic microvascular permeability and thus multiorgan failure, reduction in the incidence of chronic bacteremia, shorter hospital stay, reduced expenses, and improved survival after major thermal injury.[180] This technique, however, is associ-

TABLE 20-2. Antibiotics*

| AGENT | ACTIVITY | TECHNIQUE | SIDE EFFECTS AND COMPLICATIONS |
|---|---|---|---|
| Mafenide acetate | Broad | Open | Painful, hyperventilation |
| Silver sulfadiazine | Broad | Open | Leukopenia |
| 0.5% $AgNO_3$ | Broad | Dressings | Black stains, hyponatremia |
| Betadine | Broad | Dressings | Acidosis, elevated serum iodine |

* From Welch GW: Curr Rev Clin Anesth 1983, 4:50.

ated with the risks of removal of viable underlying tissue, multiple blood transfusions, viral or bacterial contamination of the wound, and transient bacteremia during excision. Early excision and grafting of burn wounds of less than 20% of body surface area is a generally accepted treatment; it is associated with an increased use of blood products, but no increased morbidity.[53] This technique also reduces mortality in pediatric patients with burn injuries greater than 30% TBSA.

Although various retrospective and uncontrolled studies showed that early burn wound excision improved survival after large burns in adults,[26,57,62,159] definitive work in this area has been done only recently by Herndon and associates.[76] Their findings suggest that there is no difference in the incidence of sepsis and length of hospital stay between excised and conservatively treated adult patients with burns of greater than 30% of the TBSA. However, they demonstrated that early burn wound excision reduces mortality from 45% to 9% in young adults (17 to 30 years old) with pure cutaneous injury. The survival rate of patients older than 30 years of age or those with concomitant inhalation injury did not improve. Thus, it appears that early burn wound excision should be performed after severe burn injury, at least in children and in adults between 17 and 30 years old who do not exhibit pulmonary damage.

Blood loss during excision can be significant and may be as much as 1 unit every 5 minutes, requiring preparations to be made to administer large volumes of blood and blood products. The use of tourniquets and compression dressings and a hot knife or laser, as well as performing the procedure in two stages, can reduce hemorrhage.[138,169]

Manipulation of the burn wound has been shown to result in bacteremia in approximately 20% of cases.[142] Yet, one study seems to indicate that, unless performed several weeks after injury, excision of the burned area does not result in a high incidence of bacteremia. However, serial blood cultures were not performed, and thus the reliability of these results is questionable.[130] It would appear, therefore, that prophylactic broad spectrum antibiotics should be given before and immediately after excision or manipulation of the wound.

Coverage of an excised injury can be a problem. Xenograft coverage of large excised areas is unsatisfactory. There is poor adherence, and frequently areas of suppuration develop. Autograft may be useful for temporary coverage, but will require replacement. Attempts at developing artificial skin show promise, but much remains to be done. More recently, tissue culture of the patients' own skin has allowed coverage of wounds when enough donor areas are not available for autografts.[58]

## INHALATION INJURY

Inhalation injury represents a significant insult to the patient. When combined with a cutaneous burn, there is a significant increase in mortality compared to either injury alone. Available data indicate that the presence of inhalation injury increases mortality from burn injury by 20–60%.[74,144,157] The extent of increase in mortality is related closely to the age of the patient, burn size, and development of pneumonia. Persons over 60, who also appear to sustain inhalation injury more frequently than young people, have a mortality rate close to 100% as compared to young persons who have an overall 30–50% chance of dying after a burn complicated by lung damage.[74,157] The impact of pneumonia on mortality after thermal injury has been appreciated only recently, but it appears to be highly significant. In the series of Shirani and coworkers,[144] the overall mortality increased by 20% when inhalation injury was not complicated by pneumonia; this rate increased by 60% when pneumonia developed (Fig 20-4).

Inhalation injury should be suspected whenever a burn has occurred in a confined space, and cervicofacial burns, singed nasal vibrissae, bronchorrhea, sooty sputum, sore throat, hoarseness, dysphagia, signs of upper airway obstruction, wheezing, and/or rales are observed. Many of these indirect findings, however, are not necessarily diagnostic of inhalation injury in the early phase after the accident. For example, facial burns are present in 70% of patients with inhalation injury, but 70% of patients with inhalation injury do not have facial burns.[74] Likewise, wheezing, rales, and carbonaceous sputum may not be observed for as long as 24–48 hours after injury. The most reliable indirect indicators in the early phase are occurrence of the fire in a closed space and development of unconsciousness or stupor that prevents the patient from protecting his or her own airway.

FIG. 20-4. Percent increase in mortality from inhalation injury (*left panel*), pneumonia (*middle panel*), and the combination of inhalation injury and pneumonia (*right panel*) in burn patients of various ages and burn sizes. Note the maximum increase in mortality by 20% after inhalation injury alone, by 40% after pneumonia alone, and by 60% after combined inhalation injury and pneumonia in patients in the midrange of injury severity as indexed by age and burn size. These data indicate that inhalation injury and pneumonia have independent and additive effects on mortality. (From Shirani et al[144] with permission.)

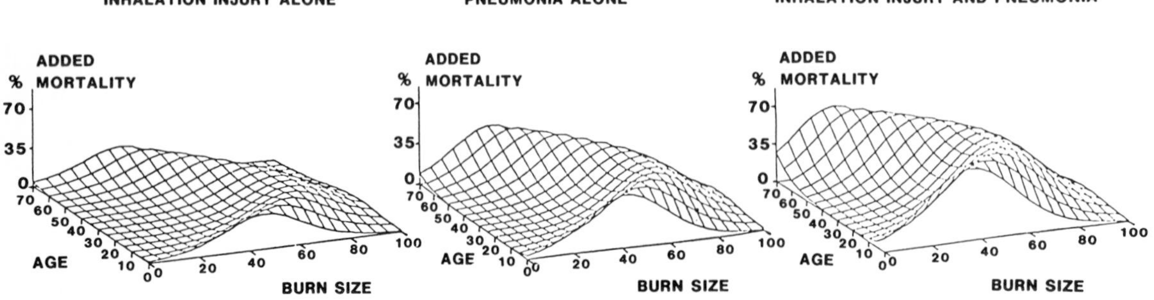

Although in clinically obvious cases, treatment of inhalation injury should be instituted immediately, certain confirmatory tests may be used before treatment when the diagnosis is equivocal. The chest X-ray is usually normal in the early phase of inhalation injury unless aspiration of gastric or pharyngeal contents occurred during the accident. The chest X-ray becomes abnormal a few days after the injury when pulmonary edema or infiltration develops. Fiberoptic nasopharyngoscopy under topical anesthesia is useful for defining the extent of upper airway injury during the early phase after burn.[78,122] Mucosal hyperemia, edema, ulceration, blisters, necrosis, abnormal cord mobility, or soot and charring in the airway suggest the presence of injury. Fiberoptic nasopharyngoscopy should be repeated at least every 6 hours for the first 24 hours after the injury if inhalation injury is suspected. Rapid progression of upper airway edema may result in sudden airway obstruction during this phase.[68] Fiberoptic bronchoscopy can also be used to define the severity of tracheal and large bronchial mucosal injury in the early phase, but diagnosis of small airway injury is not possible with this technique because the bronchoscope cannot reach these areas.

It should be emphasized that the extent of upper airway and tracheal injury during the initial stage is not predictive of the severity of subsequent pulmonary gas exchange abnormalities or of the level and duration of ventilatory support required.[14] This is probably because pulmonary parenchymal injury is not the result of heat unless steam, with its high heat capacity, has been inhaled. Because of their specific heat, hot gases administered to the trachea of experimental animals cool to 50°C by the time they reach the carina and therefore do not produce much damage to the distal airways.[118] The actual cause of parenchymal injury in most cases is inhalation of the products of incomplete combustion. The oxides of sulphur and nitrogen, and phosgene, acidic anhydrides, and acrolein produce chemical injuries resulting in denaturation and sloughing of the pulmonary mucosa, obstruction of small airways, and development of distal pneumonia. Although, as a result of the widespread use of synthetic materials chemical pulmonary injury has increased in the past few decades, many victims with upper airway injury still escape pulmonary injury. Thus, there is little correlation between the severities of upper airway and pulmonary parenchymal injury.

Small airway injury may be evaluated by three methods: $^{133}$Xe lung scanning, pulmonary function tests, and determination of extravascular lung water (EVLW). Of these, $^{133}$Xe scanning and EVLW measurement are most suitable in unconscious or agitated patients because they do not require patient cooperation. $^{133}$Xe scanning involves intravenous injection of the radioactive material and obtaining serial chest scintophotograms. Normally, $^{133}$Xe is cleared rapidly from the circulation by ventilation. In the presence of small airway obstruction caused by bronchial casts, mucosal edema, or airway sloughing, clearance of the gas from the lung decreases.[121] In uncomplicated cases, clearance returns to normal before the fifth postinjury day. Thus, the study should be performed within a few days after the injury. Hyperventilation, a history of cigarette smoking, and pre-existing pulmonary disease may result in inaccurate interpretation of the findings of this test.

Pulmonary function tests can be used to detect both upper and lower respiratory tract abnormalities. Maximum inspiratory-expiratory flow-volume loops may be useful for detection of upper airway obstruction. A sawtoothed or flattened inspiratory flow and extrathoracic obstruction pattern suggest upper airway obstruction. Damage to the lower airway is demonstrated by decreases in peak flow (PEF), forced vital capacity (FVC), and pulmonary compliance and increased respiratory resistance.[30,59] EVLW increases within hours of serious inhalation injury and thus may help identify patients who will develop respiratory failure.[129] However, this technique is seldom used clinically because of technical difficulties. With the use of fiberoptic bronchoscopy, $^{133}$Xe scanning, pulmonary function testing, and EVLW determination, inhalation injury that, based on indirect clinical signs and symptoms, was estimated to occur in between 3 and 15% of patients sustaining major burns, has been recognized in as many as 33% of victims.[74]

Clinical manifestations of inhalation injury vary according to the time after the initial insult.[151,152] The first 36 hours are characterized by varying degrees of acute pulmonary insufficiency. Patients in this stage may be hypoxic for several reasons. Fire in a closed space consumes oxygen and thus decreases the oxygen concentration in the environment. Production of carbon monoxide reduces further the availability of oxygen to the tissues of the organism. Bronchospasm, tracheobronchitis, atelectasis, coughing spells, and upper airway edema, which occur frequently during the early phase, compromise arterial oxygenation further. Hypoxia in this stage is fatal unless immediate treatment is instituted. The clinical manifestation in the second stage of inhalation injury is pulmonary edema, which occurs within 1 week after injury in as many as 30% of patients and increases mortality. The treatment of this condition is similar to that used for the acute respiratory distress syndrome. Bronchopneumonia may develop while the patient is expectorating large mucus casts formed in the tracheobronchial tree approximately 1 to 2 weeks after the initial injury and, as already mentioned, also increases the risk of mortality.

Injury to the respiratory tract can involve the upper airways, the lower airways, and the lung parenchyma. Pathologic changes vary widely, ranging from hyperemia and edema to necrosis or destruction of the respiratory epithelium. Reference has already been made to upper airway injury. In the lower airways the primary pathology is formation of pseudomembranous casts composed of damaged epithelial cells, leukocytes, and proteinaceous material. These casts produce varying degrees of bronchial obstruction, atelectasis, and increased intrapulmonary shunting. In the pulmonary parenchyma the prominent finding is interstitial edema, which results from increased capillary permeability. Increased permeability has been demonstrated in firefighters who had been intermittently exposed to smoke and had normal pulmonary function tests.[113] Several incompletely understood mechanisms are responsible for the increase in capillary permeability and other pulmonary lesions, but activation of polymorphonuclear leukocytes appears to play an important role.[72,73,161] Smoke stimulates pulmonary macrophages, which produce chemotactic substances and cause sequestration of leukocytes in the pulmonary microvasculature, lung lymph, and endobronchial exudate. These leukocytes release proteolytic enzymes that not only cause tissue destruction but also reduce the activity of $\alpha_2$-macroglobulin antiproteases. Antiproteases are also inhibited by oxygen free radicals released from polymorphonuclear cells and macrophages.[87] Activated proteases destroy pulmonary fibronectin-like substances that normally function as a glue to hold endothelial cells together. This reaction results in open gaps between the cells and permits the passage of fluid and protein into the pulmonary interstitial space. As a result, lung lymph flow increases and interstitial edema ensues within 10–12 hours.

It should be emphasized that, even in the absence of direct injury to the airway, there may be decreased pulmonary function manifested by pulmonary hypertension and hypoxia. Demling et al.[45] examined the pulmonary effects of major scald injury in sheep. They found decreased compliance, hypoxia, and pulmonary hypertension. The latter two findings correlated with venous thromboxane levels and could be partially corrected by administration of ibuprofen before and after the injury.

Even in the absence of lung damage, exposure to gaseous products of combustion may have a profound effect on respiratory function. Incomplete combustion of substances containing carbon results in the production of carbon monoxide, a colorless, odorless gas with an affinity for hemoglobin 210 times that of oxygen.[77] As a result, hemoglobin oxygen saturation is markedly reduced in spite of normal arterial oxygen pressures. Additionally, the dissociation curve for oxyhemoglobin is shifted to the left (Fig 20-5). These two effects of carbon monoxide combine to produce a profound reduction in oxygen delivery to the periphery (Fig 20-6). At one time, carbon monoxide was thought to interfere with the cytochrome system and to be directly toxic to cellular function. Geyer,[60] using a perflurochemical-type blood substitute to support oxygen delivery, appears to have proven that this effect is negligible.

In the presence of carboxyhemoglobin, monitoring of arterial oxygen saturation with a pulse oximeter may be fraught with danger. The pulse oximeter measures infrared absorbance in two wavelengths and cannot distinguish other hemoglobin species. Thus, even when carboxyhemoglobin concentration is very high, the pulse oximeter reports a normal saturation, which is actually the approximate sum of the oxyhemoglobin and carboxyhemoglobin values.[11] In contrast, transcutaneous $O_2$ tension decreases linearly with increasing carboxyhemoglobin concentration.[11]

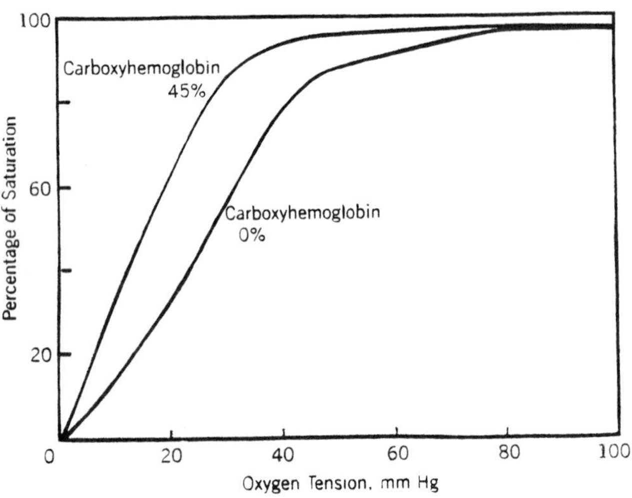


FIG. 20-5. Shift of oxyhemoglobin dissociation curve to the left by 45% carboxyhemoglobin. (From Jackson and Menges[79] with permission.)

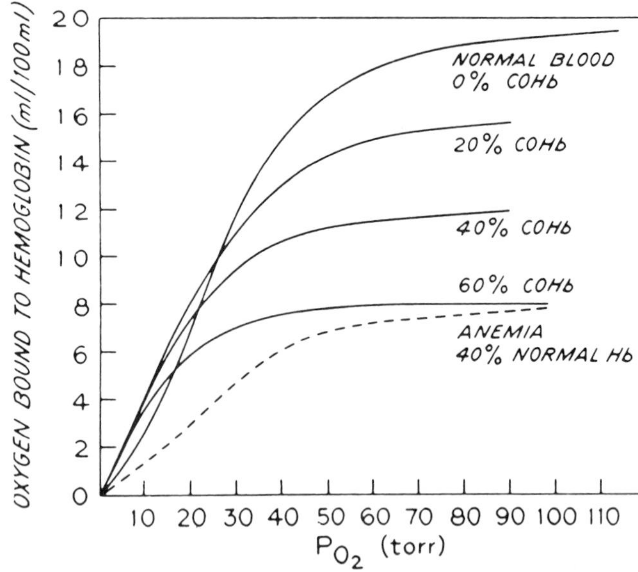


FIG. 6. Calculated absolute amounts of oxygen bound to hemoglobin for $PO_2$ levels between 0 and 110 mm Hg in human blood containing varying amounts of carboxyhemoglobin (COHb). Note that blood with 60% carboxyhemoglobin has a greater affinity for oxygen than the blood of an anemic patient with only 40% oxyhemoglobin and no carboxyhemoglobin. (From Fein et al[55] with permission.)

Initial symptoms of carbon monoxide poisoning are headache, dizziness, nausea and vomiting, and loss of manual dexterity. Since the carotid bodies are sensitive to $PaO_2$ and not to oxygen content, tachypnea is frequently absent. At carboxyhemoglobin levels approaching 50%, coma occurs. At or above 60% concentration carboxyhemoglobin is usually lethal (Table 20-3). Although much has been made of the cherry red color of carboxyhemoglobin, this is not usually seen clinically with concentrations less than 40%.[55] More frequently, the victim is cyanotic as a result of respiratory depression.

The elimination half-time of carbon monoxide from a patient breathing room air is approximately 4 hours. Adminis-

TABLE 20-3. Symptoms Produced by Different Carboxyhemoglobin Levels

| CARBOXYHEMOGLOBIN LEVEL (%) | SYMPTOMS |
|---|---|
| 0–15 | None |
| 15–20 | Headache, dizziness, confusion |
| 20–40 | Fatigue, nausea, vomiting, disorientation, visual impairment |
| 40–60 | Agitation, combativeness, hallucination, coma, shock |
| >60 | Death |

tration of 100% oxygen can reduce this time to less than an hour. Thus, oxygen should be administered as soon as possible to victims rescued from fires occurring in closed spaces and should be maintained until the carboxyhemoglobin level falls below 20%.

One of the devastating complications of carbon monoxide poisoning is coma resulting from hypoxic brain edema. Its treatment involves the rapid reduction of both the carboxyhemoglobin level and brain swelling.[88] Hyperbaric oxygen, hyperventilation, mild hypothermia, and osmotherapy may be indicated in these patients. Hyperbaric oxygen therapy is administered at 2–2.5 atmospheres for 1 hour.[147,179] Hyperventilation, although effective in reducing intracranial pressure, can cause hypotension and may further decrease oxygen delivery to tissues since it interferes with oxygen unloading by shifting the oxyhemoglobin curve to the left.[88] Thus, oxygen delivery and consumption should be serially monitored during this therapy. Some patients with severe carbon monoxide poisoning may show marked initial improvement, only to develop neurologic symptoms some days after apparent recovery.[88] This probably represents a variant of the icebox syndrome, in which victims suffering from severe hypoxia are resuscitated successfully but subsequently manifest demyelination within the central nervous system.[133] Any patient with successfully treated severe carbon monoxide poisoning should be observed for delayed effects and the family forewarned of the possibility of subsequent neurologic damage.

Treatment with hyperbaric oxygen is indicated in pregnant patients if the maternal carboxyhemoglobin level is above 20%, the mother has developed abnormal neurologic signs, and the fetus is in distress.[163] The fetus is not only more vulnerable to the deleterious effects of carbon monoxide but also develops a carboxyhemoglobin level that is 10–15% higher than that of the mother.[163] Even relatively low levels of fetal carboxyhemoglobin cause significant hypoxia in the fetus because of further leftward shift of the fetal oxyhemoglobin dissociation curve. The known toxic effects of carbon monoxide on the surviving fetus are hypotonia, persistent seizures, mental and motor disabilities, microcephaly, and teratogenicity. Fetal death may occur even when the maternal carboxyhemoglobin concentration is insufficient to produce serious symptoms. Hyperbaric oxygen therapy with 2–3 atmospheres absolute for 60–90 minutes is usually sufficient to reduce maternal and fetal carboxyhemoglobin levels and ameliorate fetal toxic effects of carbon monoxide.[163] With such therapy any deleterious effects on the fetus of high $O_2$ partial pressure—retinopathy, alterations of placental blood flow, premature closure of the ductus arteriosus, and teratogenicity—appear unlikely.[163]

Many synthetic materials release cyanide when exposed to high temperature. Inhalation of such gases results in a rapid increase of blood cyanide levels and cyanide toxicity. Hydrocyanide is also formed in fires and is absorbed along with cyanide through the skin and mucosal surfaces.[145] Blood cyanide levels greater than 0.2 mg/L are considered toxic, and a concentration greater than 1 mg/dL is lethal.[145] Although carboxyhemoglobin levels can be obtained rather quickly, blood cyanide levels usually require days to obtain. In fire victims persistent metabolic acidosis should arouse a suspicion of cyanide toxicity.[28] Clark speculates that all patients with carboxyhemoglobin levels above 15% should be considered as having elevated blood levels of cyanide and perhaps receive cyanide antidotes.[28] However, in rodents poisoned with cyanide and carbon monoxide, methemoglobin-forming cyanide antidotes (amylnitrite or sodium nitrite) caused a dose-related increase in mortality.[116] This effect was probably the result of a further leftward shift in the $O_2$ dissociation curve caused by methemoglobin, added to that already produced by carbon monoxide. Thus, treatment with oxygen and thiosulfate is preferred. Thiosulfate provides the sulfate that is necessary to enhance the normal conversion of cyanide to thiocyanate by the enzyme rhodanase in the liver. Thiocyanate is then excreted by the kidney.[145] Hydroxycobalamine (vitamin $B_{12a}$) may also be used. It is nontoxic and can reduce blood cyanide levels by half in relatively small doses.[34]

Inhalation injury is best treated with supportive therapy. As already mentioned, upper airway edema may progress rapidly and cause acute obstruction. Emergency airway management may be extremely difficult in these patients because pharyngeal swelling, cervicofacial burns, and secretions preclude visualization of the larynx by direct laryngoscopy. In centers where the upper airway cannot be evaluated with serial endoscopic examinations, prophylactic intubation of the trachea is the safest method of airway management.[166] Tracheal intubation is mandatory when coma or respiratory depression accompanies inhalation injury and there are full-thickness nasolabial or circumferential neck burns and posterior pharyngeal swelling.

For the past several decades, tracheostomy has been reserved for specific indications, such as acute upper airway edema and prolonged endotracheal intubation, because it is associated with a high rate of operative (6%) and postoperative (30%) complications in burn patients.[51,120] Operative complications include bleeding, subcutaneous emphysema, pneumothorax, and tube malposition. Postoperative complications can be divided into two categories: infections (local and pulmonary) and delayed sequelae, such as tracheal ulcerations, tracheoesophageal fistula, tracheitis, and tracheal stenosis. In a recent report from a large metropolitan burn center in which tracheostomy is performed only when the airway is acutely obstructed or has been intubated for a prolonged period, pulmonary sepsis and mortality were not increased by tracheostomy.[83] Colonization of sputum occurred in almost all patients with a tracheostomy, but this rate was not significantly different from that observed after endotracheal intubation. The most important complication of tracheostomy in this series was the development of late upper airway sequelae, such as tracheal stenosis or fistula formation between the trachea and the esophagus or a cervical vessel; these complications occurred in about 30% of patients.[83] Although the results of this study suggest that tracheostomy does not increase infectious complications and mortality, the frequent development of late airway sequelae dictates that tracheostomy should be reserved only for selected burn victims.

The inspired gases should be humidified in order to aid in clearing tracheobronchial casts and to prevent drying of secretions. Respiratory distress after inhalation injury is frequently accompanied by wheezing, which may result from peribronchial or perivascular edema, bronchospasm, or accumulation of bronchial secretions. Intravenous or aerosolized bronchodilators and removal of secretions provide dramatic relief in most of these patients.

Although myocardial depression has been documented after smoke inhalation in animals,[154] pulmonary edema is a result of increased capillary permeability in the vast majority of burned patients. Pulmonary edema without signs of cardiac failure may also develop shortly after tracheal intubation probably because the small but constant intrapulmonary pressure maintained by the glottic mechanism is abolished.[106] Low levels of prophylactic continuous positive airway pressure (CPAP) may prevent this complication. Of course, CPAP or positive end-expiratory pressure (PEEP) should be used in the presence of overt pulmonary edema.[40] Occasionally conventional techniques of mechanical ventilation may not be sufficient to improve hypercapnia and hypoxemia after inhalation injury. In a preliminary trial high-frequency percussive ventilation, which involves oscillatory PEEP during the period of interruption of pulsatile flow of high-frequency ventilation, normalized arterial oxygen and carbon dioxide tensions in these instances.[27] It has been suggested that this technique may also decrease the incidence of pneumonia and barotrauma after inhalation injury.[27] Further trials may confirm these effects.

Inhalation injury complicates fluid management of the burn victim by increasing fluid requirements approximately 50% during the first 24 hours after pulmonary insult.[123] This fact calls for modification of standard fluid resuscitation formulas. On the other hand, results of animal experiments suggest that the smoke-injured lung is susceptible to accumulation of fluid and pulmonary edema after large fluid infusion.[29] This susceptibility is mediated mainly by elevated microvascular pressure, damaged endothelial and epithelial cells, and inactivated pulmonary surfactant. Reduced plasma oncotic pressure does not appear to be responsible for it. Thus, extreme care must be used to prevent both under- and overhydration of the patient with inhalation injury. This may be achieved by monitoring pulmonary artery pressure and, if available, EVLW.

At one time, steroids were utilized to decrease the inflammatory reaction. Experimental and clinical studies, however, have demonstrated at best no benefit and at worst a deleterious effect of steroids on inhalation injury.[119,137,174] Steroids should thus be avoided in these patients.

## ELECTRICAL INJURY

Contact with a source of electrical current can produce thermal injury by two mechanisms. Flow of current through a resistance generates heat. The power generated is the product of the amperage squared and the resistance ($P = I^2R$). The amount of heat generated depends on the duration of the current flow and the power of the source. Hence, tissue damage results from the heat generated as current flows through the body to the ground. Additional damage may result from contact with a high-voltage source, which may produce an electrical arc with temperatures as high as 4,000°C[146] and can melt metals, such as belt buckles and bracelets, and ignite clothing. A 10,000 volt source can produce an arc inches in length; once a high-voltage arc occurs, it can lengthen to nearly 10 feet before breaking.[18]

The extent of major electrical injury may be difficult to diagnose. In spite of minimal cutaneous injury, there may be considerable damage to the underlying nerves, blood vessels, muscle, tendon, and bone.[67] Therefore, it has been recommended that early decompressive fasciotomies and surgical exploration be undertaken to determine the extent of such occult damage.[46,67,77]

The significant muscle damage that may occur after electric shock is very similar to a crush injury.[9] As a result, the victim may have severe myoglobinuria and, in some cases, life-threatening hyperkalemia. Acute renal failure is common, and efforts at maintaining renal function should be initiated[47,67] (see below and chapter 25). These patients frequently have excessive fluid requirements; administration of large amounts of fluid, along with osmotic or loop diuretics, may be necessary to maintain urine output. Ultimately, dialysis may be required should renal failure supervene.[67]

A number of complications have been described after electrical injury. Holliman[77] and DiVincenti[46] described abnormal ECGs in 8% of their patients. In the former study, 5% had evidence of myocardial infarction, and nearly 20% had elevated CPK-MB isoenzyme. Delayed ventricular arrhythmias may occur, especially when electrical current passes through the thorax.[81] Thus, continuous ECG monitoring for at least 24 hours has been recommended in these patients,[81] although Purdue and Hunt[135] were unable to detect serious arrhythmias in patients with normal ECGs on admission.

Neurologic injury may result from direct injury to the peripheral nerves or to the central nervous system. Spinal cord injury may also result from compression fractures.[67] A late sequela is the development of cataracts.[2]

## COMPLICATIONS

In older patients with underlying cardiac or pulmonary disease and those with associated major injuries, determination of cardiovascular status using a thermodilution pulmonary artery catheter may be critical. In at least one study, failure to develop or sustain an elevated cardiac index after resuscitation was a predictor of death.[3]

An additional advantage of monitoring physiologic profiles is to ensure adequate renal perfusion. As many as 38% of victims of major thermal injury develop renal failure.[132] Oliguria during the first 24 hours of resuscitation is most commonly secondary to inadequate fluid administration. In addition to the possibility of ischemic renal injury from low perfusion, reduced renal blood flow may make the kidneys more susceptible to damage from hemoglobin and myoglobin, which may be released into the bloodstream during crush injury, electrical injury, or extensive full-thickness burn. Although free hemoglobin is not toxic to the kidneys, it has a deleterious effect when it is produced by hemolysis. Initial attempts to maintain renal perfusion should be directed toward increasing fluid infusion. If urine output does not improve despite adequate cardiac filling pressures, osmotic or loop diuretics should be administered. Occasionally, low-dose dopamine may be of benefit (1 μg/kg/min). If the cardiac index is reduced or normal, cardiotonic support may improve renal perfusion. If hemoglobin or myoglobin is present in the urine, alkalinization should be tried in order to prevent deposition of pigment in the kidney tubules. One group has used haptoglobin therapy to clear hemoglobin from the urine of patients with massive thermal injury.[183]

A fall in urine output after the resuscitation period is frequently indicative of underlying sepsis. Polyuric renal failure may also result from sepsis or nephrotoxic drugs. The high mortality associated with renal failure makes preservation of renal function a major priority in caring for burned patients.

Nearly 60% of patients with major thermal injury develop elevation of hepatic enzymes and bilirubin.[25,38] Like renal failure, early liver dysfunction probably results from hypovolemia. Jaundice and/or liver enzyme elevation developing late in the hospital course is frequently related to sepsis.[24] Liver enzymes may remain elevated even after the patient is discharged from the hospital, but a sudden increase in serum levels of alanine and aspartate transferase after discharge may be caused by transfusion-related non-A non-B hepatitis.[24] Mortality in those patients developing acute liver injury is nine times that of patients without evidence of hepatic dysfunction.

The need for fluid replacement, intravascular monitors, and intravenous alimentation may result in suppurative thrombophlebitis. This complication occurred in 4.5% of a series of 3,751 burn patients.[91] The most frequent indication of suppurative thrombophlebitis is a positive blood culture. Additional findings are an elevated white blood cell count and persistent fever. Local evidence may not always be present, and finding the affected vein may require exploration of many sites. Therapy consists of antibiotics and excision of the involved vein.

Complex pathophysiologic changes result from major thermal injury; a great deal of recent research has been devoted to the interaction of metabolic and endocrine alterations. Of particular interest are the mediators of the hypermetabolic state that follows massive thermal injury. During the postburn period, there is a marked increase in glucose utilization.[177] Glucose is metabolized to lactate and transported to the liver, where lactate and alanine, a product of protein catabolism, are used for gluconeogenesis. This is an energy-requiring process, which results in a nitrogen loss of approximately 20–25 g/m$^2$/day and a caloric requirement of 25 kcal/kg or 40 kcal/ %burn/day.[71,149] Hyperalimentation has been used in an attempt to reduce this nitrogen loss. Administration of exogenous glucose results in increased protein synthesis.[20] There appears to be an upper limit of approximately 5 mg/kg/min above which glucose is no longer oxidized but is converted to fat.

In addition to catabolism, burn patients have a significantly negative nitrogen balance because of protein loss from the wound, which may amount to 72 g, 120 g, and 170 g per day for burns occupying 30%, 50%, and 70% of the body surface area, respectively, during the first week after injury.[171] Protein loss after the first week decreases to about 50% of these values.[171] Positive nitrogen balance can be achieved with 0.2 to 0.6 g N/kg/day, provided that energy needs are met simultaneously. Patients are usually given 250 to 300 nonprotein calories per gram of nitrogen.[107] However, because of their markedly catabolic state, this ratio should be reduced in burn patients at least to 150:1;[176] an optimal ratio for major burns appears to be 100:1.[107]

Other metabolic changes are also seen, including catecholamine-mediated hypermetabolism and hyperdynamic circulation; lipolysis may also be caused by catecholamine release.[134] There is also evidence that severe burn injury leads to carbohydrate and fat substrate cycling.[181] There is a simultaneous breakdown and resynthesis of glucose and fat without an actual change in the amount of either the substrate or the product; however, there is a net increase in energy expenditure and thermogenesis, caused by utilization of adenosine triphosphate (ATP). For example, in severe burns glucose is resynthetized after being converted to glucose-6-phosphate. Likewise, fructose-1-phosphate is converted to fructose 1.6-diphosphate and then back to fructose-1-phosphate. The breakdown of stored triglycerides to fatty acids is followed by formation of triglycerides. This substrate cycling is enhanced by 450% for fats and 250% for carbohydrates in severe burns.[181] In the absence of adequate caloric intake, the increased energy expenditure caused by these reactions ultimately results in the depletion of fat and glycogen stores.

Attempts have been made to block the metabolic and hemodynamic responses to elevated catecholamines with propranolol. At doses of 2 mg/kg/24 h for 5 days, propranolol produced a decrease in heart rate, left ventricular stroke work, and rate-pressure product in children without adversely affecting cardiac output or resting energy expenditure. Chronic propranolol infusion had little effect on plasma glucose, free fatty acid, triglyceride, or insulin levels. In addition, it produced an increase in urea production, the mechanism of which is not clear at this time.[75]

In an attempt to define the caloric requirements of burn patients, various formulas have been devised. The Curreri formula is used to calculate postburn energy requirements based on patient weight and total burn size: [25 × body weight (kg)] + [40 × % BSA burned].[36] Alternatively, a modification of the Harris-Benedict formula has been used to calculate basal energy requirements (see Chapter 22).[69] The use of a bedside indirect calorimeter, however, showed poor correlation with calculated energy requirements.[6,108,162] It has been suggested, therefore, that indirect calorimetry provides a better means of assessing energy requirements in burn patients.[108,141]

Endocrine changes follow any stress to the organism. The burn patient is no exception. Thyroid function has been extensively investigated because of the hypermetabolic state of burn patients. Paradoxically, both $T_3$ and $T_4$ levels are reduced.[10] Thyroid-stimulating hormone (TSH) levels were found to be normal and responded to administration of thyrotropin-releasing hormone (TRH). Other studies demonstrate an elevation of $T_3$, suggesting a diversion of normal synthesis to a pathway with a reduced physiologic effect.[13] These studies suggest that the hypermetabolic state is not mediated by thyroid function.

Further studies by Vaughan et al.[165] have suggested that the hypermetabolic state is mediated by anti-insulin hormones, including glucagon, norepinephrine, and cortisol. Although serum cortisol levels are closely correlated with burn size, there is a wide variation in ACTH activity, which in turn does not correlate with cortisol levels. These findings suggest that factors other than plasma ACTH determine the increase in postburn cortisol levels.[164]

Alterations in calcium and phosphate metabolism as a result of hormonal changes have also been described, although reports have been conflicting. Fenton et al.[56] found ionized calcium to be in the normal range. Szyfelbein and co-workers,[155] however, found a persistently decreased ionized calcium level in patients with large burns. Measurement of the hormones controlling calcium and phosphate metabolism revealed elevated calcitonin levels in burn patients, whereas parathormone levels were normal. The effect of calcitonin is to reduce serum levels of ionized calcium and phosphate.[92]

Other hormones regulating water and sodium balance have also been examined. There is an elevation of antidiuretic hormone, which is probably a result of the stress response.[117] Children developing hypertension after thermal injury were found to have markedly elevated plasma renin levels.[4] Elevations of plasma renin and angiotensin II have been shown to persist for some days after thermal injury.[48]

The role of these endocrine changes and the response of the patient to stress require further investigation. The question arises, however, as to the possible benefits of antagonizing some of the hormones in an attempt to reduce the stress response. As mentioned, beta-blockers inhibit the hemodynamic response to elevated catecholamines.[75] Angiotensin-converting enzymes are available to inhibit the renin response. Epidural anesthetics reduce the elevation in cortisol produced by trauma. Perhaps optimal treatment would consist of fluid replacement, pharmacologic antagonists, and regional anesthesia.[84] There is, however, no evidence at present of a beneficial effect of any of these agents in injured patients.

In addition to the metabolic and endocrine effects that occur with major thermal injury, there is depression of the patient's immune system, which affects both humoral and cellular function.[178] Cell-mediated immune responses are in part initiated by T-lymphocytes. When exposed to antigen, unsensitized T-lymphocytes are transformed, proliferate, and mature into a clone of sensitized T-lymphocytes that then protect against intracellular pathogens. T-cells can also initiate B-cell proliferation or limit the immune response by dividing into two different cell types.

B-cells mediate the humoral immune response by synthesizing and secreting specific antibodies. The function of these cells is to protect against encapsulated bacteria and to neutralize soluble toxins.

The function of T-cells appears to be more severely depressed in burned patients than is B-cell activity.[168] An indirect measurement of T-cell function is skin hypersensitivity, which is reduced in patients with thermal injury. Patients with positive delayed hypersensitivity reactions that converted to negative had a death rate over 80%.[70] Not only is function reduced but there is also a reduced number of circulating T-cells in burn patients,[124] possibly as a result of decreased interleukin-2 production.[182] Interleukin-1 and interleukin-2 are cytokines—humoral components that provide communication between components of the immune system. Interleukin-1 promotes the production of interleukin-2 from T-lymphocytes. Rapid proliferation of T-lymphocytes is in large measure controlled by interleukin-2. Although interleukin-1 levels are normal in burn patients, interleukin-2 levels are reduced.[182] In addition, it has been demonstrated that increased serum levels of interleukin-2 receptor (soluble IL-2R) interfere with IL-2-mediated cellular immune reactions in burn patients.[156] It is possible that soluble IL-2R competes with cellular IL-2R for IL-2 and thus decreases IL-2-dependent cellular immune responses. This phenomenon may be the basis of the improved cellular immune response seen after plasma exchange therapy in burn patients.[126]

In addition to the depression of lymphocyte function, there are other defects in cellular function and immune response. Experimental thermal injury has been shown to inhibit the respiratory burst in alveolar and peritoneal macrophages.[90] Although resting macrophage oxygen consumption in thermal injury is the same as in controls, it does not increase when the macrophages are challenged with latex particles. A circulating serum component has been identified that suppresses leukocyte chemotaxis and lymphocyte blastogenesis.[125] This substance was a complex of molecular weight between 1,000 and 5,000 daltons and contained protein, lipid, and carbohydrate components.

Recently, Moore et al.[115] examined the depression of neutrophil chemotaxis more closely using monoclonal antibodies to complement opsonin receptors. C5a, an activated complement fraction and a chemo-attractant, causes a tenfold increase in complement receptor sites. As a result, there is decreased chemotaxis to zymosan-activated serum.

Stratta et al. demonstrated several changes of immunologic parameters in burned patients.[153] IgG was markedly decreased, as was total protein and albumin on postburn day one compared to controls. C-reactive protein was an order of magnitude greater than normal. Fibronectin, a serum component important for phagocytic function, was slightly reduced.

It is of interest that, although neutrophils have been shown to have depressed chemotactic and bactericidal activity after an initial period of increased phagocytic capacity,[15] there is a marked increase in chromium uptake by polymorphonuclear leukocytes in burn patients.[39] Such uptake is an energy-dependent process and, in view of the otherwise depressed function of the neutrophil, may indicate an uncoupling of energy-dependent processes in the white cell.

The effect of thermal injury on the immune system is very complex, and much more work needs to be done. It would appear that the changes seen are an amplification of those that follow any significant trauma.

## SURGERY

Surgery may be required during the resuscitation, convalescence, or reconstructive phase of the patient's course. Although there are no definite boundaries between these phases, generally resuscitation occupies the first 24 hours, convalescence takes place between the first day and the second month, and the reconstruction phase extends from 2 months to 2 years after the burn. Soon after a burn injury, surgery is indicated for wound incision or excision or for exploration of an electrical injury to determine the extent of damage. After resuscitation the most common procedures are multiple debridements, further wound excision, and skin grafting. During the reconstructive phase the patient may require multiple procedures that involve skin grafts, flaps, and/or free pedicle grafts.

Surgical procedures, however, are not limited to the burned skin, but may involve other areas of the body. A significant number of patients with thermal injuries sustain concomitant injuries produced by nonthermal trauma, which may complicate management. In the early stage, signs and symptoms of these injuries may be attributed to the burn, and their diagnosis may be missed or delayed.[35] A decreasing hematocrit during resuscitation from burn shock should raise the possibility of occult bleeding. Unconsciousness in the burned patient is usually produced by hypoxia or carbon monoxide intoxication, but it can also be caused by intracranial hematoma. An inhalation injury may be erroneously blamed for respiratory distress caused by pneumothorax. Pain in an injured extremity may be attributed to the burn when it may actually be caused by a fracture of the underlying bone or by vascular occlusion. A high index of suspicion of these injuries and liberal use of radiographic imaging techniques reduce the frequency of diagnostic errors. Management of fractures needs to be individualized, but external or internal fixation may be used. External fixation allows access to the burn without risk of wound infection, although internal fixation, performed early via an incision through the burn wound, has been successful.[136,140] Compartment syndrome may develop after circumferential extremity burns. Vascular occlusion produced by this syndrome may not be relieved by simple eschar excision and may require fasciotomy.[35] Poor perfusion of an extremity may be caused by primary vascular injury and will not improve unless the damaged vessel is repaired.

Surgery may also be indicated for complications of burn injury. Of these, gastrointestinal bleeding or perforation due to stress ulceration (Curling's ulcer) was common in the past, but its frequency has decreased because of effective control of gastric pH with antacids and $H_2$-receptor blockers.[35] In burn patients the dose and/or frequency of administration of $H_2$-receptor blockers should be increased by 25–30% to obtain an adequate response. The primary cause of this increased dose requirement is a hyperdynamic circulation resulting in enhanced elimination kinetics; however, target organ sensitivity is also reduced in these patients.[105]

Other prominent surgical complications in the burn patient are acalculus cholecystitis, suppurative thrombophlebitis, ischemic enterocolitis, and abscess formation in various regions of the body. These complications usually occur 10 or more days after burn injury when the risk of sepsis is increased. Many of these patients have a tenuous nutritional status, and wound healing may be impaired. Goodwin et al.[61] reported a significant dehiscence rate in patients undergoing laparotomies. The rate was halved by the use of stainless steel retention sutures.

Infrequently a pregnant woman sustains a thermal injury. The requirement of caring for two patients, mother and fetus, complicates management. It is necessary to avoid some drugs (sulfa drugs, diuretics, vasopressors) because of their undesirable effect on the fetus or on uterine blood flow. Hemodynamic stability of the mother should be the goal since fetal survival is precisely dependent on maternal survival, especially before 28 weeks of gestation (see Chapter 19).[41]

## ANESTHESIA

Anesthetic management is affected by numerous factors, such as the age of the patient; burn size; and the presence and severity of shock, inhalation injury and pre-existing diseases. Thus, each patient presents with unique problems that require individualization of monitoring, fluid management, airway maintenance, anesthetic and adjunct drug selection, and temperature control. Certain generalizations can be made, however, for each clinical phase of burn injury.

During the early postburn period (first 24 hours) the primary objective is provision of an oxygen supply that meets organ demand. Thus, resuscitation is the hallmark of intraoperative management during this phase. As already mentioned, difficulties with the patient's airway depend upon the site of the burn and the time since the injury occurred. Burns of the upper part of the body may be particularly difficult to manage because of massive edema of the face and upper airway. Since progression of orofacial edema continues for several hours, the airway of patients undergoing surgery shortly after trauma may be easier to manage than that of victims who require intubation 3 or more hours after injury.

As stated above, venous access and obtaining blood pressure with standard cuff techniques may be difficult. A noninvasive monitor or an intra-arterial line may have to be used. Because of problems of venous access, catheters with a low degree of tissue reactivity may be used to prevent difficulties during the postoperative period.[148] Such catheters require a strict management protocol.

During resuscitation and convalescence, patients with major thermal injury are very susceptible to heat loss and therefore to cold stress. Fluids should be warmed, humidifiers added to the anesthesia circuit, and the room kept warm to prevent hypothermia.

Burn injury results in a significant alteration of response to various drugs. This alteration is most prominent during the resuscitative and convalescence phases and is affected by the multiple pathophysiologic changes that accompany thermal injury (Table 20-4). Since the direction and magnitude of change in drug response caused by each of these pathophysiologic factors vary significantly, it is difficult to predict the net effect of burn injury on the response to various drugs in an individual patient. Nevertheless, although incomplete, a significant body of research in this area, which is reviewed and summarized by Martyn and colleagues,[99,104] has provided guidelines to the use of drugs in patients with burns (Table 20-5).

The doses of intravenous anesthetics should be reduced during the resuscitation phase to prevent adverse hemodynamic responses. As in hemorrhaging patients, hypovolemia produced by thermal injury reduces the volume of distribution for these drugs.[173] In addition, crystalloid resuscitation during this phase results in decreased serum protein concentration,

TABLE 20-4. Burn-Induced Pathophysiologic Changes and Their Effects on Response to Drugs

| PATHOPHYSIOLOGIC CHANGES | EFFECT ON RESPONSE TO DRUGS | MECHANISM |
|---|---|---|
| Shock | Increased response to intravenous and inhalational agents | Decrease in the volume of distribution<br>Hypoproteinemia and acidosis causing decreased protein binding and increased availability of free drug |
| | Decreased response to drugs administered by the enteral, subcutaneous, and intramuscular routes | Decreased organ blood flow produced by hypovolemia, myocardial depression, increased blood viscosity, and catecholamine secretion, causing decreased absorption from the site of administration and thus decreased bioavailability of drug |
| Hyperdynamic circulation | Possibly increased response to flow-sensitive drugs | Increased blood flow to the brain |
| | Decreased response | Increased excretion and degradation caused by increased blood flow to the kidney and liver |
| Decreased serum albumin concentration | Increased response to albumin-bound drugs | Decreased binding to serum albumin, causing increased free fraction of drug. Decreased binding, by causing an increase in volume of distribution and in elimination of drug, may partially counter increased response. |
| Increased serum $\alpha_1$-acid glycoprotein concentration | Decreased response to $\alpha_1$-acid glycoprotein-bound drugs | Increased binding to $\alpha_1$-acid glycoprotein, causing decreased free-fraction of drug |
| Decreased sensitivity of target organ | Decreased response | Exact mechanism of this effect has not yet been elucidated |
| Other pathophysiologic changes:<br>Sepsis<br>Pre-existing diseases<br>Intake of hepatotoxic and nephrotoxic drugs<br>Intake of drugs causing hepatic microsomal enzyme induction or inhibition<br>Malnutrition<br>Parenteral nutrition | Increased or decreased response | Mechanisms remain to be elucidated in the burn patient |

increasing the free fraction of drugs.[173] Response to depolarizing and nondepolarizing muscle relaxants remains unaltered during the first 24 hours after burn injury. Thus, normal doses of a muscle relaxant should be used during a rapid sequence induction. Anesthesia is maintained using opioid and/or inhalational agents as the hemodynamic status of the patient permits. Intraoperative fluid requirements exceed those used for ordinary cases because ongoing fluid resuscitation must be carried out for the injury. Fluid infusion should be based on hemodynamic monitoring, the extent of which is based upon the severity of injury. Since up to 30% of patients with burns have coexistent inhalation injury, arterial oxygenation, acid-base status, blood carboxyhemoglobin level, and, in selected patients, blood cyanide concentration must be monitored.

In the hyperdynamic phase shock is not a concern, but some patients may be hypovolemic, requiring the infusion of fluids before anesthetic induction.[172] Orofacial edema may still be present and result in difficult airway management. During this phase patients are frequently unable to open their mouth widely enough for oral intubation to be performed. Therefore, awake, sedated, blind nasal intubation; a flexible fiberoptic laryngoscope; or a curved optical stylet may be necessary to manage the airway before surgery. During this phase, the hypermetabolic, hyperdynamic state is characterized by increased basal $O_2$ consumption ($\dot{V}O_2$) and cardiac output. Thus, the total body oxygen supply is matched to demand. Concern has arisen in the past that depression of cardiac output by anesthetics, positive pressure ventilation, and increased systemic vascular resistance may interfere with this

TABLE 20-5. Response to Various Anesthetic and Adjunct Drugs During Three Phases of Burn Injury

| DRUG | RESUSCITATION PHASE | CONVALESCENCE PHASE | RECONSTRUCTION PHASE | COMMENTS |
|---|---|---|---|---|
| Diazepam | Prolonged effect after repeated doses | Prolonged effect after repeated doses Decreased response | Normal duration Decreased response | Prolonged effect is due to impaired oxidative metabolism (phase I reaction) of the drug by the liver |
| Chlordiazepoxide | Prolonged effect after repeated doses | Prolonged effect after repeated doses | Normal duration | |
| Lorazepam | Normal duration | Normal duration | Normal duration | Lorazepam is metabolized by conjugation (phase II reaction), which is not impaired after burn |
| Optiates and opioids | Decreased or unchanged response | Decreased response | Normal response | |
| Ketamine | Increased response | Normal response | Normal response | Increased response due to hypovolemia |
| Thiopental | Increased response | Normal response | Decreased response | Increased response due to hypovolemia; decreased response during the reconstruction phase remains to be explained |
| Succinylcholine | Normal response | Contraindicated because of potentially lethal hyperkalemia; increased response | Contraindicated because of potentially lethal hyperkalemia; increased response | |
| Nondepolarizing muscle relaxants | Normal response | Decreased response | Decreased response | Decreased response mediated by both pharmacokinetic and pharcodynamic factors |

balance and result in inadequate tissue oxygenation. Results from animal and human studies using isoflurane or enflurane do not support this hypothesis.[63,64,82] Although the cardiac output decreased when these anesthetics were administered during positive pressure ventilation, they also produced a concomitant decrease in total body oxygen consumption commensurate with the degree of cardiac output depression. Thus, the oxygen supply-demand balance remained unaltered.

Although succinylcholine can safely be used during the first 24 hours after injury, it should be avoided after this period for at least 1 year because it may result in a potentially lethal increase of serum $K^+$.[65,158] The magnitude of $K^+$ elevation appears to be related to the size of the burn: large increases of $K^+$ occur when the burn size exceeds 10% of body surface area.[19] Although a moot point, it is interesting that burn victims are extremely sensitive to succinylcholine during the fourth and twelfth postburn days, and even small doses (0.1–0.2 mg/kg) result in an intense and prolonged paralysis. This sensitivity increases with increasing size of the burn (Table 20-5).[19] The availability of intermediate-acting nondepolarizing muscle relaxants has simplified tracheal intubation of these patients. The dose requirement for adequate relaxation with nondepolarizing agents, however, is higher than that recommended for patients without burns (Table 20-5).[101] Resistance to nondepolarizing muscle relaxants develops in patients with burns of more than 30% of TBSA. It is seen after the first week and peaks about 5–6 weeks after injury.[50] It is attenuated by 3 months, but some resistance may be present for as long as 2 years.[50,102] This effect has been described for d-tubocurarine, pancuronium, alcuronium, metocurine, atracurium, vecuronium, and the combination of pancuronium and dimethyltubocurarine.[50,96,97,104,111,127,143] The increase in nondepolarizing muscle relaxant requirement is not related to an increased volume of distribution or leakage from the burn wound, nor does it appear to be related to increased plasma binding.[89] Although, at least for atracurium, a contributory effect of diminished free fraction of the drug in plasma has been demonstrated,[96] there is now little doubt that pharmacodynamic mechanisms play a major role in resistance. It has been proposed that burn injury, if large enough, results in generalized denervation-like responses that are mediated, at least partly, by an increased number of acetylcholine receptors in the neuromuscular junction.[85,86] More recent data, however, fail to confirm the existence of this response or of changes in acetylcholine activity.[97] Clearly, further work is necessary to determine the exact pharmacodynamic mechanisms of resistance to nondepolarizing agents.

Often, regional anesthesia cannot be used in major thermal injury because of the location of the burn or the extent of the surgery anticipated. Burn patients generally require frequent anesthetics for serially performed wound debridements. Although the likelihood of halothane hepatitis, if it exists, appears to be decreased in these patients, other agents are probably more suitable for multiple anesthetic administration.[66] Ketamine can be very useful in anesthesia for burn patients as it allows adequate spontaneous ventilation at a surgical plane of anesthesia, does not depress hemodynamics, and has an analgesic effect. Ketamine, however, does not protect against regurgitation and aspiration; thus, patients should be kept NPO before surgery. Ketamine also produces an increase in oral secretions; a drying agent should be administered.

As stated above, early wound excision may be associated with major blood loss requiring the administration of large amounts of blood and blood products, which subjects the patient to the complications of transfusion described in Chapter 6. Although citrate-induced ionized hypocalcemia is now a rare complication of transfusion, Coté and colleagues[33] emphasized that sudden but evanescent decreases in $Ca^{++}$ occurred in all thermally injured children who received 1–2.5 mL/kg/min of fresh-frozen plasma (FFP) for 5 minutes. Changes in Q-T interval on the ECG were not predictive of hypocalcemia. Rapid infusion of FFP was occasionally associated with clinically significant hypotension that could be attenuated by the administration of calcium, although no correlation could be found between systemic hypotension and hypocalcemia. It appears that citrate-induced hypocalcemia and cardiovascular instability after massive infusion of FFP are potentiated during deep halothane anesthesia.[31] Occasionally hypotension seen in this setting may be so severe that external cardiac massage may be necessary, along with the administration of fluids, calcium, and vasopressors and discontinuation of anesthetics.

Emergence from anesthesia should be smooth in order to protect suture lines and skin grafts. Postoperatively or postinjury, patients with burns require sedation and analgesia. As has already been described, the metabolic changes that occur in these patients may alter the kinetics and dynamics of anxiolytics and analgesics. Diazepam is used frequently to provide sedation. Because of its high lipid solubility the serum concentration of this drug decreases rapidly and results in short-lived sedation if administered as a single dose.[99] On the other hand, repeated doses of the drug saturate the tissues. In this situation the duration of action of diazepam may be prolonged because biotransformation in the liver is depressed (Table 20-5).[99,103] Both diazepam and chlordiazepoxide are metabolized in the liver by cytochrome p450 oxidases (phase I reaction). The burn injury depresses the function of these enzymes and results in decreased biotransformation. Lorazepam, on the other hand, is metabolized by hepatic glucuronidation (phase II reaction), which is less impaired than the phase I reaction. Thus, the effects of lorazepam are less likely to be prolonged than those of diazepam or chlordiazepoxide after burn injury (Table 20-5).[100] Consequently lorazepam may be the preferred agent for sedation of burn victims, especially if weaning from the ventilator is contemplated. Generally, those patients are resistant to narcotics and require higher than normal doses.[99] Rather than giving predetermined doses of these agents, the dose should be titrated to its optimal effect.

Most of the anesthetic problems of the resuscitation and convalescence phases do not occur during the reconstructive phase, although airway management difficulties may be posed by cervicofacial contractures, particularly those producing neck flexion or microstomia. Generally, these patients may be intubated easily and safely with the aid of a fiberoptic bronchoscope, judicious doses of sedatives and narcotics, and topical anesthesia while the adequacy of oxygenation and spontaneous breathing is ensured. At least in children, thiopental requirements are increased by about 60% 1 or more years after recovery from a significant thermal injury.[30] Thus, these children require a thiopental dose in the range of 7–8 mg/kg, provided they have adequate intravascular volume. The mechanism of this phenomenon is unknown. As alluded to earlier, succinylcholine-induced massive hyperkalemia remains a threat to life during the reconstructive phase if this agent is administered less than 1 year after a major burn[65]; it is probably prudent to avoid succinylcholine even in patients with older injuries.

## CONCLUSION

With improved understanding of the pathophysiology of thermal injury has come an improvement in survival. Patients with injuries that once had a mortality of 100% are surviving, and the $LA_{50}$ has been increasing. Aggressive management, such as early ventilatory support, improved resuscitation, fluid therapy, early nutritional support, and early escharectomy and grafting, has also played a role in this improved survival.[42] The age of the patient and burn size, however, remain factors beyond our control.[8,130] Mortality curves developed by Curreri et al. illustrate the effect of these two factors on survival (Fig 20-7).[37] The addition of failure of other systems also has a significant impact. Cardiac failure was associated with 100% mortality, pulmonary failure with 92% mortality, and immunologic failure with 73% mortality.[98]

FIG. 20-7. Mortality curves obtained from probit analysis of 937 burn patients. TBS = Total body surface. (From Curreri et al[37] with permission.)

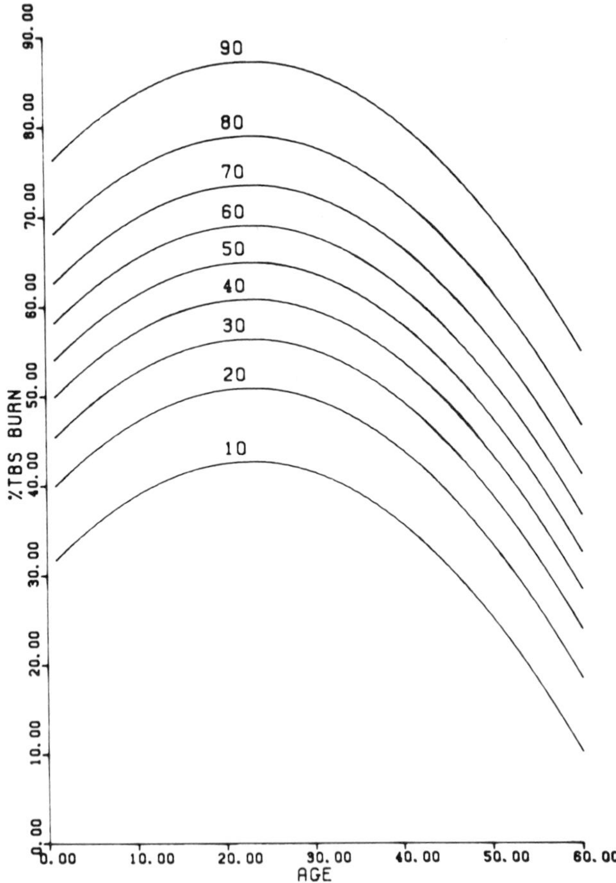

Care of patients with major thermal injury presents a challenge from the initial resuscitation to completion of reconstructive surgery. Adequate understanding of these problems will result in better anesthetic care.

## REFERENCES


1. Accident facts. Chicago: National Safety Council, 1988.
2. Adams AL, Klein M. Electrical cataract: notes on case and review of the literature. Br J Opthalmol 1945;29:169.
3. Agarwal N, Petro J, Salisbury RE. Physiologic profile monitoring in burned patients. J Trauma 1983;23:577.
4. Akrami C, Falkner B, Gould AB, et al. Plasma renin and occurrence of hypertension in children with burn injuries. J Trauma 1980;20:130.
5. Alexander JW. Burn care: a specialty in evolution. J Trauma 1986;26:1.
6. Allard JP, Jeejheebhoy KN, Whitwell J, et al. Factors influencing energy expenditure in patients with burns. J Trauma 1988;28:199.
7. Anderson G. Pathophysiology of the burn wound. Ann Clin Gynecol 1980;69:178.
8. Anous MM, Heimbach DM. Causes of death and predictors in burned patients more than 60 years of age. J Trauma 1986;26:135.
9. Artz CP. Electrical injury simulates crush injury. Surg Gynecol Obstet 1967;125:1316.
10. Balogh D, Moncayo R, Bauer M. Hormonal dysregulations in severe burns. Burns 1984;10:257.
11. Barker SJ, Tremper KK. The effect of carbon monoxide inhalation on pulse oximetry and transcutaneous $PO_2$. Anesthesiology 1987;66:677.
12. Baxter CR, Cook WA, Shires GT. Serum myocardial depressant factor of burn shock. Surg Forum 1966;17:1.
13. Becker RA, Wilmore DW, Goodwin CW, et al. Free $T_4$, free $T_3$, and reverse $T_3$ in critically ill, thermally injured patients. J Trauma 1980;20:713.
14. Bingham HG, Gallagher TJ, Powell MD. Early bronchoscopy as a predictor of ventilatory support for burned patients. J Trauma 1987;27:1286.
15. Bjerknes R, Vindenes H, Pitkänen J, et al. Altered polymorphonuclear neutrophilic granulocyte functions in patients with large burns. J Trauma 1989;29:847.
16. Boscoe MJ, deLange S. Damage to the triscuspid valve with a Swan-Ganz catheter. Br Med J 1981;283:346.
17. Bowser-Wallace BH, Cone JB, Caldwell FT Jr. Hypertonic lactated saline resuscitation of severely burned patients over 60 years of age. J Trauma 1985;25:22.
18. Brown KL, Mortiz A. Electrical injuries. J Trauma 1964;4:608.
19. Brown TCK, Bell B. Electromyographic responses to small doses of suxamethonium in children after burns. Br J Anaesth 1987;59:1017.
20. Burke JF, Wolfe RR, Mullany CJ, et al. Glucose requirements following burn injury. Ann Surg 1979;190:274.
21. Caldwell FT Jr, Bowser BH. Critical evaluation of hypertonic and hypotonic solutions to resuscitate severely burned children: a prospective study. Ann Surg 1979;189:546.
22. Carlson RG, Miller SF, Finley RK, et al. Fluid retention and burn survival. J Trauma 1987;27:127.
23. Carvajal HF, Parks DH. Optimal composition of burn resuscitation fluids. Crit Care Med 1988;16:695.
24. Chiarelli A, Casadei A, Pornaro E, et al. Alanine and aspartate aminotransferase serum levels in burned patients: a long-term study. J Trauma 1987;27:790.
25. Chiarelli A, Siliprandi L, Casadei A, et al. Aminotransferase changes in burned patients. Intens Care Med 1987;13:199.
26. Chicarilli ZN, Cruono CB, Heinrich JJ, et al: Selective aggressive burn excision for high mortality subgroups. J Trauma 1986;26:18.
27. Cioffi WG, Graves TA, McManus WF. High-frequency percussive ventilation in patients with inhalation injury. J Trauma 1989;29:350.
28. Clark GJ. Measurement of toxic combustion products in fire survivors. J Roy Soc Med 1982;75(suppl):40.
29. Clark WR, Nieman GF, Goyette D, Gryzboski D. Effects of crystalloid on lung fluid balance after smoke inhalation. Ann Surg 1988;208:56.
30. Cohen MA, Guzzardi LJ. Inhalation of products of combustion. Ann Emerg Med 1983;12:628.
31. Coté CJ. Depth of halothane anesthesia potentiates citrate-induced ionized hypocalcemia and adverse cardiovascular events in dogs. Anesthesiology 1987;67:676.
32. Coté CJ, Petkau AJ. Thiopental requirements may be increased in children reanesthetized at least one year after recovery from extensive thermal injury. Anesth Analg 1985;64:1156.
33. Coté CJ, Drop LJ, Hoaglin DC, et al. Ionized hypocalcemia after fresh frozen plasma administration to thermally injured children: effects of infusion rate, duration, and treatment with calcium chloride. Anesth Analg 1988;67:152.
34. Cottrell JE, Casthely P, Brodie JD, et al. Prevention of nitroprusside-induced cyanide toxicity with hydroxycobalamin. N Engl J Med 1978;298:809.
35. Counce JS, Cone JB, McAlister L, et al. Surgical complications of thermal injury. Am J Surg 1988;156:556.
36. Curreri PW, Richmond D, Marvin J, et al. Dietary requirements of patients with major burns. JADA 1974;65:415.
37. Curreri PW, Luterman A, Braun DW, et al. Burn injury: analysis of survival and hospitalization time for 937 patients. Ann Surg 1980;192:472.
38. Czaja AJ, Rizzo TA, Smith WR, et al. Acute liver disease after cutaneous injury. J Trauma 1975;15:887.
39. Davis JM, Illner H, Dineen P. Increased chromium uptake in polymorphonucleur leukocytes from burned patients. J Trauma 1984;24:1003.
40. Davis LK, Poulton TJ, Modell JH. Continuous positive airway pressure is beneficial in treatment of smoke inhalation. Crit Care Med 1983;11:726.
41. Deitch EA, Rightmire DA, Clothier J, Blass N. Management of burns in pregnant women. Surg Gynecol Obstet 1985;161:1.
42. Demling RH. Improved survival after massive burns. J Trauma 1983;23:179.
43. Demling RH. Burns. N Engl J Med 1985;313:1389.
44. Demling RH. Fluid replacement in burned patients. Surg Clin North Am 1987;67:15.
45. Demling RH, Wong C, Jin LJ, et al. Early lung dysfunction after major burns: role of edema and vasoactive mediators. J Trauma 1985;25:959.
46. DiVincenti FC, Moncrief JA, Pruitt BA Jr. Electrical injuries: a review of 65 cases. J Trauma 1969;9:497.
47. Dixon G. The evaluation and management of electrical injuries. Crit Care Med 1983;11:384.
48. Dolecek R, Zavoda M, Adamkova M, et al. Plasma renin-like activity (RLA) and angiotensin II levels after major burns. Acta Chir Plast 1983;15:166.
49. Dorethy JF, Welch G, Treat RC, Mason AD, Pruitt BA: Army Institute of Surgical Report progress report 1977.
50. Dwersteg JF, Pavlin EG, Heimbach DM. Patients with burns are resistant to atracurium. Anesthesiology 1986;65:517.
51. Eckhauser FE, Bullote J, Burke JF, et al. Tracheostomy com-

plicating massive burn injury: a plea for conservatism. Am J Surg 1974;127:418.
52. Ehrie M, Morgan AP, Moore FD, et al. Endocarditis with the indwelling balloon-tipped pulmonary artery catheter in burn patients. J Trauma 1978;18:664.
53. Engrav LH, Heimbach DM, Reus JL, et al. Early excision and grafting vs. nonoperative treatment of burns of indeterminant depth: a randomized prospective study. J Trauma 1984;23:1001.
54. Evans EI, Purnell OJ, Robinett WR, et al. Fluid and electrolyte requirements in severe burns. Ann Surg 1952;135:804.
55. Fein A, Leff A, Hopewell C. Pathophysiology and management of the complications resulting from fire and the inhaled products of combustion. Crit Care Med 1980;8:94.
56. Fenton JJ, Jones M, Hartford CE. Calcium fractions in serum of patients with thermal burns. J Trauma 1983;23:863.
57. Foy HM, Pavlin E, Heimbach DM. Excision and grafting of large burns: operation length not related to increased morbidity. J Trauma 1986;26:51.
58. Gallico GG, O'Connor NE, Kehinde O, et al. Permanent coverage of large burn wounds with autologous cultured human epithelium. N Engl J Med 1984;311:448.
59. Garzon AA, Seltzer B, Song IC, et al. Respiratory mechanics in patients with inhalation burns. J Trauma 1970;10:57.
60. Geyer RP. Review of perflurochemical-type blood substitutes. In: Proceedings of Tenth International Congress of Nutrition, Symposium on Perflurochemical Artificial Blood, Kyoto, Japan, 1975.
61. Goodwin CW, McManus WF, Mason AD Jr, et al. Management of abdominal wounds in thermally injured patients. J Trauma 1982;22:92.
62. Gray DT, Pine RW, Harnar TJ, et al. Early surgical excision versus conventional therapy in patients with 20 to 40 percent burns: a comparative study. Am J Surg 1982;144:76.
63. Gregoretti S, Gelman S, Dimick A, Proctor J. Effects of isoflurane on the hyperdynamic circulation of burned patients. Anesth Analg 1987;66:S74.
64. Gregoretti S, Gelman S, Dimick A, Proctor J. Total body oxygen supply-demand balance in burned patients under enflurane anesthesia. J Trauma 1987;27:158.
65. Gronert GA, Theye RA. Pathophysiology of hyperkalemia induced by succinylcholine. Anesthesiology 1975;43:89.
66. Gronert GA, Schamer PJ, Gunther RD. Multiple halothane anesthesia. Pacif Med Surg 1967;75:28.
67. Haberal M. Electrical burns: a five-year experience—1985 Evans lecture. J Trauma 1986;26:103.
68. Haponik EF, Meyers DA, Munster AM, et al. Acute upper airway injury in burn patients: serial changes of flow-volume curves and nasopharyngoscopy. Am Rev Respir Dis 1987;135:360.
69. Harris JA, Benedict FG. A biometric study of basal metabolism in man. Carnegie Institute of Washington. Philadelphia: JB Lippincott, 1919.
70. Heiber JM, McGough M, Rodeheaver G, et al. The influence of catabolism on immunocompetence in burned patients. Surgery 1979;86:242.
71. Herndon DN, Curreri PW. Metabolic response to thermal injury and its nutritional support. Cutis 1978;22:501.
72. Herndon DN, Traber DL, Niehaus GD, et al. The pathophysiology of smoke inhalation in a sheep model. J Trauma 1984;24:1044.
73. Herndon DN, Traber LD, Linares HA, et al. Etiology of the pulmonary pathophysiology associated with inhalation injury. Resuscitation 1986;14:43.
74. Herndon DN, Langner F, Thompson P, et al. Pulmonary injury in burned patients. Surg Clin North Am 1987;67:31.
75. Herndon DN, Barrow RE, Rutan TC, et al. Effect of propranolol adminstration on hemodynamic and metabolic response of burned pediatric patients. Ann Surg 1988;208:484.
76. Herndon DN, Barrow RE, Rutan RL, et al. A comparison of conservative versus early excision: therapies in severely burned patients. Ann Surg 1989;209:547.
77. Holliman CJ, Saffle JR, Kravitz M, et al. Early surgical decompression in the management of electrical injuries. Am J Surg 1982;144:733.
78. Hunt JL, Agee RN, Pruitt BA Jr. Fiberoptic bronchoscopy in acute inhalation injury. J Trauma 1975;15:641.
79. Jackson DL, Menges H. Accidental carbon monoxide poisoning. JAMA 1980;243:772.
80. Jelenko C, Williams J, Wheeler M, et al. Studies in shock and resuscitation. I: Use of hypertonic, albumin-containing, fluid demand regimen (HALFD) in resuscitation. Crit Care Med 1979;7:157.
81. Jensen PJ, Thomsen PEB, Bagger JP, et al. Electrical injury causing ventricular arrhythmias. Br Heart J 1987;57:279.
82. Jin L-J, Lalonde C, Demling RH. Effect of anesthesia and positive pressure ventilation on early postburn hemodynamic instability. J Trauma 1986;26:26.
83. Jones WG, Madden M, Finkelstein J, et al. Tracheostomies in burn patients. Ann Surg 1989;209:471.
84. Kehlet H. Should regional anesthesia and pharmacological agents such as beta blockers and opiates be utilized in modulating pain response? J Trauma 1984;24:S177.
85. Kim C, Fuke N, Martyn, JAJ. Burn injury to rat increases nicotinic acetylcholine receptors in the diaphragm. Anesthesiology 1988;68:401.
86. Kim C, Martyn JAJ, Fuke N. Burn injury to trunk of rat causes denervation-like responses in the gastrocnemius muscle. J Appl Physiol 1988;65:1745.
87. Kimura R, Traber LD, Herndon DN, et al. Treatment of smoke-induced pulmonary injury with nebulized dimethylsulfoxide. Circ Shock 1988;25:333.
88. Krantz T, Thisted B, Strom J, Sorensen MB. Acute carbon monoxide poisoning. Acta Anaesth Scand 1988;32:278.
89. Liebel WS, Martyn JAJ, Szyfelbein SK, et al: Elevated plasma binding cannot account for the burn related d-tubocurarine hyposensitivity. Anesthesiology 1981;54:378.
90. Long JM, III, Pruitt BA. Suppurative thrombophlebitis. In: Rutherford RB, ed. Vascular surgery. Philadelphia: WB Saunders, 1977:1181.
91. Loose LD, Turinsky J. Depression of the respiratory burst in alveolar and peritoneal macrophages after thermal injury. Infect Immun 1980;30:718.
92. Loven L, Nordstrom H, Lennquist S. Changes in calcium and phosphate and their regulating hormones in patients with severe burn injuries. Scand J Plast Reconstr Surg 1984;18:49.
93. Lucas CE, Denis R, Ledgerwood AM, Grabow D. The effects of hespan on serum and lymphatic albumin, globulin, and coagulant protein. Ann Surg 1988;207:416.
94. Mackay A, Halpern J, McLoughlin E, et al. A comparison of age-specific burn injury rates in five Massachusetts communities. Am J Pub Health 1979;69:1146.
95. Maher M, Anous MM, Heimbach D. Causes of death and predictors in burned patients more than 60 years of age. J Trauma 1986;26:135.
96. Marathe PH, Dwersteg JF, Pavlin EG, et al. Effect of thermal injury on the pharmacokinetics and pharmacodynamics of atracurium in humans. Anesthesiology 1989;70:752.
97. Marathe PH, Haschke RH, Slattery JT, et al. Acetylcholine receptor density and acetylcholinesterase activity in skeletal muscle of rats following thermal injury. Anesthesiology 1989;70:654.

98. Marshall WG, Dimick AR. The natural history of major burns with multiple subsystem failure. J Trauma 1983;23:102.
99. Martyn JAJ. Clinical pharmacology and drug therapy in the burned patient. Anesthesiology 1986;65:67.
100. Martyn JAJ, Greenblatt DJ. Lorazepam conjugation is unimpaired in burn trauma. Clin Pharmacol Ther 1988;43:250.
101. Martyn JAJ, Szyfelbein SK, Ali HH, et al. Increased d-tubocurarine requirements following major thermal injury. Anesthesiology 1980;52:352.
102. Martyn JAJ, Matteo RS, Szyfelbein SK, et al. Unprecedented resistance to neuromuscular blocking effects of metocurine with persistence after complete recovery in a burned patient. Anesth Analg 1982;61:614.
103. Martyn JAJ, Greenblatt DJ, Quinby WC. Diazepam kinetics in patients with severe burns. Anesth Analg 1983;62:293.
104. Martyn JAJ, Goldhill DR, Goudsouzian NG. Clinical pharmacology of muscle relaxants in patients with burns. J Clin Pharmacol 1986;26:680.
105. Martyn JAJ, Greenblatt DJ, Hagen J, Hoaglin DC. Alteration by burn injury of the pharmacokinetics and pharmacodynamics of cimetidine in children. Eur J Clin Pharmacol 1989;36:361.
106. Mathru M, Venus B, Rao TLK, et al. Noncardiac pulmonary edema precipitated by tracheal intubation in patients with inhalation injury. Crit Care Med 1983;11:804.
107. Matsuda T, Kagan J. Nutrition in the burned patient. Surg Ann 1984;16:119.
108. Matsuda T, Clark N, Hariyani GD, et al. The effect of burn wound size on resting energy expenditure. J Trauma 1987;27:115.
109. Merrell SW, Saffle JR, Sullivan JJ, et al. Fluid resuscitation in thermally injured children. Am J Surg 1986;152:664.
110. Merrell SW, Saffle JR, Sullivan JJ, et al. Increased survival after major thermal injury: a nine year review. Am J Surg 1987;154:623.
111. Mills A, Martyn JAJ. Evaluation of vecuronium neuromuscular blockade in pediatric patients with thermal injury. Anesth Analg 1987;66:S1.
112. Mills AK, Martyn JAJ. Evaluation of atracurium neuromuscular blockade in paediatric patients with burn injury. Br J Anaesth 1988;60:450.
113. Minty BD, Royston D, Jones JG, et al. Changes in permeability of the alveolar-capillary barrier in firefighters. Br J Industr Med 1985;42:631.
114. Moore DB, Rainey WC, Caldwell FT, et al. The effect of rapid resuscitation upon cardiac index following thermal trauma in a porcine model. J Trauma 1987;27:141.
115. Moore FD, Davis C, Roderick M, et al. Neutrophil activation in thermal injury as assessed by increased expression of complement receptors. N Engl J Med 1986;314:948.
116. Moore SJ, Norris JC, Walsh DA, Hume AS. Antidotal use of methemoglobin forming cyanide antagonists in concurrent carbon monoxide/cyanide intoxication. J Pharmacol Exp Ther 1987;242:70.
117. Morgan RJ, Martyn JAJ, Philbin DM, et al. Water metabolism and antidiuretic hormone (ADH) response following thermal injury. J Trauma 1980;20:468.
118. Mortiz AR, Henriques FC, McLean R. The effects of inhaled heat on the air passages and lungs. Am J Pathol 1945;21:311.
119. Moylan JA, Alexander LG. Diagnosis and treatment of inhalation injury. World J Surg 1978;2:185.
120. Moylan JA, West JT, Nash G, et al. Tracheostomy in thermally injured patients: a review of five years experience. Am J Surg 1972;38:119.
121. Moylan JA, Wilmore DW, Mouton DE, et al. Early diagnosis of inhalation injury using $^{133}$xenon lung scan. Ann Surg 1972;176:477.
122. Moylan JA, Adib K, Birnbaum M. Fiberoptic bronchoscopy following thermal injury. Surg Gynecol Obstet 1975;140:541.
123. Navar PD, Saffle JR, Warden GD. Effect of inhalation injury on fluid resuscitation requirements after thermal injury. Am J Surg 1985;150:716.
124. Neilen BA, Taddeini L, Strate RG. T lymphocyte rosette formation after major burns. JAMA 1977;238:493.
125. Ninnemann JL, Ozkan AN. Definition of a burn injury-induced immunosuppressive serum component. J Trauma 1985;25:113.
126. Ninnemann JL, Stratta RJ, Warden GD, et al. The effect of plasma exchange on lymphocyte suppression after burn. Arch Surg 1984;119:33.
127. Owen RT. Resistance to competitive neuromuscular blocking agents in burn patients. A review. Method Find Exp Clin Pharmacol 1985;7:203.
128. Pack GT, Davis AH. Burns, types, pathology and management. Philadelphia: JB Lippincott, 1930.
129. Peitzman AB, Shires T III, Carben WA, et al. Measurement of lung water in inhalation injury. Surgery 1981;90:305.
130. Petersen SR, Umphred E, Warden GD. The incidence of bacteremia following burn wound excision. J Trauma 1982;22:274.
131. Peterson VM, Murphy JR, Haddix T, et al. Identification of novel prognostic indicators in burned patients. J Trauma 1988;28:632.
132. Planas M, Watchel T, Frank H, et al. Characterization of acute renal failure in the burned patient. Arch Intern Med 1982;142:2087.
133. Plum F, Posner JB, Herin RF. Delayed neurologic deterioration after anoxia. Arch Intern Med 1982;110:56.
134. Pruitt BA Jr, Goodwin CW, Vaughan GM, et al. The metabolic problems of the burn patient. Acta Chir Scand 1985;522(suppl):119.
135. Purdue GF, Hunt JL. Electrocardiographic monitoring after electrical injury: necessity or luxury. J Trauma 1986;26:166.
136. Purdue GF, Hunt JL, Layton TR, et al. Burns in motor vehicle accidents. J Trauma 1985;25:216.
137. Robinson NB, Hudson LD, Riem M, et al. Steroid therapy following isolated smoke inhalation injury. J Trauma 1982; 22:876.
138. Rosenberg JL, Zawacki BE. Reduction of blood loss using tourniquets and "compression" dressings in excising limb burns. J Trauma 1986;26:47.
139. Rosenthal SR, Hawley PL, Hakim AA. Purified burn toxin and its composition. Surgery 1972;71:527.
140. Saffle JR, Schnelby A, Hoffmann A, et al. The management of fractures in thermally injured patients. J Trauma 1983;23:902.
141. Saffle JR, Medina E, Raymond J, et al. Use of indirect calorimetry in the nutritional management of burned patients. J Trauma 1985;25:32.
142. Sasaki TM, Welch GW, Herndon D, et al. Burn wound manipulation induced bacteremia. J Trauma 1979;19:46.
143. Satwicz PR, Martyn JAJ, Szyfelbein SK, et al. Potentiation of neuromuscular blockade using a combination of pancuronium and dimethyltubocurarine. Br J Anaesth 1984;56:479.
144. Shirani KZ, Pruitt BA, Mason AD. The influence of inhalation injury and pneumonia on burn mortality. Ann Surg 1987;205:82.
145. Silverman SH, Purdue GF, Hunt JL, Bost RO. Cyanide toxicity in burned patients. J Trauma 1988;28:171.
146. Skoog T. Electrical injuries. J Trauma 1970;10:816.
147. Smith G, Ledingham IMA, Sharp GR, et al. Treatment of coal gas poisoning with oxygen and 2 atmospheres pressure. Lancet 1962;1:816.
148. Smith RC, Hartemink RJ, Duggan D. Prolonged multipurpose

venous access in burned patients: three years' experience with Hickman right atrial catheters. J Trauma 1985;25:634.
149. Sneve H. The treatment of burns and skin grafting. JAMA 1905;45:1.
150. Soroff HS, Pearson E, Artz CP. An estimation of the nitrogen requirements for equilibrium in burned patients. Surg Gynecol Obstet 1961;112:159.
151. Stone HH, Martin JD. Pulmonary injury associated with burns. Surg Gynecol Obstet 1969;129:1242.
152. Stone HH, Rhame DW, Corbitt JD, et al. Respiratory burns: a correlation of clinical and laboratory results. Ann Surg 1967;165:157.
153. Stratta RJ, Warden GD, Ninnemann JL, et al. Immunologic parameters in burned patients: effect of therapeutic interventions. J Trauma 1986;26:7.
154. Sugi K, Newald J, Traber LD, et al. Smoke inhalation injury causes myocardial depression in sheep. Anesthesiology 1988;69:A111.
155. Szyfelbein SK, Lambertus JD, Martyn JAJ. Persistent ionized hypocalcemia in patients during resuscitation and recovery phases of body burns. Crit Care Med 1981;9:454.
156. Teodorczyk-Injeyan JA, Sparkes BG, Mills GB, et al. Increase of serum interleukin 2 receptor level in thermally injured patients. Clin Immunol Immunopathol 1989;51:205.
157. Thompson PB, Herndon DN, Traber DL, et al. Effect on mortality of inhalation injury. J Trauma 1986;26:163.
158. Tolmie JD, et al. Succinylcholine danger in the burned patient. Anesthesiology 1967;28:467.
159. Tompkins RG, Burke JF, Schoenfeld DA, et al. Prompt eschar excision: a treatment system contributing to reduced burn mortality. A statistical evaluation of burn care at the Massachusetts General Hospital (1974–1984). Ann Surg 1986;204:272.
160. Tompkins RG, Remensnyder JP, Burke JF, et al. Significant reductions in mortality for children with burn injuries through the use of prompt eschar excision. Ann Surg 1988;208:577.
161. Traber DL, Herndon DN, Stein MD, et al. The pulmonary lesion of smoke inhalation in an ovine model. Circ Shock 1986;18:311.
162. Turner WW, Ireton CS, Hunt JL, et al. Predicting energy expenditures in burned patients. J Trauma 1985;25:11.
163. Van Hoesen KB, Camporesi EM, Moon RE, et al. Should hyperbaric oxygen be used to treat the pregnant patient for acute carbon monoxide poisoning? A case report and literature review. JAMA 1989;261:1039.
164. Vaughan GM, Becker RA, Allen JP, et al. Cortisol and corticotrophin in burned patients. J Trauma 1982;22:263.
165. Vaughan GM, Becker RA, Unger RH, et al. Nonthyroidal control of metabolism after burn injury: possible role of glucagon. Metabolism 1985;34:637.
166. Venus B, Matsuda, Copozio JB, et al. Prophylactic intubation and continuous positive airway pressure in the management of inhalation injury in burn patients. Crit Care Med 1981;9:519.
167. Wang XW, Wang NZ, Zhang OZ, et al. Tissue deposition of silver following topical use of silver sulphadiazine in extensive burns. Burns 1985;11:197.
168. Warden GD, Ninnemann JL. The immune consequences of thermal injury: an overview. In: Ninnemann JL, ed. The immune consequences of thermal injury. Baltimore: Williams & Wilkins, 1981:1.
169. Warden GD, Saffle JR, Kravitz MA. A two-step technique for excision and grafting of burn wounds. J Trauma 1982;22:98.
170. Warden GD, Stratta RJ, Saffle JR. Plasma exchange in patients failing to resuscitate from burn shock. J Trauma 1983;23:945.
171. Waxman K, Rebello T, Pinderski L, et al. Protein loss across burn wounds. J Trauma 1987;27:136.
172. Waxman K, Holness R, Tominaga G, et al. Hemodynamic and oxygen transport effects of pentastarch in burn resuscitation. Ann Surg 1989;209:341.
173. Weiskopf RB, Bogetz MS. Haemorrhage decreases the anaesthetic requirement for ketamine and thiopentone in the pig. Br J Anaesth 1985;57:1022.
174. Welch GW, Lull RJ, Petroff PA, et al. The use of steroids in inhalation injury. Surg Gynecol Obstet 1977;145:539.
175. Wilmore D. Metabolic changes in burns. In: Artz C, Moncrief JA, Pruitt BA Jr, eds. Burns: a team approach. Philadelphia: WB Saunders, 1979:120.
176. Wilmore DW. Energy requirements for maximum nitrogen retention. In: Greene HL, Golliday MA, Munro HH, eds. Clinical nutrition update: amino acids. Chicago: American Medical Association, 1979:47.
177. Wilmore DW, Mason AD, Pruitt BA, Jr. Insulin response to glucose in hypermetabolic burn patients. Ann Surg 1976;183:314.
178. Winkelstein A. What are the immunologic alterations induced by burn injury? J Trauma 1984;24:S72.
179. Winter PM, Miller JN. Carbon monoxide poisoning. JAMA 1976;236:1502.
180. Wolfe RA, Roi LD, Flora JD, et al. Mortality differences and speed of wound closure among specialized burn care facilities. JAMA 1983;250:763.
181. Wolfe RR, Herndon DN, Jahoor F, et al. Effect of severe burn injury on substrate cycling by glucose and fatty acids. N Engl J Med 1987;317:403.
182. Wood JJ, Rodrick ML, O'Mahony JB, et al. Inadequate interleukin 2 production: a fundamental immunological deficiency in patients with major burns. Ann Surg 1984;200:311.
183. Yoshioka T, Sugimoto T, Ukai T, et al. Haptoglobin therapy for possible prevention of renal failure following thermal injury: a clinical study. J Trauma 1985;25:281.

# Chapter Twenty-One

Edwin A. Bowe
Elmer F. Klein, Jr.

# Near-Drowning

Drowning deaths claim an estimated 140,000 lives around the world each year.[22,25,169] Of these, nearly 5,500 occur in the United States[106,107] (accounting for approximately 2–3 deaths per 100,000 people)[76,104] and an additional 1,000–1,300 in Canada.[25] In the United States as a whole, drowning is exceeded as a cause of unintentional injury death only by motor vehicle accidents and falls.[19,107] There has been, however, a steady decrease in deaths and death rate (per 100,000 population) from this cause since 1977. A 26% decrease in deaths and a 31% decrease in the death rate were recorded in 1987 as compared to 1977.[107] The significance of drowning is greater in certain age groups. In children, drowning ranks third in deaths from any cause, being surpassed only by neonatal mortality and deaths due to motor vehicle accidents.[77,121,144] Similarly, for persons aged 5 to 44, only motor vehicle accidents claim more lives via unintentional injury than drowning.[19] The highest incidence of drowning deaths occurs in the 10- to 19-year-old group.[4,12,136,137] For the population as a whole, male drowning death rates are more than five times greater than female.[19,106] Although boys are three times more likely than girls to drown outside the home, inside the home drowning deaths among girls exceed those for boys.[77,144]

Although most drownings occur in association with recreational activities, swimming pools account for only 10% of drowning deaths in the United States.[19] However, in some areas, for example in Los Angeles, nearly half the drowning deaths occur in private swimming pools.[113] Lakes, rivers, and oceans claim more lives than swimming pools.[20] Any significant accumulation of water is a potential site for near-drowning. Bathtubs take a significant toll in the very young,[114,126] the very old,[113,137,168] and persons with epilepsy.[117,122] Even water standing in toilet bowls and buckets has claimed the lives of some toddlers.[72,148,157,166] Nonetheless, since most deaths occur during recreational activities, there is a clear-cut peak in the summer months, with most deaths occurring during daylight hours and on weekends.[1,136,167,168]

Children are especially prone to immersion episodes. The three major risk groups are teenaged boys, unsupervised toddlers (nearly 40% of childhood victims are younger than 4 years old),[125] and children with epilepsy.[44,117] A convulsion in the water may cause the victim to simply disappear from view, the seizure obliterating not only the protective airway reflexes but also the struggle that normally occurs during an immersion episode.[117] The greatest single factor contributing to drowning deaths in the pediatric population is lack of adequate adult supervision.[77,125,127,144] Often, there is confusion regarding which adult is responsible, or the designated adult is under the influence of alcohol.[77,82] The absence of barriers limiting access to swimming pools is an additional factor.[5,77,88,125,127,128,129,144] One report on 66 consecutive pool immersion incidents showed that only 1 of the 66 pools had an adequate barrier.[77,125] Reports from Australia indicate that fatal and near-fatal pool accidents can be reduced by at least 50% if adequate safety legislation is enacted.[88] One community in Australia with effective, enforced laws requiring fencing around backyard pools has not had a childhood drowning in 9,200 pool years, a significant improvement if one considers that the annual pool:accident ratio in subtropical Australia is 470:1.[88]

## PREVENTION

The common thread that runs through most case histories of drowning victims is preventability. Alcohol consumption, a key contributing factor, is present in 47% of adults who drown.[19] Data from Australia suggest that the problem of alcohol consumption involves men, particularly in the 30- to 64-year-old group.[132] Education of the population at risk may be helpful in reducing mortality and morbidity from alcohol-related immersion events.[124] Risk for all accidents, including drowning, increases rapidly as blood alcohol concentrations rise to 0.05 g/100 mL.[131] At these levels swimming performance is impaired, causing the individual to function suboptimally in the water.[154]

Swimming ability, although touted by many as an effective preventive measure, is not a panacea. It was offset in the 35% of drowning victims who could swim by overconfidence, attempts to show off, or attempts to swim long distances.[136,137] Finally, in the adult population, inadequate or improperly used personal flotation devices are a key factor contributing to drowning deaths while boating. Although Coast Guard data showed that only 7% of boats involved in drownings lacked appropriate life preservers, these boats accounted for 29% of fatalities.[20] A second study revealed that, of 166 persons who drowned while boating, only 5 wore any kind of life preserver and remained with the boat and 3 of the 5 used their life preservers improperly.[136] Nearly one-fifth of yearly drowning deaths result from recreational boating.[162] Alcohol is a well-recognized contributing factor in this type of accident.[105]

For the most part the data presented above deal only with individuals who died as a result of immersion. They do not include other forms of injury (including spinal cord injuries incurred while surfing or diving) or individuals who survived a near-drowning incident.

## SEQUENCE OF EVENTS

Controlled studies and reports of disinterested observers of human drownings and near-drownings are obviously in short supply. However, some conclusions regarding the sequence of events may be drawn from experiments involving rodents[67,88] and dogs,[78] reconstruction of events observed in human victims,[90,108] and even one personal account of a near-drowning episode[79] in the medical literature. From these sources, the following sequence of events may be hypothesized. Initially the victim panics and holds his or her breath while struggling violently; some automatic swimming motions are made; movement is terminated and small amounts of air are exhaled while large amounts of water are being swallowed; emesis commonly occurs, at least partly in response to the volume of water ingested; spasmodic movements resembling convulsions occur while the victim aspirates water and/or regurgitated gastric contents during terminal gasping respirations (at times laryngeal spasm occurs, preventing aspiration); all airway reflexes disappear and water passively enters the trachea; and finally the patient succumbs.[77,90]

This reconstruction is probably applicable to most victims of drowning, but significant variations may occur from individual to individual. For example, some elderly patients may experience the immersion episode as a result of cardiovascular collapse and thereby lack any protective reflexes as soon as they become submerged.[136] Alternatively, immersion of the face in cold water (less than 20°C) may stimulate the diving reflex. The resultant severe bradycardia and shunting of blood to the brain and heart may prolong the duration of hypoxemia that may be tolerated before irreversible brain damage occurs.[25,39,90] On the other hand, contact with extremely cold water has been reported to produce a vagally mediated cardiac arrest resulting in sudden death (immersion syndrome).[47,48,68,77] Perhaps the most common variation, however, is the occurrence of drowning (or near-drowning) without aspiration. This syndrome, reported in 10% of drowning victims,[28,90,99,102,155] is presumably the result of laryngospasm. Under these circumstances no water is actually aspirated, even though the victim remains submerged. It should be obvious considering the different responses to submersion, as well as the possible presence of pre-existing disease, that each victim is unique. Accordingly, therapy must be based on the condition of each specific victim, rather than on the use of "cookbook" maneuvers applied to all patients.

Despite the uniqueness of each victim, attempts have been made to categorize patients for the purposes of evaluating and reporting therapies, as well as to allow the development of some kind of rational approach to drowning. Currently, most studies divide patients into groups depending on whether or not they survive the first 24 hours ("drowned" versus "near-drowned") and whether or not they aspirate (sometimes termed "wet" versus "dry").[90] Further categorization is made on the basis of the medium in which they were immersed (salt water versus fresh water). An additional group, termed "secondary drowning"[77] or "delayed death subsequent to near-drowning,"[95] comprises those patients who develop delayed respiratory deterioration[123] or die during therapy despite survival for the first 24 hours and apparently successful resuscitation. Table 21-1 presents the most commonly used terminology, as initially proposed by Modell.[90,91]

TABLE 21-1. Nomenclature

| | |
|---|---|
| Drown with aspiration | Death within 24 hours with aspirated fluid material in the lungs |
| Near-drowning with aspiration | Immersion episode in which patient aspirates fluid material but survives for at least 24 hours |
| Drown without aspiration | Death within 24 hours after immersion in which aspiration did not occur |
| Near-drowning without aspiration | Immersion episode without associated aspiration in which patient survives the first 24 hours |
| Delayed death subsequent to near-drowning | Death more than 24 hours after immersion episode |

## PATHOPHYSIOLOGY

Although early papers dealing with the treatment of near-drowning victims emphasized changes in blood volume and serum electrolytes,[158] more recent work has made it clear that the most important pathophysiologic event produced by immersion (whether in fresh water or sea water) is the development of arterial hypoxemia.[71,90] Experiments in which the endotracheal tubes of intubated dogs were occluded (basically simulating near-drowning without aspiration) demonstrated that $PaO_2$ fell from a value of 92 mm Hg before tracheal obstruction to 40 mm Hg in the first 60 seconds and to 10 mm Hg by the end of 3 minutes.[92] After the same time interval, $PaCO_2$ had increased by only 12 mm Hg, and pH had decreased only to 7.32.[90] Although a $PaO_2$ level of 10–15 mm Hg is uniformly fatal, lethal levels of hypercarbia and acidosis were not attained under the circumstances of near-drowning without aspiration.[71] Numerous studies have documented that aspiration of salt or fresh water produces almost immediate hypoxemia.[23,52,93,97]

The type and quantity of fluid aspirated determine the pathophysiology of drowning and near-drowning. Because sea water osmolaity is roughly three to four times that of plasma, the presence of sea water in the lung should produce a flow of plasma from the vascular space into the alveoli. Intravascular hypovolemia with hemoconcentration and increased serum electrolyte concentrations should result. By contrast, aspiration of fresh water should produce hemodilution (with decreased concentrations of hemoglobin and electrolytes) and intravascular hypervolemia due to the rapid absorption of aspirated fluid into the circulation. The influx of large quantities of hypotonic fluid has been postulated to produce lysis of red blood cells by virtue of a pronounced reduction in serum osmolality.[77,99] Although these changes have been documented in laboratory experiments and may well occur in at least some of the human victims who die, they are rarely seen in patients who survive long enough to reach the hospital because the quantity of water necessary to produce these changes is so great.[77,99] Indeed, roughly 10% of patients do not aspirate any water at all,[99,102] and the majority of those who do aspirate inhale less than 22 mL/kg.[89,94,99,155] Thus, the major pathophysiologic event in drowning and near-drowning is hypoxemia, rather than the complex electrolyte imbalances predicted by previous studies. Indeed, the cause of death in many drowning victims is an inability to re-establish spontaneous circulation at the scene of the accident due to the severity of the asphyxia. By the same token, hypoxic damage to the central nervous system accounts for almost all *late* morbidity and mortality in near-drowning victims.[112]

Although their manifestations are the same, the pulmonary injuries resulting from fresh or salt water are different. Atelectasis after fresh water aspiration results from surfactant washout or inactivation by the fluid entering the lung.[77,99,123,145] The regeneration of surfactant usually requires 24–48 hours.[123] Salt water, on the other hand, does not alter surfactant.[123] Instead, the major pulmonary lesion associated with sea water aspiration is filling of the alveoli not only with the initially aspirated fluid but also by pulmonary edema, a result of alveolar membrane disruption.[77,99] In either case, the hypoxemia results from intrapulmonary shunt caused by continued perfusion of unventilated or inadequately ventilated alveoli.[77,99,145,155]

Morphologic abnormalities in the lung are not limited to the alveoli; mitochondrial swelling develops in the animal pulmonary vascular endothelium. This swelling is more likely to be caused by excessive catecholamine secretion than by the effect of water inhalation.[66] In fact, pathologic findings consistent with catecholamine release have been demonstrated in the hearts of animal and human drowning victims.[65,80] These findings include smooth muscle contraction banding within the media of the major coronary arteries, focal myocardial necrosis, and ventricular myocyte contraction banding. Smooth muscle contraction banding in the coronaries suggests spasm. Thus, many drowning victims probably die from complications of decreased or abolished myocardial perfusion, rather than from inhalation of water during the initial stage.

The patient who has aspirated significant quantities of water during an immersion episode presents with tachypnea (often 60–80 breaths/min), decreased lung compliance, increased work of breathing, increased $O_2$ consumption, hypoxemia, and hypocarbia.[25] Metabolic acidosis, probably due to tissue hypoxia, is generally present.[99] Studies with dogs demonstrate that aspiration of 22 mL/kg of fresh water produces a fall in $P_aO_2$ to 60 mm Hg within 3 minutes of aspiration. Salt water is even more damaging, with $P_aO_2$ decreasing to 40 mm Hg in the same time interval.[99] Given these studies, it is generally accepted that patients who present with normal $P_aO_2$ (>80 mm Hg) while spontaneously breathing room air are examples of near-drowning without aspiration.[99] Delayed pulmonary manifestations may be explained by superimposed bacterial pneumonia, pulmonary barotrauma, mechanical lung damage from resuscitation, foreign body or chemical pneumonitis, inadequate ventilation, apnea secondary to central nervous system (CNS) damage, $O_2$ toxicity, or neurogenic pulmonary edema.[123]

As previously noted, most delayed morbidity and mortality result from asphyxial damage to the brain. The etiology of the CNS lesion is both simple and complex. The hypoxemic episode suffered during and after submersion is, in itself, capable of causing severe CNS damage. Other factors related to the pathophysiology of the immersion episode and to resuscitation may interact to alter the final cerebral insult. During immersion, victims take in large quantities of water, both by aspiration and by ingestion. This creates a hypervolemia that, especially in the case of hypotonic fresh water, is capable of producing cerebral edema. Resuscitation often involves infusion of large quantities of salt-containing fluids, which further increases blood volume. Cerebral edema may also be exacerbated by a postasphyxial increase in capillary permeability that allows fluid to leak into the tissues, including the brain.[169] This excess fluid aggravates the cerebral edema that may have been initiated by asphyxia.

Cerebral ischemia may also result from loss of autoregulation and increased intracranial pressure caused by cerebral edema. Although some neuronal destruction occurs at the time of the insult, other cells may be either incompletely damaged or initially escape damage altogether. Following the reestablishment of cerebral perfusion, the damage to some neurons may progress. Also, if impaired cerebral perfusion results from intracranial hypertension, neurons that escaped initial injury may suffer sufficient insult to affect their functional status.[169] Long-term CNS morbidity, then, may be determined not only by the magnitude of the initial damage but also by the severity of any postresuscitation insult. Nevertheless, much of the damage in near-drowning occurs during the initial hypoxic insult; secondary injury is a rare occurrence.

Two additional factors may in certain circumstances ameliorate the degree of cerebral damage: the "diving reflex" and "immersion hypothermia." As mentioned, the diving reflex is a neurogenic response that diverts blood from "nonessential" organs to the heart and brain. Independent of chemoreceptors or baroreceptors,[25,46] it is stimulated by facial immersion and reflex or voluntary breath-holding. It is potentiated by cold water and fear and is probably more active in young children.[25,41,46,155] Some authors believe that outcome, even after a period of cardiac arrest, is much better in patients in whom the diving reflex is activated.[25] Because this reflex may close vascular beds other than those of the heart and brain so effectively, the patient's appearance (cold, profoundly vasoconstricted, and with marked bradycardia) can easily be misinterpreted as signifying irreversible cardiac depression, and resuscitative efforts may be stopped prematurely.[155]

## HYPOTHERMIA

Hypothermia, a core temperature of less than 35° C,[139] commonly results from submersion episodes. Water temperature is significantly lower than body temperature during most submersions. Also, conductive heat loss is very rapid during submersion since the thermal conductivity of water is 32 times greater than that of air.[139] Alcohol, one of the most common factors contributing to hypothermia of all causes,[171] enhances the likelihood of hypothermia by producing cutaneous vasodilation and further accelerating heat loss.

Three stages of hypothermia have been described.[85] The responsive phase (core temperature 32°–35°C) is characterized by an attempt on the part of the patient to maintain body temperature. Shivering, hypertension, tachycardia, and cutaneous vasoconstriction are evident. The increase in central blood volume induced by vasoconstriction produces a diuresis that may cause clinically significant hypovolemia in later stages. During the slowing phase (core temperature 23°–32°C), enzyme kinetics slow; shivering may be manifest only as a fine tremor; and heart rate, respiratory rate, and blood pressure are decreased. Patients in the poikilothermic phase (core temperature less than 23°C) have no effective way of preventing heat loss.

Hypothermia produces a decrease in basal metabolic rate of approximately 7% per degree C (51% of normal at a core temperature of 28°C),[8,34,38,139,143,164] with a concomitant decrease in oxygen consumption and $CO_2$ production. This decreases the respiratory quotient from 0.82 to 0.65 at 30°C.[139] Initially, blood pressure increases because normal cardiac output is maintained in the presence of the increased systemic vascular resistance resulting from the intense peripheral vasoconstriction. Hypotension then occurs as cardiac output decreases due to hypovolemia, bradycardia, and decreased tissue $O_2$ requirement. Animal experiments document reproducible bradycardia below 32°C, which is replaced by atrial fibrillation secondary to atrial distention[87,164] at 26°–29°C. Ventricular fibrillation or asystole occurs at temperatures less than 28°C.[58,87,164] Sinus bradycardia, prolonged P-R interval, prolonged Q-T interval, T-wave inversion, nodal rhythm, and Osborn's J wave (a secondary wave in such close proximity to the S wave that it may be difficult to distinguish from the QRS complex) all have been described (see Fig 6-11).[38,51,83,119,139,147,161]

Respiratory depression (decreased respiratory rate), classically described in hypothermia from other causes, is commonly masked in the near-drowning victim by manifestations of aspiration. Cold bronchorrhea, the respiratory tract response to hypothermia, is manifested by the production of copious thick secretions[171] and may adversely affect those victims who have not already aspirated. Additionally, hypothermia decreases the cough reflex[8] and reduces vital capacity,[59] both of which predispose to atelectasis.[38] Although temperature correction of blood gas values has historically been advocated,[13,38,69,139,150,151] more recent work seems to indicate that these corrections are unnecessary for pH and $PCO_2$; maintenance of normal values as measured by the blood gas analyzer at 37°C provides optimal metabolic status.[138]

Blood viscosity increases with decreased core temperature as a result of an increase in plasma viscosity[134] in combination with the hematocrit increase resulting from diuresis. Platelets and leukocytes may be sequestered in the spleen or liver, resulting in laboratory values lower than normal.[139] Intestinal motility is decreased at temperatures below 34°C, and hepatic conjugation and detoxification diminish.[8,15,38,139,140] Hyperglycemia may result from decreased insulin release from the pancreas,[29,38,85,139] inhibition of peripheral glucose utilization,[29,139] and altered hepatic carbohydrate metabolism.[37,38,43] Hypoglycemia, however, is not an uncommon finding in near-drowning victims who present with or without hypothermia; a 22% incidence was reported in a recent communication.[11] Acute alcohol intoxication, exhaustion from struggling, and a prolonged stay in the water may be causative in its development. These patients should be treated with glucose, but hyperglycemia should be avoided since it may worsen neurologic outcome.[74]

Urine volume increases and specific gravity decreases due to the reduction of salt and water reabsorption induced by depressed tubular oxidative activity.[38,64,103,139,149] Renal tubular glucosuria may also result.[8,38]

Deep tendon reflexes,[38,84,153] peripheral nerve conduction,[36,38,40] and pain sensitivity[36,38] may be depressed by hypothermia. Pupillary dilation is commonly present below 30°C, and the electroencephalogram is generally flat when the core temperature is lower than 20°C. Although cooling lags behind hypoxic effects, the occurrence of immersion hypothermia before asphyxia may protect the brain from anoxic damage to some degree.[25,41]

Finally, although not proven in drowning victims, some hemodynamic adjustments may occur during immersion. Hydrostatic pressure on the body by the surrounding water may increase venous return and cause a rise in cardiac output.[3,6] In young healthy patients this hemodynamic adjustment may be of little clinical importance. However, in individuals with limited cardiac function, an increase in preload, whether resulting from hydrostatic squeeze, absorption of water from the lungs and gastrointestinal tract, or hypothermia-induced redistribution, may have deleterious consequences. Also, after removal from the water, the sudden reduction in venous return may result in decreased cardiac output and hypotension. This mechanism is suggested to be at least partly responsible for the postrescue collapse frequently described in shipwreck survivors.[46]

## TREATMENT

In keeping with the current understanding that asphyxia is the primary factor producing both short- and long-term morbidity and mortality, the first thrust of resuscitative efforts at the scene of the accident should be to correct hypoxemia and restore adequate perfusion. Virtually every author describing initial management of the immersion victim stresses the importance of prompt, effective cardiopulmonary resuscitation (CPR), to the point of advocating that mouth-to-mouth resuscitation and external cardiac massage be started in the water if feasible.[25,77] It should be emphasized that vomiting may occur in up to 50% of drowning victims during resuscitation.[53] Airway obstruction with either sand or regurgitated particulate matter is common and should be cleared before attempting ventilation with any technique.[53] Standard American Heart Association guidelines for managing cardiac arrest are reasonable for treatment at the scene of the accident.[46] It is worth noting that the need for drainage of water from the lungs is a debatable aspect of care for the near-drowning victim.[77,155,170] All authors agree, however, that supplemental $O_2$ should be administered in as high a concentration as possible, even in spontaneously breathing patients, during transportation to the hospital.[53,77,99,155] Many authors stress that adequate CPR after near-drowning is one of the major determinants of survival without neurologic sequelae.[24,77] One study showed that 93% of patients who arrived in the emergency department with a spontaneous heartbeat survived without neurologic problems.[99] Neurologic and respiratory considerations dictate care, not only at the scene of the accident and in the emergency department but also in the intensive care unit (ICU).[123]

In the emergency department, resuscitative measures should be continued until effective spontaneous circulation is re-established or until the decision is made to terminate resuscitation. It is important to note that, in the presence of hypothermia, conventional time limits for resuscitation should be ignored until the core temperature reaches 30°C.[24] In children especially, time limits become meaningless: complete neurologic recovery has been documented after prolonged (>40 minutes) submersion time.[60,77,109,116] Even in normothermic children spontaneous cardiac activity has been reestablished after as much as 45 minutes of submersion.[25] Respiratory support must also be maintained until adequate blood gas values have been obtained on room air.

Some authors suggest that all patients should be admitted to the hospital for at least 24–48 hours of observation, even if blood gases are adequate during spontaneous room air ventilation, because of the possibility of significant acute respiratory deterioration at some time after the immersion episode.[77,123,155] This concept, however, has been questioned: none of the 52 swimmers involved in sea water submersion developed symptoms of respiratory distress after an asymptomatic period, and in all patients who required hospital admission, respiratory deterioration occurred within 4 hours after the accident.[135] Thus, observation in the emergency department for 4–6 hours may be sufficient. A recent review summarizes the criteria for hospital admission as follows[152]: (a) history of apnea, cyanosis, loss of consciousness, and cardiopulmonary resuscitation (CPR) after the accident; (b) hypoxemia; (c) acidosis; (d) abnormal chest X-ray; and (e) abnormal physical examination. All patients who require assisted ventilation, have altered mental status, and required prolonged resuscitation should be admitted to the ICU.[152]

### EVALUATION

Admission laboratory studies should include chest X-ray, arterial blood gases, serum electrolytes (sodium, potassium, chloride, glucose, calcium, BUN, creatinine, and osmolality), urinalysis, complete blood count including a differential leukocyte count, and an electrocardiogram. If the patient's condition necessitates mechanical ventilation and admission to an intensive care unit, the following parameters should be monitored continuously: heart rate, respiratory rate, blood pressure (via indwelling arterial catheter), central venous or pulmonary artery pressure, and fluid intake and output. Additionally, physical examination should be repeated periodically; specifically, one should look for evidence of further respiratory compromise (diminished tidal volume, dyspnea, retractions, wheezing, or cyanosis), neurologic deterioration (ocular reflexes, state of consciousness, motor responses to noxious stimuli, and response to spoken commands), elevation of intracranial pressure (papilledema or loss of venous pulsations on funduscopic exam), and evidence of circulatory compromise (capillary refill, skin color, urine output, temperature, and recurrence of metabolic acidosis).[77] In addition to periodic sputum cultures, the immersion medium itself should be cultured if possible.

### BASIC THERAPY

Therapeutic maneuvers after admission to the ICU should include correction of abnormal electrolytes and normalization of intravascular volume by appropriate measures. The stomach should be emptied to prevent further absorption of swallowed water and diminish the likelihood of further regurgitation. Attention should also be paid to the patient's temperature. Arrhythmias—most frequently caused by hypoxia or acidosis—and hypotension should be treated appropriately.

Earlier articles directed therapy toward correction of electrolyte abnormalities based on the results of experiments in animals that showed different patterns of abnormality depending on the type of fluid aspirated.[158] They emphasized the occurrence of ventricular fibrillation due to electrolyte abnormalities as a major cause of death in drowning patients. Subsequent research on animals has shown that the tonicity of fluid is not important, and both fresh and salt water aspiration may cause mild to moderate depletion of intravascular volume within 1 hour because of increased capillary permeability from anoxia and a loss of protein in the pulmonary edema fluid.[159] With such a fluid shift hypoproteinemia, hypernatremia, and hemoconcentration may also occur in experimental animals if the aspirate volume exceeds 10 mL/kg, but even after aspiration of large volumes, blood chemistries are usually normal.[118] Studies on drowning and near-drowning victims have shown that humans aspirate a relatively small amount of water during immersion incidents.[94,99] Analysis of left ventricular blood from drowning victims has shown that only 15% of those who die in the water aspirate more than 10 mL/kg.[94] In a series of near-drowning patients, not a single one had an electrolyte disturbance significant enough to require emergency therapy.[99] Thus, near-drowning victims do not require specific fluid therapy with hypotonic or hypertonic solutions. Treatment is initiated with lactated Ringer's solution (10–15 mL/kg) and maintained according to hemodynamic status, serum electrolytes, and hematocrit.

## BASIC PULMONARY THERAPY

After near-drowning, patients are likely to fall into one of three categories regarding their need for pulmonary therapy. At one extreme are those who have not aspirated gastric contents or any appreciable quantity of water. Arterial blood gases reveal a normal $P_aO_2$ while spontaneously breathing room air. For these patients, no further therapy, except perhaps admission and overnight observation with repeated arterial blood gas determinations, is indicated.[99] At the other extreme are those patients who require mechanical ventilation and in whom there is no doubt about the need to provide optimal ventilatory therapy. The third group of patients generally present with hypoxemia and a normal chest X-ray and require only enhancement of $F_IO_2$. However, a normal chest X-ray does not necessarily indicate that no pulmonary damage has been sustained or that supplemental oxygen is unnecessary.[77] These patients should have repeated determination of arterial blood gases, continued supplemental oxygen, treatment of metabolic acidosis if present, and encouragement to cough and deep breathe. Deterioration of ventilation to the point where more than 40% oxygen is necessary to sustain an adequate $P_aO_2$ is an indication for more intensive pulmonary therapy.[99] Additional indications for airway intervention and/or mechanical ventilation include severe neurologic compromise, respiratory acidosis, and inability to clear pulmonary secretions.[77] Ventilatory assistance for prolonged periods of time may be required in these individuals.[77] Appropriate suctioning and position change are also important aspects of pulmonary therapy.[81]

Prophylactic steroids have no effect on survival rates, oxygenation, or intrapulmonary shunt[17,100] and may blunt hypoxic pulmonary vasoconstriction.[163] Consequently, the majority of authors no longer recommend routine steroid administration. The role of prophylactic antibiotics has also been debated. In this circumstance, both antibiotics and steroids may make infection with an opportunistic organism more likely.[100] Most authors now recommend withholding antibiotics until a specific organism is documented by repeated sputum cultures.

## VENTILATORY THERAPY

Adult respiratory distress syndrome (ARDS) subsequent to near-drowning results from aspiration of gastric contents or submersion medium. Many studies have shown that near-drowning is one of the more common causes of ARDS and was, in fact, the most common etiology of ARDS in one group of children admitted to a pediatric intensive care unit.[81] Ventilatory therapy of ARDS has been a subject of ongoing controversy. Articles have appeared from a multitude of groups, with each group espousing the virtues of one particular ventilatory device or technique over all others. A comprehensive discussion of the proposed merits of each technique is beyond the scope of this chapter. What is presented instead is a brief explanation of the rationale behind some of the therapeutic modalities. A more complete discussion of ARDS is presented in Chapter 24.

Failure to provide adequate arterial oxygenation by simple elevation of inspired oxygen concentration is an indication for more aggressive therapy, ie, mechanical ventilation or expiratory distending pressure—positive end-expiratory pressure (PEEP), continuous positive airway pressure (CPAP), or expiratory positive airway pressure (EPAP). In addition, pulmonary edema is a generally accepted indication for intervention. Many authors advocate the establishment of specific arterial blood gas criteria—for instance the inability to maintain an acceptable $P_aO_2$ on more than 40% oxygen[99]—for instituting some form of intervention.

Although the precise levels required, the devices used to attain them, and the waveforms generated may be argued, application of some form of expiratory distending pressure is a generally accepted treatment for severe hypoxemia resulting from near-drowning. Animal experiments have reported that expiratory distending pressure, with or without mechanical ventilation, was effective in resolving the hypoxemia of near-drowning in salt water.[98] The same laboratory was, however, unable to achieve adequate resolution of arterial hypoxemia after fresh water near-drowning unless mechanical ventilation was combined with the expiratory distending pressure.[7] In neither group was mechanical ventilation alone as effective in resolving hypoxemia as combining it with expiratory distending pressure.

The difference in responsiveness of these two apparently similar situations has been attributed to the effects of the different aspirates on pulmonary surfactant. Although aspiration of fresh water alters significantly the surface tension characteristics of pulmonary surfactant,[45] aspiration of salt water appears to reduce its quantity without altering its quality. The thesis advanced is that large tidal volume mechanical breaths are necessary to recruit atelectatic alveoli after fresh water near-drowning. Expiratory distending pressure is necessary to maintain patency of those alveoli. In salt water near-drowning, however, because the remaining surfactant is normal in its functional characteristics, expiratory positive pressure alone is adequate to prevent airway closure.

Expiratory distending pressure is not without disadvantages. Pulmonary barotrauma (pneumothorax, pneumomediastinum, etc.) and increased intracranial pressure may result from the use of this modality; however, the most commonly seen and uniformly agreed-upon complication is a decrease in cardiac output. Although both reflex[18,95] and humoral mechanisms[86] have been proposed, a simple decrease in venous return to the right heart resulting from the increased intrathoracic pressure generated by the combination of mechanical ventilation and expiratory distending pressure is the most widely accepted cause. For this reason, many physicians prefer to use intermittent mandatory ventilation (IMV) to allow spontaneous ventilation and to provide only enough machine breaths to maintain normal pH and/or to facilitate the resolution of hypoxemia by alveolar recruitment. The theory behind this approach is that the decrease in airway pressure during spontaneous inspiration will result in a higher cardiac output than if ventilation is totally controlled. Opponents of IMV, however, argue that the increase in oxygen consumption produced by spontaneous inspiratory efforts tends to offset any benefit of increased cardiac output.

Clinically it appears that ventilator rate and level of distending pressure work synergistically. Higher levels of expiratory pressure work best with lower rates of ventilation, whereas lower distending pressures commonly require higher ventilator rates to maintain equivalent $P_aO_2$. Although there may be a rate of mechanical ventilation that produces optimal $O_2$ delivery, pulmonary barotrauma and depression of cardiac output are a greater problem at higher rates.

Obviously, the severity of the near-drowning incident dictates the magnitude of ventilatory intervention. Routine institution of expiratory distending pressure alone in salt water near-drownings or expiratory distending pressure combined with mechanical ventilation in fresh water incidents does not take into account the wide range of severity of the pulmonary insult. Rather than proposing a rigid set of guidelines, the intent of this chapter is to indicate the need for individualizing therapy based on the severity of the pulmonary lesion. We would, however, propose that IMV at a rate sufficient to maintain normocarbia combined with some form of expiratory distending pressure is a generally acceptable approach in both groups.

Whatever combination of mechanical ventilation and expiratory distending pressure is ultimately utilized, most authors advocate placement of a thermodilution pulmonary artery catheter when levels of expiratory distending pressure exceed 15 cm of $H_2O$. This catheter ensures the ability to monitor cardiac output and its adequacy reflected in the mixed venous $PO_2$. It also allows the calculation of intrapulmonary shunt and facilitates monitoring of the efficacy of maneuvers used to decrease it (increased expiratory distending pressure, increased ventilator rate, increased tidal volume) or to increase cardiac output (volume expansion, administration of inotropic agents or vasodilators).[109]

## THERAPY FOR THE CENTRAL NERVOUS SYSTEM

Neurologic status after near-drowning has been classified as awake (alert and oriented), blunted (lethargic, semicomatose, combative, agitated, disoriented, or confused), or comatose (decorticate, decerebrate, or flaccid)[26,27,100] on the basis of physical examination in the ICU 1–2 hours after rescue (Table 21-2). It has recently been recommended that patient classification be done immediately upon admission to the emergency department and "deceased" be added to the classification.[24]

Both prospective and retrospective analyses have shown that virtually no neurologic deaths occur in patients classified as awake or blunted.[24,146] Consequently, these patients do not require aggressive cerebral resuscitation, although close observation for 24 hours, preferably in the ICU, is indicated.[24,166]

Comatose patients are candidates for cerebral resuscitation; however, the extent of treatment required has not been defined clearly. The pathophysiologic aspects of cerebral injury have been given the acronym "HYPER" to represent the HyperHydration, HyperVentilation, HyperPyrexia, HyperExcitability, and HyperRigidity present in near-drowned patients.[25,41] In 1978 Conn et al.[25] suggested that cerebral salvage might be improved if the treatment was directed to each component of HYPER: mild dehydration, paralysis and mechanical ventilation, maintenance of stable blood pressure by means of fluids and/or dopamine, maintenance of normothermia or intentional hypothermia when necessary, sedation, steroid therapy, head elevation, and barbiturate coma. Several reports appeared in the literature about the beneficial effects of this therapy,[101,130,169] but the fact remained that overall survival with normal neurologic function in the series of Conn et al.[25] did not differ from that of Modell et al.[99] who treated their patients similarly except without the use of hypothermia or barbiturate coma (Tables 21-3 and 21-4). The following discussion is based on each component of HYPER therapy, although it should be emphasized that most centers currently involved in management of near-drowning do not employ the complete protocol. The therapeutic efficacy and side effects of some components of this therapy, especially hypothermia and barbiturates, must be evaluated further before they can be definitively recommended.

### *Fluid Management*

As has already been mentioned, humans aspirate a relatively small amount of water and thus do not develop severe elec-

TABLE 21-2. Criteria for Neurologic Classification of Near-Drowning Patients in the Emergency Department and Correlation of the Classification with the Glasgow Coma Scale*

| GROUP | GLASGOW COMA SCORE | CRITERIA |
|---|---|---|
| A (Awake) | 15 | Alert, oriented, and conscious |
| B (Blunted) | 10–13 | Lethargic, semicomatose, combative, agitated, obtunded, disoriented, confused, purposeful response to pain, normal breathing |
| C (Comatose) | 3–5 | Unresponsive, abnormal response to pain, abnormal respirations |
| Subgroups | | |
| C1 (Decorticate) | 5 | Flexor response to noxious stimuli, Cheyne-Stokes respiration |
| C2 (Decerebrate) | 4 | Extensor response to pain |
| C3 (Flaccid) | 3 | No response to pain, absent or irregular breathing |
| C4 (Decreased) | <3 | Dead |

* From Modell et al[99] and Conn et al.[26]

TABLE 21-3. Outcome of Fresh Water Drowning and Near-Drowning Victims in Each Neurologic Classification Group*

| NEUROLOGIC CLASSIFICATION GROUP | NUMBER OF PATIENTS | % DEATH | % WITH NEUROLOGIC DYSFUNCTION | % WITH NORMAL NEUROLOGIC FUNCTION |
|---|---|---|---|---|
| A | 56 | 0 | 0 | 100 |
| B | 19 | 5 | 0 | 95 |
| C | 65 | 38.5 | 14 | 48 |
| TOTAL | 140 | 19 | 6 | 75 |
| Subgroups | | | | |
| C1 | 5 | 0 | 0 | 100 |
| C2 | 14 | 7 | 7 | 86 |
| C3 | 6 | 17 | 17 | 25 |
| C4 | 40 | 58 | 18 | 25 |
| | 65 | 39 | 14 | 48 |

* From Conn et al.[25]

trolyte abnormalities, although they may be hypovolemic because of fluid loss into tissues.[94,99,159] Fluid therapy with lactated Ringer's (10–15 mL/kg) can be initiated and followed by adjustment of infusion according to the intravascular volume. Careful assessment of hemodynamic status with appropriate monitoring is necessary since in addition to hypovolemia, PEEP and barbiturate coma, if used, may impair cardiovascular function.[61]

After initial hydration of the near-drowning victim, fluid restriction and diuretic therapy may be indicated to reduce brain edema.[24,26,77,97] Increasing serum osmolality by administration of osmotic diuretics should be effective in removing some of the edema fluid. Furosemide may have deleterious effects in a patient already suffering from hypovolemia, but may be indicated in normovolemic patients with intracranial hypertension.

### *Control of Ventilation*

Maintenance of spontaneous ventilation is associated with lower mean intrathoracic pressure and higher cardiac output,[33,70] as well as better matching of ventilation and perfusion, than controlled mechanical ventilation of a paralyzed patient.[16,42,57,142] For these reasons we favor maintenance of as much spontaneous ventilation as possible in the near-drowning victim suffering primarily from lung injury. However, when there is documented elevation of ICP and the neurologic injury is paramount, these principles must be sacrificed in order to prevent or treat further increases in ICP. Paralysis with long-acting muscle relaxants (eg, pancuronium, .05–.15 mg/kg) will allow control of ventilation in the rare patient who will not breathe in synchrony with the IMV mode of the ventilator despite adequate blood gases. Paralysis is also effective in preventing coughing and bucking and the attendant increase in ICP associated with suctioning or other pulmonary maneuvers. On the other hand, muscle relaxation makes a complete neurologic examination impossible. Accordingly, we believe that muscle relaxants should be reserved for those patients with an ICP monitor already in place or for those in whom control of ventilation before insertion of an ICP monitor is indicated.

Maintenance of adequate oxygenation is imperative in all patients, whether they are initially comatose or not. It may be necessary to increase $F_IO_2$ above normally acceptable levels in patients with increased ICP who cannot tolerate expiratory distending pressure.

In the patient who is treated aggressively for increased ICP, some degree of controlled hyperventilation is necessary.[10,24,101] The optimal level of $P_aCO_2$ is not known and may vary with the presence of pre-existing cerebrovascular disease, as well as with the duration and magnitude of the spontaneous hyperventilation that the near-drowned patient may develop as a result of arterial hypoxemia or inadequate cerebral per-

TABLE 21-4. Outcome of Near-Drowned Patients in Each Neurologic Classification Group*

| NEUROLOGIC CLASSIFICATION GROUP | NUMBER OF PATIENTS | % DEATH | % WITH NEUROLOGIC DYSFUNCTION | % WITH NORMAL NEUROLOGIC FUNCTION |
|---|---|---|---|---|
| A | 61 | 0 | 0 | 100 |
| B | 31 | 10 | 0 | 90 |
| C | 29 | 34 | 10 | 55 |
| TOTAL | 105 | 11 | 2 | 87 |

* From Modell et al.[99]

fusion. Controlled hyperventilation decreases ICP primarily by reducing cerebral blood flow, which may result in a decrease in cerebral perfusion. Thus, attempts to decrease ICP by hyperventilation must also take into account the effect of this maneuver on cerebral perfusion pressure (CPP). Since optimal CPP is essential, controlled hyperventilation should probably be instituted under careful ICP monitoring.[92,110]

### Control of Temperature

Most near-drowning victims are hypothermic; however, in some patients hyperpyrexia may develop. Core temperature should be monitored and normothermia maintained using cooling mattresses, muscle relaxants, low ambient temperature, and antipyretics. Hypothermia to temperatures of 30°–32°C was, and probably still is, used in some institutions when ICP could not be controlled by other maneuvers.[24,111] In a retrospective analysis Conn's group,[10] who had recommended this therapy in the late 1970s, has demonstrated that hypothermia is not only ineffective in improving neurologically intact survival but also may be associated with significant complications. In addition to cardiovascular complications, long-term hypothermia is associated with neutropenia or immune suppression predisposing the patient to infection.[10] If this therapy is instituted, care must be taken during rewarming of patients surviving the treatment lest ICP increase again.

### Control of Hyperexcitability and Hyperrigidity

Sedation with benzodiazepines and/or narcotics and relaxation can be used to control flexor-extensor spasms and combative behavior. Anticonvulsants (barbiturates, phenytoin) are indicated for prevention or treatment of convulsions. Thiopental, 75–150 mg IV, can be administered for immediate control if convulsions occur. Phenobarbital is administered intramuscularly in a dose of 100–200 mg in adults. Intravenously the drug can be given as a slow intravenous infusion at a dose of 1 mg/kg; this may be increased to 500 mg in adults with careful monitoring of systemic blood pressure. Phenytoin is given in intravenous doses of 2–3 mg/kg, slowly and under ECG control since it may produce ventricular arrhythmias. The usual intramuscular dose is 100–200 mg every 6–12 hours.

Large doses of barbiturates have been used to induce or maintain "coma" and lower ICP. Although initial reports[9] that barbiturates were capable of providing some degree of cerebral protection after a global hypoxic/ischemic insult have been disproven,[14,50,156,160] their efficacy in decreasing ICP remains unchallenged. There are numerous protocols for maintenance of barbiturate coma. Although some advocate phenobarbital,[130,169] others recommend pentobarbital[25,146] or thiopental.[130] Even the method of evaluating the depth of coma is not agreed upon. Some advocate following serum levels[25,101,112] whereas others argue that tachyphylaxis or resistance may develop and that the only way to gauge truly the depth of coma is by following the electroencephalogram (EEG) and titrating dosage to a specific level[112]—three-second burst-suppression, flat line, etc. There are even those who have continued administration of barbiturates despite a continuing increase in intracranial pressure,[146] believing that direct cerebral vasoconstriction may ultimately, in some circumstances, lower ICP.

Barbiturate therapy does not seem to have any beneficial effect on the brain after near-drowning.[10,31,111,141] It may control ICP, but it has not been established that ICP control in this setting improves outcome. In near-drowning, elevated ICP results from ischemia. Consequently the damage, which is global, usually is established by the time that barbiturate therapy is initiated. This is unlike the situation in head injury in which the primary event is the ICP elevation and ischemia is a secondary phenomenon. Thus, ICP control with barbiturates may prevent secondary brain ischemia and injury in head trauma, whereas it is, as demonstrated by many clinical trials, of little value in near-drowning.[10,31,111,141]

The use of corticosteroids, a treatment recommended by some authors in the 1970s to reduce brain edema after near-drowning,[26] also has been shown to be ineffective. In addition it may increase the danger of disseminated infection.

## ICP MONITORING AND CONTROL

Repeated assessment is the key to detecting neurologic deterioration in those near-drowning patients presenting in an awake or blunted state. On the other hand, repeated evaluations of responses to noxious stimuli are associated with increases in intracranial pressure[165] and are not warranted in patients with documented intracranial hypertension. Muscle relaxation, sedation, and barbiturate coma make clinical assessment of neurologic function difficult, impossible, or unnecessary. Funduscopic evidence (papilledema, loss of venous pulsations) of increased ICP is notoriously unreliable.[54–56] Since intraocular venous pressure is almost 40 mm Hg, loss of venous pulsations is a late finding.

Although direct monitoring of ICP in comatose near-drowning victims has been recommended by some authors,[21,25,92,109,110] others believe that ICP monitoring does not improve neurologic outcome because intracranial hypertension is rarely observed in the absence of brain death.[10,24,146] Indeed in most comatose near-drowning victims, ICP during the first 48–72 hours postimmersion generally remains below 15 mm Hg.[31,146] Brief, nonrepetitive elevations in ICP may occur, but they respond readily to hyperventilation. However, after the second or third day, there may be ICP elevation above 20 mm Hg.[146] ICP monitoring may be useful in detecting early and late elevation of intracranial pressure and promoting institution of simple measures, such as 10°–15° head elevation or administration of muscle relaxants to control ICP. As was mentioned, ICP monitoring may also be useful in adjusting $P_aCO_2$ to an optimal ICP and CPP during hyperventilation.

At present there is no prospective well-controlled study that evaluates the effect of ICP monitoring and aggressive therapy to control ICP. Opinions about ICP control in near-drowning are divided. Some suggest that maintenance of ICP below 20 mm Hg and CPP above 50 mm Hg may improve survival,[110] whereas others have noted only equivocally beneficial effects of these maneuvers on residual brain function in surviving decorticate or decerebrate comatose patients.[2,146] Thus, until further experience is obtained, monitoring of ICP, a relatively low-risk procedure, and control of ICP and CPP by the usual therapeutic modalities seem reasonable in near-drowning victims who present in coma or who progress to that level after admission.

## COMPLICATIONS OF NEAR-DROWNING

Up to this point little or no mention has been made of other injuries that may result from the immersion incident or from initial resuscitation and stabilization. Perhaps the most common and dramatic catastrophic injuries occurring during immersion are to the spinal cord. Seventy-seven percent of all sports-related cervical spinal cord injuries are due to diving, surfing, or water-skiing. The number of injuries to the cord from diving alone exceeds the total of all other sports-related spinal cord trauma. The majority of these injuries associated with aquatic accidents are sufficiently serious to cause permanent paralysis.[19]

Other possibilities include trauma to the head, viscera, or skeleton. That a medical illness may precipitate the immersion episode (myocardial infarction, cerebrovascular accident, convulsion)[44,46,117,136] has been alluded to above. Consideration must be given to the possibility of a coexisting medical illness, especially in the elderly, with appropriate measures taken to exclude them or establish a definitive diagnosis.

Immediately after retrieval of the patient from the water, attention should be focused on resuscitation and stabilization. On admission to the emergency department and again upon transfer to the ICU, the possibility must be considered not only that concomitant trauma may be present but also that initial efforts at resuscitation may have introduced another complication. Cardiopulmonary resuscitation has been reported to produce numerous medical problems,[35,53,120] any of which may occur in near-drowning patients subjected to it.

Other complications may not develop or be evident until later in the hospitalization. Careful monitoring for evidence of renal compromise may permit early recognition of this relatively uncommon complication of near-drowning.[49] Although hemoglobinuria or myoglobinuria are potential causes of renal failure associated with near-drowning, most renal tubular damage occurs as a result of asphyxia.[77,103] Sepsis may result not only from indwelling lines but also from an unrecognized perforated viscus or from pneumonia, possibly secondary to aspiration of polluted water.[46] Disseminated intravascular coagulation has also been reported in near-drowning victims.[133]

The issue of pulmonary sequelae should be clarified. Pulmonary function tests in survivors of near-drowning episodes show an initial period of restrictive lung disease with decreased forced vital capacity and total lung capacity that return to normal within several months.[63,75] More recent studies have shown residual hyperreactivity of both large and small airways[75] believed to be a result of aspiration. The significance of these findings in otherwise healthy individuals remains to be determined, but it is postulated that bronchial hyperreactivity and small airway dysfunction may signify the development and progression of chronic obstructive pulmonary disease.[75] However, individuals suffering from ARDS from other causes suffer minimal long-term pulmonary consequences when managed with IMV and PEEP.[32]

## PROGNOSIS

Ultimate recovery and restoration to preaccident status after an immersion episode depend primarily on the development of residual neurologic deficits.[77] Not only is neurologic damage often the etiologic factor in the victim's ultimate death but it is also the single most significant determining aspect of the long-term prognosis of these patients.[30] The severity of the initial cerebral injury depends on several factors, the most significant of which are duration of submersion, water temperature, and efficacy of resuscitative efforts.[112] The importance of water temperature to severity of brain damage has only recently been appreciated. Recent reports have documented that patients who have sustained prolonged immersion in cold water and appear clinically dead on arrival in the emergency department have responded favorably to rewarming while CPR and ventilation are continued.[41] Nonetheless, there is little doubt that, even in very cold water, prolonged submersion is associated with a poor prognosis.[25] Of those individuals surviving a near-drowning episode, up to 21% have residual incapacitating brain damage.[100]

Initial attempts to predict outcome in near-drowning victims were based primarily on historical facts (immersion interval, CPR efficacy, etc.). Unfortunately, because of interobserver variability, it has been repeatedly shown that none of these variables could be accurately determined from individuals at the scene.[112] Subsequent attempts at predicting outcome were based on the patient's condition in the emergency department. Commonly used discriminators were continued need for CPR in the emergency department,[41,77,99,112] significant acidosis,[30,77,110,112] fixed dilated pupils,[41,77] and coma.[30,41,100] Other individuals have attempted to correlate age,[99] hyperkalemia,[112] the presence of an early first gasp,[62,123] or maintenance of only gasping respiration[73] after institution of CPR. Recently, several papers have been published using more detailed assessment of neurologic status in an attempt to discriminate in a meaningful manner.[26,96,100] The previously mentioned study that categorized the patient's neurologic status as "A" (awake), "B" (blunted), or "C" (comatose) reports improved survival in awake patients compared with those who present with a blunted neurologic status and in blunted patients compared with those in coma.[100] Furthermore, the subdivisions of the comatose category have also been shown to correlate with survival, ie, patients who are decorticate have a higher survival rate than those who are decerebrate who in turn have a higher survival rate than those who are flaccid (Tables 21-3 and 21-4).[24,100] Orlowski[115] described five unfavorable prognostic factors in pediatric near-drowning and proposed a predictive scoring system. Age less than 3 years, submersion time longer than 5 minutes, delay of resuscitation for 10 minutes after rescue, coma on admission to the emergency department, and pH less than 7.1 were each given a score of one. A 90% chance of good recovery with standard therapy was observed in patients with a total score of 2 or less. The corresponding rate was only 5% for those who had a score of 3 or more. Other authors have reported that use of the Glasgow coma scale (GCS) has been successful in defining a group of individuals at high risk of death or permanent neurologic sequelae (a GCS score of 5 or less; no patient who died or survived with permanent neurologic sequelae scored higher than 4 on this scale). The authors additionally point out, however, that the GCS correlates very well with the "A,B,C" system and Orlowski score just described.[30] Finally, attempts have been made to correlate intracranial pressure (ICP) and cerebral perfusion pressure (CPP) with survival and neurologic outcome.[110] Although these measurements were useful in discriminating those patients who would ultimately die (100% of patients with ICP greater than 20 mm Hg and CPP less than 50 mm Hg died) from those who would survive (ICP less than or equal to 20 mm Hg, CPP greater than or equal to 50 mm Hg resulted in 92% survival), it was unsuccessful in predicting neurologic outcome.[110]

Although many reports have purported to show factors that were 100% successful in discriminating survivors from nonsurvivors, subsequent analysis of these discriminatory factors has shown that no system was absolutely reliable in determining which patients would succumb or which would survive with significant neurologic residual.[30,110] Accordingly, the conclusion has been that there is no justification for withholding resuscitative efforts in the near-drowned patient.[30]

Since the determination of factors that allow us to discriminate survivors from nonsurvivors and damaged patients from neurologically intact patients is very important, the development of accurate outcome prediction would allow physicians to withhold therapy from patients who could not survive and to plan appropriate therapy for those who would. Unfortunately, there is no prognostic indicator or set of indicators that allow complete discrimination between patient subsets. In any group of patients there is an exceptional one whose demise would be predicted but who survives and recovers complete neurologic function despite the presence of these indicators.[30]

## CONCLUSION

Both drowning and near-drowning are preventable in most circumstances. Although the precise sequence of events is not known fully, most victims, whether they aspirate fluid or not, exhibit hypoxemia as the major pathologic feature. Pulmonary and central nervous system pathology account for most of the morbidity and mortality associated with near-drowning. Hypothermia may complicate the initial presentation and evaluation of victims of immersion episodes.

Initial treatment consists of oxygen administration and stabilization in accordance with American Heart Association guidelines. Pulmonary therapy should be individualized on the basis of the patient's respiratory status. In some instances nothing more than supplemental $O_2$ administration is necessary, whereas in others aggressive ventilatory assistance combining mechanical ventilation and expiratory distending pressure is required. Aggressive CNS therapy may be necessary in some patients, but no beneficial effect from hypothermia and barbiturate coma has been demonstrated. In fact, these measures may be harmful. Although there is no good way to predict neurologic outcome, it appears that most patients who survive even the most severe pulmonary dysfunction will be left without significant long-term pulmonary residual.

## REFERENCES


1. Adams AI. The descriptive epidemiology of drowning accidents. Med J Aust 1966;2:1257.
2. Allman FD, Nelson WB, Pacentine GA, McComb G. Outcome following cardiopulmonary resuscitation in severe pediatric near-drowning. Am J Dis Child 1986;140:571.
3. Arborelius M, Baldin UI, Lilja B, et al. Hemodynamic changes in man during immersion with the head above water. Aerospace Med 1972;43:592.
4. Arkansas Public Health at a glance: deaths from accidental drowning. Arkansas Med Soc 1961;58:65.
5. Barry W, Little TM. Childhood drownings in private swimming pools: an avoidable cause of death. Br Med J 1982;285:542.
6. Begin R, Epstein M, Sackner MA, et al. Effects of water immersion to the neck on pulmonary circulation and tissue volume in man. J Appl Physiol 1976;40:293.
7. Berguist RG, Vogelhut MM, Modell JH, et al. Comparison of ventilatory patterns in the treatment of freshwater near-drowning in dogs. Anesthesiology 1980;52:142.
8. Blair E. Clinical hypothermia. New York: McGraw-Hill, 1964.
9. Bleyaert AL, Nemoto EM, Safar P. Thiopental amelioration of postischemic encephalopathy in monkeys. Physiologist 1975;18:145.
10. Bohn DJ, Biggar WD, Smith CR, et al. Influence of hypothermia, barbiturate therapy, and intracranial pressure monitoring on morbidity and mortality after near-drowning. Crit Care Med 1986;14:529.
11. Boles JM, Mabille S, Scheydecker JL, et al. Hypoglycaemia in salt water near-drowning victims. Intens Care Med 1988;14:80.
12. Boucher CA. Drowning. Monthly Bull Minist Health (London) 1962;21:114.
13. Bradley AF, Stupfel M, Severinghaus JW. Effect of temperature on $PCO_2$ and $PO_2$ of blood in vitro. J Appl Physiol 1956;9:201.
14. Brain Resuscitation Clinical Trial I Study Group. Randomized clinical study of thiopental loading in comatose survivors of cardiac arrest. N Engl J Med 1986;314:397.
15. Brauer RW, Hollway RJ, Krebs JS, et al. The liver in hypothermia. Ann NY Acad Sci 1959;80:395.
16. Bynum LJ, Wilson JE, Pierce AK. Comparison of spontaneous and positive pressure breathing in supine normal subjects. J Appl Physiol 1976;41:341.
17. Calderwood HW, Modell JH, Ruiz BC. The ineffectiveness of steroid therapy for treatment of fresh-water near-drowning. Anesthesiology 1975;43:642.
18. Cassidy SS, Eschenbacher WL, Johnson RL. Reflex cardiovascular depression during unilateral lung hyperinflation in dog. J Clin Invest 1979;64:620.
19. Centers for Disease Control. Aquatic deaths and injuries. Morb Mort Weekly Rep 1982;31:417.
20. Center for Environmental Health. Report: a model state recreational injury control program. Atlanta: Centers for Disease Control, 1981.
21. Chandler WF, Kindt GW. Monitoring and control of intracranial pressure in non-traumatic encephalopathies. Surg Neurol 1976;5:311.
22. Clarke EB, Niggeman EH. Near drowning. Heart Lung 1975;4:946.
23. Colebatch HJH, Halmagyi DFJ. Lung mechanics and resuscitation after fluid aspiration. J Appl Physiol 1961;16:684.
24. Conn AW, Barker GA. Fresh water drowning and near drowning. An update. Can Anaesth Soc J 1984;31:S38.
25. Conn AW, Edmonds JF, Barker GA. Near-drowning in cold fresh water: current treatment regimen. Can Anaesth Soc J 1978;25:259.
26. Conn AW, Montes JE, Barker GA, et al. Cerebral salvage in near-

drowning following neurological classification by triage. Can Anaesth Soc J 1980;27:201.

27. Conn AW, Barker GA, Edmonds JF, et al. Submersion hypothermia and near-drowning. In: Pozos RS. Wittmers LE, eds. The nature and treatment of hypothermia. Minneapolis: University of Minnesota Press, 1983:152.
28. Cot C. Les asphyxies accidentalles (submersion, electrocution, intoxication oxycarbonique): etude clinique, therapeutique et preventive. Paris: Editions Medicales N. Maloine, 1931.
29. Curry DL, Curry KP. Hypothermia and insulin secretion. Endocrinology 1970;81:750.
30. Dean JM, Kaufman NS. Prognostic indicators in pediatric near-drowning: the Glasgow Coma Scale. Crit Care Med 1981;9:536.
31. Dean JM, McComb JG. Intracranial pressure monitoring in severe pediatric near-drowning. Neurosurgery 1981;9:627.
32. Douglas ME, Downs JB. Pulmonary function following severe acute respiratory failure and high levels of positive end-expiratory pressure. Chest 1977;71:18.
33. Downs JB, Douglas ME, Sanfelippo PM, et al. Ventilatory pattern, intrapleural pressure, and cardiac output. Anesth Analg 1977;56:88.
34. Ehrmantraut WR, Ticktin HE, Fazekas JF. Cerebral hemodynamics and metabolism in accidental hypothermia. Arch Intern Med 1957;99:57.
35. Fandel I, Bancalari E. Near-drowning in children: clinical aspects. Pediatrics 1976;58:573.
36. Fay T, Smith GW. Observations on reflex responses during prolonged periods of human refrigeration. Arch Neurol Psychiatr 1941;42:215.
37. Fisher B, Fedor EJ, Lee SH, et al. Some physiologic effects of short and long term hypothermia upon the liver. Surgery 1956;40:862.
38. Fitzgerald FT, Jessop C. Accidental hypothermia: a report of 22 cases and review of the literature. Adv Intern Med 1982;27:128.
39. Fleetham JA, Munt PW. Near-drowning in Canadian waters. Can Med Assoc J 1978;118:914.
40. Forbes A, Ray LH. Conditions of survival of mammalian nerve trunks. Am J Physiol 1923;64:435.
41. Frates RC. Analysis of the predictive factors in the assessment of warm-water near-drowning in children. Am J Dis Child 1981;135:1006.
42. Froese AB, Bryan AC. Effects of anesthesia and paralysis on diaphragmatic mechanics in man. Anesthesiology 1974;41:242.
43. Fuhrman FA, Crismon JM. The influence of acute hypothermia on the rate of oxygen consumption and glycogen content of the liver and on the blood glucose. Am J Physiol 1947;149:552.
44. Giamonna ST. Drowning: pathophysiology and management. Curr Probl Pediatr 1971;1:1.
45. Giamonna ST, Modell JH. Drowning by total immersion. Effects on pulmonary surfactant of distilled water, isotonic saline and sea water. Am J Dis Child 1967;114:612.
46. Golden FSTC. Problems of immersion. Br J Hosp Med 1980;23:371.
47. Goode RC, Duffin J, Miller R, et al. Sudden cold water immersion. Respr Physiol 1975;23:301.
48. Graham JM, Keatinge WR. Deaths in cold water. Br Med J 1978;2:18.
49. Grausz H, Amend WJC, Earley LE. Renal failure complicating drowning. JAMA 1971;217:207.
50. Grisvold SE, Safar P, Hendricks HHL, et al. Thiopental treatment after global brain ischemia in pigtail monkeys. Anesthesiology 1984;60:88.
51. Gunton RW, Scott JW, Lougheed WN, et al. Changes in cardiac rhythm and in the form of the electrocardiogram resulting from induced hypothermia in man. Am Heart J 1956;52:419.
52. Halmagyi DFJ, Colebatch HJH. Ventilation and circulation after fluid aspiration. J Appl Physiol 1961;16:35.
53. Harries MG. Drowning in man. Crit Care Med 1981;9:407.
54. Hayreh MS, Hayreh SS. Optic disc edema in raised intracranial pressure I. Arch Ophthalmol 1977;95:237.
55. Hayreh MS, Hayreh SS. Optic disc edema in raised intracranial pressure II. Arch Ophthalmol 1977;95:1245.
56. Hayreh MS, Hayreh SS. Optic disc edema in raised intracranial pressure III. Arch Opthalmol 1977;95:1553.
57. Hedenstierna G, Santesson J. Studies on intrapulmonary gas distribution in the normal subject: influence of anaesthesia and artificial ventilation. Acta Anaesth Scand 1979;23:291.
58. Hegnauer AH, Shriber WJ, Haterius HO. Cardiovascular response of the dog to immersion hypothermia. Am J Physiol 1950;161:455.
59. Hervey GR. Hypothermia: physiologic changes encountered in hypothermia. Proc Roy Soc Med 1973;66:1053.
60. Herz BL, Coville FA, Kocsis CA. Management of submersion hypothermia: successful resuscitation of a 14-year-old girl. NY State J Med 1988;88:434.
61. Hildebrand CA, Hartmann AG, Arcinue EL, et al. Cardiac performance in pediatric near-drowning. Crit Care Med 1988;16:331.
62. Jacobsen WR, Mason LJ, Briggs BA, et al. Correlation of spontaneous respiration and neurologic damage in near-drowning. Crit Care Med 1983;11:487.
63. Jenkinson SG, George RB. Serial pulmonary function studies in survivors of near drowning. Chest 1980;77:777.
64. Kanter GS. Renal clearance of glucose in hypothermic dogs. Am J Physiol 1959;196:366.
65. Karch SB. The pathology of the heart in drowning. Arch Pathol Lab Med 1985;109:176.
66. Karch SB. Pathology of the lung in near-drowning. Am J Emerg Med 1986;4:4.
67. Karpovich PV. Water in the lungs of drowned animals. Arch Pathol 1933;15:828.
68. Keatinge WR. Accidental immersion hypothermia and drowning. Practitioner 1977;219:183.
69. Kelman GR, Nunn JF. Nomograms for correction of blood $PO_2$, $PCO_2$, pH, and base excess for time and temperature. J Appl Physiol 1966;21:1484.
70. Kirby RR, Downs JB, Civetta JM, et al. High level positive end expiratory pressure (PEEP) in acute respiratory insufficiency. Chest 1975;67:156.
71. Kristofferson MB, Rattenborg CC, Holaday DA. Asphyxial death: the roles of acute anoxia, hypercarbia and acidosis. Anesthesiology 1967;28:488.
72. Kruus S, Bergstrom L, Suutarinen T, Hayvonen R. The prognosis of near-drowned children. Acta Paediatr Scand 1979;68:315.
73. Lacroix J, Gagne M. Correlation of respiration and prognosis in near-drowning. Crit Care Med 1984;12:540.
74. Lanier WL, Stangland KJ, Scheithauer BW, et al. The effects of dextrose infusion and head position on neurologic outcome after complete cerebral ischemia in primates: examination of a model. Anesthesiology 1987;66:39.
75. Laughlin JJ, Eigen H. Pulmonary function abnormalities in survivors of near drowning. J Pediatr 1982;100:26.
76. Leads from the MMWR. Progress toward achieving the national 1990 objectives for injury prevention and control. JAMA 1988;259:2069.
77. Levin DL. Near-drowning. Crit Care Med 1980;8:590.
78. Lougheed DW, Janes JM, Hall GE. Physiological studies in experimental asphyxia and drowning. Can Med Assoc J 1939;40:423.

79. Lowson JA. Sensations in drowning. Edinburgh Med J 1903;13:41.
80. Lunt DWR, Rose AG. Pathology of the human heart in drowning. Arch Pathol Lab Med 1987;111:939.
81. Lyrene RK, Truog WE. Adult respiratory distress syndrome in a pediatric intensive care unit: predisposing conditions, clinical course, and outcome. Pediatrics 1981;67:790.
82. Mackie I. Alcohol and aquatic disasters. Med J Aust 1978;12:652.
83. Maclean D, Griffiths PD, Emslie-Smith D. Serum enzymes in relation to electrocardiographic changes in accidental hypothermia. Lancet 1968;2:1266.
84. Maclean D, Taig DR, Emslie-Smith D. Achilles tendon reflex in accidental hypothermia and hypothermic myxedema. Br Med J 1973;2:87.
85. Maclean D, Murison J, Griffiths PD. Acute pancreatitis and diabetic ketoacidosis in hypothermia. Br Med J 1974;2:58.
86. Manny J, Gringlinger G, Mathe AA, et al. Positive end-expiratory pressure, lung stretch and decreased myocardial contractility. Surgery 1978;84:127.
87. Mauritzen CV, Andersen MN. Myocardial temperature gradients and ventricular fibrillation during hypothermia. J Thorac Cardiovasc Surg 1965;49:937.
88. Milliner N, Pearn J, Guard R. Will fenced pools save lives? A 10-year study from Mulgrave Shire, Queensland. Med J Aust 1980;2:510.
89. Modell JH. Die physiologischen Grundlagen fur die Behandlung von Ertrunkenen. Ther Woche 1968;43:1928.
90. Modell JH. Pathophysiology and treatment of drowning and near drowning. Springfield, IL: Charles C Thomas, 1971.
91. Modell JH. Drown versus near-drown: a discussion of definition. Crit Care Med 1981;9:351.
92. Modell JH. Treatment of near-drowning: is there a role for H.Y.P.E.R. therapy? Crit Care Med 1986;14:593.
93. Modell JH, Moya F. Effects of volume of aspirated fluid during chlorinated fresh water drowning. Anesthesiology 1966;27:662.
94. Modell JH, Davis JH. Electrolyte changes in human drowning victims. Anesthesiology 1969;30:414.
95. Modell JH, Boysen PG. Respiratory crises. The Society of Critical Care Medicine, Critical Care: State of the Art, 1: March, 1980.
96. Modell JH, Conn AW. Current neurological considerations in near-drowning. Can Anaesth Soc J 1980;27:197.
97. Modell JH, Moya F, Newby EJ, et al. The effects of fluid volume in seawater drowning. Ann Intern Med 1967;67:68.
98. Modell JH, Calderwood HW, Ruiz BC. Effects of ventilatory patterns on arterial oxygenation after near-drowning in sea water. Anesthesiology 1974;40:376.
99. Modell JH, Graves SA, Ketover A. Clinical course of 91 consecutive near-drowning victims. Chest 1976;70:231.
100. Modell JH, Graves SA, Kuck EJ. Near-drowning: correlation of level of consciousness and survival. Can Anaesth Soc J 1980;27:211.
101. Montes JE, Conn AW. Near-drowning: an unusual case. Can Anaesth Soc J 1980;27:172.
102. Moritz AR. Chemical methods for the determination of death by drowning. Physiol Rev 1944;24:70.
103. Moyer JH, Morris G, DeBakey ME. Hypothermia: 1. effect on renal hemodynamics and on excretion of water and electrolytes in dog and man. Ann Surg 1957;145:26.
104. National Center for Health Statistics: Annual report. Washington, DC: National Center for Health Statistics, 1982.
105. National Research Council. Proceedings of the workshop on alcohol-related accidents in recreational boating. Washington DC: Transportation Research Board, National Research Council, 1986.
106. National Safety Council. Accident facts, 1987. Chicago: National Safety Council, 1987.
107. National Safety Council. Accident facts, 1988. Chicago: National Safety Council, 1988.
108. Noble CS, Sharpe N. Drowning: its mechanism and treatment. Can Med Assoc J 1963;89:402.
109. Nugent SK, Rogers MC. Resuscitation and intensive care monitoring following immersion hypothermia. J Trauma 1980;20:814.
110. Nussbaum E, Galant SP. Intracranial pressure monitoring as a guide to prognosis in the nearly drowned, severely comatose child. J Pediatr 1983;102:215.
111. Nussbaum E, Maggi JC. Pentobarbital therapy does not improve neurologic outcome in nearly drowned, flaccid-comatose children. Pediatrics 1988;81:630.
112. Oakes DD, Sherck JP, Maloney JR, et al. Prognosis and management of victims of near-drowning. J Trauma 1977;22:544.
113. O'Carroll PW, Alkon E, Weiss B. Drowning mortality in Los Angeles County, 1976 to 1984. JAMA 1988;260:380.
114. Orlowski JP. Prognostic factors in drowning and the post-submersion syndrome. Crit Care Med 1978;6:94.
115. Orlowski JP. Prognostic factors in pediatric cases of drowning and near-drowning. Ann Emerg Med 1979;8:176.
116. Orlowski JP. Drowning, near-drowning, and ice-water submersions. Pediatr Clin North Am 1987;34:75.
117. Orlowski JP, Rothner AD, Lueders H. Submersion accidents in children with epilepsy. Am J Dis Child 1982;136:777.
118. Orlowski JP, Abulleil MM, Phillips JM. Effects of tonicities of saline solutions on pulmonary injury in drowning. Crit Care Med 1987;15:126.
119. Osborn JJ. Experimental hypothermia: respiratory and blood pH changes in relation to cardiac function. Am J Physiol 1953;175:389.
120. Paterson B. Morbidity of childhood near-drowning. Pediatrics 1977;59:364.
121. Pearn JH. Drowning in Australia: A national approach with particular reference to children. Med J Aust 1977;2:770.
122. Pearn JH. Epilepsy and drowning in childhood. Br Med J 1977;1:1510.
123. Pearn JH. Secondary drowning in children. Br Med J 1980;281:1103.
124. Pearn JH. Drowning and alcohol. Med J Aust 1984;2:6.
125. Pearn JH, Nixon J. Are swimming pools becoming more dangerous? Med J Aust 1977;2:702.
126. Pearn JH, Nixon J. Bathtub immersion accidents involving children. Med J Aust 1977;1:211.
127. Pearn JH, Nixon J. Swimming pool immersion accidents on analysis from the Brisbane drowning study. Med J Aust 1977;1:432.
128. Pearn JH, Wong R, Brown J, Ching Y, et al. Drowning and near-drowning involving children: a five-year total population study from the city and county of Honolulu. Am J Public Health 1979;69:450.
129. Pearn JH, Brown J, Hsia E. Swimming pool drowning and near-drowning involving children. A total population study from Hawaii. Milit Med 1980;145:15.
130. Pfenninger J, Sutter M. Intensive care after fresh water immersion accidents in children. Anaesthesia 1982;37:1157.
131. Plueckhahn VD. Ethics, legal medicine and forensic pathology. Melbourne: Melbourne University Press, 1983.
132. Plueckhahn VD. Alcohol and accidental drowning. A 25 year study. Med J Aust 1984;2:22.
133. Ports TA, Deuel TF. Intravascular coagulation in fresh-water submersion. Ann Intern Med 1977;87:60.

134. Postlethy JC, Dorm J. Hypothermia, thrombosis, and acute pancreatitis. Br Med J 1974;2:446.
135. Pratt FD, Haynes BE. Incidence of "secondary drowning" after saltwater submersion. Ann Emerg Med 1986;15:1084.
136. Press E, Walker J, Crawford I. An interstate drowning study. Am J Public Health 1968;58:2275.
137. Press E, Walker J, Crawford I. Preliminary study of Illinois drownings. Illinois Med J 1965;127:577.
138. Ream AK, Reitz BA, Silverberg G. Temperature correction of $PCO_2$ and pH in estimating acid-base status: an example of the Emperor's new clothes? Anesthesiology 1982;56:41.
139. Reuler JB. Hypothermia: pathophysiology, clinical settings and management. Ann Intern Med 1978;89:519.
140. Rink RA, Gray I, Ruekert RR, et al. The effect of hypothermia on morphine metabolism in an isolated perfused liver. Anesthesiology 1956;17:377.
141. Rockoff MA, Marshall LF, Shapiro HM. High-dose barbiturate therapy in humans: a clinical review of 60 patients. Ann Neurol 1979;6:194.
142. Rose DK, Froese AB. Changes in respiratory pattern affect dead space/tidal volume ratio during spontaneous but not during controlled ventilation: a study in pediatric patients. Anesth Analg 1980;59:341.
143. Rosomoff HL. The effects of hypothermia on the physiology of the nervous system. Surgery 1956;40:328.
144. Rowe MI, Arango A, Allington G. Profile of pediatric drowning victims in a water-oriented society. J Trauma 1977;17:587.
145. Ruiz BC, Calderwood HW, Modell JH, Brogdon JE. Effect of ventilatory patterns on arterial oxygenation after near-drowning with fresh water: a comparative study in dogs. Anesth Analg 1973;52:570.
146. Sarnaik AP, Preston G, Liehlai M, et al. Intracranial pressure and cerebral perfusion pressure in near-drowning. Crit Care Med 1985;13:224.
147. Schwab RH, Lewis DW, Killough JH, et al. Electrocardiographic changes occurring in rapidly induced deep hypothermia. Am J Med Sci 1964;248:290.
148. Scott PH, Eigen H. Immersion accidents involving pails of water in the home. J Pediatr 1980;96:282.
149. Segar WE, Riley PA, Barila TG. Urinary composition during hypothermia. Am J Physiol 1956;185:528.
150. Severinghaus JW. Oxyhemoglobin dissociation curve correction for temperature and pH variation in human blood. J Appl Physiol 1958;12:485.
151. Severinghaus JW, Stupfel M, Bradley AF. Variations of serum carbonic acid pK with pH and temperature. J Appl Physiol 1956;9:197.
152. Shaw KN, Briede CA. Submersion injuries: drowning and near-drowning. Emerg Med Clin North Am 1989;7:355.
153. Simpson S, Herring PT. The effect of cold narcosis on reflex actions in warm-blooded animals. J Physiol 1905;32:305.
154. Starmer G. The effects of alcohol on swimming performance. In: Drink and Drown: The Fourth Water Safety Symposium. Sydney: Department of Leisure, Sport and Recreation, 1980.
155. Stathers GM. Near-drowning: principles of emergency care. Aust Fam Physician 1981;10:943.
156. Steen PA, Milde JH, Michenfelder JD. No barbiturate protection in a dog model of complete cerebral ischemia. Ann Neurol 1979;5:343.
157. Sturner WQ, Spruill FG, Smith RA, et al. Accidental asphyxial deaths involving infants and young children. J Forensic Sci 1976;21:483.
158. Swann HG, Spafford NR. Body salt and water changes during fresh and sea water drowning. Tex Rep Biol Med 1951;9:356.
159. Tabeling BB, Modell JH. Fluid administration increases oxygen delivery during continuous positive pressure ventilation after freshwater near-drowning. Crit Care Med 1983;11:693.
160. Todd MM, Chadwick HS, Shapiro HM, et al. The neurologic effects of thiopental therapy following experimental cardiac arrest in cats. Anesthesiology 1982;57:76.
161. Trevino A, Razi B, Beller BM. The characteristic electrocardiogram of accidental hypothermia. Arch Intern Med 1971;127:470.
162. U.S. Coast Guard. Boating statistics 1985. Washington DC: US Department of Transportation 1986, Publ No. COMDTINST M16754.IG.
163. Vaage J, Bugge-Aperheim B, Svennevig JL. Hypoxic pulmonary vasoconstriction in post-traumatic pulmonary insufficiency: The effect of methylprednisolone. Acta Chir Scand 1980;499(Suppl):93.
164. Vandam LD, Burnap TK. Hypothermia. N Engl J Med 1959;261:546 and 595.
165. Venes JL, Bennett AS, Spencer DD. Management of severe cerebral edema in the metabolic encephalopathy of Reyes-Johnson syndrome. J Neurosurg 1978;48:903.
166. Walker S, Middlekamp JN. Pail immersion accidents. Clin Pediatr 1981;20:341.
167. Webster DP. Skin and scuba diving fatalities in the United States. Public Health Rep 1966;81:703.
168. Webster DP. Pool drownings and their prevention. Public Health Rep 1967;82:587.
169. Wegener FH, Edwards RM. Cerebral support for near-drowned children in a temperature environment. Med J Aust 1980;2:135.
170. Werner JZ, Safar P, Bircher NG, et al. No improvement in pulmonary status by gravity drainage or abdominal thrusts. Anesthesiology 1982;57:A81.
171. Weyman AE, Greenbaum DM, Grace WJ. Accidental hypothermia in an alcoholic population. Am J Med 1974;56:13.

# Section Three

# Complications

Chapter Twenty-Two

Alexander Nacht
Roberta C. Kahn
Sivam Ramanathan

# Metabolic-Endocrine Response to Trauma and Nutritional Support

Acute trauma induces metabolic and nutritional stress in the patient. This chapter reviews (a) normal regulation of metabolism; (b) carbohydrate, fat, and protein metabolism; (c) metabolic changes in starvation; (d) metabolic responses to trauma and stress; (e) nutritional assessment and treatment after trauma; and (f) effects of trauma, stress, and nutritional support on organ function.

Frequently the person who sustains an injury is in an altered metabolic state before the traumatic event. For instance, the use of alcohol and/or tobacco is likely to produce significant metabolic effects.[74,79] Alcohol interferes with the metabolism of catecholamines and hepatic utilization of lactate.[49,74] Smoking not only mobilizes free fatty acids but also causes an elevation of urinary catecholamine and serum 11-hydroxycorticosteroid levels. Prolonged starvation can occur in entrapped victims and may further complicate the metabolic and endocrine alterations caused by trauma. At the other extreme, ingestion of a diet rich in carbohydrates shortly before an injury alters the insulin/glucagon ratio in blood and may affect carbohydrate, fat, and protein metabolism. Obviously, any pre-existing disease is also likely to have a major impact on the metabolic response to trauma. Nevertheless, despite this wide array of factors that are likely to alter the metabolic responses of different individuals, it has often been noted that the pattern of metabolic-endocrine responses is surprisingly uniform after trauma. Furthermore, it appears that the metabolic changes that follow severe trauma are in general similar to those seen in other critically ill patients suffering from sepsis, pancreatitis, ruptured aortic aneurysm, etc.[93,94,110] Thus, these changes actually occur in response to stress and not specifically to trauma.

## REGULATION OF METABOLISM

Metabolism is regulated by both neural and hormonal factors. The hypothalamus is responsible for orchestrating the neurohumoral response to trauma. The nervous system's major role in regulating the metabolic responses of the injured organism was demonstrated by the elegant experiments of Egdahl.[32] He showed that, when the nerve supply to the lower extremity was severed, the increase in cortisol and adrenocorticotrophic hormone (ACTH) following trauma to this extremity was not as pronounced as it was when the nerve supply was intact. In fact, these experiments led to our current understanding that a sufficiently high level of epidural or spinal anesthesia can block, or at least attenuate, the stress response to injury.[17,105]

Neural control of metabolism is regulated by the ventromedial hypothalamic nucleus, which is connected to and modulated by several other areas of the brain. The hypothalamus is also directly exposed to various metabolic substrates since the blood-brain barrier is absent in this region of the central nervous system.[74] This area also responds to impulses from the carotid sinus, aortic baroreceptors, and the renal nerves. Increased activity of the paraventricular nucleus causes both sympathetic and parasympathetic excitation. Sympathetic activity mobilizes substrate, increases cardiac output, and produces peripheral vasoconstriction. Activation of the sympathetic system is also responsible for regulating hormone release from the pancreas. The parasympathetic system promotes absorption of nutrients from the gastrointestinal tract.

Neurohormones are synthesized in the neurosecretory cells of the hypothalamus and reach the anterior pituitary gland via its specialized portal vascular system (Fig 22-1). The posterior lobe of the pituitary is an extension of the ventral hypothalamus and receives direct neural (not vascular) connections from it.

The anterior pituitary releases ACTH, somatotrophic hormone (STH), thyroid-stimulating hormone (TSH), prolactin, luteinizing hormone, and follicle-stimulating hormone. ACTH is derived from a large precursor molecule, which is also the core structure for melanocyte-stimulating hormone, beta-lipoprotein, and beta-endorphin.[33] Synthesis and secretion of ACTH are controlled by corticotropin-releasing hormone (CRH) produced in the supraoptic and paraventricular nuclei of the hypothalamus (Fig 22-1). CRH neurosecretory cells are stimulated by a number of central afferent nerve pathways and by several neurotransmitters, including epinephrine and norepinephrine. The CRH-ACTH-cortisol axis is essential for the integrated response to stress.

The autonomic nervous system can be stimulated both indirectly by the CRH axis and directly by the paraventricular nucleus. These neurons have direct connections with cells in the brainstem and spinal cord that activate preganglionic sympathetic and parasympathetic neurons throughout the autonomic nervous system. Thus, the hypothalamus can influence both anterior and posterior hypophyses, as well as the autonomic nervous system. In addition, since the adrenal medulla is an extension of the central nervous system, it is directly influenced by the hypothalamus via the great splanchnic nerve.[62,99]

FIG. 22-1. Organization of neuroendocrine mechanisms. Note the direct neural connections between paraventricular nucleus and the posterior hypophysis. Also note the rich portal vascular supply of the anterior hypophysis.

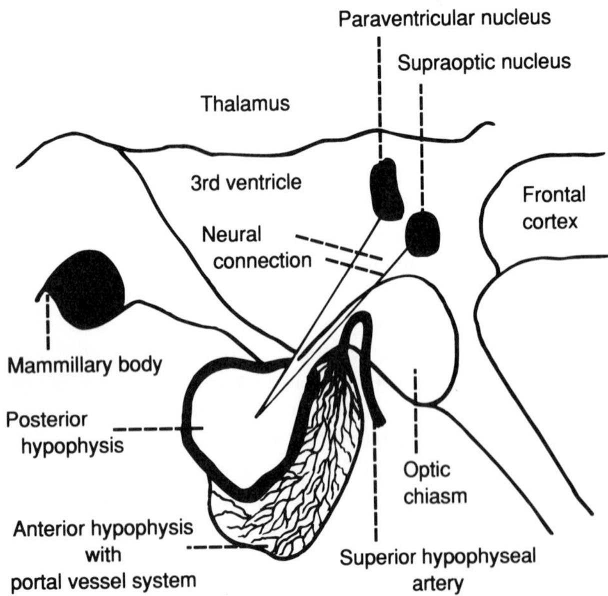


The posterior pituitary hormones—antidiuretic hormone (ADH) and oxytocin—are actually produced in the supraoptic and paraventricular nuclei of the hypothalamus; the posterior pituitary is merely a storage site. ADH is responsible for maintaining vascular and cellular hydration (normal fluid homeostasis) by causing water retention and for maintaining systemic blood pressure by producing vasoconstriction. A 1 to 2% increase in plasma osmolality is sufficient to trigger ADH release. Other stimuli of ADH secretion include stress, hypoglycemia, and pain. Elevated blood levels of ADH may stimulate production of CRH and thus of ACTH.[44]

Insulin and glucagon, which are released directly into the hepatic circulation from the pancreas, have important regulatory effects on substrate metabolism. Because these hormones are utilized extensively by the liver, their portal venous blood concentrations are higher than their levels in systemic blood. The hypothalamic nuclei control pancreatic islet cells by augmenting catecholamine output from the adrenal medulla. Catecholamines inhibit insulin secretion and stimulate glucagon release. Mobilization of fatty acids and glycerol from adipose tissue is controlled by ACTH, glucocorticoids, catecholamines, and glucagon. Antidiuretic hormone (ADH), the renin-angiotensin system, and mineralocorticoid activity are also subject to sympathetic control. ADH and mineralocorticoids have important roles to play in regulation of circulating fluid volume. The renin-angiotensin system is vital to the maintenance of systemic perfusion pressure in the event of sudden hypovolemia.

## SUBSTRATE METABOLISM

### CARBOHYDRATE METABOLISM

Carbohydrate metabolism is controlled by both insulin and glucagon. Insulin lowers blood glucose and amino acid levels and prevents gluconeogenesis—the synthesis of glucose from lactate and amino acids—by promoting lipogenesis and protein synthesis.[43] It is thus an anabolic hormone.[49,74,88] Glucagon stimulates hepatic glycogenolysis, converts muscle proteins to amino acids, and causes a breakdown of body fat. This hormone also facilitates gluconeogenesis. The insulin/glucagon ratio (I/G ratio) is a major determinant of the rapidity with which a trauma victim will be able to mobilize energy sources.[74,88] A low I/G ratio indicates the presence of a catabolic state.

The body has four sources of glucose: ingested food, glycogen, adipose tissue, and proteins. Glucose must be oxidized to $CO_2$ and water for maximum energy liberation to occur. Glucose is converted to pyruvate via the Embden-Meyerhof pathway. Pyruvate is then oxidatively decarboxylated to acetyl coenzyme A (acetyl-CoA) by the enzymes known as the pyruvate-dehydrogenase complex.[49,96] Acetyl-CoA enters the citric acid cycle within the mitochondria. Oxidation of glucose via the citric acid cycle produces 38 high-energy phosphate bonds with an energy equivalent of 288,800 calories per mole of glucose.

Carbohydrate metabolism is the common metabolic pathway for all the body's nutrients (Fig 22-2). Fatty acids are linked with carbohydrate metabolism via acetyl-CoA. Glycerol is linked with the Embden-Meyerhof pathway via glyceraldehyde-3-phosphate. The linkage of amino acid and carbohydrate metabolism occurs at the following steps: at pyruvate, at acetyl-CoA, at alpha-ketoglutarate (Krebs cycle), at fumarate, and at succinyl-CoA (Fig 22-2). Thus, one can say that fats and proteins burn in the hearth of carbohydrates. The byproducts of fat and protein metabolism are ketone bodies and urea (from deamination of amino acids), respectively. This coupling among the different metabolic pathways facilitates the efficient utilization of all possible resources at the time of trauma and during repair of injured tissues.

The first available fuel is glucose, but carbohydrate reserves are quite limited, with about 300–400 g of glycogen stored in the liver and muscle. Although glucose has a thermodynamic value of 4 kcal/g, glycogen is inefficiently stored in the hydrated state, yielding only 1 to 2 kcal/g.[84] Certain body tissues—the central nervous system, the renal medulla, the formed elements of the blood, and the fibroblasts—are obligate glucose users and require 600 to 1000 kcal/day for their energy needs.[59] During starvation, available carbohydrate is utilized preferentially by these tissues, and the remainder of the body relies on lipid. Even after a simple overnight fast, as much as 50% of the total expired $CO_2$ may be produced by fatty acid oxidation.[43] In summary, the limited available glycogen stores may be depleted within 24 hours, and the continued need for glucose by the tissues requires ongoing gluconeogenesis.

## FAT METABOLISM

Excess glucose can be converted into fat and stored in adipose tissue. Insulin inhibits lipolysis, whereas glucagon, catecholamines, and STH promote it. Glucocorticoids increase the lipolytic effect of catecholamines. There are two types of lipases: hormone-sensitive lipase and lipoprotein lipase. Hormone-sensitive lipase degrades lipids to fatty acids and glycerol. This enzyme is activated by a cyclic-AMP pathway triggered by a catecholamine-receptor interaction on the surface of the adipocyte.[97] Some of the free fatty acid formed as a result of hydrolysis is reabsorbed by the adipocyte. The remainder is oxidized via the Krebs cycle to produce energy (Fig 22-2). Glycerol, on the other hand, is not reabsorbed, and therefore its blood level reflects the true extent of triglyceride breakdown.[97] The released glycerol can be converted either to glucose or to triglycerides in the liver. Lipoprotein lipase is responsible for catalyzing the uptake of triglycerides from chylomicra and low-density lipoproteins.[97] Its effects are thus opposite to those of hormone-sensitive lipase. Insulin and glucose increase and catecholamines decrease its activity.

Energy is stored most efficiently as fat in the form of triglycerides. One gram of fat yields 9 kcal when completely oxidized, whereas 1 g of hydrated glucose or protein yields 3.3 to 4.0 kcal.[37] The average 70-kg man has 15 to 20 kg of

FIG. 22-2. The pathways of the three major metabolic substrates. Meth = methionine; Ala = alanine; Trypto = tryptophan; Ser = serine; Gly = glycine; Pro = proline; Phen = phenylalanine; Tyr = tyrosine; Val = valine; Threo = threonine; Orn = ornithine; His = histidine; Glu = glutamic acid.

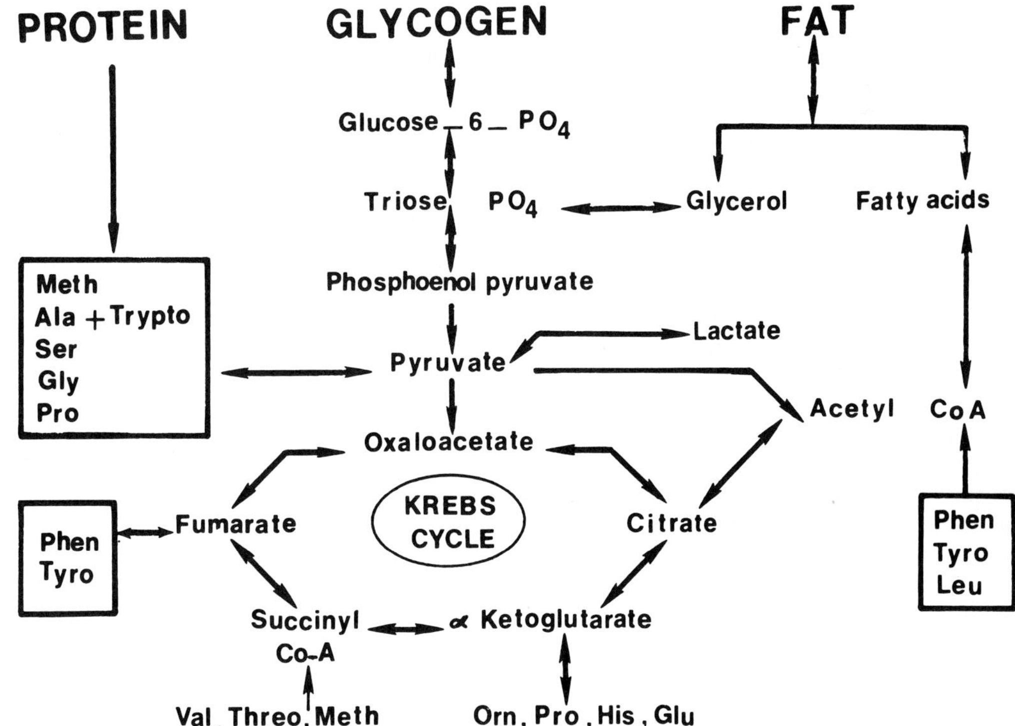

adipose tissue, with a potential energy yield of approximately 140,000 kcal. During starvation fat becomes the principal source of energy[84]; utilization of lipid as a primary fuel source is the major adaptive response that helps conserve protein during prolonged starvation. Yet, as was noted, some tissues are obligate glucose users, and fat cannot be effectively converted to glucose; it has a limited capacity to serve as a gluconeogenic substrate since only the glycerol component of the molecule is available (Fig 22-2).[20,104,118] Thus, the carbon needed for hepatic gluconeogenesis must come primarily from amino acids, which implies a need for catabolism of muscle protein.

The maintenance of normal glucose levels in body fluids under all conditions is essential for brain survival. This is accomplished by a balance between insulin and glucagon secretion. Depletion of glycogen stores results in a reduced level of the main anabolic hormone, insulin, and increased secretion of glucagon, to which the liver responds by stimulating gluconeogenesis. Glucagon activates catecholamine-sensitive lipases in adipose tissue, thus promoting breakdown of triglycerides and increasing circulating free fatty acids and glycerol.[43] "Ketoadaptation" occurs.[18,84] The liver catabolizes the fatty acids to ketones, and as the concentration of these substances increases in the bloodstream, they become an oxidative fuel source and substitute for glucose as a main source of energy in most of the tissues.[10,20,43,118] Most importantly, the brain gradually adapts to utilization of ketones instead of glucose for part of its fuel requirement. The mechanism of this progressive increase in cerebral ketone utilization is thought to be an increase in arterial ketone concentration to a level sufficient to allow these substances to cross the blood-brain barrier. This is probably caused by a gradually decreased extracerebral utilization of ketones and diminished urinary losses. Excess ketones are secreted by the kidney where, since they are acid, they are bound to cations, lowering the pH of body fluids and producing the acidotic state typical of starvation.[43,47,59]

One of the results of lipolysis is the changed respiratory quotient (RQ) typical of starvation. RQ is obtained by dividing carbon dioxide production by oxygen consumption. Each substrate is associated with its own RQ—carbohydrate, 1.00; fat, 0.70; protein, 0.82. The conversion of glucose to fat, or lipogenesis, may have an RQ greater than 8.0, depending on which fat is synthesized. In any case, a whole-body RQ greater than 1.0 would imply net lipogenesis. During prolonged starvation, the whole-body RQ approaches 0.7, as fat and fat-derived fuels serve as major substrates for the body's energy needs.[84] Changes in RQ affect alveolar $PO_2$; at any given level of $PCO_2$ alveolar $PO_2$ decreases with decreasing RQ (Fig 22-3). This may not be clinically significant when the patient is breathing high inspired concentrations of $O_2$, but can result in hypoxemia in hypercapneic marginally oxygenated patients who are breathing room air.

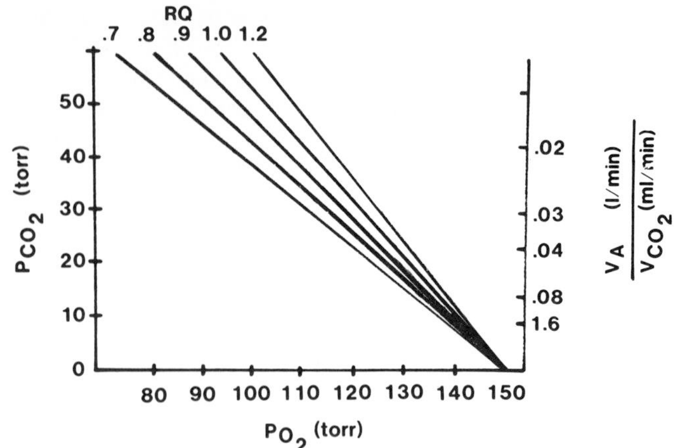


FIG. 22-3. Alveolar $PO_2$ at a given level of $CO_2$ tension varies according to the respiratory quotient (RQ). With decreasing RQ the alveolar $PO_2$ also decreases. (From Askanazi et al,[7] with permission.)

## PROTEIN METABOLISM

When the demand for glucose cannot be met by the usual means, mobilization of amino acids from the muscles takes place. Generally, glucocorticoids cause breakdown of muscle proteins, whereas insulin and STH increase their production.

Protein is present in lean body tissue, the bulk of which consists of skeletal muscle and visceral organs. Unlike fat and glycogen, the function of protein is not energy storage; however, once glycogen stores are depleted proteins can be oxidized for energy.[84] The breakdown products of protein, the amino acids, are transported to the liver where they are deaminated, the nitrogen being excreted as ammonia and urea while the carbon skeletons are converted to glucose. The blood level of urea is the classic indicator of the degree of catabolism. It should be noted that increased protein breakdown and thus increased excretion of urea—and in severe cases, creatinine—also result from severe injury to skeletal muscles. The branched chain amino acids are metabolized in a different manner: they are largely degraded in muscle, with their nitrogen transaminated to form alanine and glutamine.[10,118]

Protein catabolism results in the loss of lean body mass and negative nitrogen balance, or nitrogen excretion in excess of intake. The initial reaction of the body, once glucose is no longer directly available as an energy source, is to break down protein as a source for gluconeogenesis. Organ function is affected, including that of the lungs and heart. In general, the proteins essential to life are preferentially maintained while less vital substances are not replaced. Thus, the liver and intestinal tract normally have a high turnover of their constituents because enzymes must be synthesized in order to utilize the constant inflow of nutrients. When the flow of nutrients is interrupted, this turnover ceases.[43,83]

# METABOLIC CHANGES IN STARVATION

If adequate calories are not supplied to the body, a state of starvation exists. The average man needs about 2,000 cal/day under ordinary resting conditions; the average woman, about 1,800 Cal/day. Any heavy energy demand on the individual can increase this requirement to 2,800 Cal/day or more. Fever, for example, increases caloric needs by 7 to 10% per degree Fahrenheit.[37]

In starvation—whether partial or total—the problem is simply a lack of adequate nutrient input. At the cellular level the ability to utilize nutrients is normal, there is little or no ac-

TABLE 22-1. Demonstrable End-Organ Alterations in Malnutrition

| ORGAN | ANATOMIC ALTERATIONS | PHYSIOLOGIC ALTERATIONS |
|---|---|---|
| Heart | Four-chamber dilation<br>Atrophic degeneration with necrosis and fibrosis<br>Myofibrillar disruption | QR prolongation, low voltage, bradycardia; decreased cardiac output, stroke volume, and contractility<br>Preload intolerance<br>Diminished responsiveness to drugs |
| Lung | Emphysematous changes<br>Pulmonary infarcts<br>Reduced bacterial clearance<br>Muscle atrophy | Pneumonia<br>Decreases in functional residual capacity, vital capacity, and maximum breathing capacity<br>Depressed hypoxic/hypercarbic drives |
| Blood | Stem-cell failure<br>Depressed erythropoietin synthesis | Anemia |
| Kidney | Epithelial swelling<br>Atrophy<br>Mild cortical calcification | Reduced GFR and ability to handle sodium loads<br>Polyuria<br>Metabolic acidosis |
| Gut | Disproportionate loss of mass<br>Hypoplastic and atrophic changes<br>Decrease in total mucosal thickness | Depressed enzymatic activity<br>Shortened transit time<br>Impaired motility<br>Propensity for bacterial growth<br>Maldigestion and malabsorption |
| Liver | Loss of mass<br>Periportal fat accumulation | Decreased visceral protein synthesis<br>Eventual hepatic insufficiency |
| White Blood Cells | Decreased PMN chemotaxis<br>Decreased lymphocyte count, with reduced T-helper cells and increased T-suppressor and killer cells<br>Decreased blastogenesis in response to PHA and MLC | Anergy<br>Decreased granuloma formation<br>Impaired response to chemotherapy<br>Increased infection rate |

(From Cerra F[20] with permission.)
GFR = glomerular filtration rate; PMN = polymorphonuclear leukocyte; PHA = phytohemagglutinin; MLC = mixed lymphocyte culture.

tivation of metabolic mediators, and the system responds rapidly to replacement of proteins and sugar.[20]

The initial response to starvation aims at adapting the body to the utilization of alternative fuel sources. These include maximum utilization of the major storage fuel (fat), maintaining glucose availability to obligate glucose-consuming tissues, and minimizing protein breakdown.[59] As starvation continues, there is an attempt to conserve body mass by minimizing energy expenditure. There is a gradual decrease in the basal metabolic rate along with decreased activity, mild lethargy, decreased body core temperature, decreased cardiac rate and output, and decreased respiratory rate. Energy requirement and nitrogen excretion are thus reduced, but this response is limited in extent.[47] Minimal energy is available from circulating substrates; rather, tissue stores constitute the major source of fuel during periods of starvation, and the body adapts to this state by mobilizing these stores and thus essentially cannibalizing itself to meet the metabolic needs of various organs.[47,84]

Initially, the major response to simple starvation is to maintain the supply of glucose as an energy source. During the first few days this is accomplished at the expense of major protein loss. As starvation continues, there is an attempt to maintain protein economy by shifting to fat as a fuel source and by decreasing the metabolic expenditure. This is reflected in a decline in nitrogen excretion after the first week. There is also more efficient utilization of amino acids released by tissue breakdown and a disproportionate loss of tissue from systems not vital for survival. Extracellular fluid volume is essentially unchanged, but increases in proportion to the declining body weight. This reduction in body processes and weight loss means that there is a widespread loss of reserve capacity, which may occur without the obvious failure of any specific organ or tissue. The malnourished individual cannot respond appropriately to sudden stress of any kind. There is depression of the inflammatory response and weakening of tissue immunity, there may be an overgrowth of native bacteria, and there are persistent sores and poor wound healing. There is an overall loss of the "capacity for homeostasis" (Table 22-1).[59]

In contrast to the stress reaction (see below), an exogenous supply of glucose has a marked protein-sparing effect in simple starvation. The obligatory metabolic requirements of the brain can be met by supplying 150 g of glucose (3 L of 5% dextrose), which spares 75 g of protein. In response to this increase in glucose, increased insulin secretion inhibits proteolysis and gluconeogenesis. Further glucose does not spare more protein; rather, total parenteral nutrition (TPN) is necessary.[55] Indeed, excess glucose in the absence of adequate protein intake may lead to conservation of muscle protein at the expense of visceral and blood proteins and may also increase extracellular water. Exogenously supplied protein may also have a protein-sparing effect by serving as a substrate for gluconeogenesis. Dietary fat (in the form of intravenous emulsions) does not have this effect, except to the extent that its glycerol can be converted to glucose.[30,104] In any case, the major goal of nutritional therapy and a readily achievable one in simple starvation is to prevent the loss of body protein and maintain metabolic balance.

## METABOLISM IN THE STRESSED PATIENT

In the trauma patient, the picture is radically different. In starvation, the body responds to a lack of nutrients by minimizing energy expenditure and vital tissue breakdown. In trauma, the body mobilizes its resources to deal with the injury. A hypercatabolic state is induced and sustained by a series of hormonal and adrenergic responses distinct from those seen during acute starvation.[27,43,63,118] In addition, the adaptive mechanisms present in chronic nutrient restriction are not seen.[13] Rather, the severely stressed patient cannibalizes visceral and skeletal muscle protein, thereby aggravating multisystem organ failure.[92]

Cuthbertson divided the metabolic responses of the traumatized patient into two phases: the first, *the ebb phase,*[26,30,74,88] which may last up to 24–48 hours, is characterized by circulatory and metabolic depression. If the patient is resuscitated successfully, the ebb phase usually merges into a metabolically active *flow phase,* which may be subdivided into two stages. The first stage is characterized by hypercatabolism and maximum mobilization of nutrients. In the adaptive stage of the flow phase anabolism and reparative processes take place (Fig 22-4).

## THE EBB PHASE

Based on data from a small number of patients, it is generally accepted that immediately after a major injury the body enters a lag or "ebb" state. This phase includes the period of initial resuscitation. It is characterized by a low metabolic rate, diminished cardiac output, decreased body temperature and blood volume, elevated blood lactate level, and increased body weight (Fig 22-4).[26,30] It is believed that this state is associated with massive epinephrine and norepinephrine release.[43,55] Thus, the severity of trauma dictates the course of events during this phase, the duration of which depends on how quickly the patient is resuscitated.

More recent findings dispute the presence of an ebb phase. Edwards and co-workers[31] have measured $O_2$ consumption ($\dot{V}O_2$) within about 1.6 hours (range, 0.8–9 hours) after trauma and found that $\dot{V}O_2$ was low in only 2, unchanged in 4, and above normal in 10 of 16 patients. Of the two patients with reduced $\dot{V}O_2$, one had a high blood alcohol level (356 mg%), and in the other, $O_2$ delivery ($DO_2$) to tissues was extremely low. In several other patients in whom $DO_2$ was low, $\dot{V}O_2$ was maintained at near normal levels by increased $O_2$ extraction from arterial blood, as evidenced by reduced mixed venous $O_2$ saturation ($S_vO_2$). Their conclusion that "there is no evidence for an ebb phase response in man"[31] may alter the classical concept.[26]

## ACTIVE FLOW PHASE

The flow phase is so called because the flow of substrates is in excess of energy requirements.[84] It is characterized by hypermetabolism and hypercatabolism, with massive mobilization of body fuels from energy depots into the bloodstream, to the site of injury, and to the vital organs (Fig 22-4). In addition to the increased availability of nutrients, the hypercatabolic response is also characterized by changes in sensitivity to hormones and substrates. This condition results in a change in the proportion of fuels oxidized by different tissues.[30]

Teleologically, this response may originally have had an adaptive value, in that an injured animal would not be able to forage actively for food but would need increased nutrients for wound healing. Thus, the body may be said to have developed a set of mechanisms that allow it to consume itself for brief periods of time in order to promote rapid repair and recovery.[30] and to maintain a relative abundance of circulating substrates to meet the varying requirements of different cells.[15] The aim is not only to provide energy sources but also to make amino acids available in order to maximize the protein synthesis and cell replication required to respond appropriately to the traumatic insult.

Although recent data have failed to demonstrate a correlation between the injury severity score and the degree of metabolic abnormality,[94] it is generally believed that the trauma-related increase in metabolic rate in this phase is proportional to the severity of injury.[39] It is also related in length and severity to the patient's nutritional status before injury.[63] It should be noted that this is a generalized systemic response, not a localized one. $O_2$ consumption, for example, increases in proportion to the degree of injury because of increased whole-body consumption; it is not a direct function of in-

INJURY

| EBB PHASE | FLOW PHASE | |
|---|---|---|
| | ACUTE PHASE | ADAPTIVE PHASE |
| Low C.O. Shock | ↑ C.O. | ↑ Glucocorticoid |
| Low BMR | ↑ BMR | Hyperglycemia |
| Low Body Temperature | ↑ Catechols | Normalizing I / G ratio |
| Acidosis | Hyperglycemia | ↓ Lypolysis |
| Hyperlactacidemia | Low I/G ratio | Anabolic |
| | ↑ Lipolysis | |
| | Catabolic | |

FIG. 22-4. The metabolic tide following trauma. C.O. = cardiac output; BMR = basal metabolic rate, I/G ratio = insulin/glucagon ratio.

creased uptake by the wound.[8] These processes usually peak between the third and tenth days after injury; they then abate over another 3 or 4 days unless a complication ensues. In the latter case, the process reactivates and may reach a new peak. Mediator systems are activated; how much and for how long will determine the extent and duration of the flow or stress response.[20] Activated white cells of different types are known to release products, such as leukocyte endogenous mediator (LEM), lymphocyte activating factor (LAF), leukocyte pyrogen (interleukin-1), and tumor necrosis factor/cachectin, in response to trauma and immunologic challenge. These have catabolic effects possibly mediated by prostaglandin $E_2$.[20,39,43] Thus, necrotic tissue, septic foci, severe perfusion deficits, end-organ failure, persistent hematomas, or nonhealing wounds activate these mediator systems and may prolong this phase for days or weeks, preventing the transition to the anabolic or recovery phase.

As mentioned, the increased metabolic rate represents a major difference from the energy- and protein-conserving adaptation to starvation that occurs in healthy humans (Figs 22-5 and 22-6).[42,118] In uncomplicated hospitalized patients, resting energy expenditure (measured caloric utilization) does not exceed the predicted basal metabolic rate by more than approximately 10%. Elective surgery, even such extensive procedures as total hip replacement, does not normally increase caloric requirement beyond this level. Major injury, however, may increase energy expenditure by 10 to 30% above resting levels. Septic complications, such as peritonitis, may increase metabolism by over 40%, and burns, depending on their severity, may increase energy requirements by over 80% (Table 22-2).[30,66,118] To the extent that the stress response is controlled, some aspects of this metabolic overdemand may be reduced by anesthesia, at least temporarily.[43,70,101,115]

Perhaps the most important immediate response to trauma is the outpouring of epinephrine and norepinephrine from the sympathetic nerves and adrenal medulla mediated through the ventromedial (paraventricular) nucleus of the hypothalamus. Both norepinephrine and epinephrine increase within 5 minutes of trauma.[23] Plasma norepinephrine increases as rapidly as the epinephrine concentration, but not to the same extent (Fig 22-7). The degree of increase in catecholamine levels has been shown to correlate with the severity of the injury (Fig 22-8).[28]

FIG. 22-5. Percent change from normal of resting metabolism as a function of time in patients with major burn, peritonitis, fracture, and total and partial starvation. (From Long et al[66] with permission.)

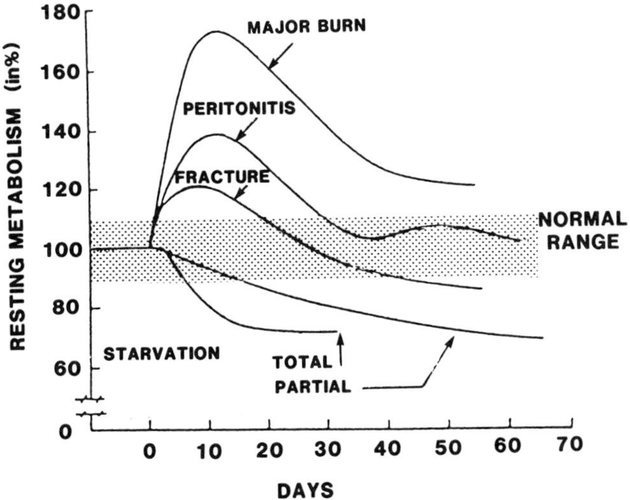


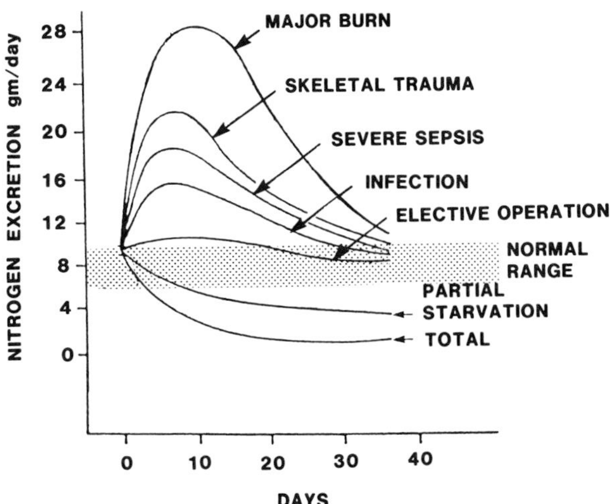


FIG. 22-6. Nitrogen excretion as a function of time in conditions of major burn, skeletal trauma, severe sepsis, infection, elective surgery, and partial and total starvation. (From Long et al[66] with permission.)

Catecholamines have an important role to play in orchestrating the endocrine responses to trauma. They stimulate glucagon release from the alpha cells of the pancreatic islets of Langerhans and inhibit insulin release from beta cells. It appears rather odd that insulin levels should be decreased at a time when all other hormone concentrations increase. However, from a teleologic point of view such a decrease in insulin is appropriate since it will ensure an adequate supply of glucose (a readily utilizable substrate) to all vital areas. Increased glucose concentration causes increased serum osmolarity, which has been shown to correlate with the severity of injury.[58] This osmotic effect may help augment blood volume by absorption of extravascular fluid into the intravascular compartment, since fed animals have been observed to refill plasma volume more effectively after hemorrhage than fasted animals. Hematocrit decreases after hemorrhage by as much as 10% in fed animals and changes only negligibly in fasted animals (Fig 22-9)[41] because of an inability to affect plasma refill. Because of this, the ability of fasted animals to survive hemorrhage is curtailed severely.

There is a possibility that reduced insulin levels may interfere with the entry of glucose into the cells. However, it has been shown that glucose can enter hypoxic cells without the need for insulin.[82,100] In fact, hypovolemia augments the rate of disappearance of glucose from the peripheral circulation in eviscerated animal preparations.[87]

The hyperglycemic response to trauma is so typical that it is called the "diabetes of injury." Although high catecholamine levels may inhibit insulin release initially, with volume repletion, increasing levels of catabolic or counterregulatory hormones, and hyperglycemia, insulin levels increase markedly.[94] Nevertheless, hyperglycemia persists in spite of these high levels of insulin.[94] In general, hormones may affect the

TABLE 22-2. Resting Metabolic Expenditure in Surgical Patients*

| CONDITION | NORMAL BMR** (kcal/day) | STRESS INCREASE (%) | ACUTE EXPENDITURE kcal/day | ACUTE EXPENDITURE kcal/kg/day |
|---|---|---|---|---|
| Normal | 1800 | | | 26 |
| Postoperative | 1800 | 0%† | 1800 | 26 |
| Multiple fractures | 1800 | +20% | 2160 | 31 |
| Major sepsis | 1800 | +40% | 2520 | 36 |
| Major burn | 1800 | +80% | 3240 | 46 |

* From Wolfe et al[118] with permission.
** Basal metabolic rate.
† Will increase significantly after extensive major procedures, eg, abdominoperineal resection, pancreatic resection with reconstructions.

action of other hormones by changing the affinity or number of their receptors. Both cortisol and growth hormone alter insulin receptors and insulin can "down-regulate" its own receptors, thus leading to peripheral tissue resistance to insulin,[94,115] although the primary defect here may also be at a postreceptor site.

The hallmark of this stage is thus a persistent hyperglycemia that is resistant to insulin.[94,119] In addition and contributing to this state, the entire hormonal environment leads to an increased rate of gluconeogenesis, despite higher than normal basal insulin levels. The increased pancreatic secretion of glucagon leads to a decrease or reversal of the normal I/G ratio (Fig 22-4). Combined with increased levels of catecholamines and glucocorticoids, this leads to an acceleration of hepatic production and release of glucose by glycogenolysis and by activation of hepatic adenylcyclase.[11,91] Peripherally, there may be a greater, although less efficient, clearance of glucose by muscle. That is, the fraction of glucose uptake actually oxidized to provide energy is abnormally low.[94] In stressed individuals there may be a defect in pyruvate entry into the Krebs cycle because of enzyme inhibition. The result is an increased production of the end products of anaerobic glycolysis, namely pyruvate and lactate, and to a lesser extent, alanine and glutamine. These compounds are eventually returned to the liver where they serve as substrates for glucose resynthesis via the Cori cycle.[11,30,118] Glucose is thus essentially recycled.[94] One of the consequences of this self-perpetuating cycle is that exogenous glucose, which if administered in sufficient quantity (150 g/70 kg/day) can suppress gluconeogenesis in simple starvation, cannot inhibit glucose synthesis in traumatized individuals,[94] although there is some evidence that very high infusion rates may do so.[91] It should also be noted that catecholamine infusions used for circulatory support may also have the effect of aggravating this situation.

The abnormality in glucose metabolism results in a shift to free fatty acids as a primary source of energy in the stressed individual, although their utilization is variable. Release from fat depots (lipolysis) occurs in spite of high glucose and insulin levels, probably because of elevated catecholamines; thus, adipose tissue also exhibits insulin resistance. Yet, the ability of certain tissues to oxidize free fatty acids and therefore to use them as a metabolizable fuel source may be limited. Thus, there may be an increased degree of "futile" cycling of triglycerides in critical disease states. That is, triglyceride re-

FIG. 22-7. Plasma catecholamine levels after hemorrhage in the subhuman primate. (•) denotes statistical difference from control. (Adapted from Chernow et al[23] with permission.)

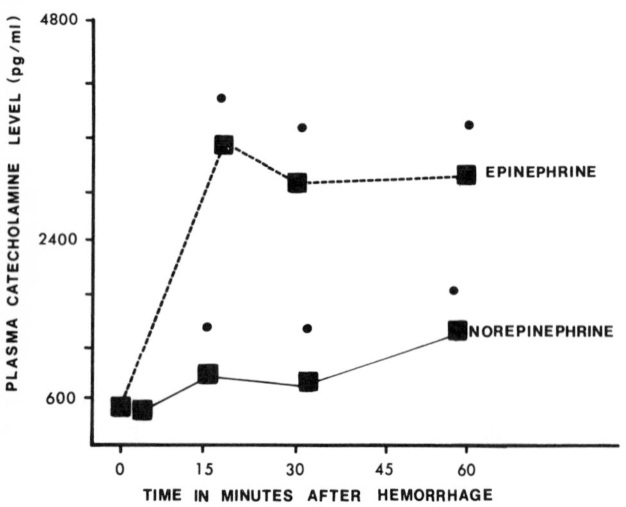


FIG. 22-8. Relationship between plasma adrenaline levels and injury severity scores. (Adapted from Davies et al[28] with permission.)

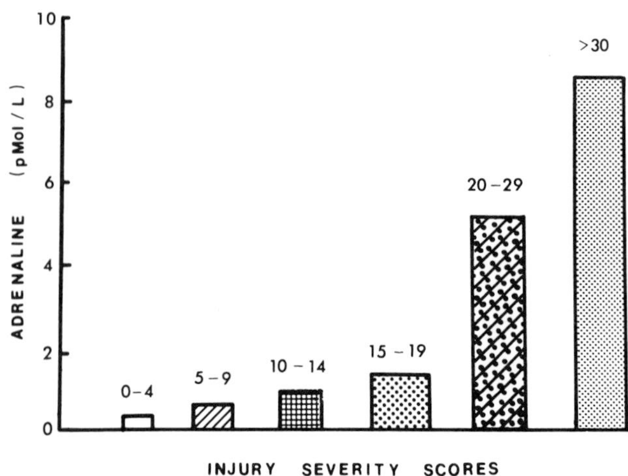

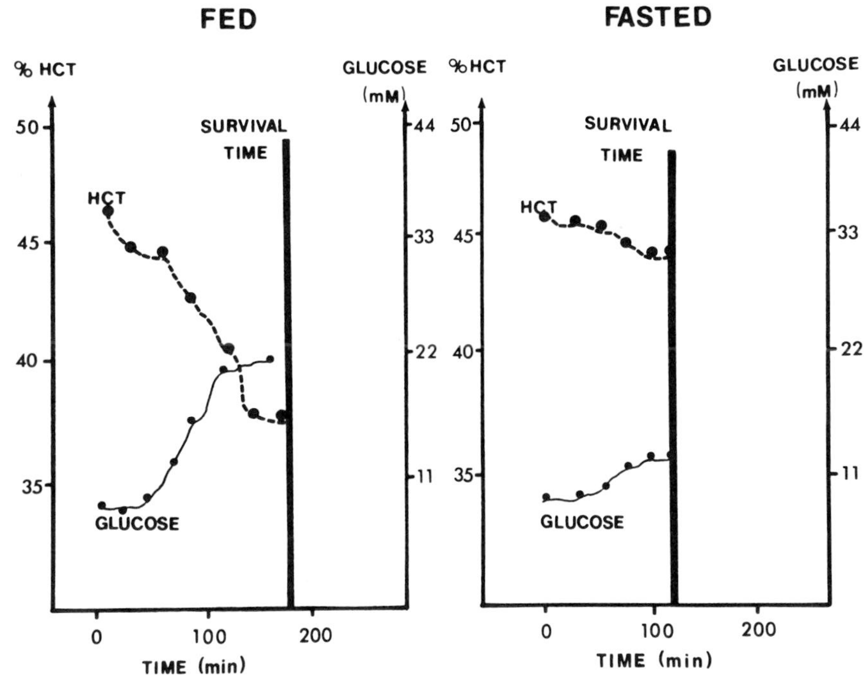


FIG. 22-9. Hematocrit and plasma glucose values in fed and fasted animals during hemorrhage. Normalized time is shown on the x-axis. (Adapted from Friedman et al[41] with permission.)

synthesis or lipogenesis is seen simultaneously with lipolysis, and indeed, hepatic steatosis is not uncommon in this setting. It is most probably secondary to increased levels of glucose and insulin; consistent with this hypothesis is the suppression of hepatic ketogenesis in stress states.[11,20,39,91,114,118]

One of the major metabolic problems in the trauma patient is the increased rate of protein turnover, which may result in major losses of lean body mass and emaciation.[94] The purpose of this catabolic response, which appears to occur predominantly at the expense of skeletal muscle (although there has been some controversy on this point),[83] would seem to be to increase the available amino acid pool. Although some of these mobilized amino acids are oxidized directly for fuel or used for gluconeogenesis, the major effect is to make more precursors available for synthesis of visceral proteins, acute phase reactants, and proteins of tissue repair. The major organ of protein synthesis is the liver, which responds in trauma and sepsis by increasing its metabolic rate and therefore its extraction of amino acids from the circulation.[50] In the acutely ill patient then, the breakdown of lean body mass may serve as an adaptive phenomenon to redistribute the amino acid pool.[84] Yet, depending on the severity of trauma or sepsis, this can lead to the catabolism of 75–150 g/day of body protein, resulting in a lean body mass loss of 300–600 g/day.[39] The problem is that much of this loss is obligate. In the stressed patient, protein synthesis and breakdown increase, but the latter is increased disproportionately.[94] There is evidence that this effect is driven or potentiated by humoral mediators released by leukocytes in response to stress.[20,25,63,118] Since proteolysis is not a response to energy needs, as in simple starvation, it is not suppressible by infusion of glucose. Similarly, protein (amino acid) infusions, although providing substrates for synthetic needs, do not serve to prevent continued tissue breakdown, since this is not a feedback mechanism.

There is evidence, however, that provision of the branched chain amino acids (valine, leucine, isoleucine) may ameliorate protein loss. The branched chain amino acids (BCCAs) are the only ones oxidized principally by skeletal muscle, and their rate of oxidation is increased by fasting, hormones, stress, diabetes, and conditions associated with muscle wasting and negative nitrogen balance. Their utilization supplies not only energy but also nitrogen and possibly carbon skeletons for intramuscular synthetic processes.[35,39] During stress states, muscle tissue may have difficulty utilizing exogenous fuel sources because of insulin deficiency or enzyme malfunction. There may therefore be a fuel deficit that can be filled only by the BCAAs, thus further stimulating muscle proteolysis.[81,91,118] Amino acids that are not used for protein synthesis are deaminated in the liver; their carbon skeletons become substrates for gluconeogenesis while the nitrogen released is converted into urea and excreted in the urine. The level of urea thus serves as a marker of protein loss.[11]

Shortly after the traumatic event, hepatic blood flow must increase considerably to cope with the increasing metabolic demand. This can occur only if blood volume is restored without delay. In the presence of adequate circulatory volume, hepatic blood flow index and hepatic flow/cardiac output ratio increase (Fig 22-10).[46] Concomitant with the increase in hepatic blood flow is an increase in hepatic oxygen consumption.[46] In addition to perfusion, the extent of substrate mobilization from the liver also depends on the nutritional status of the individual at the time of injury.

During the metabolic tide the plasma concentrations of ADH, ACTH, STH, and thyroid hormones are increased.[74] The stimuli for ADH release come from osmoreceptors and low-pressure/volume receptors located in the left atrium. The adrenal venous cortisol concentration starts increasing soon after significant blood loss.[64] The cortisol response is even more dramatic if the organism has experienced another traumatic event in the recent past. It has been shown in animal

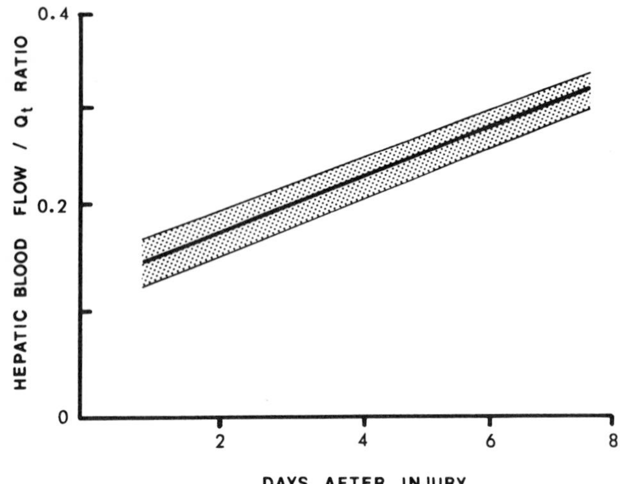


FIG. 22-10. Hepatic blood flow/total cardiac output ($Q_t$) ratio in trauma patients. (Adapted from Gottlieb et al[46] with permission.)

experiments that the response of both cortisol and catecholamines to hemorrhage is greater after a second injury than after a first episode occurring on the previous day.[64] The increased concentrations of ADH, STH, and ACTH, together with the elevation in catecholamine levels already described, stimulate the adrenal cortex to produce more cortisol. Elevated levels of glucagon, catecholamines, STH and glucocorticoids cause increased breakdown of triglycerides to fatty acids and glycerol.

The normal thyroid gland produces the hormones, thyroxine ($T_4$) and tri-iodothyronine ($T_3$). Deiodination of $T_4$ to form $T_3$ and reverse $T_3$ (r-T3) takes place in both thyroid and extrathyroid tissues. Biologically, $T_3$ is many times more active than $T_4$, while r-$T_3$ is inactive. In trauma victims and in patients with acute medical illness, peripheral conversion of $T_4$ to $T_3$ is diminished and to r-$T_3$ is increased.[9,76] The significance of reduced $T_3$ levels is not clear. Presumably it reflects an altered metabolic state in response to the metabolic tide of the flow phase. The diminished formation of the biologically active $T_3$ is implicated in the posttraumatic pseudodiabetic state.

A number of publications[36,48,89] have implicated increased circulating β-endorphins in the pathogenesis of hypovolemic shock. The evidence for this is mainly indirect. It has been shown that administration of naloxone not only improves cardiovascular performance in severely hypovolemic animals but also improves the survival rate. The dose of naloxone required to produce any sustained effect on cardiovascular performance is about 2 mg/kg. Although there is considerable beneficial effect on the mean arterial pressure, cardiac output improves only minimally. Until further data become available, we cannot recommend the routine use of high-dose naloxone for treatment of hypovolemic shock. A summary of metabolic changes during the active flow phase that ensure adequate nutrient supply to various organs is depicted in Figure 22-11.

The success of the metabolic tide depends on many factors. Severe hypovolemia, by reducing cardiac output and hepatic and muscle blood flow, counteracts the beneficial effects of this phenomenon. The extent and severity of muscle injury may also affect the magnitude of substrate mobilization. Likewise, the degree of muscular development determines the level of the metabolic tide. Well-developed persons lose more muscle mass during the posttraumatic catabolic response than poorly developed individuals. By the same token, women lose less muscle mass than men.

Nutritional intervention in the acute stage has limited effects. An increase in plasma glucose oxidation, a decrease in fat oxidation, and an increase in protein synthesis may be noted. However, nutritional support cannot completely eliminate the protein loss.[94] Patients who are nutritionally depleted before trauma actually have a lower rate of catabolism,[21,43] but also tend to do worse. Support at this time is largely limited to preservation of the patient's nutritional status—to ensuring that adequate substrates are present to meet requirements for energy and protein synthesis. Although this does not affect the catabolic process, it helps the patient respond appropriately to whatever insult has been sustained, especially if the duration of the stress response is prolonged by recurrent complications. In addition, proper attention to cardiovascular support, fluid resuscitation, and appropriate surgical intervention is obviously critical.

## THE ADAPTIVE PHASE

During this part of the flow phase, improvement in the organization of metabolic processes results in tissue repair and stimulation of the immune system.[55] It is during this stage that nutritional support is most effective.[15,83] The body is able to respond to exogenous nutritional intervention by restoration of cell mass, not merely by minimizing losses. Body mechanisms now turn to different sources of energy, and the organism seeks to adapt its metabolism to changes in the nature

FIG. 22-11. Metabolic changes in the active flow phase. Note that the body tries to maximize gluconeogenesis from all available sources. Juxtaglom = juxtaglomerular.

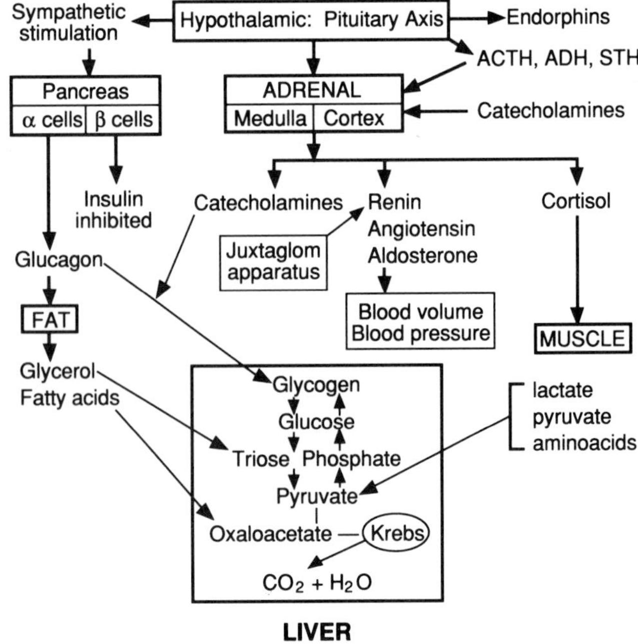

and source of nutrition. It is important to understand the underlying metabolic processes so that nutritional intervention can be appropriate.[15,55,83]

During this stage body temperature may be elevated, and leukocytosis and elevated erythrocyte sedimentation rate are common. Impulses originating in the paraventricular nucleus of the hypothalamus decrease in intensity, with the result that sympathetic activity begins to return to pretrauma levels and urinary catecholamine excretion falls, although they remain somewhat above normal. Serum glucose and glucocorticoid concentrations decrease, and the insulin/glucagon ratio becomes more appropriate to the circulating blood sugar level, although it remains smaller than the physiologic ratio (Fig 22-4). Administration of exogenous glucose may sometimes prevent the recognition of a decreased serum glucose level. Ketosis and ketonuria may occur during this phase. The body weight may drop as less fluid is retained, and urinary nitrogen excretion (urea) may begin to fall.

Decreasing urinary nitrogen signifies the onset of a trend toward positive nitrogen balance. Urinary nitrogen loss can be stopped completely by providing exogenous glucose during this period. Approximately 70% more glucose than the usual daily requirement is needed to accomplish this.[15] Because the insulin/glucagon ratio remains below the physiologic range, exogenously administered amino acids are still likely to augment glucose output from the liver and thus the negative nitrogen balance, a fact to be remembered when tailoring a hyperalimentation regimen for the individual trauma victim.

During the adaptive phase the patient's metabolism becomes gradually anabolic. However, in the early stages of this phase there is increased hepatic protein synthesis and breakdown of muscle proteins. Although there is some evidence to suggest that protein metabolism in the muscle and liver may be regulated by different mechanisms,[50] it is generally believed that increased proteolysis in the muscle serves to provide amino acids for protein synthesis in the liver. Sepsis causes further augmentation of liver protein synthesis, but this does not alter trauma-induced reduction of muscle protein synthesis.[50] In fact muscle protein degradation is enhanced when infection complicates injury. Increased muscle breakdown in sepsis results in increased serum levels of alanine, phenylalanine, ornithine, histidine, and arginine. An increased phenylalanine/tyrosine ratio is an indicator of the degree of muscle wasting. Increased alanine levels are believed to be a potent stimulus for hepatic protein synthesis. The amino acid leucine is also important in this regard.[15] Irreversible combustion of this amino acid occurs in muscles and fat during trauma and sepsis. Leucine is essential for the utilization of many amino acids by the liver. When leucine is lacking, it is conceivable that many other amino acids cannot be utilized by the liver, resulting in their excretion by the kidney. Those essential amino acids that cannot be synthesized by the body must be supplied exogenously at this stage.

## NUTRITIONAL ASSESSMENT AND THERAPY

In guiding nutritional therapy, two major issues must be addressed: the nutritional status of the patient and the degree of stress and special needs imposed by the trauma and its complications.[63,81] A number of parameters have been suggested for assessment of nutritional status. They include measurement of height and weight, triceps skinfold thickness, arm muscle circumference, or creatinine-height index; measures of immune competence, such as total lymphocyte count or delayed cutaneous hypersensitivity; levels of various visceral proteins, such as serum albumin, retinol-binding protein, serum transferrin, ceruloplasmin, plasma cholinesterase, and plasma thyroxine-binding prealbumin; measurements of skeletal muscle function; and others.[45,59,61,63] Characteristics and clinical utility of each of these parameters are summarized in Table 22-3. Unfortunately, these indices are neither sensitive nor specific in quantitating nutritional status; they are often inaccurate as whole-body parameters and do not give adequate information about specific organs or compartments. Moreover, most of these parameters do not necessarily reflect the magnitude or even direction of change of nutritional status.[91,106] This is especially true in the acute and/or unstable trauma patient in whom they are affected by events other than nutritional status: fluid resuscitation, stress response, extensive surgery, and septic complications. For instance, fluid leakage into tissues and altered immune response, which are not uncommon after severe trauma, may result in misinterpretation of these parameters. Indeed, many of these markers may be useful only when the stress period is over and the patient is already stable and recovering.[1,52,63]

In planning nutritional support, caloric guidelines are usually derived from the Harris-Benedict equations for estimating basal energy expenditure (BEE):

$$\text{Male, kcal/24 h} = 66.5 + 13.76 \times \text{wt (kg)} + 5 \times \text{ht (cm)} - 6.76 \times \text{age (yr)}$$

$$\text{Female, kcal/24 h} = 655.1 + 9.56 \times \text{wt (kg)} + 1.8 \times \text{ht (cm)} - 4.7 \times \text{age (yr)}$$

Resting energy expenditure (REE) in the bedridden patient is usually 10% higher than that estimated from these equations. Estimates of requirements above REE can then be added, depending on the severity of injury, to arrive at the nutritional goal.[65,72,75] These estimates are arrived at by multiplying the REE by a "stress factor" (Table 22-4). Recent data, however, suggest that this approach may underestimate or, just as dangerously, significantly overestimate the caloric requirements of critically ill patients with multiple organ damage or failure.[70,109,112,113] Moreover, they may not accurately predict changing needs at different times in the course of illness. More precise measurements can be achieved at the bedside via indirect calorimetry with gas-exchange techniques to measure oxygen consumption and carbon dioxide production. Wherever possible, this is the preferred method; metabolic carts are available for this purpose.[34,63,91,111]

The hypercatabolism that accompanies the posttraumatic state results in excessive nitrogen loss, which is reflected in increased urinary creatinine and urea excretion. Nitrogen balance can most easily be monitored by measuring 24-hour urine urea nitrogen loss (UUN) and comparing this value to nitrogen intake. Urine urea nitrogen represents about 80% of urinary nitrogen excretion; in addition to the urine loss approximately 1.5–3 g are lost via skin and stool. Thus,

TABLE 22-3. Clinical Utility of Nutritional Assessment Parameters Used in the ICU Population*

| | |
|---|---|
| Serum albumin | Correlates with body cell mass in large populations, but is nonsensitive, nonspecific for individual patients. Remains normal in malnourished patients with anorexia nervosa, but may fall rapidly during critical illness before significant malnutrition has occurred. Rises slowly during nutritional repletion. |
| Serum transferrin | Correlates with body cell mass in large populations, but is nonsensitive, nonspecific for individual patients. Rises during iron deficiency. Rises earlier than albumin during nutritional repletion of unstressed patients. |
| Retinol-binding protein | More sensitive than albumin or transferrin to nutritional repletion; unclear role in assessment of ICU patients |
| Thyroxine-binding prealbumin | More sensitive than albumin or transferrin to nutritional repletion; decline during critical illness may be related to thyroxine homeostatic function, rather than to nutritional change |
| Fibronectin | Very sensitive to nutritional depletion and repletion during health and critical illness. Consumed rapidly during acute illness. Peaks early during nutritional repletion, does not track positive nitrogen balance after 1 week |
| Somatomedin C | May be related to hormonal adaptation to nutrient restriction. More sensitive to nutritional repletion than prealbumin, albumin, retinol-binding protein, or transferrin in nonacutely ill patients. Unclear role in the ICU population |
| Midarm muscle circumference | Cumbersome method, requires experience, may be influenced by skin edema |
| Creatinine-height index | May grossly overestimate muscle mass of critically ill patients |
| Skinfold thickness | Assesses adiposity; serial measurements reflect positive or negative caloric balance. Measurement influenced by skin edema |
| Cutaneous reactivity | Poor measure of either total body nutritional status or of nutritional integrity of the immune system |
| Lymphocyte count | Nonsensitive, nonspecific. Unclear role in tracking nutritional progression |
| Urinary nitrogen | Useful for assessing catabolic rate |
| Nitrogen balance | Useful for assessing adequacy of nutritional formula |
| Subjective global assessment | Easy to perform, best predictor of nutrition-related complications. Nonsensitive for following nutritional progression |

* (From Schlichtig and Ayres[91] with permission.)

$$\text{Total N loss (g/day)} = \frac{\text{24 h UUN}}{0.8} + 3\text{ g}.$$

Since about 6.25 g of protein yields 1 g of nitrogen,

$$\text{N intake} = \frac{\text{Protein intake}}{6.25}$$

In general, enteral feeding is preferred when possible. It avoids some of the septic complications of central venous cannulation and is more "physiologic." Using the gut, moreover, preserves its motility and stimulates the synthesis of appropriate visceral proteins, thus maintaining its barrier function and possibly decreasing the incidence of infections from intestinal flora. Major problems are diarrhea and pulmonary aspiration, although the latter can be largely eliminated when small-lumen feeding tubes are used and food is infused distal to the pylorus. Continuous rather than bolus or intermittent infusion is necessary with this technique. Feeding jejunostomies have become popular because they offer these advantages: ease of insertion and reduced risk of aspiration and gastric atony. When enteral feeding is started early, it may speed healing in abdominal trauma.[2,71] Metabolic complications are rare with this route, but it may take longer to achieve positive nitrogen balance because diarrhea may limit the rate of infusion and initially prevent the use of full-strength solutions.

In some patients who are only moderately stressed, peripheral intravenous alimentation may be efficacious. In already well-nourished individuals who are not in a hypercatabolic state and need support for only a few days until they can resume oral intake, this route can be used for "protein-sparing therapy." Clinical evidence of response is the development of ketonuria after administration of hypocaloric amino acid. Fat emulsions may be given peripherally, and this route may also be used to supplement enteral feeding. The problem is that solutions of greater than 600 mosm are poorly tolerated by

TABLE 22-4. The Effect of Different Degrees of Injury on the Metabolic Activity*

| | % INCREASE IN METABOLIC RATE | NITROGEN BALANCE (g/day) | "STRESS FACTOR" |
|---|---|---|---|
| Hernia repair | 0–5 | (−2)–(−3) | 1–1.05 |
| Peritonitis | 5–25 | (−12)–(−15) | 1.05–1.25 |
| Long bone fracture | 15–30 | (−12)–(−15) | 1.15–1.30 |
| Multiple trauma | 30–55 | (−15)–(−16) | 1.30–1.55 |
| Burn 20% | 50 | (−16)–(−18) | 1.50 |
| Severe head injury | 30–50 | (−20) | 1.30–1.5 |
| Multiple trauma & sepsis | 50–75 | (−25) | 1.50–1.75 |
| Burn 30% | 70 | (−25) | 1.70 |
| Burn 50% | 100 | (−40) | 2.0 |
| Burn 75% | 100–110 | (−50) | 2.0–2.1 |

* (From Freund[39] with permission.)

**BELLEVUE HOSPITAL CENTER — ENTERAL PRODUCT FORMULARY**

| PRODUCT CATEGORY | STANDARD FORMULAS | | | CALORIE/PROTEIN DENSE FORMULAS | | DISEASE SPECIFIC FORMULAS | |
|---|---|---|---|---|---|---|---|
| PRODUCT NAME | OSMOLITE® | SUSTACAL | COMPLETE MODIFIED | TWO CAL HN | ISOTEIN HN | AMIN-AID | HEPATIC-AID II |
| Calories/cc | 1 | 1 | 1.07 | 2 | 1.2 | 2 | 1.2 |
| gm Protein/L | 37 | 61 | 43 | 83.7 | 68 | 19.4 EAA | 44 BCAA |
| gm Carbohydrate/L | 145 | 140 | 140 | 217.3 | 156 | 366 | 169 |
| gm Fat/L | 39 | 23 | 37 | 90.9 | 34 | 46 | 36 |
| non Pro Kcal:N | 144:1 | 79:1 | 131:1 | 125:1 | 85:1 | 830:1 | 147:1 |
| Na/K (mg/L) | 549/1014 | 940/2100 | 680/1400 | 1052/2316 | 620/1007 | 320/ negligible | 320/ negligible |
| Osmolality | 300 | 625 | 300 | 690 | 300 | 700 | 560 |
| 100% RDA in - cc | 2000 | 1080 | 1500 | 947 | 1770 | no vits added | no vits added |
| Route | tube (or oral) | oral (or tube) | tube | tube (or oral) | tube (or oral) | tube (or oral) | tube (or oral) |
| Indications and Features | Isotonic, lactose free, low residue, low sodium, requires digestion. | Lactose free, low residue | Blenderized foods, isotonic, lactose free, low sodium, requires digestion | High calorie, high protein, lactose free. For patients on fluid restrictions. | High protein, isotonic, lactose free, low residue. | Calorically dense, low electrolyte formula with EAA. For patients with renal failure. | Calorically dense, high BCAA formula. For patients with hepatic encephalopathy or coma. |

FIG. 22-12. Standard calorie/protein dense and disease-specific enteral alimentation formulas available in Bellevue Hospital Center, New York City.

peripheral veins, thus limiting the concentration of nutrients that can be delivered. This route should therefore not be the major one in patients who cannot tolerate large fluid loads or who are under severe stress.[1,54,60,108]

Total parenteral nutrition (TPN) involves central venous access with its attendant risks. The major complication, of course, is sepsis,[116] although the risk of this has been considerably reduced in recent years by careful attention to technique and by the use of special teams to manage TPN catheters. Other complications are technical or metabolic.[14,55,111]

With enteral feeding, premixed solutions are available for various situations; supplements may be added as needed (Figs 22-12 and 22-13). If TPN is used, the formulas are aseptically prepared by the hospital pharmacy on a daily basis; therefore, orders must be written daily based on the patient's changing needs. The form used for this purpose at our institution is shown in Figure 22-14. An attached page describes the available formulations (Fig 22-15).

Whichever route is used, certain nutritional goals must be met. The first is meeting energy or caloric requirements. The

FIG. 22-13. Special enteral alimentation formulas included in Bellevue Hospital Center formulary. Note the high concentration of branched chain amino acids (BCAAS) in the formula used in polytrauma patients.

**BELLEVUE HOSPITAL CENTER — ENTERAL PRODUCT FORMULARY**

| PRODUCT CATEGORY | CHEMICALLY DEFINED | LOW RESIDUE | STRESS | MODULAR COMPONENTS | | |
|---|---|---|---|---|---|---|
| PRODUCT NAME | CRITICARE HN | CITROTEIN | STRESSTEIN | POLYCOSE (POWDER) | CASEC (POWDER) | MEDIUM CHAIN TRIGLYCERIDE |
| Calories/cc | 1 | .66 | 1.2 | 380 cal/100gm | 370 cal/100 gm | 115 cal/15 ml (1 Tbsp.) |
| gm Protein/L | 38 | 41 | 70 (44% BCAA) | — | 88 gm/100 gm | — |
| gm Carbohydrate/L | 222 | 122 | 170 | 94 gm/100 gm | — | — |
| gm Fat/L | 3 | 1.6 | 28 | — | 2 gm/100 gm | 14 gm/15 ml (Tbsp) |
| non Pro Kcal:N | 148:1 | 76:1 | 97:1 | — | — | — |
| Na/K (mg/L) | 630/1320 | 710/710 | 650/1100 | 110 mg Na/100 gm 10 mg K/100 gm | 150 mg Na/100 gm 10 mg K/100gm | — |
| Osmolality | 650 | 480-510 | 910 | 850 | — | — |
| 100% RDA in - cc | 1890 | 1270 | 2000 | — | — | — |
| Route | tube (or oral) | oral | tube only | component of oral or tube feeding | component of oral or tube feeding | component of oral or tube feeding |
| Indications and Features | Elemental, lactose free, low fat, low sodium, minimum residue. For patients with malabsorption/ maldigestion. | Lactose free, low residue. For bowel prep or clear liquid diet supplement. | High BCAA, low residue. For catabolic states, sepsis or polytrauma. | Carbohydrate supplement to increase calorie intake without increasing protein, fat and/or electrolyte intake. | Protein supplement to increase protein intake. Low sodium, low fat, requires digestion. | Fat source for those with impaired absorption or digestion of LCFA. |

formu-130 93231a 7/86

**BELLEVUE HOSPITAL CENTER**
**PHARMACY DEPARTMENT**

Patient Name ___ Nursing Unit ___
Chart # ___ Age ___

(IMPRINT NAME PLATE OR PRINT INFO ABOVE)

**DOCTOR:**
1. Fill out either SECTION 1 or SECTION 2.
2. Daily Iv fat is recommended for TPN patients; especially those receiving peripheral formulations. Order separately on Standard Doctor's Order form.
3. Orders received after 12 Noon will be prepared for the following day. See SECTION 3 for information on Standing Orders.

TOTAL PARENTERAL NUTRITION (TPN) FORM
ADULT

DATE ______ TIME ______

Solution to be administered through: CENTRAL VEIN ☐ ______ PERIPHERAL VEIN ☐ ______

SECTION 1. Standard Solutions - See reverse side for complete information on formulas.

| STANDARD CENTRAL ☐ | | STANDARD PERIPHERAL ☐ | |
|---|---|---|---|
| Amino Acid Soln. 8.5% | 500ml/L | Amino Acid Soln. 8.5% | 500ml/L |
| Dextrose Inj. 50% | 500ml/L | Dextrose Inj. 10% | 500ml/L |
| Standard Electrolytes | 25 ml/L | Standard Electrolytes | 25 ml/L |
| Potassium Phosphate (per day) | 15mM | Potassium Phosphate (per day) | 15mM |
| MVI—12 (per day) | l0ml | MVI—12 (per day) | l0ml |
| Trace Elements (per day) | 1ml | Trace Elements (per day) | 1ml |
| Other______ | per/L | Other______ | per/L |
| Number of liters per day ______ | L | Number of liters per day ______ | L |
| Administration Rate ______ | ml/hr | Administration Rate ______ | ml/hr |

SECTION 2. If standard Solutions are not appropriate, SPECIAL FORMULAS may be ordered as:

| | | | EACH DAY'S THERAPY TO CONTAIN: |
|---|---|---|---|
| PROTEIN | ☐ Amino Acid Soln. 10%<br>☐ Amino Acid Soln. 8.5% | Special Amino Acid Soln.: | ml/day |
| DEXTROSE | ____70% ____50%<br>____20% ____10% | | ml/day |
| STANDARD ELECTROLYTES (See Reverse Side) | | 25ml recommended | ml/day |
| SODIUM | ______ | Chloride | mEq/day |
| | ______ | Acetate | mEq/day |
| POTASSIUM | ______ | Chloride | mEq/day |
| | ______ | Acetate | mEq/day |
| | ______ | Phosphate (3mM P/ml; 4.4mEq K/ml) | mM/day |
| CALCIUM | ______ | Chloride (10ml=1gm=13.5mEq Ca) | mEq/day |
| | ______ | Gluconate (10ml=1gm=4.7mEq Ca) | mEq/day |
| MAGNESIUM | ______ | Sulfate (2ml =1gm=8.1mEq Mg) | mEq/day |
| INSULIN | | | units/day |
| MULTIVITAMINS | | (10ml per day recommended) | ml/day |
| TRACE ELEMENTS | | (1ml per day recommended) | ml/day |
| OTHER | ______ | | |
| | ______ | | |
| | ______ | | |
| | ______ | | |

Administration Rate: ______ml/hr    Approximate Number of Liters/Day:______

SECTION 3. Standing Orders:

If stable patients have received a central TPN formulation for one week, physician may issue Standing Order for 3 DAYS at a time. Order written above will be prepared by Pharmacy (Standing Orders may not be written for peripheral TPN formulations.)

______ Date TPN started    DAY 1.______ DAY 2.______ DAY 3.______ Dates of Standing Orders

Signature:______M.D.    Print Name (required)______
Beeper Number

Retain top copy for chart. Send other copy to Pharmacy.

FIG. 22-14. Request form used for total parenteral nutrition (TPN) of critically ill patients in Bellevue Hospital Center, New York.

**FORMULATIONS - PER LITER CONTENTS**

| | | Standard Central | Standard Peripheral | * Liver Failure | ** Renal Failure |
|---|---|---|---|---|---|
| **PROTEIN** | | | | | |
| | Nitrogen (gm/L) | 7 | 7 | 6 | 1.6 |
| | Protein (gm/L) | 42.5 | 42.5 | 38 | 10 |
| **CARBOHYDRATE** | | | | | |
| | Glucose (% L) | 25 | 5 | 25 | 47 |
| **ELECTROLYTES** (mEq/L) | | | | | |
| | Sodium | 25 | 25 | 30 | 30 |
| | Potassium *** | 40.5 | 40.5 | 40.5 | 40.5 |
| | Calcium | 5 | 5 | 5 | 5 |
| | Magnesium | 8 | 8 | 8 | 8 |
| | Acetate | 77.1 | 77.1 | 31 | 84.6 |
| | Phosphate *** | — | — | 10 | — |
| | Chloride | 50.5 | 50.5 | 33.5 | 33.5 |
| | Gluconate | 5 | 5 | 5 | 5 |
| **VITAMINS** | See Below | | | | |
| **TRACE ELEMENTS** | See Below | | | | |
| **OSMOLARITY** | (mOsm/L) | 1859 | 848 | 1805 | 2024 |
| **TOTAL CALORIES** | | 1020 | 340 | 1002 | 1230 |

**STANDARD ADULT FORMULAS - PER DAY ADDITIONS**

**MVI-12/10ml**

| | | | |
|---|---|---|---|
| Ascorbic Acid | 100mg | Niacinamide | 40mg |
| Vitamin A | 3,300IU | Dexpanthenol | 15mg |
| Vitamin D | 200IU | Vitamin E | 10IU |
| Thiamine | 3mg | Biotin | 60mcg |
| Riboflavin | 3.6mg | Folic Acid | 400mcg |
| Pyridoxine | 4mg | Cyanocobolamin | 5mcg |

*** Potassium Phosphate 15mM Phosphate; 22mEq Potassium Per Day

**TRACE ELEMENTS**

| | |
|---|---|
| Manganese | 0.5mg |
| Copper | 1mg |
| Zinc | 4mg |
| Chromium | 10mcg |

**STANDARD ELECTROLYTES (25ml)**

| | | | |
|---|---|---|---|
| Sodium | 25mEq | Potassium | 40.5mEq |
| Calcium | 5mEq | Magnesium | 8mEq |
| Gluconate | 5mEq | Chloride | 33.5mEq |
| Acetate | 40.6mEq | | |

**10mEq CALCIUM PRECIPITATES WITH MORE THAN 30mEq POTASSIUM PHOSPHATE**

**15mEq CALCIUM PRECIPITATES WITH MORE THAN 20mEq POTASSIUM PHOSPHATE**

| * Liver Failure Formula (suggested) | |
|---|---|
| Amino Acid Soln. 8% (HepatAmine) | 500ml/L |
| Dextrose Inj. 50% | 500ml/L |
| Standard Electrolytes | 25ml/L |
| MVI-12 (per day) | 10ml |
| Trace Elements (per day) | 1ml |

| ** Renal Failure Formula (suggested) | |
|---|---|
| Amino Acid Soln. 5.4% (NephrAmine) | 250ml/750ml |
| Dextrose Inj. 70% | 500ml/750ml |
| Standard Electrolytes | 25ml/750ml |
| MVI-12 (per day) | 10ml |

For further information on formulations or procedures, please contact the following areas 9 AM to 5 PM daily:

Department of Pharmacy - Hyperalimentation Services Ext. 2932

Food Service - Dietitians Office Ext. 4838

FIG. 22-15. Information page attached to the total parenteral nutrition (TPN) request form used in Bellevue Hospital Center, New York.

increase in energy expenditure varies directly with the extent and nature of the injury. When designing a nutritional support regimen, however, care must be taken not only to supply the calories needed but also to avoid overfeeding. Excess calories not only do not help, but they may actually be harmful. The administration of glucose in amounts exceeding immediate energy requirements leads to an increased metabolic rate and therefore increased energy expenditure, mainly because of the energy cost of glycogen synthesis. Conversion of glucose to fat is not likely to occur to any significant degree.

Instead, the result will be excessive glycogen deposition, increased sympathetic activity due mainly to norepinephrine secretion, increased heat production, hyperglycemia, increased carbon dioxide production,[30,73] and hepatic abnormalities. Although there is some evidence that increased insulin levels may diminish protein loss,[53,120] "force feeding" of glucose may worsen some of these effects, especially respiratory failure, even when insulin is given.[4,5] Moreover, elevated protein turnover is not reduced to any substantial degree by glucose loading; indeed, visceral protein losses may actually increase, as glucose may induce a shift of amino acids to the skeletal muscles.[15]

Most authorities therefore recommend a mixed energy source, with 50% of caloric intake being provided as fat and 50% as glucose. This approach combines the advantages and reduces the disadvantages of each.[69,113] In addition to providing the requirements for essential fatty acids, a smaller volume of fluid is needed to deliver the same amount of calories. Glucose is required by the obligate glucose-utilizing tissues, but fat remains the major energy source in the stressed patient. Supplying lipid as a major component of TPN therefore preserves endogenous fat stores. Lipid clearance should be monitored by assaying serum triglyceride levels, since hypertriglyceridemia can potentially occur in sepsis due to depressed lipoprotein lipase activity in muscle and adipose tissue.[85]

The other major goal of nutritional therapy is maintenance of lean body mass by providing a positive nitrogen balance. Daily protein requirements in the nonstressed, well-nourished individual are about 0.5 g/kg/day. This is inadequate in trauma patients because of the enormous metabolic response to stress. The common practice is to start with 1.5 g/kg/day protein and increase to 2.5 g/kg/day (equivalent to 0.4 g/kg/day of N) or more in severely stressed patients. In optimal states of metabolic support, a 3 to 5 g positive nitrogen balance can be expected.[47] Although maintenance of specific nonprotein calorie-to-nitrogen ratios is sometimes recommended, it is not clear that doing so has any importance[56] as long as caloric needs are met. However, excess amino acid administration can be detrimental, resulting in an increased metabolic rate, hypercalciuria, and neurotoxicity. Renal and hepatic dysfunction may further limit the amount of protein that can be given safely.[30,64] In spite of aggressive nutritional support, however, the catabolic process proceeds unabated, and substantial losses in body protein may continue to occur,[93,98] especially in severely septic patients. Weight loss or gain is not a good guide in this situation since these changes may be due to alterations in fat and/or water content.

Some patients exhibit a progressive autocannibalism that seems to lead inevitably to death.[20,21] In highly stressed patients, serum assays have demonstrated inappropriately high concentrations of circulating aromatic and sulfurated amino acids and depressed levels of BCAAs. It would appear that the latter are utilized by muscle as direct oxidative fuels in spite of the availability of glucose and fatty acids. As a result, the liver is unable to extract a balanced mixture of amino acids from the plasma for protein synthesis.[43] This may result in a vicious cycle of increased catabolism and may contribute to end-organ failure from lack of proper anabolic substrates. Several studies have provided strong evidence that the use of a 45–50% BCAA-enriched amino acid formulation results in improved nitrogen balance, improved visceral protein status, and better overall status as reflected in measures of immunocompetence.[19,20,22,39]

Mention should also be made of additives that must be included in nutritional preparations: electrolytes, which should be monitored and adjusted on a regular basis; trace elements,[68] which may be lost from the gastrointestinal tract; and vitamins.[3]

## NUTRITIONAL SUPPORT AND ORGAN FAILURE

Hypercatabolism and nutritional problems may contribute to the development of the multisystem organ failure syndrome in the trauma patient.[16,29,51] In addition, specific organs pose specific problems for nutritional support. Of these, the impact of nutritional care on respiratory function has been studied most extensively.[7,12,77,86,112,117] Insufficient nutrition does not spare the respiratory system. Glycogen stores are depleted within a few hours, and the diaphragm and accessory muscles then become dependent on glucose delivery via the blood. Although there is a preferential flow of cardiac output to the diaphragm, if caloric intake drops, increased flow cannot compensate for this decrease. Free fatty acids can be utilized as fuel, but are inadequate unless workloads are low. However, the trauma patient often has maximal respiratory requirements because of infection, ARDS, chest injury, etc. Thus, the respiratory muscles must be able to support prolonged, elevated demands. In addition, these muscles are subject to the same hypercatabolic processes as other skeletal muscles. Therefore, there may be a rapid development of respiratory fatigue and failure. With time, unless proper support is provided, loss of muscle mass may occur; this loss is difficult to correct and increases the difficulty of weaning from respiratory support.

The metabolic activity of the lung itself is also affected, resulting in decreased production of airway surfactant. Although this decrease may not itself be significant, the trauma patient is already at high risk of development of ARDS, and this may make recovery more difficult. Pulmonary defense mechanisms—immune function, the ability of damaged epithelium to replicate itself, and mucociliary and other mechanical functions of the lung—are also affected. Finally, starvation reduces the central ventilatory drive and thus affects the patient's ability to respond to stress situations that may increase oxygen demand (Table 22-1).

Nutritional support can also create respiratory problems if not managed carefully. Attention must be paid to electrolyte balance; hypophosphatemia, for example, can markedly affect respiratory muscle function. Use of the enteral route for feeding carries the risk of aspiration, which, in an already compromised patient, increases the possibility of respiratory infection and failure. The large volumes of fluid required in TPN may make management of ARDS more difficult, especially since the trauma patient is likely to be fluid overloaded. Use of high glucose loads in TPN results in marked increases in $CO_2$ production and thus in increased ventilatory demand. In a compromised patient this may precipitate respiratory failure, whereas in the already intubated patient weaning may be more difficult. Use of lipids as a major component of nutritional support can reduce this problem significantly because of the lower respiratory quotient (Fig 22-3).

Infusion of amino acids also increases metabolic work and ventilatory drive. Interestingly, however, BCAAs may increase the ventilatory response to $CO_2$ and hence respiratory work disproportionately. Although this may be a stimulus to breathing, it may also be detrimental to patients with compromised respiratory status. This risk has to be balanced against the potentially beneficial anticatabolic effects of BCAA administration.[103]

Although not common, cardiac dysfunction can occur in trauma patients secondary to myocardial contusion or to an inability to sustain the high outputs imposed by stress or fluid overload.[1] Normally, free fatty acids are preferentially utilized, although glucose is an important fuel under anaerobic conditions. With prolonged malnutrition, cardiac wasting may occur, and abrupt refeeding may lead to congestive failure. In a patient with cardiac failure, careful attention must be paid to limiting sodium intake and avoiding fluid overload.[80]

Liver and cerebral dysfunction may occur from a number of causes: multiorgan failure syndrome, hypotension and hypoperfusion, and alcoholism. The main problem is a decreased ability to process certain amino acids. Unlike the aromatic amino acids, BCAAs are not significantly metabolized by the liver. The two types of compounds compete for transport across the blood-brain barrier. When BCAAs decrease, aromatic amino acids accumulate in the brain and induce the synthesis of the false neurotransmitters, octopamine and phenylethanolamine, which may precipitate metabolic encephalopathy. Preferential infusion of BCAAs may ameliorate this complication.[38,40]

Renal failure poses its own problems. Where dialysis is available, full nutritional support should not be problematic. If some form of dialysis is not possible, fluid restriction is necessary; calories must then be supplied by concentrated solutions of dextrose and lipids. In such a situation uremia may develop. It may be possible to prevent this complication by restricting protein input to the essential amino acids, thereby allowing the liver to utilize urea nitrogen to synthesize the nonessential amino acids.[102] It should also be noted that in the presence of renal failure, urinary nitrogen excretion does not accurately reflect ongoing catabolism; the extent of nitrogen retention must be taken into account (see also Chapter 25).[24]

Patients with brain trauma may have higher than expected nutritional needs. Caloric requirements and urinary nitrogen excretion increase for an extended period of time. The severely brain-injured patient is hypercatabolic and hypermetabolic to an extent comparable to one with major systemic trauma. High protein intake is required since protein appears to be the preferred metabolic fuel. In patients with ischemic brain damage, glucose levels should be monitored carefully.[95,107,121] Hyperglycemia in these patients may worsen the outcome by increasing cerebral metabolism. There is inconclusive evidence that hyperglycemia may cause similar effects in brain-injured patients.[78]

## CONCLUSION

Acute trauma induces a metabolic stress in the organism. An elevation in caloric expenditure and nitrogen requirement occurs rapidly in response to injury, and this increased need can be met only initially and to a limited extent by the body's own available substrates. Failure to recognize and supply the nutritional needs of the critically ill patient results in marked depletion of lean body mass and serious compromise of wound healing, vital organ function, immune response, and level of consciousness. Indeed, once malnutrition develops, virtually all organ systems can be affected. They suffer a loss of mass, of function, and, most importantly, of capacity to respond to additional or sustained stress. It is especially in these circumstances that malnutrition can become a major contributing factor to prolongation of recovery and increased morbidity and mortality.[19] The nutritional support regimen must be tailored to specific demands and must be re-evaluated and adjusted repeatedly. Close attention to these changing requirements in a dynamic situation may help reduce some of the morbidity and complications that commonly follow trauma.

## REFERENCES


1. Abbott WC, Echenique MM, Bistrian BR, et al. Nutritional care of the trauma patient. Surg Gynecol Obstet 1983;157:585.
2. Adams S, Dellinger EP, Wertz WJ, et al. Enteral vs parenteral nutritional support following laparotomy for trauma. J Trauma 1986;26:882.
3. Alperin JB. Coagulopathy caused by vitamin K deficiency in critically ill, hospitalized patients. JAMA 1987;258:1916.
4. Askanazi J, Elwyn DH, Silverberg PA, et al. Respiratory distress secondary to the high carbohydrate load of TPN. Surgery 1980;87:596.
5. Askanazi J, Rosenbaum SH, Hyman AI, et al. Respiratory changes induced by the large glucose loads of total parenteral nutrition. JAMA 1980;243:1444.
6. Askanazi J, Nordenstrom J, Rosenbaum SH, et al. Nutrition for the patient with respiratory failure: glucose vs fat. Anesthesiology 1981;54:373.
7. Askanazi J, Weissman C, Rosenbaum H, et al. Nutrition and the respiratory system. Crit Care Med 1982;10:163.
8. Askanazi J, Kvetan V, Goldiner P. Nutrition in the acutely ill. Anesth Clin North Am 1988;6:49.
9. Aun F, Medieros-Neto GA, Younes RN, et al. The effects of major trauma on the pathways of thyroid hormone metabolism. J. Trauma 1983;23:1048.
10. Baker JP, Lemoyne M. Nutritional support in the critically ill patient. Crit Care Clin 1987;3:97.
11. Beisel WR, Wannemacher RW. Gluconeogenesis, ureagenesis, and ketogenesis during sepsis. JPEN 1980;4:277.
12. Bell RM, Bynoe RP. Nutrition and respiration. Prob Crit Care 1987;1:413.
13. Benotti P, Blackburn GL. Protein and caloric macro-nutrient metabolic management of the critically ill patient. Crit Care Med 1979;7:520.
14. Benotti PN, Bistrian BR. Practical aspects and complications of total parenteral nutrition. Crit Care Clin 1987;3:115.
15. Blackburn GL, Bistrian BR. Nutritional care of the injured and/or septic patient. Surg Clin North Am 1976;56:1195.
16. Border JR, Hassett JM. Multiple system organ failure. In: Clowes GHA Jr., ed. Trauma, sepsis and shock. New York: Marcel Dekker, 1988:335.
17. Brandt RM, Fernandes A, Mordhorst E, Kehlet H. Epidural analgesia improves postoperative nitrogen balance. Br Med J 1978;1:1106.
18. Cahill GF Jr. Ketosis. JPEN 1981;5:281.

19. Cerra FB. Nutrition in the critically ill: modern metabolic support in the intensive care unit. Crit Care: State Art 1986;7:1.
20. Cerra FB. The role of nutrition in the management of metabolic stress. Crit Care Clin 1986;2:807.
21. Cerra FB, Siegel JH, Coleman B, et al. Septic autocannibalism: a failure of exogenous nutritional support. Ann Surg 1980;192:570.
22. Cerra FB, Blackburn G, Hirsch J, et al. The effect of stress level, amino acid formula, and nitrogen dose on nitrogen retention in traumatic and septic stress. Ann Surg 1987;205:282.
23. Chernow B, Lake R, Barton M, et al. Sympathetic nervous system sensitivity to hemorrhagic hypotension in the subhuman primate. J Trauma 1984;24:229.
24. Clemmer TP, Orme JF Jr. Nutritional support in the adult respiratory distress syndrome. Clin Chest Med 1982;1:101.
25. Clowes GH, George BC, Villee CA, et al. Muscle proteolysis induced by a circulating peptide in patients with sepsis or trauma. N Engl J Med 1983;308:545.
26. Cuthbertson DP. The metabolic response to injury and its nutritional implications. JPEN 1979;3:108.
27. Damask MC, Weissman C, Askanazi J, et al. A systematic method for validating gas exchange measurements. Anesthesiology 1982;57:213.
28. Davies CL, Newman RJ, Molyneux SG, et al. The relationship between plasma catecholamines and the severity of injury in man. J Trauma 1984;24:99.
29. De Camp MM, Demling RH. Post-traumatic multisystem organ failure. JAMA 1988;260:530.
30. Edens NK, Gil KM, Elwyn DH. The effects of varying energy and nitrogen intake on nitrogen balance, body composition, and metabolic rate. Clin Chest Med 1986;7:3.
31. Edwards JD, Redmond AD, Nightingale P, Wilkins RG. Oxygen consumption following trauma: a reappraisal in severely injured patients requiring mechanical ventilation. Br J Surg 1988;75:690.
32. Egdahl RH. Pituitary-adrenal response following trauma to the isolated leg. Surgery 1959;46:9.
33. Eiper BA, Mains RE. Structure and biosynthesis of proadrenocorticotropin/endorphin and related peptides. Endocr Rev 1980;1:1.
34. Elwyn DH. Nutritional requirements of adult surgical patients. Crit Care Med 1980;8:9.
35. Elwyn DH. Protein metabolism and requirements in the critically ill patient. Crit Care Clin 1987;3:57.
36. Faden AJ, Holaday JW. Opiate antagonists: a role in the treatment of hypovolemic shock. Science 1979;205:317.
37. Fischer JE. Nutritional support in the seriously ill patient. Curr Prob Surg 1980;17:466.
38. Fischer JE, Rosen HM, Ebeid AM, et al. The effect of normalization of plasma amino acids on hepatic encephalopathy in man. Surgery 1976;80:77.
39. Freund HR. Nutritional support of the trauma patient. Prob Crit Care 1987;1:651.
40. Freund HR, Ryan JA, Fischer JE. Amino acid derangements in patients with sepsis: treatment with branched chain amino acids. Ann Surg 1978;188:423.
41. Friedman SG, Pearce FJ, Drucker WR. The role of blood glucose in defense of plasma volume. J Trauma 1982;22:86.
42. Gil KM, Askanazi J, Hyman AI. Substrate utilization in the acutely ill: implications for nutritional support. Crit Care: State Art 1984;5:C1–C45.
43. Gilder H. Parenteral nourishment of patients undergoing surgical or traumatic stress. JPEN 1986;10:88.
44. Gill GG, Bardin CW. The hypothalamic-pituitary control system. In: West JP, ed. Best and Taylor's physiologic basis of medical practice. Baltimore: Williams & Wilkins, 1985:854.
45. Goode AW. The scientific basis of nutritional assessment. Br J Anaesth 1981;53:161.
46. Gottlieb ME, Sarfeh J, Stratton H, et al. Hepatic perfusion and splanchnic oxygen consumption in patient postinjury. J Trauma 1983;23:836.
47. Grant JP. Nutrition in the trauma patient: In: Moylan JA, ed. Trauma surgery. Philadelphia: JB Lippincott, 1988:501.
48. Gurll NJ, Vargish T, Reynolds DG, et al. Opiate receptors and endorphins in the pathophysiology of hemorrhagic shock. Surgery 1981;89:364.
49. Harper HA. Review of physiological chemistry. Los Altos, CA: Lange Medical Publications, 1984.
50. Hasselgren PO, Jagenburg R, Karlstrom L, et al. Changes of protein metabolism in liver and skeletal muscle following trauma complicated by sepsis. J Trauma 1984;24:224.
51. Hassett J, Cerra FB, Siegel J, et al. Multiple systems organ failure—a very brief summary. Injury 1983;14:93.
52. Hershey SD, Moore EE, Jones TN. Nutritional care of the acutely injured. Adv Trauma 1986;1:21.
53. Herve P, Simonneau G, Girard P, et al. Hypercapnic acidosis induced by nutrition in mechanically ventilated patients: glucose versus fat. Crit Care Med 1985;13:537.
54. Heymsfield SB, Erbland M, Casper K, et al. Enteral nutritional support. Clin Chest Med 1986;7:41.
55. Hyman AI, Rodriquez J, Weissman C. Nutritional support of the critically ill patient. Semin Anesth 1982;1:354.
56. Iapichino G, Radrizzani D, Soka M, et al. The basic determinants of nitrogen balance during total parenteral nutrition in critically ill patients. Intens Care Med 1984;10:251.
57. Jaksic T, Blackburn GL. Nutritional support. In: Clowes GHA Jr, ed. Trauma, sepsis and shock. New York: Marcel Dekker, 1988:493.
58. Kenney PR, Allen CF, Rowlands A. Glucose and osmolality as predictors of injury severity. J Trauma 1983;23:712.
59. Kinney JM, Weissman C. Forms of malnutrition in stressed and unstressed patients. Clin Chest Med 1986;7:19.
60. Koruda MJ, Guenter P, Rombeau JL. Enteral nutrition in the critically ill. Crit Care Clin 1987;3:133.
61. Lakshman K, Blackburn GL. Monitoring nutritional status in the critically ill adult. J Clin Monitoring 1986;2:114.
62. Livingston RL. Visceral control mechanisms. In: West JB, ed. Best and Taylor's physiologic basis of medical practice. Baltimore: Williams & Wilkins, 1985:1211.
63. Lemoyne M, Jeejeebhoy KN. Total parenteral nutrition in the critically ill patient. Chest 1986;89:568.
64. Lilly M, Engeland WC, Cann DS. Adrenal response to repeated hemorrhage: implications for studies of trauma. J Trauma 1982;22:809.
65. Long CL. Energy balance and carbohydrate metabolism in infection and sepsis. Am J Clin Nutr 1977;30:1301.
66. Long CL, Schaffel N, Geiger JW, et al. Metabolic response to injury and illness. JPEN 1979;3:452.
67. Mann S, Westenskow DR, Houtchens BA. Measured and predicted caloric expenditure in the acutely ill. Crit Care Med 1985;13:173.
68. McClain CJ. Trace metal abnormalities in adults during hyperalimentation. JPEN 1981;5:424.
69. Meguid MM, Akahoshi MP, Debonis D, et al. Use of 20% fat emulsions in total parenteral nutrition. Crit Care Med 1986;14:29.
70. Merin RG, Samuelson PN, Schalch DS. Major inhalation anesthetics and carbohydrate metabolism. Anesth Analg 1971;50:625.
71. Moore EE, Jones TM. Benefits of immediate jejunostomy feeding after major abdominal trauma. J Trauma 1986;26:874.

72. Munro H. Nutritional requirements in health. Crit Care Med 1980;8:2.
73. Nordenstrom J, Jeevandaum M, Elwyn DH, et al. Increasing glucose intake during total parenteral nutrition increases norepinephrine secretion in trauma and sepsis. Clin Physiol 1981;1:525.
74. Odling-Smee GW. The metabolic response to injury. In: Odling-Smee W, Crockard A, eds. Trauma care. London: Academic Press, 1981:33.
75. Owen OE. Resting metabolic requirements of men and women. Mayo Clin Proc 1988;63:605.
76. Phillips RH, Valente WA, Caplan ES. Circulating thyroid hormone changes in acute trauma: prognostic implications on clinical outcome. J Trauma 1984;24:116.
77. Pingleton SK, Harmon GS. Nutritional management in acute respiratory failure. JAMA 1987;257:3094.
78. Prough DS, Coker LH, Lee S, et al. Hyperglycemia and neurologic outcome in patients with closed head injury. Anesthesiology 1988;69A:A584.
79. Pruitt BA. Forces and factors influencing trauma care. J Trauma 1984;24:463.
80. Quinn T, Askanazi J. Nutrition and cardiac disease. Crit Care Clin 1987;3:167.
81. Randall S, Blackburn GL. Nutritional therapy in trauma and sepsis. In: Siegel JH, ed. Trauma, emergency surgery and critical care. New York: Churchill Livingstone, 1987:543.
82. Randle PJ, Smith GH. Regulation of glucose uptake by muscle: (1) The effects of insulin, anaerobiosis and cell poisons on the uptake of glucose and release of potassium by isolated rat diaphragm. Biochem J 1958;70:490.
83. Rennie MJ, Harrison R. Effects of injury, disease, and malnutrition on protein metabolism in man. Lancet 1984;1:323.
84. Robin AP, Grieg PD. Basic principles of intravenous nutritional support. Clin Chest Med 1986;7:29.
85. Robin AP, Askanazi J, Greenwood RC, et al. Lipoprotein lipase activity in surgical patients: influence of trauma and infection. Surgery 1981;90:401.
86. Rochester DF, Esau SA. Malnutrition and the respiratory system. Chest 1984;85:411.
87. Russell JA, Long CNH, Engel FL. Biochemical studies on shock: (II) The role of peripheral tissue on the metabolism of protein and carbohydrate during hemorrhagic shock in the rat. J Exp Med 1944;79:1.
88. Ryan NT. Metabolic adaptations of energy production during trauma and sepsis. Surg Clin North Am 1976;56:1073.
89. Salerno TA, Miline B, Jhamandas KH. Hemodynamic effects of naloxone in hemorrhagic shock in pigs. Surg Gynecol Obstet 1981;152:773.
90. Savino JA, Dawson JA, Agerwai N, et al. The metabolic cost of breathing in critical surgical patients. J Trauma 1985;25:1126.
91. Schlichtig R, Ayres SM. Nutritional support of the critically ill. Chicago: Year Book Medical Publishers, 1988.
92. Schummer W. The metabolic effects of trauma. Contemp Surg 1972;1:39.
93. Shaw JHF, Wildbore M, Wolfe RR. Whole body protein kinetics in severely septic patients. Ann Surg 1987;205:288.
94. Shaw JHF, Wolfe RR. An integrated analysis of glucose, fat, and protein metabolism in severely traumatized patients. Studies in the basal state and the response to total parenteral nutrition. Ann Surg 1989;209:63.
95. Sieber F, Smith DS, Kupferberg J, et al. Effect of intraoperative glucose on protein catabolism and plasma glucose levels in patients with supratentorial tumors. Anesthesiology 1986;64:453.
96. Steinberg DL. Regulation of carbohydrate metabolism. In: West JB, ed. Best and Taylor's physiologic basis of medical practice. Baltimore: Williams & Wilkins, 1985:792.
97. Steinberg DL. Regulation of lipid and lipoprotein metabolism. In: West JB, ed. Best and Taylor's physiologic basis of medical practice. Baltimore: Williams & Wilkins, 1985:805.
98. Streat SJ, Beddoe AH, Hill GH. Aggressive nutritional support does not prevent protein loss despite fat gain in septic intensive care patients. J Trauma 1987;27:262.
99. Swanson SW, Sawchenko PE. Hypothalamic integration. Organization of the paraventricular and supraoptic nuclei. Ann Rev Neurosci 1983;6:269.
100. Swerlick RA, Drucker NA, McKoy S, et al. Insulin effectiveness in hypovolemic dogs. J Trauma 1981;21:1013.
101. Swinamer DL, Phang PT, Jones RL, et al. Effect of routine administration of analgesia on energy expenditure in critically ill patients. Chest 1988;92:4.
102. Takala J. Nutrition in acute renal failure. Crit Care Clin 1987;3:155.
103. Takala J, Askanazi J, Weissman C, et al. Changes in respiratory control induced by amino acid infusions. Crit Care Med 1988;16:465.
104. Tao RC, Kelley RE, Yoshimura NY, et al. Glycerol: its metabolism and use as an intravenous energy source. JPEN 1983;7:479.
105. Tsuji H, Shirasaka C, Asoh T, Uchida I. Effects of epidural administration of local anesthetics or morphine on postoperative nitrogen loss and catabolic hormones. Br J Surg 1987;74:421.
106. Twomey P, Ziegler D, Rombeau J. Utility of skin testing in nutritional assessment: a critical review. JPEN 1982;6:50.
107. Twyman DL, Bivins BA. Nutritional support of the brain injured patient. Henry Ford Hosp Med J 1986;34:41.
108. Van Landingham SB, Key JC, Symmonds RE. Nutritional support of the surgical patient. Surg Clin North Am 1982;62:321.
109. Van Lanschot JJB, Feenstra BWA, Vermeij CG, et al. Calculation versus measurement of total energy expenditure. Crit Care Med 1986;14:981.
110. Vente JP, Von Meyenfeldt MF, Van Eijk HMH, et al. Plasma-amino acid profiles in sepsis and stress. Ann Surg 1989;209:57.
111. Vestrup JA. Nutrition in the surgical patient. Can J Anaesth 1987;34:516.
112. Weissman C, Hyman AI. Nutritional care of the critically ill patient with respiratory failure. Crit Care Clin 1987;3:185.
113. Weissman C, Kemper M, Askanazi J, et al. Resting metabolic rate of the critically ill patient: measured versus predicted. Anesthesiology 1986;64:673.
114. Wiener M, Rothkopf MM, Rothkopf G, Askanazi J. Fat metabolism in injury and stress. Crit Care Clin 1987;3:25.
115. Willatts SM. Nutrition. Br J Anaesth 1986;58:201.
116. Williams WW. Infection control during parenteral nutrition therapy. JPEN 1985;9:735.
117. Wilson DO, Rogers RM, Hoffman RM. Nutrition and chronic lung disease. Am Rev Respir Dis 1985;132, 1347.
118. Wolfe BM, Ruderman RL, Pollard A. Basic principles of surgical nutrition: metabolic responses to starvation, trauma and sepsis. In: Dietel M, ed. Nutrition in clinical surgery. 2nd ed. Baltimore: Williams & Wilkins, 1985:14.
119. Wolfe RR. Carbohydrate metabolism in the critically ill patient. Crit Care Clin 1987;3:11.
120. Woolfson AMJ, Heatley RV, Allison SP. Insulin to inhibit protein catabolism after injury. N Engl J Med 1979;300:14.
121. Young B, Ott L, Rapp R, Roston J. The patient with critical neurological disease. Crit Care Clin 1987;3:217.

# Chapter Twenty-Three

*P. Prithvi Raj*
*Craig Hartrick*
*Charles E. Pither*

# Pain Management of the Injured

In the United States about 60 million accidental injuries occur annually, resulting in approximately 95,000 deaths, 350,000 permanent disabilities, and 8.5 million temporary disabilities.[2] The cost of accidents to the United States is enormous, reaching $133 billion in 1987.[2] In addition, homicides and suicides result in the loss of 50,000 lives and cause at least 100,000 permanent disabilities every year.[2]

The impact of pain from all causes on human suffering, productivity, and the national economy is on a par with that of trauma. Accurate statistics from national epidemiologic studies on the prevalence of pain and its effect on the national economy are not easy to find. However, estimates can be made from local and regional surveys. In a community survey, Crook et al.[99] demonstrated that 16% of the individuals from a small sample of the general population complained of pain within a given 2-week period: 11% had persistent pain, whereas in 5% pain was temporary. The patients in the persistent pain group were disabled for an average of 3 days, and those who had temporary pain were unproductive for 4 days during the 2-week period. Accidents accounted for 19% of acute pain and 26% of persistent pain. Obviously, inclusion of hospitalized patients with various types of acute pain and those actively treated for chronic pain would have resulted in a higher prevalence rate. Bonica,[39,40] based on data gathered from a variety of sources, estimates that annually about 15 to 20% of people in industrialized nations experience acute painful conditions requiring treatment and about 25 to 30% have chronic pain. Nearly one-half to two-thirds of patients with chronic pain are partially or totally disabled for a period ranging from days to years.[39,40] For these patients pain, not the underlying pathology, is the primary disabling factor. Thus, in addition to causing unnecessary suffering, pain is an important factor in inhibiting or abolishing people's productivity. The cost of pain from all causes to the American society in workdays lost, health care expenses, and compensation was estimated to be $60 billion in 1980 and nearly $70–80 billion in 1983.[40,74] Epidemiologic data collected by Louis Harris from a survey of 1,254 people across the United States are shown in Table 23-1.[293]

Although precise figures on the proportion of injured patients with disabling pain are lacking, we estimate that nearly one-third of the 60 million accidental injuries that occur annually are associated with acute, moderate to severe pain. Acute and chronic pain from sports injuries is becoming increasingly significant, the highest injury rate occurring in contact sports, such as football, soccer, and rugby (4.9 per 100 participants).[393] Skiing is another common cause of injury. Almost 500,000 persons are injured and 250,000 fractures occur each year from this sport alone.[298]

Pain management may be needed in three phases after injury. First, it is needed for the acute pain that is caused by the injury itself. Various specialists, including paramedics, emergency department physicians, surgeons, and anesthesiologists, are involved in pain treatment during this phase. Second, pain management is needed for postoperative pain, which involves a period of 7 to 10 days after surgery. Anesthesiologists are actively involved in treating pain during this phase. Some anesthesia departments now have teams to provide acute and postoperative pain relief in critical care areas. The need for proper use of the various methods that produce

TABLE 23-1. Epidemiology of Pain*

| | |
|---|---|
| Pain | Number one health complaint |
| Headaches | The most common pain complaint |
| Backaches | 56% |
| Muscle pains | 53% |
| Joint pains | 51% |
| Stomach pains | 46% |
| Menstrual pains | 40% |
| Arthritis | Most common medical condition cited for pain |
| People under stress | Report more aches and pains |
| Working women | Have more complaints than homemakers |
| Doctor consulted | If the pain was felt more than six times a year in 88% of pain complainers |
| Pain killers prescribed | 42% of patients consulted |
| Nonprescription drugs | Taken by 17% of patients |
| Exercises useful | In 18% of patients |
| People who exercise, don't smoke, or drink moderately | Have less pain than their counterparts |
| People who exercise strenuously | Complain of more muscle pain but fewer backaches and joint pains |

* Statistics from survey of 1,254 people across the United States by Louis Harris and Associates. Published in *USA Today*, October 23, 1985.

postoperative analgesia is well acknowledged, and research in this realm has been encouraged by various medical specialties, including anesthesiology, critical care medicine, and surgery. The third phase involves the management of chronic pain, which is usually treated 2 months or more after injury. In this chapter is presented a discussion of the effect of pain and its treatment on organ function, which is followed by a detailed examination of analgesic techniques during each of these three phases of pain management.

## PATHOPHYSIOLOGY OF ORGAN FUNCTION AND PAIN IN THE INJURED

Pain sensation usually serves a protective function. Although withdrawal reflexes and muscle guarding act initially to avoid further injury, the perception of pain permits learned avoidance behavior. Diagnostically, pain helps identify sites of somatic or visceral anatomic disruption and the topography of physiologic dysfunction. Pathophysiologically, tissue injury and concomitant pain evoke an endocrine-metabolic response. The stress response is characterized by increased catecholamine and cortisol levels, which can be essential to the maintenance of homeostasis in the absence of appropriate intervention.

Once the process of injury has been identified and halted, and diagnostic delineation of the injury is complete, further nociceptive information serves no protective role. In fact, continued pain may serve only to increase anxiety and the stress response, which taxes physiologic reserves.

The rationale for treatment of posttraumatic and postoperative pain therefore must encompass more than humanitarian considerations if morbidity secondary to trauma is to be reduced. Reduction of stress, restoration of function, and prevention of subsequent complications are all intimately related to posttraumatic analgesia and must be addressed.

### ACUTE INJURY

When the traumatized patient arrives in the emergency department, attention should be directed first toward initial resuscitation and stabilization. Priority should be given to establishing ventilatory and cardiovascular stability, controlling the external hemorrhage, and restoring fluid and blood volume. Attention then should be shifted to determining the site of injury in order to plan for appropriate therapeutic intervention. After this, consideration should be given to providing adequate pain relief. Analgesics, if needed, should be administered without delay when initial assessment and resuscitation are completed. The analgesic agent, its dose, and its route of administration must be selected carefully with due consideration to the patient's hemodynamic, respiratory, and neurologic status and the possibility of regurgitation and aspiration of gastric contents.

Although most preliminary diagnostic and therapeutic procedures (tracheal intubation, paracentesis, chest tube insertion, etc.) can be performed with local or topical anesthetics, systemic or regional analgesic or anesthetic techniques may be required for optimal performance of certain radiologic or CT scanning studies and such painful procedures as fracture splinting or reduction. In addition to facilitating specific diagnostic therapeutic interventions, there is now ample evidence that pain relief can decrease both patient anxiety and the stress response.[27,45,51,53,193,194,245,285,399]

### STRESS RESPONSE TO INJURY AND PAIN

The stress response is a complex hormonal and neurologic sequence mediated via adrenergic sympathetic pathways. This response may help promote survival. It is triggered by a variety of factors associated with injury, including the release of humoral substances from the traumatized area, hemorrhage, pain, fear, hypoxia, hypercarbia, acidosis, and changes in body temperature.[136,169,403] Increased sympathetic efferent activity, along with elevated serum levels of epinephrine, norepinephrine, growth hormone, cortisol, renin, aldosterone, antidiuretic hormone (ADH), enkephalin, and endorphin, results in tachycardia, hypertension, decreased renal and splanchnic blood flow, decreased glomerular filtration, and sodium and water retention.[136] The predominant catabolic response leads to hyperglycemia, which is caused by increased glycogenolysis, lipolysis, and proteinolysis in the presence of decreased glucose turnover (see also Chapter 22). Vasoconstriction and tachycardia associated with the stress response are important compensatory life-sustaining mechanisms before therapeutic intervention. However, once treatment is initiated, further stress or amplification of existing stress is unnecessary and can be deleterious to patients at risk for end-organ ischemia or infarction.[54,122,194,197,370]

Pain is considered to be an important factor in the production of the stress response to surgery.[325] Although its exact role in the neuroendocrine response of the multiple trauma patient is not clearly defined, in animals the ACTH response to hemorrhage is potentiated by noxious stimulation (Fig. 23-

1).[28] In addition, pain alone causes release of endorphins, enkephalins, catecholamines, ACTH, ADH, and other hormones to maintain life during acute stress.[136] Nevertheless, suppression of this endocrine response by alleviation of pain should be considered beneficial rather than deleterious as long as the pain treatment modalities do not cause uncontrollable hemodynamic alteration and adrenocortical hormone depletion. For instance, administration of epidural or spinal analgesia to a hemorrhaging patient to control pain will result in significant hypotension that may be difficult to correct.[44] Likewise, etomidate infusion to provide sedation and reduce anxiety in critically ill ICU patients may be fraught with danger. Etomidate, once frequently used in Europe, has been implicated in increasing the mortality rate of critically ill trauma patients.[205,206] This drug inhibits the activity of the enzymes, 17-alpha and 11-beta hydroxylase, which catalyze the conversion of 11-deoxycortisol to active cortisol.[276,382] Fortunately, however, drugs generally used to treat acute traumatic or surgical pain or to relieve anxiety do not interfere with steroidogenesis.

Considerable work has been done on modifying the stress response to anesthesia and surgery. Although most of the available data in this area pertains to patients undergoing various types of elective surgical operations and may not exactly reflect the response of the traumatized patient, some similarities may exist between the two patient populations.

The stress response to surgery may be modified by three different techniques: parenterally administered narcotic agents, spinally administered narcotic agents, and afferent neuronal blockade by local anesthetics. Although all of these methods are commonly used to control pain and abolish endocrine and metabolic responses to accidental or surgical trauma, a significant endocrine response in the absence of pain may be observed after surgery.[60,78,173] The cause of the neuroendocrine response to trauma in these circumstances was at one time thought to be the release of humoral substances from surgical or traumatic wounds. This concept was refuted by Egdahl's classical experiments in 1959.[118] He and his co-worker Hume emphasized the importance of an intact nervous system in mediating the adrenocortical response to trauma. Although later Wilmore et al.[403] suggested that humoral substances could be responsible for initiating the metabolic and hormonal response to severe trauma and burns, the importance of intact afferent pathways as a release mechanism has been well accepted.[196]

FIG. 23-1. Potentiation of ACTH response to hemorrhage by pain in cats. H = hemorrhage; TP = pain produced by tooth pulp stimulation; H + TP = hemorrhage and tooth pulp stimulation. * $p < 0.05$ vs. baseline; ** $p < 0.01$ vs. baseline. Letters a, b, c, and d above each sample time point represent the statistical significance of differences between H + TP and H or TP alone. (From Bereiter et al[28] with permission.)

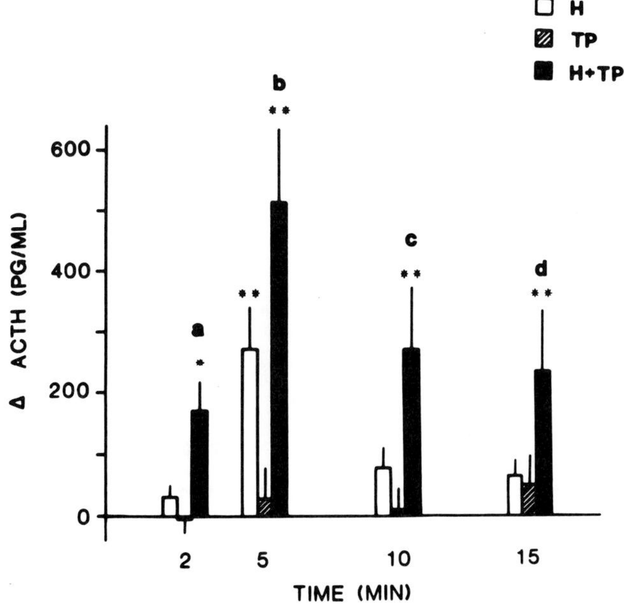


## *Effect of Parenterally Administered Narcotic Agents on Pain and the Stress Response*

During surgery, the extent of inhibition of the stress response by parenterally administered narcotic agents depends upon the narcotic used, its dose, the type of surgery, and the extent of physiologic disturbances associated with the procedure. For instance, relatively small intraoperative doses of morphine (1 mg/kg) are capable of inhibiting ACTH release, blocking the pituitary-adrenal axis, and preventing the substrate mobilization response to noncardiac surgery.[139] Equal doses of morphine, however, cannot prevent the rise of plasma catecholamines during cardiac surgery.[17] Higher doses of morphine (4 mg/kg)[52,139] fentanyl (75 μg/kg)[331,352,389] and sufentanil (20 μg/kg)[48] can at least partially prevent the endocrine-metabolic response to cardiac surgery until the initiation of cardiopulmonary bypass. After this period, however, plasma cortisol, adrenaline, noradrenaline, and ADH levels rise. Still higher doses of these narcotics may perhaps block the stress response during and after cardiopulmonary bypass, but the resulting prolonged respiratory depression would negate their beneficial effects. Modification of the stress response during noncardiac surgery by morphine (1 mg/kg),[139] fentanyl (50 μg/kg),[86,163] alfentanil (150 μg/kg followed by 3 μg/kg/min infusion),[244] and fentanyl infusion (1.5–2.5 μg/kg/min)[281] has been described. Although it is difficult to assess the relationship between the narcotic doses required to abolish pain and those needed to blunt the stress response during anesthesia, it appears that stress response inhibition requires higher doses of narcotics than those required to control pain.

Postoperatively, both pain and the stress response to surgery continue. High-dose narcotic agents used during surgery can prevent the rise of plasma cortisol and glucose concentrations only during the first few postoperative hours.[244] After this period, surgically induced endocrine-metabolic changes become apparent. Systemically administered opiates in their usual doses may provide partial pain relief during the postoperative period, but they cannot adequately block endocrine and metabolic responses.[78,173,228,415]

## *Effect of Spinally Administered Narcotic Agents on Pain and the Stress Response*

Spinally administered narcotics are effective in eliminating pain after surgical and accidental trauma.[78,325,347] However, both epidural and intrathecal opiates, with the possible exception of meperidine,[96] have been shown to be ineffective in blocking the stress response during surgery.[77,78,115,173,186,325,332] Postoperatively, however, plasma glucose and cortisol levels with these agents are lower than those seen after general anesthesia and parenteral opiates, although they are still higher than in patients receiving epidural local anesthetics.[78] The inability of spinal opiates to suppress the stress response completely may be due to their lack of effect on pain pathways dependent on γ-aminobutyric acid (GABA) and sympathetic or proprioceptive afferents. It has been shown that intrathecal/epidural narcotics block C-fiber nociceptive discharge preferentially, and thus they are more effective for relief of dull postoperative pain than surgical pain.[196]

### *Effect of Epidurally Administered Local Anesthetics on Pain and the Stress Response*

Since the endocrine-metabolic response to surgery is mainly initiated via afferent neurogenic stimuli (somatic and sympathetic pathways), neural blockade with local anesthetic agents should abolish both pain and the stress response by interrupting these pathways.[195,245] In fact, epidural analgesia with local anesthetic agents, including T6 through L2 spinal segments, has been particularly effective in abolishing the stress response during and after lower abdominal surgery.[27,37,51,193,197,245] This effect of epidural analgesia results from its inhibition of catecholamine discharge from the adrenal glands, which are innervated by these segments. However, epidural blockade (T5 sensory level) has been less effective in abolishing the stress response during upper abdominal as compared to lower abdominal surgery.[60,325] Although this is thought to be due to unblocked afferent pathways transmitted via the vagus, a study by Traynor and coworkers disputes this mechanism.[371] Ligation or infiltration of the vagus nerve with local anesthetic agents had no effect on the stress response.

Brandt et al.[51] found that postoperative epidural analgesia with local anesthetic agents maintained for 24 hours was associated with a reduction of negative nitrogen balance during the subsequent 4 postoperative days. Reduced plasma glucose and cortisol levels were presumed to account for the relative improvement in nitrogen balance in these patients. There is evidence that suppression of blood glucose concentrations may be related to reduced splanchnic release of glucose. This would diminish the splanchnic uptake of gluconeogenic substrates, thereby producing an improvement in nitrogen balance.[212]

Although epidural blockade with local anesthetics suppresses endocrine and metabolic responses to surgery more than systemically or spinally administered narcotics, it cannot reverse the moderate rise of plasma cortisol levels seen immediately after the initiation of surgery (Fig. 23-2).[12,162,245,325] Since all patients receiving epidural analgesia have excellent pain relief, it is obvious from these results that the catabolic response to surgery cannot be entirely prevented by analgesia.[173]

### *Modification of the Stress Response by Pain Relief in Acutely Traumatized Patients*

The stress response after acute multiple trauma and burn injuries is far greater than that observed after elective surgery (see Chapters 20 and 22). As many of these patients are also in severe pain, analgesia may provide greater attenuation of the stress response and a better outcome compared to those

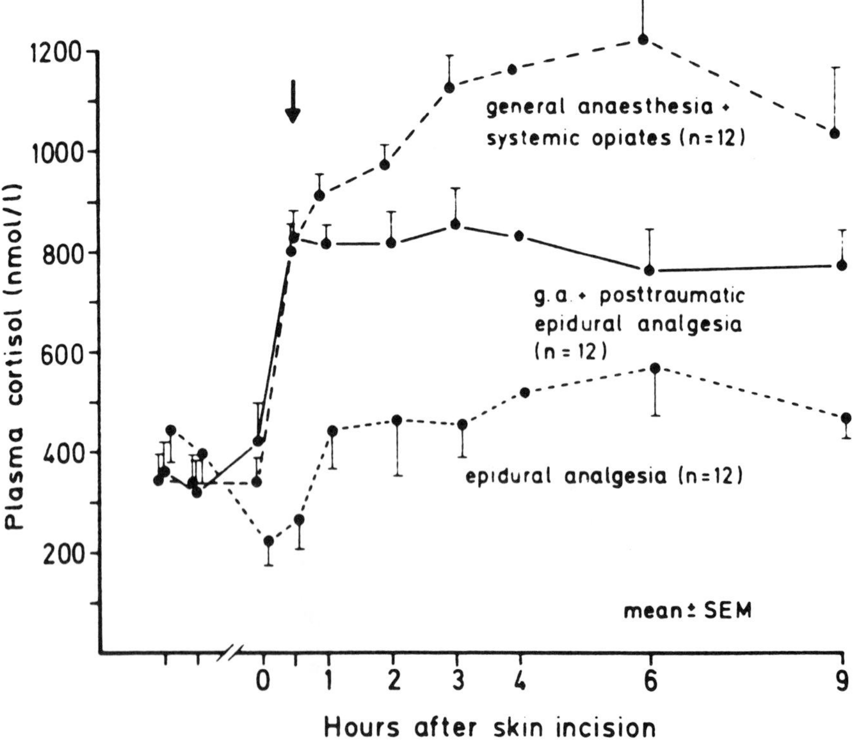


FIG. 23-2. Graph showing the influence of posttraumatic (surgical) neurogenic blockade on plasma cortisol response. The arrow indicates the commencement of epidural blockade 30 minutes after skin incision (*middle trace*). It is obvious that posttraumatic epidural blockade inhibits a further rise in the plasma cortisol level, although it cannot return it to baseline. General anesthesia alone (*uppermost trace*) cannot prevent the cortisol rise caused by surgical trauma, whereas epidural analgesia administered before surgery (*lowermost trace*) blunts this response. (From Moller et al[245] with permission.)

with postoperative pain. Unfortunately, the available data on this subject are too scanty and are mostly limited to burn injuries. Taylor et al.,[364] using high doses of morphine, were able to demonstrate a reduction in oxygen consumption, temperature, catecholamine, and nitrogen excretion in burn patients. Demling,[105] in a review article on burn injuries, suggested that afferent responses to increased metabolism can be accentuated by the brain, especially when pain and anxiety are present. However, pain relief by spinal anesthesia in one patient and by topically applied local anesthetics in three burn patients failed to attenuate the stress response.[402] In a preliminary study, Demling[104] demonstrated that burn patients with high plasma levels of beta-endorphin developed sepsis. Administration of opiates and sedatives produced decreased beta-endorphin levels, and these patients appeared to do well during the postinjury period. However, the question was raised whether increased beta-endorphin levels indeed contributed to sepsis and death in the group with poor outcome. More recently, a temporal association has been established between depressed immune parameters and elevated beta-endorphin levels after multiple trauma.[208] Finally, Szyfelbein et al.[363] demonstrated an inverse relationship between the severity of pain and plasma endorphin immunoreactivity during dressing changes in burned children. Clearly, further well-controlled studies are needed to determine the effect of pain relief on the stress response in acutely traumatized patients. However, it appears that adequate pain control in this group of patients modifies the stress response and probably improves outcome.

### *Stress Response in Chronic Pain Patients*

Chronic pain, like acute pain, may lead to episodic cortisol release. There seems to be a correlation between the intensity of pain and increased plasma cortisol levels.[113] However, information on this subject is far from conclusive.

## EFFECT OF INJURY AND PAIN ON RESPIRATORY FUNCTION

Oxygenation can be impaired in the trauma patient for a variety of reasons. Pulmonary injury as a result of direct penetrating wounds or parenchymal contusion, aspiration of gastric contents, or parenchymal compression due to hemothorax or pneumothorax occurs frequently. Hypoventilation and atelectasis caused by reduced chest wall and diaphragmatic movement can result from (a) pain and resulting chest wall and thoracoabdominal muscle spasm and (b) the anatomic disruption of chest wall mechanics secondary to surgery and/or rib or sternal fractures. In addition, anxiety, neuroticism, and fear, frequently observed in traumatized patients, may potentiate pain and pulmonary morbidity.[279,329] Parbrook et al.[279] found a significant correlation between neuroticism, postoperative pain, and pulmonary morbidity in 50 male patients undergoing elective gastric surgery.

On the first day after elective surgery, FVC and $FEV_1$ may decrease 75% for thoracic, 68% for xyphoid-to-pubis abdominal, 61% for paramedian upper abdominal, 53% for subcostal, and 38% for midline lower abdominal incisions.[183] These changes, albeit with gradual improvement, frequently continue for up to 2 weeks after surgery.[97] Postanesthetic respiratory failure is most common when these insults are complicated by pre-existing chronic obstructive pulmonary disease.[137] Posttraumatic and postoperative pain relief in these patients often facilitates the institution of chest physiotherapy, restoration of pulmonary function, prevention of further deterioration, and weaning from mechanical ventilatory support.

### *Effect of Various Pain Treatment Modalities on Postoperative Pulmonary Function*

There has been a great effort to discover new pain treatment modalities to improve pulmonary function during the postoperative period. Indeed, some analgesic methods appear to result in better lung function than others, although considerable discordance among the results of various studies exists. Many factors play a role in this discrepancy; most notable are differences in patient population and study design. It is important to remember that postoperative pain per se is not the sole factor producing pulmonary dysfunction.[97] Consequently, it is not surprising that, even in the presence of excellent postoperative pain relief, respiratory dysfunction remains, although decreased in magnitude. In general, the difference in lung function among techniques producing adequate and inadequate pain relief does not seem to be more than 20–25%. For example, if, with a relatively ineffective analgesic method, a given respiratory function test is 40% of the preoperative value on the first postoperative day, effective analgesia will only bring this value up to 60% or 65%; complete reversal of respiratory dysfunction is not possible with any analgesic method.[11] Not infrequently, however, even a small improvement in pulmonary function may be beneficial since the increase in ventilation and oxygenation may be sufficient to avoid mechanical ventilation. Of course, serious abnormalities in respiratory function usually occur after upper abdominal and thoracic surgery; they are uncommon in other types of procedures, with the possible exception of some lower abdominal and hip surgery.

Spence[348] suggests that pulmonary sequelae of abdominal surgery occur in two phases. Phase I, which lasts approximately 24 hours, is characterized by a reduction in functional residual capacity (FRC), shallow breathing, and consequent arterial hypoxemia. In phase II, which lasts 48 hours or more, phase I changes combine with the retention of secretions and inability to cough, resulting in atelectasis. He further suggests that postoperative pneumonia is a consequence of phase I changes, and thus improvement in FRC during the first 24 hours of the postoperative period should minimize the late pulmonary sequelae of anesthesia or surgery. Nerve blocks with intercostal or epidural techniques have little value in improving FRC and the consequent hypoxemia, but they do have a beneficial effect on phase II changes. Bromage[58] demonstrated that end-expiratory intrathoracic pressure in patients with postoperative pain is more positive than that seen in patients without pain. This effect is accentuated during deep breathing, resulting in glottic closure, abdominal splinting, and grunting respiration. Parenterally administered narcotics are effective in improving end-expiratory pressure, but they also decrease tidal volume. Thus, the resulting decrease in grunting is an apparent but deceptive improvement. Segmental thoracic epidural analgesia, on the other hand, causes both a reduction in positive pressure and increased tidal volume, an obvious advantage over parenteral analgesics (Fig. 23-3).

More recently, Simonneau et al.,[340] by measuring abdominal and rib cage movements separately, demonstrated significant diaphragmatic dysfunction lasting about 1 week after upper abdominal surgery (Fig. 23-4). Interestingly, this dysfunction remained unchanged after analgesia provided by epidurally administered fentanyl, suggesting that chest and abdominal wall instability, rather than pain, is the prime factor in the pathogenesis of this problem. Thoracic epidural block with 0.5% bupivacaine up to the T4 segment, however, causes partial reversal of diaphragmatic dysfunction.[217] Thus, it appears that diaphragmatic dysfunction after upper abdominal surgery results from reflex inhibition of phrenic nerve activity by the abdominal compartment.[217]

As noted above, the degree of improvement in pulmonary function produced by analgesia depends upon the type of pain treatment used. Intramuscular morphine or meperidine, given at preset intervals or on demand, is still the most widely used method for postoperative analgesia and is the standard against which almost all more recently introduced methods of acute pain therapy are compared. Although some studies have demonstrated that postoperative lung function after the administration of intramuscular narcotics is comparable with that after other acute pain treatment methods,[240,284,317,350] it is well established that the ventilatory improvement offered by this method is less than that obtained by regional anesthetic techniques.[101,120,121,237,240,284,301,303,326,349] Postoperative respiratory function tests—peak expiratory flow rate (PEFR), forced vital capacity (FVC), forced expiratory volume (FEV), and FRC—are more depressed after parenteral opiates than after epidural analgesia (local anesthetics or narcotics) or intercostal blocks,[120,121,237,301,303] resulting in lower $PaO_2$[101,237,301,303,326]; less efficient coughing, deep breathing, and removal of bronchial secretions[240]; and an increased incidence of atelectasis and pulmonary infections.[101,284,326] Little difference in postoperative pulmonary function has been noted among studies comparing the administration of narcotics (a) intravenously (intermittent bolus or infusion) and intramuscularly,[4,24,101,253,317,337] (b) at regular intervals and on demand,[5] (c) with "patient-controlled" intravenous and conventional intramuscular injections,[317,397] and (d) by intramuscular or the more recently introduced "slow-release oral morphine."[127]

Transcutaneous electrical nerve stimulation (TENS) has been shown to minimize the tendency to altered respiratory mechanics and to decrease the incidence of pulmonary complications after elective cholecystectomy[5] and rib fractures.[345] TENS, when used alone, is usually not effective in abolishing

FIG. 23-3. Graphs showing thoracic pressure-tidal volume relationships during quiet breathing (*left panel*) and deep breathing (*right panel*) with untreated pain and after treatment of pain with meperidine or epidural analgesia. Note that end-expiratory esophageal pressure is more positive with pain than without pain and that this effect is accentuated during deep breathing. Both meperidine and epidural analgesia shift the end-expiratory pressure toward a less positive value, but the tidal volume decreases with meperidine whereas it increases with epidural analgesia. (From Bromage PR. Philadelphia: WB Saunders, 1978, with permission.)

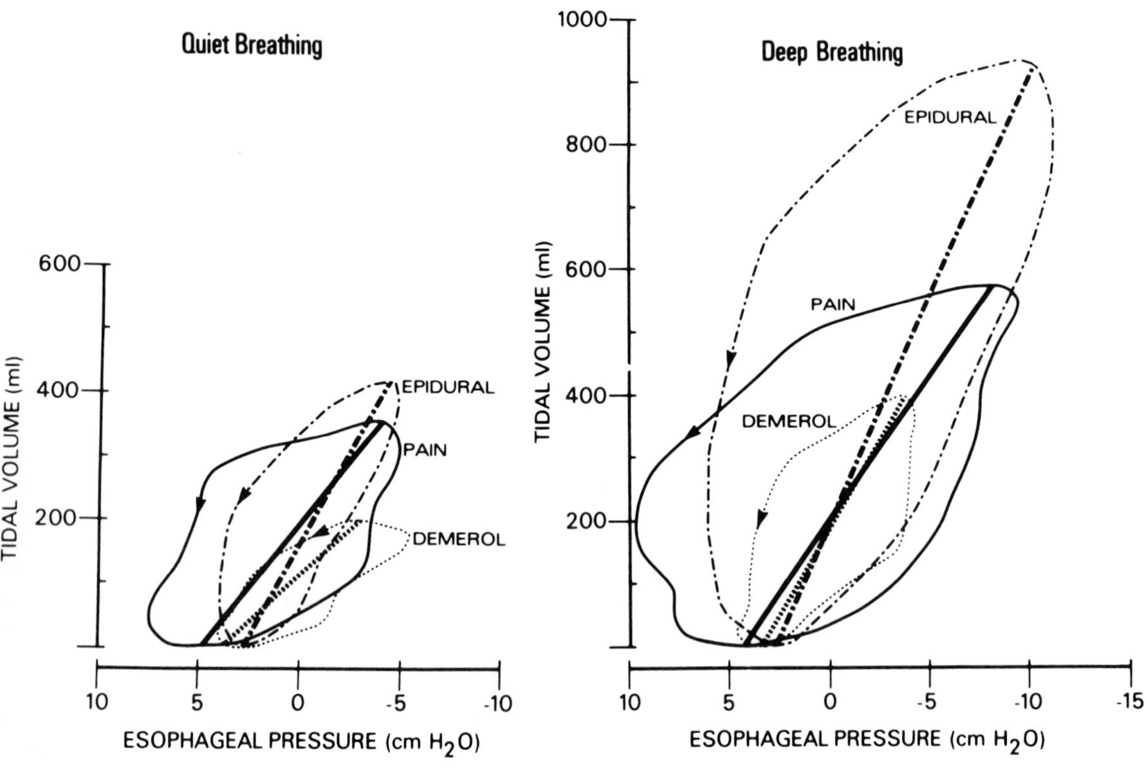

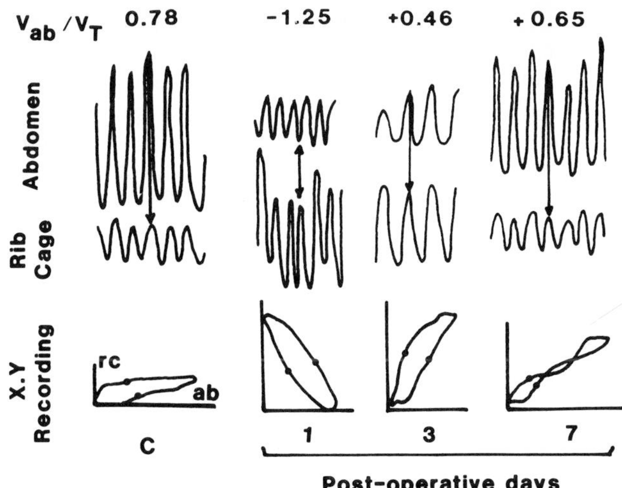


FIG. 23-4. Simultaneous recordings of abdominal and rib cage displacements within tidal breathing preoperatively (C) and 1, 3, and 7 days postoperatively (*upper panel*). $V_{ab}/V_T$ is the ratio between abdominal displacement and tidal volume. Note that the ratio decreases to a negative value on the first postoperative day, suggesting an inward instead of a normal outward movement of the anterior abdominal wall during inspiration. During the preoperative (C) period, abdominal and rib cage circumferences increased synchronously during inspiration as indicated by the arrow. On the first postoperative day abdominal wall and rib cage movements are asynchronous (*arrow*). Also, the amplitude of abdominal wall movement is decreased. The asynchrony reverts to normal on the third postoperative day. In the lower panel, the rib cage (rc) and abdominal displacements (ab) are plotted on an X-Y recorder. Note again the reversal of the loop on the first postoperative day and gradual normalization until the seventh postoperative day. Relief of postoperative pain by epidural fentanyl produced no improvement in these changes. (From Simonneau et al[340] with permission.)

postoperative pain, but with small doses of parenterally administered narcotic agents, it may reduce both pain and postoperative respiratory dysfunction.

Infiltration or continuous infusion of the surgical wound with local anesthetic agents produces postoperative pain relief and improvement in pulmonary function tests (FVC and $FEV_1$).[280] Although a significant reduction in pulmonary function remains, the amount of improvement by this method is shown to be adequate to increase arterial oxygenation and reduce the incidence of radiologically detected atelectasis.[280]

Multilevel intercostal blocks have been described by Moore as an excellent method of postoperative analgesia.[247] Their effects on various pulmonary function tests have been evaluated in normal and postoperative patients. Chest wall motor blockade produced by bilateral intercostal nerve block (T5–T11) may change the relationship between closing capacity and FRC, potentially causing hypoxemia and hypercarbia.[88,89] However, these complications are likely to occur only in elderly patients with high body mass indices (weight/height$^2$)[88]; in an otherwise healthy patient, the negative impact of intercostal block on respiratory function is probably negligible.[166] Several studies have demonstrated no difference in pulmonary function between patients receiving narcotics and those given intercostal blocks after thoracic or upper abdominal surgery.[120,121,317,409] However, unilateral intercostal block, given at multiple levels for a subcostal incision, caused a significant improvement in lung function, which became more pronounced if a second block was administered 8 hours later.[120,121] The results of many other studies also are consistent with improvement in pulmonary function and arterial blood gases with intercostal block after upper abdominal surgery.[57,254,301] We therefore believe that intercostal block using local anesthetic agents produces improvement, albeit incomplete, in pulmonary function tests (especially PEFR) and arterial blood gases. Since the duration of this block is not more than 12–16 hours, the procedure should be repeated at least twice during the postoperative period.

In an interesting randomized study, intraoperative injection of 6% phenol in glycerine (1 mL) into three intercostal nerves adjacent to the thoracotomy incision site produced good pain relief and significant improvement in inspiratory reserve volume and vital capacity.[322] The long term follow-up of these patients did not find that intercostal neuralgia was caused by phenol. We believe that several other series should document the beneficial effect of intraoperative intercostal phenol block before the method is recommended.

Intraoperative freezing of the intercostal nerves with a cryoprobe is another method of producing pain relief for 1 to 2 weeks after thoracotomy.[191] Analgesia produced by this method, however, does not appear to improve forced vital capacity during the postoperative period.[191]

It is clear that the lung function of patients with chronic lung disease can be improved when continuous segmental epidural analgesia with local anesthetic agents is used during the postoperative period.[339] In this group of patients, epidural analgesia may prevent respiratory failure and the consequent need for mechanical ventilation.[350] Until recently, however, the effect of this method on pulmonary function and arterial oxygenation, as compared with parenterally administered opioids, in patients without preoperative lung disease was somewhat less clear, since earlier reports could document little difference in their effects.[253,344,350] More recent data, however, suggest a definite improvement in lung function during segmental epidural analgesia.[24,100,101,237]

In healthy volunteers, segmental epidural analgesia limited to thoracic segments below T4 causes no significant change in FRC, $FEV_1$, FVC, $A\text{-}aDO_2$, $\dot{Q}_s/\dot{Q}_t$, or cardiac output.[383] The relationship between FRC and closing volume is also unchanged during this block. Thus, unlike general anesthesia, it does not affect airway closure or cause $\dot{V}/\dot{Q}$ abnormality.[213] During the first day after thoracic or upper abdominal surgery, epidural block, despite producing pain relief and improving mechanical parameters, has little effect on $PaO_2$ or $A\text{-}aDO_2$.[49] A rise in $PaO_2$ is observed after this period, which continues until the third or fourth postoperative day. Functional residual capacity may be restored to a moderate extent with epidural analgesia in operated patients, but this effect is variable, ranging from a moderate increase to no change.[384] The vital capacity increases by 30–40%, and the improvement is more pronounced in patients with chronic lung disease, reaching up to 50%.[49,339] The peak expiratory flow rate (PEFR) and the $FEV_1$ are markedly improved by thoracic and lumbar epidural analgesia, which facilitates coughing, deep breathing, and removal of secretions.[49,339] At least two reports have shown that the incidence of postoperative pulmonary complications, including chest infections, was decreased when epidural analgesia was employed.[110,284] Epidural analgesia is also shown to facilitate ambulation after surgery,[284] by which mechanism it may also decrease postoperative pulmonary complications.

Epidural or intrathecal opiates have been used extensively to relieve pain from various causes, including surgery. Some studies showed no change in pulmonary function when narcotics were administered epidurally after upper abdominal surgery.[46,317,340] They suggested that pain was not an important factor in diminished postoperative respiratory dysfunction. Although it is true that pain is not the only factor producing this complication, available data suggest that its treatment with epidurally or intrathecally administered opiates results in partial improvement of pulmonary function.

Bromage et al.[61] have demonstrated improved $FEV_1$ postoperatively with segmental analgesia produced by epidural narcotics. Benhamou et al.[24] demonstrated that intravenous morphine was unable to alter any objective pulmonary function in high-risk patients with respiratory disease after upper abdominal surgery. However, epidural morphine or epidural lidocaine was able to partially restore VC and $FEV_1$ to preoperative levels. The other effort-dependent ventilatory parameters, however, remained unaffected, suggesting a contribution from nonanalgesic factors. Rybro et al.[326] compared morphine administered on demand after upper abdominal surgery via the intramuscular and epidural routes. The epidural morphine group demonstrated a significant reduction in radiographic pulmonary changes and significantly higher $PaO_2$, with a slower rise in the alveolar-arterial oxygen gradient. Although $PaCO_2$ levels were similar in both groups, the amount of morphine required was far less via the epidural route. Other studies confirm that postoperatively FVC, $FEV_1$, and PEFR are less depressed with epidural than with parenteral morphine.[301,303,337] These findings suggest that regional anesthesia may modify the deterioration of pulmonary function frequently seen in the postoperative period. However, it is not clearly known whether the postoperative pulmonary infection rate is reduced by this method. Kehlet,[195] after cumulating data from several studies, suggested that postoperative pulmonary infections may be reduced by approximately 30% when regional anesthesia is used.

### *Effect of Pain and Analgesia on Pulmonary Function After Trauma*

The foregoing discussion has focused on the effect of pain and its relief on postoperative pulmonary function after elective upper abdominal and thoracic surgery. Except for thoracic injuries, there is little information specifically describing the relationship between postoperative pain and pulmonary dysfunction in spontaneously breathing traumatized patients. It is probably reasonable to assume that, in this group of patients, postoperative pain and its relief will affect pulmonary function in the same way as after elective surgery. However, in injured patients there may be additional factors increasing the severity of dysfunction. Pneumothorax, hemothorax, diaphragmatic injury, pulmonary aspiration, and neurally mediated parenchymal abnormalities are some of the complicating features that may nullify the effects of postoperative pain relief on pulmonary function and oxygenation.

Pain relief for the injured patient is required not only for alleviation of postoperative pain but also for pain produced directly by trauma. Classically, injuries to the chest resulting in rib and/or sternal fractures produce severe pain and impairment in pulmonary function, often necessitating mechanical ventilation during the immediate posttrauma period.[111,112,143,273] In conventional doses, parenterally administered narcotic agents are usually ineffective in relieving the pain and improving pulmonary function.[111,112,143] Increasing the dose until pain relief is obtained results in excessive sedation and respiratory depression.[143] Most patients treated with this method may need mechanical ventilation because of narcotic-induced respiratory failure. However, analgesia provided by continuous intercostal nerve block at the affected site produces remarkable improvement in spirometric volumes and arterial blood gases.[214,273] Likewise, pain relief with continuous segmental epidural analgesia with bupivacaine, 0.5% with 1/200,000 epinephrine, has been shown to produce a more than twofold increase in vital capacity and significant improvement in arterial blood gases.[411] Epidural (4–5 mg) or intrathecal (1 mg) morphine injection produces pain relief and improvement in pulmonary function in some patients during normal breathing,[109,198] but patients may be uncomfortable during pulmonary physiotherapy.[300] The use of epidural bupivacaine, 0.5% with 1/200,000 epinephrine, to provide analgesia for chest physiotherapy and of epidural morphine (3 mg) to produce patient comfort during the intervening period resulted in improved arterial blood gases and recovery without ventilatory support in 43 of 50 patients.[300] Mechanical ventilation was indicated in only two of the remaining patients because of inadequate pain relief and lack of improvement in lung function. Acute respiratory distress and myocardial infarction were the causes of mechanical ventilation in the other patients. We believe, as do others, that continuous epidural analgesia with local anesthetic agents is the first choice in treating pain and improving pulmonary function after chest trauma.[109]

Although the effects of various pain treatment modalities on pulmonary function in posttraumatic pain syndromes have not been studied as extensively as in postoperative pain, available data suggest that improvement in pulmonary function and oxygenation with pain relief in this group of patients is more prompt and greater than that obtained for postoperative pain. This effect is probably the result of a more limited abdominal and/or chest wall disruption in trauma victims who have not had surgery than in postoperative patients.

## EFFECT OF PAIN AND ANALGESIA ON CARDIOVASCULAR FUNCTION

Trauma, surgical or accidental, produces increased sympathetic activity resulting in hyperkinetic circulation. Pain associated with trauma contributes to this response, so that its elimination may result in decreased heart rate, blood pressure, cardiac output, and peripheral vascular resistance. Almost any analgesic method, with the exception of TENS, may cause hypotension if the patient's circulating blood volume is depleted enough and he or she is placed in the upright position.

However, the likelihood of hypotension varies with the analgesic technique. Analgesia produced by epidurally injected local anesthetic agents is more likely to produce hypotension than that produced by parenteral or spinal opioids or intercostal block. Parenteral opiates may produce hypotension by causing arterial and venous dilation (histamine release), by blunting cardiovascular responses to postural changes, and, at very high doses, by reducing coronary blood flow.[225] At clinically used doses, narcotic agents usually have negligible myocardial depressant effects.[225] Fentanyl, sufentanil, alfentanil, and probably methadone have the least potential, among agonist narcotic agents, of producing cardiovascular depression. Likewise, nalbuphine and other agonist-antagonist opioids may have minimal cardiovascular effects.[225] Meperidine, especially at high doses, produces the greatest cardiovascular depression and should be avoided in critically ill hypovolemic patients. In general, parenterally administered opioid agents produce less severe hemodynamic alterations than epidural analgesia.

Although there are only limited data about the cardiovascular effects of intercostal blockade, this method is seldom accompanied by clinically significant hemodynamic changes. Occasionally, however, it may produce severe hypotension. The mechanism of this effect is not clear. Nunn and Slavin,[270] after showing a free subpleural distribution of local anesthetic solution, speculated that the drug can spread medially to the anterolateral portion of the thoracic vertebra and produce sympathetic blockade. In contrast, Moore's group demonstrated that the endothoracic fascia fuses with the periosteum at the posterior aspect of the thoracic vertebral body, preventing spread to the sympathetic chain.[248,249] Middaugh et al.,[234] by using radionuclides in one patient, showed the paravertebral spread of local anesthetic solution, which could potentially produce epidural blockade of multiple dermatomes (Fig. 23-5). Later, these authors, after studying 15 additional patients, confirmed their findings, but they stated that the pattern of spread is variable[235] and epidural spread did not occur in all patients (Middaugh et al., personal communication). The finding of paravertebral spread of local anesthetic has been corraborated by Mowbray et al.[251] who have also demonstrated that occasionally the drug can spread to the contralateral side over the anterior surface of the vertebral body. Murphy,[256] who introduced the technique of continuous intercostal nerve blockade, demonstrated in cadavers that epidural spread does not occur. In view of this controversy, it is difficult to state that sympathetic and epidural blockades are the only causes of hypotension, even though total spinal anesthesia has been described after intercostal nerve blocks.[138] This complication, which usually occurs after an intrathoracic approach, may be caused by injection of local anesthetic directly into the dural cuff. It is also possible that the notoriously high systemic blood concentration of local anesthetic that occurs after intercostal blockade may contribute to the occasional development of hypotension.

Hemodynamic alterations produced by epidural analgesia with local anesthetic agents depend on (a) the region, extent, and level of the block; (b) the use of vasoconstrictor agents; (c) the presence of pain and the degree of sympathetic overactivity before the block; and (d) the intravascular volume before administration of epidural analgesia.

FIG. 23-5. Upper images show a radionuclide scan of a patient before (A) and after (B, C, and D) receiving a continuous intercostal nerve block with divided doses of bupivacaine 0.5%, 13 mL, mixed with 500 uCi technetium-99-m diethylenetriamminepenta-acetic acid (DTPA). Lower images (B, C, and D) represent radioactivity associated with local anesthetic only, the bony elements having been subtracted. The subtraction image in A is blank since no anesthetic is given. In B, 3 mL of bupivacaine 0.5% is given, 5 mL in C, and an additional 5 mL in D. Note the increasing paravertebral spread of anesthetic in B, C, and D as shown by arrows on the upper images and by gradually enhanced radioactivity in the lower images. (From Middaugh et al[234] with permission.)

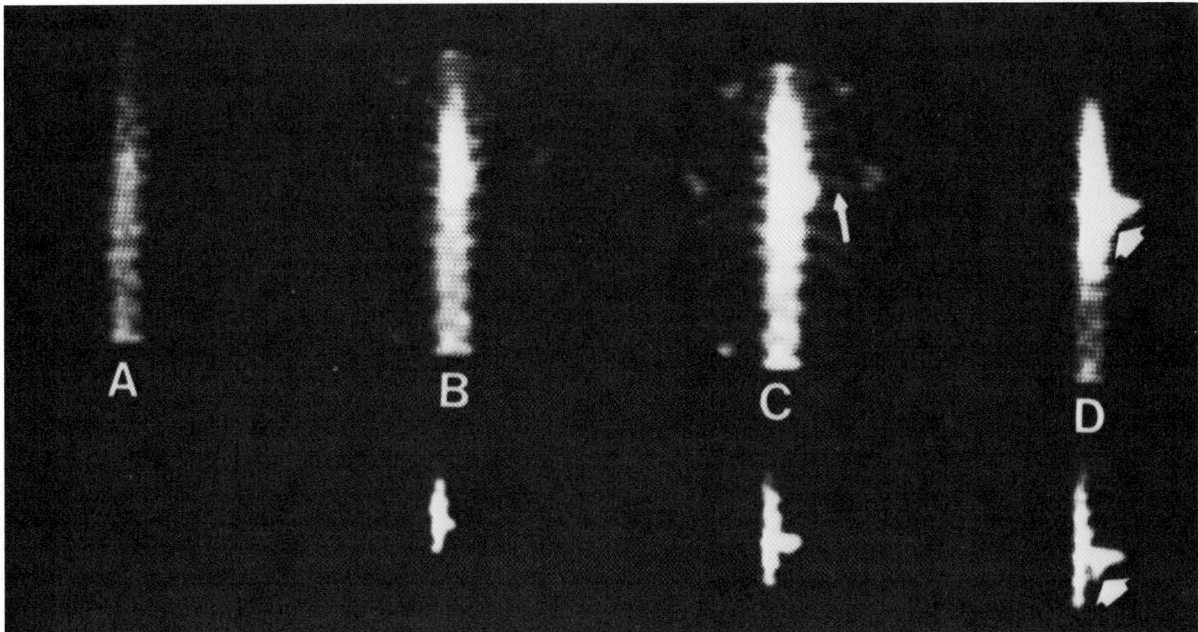

Lumbar epidural analgesia with lidocaine at levels below T6 in healthy, normovolemic volunteers without pain results in only minor hemodynamic changes.[42] The resistance of lower extremity vessels decreases while upper extremity vessels constrict, resulting in unchanged total systemic vascular resistance (TSVR). Raising the sensory block to higher levels (T3–4) causes a 15–20% decrease in TSVR and a comparable increase in cardiac output ($\dot{Q}_t$); thus, the mean arterial pressure (MAP) remains unaltered. Thoracic epidural analgesia limited to the region between T3 and T12, a technique that is used frequently to relieve postoperative pain from thoracic and upper abdominal surgery or chest injuries, causes a decrease in MAP (10–15%) by reducing the TSVR in healthy and normovolemic patients.[343] A slight decrease in heart rate (7–10%) is usually compensated for by an equal increase in stroke volume; thus, the $\dot{Q}_t$ remains unchanged.[343] Addition of epinephrine (1/200,000) to local anesthetic agents causes an increase in heart rate and $\dot{Q}_t$ and a decrease in TSVR by beta-adrenergic stimulation.[43] As the decrease in TSVR is usually greater than the increase in $\dot{Q}_t$, the overall effect on MAP is a 5–10% reduction. In hypovolemic patients (greater than 5–10% blood volume depletion), these relatively benign hemodynamic effects of epidural analgesia are replaced by severe decreases in heart rate, MAP, and $\dot{Q}_t$.[44] These changes occur frequently with sensory blocks extending to T4–5 levels, but may also be seen with blocks involving lower spinal segments. The decreased heart rate that usually occurs with high sensory analgesia is probably caused by unopposed vagal activity. It appears that the addition of epinephrine to local anesthetic solution can partially prevent these hemodynamic effects (Fig. 23-6).

In addition to the above well-known facts, the hemodynamic response to epidural analgesia in accidentally and/or surgically injured patients depends upon the degree of increased sympathetic tone before the blockade and the cause of this increase. If the increased sympathetic tone is a result of pain, analgesia and the associated sympathetic blockade produced by epidural block will decrease heart rate, $\dot{Q}_t$, and MAP to normal levels, diminishing unnecessary cardiac work. On the other hand, if the sympathetic tone is required primarily to maintain circulatory homeostasis in the face of hypovolemia, epidural analgesia will result in severe hypotension or even cardiac arrest.[44,212]

Sjögren and Wright[343] evaluated the effects of pain and its treatment by thoracic epidural analgesia on hemodynamic responses in healthy patients after elective upper abdominal surgery. Postoperative pain caused increases in TSVR, MAP, heart rate, $\dot{Q}_t$, oxygen consumption, and left ventricular work. These changes were restored by thoracic epidural analgesia to levels comparable to those observed before the development of pain (Fig. 23-7). These findings are consistent with the notion that postoperative pain relief with epidural analgesia has beneficial effects on heart function.

However, significant hypotension may occur after thoracic

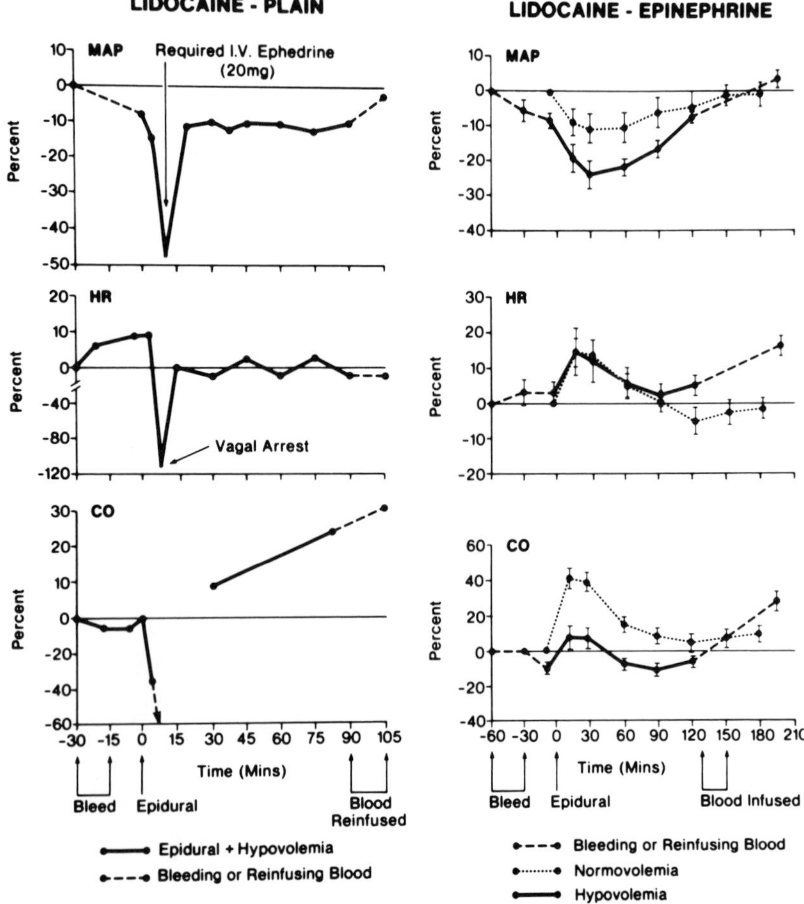


FIG. 23-6. Left, percent changes of mean arterial pressure (MAP), heart rate (HR), and cardiac output (CO) during epidural blockade ($T_5$) with plain lidocaine in a hypovolemic volunteer. Epidural blockade with plain lidocaine produces severe bradycardia and hypotension causing vagal arrest in some patients. Right, addition of epinephrine to lidocaine did not prevent the hypotension (25%), but the reduction in MAP was less than that produced by plain lidocaine. Heart rate elevation was responsible for the maintenance of CO and relatively smaller decrease in MAP with lidocaine-epinephrine solution than with plain lidocaine. Note also that in hypovolemic patients receiving lidocaine with epinephrine, hypotension was more pronounced than in those with normal blood volume. (From Cousins MJ, Bridenbaugh PO,[91] with permission.)

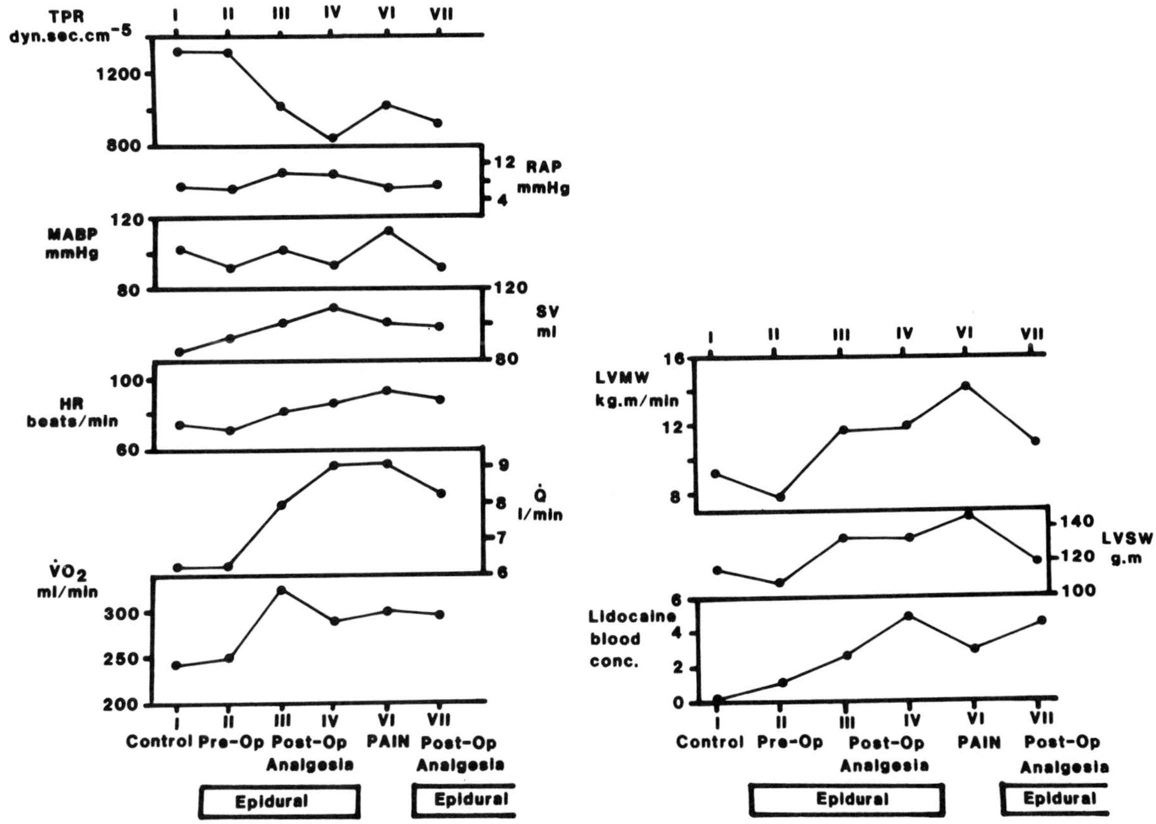


FIG. 23-7. Effect of postoperative pain relief with thoracic epidural analgesia produced by lidocaine (8 mL), on total peripheral resistance (TPR), right atrial pressure (RAP), mean arterial blood pressure (MABP), stroke volume (SV), heart rate (HR), cardiac output ($\dot{Q}$), oxygen consumption ($\dot{V}O_2$), left ventricular minute work (LVMW), left ventricular stroke work (LVSW), and blood lidocaine concentrations. The cardiovascular variables were measured before administration of epidural analgesia (I), one half-hour after administration of epidural block (II), 1 hour after cholecystectomy while postoperative analgesia was maintained with epidural lidocaine infusion (III), the morning after surgery while continuous epidural lidocaine infusion and analgesia were maintained (IV), 30–60 minutes after discontinuing the infusion and allowing the pain to return (V not shown), 60–90 minutes after discontinuing the infusion while severe pain was present (VI), and 90 minutes after re-establishing the epidural analgesia. Note the difference in TPR, MABP, $\dot{Q}$, LVMW, and LVSW between steps VI and VII. (From Sjögren S and Wright B: Acta Anaesth Scand 1972;16:5 and Cousins MJ, Phillips GD: Acute pain management, New York: Churchill Livingstone, 1986, with permission.)

epidural analgesia in patients with recent chest injuries and thoracotomies.[85,142,143,158,339,411] The incidence of this complication in published reports varies from 25 to 80%. Hypotension was at times persistent, and some patients progressed to cardiac arrest.[85,143,158,411] As the MAP was restored to normal levels with rapid fluid infusion in the majority of these patients, there is little doubt that the presence of hypovolemia before the administration of epidural block played an important role in the development of hypotension. However, hypotension occurs commonly after thoracic epidural analgesia, even without intravascular volume depletion, if the patient is placed in a sitting position shortly after injection of the local anesthetic agent. This is probably caused by sudden vagal overactivity (vasovagal attack) and can be prevented by keeping the patient supine for about 30 minutes after administration of the drug. Likewise, infusion of fluids and administration of vasopressor agents before elevation of the head may prevent this complication.[49]

Should thoracic epidural analgesia be given to patients with severe coronary artery disease? There is no definite answer to this question at present. Hypotension caused by this technique may result in severe impairment of cardiac performance, leading potentially to the development of myocardial infarction. On the other hand, epidural analgesia may produce coronary vasodilation and decreased myocardial $O_2$ consumption. Reiz et al.,[307] after administering thoracic epidural block (T1 to T12) to four patients with coronary artery disease, found a marked reduction in MAP and coronary vascular resistance and a moderate decrease in heart rate and coronary sinus blood flow. The decrease in myocardial $O_2$ and lactate utilization was commensurate with the decrease in cardiac work. Epidural analgesia did not result in arrhythmias or ST-T segment changes on the ECG, but the absence of regional dysoxia could not be proven. In a separate study Reiz et al.[308] demonstrated that epidural analgesia combined with light general anesthesia in patients undergoing major vascular surgery within 3 months after myocardial infarction resulted in a lower incidence of intraoperative myocardial ischemic events and of infarction rate (4 versus 23%) as compared to neuroleptanesthesia. There was, however, no difference in postoperative mortality rates. In view of these results, carefully administered thoracic epidural analgesia, if hypotension is avoided, may be beneficial in patients with coronary artery disease. However, this method must be tested further in these patients.

Hypotension caused by epidural analgesia may also be deleterious to patients with head injury. The decreased cerebral perfusion caused by hypotension may lead to serious cerebral hypoxia. In addition, injection of local anesthetic solution into the epidural space can produce a transient but clinically significant increase in intracranial pressure,[171] and incidental dural tap may be potentially fatal.

The effects of spinal anesthesia, which are probably comparable to those of epidural analgesia, on liver and kidney blood flow have been studied extensively by Mather and his colleagues in the sheep model.[224,323,324] These authors have demonstrated that, after adequate hydration, spinal anesthesia (T4 level) had little effect on hepatic and renal blood flow and drug clearance. In contrast, general anesthesia with thiopental and halothane caused a significant reduction of blood flow to these organs.

It is well established that epidurally or intrathecally administered opioid agents produce little hemodynamic alteration. There are, however, isolated reports describing hypertension or hypotension immediately after the injection of endogenous or exogenous opioid agents to animals or humans. In one report, injection of meperidine, 50 mg epidurally, to an elderly patient with chest injury produced severe hypertension.[314] Hypotension after intrathecal administration of meperidine to produce spinal anesthesia for surgery results primarily from decreased TSVR.[96] Thus, one cannot be assured that cardiovascular stability is a constant characteristic of this method, and periodic measurement of blood pressure should be carried out in all patients.

## EFFECT OF PAIN AND ANALGESIA ON THE FUNCTION OF THE DIGESTIVE TRACT

Gastrointestinal motility is diminished after major abdominal surgery. The role of postoperative pain in producing ileus has not been clearly established, but pain may exacerbate intestinal hypomotility by augmenting efferent sympathetic tone. In fact, the most popular hypothesis explaining the pathogenesis of postoperative ileus is based on the activation of spinal reflexes.[135] The afferent arc of these reflexes originates from the abdominal cavity, and the efferent arc involves the sympathetic efferent fibers to the intestines. Given this explanation, analgesia provided by epidural blockade should accelerate the return of gastrointestinal motility during the postoperative period. Although some studies showed such acceleration with postoperative epidural analgesia,[265,391] others show no such effect.[388] It should be remembered that return of bowel sounds may not necessarily imply adequate gastrointestinal function. Intestinal motility should be propulsive in order to be effective.

Narcotic agents, particularly morphine, produce an increase in intracolonic pressure by inducing nonpropulsive contractions in colonic smooth muscle.[3] Meperidine is thought to be more advantageous than morphine as it decreases intracolonic pressure and possibly reduces the incidence of anastomotic disruption.[3]

Certainly there are factors other than pain and the analgesic method that determine the length of postoperative ileus and the fate of the gastrointestinal anastomosis. Thus, selection of the analgesic method should not be based only on consideration of postoperative bowel function.

Another clinically important issue involves the effect of various analgesic drugs on intrabiliary pressure. Whether used subcutaneously, intramuscularly, or intravenously, clinical doses of agonist opiates can produce marked pressure increases in the common bile duct and result in epigastric distress and biliary colic.[227,292] This increase in intrabiliary pressure can be inhibited by naloxone (Fig. 23-8).[292] Narcotic agents with agonist-antagonist action (nalbuphin, butorphanol) cause only minimal increases of common bile duct pressure (Fig. 23-8).[227,292,380] It has been demonstrated that in animals intrathecally or epidurally administered agonist opiates do not increase pressure in the common bile duct.[381] Likewise, epidural analgesia with local anesthetic agents has little effect on biliary pressure.

## EFFECT OF REGIONAL ANESTHESIA ON THROMBOEMBOLISM

Regional anesthetic techniques decrease thromboembolic phenomena by increasing blood flow to the lower extremity, increasing fibrinolysis, and decreasing coagulation.[241] Inhibition of white blood cell invasion and preservation of endothelial cells in autogenous vein grafts by this method have also been demonstrated.[72,145,357] These effects, combined with early patient mobilization as provided by regional anesthesia, decrease the posttraumatic and postoperative incidence of thromboembolism (see also Chapter 28).[242] An increase in graft blood flow after vascular surgery has been demonstrated by Cousins et al.[90] with lumbar epidural an-

FIG. 23-8. The effect of narcotics and placebo on common bile duct pressure over a period of 20 minutes and the response to naloxone administered at 20 minutes. (From Radnay et al[292] with permission.)

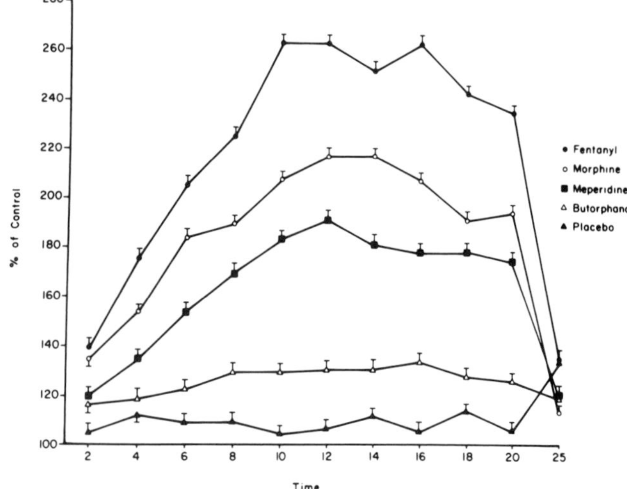

algesia. These results, combined with more recent reports describing the prevention of thromboembolism, should encourage the use of epidural analgesia for pain relief after lower extremity surgery.

## RATIONALE FOR MANAGEMENT

### RESTORATION OF FUNCTION

An important goal of posttraumatic pain management is early restoration of function. Cellular function depends upon blood flow for delivery of nutrients to the tissues. Vasoconstriction, whether secondary to pain or to direct vascular injury by trauma or surgical manipulation, interferes with nutrient supply. Sympathetic blockade can be employed to decrease vascular resistance and improve skin and vascular graft flow while decreasing pain-mediated vasoconstriction.[90] Regional blocks, by relieving pain, result in improved mobilization of injured parts.[56,267,284] Early mobilization contributes to preservation of normal musculoskeletal and gastrointestinal function.[265]

### PREVENTION OF DELAYED SEQUELAE OF INJURY BY EARLY PAIN RELIEF

The development of late posttraumatic pain syndromes may be partially dependent upon initial pain management. Myofascial pain syndromes resulting from injury to musculoskeletal structures and disuse secondary to pain and muscle spasm might well be minimized with early ambulation and mobilization of injured regions. Although sympathetic blockade is beneficial for causalgia and reflex sympathetic dystrophy, whether pre- or early posttraumatic blockade of sympathetic pathways tends to prevent the subsequent occurrence of these syndromes requires further study. There is some evidence that pretraumatic sympathectomy may prevent the development of phantom limb pain after amputation.[16,93]

## METHODS OF PAIN MANAGEMENT

Pain is an extremely common finding immediately after trauma. It occurs frequently with fractures, sprains, lacerations, cuts, and blunt abdominal and thoracic injuries. There are, however, some injuries that are not associated with significant degrees of pain. Patients with third-degree burns, for instance, complain very little of pain.[373] First- and second-degree burns are associated with severe pain that should be treated immediately.[373]

Evaluation of pain in patients with multiple trauma may be difficult. The associated confusion caused by cerebral hypoxia, fear, behavioral disturbances, and intoxication may result either in an exaggerated response manifested by agitation, moaning, groaning, and crying or in a state of apathy. Patients with relatively minor injuries, such as those limited to skin and/or musculoskeletal structures, may have a delay in the onset of pain, usually for 1, but sometimes for as long as 9 hours after injury.[233]

Wall[385] divides the posttrauma period into three stages: immediate, acute, and chronic. During the immediate stage, which lasts about 1 to 5 hours after injury, many patients feel very little pain. In the acute stage, lasting several days, pain is a prominent feature. The chronic stage is characterized by complex behavioral disturbances in conjunction with pain. Chronic pain develops in a relatively small fraction of injured patients. It usually follows musculoskeletal injury and may be difficult to treat. Various management modalities for acute and chronic pain are shown in Table 23-2.

### ACUTE PAIN MANAGEMENT

#### *General Principles*

Although patients in acute pain form a large group comprising not only those with severe trauma but also those with minor sprains and injuries, the latter segment is not discussed here as they can be managed with simple analgesic therapy familiar to all clinicians. Severely injured patients, on the other hand, present a very different picture. This group, as has been discussed in the previous section, may need analgesia both to provide comfort and minimize end-organ damage. They often need pain relief to tolerate simple diagnostic tests, such as radiography or a CT scan. Occasionally, analgesia may form the basis of treatment; for instance, in the reduction of a dislocated shoulder or during manipulation of a fractured femur.

It must be emphasized that analgesic therapy of the injured patient is not a major priority until primary resuscitative measures have been applied. It is, however, all too often ignored completely even when the patient has been adequately stabilized. Although this is often rationalized in terms of the basic principles of management of the traumatized patient, these principles are often wrongly applied. The patient with a severe fracture who is denied analgesia because of a minor head in-

TABLE 23-2. Methods Used for Traumatic Pain Management

- Acute Pain Management
  - Medications
    - Narcotics
      - Intravenous
      - Intramuscular
      - Oral
      - Sublingual
      - Spinal
    - Nonsteroid anti-inflammatory drugs
    - Inhalational agents
    - Local anesthetics
      - Infiltration
      - Nerve block
      - Spinal and epidural
- Chronic Pain Management
  - Medications
  - Nerve blocks
  - Stimulation-produced analgesia
  - Ablative neurosurgery
  - Physical therapy
  - Psychological techniques

jury or the patient awaiting surgery who is frightened and in pain without the benefit of analgesia is familiar to all who have been asked to evaluate patients in the emergency department.

The principles and rationale of analgesic management of this group of patients are as follows. The goal is to reduce pain intensity to tolerable levels. The treatment must be compatible with the altered physiology of vital organ systems.

CARDIOVASCULAR SYSTEM. The circulation may be severely deranged because of hypovolemia. Drugs given systemically must not interfere with normal physiologic responses. Reduced cardiac output and plasma volume may considerably alter the pharmacokinetics of administered drugs. Normal doses of drugs given at conventional rates may produce extremely high plasma levels, causing undesirable side effects. Similarly, muscle blood flow may be seriously impaired, thus preventing the uptake of drugs administered by this route. Organ perfusion may also be altered, which can affect the clearance and elimination of analgesics, causing them to have prolonged effects.

RESPIRATORY SYSTEM. Oxygenation may be compromised at several levels in the oxygen cascade. Therapy that interferes with the mechanics of respiration (chest muscle function, airway patency, etc.) or central control should be avoided. A rise in $PaCO_2$ caused by hypoventilation will cause cerebral vasodilation; this is of critical importance in cases where the intracranial pressure is already elevated.

CENTRAL NERVOUS SYSTEM. The conscious state may be altered, and intracranial pathology may be present. Drugs either masking or imitating the signs of raised intracranial pressure—sedation, vomiting, or pupillary dysfunction—should be avoided. Epidural anesthesia, which carries the risk of dural puncture, may result in brain herniation. In addition, as was mentioned, deposition of local anesthetic agents into the epidural space can cause a considerable increase in intracranial pressure.[171] Therefore, this form of therapy is contraindicated.

GASTROINTESTINAL SYSTEM. The stomach may be full, and gastric emptying may be delayed. Thus, drugs should not be given by the oral route. Narcotics can cause vomiting and delay gastric emptying even further. This may be particularly inappropriate in elderly patients with decreased tracheobronchial reflexes.

OTHER PRINCIPLES OF MANAGEMENT. The patient may have pain in more than one site. Thus, an appropriate pain treatment modality should be selected to provide analgesia with the least amount of drug and the fewest procedures.

The patient may be intoxicated or under the influence of other drugs, which may interact with analgesic medications. Adequate knowledge of drug interactions, the careful search for such potential problems, and the use of appropriate methods of analgesia will minimize adverse drug effects.

Analgesic management should be based on an individually tailored regimen in a well-monitored environment. Administration of potent analgesic drugs or sophisticated regional anesthetic procedures without appropriate monitoring and supervision may result in either inadequate pain relief or catastrophic complications.

## ACUTE POSTTRAUMATIC PAIN MANAGEMENT

### *Medications*

SYSTEMIC ANALGESICS. The narcotic analgesics are still the mainstay of the analgesic armamentarium for the trauma victim. Many injuries are associated with severe pain requiring the use of powerful analgesics.

The intramuscular route is not suitable, particularly for the patient with diminished tissue perfusion, as absorption of the drug is poor. Analgesic drugs given by this route even to patients without perfusion abnormalities may produce unstable plasma concentrations (Fig. 23-9). In practice, the drug level in the blood will reach or exceed minimal analgesic concentration during only 35% of the dosing interval.[14] This is caused by several factors:[14,15] (a) the minimum analgesic blood concentration is highly variable among patients, (b) small changes in blood concentration are associated with important effects in pain relief since the plasma concentration-response curve of the drug is steep, and (c) the absorption of the drug is so unreliable that there is a significant variation in peak plasma concentrations and the time required to reach these blood levels (Fig. 23-10).

Morphine, in spite of its disorderly kinetics and undesirable pharmacodynamic properties, is probably the drug most commonly used to treat acute pain. Its principal disadvantage is that analgesia after an intravenous dose is delayed for at least 15–20 minutes, a property that is reproducible by pharmacokinetic and pharmacodynamic studies. After injection of this drug, CSF concentration rises fairly rapidly; however there is a delay of approximately 1 hour between the time of administration of morphine and its peak effect, measured by elevation of end-tidal carbon dioxide.[175] The delay in attaining peak effect also accounts for the late respiratory depression occasionally seen with this drug. Morphine is usually administered intravenously in doses of up to 10 mg. Small doses are given every 10 minutes until analgesia is adequate.[80] Not infrequently, doses as high as 30 mg of morphine are needed, a phenomenon confirmed in battle casualties.[187]

Meperidine is another drug commonly used to relieve acute pain. It has been demonstrated that its pharmacokinetics are not significantly changed after trauma provided that renal and hepatic functions are intact.[202] Intravenous doses of 10–20 mg may be administered every 5 to 10 minutes to reach adequate analgesia. Pain relief is usually obtained by a total dose of 75 to 100 mg, but larger doses may be needed. Among all narcotic agents, meperidine is the most powerful cardiovascular depressant; thus, it should be used with great caution in the hypovolemic trauma victim.[225]

Fentanyl and alfentanil are probably the most suitable drugs for relief of acute pain.[328,353] Unlike morphine, fentanyl has an extremely rapid onset, producing EEG slowing within 2 minutes.[328] Under close monitoring of airway and ventilation, an initial loading dose of fentanyl, 2 to 4 μg/kg, over a 20-minute period followed by a 1–1.5 μg/kg/h infusion, may provide rapid and effective pain control. Alfentanil may be

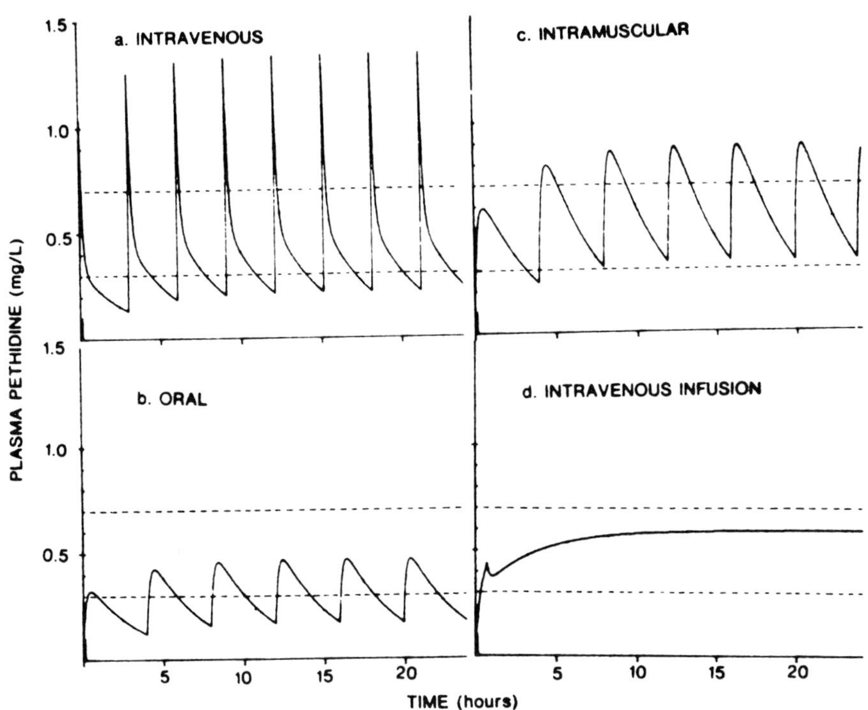


FIG. 23-9. Graph showing computer-simulated plasma meperidine levels after four different routes of administration. The dotted lines represent a therapeutic range above which toxic effects are likely and below which analgesia is unlikely to be adequate. The doses are (a) intravenous injections, 50 mg, three hourly; (b) oral 100 mg, four hourly; (c) intramuscular 100 mg, four hourly; and (d) infusion 50 mg in 45 minutes, then 25 mg/h. (From Cousins MJ, Bridenbaugh PO[91] with permission.)

given as a 20 μg/kg/h infusion. Doses of this magnitude produced depression of the carbon dioxide response curve, but had only moderate effects on minute volume and $PaCO_2$ in postoperative patients.[8,271] Respiratory function returns to normal within 1 hour after discontinuing alfentanil.[8,271] These drugs, however, are seldom used in the preoperative period to control pain probably because of the need for intense patient supervision and monitoring. Narcotics with agonist-antagonist action may be advantageous in trauma patients because of their ceiling effect on respiratory depression. However, a significant number of these patients may be intoxicated by narcotic drugs, in which case agonist-antagonist agents may produce severe agitation.[266]

FIG. 23-10. Blood meperidine concentration-response curves from three patients (A, B, and C) who received meperidine 75–100 mg on demand with a minimum dosing interval of 90 minutes. Note the steep blood concentration-response curve: small changes in blood concentration of meperidine produce major differences in pain scores. Note also the wide interindividual differences in terms of response to blood concentration. The minimum analgesic blood meperidine concentration for patient A is 0.18 μg/mL. The corresponding values for patient B and C are 0.48 μg/mL and 0.8 μg/mL, respectively. (From Austin et al[15] with permission.)

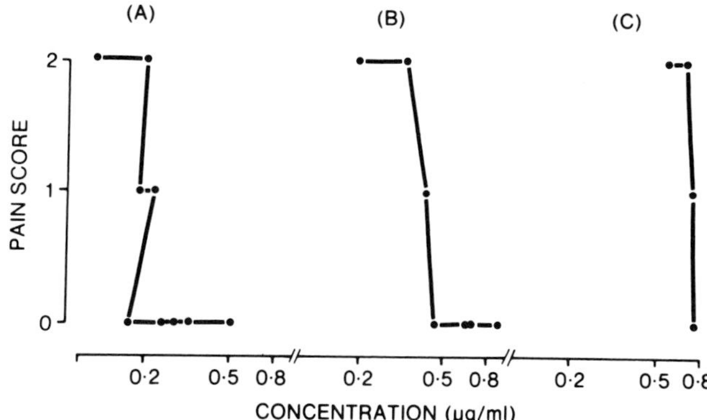


In head injury patients, all narcotics have undesirable side effects. These drugs should be avoided in all but the most trivial head trauma. Less efficacious drugs, such as codeine phosphate, 30–60 mg, have been used in an attempt to reduce the side effects of more potent opiates, such as respiratory depression and pupillary constriction. However, all too often, such agents produce only minimal analgesia even in modest doses; analgesia for this group is best provided by alternative methods.

Ketamine produces profound analgesia and may be used in a high dosage (1–2 mg/kg IV) as the sole anesthetic induction agent for emergency and trauma surgery.[34,87] At lower doses (0.2–0.3 mg/kg IV, or 1 mg/kg IM) it can be used as an analgesic.[154,172] This agent has the advantage of having a sympathomimetic action, which may be beneficial in injured patients with cardiovascular depression caused by shock.[87] After an initial bolus dose, an infusion may be started (0.2–0.3 mg/kg/h) to obtain continuous analgesia.[33] Ketamine, however, increases intracranial pressure and is contraindicated in patients with head injuries. Pentazocine also has been used to provide analgesia in war injuries. The initial dose of 10–30 mg IV may be followed by an infusion of 10–30 mg/h in adults.[33]

INHALATIONAL AGENTS. Nitrous oxide is a powerful analgesic, and at inspired concentrations of 20–40% it can produce pain relief equivalent to 10–15 mg of morphine.[277] In some centers, it is often available premixed with oxygen 50:50 as entonox. Administration is simple via a face mask or nasal prongs, and its use is a safe and effective way of producing analgesia for trauma victims.[272,278,358] In many countries, entonox is available in ambulances for administration by paramedics.[358] Although some cardiodepressant action has been demonstrated with 60% $N_2O$,[119] its principal advantage is that any clinical deterioration can be treated by removal of the agent with very rapid reversal of effects. Nitrous oxide, however, also causes an increase in intracranial pressure[250]; thus, it should not be used in head-injured patients.

## Nerve Blocks

USE OF LOCAL ANESTHETIC AGENTS FOR NERVE BLOCK. Many of the general constraints discussed above apply equally well to the use of local anesthetic agents. In the patient with compromised cardiovascular function, care must be exercised when administering drugs that have further depressant effects on cardiac or cerebral functions. Routes of administration that produce sympathetic blockade are inappropriate in the hypovolemic patient; therefore, spinal or epidural analgesia is precluded until blood volume is restored to normal. Equally inappropriate are long-acting peripheral nerve blocks when assessment of limb function and of pain is important for diagnostic purposes (compartment syndromes, plaster casts, etc.). However, the use of regional anesthesia in trauma victims not only avoids the systemic effects of narcotics (sedation, vomiting, etc.) but also diminishes the stress response and avoids the problems of a full stomach. These facts, combined with the complete pain relief afforded by the placement of only a few milliliters of local anesthetic on a nerve, confer immutable advantages on this technique in the injured patient. Local anesthetics can be administered by the following routes: infiltration, peripheral nerve block, and conduction blockade.

INFILTRATION. Local anesthetics can be administered by subcutaneous infiltration for analgesia of minor wounds or by injection into a fracture hematoma for reduction of fractures, eg, for Colles fracture, 5–10 mL of 1% lidocaine is injected into the hematoma. The technique does not always produce perfect analgesia, but can be used in situations where staff or resources are limited.[13]

PERIPHERAL NERVE BLOCKS. The benefits of peripheral nerve block to trauma patients are often not fully exploited either because of inexperience of the available personnel in performing blocks or of surgical time constraints. These techniques deserve wider utilization since they usually produce total and long-lasting analgesia with minimal side effects. Further, therapeutic measures including surgery can often be carried out with this technique alone. This obviates the need for general anesthesia, avoids potential hazards in a patient with full stomach, and, in fact, shortens the patient's hospital stay.[56] The use of regional anesthesia has been recommended for disaster situations.[395] Of course, patient selection is an important consideration; patients with multiple trauma and a high level of anxiety and/or coagulation abnormalities are not candidates for this type of treatment.

*Techniques for Upper Limbs.* Brachial plexus block can be performed by the axillary,[103,406] infraclavicular,[294] subclavian perivascular,[406] interscalene,[405,406] and supraclavicular routes.[246] A different approach to the brachial plexus involves insertion of a catheter about 4 cm distal to the humeral insertion of the pectoralis major muscle at the medial aspect of the arm in the groove between the biceps and triceps muscles.[9] Advancing the catheter for about 3 to 4 cm proximally within a well-defined fascial space and injecting approximately 40 mL of local anesthetic solution will produce satisfactory analgesia. Techniques for providing continuous brachial plexus analgesia with axillary, supraclavicular, and interscalene approaches are also available.[168,218,334]

The choice of technique depends upon the site of injury, the patient's ability to abduct the arm, and the presence of head injury requiring observation. The axillary route has been used with success in both adults[392] and children.[82,123] In general, higher lesions (upper arm injuries, dislocated shoulder, etc.) require analgesia extending to the C5 dermatome, which is best achieved with an interscalene block.[167,176] This technique is also perhaps the most suitable for Colles fracture,[168,176] as the anatomic snuff box is often difficult to anesthetize adequately with lower approaches to the brachial plexus. When upper extremity injuries are associated with head injuries that do not require immediate neurosurgical intervention, the axillary approach to the brachial plexus may be preferable to the interscalene technique.[7] Horner's syndrome is commonly associated with the interscalene approach (18.5% incidence) and may interfere with accurate assessment and follow-up of the head injury.[7] Patchy analgesia in the hand with any of the above techniques can often be remedied by blockade of the individual nerves at the elbow or wrist.

The use of the peripheral nerve stimulator has greatly facilitated the performance of all of these blocks.[287,296] Although uninsulated needles have been used to locate the nerve or plexus to be blocked, insulated needles with only the tip uncovered localize the neural tissue more precisely.[20,129] The usual minimum stimulation current by which proximity of the needle to the nerve is ensured is about 0.5–0.7 mA.[287] Much smaller currents (0.09 mA) have been described,[414] but these values were probably obtained by long pulse width (5 ms). Stimulation of motor fibers results in a characteristic twitch of the respective muscle groups. Thus, the method is especially useful in traumatized patients who may not cooperate because of injury and/or effects of alcohol and drugs.

*Techniques for Lower Limbs.* Although the lower limb is more difficult to block with a single injection, worthwhile techniques are still available. In particular, femoral nerve block can be easily performed and can provide excellent analgesia for femoral fractures.[29] The exact extent of analgesia depends on the fracture site; excellent relief can be obtained for midshaft fractures, good relief for the lower third, and partial relief for the upper third.[367] The method is also recommended for children[159] and can be extended to give continuous analgesia for several days by insertion of a catheter.[319] By increasing the volume of injectate and encouraging its cephalad spread, femoral nerve block can be extended to include the lateral femoral cutaneous nerve and the obturator nerve, thus providing more complete analgesia for the thigh.[407]

Blockade of the sciatic nerve alone is of little value in providing analgesia for the traumatized patient, and the traditional (Labat) approach requires the patient to adopt the Sims position, which is not always possible with an injured limb. Likewise, the approach described by Raj et al.,[295] in which the patient is in the supine position, requires flexion of the hip and knee and may not be tolerated by patients with severe extremity fractures. The anterior approach is less reliable, but is suitable for the trauma patient.[21] The lateral approach may be tolerated better by the traumatized patient since it does not necessitate extensive positioning.[178] A technique for continuous sciatic nerve block is described,[346] but is rarely needed in traumatized patients with the possible exception of those with frostbite injuries.

Combined femoral-sciatic nerve block can provide excellent analgesia below the knee and can be used for Pott's fractures and dislocations around the ankle.[30] Blockade of the saphenous, common peroneal, and tibial nerves at the knee, a rather neglected technique, can produce excellent analgesia below the upper third of the leg.[316]

Sympathetic blockade of the extremities by peripheral nerve, stellate ganglion, lumbar sympathetic, or epidural blocks may be extremely useful in providing pain relief and improving blood flow, viability, and function of the limbs after frostbite injuries.[6] Sympathetic blockade should be performed as soon after injury as possible and continued for 3 or 4 days. The use of long-acting local anesthetic agents (bupivacaine or etidocaine) and catheter techniques allowing intermittent or continuous injections may facilitate the management of these injuries.

*Techniques for Traumatic Chest Pain.* Tracheal intubation and ventilation may be required in the management of rib fractures because of inadequate breathing caused by chest wall instability and splinting due to pain. Parenteral opiate analgesia is not desirable in these patients because of its respiratory depressant and cough suppressant actions. Epidural blockade can provide complete analgesia, preventing atelectasis, while the patient is awake and cooperative. Initially, thoracic epidural analgesia was recommended entirely for its ability to relieve pain,[143] but it is now also appreciated that epidural blockade can improve chest compliance, increase vital capacity and functional residual capacity, and decrease the high bronchial resistance seen in these patients.[111,211] Thus, the recognition that the problem is primarily a functional rather than an anatomic derangement led to more liberal use of epidural analgesia in the treatment of these fractures.[112] Dittman et al.[112] recommended that all patients with multiple rib fractures should have thoracic epidural analgesia provided the patient is conscious and has no associated head injury, has a vital capacity greater than 15 mL/kg, and has a $PaO_2$ greater than 60 mm Hg while breathing room air. This regime was highly effective in alleviating pain and associated pulmonary complications in a series of about 250 patients. By using this method and providing complete analgesia, Worthley[411] also demonstrated that only 9% of his patients required mechanical ventilation; previously all of his patients needed ventilatory support. It is, however, important to realize that epidural analgesia should not be used indiscriminately as the sole treatment modality; mechanical ventilation should be initiated without delay when indicated.

Insertion of a thoracic epidural catheter should be undertaken with care in a patient who has other injuries and should not be performed until hypovolemia has been corrected.[411] No more than five or six dermatomes should be blocked. If more than this number of ribs are fractured, the lower ribs should be blocked preferentially since these tend to be more painful and a lower block interferes less with the cardioaccelerator fibers.[211] The epidural catheter should be placed at a thoracic level halfway between the upper and lower border of the area planned for analgesia. The initial dose of local anesthetic agent (bupivacaine 0.5%) should not exceed 25–30 mg, and the pain level, blood pressure, and pulse rate should be assessed every 5 minutes for 30 minutes. If pain relief is not adequate at the end of this period and a significant fall in blood pressure (more than 30 mm Hg or systolic BP below 80 mm Hg) is not recorded, additional doses of bupivacaine in 10-mg (2-mL) increments, up to 30 mg, can be administered. Blockade can be maintained with intermittent doses or continuous infusion of the agent; the latter approach has many advantages. Continuous infusion techniques are discussed in the section on postoperative pain.

Patients who are given epidural analgesia should be managed in special care units, eg, the recovery room, ICU, or postoperative unit. These patients require an average dose of 200–300 mg bupivacaine every day for 5 or 6 days and sometimes longer. As mentioned above, hypotension and even cardiac arrest may occur, especially in hypovolemic patients, after the injection of local anesthetics into the thoracic epidural space.[85,143,158,411] Local anesthetic toxicity involving the CNS or cardiovascular system may occur if the epidural catheter migrates into an epidural vein and the drug is injected intravascularly. The absence of valves within the epidural venous system may result in direct transport of the anesthetic into the brain. A rare complication of epidural analgesia is development of epidural abscess.[411] Thus, patients should be examined at least daily for back pain and tenderness. Epidural analgesia should not be given to those patients who have a skin infection, abrasion, or wound overlying the area required for insertion of the epidural catheter. Patients with severe multiple trauma may also develop coagulation abnormalities shortly after injury.[312] Therefore, an epidural hematoma may develop after placement of an epidural catheter. A careful evaluation of patients for coagulation abnormalities before initiating epidural analgesia will reduce the incidence of this complication. Other complications of epidural analgesia include dural puncture and urinary retention.

In order to overcome the problems of sympathetic blockade and resultant hypotension, narcotic agents have been used in the epidural and intrathecal spaces with some success.[75,79,114,116,182,198,347] Morphine sulfate (3–5 mg epidurally, 0.5 mg intrathecally) is probably the most commonly used drug for this purpose, although fentanyl, 1 μg/kg bolus dose followed by 1–2 μg/kg/h infusion from a reservoir containing the narcotic at a concentration of 5–10 μg/mL, produces satisfactory analgesia and improvement of pulmonary function in between 85 and 100% of patients.[116,215] Continuous thoracic epidural morphine infusion (5-mg loading dose followed by 0.7–1 mg/h) also reduces the pain, the incidence of tracheostomy, and the length of ICU and total hospital stay of patients with rib fractures.[375] However, it is not necessary to inject these drugs into the thoracic epidural space as injection into the lumbar region results in pain relief to the level of the thoracic dermatomes.[132,215,337] Neither epidural nor intrathecal morphine appears to be as effective as epidural local anesthetic agents in alleviating the pain or improving the pulmonary function after chest wall injuries.[81,109] As mentioned earlier, combinations of narcotics and local anesthetic agents have also been used.[300] Administration of morphine, 3 mg epidurally, while the patient is resting provides adequate pain relief, but cannot prevent pain during chest physiotherapy or other activities requiring movement. Epidural injection of a local anesthetic agent in these circumstances will decrease the pain and allow the patient to cooperate. Further discussion of epidural and intrathecal narcotics is offered in the section on postoperative pain treatment.

A frequently used method to relieve pain from chest injuries is intercostal block.[255,273] In the traditional approach, each intercostal nerve responsible for pain is blocked individually by inserting a needle in the region of the lower border of the fractured rib and injecting a local anesthetic between the internal intercostal and intercostalis intimus muscles.[57,247] The block is performed anywhere in the area between the paravertebral and posterior axillary lines; for each nerve, 3 to 5 mL of local anesthetic solution (bupivacaine 0.25% or 0.5% with epinephrine 1/200,000 is preferred) is deposited. Usually these blocks have to be repeated as the pain returns, although by using bupivacaine, analgesia as long as 16 hours has been obtained.[365] There is also a risk of causing pneumothorax by advancing the block needle into the visceral pleura. Patient discomfort caused by repeated blocks and the possibility of pneumothorax in patients who may already have a compromised respiratory function are significant disadvantages of this technique.

In a more recently described technique, a catheter is inserted into the intercostal space, and by injecting an adequate volume of local anesthetic solution (about 20 mL), several intercostal segments are blocked.[254] The technique involves insertion of a Tuohy needle and threading of an epidural catheter through this needle into the appropriate intercostal space. As discussed earlier, large volumes of local anesthetic injected in this area may produce analgesia by subpleural diffusion into other intercostal spaces,[254,270] perivertebral or epidural spread,[234,235,251] or diffusion to the sympathetic chain located at the anterolateral aspect of the body of the vertebra.[270] Whatever the mechanism, the method is shown to produce satisfactory analgesia in patients with rib fractures.[214,255,273] The possibility of pneumothorax with this method remains and may be more severe than that caused by the traditional technique, as the Tuohy needle produces greater damage than the usual intercostal block needles. The block, however, is quite safe in patients who already have a chest tube in place.

Injection of local anesthetic solution (bupivacaine 0.5%, 20 mL) into the intrapleural space has been shown to provide good relief of acute pain produced by multiple rib fractures.[315] Analgesia with this technique can be maintained by continuous infusion of lidocaine, 1–2 mg/min.[288] Serum lidocaine level should be monitored and maintained below 5 μg/mL by adjusting the rate of infusion. Since intrapleural local anesthetic can mask the pain of associated intra-abdominal injuries and result in a delayed or missed diagnosis,[288] the block should be administered only after excluding such injuries with abdominal CT scan. Further discussion on this technique is offered under the section of postoperative pain.

*Techniques for Abdomen and Pelvis.* Abdominal and pelvic pain can be alleviated by the use of continuous epidural analgesia. However, there is little place for this technique in the acute phase of trauma management since it causes extensive sympathetic block and hypotension in the hypovolemic patient. In addition, there is the problem of positioning the injured patient for this procedure. Thus, it should be reserved for pain control after the patient has been stabilized.

## POSTOPERATIVE PAIN MANAGEMENT

Analgesia is needed in patients who have prolonged pain after the initial injury (burns, fractures, crush injuries, etc.) or who have pain secondary to operative intervention. Some similarities of pain mechanisms between these two groups of patients allow the use of the same pain management methods. It should be emphasized that, despite the abundant literature relating to the management of postoperative pain after elective surgery, only a few studies have investigated the efficacy of analgesic methods in traumatized patients after surgery. Thus, our discussion in this section is generally based on data obtained from electively operated patients. Studies on postoperative pain management in traumatized patients are urgently needed.

Injured patients with prolonged or postoperative pain differ in many respects from patients seen immediately after trauma:

- Abolition of pain is a realistic goal.
- In general, the cardiovascular system is stable. Although blood transfusions may still be required, large volume deficits will have been corrected and tissue perfusion will be returning to normal.
- Diagnosis for the most part will have been confirmed. Blunting of signs and symptoms, although not desirable, is no longer a critical problem in the management of the patient.
- The patient probably is not in a high-dependency zone, and thus, the analgesic regime must fit into the practical situation of limited manpower.
- Pain is diminishing as healing progresses. Thus, potent analgesia, which is required for only a few days, needs to be tapered while the patient's response is monitored.

The following methods are available for providing postoperative analgesia for these patients.

### *Intramuscular Narcotics*

The use of narcotic analgesics by the intramuscular route is the most common method of providing postoperative analgesia. This method, however, often provides inadequate analgesia of too short a duration.[14,15,379] This phenomenon has many contributory factors, among which are poor prescribing by physicians[219,351,394] (poor choice of drug, inadequate dose, inappropriate dosing interval), inadequacies in administering the prescribed drugs[83,351,394] (personnel limitations, fear of addiction and respiratory depression), the reluctance of patients to ask for drugs,[83,351] the steep dose-response curve of intramuscularly administered narcotics, and variations among patients in drug absorption rate and therapeutic response (Figs. 23-9 and 23-10).[14,15] Intramuscular regimes can be considerably improved by giving consideration to these basic problems.

The physician should administer the first dose of an appropriate drug and monitor its effect. He or she can then decide upon a suitable dose to be given at a suitable dosing interval, within the confines of tolerable side effects, for at least the first 24 hours.

Morphine sulfate (10–12 mg) and meperidine (80–100 mg) are the most commonly used narcotic agents. However, new narcotic agents are being used increasingly. The usual intramuscular doses of these agents are shown in Table 23-3.

### *Intravenous Narcotics*

The intravenous route gives immediate access to the circulation, and this rapidity of onset is most useful in the recovery room or when an immediate effect is needed. The initial intravenous bolus doses of various narcotics used for postoperative pain are shown in Table 23-4. The rapid distribution and elimination of drugs given by this route may, however, produce an effect of shorter duration than the same dose given intramuscularly. To overcome this problem, drugs can be given in an infusion. Many drugs have been administered by this route, including fentanyl,[117,264] alfentanil,[8,271,415] lysine acetylsalicylate,[70,184] meperidine,[354] papaveratum,[133] and morphine[275]; there is little doubt as to the vastly improved analgesia produced by this method.[223] The usual infusion rates of analgesic agents administered for postoperative pain relief are shown in Table 23-5. A steady state can be achieved rapidly either with an initial bolus dose or a two-rate infusion. However, the infusion technique may be associated in the postoperative period with episodic oxygen desaturation, especially during sleep.[71] These changes have been shown to be caused by an altered ventilatory pattern—central apnea, obstructive apnea, or paradoxical breathing.[71] Thus, although the method is safe and decreases the oxygen demand of organs in mechanically ventilated patients,[321] the infusion technique is associated with some risk in those who are breathing spontaneously. These patients should be attended at all times and monitored continuously with a pulse oximeter.

A different approach for intravenous narcotic analgesia has been suggested by Gourlay et al.[150–152] They administered methadone (20 mg IV) shortly after induction of anesthesia during elective surgery. Forty percent of the patients did not require any postoperative analgesia. In the remaining patients, methadone (2.5–5.0 mg IV) given two or three times provided good pain relief. Methadone has a prolonged elimination half-life (35 hours), and the mean duration of analgesia is about 21 hours (Fig. 23-11). If satisfactory analgesia is *not* obtained with the initial dose, additional doses should be given with care to avoid accumulation and dangerous respiratory depression.

Further refinements of intravenous analgesia techniques have led to the use of patient-controlled demand systems.[25,125,144,155,177,397,398] These devices consist of an electromechanical apparatus that administers a preset bolus of the drug when the patient presses a bedside button. The complexity of the machines varies, but all include safeguards to prevent the patient from receiving more than a preset number of doses per hour. Recommended bolus dosages and lockout intervals of various parenteral analgesics with this technique are shown in Table 23-6. These machines work well, as most patients maintain their own level of analgesia and do not utilize the maximum available dose. Many manufacturers now are also offering patient-controlled analgesia devices that are capable of delivering continuous infusion of narcotics, in addition to bolus doses. The safety record of patient-controlled analgesia machines is excellent, and few complications have been reported. However, the high cost of equipment and the

TABLE 23-3. Usual Intramuscular Doses of Newer Narcotics Agents for Adults*

| AGENT | DOSE |
|---|---|
| Buprenorphine | 0.2–0.4 mg |
| Ciramadol | 45–60 mg |
| Slow-release morphine preparation* | 1.0 mL |
| Dezocine | 10–15 mg |
| Butorphanol | 1–3 mg |
| Nalbuphine | 20–30 mg |

* Slow-release Morphine contains morphine base, 64 mg in 1 mL; approximately 3.0 mg is present as free morphine and the remainder as crystals, from which the drug is slowly released over 9–12 hours.

TABLE 23-4. Usual Bolus Intravenous Doses of Various Narcotic Agents Used for Postoperative Pain in Adults*

| AGENT | BOLUS IV DOSE |
|---|---|
| Morphine sulfate | 2–4 mg |
| Meperidine hydrochloride | 20–40 mg |
| Fentanyl | 0.05–0.1 mg |
| Alfentanil | 6 μg/kg |
| Nalbuphine | 3–5 mg |
| Butorphanol | 1–2 mg |
| Buprenorphine | 0.1–0.2 mg |
| Dezocine | 0.1–0.15 mg/kg |

* These doses can be repeated within 15–20 minutes after the initial administration according to the degree of pain relief and respiratory depression.

TABLE 23-5. Usual Intravenous Infusion Rates of Analgesic Agents Administered for Postoperative Pain Relief in Adults*

| AGENT | INFUSION RATE |
|---|---|
| Morphine sulfate | 1.0–1.5 mg/h |
| Fentanyl | 0.5–1.5 μg/kg/h |
| Alfentanil | 10–20 μg/kg/h |
| Meperidine | 7–10 mg/h |
| Lysine acetyl salicylate | 0.3 mg/h |

* The infusion rates specified are administered after a loading dose.

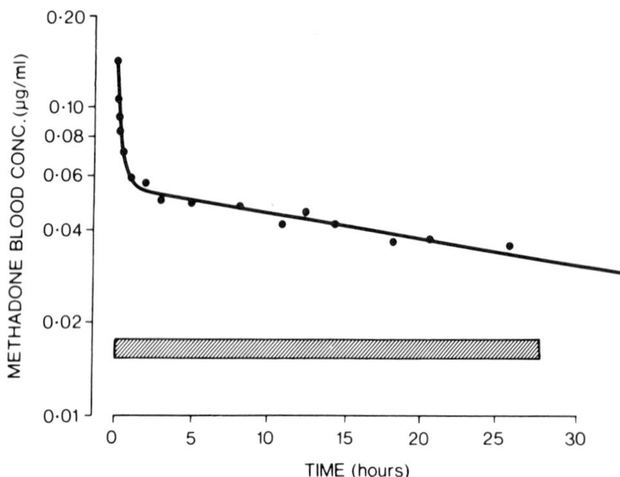


FIG. 23-11. Blood methadone concentration decay curve of a patient who received intravenous injection of 20 mg methadone shortly after induction of anesthesia. The patient was pain free for a period of 28 hours as demonstrated by the shaded area. Black circles represent the blood methadone concentration. (From Gourlay et al[150] with permission.)

need for reliance on electronic components detract somewhat from this technique.

Agitation occurs frequently in the postoperative period, and pain is one of the factors promoting its development. Increasing the narcotic dose usually provides adequate pain relief and sedation, but may also produce prolonged respiratory depression. Sedative agents are being used with increasing frequency in intensive care units to provide sedation without excessive doses of narcotic agents. Midazolam appears to be a desirable drug for this purpose because it has a rapid onset of action and short elimination half-life compared with other benzodiazepines. It can be administered intramuscularly (0.05 mg/kg)[10] or as an intravenous infusion (loading dose, 0.15–0.5 mg/kg followed by infusion at a rate of 0.1–20.0 µg/kg/min depending on the response).[336] A marked individual

TABLE 23-6. Recommended Bolus Dosages for Lockout Intervals of Various Narcotics Used for Patient-Controlled Analgesia*

| NARCOTIC | BOLUS DOSE (mg) | LOCKOUT INTERVAL (min) |
|---|---|---|
| Agonists | | |
| Fentanyl citrate | 0.02–0.1 | 3–10 |
| Hydromorphone hydrochloride | 0.1–0.5 | 5–15 |
| Meperidine hydrochloride | 5–30 | 5–15 |
| Methadone hydrochloride | 0.5–3.0 | 10–20 |
| Morphine sulfate | 0.5–3.0 | 5–20 |
| Oxymorphone hydrochloride | 0.2–0.8 | 5–15 |
| Sulfentanil citrate | 0.003–0.015 | 3–10 |
| Agonist-Antagonists | | |
| Buprenorphine hydrochloride | 0.03–0.2 | 10–20 |
| Nalbuphine hydrochloride | 1–5 | 5–15 |
| Pentazocine hydrochloride | 5–30 | 5–15 |

* From White[398] with permission.

variation of response to the drug necessitates careful titration. Etomidate also had been used for this purpose, but it has been abandoned because of its inhibitory effect on steroidogenesis.[276,383]

## *Spinal Opiates*

Since the first report in 1979,[22] the introduction of opiates into the subarachnoid and extradural spaces has become commonplace. There has been a profusion of clinical and experimental reports, including controlled trials elucidating the basic pharmacology, pharmacokinetics, mechanism of action, and effects of spinal drugs. Excellent reviews published during the past several years have enhanced the understanding and enthusiasm of clinicians for this method.[32,92,93,114,243,268,413] There is no doubt that good analgesia can be produced by this route, although it is not as free from side effects as had been hoped.[229,356] The side effects, however, are generally not unduly troublesome. When this technique is compared with epidural analgesia produced by local anesthetic agents, it appears that pain relief is better with local anesthetics, but the duration of analgesia is longer with morphine.[368] In addition, the hypotension frequently produced by epidural local anesthetic agents is extremely uncommon with spinal narcotics.[368]

Several opiates have been used epidurally or intrathecally to produce postoperative pain relief, but morphine has been studied most extensively. The physical and clinical characteristics of various agents are shown in Table 23-7. Nonopiate agents such as ketamine (30 mg)[179,258] have also been used, but experience with these is limited. Epidural and intrathecal opiates produce analgesia primarily by acting on the spinal cord, most probably at the substantia gelatinosa.[400,401] As with local anesthetic agents, the dose of epidural opiates is greater than that required for intrathecal injection. Thus, it is important to ensure correct placement of the needle or catheter tip during epidural administration of drugs. This can be attained by careful aspiration of the catheter or by injection of a test dose of local anesthetic agent before opiate administration.

In general, the lipid solubility of the opiate determines the onset and duration of its effects. Morphine has poor lipid solubility, and therefore its onset and duration are prolonged since it remains within the CSF for a long time. On the other hand, fentanyl is highly lipid soluble and enters the spinal cord easily, explaining its short onset and duration compared to morphine. Lipid solubility also determines the tendency of the drug to spread cephalad. Cephalad spread with morphine is greater than with fentanyl, explaining the more frequent occurrence of late respiratory depression with this drug.[92,124] Respiratory depression with fentanyl or other lipophilic opioids usually occurs soon after administration of a single dose.[95,124]

Several studies have investigated the dose-response relationship of epidural morphine.[222,269,291] Increasing the dose of morphine enhances the intensity and prolongs the duration of analgesia. However, beyond a dose of 4 or 5 mg, the intensity of analgesia seems to plateau, whereas the relationship between dose and duration of analgesia continues until higher doses (7–8 mg) are given (Fig. 23-12). Thus, once satisfactory

TABLE 23-7. Physical and Clinical Characteristics of Epidurally Used Opioid Agents*

| AGENT | PARTITION COEFFICIENT | MOLECULAR WEIGHT | pKa | ONSET (min) | DURATION (h) | BOLUS DOSE |
|---|---|---|---|---|---|---|
| Morphine | 1.40 | 280 | 7.6 | 30–60 | 15–20 | 3–6 mg |
| Methadone | 116 | 300 | 9.2 | 15–20 | 6–8 | 3–6 mg |
| Meperidine | 38 | 247 | 8.5 | 10–25 | 6–8 | 40–80 mg |
| Hydromorphone | 0.316 | — | 8.0 | 15–30 | 10–12 | 1 mg |
| Fentanyl | 813 | 335 | 8.4 | 5–10 | 3–4 | 50–150 μg |
| Alfentanil | 126 | — | — | 10–15 | 0.75–1.25 | 15–30 μg/kg |
| Lofentanil | 1450 | 405 | 7.8 | 8–10 | 8–10 | 1–5 μg |
| Sufentanil | 1778 | 386 | 8.0 | 2–8 | 4–6 | 50–75 μg |
| Butorphanol | 100 | 270 | — | 10–15 | 6–12 | 1–3 mg |
| Nalbuphine | — | — | — | 15–45 | 7–21 | 10 mg |
| Buprenorphine | — | — | — | 8–10 | 6–8 | 0.15–0.30 mg |
| Somatostatin | — | — | — | 10–15 | bolus dose 0.5–1 | 250 μg + infusion of 125 μg/h |

* Data gathered from following sources: Cousins MJ, Mather LE: Anesthesiology 1984, 61:276; Mok et al: Anesthesiology 1984, 61:A187; Chrubasik et al: Anesth Analg 1985, 64:1085; Bilsback et al: Br J Anaesth 1985, 57:943; Coyle et al: Anesthesiology 1984, 61:A240; Chauvin et al: Br J Anaesth 1985, 57:886; Donadoni et al: Anaesthesia 1985, 40:634.

analgesia is obtained, increasing the dose of morphine will produce only prolongation of pain relief.

Some of the clinical characteristics of epidural morphine are as follows:

- Initial segmental analgesia at the site of injection, ascending cephalad over several hours[63]
- Absence of motor or sympathetic blockade and thus minimal fall in blood pressure after injection
- Analgesia of longer duration than that produced by systemic administration; the duration is longer for drugs of low lipid solubility, such as morphine
- Although plasma levels can be high enough to contribute to the initial analgesic effect, this does not account for the duration of analgesia[268]

FIG. 23-12. Relationship between log dose epidural morphine and duration of analgesia. Although analgesia is prolonged with increasing doses of morphine, the correlation coefficient (r) is only 0.40. (From Nordberg et al[269] with permission.)

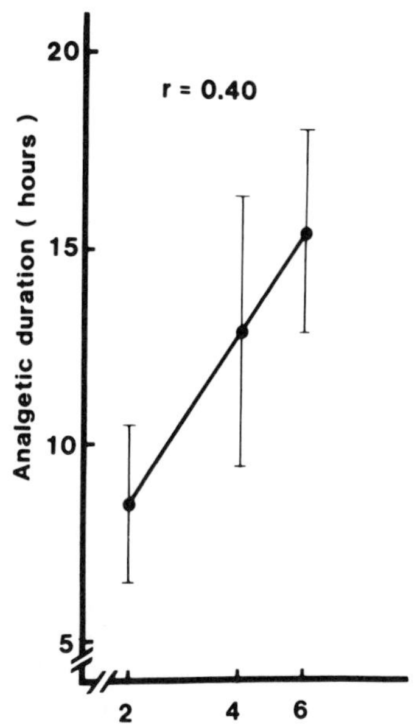


- A decreased sensitivity to $CO_2$ starting soon after injection and peaking 6–10 hours after injection,[68,188] with frank respiratory depression occurring in 0.36–5.0% of intrathecal and 0.1–0.4% of extradural morphine administrations[161,304]; fentanyl via this route also decreases the sensitivity to $CO_2$ but only rarely results in frank respiratory depression[309]; systemic naloxone (0.2–0.4 mg), sometimes in repeated doses or as an infusion (5–10 μg/kg/h), reverses the respiratory depression,[160] although the first measure is to ventilate the lung with oxygen in the apneic patient
- Other side effects, such as nausea and vomiting, itching, and urinary retention, occur commonly,[62] but respond to systemic naloxone (0.2–0.4 mg).[302] For pruritus, diphenhydramine and, for nausea, dimenhydrinate 25–50 mg, IV or IM, every 4–6 hours, may be preferred since naloxone decreases the quality of analgesia.

The indications for the technique, the choice of drug, and the site and mode of administration (thoracic, lumbar, extradural, intrathecal, continuous, bolus, etc.) remain a matter of individual preference. Let it suffice to say that the epidural route is probably used more frequently at present. This approach has the advantage that drugs may be administered over a period of several days.

The dangers of respiratory depression must always be considered, especially in (a) the elderly (over age 70), (b) those with poor respiratory function, (c) those who have had concomitant systemic narcotics and other sedatives or tranquilizers, and (d) those receiving the drug intrathecally at the lumbar or epidurally at the thoracic level.[124,161,304]

Administration of spinal opiates, especially to the above groups of patients, should be undertaken only in a high-dependency zone, such as an ICU or recovery room or in specialized units where respiratory function can be monitored. Apnea can occur suddenly without prior significant decrease of respiratory rate.

SUBLINGUAL AND ORAL NARCOTICS. Buprenorphine, a relatively new partial agonist analgesic with a long duration of action (6–8 hours), can be given sublingually. It has obvious advantages for both the patient and nursing staff and has been shown to produce effective postoperative analgesia.[66,67] A troublesome side effect of this drug is persistent nausea, which at times may be unresponsive to conventional antiemetics, including naloxone.[67] Plasma buprenorphine concentration after a 0.4 mg sublingual dose rises slowly and reaches a peak in about 3 hours.[66,67] The drug is given on a regular basis every 8 hours for 3 or 4 days postoperatively.

Controlled-release oral morphine, given in a dose of 20–30 mg every 8 hours, has been recommended as an effective and convenient postoperative analgesic.[127] However, more recent data show that 70% of patients needed rescue analgesics within 6 hours of surgery, and the drug was inferior to intramuscular or epidural morphine in providing postoperative analgesia.[18,106] The prolonged gastric emptying time after surgery may prevent sufficient absorption of this drug from the gastrointestinal tract, explaining the poor results. The drug may be effective after the second or third postoperative day when gastrointestinal function has recovered.

Buccal morphine (13.3 mg) is a relatively new preparation used in Europe. Preliminary studies suggest that it produces postoperative analgesia comparable to an equal dose of intramuscular morphine.[23]

None of the preparations described above appears to provide as powerful postoperative analgesia as intravenous or epidural opiates. Thus, their use is limited to relatively minor postoperative pain.

### *Nerve Blocks*

INFILTRATION. Infiltration of wound edges with a long-acting local anesthetic agent, such as bupivacaine, has been practiced by orthopedists and neurosurgeons for some time,[110,252] and the technique has been advocated to produce postoperative analgesia for other incisions.[280,342] The concept has been extended to leaving a catheter in the wound and infusing 0.5% bupivacaine, 10 mL, twice daily, to provide analgesia for complex incisions, such as laparotomy and thoracotomy.[207,274,280,366] It should be noted that reasonable analgesia can be produced by infusion of normal saline into surgical wounds,[366] probably by washing pain-producing substances away from the site of injury.

PERIPHERAL NERVE BLOCK. Peripheral nerve block can be administered either by single injection or a continuous catheter technique. With the single injection technique, a long-acting local anesthetic agent is used, and the block is repeated as required. With the continuous technique, a catheter is inserted adjacent to the nerve(s), and either intermittent doses or continuous infusion of local anesthetic agent can be administered. When continuous infusion is used, following an initial bolus dose, bupivacaine, 0.25%, 0.1–0.25 mg/kg/h (approximately 5 mL/hr), produces adequate analgesia with plasma bupivacaine levels maintained below the toxic range (1.5–1.7 μg/mL).[201,372] In practice, these techniques have been performed primarily to produce anesthesia for surgery and have been continued postoperatively to provide analgesia. Thus, analgesia by this method is usually confined to the limbs; the brachial plexus,[296] femoral nerve,[319] and the lumbar plexus[50] are blocked most frequently. Occasionally, the trauma patient may pose some limitations for these blocks; time constraints may not permit the insertion of a preoperative catheter, and the need for surgical assessment of the limb postoperatively may preclude prolonged blockade. In the absence of these conditions, however, peripheral nerve blocks, by providing excellent analgesia, improving the mobilization of the injured limb, and augmenting the blood flow to the extremity, not only speed the return to function but probably lessen the risk of reflex sympathetic changes.

Some peripheral nerve blocks can be performed easily in the operating room after surgery is completed. The lateral femoral cutaneous nerve can be blocked by fan-wise injection of local anesthetic agents under Poupart's ligament slightly anterior and 1 cm inferior to the anterior superior iliac spine. This block can reduce the postoperative narcotic requirement of patients having surgery for femoral neck fractures with a lateral thigh incision.[185]

INTERCOSTAL BLOCKS. Although much has been written about the advantages and feasibility of performing repeated intercostal blocks for postoperative analgesia,[57,247] the technique has not found much favor. Although bupivacaine can produce blockade for as long as 16 hours, this is still not long enough for most abdominal and thoracic incisions. Also, the inability of physicians to be present immediately at the time the patient complains of pain detracts from the method. As discussed earlier, the technique described by Murphy[254–256] of using a percutaneously inserted intercostal catheter allows repeated injections or continuous infusion of local anesthetic agents without pain or discomfort.

A more recently described method of postoperative analgesia involves insertion of an epidural catheter into the pleural space and injection of 0.5% bupivacaine (20 mL).[204,306] A Tuohy needle is inserted into the eighth intercostal space about 10 cm lateral to the spinous process of the corresponding vertebra and angled 45° to the skin. After perforating the intercostal membrane, the stylet is removed, and a 5-mL syringe is attached to the hub of the needle. The syringe and needle are then carefully advanced until a "clicking" perforation of parietal pleura is felt, and the loss of resistance produced by intrapleural negative pressure surges the plunger of the syringe forward. An extradural catheter is inserted through the Tuohy needle 5–6 cm into the pleural space, and after removing the needle, it is secured with tape. Addition of epinephrine to the bupivacaine limits local anesthetic absorption from the pleural space.[190] Intrapleural bupivacaine appears to provide prolonged analgesia for between 5 and 7 hours without opiate supplementation.[204] The method has been used successfully to provide postoperative analgesia after cholecystectomy by the subcostal approach,[359] renal surgery, and mastectomy. However, pain relief produced by this technique after thoracotomy is less profound and of shorter duration than that in patients with intact closed chest.[315] This has been attributed to the loss of local anesthetic from the chest drains. Clamping of chest tubes and discontinuing pleural suction for 10–15 minutes after the local anesthetic bolus injection, however, provided only limited success in some studies.[327,362] Rapid absorption of local anesthetic through the injured pleural surface and dilution by the residual irrigation fluid and/or blood may also be responsible for the decreased efficacy.[190] An important complication of this technique is pneumothorax, sometimes under tension, especially when insertion of the catheter is followed by ventilation of the patient with positive pressure. In one series nearly half of the catheters inserted in this fashion were malpositioned, and one-third were found within the lung parenchyma, resulting in a 14% incidence of pneumothorax.[361]

Two other invasive techniques described to relieve thoracotomy pain involve intraoperative cryoanalgesia[147,191,192,216] and injection of phenol into the intercostal nerves.[322] In the former technique, a cryoprobe freezes the dissected intercostal nerves at a site close to the intervertebral foramen twice within an interval of a few minutes for 30 seconds at a time. The technique is reported to produce excellent postoperative pain relief in 80% of patients undergoing elective thoracotomy.[216] Refinement of the method also allows the performance of cryoanalgesia percutaneously, but experience with this method is limited. The second technique involves injection of 1 mL phenol (6% in glycerine) into the dissected nerves involved in the incision.[322] The technique is reported to be effective in producing postoperative pain relief in patients undergoing elective thoracotomy, and intercostal neuralgia due to irritation of the nerve by phenol does not appear to be a problem.[322]

EPIDURAL BLOCKADE. Reference has already been made to the use of thoracic epidural local anesthetics for the treatment of fractured ribs and also to the use of opiates by this route. The technique can be applied to all abdominal and thoracic incisions, as well as for pelvic and lower limb surgery. The advantages of the technique are complete pain relief, even for coughing and physical therapy; freedom from detrimental effects of opiates—sedation, respiratory depression, and possibly decreased intestinal function; and earlier ambulation and better restoration of the FRC than after systemic narcotics.[58]

This technique is not without side effects. The most notable are hypotension, urinary retention, and motor blockade, and these, combined with the complexities of the technique, account for its limited use. However, those workers who have persevered and attained a high rate of success have been uniformly enthusiastic about the method and its advantages.[156,284,341] One of the reasons for the high incidence of side effects would seem to be the use of intermittent injections. Not only is the intermittent technique unsatisfactory because of breakthrough pain every few hours but intermittent sympathetic blockade also causes hypotension and the development of tachyphylaxis.[59] Furthermore, the necessity for repeated injections followed by an hour of close monitoring places a heavy burden on the medical staff.

Continuous infusions offer a much more logical approach from both the pharmacologic and manpower viewpoints.[298] By adjusting the concentration and volume of the infusate one can alter the intensity and extent of the blockade. Once the block has been established, it is often possible to maintain it with a relatively weak anesthetic solution, which diminishes the likelihood of toxicity. For lower limb and perineal wounds it is usually possible to obtain good analgesia with 0.1–0.2% solutions of bupivacaine, which do not produce significant motor blockade. Higher incisions, such as abdominal or thoracic, often require larger volumes of stronger solutions at least initially, and positioning the catheter at the level of the center of the wound is more critical in these patients. Once the infusion is underway, the patient requires only routine observation, as the infusate is changed only once a day or whenever a change in concentration is required. Pain relief with the continuous infusion technique is also possible via paravertebrally placed catheters if the postoperative pain is unilateral. Hypotension and urinary retention are less likely with this approach than with continuous epidural analgesia.[226]

With thoracic and abdominal incisions, severe pain can be engendered by regression of the block by as little as one segment: in the early stages this may occur very rapidly. In these situations there may be a case for adding a narcotic (meperidine, 5–10 mg/h, morphine 0.5–1.0 mg/h, or fentanyl 35–50 μg/h) to the infusate.[330] In this way the advantages of the local anesthetic agent are supplemented by an analgesic safety net that closes any gaps in the block and covers other pains not adequately treated by a limited segmental blockade.

## CHRONIC PAIN AFTER TRAUMA AND ITS MANAGEMENT

Pain persisting longer than the normal recovery period, often greatly exceeding that which might be anticipated in the light of the residual pathology, can be considered chronic posttraumatic pain.

### *General Principles*

The treatment of persistent posttraumatic pain that results from deranged patterns of healing, the development of altered pain pathways, chronic ischemia, and/or misuse or disuse of myofascial structures is far more complex than the management of acute pain syndromes. Contributing psychosocial and stress factors in the interpretation and outward expression of pain must always be considered in the chronic pain patient; resultant cognitive, affective, and/or behavioral changes often contribute to the perpetuation of pain.[134,146,257] Consequently, a multidisciplinary approach as proposed by Bonica should be utilized if consistent success is to be realized.[36,38] This approach requires not only accurate medical diagnosis but also behavioral and functional therapy utilized *in concert* with medical and physical treatment. No single therapeutic mode can be expected to provide consistently satisfactory results.

The complexity of chronic pain mechanisms is such that, when compared to the acute pain syndromes previously described, one is generally forced to accept lesser degrees of therapeutic success. Reasonable goals need to be discussed frankly with the patient at the onset of treatment and frequently reiterated. Chronic pain management should be directed toward pain control, rather than cure, with specific goals that include

- Reduction of pain and elevation of pain threshold
- Emphasis on improved function and rehabilitation
- Reduction of reliance upon medication, with elimination of potentially addictive drugs

## *Chronic Pain Syndromes and their Mechanisms*

PERIPHERAL MECHANISMS. *Myofascial Pain.* Perhaps the most common persistent pain after trauma is that emanating from myofascial (musculoskeletal) structures: muscle, bone, tendon, ligament, and other soft tissues of mesodermal origin. Myofascial pain may be due to one or more of the following causes: (a) reflex muscle spasm, (b) ischemia of the myofascial structures, (c) decreased nutrition, (d) muscle fatigue due to excessive use, and (e) muscle injury.[153,412] In most instances, pain is caused by interference with oxidative processes in the muscle due to decreases in oxygen, enzymes, and nutrients necessary for muscle metabolism. When fatigue follows overexertion, pain and soreness are experienced hours or days later. They may be caused by increased levels of cellular metabolites and water, which stimulate nociceptive nerve endings. Once the painful state is produced, it can be perpetuated by feedback cycles from myofascial trigger points.[297]

Afferent pain signals from spastic muscle enter the spinal cord through the dorsal root, where communication via internuncial neurons leads to hyperactivity in the anterior and anterolateral horn cells. As a result of this hyperactivity, efferent impulses cause more muscle spasm and vasoconstriction. Exercise exaggerates this relative ischemia, intensifying the pain.[36] Long-standing persistence of this positive feedback cycle can lead to sympathalgia with vasomotor disturbance.

Trigger points are regions of hyperirritability within myofascial structures that, when stimulated by direct pressure, elicit tenderness and, if severe, referred pain.[412] These regions of focal muscle spasm limit active and passive motion, producing apparent shortening and weakening of the involved musculature. Pain from deep somatic structures is typically dull and diffuse in character. The ability to localize precise trigger areas decreases with increasing depth. Diffusion and radiation can be indicators of severity, with muscle spasm and tenderness in zones of reference (to be distinguished from trigger point) often appearing at sites distant from the lesion. The intensity of the hyperirritability makes it relatively resistant to systemic muscle relaxants or analgesics. Injection of local anesthetic agents into specific zones of reference will decrease tenderness in that region. However, injection of trigger points not only decreases tenderness but also reduces muscle spasm and spontaneous pain.[153,412]

Fibrositis is a term used to characterize the chronic aseptic inflammatory reaction within soft tissues that can result in fibrosis and contracture. The importance of maintaining function as a means of ultimately reducing pain cannot be overemphasized. Yet, mobilization of the affected body parts and physical therapy are often difficult or impossible without first alleviating the attendant pain (Fig. 23-13).

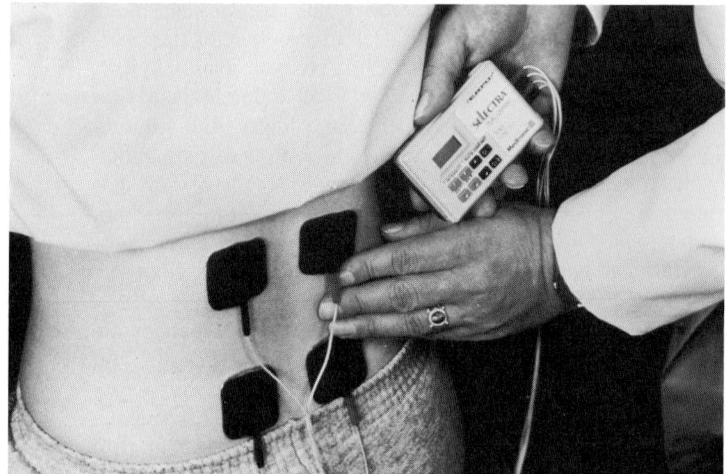
A

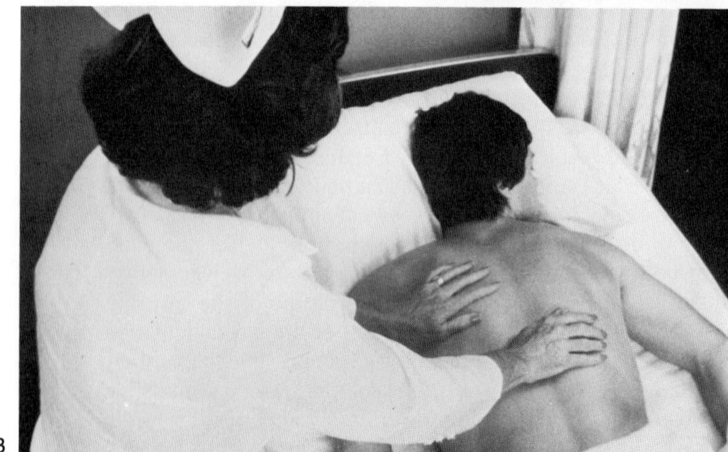
B

FIG. 23-13. Myofascial pain: The treatment of myofascial pain should emphasize return of function. The photographs shown depict four of the commonly used modalities to facilitate this goal: transcutaneous electrical nerve stimulation (TENS) (A); physical therapy (B); fluorimethane spray and muscle stretching (C); and myoneural injection (D).

Nonmuscular structures, such as tendon, ligament, and fascia, are also common sources of myofascial pain. Thoracic fasciitis after thoracotomy, bursitis, tenosynovitis, and traumatic arthritis, as well as ligamentous strains and sprains, are but a few of the myriad of common examples.

*Sympathalgia.* This syndrome is characterized by hyperactivity of either afferent or efferent C fibers or both. It is generally classified into two syndromes: causalgia and reflex sympathetic dystrophy. There are three theories that attempt to explain the pain associated with these syndromes: (1) gate control theory, (2) vicious cycle of reflexes theory, and (3) artificial synapse theory. The most credible of the three is the last one.[238,313] It is based on the fact that, when a lesion destroys the electrical insulation between different adjacent nerve fibers or otherwise alters the anatomy, efferent C fibers may directly stimulate afferent somatic fibers. Constant orthodromic bombardment is interpreted as pain. In addition, antidromic depolarization sensitizes peripheral nerve endings. This too results in increased impulse transmission that also is interpreted as pain. Thus, the classic nociceptive model that has been described for acute pain does not necessarily apply in chronic pain states. In fact, chronic pain information may be transmitted in the fashion described, even over the very large A-alpha fibers if afferent traffic is sufficiently intense. These pathways can be delineated by differential nerve blocking techniques to provide a focus for therapeutic intervention.

Reflex sympathetic dystrophies are sometimes categorized according to predominant symptoms. However, certain features are characteristic. Burning and aching pain—initially localized but later spreading proximally—cold sensitivity, hyperesthesia, and vasomotor and sudomotor disturbances are typical. When occurring as the result of traumatic insult, the onset of such changes is usually relatively rapid, often beginning within days or weeks of the injury (Fig. 23-14).[107,283]

Early signs include vasodilation with resultant rubor and edema. Sudomotor changes, such as hyperhidrosis, also occur, but are somewhat less constant. Later signs result from vasoconstriction, ie, cyanosis and cold skin distally. Trophic changes—thin glossy skin, nutritional nail changes, coarse-appearing hair or loss of hair, muscle atrophy, and bone demineralization—are noted late in the course of the disease. As these changes are essentially the result of a nutritional deficit imposed by perpetual vasoconstriction, they tend to be present distally since these tissues are most vulnerable to ischemic insult.

Clinical presentation of reflex sympathetic dystrophy varies widely, and clear-cut signs and symptoms of the disease are lacking in many patients. As laboratory and routine radiographic tests are of little value, in many instances sympathetic

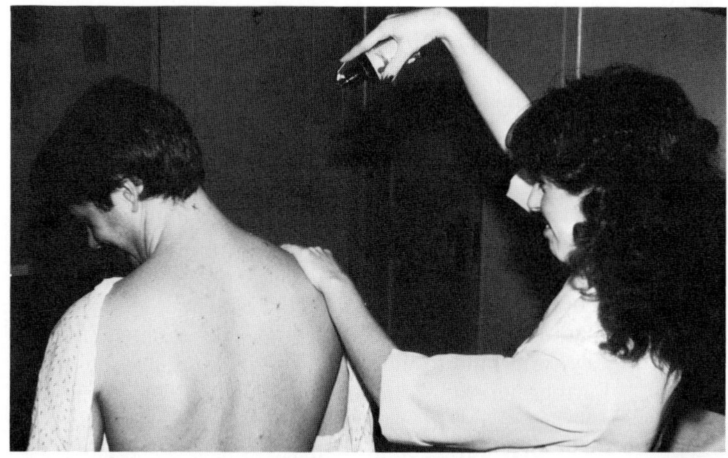

C

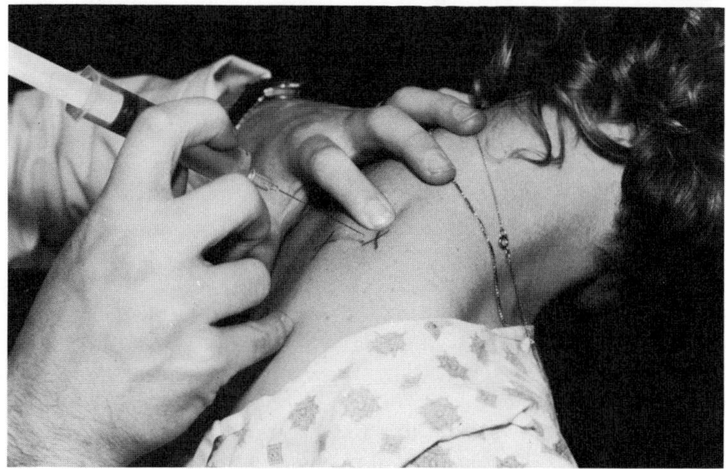

D

FIG. 23-13. Continued.

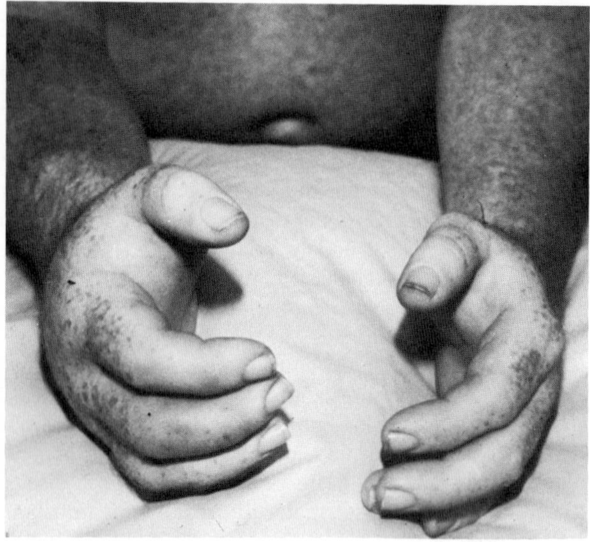

FIG. 23-14. Reflex sympathetic dystrophy: The photograph shows the hands of a 30-year-old man who suffered a scaphoid fracture of the right wrist. Subsequently, he developed burning pain in the hand appearing at the time of cast removal. The pain was associated with hyperesthesia, cold sensitivity, edema, and hyperhidrosis, suggesting the diagnosis of reflex sympathetic dystrophy. All symptoms resolved after a series of three stellate ganglion blocks, but recurred promptly when the hand was reinjured several months later. The response to sympathetic blockade was less pronounced when repeated. However, the patient responded favorably to a continuous brachial plexus infusion.

nerve blocks have been performed partly as a diagnostic measure.[283] However, triple-phase radionuclide bone scanning has been shown to be a reliable test, with a sensitivity of 96%, a specificity of 97%, and a negative predictive value of 99% in diagnosing reflex sympathetic dystrophy.[174] This test may be particularly useful in differentiating the pain produced by reflex sympathetic dystrophy from that caused by central mechanisms; for example, in patients with recent spinal cord injury.[98]

Although sympathetic blockade and aggressive physical therapy are well-proven techniques for promoting repair and decreasing pain after the development of reflex sympathetic dystrophy, the notion that early analgesic and sympathetic blocks in conjunction with early active motion might prevent the development of the syndrome holds tremendous logical appeal.[31,283,374,390] Controlled studies, however, have yet to be completed.

The term "causalgia" describes a similar syndrome of burning pain with hyperesthesia and accompanying vasomotor and sudomotor disturbances occurring soon after a partial nerve injury.[180,338] Penetrating wounds, especially from high-velocity missiles, seem to predispose to causalgia, but other forms of nerve injury may also produce the syndrome. The pain is usually constant, severe, and spontaneous, but can be precipitated by emotional stress or peripheral stimuli and relieved by sympathetic blockade.[180,338] Often, an extreme degree of hyperesthesia—hyperpathia—is seen. Pathologically, ruptured axons seem to heal with endoneural fibrosis, rather than discrete neuromas. Why some partial nerve injuries result in neuritis and others in causalgia is not known. Whether the nature of the insult affects either the mode of healing or the subsequent symptomatology is also unclear.

*Neuralgias and Neuromas.* Partial nerve injuries resulting from mechanical trauma sometimes result, as previously mentioned, in an irritative state associated with perineuritis or neuritis. Typical neuritic pain is burning, lancinating, worse at night, and aggravated by stretching of the affected nerve. Other irritative phenomena, such as fascicular muscle twitching or spasm, hyperesthesia, paresthesia, or dysesthesia, may be present. Vasomotor or sudomotor changes are not seen in the absence of significant sympathalgia (Fig. 23-15).

There are numerous examples of postoperative and posttraumatic injuries to peripheral nerves resulting in mononeuritides. The host of postoperative neuralgias caused by mechanical nerve trauma in the form of pressure resulting from improper patient positioning on the operating room table have been well described. Intercostal neuralgia after thoracotomy or chest wall injury is particularly common. Nerve entrapment or involvement in scar tissue also gives rise to pain. Irritation of sympathetic fibers around the spermatic cord or injury to the genitofemoral nerve during herniorrhaphy or other inguinal surgery is often unusually resistant to treatment.

Plexalgias occur posttraumatically in both upper and lower extremities. Cervical plexalgia can give rise to extensive myofascial neck and shoulder pain. Sudden stretching of the upper extremity at the shoulder can cause brachial plexalgia. Lumbar plexalgia, although usually of viral origin, can occur after trauma because of the considerable mobility of the lumbar spine. Early sympathetic blockade is probably useful in the prevention of sympathalgias after these injuries.

After complete disruption of a peripheral nerve, the severed ends of the axons grow in an effort to reunite. Anatomic disruption often precludes proper realignment of the proximal axon with its corresponding distal component. This may result in dysesthesias. Additionally, abnormal afferent impulses emanating from the dorsal root ganglion after nerve injury probably contribute to the production of abnormal sensations.[387] Furthermore, after trauma or amputation, the cut ends of the neurons search in vain for the missing nerve trunk and eventually may curl around themselves or become embedded in scar or other soft tissue. These bulbous collections of nonmyelinated neurons are called neuromas. Neuromata do not behave like normal sensory receptors, but instead, when appropriately stimulated, often generate an exaggerated response with sharp lancinating pain in the distribution of the affected nerve.[404] Protracted, often chronic muscular contractions of the affected stump can result. Neuromas can be quite labile, giving rise to spontaneous discharge, especially when large and tender, as can be the case when infection complicates the postamputation period.

CENTRAL MECHANISMS. *Deafferentation and Phantom Limb Pain.* Dysesthesia after denervation is thought to be caused by abnormal neuronal activity at central sites resulting from either the loss or relative imbalance of afferent input.[232] It may be related to a relative predominance of small fibers in the absence of input from larger fibers.[263] As in other cen-

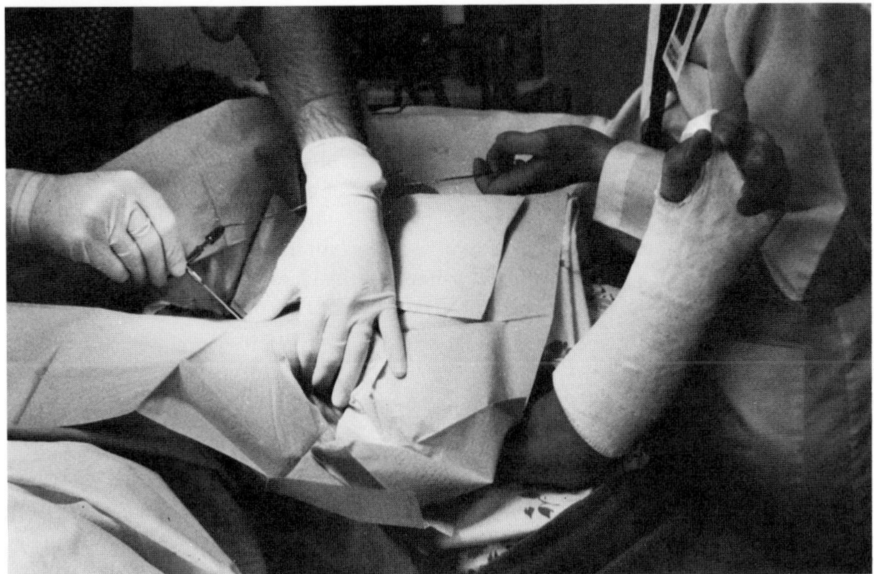

FIG. 23-15. Neuritis: The patient shown is a 54-year-old woman who suffered a Colles fracture with median nerve contusion requiring open reduction and internal fixation with exploration of the median nerve. She experienced burning pain secondary to median nerve neuritis initially, with the subsequent development of dystrophic changes 6 weeks after the injury. Here a brachial plexus catheter is being placed for continuous infusion with the aid of a nerve stimulator using the infraclavicular approach. The patient responded very well to 7 days of continuous analgesia and intensive physical therapy.

tral pain states, therapies resulting in further peripheral denervation are generally of no value.

Postamputation phantom sensations occur in most amputees; however, only 5 to 10% report associated pain. It has been suggested that the incidence of pain may in fact be much higher (72%).[181] The pain may be burning, crushing, shooting, throbbing, or related to the impression that the missing part is fixed in an abnormal and uncomfortable position. This is particularly true if the pain or abnormal posture was present before the amputation.[231,311]

Despite the appearance of vasomotor and sudomotor changes in some patients with phantom limb pain, sympathetic interruption rarely is of lasting value.[189] Further, although these painful sensations can be aggravated by irritation of neuromas within the stump, clearly such peripheral mechanisms cannot fully explain this form of deafferentation pain. Neither the time course of neuroma formation nor the anatomic distribution of the affected nerves is consistent with phantom sensation. Phantom sensations usually correspond to the areas with the greatest representation in the sensory cortex, with an impression of gradual shortening of the phantom limb until only the hand or foot remains attached to the stump just before resolution. The presence of pain prevents this apparent shrinkage. Emotional upset and fatigue can trigger phantom pain.

Increasing evidence now suggests that reorganization of neural pathways at spinal as well as thalamic and cortical levels takes place after peripheral deafferentation.[108,386] Melzack proposed a central biasing mechanism.[230] This concept is similar to the central mechanism of deafferentation mentioned above. Sensory loss creates a relative predominance of small fibers, which results in release of normal tonic inhibition from central sites. This release presumably predisposes to self-perpetuating neuronal activity at spinal and higher centers in the central nervous system. This line of thinking is consistent with the development of phantom limb pain in previous amputees following a sufficiently high level of spinal or epidural anesthesia.[203] Presumably, anesthesia-induced loss of somatic input to the spinal cord causes decreased inhibition from central sites, resulting in the increase of self-sustaining neural firing by the small fibers in the unblocked spinal cord or higher levels of the central nervous system. Phantom limb pain precipitated by spinal anesthesia can be abolished by intravenous administration of subanesthetic doses of thiopental or benzodiazepines.[203]

### *Treatment of Chronic Pain*

ORAL MEDICATIONS. The treatment of chronic pain by oral analgesics is very much a two-edged sword; although symptomatic relief can often be obtained, especially by using the more potent analgesics, they do nothing to modify the pain in the long term. Furthermore, the more potent the drug, the greater the likelihood of dependence. The less potent agents, although less troublesome in this respect, often do little to relieve the pain.

Most physicians involved in chronic pain treatment are reluctant to prescribe narcotics, although they often see patients who are taking these drugs at the time of referral. Some believe there is a population who can be managed satisfactorily with long-term narcotics,[289,378] but for most, the goal remains the elimination of drugs with the potential for abuse or addiction, a group that includes all the opiates.

Simple anti-inflammatory drugs, such as acetaminophen and aspirin, can be effective, especially in those syndromes where the tissue prostaglandin system may be incriminated.[200,310] However, in this situation the more potent nonsteroidal anti-inflammatory agents, such as indomethacin, ibuprophen, naprosyn, etc., are probably more effective and have been used with success in posttraumatic syndromes, especially the neuralgias and myofascial pain.[149,200,310]

All these drugs should be given on a regular basis, rather than when the pain requires it. The latter regimen not only fails to maintain adequate plasma levels but also tends to reinforce the behavioral component of the pain process, a phenomenon that must be eliminated as soon as possible.

Inadequate sleep and depression, either masked or overt, are problems common to many pain sufferers.[286] These two problems are amenable to pharmacologic intervention. Tricyclic antidepressants, such as amitriptyline (50–150 mg/day), desipramine (50–150 mg/day), and doxepin (75–150 mg/day), are particularly useful in this context; their central effect on serotoninergic pathways gives them a direct influence on pain transmission.[47,64,128] In addition, a small dose given at bedtime can provide enough sedation to aid sleep, as well as improve depressive symptoms.[164,320] Long-term use of a narcotic-antidepressant combination has been recommended for the treatment of intractable phantom limb pain.[378] Frank depression requires more aggressive treatment with larger doses of tricyclic or tetracyclic antidepressants or monoamine oxidase inhibitors in close liaison with skilled psychiatric staff.

Psychotropic drugs, such as fluphenazine (1 mg/day), can be of value when combined with tricyclic antidepressants in the treatment of neuropathies and phantom limb pain.

Muscle relaxants, such as carisoprodol (Soma®), methocarbamol (Robaxin®), cyclobenzaprine (Flexeril®), and chlorozoxazone (Paraflex®), are often prescribed in myofascial pain syndromes, although this therapy seldom provides anything more than minimal help. Diazepam (2.5–10 mg/day) and baclofen both have muscle relaxant actions due to their interactions with GABA. The former, although a drug with dependence and abuse potential, is useful in the more anxious personality, whereas the latter is beneficial for painful muscle spasms, especially those associated with traumatic paraplegia. Baclofen should be started in small doses (5 mg × 3) and gradually increased until adequate response is obtained. The usual daily dose is between 40–80 mg.

Carbamazepin (Tegretol), 400–800 mg/day in three divided doses, has a specific use in trigeminal neuralgia, but can also be of benefit in other neuralgias.[360] This drug may cause bone marrow depression; thus hematocrit, leucocyte, platelet, and reticulocyte counts should be monitored on a weekly or biweekly basis. Phenytoin (300–500 mg/day) has also been found useful in some patients with chronic pain.[360] A combination of tricyclic antidepressants and antiepileptic drugs may be useful in reducing persistent neuralgic pain, such as traumatic brachial plexalgia.[65]

L-tryptophan, the amino acid precursor of serotonin, has been advocated for use in chronic pain. This drug, by increasing brain serotonin levels, may reduce depression and increase pain tolerance in chronic pain patients.[334] L-tryptophan is also a mild sedative and may aid sleep if it is given at bedtime. Ketanserin, a specific 5-hydroxy tryptamine antagonist, may be beneficial in the treatment of pain of causalgia. In one patient oral ketanserin, 60–80 mg/day in divided doses after a single 14-mg intravenous dose, provided pain relief for at least 1 year.[102]

Various sympathetic blocking agents have been used with success in a few patients with phantom limb pain,[220] but the overall results are not encouraging. However, nifedipine, 30–60 mg/day given orally for 2 weeks, produced satisfactory pain relief in a small group of patients with reflex sympathetic dystrophy.[290] Phenoxybenzamine, a pre- and postsynaptic alpha-adrenergic blocking agent, has been used with success in patients with causalgia.[141] In one clinical trial, treatment with this drug (40–120 mg/day, orally) for 6 to 8 weeks produced a total resolution of pain in all patients.[141] These preliminary results are encouraging, but further trials are needed to confirm these findings.

NERVE BLOCKS. Neural blockade with local anesthetic agents is often the only way of actually abolishing a patient's pain.[36,91,299] Blocks can be *diagnostic* where blockade of particular nerves can give important information about pain pathways, *prognostic* where the block is performed to predict the analgesia from more permanent therapy, or *therapeutic* where the block has beneficial effects by either permanently diminishing the nociception, or secondarily by increasing blood flow to the tissues. Blocks can be central (subarachnoid or extradural), peripheral, or sympathetic (stellate ganglion[69] or lumbar paravertebral sympathetic[165]).

In general, a block is first performed as a diagnostic or prognostic maneuver with a local anesthetic agent. Frequently, in certain syndromes—phantom limb pain, causalgia, and sympathetic dystrophy—such a block, usually of the sympathetic system, will provide relief of longer duration than the action of the agent used. This relief can be extended further by repeating the block or by using continuous analgesia techniques. It should be noted that with most of the syndromes where blocks have been shown to be of value, results are usually better if the block is performed relatively early after the injury.[1,282] Sometimes blocks with reversible agents provide only transient relief, and one needs to contemplate the use of a neurolytic agent. The two most commonly used neurolytic agents are phenol (6–12%)[410] and absolute ethyl alcohol. These agents are relatively effective for chemical sympathectomy or rhizotomy, but are less satisfactory for lysis of peripheral nerves because of the possibility of neuritis. Alcohol and phenol have both been used in the treatment of pain and contractures secondary to paraplegia as intrathecal, perineural, or local neurolytic agents. The effect of neurolytic agents tends not to be permanent, since some function may return after 3 or 4 months.

In myofascial dysfunction, the use of nerve blocks can relieve muscle spasm, increase blood flow by sympathetic blockade, relieve pain, and allow aggressive physical therapy. In severe cases such blocks are often needed, at least initially. Milder cases can be managed with local anesthetic trigger point injections[153,412] using either a conventional needle-syringe system or a jet injector. The latter has been shown to produce less pain during treatment.[305] A variety of agents have been used for trigger point injections including most local anesthetic agents, serapin, saline, and even dry needles.[369]

Steroids, usually in the form of depo-medrol (40–80 mg), have been used extensively in the treatment of neuralgias, neuromas, myofascial pain, sympathetic dystrophies and most other posttraumatic pain syndromes. However, the precise indication for and results of their use remain poorly elucidated.

A further method of considerable value in the treatment of sympathetic dysfunction in limbs is an intravenous regional technique using either guanethidine (10–20 mg), reserpine (1–2.5 mg), or bretylium (1 mg/kg) in 50 mL of saline solution.[26,130,148,199] These agents deplete adrenergic neurons and thus provide sympathetic blockade for 1–2 weeks, a period often long enough to produce sustained relief in sympathalgias and phantom limb pain.[210] In patients with reflex sympathetic dystrophy, Bonelli et al.[35] showed more persistent increases in skin temperature after intravenous guanethidine regional analgesia performed at 4-day intervals than after stellate ganglion block administered at 1-day intervals. Although this method appears to be effective, it is not free of complications. Apnea and syncope may occur upon injection of the drug[221] or deflation of the tourniquet, probably because of the escape of guanethidine into the systemic circulation. Injection of the drug into a distal vein of the extremity, rather than into a more proximal vein, over at least 90 seconds with the use of a tourniquet pressure of at least 300 mm Hg may prevent this complication.[157] Exsanguination of the extremity with an Esmarch bandage before tourniquet inflation is another preventive measure,[157] but this maneuver may be difficult in some patients with painful extremities. Although used in Europe, neither guanethidine nor reserpine is available for intravenous use in the United States. Therefore, presently, this type of block can be performed only with bretylium with which experience is yet limited.

STIMULATION-PRODUCED ANALGESIA.[236,396] It has long been realized that rubbing or stimulating the skin adjacent to a painful area could relieve the pain, but it was not until the introduction of the gate control theory that this phenomenon could be explained at the spinal level.[232] Publication of this theory led to renewed interest in the possibilities of stimulation-produced analgesia and initiated the necessary research for the development of clinical transcutaneous nerve stimulation (TENS). A small battery-operated device that produces high-frequency (2–100 hz) alternating current is attached to the skin by adhesive electrodes. There are no rigid criteria for electrode placement as long as the painful area is stimulated.[408] These devices have proven to be of value in many types of pain, but they are particularly useful in posttraumatic pain syndromes, such as phantom limb pain and myofascial dysfunction. In the former, notoriously difficult condition, TENS can often provide some pain relief even when other maneuvers have been unsuccessful.[355] The unit is generally worn inconspicuously under clothing for 3 to 5 hours a day periodically (Fig. 23-16).[140]

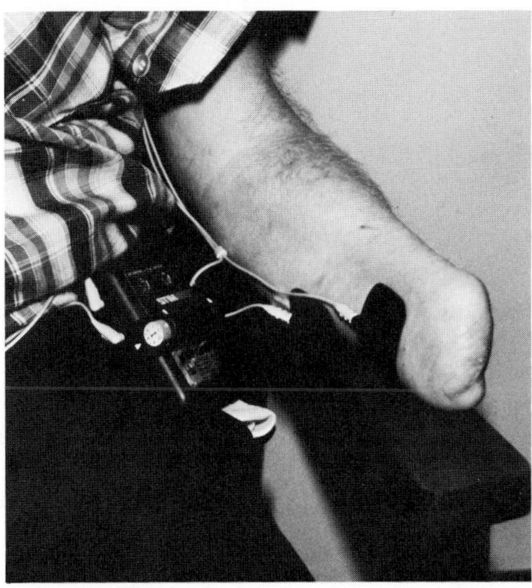

FIG. 23-16. The patient shown developed stump pain and phantom sensation after amputation. He was initially treated with stellate ganglion blocks. TENS provided prolonged relief and enabled him to tolerate his prosthesis.

Acupuncture, although of much greater antiquity, is thought to work in a similar fashion by stimulating the larger cutaneous sensory fibers and thus activating the spinal endorphin-gating mechanism that antagonizes the nociceptive traffic via the smaller A and C fibers. Acupuncture has been used in many pain syndromes, including posttraumatic sympathetic dystrophy[73] but, although effective,[55] is less practical than TENS.

Experimentally electrical stimulation of certain areas of the brain (in particular, the pariaqueductal gray area and the thalamus)[417,418] and the dorsal columns of the spinal cord[376] can produce analgesia, presumably because of stimulation of descending inhibitory pathways. Dorsal column stimulators can be inserted into the epidural space percutaneously via a Tuohy needle.[376] Such devices have been used for intractable posttraumatic pain, but analgesia with this technique is all too frequently of short duration, with pain returning to previous levels after 3 to 6 months. Another important disadvantage of this technique is paresthesias produced by stimulation and referred to the painful part of the body. However, simultaneous stimulation of the appropriate paravertebral nerve with a separately introduced percutaneous electrode may reduce the intensity of this discomfort.[377]

ABLATIVE NEUROSURGERY. Various neurosurgical techniques have been devised primarily for the treatment of pain produced by malignant tumors,[416] but some of these have been applied to persistent severe posttraumatic pain as well.[236] In general, the approach that patients often suggest of "cutting the nerves" seldom produces pain relief and can produce a sensory deficit with deafferentation pain that is worse or, at best, no better than the original discomfort.

Surgical sympathectomy in selected patients with causalgia produces a dramatic and lasting pain relief.[180,239] Postsympathectomy neuralgia may develop in about 50% of these patients, but it disappears within 2 months.[239] Among many central neuroablative procedures, chordotomy is probably the most satisfactory. However, as an open procedure this operation is associated with a high complication rate, including motor weakness, sensory loss, failure to relieve pain, and disturbance of bladder and bowel function. The development of a percutaneous approach using a radiofrequency coagulator has improved this record, but even so, the applications of chordotomy in nonmalignant pain are limited to those patients for whom conventional less invasive techniques have brought no relief and who are completely debilitated by pain.

Destruction of the dorsal root entry zone (DREZ lesion) has been used in persistent phantom limb pain with some success.[262] This procedure also has been used to treat pain caused by brachial plexus avulsion and spinal cord trauma, with results of long-term pain relief of 50% or more in almost 90% of patients.[65,260,261] Percutaneous radiofrequency lysis of dorsal root ganglia has also been tried in a few patients with posttraumatic pain. The procedure appears to be of value in posttraumatic neuralgia and peripheral nerve injuries, but is ineffective for phantom limb and stump pain.[259]

PHYSICAL THERAPY. Physical therapy is of major therapeutic value to many trauma victims who need rehabilitation of stiff and painful joints and muscles after injury. In particular, myofascial dysfunction is best treated in the long term with vigorous exercise once the cycle of pain has been broken. Physical therapy in this context not only utilizes active and passive exercise programs but also the application of heat and cold.

Heat can be applied with hot packs for surface warmth and ultrasound for deeper tissues. Likewise, cold can be applied with either ice packs or fluorimethane spray. This latter technique, especially when combined with passive and active stretching of the muscles, is of great value in treating myofascial pain. Not only does this treatment produce analgesia by cooling but, like ultrasound, it is also followed by reflex vasodilation that improves muscle blood flow, removes metabolites, and restores function.

Once initial assessment and treatment have been carried out in the clinic, patients are given a home exercise program of progressive rigor; they need only occasional return visits to treat exacerbations of pain or stiffness. Likewise, family or friends can be taught to administer fluorimethane spray, often with considerable benefit.[369]

PSYCHOLOGICAL TECHNIQUES. The importance of the psyche in chronic pain of any origin is now recognized by all workers in the field, not only in the development of pain behavior but also in its treatment.[19]

Treatment is directed along two main avenues—cognitive therapy and behavioral therapy—with the aims being to alter the way the patient perceives the sensory input that is interpreted as pain and the emotive and behavioral patterns that reinforce that perception. The most commonly utilized techniques are psychotherapy, biofeedback, relaxation, hypnosis, and operant conditioning.

Psychotherapy in the pain clinic is offered at two levels. The first utilizes formal sessions with the psychologist as a definitive treatment modality in an attempt to modify the patient's attitude to pain, and the second is used by the other pain control center workers in day-to-day patient contact. The importance of this latter aspect should not be underestimated, as the attitudes of the clinic personnel and their understanding of the complexities of pain syndromes, their mechanisms, and the associated behavior patterns can make a considerable difference to the patient who has previously only been seen in routine outpatient clinics. Thus, the mere fact that the patient is attending a clinic in which the staff have an appreciation of the problems of chronic pain can improve the outlook and symptoms of the patient who feels that at last something helpful can be done. In fact, subliminal psychotherapy applied by the members of the multidisciplinary team is often of paramount importance in the successful treatment of these patients.

In biofeedback, the patient learns to modify such physiologic parameters as skin blood flow by the use of a simple feedback apparatus, such as a temperature monitor, and then applies this skill to relieve pain by similar mechanisms. Although recent reports have demonstrated mixed results from the use of biofeedback,[209] the technique may be of value in such syndromes as myofascial pain or sympathetic dystrophy, in which diminishing sympathetic overactivity can improve symptoms.[419]

Relaxation techniques offer a similar approach and are again of most use where there is an anxiety component to the pain syndrome that worsens symptoms by increasing catecholamine levels. The patient is instructed to relax with the help of breathing exercises and the suggestions of the psychologist and can then apply this subsequently on a daily basis as a method of lessening pain. Relaxation techniques are used widely at present because they result in a significant reduction in pain complaints and drug intake.[209] Improvements in mood and activity have also been noted with this treatment modality.[209]

Hypnosis[76,170] takes relaxation a stage further and, although suitable only for certain susceptible individuals, has been used in various ways to help control chronic pain. Various modes of therapy exist: symptom suppression and substitution, time dissolution, age regression, and guided imagery all can be of use in modifying the patient's outlook, which may not only decrease pain but also improve his or her response to other therapeutic maneuvers.

Operant conditioning[131] is based on the concept that pain patients learn abnormal behavior that reinforces their pain and that this behavior can be unlearned, with a concomitant diminution of distress, in a suitable environment. The treatment generally requires an inpatient facility in which patients are placed for a period of time in an atmosphere where any "pain behavior" is negatively reinforced. This approach is the basis for most inpatient pain units and can be successful in those patients for whom abnormal behavior or an adverse environment, rather than organic pathology, is a predominant component of the syndrome. Controlled studies have demonstrated that operant procedures are valuable techniques in behavioral remediation of chronic pain, especially when treatment objectives are to increase activity levels and decrease the consumption of medication.[209]

## CONCLUSION

Posttraumatic pain encompasses acute posttraumatic pain, postoperative pain, and subsequent chronic pain states. The pathophysiology of pain varies with its chronicity. Appropriate therapeutic intervention in acute posttraumatic and postoperative pain requires consideration of the perturbations in both hemodynamic and respiratory physiology, as well as the resultant alterations in pain mechanisms. Posttraumatic complications and the late development of chronic pain states can be altered by the choice of analgesic technique during the early stages after injury. Acute pain management should promote early mobilization and thereby reduce posttraumatic and postoperative complications. Although substantial information is available on the management of acute postoperative pain in electively operated patients, data regarding the management of acute pain after trauma and associated surgery are relatively scarce. Thus, studies in this area are urgently needed. The complexity of posttraumatic chronic pain is such that a multidisciplinary approach to management is required, with emphasis on improved function and rehabilitation.

## REFERENCES


1. Abram SE, Anderson RA, Maitra-D'Cruze AM. Factors predicting short-term outcome of nerve blocks in the management of chronic pain. Pain 1981;10:323.
2. Accident Facts. National Safety Council. Chicago: National Safety Council, 1988:2.
3. Aitkenhead AR. Anaesthesia for bowel surgery. Ann Chir Gynaecol 1984;73:177.
4. Alexander JI, Parikh RK, Spence AA. Postoperative analgesia and lung function: a comparison of narcotic analgesic regimen. Br J Anaesth 1973;45:346.
5. Ali J, Yaffe CS, Serrette C. The effect of transcutaneous electric nerve stimulation on postoperative pain and pulmonary function. Surgery 1981;89:507.
6. Ali NMK, Green L, Buckwalter JA. Effective management of frostbite with sympathetic blockade. Regional Anesth 1982;7:128.
7. Al-Khafaji JM, Ellias MAY. (Letter to the Editor) Incidence of Horner's syndrome with interscalene brachial plexus block and its importance in the management of head injury. Anesthesiology 1986;64:127.
8. Andrews CJH, Sinclair M, Prys-Roberts C, Dye A. Ventilatory effects during and after continuous infusion of fentanyl or alfentanil. Br J Anaesth 1983;55:211S.
9. Ang ET, Lassale B, Goldfarb G. Continuous axillary brachial plexus block—a clinical and anatomical study. Anesth Analg 1984;63:680.
10. Artru AA. Midazolam potentiates the analgesic effect of morphine in patients with postoperative pain. Clin J Pain 1986;2:93.
11. Asantila R, Rosenberg PH, Scheinin B. Comparison of different methods of postoperative analgesia after thoracotomy. Acta Anaesth Scand 1986;30:421.
12. Asoh T, Tsuji H, Shirasaka C, Takeuchi Y. Effect of epidural analgesia on metabolic response to major upper abdominal surgery. Acta Anaesth Scand 1983;27:233.
13. Atkinson RJ, Rushman GB, Lee JA. A synopsis of anaesthesia. 8th ed. Bristol: John Wright & Sons, 1977:417.
14. Austin KL, Stapleton JV, Mather LE. Multiple intramuscular injections, a major source of variables in analgesic responses to meperidine. Pain 1980;8:47.
15. Austin KL, Stapleton JV, Mather LE. Relationship between blood meperidine concentrations and analgesic response. Anesthesiology 1980;53:460.
16. Bach S, Noreng M, Tjellden N. Phantom limb pain in amputees during the first 12 months following limb amputation, after preoperative lumbar epidural blockade. Pain 1988;33:297.
17. Balasaraswathi K, Gilsson SN, EL-Etr AA, et al. Serum epinephrine and norepinephrine during valve replacement and aorto-coronary bypass. Can Anaesth Soc J 1978;25:198.
18. Banning AM, Schmidt JF, Chraemmer-Jorgensen B, Risbo A. Comparison of oral controlled release morphine and epidural morphine in the management of postoperative pain. Anesth Analg 1986;65:385.
19. Barber J, Adrian C. Psychological approaches to the management of pain. New York: Brunner/Mazer, 1982.
20. Bashein G, Haschke RH, Ready LB. Electrical nerve location: numerical and electrophoretic comparison of insulated vs uninsulated needles. Anesth Analg 1984;63:919.
21. Beck GP. Anterior approach to sciatic nerve block. Anesthesiology 1963;26:222.
22. Behar M, Magora F, Olshwang D, Davidson J. Epidural morphine in the treatment of pain. Lancet 1977;1:527.
23. Bell MDD, Murray GR, Mishra P, et al. Buccal morphine—a new route for analgesia? Lancet 1985;1:71.
24. Benhamou D, Samii K, Noviant Y. Effect of analgesia on respiratory muscle function after upper abdominal surgery. Acta Anaesth Scand 1983;27:22.
25. Bennett RL, Batenhorst RL, Bivins BA, et al. Patient-controlled analgesia. A new concept of postoperative pain relief. Ann Surg 1982;195:700.
26. Benzon HT, Chomka CM, Brunner EA. Treatment of reflex sympathetic dystrophy with regional intravenous reserpine. Anesth Analg 1980;59:500.
27. Beran DR. Modification of the metabolic response to trauma under extradural analgesia. Anaesthesia 1971;26:188.
28. Bereiter DA, Plotsky PM, Gann DS. Tooth pulp stimulation potentiates the ACTH response to hemorrhage in cats. Endocrinology 1982;111:1127.
29. Berry FR. Analgesia in patients with fractured shaft of femur. Anaesthesia 1977;32:576.
30. Berry FR, Kirchoff JA. Neural blockade in the outpatient clinic, emergency room and private office. In: Cousins MJ, Bridenbaugh PO, eds. Neural blockade. Philadelphia: JB Lippincott, 1980:501.
31. Betcher AM, Bean G, Casten DR. Continuous procaine block of paravertebral sympathetic. JAMA 1953;151:288.
32. Bilsback P, Rolly G, Tampubolon O. Efficacy of the extradural administration of lofentanil, buprenorphine or saline in the management of postoperative pain. A double-blind study. Br J Anaesth 1985;57:943.
33. Bion JF. Infusion analgesia for acute war injuries. A comparison of pentazocine and ketamine. Anaesthesia 1984;39:560.
34. Bond AC, Davies CK. Ketamine and pancuronium for the shocked patient. Anaesthesia 1974;29:59.
35. Bonelli S, Conoscente F, Movilia PG et al. Regional intravenous guanethidine vs. stellate ganglion block in reflex sympathetic dystrophies: A randomized trial. Pain 1983;16:297.
36. Bonica JJ. The management of pain. Philadelphia: Lea & Febiger, 1953.
37. Bonica JJ. Autonomic innervation of viscera in relation to nerve block. Anesthesiology 1968;29:793.
38. Bonica JJ. Basic principles in managing chronic pain. Arch Surg 1977;112:783.
39. Bonica JJ. Pain research and therapy: past and current status and future needs. In: Nh LKY, Bonica JJ, eds. Pain, discomfort and humanitarian care. New York: Elsevier, 1980:1.
40. Bonica JJ. History of pain concepts and pain therapy. Semin Anesth 1985;4:189.
41. Bonica JJ, Benedetti C. Postoperative pain. In: Condon RE, Decosse JJ, eds. Surgical care: a physiologic approach to clinical management. Philadelphia: Lea & Febiger, 1980:394.
42. Bonica JJ, Berges PU, Morikawa K. Circulatory effects of peridural block. I: Effects of level of analgesia and dose of lidocaine. Anesthesiology 1970;33:619.
43. Bonica JJ, Akamatsu TJ, Berges PU, et al. Circulatory effects of epidural block. II: Effects of epinephrine. Anesthesiology 1971;34:514.
44. Bonica JJ, Kennedy WF, Akamatsu TJ, Gerbershagen HU. Circulatory effects of peridural block. III: Effects of acute blood loss. Anesthesiology 1972;36:219.
45. Bonnett F, Harari A, Thibonnier M, Viars P. Suppression of antidiuretic hormone hypersecretion during surgery by extradural anaesthesia. Br J Anaesth 1982;54:29.
46. Bonnet F, Blery CH, Zatan M, et al. Effect of epidural morphine on postoperative pulmonary dysfunction. Acta Anaesth Scand 1984;28:147.

47. Botney M, Fields HL. Amitriptyline potentiates morphine analgesia by a direct action on the central nervous system. Ann Neurol 1983;13:160.
48. Bovill JG, Sebel PS, Fiolet JWT. The influence of sufentanil on endocrine and metabolic responses to cardiac surgery. Anesth Analg 1983;62:391.
49. Bowler GMR, Wildsmith JA, Scott DB. Epidural administration of local anesthetics. Clin Crit Care Med 1986;187.
50. Brands E, Callanan VI. Continuous lumbar plexus block analgesia for femoral neck fractures. Anaesth Intens Care 1978;6:256.
51. Brandt MR, Fernades A, Mordhorst R, Kehlet H. Epidural analgesia improves postoperative nitrogen balance. Br Med J 1978;1:1106.
52. Brandt MR, Korshin J, Prange H, et al. Influence of morphine anesthesia on the endocrine-metabolic response to open-heart surgery. Acta Anaesth Scand 1978;22:400.
53. Brandt MR, Olgaard K, Kehlet H. Epidural analgesia inhibits the renin and aldosterone response to surgery. Acta Anaesth Scand 1979;23:267.
54. Braunwald E, Maroko PR. Protection of the ischemic myocardium. In: Braunwald E, ed. The myocardium: failure and infarction. New York: H.P. Publishing, 1974:329.
55. Bresler DE, Katz RL. Chronic pain and alternatives to neural blockade. In: Cousins MJ, Bridenbaugh PO, eds Neural blockade. Philadelphia: JB Lippincott, 1980:651.
56. Bridenbaugh PO. Anesthesia and influence on hospitalization time. Regional Anesth 1982;7(suppl):5151.
57. Bridenbaugh PO, Dupen SL, Moore DC, et al. Postoperative intercostal nerve block analgesia versus narcotic analgesia. Anesth Analg 1972;52:81.
58. Bromage PR. Extradural analgesia for pain relief. Br J Anaesth 1967;39:721.
59. Bromage PR, Pettigrew RT, Crowell DE. Tachyphylaxis in epidural analgesia. Augmentation and decay of local analgesia. J Clin Pharmacol 1969;9:30.
60. Bromage PR, Shibata HR, Wiloughby HW. Influence of prolonged epidural blockade on blood sugar and cortisol responses to operations upon the upper part of the abdomen and the thorax. Surg Gynecol Obstet 1971;132:1051.
61. Bromage PR, Camporesi EM, Chestnut D. Epidural narcotics for postoperative analgesia. Anesth Analg 1980;59:473.
62. Bromage PR, Camporesi EM, Durant PAC, Nielsen CH. Nonrespiratory side effects of epidural morphine. Anesth Analg 1982;61:490.
63. Bromage PR, Camporesi EM, Durant PAC, Nielsen CH. Rostral spread of epidural morphine. Anesthesiology 1982;56:431.
64. Bromm B, Meier W, Scharein E. Imipramine reduces experimental pain. Pain 1986;25:245.
65. Bruxelle J, Travers V, Thiebaut JB. Occurence and treatment of pain after brachial plexus injury. Clin Orthop 1988;237:87.
66. Bullingham RES, McQuay HJ, Dwyer D, et al. Sublingual buprenorphine used postoperatively: clinical observations and preliminary pharmacokinetic analysis. Br J Clin Pharmacol 1981;12:117.
67. Bullingham RES, O'Sullivan G, McQuay HJ, et al. Mandatory sublingual buprenorphine for postoperative pain. Anaesthesia 1984;39:329.
68. Camporesi EM, Nielsen CH, Bromage PR, Durant PAC. Ventilatory $CO_2$ sensitivity after intravenous and epidural morphine in volunteers. Anesth Analg 1983;62:633.
69. Carron H, Litwiller R. Stellate ganglion block. Anesth Analg 1975;54:567.
70. Cashman JN, Jones RM, Foster JMG, Adams AP. Comparison of infusions of morphine and lysine acetyl salicylate for the relief of pain after surgery. Br J Anaesth 1985;57:255.
71. Catley DM, Thornton C, Jordan C, et al. Pronounced, episodic oxygen desaturation in the postoperative period: its association with ventilatory pattern and analgesic regimen. Anesthesiology 1985;63:20.
72. Cazenave JP, Benveniste J, Mustard JF. Aggregation of rabbit platelets by platelet-activating factor is independent of the release reaction and the arachidonate pathway and inhibited by membrane active drugs. Lab Invest 1979;41:275.
73. Chan CS, Chow SP. Electroacupuncture in the treatment of post-traumatic sympathetic dystrophy (sudeck's atrophy). Br J Anaesth 1981;53:899.
74. Chapman CR, Bonica JJ. Acute pain. Current concepts. Scope Monograph, Upjohn Company, 1983.
75. Chauvin M, Salbaing J, Perrin D, et al. Clinical assessment and plasma pharmocokinetics associated with intramuscular or extradural alfentanil. Br J Anaesth 1985;57:886.
76. Cheek DB, LeCron LM. Clinical hypnotherapy. New York: Grune & Stratton, 1968.
77. Child CS, Kaufman L. Effect of intrathecal diamorphine on the adrenocortical, hyperglycaemic and cardiovascular responses to major colonic surgery. Br J Anaesth 1985;57:389.
78. Christensen P, Brandt MR, Rem J, et al. Influence of extradural morphine on the adrenocortical and hyperglycaemic response to surgery. Br J Anaesth 1982;54:23.
79. Chrubasik J, Meynadier J, Scherpereel P, Wunsch E. The effect of epidural somatostatin on postoperative pain. Anesth Analg 1985;64:1085.
80. Churchill-Davidson HC. Pain and the analgesic drugs. In: Churchill-Davidson HC, ed. A practice of anaesthesia. 5th ed. Chicago: Year Book Medical Publishers, 1984:800.
81. Cicala R, Voeller G, Fox T, et al. Epidural analgesia in thoracic trauma: effects of lumbar morphine and thoracic bupivacaine on pulmonary function. Crit Care Med 1989;17:S39.
82. Clayton ML, Turner DA. Upper arm block anaesthesia for children with fractures. JAMA 1959;169:327.
83. Cohen FL. Postsurgical pain relief: patients' status and nurses' medication choices. Pain 1980;9:265.
84. Collins WF, Ranch CT. Midbrain evoked responses relating to peripheral unmyelinated or "C" fibers in cat. J Neurophysiol 1960;23:47.
85. Conacher ID, Paes ML, Jacobson L, et al. Epidural analgesia following thoracic surgery. A review of 2 years' experience. Anaesthesia 1983;38:546.
86. Cooper GM, Paterson JL, Ward LD, et al. Fentanyl and the metabolic response to gastric surgery. Anaesthesia 1981;36:667.
87. Corssen G, Domino FF. Dissociative anaesthesia: further studies and first clinical experience with the phencyclidine derivative CI 581. Anesth Analg 1966;45:29.
88. Cory PC, Horton WG. Lung volume changes produced by intercostal nerve block with 0.5% bupivacaine. Anesthesiology 1981;55:A144.
89. Cory PC, Mulroy MF. Postoperative respiratory failure following intercostal block. Anesthesiology 1981;54:418.
90. Cousins MJ, Wright CFJ. Graft, muscle, skin blood flow after epidural block in vascular surgical procedures. Surg Gynec Obstet 1971;133:59.
91. Cousins MJ, Bridenbaugh PO. Neural blockade in clinical anaesthesia and management of pain. Philadelphia: JB Lippincott, 1988.
92. Cousins MJ, Mather LE. Intrathecal and epidural administration of opioids. Anesthesiology 1984;61:276.
93. Cousins MJ, Bridenbaugh PO. Spinal opioids and pain relief in acute care. Clin Crit Care Med 1986;8:151.
94. Cousins MJ, Reeve TS, Glynn CJ, et al. Neurolytic lumbar sympathetic blockade: duration of denervation and relief of rest pain. Anaesth Intens Care 1979;7:121.
95. Coyle DE, Parab PV, Streng WH, et al. Is hydromorphone more lipid soluble than morphine? Anesthesiology 1984;61:A240.

96. Cozian A, Pinaud M, Lepage JY, et al. Effects of meperidine spinal anesthesia on hemodynamics, plasma catecholamines, angiotensin I, aldosterone, and histamine concentrations in elderly men. Anesthesiology 1986;64:815.
97. Craig DB. Postoperative recovery of pulmonary function. Anesth Analg 1981;60:46.
98. Cremer SA, Maynard F, Davidoff G. The reflex sympathetic dystrophy syndrome associated with traumatic myelopathy: report of 5 cases. Pain 1989;37:187.
99. Crook J, Rideout E, Browne G. The prevalence of pain complaints in a general population. Pain 1984;18:299.
100. Cullen ML, Staren ED, El-Ganzouri A, et al. Continuous epidural infusion for analgesia after major abdominal operations: a randomized, prospective, double-blind study. Surgery 1985;98:718.
101. Cuschieri RJ, Morran CG, Howie JC, McArdle CS. Postoperative pain and pulmonary complications: comparison of three analgesic regimens. Br J Surg 1985;72:495.
102. Davies JAH, Beswick T, Dickson G. Ketanserin and guanethidine in the treatment of causalgia. Anesth Analg 1987;66:575.
103. deJong RH. Axillary block of the brachial plexus. Anesthesiology 1961;22:215.
104. Demling RH. What are the functions of endorphins following thermal injury? J Trauma 1984;24:S172.
105. Demling RH. Burns. N Engl J Med 1985;313:1389.
106. Derbyshire DR, Bell A, Parry B, Smith G. Morphine sulphate slow release. Comparison with i.m. morphine for postoperative analgesia. Br J Anaesth 1985;57:858.
107. DeTakats G. Nature of painful vasodilation in causalgic state. Arch Neurol Psychiatr 1943;50:318.
108. Devor M, Wall PD. Reorganization of spinal cord sensory map after peripheral nerve injury. Nature (Lond.) 1978;276:75.
109. Dickson GR, Sutcliffe AJ. Intrathecal morphine and multiple fractured ribs. Br J Anaesth 1986;58:1342.
110. Dinley J, Dickson RA. The control of pain after Kellers operation by the instillation of anaesthetic before closure. J Bone Joint Surg 1976;58B:356.
111. Dittman M, Keller R, Wolff G. A rationale for epidural analgesia in the treatment of multiple rib fractures. Intens Care Med 1976;4:193.
112. Dittman M, Steenblock G, Krazlin M, Wolff G. Epidural analgesia or mechanical ventilation for multiple rib fractures. Intens Care Med 1982;8:89.
113. Domazal T, Szczudlik A, Kwasucki J, et al. Plasma cortisol concentrations in patients with different circadian pain rhythm. Pain 1983;17:67.
114. Donadoni R, Rolly G, Noorduin H, Vanden Bussche G. Epidural sufentanil for postoperative pain relief. Anaesthesia 1985;40:634.
115. Downing B, Davis J, Black J, Windsor CWO. Effect of intrathecal morphine on the adrenocortical and hyperglycaemic responses to upper abdominal surgery. Br J Anaesth 1986; 58:858.
116. Downs DL, Eisele JH. Continuous epidural analgesia with fentanyl in trauma patients. Anesthesiology 1988;69:A180.
117. Duthie DJR, McLaren AD, Nimmo WS. Pharmacokinetics of fentanyl during constant rate I.V. infusion for the relief of pain after surgery. Br J Anaesth 1986;58:950.
118. Egdahl RH. Pituitary-adrenal response following trauma to the isolated leg. Surgery 1959;46:9.
119. Eisele JH, Trenchard D, Stubb J, Guz A. The immediate cardiac depression by anaesthetics in conscious dogs. Br J Anaesth 1969;41:86.
120. Engberg G. Relief of postoperative pain with intercostal blockade compared with the use of narcotic drugs. Acta Anaesth Scand 1978;70(suppl):36.
121. Engberg G. Respiratory performance after upper abdominal surgery. A comparison of pain relief with intercostal blocks and centrally acting analgesics. Acta Anaesth Scand 1985;29:427.
122. Epstein SE, Redwood DR, Goldstein RE, et al. Angina pectoris: pathophysiology, evaluation and treatment. Ann Intern Med 1971;75:263.
123. Eriksson E. Axillary brachial plexus anaesthesia in children with citanest. Acta Anaesth Scand 1965;16(suppl):281.
124. Etches RC, Sandler AN, Daley MD. Respiratory depression and spinal opioids. Can J Anaesth 1989;36:165.
125. Evans JM, MacCarthy J, Rosen M, Hogg MIJ. Apparatus for patient controlled administration of intravenous narcotics during labor. Lancet 1976;1:17.
126. Eysenck SB, Eysenck HJ. The measurement of psychoticism: a study of factor stability and reliability. Br J Soc Clin Psychol 1968;7:286.
127. Fell D, Chmielewski A, Smith G. Postoperative analgesia with controlled-release morphine sulphate: comparison with intramuscular morphine. Br Med J (Clin Res) 1982;285:92.
128. Fienmann C. Pain relief by antidepressants: possible modes of action. Pain 1985;23:1.
129. Ford DJ, Pither C, Raj PP. Comparison of insulated and uninsulated needles for locating peripheral nerves with a peripheral nerve stimulator. Anesth Analg 1984;63:925.
130. Ford SR, Forrest WH, Eltherington L. The treatment of reflex sympathetic dystrophy with intravenous regional bretylium. Anesthesiology 1988;68:137.
131. Fordyce WE. Behavioral methods for chronic pain and illness. St. Louis: CV Mosby, 1976.
132. Fromme GA, Steidl LJ, Danielson DR. Comparison of lumbar and thoracic epidural morphine for relief of postthoracotomy pain. Anesth Analg 1985;64:454.
133. Fry EN. Postoperative analgesia using continuous infusions of papaveratum. Ann Roy Coll Surg 1979;61:371.
134. Fulton WM. Psychological strategies and techniques in pain management. Semin Anesth 1985;4:247.
135. Furness JB, Costa M. Adynamic ileus, its pathogenesis and treatment. Med Biol 1974;52:82.
136. Gann DS, Amaral JF. Pathophysiology of trauma and shock. In: Zuidema GD, Rutherford RB, Ballinger WF, Eds. The management of trauma. 4th ed. Philadelphia: WB Saunders, 1985:37.
137. Gass GD, Olsen GN. Clinical significance of pulmonary function tests. Preoperative pulmonary function testing to predict postoperative morbidity and mortality. Chest 1986;89:127.
138. Gauntlett IS. Total spinal anesthesia following intercostal nerve block. Anesthesiology 1986;65:82.
139. George JM, Reier CE, Lanese RR, et al. Morphine anesthesia blocks cortisol and growth hormone response to surgical stress in humans. J Clin Endocrinol Metab 1974;38:736.
140. Gersh M. Application of TENS in the treatment of patients with musculoskeletal and neurologic disorders. Clin Phys Med 1981;2:155.
141. Ghostine SY, Comair YG, Turner DM, et al. Phenoxybenzamine in the treatment of causalgia. J Neurosurg 1984;60:1263.
142. Gibbons J, James O, Quail A. Management of 130 cases of chest injury with respiratory failure. Br J Anaesth 1973;45:1130.
143. Gibbons J, James O, Quail A. The relief of pain in chest injury. Br J Anaesth 1973;45:1136.
144. Gibbs JM, Johnson HD, Davis FM. Patient administration of I.V. buprenorphine for postoperative pain relief using the "Cardiff" demand analgesia apparatus. Br J Anaesth 1982;54:279.
145. Giddon DB, Lindhe J. In vivo quantitation of local anesthetic suppression of leukocyte adherence. Am J Pathol 1972;68:327.
146. Giddon DB, Rabinovitz SL. The psychological aspects of treatments of chronic pain patients. Regional Anesth 1980;5:16.
147. Glynn CJ, Lloyd JW, Barnard JDW. Cryoanalgesia in the management of pain after thoracotomy. Thorax 1980;35:325.
148. Glynn CJ, Basedow RW, Walsh JA. Pain relief following post-

ganglionic sympathetic blockade with IV guanethidine. Br J Anaesth 1981;53:1297.
149. Goodwin JS. Mechanism of action of nonsteroidal antiinflammatory agents. Am J Med 1984;13:57.
150. Gourlay GK, Wilson PR, Glynn CJ. Pharmacodynamics and pharmacokinetics of methadone during the postoperative period. Anesthesiology 1982;57:458.
151. Gourlay GK, Willis RJ, Wilson PR. Postoperative pain control with methadone: influence of supplementary methadone doses and blood concentration-response relationship. Anesthesiology 1984;61:19.
152. Gourlay GK, Willis RJ, Lamberty J. A double-blind comparison of the efficacy of methadone and morphine in postoperative pain control. Anesthesiology 1986;64:322.
153. Graff-Radford SB. Myofascial pain: an overview. Semin Anesth 1985;4:281.
154. Grant IS, Nimmo WC, Clements JH. Pharmacokinetics and analgesic effects of i.m. and oral ketamine. Br J Anaesth 1981;53:805.
155. Graves DA, Foster TS, Batenhorst RL, et al. Patient-controlled analgesia. Ann Intern Med 1983;99:360.
156. Green R, Dawkins CJM. Postoperative analgesia: the use of a continuous drip epidural block. Anaesthesia 1966;21:312.
157. Grice SC, Morell RC, Balestrieri FJ, et al. Intravenous regional anesthesia: evaluation and prevention of leakage under tourniquet. Anesthesiology 1986;65:316.
158. Griffiths DPG, Diamond AW, Cameron JD. Postoperative extradural analgesia following thoracic surgery: a feasibility study. Br J Anaesth 1975;47:48.
159. Grossbard GD, Love BRT. Femoral nerve block: a simple and safe method of instant analgesia for femoral fractures in children. Aust NZ J Surg 1979;49:592.
160. Gueneron JP, Ecoffey CL, Carli P, et al. Effect of naloxone infusion on analgesia and respiratory depression after epidural fentanyl. Anesth Analg 1988;67:35.
161. Gustafsson LL, Schildt B, Jacobsen K. Adverse effects of extradural and intrathecal opiates: report of a nationwide survey in Sweden. Br J Anaesth 1982;54:479.
162. Hakanson E, Rutberg H, Jorfeldt L, Martensson J. Effects of the extradural administration of morphine or bupivacaine on the metabolic response to upper abdominal surgery. Br J Anaesth 1985;57:394.
163. Hall GM, Young C, Holdcroft A, et al. Substrate mobilization during surgery—a comparison between halothane and fentanyl anaesthesia. Anaesthesia 1978;33:924.
164. Hameroff SR, Cork RC, Weiss JL, et al. Doxepin effects on chronic pain and depression: a controlled study. Clin J Pain 1985;1:171.
165. Hatangdi VS, Boas RA. Lumbar sympathectomy: a single needle technique. Br J Anaesth 1985;57:285.
166. Hecker BR, Bjurstrom R, Schoene RB. Effect of intercostal nerve blockade on respiratory mechanics and $CO_2$ chemosensitivity at rest and exercise. Anesthesiology 1989;70:13.
167. Hefington CA, Thompson RC. The use of interscalene block anesthesia for manipulative reduction of fractures and dislocations of the upper extremity. J Bone Joint Surg 1973;55A:836.
168. Hempel V, van Finck M, Baumgartner E. A longitudinal supraclavicular approach to the brachial plexus for the insertion of plastic cannulas. Anesth Analg 1981;60:352.
169. Herrmann JM, Schoenecke OW, Wagner H, et al. Different endocrinal and hemodynamic response patterns to various noxious stimuli. Psychother Psychosom 1980;33:160.
170. Hilgard ER, Hilgard JR. The alleviation of pain by hypnosis. Pain 1975;1:213.
171. Hilt H, Gramm HJ, Link J. Changes in intracranial pressure associated with extradural anaesthesia. Br J Anaesth 1986;58:676.
172. Hirlinger WK, Pfenninger E. Intravenöse analgesie mit ketamin bei notfallpatienten. Anaesthesist 1987;36:140.
173. Hjortso NC, Christensen NJ, Andersen T, et al. Effects of the extradural administration of local anesthetic agents and morphine on the urinary excretion of cortisol, catecholamines and nitrogen following abdominal surgery. Br J Anaesth 1985;57:400.
174. Holder LE, MacKinnon SE. Reflex sympathetic dystrophy in the hands: clinical and scintigraphic criteria. Radiology 1984;152:517.
175. Hug CC Jr, Murphy MR, Rigel EP, et al. Pharmacokinetics of morphine injected intravenously into the anesthetized dog. Anesthesiology 1981;54:38.
176. Hughes TJ, Desgrand DA. Interscalene block for Colles fracture. Anaesthesia 1983;38:149.
177. Hull CJ, Sibbald A. Control of postoperative pain by interactive demand analgesia. Br J Anaesth 1981;53:385.
178. Ichiyanagi G. Sciatic nerve block: lateral approach with the patient supine. Anesthesiology 1959;20:601.
179. Islas JA, Astorga J, Laredo M. Epidural ketamine for control of postoperative pain. Anesth Analg 1985;64:1161.
180. Jebara VA, Saade B. Causalgia: a wartime experience—report of twenty treated cases. J Trauma 1987;27:519.
181. Jensen TS, Krebs B, Nielsen J, Rassmussen P. Phantom limb, phantom pain and stump pain in amputees during the first 6 months following amputation. Pain 1983;17:243.
182. Johnson JR, McCaughey GJ. Epidural morphine: a method of management of multiple fractured ribs. Anaesthesia 1980;35:155.
183. Johnson WC. Postoperative ventilatory performance: dependence upon surgical incision. Am Surg 1975;41:615.
184. Jones RM, Cashman JN, Foster JMG, et al. Comparison of infusions of morphine and lysine acetyl salicylate for the relief of pain following thoracic surgery. Br J Anaesth 1985;57:259.
185. Jones SF, White A. Analgesia following femoral neck surgery. Lateral cutaneous nerve block as an alternative to narcotics in the elderly. Anaesthesia 1985;40:682.
186. Jorgensen BC, Andersen HB, Engquist A. Influence of epidural morphine on postoperative pain, endocrine-metabolic and renal responses to surgery: a controlled study. Acta Anaesth Scand 1982;26:63.
187. Jowitt MD, Knight RJ. Anaesthesia during the Falklands campaign. Anaesthesia 1983;38:776.
188. Kafer ER, Brown JT, Scott D, et al. Biphasic depression of ventilatory responses to $CO_2$ following epidural morphine. Anesthesiology 1983;58:418.
189. Kallio KE. Permanency of results obtained by sympathetic surgery in the treatment of phantom pain. Acta Orthop Scand 1950;19:391.
190. Kambam JR, Hammon J, Parris WCV, Lupinetti FM. Intrapleural analgesia for postthoracotomy pain and blood levels of bupivacaine following intrapleural injection. Can J Anaesth 1989;36:106.
191. Katz J, Nelson WL, Forest R, et al. Prolonged postthoracotomy analgesia by cryoprobe nerve block. Anesthesiology 1979;51:S233.
192. Keenan DJM, Cave K, Langdon L, Lea RE. Comparative trial of rectal indomethacin and cryoanalgesia for control of early postthoracotomy pain. Br Med J 1983;287:1335.
193. Kehlet H. The endocrine-metabolic response to postoperative pain. Acta Anaesth Scand 1982;74(suppl):173.
194. Kehlet H. The modifying effect of general and regional anesthesia on the endocrine-metabolic response to surgery. Regional Anesth 1982;7(suppl):S38.
195. Kehlet H. Does regional anesthesia reduce postoperative morbidity? Intens Care Med 1984;10:165.

196. Kehlet H: Pain relief and modification of the stress response. Clin Crit Care Med 1986;8:49.
197. Kehlet H, Brandt MR, Rem J. Role of neurogenic stimuli in mediating the endocrine-metabolic response to surgery. JPEN 1980;4:152.
198. Kennedy BM. Intrathecal morphine and multiple fractured ribs. Br J Anaesth 1985;57:1266.
199. Kepes ER, Raj SS, Vemulapalli R, et al. Regional intravenous guanethidine for sympathetic blockade. Report of ten cases. Regional Anesth 1982;7:52.
200. Khoury GF. Therapeutic use of pain relieving drugs in chronic pain patients. Semin Anesth 1985;4:300.
201. Kirkpatrick AF, Bednarczyk LR, Hime GW, et al. Bupivacaine blood levels during continuous interscalene block. Anesthesiology 1985;62:65.
202. Kirkwood CF, Edwards DJ, Lalka D, et al. The pharmacokinetics of meperidine in acute trauma patients. J Trauma 1986;26:1090.
203. Koyama K, Watanabe S, Tsuneto S, et al. Thiopental for phantom limb pain during spinal anesthesia. Anesthesiology 1988;69:598.
204. Kvalheim L, Reiestad F. Interpleural catheter in the management of postoperative pain. Anesthesiology 1984;61:A231.
205. Ledingham I McA, Watt I. Influence of sedation on mortality in critically ill multiple trauma patients. Lancet 1983;1:1270.
206. Ledingham I McA, Finlay WE, Watt I, et al. Etomidate and adrenocortical function. Lancet 1983;1:1434.
207. Levack ID, Holmes JD, Robertson GS. Abdominal wound perfusion for the relief of postoperative pain. Br J Anaesth 1986;58:615.
208. Levy EM, McIntosh T, Black PH. Elevation of circulating beta-endorphin levels with concomitant depression of immune parameters after traumatic injury. J Trauma 1986;26:246.
209. Linton SJ. Behavioral remediation of chronic pain: a status report. Pain 1986;24:125.
210. Loh L, Nathan PW. Painful peripheral states and sympathetic blocks. J Neurol Neurosurg Psychiatry 1978;41:664.
211. Loyd JW, Rucklidge MA. The management of closed chest injuries. Br J Surg 1969;56:721.
212. Lund J, Stjernstrom H, Jorfeldt L, Wiklund L. Effect of extradural analgesia on glucose metabolism and gluconeogenesis. Br J Anaesth 1986;58:851.
213. Lundh R, Hedenstierna G, Johansson H. Ventilation-perfusion relationships during epidural analgesia. Acta Anaesth Scand 1983;27:410.
214. Lyles R, Skurdal D, Stene J, Jaberi M. Continuous intercostal catheter techniques for treatment of post-traumatic thoracic pain. Anesthesiology 1986;65:A205.
215. Mackersie RC, Shackford SR, Hoyt DB, Karagianes TG. Continuous epidural fentanyl analgesia: ventilatory function improvement with routine use in treatment of blunt chest injury. J Trauma 1987;27:1207.
216. Maiwand O, Makey AR. Cryoanalgesia for relief of pain after thoracotomy. Br Med J 1981;282:1749.
217. Mankikian B, Cantineau JP, Bertrand M, et al. Improvement of diaphragmatic function by a thoracic extradural block after upper abdominal surgery. Anesthesiology 1988;68:379.
218. Manriquez RG, Pallares VS. Continuous brachial plexus block for prolonged sympathetectomy and control of pain. Anesth Analg 1978;57:128.
219. Marks BM, Sachar EJ. Undertreatment of medical inpatients with narcotic analgesics. Ann Intern Med 1973;78:173.
220. Marsland AR, Weekes JWN, Atkinson RL, Leong MG. Phantom limb pain: a case for beta blockers? Pain 1982;12:295.
221. Martin RL, Abram SE. Apnea following intravenous regional guanethidine blockade. Regional Anesth 1986;11:39.
222. Martin RL, Salbaing J, Blaise G, et al. Epidural morphine for postoperative pain relief, a dose response curve. Anesthesiology 1982;56:423.
223. Mather LE. Parenteral opiates for postoperative analgesia. Regional Anesth 1982;7:144.
224. Mather LE, Runciman WB, Ilsley AH. Anesthesia induced changes in regional blood flow. Implications for drug disposition. Regional Anesth 1982;7:S24.
225. Mather LE, Phillips GD. Opioids and adjuvants: principles of use. Clin Crit Care Med 1986;8:77.
226. Matthews PJ, Govenden V. Comparison of continuous paravertebral and extradural infusions of bupivacaine for pain relief after thoracotomy. Br J Anaesth 1989;62:204.
227. McCammon RL, Stoelting RK, Madura JA. Effects of butorphanol, nalbuphine, and fentanyl on intrabiliary tract dynamics. Anesth Analg 1984;63:139.
228. McQuay HJ, Bullingham RES, Paterson GMC, Moore RA. Clinical effects of buprenorphine during and after operation. Br J Anaesth 1980;52:1013.
229. Mehnert JH, Dupont TJ, Rose DH. Intermittent epidural morphine instillation for control of postoperative pain. Am J Surg 1983;146:145.
230. Melzack J. Central neural mechanisms in phantom limb pain. In: Advances in neurology. vol 4. New York: Raven Press, 1974.
231. Melzack R. Phantom limb pain: implications for treatment of pathologic pain. Anesthesiology 1971;35:409.
232. Melzack R, Wall PD. Pain mechanisms: a new theory. Science 1965;150:971.
233. Melzack R, Wall PD, Ty TC. Acute pain in an emergency clinic: latency of onset and descriptor patterns related to different injuries. Pain 1982;14:33.
234. Middaugh RE, Menk EJ, Reynolds WJ, et al. Epidural block using large volumes of local anesthetic solution for intercostal block. Anesthesiology 1985;63:214.
235. Middaugh RE, Bauman JM, Menk E. (Reply) Continuous intercostal nerve block. Anesthesiology 1986;64:670.
236. Miles JB. Surgery for the relief of pain. In: Lipton S, ed. Persistent pain: modern methods of treatment. London: Academic Press, 1977;1:129.
237. Miller L, Gertel M, Fox GS, MacLean LD. Comparison of effect of narcotic and epidural analgesia on postoperative respiratory function. Am J Surg 1976;131:291.
238. Miller RD, Munger WL, Powell PE. Chronic pain and local anesthetic. In: Cousins MJ, Bridenbaugh PO, eds. Neural blockade. Philadelphia: JB Lippincott, 1980:616.
239. Mockus MB, Rutherford RB, Rosales C, Pearce WH. Sympathectomy for causalgia. Arch Surg 1987;122:668.
240. Modig J. Lumbar epidural nerve blockade versus parenteral analgesics. Acta Anaesth Scand 1978;70(suppl):30.
241. Modig J, Malmberg P, Karlstrom G. Effect of epidural versus general anaesthetic on calf blood flow. Acta Anaesth Scand 1980;24:305.
242. Modig J, Hjelmstedt A, Sahlstedt B. Comparative influences of epidural and general anaesthesia on deep venous thrombosis and pulmonary embolism after total hip replacement. Acta Chir Scand 1981;147:125.
243. Mok MS, Lipmann M, Wang JJ. Efficacy of epidural nalbuphine in postoperative pain control. Anesthesiology 1984;61:A187.
244. Moller IW, Krantz T, Wandall E, et al. Effect of alfentanil anaesthesia on the adrenocortical and hyperglycemic response to abdominal surgery. Br J Anaesth 1985;57:591.
245. Moller IW, Rem J, Brandt MR, Kehlet H. Effect of posttraumatic epidural analgesia on the cortisol and hyperglycemic response to surgery. Acta Anaesth Scand 1982;26:56.
246. Moore DC. Regional block. 4th ed. Springfield, IL: Charles C Thomas, 1971.
247. Moore DC. Intercostal nerve block for postoperative somatic

pain following surgery of thorax and upper abdomen. Br J Anaesth 1975;47:284.
248. Moore DC. Intercostal nerve block: spread of India ink injected to the ribs' costal groove. Br J Anaesth 1981;53:325.
249. Moore DC, Bush W, Burnett LL. Intercostal nerve block: a roentgenographic anatomic study of technique and absorption of solution in humans. Anesth Analg 1980;59:815.
250. Moss E, McDowall DG. ICP increases with 50% nitrous oxide in oxygen in severe head injuries during controlled ventilation. Br J Anaesth 1979;51:757.
251. Mowbray A, Wong KKS, Murray JM. Intercostal catheterisation: an alternative approach to the paravertebral space. Anaesthesia 1987;42:958.
252. Mullen JB, Cook WA. Reduction of postoperative lumbar hemilaminectomy pain with marcaine. J Neurosurg 1979;51:126.
253. Muneyuki M, Ueda Y, Urabe N, et al. Postoperative pain relief and respiratory function in man: comparison between intermittent intravenous injections of meperidine and continuous lumbar epidural analgesia. Anesthesiology 1968;29:304.
254. Murphy DF. Continuous intercostal nerve blockade for pain relief following cholecystectomy. Br J Anaesth 1983;55:521.
255. Murphy DF. Intercostal nerve blockade for fractured ribs and postoperative analgesia. Regional Anesth 1983;8:151.
256. Murphy DF. Continuous intercostal nerve blockade. Br J Anaesth 1984;56:627.
257. Muse M. Stress-related, posttraumatic chronic pain syndrome: criteria for diagnosis, and preliminary report on prevalence. Pain 1985;23:295.
258. Naguib M, Adu-Gyamfi Y, Absood GH, et al. Epidural ketamine for postoperative analgesia. Can Anaesth Soc J 1986;33:16.
259. Nash TP. Percutaneous radiofrequency lesioning of dorsal root ganglia for intractable pain. Pain 1986;24:67.
260. Nashold BS, Ostdahl RH. Dorsal root entry zone lesions for pain relief. J Neurosurg 1979;51:59.
261. Nashold BS, Bullitt E. Dorsal root entry zone lesions to control central pain in paraplegics. J Neurosurg 1981;55:414.
262. Nashold BS, Urban B, Zorub DS. Phantom pain relief by focal destruction of the substantia gelatinosa of Rolando. In: Bonica J, AlbeFessard D, eds. Advances in pain research and surgery. vol I. New York: Raven Press, 1976:959.
263. Nathan PW, Noordenbos W, Wall PD. Ongoing activity in peripheral nerve: interactions between electrical stimulation and ongoing activity. Exp Neurol 1973;38:90.
264. Nimmo WS, Todd JG. Fentanyl by constant rate I.V. infusion for postoperative analgesia. Br J Anaesth 1985;57:250.
265. Nimmo WS, Littlewood DS, Scott DB, Prescott LF. Gastric emptying following hysterectomy with extradural analgesia. Br J Anaesth 1978;50:559.
266. Nimmo WS, Duthie DJR, Clark C. Therapeutic drug interactions. Clin Crit Care Med 1986;8:133.
267. Noller DW, Gillenwater JY, Howards SS, Vaughn ED. Intercostal nerve block with flank incision. J Urol 1977;117:759.
268. Nordberg G. Pharmacokinetic aspects of spinal morphine analgesia. Acta Anaesth Scand 1984;29(suppl 79):6.
269. Nordberg G, Hedner T, Mellstrand T, Dahlstrom B. Pharmacokinetic aspects of epidural morphine analgesia. Anesthesiology 1983;58:545.
270. Nunn JF, Slavin G. Posterior intercostal nerve block for pain relief after cholecystectomy. Br J Anaesth 1980;52:253.
271. O'Connor M, Escarpa A, Prys-Roberts C. Ventilatory depression during and after infusion of alfentanil in man. Br J Anaesth 1983;55:217S.
272. Oji A. Entonox for casualties at 1000 m: use of nitrous oxide analgesia in Nigeria at moderate altitude. Anaesthesia 1984;39:1127.
273. O'Kelly E, Garry B. Continuous pain relief for multiple fractured ribs. Br J Anaesth 1981;53:987.
274. Olivet RT, Nauss LA, Payne WS. A technique for continuous intercostal nerve block analgesia following thoracotomy. J Thorac Cardiovasc Surg 1980;80:308.
275. Orr IA, Keenan DJ, Dundee JW. Improved pain relief after thoracotomy: use of cryoprobe and morphine infusion. Br Med J (Clin Res) 1981;283:945.
276. Owen H, Spence AA. Etomidate (editorial). Br J Anaesth 1984;56:555.
277. Parbrook GD. Technique of inhalation analgesia in the postoperative period. Br J Anaesth 1967;39:730.
278. Parbrook GD. Therapeutic uses of $N_2O$. Br J Anaesth 1968;40:365.
279. Parbrook GD, Steel GF, Dacrymple FG. Factors predisposing to postoperative pain and pulmonary complications. Br J Anaesth 1973;45:21.
280. Patel JM, Lanzafame RJ, Williams JS, et al. The effect of incisional infiltration of bupivacaine hydrochloride upon pulmonary functions, atelectasis and narcotic need following elective cholecystectomy. Surg Gynecol Obstet 1983;157:338.
281. Pathak KS, Anton AH, Sutheimer CA. Effects of low-dose morphine and fentanyl infusions on urinary and plasma catecholamine concentrations during scoliosis surgery. Anesth Analg 1985;64:509.
282. Patman RD, Thompson JE, Persson AV. Management of posttraumatic pain syndromes: report of 113 cases. Ann Surg 1973;117:780.
283. Payne R. Neuropathic pain syndromes with special reference to causalgia and reflex sympathetic dystrophy. Clin J Pain 1986;2:59.
284. Pflug AE, Murphy TM, Butler SH, et al. The effects of postoperative peridural analgesia on pulmonary therapy and pulmonary complications. Anesthesiology 1974;41:8.
285. Pflug AE, Halter JB, Tolas AG. Plasma catecholamine levels during anesthesia and surgical stress. Regional Anesth 1982;7(suppl):S49.
286. Pilowsky I, Crettenden I, Townley M. Sleep disturbances in pain clinic patients. Pain 1985;23:27.
287. Pither CE, Raj PP, Ford DJ. The use of peripheral nerve stimulators for regional anesthesia. A review of experimental characteristics, technique, and clinical applications. Regional Anesth 1985;10:49.
288. Pond WW, Somerville GM, Thong SH, et al. Pain of delayed traumatic splenic rupture masked by intrapleural lidocaine. Anesthesiology 1989;70:154.
289. Portenoy RK, Foley KM. Chronic use of opioid analgesics in nonmalignant pain: report of 38 cases. Pain 1986;25:171.
290. Prough DS, McLeskey CH, Poehling GG, et al. Efficacy of oral nifedipine in the treatment of reflex sympathetic dystrophy. Anesthesiology 1985;62:796.
291. Pybus DA, Torda TA. Dose-effect relationships of extradural morphine. Br J Anaesth 1982;54:1259.
292. Radnay PA, Duncalf D, Novakovic M, Lesser ML. Common bile duct pressure changes after fentanyl, morphine, meperidine, butorphanol, and naloxone. Anesth Analg 1984;63:441.
293. Raj PP. Epidemiology of pain. In: Raj PP, ed. Practical management of pain. Chicago: Year Book Medical Publishers, 1986:2.
294. Raj PP, Montgomery SJ, Nettles D, Jenkins MT. Infraclavicular brachial plexus block—a new approach. Anesth Analg 1973;52:897.
295. Raj PP, Parks RI, Watson TD, Jenkins MT. A new single-position supine approach to sciatic-femoral nerve block. Anesth Analg 1975;54:489.
296. Raj PP, Rosenblatt R, Montgomery SJ. Use of the nerve stimulator for peripheral blocks. Regional Anesth 1980;5:14.
297. Raj PP, McLennan JE, Phero JC. Assessment and management planning of chronic low back pain. In: Stanton-Hicks & Boas

R, Eds. Chronic low back pain. New York: Raven Press, 1982:71.
298. Raj PP, Finnsson R, Denson D. Epidural analgesia—intermittent or continuous? In: Meyer J, Nolte H, eds. Die Kontinuierliche periduralanesthesie. Stuttgart: Georg Thieme Verlag, 1983:26.
299. Ramamurthy S, Winnie AP. Regional anesthetic techniques for pain relief. Semin Anesth 1985;4:237.
300. Rankin APN, Comber REH. Management of fifty cases of chest injury with a regimen of epidural bupivacaine and morphine. Anaesth Intens Care 1984;12:311.
301. Rawal N, Sjostrand UH, Dahlstrom B, et al. Epidural morphine for postoperative pain relief: a comparative study with intramuscular narcotic and intercostal nerve block. Anesth Analg 1982;61:93.
302. Rawal N, Mollefors, Axelsson K, et al. An experimental study of urodynamic effects of epidural morphine and of naloxone reversal. Anesth Analg 1983;62:641.
303. Rawal N, Sjostrand UH, Christoffersson E, et al. Comparison of intramuscular and epidural morphine for postoperative analgesia in the grossly obese: influence on postoperative ambulation and pulmonary function. Anesth Analg 1984;63:583.
304. Rawal N, Arnér S, Gustafsson LL, Allvin R. Present state of extradural and intrathecal opioid analgesia in Sweden. A nationwide follow-up survey. Br J Anaesth 1987;59:791.
305. Ready LB, Kozody R, Barsa JE, Murphy TM. Trigger point injection vs. jet injection in the treatment of myofascial pain. Pain 1983;15:201.
306. Reiestad F, Stromskag KE. Intrapleural catheter in the management of postoperative pain. A preliminary report. Regional Anesth 1986;11:89.
307. Reiz S, Nath S, Rais O. Effects of thoracic epidural block and prenalterol on coronary vascular resistance and myocardial metabolism in patients with coronary artery disease. Acta Anesth Scand 1980;24:11.
308. Reiz S, Balfors E, Sorensen MB, et al. Coronary hemodynamic effects of general anesthesia and surgery. Modification by epidural analgesia in patients with ischemic heart disease. Regional Anesth 1982;7:S24.
309. Renaud B, Brichant JF, Clergue F, et al. Ventilatory effects of continuous epidural infusion of fentanyl. Anesth Analg 1988;67:971.
310. Richlin DM, Brand L. The use of oral analgesics for chronic pain. Hosp Formulary 1982;17:32.
311. Riddock GP. Phantom limbs and body shape. Brain 1941;64:197.
312. Risberg B, Medegard A, Heideman M, et al. Early activation of humoral proteolytic systems in patients with multiple trauma. Crit Care Med 1986;14:917.
313. Roberts WJ. A hypothesis on the physiological basis for causalgia and related pains. Pain 1986;24:297.
314. Robinson RJS, Metcalf IR. Hypertension after epidural meperidine. Can Anaesth Soc J 1985;32:658.
315. Rocco A, Reiestad F, Gudman J, McKay W. Intrapleural administration of local anesthetic for pain relief in patients with multiple rib fractures. A preliminary report. Regional Anesth 1987;12:10.
316. Rorie DK, Byer DE, Nelson DO, et al. Assessment of block of the sciatic nerve in the popliteal fossa. Anesth Analg 1980;59:371.
317. Rosenberg PH, Heino A, Scheinin B. Comparison of intramuscular analgesia, intercostal block, epidural morphine and on-demand-i.v.-fentanyl in the control of pain after upper abdominal surgery. Acta Anaesth Scand 1984;28:603.
318. Rosenberg PH, Scheinin BM-A, Lepantalo MJA, Lindfors O. Continuous intrapleural infusion of bupivacaine for analgesia after thoracotomy. Anesthesiology 1987;67:811.
319. Rosenblatt RM. Continuous femoral anesthesia for lower extremity surgery. Anesth Analg 1980;59:631.
320. Rosenblatt RM, Reich J, Dehring D. Tricyclic antidepressants in treatment of depression and chronic pain: analysis of the supporting evidence. Anesth Analg 1984;63:1025.
321. Rouby JJ, Eurin B, Glaser P, et al. Hemodynamic and metabolic effects of morphine in the critically ill. Circulation 1981;64:53.
322. Roviaro GC, Varoli R, Fascianella A, et al. Intrathoracic intercostal nerve block with phenol in open chest surgery: a randomized study with statistical evaluation of respiratory parameters. Chest 1986;90:64.
323. Runciman WB, Mather LE, Ilsley AH, et al. A sheep preparation for studying the interaction of regional blood flow and drug disposition. III: Effects of general and spinal anesthesia. Br J Anaesth 1984;56:1247.
324. Runciman WB, Mather LE, Ilsley AH, et al. A sheep preparation for studying interactions between blood flow and drug disposition. IV: The effects of general and spinal anaesthesia on blood flow and cefoxitin disposition. Br J Anaesth 1985;57:1239.
325. Rutberg H, Hakanson E, Anderberg B, et al. Effects of the extradural administration of morphine or bupivacaine on the endocrine response to upper abdominal surgery. Br J Anaesth 1984;56:233.
326. Rybro L, Schurizer BA, Petersen TK, Wernberg M. Postoperative analgesia and lung function: a comparison of intramuscular with epidural morphine. Acta Anaesth Scand 1982;26:514.
327. Scheinin B, Lindgren L, Rosenberg PH. Treatment of post-thoracotomy pain with intermittent instillations of intrapleural bupivacaine. Acta Anesth Scand 1989;33:156.
328. Scott JC, Stanski DR, Ponganis KV. Quantitation of fentanyl's effect on the brain using the EEG. Anesthesiology 1983;59:A370.
329. Scott LE, Clum GA, Peoples JB. Preoperative predictors of post-operative pain. Pain 1983;15:283.
330. Scott NB, Mogensen T, Bigler D, et al. Continuous thoracic extradural 0.5% bupivacaine with or without morphine: effect on quality of blockade, lung function and the surgical stress response. Br J Anaesth 1989;62:253.
331. Sebel PS, Bovill JG, Schellekens APM, et al. Hormonal responses to high-dose fentanyl anaesthesia. Br J Anaesth 1981;53:941.
332. Sebel PS, Aun C, Fiolet J, et al. Endocrinological effects of intrathecal morphine. Eur J Anaesthesiol 1985;2:291.
333. Selander D. Catheter technique in axillary plexus block. Presentation of a new method. Acta Anaesth Scand 1977;21:324.
334. Seltzer S, Marcus R, Stoch R. Perspectives in the control of chronic pain by nutritional manipulation. Pain 1981;11:141.
335. Selzer M, Spencer WA. Convergence of visceral and cutaneous afferent pathways in the lumbar spinal cord. Brain Res 1969;14:331.
336. Shapiro JM, Westphal LM, White PF, et al. Midazolam infusion for sedation in the intensive care unit: effect on adrenal function. Anesthesiology 1986;64:394.
337. Shulman M, Sandler AN, Bradley JW, et al. Postthoracotomy pain and pulmonary function following epidural and systemic morphine. Anesthesiology 1984;61:569.
338. Shumacker HB. A personal overview of causalgia and other reflex dystrophies. Ann Surg 1985;201:278.
339. Shuman RL, Peters RM. Epidural anesthesia following thoracotomy in patients with chronic obstructive airway disease. J Thorac Cardiovasc Surg 1976;71:82.
340. Simonneau G, Vivien A, Sartene R, et al. Diaphragm dysfunction induced by upper abdominal surgery. Am Rev Respir Dis 1983;128:899.
341. Simpson BRJ, Parkhouse J, Marshall R, Lambrechts W. Extradural analgesia and the prevention of respiratory complications. Br J Anaesth 1961;33:638.
342. Simpson PJ, Hughes DR, Long DH. Prolonged local analgesia

for inguinal herniorrhaphy with bupivacaine and dextran. Ann Roy Coll Surg (Engl) 1982;64:238.

343. Sjögren S, Wright B. Circulatory changes during continuous epidural blockade. Acta Anaesth Scand 1972;16:5.
344. Sjögren S, Wright B. Respiratory changes during continuous epidural blockade. Acta Anaesth Scand 1972;16:27.
345. Sloan JP, Muwanga CL, Waters EA, et al. Multiple rib fractures: transcutaneous nerve stimulation versus conventional analgesia. J Trauma 1986;26:1120.
346. Smith BE, Fischer HBJ, Scott PV. Continuous sciatic nerve block. Anaesthesia 1984;39:155.
347. Soliman IE, Safwat A. Successful management of an elderly patient with multiple trauma. J Trauma 1985;25:806.
348. Spence AA. Pulmonary changes after surgery. Regional Anesth 1982;7(suppl):S119.
349. Spence AA, Smith G. Postoperative analgesia and lung function: a comparison of morphine with extradural block. Br J Anaesth 1971;43:146.
350. Spence AA, Logan DA. Respiratory effects of extradural nerve block in the postoperative period. Br J Anaesth 1975;47:281.
351. Sriwatanakul K, Weis OF, Alloza JL, et al. Analysis of narcotic analgesic usage in the treatment of postoperative pain. JAMA 1983;250:926.
352. Stanley TH, Philbin DM, Coggins CH. Fentanyl oxygen anaesthesia for coronary artery surgery: cardiovascular and ADH responses. Can Anaesth Soc J 1979;26:168.
353. Stanski Dr, Hug CC JR. Alfentanil—a kinetically predictable narcotic analgesic. Anesthesiology 1982;57:435.
354. Stapleton JV, Austin KL, Mather LE. A pharmacokinetic approach to postoperative pain: continuous infusion of pethidine. Anaesth Intens Care 1979;7:25.
355. Stein JM, Warfield CA. Phantom limb pain. Hosp Pract 1982;2:166.
356. Stenstheth R, Sellevold O, Breivik H. Epidural morphine for postoperative pain: experience with 1085 patients. Acta Anaesth Scand 1985;29:148.
357. Stewart GJ, Ritchie WG, Lynch PR. Venous endothelial damage produced by massive sticking and emigration of leukocytes. Am J Pathol 1974;74:507.
358. Stewart RD, Paris PM, Stoy WA, Cannon G. Patient-controlled inhalational analgesia in prehospital care: a study of side-effects feasibility. Crit Care Med 1983;11:851.
359. Strömskag KE, Reiestad F, Holmqvist ELO, Ogenstad S. Intrapleural administration of 0.25%, 0.375%, and 0.5% bupivacaine with epinephrine after cholecystectomy. Anesth Analg 1988;67:430.
360. Swerdlow M. Anticonvulsant drugs and chronic pain. Clin Neuropharmacol 1984;7:51.
361. Symreng T, Gomez MN, Johnson B, et al. Intrapleural bupivacaine—technical considerations and intraoperative use. J Cardiothorac Anesth 1989;3:139.
362. Symreng T, Gomez MN, Rossi N. Intrapleural bupivacaine vs saline after thoracotomy—effects on pain and lung function—a double blind study. J Cardiothorac Anesth 1989;3:144.
363. Szyfelbein SK, Osgood PF, Carr DB. The assessment of pain and plasma beta-endorphin immunoactivity in burned children. Pain 1985;22:173.
364. Taylor JW, Hander EW, Skreen R, Wilmore DW. The effect of central nervous system narcosis on the sympathetic response to stress. J Surg Res 1976;20:313.
365. Telivoo L, Perttala Y. Use of x-ray contrast medium to control intervertebral nerve blocks. Ann Chir Gynaecol 1966;55:185.
366. Thomas OFM, Lambert WG, Lloyd-Williams K. The direct perfusion of surgical wounds and local anaesthetic solution: an approach to postoperative pain. Ann Roy Coll Surg (Engl) 1983;65:226.
367. Tondare AS, Nadkarni AV. Femoral nerve block for fractured shaft of femur. Can Anaesth Soc J 1982;29:270.
368. Torda TA, Pybus DA. Extradural administration of morphine and bupivacaine. A controlled comparison. Br J Anaesth 1984;56:141.
369. Travell JG, Simons DG. Myofascial pain and dysfunction. Baltimore: Williams & Wilkins, 1983.
370. Traynor C, Hall GM. Endocrine and metabolic changes during surgery: anesthetic implications. Br J Anaesth 1981;53:153.
371. Traynor C, Paterson JL, Ward ID, et al. Effects of extradural analgesia and vagal blockade on the metabolic and endocrine response to upper abdominal surgery. Br J Anaesth 1982;54:319.
372. Tuominen M, Haasio J, Hekali R, Rosenberg PH. Continuous interscalene brachial plexus block: clinical efficacy, technical problems and bupivacaine plasma concentrations. Acta Anaesth Scand 1989;33:84.
373. Ty TC, Melzack R, Wall PD. Acute trauma. In: Wall P, Melzack R, eds. Textbook of pain. New York: Churchill Livingstone, 1985:209.
374. Tyson MD, Gaynor JS. Interruption of the sympathetic nervous system in relation to trauma. Surgery 1946;19:167.
375. Ullman DA, Fortune JB, Greenhouse BB, et al. The treatment of patients with multiple rib fractures using continuous thoracic epidural narcotic infusion. Regional Anesth 1989;14:43.
376. Urban BJ, Nashold BS. Percutaneous epidural stimulation of the spinal cord for relief of pain. Long-term results. J Neurosurg 1978;48:323.
377. Urban BJ, Nashold BS. Combined epidural and peripheral nerve stimulation for relief of pain. Description of technique and preliminary results. J Neurosurg 1982;57:365.
378. Urban BJ, France RD, Steinberger EK, et al. Long-term use of narcotic/antidepressant in the management of phantom limb pain. Pain 1986;24:191.
379. Utting JE, Smith JM. Postoperative analgesia. Anaesthesia 1979;34:320.
380. Vatashsky E, Haskel Y. Effect of nalbuphine on intrabiliary pressure in the early postoperative period. Can Anaesth Soc J 1986;33:433.
381. Vatashsky E, Haskel Y, Beilin B, Aronson HB. Common bile duct pressure in dogs after opiate injection—epidural versus intravenous route. Can Anaesth Soc J 1984;31:650.
382. Wagner RL, White PF, Kan PB, et al. Inhibition of adrenal steroidogenesis by the anesthetic etomidate. N Engl J Med 1984;310:1415.
383. Wahba WM, Craig DB, Don HF, Becklake MR. The cardiorespiratory effects of thoracic epidural anaesthesia. Can Anaesth Soc J 1972;19:8.
384. Wahba WM, Don HF, Craig DB. Post-operative epidural analgesia: effects on lung volumes. Can Anaesth Soc J 1975;22:519.
385. Wall PD. On the relation of injury to pain. Pain 1979;6:253.
386. Wall PD, Eggerr MD. Formation of new connections in adult rat brain after partial deafferentation. Nature (Lond) 1971;232:542.
387. Wall PD, Devor M. Sensory afferent impulses originate from dorsal root ganglia as well as from the periphery in normal and nerve injured rats. Pain 1983;17:321.
388. Wallin G, Cassuto J, Högström S, et al. Failure of epidural anesthesia to prevent postoperative paralytic ileus. Anesthesiology 1986;65:292.
389. Walsh ES, Paterson JL, O'Riordan JBA. Effect of high dose fentanyl anesthesia on the metabolic and endocrine response to cardiac surgery. Br J Anaesth 1981;53:1155.
390. Wang JK, Johnson KA, Ilstrup DM. Sympathetic blocks for reflex sympathetic dystrophy. Pain 1985;23:13.
391. Wattwil M, Thorén T, Hennerdal S, Garvill JE. Epidural anal-

gesia with bupivacaine reduces postoperative paralytic ileus after hysterectomy. Anesth Analg 1989;68:353.

392. Webling DD. Anaesthesia of the upper arm for casualty procedures. Med J Aust 1960;2:496.
393. Weightman D, Browne RC. Injuries in eleven selected sports. Br J Sports Med 1975;9:136.
394. Weis OF, Sriwatanakul K, Alloza JL, et al. Attitudes of patients, house staff and nurses towards postoperative analgesic care. Anesth Analg 1983;62:70.
395. Whifler K, Leiman BC. The application of regional anaesthesia in a disaster situation. S Afr Med J 1983;63:409.
396. White JG, Sweet WH. Pain and the neurosurgeon. Springfield, IL: Charles C. Thomas, 1969.
397. White PF. Patient-controlled analgesia: a new approach to the management of postoperative pain. Semin Anesth 1985;4:255.
398. White PF. Use of patient-controlled analgesia for management of acute pain. JAMA 1988;259:243.
399. Wikland C. Regional blockade versus analgesic therapy. Acta Anaesth Scand 1982;74(suppl):169.
400. Willer JC. Studies on pain. Effects of morphine on a spinal nociceptive flexion reflex and related pain sensation in man. Brain Res 1985;331:105.
401. Willer JC, Bergeret S, Gaudy JH. Epidural morphine strongly depresses nociceptive flexion reflexes in patients with postoperative pain. Anesthesiology 1985;63:675.
402. Wilmore DW. Hormonal responses and their effect on metabolism. Surg Clin North Am 1976;56:999.
403. Wilmore DW, Long JM, Mason ED, et al. Stress in surgical patients as a neurophysiologic stress response. Surg Gynecol Obstet 1976;142:257.
404. Wilson RL. Management of pain following peripheral nerve injuries. Orthop Clin North Am 1981;12:343.
405. Winnie AP. Interscalene brachial plexus block. Anesth Analg 1970;47:455.
406. Winnie AP. Plexus anesthesia. Perivascular techniques of brachial plexus block. Philadelphia: WB Saunders, 1983:117.
407. Winnie AP, Ramamurthy S, Durani Z. The inguinal perivascular technique of lumbar plexus anesthesia. The 3 in 1 block. Anaesth Analg 1973;52:989.
408. Wolf SL, Gersh MR, Rao VR. Examination of electrode placements and stimulating parameters in treating chronic pain with conventional transcutaneous electrical nerve stimulation (TENS). Pain 1981;11:37.
409. Woltering EA, Flye MW, Huntley S, et al. Evaluation of bupivacaine nerve blocks in the modification of pain and pulmonary function changes after thoracotomy. Ann Thorac Surg 1980;30:122.
410. Wood M. The use of phenol as a neurolytic agent: a review. Pain 1978;5:205.
411. Worthley LIG. Thoracic epidural in the management of chest trauma. A study of 161 cases. Intens Care Med 1985;11:312.
412. Wyant GM. Chronic pain syndromes and their treatment. II. Trigger points. Can Anaesth Soc J 1979;26:216.
413. Yaksh TL. Spinal opiate analgesia: characteristics and principles of action. Pain 1981;11:293.
414. Yasuda I, Hirano T, Ojima T, et al. Supraclavicular brachial plexus block using a nerve stimulator and an insulated needle. Br J Anaesth 1980;52:409.
415. Yate PM, Thomas D, Short SM, et al. Comparison of infusions of alfentanil or pethidine for sedation of ventilated patients of the ITU. Br J Anaesth 1986;58:1091.
416. Young RF. Surgical role in relief of pain. Semin Anesth 1985;4:323.
417. Young RF, Brechner T. Electrical stimulation of the brain for relief of intractable pain due to cancer. Cancer 1986;57:1266.
418. Young RF, Kroening R, Fulton W, et al. Electrical stimulation of the brain in treatment of chronic pain. Experience over 5 years. J Neurosurg 1985;62:389.
419. Zitman FG. Biofeedback, relaxation therapy and chronic pain. In: Lipton S, Miles J, eds. Persistent pain: modern methods of treatment. vol 3. New York: Academic Press, 1981:99.

# Chapter Twenty-Four

*Alexander Nacht*
*Roberta C. Kahn*
*Sanford M. Miller*

# *Adult Respiratory Distress Syndrome and Its Management*

Respiratory failure is the clinical state in which pulmonary gas exchange is inadequate to maintain body function without mechanical support.[76] It is not uncommon after trauma. Aspiration of gastric contents, chest trauma, fat embolism, thromboembolism, central nervous system injury, fluid overload, cardiac failure, pain, respiratory muscle fatigue, residual postoperative paralysis, and respiratory depression by anesthetic drugs and opiates are among the major causes of this complication (Fig 24-1).[14] Fortunately, in most cases the etiology is obvious, mechanical support is adequate to maintain the patient's respiratory needs, and oxygenation is not a progressively worsening problem. However, this is typically not the case in the adult respiratory distress syndrome (ARDS), a form of acute respiratory failure that is essentially a secondary and nonspecific response of the lungs to a variety of diseases and accidental events, most of which do not in fact affect the pulmonary parenchyma or thoracic cavity directly. ARDS should not be thought of as a specific disease, but rather as a *clinical syndrome* of diffuse lung injury and destruction,[190] which may lead to respiratory failure or may follow respiratory failure from other causes.

ARDS has been recognized in one form or another at least since World WAR I[243] and has been referred to by a variety of names (Table 24-1).[250] As this table indicates, there has been a good deal of confusion about the syndrome, although there has been agreement that it represents a more ominous development than simple respiratory failure. It was not until 1967 that this diversity of observations was unified into one conceptual entity, and the terms of discussion were defined.[5] The term "adult respiratory distress syndrome" was derived by analogy from the infant respiratory distress syndrome (IRDS). Yet, the comparison is incorrect because in the latter there is a primary surfactant deficiency,[58,91,254] whereas in the adult syndrome surfactant depletion follows and is part of a more generalized process. Given the same initiating events, ARDS is as likely to develop in the young and vigorous as it is in the aged with decreased reserve,[251] and it can also occur in children.[89,139,254]

Much of the difficulty in assessing the risk of ARDS from available information is that most studies are retrospective and consider only cases in which the full syndrome has developed. Even the two major prospective series by Pepe,[245] Fowler,[104] and their co-workers differed significantly in their criteria of inclusion. As a result, published incidence rates and descriptions of ARDS severity show a great deal of variation. However, one consistent finding in the above studies[104,245] and in a more recent follow-up study[204] is that there is a markedly higher incidence of ARDS in patients with multiple risk factors than in those presenting with a single risk condition (Table 24-2). In addition, and probably related to this finding, there is a definite relationship between the severity of injury in traumatized patients and the likelihood of the subsequent occurrence of ARDS (Fig 24-2).[9]

Between 150,000 and 200,000 cases of ARDS occur in the United States each year. The number may be increasing since more victims and more severely injured victims of acute trauma may be surviving as a result of improved initial therapy.[151] However, the mortality rate of approximately 50% has not changed in the last 20 years despite advances in care.[355,356] This mortality rate translates to 75,000 to 100,000

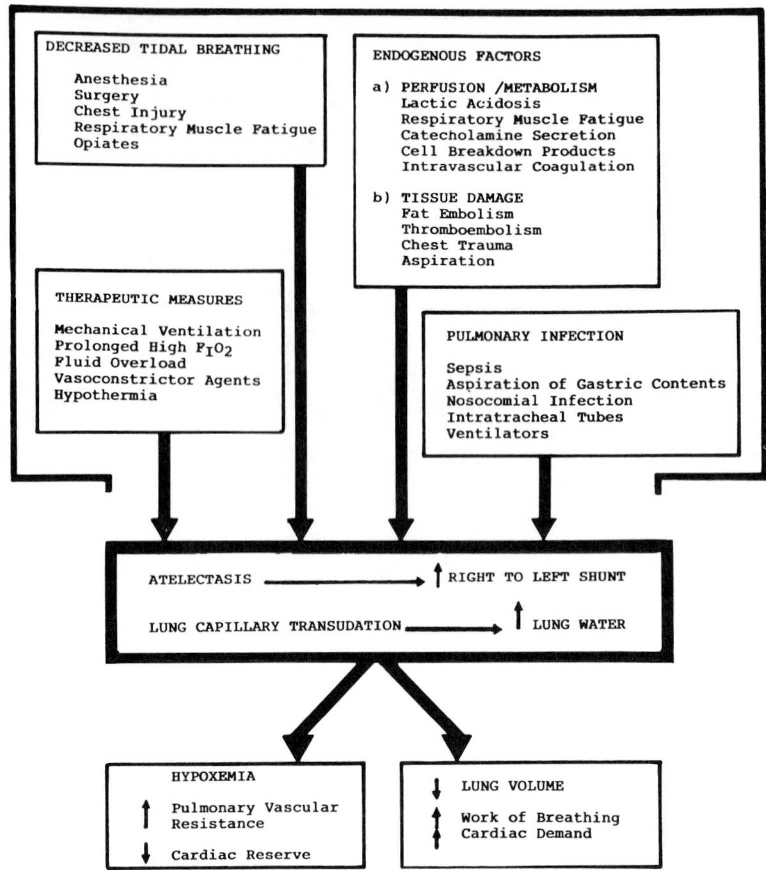


FIG. 24-1. Factors associated with posttraumatic and postsurgical respiratory failure. (Adapted from Bartlett RH, Surg Ann 1971;3:1, with permission.)

deaths per year associated with ARDS from all causes. Claiming that changing criteria of selection may account for this apparent lack of progress, one authority has recently argued that these numbers are deceptive and lead us to an attitude of "inappropriate pessimism" with regard to therapeutic progress.[271]

TABLE 24-1. Names Used for Acute Respiratory Distress Syndrome (ARDS)

| |
|---|
| Da Nang lung |
| Shock lung |
| Traumatic wet lung |
| Capillary leak syndrome |
| White lung syndrome |
| Acute alveolar failure |
| Stiff lung syndrome |
| Postperfusion lung |
| Congestive atelectasis |
| Adult hyaline membrane disease |
| Posttransfusion lung |
| Hemorrhagic lung |
| Permeability pulmonary edema |
| Low-pressure pulmonary edema |
| Pump lung |
| Respirator lung |
| Noncardiac pulmonary edema |
| Progressive pulmonary failure |
| Progressive pulmonary consolidation |

One of the major problems in studying ARDS is the vast range of disorders in which it is seen (Table 24-3). Moreover, because reports tend to be anecdotal and studies tend to be retrospective and variable in their inclusion criteria, there has been controversy over whether the term should be used as broadly as it is.[98,222,249,281] As a result, assigning causes and making predictions of outcome based on these causes can be problematic. In discussing ARDS, cause can refer either to a clinical event that initiates the syndrome or a mechanism that mediates the actual lung injury.[145] Since the lung has a limited repertoire of responses, what we see clinically may represent a final common pathway for a variety of insults. It is necessary to understand the relationship between these two levels in order to guide therapeutic intervention effectively. Thus, rather than thinking in terms of causes, it is more appropriate to consider conditions associated to varying degrees with the development of ARDS. Some of these conditions, such as aspiration of gastric contents, may injure the lung directly, whereas others may affect pulmonary function only through humoral mediators.

## CONDITIONS ASSOCIATED WITH ARDS

The clinical "causes" of ARDS in the trauma patient may be categorized as primarily direct or indirect,[230] although this classification should not be taken as a hard-and-fast distinction since some conditions have aspects of both. The initial

TABLE 24-2. Incidence of ARDS After One of the Specified Clinical Conditions and When Simultaneously Combined With Other Specified Conditions*

| CLINICAL CONDITIONS | ALONE | | WITH ONE OTHER CONDITION | | WITH TWO OTHER CONDITIONS | | TOTAL | |
|---|---|---|---|---|---|---|---|---|
| | *n* | % | *n* | % | *n* | % | *n* | % |
| Sepsis syndrome | 5/13 | 38 | 2/4 | . . . | 2/2 | . . . | 9/19 | 47 |
| Aspiration of gastric contents | 7/23 | 30 | 3/9 | 33 | 0/0 | . . . | 10/32 | 31 |
| Pulmonary contusion | 5/29 | 17 | 7/12 | 58 | 7/9 | 78 | 19/50 | 38 |
| Multiple emergency transfusions | 4/17 | 24 | 3/11 | 27 | 12/14 | 86 | 19/42 | 43 |
| Multiple major fractures | 1/12 | 8 | 4/10 | 40 | 10/12 | 83 | 15/34 | 44 |
| Near-drowning | 2/3 | . . . | 1/1 | . . . | 0/0 | . . . | 3/4 | . . . |
| Pancreatitis | 1/1 | . . . | 0/0 | . . . | 0/0 | . . . | 1/1 | . . . |
| Prolonged hypotension | 0/1 | . . . | 0/1 | . . . | 2/2 | . . . | 2/4 | . . . |
| Overall risk | | 25 | | 42 | | 85 | | |

*From Pepe et al[245] with permission.

lung injury is usually at the capillary rather than the alveolar level. However, once set into motion, the pathologic evolution of the two may be indistinguishable. The major direct cause is aspiration of gastric contents.[104,204,245] It is important to note that gastric aspirates with a pH greater than 2.5 are quite capable of producing ARDS,[294] especially if large volumes of fluid containing particulate matter are aspirated. The major initial damage is to the pulmonary epithelial surface with alveolar flooding and collapse, but eventually the capillary endothelium may also be involved. When there are no other medical problems or complications, the prognosis is quite good.[34] On the other hand, if bacterial infection supervenes or if the patient is otherwise debilitated, the outlook becomes grim. In near-drowning, edema probably results from osmotic imbalance and surfactant washout.[202,216] Although edema may worsen after initial presentation, resolution should be rapid unless there has also been endothelial injury.[164] Aspiration of blood after craniofacial injuries can result in severe hypoxemia, but unless there is concomitant aspiration of gastric contents, the pulmonary parenchyma is little affected and symptoms disappear within a few days.

Delayed pulmonary edema is said to follow smoke inhalation, although this has been disputed on the basis of both clinical experience and laboratory experiments.[92,145,340] Such inhalation of toxic gases as phosgene, ammonia, ozone, nitrogen dioxide, and sulfur dioxide may result in ARDS; the

FIG. 24-2. Relationship between injury severity score on admission and subsequent development of ARDS. (Adapted from Maunder[204] with permission.)

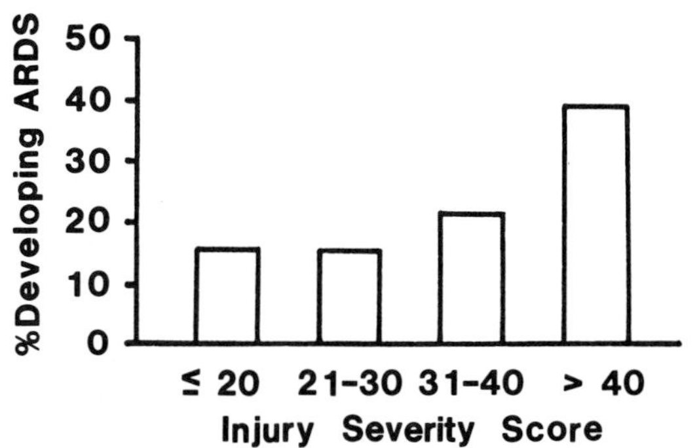


TABLE 24-3. Trauma-Associated Conditions That Have the Potential of Producing ARDS*

| | |
|---|---|
| Shock | Disseminated intravascular coagulation |
| Septic (including toxic shock syndrome) | Bowel infarction |
| Hemorrhagic | Irritant gas or chemical inhalation ($NO_2$, $CL_2$, $SO_2$, $NH_3$, $H_2SO_4$, phosgene, mercury, cadmium, perchlorethylene, organophosphates) |
| Cardiogenic | Smoke inhalation |
| Anaphylactic | $O_2$ toxicity |
| Trauma** | Drug overdose |
| Direct pulmonary contusion/ concussion | Heroin, methadone |
| Nonpulmonary, multisystem | Ethchlorvynol, acetylsalicylic acid, proproxyphene, tricyclic antidepressants |
| Multiple major fractures | Drug idiosyncratic reaction (colchicine, hydrochlorothiazide, ampicillin) |
| Fat embolism syndrome | Venous air embolism |
| Severe head injury/intracranial bleeding | Hemodialysis |
| Surface burns | Cardiopulmonary bypass |
| Aspiration of gastric contents (especially low pH) | Toxic ingestion (ethylene glycol, paraquat, kerosene) |
| Near-drowning** | Radiation |
| Lung infection** | Strangulation |
| Bacterial pneumonia (staphylococcal, streptococcal, *Klebsiella*, pneumococcal, enterococcal, *Pseudomonas*) | Re-expansion of collapsed lung |
| Sepsis** (Gram-negative rods most common, but also other Gram-negative and postive organisms, including clostridial and gonococcal septicemia) | Uremia |
| Pancreatitis | Liver failure |
| Multiple (massive) transfusions | Heat stroke |
| | Transfusion reaction |
| | Postpartum complications |
| | Diabetic ketoacidosis |

* From Pepe[243] with permission.
** Common risk of ARDS.

most common setting for this is an industrial accident.[329] ARDS may also occur in the presence of pneumonia, especially diffuse viral pneumonia. Influenza, *Mycoplasma, Rickettsia,* cytomegalovirus, and *Pneumocystis* (especially in patients with acquired immune deficiency syndrome)[15] have all been implicated, as have, less commonly, bacterial and fungal agents.[158] The etiology may be widespread inflammation or activation of blood-borne mediators. Indeed, even in localized pneumonias, peripneumonic areas probably have some degree of inflammation and increased permeability.[190]

This last point is important because permeability edema is not necessarily identical with ARDS.[321] Pulmonary capillary permeability may also increase after severe head and spinal cord injury (see Chapter 10).[100,186,210] The mechanism is not fully understood, but is thought to be related to increased pulmonary arteriolar and venular tone resulting from massive sympathetic discharge. The effect of venoconstriction is to raise vascular hydrostatic pressure and thus cause noncardiogenic pulmonary edema.[61,62,96,197,338,366] Actually, transient inotropic depression may also be present at this time. It should be noted that these effects are usually of only brief duration. However, they cause cellular damage that may last for days. There is some question as to whether edema resulting from this and other causes (high altitude,[292] lung reexpansion, strangulation) can properly be called ARDS. Even though there is some opening of vascular pores with resultant high-permeability edema, there is really no progressive syndrome. It may then be more appropriate to speak of a spectrum of low-pressure edema, with ARDS representing only the most severe end.[317]

ARDS has been attributed to fluid overload from massive volume resuscitation in shock or to hemorrhagic shock itself ("shock lung"), but there is simply no evidence to support these contentions.[76,299] Several studies have shown that hemorrhagic shock and hypotension alone are not important risk factors for ARDS.[57,73–77,110,143,145,221] Hypovolemic patients who develop the syndrome most often have other predisposing problems. ARDS has also been thought to be the result of pulmonary microemboli of red cell clumps during multiple transfusions of unfiltered blood.[43] Other possibilities include capillary flow reduction from the high viscosity and tissue hypoxia from the low $P_{50}$ of packed red blood cells.[282] Studies on micropore filtration have failed to demonstrate that these problems really exist,[88] although passive transfer of immune factors may occur, with effects on the lung.[72,260] Although massive transfusion may cause transient abnormalities of pulmonary function, the evidence that it in and of itself leads to ARDS is weak.[169] In one study, patients receiving *over* 22 units of blood within a 12-hour period had a higher incidence of ARDS without other predisposing factors.[245] Since these cases were few in number and not described in sufficient detail, it is difficult to know whether they represent a real effect. In any event, these conditions should be viewed not as causes of ARDS, but as concomitant factors or markers for more profound underlying conditions that may precipitate the pathophysiologic cascade producing the syndrome.

The one known major predisposing factor is sepsis or, more specifically, the sepsis syndrome.[56,204,245,261,351] This is an important distinction because patients with the sepsis syndrome may not have positive blood cultures or obvious source of infection, but will behave as if they are septic, ie, hypotension, lowered systemic vascular resistance, persistent unexplained metabolic acidosis. Prognostically this is in fact a more ominous picture than bacteremia, and these patients do poorly. In one study, 18% of all patients admitted with septicemia documented by positive blood cultures developed ARDS.[93] In another, 23% of patients with Gram-negative sepsis had ARDS with 90% mortality.[163] In a third series, 38% of those with the sepsis syndrome developed ARDS.[245] The clinical picture of sepsis without positive blood cultures is more likely to occur in trauma patients than in any other group, possibly secondary to prophylactic antibiotic coverage[145] or to the presence of a walled-off infection with intermittent seeding. It is quite possible that bacteremia may never be present; what one may be dealing with in this situation is endotoxemia from an isolated abscess.[227] Thus, it is not bacteremia per se that leads to ARDS; instead the syndrome may be an inflammatory response to endotoxin. This can be a devastating situation because the pulmonary problems cannot be resolved unless the source of sepsis is eliminated.[110]

The oleic acid infusion model of lung injury is often used as the prototype for animal research into ARDS. Yet, simple injury to the lung may have relatively mild consequences and a good outlook for rapid resolution. However, superimposed infection of the lung or elsewhere after lung injury may produce marked deterioration,[49] probably because a second injury produces a continuing insult. For the most part, sepsis leading to ARDS originates in an extrapulmonary source, usually the abdomen. Direct infection of the lung resulting in ARDS is the exception, rather than the rule. Pulmonary sources of systemic sepsis actually tend to develop after the onset of ARDS.[218] Direct injury of the lung, as in acid aspiration, can result in ARDS, but the parenchymal damage also increases the likelihood of supervening pneumonia that may not cause but will exacerbate the course of the already existing ARDS.

Additional causes of ARDS that should be noted are dialysis; cardiopulmonary bypass;[196,362] pre-existing autoimmune disorders, such as Goodpasture's syndrome or systemic lupus erythematosus; pancreatitis[50,170,287]; fat embolism (secondary to pelvic and long bone fractures)[159,242,275]; amniotic fluid embolism; air embolism[248]; and drug overdose.[118,166] What these and other causes have in common is that, like the sepsis syndrome, they do not necessarily involve direct lung injury. Rather, they are initiating events that set off some sort of pathophysiologic cascade, which involves more than one possible mechanism. The prognosis and outcome of ARDS depend very strongly on whether the cause or initiating event is a transient or persistent phenomenon.

ARDS usually develops within 3 days of the initiating event, especially if multiple risk factors are present (Fig 24-3).[104] Early posttraumatic death (within 72 hours) is generally due to the initial insult. Mortality after 72 hours is most commonly secondary to the sepsis syndrome; indeed, in one study six times as many ARDS patients had sepsis syndrome as patients with similar risk factors who did not develop ARDS.[218] The overwhelming majority of deaths associated with ARDS take place within 2 weeks of onset (Fig 24-4). These numbers can be misleading, however. The most important point to be made in this context is that very few patients actually die *from*

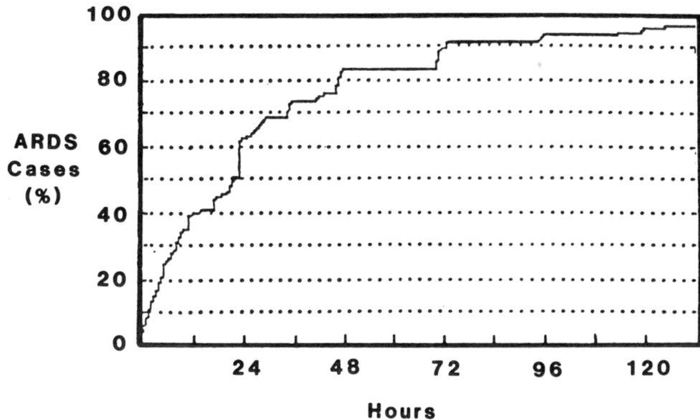


FIG. 24-3. Cumulative onset time of ARDS after a predisposing insult. Note that 80% of patients developed the syndrome within 72 hours of insult and 96.5% within 132 hours. Of the remaining five patients (3.5%), three had onset times 134, 264, and 303 hours after injury. In two patients onset time was missed. (From Fowler et al[104] with permission.)

ARDS; they die *with* it.[184] That is, hypoxemia is not a major cause of death in ARDS, a finding on which several authors agree.[197,218,266] Although patients requiring ventilation may have an increased mortality, the death rate is not significantly increased by the duration of respiratory support.[188] One characteristic of nonsurvivors, however, is lack of pulmonary improvement over time. Generally, then, death is most often due to the inability to control an underlying disease process. Usually it results from an untreated or untreatable infection—an abscess needing drainage or pneumonia causing nonbacteremic sepsis.[16] Multiple organ failure is especially common in such infected patients (see Chapter 27).

## PATHOPHYSIOLOGY

The major lesion in ARDS is increased alveolar-capillary permeability, which is actually the common denominator of a heterogeneous disease process. The syndrome may be viewed as a clinical constellation that is the end result of a complex sequence of cellular and biochemical events following systemic or pulmonary injury.[95] These events may have different degrees of significance in different forms of ARDS. The search for a single mechanism has been unsuccessful, but an understanding of how these processes interact may lead to more successful early intervention (Table 24-4).

FIG. 24-4. Survival rate after onset of ARDS. Median survival time of the 88 patients was 13.3 days, and overall mortality approached 65%. Vertical bars represent standard error. (From Fowler et al[104] with permission.)

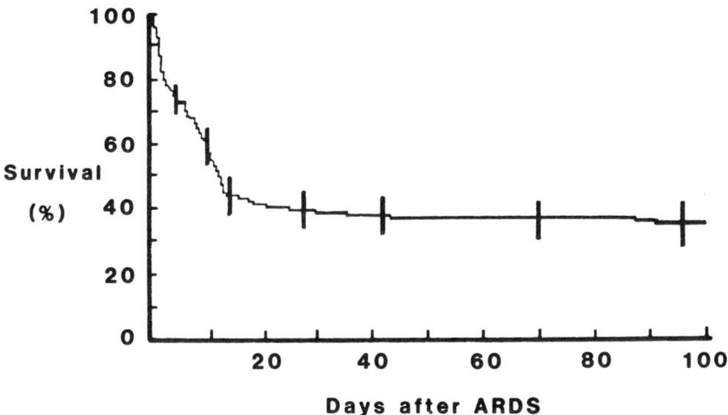


In recent years, one major focus of research has been on the role of leukocytes in lung injury. The earliest pathologic sections from the lungs of patients dying with "shock lung" showed massive granulocyte infiltration, packing capillaries and occasionally passing into the lung interstitium.[20] In 1968, in patients undergoing cellophane membrane hemodialysis, the phenomenon of sudden but transient neutropenia was noted. Further investigation of this process disclosed aggregation and deposition of neutrophils in the pulmonary vasculature during the neutropenic interval.[20,274] Similarly, transient neutropenia is often noted just before the development of ARDS.

Subsequent evidence pointed to an important role for complement in this phenomenon. Activation of the complement cascade produced the same effect; the leukocyte-aggregating factor was shown to be peptide fragment C5a or one of its metabolites, C5a des arginine. C5a has both anaphylatoxin and chemotactic activity, whereas C5a des arginine has only chemotactic activity. The C3a fragment has also been implicated in leukocyte aggregation, although it appears to be of lesser importance. When activated complement was infused into experimental animals, an ARDS-like syndrome resulted. Major studies reported significant correlation between neutrophil-aggregating activity in plasma and subsequent development of ARDS in patients with a variety of predisposing insults.[126,152,274] Studies of bronchoalveolar lavage fluid have shown the presence of chemotactic factors[237] and increased elastase, a leukocyte-elaborated proteolytic enzyme that cleaves complement.[185]

The complement hypothesis holds that acute lung injury is caused by leukocyte stimulation by complement compo-

TABLE 24-4. Proposed Mediators or Markers of Acute Lung Injury*

| |
|---|
| Formed blood elements |
| Neutrophila |
| Platelets |
| Chemoattractants |
| Complement fragments |
| Leukotriene $B_4$ |
| Platelet-activating factor |
| Bacterial peptides |
| Mediators of cell damage |
| Oxygen radicals ($H_2O_2$, $O_2^-$, HO·) |
| Proteolytic enzymes |
| Phospholipase products |
| Markers of cell damage |
| Prostacyclin |
| Factor VIII |
| Miscellaneous markers |
| Angiotensin-converting enzyme |
| Fibronectin |
| Fibrin degradation products |
| Phospholipase $A_2$ |

* From Maunder[204] with permission.

nents. Activation of the complement system results in production of small molecular weight fragments, especially C5-derived peptides that are recognized by and activate polymorphonuclear cells (PMNs).[101] Neutrophils may indeed have specific receptors that bind, internalize, and ultimately control the degradation of C5a.[107,314] C5-derived peptides are generated either by complement activation or by direct proteolytic cleavage (by elastin or plasmin) of C5. Trauma, sepsis, and other events associated with ARDS are known to activate the complement pathway. The components of the complement system are found in the lung, and lung macrophages release proteases that cleave them to their active form.[136] These fragments are able to stimulate PMNs to migrate in a directed fashion (respond chemotactically), to release lysosomal contents (degranulate), and to increase their oxygen metabolism (respiratory burst that generates superoxide anion radical). They also enhance the adhesiveness of PMNs, resulting in the development of leukocyte clumps and emboli.[101,124] Although complement may directly increase the permeability of capillary endothelium and cause vasoconstriction, these actions are not considered significant. Its major action occurs through its effects on white blood cells.

The complement hypothesis is a highly attractive theory that would appear to tie a number of processes together neatly. Unfortunately, recent studies do not confirm it. In one study, although C5a activity was present in 81% of patients developing ARDS, it was also present in patients at risk who did not develop the syndrome.[86] No consistent relation between complement fragment levels and the subsequent development of ARDS has been shown; thus, there is no support for the use of these measurements as clinically valuable predictors.[289,358] In addition, when activated complement is infused into animals, the pulmonary reaction that occurs is only transient.[150,211,212] When major lung inflammation does result, it seems to require an additional stress, such as hypoxia or prostaglandin $E_2$ infusion. Severe lung injury has been demonstrated in C5-depleted animals, and leukocyte aggregation in the lungs has been shown to occur secondary to other mechanisms. Thus, although in some forms of lung injury complement activation may indeed be necessary to start the process, it has not yet been shown to be a necessary or sufficient condition in all cases.[337]

The role of the white blood cell in the development of ARDS is also controversial. However, a good deal of experimental evidence supports the hypothesis that lung injury is caused by activation of leukocytes and their subsequent release of toxic products. In addition to the possible role of complement, alveolar macrophages also elaborate chemotaxins and specific factors that increase neutrophil adhesion to endothelium. Mechanisms of recruitment of neutrophils to the lungs have thus been demonstrated. Studies have also shown that neutrophils can cause or at least contribute to the development of pulmonary edema. Basically, these studies consist of introducing a stimulus known to cause increased pulmonary permeability and then showing that rendering experimental animals neutropenic attenuates this response.[334]

The mechanism of leukocyte activation seems to be a stimulus-response coupling, with the response depending on the nature of the stimulus and the involved inflammatory cell. The ligand-receptor complex enhances the activity of a membrane-bound guanine nucleotide regulatory protein (GNRP), which in turn increases phospholipase C (PLC) activity as shown in Figures 24-5 and 24-6.[90] Three types of products are thought to be elaborated, any of which may injure the lung: (1) toxic oxygen free radicals; (2) neutral proteases, especially elastase; and (3) arachidonic acid metabolites.

## OXYGEN FREE RADICALS

There are a number of toxic oxygen products—free radical derivatives of molecular oxygen. They include superoxide anion ($O_2$), hydrogen peroxide ($H_2O_2$), hydroxyl radical (HO·), and peroxide radical (ROO·). A free radical has an unpaired electron in its outer orbit; it is therefore unstable and will tend to give up its electron and act as a reducing agent or accept another electron and act as an oxidizing agent. $O_2^-$ is moderately unstable and with the addition of an electron and two H+ ions is converted to $H_2O_2$, which is freely diffusable. In the presence of $Fe^{2+}$ it produces the extremely unstable HO· radical, which may accept a proton ($H^+$ ion) to yield $H_2O$ (Table 24-5). HO· is so unstable indeed that it can induce damage only if it is close to its target. $H_2O_2$, in the presence of $Cl^-$ ion and the lysosomal enzyme myeloperoxidase, may be converted to hypochlorous acid, another powerful oxidant.[354]

Large amounts of superoxide anions are generated during the respiratory burst that accompanies phagocytosis.[20] In the normal course of events, these reactive oxygen intermediaries cause little problem since they are neutralized rapidly by endogenous defense systems that protect the integrity of cells and tissues.[24] These include superoxide dismutase, which catalyzes the conversion of superoxide radicals to hydrogen peroxide; catalases and oxidases, which detoxify hydrogen peroxide to $H_2O$ and $O_2$; glutathione peroxidase and glutathione reductase, which alter cellular susceptibility to oxidants; and a variety of scavengers that absorb free electrons. However, when oxygen metabolites are released in massive amounts, intracellular defenses are overcome, and they may enter the extracellular space where defenses are weaker; extensive tissue damage may result. Further, NADPH oxidase, which is localized in the membrane of phagocytic cells, is activated when these cells are stimulated; its reactive products are released directly into the extracellular environment (Fig 24-6).[353]

Stimulated granulocytes probably must be closely apposed to endothelial cells in order to cause damage through a free radical dependent mechanism. In isolated preparations in which the cells are pretreated to decrease adherence, this effect is markedly reduced.[150,368] The effects of oxygen radicals are diverse because of the wide range of chemical reactions in which they may participate. These effects range from cell dysfunction secondary to cross-linking of membrane proteins to cell necrosis, which in turn may produce increased vascular permeability in the lung with intraalveolar edema, hemorrhage, and fibrin deposition, and may result in progressive interstitial fibrosis if damage is sufficiently widespread. Clinically, these effects are seen as defects in gas exchange, increased pulmonary artery pressure, and decreased lung compliance.[90]

Oxygen radicals usually cause damage by lipid peroxidation

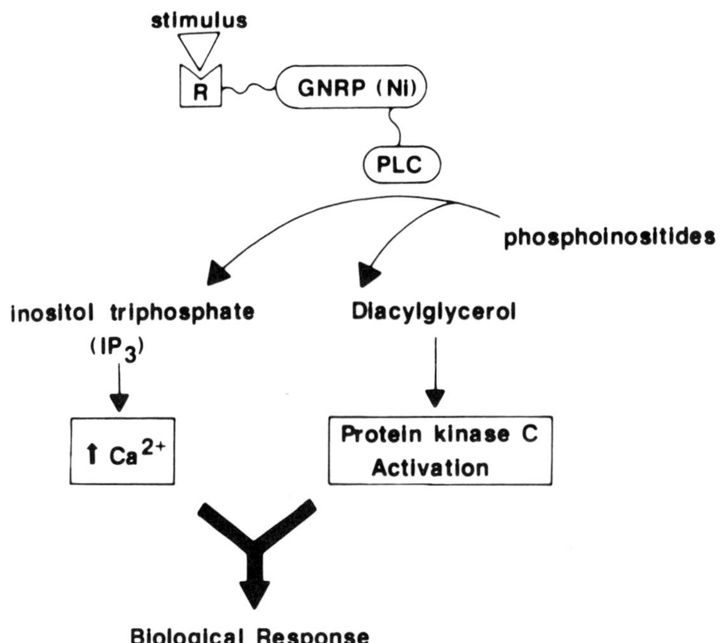


FIG. 24-5. Biochemical consequences of stimulus-response coupling in an inflammatory cell. The ligand-receptor complex enhances the activity of inhibitory guanine nucleotide regulatory protein (GNRP NI) in the cell. The result is increased phospholipase C (PLC) aactivity with enhanced turnover of phosphoinositides and the generation of inositol triphosphate and diacylglycerol. Inositol triphosphate stimulates the release of membrane-bound $Ca^{2+}$ from intracellular stores, causing a net increase in free intracellular calcium concentration. Diacylglycerol activates protein kinase C, which in turn is capable of phosphorylating substrate proteins in the cell. Increased intracellular calcium and activated protein kinase C then produce a number of cellular responses that differ depending on the cell in which the reaction takes place. $TxA_2$ = thromboxane, LT = leukotriene. (From Fantone et al[90] with permission.)

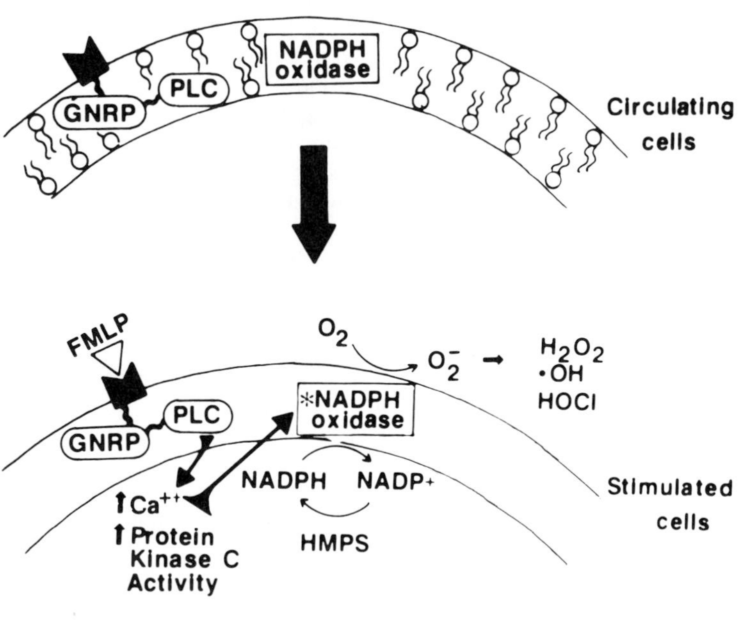


FIG. 24-6. Generation of oxygen radicals by phagocytic cells (neutrophils, eosinophils, monocytes, or macrophages): NADPH oxidase enzyme activation. After a stimulus-response coupling in the cell membrane, activated guanine nucleotide regulatory protein (GNRP) increases phospholipase C (PLC) activity. The resulting increase in intracellular $Ca^{2+}$ and protein kinase C causes activation of NADPH oxidase, which, using NADPH as substrate and source of electrons, reduces molecular oxygen to $O_2^-$. The sequential addition of single electrons to $O_2^-$ then results in the hydrogen peroxide ($H_2O_2$), hydroxyl radical (.OH), and hypochlorous acid (HOCl). Formylmethionyl-leucyl-phenylalanine (FMLP) is the chemotactic stimulus binding to a specific receptor on the cell membrane. (From Fantone et al[90] with permission.)

TABLE 24-5. Sequential Production of Oxygen Free Radicals

$$O_2 + e^- \rightarrow O_2^-$$

$$O_2^- + e^- + 2H^+ \rightarrow H_2O_2$$

$$H_2O_2 + e^- \rightarrow HO\cdot + OH^-$$

$$HO\cdot + e^- + H^+ \rightarrow H_2O$$

in biologic membranes, with resultant alteration of the physical properties of membrane phospholipids. The structure of the cell wall is altered, and membrane-bound enzymes, such as Na-K ATPase, adenylate cyclase, and cytochrome oxidase, are inactivated. Membrane fluidity is decreased, favoring entrapment of such cells as platelets and leukocytes on endothelial surfaces. Loss of functional integrity results in increased permeability. Lipid peroxidation results in the production of reactive fatty acid hydroperoxides that are also toxic to plasma membranes. Eventually, intracellular lysosomal enzymes may be released into the extracellular space with further destructive consequences.

One of the most important cellular membrane fatty acids is arachidonic acid, which can undergo peroxidative degradation. Thus, lipid peroxidation may be the first step in the generation of arachidonic acid metabolites (see below). Free radicals may also degrade hyaluronic acid and cellular fibronectin, two essential structural components, resulting in a loss of interstitial integrity.[24] Superoxide anions can also react with arachidonic acid or with a lipid component bound to serum albumin to produce chemotactic factors that attract more neutrophils and thus amplify the inflammatory response.[101,334]

Oxygen radicals have been shown to inactivate $\alpha_1$- antiproteinase, an important protective enzyme in the lung. They also potentiate the activity of leukocyte proteases by damaging protein substrates, such as elastin and collagen, producing further compromise of tissue integrity. Protease activation may cause a marked increase in the quantity of oxygen metabolites generated so there may actually be a synergism between these two factors. Further, some proteases may be converted to their active forms by oxygen products.[27,90,352]

Many of the characteristic signs of oxygen toxicity are similar to those seen in ARDS—atelectasis, edema, alveolar hemorrhage, inflammation, fibrin deposition, and hyalinization of alveolar membranes. The mechanism of these effects is the same as that described above—lipid peroxidation, oxidation of protein sulfhydryls and nucleic acids, and enzyme inactivation—since increased partial pressure of oxygen produces accelerated intracellular metabolic processes that generate free radicals and peroxidases.[78,79,106,156,320] Interestingly, however, ARDS and septic shock may provide some protection against oxygen toxicity. Presumably this is because elaboration of oxygen metabolites has already occurred, and there has been a corresponding increase in the production of antioxidant enzymes.[212,241,309] Whether or not this proves to be true, patients with diseased lungs probably do have an altered response to hyperoxia.[156,323]

Although there is no doubt that oxygen products can and in some circumstances do cause severe damage, it is not clear that this is a major mechanism of leukocyte-mediated cytotoxicity. Some in vivo modulating mechanisms may limit damage. Endothelial cell surface membranes may interact with activated neutrophils to inhibit the respiratory burst and thus limit damage. Erythrocytes contain glutathione, which even in minute quantities is a very potent scavenger of oxygen radicals. Indeed, the oxygen radical mediated acute lung injury caused by complement-activated phagocytes may be evanescent and self-limited. Thus, this mechanism may not be injurious to normal pulmonary endothelium, but may become important only when prior injury is present.[270]

## NEUTRAL PROTEASES

Acute inflammatory lung injury is also associated with the release of protease enzymes, such as elastase, β-glucuronidase, cathepsin G, and collagenase, which can destroy the components of the vascular basement membrane.[361] Some of these enzymes have been found, accompanied by reduced levels of protective factors, in bronchoalveolar lavage fluid of patients with ARDS, although the exact meaning of these findings is not clear.[59,185] Of note, however, is that these proteases also cleave fibrinogen, Hageman factor, complement, and other plasma proteins. Therefore, they may not only destroy interstitial architecture but may also amplify lung injury by activating agents that cause further leukocyte aggregation and intravascular coagulation.[274]

## ARACHIDONIC ACID METABOLITES

Arachidonate normally exists as a component of cell membranes bound to phospholipids. When injury occurs and neutrophils are activated, there is an increase in intracellular calcium and in phospholipase activity, resulting in the release of free arachidonic acid from the membrane. Other mechanisms may also be involved in this process, including, as discussed above, oxygen free radical activity.[10,36,90,295] Arachidonic acid, once released, serves as the substrate for the production of several substances that are thought to play a major role in the pathophysiology of ARDS.

These lipid mediators have effects on pulmonary vascular and airway smooth muscle and on vascular permeability. In certain cells, such as platelets, basophils, mast cells, and neutrophils, the metabolism of arachidonic acid is fairly specific. Mononuclear phagocytic cells—circulating monocytes, macrophages, and pulmonary alveolar macrophages—are able to synthesize and secrete various products of arachidonic acid metabolism. Production of these metabolites is quantitatively and qualitatively a function of the nature of the stimulus and the state of activation of the cell, as well as the source—endogenous or exogenous—of the arachidonic acid. Why and when specific metabolites are produced during the course of lung injury is still not clear.[90]

Once released, arachidonic acid is metabolized via one of two pathways mediated by two different enzymes: cyclo-oxygenase or lipooxygenase (Fig 24-7). The cyclo-oxygenase pathway leads to the production of prostaglandins $PGE_2$, $PGD_2$ and most important, $PGI_2$ or prostacyclin. These products are vasodilators and inhibitors of platelet aggregation.

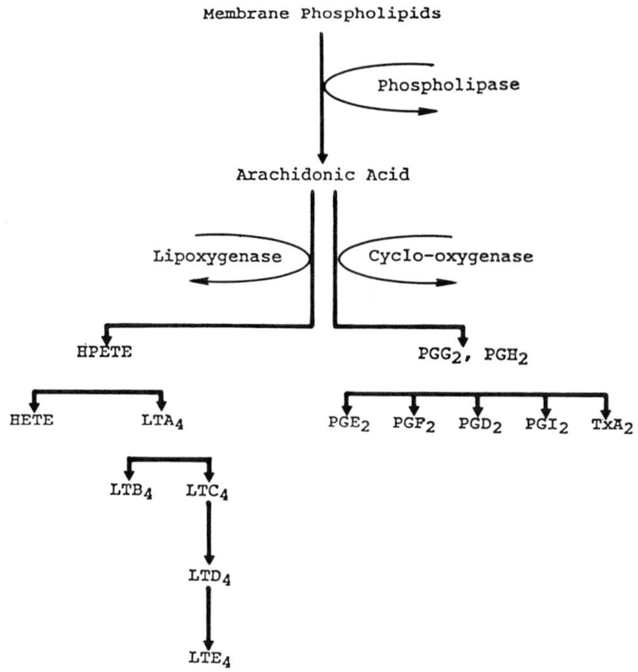


FIG. 24-7. The metabolism of cellular membrane phospholipids and arachidonic acid. HPETE = hydroperoxyeicosatetraenoic acid, LT = leukotriene, PG = prostaglandin.

They also increase vascular permeability. $PGI_2$ is probably the most potent vasodilator in the pulmonary circulation; it inhibits hypoxic pulmonary vasoconstriction and may affect inflammatory cell function. $PGF_2$ and $TxA_2$ (thromboxane) are vasoconstrictors, affecting both microvascular and pulmonary smooth muscle tone. $TxA_2$ also enhances platelet aggregation. The ratio of $PGI_2$ to $TxA_2$ production determines the ultimate effects of cyclo-oxygenase metabolism.

The lipoxygenase pathway leads to production of the leukotrienes, especially leukotriene $B_4$ ($LTB_4$) (Fig 24-7). In this pathway hydroperoxyeicosatetraenoic acid (HPETE) is rapidly converted to hydroxyeicosatetraenoic acid (HETE) and leukotriene $A_4$ ($LTA_4$). HETE is chemotactic and $LTB_4$ aggregates white cells and stimulates them to release lysosomal products. The leukotrienes are smooth muscle constrictors and increase vascular permeability, thus possibly contributing to the edema associated with lung injury.[10,76,85,113,121,132,133] $LTC_4$, $LTD_4$, and $LTE_4$ have also been shown to be the slow-reacting substances of anaphylaxis (SRS-A).

Corticosteroids stabilize cell membranes and inhibit phospholipase activity. Nonsteroidal anti-inflammatory agents have more specific effects. Thus, aspirin, indomethacin, ibuprofen, and meclofenamate inhibit reactions in the cyclo-oxygenase pathway, possibly shifting arachidonate metabolism to the lipoxygenase pathway, whereas imidazole acts to inhibit the activity of thromboxane synthetase, thus preventing the formation of $TxA_2$ and shifting the balance to the prostaglandins.[10,36,90,133,233]

Although there is evidence from animal experiments that arachidonic acid metabolites may play a significant role in ARDS and clinical shock, the evidence in humans is less clear cut. Whether these products play a direct contributory role in the pathogenesis of ARDS and shock or are simply markers and secondary products that may exacerbate the primary injury remains to be established. Animal studies have shown that some of the effects of endotoxin administration are significantly mitigated if inhibitors of arachidonic acid metabolism are administered first.[10,227] Whether prophylactic administration of these agents may benefit humans is an unanswered question.

Other factors may play a role in the development of ARDS. Fibrin degradation products may be related to ARDS; elevated levels of factors VIII[53] and XIII[207] and of fragment D[199] have been noted. Again, whether these are modulators or markers of an ongoing process remains unclear.[368] Platelet-activating factor (PAF), a product of alveolar macrophages, may have a role in the aggregation and activation of leukocytes and platelets, as well as in smooth muscle constriction. In the ARDS model produced by microembolism,[28,284,285,290] both inhibition of fibrinolysis and arachidonic acid metabolites may have important roles; platelets may also play an active role.[135] The key factor in experimental production of ARDS may depend on the model used: hemorrhagic, septic, microembolism, neurogenic, acid aspiration, drug related, oxygen toxicity, or air embolism.[320] Thus a common pathway may not exist. Different insults may activate different mechanisms that eventuate in a final common clinical picture.

Recently, some doubt has also been cast on the role of neutrophils in the development of ARDS. Cases have been reported of neutropenic patients who have clearly developed the syndrome.[35,181,205,234] Thus in sepsis, endotoxin injury may be adequate in itself to produce ARDS. Once the pulmonary endothelium has been damaged by neutrophil-independent mechanisms, however, the reappearance of circulating neutrophils in neutropenic patients coincides with worsening of the syndrome.[272] Much of the clinical evidence for the role of neutrophils rests on demonstrating their presence and that of their products in the lungs of patients with ARDS.[8,207,370,371] This does not necessarily demonstrate causation, however, since it may be a nonspecific finding.[272] What we are left with, then, is a number of factors that, to different degrees, may be important in different forms of ARDS not as causes, but as aggravators—agents that may make a bad situation worse. An understanding of these factors is important not so much for preventing ARDS as for mitigating it.

## PREDICTION AND DIAGNOSIS

The diagnosis of full-blown ARDS is rarely a problem. The patient is almost always in obvious respiratory failure, and tracheal intubation and mechanical ventilation are either established or must be initiated. The major diagnostic goal must be to identify ARDS as early in its development as possible. It is generally held that, if any successful therapy for ARDS exists, it will certainly be most effective if given early in the process, ideally before respiratory distress is evident.[21]

ARDS has most often been described as "normal pressure" or "high-permeability" lung edema. Unfortunately, clinically available methods are not sufficiently sensitive or noninvasive to allow this diagnosis in its earliest stage. Monitoring of lung water in conjunction with pulmonary artery pressures and careful clinical evaluation might be appropriate for early diagnosis, but currently available methods of measuring lung water (thermal dye dilution technique, soluble inert gas technique, and chest roentgenography) have severe limitations and have not been very useful clinically.[66] Other methods, such as measurement of lung density, nuclear magnetic resonance, positron emission tomography, and microwave techniques, either cannot be used at the bedside or have not yet been proven reliable.[66] The need for pulmonary artery catheterization is usually recognized only during relatively advanced stages of ARDS when it is already clinically obvious. By this time filling pressures are low or normal, and the acute events have already taken place. Relying on invasive means for diagnosis may lead us to overlook less severe cases that do not require admission to the intensive care unit[94,271,273] and are therefore not often included in formal studies.

The definition of ARDS as "high-permeability edema" is too general and does not differentiate among types of permeability lesions. There is significant variation in microvascular permeability lesions in ARDS with respect to their intensity, localization in the lung, and time of appearance. In some cases, such as neurogenic edema, the pathologic alteration is limited to transient central fluid overload and generalized "stretching" of vascular pores. In other cases, light and electron microscopy studies show a severely deranged, often necrotic capillary bed.[21] ARDS is often described as a diffuse disease, an impression based largely on the chest X-ray appearance. Yet, recent studies utilizing CT scans show remarkable regional variation, with normal areas adjacent to areas of severely damaged lung.[204] Sepsis has been discussed as a cause of ARDS, but there is evidence that in trauma patients increased pulmonary capillary permeability may be present early and precede the development of sepsis.[327] This may indicate that certain "causes" of ARDS require an already susceptible lung as a predisposing or necessary condition. Thus, although disruption of the alveolar-capillary membrane is a constant aspect of ARDS,[364] the architecture and extent of disruption can vary quite considerably.

Labeled isotope tracers have been used to evaluate fluid balance and movements in the lung.[3,190,315] A study of radioaerosol lung clearance in multitrauma and septic patients showed that the predictive value of this technique for ARDS was at least as good as and possibly better than prediction based on clinical risk indices. Most high-risk patients had early evidence of increased permeability even though they were clinically stable. Those who went on to develop the full-blown syndrome, however, had increasing permeability over time, implying an additional, possibly ongoing insult.[336] In another study employing labeled albumin, it was found that patients with low-pressure edema had different degrees of leakage. Patients with drug overdose had none, implying a transient event that had passed even though edema was still present, whereas some patients who had clearly documented hydrostatic edema also had some degree of permeability leak.[214] Permeability edema thus appears to represent a wide spectrum of endothelial damage and pulmonary dysfunction, much of which may remain in a subclinical state.

The above studies indicate that significant permeability changes may occur long before there is any clinical evidence of disease. Similarly, lung edema does not necessarily correlate well with clinical changes. In the first place, the pulmonary lymphatics are able to compensate for a severe degree of increased permeability. Studies have shown a marked increase in lung lymph flow before extravascular lung water rises. The lymphatics may be overwhelmed by sudden massive extravasation of fluid; if this is transient, edema will be cleared rapidly. In ARDS, however, lung damage grows progressively worse over hours or days until the lymphatics can no longer compensate and significant edema begins to accumulate (Fig 24-8). It is notable that a pulmonary weight increase of as much as 50% is required before arterial blood gas values change on the basis of edema alone. Moreover, the relationship between measured lung water and the subsequent clinical course is not predictable.[307,322] For instance, there is no correlation between the severity of the oxygenation deficit (alveolar-arterial $O_2$ gradient) and the amount of edema in the lungs (Fig 24-9). Not only may hypoxemia occur before significant pulmonary edema, but the oxygen deficit may also not respond well to attempts to reduce lung water. In sepsis, derangements in gas exchange occur in the absence of chest roentgenographic changes, which may develop later or not at all.[21,37,40] This is a considerably different picture from hydrostatic pulmonary edema in which gas exchange abnormalities and hypoxemia correlate better with the increase in lung water.[227] Thus, although fluid in the lungs is one of the more dramatic phenomena associated with ARDS, it may actually play only a secondary role in the pathophysiology and progression of the disease. The primary changes occur in the airways and the vascular endothelium.

Nevertheless, clinical assessment is the mainstay of diagnosis (Table 24-6). Hypoxemia is an early sign, often occurring before the spontaneously breathing patient experiences respiratory distress. The patient then becomes dyspneic, tachypneic, agitated, possibly confused, and anxious and may be frankly cyanotic or exhibit an ashen gray appearance. In some

FIG. 24-8. The relationship between lung lymph flow and extravascular lung water. Note that up to a certain point increased lung lymph flow prevents the increase in extravascular lung water. Beyond this point lymph flow cannot compensate for the increase in pulmonary interstitial fluid, and fluid accumulation occurs. This relationship between lymph flow and lung water is similar whether vascular permeability is normal or increased. With normal permeability, large increases in intravascular pressure are required for edema formation and lymph flow is also high. When vascular permeability is increased, fluid efflux occurs at low intravascular pressures; lymph flow is, however, very high. Thus, the relationship between lymph flow and lung water is unchanged. See also Fig 24-10. (From Brigham[37] with permission.)

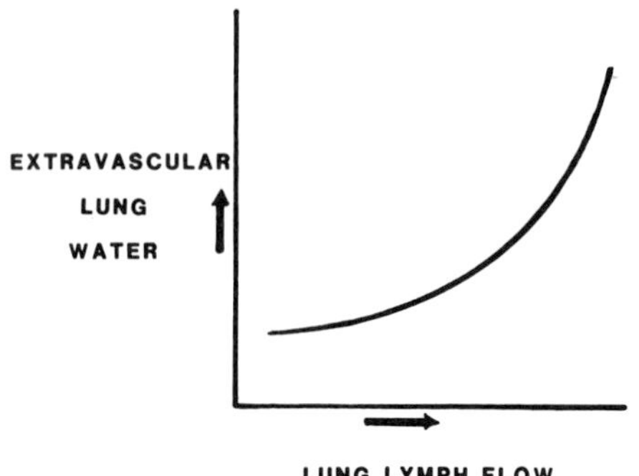

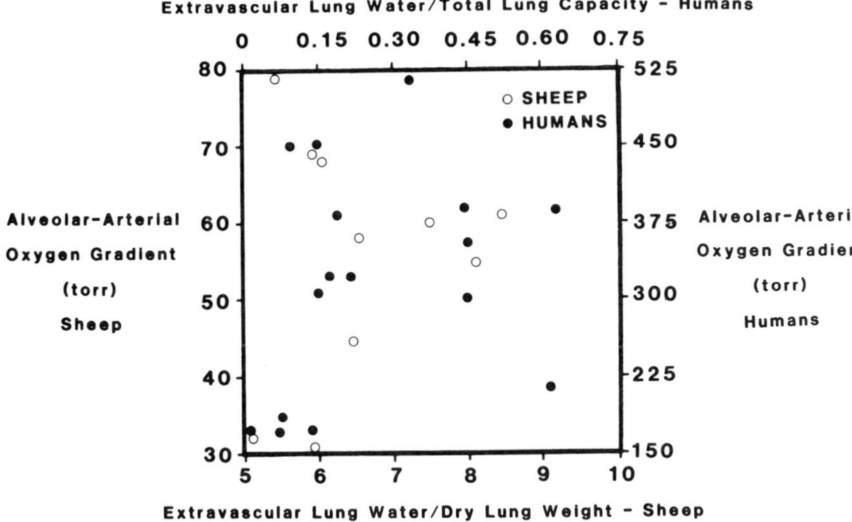


FIG. 24-9. Relationship between lung water and alveolar-arterial $O_2$ gradient (A-a $DO_2$) in patients with ARDS and in a group of sheep given *E. coli* to produce pulmonary edema and respiratory failure. Note the poor correlation between the severity of the oxygenation defect and the amount of edema in the lungs. These data suggest that failure of oxygenation is not due simply to water in the lungs. Abnormalities in airway function and pulmonary circulation contribute greatly to failure of oxygenation in patients with high permeability edema or ARDS. (From Brigham[37] with permission.)

ways this presentation is similar to that of patients who are septic and about to go into frank shock. Indeed, ARDS has been called "sepsis of the lung" and has been viewed by some as part of the multiorgan failure syndrome.[243] Although hypoxemia is undoubtedly responsible for the above symptoms, it is difficult to explain why most patients continue to be dyspneic and to hyperventilate even after administration of sufficient oxygen to correct arterial desaturation. A possible mechanism for this may be stimulation of J-receptors in the pulmonary interstitium as a consequence of interstitial edema or disturbance of normal length-tension relationships; that is, decreased lung expansion for a given amount of pleural pressure generation.[21,225] The increased work of breathing absorbs a larger percentage of the cardiac output and the available oxygen and may result in lactic acidosis and rapid depletion of energy stores.[6,115] The patient may require mechanical ventilation because of fatigue.[60] This picture is consistent with extensive ventilation-perfusion ($\dot{V}/\dot{Q}$) mismatch and may occur before changes are visible on the chest X-ray. Another possible mechanism of this syndrome is a hyperdynamic state with increased cardiac output and regional perfusion shifts.[306] It should be noted that these two mechanisms are not mutually exclusive; both may be involved in the production of dyspnea, hyperventilation, and increased work of breathing in the presence of reasonable arterial oxygen saturation.

TABLE 24-6. Diagnostic Criteria of ARDS*

Clinical history of catastrophic event
  Pulmonary (aspiration, massive infection, contusion)
  Nonpulmonary (shock, multisystem trauma)
But excluding
  Chronic pulmonary disease
  Left ventricular failure (wedge pressure $\geq$16 cm $H_2O$)
Clinical respiratory distress
  Tachypnea >20 breaths/min
  Labored breathing
With chest radiograph showing
  Diffuse pulmonary infiltrates
  (Early interstitial, later alveolar)
And physiologic measurements of
  $PaO_2$ <50 mm Hg when $FIO_2$ >0.6
  Total respiratory compliance $\leq$50 mL/cm $H_2O$ (usually 20 to 30)
Increased shunt fraction and dead space ventilation

* From Petty[250] with permission.

Eventually a second stage develops that is characterized by alveolar flooding, atelectasis, and decreased functional residual capacity. Compensatory hypoxic pulmonary vasoconstriction is lost, and pulmonary hypertension may occur.[369] At this point, there is massive intrapulmonary shunting and lack of response to increased oxygen.[42,56,57,81]

Prediction of ARDS remains problematic. Pepe[246] developed a risk index on the basis of prospective studies. He was able to predict the onset of ARDS in 50% of patients with 80% accuracy. Four major risk factors were identified: injury severity score, multiple transfusions, sepsis syndrome, and an initial $PaO_2/FIO_2$ ratio of less than 200 in patients on mechanical ventilation.[246] The major goal of prediction, however, must be early assessment in order that therapy can begin before multiple organ involvement occurs.[4] Unfortunately, the advantage of early evaluation is more theoretic than real because there is no effective early therapy for ARDS.

Nevertheless, interest has focused on early identification of patients who are developing ARDS by testing for alterations in blood levels of various cellular and biochemical markers (Table 4).[204] Many of these substances are mediators of acute lung injury; thus, their levels or activity should correlate with the development of ARDS. Some of the proposed markers include changes in leukocyte[339] or platelet[95,291] counts, changes in neutrophil activity,[370,371] levels of such granulocyte enzymes as elastase,[232] increased complement levels and activity,[86,358] release of such products as factor VIII and prostacyclin from damaged endothelial cells, and pulmonary extraction of serotonin and propranolol as a function of endothelial metabolic activity.[219] Although some of the results show promise, there is wide variability among individual patients and a lack of specificity. Perhaps one reason for this is that different mechanisms of injury may be more or less prominent in different forms of ARDS. If so, attempts to find global indicators will be unavailing as markers must be tied to the specific type of damage that is taking place. At present, therefore, the clinical picture remains the basis of prediction.

## EVOLUTION OF PULMONARY PATHOLOGY

One of the diagnostic features of ARDS is significant hypoxemia that is relatively unresponsive to supplemental oxygen.[266] All attempts to understand and treat the syndrome must focus on this abnormality in gas exchange. Although there is considerable variation in both the etiology of ARDS and the mechanisms of lung injury, once injury occurs the subsequent progression of pulmonary pathology tends to be remarkably constant.

On the cellular level, changes are usually divided into three phases: the acute or exudative phase (up to 6 days), the subacute or proliferative phase (4 to 10 days), and the chronic or fibrotic phase (after 8 days). The timing of these phases may vary.[212] Within 24 hours of injury, an acute inflammatory reaction appears in the lung. Interstitial and then alveolar edema develop, thickening the walls and septa with fluid. Inflammatory cells—lymphocytes and other mononuclear cells—migrate into lung tissue and alveoli. Overloaded macrophages are present, clearing away debris. There is fluid leakage, mainly peribronchial, and destruction of Type I alveolar cells, leaving a denuded basement membrane. Eosinophilic hyaline membranes—the hallmark of this phase—are usually found along the alveolar ducts. These consist of proteinaceous fluid, cellular fragments and debris, fibrin strands, and remnants of surfactant.[63,104,256,290,335] It is important to note that involvement can be very patchy; normal areas may be intermingled with damaged ones.[206] Involvement tends to be greater in gravity-dependent areas, and oddly enough, hyaline membranes may be more prominent in regions that do not suffer direct injury.[262] Finally, capillary congestion and vascular obstruction by leukocytes and platelets occur. There appears to be greater destruction of the epithelial than of the endothelial surface, possibly because of the greater reparative ability of the latter.[2,8]

If the syndrome progresses, there is proliferation of cuboidal Type II pneumocytes that line the alveoli, essentially transforming the epithelium. The interstitium remains thickened, and there is an increase in fibroblasts and mild interstitial fibrosis. Hyaline membranes may appear to resolve, but they are actually becoming more organized and fibrin strands appear in the protein-rich edema fluid. Capillary endothelial cells begin to show more damage with focal swelling, and there is some evidence of increased immunologic activity as shown by infiltration of eosinophils and plasma cells.

The third stage, if the syndrome continues to progress, is essentially one of progressive fibrosis of the interstitium and intra-alveolar spaces, with obliteration of the alveolar structure.

The pulmonary vasculature is affected in several ways. First, pulmonary hypertension is common in ARDS, although the extent may vary with its etiology. There has been speculation about the role of humoral mediators, such as thromboxane $A_2$ or serotonin, in the development of pulmonary hypertension, but it is difficult to apply animal models to human ARDS. Obstruction of the pulmonary microvasculature with particulate microemboli, such as neutrophils or platelets, may play a role. Perivascular "cuffing" by edema fluid in the interstitium may reduce vascular compliance and increase right ventricular afterload, depressing cardiac output and therefore the delivery of oxygen to peripheral tissues. This may contribute significantly to multisystem organ failure, which is often the terminal manifestation of ARDS.[300] Indeed, as ARDS progresses, there is physical remodeling of the pulmonary vasculature; much of the vascular bed is disrupted or obliterated, and the rest adapts to the relatively increased blood flow with increased tortuosity, dilation, possibly appearance of new vessels, and also an extension of smooth muscle into the smaller, normally nonmuscular pulmonary arterioles.[313] This remodeling is probably part of the structural basis of persistent pulmonary hypertension. Hypoxia, hyperoxia, and irregular repair also contribute to this effect. In addition, vascular thrombosis is found in many patients. Whether this is a primary or a secondary phenomenon is not clear,[212] but it contributes to the development of ischemic and necrotic pulmonary lesions.[342] At the same time, there is loss of the hypoxic vasoconstriction response, resulting in increased shunting through atelectatic areas of the lung.[7,13,97,99,130,226] This effect may be secondary to endotoxin and/or the production of vasodilator prostaglandins.[21,121]

As discussed above, the most notable pathologic event in ARDS is leakage of fluid into the lungs. The primary injury may be on the endothelial side as in sepsis, or on the alveolar epithelial side, as in aspiration, but the ultimate pathology is the same.[208,344] Normally, fluid flow across the capillary membrane into the interstitium is governed by the sum of the Starling forces, ie, tissue and blood hydrostatic and oncotic pressures. In ARDS this principle still applies, but new factors are also at work. The normal pulmonary interstitium is not water- or protein-free; a net influx of fluid and protein occurs across the microvascular membrane. Channels or pores are present whose number (and therefore the leakiness of the endothelium) increases from the arteriolar to the venular side of the pulmonary vasculature. In fact, many agents that cause edema are thought to act on the pulmonary venules. Channels exist at intercellular gaps, and only a slight increase in the size of these gaps is needed to allow increased protein flow. Once this injury to the microvascular membrane occurs, efflux of fluid from intravascular space requires only a minimal increase in intravascular pressure. (Fig 24-10).[76]

The pulmonary interstitium can function as a reservoir.[129] Once fluid enters the interstitial space it moves proximally toward the peribronchial and perivascular spaces in the extraalveolar interstitium; pressure in this region is negative relative to that in the alveolar interstitial space. Thus, a pressure gradient exists from the lung periphery to the hilum. The loose connective tissue can therefore act as a capacitance bed and drain fluid from the alveolar interstitium.[203] Lung water may increase by 70 to 100% before changes in arterial blood gas values are detectable, which is probably why clinical symptoms may precede laboratory signs of ARDS. Edema first becomes apparent in the peribronchial area.[64,211,236,290,363] Alveolar flooding is a late sign and occurs when the capacity of the lymphatics to filter fluid has been exceeded. It should be noted that any increase in venous pressure, as in right heart

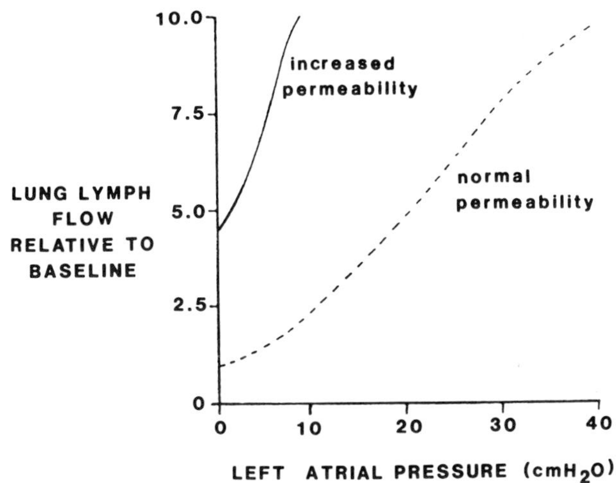


FIG. 24-10. Relationship between left atrial pressure and lung lymph flow, a marker of interstitial fluid, during increased and normal pulmonary vascular permeability. Note that, despite a significant difference in left atrial pressures, lung lymph flow is similarly increased in both conditions. (From Brigham[37] with permission.)

failure, decreases lymphatic flow and, especially in the face of an increased capillary filtration rate, increases edema formation. In addition, an increase in the size of the effective vascular surface will increase filtration;[39] this is especially likely to happen in the high cardiac output states associated with sepsis. Thus although increased permeability is certainly central to fluid leakage in ARDS, pressure factors are also critical.

It is important to keep in mind that edema is a consequence of lung injury and that many changes in airway function are unrelated to pulmonary edema.[38] Alterations in lung mechanics are also part of the ARDS and tend to be much more marked than those observed in cardiogenic pulmonary edema. As already noted, several studies have shown that, in contrast to cardiogenic pulmonary edema, there is no correlation between the amount of lung water and the degree of hypoxia or shunt.[39,103,131,177,182] Peribronchial edema can cause airway constriction with wheezing, decreased $\dot{V}/\dot{Q}$ ratio, and increased airway pressures. In both cardiogenic and noncardiogenic edema, this effect results from passive narrowing of the airways, does not indicate the presence of airway hyperreactivity, and is usually relatively transient and responsive to therapy. In ARDS, however, there is also evidence of significant release of humoral mediators, with increased airway responsiveness and active bronchoconstriction. Although the exact mechanism of these changes is not known, it probably involves an inflammatory reaction and subsequent damage. Survivors of ARDS may recover with generally normal lung function, but they are often found to have increased airway reactivity long after the episode.[297,311,312]

There is also a change in lung mechanics as a result of alveolar flooding. The edema fluid itself is rich not only in protein but also in the mediators of lung injury and inflammatory cells and may cause severe and refractory alteration in surfactant.[312] Indeed, the chemical composition of surfactant in ARDS patients has been found to be altered and to demonstrate increased compressibility and reduced minimum surface tension.[125,251–253,335] Alveolar type II cells are responsible for the production of surfactant and also serve as stem cells for the regeneration of type I pneumocytes; there is a rapid increase in their number in response to lung injury. There may be some change or specific biochemical abnormality in these cells.[95] On the other hand, the reserve pool of surfactant is not large, and it is normally recycled.[367] It would appear then that surfactant is not simply washed out by edema fluid, but is chemically changed in the course of ARDS. This may explain the fact that some patients seem to recover from their initial injury or the acute phase of their illness, but continue to remain ventilator dependent with persistent stiff lungs and severe, although manageable hypoxemia. In any case, these changes lead to alveolar collapse, decreased functional residual capacity, decreased compliance, and therefore decreased functional lung volume.

Intrapulmonary shunt is central to functional disturbances caused by ARDS. Although interstitial edema and the consequent thickening of the alveolar-capillary membrane do increase the diffusion distance for gases, there is no evidence that this barrier is severe enough to limit gas exchange and therefore to play any significant role in the hypoxemia of ARDS. $\dot{V}/\dot{Q}$ abnormality probably plays some role in ARDS, although there is some question about its importance.[180] It probably plays a key role early in the course of the disease when bronchoconstriction is present. However, the most severe hypoxemia occurs only after frank alveolar flooding. Before this, there may be a dramatic response of $PaO_2$ to increased inspired oxygen, but once the chest X-ray starts showing signs of alveolar edema this responsiveness dramatically declines. Lack of improvement in arterial oxygenation with increased $FIO_2$ is the major characteristic of shunt. Thus, the progression from interstitial to intra-alveolar edema marks a significant turning point in the course of the syndrome. It means that the lymphatic defenses have been overwhelmed by leakage of fluid and proteins and alveolar collapse with intrapulmonary shunting has begun.

Although ARDS has often been described as a diffuse disease of the lung, recent investigations have shown that this is not the case. First, as has already been discussed, normal regions appear to be interspersed with diseased areas.[206] The reason for this is not clear, although it is possible that the disease may be heterogeneous in impact. Thus, damage may be widespread but nonuniform, with some areas not affected severely enough to progress to alveolar edema and atelectasis. Second, gravity causes both higher capillary pressure and compression by more superior structures in dependent portions of the lung, which may in part account for the development of localized areas of increased density. Even though microvascular damage may be the same in nondependent regions, detectable alveolar edema may not appear.[114] Indeed, edema appears to be more common in dependent areas of the lung. On chest X-ray, the first appearance of edema tends to be peripheral rather than central as in hydrostatic pulmonary edema.[258] In addition, changing the patient's position often (but not always) changes the pattern or distribution of edema. In any case, once this stage is reached, lung units tend to behave in an all-or-none manner, either normally ventilated and perfused or totally unventilated, as if alveolar flooding is either total or absent. In addition, there may also be a third type of lung unit that is flooded but open during part of the respiratory cycle and therefore functioning at a very low $\dot{V}/\dot{Q}$.[42,68,69,87] These areas may be recruitable with PEEP, but the extent of this recruitment diminishes as consolidation replaces alveolar edema.

In this situation, the $PaO_2$ or the A-$aDO_2$ may not be good markers of the degree of lung injury.[293] A major consequence of shunt as the predominant cause of abnormal gas exchange is that $PaO_2$ is markedly influenced by alterations in the mixed venous $PO_2$ ($P\bar{v}O_2$). In the normal lung a low $P\bar{v}O_2$ has a minimal adverse effect on the end-capillary $PO_2$ of lung units; in the presence of shunt this effect increases markedly since there is direct admixture of venous with arterial blood. Normally ventilated alveoli cannot increase oxygen exchange to compensate for atelectatic areas since postcapillary saturation is already maximal. Thus, the lower the $P\bar{v}O_2$, the lower the $PaO_2$. A low $P\bar{v}O_2$ results from the imbalance between $O_2$ demand and delivery, which may be caused by low arterial $O_2$ saturation, low hemoglobin concentration, or low cardiac output and, from the demand side, by increased $O_2$ consumption. It is therefore important not to mistake a fall in $PaO_2$ for increased pulmonary edema when it may be caused by one or more other factors.[69]

The relation between respiratory and hemodynamic function in ARDS is even more complex—it is not linearly related—and has been studied since the first research on respiratory failure.[134,153,187,191,255,261,331] An increase in cardiac output may paradoxically increase the degree of shunt.[55] One reason is that diseased areas may be preferentially perfused. Pathologic changes in these areas often include microvascular occlusion by fibrin and thrombi, which causes mechanical differences from normal areas. If critical narrowing of vessels occurs in the more severely affected areas of the lung, further reduction in perfusion pressure with decreased cardiac output may cause the vessels to collapse completely, resulting in decreased shunt. Conversely, increases in cardiac output may recruit these vessels and increase shunt.[195] Similarly, if hypoxic vasoconstriction is still operative in these areas (it may not be),[227] an increase in $P\bar{v}O_2$ may cause vasodilation, thus increasing perfusion of these areas and increasing effective shunt.[17,18,286,310] This is especially likely to occur in a hyperdynamic state when the patient is hypovolemic; for instance, after hemorrhage,[298] in sepsis,[304–306] or when cardiac output has been markedly augmented with inotropes without volume loading.[266] In all these circumstances there is preferential perfusion of dependent areas where alveolar collapse is more likely to be present. When PEEP is used in the treatment of ARDS, there may appear to be an improvement in intrapulmonary shunting and arterial oxygenation as cardiac output is depressed. However, oxygen delivery and overall tissue oxygenation may actually be falling, and the patient's condition may worsen even though the pulmonary status may appear to improve. Thus, any interpretation of changes in gas exchange in ARDS must take into account accompanying hemodynamic alterations.[71]

A peripheral defect in oxygen utilization has become increasingly apparent with advances in research on ARDS. In several studies,[67,146,217,244] it has been shown that decreased oxygen supply to peripheral tissues is not, as one would expect, accompanied by increased extraction. Rather, below a critical threshold there is a decrease in oxygen uptake or utilization without a shift to anaerobic metabolism. This is a pathologic oxygen supply dependency that does not take place in non-ARDS patients. There is no increase in lactate production and no predictable change in the $P\bar{v}O_2$, indicating that the mixed venous gas may not be a reliable indicator of ongoing tissue hypoxia or hypoperfusion.[46] The mechanism of this abnormality is not known. There may be disordered peripheral vasoregulation with shunting of blood to organs with low $O_2$ requirement or a diffuse cellular dysfunction resulting in the inability to extract or utilize oxygen efficiently. More likely, the endothelial injury, a characteristic feature of ARDS, is not restricted solely to the pulmonary vasculature, but may be present in the periphery as well. This is most apparent in sepsis in which peripheral interstitial edema is likely to develop and interfere with oxygen delivery to the tissues. The issue is critical because death in ARDS most often comes not from respiratory failure, but from multisystem organ failure, and peripheral tissue hypoxia may be one of the causes of this syndrome.[300]

## THERAPEUTIC GOALS

ARDS is not a primary disease; it is always secondary to some other insult. As such, one of the primary goals in the treatment of ARDS is to control the underlying pathology. The importance of this aspect of care cannot be overemphasized. Mortality from ARDS does not correlate with what would appear to be indicators of the extent of lung injury, such as degree of shunt or extent of extravascular lung water.[22] Instead, it correlates with signs of persistent and uncontrolled sepsis, such as hypotension and continuing metabolic acidosis.[218] Sepsis generally is a multiorgan disease and therefore can lead to multisystem organ failure,[192] the major cause of death in uncontrolled infections.[109,176] The sepsis syndrome, the major cause of death in ARDS, may often be suspected clinically even when no site of infection has been identified, and in fact often it is difficult to identify such a source. Nevertheless, aggressive diagnostic maneuvers are imperative since the chances of survival are minimal unless the source is found. Once diagnosed it may very often be treated simply and effectively by drainage.[16]

### VENTILATORY THERAPY

Until the underlying cause is resolved, however, the main goal of therapy is support of the vital systems since there is no "cure" for ARDS. From a respiratory point of view, this means maintaining a viable $PaO_2$ at a nontoxic $FIO_2$. The usual values given are an $FIO_2$ of 0.5 or less and a $PaO_2$ of at least 60 mm Hg (90% saturation) or preferably 70 mm Hg to allow for some reserve. Although these are the standard guidelines, it is important to keep in mind that one should not be interested in arterial oxygenation only, but also in oxygen delivery and utilization; therefore, this $PaO_2$ value assumes adequate hemoglobin concentration, peripheral organ perfusion, and $O_2$ extraction by the tissues. An $FIO_2$ of less than 0.5 is generally considered to be nontoxic, yet, as has been mentioned, ARDS patients often tolerate much higher levels for prolonged periods without developing signs of oxygen toxicity. Concern about oxygen toxicity should not prevent the administration of high levels of oxygen if this is the only way to maintain adequate arterial oxygenation.

When intrapulmonary shunt is more than 25%, however, high $FIO_2$ offers little or no benefit; in order to improve oxygenation, shunt must be reduced (Fig 24-11).[183] The cause of increased intrapulmonary shunt in ARDS is alveolar collapse secondary to surfactant washout. Typically atelectasis occurs first in small alveoli with already low $\dot{V}/\dot{Q}$ ratios. High surface tension renders these airway units prone to collapse with even minor reductions in surfactant activity. Many of these alveoli are at the base of the lungs where most of the pulmonary blood flow is distributed. As the surface tension increases, small alveoli empty into larger ones with already high $\dot{V}/\dot{Q}$ ratios, increasing their size further. The oxygenation, however, does not improve unless blood flow is also redirected to these large alveoli by vasoconstriction in hypoxic lung units. Increasing the $FIO_2$ in this situation may actually worsen oxygenation because the rapid absorption of oxygen facilitates the collapse of unstable airway units with low $\dot{V}/\dot{Q}$ ratio. Additionally, in those low $\dot{V}/\dot{Q}$ airway units that remain open, high $FIO_2$ may impede the physiologically adaptive vasoconstrictive response to hypoxia and thereby the redirection of blood flow to better ventilated alveoli.

Positive end-expiratory pressure (PEEP) is the mainstay of therapy in these circumstances.[70,267,296,345,359] It has many effects; some are beneficial, whereas others may be deleterious. Therapy involves setting priorities and balancing these effects to achieve the most favorable overall outcome. PEEP reduces intrapulmonary shunt and ameliorates hypoxemia unresponsive to high $FIO_2$ by recruiting or reopening previously collapsed alveoli. Reopening alveoli cannot be accomplished by simply ventilating the lungs with large tidal volumes because collapsed alveoli are on a flat compliance curve (Fig 24-12),[231] and their re-expansion requires not only elevated airway pressures but also prolonged maintenance of these pressures.[167] Even with the use of PEEP several breaths are needed to recruit a collapsed alveolus.[167] The second role of PEEP is to "splint" the lung in an inflated state. By this effect it keeps the unstable alveoli open at end-expiration when they are most vulnerable to collapse.[165,172] The third role of PEEP is to improve lung compliance and thereby facilitate ventilation. The work required for re-expansion of alveoli during each inspiration is less when PEEP increases FRC; since less effort must be spent to open up alveoli on the flat portion of the compliance curve, lung expansion per unit of alveolar distending pressure increases. Finally, PEEP expands alveoli with low or normal $\dot{V}/\dot{Q}$ ratios, with the result that fluid in these alveoli tends to "spread out" into a larger space.[318,319] Thus, PEEP improves oxygenation by reducing shunt, minimizing $\dot{V}/\dot{Q}$ mismatch, and increasing FRC.

It is also important to understand the limitations of PEEP. Although it may reduce the work of breathing and prevent atelectasis, PEEP has *no* prophylactic value; it does not prevent ARDS or reduce its incidence.[247] Further, there is no evidence that PEEP alters the course or the outcome of the disease.[194,316] It is only a means of maintaining oxygenation while the underlying etiology of the disease is treated and the lung injury resolves with time. Thus, there is no justification for instituting more than "physiologic" levels of PEEP unless it is clinically indicated by developing hypoxemia. There is also substantial evidence that PEEP does not decrease extravascular lung water, but may actually increase it.[1,47,137,142,235] Increasing lung volume and airway pressure by the use of PEEP results in a shift of fluid from alveolar to extra-alveolar vessels, which increase in size. There is also a decrease in extra-alveolar interstitial hydrostatic pressure, promoting the

FIG. 24-11. Isoshunt diagram indicating the relationship between $FIO_2$ and $PaO_2$ for intrapulmonary shunt values from 0% to 50%. Note that above 30% shunt, increasing $FIO_2$ has very little effect on $PaO_2$. The shaded areas define the limits of the relationship for each level of shunt. (From Lawler, Nunn[183] with permission.)

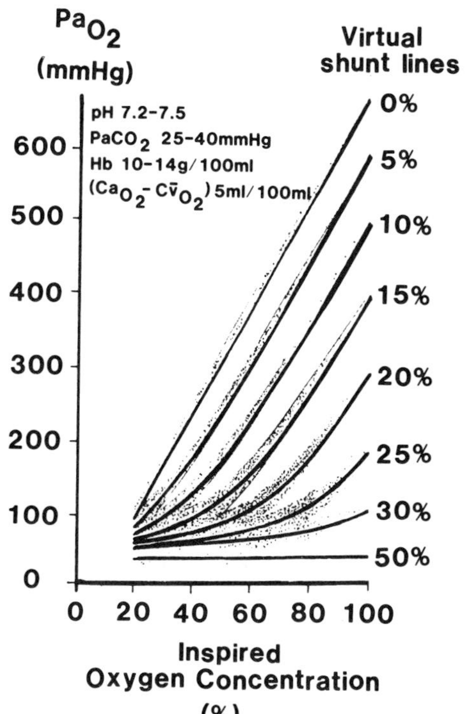


FIG. 24-12. Pulmonary pressure-volume (compliance) curves of (a) normal lung, (b) ARDS lung, and (c) ARDS lung treated with PEEP. In the normal lung, a small change in pressure results in a large increase in volume. In the untreated ARDS lung the curve is flat, and only a small increase in lung volume is noted after a large increase in pressure (*solid line*). Application of PEEP shifts the compliance curve upward, resulting in a relatively larger increase in lung volume than that produced in the untreated lung (*dotted line*). (From Norwood, Civetta[231] with permission.)

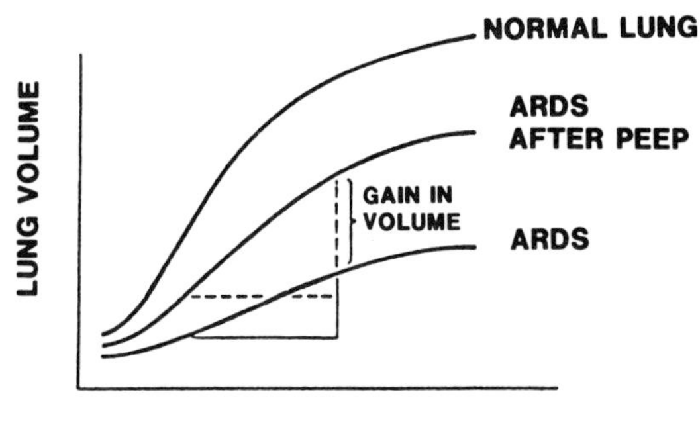

accumulation of fluid. In addition, lymphatic drainage may be blocked.[1,47,137,142,235] Finally, PEEP may compress capillaries of the compliant alveoli, shifting blood from these vessels to those perfusing noncompliant, poorly ventilated alveoli. This effect of PEEP may result in paradoxical increase of intrapulmonary shunt and decrease of $PaO_2$.

PEEP is usually instituted in 2.5- to 5.0-cm $H_2O$ increments. Changes can be made fairly rapidly; it takes about 15 or 20 minutes to evaluate the effect of PEEP on oxygenation, and if improvement is not adequate, a further upward titration can be made. Simultaneous monitoring of $SaO_2$ by pulse oximeter and $S\bar{v}O_2$ by a continuous mixed venous oximetry catheter may expedite estimation of intrapulmonary shunt ($\dot{Q}_s/\dot{Q}_t$), oxygen utilization, and oxygen extraction, facilitating the titration of PEEP or CPAP.[268,269] These indices may be calculated as follows:

$$\dot{Q}_s/\dot{Q}_t = 1\text{-}SaO2 \ / \ 1\text{-}S\bar{v}O_2$$

$$O_2 \text{ utilization} = CaO_2\text{-}C\bar{v}O_2 \ /CaO_2$$

$$O_2 \text{ extraction} = SaO_2\text{-}S\bar{v}O_2 \ /SaO_2$$

In patients with low $\dot{Q}_s/\dot{Q}_t$ and high $PaO_2$, $SaO_2$ approaches 100%, and the shunt equation becomes less accurate, but these patients have at most minimal lung dysfunction. When there is coexisting sepsis, microcirculatory disturbances in the periphery may result in a misleadingly high $S\bar{v}O_2$, rendering these calculations inaccurate.

What is the endpoint of therapy with PEEP? All clinicians agree that adequate oxygenation at a nontoxic $FIO_2$ should be achieved. Beyond this, controversy rages over how to define "optimal" PEEP. Several approaches have been advocated, and goals that have been emphasized as therapeutic endpoints include maximizing pulmonary compliance,[141,330] reducing pulmonary shunt to less than 15 or 20% by using "super PEEP" levels,[84,171,173] decreasing dead space by monitoring arterial to end-tidal $CO_2$ gradient,[155,223,329] maximizing $O_2$ transport or delivery to the periphery,[217,331] achieving a $PaO_2/FIO_2$ ratio greater than 200,[29] and using the "least PEEP" to minimize complications.[1]

There is probably no single criterion for optimal PEEP. Balancing of benefits and adverse effects from PEEP with constant reassessment of cardiorespiratory variables, organ perfusion, and oxygen delivery and utilization is the key to optimal management (Fig 24-13). PEEP initially acts on airways that exert the least resistance to inspired gas flow; that is, alveoli that are already open. These alveoli become overdistended before reinflation of collapsed lung segments occurs with increasing PEEP. Recruitment of new alveoli results in improvement in lung compliance, which should correlate with improvement in oxygenation. If too much PEEP is applied, however, the upper flat portion of the pulmonary pressure-volume curve is approached in which there is little gain in lung volume for additional applied pressure. Similar changes are noted in dead space with increasing levels of PEEP. Initially, when low levels of PEEP produce overdistention of poorly perfused alveoli in the nondependent zone of the lung and other already open alveoli, a slight increase in dead space is noted. As new well-perfused alveoli are recruited, dead space decreases. A further increase in PEEP beyond the point where recruitment of new alveoli ceases results in the increase of dead space (Fig 24-13).[330]

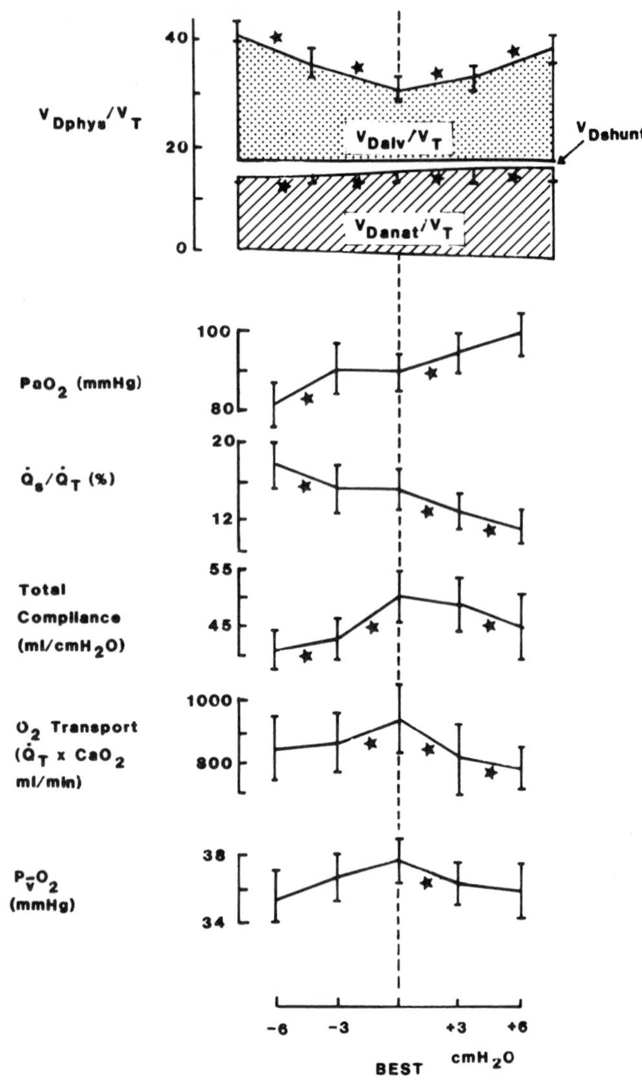


FIG. 24-13. Changes in physiologic dead space ($V_D$ phys) and its components: alveolar ($V_D$ alv), shunt ($V_D$ shunt), and anatomic ($V_D$ anat) dead spaces; arterial oxygen tension ($PaO_2$); intrapulmonary shunting ($\dot{Q}_s/\dot{Q}_t$); total lung compliance; $O_2$ transport and mixed venous oxygen tension ($P_{\bar{v}}O_2$) at 3 and 6 cm $H_2O$ PEEP below and above "best PEEP." Best PEEP is defined as the PEEP resulting in maximum oxygen transport. Asterisks indicate difference ($P < 0.05$) as compared to values obtained with "best PEEP." (From Suter et al[330] with permission.)

The major detrimental effect of PEEP is on cardiac output, especially when levels above 10–15 cm $H_2O$ are used. The relationship between PEEP and cardiac output is not simple and is determined by several mechanisms.[54,154,257,276,301,303,350] PEEP increases intrathoracic pressure, which in turn decreases venous return to the heart. This is probably the major mechanism by which PEEP reduces cardiac output, and to some extent this effect can be attenuated by increased intravascular volume. PEEP also increases pulmonary vascular resistance, which may already be elevated in ARDS. By this mechanism, PEEP essentially increases right ventricular afterload. Apparently PEEP does not cause sufficient right ventricular dilation to impinge on the left ventricle and impede its filling, thus decreasing cardiac output; nor does it cause a significant decrease in left ventricular compliance[41] although these issues have been matters of some debate.[48,65,80,184,189,200,263,264,288]

When cardiac output is depressed by PEEP, fluids should be infused as a first maneuver, especially if the patient is hypovolemic. Among other indicators, hypovolemia should be suspected in patients in whom small doses of PEEP result in depression of cardiac output and blood pressure. However, overzealous volume loading in a patient who is not hypovolemic may be deleterious and result in cardiac failure and further depression of cardiac output. In such a patient inotropic support may be the appropriate therapy.[41] Invasive hemodynamic monitoring is essential in these circumstances as it allows constant assessment of the relationship between cardiac output and filling pressures and thereby helps in selection of appropriate therapy. In the early phase after trauma, patients may be hypovolemic, but this may be masked by compensatory vasoconstriction. On the other hand, septic patients in the late phases of trauma may be vasodilated and require an inordinate amount of fluids. Increasing cardiac output by inotropes in a hypovolemic patient may increase pulmonary shunt and result in inadequate regional perfusion.[63,306] Excessive volume, on the other hand, may worsen pulmonary and peripheral edema, interfering with arterial and tissue oxygenation. In summary, it is desirable to minimize fluid intake in patients with ARDS. However, this should not be done to the point of jeopardizing the adequacy of organ perfusion. The use of invasive monitoring in these circumstances will help the clinician in balancing fluid management. The type of fluid used to restore intravascular volume is probably less important since little difference in terms of outcome has been demonstrated between colloid and crystalloid solutions.[11,251,259,302]

Although maintaining adequate arterial oxygenation is the primary goal, ensuring adequate oxygen delivery to and utilization by tissues is equally important. PEEP may actually improve shunt by depressing cardiac output and thus reducing blood flow to unventilated alveoli. This, however, is not a desirable result since a similar reduction in peripheral organ perfusion and oxygenation will occur. Unfortunately, the assessment of tissue oxygen delivery may be difficult since measurement of mixed venous $O_2$ saturation ($S\bar{v}O_2$) may not always indicate inadequacies of tissue oxygenation (see also Chapter 5).[186] However, serum lactate concentration (normally less than 2 mEq/L), when used in conjunction with $S\bar{v}O_2$ provides a reasonable estimate of organ perfusion and oxygenation.[215]

The criterion used for titration of PEEP has little importance so long as the goals described above are met.[175,224] Initially, overdistention of normal alveoli may be necessary in order to administer an airway pressure high enough to open up collapsed alveoli. After expansion, alveoli function on a different pressure-volume curve and require lower pressures to remain inflated. Once adequate oxygenation is attained there is often a tendency to lower PEEP in order to prevent barotrauma to the lung. $FIO_2$ should first be lowered to nontoxic levels, and if the $PaO_2$ becomes only barely adequate, PEEP should not be decreased. If an improvement in $PaO_2$ sufficient to provide a safety margin is noted, PEEP can be lowered in small decrements, usually no more than 10 cm $H_2O$ in 24 hours. Adequate time should be allowed between changes in order to assess the effect on oxygenation.

When high levels of PEEP are utilized, even transient disconnection of the ventilator can lead to rapid alveolar collapse and hypoxemia. Re-expansion of collapsed alveoli in these instances may take several hours. Thus, the patient should not be disconnected from the ventilator during measurement of pulmonary capillary wedge pressure.[82] The duration of tracheal suctioning should be minimized, and the patient must be ventilated adequately before and after each suctioning episode with an Ambu bag supplied with a special PEEP attachment. The level of PEEP used should be recorded on each follow-up chest X-ray in order to provide a rational assessment of pulmonary parenchymal changes.[160,258]

Barotrauma to the lungs during artificial ventilation is a definite concern, but the contribution of PEEP to this complication is controversial. It occurs more frequently in patients with infected lungs and chronic pre-existing lung disease and may be related to the extent and duration of lung expansion.[122,144,365]

Efforts have been made to improve oxygenation and reduce the complications of PEEP by using high-frequency jet ventilation (HFJV), but its use has not gained wide acceptance.[148] During comparable ventilation HFJV produces a lower peak airway pressure than conventional ventilation, but the mean airway pressures are similar with both ventilatory modes.[308] Oxygenation in patients with ARDS is similar whether HFJV or conventional ventilation is used.[148,308] Animal and human studies suggest that PEEP, whether used with conventional ventilation or HFJV, produces similar hemodynamic changes.[308] Air trapping during HFJV is an important drawback and may result in barotrauma.[108] Finally, humidification of inspired gases during HFJV is difficult, and prolonged ventilation with dry inspired gases may lead to serious tracheobronchial injuries.[108,111,112,213,278] Several modifications of high-frequency ventilation introduced during recent years may offer advantages in ventilatory support of patients with ARDS, but currently little benefit over conventional ventilation is obtained with this technique.

Several attempts have been made to use extracorporeal membrane oxygenation (ECMO) to improve gas exchange. Although initial trials showed no improvement in survival, some recent studies have produced encouraging results.[312a] Clinical use of ECMO as a treatment of ARDS in trauma awaits the results of careful trials.

## WEANING FROM MECHANICAL VENTILATION

Although the main purpose of mechanical ventilation with PEEP in patients with ARDS is to recruit collapsed alveoli and possibly redistribute alveolar fluid, the patient who develops ARDS after trauma often has additional problems which require continuation of ventilatory therapy after the reopening of alveoli. Results from animal studies suggest that spontaneous breathing in the presence of circulatory shock is associated with increased diaphragmatic blood flow, which reduces blood supply to vital organs. By redistributing blood to vital organs, mechanical ventilation may be beneficial in these instances.[149,349] Alveolar hypoventilation caused by diminished respiratory drive (head injury, residual effects of depressant drugs), neurogenic weakness of respiratory muscles (high spinal cord injury, phrenic nerve paralysis), dysfunction of the neuromuscular junction (residual muscle relaxants), disruption of the musculoskeletal integrity of the chest wall (flail chest), and pre-existing or posttraumatic nutritional defects or electrolyte abnormalities (hypokalemia, hypomagnesemia, hypophosphatemia) may also necessitate the prolongation of ventilatory support. Finally, obesity, recent abdominal surgery, smoking history, and fluid overload may contribute to the need for controlled mechanical ventilation. Thus, consideration must be given to all of these coexisting factors when weaning of the patient with posttraumatic ARDS from mechanical ventilation is contemplated.

Generally, when intrapulmonary shunt is reduced to less than 20% of total pulmonary blood flow, $PaO_2$ is adequate with $FIO_2$ less than 0.4 and PEEP is less than 5cm $H_2O$, there is no other major organ insufficiency, hemodynamic status is optimized, the patient is alert, and respiratory drive and muscle function are adequate, weaning from mechanical ventilation may be attempted.[123] Although in most patients successful weaning is not a problem, in up to 19% of patients long-term spontaneous ventilation is inadequate and mechanical support must be resumed.[333] The most valid predictors of successful weaning from mechanical ventilation are tidal volume >5 mL/kg, forced vital capacity >10–15 mL/kg, maximal inspiratory pressure $\geq -$ 20 cm $H_2O$, dead space/tidal volume ratio < 0.6, and alveolar to arterial $PO_2$ gradient on $FIO_2$ = 1.0 <350 mm Hg.[119,138,201,220,283] There is some evidence that the oxygen cost of spontaneous breathing may predict the duration of weaning from mechanical ventilation. Patients could be weaned within 3 days if the oxygen cost of breathing was less than 10% of total oxygen consumption ($\dot{V}O_2$) during spontaneous breathing, whereas those with a value of more than 10% had a mean weaning time of 36 days.[128] However, this test may not have the same predictive value in all types of patients; in comatose and hyperventilating neurosurgical patients it has not been found to be useful (Kahn RC and Koslow M, unpublished data).

Respiratory muscle fatigue is considered the principal cause of failure to sustain spontaneous breathing after the cessation of mechanical ventilation.[120,280] One index that has been devised to predict diaphragmatic fatigue is the ratio between the diaphragmatic pressure generated during each spontaneous breath ($P_{di}$), and the maximum the patient can achieve ($P_{dimax}$). Clinically, $P_{di}$ represents the combined resistive and elastic load of the lung imposed on the diaphragm, whereas $P_{dimax}$ is the maximum inspiratory pressure. $P_{di}$ can be determined by allowing the patient to breath spontaneously for a short period of time during which tidal volume and respiratory rate are measured. The patient is then ventilated mechanically at a tidal volume equal to and respiratory rate slightly above that of the patient's spontaneous breathing in order to ensure cessation of spontaneous respiration. The peak airway pressure measured during this period is $P_{di}$. $P_{dimax}$ can easily be determined by measuring inspiratory pressure during a maximal breath against a closed airway. In healthy volunteers in whom $P_{di}/P_{dimax}$ is greater than 0.4, diaphragmatic fatigue and thus respiratory failure occur within a short time after the resumption of spontaneous breathing, whereas $P_{di}/P_{dimax}$ <0.4 is not associated with diaphragmatic fatigue (Fig 24-14).[279] Although the critical value for $P_{di}/P_{dimax}$ is unknown for patients with respiratory failure, Hall and Wood[123] suggest that a value of 0.25–0.3 or less for this simple bedside test is a predictor of successful weaning from the ventilator.

The basic purpose of any weaning protocol is to exercise respiratory muscles gradually to a level of strength at which spontaneous breathing is possible without fatigue. This goal is accomplished by allowing the patient to breathe spontaneously for regular, but gradually prolonged periods and to rest between these intervals. The traditionally used T-piece technique, in which the patient is allowed to breathe spontaneously for a gradually increasing duration and is mechanically ventilated between trials, may produce tachycardia, dysrhythmias, hypertension, diaphoresis, and agitation upon

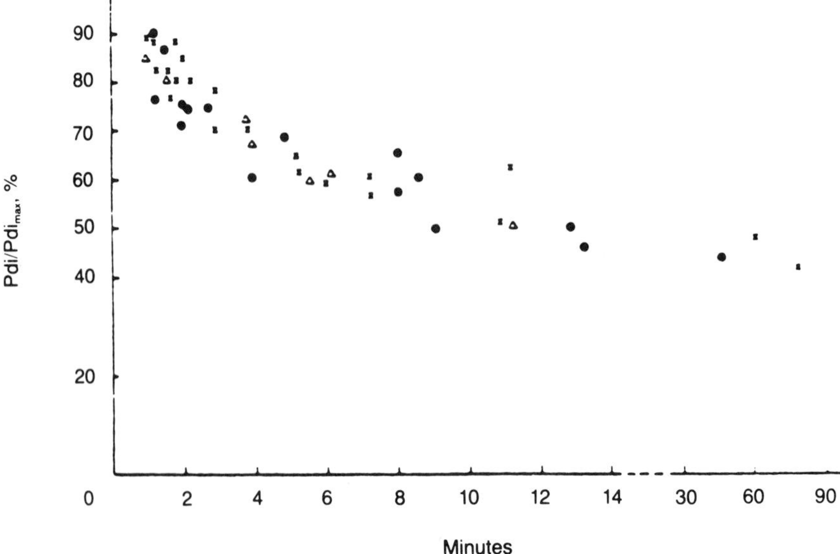


FIG. 24-14. Relationship between the ratio $P_{di}/Pdi_{max}$ and duration of tolerance to spontaneous breathing. Data are obtained from three healthy volunteers in whom the ratio of $P_{di}/Pdi_{max}$ was changed by adding varying levels of inspiratory resistance. In the diagram each volunteer is represented by open triangles, open circles, and solid circles; each point represents an individual determination from each subject. Note that the relationship is curvilinear, and the critical value for $p_{di}/Pdi_{max}$ ratio is 0.4; below this, the endurance time for spontaneous breathing is >90 min, whereas above this value diaphragmatic fatigue occurs within a few minutes. $P_{di}$ = transdiaphragmatic pressure, $Pdi_{max}$ = maximum inspiratory diaphragmatic pressure. (From Roussos, Macklem[279] with permission.)

sudden withdrawal from the ventilator.[123] Intermittent mandatory ventilation (IMV) is the maneuver most commonly used in the United States for weaning patients from mechanical ventilation.[346] Although IMV was originally developed as a weaning technique, it is often used as a primary ventilatory mode. When patients are on controlled ventilation or paralyzed for a prolonged period of time, they may have to "relearn" how to breathe. IMV allows the patient to breathe spontaneously between a predetermined number of mechanically supported breaths, which is gradually reduced to zero. Several advantages of this maneuver are (a) reduced need for sedation or muscle relaxants for ventilator synchrony, (b) lower mean airway pressures with decreased risk of barotrauma and cardiovascular depression, (c) possible avoidance of respiratory alkalosis and (d) improved intrapulmonary gas distribution.[360] However, it can promote discoordinate breathing[116] and may increase the work of breathing in unstable patients.[209,326] This problem can be overcome by using an assist-control mode of ventilation in which inadequate spontaneous breaths are supported with mechanical breaths when the inspiratory pressure falls to a range between one-fourth and one-third of the maximum inspiratory pressure.[123]

A relatively new technique is pressure-support ventilation in which an additional gas flow through a demand valve, in response to the patient's spontaneous breath, produces an increase in airway pressure during inspiration. When the patient's respiratory flow rate diminishes to a predetermined level, the inspiratory gas flow ceases. By decreasing respiratory work, pressure-support ventilation may be more comfortable for the patient than IMV.[12,162]

Progressive alveolar collapse develops in patients recovering from ARDS if the ventilatory modes described above are applied without end-expiratory distending pressures. Hypoxemia, decreased compliance, and increased respiratory work result in recurrence of respiratory failure and necessitate the resumption of mechanical ventilation. Continuous positive airway pressure (CPAP) should be used to prevent these complications.[172] In patients with ARDS, CPAP reduces the elastic load on the respiratory muscles and thus respiratory work by increasing FRC and lung compliance toward normal,[147,165] therapy improving tidal volume and $PaO_2$. The level of CPAP, however, must be adjusted carefully in patients with ARDS since overdistention of the lung can increase the work of breathing, and inadequate levels of CPAP do not improve FRC or oxygenation. While reducing inspiratory effort, CPAP can increase expiratory effort, which may not be tolerated by a weak patient.

A recently introduced mode of ventilatory support, airway pressure release ventilation (APRV), is capable of delivering CPAP when needed without causing an excessive increase in mean airway pressure.[83] An APRV valve, positioned over an outlet added to a T-piece system equipped with a CPAP valve, is released when mechanically assisted ventilation is required.[83,325] Thus, a brief reduction in airway pressure allows the lungs to deflate passively, thereby eliminating $CO_2$ and reducing expiratory effort. This system is still being studied, but it may be useful during the weaning phase of mechanical ventilation since it allows unrestricted spontaneous ventilation with maintenance of optimal FRC and $CO_2$ elimination without an increase in mean airway pressure.

Equipment design also influences the inspiratory work of breathing. A valveless continuous flow system, although less economical in gas consumption, has significantly less effect on the work of breathing than demand valve systems.[117,168,348] Considerable differences in respiratory work have also been noted among various demand valve systems.[168,326] The flow resistance of commercially available system humidifiers also varies significantly and may influence the success of the weaning procedure.[209] Thus, IMV and CPAP systems must be evaluated carefully, and those that provide the least fluctuation in airway pressure (less than 2.5 $cmH_2O$) should be used.[326]

## TREATMENT OF LUNG INJURY

In recent years progress in understanding the pathophysiology of ARDS has led to the introduction of several new treatments of the underlying lung injury. The use of high-dose corticosteroids in ARDS was partly derived from numerous attempts at using the drug in the treatment of sepsis and septic shock, an application that has not been shown to confer no benefit and possibly to be associated with considerable risk.[32,347] On a theoretical basis, corticosteroids would appear to be of benefit in curbing the underlying inflammatory reaction and interfering with the mechanisms of lung injury. Such benefits would include inhibition of complement-induced neutrophil aggregation, impairment of neutrophil chemotaxis, preservation of vascular tone and endothelial integrity, inhibition of the complement cascade and of arachidonic acid production, and reduction of pulmonary vascular resistance.[161,357] Nevertheless, there is no indication for corticosteroids in ARDS because no beneficial effect has been demonstrated from this drug and the risk in terms of secondary infection and poor tissue healing is considerable.[23,33,102,193,228,229]

Prostaglandin $E_1$ is currently being studied. It blocks coagulation and the inflammatory response by inhibiting platelet aggregation, macrophage activation, neutrophil chemotaxis, and neutrophil release of oxygen radicals and lysosomal enzymes. These effects are dose dependent; in high doses it blocks the inflammatory response, whereas in low doses it may augment it. Most of the administered agent is metabolized after a first pass through the lungs so that even high-dose infusions result in relatively low concentrations in the systemic circulation. Prostaglandin $E_1$ dilates pulmonary as well as systemic vessels, but has minimal effects on pulmonary hypoxic vasoconstriction.[140,341] Preliminary results with prostaglandin $E_1$ are encouraging, but more extensive studies are needed to confirm these findings.

Attempts have been made to inhibit the production of arachidonic acid metabolites. Ibuprofen, meclofenamate, and indomethacin inhibit the degradation of arachidonic acid via the cyclo-oxygenase pathway and may thus improve pulmonary function. For instance, indomethacin (1 mg/kg) may improve $PaO_2$ in patients with severe bacterial pneumonia.[127] Dazoxiben is more specific and acts further down the cyclo-oxygenase pathway to inhibit thromboxane synthetase. Specific inhibitors of the lipoxygenase pathway have also been developed. Prostacyclin ($PGI_2$) is a vasodilator, but it also inhibits platelet and leukocyte adhesion and stabilizes cell membranes. Prostacyclin infusions have been used in ARDS, but currently the drug cannot be recommended for clinical use.[31,45,161,265] In a preliminary study in primates, pretreatment with anti-C5a des arginine antibody infusion protected the animals against subsequently infused *E. coli*.[324] Arterial blood pressure decreased little, but there was no evidence of respiratory failure despite the development of profound and sustained neutropenia. In the future, antibodies not only for C5a but for other mediators of ARDS, including endotoxin, may help prevent or treat this disease. Antioxidant agents, such as glutathione reductase and superoxide dismutase, have been used to protect the lung against toxic oxygen radicals, but experience with these agents in humans is limited. Likewise, fibronectin repletion has been investigated as a possible therapeutic modality for ARDS.[30,31,161]

Most recently, interest has focused on a newly isolated mediator of endotoxin activity: cachectin or tumor necrosis factor. This is a macrophage-produced polypeptide hormone with a subunit size of 17 kilodaltons. In animals it mediates hemorrhagic tumor necrosis, cachexia, and endotoxic shock. The development of antibodies or receptor antagonists to this substance may have important implications in the treatment of sepsis and thereby of ARDS.[25,26,343] In neonates with respiratory distress syndrome, aerosolized surfactant repletion via the endotracheal tube has met with success.[157,332] Whether this type of therapy is applicable in adults in whom surfactant depletion is a secondary phenomenon remains to be seen.

## ANESTHETIC CONSIDERATIONS

In 76% of patients who develop ARDS, clinical and roentgenographic findings begin to appear within 2 to 24 hours after trauma.[104,238] Thus, in a significant percentage of patients, this complication may develop during anesthesia for initial emergency surgery. Progressive decline in $PaO_2$, decreased lung compliance, and development of rhonchi and rales are the most common clinical signs suggesting the development of ARDS at this stage. Since many of these patients receive large amounts of intravenous fluid during the early phase after injury, it is not uncommon to ascribe these findings to fluid overload, rather than to ARDS. This is especially true in elderly trauma patients in whom there is concern for cardiac dysfunction. Reducing the flow rate of intravenous fluids frequently results in hypotension without improvement in $PaO_2$, lung compliance, or breath sounds if bleeding is continuing. Placement of a Swan-Ganz catheter and sequential measurements of pulmonary artery pressure, pulmonary artery wedge pressure, and cardiac output in order to construct a ventricular function curve may alleviate these diagnostic difficulties. The patient with myocardial failure whose bleeding is controlled may have elevated pulmonary artery and pulmonary artery wedge pressures that increase further without an increase in cardiac output or left ventricular stroke work index, when 250–500 mL of lactated Ringer solution is infused within 15 minutes. Such a response to a fluid challenge implies a flat ventricular function curve. On the other hand, the patient with pulmonary dysfunction may also have elevated pulmonary artery pressure, but normal or low pulmonary artery wedge pressure. Fluid challenge in this patient results in increased cardiac output and left ventricular stroke work index without a significant increase in pulmonary arterial wedge pressure, implying a steep ventricular function curve (see Fig. 4-10, Chapter 4). This differential diagnosis may be difficult when there is concomitant myocardial and pulmonary dysfunction. In these circumstances fluid and inotropic therapy should be adjusted carefully according to arterial blood pressure, cardiac filling pressures, cardiac output, and $S\bar{v}O_2$. Of course, causes other than ARDS and myocardial dysfunction that may produce hypoxemia, decreased lung compliance, and changes in breath sounds should also be ruled out before deciding to institute PEEP therapy for ARDS.

A small percentage of patients who develop ARDS after trauma and are already receiving ventilatory therapy may require delayed surgery. The majority of these patients require surgery for drainage of a septic focus. Thus, the guidelines described in Chapter 27 for anesthetic management of septic patients also apply to most of these patients. Preoperative assessment of organ function, particularly the lungs, heart, kidney, liver, and brain, is important since many of these patients develop multiorgan failure syndrome. Evaluation of the chest radiogram, arterial and mixed venous blood gases, and the level of PEEP and other ventilatory parameters will give an idea of the patient's oxygenation and aid in determining intraoperative ventilatory management. The doses of any vasoactive agents administered in the intensive care unit must be recorded as they provide information about the patient's hemodynamic condition and will give a rough estimate of the types and doses of these agents that may be required intraoperatively.

Transportation of these patients to the operating room requires careful planning, adequate monitoring, and appropriate ventilatory equipment. A functioning Ambu bag with PEEP attachment and an adequate supply of $O_2$, a battery-operated ECG and two-channel intravascular pressure monitoring device, pulse oximeter, appropriate infusion pumps for vasoactive agents, and necessary resuscitative drugs must be available. At least one physician and a nurse should accompany the patient to ensure adequate monitoring, ventilation, and appropriate resuscitation if deterioration in hemodynamics or gas exchange occurs en route. The operating room and anesthetic equipment must be prepared in advance to avoid the patient's waiting in the holding area, which in most operating rooms is not equipped to care for such seriously ill patients.

Since all critically ill ARDS patients arrive in the operating room with their tracheas intubated, anesthetic induction usually involves administration of incremental doses of anesthetic and adjunct drugs. Anesthesia can be maintained with narcotics and/or low concentrations of inhalational anesthetics. There is little information about the effect of anesthesia on gas exchange in patients with ARDS. Paralysis of respiratory muscles, by producing the upward movement of intra-abdominal contents, and high inspired oxygen concentrations, by producing absorption atelectasis, increase intrapulmonary shunting and interfere with oxygenation in normal patients. Similar adverse effects on oxygenation probably occur in patients with ARDS. In addition, hypocapnia, inhalation anesthetics, vasodilator agents, and intraoperative events that cause an increase in pulmonary artery pressure may increase intrapulmonary shunt and reduce arterial oxygenation by interfering with hypoxic pulmonary vasoconstriction in atelectatic areas of the lung.[19] Although recent findings in humans with normal lungs demonstrate that inhalation anesthetics in concentrations of up to 1 MAC, in the presence of acutely induced regional alveolar hypoxia, have little effect on hypoxic pulmonary vasoconstriction,[51,52] in an animal model of ARDS Pavlin et al[238–240] demonstrated a doubling of right-to-left shunt with halothane, enflurane, and isoflurane, underscoring the importance of monitoring oxygenation. Monitoring of $S\bar{v}O_2$ and, if available, measurement of blood lactate concentration may be invaluable in assessing tissue oxygenation and adjusting hemodynamic and ventilatory therapy.

Unlike critical care unit ventilators, most anesthesia ventilators are incapable of generating high enough peak inspiratory pressures (PIP) and PEEP to satisfy the ventilatory needs of some of these patients. Maximal PIP and PEEP generated by critical care ventilators are in the range of 150 cm $H_2O$ and 50 cm $H_2O$, respectively. Among commercially available anesthesia ventilators only the Siemens 900C and 900D (Elk Grove Village, IL.) can meet these performance characteristics. Brown and co-workers[44] modified an Emerson 3MV (Cambridge, MA.) critical care ventilator for use during anesthetic management of patients with pulmonary injury (Fig 24-15). This ventilator is capable of generating high levels of PIP (up to 160 cm $H_2O$) and PEEP (up to 50 cm $H_2O$) and delivering inhalation anesthetics at concentrations similar to those indicated on the vaporizer dial if fresh gas flow rates between 12.5 and 20 L/min are used. At flow rates higher or lower than these, concentrations of anesthetics delivered are lower than the vaporizer settings.

FIG. 24-15. Emerson 3 MV ventilator modified for anesthesia use. The location of the PEEP column and the inspiratory limb connection has been reversed to ease interpretation. Arrows indicate the direction of gas flow. $B_1$ = ventilator reservoir bag (5L), $B_2$ = spontaneous breathing reservoir bag (5L), E = entrainment valve, EXP = expiratory tubing, $F_1$ = $O_2$/air flowmeters, $F_2$ = $N_2O$ flowmeter, H = humidifier, INSP = inspiratory tubing, $N_2O$ = $N_2O/O_2$ blender, $O_2$ = $O_2$/air blender, PAP = proximal airway pressure line, PEEP = PEEP column, R = exhaust gas reservoir, S = suction connection for scavenging, V = vaporizer, W = one-way valve. (From Brown et al[44] with permission.)

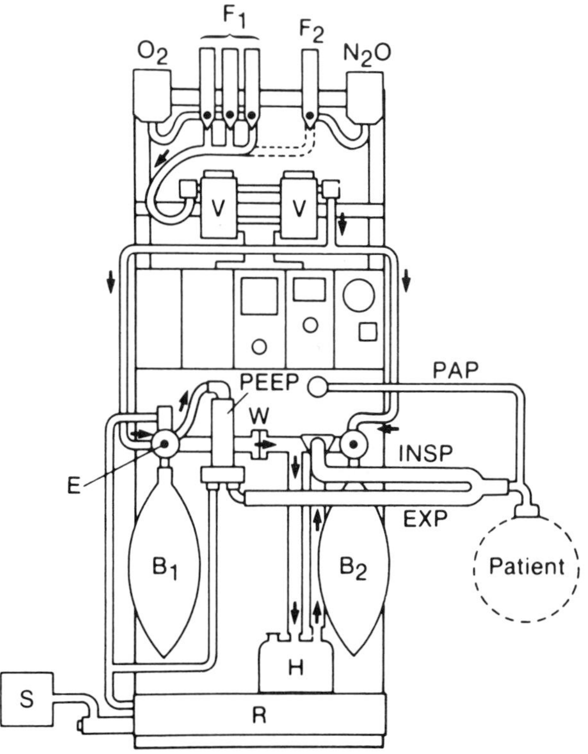


## CONCLUSION

The adult respiratory distress syndrome is a serious complication of major trauma. It may be secondary to tissue destruction, direct lung injury, massive transfusions, aspiration of gastric contents, sepsis, and many other events associated with trauma. Sepsis is an important cause of ARDS, and its source should be diagnosed and treated aggressively, for if the underlying cause is not eliminated, ARDS will not resolve. Moreover, sepsis provokes the development of the multisystem organ failure syndrome. Once this complication supervenes, the prognosis of ARDS worsens precipitously.[16,105,109,176,198,218] After 20 years of investigation, the survival rate of patients with ARDS has not improved. With advances in ventilatory methods we may be able to improve respiratory support for victims, but we still have no effective direct treatment for ARDS. Progress in understanding the pathophysiology of ARDS has led to trials of therapeutic agents, including prostaglandin $E_1$, ibuprofen, meclofenamate, indomethacin, dazoxiben, prostacyclin ($PGI_2$), free oxygen radical scavengers, and fibronectin, but none can be recommended for clinical use at this time. On the other hand, those patients who survive have minimal impairment of pulmonary function.[174,178,179,277] Even when fibrotic changes are produced by ARDS, gradual improvement in lung function is common. This is encouraging since it means that, if the underlying cause of the complication can be treated and the patient can be sustained, the ultimate outcome is worth striving for.

## REFERENCES

1. Albert RK. Least PEEP: primum non nocere. Chest 1985;87:2.
2. Albertine KH. Ultrastructural abnormalities in increased permeability pulmonary edema. Clin Chest Med 1985;6:345.
3. Anderson RR, Holiday RL, Driedger AA, et al. Documentation of pulmonary capillary permeability in the adult respiratory distress syndrome accompanying human sepsis. Am Rev Respir Dis 1979;119:869.
4. Andreadis N, Petty TL. Adult respiratory distress syndrome: problems and progress. Am Rev Respir Dis 1985;132:1344.
5. Ashbaugh DG, Bigelow DB, Petty TL, et al. Acute respiratory distress in adults. Lancet 1967;2:319.
6. Aubier M, Viires N, Syllie G, et al. Respiratory muscle contribution to lactic acidosis in low cardiac output. Am Rev Respir Dis 1982;126:648.
7. Bachofen M, Weibel ER. Alterations of the gas exchange apparatus in adult respiratory insufficiency associated with septicemia. Am Rev Respir Dis 1977;116:589.
8. Bachofen M, Weibel ER. Structural alterations of lung parenchyma in the adult respiratory distress syndrome. Clin Chest Med 1982;3:35.

9. Baker SP, O'Neill B, Haddox W, et al. The injury severity score: a method for describing patients with multiple injuries and evaluating emergency care. J Trauma 1974;14:187.
10. Ball HA, Cook JA, Wise WC, et al. Role of thromboxane, prostaglandins and leukotrienes in endotoxic and septic shock. Intens Care Med 1986;12:116.
11. Bandendistel L, Dahms TE, Kaminski DL. The effect of albumin on extravascular lung water in animals and patients with low-pressure pulmonary edema. J Surg Res 1982;33:328.
12. Banner MJ, Kirby RR. Pressure support ventilation. Crit Care Med 1986;14:666.
13. Barer G. Reactivity of the vessels of collapsed and ventilated lungs to drugs and hypoxia. Circ Res 1966;18:366.
14. Bartlett RH. Respiratory care of the surgical or traumatized patient. In: Burton G, ed. Respiratory care—a guide to clinical practice. Philadelphia: JB Lippincott, 1977:874.
15. Baumann WR, Jung RC, Koss M, et al. Incidence and mortality of adult respiratory distress syndrome: a prospective analysis from a large metropolitan hospital. Crit Care Med 1986;14:1.
16. Bell RC, Coalson JJ, Smith JD, et al. Multiple organ failure and infection in the adult respiratory distress syndrome. Ann Intern Med 1983;99:293.
17. Benumof JL, Wahrenbrock EA. Blunted hypoxic pulmonary vasoconstriction by increased lung vascular pressures. J Appl Physiol 1975;38:846.
18. Benumof JL, Prilo AF, Johanson I, et al. Interaction of $P\bar{v}O_2$ with $P_AO_2$ on hypoxic pulmonary vasoconstriction. J Appl Physiol 1981;51:871.
19. Bergman NA. Hypoxic pulmonary vasoconstriction. Semin Anesth 1987;6:188.
20. Bernard GR. Granulocytes as mediators in pulmonary edema. Semin Respir Med 1983;4:308.
21. Bernard GR, Brigham KL. Pulmonary edema: pathophysiologic mechanisms and new approaches to therapy. Chest 1986;89:594.
22. Bernard GR, Rinaldo J, Harris T, et al. Early predictors of ARDS reversal in patients with established ARDS (Abstr). Am Rev Respir Dis 1985;131:A143.
23. Bernard GR, Luce JM, Sprung CL, et al. High-dose corticosteroids in patients with the adult respiratory distress syndrome. N Engl J Med 1987;317:1565.
24. Bertrand Y. Oxygen-free radicals and lipid peroxidation in adult respiratory distress syndrome. Intens Care Med 1985;11:56.
25. Beutler B, Cerami A. Cachectin: more than a tumor necrosis factor. N Engl J Med 1987;316:379.
26. Beutler B, Milsark IW, Cerami A. Passive immunization against cachectin/tumor necrosis factor protects mice from lethal effects of endotoxin. Science 1985;229:869.
27. Bigelow DB, Iannuzzi M. Adult respiratory distress syndrome in the trauma patient: current concepts and controversies. In: Maull KI, ed.Advances in trauma. vol I. Chicago: YearBook Publishers, 1986:85.
28. Blaisdell FW. Pathophysiology of the respiratory distress syndrome. Arch Surg 1974;108:44.
29. Bolin RW, Pierson DJ. Ventilatory management in acute lung injury. Crit Care Clin 1986;2:585.
30. Bone RC, Jacobs ER. Research on ibuprofen for sepsis and respiratory failure. Am J Med 1984;July 13:114.
31. Bone RC, Jacobs ER. Advances in pharmacologic treatment of acute lung injury and septic shock. Adv Anesth 1987;4:327.
32. Bone RC, Fisher CJ Jr, Clemmer TP, et al. A controlled clinical trial of high-dose methylprednisolone in the treatment of severe sepsis and septic shock. N Engl J Med 1987;317:653.
33. Bone RC, Fisher CJ Jr, Clemmer TP, et al. Early methylprednisolone treatment for septic syndrome and the adult respiratory distress syndrome. Chest 1987;92:1032.
34. Brandstetter RD, Conetta R, Sander NW, et al. Adult respiratory distress syndrome in adolescents due to aspiration of gastric contents. NY State J Med 1986;86:513.
35. Braude S, Apperley V, Krausz T, et al. Adult respiratory distress syndrome after allogenic bone marrow transplantation: evidence for a neutrophil-independent mechanism. Lancet 1985;1:1239.
36. Brigham KL. Mechanisms of lung injury. Clin Chest Med 1982;3:9.
37. Brigham KL. Primary (high permeability) pulmonary edema. Semin Respir Med 1983;4:285.
38. Brigham KL, Meyrick B. Endotoxin and lung injury. Am Rev Respir Dis 1986;133:913.
39. Brigham KL, Kariman K, Harris T, et al. Lung water and vascular permeability surface area in humans during respiratory failure. Am Rev Respir Dis 1980;121:426.
40. Brigham KL, Kariman K, Harris T, et al. Correlation of oxygenation with vascular permeability surface area but not with lung water in humans with acute respiratory failure and pulmonary edema. J Clin Invest 1983;72:339.
41. Broaddus VC, Berthiaume Y, Biondi JW, et al. Hemodynamic management of the adult respiratory distress syndrome. J Intens Care Med 1987;2:190.
42. Brook CJ, DeHart P, Weg JG, et al. Ventilation-perfusion distribution in acute respiratory failure. Am Rev Respir Dis 1977;115(suppl):310.
43. Brown C, Dhiviandhar HN, Barrett J, et al. Progression and resolution of changes in pulmonary function and structure due to pulmonary microembolism and blood transfusion. Ann Surg 1977;185:92.
44. Brown DL, Schulz J, Kirby RR. Modification of a critical care ventilator for anesthesia use. Crit Care Med 1987;15:1055.
45. Buchman SR, Sugarman HJ, Tatum JL, et al. Failure of methylprednisolone, ibuprofen, or prostacyclin to reduce HCL-induced pulmonary albumin leak in dogs. Surgery 1984; 96:163.
46. Cain SM. Assessment of tissue oxygenation. Crit Care Clin 1986;2:537.
47. Caldini P, Leith D, Brennan M. Effects of continuous positive pressure ventilation on edema formation in dog lung. J Appl Physiol 1975;39:672.
48. Calvin JE, Driedger AA, Sibbald WJ. Positive end-expiratory pressure (PEEP) does not depress left ventricular function in patients with pulmonary edema. Am Rev Respir Dis 1981;124:121.
49. Campbell GD, Coalson JJ, Johanson WG. The effect of bacterial superinfection on lung function after diffuse alveolar damage. Am Rev Respir Dis 1984;129:974.
50. Carey LC. Extra-abdominal manifestations of acute pancreatitis. Surgery 1980;87:509.
51. Carlsson AJ, Binslev L, Hedenstierna G. Hypoxia-induced pulmonary vasoconstriction in the human lung. The effect of isoflurane anesthesia. Anesthesiology 1987;66:312.
52. Carlsson AJ, Hedenstierna G, Bindslev L. Hypoxia-induced vasoconstriction in human lung exposed to enflurane anaesthesia. Acta Anaesth Scand 1987;31:57.
53. Carvalho A, Bellman SM, Saullo V, et al. Altered factor VIII in acute respiratory failure. N Engl J Med 1982;307:1113.
54. Cassidy SS, Roberts CH, Piere AK, et al. Cardiovascular effects of positive end-expiratory pressure in dogs. J Appl Physiol 1978;44:743.
55. Cheney F, Colley PS. The effect of cardiac output on arterial blood oxygentation. Anesthesiology 1980;52:496.
56. Clowes GHA Jr, Zuschneid W, Dragacevic S, et al. The nonspecific pulmonary inflammatory reactions leading to respiratory failure after shock, gangrene and sepsis. J Trauma 1968;8:899.

57. Clowes GHA Jr, Hirsch E, Williams L, et al. Septic lung and shock lung in man. Ann Surg 1975;181:681.
58. Coalson JJ. Pathophysiologic features of respiratory distress in the infant and adult. Critical Care: State of the Art 1982;3:A1.
59. Cochrane CG, Spragg R, Revak SD. Pathogenesis of the adult respiratory distress syndrome. Evidence of oxidant activity in bronchoalveolar lavage fluid. J Clin Invest 1983;71:754.
60. Cohen CA, Zagelbaum G, Gross D, et al. Clinical manifestations of inspiratory muscle fatigue. Am J Med 1982;73:308.
61. Colice GL. Neurogenic pulmonary edema. Clin Chest Med 1985;6:473.
62. Colice GL, Matthay MA, Bass E, et al. Neurogenic pulmonary edema. Am Rev Respir Dis 1984;130:941.
63. Connors AF, McCaffree DR, Rogers RM. The adult respiratory distress syndrome. Disease-a-Month 1981;27:1.
64. Crandall ED, Staub NC, Goldberg HS, et al. Recent developments in pulmonary edema. Ann Intern Med 1983;99:808.
65. Culver BH, Marini JJ, Butler J. Lung volume and pleural pressure effects on ventricular function. J Appl Physiol 1981;50:630.
66. Cutillo AG. The clinical assessment of lung water. Chest 1987;92:319.
67. Danek SJ, Lynch JP, Weg JG, et al. The dependence of oxygen uptake on oxygen delivery in the adult respiratory distress syndrome. Am Rev Respir Dis 1980;122:387.
68. Dantzker DR. Gas exchange in the adult respiratory distress syndrome. Clin Chest Med 1982;3:57.
69. Dantzker DR. Gas exchange in acute lung injury. Crit Care Clin 1986;2:527.
70. Dantzker DR, Brook CJ, Dehart P, et al. Ventilation-perfusion distributions in the adult respiratory distress syndrome. Am Rev Respir Dis 1979;120:1039.
71. Dantzker DR, Lynch JP, Weg JC. Depression of cardiac output is a mechanism of shunt reduction in the therapy of acute respiratory failure. Chest 1980;77:636.
72. Dean NC, Amend WC, Matthay MA. Adult respiratory distress syndrome related to antilymphocyte globulin therapy. Chest 1987;91:619.
73. Demling RH. Lung fluid and protein dynamics during hemorrhagic shock resuscitation and recovery. Circ Shock 1980;7:149.
74. Demling RH. The pathogenesis of respiratory failure after trauma and sepsis. Surg Clin North Am 1981;60:1373.
75. Demling RH. Traumatic pulmonary edema. Semin Respir Med 1981;3:97.
76. Demling RH. Respiratory failure from trauma and sepsis (ARDS). In: Zuidema GD, Rutherford RB, Ballinger RF, eds. The Management of trauma 4th ed. Philadelphia: WB Saunders, 1985:137.
77. Demling RH, Niehaus G, Will JA. Pulmonary microvascular response to hemorrhagic shock, resuscitation and recovery. J Appl Physiol 1979;46:498.
78. Deneke SM, Fanburg BL. Normobaric oxygen toxicity of the lung. N Engl J Med 1980;303:76.
79. Deneke SM, Fanburg BL. Oxygen toxicity of the lung: an update. Br J Anaesth 1982;54:737.
80. Dhainaut JF, Devaux JY, Monsallier JF, et al. Mechanisms of decreased left ventricular preload during continuous positive pressure ventilation in ARDS. Chest 1986;90:74.
81. Divertie MB. The adult respiratory distress syndrome. Mayo Clin Proc 1982;57:371.
82. Divertie MB, McMichan JC, Michal L, et al. Avoidance of aggravated hypoxemia during measurement of mean pulmonary artery wedge pressure in ARDS. Chest 1983;83:70.
83. Downs JB, Stock MC. Airway pressure release ventilation: a new concept in ventilatory support. Crit Care Med 1987; 15:459.
84. Downs JB, Klein EF Jr, Modell JH. The effect of incremental PEEP on $P_aO_2$ in patients with respiratory failure. Anesth Analg 1973;52:210.
85. Drazen JM, Austen KF. Leukotrienes and airway responses. Am Rev Respir Dis 1987;136:985.
86. Duchateau J, Haas M, Schreyen H, et al. Complement activation in patients at risk of developing the adult respiratory distress syndrome. Am Rev Respir Dis 1984;130:1058.
87. Dueck R, Wagner PD, West JB. Effects of positive end-expiratory pressure or gas exchange in dogs with normal and edematous lungs. Anesthesiology 1977;47:359.
88. Durtschi MB, Haisch CE, Reynolds L, et al. Effect of micropore filtration on pulmonary functions after massive transfusion. Am J Surg 1979;138:8.
89. Fanconi S, Kraemer R, Weber J, et al. Long term sequelae in children surviving adult respiratory distress syndrome. J Pediatr 1985;106:218.
90. Fantone JC, Feltner DE, Brieland JK, et al. Phagocytic cell-derived inflammatory mediators and lung disease. Chest 1987;91:428.
91. Farrell PM, Avery ME. Hyaline membrane disease. Am Rev Respir Dis 1975;111:657.
92. Fein AM, Leff A, Hopewell PC. Pathophysiology and management of the complications resulting from fire and the inhaled products of combustion: review of the literature. Crit Care Med 1980;8:94.
93. Fein AM, Lippmann M, Holtzman H, et al. The risk factors, incidence, and prognosis of ARDS following septicemia. Chest 1983;83:40.
94. Fein AM, Goldberg SK, Walkenstein MD, et al. Is pulmonary artery catheterization necessary for the diagnosis of pulmonary edema? Am Rev Respir Dis 1984;129:1006.
95. Fein AM, Wiener-Kronish JP, Niederman M, et al. Pathophysiology of the adult respiratory distress syndrome. Crit Care Clin 1986;2:429.
96. Fein IA, Rackow EC. Neurogenic pulmonary edema. 1982; Chest 81:318.
97. Fishman AP. Respiratory gases in the regulation of the pulmonary circulation. Physiol Rev 1961;41:214.
98. Fishman AP. Shock lung (a distinctive non-entity). Circulation 1973;47:921.
99. Fishman AP. Hypoxia in the pulmonary circulation. How and where it works. Circ Res 1976;38:221.
100. Fishman AP, Pietra GG. Stretched pores, blunt injury and neurohemodynamic pulmonary edema. Physiologist 1980;23:53.
101. Flick MR. Mechanism of acute lung injury. Crit Care Clin 1986;2:455.
102. Flick MR, Murray JF. High dose corticosteroid therapy in the adult respiratory distress syndrome. JAMA 1984;251:1054.
103. Forsgren P, Wegenius G, Modig J. Pulmonary function, extravascular lung water and chest radiography in a porcine model of adult respiratory distress syndrome. Acta Anaesth Scand 1986;30:463.
104. Fowler AA, Hamman RF, Good JT, et al. Adult respiratory distress syndrome: risk with common predispositions. Ann Intern Med 1983;98:593.
105. Fowler AA, Hamman RF, Zerbe GO, et al. Adult respiratory distress syndrome: prognosis after onset. Am Rev Respir Dis 1985;132:472.
106. Frank L, Massaro D. Oxygen toxicity. Am J Med 1980;69:117.
107. Frank MM. Complement in the pathophysiology of human disease. N Engl J Med 1987;316:1525.
108. Froese AB, Bryan AC. High frequency ventilation. Am Rev Respir Dis 1987;135:1363.
109. Fry DE, Pearlstein L, Fulton RL, et al. Multiple system organ failure. The role of uncontrolled infection. Arch Surg 1980;115:136.

110. Fulton RL, Jones CE. The course of post-traumatic pulmonary insufficiency in man. Surg Gynecol Obstet 1975;140:179.
111. Fusciardi J, Rouby JJ, Barakat T, et al. Hemodynamic effects of high-frequency jet ventilation in patients with and without circulatory shock. Anesthesiology 1986;65:485.
112. Gallagher TJ, Klein MM, Carlon GC. Present status of high frequency ventilation. Crit Care Med 1982;10:613.
113. Garcia JGN, Noonan TC, Jubiz W, Malik AB. Leukotrienes and the pulmonary microcirculation. Am Rev Respir Dis 1987;136:161.
114. Gattinoni L, Pesouti A. ARDS: the non-homogeneous lung; facts and hypothesis. Intens Crit Care Dig 1987;6:1.
115. Gelb AW. Pulmonary dysfunction in trauma. Can Anaesth Soc J 1985;32:235.
116. Gibbons WJ, Rotaple MJ, Newman SL. Effect of intermittent mandatory ventilation on inspiratory muscle coordination in prolonged mechanically-ventilated patients. Am Rev Respir Dis 1986;133:A123.
117. Gibney RTN, Wilson RS, Pontoppidan H. Comparison of work of breathing in high gas flow and demand valve continuous positive airway pressure systems. Chest 1982;82:692.
118. Glassroth J, Adams GD, Schnoll S. The impact of substance abuse on the respiratory system. Chest 1987;91:596.
119. Gottfried SB, Rossi A, Higgs BD, et al. Noninvasive determination of respiratory system mechanics during mechanical ventilation for acute respiratory failure. Am Rev Respir Dis 1985;131:414.
120. Grassino A, Macklem PT. Respiratory muscle fatigue and ventilatory failure. Annu Rev Med 1984;35:625.
121. Grover RF. The fascination of the hypoxic lung. Anesthesiology 1985;63:580.
122. Haake R, Schlichtig R, Ulstad DR, Henschen RR. Barotrauma. Pathophysiology, risk factors, and prevention. Chest 1987;91:608.
123. Hall JB, Wood LDH. Liberation of the patient from mechanical ventilation. JAMA 1987;257:1621.
124. Hallgren R, Borg T, Venge P, et al. Signs of neutrophil and eosinophil activation in adult respiratory distress syndrome. Crit Care Med 1984;12:14.
125. Hallman M, Spragg R, Harrell JH, et al. Evidence of lung surfactant abnormality in respiratory failure. J Clin Invest 1982;70:673.
126. Hammerschmidt DE, Weaver LJ, Hudson LD, et al. Association of complement activation and elevated plasma-C5a with adult respiratory distress syndrome: pathophysiologic relevance and possible prognostic value. Lancet 1980;1:947.
127. Hanly PJ, Dobson K, Roberts D, Bruce Light R. Effect of indomethacin on arterial oxygenation in critically ill patients with severe bacterial pneumonia. Lancet 1987;1:351.
128. Harpin RP, Baker JP, Downer JP, et al. Correlation of the oxygen cost of breathing and length of weaning from mechanical ventilation. Crit Care Med 1987;15:807.
129. Harris TR. Basics of lung fluid balance. Semin Respir Med 1983;4:274.
130. Hauge A. Hypoxia and pulmonary vascular resistance. The relative effects of pulmonary arterial and alveolar $PO_2$. Acta Physiol Scand 1969;76:121.
131. Hechtman HB, Weisel RD, Vito L, et al. The independence of pulmonary shunting and pulmonary edema. Surgery 1973;74:300.
132. Hechtman HB, Weisel RD, Vito L, et al. Role of humoral mediators in adult respiratory distress syndrome. Chest 1984;86:623.
133. Hechtman HB, Lelcuk S, Alexander F, et al: Humoral mediators in adult respiratory distress syndrome. In: Siegel J, ed. Trauma: emergency surgery and critical care. New York: Churchill Livingstone. 1987:565.
134. Hedley-White J, Pontoppidan H, Morris MJ. The response of patients with respiratory failure and cardiopulmonary disease to different levels of constant volume ventilation. J Clin Invest 1966;45:1543.
135. Heffner JE, Sahn SA, Repine JE. The role of platelets in the adult respiratory distress syndrome. Am Rev Respir Dis 1987;135:482.
136. Hempel FG, Lenfant CJM. Current and future research on adult respiratory distress syndrome. Semin Respir Med 1981;2:165.
137. Henning RJ, Heyman V, Alcover I, et al. Cardiopulmonary effects of oleic acid induced pulmonary edema and mechanical ventilation. Anesth Analg 1986;65:925.
138. Hodgkin JE, Bowser MA, Burton GG. Respiratory weaning. Crit Care Med 1974;2:96.
139. Holbrook PR, Taylor G, Pollack MM, et al. Adult respiratory distress syndrome in children. Pediatr Clin North Am 1980;27:677.
140. Holcroft JW, Vassar MJ, Weber CJ. Prostaglandin $E_1$ and survival in patients with the adult respiratory distress syndrome. Ann Surg 1986;203:371.
141. Holzapfel L, Dominique R, Francois P, et al. Static pressure-volume curves and effect of positive end-expiratory pressure on gas exchange in the respiratory distress syndrome. Crit Care Med 1983;11:591.
142. Hopewell PC. Failure of positive end-expiratory pressure to decrease lung water content in alloxan induced pulmonary edema. Am Rev Respir Dis 1979;120:813.
143. Horovitz JH, Carrico CJ, Shires GT. Pulmonary response to major injury. Arch Surg 1974;108:349.
144. Hudson LD. Ventilatory management of patients with adult respiratory distress syndrome. Semin Respir Med 1981;2:128.
145. Hudson LD. Causes of the adult respiratory distress syndrome—clinical recognition. Clin Chest Med 1982;3:195.
146. Hudson LD. Getting oxygen to the tissues. In: O'Donohue WJ Jr, ed. Current advances in respiratory care. American Collage of Chest Physicians, Park Ridge: 1984:120.
147. Hurst JM, De Haven CB, Branson RD. Use of CPAP mask as the sole mode of ventilatory support in trauma patients with mild to moderate respiratory insufficiency. J Trauma 1985;25:1065.
148. Hurst JM, Branson RD, DeHaven CB. The role of high frequency ventilation in post-traumatic respiratory insufficiency. J Trauma 1987;27:236.
149. Hussain SNA, Roussos C. Distribution of respiratory muscle and organ blood flow during endotoxic shock in dogs. J Appl Physiol 1985;59:1802.
150. Hyers TM. Pathogenesis of adult respiratory distress syndrome: current concepts. Sem Respir Med 1981;2:104.
151. Ingbar DH, Matthay RA. Pulmonary sequelae and lung repair in survivors of the adult respiratory distress syndrome. Crit Care Clin 1986;2:629.
152. Jacobs H, Craddock P, Hammerschmidt D, et al. Complement induced granulocyte aggregation: an unsuspected mechanism of disease. N Engl J Med 1980;302:789.
153. Jardin F, Gurdjian F, Desfonds P, et al. Effect of dopamine on intrapulmonary shunt fraction and oxygen transport in severe sepsis with circulatory and respiratory failure. Crit Care Med 1979;7:273.
154. Jardin F, Farcot JC, Boisante L, et al. Influence of positive end-expiratory pressure on left ventricular performance. N Engl J Med 1981;304:387.
155. Jardin F, Genevroy B, Pazin M, et al. Inability to titrate PEEP in patients with acute respiratory failure using end-tidal carbon dioxide measurements. Anesthesiology 1985;62:530.
156. Jenkinson SG. Pulmonary oxygen toxicity. Clin Chest Med 1982;3:109.

157. Jobe A, Ikegami M. Surfactant for the treatment of respiratory distress syndrome. Am Rev Respir Dis 1987;136:1256.
158. Johanson WG. Bacterial infection in ARDS. Pathogenic mechanisms and consequences. Critical Care: State of the Art 1984;5:H1.
159. Johnson KD, Cadambi A, Seibert GB. Incidence of adult respiratory distress syndrome in patients with multiple musculoskeletal injuries: effects of early operative stabilization of fractures. J Trauma 1985;25:375.
160. Johnson TH, Altman AR, McCaffree RD. Radiologic considerations in the adult respiratory distress syndrome treated with positive end-expiratory pressure (PEEP). Clin Chest Med 1982;3:89.
161. Judson MA. Pharmacotherapy of ARDS. Probl Crit Care 1987;1:401.
162. Kanak R, Fahey PJ, Vaderwarf C. Oxygen cost of breathing. Changes dependent upon mode of mechanical ventilation. Chest 1985;87:126.
163. Kaplan RL, Sahn SA, Petty TL. Incidence and outcome of the respiratory distress syndrome in gram-negative sepsis. Arch Intern Med 1979;139:867.
164. Karch SB. Pathology of the lung in near-drowning. Am J Emerg Med 1986;4:4.
165. Katz JA, Marks JD. Inspiratory work with and without continuous positive airway pressure in patients with acute respiratory failure. Anesthesiology 1985;63:598.
166. Katz JA, Aberman A, Frand V, et al. Heroin pulmonary edema: evidence for increased pulmonary capillary permeability. Am Rev Respir Dis 1972;106:472.
167. Katz JA, Ozanne GM, Zinn SE, Fairley HB. Time course and mechanisms of lung-volume increase with PEEP in acute pulmonary failure. Anesthesiology 1981;54:9.
168. Katz JA, Roger WK, Gjerde GE. Inspiratory work and airway pressure with continuous positive airway pressure delivery systems. Chest 1985;88:519.
169. Ketai LH, Grum CM. C3a and adult respiratory distress syndrome after massive transfusion. Crit Care Med 1986; 14:1001.
170. Kimura T, Toung JR, Margolis S, et al. Respiratory failure in acute pancreatitis; the role of free fatty acids. Surgery 1980;87:509.
171. Kirby RR. The treatment of adult respiratory distress syndrome (ARDS). Semin Anesth 1982;1:312.
172. Kirby RR. Continuous positive airway pressure. To breathe or not to breathe. Anesthesiology 1985;63:578.
173. Kirby RR, Downs JB, Civetta JM, et al. High level positive end-expiratory pressure (PEEP) in acute respiratory insufficiency. Chest 1975;67:156.
174. Klein JJ, van Haeringen JR, Sluiter HJ, et al. Pulmonary function after recovery from the adult respiratory distress syndrome. Chest 1976;69:350.
175. Klose R, Osswald PM. Effects of PEEP on pulmonary mechanics and oxygen transport in the late stages of acute pulmonary failure. Intens Care Med 1981;7:165.
176. Knaus WA, Draper EA, Wagner DP, et al. Prognosis in acute organ-system failure. Ann Surg 1985;202:685.
177. Krausz M, Perel A, Eimerl D, et al. Cardiopulmonary effects of volume loading in patients in septic shock. Ann Surg 1977;183:249.
178. Lakshminarayan S, Hudson LD. Pulmonary function following adult respiratory distress syndrome. Sem Respir Med 1981;2:160.
179. Lakshminarayan S, Stanford RE, Petty TL. Prognosis after recovery from adult respiratory distress syndrome. Am Rev Respir Dis 1976;113:7.
180. Lamy M, Fallat RJ, Koeniger E, et al. Pathologic features and mechanisms of hypoxemia in adult respiratory distress syndrome. Am Rev Respir Dis 1976;114:267.
181. Laufe MD, Simon RH, Flint A, et al. Adult respiratory distress syndrome in neutropenic patients. Am J Med 1986;80:1022.
182. Lava J, Rice C, Moss G, et al. Pulmonary dysfunction in sepsis. Is pulmonary edema the culprit? J Trauma 1982;22:280.
183. Lawler PGP, Nunn JF. A reassessment of the validity of the iso-shunt graph. Br J Anaesth 1984;56:1325.
184. Lazar NM, Luce JM. Hemodynamic assessment and management of patients with the adult respiratory distress syndrome. Crit Care Clin 1986;2:601.
185. Lee CT, Fein AM, Lippman M, et al. Elastolytic activity in pulmonary lavage fluid from patients with the adult respiratory distress syndrome. N Engl J Med 1981;304:192.
186. Lee DS, Kobrine A. Neurogenic pulmonary edema associated with ruptured spinal cord arteriovenous malformation. Neurosurgery 1983;12:691.
187. Lemaire F, Gastine H, Regnier B, et al. Perfusion changes modify intrapulmonary shunting (Qs/Qt) in patients with adult respiratory distress syndrome (ARDS). Am Rev Respir Dis 1978;117(suppl):144.
188. Lewis FR, Blaisdell FW, Scholbohm RM. Incidence and outcome of post-traumatic respiratory failure. Arch Surg 1977;112:436.
189. Liebman PR, Patten MT, Manny J, et al. The mechanism of depressed cardiac output on positive end-expiratory pressure (PEEP). Surgery 1978;83:594.
190. Loyd JE, Newman JH, Brigham KL. Permeability pulmonary edema. Diagnosis and management. Arch Intern Med 1984;144:143.
191. Lucas CE, Ross M, Wilson FR. Physiologic shunting in the lungs in shock or trauma. Surg Forum 1968;19:35.
192. Luce JM. Pathogenesis and management of septic shock. Chest 1987;91:883.
193. Luce JM, Pierson DJ. Corticosteroids and antibiotics in adult respiratory distress syndrome: a review. Semin Respir Med 1981;2:151.
194. Luce JM, Robertson HT, Huang T, et al. The effects of expiratory positive airway pressure on the resolution of oleic acid induced lung injury in dogs. Am Rev Respir Dis 1985;125:716.
195. Lynch JP, Mhyre JG, Dantzker DR. Influence of cardiac output on intrapulmonary shunt. J Appl Physiol 1979;46:315.
196. Maggart M, Stewart S. The mechanisms and management of noncardiogenic pulmonary edema following cardiopulmonary bypass. Ann Thorac Surg 1987;43:231.
197. Malik AB. Pulmonary vascular response to increase in intracranial pressure. Role of sympathetic mechanisms. J Appl Physiol 1977;42:335.
198. Mancebo J, Artigas A. A clinical study of the adult respiratory distress syndrome. Crit Care Med 1987;15:243.
199. Manwaring D, Curreri PW. Platelet and neutrophil sequestration after fragment D-induced respiratory distress. Circ Shock 1982;9:75.
200. Marini JJ, Culver BH, Butler J. Effect of positive end-expiratory pressure on canine ventricular function curves. J Appl Physiol 1981;51:1367.
201. Marini JJ, Rodriguez M, Lamb V. Bedside estimation of the inspiratory work of breathing during mechanical ventilation. Chest 1986;89:56.
202. Martin TG. Near drowning and cold water immersion. Ann Emerg Med 1984;13:263.
203. Matthay MA. Pathophysiology of pulmonary edema. Clin Chest Med 1985;6:301.
204. Maunder RJ. Clinical prediction of the adult respiratory distress syndrome. Clin Chest Med 1985;6:413.
205. Maunder RJ, Hackman RC, Riff E, et al. Occurrence of the adult

respiratory distress syndrome in neutropenic patients. Am Rev Respir Dis 1986;133:313.
206. Maunder RJ, Shuman WP, McHugh JW, et al. Preservation of normal lung regions in the adult respiratory distress syndrome: analysis by computed tomography. JAMA 1986;255:1463.
207. McGuire W, Spragg R, Cohen A, et al. Studies on the pathogenesis of the adult respiratory distress syndrome. J Clin Invest 1982;69:543.
208. Mecca RS. Clinical aspects of pulmonary edema. In: Kirby RR, Taylor RW, eds. Respiratory failure. Yearbook Medical Publishers, Chicago: 1986:191.
209. Mecklenburgh JS, Latto IP, Al-Obaidi TAA, et al. Excessive work of breathing during intermittent mandatory ventilation. Br J Anaesth 1986;58:1048.
210. Melon E, Bonnet F, Lepresle E, et al. Altered capillary permeability in neurogenic pulmonary edema. Intens Care Med 1985;11:323.
211. Meyrick BO. Pathology of pulmonary edema. Semin Respir Med 1983;4:267.
212. Meyrick BO. Pathology of the adult respiratory distress syndrome. Crit Care Clin 1986;2:405.
213. Mikhail MS, Banner MJ, Gallagher TJ. Hemodynamic effects of positive end-expiratory pressure during high-frequency ventilation. Crit Care Med 1985;13:733.
214. Mishkin FS, Niden A, Kumar A, et al. Albumin lung/heart ratio change. A simple clinical means of documenting increased pulmonary endothelial permeability to protein. JAMA 1987;257:953.
215. Mizock BA. Controversies in lactic acidosis. Implications in critically ill patients. JAMA 1987;258:497.
216. Modell JH. Biology of drowning. Annu Rev Med 1978;29:1.
217. Mohsenifar Z, Goldbach P, Tashkin DP, et al. Relationship between $O_2$ delivery and $O_2$ consumption in the adult respiratory distress syndrome. Chest 1983;84:267.
218. Montgomery AB, Stager MA, Carrico CJ, et al. Causes of mortality in patients with the adult respiratory distress syndrome. Am Rev Respir Dis 1985;132:485.
219. Morel DR, Dargent F, Bachman M, et al. Pulmonary extraction of serotonin and propranolol in patients with adult respiratory distress syndrome. Am Rev Respir Dis 1985;132:479.
220. Morganroth ML, Morganroth JL, Nett LM, et al. Criteria for weaning from prolonged mechanical ventilation. Arch Intern Med 1984;144:1012.
221. Moss GS. Pulmonary involvement in hypovolemic shock. Annu Rev Med 1972;23:201.
222. Murray JF. The adult respiratory distress syndrome (may it rest in peace). Am Rev Respir Dis 1975;111:716.
223. Murray IP, Modell JH, Gallagher TJ, et al. Titration of PEEP by the arterial minus end-tidal carbon dioxide gradient. Chest 1984;85:100.
224. Nelson LD, Civetta JM, Hudson-Civetta J. Titrating positive end-expiratory pressure therapy in patients with early moderate arterial hypoxemia. Crit Care Med 1987;15:14.
225. Newman JH. ARDS: new insights and unresolved problems. Intens Care Med 1983;9:303.
226. Newman JH. Pulmonary vascular reactivity in primary pulmonary edema. Semin Respir Med 1983;4:296.
227. Newman JH. Sepsis and pulmonary edema. Clin Chest Med 1985;6:371.
228. Nicholson DP. Corticosteroids in the treatment of septic shock and the adult respiratory distress syndrome. Med Clin North Am 1983;67:717.
229. Nicholson DP. Glucocorticoids in the treatment of shock and the adult respiratory distress syndrome. Clin Chest Med 1983;3:558.
230. Norwood SH, Civetta JM. The adult respiratory distress syndrome. Surg Gynecol Obstet 1985;161:497.
231. Norwood SH, Civetta JM. Ventilatory support in patients with ARDS. Surg Clin North Am 1985;65:895.
232. Nuytinck J, Goris R, Redl H, et al. Post-traumatic complications and inflammatory mediators. Arch Surg 1986;121:886.
233. Ogletree ML. Roles of arachidonic acid metabolites in endotoxin-induced pulmonary edema. Semin Respir Med 1983;4:303.
234. Ognibene FP, Martin SE, Parker MM, et al. Adult respiratory distress syndrome in patients with severe neutropenia. N Engl J Med 1986;315:547.
235. Pare PD, Warriner B, Baile EM, et al. Redistribution of pulmonary extra-vascular lung water with positive end-expiratory pressure in canine pulmonary edema. Am Rev Respir Dis 1983;127:590.
236. Parker RE. Secondary pulmonary edema. Semin Respir Med 1983;4:279.
237. Parsons PE, Fowler AA, Hyers TM, et al. Chemotactic activity in bronchoalveolar lavage fluid from patients with adult respiratory distress syndrome. Am Rev Respir Dis 1985;132:490.
238. Pavlin EG. Anesthesia for the traumatized patient. Can Anaesth Soc J 1983;30:S27.
239. Pavlin EG, Yazaki S, Winn R, et al. Ethrane and halothane anesthesia increases shunt ($\dot{Q}_s/\dot{Q}_t$) in goats following acid aspiration. Anesthesiology 1981;55:A382.
240. Pavlin EG, Yazaki S, Winn R, et al. The effect of isoflurane and ketamine anesthesia on pulmonary shunt ($\dot{Q}_s/\dot{Q}_t$) in goats following acid aspiration. Anesthesiology 1983;59:A509.
241. Pavlin DJ, Tyler D, Nessly ML, et al. Effects of breathing 80% oxygen on water and albumin accumulation in oleic acid injured rabbit lungs. Crit Care Med 1987;15:204.
242. Peltier LF. Fat embolism. Clin Orthop 1984;187:3.
243. Pepe PE. The clinical entity of adult respiratory distress syndrome. Definition, prediction and prognosis. Crit Care Clin 1986;2:377.
244. Pepe PE, Culver BH. Independently measured oxygen consumption during reduction of oxygen delivery by positive end-expiratory pressure. Am Rev Respir Dis 1985;132:788.
245. Pepe PE, Potkin RT, Reus DH, et al. Clinical predictors of the adult respiratory distress syndrome. Am J Surg 1982;144:124.
246. Pepe PE, Thomas RG, Stager MA, et al. Early prediction of the adult respiratory distress syndrome by a simple scoring method. Ann Emerg Med 1983;12:749.
247. Pepe PE, Hudson LD, Carrico CJ. Early application of positive end-expiratory pressure in patients at risk for the adult respiratory distress syndrome. N Engl J Med 1984;311:281.
248. Perschan RA, Munson ES, Chapin JC. Pulmonary interstitial edema after multiple venous air emboli. Anesthesiology 1976;45:364.
249. Petty TL. The adult respiratory distress syndrome. Confessions of a "lumper". Am Rev Respir Dis 1975;111:713.
250. Petty TL. Adult respiratory distress syndrome: historical perspective and definition. Semin Respir Med 1981;2:99.
251. Petty TL, Fowler AA. Another look at ARDS. Chest 1982;82:98.
252. Petty TL, Reiss OK, Paul GW, et al. Characteristics of pulmonary surfactant in adult respiratory distress syndrome associated with trauma and shock. Am Rev Respir Dis 1977;115:531.
253. Petty TL, Silvers GW, Paul GW, et al. Abnormalities in lung elastic properties and surfactant function in adult respiratory distress syndrome. Chest 1979;75:571.
254. Pfenninger J, Gerber A, Tschappeler H, et al. Adult respiratory distress syndrome in children. J Pediatr 1982;101:352.
255. Philbin DM, Sullivan SF, Bowman FO, et al. Post-operative hypoxemia: contribution of the cardiac output. Anesthesiology 1970;32:136.
256. Pietra GG, Ruttner JR, Wust W, et al. The lung after trauma and shock: fine structure of the alveolar capillary barrier in 23 autopsies. J Trauma 1981;21:454.

257. Pinsky MR. The influence of positive pressure ventilation on cardiovascular function in the critically ill. Crit Care Clin 1985;1:699.
258. Pistolesi M, Miniati M, Milne E, et al. The chest roentgenogram in pulmonary edema. Clin Chest Med 1985;6:315.
259. Poole GV, Meredith JW, Pennall T, et al. Comparison of colloids and crystalloids in resuscitation from hemorrhagic shock. Surg Gynecol Obstet 1982;154:577.
260. Popovsky MA, Abel MD, Moore SB. Transfusion related acute lung injury associated with passive transfer of antileukocyte antibodies. Am Rev Respir Dis 1983;128:689.
261. Powers SR, Burdge R, Leather R, et al. Studies of pulmonary insufficiency in non-thoracic trauma. J Trauma 1972;12:1.
262. Pratt PC. Pathology of adult respiratory distress syndrome: implications regarding therapy. Semin Respir Med 1982;4:79.
263. Prewitt RM, Oppenheimer L, Sutherland JB, et al. Effect of positive end-expiratory pressure on left ventricular mechanics in patients with hypoxemic respiratory failure. Anesthesiology 1981;55:409.
264. Qvist J, Pontoppidan H, Wilson RS, et al. Hemodynamic responses to mechanical ventilation with PEEP: the effect of hypervolemia. Anesthesiology 1975;42:45.
265. Raffin TA. Novel approaches to ARDS and sepsis. Crit Care: State Art 1986;7:247.
266. Ralph DD, Robertson HT. Respiratory gas exchange in adult respiratory distress syndrome. Semin Respir Med 1981; 2:114.
267. Ralph DD, Robertson HT, Weaver LJ, et al. Distribution of ventilation and perfusion during positive end-expiratory pressure in the adult respiratory distress syndrome. Am Rev Respir Dis 1985;131:54.
268. Rasanen J, Downs JB, DeHaven B. Titration of continuous positive airway pressure by real-time dual oximetry. Chest 1987;92:853.
269. Rasanen J, Downs JB, Malec DJ, et al. Estimation of oxygen utilization by dual oximetry. Ann Surg 1987;206:621.
270. Rinaldo JE. Mediation of ARDS by leukocytes: clinical evidence and implications for therapy. Chest 1986;89:590.
271. Rinaldo JE. The prognosis of the adult respiratory distress syndrome: inappropriate pessimism? Chest 1986;90:470.
272. Rinaldo JE, Rogers RM. Adult respiratory distress syndrome. N Engl J Med 1986;315:578.
273. Rinaldo JE, Petty TL. Indicators of risk, course, and prognosis in adult respiratory distress syndrome. Am Rev Respir Dis 1986;133:343.
274. Rinaldo JE, Rogers RM. Adult respiratory distress syndrome: changing concepts of lung injury and repair. N Engl J Med 1982;306:900.
275. Riska EB, Myllynen P. Fat embolism in patients with multiple injuries. J Trauma 1982;22:891.
276. Robotham JL, Bell RC, Bodke FR, et al. Left ventricular geometry during positive end-expiratory pressure in dogs. Crit Care Med 1985;13:617.
277. Rotman HH, Lavelle TF, Dimcheff DG, et al. Long term physiological consequences of the adult respiratory distress syndrome. Chest 1977;72:190.
278. Rouby JJ, Simonneau G, Benhamou D, et al. Factors influencing pulmonary volumes and $CO_2$ elimination during high frequency jet ventilation. Anesthesiology 1985;63:473.
279. Roussos C, Macklem PT. Diaphragmatic fatigue in man. J Appl Physiol 1977;43:189.
280. Roussos C, Macklem PT. The respiratory muscles. N Engl J Med 1982;307:786.
281. Royston D. A sideways look at ARDS. Br J Anaesth 1986; 58:1207.
282. Rutledge R, Sheldon GF, Collins ML. Massive transfusion. Crit Care Clin 1986;2:791.
283. Sahn SA, Lakshminarayan S. Bedside criteria for discontinuation of mechanical ventilation. Chest 1973;63:1002.
284. Saldeen T. The microembolism syndrome. Microvasc Res 1976;11:227.
285. Saldeen T. Clotting, microembolism, and inhibition of fibrinolysis in adult respiratory distress. Surg Clin North Am 1983;63:285.
286. Sandoval J, Long GR, Skoog C, et al. Independent influence of blood flow rate and mixed venous $PO_2$ on shunt fraction. J Appl Physiol 1983;55:1128.
287. Sanfrez H, Buckley GB, Cameron JL. The role of oxygen derived free radicals in the pathogenesis of acute pancreatitis. Ann Surg 1984;200:405.
288. Scharf SM, Brown R. Influence of the right ventricle on canine left ventricular function with PEEP. J Appl Physiol 1982;52:254.
289. Schein R, Bergman R, Marcial E, et al. Complement activation and corticosteroid therapy in the development of the adult respiratory distress syndrome. Chest 1987;91:850.
290. Schlag G, Redl HR. Morphology of the human lung after traumatic injury. In: Zapol WM, Falke KJ, eds. Acute respiratory failure. New York: Marcel Dekker, 1985:161.
291. Schneider RC, Zápol WM, Carvalho AC. Platelet consumption and sequestration in severe acute respiratory failure. Am Rev Respir Dis 1980;122:445.
292. Schoene RB. Pulmonary edema at high altitudes. Clin Chest Med 1985;6:491.
293. Schuster DP, Trulock EP. Correlation of changes in oxygenation, lung water and hemodynamics after oleic acid-induced acute lung injury in dogs. Crit Care Med 1984;12:1044.
294. Schwartz DJ, Wynne JW, Gibbs CP, et al. The pulmonary consequences of aspiration of gastric contents at pH values greater than 2.5. Am Rev Respir Dis 1980;121:119.
295. Serafin WE, Austen KF. Mediators of immediate hypersensitivity reactions. N Engl J Med 1987;317:30.
296. Shapiro BA, Cane RD, Harrison RA. Positive end-expiratory pressure therapy in adults with special reference to acute lung injury. Crit Care Med 1984;12:127.
297. Sheller JR, Snapper JR. Effects of pulmonary edema on airway reactivity. Semin Respir Med 1983;4:293.
298. Shoemaker WC. Circulatory pathophysiology of ARDS and its fluid management. In: Shoemaker WC, Thompson WL, Holbrook PR, eds. Textbook of critical care. Philadelphia: WB Saunders, 1984:310.
299. Shoemaker WC, Appel P, Czer LSC, et al. Pathogenesis of respiratory failure (ARDS) after hemorrhage and trauma. Crit Care Med 1980;8:504.
300. Sibbald WJ, Bone RC. The adult respiratory distress in 1987: is it a systemic disease? Crit Care: State Art 1987;8:279.
301. Sibbald WJ, Driedger AA, Myers AL, et al. Biventricular function in the adult respiratory distress syndrome. Chest 1983;84:126.
302. Sibbald WJ, Driedger AA, Wells GA, et al. The short term effects of increasing plasma colloid pressure in patients with noncardiac pulmonary edema. Surgery 1983;93:620.
303. Sibbald WJ, Driedger AA, Cunningham DG, et al. Right and left ventricular performance in acute hypoxemic respiratory failure. Crit Care Med 1986;14:852.
304. Siegel JH, Greenspan M, Del Guerico LRM. Abnormal vascular tone, defective oxygen transport and myocardial failure in human septic shock. Ann Surg 1967;165:504.
305. Siegel JH, Giovannini I, Coleman B. Ventilation: perfusion maldistribution secondary to the hyperdynamic cardiovascular state as the major cause of increased pulmonary shunting in human sepsis. J Trauma 1979;19:432.
306. Siegel JH, Stoklosa JC, Borg U. Cardiorespiratory management of the adult respiratory distress syndrome. In: Siegel JH, ed. Trauma: emergency surgery and critical care. New York: Churchill Livingstone, 1987:581.

307. Sivak ED, Wiedemann HP. Clinical measurement of extravascular lung water. Crit Care Clin 1986;2:511.
308. Sladen A. High-frequency jet ventilation in trauma. In: Maull KI, Cleveland HC, Strauch GO, Wolferth CC, eds. Advances in trauma. Chicago: Year Book Medical Publishers, 1986:167.
309. Smith G, Winter PM, Wheelis RF. Increased normobaric oxygen tolerance of rabbits following oleic acid-induced lung damage. J Appl Physiol 1973;35:395.
310. Smith G, Cheney FW, Winter PM. The effect of change in cardiac output on intrapulmonary shunting. Br J Anaesth 1974;46:337.
311. Snapper JR, Sheller JR. Effects of pulmonary edema on lung mechanics. Semin Respir Med 1983;4:289.
312. Snapper JR, Hutchison AA, Ogletree ML, et al. Lung mechanics in pulmonary edema. Clin Chest Med 1985;6:393.
312a. Snider M. Adult respiratory distress syndrome in the trauma patient. Crit Care Clin 1990;6:103.
313. Snow RL, Davies P, Pontoppidan H, et al. Pulmonary vascular remodeling in adult respiratory distress syndrome. Am Rev Respir Dis 1982;126:887.
314. Solomkin JS, Cotta LA, Satoh PS, et al. Complement activation and clearance in acute illness and injury: evidence for $C5_a$ as a cell-directed mediator of the adult respiratory distress syndrome in man. Surgery 1985;97:668.
315. Spicer KM, Reines DH, Frey GD. Diagnosis of adult respiratory distress syndrome with Tc-99m human serum albumin and portable probe. Crit Care Med 1986;14:669.
316. Springer RR, Stevens DM. The influence of PEEP on survival of patients in respiratory failure. Am J Med 1979;66:196.
317. Sprung CL, Rackow EC, Fein IA, et al: The spectrum of pulmonary edema. Am Rev Respir Dis 1981;124:718.
318. Staub NC. Pathogenesis of pulmonary edema. Am Rev Respir Dis 1974;109:318.
319. Staub NC. Pulmonary edema. Physiol Rev 1974;54:678.
320. Staub NC. Pulmonary edema due to increased microvascular permeability. Annu Rev Med 1981;32:291.
321. Staub NC. Pathophysiology of pulmonary edema. In: Staub NC, Taylor AE, eds. Edema. New York: Raven Press, 1984:719.
322. Staub NC. Clinical use of lung water measurements. Chest 1986;90:589.
323. Stevens JH, Raffin TA. Adult respiratory distress syndrome. Postgrad Med J 1984;60:505 and 1984;60:573.
324. Stevens JH, O'Hanley P, Shapiro JM, et al. Effects of anti-C5a antibodies on the adult respiratory distress syndrome in septic primates. J Clin Invest 1986;77:1812.
325. Stock MC, Downs JB, Frolicher DA. Airway pressure release ventilation. Crit Care Med 1987;15:462.
326. Street MK, Hopkinson RB. Evaluation of the comfort of spontaneous respiration through three ventilator systems. Intens Care Med 1987;13:405.
327. Sturm JA, Wisner DH, Oestern HJ, et al. Increased lung capillary permeability after trauma. A prospective clinical study. J Trauma 1986;26:409.
328. Summer W, Haponik E. Inhalation of irritant gases. Clin Chest Med 1981;2:273.
329. Suter PM. Appropriate lung distension for gas exchange in ARDS. Chest 1984;85:4.
330. Suter PM, Fairley HB, Isenberg MD. Optimum end-expiratory airway pressure in patients with acute pulmonary failure. N Engl J Med 1975;292:284.
331. Suter PM, Fairley HB, Schlobohm RM. Shunt, lung volume and perfusion during short periods of ventilation with oxygen. Anesthesiology 1975;43:617.
332. Svenningsen N, Robertson B, Andreason B, et al. Endotracheal administration of surfactant in very low birth weight infants with respiratory distress syndrome. Crit Care Med 1987;15:918.
333. Tahvanainen J, Salmenpera M, Nikki P. Extubation criteria after weaning from intermittent mandatory ventilation and continuous positive airway pressure. Crit Care Med 1983;11:702.
334. Tate RM, Repine JE. Neutrophils and the adult respiratory distress syndrome. Am Rev Respir Dis 1983;128:552.
335. Taylor RW. The adult respiratory distress syndrome. In: Kirby RR, Taylor RW, eds. Respiratory failure. Chicago: Year Book Medical Publishers, 1986:208.
336. Tennenberg SD, Jacobs MP, Solomkin JS, et al. Increased pulmonary alveolar capillary permeability in patients at risk for adult respiratory distress syndrome. Crit Care Med 1987; 15:289.
337. Tennenberg SD, Jacobs MP, Solomkin JS. Complement-mediated neutrophil activation in sepsis- and trauma-related adult respiratory distress syndrome. Arch Surg 1987;122:26.
338. Theodore J, Robin ED. Speculations on neurogenic pulmonary edema. Am Rev Respir Dis 1976;113:405.
339. Thommasen HV, Russel JA, Boyko WJ, et al. Transient leukopenia associated with adult respiratory distress syndrome. Lancet 1984;1:809.
340. Thorning DR, Howard ML, Hudson LD, et al. Pulmonary responses to smoke inhalation. Human Pathol 1982;13:355.
341. Tokioka H, Kobayashi O, Ohta Y, et al. The acute effects of prostaglandin $E_1$ on the pulmonary circulation and oxygen delivery in patients with the adult respiratory distress syndrome. Intens Care Med 1985;11:61.
342. Tomashefski JF, Davies P, Boggis C, et al. The pulmonary vascular lesions of the adult respiratory distress syndrome. Am J Pathol 1983;112:112.
343. Tracey KJ, Beutler B, Lowry SF, et al. Shock and tissue injury induced by recombinant human cachectin. Science 1986;244:470.
344. Tranbaugh RF, Lewis FR. Mechanisms and etiologic factors of pulmonary edema. Surg Gynecol Obstet 1984;158:193.
345. Tyler DC. Positive end-expiratory pressure: a review. Crit Care Med 1983;11:300.
346. Venus B, Smith RA, Mathru M. National survey of methods and criteria used for weaning from mechanical ventilation. Crit Care Med 1987;15:530.
347. Veterans Administration Systemic Sepsis Cooperative Study Group: Effect of high-dose glucocorticoid therapy on mortality in patients with clinical signs of systemic sepsis. N Engl J Med 1987;317:659.
348. Viale JP, Annat G, Bertrand O, et al. Additional inspiratory work in intubated patients breathing with continuous positive airway pressure systems. Anesthesiology 1985;63:536.
349. Viires N, Sillye G, Aubier M, et al. Regional blood flow distribution in the dog during induced hypotension and low cardiac output. J Clin Invest 1983;72:935.
350. Viquerat CE, Righetti A, Suter PM. Biventricular volumes and function in patients with adult respiratory distress syndrome ventilated with PEEP. Chest 1983;83:509.
351. Vito L, Dennis RC, Weisel RD. Sepsis presenting as acute respiratory insufficiency. Surg Gynecol Obstet 1974;138:896.
352. Ward PA, Johnson KJ, Till GO, et al. Current concepts regarding adult respiratory distress syndrome. Ann Emerg Med 1985;14:725.
353. Ward PA, Till GO, Hatherill JR, et al. Systemic complement activation, lung injury and products of lipid peroxidation. J Clin Invest 1985;76:517.
354. Ward PA, Johnson KJ, Till GO. Complement and experimental respiratory failure. Intens Care Med 1986;12:17.
355. Waxman K, Shoemaker WC. Management of postoperative and posttraumatic respiratory failure in the intensive care unit. Surg Clin North Am 1980;60:1413.
356. Weigelt J, Mitchell RA, Snyder WH. Early identification of pa-

tients prone to develop the respiratory distress syndrome. Am J Surg 1981;142:687.

357. Weigelt J, Norcross J, Snyder W, et al. Early steroid therapy for respiratory failure. Arch Surg 1986;120:536.
358. Weinberg P, Matthay M, Webster R, et al. Biologically active products of complement and acute lung injury in patients with the sepsis syndrome. Am Rev Respir Dis 1984;130:791.
359. Weisman IM, Rinaldo JE, Rogers RM. Positive end-expiratory pressure in adult respiratory distress syndrome. N Engl J Med 1982;307:1381.
360. Weisman IM, Rinaldo JE, Rogers RM, et al. Intermittent mandatory ventilation. Am Rev Respir Dis 1983;127:641.
361. Westaby S. Mechanism of membrane damage and surfactant depletion in acute lung injury. Intens Care Med 1986;12:2.
362. Westaby S. Organ dysfunction after cardiopulmonary bypass. A systemic inflammatory reaction initiated by the extracorporeal circuit. Intens Care Med 1987;13:89.
363. Wiener-Kronish JP, Berthiaume Y, Albertine K. Pleural effusion and pulmonary edema. Clin Chest Med 1985;6:509.
364. Wilson RS, Pontoppidan H. Acute respiratory failure: diagnostic and therapeutic criteria. Crit Care Med 1974;2:293.
365. Woodring JH. Pulmonary interstitial emphysema in the adult respiratory distress syndrome. Crit Care Med 1985;13:786.
366. Wray NP, Nicotra MB. Pathogenesis of neurogenic pulmonary edema. Am Rev Respir Dis 1978;118:783.
367. Wright JR, Clements JA. Metabolism and turnover of lung surfactant. Am Rev Respir Dis 1987;135:426.
368. Yeston NS, Niehoff JM. Trauma and pulmonary insufficiency: mediators and modulators of adult respiratory distress syndrome. Int Anesth Clin 1987;25:91.
369. Zapol WM, Snider MT. Pulmonary hypertension in severe acute respiratory failure. N Engl J Med 1977;296:476.
370. Zimmerman GA, Renzetti AD, Hill HR. Circulatory polymorphonuclear leukocyte activity in patients with the adult respiratory distress syndrome. Chest 1983;83:87S.
371. Zimmerman GA, Renzetti AD, Hill HR. Functional and metabolic activity of granulocytes from patients with adult respiratory distress syndrome. Am Rev Respir Dis 1983;127:290.

# Chapter Twenty-Five

M. Donald McGoldrick
Levon M. Capan

# Acute Renal Failure in the Injured

Acute renal failure (ARF), the abrupt decline of renal function, may be accompanied by normal urine volume, oliguria, (urine volume <400 mL/day) or anuria. It always results in retention of nitrogenous waste products, with a resultant increase in blood urea nitrogen (BUN) and serum creatinine. Posttraumatic ARF was first well documented during World War II.[39,49] During the 1940s the mortality rate from renal failure was 90%, but hemodialysis has since decreased this rate to 50%.[52] The incidence of posttraumatic ARF has also decreased over the years. In the 1940s ARF occurred in 33% of seriously injured American soldiers. The incidence decreased to 0.5% in the 1950s and to approximately 0.2% during the 1960s.[259] Most of this decline is related to the early availability of medical and surgical care. However, improved care has introduced the risks of drug- and radiocontrast dye-induced ARF. Up to 27% of today's ARF cases occur in a hospital setting.[172]

## ETIOLOGY OF RENAL DYSFUNCTION IN THE INJURED PATIENT

Although acute tubular necrosis (ATN) is the most serious cause of renal dysfunction, other possibilities should be considered before initiating treatment. The most common causes of renal dysfunction within the first few days after trauma are prerenal azotemia, ATN, obstructive uropathy, and renal vascular injury. Renal dysfunction that develops 1 to 2 weeks after trauma is usually caused by (a) ATN secondary to drug- or radiocontrast dye-induced ischemia, (b) acute tubular interstitial nephritis (ATIN), most frequently drug-induced, (c) postinfectious glomerulonephritis, or (d) prerenal azotemia.

### PRERENAL AZOTEMIA

Prerenal azotemia is the most common cause of oliguria.[11] Suboptimal perfusion of the nephrons due to extracellular fluid (ECF) depletion and cardiac output reduction is the primary cause of this disorder. Prerenal azotemia develops only after renal responses to decreased glomerular blood flow fail to maintain normal kidney perfusion, filtration, and reabsorption. The compensatory mechanisms utilized by the healthy kidney are autoregulatory dilation of the afferent arterioles, tubuloglomerular feedback, modulation of the actions of systemic vasoconstrictors by intrarenal vasodilator prostaglandins, constriction of the efferent arterioles, and the fluid-retaining ability of the kidney.[19] Clinically, these patients are dehydrated and may show signs of hypovolemia. Prerenal azotemia can be differentiated from ATN by clinical signs and by blood and urine findings described later in this chapter. The urine concentrating function of the kidneys remains intact in prerenal azotemia, whereas it is lost in ATN. Appropriate fluid therapy is required to prevent or treat posttraumatic prerenal azotemia.

### POSTRENAL OBSTRUCTION

After abdominal and/or pelvic injuries, the anatomic integrity of the entire urinary tract should be assessed carefully. Blunt or penetrating trauma to any portion of the urinary tract may result in oliguria or renal dysfunction. Renal failure may occur due to the obstruction of urinary passages by extrinsic compression from hematomas,[124] displaced bony fragments, or massive intraluminal blood clots. Disruption of urinary conduits or rupture of the urinary bladder may cause extravasation of urine and may produce a clinical picture of ARF in spite of normal renal function.

Obstruction at or below the level of the bladder may be ruled out by inserting a urinary catheter. If the possibility of obstructive uropathy still cannot be excluded, renal ultrasound imaging should be performed. B-mode scanning provides the most reliable confirmatory test, with an accuracy greater than 90%.[239] Real-time ultrasonography is equally sensitive and can shorten the examination time considerably.[146] Thus, it is potentially useful in the seriously injured patient (Table 25-1).

Obstructive renal failure is treated by relieving the obstruction. Percutaneous nephrostomy, double-J ureteral stent, or surgical bypass of the obstruction is usually necessary. Introduction of indwelling Silastic ureteral stents, which can remain in place for a long time, has solved the problem of long-term external drainage. These techniques can be applied successfully for temporary or permanent relief of obstruction and, hence, prevention of ARF.

## VASCULAR INJURY

Injury to renal vessels can result in gross hematuria and retroperitoneal bleeding, but ARF after isolated renal vascular injury is uncommon. Traumatic renal artery thrombosis requires early diagnosis and treatment to avoid possible renal infarction.[160] Similarly, the prognosis of renal vein thrombosis is improved if the condition is diagnosed and treated without delay (Table 25-1). Most patients with renal vein thrombosis have severe nephrotic syndrome, but only 30% develop ARF.

Fulminant ischemic cortical necrosis is distinguishable from ATN pathologically, but not clinically. Cortical necrosis classically occurs as an obstetric complication, but has also been encountered after severe hemorrhage and trauma.[160] Occasionally a renal biopsy may be necessary for a definitive diagnosis, especially when oliguria or anuria has not responded to treatment after a few weeks of therapy.

## ACUTE TUBULAR INTERSTITIAL NEPHRITIS (ATIN)

Acute tubular interstitial nephritis usually presents as oliguric ARF without a history suggesting acute glomerulonephritis or ATN. In the trauma patient, it is almost invariably drug-induced. The drugs that most commonly cause this entity are (a) antibiotics (penicillins, sulfadiazines, and cephalosporins),

TABLE 25-1. History, Physical Findings, Diagnosis, and Treatment of ARF Caused by ATIN, Vascular Disease, and Urinary Outflow Obstruction*

| | RENAL | VASCULAR DISEASE | | POSTRENAL |
|---|---|---|---|---|
| | *ATIN* | *Venous* | *Arterial* | *Urinary Outflow Obstruction* |
| History and physical findings | Drug- or infection-induced | Pre-existing GN | Atheroembolic | Anuria |
| | | 4+ proteinuria (>10 g) | Left-sided valvular lesions of the heart | Men with prostatic disease<br>Women with cancer of cervix |
| | +/− oliguria<br>Findings similar to ATN except history | Severe nephrosis | Arteriosclerotic abdominal aorta<br>Malignant hypertension | Calculi |
| | Eosinophilia<br>Elevated serum IgE levels | Flank pain | Postangiogram | Retroperitoneal trauma and/or surgery |
| | Wright's stain of urine sediment showing eosinopilic casts (eosinophiliuria)<br>Other evidence of drug reaction | | Traumatic renal artery thrombosis, abruptio placentae<br>Flank pain<br>Hematuria<br>Hypertension | |
| Diagnosis and treatment | Dx: + gallium scan, renal biopsy | Dx: IVP, renal venogram | Dx: renal flow scan, renal angiogram | Dx: renal ultrasound, real time ultrasonography, retrograde urogram |
| | Rx: stop the drugs; administer steroids? | Rx: anticogulants and/or streptokinase, treatment of underlying GN | Rx: control BP, embolectomy, surgical repair, anticoagulants and/or streptokinase | Rx: relieve the obstruction |

* From McGoldrick[173] with permission.
ATIN: acute tubular interstitial nephritis; GN: glomerulonephritis; Dx: diagnosis; Rx: treatment.

(b) nonsteroidal anti-inflammatory agents (with the possible exception of Sulindac), (c) diuretics, and (d) others, including cimetidine, allopurinol, and diphenylhydantoin. Many systemic infections may also cause ATIN. A minority of patients with ATIN manifest the classic features of rash, arthralgias, and fever in association with ARF. Peripheral blood eosinophilia and elevated serum IgE levels can help confirm the diagnosis of ATIN, but their absence does not exclude this disorder. Eosinophiliuria is the most useful indicator of ATIN.[164] Improvement in urine output and renal function within several days of removing the offending drug or agent is also suggestive of the diagnosis. The renal uptake of gallium citrate as quantitated by scanning is markedly increased only in ATIN and not in ATN, vasculitis, or pyelonephritis (Table 25-1).[153] This test offers a promising noninvasive method of confirming the diagnosis of ATIN. The diagnosis of ATIN can be made by renal biopsy, if necessary. Although most patients make a good recovery after withdrawal of the offending agent, some patients may deteriorate and develop advanced renal failure requiring dialysis. Corticosteroids seem to shorten the azotemic phase of ATIN[247] and have been recommended for treatment of this disease, provided there is no contraindication to their use.

## ACUTE GLOMERULONEPHRITIS (AGN)

Postinfectious glomerulonephritis can give rise to acute renal failure. The usual histologic picture in such cases is crescentic glomerular inflammation. Visceral abscesses and bacterial endocarditis are the two conditions that may be associated with this disease in trauma victims.

### *Glomerulonephritis with Visceral Abscesses*

Acute glomerulonephritis and ARF may be associated with pyogenic visceral abscesses.[28] The common sites of infection are the respiratory tract and the abdominal organs, but AGN has also been reported to occur with uterine infections and infected vascular prosthetic grafts.[29] Almost any type of bacteria may precipitate glomerulonephritis.[29] Cryoglobulins and circulating immune complexes may be detected. Treatment involves eradication of the underlying infection.

### *Glomerulonephritis Associated with Bacterial Endocarditis*

Infectious endocarditis is not a rare occurrence in the septic trauma patient. The primary source of infection may be the injury site, and secondary sources may be intravenous lines, especially a subclavian hyperalimentation catheter, Hickman catheter, dialysis catheter, or heparin lock. Up to 70% of these patients develop proteinuria and/or hematuria and, on rare occasions, ARF.[103] Frequently, serum complement levels (C3, C5) are depressed. Other abnormal laboratory findings are cryoglobulinemia, rheumatoid factor, hypergammaglobulinemia, and elevated levels of circulating immune complexes. Renal function may improve after the infection is treated. Methylprednisolone has been used successfully in these patients (Table 25-2).[266]

## ACUTE TUBULAR NECROSIS (ATN)

The most common cause of ARF after trauma is ATN. Injured patients with any of the following conditions are likely to develop ATN[23,87,260]:

TABLE 25-2. History, Physical Findings, Diagnosis, and Treatment of Renal Dysfunction Caused by Prerenal Factors, AGN, and ATN*

| | | RENAL | |
|---|---|---|---|
| | PRERENAL FACTORS | *AGN* | *ATN* |
| History and physical findings | ECF volume changes<br>CHF<br>High BUN/creatinine ratio (>10:1)<br>High urinary specific gravity (>1.015)<br>Urine sediment unremarkable<br>Low urine sodium (<10 mEq/L)<br>U/P creatinine >40/1<br>RFI <1<br>Fractional excretion of filtered sodium <1 | Infection exposure<br>Proteinuria<br>Hematuria<br>RBC casts<br>Edema<br>Hypertension<br>Low C3 and C5 levels<br>Elevated levels of ANA, ASO | Ischemia and/or toxin<br>Oliguria<br>Specific gravity ~1.010<br>Brown granular casts<br>$U_{NA}$ >10–20 mEq/L<br>U/P creatinine <20/1<br>RFI >1–2<br>Fractional excretion of filtered Na >1–2 |
| Diagnosis and treatment | Dx: hemodynamic and laboratory findings<br>Rx: treat prerenal problem(s) | Dx: history, laboratory findings, kidney biopsy<br>Rx: observation, steroids, immunosuppressives, pheresis | Dx: renal flow scan, renal ultrasound, ? biopsy<br>Rx: furosemide, mannitol, dopamine, dialysis (if needed) |

* From McGoldrick[173] with permission.

ATN = acute tubular necrosis; ECF = extracellular fluid; ANA = antinuclear antibody; RBC = red blood cell; BUN = blood urea nitrogen; IVP = intravenous pyelogram; BP = blood pressure; AGN = acute glomerulonephritis; CHF = congestive heart failure; U/P = urinary to plasma; RFI = renal failure index; ASO = antistreptylosine O; $U_{NA}$ = urinary sodium.

- A prolonged period of systemic hypotension
- A need for cardiopulmonary resuscitation with or without temporary aortic cross-clamping
- Extensive muscle damage with resultant myoglobinuria
- Second- and third-degree burns involving greater than 40% of the body surface area
- Multiple organ failure
- Disseminated intravascular coagulation (DIC)[104]
- Gram-negative sepsis[92]
- Large bowel injury or gangrene with intra-abdominal abscess and systemic sepsis
- Severe gunshot injuries, stabbings, or vehicular accidents
- Mismatched blood transfusions

Such conditions as advanced age, pre-existing renal or aortorenal vascular disease, perioperative hypotension in a previously hypertensive patient, excessive aminoglycoside therapy, and radiocontrast dye studies are important factors that may contribute to the development of ATN.[207,256]

## PATHOPHYSIOLOGY OF ACUTE TUBULAR NECROSIS

In most cases, ATN is caused by one of two types of injuries: ischemic or nephrotoxic. Ischemic ATN may be caused by trauma, hemorrhage, sepsis, and pigmenturia (hemoglobin or myoglobin). Nephrotoxic disorders may follow the use of aminoglycoside antibiotics, radiocontrast agents, heavy metals, and a variety of other medications. The results of experimental studies suggest that in renal failure renal blood flow (RBF) is reduced to 50–60% of normal, renal solute and water excretion remains depressed after the restoration of RBF, and there is a varying degree of tubular destruction, with proximal tubular injury being the most common abnormal histologic finding.[64]

Data from animal models have led to the development of several theories to explain the pathogenesis of ARF: tubular obstruction, back-leak of filtrate, vasomotor mechanisms, and tubuloglomerular feedback. Unfortunately, none of these mechanisms explains all the defects seen in ARF. However, it appears that in the injured patient, tubular obstruction, vasomotor mechanisms, and back-leak of filtrate may play a major role in the development and maintenance of ARF.

The tubular obstruction theory proposes that necrotic cell debris and precipitated proteins obstruct the renal tubular lumen, raising intratubular pressure and thus decreasing the glomerular filtration rate (GFR).[240] In ARF, even when the glomeruli appear normal under light microscopy, tubular morphology is quite distorted.[188] The basement membrane of the tubule is separated from its underlying wall, and casts and debris formed within the lumen may cause intraluminal obstruction. One striking feature of the tubular lesions is that they are patchy in distribution. The proximal tubules seem to bear the brunt of the attack, with debris blocking the straight terminal segment. Later in the course of ARF, more and more distal portions of the nephron are blocked with intraluminal debris.[188,190]

Back-leak of filtrate across damaged proximal and distal tubular epithelial cells is another factor proposed for the pathogenesis of postischemic ARF.[78] Increasing tubular back pressure eventually produces reverse flow into the interstitium, thus accounting for loss of urine production. The magnitude of the back-leak appears to be proportional to the duration of ischemia.[77] However, the existence and importance of tubular leakage are controversial. The presence or absence of this phenomenon appears largely to be a function of the model used in the study.[190]

Proponents of the vasomotor theory contend that the mechanism of ARF may be explained solely on the basis of vascular phenomena without invoking other mechanisms.[190] This is based on the finding that four features are of importance in human oliguric ARF: (1) GFR is reduced to 10% of normal, (2) blood flow to the renal cortex is reduced by 50–70%, (3) the proximal tubular pressure is normal, and (4) tubular histologic abnormalities are minimal.[190] Because renal blood flow is consistently reduced, the condition is termed vasomotor nephropathy. Figure 25-1 shows the renal angiogram of a patient who ingested large amounts of mercuric chloride. One can see a dramatic reduction in cortical blood flow, which is characteristic of vasomotor nephropathy resulting in near-total filtration failure.

Clamping of renal vessels for 1 hour in the rat results in oliguria lasting for 1 week.[240] Likewise, glomerular filtration rate (GFR) and renal blood flow (RBF) may remain depressed long after release of the vascular occlusion. The fact that renal blood flow remains reduced in spite of normal systemic blood pressure indicates that total renal vascular resistance remains high after declamping. An early hypothesis suggested that ischemia leads to persistent endothelial cell swelling that prevents the restoration of RBF, the so called no-reflow phenomenon.[238] This hypothesis was subsequently rejected because it was shown that endothelial swelling was only patchy and disappeared promptly after reversal of the occlusion. The increased renovascular resistance appears to be due to afferent arteriolar vasoconstriction, resulting in a disproportionate reduction in outer cortical blood flow.[190] The mechanism of this increased resistance is a subject of debate. Increased solute delivery to the macula densa may produce an increased release of renin from its storage sites in the juxtaglomerular apparatus, resulting in a local increase in angiotensin II production.[242] Plasma renin activity is elevated in ARF, but this mechanism is unlikely to play a significant role in decreasing the GFR, because depletion of intrarenal renin experimentally does not seem to provide protection against ARF.[37] A tubuloglomerular feedback mechanism causing afferent arteriolar obstruction may also be responsible for the increased renal vascular resistance. This mechanism may be activated by the increased delivery of proximal tubular fluid to distal segments of incompletely obstructed tubules.[188]

Although there is no consensus of opinion, both tubular injury and abnormal glomerular perfusion appear to play a role in the pathogenesis of ARF.[148,187] Figure 25-2 presents a simplified approach to understanding the interaction between tubular pressure (TP) and glomerular hydraulic pressure (HP). The HP is dependent on the tone and caliber of the afferent and efferent arterioles. However, it is believed that efferent arteriolar resistance plays only a minor role in determining the glomerular perfusion pressure.[188,190] The net

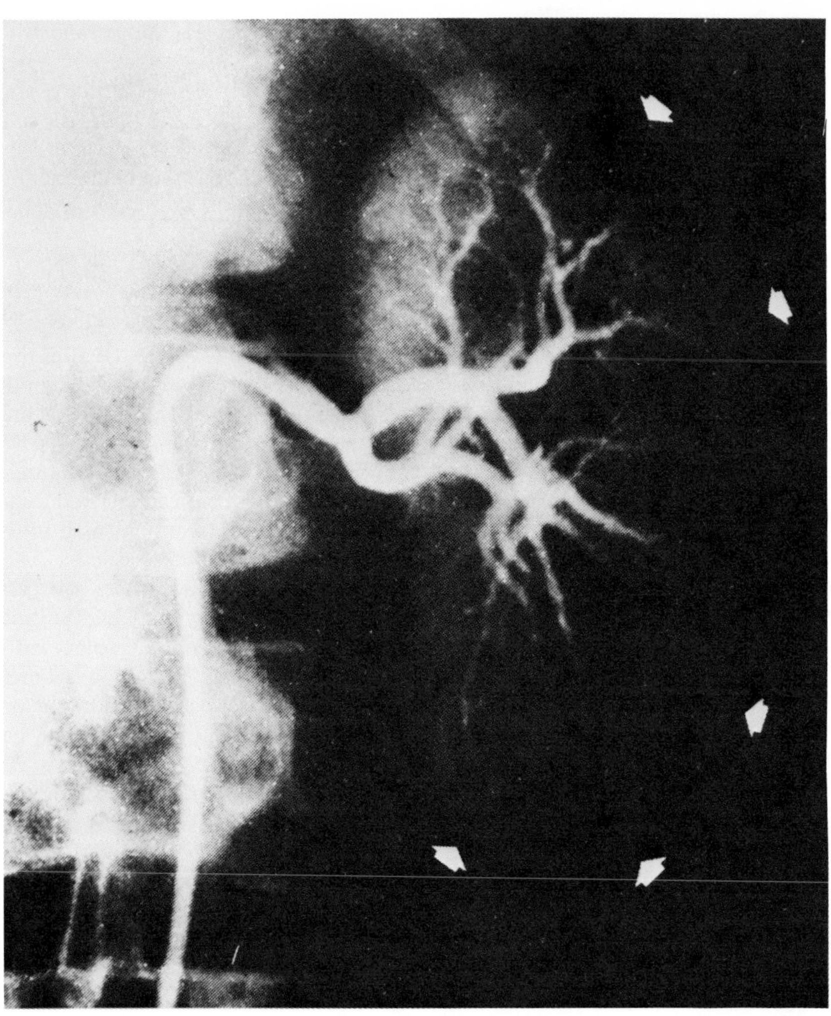

FIG. 25-1. The arterial phase of an angiogram of a 19-year-old woman with vasomotor nephropathy after ingesting mercuric chloride. The cortical margin is marked with arrows. The virtual disappearance of the outer cortical vessels is characteristic of this syndrome. (From Oken[190] with permission.)

FIG. 25-2. Vasomotor mechanism in acute renal failure. NFP = net filtration pressure [NFP = glomerular hydraulic pressure (HP) − plasma oncotic pressure]. EFP = effective filtration pressure [EFP = NFP − tubular pressure (TP)]. JGA = juxtaglomerular apparatus. Note in *3* that the caliber of the afferent arteriole is reduced by the tubular feedback mechanism. NFP has decreased to 30 torr and EFP to zero with the result that urine formation has ceased.

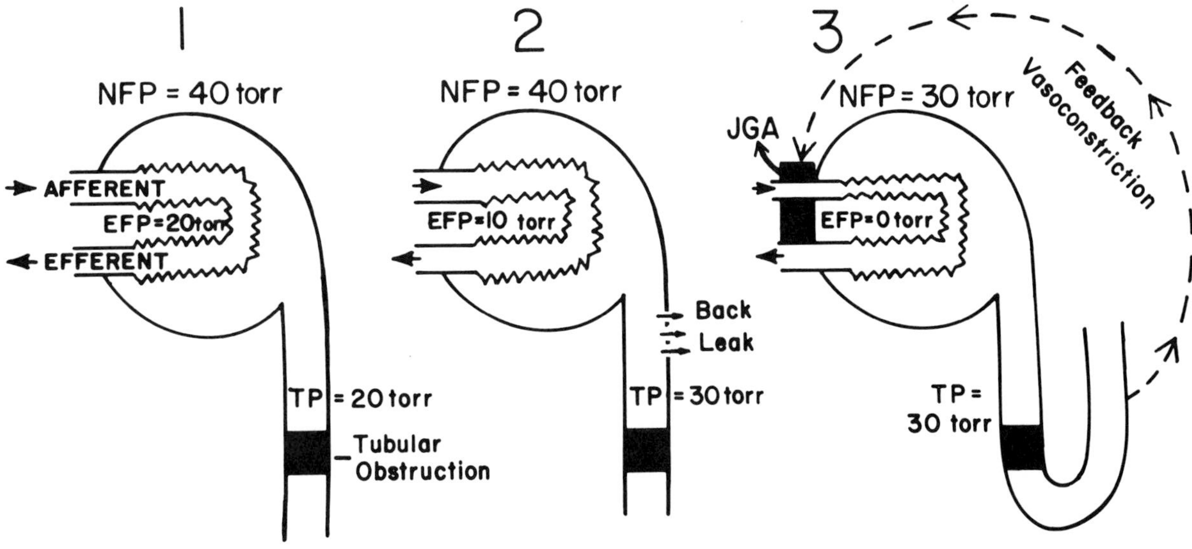

filtration pressure (NFP) is the difference between HP and the plasma oncotic pressure. Effective filtration pressure (EFP) is the difference between NFP and TP. Thus, the higher the tubular back pressure, the less will be the EFP. When NFP is decreased sufficiently by arteriolar vasoconstriction, the increased TP will stop all filtration. Obviously, any reduction in HP due to systemic hypotension will diminish EFP further. An increase in TP and a decrease in EFP may also result in back-leak of ultrafiltrate into the interstitial tissue through the damaged tubular wall. Finally, afferent arteriolar vasoconstriction caused by tubuloglomerular feedback may result in equalization of NFP and TP and thus prevent glomerular filtration.[188]

At a molecular level several factors including hypoxia, lysomal enzyme release, endotoxins and kinins have been involved in the pathogenesis of ARF.[57a] Hypoxia initiates a series of biochemical reactions which culminate in the production of oxidative radicals, such as superoxide ions ($O_2-$). These free radical substances can injure cells by peroxidating the lipid membranes. In the experimental animal, the prevention of free radical formation and their accelerated removal has been demonstrated to be beneficial. However these findings have not yet been substantiated in the clinical setting.

In summary, although persistent vasoconstriction and suppressed renal blood flow are present during the early phases of ARF in the ischemic rat model, they appear to be only two of several contributing factors to decreased GFR. Tubular obstruction and abnormal tubular leakage may be important factors in initiating and maintaining ARF.

## INTERVENTION AND REVERSIBILITY IN ACUTE TUBULAR NECROSIS

Oliguria is a common finding in ARF and attempts to reverse it date back to the early 1940s. More recent findings that indicate that nonoliguric ARF has a better prognosis than the oliguric form have lent support to the use of mannitol and loop diuretics.[8] These measures may be beneficial in the management of ARF by the following mechanisms. They inhibit salt and water reabsorption in the renal tubule, increasing intratubular flow and pressure, thus preventing intratubular obstruction. By this mechanism, they convert acute oliguric renal failure to nonoliguric failure without necessarily improving renal function. Mannitol limits cell injury by minimizing cell swelling because it is hypertonic. Furosemide also inhibits tubuloglomerular feedback, which reduces glomerular filtration when the solute flow at the macula densa is high. Both mannitol and loop diuretics reverse vasoconstriction by increasing intrarenal vasodilator prostaglandin synthesis or decreasing renin secretion in some instances. A similar effect is also attributed to other vasodilators. Thus diuretics have the potential to alter the course of ARF[149]: they may prevent ARF in those patients at risk, they may halt progression of ARF after it has developed, and they may accelerate recovery in well-established ARF.

## PROPHYLAXIS

Mannitol and/or furosemide are known to be effective in preventing ARF in jaundiced patients undergoing surgery,[15] in patients receiving certain drugs, such as amphotericin B[192] or radiocontrast media,[13] in patients with pigmenturia,[95] and in patients with acute severe hyperuricemia (urinary uric acid/urinary creatinine ratio >1).[112,129] In the high risk surgical patient, however, prophylactic administration of diuretics is generally no more effective than repletion of circulating volume, and under no circumstances should diuretics be administered in the presence of hypovolemia.

### EARLY ACUTE TUBULAR NECROSIS

Early ATN usually causes ARF within 24–48 hours after the causative episode. Levinsky et al.[149] reviewed 161 patients treated with furosemide or mannitol soon after the insult. One hundred eight patients responded to therapy, and of these 82 (76%) survived. Of the 53 patients who remained oliguric, only 31 (58%) survived. Although these data are derived from several studies, they suggest that early treatment with furosemide or mannitol may have a beneficial role.

Furosemide is administered intravenously in doses between 40–100 mg. If no response occurs, an additional 240 mg is given over a 1-hour period. Ototoxicity is not a problem with high doses of furosemide if the rate of administration is 4 mg/min or less. If ototoxicity is of real concern, as it might be with patients receiving aminoglycosides, bumetanide can be substituted. One milligram IV bumetanide is equivalent to 20 mg IV furosemide (one milligram PO bumetanide is equivalent to 40 mg PO furosemide). Mannitol is administered intravenously in an initial dose of 25 g. If this produces increased urinary output, a maintenance dose of 5–10 g/h is administered.

Experimentally, vasodilator prostaglandins ($E_2$, $D_2$, $I_2$, and $E_1$ series)[40,127,244], thromboxane inhibitors,[128] and cryoprecipitate[12] have been used for prevention of ARF after ischemic injury. Initial animal work with prostacyclin and prostaglandin $E_1$ as protective agents against ARF is encouraging. Prostacyclin ($PGI_2$) is a potent renal cortical vasodilator. Its infusion in experimental ischemic ARF results in elevation of the prostacyclin to thromboxane $A_2$ ratio, thereby protecting the kidney. This agent also raises platelet and leukocyte cyclic AMP, thereby minimizing cell damage. Unfortunately, $PGI_2$ is very unstable at physiologic pH and temperature.[244] A new stable analog of $PGI_2$ has been synthesized and shown to be protective of renal function in animals. It may prove beneficial in clinical ARF.[244] More recently atrial natiuretic peptide and calcium entry blockers have been shown to be beneficial in ischemic acute renal failure.[214a,218a]

### ESTABLISHED ACUTE TUBULAR NECROSIS

#### *Diuretics*

Levinsky et al.[149] reviewed 19 studies in which diuretics were administered more than 48 hours after the onset of ARF. Furosemide was used in 18 studies; 9 reported no improvement, 2 showed equivocal effects, and 7 reported a favorable outcome. In 14 studies evaluating the effect of diuretic administration on the need for hemodialysis, 5 reported no effect, 2 showed equivocal effects, and 7 reported a reduced need for dialysis. The effect on survival was reviewed in 15 reports.

Fourteen of these showed no improvement, and only one reported a lower mortality rate. The above data suggest that there may be little, if any, benefit in treating established acute renal failure with furosemide and/or mannitol.

### *Dopamine*

This naturally occurring catecholamine is a potent inotrope causing renal vasodilation, diuresis, and natriuresis. Dopamine in small doses (1–3 μg/kg/min) has no significant systemic hemodynamic effect, but has a renal effect and has been used to treat ARF in patients who have been resistant to furosemide or mannitol therapy.[195] Some patients in ARF may convert from oliguric to nonoliguric renal failure and others may show prompt improvement in renal function.[116] Although no definite indication can be given for using dopamine, it seems reasonable to try it in difficult situations, especially when mannitol and/or furosemide have failed. There is some evidence to suggest that the combination of dopamine infusion (2 μg/kg/min) and furosemide, 200 mg every 6 hours, may be more effective than either of these agents used alone.[150] With the recent clinical availability of the non-invasive duplex doppler it is now possible to monitor and analyze the renal vascular response to low-dose dopamine in the critically ill patient and consequently adjust the infusion rate to optimize renal blood flow.[237a]

## VARIANTS OF ACUTE TUBULAR NECROSIS IN THE INJURED

### RHABDOMYOLYSIS AND MYOGLOBINURIA

Whenever skeletal muscle cells are injured, cell contents escape. Each kilogram of skeletal muscle contains 110 mEq of potassium, 500–750 mL of $H_2O$, 0.75 mmol (2.25 g) of phosphate, and 4 g of myoglobin.[137] The clinical indicators of "crush injury" are thus hyperkalemia, hyperphosphatemia, disproportionate elevation of serum creatinine, hyperuricemia, hypocalcemia, disseminated intravascular coagulopathy, systemic hypotension, and myoglobinuria. Identifiable blood markers of skeletal muscle injury include creatine phosphokinase (CPK), aldolase, glutamic-oxaloacetic transaminase, lactic dehydrogenase, myoglobin, and electrolytes.

Myoglobin has a half-life of 1 to 3 hours and disappears from the plasma in less than 6 hours.[143] Its volume of distribution in an average adult is 28 liters. Concentrations of 100 mg/dL are necessary to produce discoloration of plasma or urine. Since myoglobin (unlike hemoglobin) is not bound to any specific serum protein, it is readily excreted in the urine, which is consequently stained reddish-brown while the plasma remains clear. Myoglobin is not excreted in the urine at plasma myoglobin concentrations less than 1.5 mg/dL. The muscle myoglobin content is 4 mg/dL; therefore, injury to a muscle mass of about 112 g is necessary to release enough myoglobin to exceed the renal threshold. Although benzidine, guaiac, or orthotoluidine (dipstick) are used to demonstrate myoglobin in the urine, immunodiffusion is the most sensitive test of myoglobinuria. Myoglobin is pink in freshly voided neutral or slightly alkaline urine. In acidic urine, it is brown due to the spontaneous conversion of myoglobin to hematin and globin. Myoglobin nephrotoxicity is unlikely to occur in the absence of hypovolemia or when urine pH exceeds 5.6. ARF is the result of a dose-dependent tubular toxicity of ferrihemate in the presence of hypotension and acidic urine.[137]

An important phenomenon called the "second wave phenomenon" often occurs with crush injuries.[137] Creatine phosphokinase (CPK) is released from damaged muscles, and its plasma concentration reaches a maximum 24–36 hours after the injury. Without further muscle injury, CPK should decline by 50% each 48 hours thereafter. If there is an increase in CPK during this time, one should suspect extension or recurrence of muscle necrosis and associated ARF. If fasciotomy is not performed immediately, vascular compression may result in gangrene. This second wave phenomenon occurs after fluid resuscitation and is the result of decomposition of damaged muscle into smaller proteins and amino acid fragments, which increases the intracellular oncotic pressure and thus shifts fluids to this compartment.

Acute renal failure caused by rhabdomyolysis and myoglobinuria is treated with mannitol and sodium bicarbonate.[84] Particular attention should be given to life-threatening hyperkalemia.

Transient hypercalcemia may be seen in the polyuric recovery phase of rhabdomyolysis-induced ARF. It was originally thought that this hypercalcemia was caused by the release of calcium deposits from the muscle. However, it has been shown that it is, at least partly, due to elevated levels of 1,25-dihydroxyvitamin D [1,25-$(OH)_2D$].[154] In contrast, during the oliguric phase of rhabdomyolysis-induced ARF, hypocalcemia may occur secondary to the decreased synthesis of 1,25-$(OH)_2D$ and hyperphosphatemia.[154] The overall mortality rate of rhabdomyolysis-induced ARF is 15%.[57]

### HEMOGLOBIN-INDUCED ACUTE RENAL FAILURE

Release of free hemoglobin from hemolyzed red blood cells can result in ARF, especially when associated with hypotension and ischemia.[123] Incompatible blood transfusion and thermal injury are the most common causes of hemoglobinuria in the trauma patient.[120,121] Advances in blood banking techniques have decreased the frequency of primary hemolytic reactions.[120] However, delayed transfusion reactions that occur between 4 and 14 days after transfusion may also result in hemoglobinuric ARF (see Chapter 6).[120]

The initial symptoms of hemoglobinuric ARF include fever and urticaria. Hemoglobinuria, oliguria, and hemolytic anemia occur rapidly. Administration of mannitol immediately after detection of hemoglobinuria may be beneficial. Recovery from transfusion-reaction-induced ARF, especially when it occurs 1–3 weeks after the transfusion, is very common.[176]

### AMINOGLYCOSIDE NEPHROTOXICITY

Aminoglycosides carry a cationic charge in solution and therefore penetrate membrane barriers poorly. Their distribution volume is thus essentially limited to the ECF. A major reduction in ECF volume due to hemorrhage and shock significantly increases aminoglycoside concentration.[31]

Azotemia (serum creatinine concentration greater than 1.3 mg/dL) occurs in 8–11% of all hospitalized patients on aminoglycoside therapy.[31] Clinically significant ARF (serum creatinine concentration greater than 2.0 mg/dL) occurs in only 3–5% of patients.[31] If the serum creatinine concentration before aminoglycoside therapy is greater than 2 mg/dL, the incidence of ARF rises to 20%.[268] The concomitant use of aminoglycosides and cephalosporins results in nephrotoxicity in 20% of patients.[217] The nephrotoxicity of aminoglycosides is also increased in elderly patients and when they are used concurrently with diuretics, X-ray contrast media, or antifungal agents. Generally, the nephrotoxic potential of aminoglycosides is increased when (a) the number of ionizable amino groups is increased (for instance, neomycin with six amino groups is more nephrotoxic than streptomycin, which has only two), (b) trough serum levels are greater than 2 μg/mL, (c) peak serum levels are greater than 12–15 μg/mL, and (d) the drug is used for longer than 2 weeks.

The major lesion in aminoglycoside-induced ARF is proximal tubular necrosis with relative sparing of the glomeruli and blood vessels.[268] Aminoglycosides also inhibit phospholipase activity in the $Na^+ - K^+$ pump of the inner mitochondrial membrane.[64] Aminoglycoside nephrotoxicity presents as nonoliguric ARF that may be delayed for several days.[63] The first functional defect is a decrease in urine concentrating ability, resulting in polyuria. Before the onset of azotemia, there is an increase in urinary microglobulins, muramidase, beta-glucuronidase, and N-acetyl hexosaminidase. However, these tubular proteins are not pathognomonic of ARF. The appearance of mild proteinuria and granular casts precedes the development of azotemia. After the discontinuation of aminoglycosides, resolution of ARF takes several weeks.[16]

In summary, aminoglycosides are frequently used in the trauma patient and can be associated with ARF. If possible, the combined use of potentially nephrotoxic drugs should be avoided. Serum levels of aminoglycosides should be measured frequently. Any unexpected increase in urinary output during aminoglycoside therapy must be investigated at the earliest opportunity.

## NONOLIGURIC ACUTE RENAL FAILURE

The incidence of nonoliguric ATN (urine volume >1 L/day) is increasing. Before 1970, fewer than 5% of patients with ATN were nonoliguric. In recent years the overall incidence in trauma patients has risen to approximately 50%.[156,225] This increase is probably related to the following factors. Trauma victims receive early and appropriate fluid resuscitation. Nephrotoxin-induced ATN has become more frequent, and it is often nonoliguric. With the frequent monitoring of blood levels of nephrotoxic substances, milder forms of nonoliguric ARF are diagnosed with greater accuracy. The use of diuretics may convert early oliguric ATN to a nonoliguric form.

Generally, management of these patients is easier than of those with oliguric ARF because they have fewer fluid, electrolyte, and acid-base abnormalities.[9] Indeed, few of these patients require dialysis. Nonoliguric ATN has a mortality rate of only 26–32%, whereas oliguric ATN is associated with a 50% mortality.[8,10]

## RADIOCONTRAST DYE-INDUCED NEPHROPATHY

The trauma patient is often exposed to radiographic contrast media during tomographic scans and angiograms. In certain situations, these agents may be nephrotoxic.[81] Two medical centers have reported that 9–11% of all ARF is caused by radiocontrast media.[122,172] The most commonly used contrast agents are 2, 4, 6-triiodinated benzoic acid derivatives. These preparations are markedly hyperosmolar and contain 26–37% iodine by weight. They are excreted entirely by the kidney, and their serum half-life is 30 to 60 minutes in patients with normal renal function. They increase the urinary excretion of uric acid and oxalate and also stimulate ADH production. According to retrospective studies the incidence of contrast media-induced nephropathy after angiography varies from 1.5%[144] in a random population to as high as 92%[256] in diabetic patients with advanced nephropathy. However, two more recent prospective studies suggest that this complication occurs less frequently than previously reported; the incidence of renal insufficiency ranged from 1.5 to 5% in low-risk patients to 9 to 16% in high–risk patients.[194,219] These rates are not decreased by the use of nonionic low osmolality radiocontrast agents.[194,219] The two most important risk factors for contrast medium-induced ARF are pre-existing renal impairment and diabetic nephropathy. Other risk factors include peripheral vascular disease, dehydration, multiple myeloma, hypertension, and age over 60.

Contrast medium-induced nephropathy is diagnosed by elevation of serum creatinine levels. This occurs 24 hours after dye injection, and peak levels are reached between the third and fifth day. It may or may not be accompanied by oliguria. Urine specific gravity is often high initially (greater than 1.025) secondary to the high osmolarity of the contrast medium. The urine sodium level and the 24-hour urinary sodium excretion may be quite low. In most instances, serum creatinine concentration returns to baseline in less than 10 days. When renal failure is accompanied by oliguria, however, there is often only a partial return of renal function. Irreversible renal failure is uncommon as is the need for acute hemodialysis.[194,219] The pathogenesis of contrast medium-induced renal nephropathy is unclear, but possible mechanisms include tubular toxicity, renal ischemia, intratubular obstruction and, least likely, immunologic abnormality.

### *Prevention of Radiocontrast Dye-Induced Acute Renal Failure*

Anto and colleagues[14] have proposed the following regimen for protection against contrast medium-induced renal failure: intravenous infusion of 250 mL of 20% mannitol over 1 hour after contrast administration, followed by infusion of 0.45% saline in 5% dextrose at a rate equal to urine output. Berksett and Kjellstrand[33] have proposed that all patients with serum creatinine levels greater than 2 mg/dL receive 500 mL of 20% mannitol. In addition, furosemide is administered at a dose of 100 mg for each mg/dL elevation of serum creatinine. Prophylactic mannitol infusion is given at a rate of 20 mL/h starting 1 hour before the administration of contrast media and continuing during the procedure and for 6 hours thereafter. An infusion of 5% dextrose in 0.45% NaCl containing KCl, 30mEq/L, is used to replace fluid volume lost during diuresis. With this prophylaxis Shafi and co-workers[221] and Anto et al.[13] have shown that the incidence of contrast-induced renal failure in patients with chronic preexisting renal insufficiency was reduced from 61 to 18% and in diabetics from 92 to 33%.

Although there is no direct proof that such a regimen will be useful in trauma patients, one may still use these measures if the patient is at high risk for developing ARF.

## RISK FACTORS AND OUTCOME IN PATIENTS WITH ACUTE RENAL FAILURE

A number of prognostic indicators can help in planning the patient's hospitalization and treatment. Bullock et al.[47] analyzed risk factors and outcome in 462 patients with ARF. Pulmonary complications, including aspiration pneumonia, respiratory failure, respiratory arrest, or adult respiratory distress syndrome, cause an eightfold increase in ARF mortality. Hepatic impairment, defined as a bilirubin level of 2.5 mg/dL or greater, causes a fourfold increase. Urine output less than 50 mL/day has a similar effect. Oliguria less than 400 mL/day has been shown to increase mortality 1.5 times. Cardiovascular complications, including congestive heart failure, pulmonary edema, acute myocardial infarction, cardiac arrest, and cardiac arrhythmias (ventricular tachycardia and fibrillation), increase mortality threefold. Hypercatabolism, as evidenced by a daily increase of BUN > 30 mg/dL, serum $K^+$ > 2 mEq/L, and weight loss > 1 kg, doubles mortality. Advanced age also plays a role. Mortality from ARF increases by 1.65% for every 10-year increase in age. The development of a second episode of ATN during the course of recovery from the first one carries a poor prognosis.[38] Acute renal failure associated with burns or severe trauma seems to carry a worse prognosis than that secondary to nephrotoxins, rhabdomyolysis, or obstetric complications,[10] although Bullock et al.[47] were unable to confirm these conclusions. That study also indicated that septicemia did not increase mortality if other risk factors were not present. However, most septicemic patients develop such risk factors.

## DIAGNOSIS OF ACUTE RENAL FAILURE AFTER TRAUMA AND SURGERY

After stabilizing the patient's hemodynamic condition the potential for renal dysfunction should be recognized and appropriate clinical and laboratory tests utilized to diagnose it as early as possible. Although specific treatment for ARF is not available, the measures described above may be employed to convert oliguric renal failure to a nonoliguric form.[12,40,116,149,150] As mentioned previously, renal failure is easier to manage when urine output is adequate, since there are fewer fluid and electrolyte problems and lower morbidity and mortality.[8,10]

### CLINICAL DIAGNOSIS

The diagnosis of ARF is made primarily by exclusion.[2] Oliguria is a frequent finding in the severely injured patient. It may be caused, as noted above, by prerenal, renal, or postrenal factors. The most common cause of oliguria in the trauma victim is hypovolemia. Oliguria due to congestive heart failure occurs infrequently in the trauma patient and is mainly caused by pre-existing heart disease or cardiac trauma. Clinically, prerenal causes of oliguria can be diagnosed by measuring systemic, central venous, pulmonary artery, and pulmonary artery wedge pressures and cardiac output. Prerenal oliguria due to hypovolemia is associated with diminished systemic and central filling pressures and cardiac output, whereas that caused by pump failure is characterized by decreased or normal blood pressure, elevated central filling pressures and diminished cardiac output. Oliguria caused by renal or postrenal factors is associated with normal systemic and central filling pressures and cardiac output; however, these may be reduced by ongoing blood loss and fluid sequestration into the third space. In these instances, the diagnosis may be established by infusion of fluids to restore intravascular blood volume and improve filling pressures.[42] If oliguria continues after these values are restored, renal or postrenal factors should be suspected.

Postrenal causes of oliguria or anuria can be ruled out by evaluation of the traumatic injury, catheterization of the urinary tract, and radiographic studies. Pelvic injuries are likely to be associated with urethral and urinary bladder disruption. Unless contraindicated all trauma patients with major injuries should be catheterized not only to monitor urine output but also to ensure the integrity of the lower urinary tract. In addition, a urinary catheter enables one to obtain a cystogram when indicated. When urethral injury is suspected, catheterization should be performed only after a urethrogram.

Oliguria due to upper urinary tract disruption is rare because this complication results only from bilateral injury or obstruction of the ureters or kidneys; for instance, as a result of major retroperitoneal bleeding[124] or direct trauma. A definitive diagnosis of postrenal oliguria may be made by intravenous urography, cystography, CT scanning, sonography, radioisotope renograms, and/or renal perfusion scans.[51,223,239]

Occasionally, renal dysfunction may have been present before the traumatic event. Pre-existing renal failure may usually be diagnosed by a careful history. The finding of small kidneys on abdominal X-rays or during surgery and the presence of uremic osteodystrophy and neuropathy suggest pre-existing kidney disease. Although anemia is a common manifestation of chronic renal failure, it has little diagnostic value in the severely traumatized patient.

### LABORATORY DIAGNOSIS

Many ARF patients are not oliguric,[225] and oliguria does not necessarily occur immediately after the traumatic event. It may develop over a period of several hours or even a day, during which time clinical findings alone may not be sufficient to establish the diagnosis. Laboratory analysis of blood and urine, and renal function tests, may facilitate the diagnosis of renal dysfunction and early prediction of ARF in these circumstances.

Microscopic examination of urinary sediment in prerenal or postrenal oliguria shows few formed elements and hyaline casts. If there is a direct injury to the genitourinary tract, analysis of the urinary sediment may not be helpful because the urine is usually contaminated by blood cells and tissue particles. In acute renal failure, the sediment may show brownish pigmented cellular casts and many renal tubular epithelial cells. Dark-colored urine containing brownish pigmented granular casts suggests hemoglobinuria or myoglobinuria. Both hemoglobin and myoglobin react strongly with benzidine or with other reagents that detect blood. However, a negative benzidine test in the presence of obvious muscle injury does not exclude myoglobinuria.[87] In these instances elevation of serum CPK and uric acid is indicative of myoglobinuria. A urine specimen should be sent for myoglobin determination and an alkalinizing regimen initiated. In chronic renal failure, the urine sediment shows many broad casts.

Biochemical analysis of urine and blood and kidney function tests are useful in differentiating prerenal from renal azotemia (Table 25–3).[191] The rationale for performing these tests is based on the difference between responses of the normal and malfunctioning kidney to inadequate perfusion. Normal kidneys respond to diminished RBF by conserving water and $Na^+$; the urine is decreased and concentrated, and urine flow and urinary $Na^+$ excretion are low. In ARF, the ability of the kidney to concentrate urine and conserve $Na^+$ is decreased or lost, and the glomerular filtration rate (GFR) is decreased significantly. The most prominent effect of filtration failure on blood chemistry is retention of catabolic end-products: urea and creatinine. Thus, measurement of urinary and plasma concentrations of urea and creatinine and the calculation of their clearances from plasma, together with tests measuring the kidney's capacity to handle $Na^+$ and water, yield valuable information about kidney function.

The kidneys excrete creatinine mainly by glomerular filtration. Under normal circumstances, creatinine is neither reabsorbed nor secreted by the renal tubules. Diminished GFR, a common finding in ARF, results in decreased excretion of creatinine. Thus, plasma creatinine rises at a rate equal to creatinine production minus the remaining glomerular filtration and urinary excretion capacity. When there is no excessive catabolism and creatinine production, the daily rate of plasma creatinine rise is approximately 0.5–1 mg/dL. In severely traumatized patients with ARF, the daily rate of creatinine rise may be as high as 2–5 mg/dL because of excessive tissue catabolism.[9,87] Urea is also excreted by glomerular filtration, and thus a decrease in GFR results in urea retention. Unlike creatinine, however, a significant portion of the filtered urea undergoes tubular reabsorption. Therefore, in the catabolic traumatized patient with diminished GFR, the daily rate of plasma urea rise is greater than that of creatinine.

Normally, the BUN to plasma creatinine ratio is between 10 and 15. In the presence of accelerated tissue catabolism, this ratio may be increased. Conversely, when there is significant rhabdomyolysis the ratio decreases because muscle creatine is converted to creatinine, resulting in a disproportionately greater increase in plasma creatinine over BUN.

At very low glomerular filtration rates, there is tubular excretion of creatinine by the acutely damaged tubular epithelium.[132,189] The creatinine clearance test in these instances overestimates GFR by approximately 100%.[132] However, the difference between the actual GFR and creatinine clearance does not diminish the value of this diagnostic test, because creatinine clearance varies in parallel with changes in GFR.[132] In addition, overestimation of GFR by the creatinine clearance test is not clinically important, because even the measured GFR remains below normal. For instance, when the actual GFR is 15 mL/min, the creatinine clearance would be 30 mL/min, a value that is still below the normal range. Creatinine clearance is calculated using the equation

$$C_{cr} = U_{cr} \times V/P_{cr}$$

where $C_{cr}$ is the creatinine clearance; $U_{cr}$, the urinary creatinine concentration in mg/dL; V, the urinary flow in mL/min; and $P_{cr}$ the plasma creatinine concentration. Ideally, the urine should be collected for 24 hours and V derived from this value. In the setting of trauma where rapid diagnosis of ARF is desirable, the use of a 1- or 2-hour creatinine clearance test may be employed with reasonable accuracy, provided that $C_{cr}$

TABLE 25-3. Differences Between Acute Tubular Necrosis and Prerenal Azotemia

| FEATURE | ATN | PRERENAL AZOTEMIA |
|---|---|---|
| Urine odor | Odorless | Characteristic urine odor |
| Specific gravity | <1.015 | >1.020 |
| Urine sediment | "Dirty" brown granular casts | Unremarkable |
| Urine Osmolality (mosm/L) | <350 | >500 |
| U/P osmolar ratio | <1.1 | >1.1 |
| U/P urea ratio | <4 | >7 |
| U/P creatinine ratio | <20 | >20–40 |
| Urine sodium (mEq/L) | >20–40 | <10 |
| Free water clearance (mL/h) | Rising to > −15 | < −20 |
| 2-hour creatinine clearance | Decreases | Remains stable |
| $FE_{Na}$ (%) | 1–2 | <1 |
| Renal failure index (RFI) | >1–2 | <1 |

U/P = urine/plasma.

$FE_{Na}$ = Fractional excretion of filtered sodium

$$= \frac{\text{U/P sodium}}{\text{U/P creatinine}} \times 100$$

$$\text{RFI} = \frac{U_{Na}}{\text{U/P creatinine}}$$

is determined sequentially and the values obtained are compared with each other.[233,265] Shin et al.,[226] using this method in acutely traumatized patients, demonstrated that $C_{cr}$ values less than 25 mL/min within 6 hours after trauma or surgery were predictive of posttraumatic renal failure (Fig 25–3). The BUN, urine flow rate, and mean blood pressure during the first 6 hours after trauma or surgery had no predictive value.

FIG. 25-3. Sequential changes in BUN, free water clearance, creatinine clearance, urine flow rate, and mean blood pressure in patients who developed renal dysfunction (*solid lines*) and in those who maintained normal renal function after surgery for trauma. Note that BUN, urine flow rate, and blood pressure are well maintained during the first postoperative day. * Indicates that the values are the mean ± SE of five instead of seven patients who developed renal dysfunction. (From Shin et al[226] with permission.)

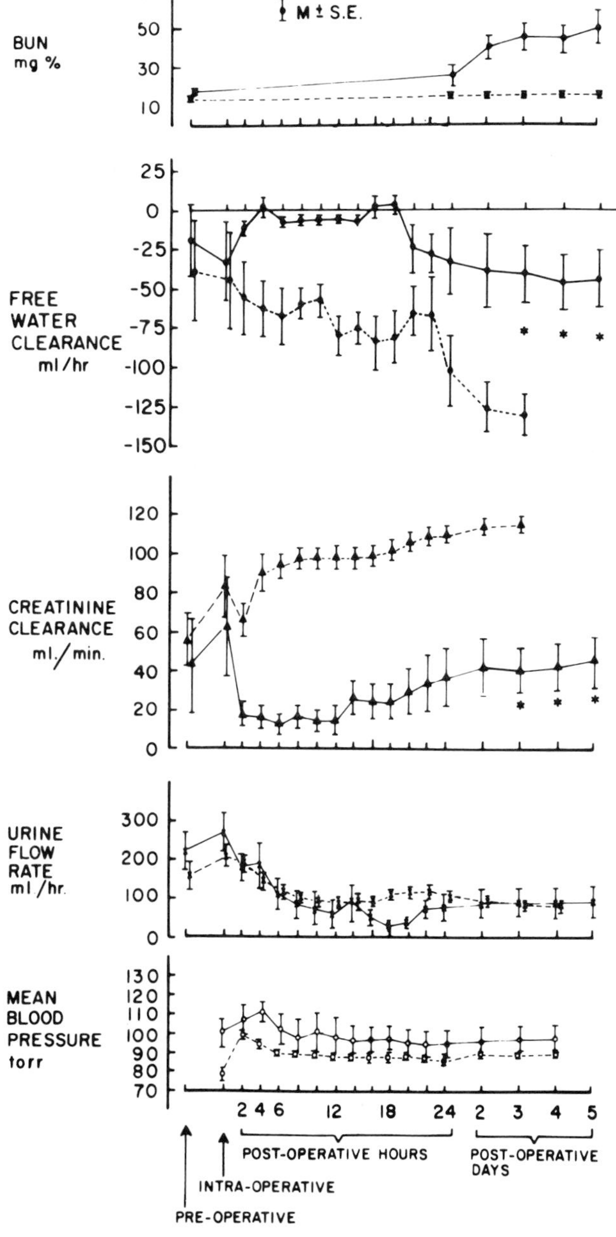


The ratios of urinary to plasma creatinine ($U/P_{cr}$) and urea ($U/P_{urea}$) concentrations may allow for differential diagnosis between prerenal and renal azotemia.[191] In prerenal azotemia, the kidney is capable of excreting the maximum amount of creatinine or urea; therefore, both $U/P_{cr}$ and $U/P_{urea}$ ratios increase. However, $U/P_{cr}$ is a more reliable index than $U/P_{urea}$, because part of the filtered urea is reabsorbed by the renal tubules. Normal $U/P_{cr}$ is greater than 20 to 30, and $U/P_{urea}$ is greater than 5 to 10.[87] In ARF, the $U/P_{cr}$ and $U/P_{urea}$ fall below 20 and 4, respectively (Table 25-3). $U/P_{urea}$ between 8 and 10 may be observed in patients who are developing renal dysfunction. An infusion of 500–1000 mL crystalloid solution results in normalization of $U/P_{urea}$ in patients who do not have renal impairment. The ratio remains unaltered or falls in those who have already developed ARF.

The urinary sodium concentration ($U_{Na}$) is elevated in ARF because the renal tubules are unable to reabsorb sodium. $U_{Na}$ in excess of 40 mEq/L is common in patients with established ARF. In contrast, in prerenal azotemia, sodium is conserved by the kidney, and $U_{Na}$ does not exceed 20 mEq/L. The fractional excretion of sodium ($FE_{Na}$) is an index of tubular $Na^+$ reabsorption and glomerular filtration. It represents the fraction of the total filtered $Na^+$ load that is excreted in the urine. This index is calculated according to the following equation:

$$FE_{Na}\ (\%) = \left[ (U_{Na}/P_{Na}) \Big/ (U_{cr}/P_{cr}) \right] \times 100$$

An $FE_{Na}$ value less than 1% is consistent with prerenal azotemia, whereas greater values suggest renal parenchymal damage (Table 25-3). This test requires only simultaneously collected "spot urine" and blood samples. Espinel and Gregory[86] were able to make an accurate diagnosis of renal failure in 86 of 87 patients solely on the basis of $FE_{Na}$ values. Occasionally, however, $FE_{Na}$ may be less than 1% in patients with ARF, especially after burn injury.[74,133] Also, $FE_{Na}$ may not detect renal dysfunction in nonoliguric patients.[184,226]

Simultaneous determination of $U_{Na}$ and $U/P_{cr}$ may provide a more accurate differential diagnosis between prerenal azotemia and ARF than either test alone. Handa and Morrin[113] described the "renal failure index" in which the urinary sodium concentration is divided by $U/P_{cr}$. A value greater than 1 suggests ATN, whereas a value below 1 indicates prerenal azotemia (Table 25-3).

The injured kidney is defective in handling water as well. Impairment of water reabsorption by the tubular epithelium results in an isosthenuric urine (specific gravity 1.010). Renal water excretion serves to eliminate both solutes and water from the body. The amount of excreted water that carries the solutes is referred to as osmolar clearance ($C_{osm}$); the remainder is the free water clearance ($C_{H2O} = V - C_{osm}$). Simultaneous measurement of urinary and plasma osmolality is used to determine osmolar clearance, which may be calculated as

$$C_{osm} = U_{osm} \times V/P_{osm}$$

where $U_{osm}$ is the urinary osmolality, V is the urinary flow in mL/min, and $P_{osm}$ is the plasma osmolality. $C_{H2O}$ has a negative value when the urine is hypertonic, and a positive value when the urine is hypotonic. In a normally functioning kidney the value of $C_{osm}$ is greater than that of urinary volume (V). Thus, the normal $C_{H2O}$ is between −15 and −50. In ARF, $C_{osm}$ decreases, and the $C_{H2O}$ moves toward a positive value. Monitoring of $C_{H2O}$ and $C_{osm}$ in the traumatized patient during the early postoperative period may predict the development of ARF. By using this test, Baek and co-workers[20,21] were able to predict ARF in 93% of their patients 48 hours before establishment of the diagnosis. $C_{H2O}$ in ARF usually ranges between −15 and +15 mL/h. A markedly positive $C_{H2O}$ value (> +60 mL/h) may be observed immediately after reversal of shock: it is not predictive of ARF.

The observation that free water clearance can be used to predict the onset of ARF before the development of oliguria has been supported by several studies.[45,142,145] However, Shin et al.[224,226] demonstrated in severely injured patients that the $C_{cr}$ during the first 6 hours after surgery was a more sensitive index than the $C_{H2O}$ (Fig 25-3). Simultaneous measurement of $C_{cr}$ and $C_{H2O}$ has been suggested to reinforce the reliability of $C_{H2O}$ as an early predictor of ARF.[45,46]

Considerable differences exist between urinary indices in oliguric and nonoliguric ARF.[10] In nonoliguric ARF, $U_{Na}$ is usually lower than that observed in the oliguric form. Likewise, $FE_{Na}$ and $U/P_{urea}$ values are higher in nonoliguric ARF.[10]

The differentiation of prerenal azotemia from acute renal parenchymal disease is usually possible with renal function indices. It has been suggested that diagnosis can be established with these tests in 80% of patients.[218] However, interpretation of these results requires caution. None of them is diagnostic in isolation. Thus, they should be evaluated along with other clinical and laboratory findings. Also, these tests may become nondiagnostic in the presence of underlying chronic renal disease, glycosuria, and the recent administration of diuretic or radiocontrast agents.[72] Ideally, blood and urine specimens should be obtained before administration of these agents.

It is important to remember that a single laboratory determination of blood and urinary indices may be misleading. These tests should be performed at 2- to 4-hour intervals to ensure an accurate diagnosis.[45,226] Measurements of serum creatinine or BUN taken immediately after an abrupt drop in GFR, such as after hemorrhagic shock, will give misleading overestimates of this value. BUN and plasma creatinine rise very slowly after a sudden decline in GFR, and it takes several hours for these indices to reflect the new steady-state GFR.

## GENERAL MANAGEMENT OF ACUTE RENAL FAILURE

Management of ARF may be divided into five phases (Table 25-4). In Phase I the extent of trauma is evaluated, and the patient is stabilized hemodynamically. In Phase II the diagnosis of ARF is established. Attention is given to all reversible causes of ARF, and appropriate treatment is instituted. Phase III focuses on treatment of fluid-electrolyte and acid-base problems and on therapy of infections. It is important to concentrate on life-threatening problems, such as hyperkalemia, during this phase. Phase IV deals with management of dialysis and the problems associated with it. Phase V is concerned with recovery from ARF. Phase I is discussed in Chapter 4. Phase II has already been discussed at length in this chapter. Phases III, IV, and V are discussed in the following sections.

### MANAGEMENT OF PHASE III

Several potentially serious clinical issues must be dealt with in Phase III of ARF management.

#### *Fluid Overload*

This is often caused by vigorous administration of fluids during the preceding phases, especially when the traumatized patient is oliguric. A mild degree of fluid overload may be treated with fluid restriction. In more urgent situations, large doses of loop diuretics may be necessary to prevent pulmonary edema. A less frequently used therapy is oral sorbitol 70% (2 mL/kg) or rectal sorbitol 20% (10 mL/kg) provided that there is no trauma to the gastrointestinal tract.[7] If the above treatment is not effective, emergency isolated ultrafiltration with or without dialysis or continuous arteriovenous hemofiltration (CAVH) may be necessary.

#### *Hyperkalemia*

Five to ten percent of all deaths in patients with ARF are related to hyperkalemia. In addition to a high serum potassium level ($K^+ > 5.5$ mEq/L), the physician should look for a hyperkalemic pattern on the ECG: peaked T waves, prolongation of PR and QRS intervals, and, at high serum $K^+$ concentrations, ventricular fibrillation and sine wave. Early ECG changes of hyperkalemia should be recognized and treated promptly. The treatment of hyperkalemia is aimed at antagonizing the effect of $K^+$ on the cardiac conduction system, shifting $K^+$ intracellularly and removing it from the body. Table 25-5 lists the treatment modalities for hyperkalemia. The following are a few points of clinical interest in caring for such patients.

Acidosis caused by the accumulation of inorganic acids (hyperchloremic metabolic acidosis) has a greater hyperkalemic effect (for every 0.1 unit decrease in pH, serum $K^+$ increases 1.6 mEq/L) than that of organic acids (for every 0.1 unit decrease in pH, serum $K^+$ increases 0.7 mEq/L).[111] In ARF, metabolic acidosis is mainly caused by the accumulation of organic acids. It is important to remember that metabolic acidosis may still cause hyperkalemia even though pH is normal.[96] An increase in serum $K^+$ may also result from increasing serum osmolality: a rise of 10 mosm/kg will increase serum $K^+$ 0.1–0.6 mEq/L. Thus, hyperkalemia may result from the mannitol used to reduce ICP in oliguric patients with acute head injury. Other therapeutic measures may also produce hyperkalemia: beta-adrenergic receptor blockers, potassium-sparing diuretics, blood transfusions (especially of stored blood), salt substitutes, captopril, nonsteroidal anti-inflammatory drugs, and administration of glucose to insulin-deficient patients.

Increased serum calcium levels antagonize the effects of $K^+$ on cardiac conduction without lowering serum $K^+$. However, exogenously administered $CaCl_2$ produces only a transient elevation of serum $Ca^{++}$.[85] Thus, in addition to admin-

TABLE 25-4. Guidelines for Management of Acute Renal Failure (ARF)

| PHASE I | PHASE II | PHASE III | PHASE IV | PHASE V |
|---|---|---|---|---|
| *Immediately* | *Day 1* | *Days 1–3* | *Days 3–7* | *Days 7–30* |
| Evaluation and stabilization of the injured patient | Diagnosis<br>Reversibility<br>Treatment | Control of fluid, electrolyte, and acid-base derangements<br>Adjustment of medication dose<br>Treatment of infection<br>Dialysis may be needed to treat hyperkalemia and congestive heart failure | Treatment of uremia<br>Dialysis—peritoneal, hemodialysis<br>Nutrition<br>Continuous AV hemofiltration or hemodialysis and isolated ultrafiltration | Monitoring of recovery<br>Specific attention to infection, nutrition, fluid & electrolytes, ambulation<br>Care of the primary injury |

istering calcium salts, other measures that lower serum $K^+$ should be instituted. Potassium can be shifted into cells by administration of alkali ($NaHCO_3$ 8.4%, 50–100 mL) or a combination of glucose and insulin. The hypokalemic effect of insulin is concentration dependent[109]; therefore, the authors favor intermittent bolus insulin injections (plus glucose) every few hours or as needed. Serum $K^+$ can also be reduced by inducing respiratory alkalosis; for each 0.1 unit increase in pH, a decrease in $K^+$ of 0.6–0.8 mEq/L is noted. Although dialysis removes 100–200 mEq/L of $K^+$ in 4 hours, it may not be adequate for handling the $K^+$ shifts that may occur in catabolic and acidotic patients. Consequently, these patients will require serial serum $K^+$ measurements after dialysis, and if they are still hyperkalemic, appropriate therapy must be instituted as outlined in Table 25-5.

### *Infections*

Thirty percent of patients with ATN present with septicemia, and 15% with positive bacterial blood cultures.[6] Sepsis is likely to occur after severe trauma, particularly after prolonged shock and multiple transfusions. Sepsis and associated multiple organ failure account for most of the deaths of trauma victims who live 48 hours or longer.[97] Unfortunately, the diagnosis of sepsis may be difficult because severe trauma, especially burns, and ARF impair host defenses. Consequently, the usual signs of infection, such as fever, leukocytosis, and local inflammation, may be minimal or absent. Sometimes the only indication of sepsis is progressive multiorgan failure. Septic patients have an opsonic fibronectin deficiency that may not only impair host defenses but also alter vascular permeability.[216] Cryoprecipitate administration to these fibronectin-deficient patients may sometimes markedly improve their condition by correcting cardiovascular, pulmonary, and renal functions. (see Chapter 26).[12]

Urinary tract and pulmonary infections occur in about 60% of patients with ARF. Consequently, indwelling bladder catheters must be removed at the earliest opportunity. Likewise, good pulmonary physiotherapy is essential.

The other major source of infection is intravenous lines, especially central venous cannulae. The pathogen is usually *Staphylococcus aureus*. This puts a major onus on the medical

TABLE 25-5. Guidelines for Management of Hyperkalemia*

| SEVERITY | TREATMENT | ONSET OF ACTION/ DURATION | COMMENTS |
|---|---|---|---|
| Life threatening | Calcium chloride (10%) 10 mL (Repeat if necessary 1–3 times every 7–10 min) Monitor ECG. | Immediately (duration usually 10–15 min) | Raises threshold. Avoid in patients on digitalis. |
| Acute | Regular insulin, IV, 15 units plus glucose 50%, 50–100 mL | ~5 minutes, (duration 1–3 h) | Intracellular $K^+$ shift. Repeat as often as needed. Check serum $K^+$ and blood glucose levels frequently. |
| | Sodium bicarbonate (40–80 mEq) (particularly effective in acidotic patients) | Minutes, (duration ½–1 h) | Intracellular $K^+$ shift. For each ↑ 0.1 pH, ↓ 0.8 mEq $K^+$/L.<br>Be careful of sodium load, and if large quantities are used, check serum sodium (to avoid hypernatremia). |
| Less severe | Sodium polystyrene sulfonate (SPS) 30 g orally + 200 mL 20% sorbitol orally or SPS 50 g + 200–500 mL 10% sorbitol as an enema | 2–3 h, (duration 6–8 h) | Removes $K^+$ via GI tract. 1 mEq $K^+$ is removed for each gram of SPS. Beware of sodium load, especially in patients with CHF. Each 16 g of SPS contains 65 mEq $Na^+$. |
| | Dialysis | Minutes to an hour (duration 2–3 days) | Acute peritoneal dialysis removes ~10 mEq $K^+$/h<br>Acute hemodialysis removes ~25–50 mEq $K^+$/h |

* From McGoldrick[173] with permission.
ECG = Electrocardiogram; GI = gastrointestinal; CHF = congestive heart failure.

team to check intravenous lines carefully every day. Any evidence of infection at the site of entry warrants removal of the cannula and appropriate culturing. This also applies to temporary hemodialysis catheters.

Renal function may be impaired in patients who develop tetanus after trauma. Sympathetic nervous system instability, a common finding in tetanus resulting in wide swings in blood pressure and changes in renal blood flow, appears to be an important factor in the development of renal dysfunction.[114] Other factors include hypovolemia and septicemia from the original wound. Overt ARF in this condition may be prevented by adequate control of sympathetic overactivity (see Chapter 26).

### *Management of Other Complications*

GASTROINTESTINAL COMPLICATIONS. Gastrointestinal stress ulcers occur in up to 20% of ARF patients and contribute to the mortality from this disease.[136] They may result from elevated gastrin levels.[232] Aluminum hydroxide antacids not only decrease gastric acidity and the risk of peptic ulcer disease but also control hyperphosphatemia, which is a common finding in ARF. Constipation caused by aluminum-containing antacids may be minimized by administering them with sorbitol. Magnesium-containing antacids should not be given because of their potential for causing magnesium toxicity. Cimetidine can also prevent stress ulceration, although it appears to be less effective than antacids.[202] In addition to nephrotoxicity, cimetidine may cause mental confusion and encephalopathy, especially in elderly patients in ARF.[255] It should be noted that early dialysis decreases the risk of major gastrointestinal complications.[136]

HEMATOLOGIC COMPLICATIONS. Anemia develops in severe oliguric ATN because of a reduced serum erythropoietin level. Other factors, such as gastrointestinal bleeding and hemolysis, may also contribute to anemia. It has been suggested that the optimal hematocrit level in the critically ill patient should be 32% or greater.[67] Thus, hematocrit should be measured frequently and anemia corrected with packed red cell transfusions. With the recent introduction of erythropoietin (EPO) as clinical therapy for the anemia of chronic renal failure, there is reason to believe that the need for blood transfusions will decrease in anemic patients with acute renal failure treated with this agent.

Bleeding secondary to platelet defects is common in ARF patients; dialysis may partly correct this problem.[82,121,210] The bleeding time must be measured before any invasive or surgical procedure is undertaken. If prolonged, the patient should receive cryoprecipitate[125] or 1-deamino-8-D-arginine vasopressin (DDAVP) infusion (0.3 μg/kg in 50 mL normal saline over a period of 30 minutes) before the procedure.[161] With the use of these agents bleeding time in uremic patients normalizes within 1 to 2 hours of infusion and remains normal for 12–24 hours.[125] Trauma victims often receive massive transfusions, which may cause thrombocytopenia.[58,208] Thrombocytopenia further compounds the coagulation abnormalities seen in ARF. After 15 units of blood, one-half of these patients have platelet counts of 50,000/μL or less.[58,208,264] Thus, posttraumatic ARF patients frequently have both qualitative and quantitative platelet defects. Transfusion of platelet concentrates may be necessary to correct this complication. Some success has been reported with the use of IV estrogens in uremic bleeding.

CARDIOVASCULAR COMPLICATIONS. Patients with ARF may develop congestive heart failure, primarily from salt and water overload. Consequently, body weight must be measured daily. The diet should contain 2 g of sodium and 2 g of potassium. The total administered fluid volume must be equal to the insensible loss plus 600 mL. In cases of life-threatening congestive heart failure that is unresponsive to these conservative measures, CAVH or dialysis may be needed. Indeed, it may not be practical to restrict fluid in catabolic trauma patients as they have high caloric and protein needs; thus dialytic therapy may be necessary even early in Phase III (Table 25-4).

Pericarditis, with or without pleuritis or pleural effusion,[241] occurs in 10–18% of patients with ARF.[251] Acute pericarditis secondary to ARF has a wide clinical spectrum ranging from asymptomatic disease to cardiac tamponade with severe hemodynamic alterations. A pericardial friction rub is the most common clinical finding. Chest pain is usually not a dominant feature, but the patient may have a low-grade fever with or without leukocytosis.

Pericardial tamponade is a well-recognized complication of ARF. It was reported in 10–24% of patients in earlier studies.[27] Because of aggressive dialysis therapy, it now occurs less frequently. Uremic pericardial tamponade causes acute right-sided heart failure with elevated jugular venous pressure, hepatic enlargement, and generalized edema. Pulsus paradoxus and systemic hypotension producing cerebral ischemia may be present. The clinical picture may actually deteriorate after vigorous dialysis with ultrafiltration. Hemodialysis may carry the risk of hemopericardium if the patient has been on anticoagulant therapy. Treatment of uremic pericarditis is generally directed toward treating the uremia. If cardiac tamponade occurs, a pericardial window and/or pericardiectomy may be required in addition to supportive therapy.

Patients with ARF may develop acute myocardial infarction, especially if they have an underlying generalized arteriosclerosis.[175] In one study, 6% of deaths in patients with ARF were attributed to myocardial infarction.[136] Diskin et al.[75] observed that asymptomatic ECG changes suggestive of ischemia are common immediately after dialysis. ST-segment depression occurred in 45%, T-wave inversion in 30%, and an increase in R-wave amplitude over the left ventricle in 75% of their patients. Caution must be exercised in interpreting these ECG changes as indicators of myocardial infarction.

Supraventricular arrhythmias may occur in patients in ARF secondary to congestive heart failure or as a result of dialysis.[237] Management in these instances is again directed toward treating the heart failure and using low-flow dialysis with the patient receiving oxygen. In some situations, because of its simplicity, CAVH or peritoneal dialysis may be more suitable than standard hemodialysis.

METABOLIC COMPLICATIONS. *Fluid and Electrolyte Abnormalities*. Major fluid and electrolyte changes occur immediately after acute injury. Salt and water are retained, especially in the ECF, and the total body sodium increases.

However, despite this sodium increase, serum sodium may be decreased because of dilution.[227] Maximum water and sodium retention usually occurs on the first and second day and persists for 4 to 7 days.[249] In most hyponatremic patients, no specific therapy is needed unless the serum sodium level falls below 125 mEq/L. When the patient begins to recover from the traumatic event, water excretion increases slowly, and consequently hyponatremia improves within 7 to 10 days. In the rare cases in which serum sodium concentration declines below 125 mEq/L, a combination of furosemide (5–20 mg) and hypertonic saline infusion guided by frequent serum electrolyte measurement may be required. Another metabolic complication, hyperkalemia, has been previously discussed.[228]

Shortly after the onset of ARF, plasma $Ca^{++}$ levels start to decline. Calcitonin and parathyroid hormone concentrations begin to rise in response to hypocalcemia.[17] Tetany is an uncommon finding in ARF patients with hypocalcemia unless serum calcium is below 6 mg/dL. Metabolic acidosis increases the concentration of serum $Ca^{++}$ and thus offers some protection against tetany. Many metabolic disorders (hypocalcemia, hyperphosphatemia, hypermagnesemia, and hyperuricemia) respond to dialysis.

*Metabolic Acidosis.* In normal adults who consume an average diet, approximately 1 mEq/kg of hydrogen ions are produced daily by metabolism. However, in the catabolic patient with ARF, especially in association with traumatic injury or sepsis, a large acid load is generated. Thus, serum $HCO_3^-$ declines rapidly and the pH decreases. The specific cations released during catabolism are sulfate and a number of organic acids, including lactic acid. The accumulation of these ions in the body results in the development of anion gap acidosis. Metabolic acidosis is associated with many deleterious effects, which are listed in Table 25-6. Reversal of acidosis is associated with improvement in all of these problems. However, the abrupt correction of acidosis in patients with hypocalcemia can precipitate tetany. Therefore, acidosis should be corrected gradually, or supplemental calcium should be administered simultaneously.

## DRUGS AND ACUTE RENAL FAILURE

Since the kidney is a major route of elimination for drugs, it is not surprising that the side effects of many therapeutic agents are markedly increased in patients with ARF. Doses of these drugs must be adjusted carefully and their dosage interval extended. In stable renal failure these adjustments may be guided by calculating creatinine clearance ($C_{cr}$) using the equation[54]:

$$C_{cr} = \frac{(140 - \text{age}) \times \text{weight (kg)}}{72 \times \text{serum creatinine}}$$

This formula applies to male patients. In women creatinine clearance is calculated by multiplying the result for male patients by 0.85.[54]

Appendix I lists some commonly used drugs, their biologic half-lives, sites of elimination, dose modification in renal failure, and the effect of dialysis in removing each drug from the body.[32] It is important to measure both peak and trough serum levels of certain drugs; if this is not possible random blood levels should be obtained to determine appropriate dosages.

TABLE 25-6. Deleterious Effects of Metabolic Acidosis*

| |
|---|
| Decreased threshold for ventricular ectopy |
| Cerebral dysfunction |
| Pulmonary hypertension |
| Nausea and vomiting |
| Insulin resistance |
| Impaired carbohydrate utilization and ATP production |
| Hyperkalemia |
| Decreased phosphofructokinase activity resulting in substantial reduction of energy production by glycolysis |
| Negative inotropic effect on the myocardium |
| Increased central or intrathoracic fluid volume |
| Decreased sensitivity to catecholamines |

* From Relman[209] with permission.

## NUTRITION OF PATIENTS WITH ACUTE RENAL FAILURE

Increased attention has been paid to nutrition of patients with ARF since the work of Abel and co-workers.[1] They showed more rapid recovery of renal function and increased survival when glucose solutions and essential amino acids were given. Although subsequent workers have not demonstrated similar dramatic effects on survival, most authorities follow the intensive nutritional support suggested by Abel et al. for ARF patients.[140,258]

All nutritional solutions must be administered orally whenever possible. The required calories and amino acids should be given in a minimal amount of fluid to prevent volume overload. It is desirable to maintain a neutral or slightly positive nitrogen balance while keeping the BUN less than 100 mg/dL. Unless the patient is edematous or has a contracted ECF volume, sodium intake should equal losses. Thus, sodium loss from various routes should be measured. Blood levels of potassium, magnesium, and phosphate should be monitored frequently.

Unless the patient had nutritional problems before the onset of ARF or is markedly catabolic at the time of evaluation, hyperalimentation should be delayed for several days. Each 6.25 g of protein contains a gram of nitrogen. Thus, patients with severe ARF may accumulate significant amounts of nitrogenous waste products. On the other hand, amino acid loss during hemodialysis amounts to 10–15 g per run, and the loss during CAVH is 6 g in every 12–14 hours. Additional nitrogen loss in patients with burns, peritonitis, or sepsis requires a minimum of 1.5 g/kg/day protein administration for nutritional support.

The urea nitrogen appearance (UNa) test must be used whenever there is a question about the administration of amino acids in posttraumatic ARF. Urea nitrogen appearance (UNa) is equal to urinary urea nitrogen plus dialysate urea nitrogen plus the change in body urea nitrogen. Change in body urea nitrogen can be calculated as follows:

Change in body urea nitrogen =

$$[(BUN_F - BUN_I)\,BW_I \times 0.06] + [(BW_F - BW_I)BUN_F]$$

TABLE 25-7. Typical Dietary Prescriptions for Patients with Acute Renal Failure

| | CATABOLIC STATUS | |
|---|---|---|
| | *Mild* | *Severe* |
| Route | PO (GI tract) | Central IV |
| Fluids | 600–1,000 mL | 2,000–4,000 mL |
| Caloric requirement | 2,500 kcal (>100 g carbohydrate, the rest as fat) | 3,500–4,000 kcal (70% as carbohydrate, the rest as fat) |
| Protein | 40 g protein (high biologic value) | 1.0–1.2 g/kg<br>10–15 g of essential and 5 g of nonessential amino acids |
| Solution | Amin-Aid, Travasorb, Renal Powder | Freamine III 8.5% in 20–60% Dextrose<br>+ Insulin 20 units/L<br>+ Vitamins, electrolytes, acetate, trace elements<br>+ 10–20% Intra-lipid two times a week |

where $BUN_F$ = blood urea nitrogen at the end of the measurement period, $BUN_I$ = blood urea nitrogen in the beginning of the measurement period, and $BW_I$ and $BW_F$ are body weights before and after dialysis. When UNa is less than 4 g/day, 0.3–0.5 g/kg of high biologic protein (or amino acid) should be given daily. When UNa is greater than 5 g/day, 1.0–1.2 g/kg high biologic protein or amino acid should be given. Typical dietary prescription for patients with ARF are shown in Table 25-7.

Since water-soluble vitamins are eliminated in the dialysate outflow, they must be replaced during dialysis. When glucose-free dialysate is used, approximately 20–50 g of glucose is lost with each treatment. Many centers use a bath containing 200 mg/dL of glucose to avoid this problem. Hyperglycemia may occur in some patients with ARF, especially in those receiving hypertonic glucose solutions. These patients should receive appropriate insulin therapy to achieve normal blood glucose levels. Large volumes of hyperalimentation solutions may be required in severely catabolic patients. To maintain fluid balance in these patients, daily ultrafiltration or CAVH may be necessary. The injured patient with ARF may develop phosphate, potassium, and magnesium depletion requiring dietary supplementation of these electrolytes. In the catabolic patient intralipid infusions are necessary two to three times per week.[258]

## DIALYSIS (PHASE IV)

Approximately 30–60 patients per one million population require hemodialysis for treatment of ARF.[135,173] Dialysis or ultrafiltration is urgently needed in the following situations[110]: (a) life-threatening pulmonary edema that is unresponsive to usual therapy; (b) life-threatening hyperkalemia when serum potassium levels are > 7mEq/L and/or are unresponsive to initial treatment; (c) uremic encephalopathy (mental confusion, lethargy, seizures, etc.); and (d) BUN > 150–200 mg/dL, serum creatinine > 10–15 mg/dL, and/or serum bicarbonate < 10–12 mEq/L.

A beneficial role of dialysis in ARF is confirmed by an epidemiologic study that showed a mortality rate of 25% in adequately dialyzed patients versus 73% in those inadequately dialyzed and almost 90% in patients who were not dialyzed at all.[83] There are four methods available for acute dialysis: hemodialysis, peritoneal dialysis, CAVH, and hemoperfusion. Hemodialysis is the fastest of all. It rapidly corrects uremia, fluid and electrolyte disturbances, and acidosis. However, in part because of the nature of the dialysis membrane, reduction in $PaO_2$ (~ 20 mm Hg) and platelet count (~ 30%) may occur in the first hour of dialysis.[62] Both $PaO_2$ and platelet count return to baseline levels within 1 to 2 hours after the start of the treatment.

Complications of hemodialysis are the disequilibrium syndrome, hypotension, hypoxemia, hemorrhage, arrhythmias, and problems related to technical errors (air embolism, dialysate contamination, etc.) (Table 25-8). The disequilibrium syndrome is manifested by headache, nausea, vomiting, disorientation, tremors, increased CSF pressure, and EEG abnormalities. Seizures and coma may occur in severe cases. These symptoms are probably caused by cerebral edema secondary to sudden osmotic gradient changes between the brain and blood during hemodialysis.[252] Paradoxical acidosis may develop in the CSF during hemodialysis and can also cause these symptoms.[18] Elevation of intracranial pressure has been described in head-injured patients during dialysis.[34] Thus, intracranial pressure monitoring may be necessary in these patients.

Hypotension, which occurs in approximately 35% of patients during hemodialysis, is often secondary to excessive fluid removal, but may also be related to changes in osmolarity, plasticizer infusion, blood-membrane incompatibility, or acetate toxicity.[5] Acetate, the cation used in the dialysis bath fluid, is metabolized by the liver. In patients in whom a large dialysis membrane is used or in those who have decreased cardiac output or liver impairment, acetate toxicity may occur. Hypotension from this cause is a result of peripheral vasodilation and myocardial depression. Bicarbonate

TABLE 25-8. Problems Associated with Hemodialysis

| | EXPECTED | UNEXPECTED |
|---|---|---|
| Dialyzer membrane-related | Hypoxemia<br>Leukopenia<br>Thrombocytopenia | Dialyzer leak |
| Dialysate compartment-related | Water-soluble vitamin loss<br>Bicarbonate loss | Errors in dialysate composition<br>Contamination of dialysate (formaldehyde, nitrate, aluminum)<br>Acetate toxicity |
| Blood compartment-related | Prolonged clotting time | Bleeding—GI tract, subdural, hemopericardium<br>Air embolism |
| Combined compartment-related | Hypotension | Disequilibrium syndrome |

baths are preferable in patients who do not tolerate acetate dialysis.

Hypoxemia may be caused by hypoventilation, increased oxygen consumption, or pulmonary microembolism by blood clots or fibrin. This complication is usually seen when acetate is used in the dialysate; the problem appears to be averted by using bicarbonate.[203] Bleeding from heparin anticoagulation can be minimized by using a constant low-dose heparin infusion to maintain a clotting time twice normal. Occasionally, it may be necessary to use protamine in the venous return channel of the dialysis system. The use of prostacyclin as an anticoagulant during hemodialysis is under investigation.[269] Despite these problems, hemodialysis remains the mainstay of dialysis therapy for ARF.

Peritoneal dialysis is the slowest dialysis technique, but has a low incidence of side effects. It is contraindicated in patients with abdominal sepsis or in those who require laparotomy for abdominal trauma. In addition, patients who are catabolic may be underdialysed when this method is used. Currently, peritoneal dialysis does not enjoy widespread popularity for ARF treatment in trauma patients.

Continuous AV hemofiltration (CAVH) using small hollow-fiber hemofilters without pumps is an alternative to conventional acute dialysis methods. (Fig 25-4).[126,159] There is little hemodynamic interference when this method is employed; thus, it is particularly useful in ARF patients who are likely to develop hypotension during standard hemodialysis therapy. CAVH provides smooth continuous treatment of uremia without causing a disequilibrium state. Another important advantage of this method is that filtrate removal (500–800 mL/h) permits administration of the large volumes of parenteral nutrition solutions needed by the injured oliguric patient without the risk of volume overload. The problems associated with CAVH are the needs for continuous heparinization and for constant supervision. CAVH also may impose difficulties in mobilizing and transporting these patients.

Vascular access for venovenous shunts is usually achieved with a double-lumen catheter via either the subclavian or femoral vein (Table 25-9). Femoral catheters can be left in place for at least 1 week and subclavian catheters for as long as 3 weeks. A Scribner shunt (radial artery to vein or femoral artery to vein) is especially useful in CAVH. Unfortunately, the use of this shunt makes an important artery unavailable for further use if the patient requires long-term dialysis.

TABLE 25-9. Vascular Access for Hemodialysis and Hemofiltration

| TRANSIENT ACUTE RENAL FAILURE | PERMANENT OR CHRONIC RENAL FAILURE |
|---|---|
| Venovenous | Artery to vein |
| Femoral or subclavian veins (double-lumen catheters) | Femoral artery to vein (CAVH)<br>Scribner shunt (radial artery to radial vein)<br>AV fistula |
| Artery to vein | |
| Femoral artery to vein (continuous arteriovenous hemofiltration) | Gortex graft |

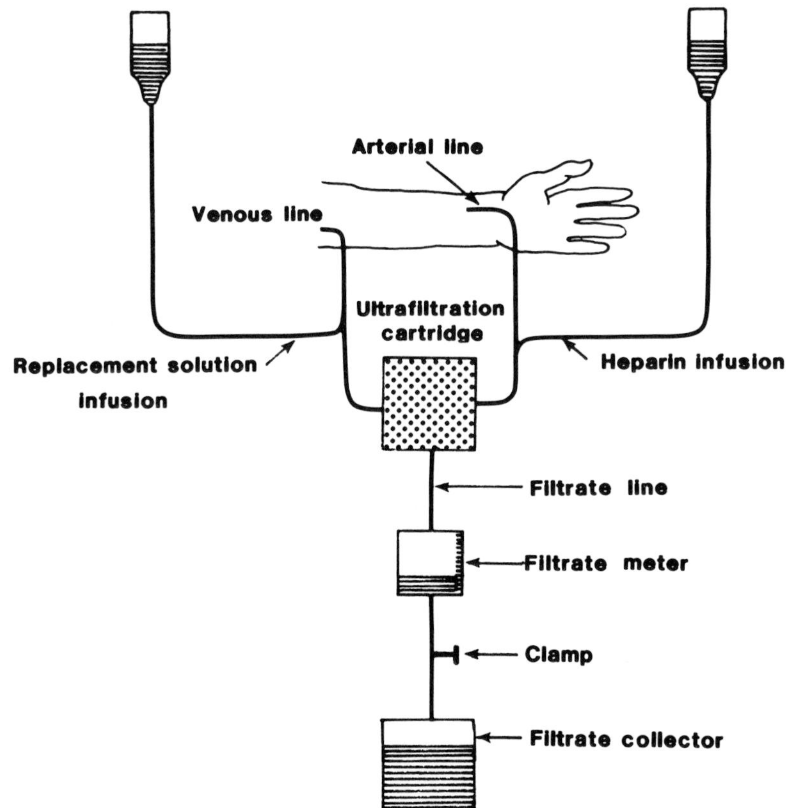


FIG. 25-4. Continuous AV hemofiltration (CAVH) system.

Charcoal hemoperfusion is used infrequently in the treatment of ARF. However, impressive results have been obtained in patients with fulminant hepatic failure (hepatorenal syndrome) by this method and by the use of prostacyclin to prevent platelet activation.[102]

## RECOVERY (PHASE V)

Fifty percent of patients who survive ARF can expect the return of adequate renal function. After recovery, the oliguric ARF patient experiences some reduction in urine volume for about 10 to 23 days.[151] The onset of diuresis should not prompt the physician to relax close supervision as significant mortality can still occur during this period. The homeostatic regulation of fluid and electrolytes is often diminished during this phase, and sodium wasting may occur. If there is polyuria, daily serum and urinary electrolytes and body weight must be measured. In most cases diuresis and natriuresis appear to be secondary to excretion of edema fluid. Large urinary potassium losses can occur during the polyuric phase, requiring potassium supplementation if the serum $K^+$ is less than 3 mEq/L.

Within the first month, more than 90% of patients with ARF have either regained adequate renal function or have died.[134] The longest reported dialysis time after which the patient recovered normal kidney function is 88 days.[134] Renal function usually continues to improve over the first month after the final dialysis. Although the duration of dialysis does not appear to correlate with the degree of functional recovery, the patient's age does. Older patients progress to chronic renal failure more often and rarely make a complete recovery.[91] The renal consequences in the 50% of the patients who survive are as follows: 15% recover completely; 25% have an incomplete recovery but renal function is stable for the rest of their lives, 5% have no renal recovery and exhibit end-stage renal disease, and 5% have partial recovery but progress slowly to end-stage renal disease.

### PROGNOSIS

The overall mortality rate from posttraumatic ARF is 50%,[91] which is an improvement over the 67% mortality observed in similar trauma patients in the 1960s. Of these, 50% die of infection, 20% of congestive heart failure, 10% of hyperkalemia, 10% of gastrointestinal bleeding, and 10% of respiratory failure.[91]

## ANESTHETIC CARE OF THE PATIENT WITH ACUTE RENAL FAILURE

During the course of their disease, many trauma victims with ARF require surgery, often more than once. Creation of an arteriovenous fistula in the upper extremity for hemodialysis is generally an elective procedure. Emergency surgery usually involves exploratory laparotomy for drainage of intra-abdominal abscesses, debridement of extremity wounds, or operation for gastrointestinal bleeding. Marshall[162] re-explored 18 patients who had ARF and had developed complications after abdominal surgery. He noted major surgical complications in 17 of these patients and commented on the seriousness of their condition. As mentioned earlier, any additional insult to the kidney during the course of ARF carries a poor prognosis.[38] Therefore, extreme care should be exercised during anesthetic management of these patients to prevent unfavorable sequelae.

### PREOPERATIVE EVALUATION AND PREPARATION

Trauma patients with ARF may undergo surgery in different phases of the disease. Although the basic pathophysiology is the same, the clinical manifestations of the disease may vary during each of these phases. For instance, early in ARF, especially when the patient is oliguric, hypervolemia is a common problem, and its preoperative recognition and treatment are prime considerations. Later, in the diuretic phase, hypovolemia may be prominent, and fluid replacement based on the patient's intake, output, and hemodynamic condition may be necessary. Accordingly, preoperative fluid and electrolyte therapy for the patient with acute renal failure varies considerably with the phase of the disease.

Another important consideration during preoperative evaluation is the type of ARF. As mentioned earlier, fluid and electrolyte abnormalities and acid-base disturbances occur more slowly in the nonoliguric than in the oliguric form of the disease. Finally, the surgical problem may confuse the preoperative assessment of the patient with renal failure. For instance, metabolic acidosis caused by hypovolemia and decreased tissue perfusion during hemorrhage or sepsis may be interpreted as being caused by ARF, resulting in a delay in instituting appropriate treatment.

A systematic approach, which places emphasis on fluid and electrolyte status, acid-base balance, hematologic abnormalities, and other systemic disturbances, is probably the best way to evaluate these patients preoperatively. The wide variation of urine output, insensible water loss, fluid sequestration, and prior fluid infusion makes prediction of net intravascular volume status difficult; an active search for clinical signs of hypovolemia or hypervolemia and, at times, invasive preoperative measurement of hemodynamic indices may be necessary. Electrolytes must be measured shortly before surgery since a rapid elevation of serum $K^+$, decline of serum $Na^+$, and elevation or decline of serum $Ca^{++}$ may occur. Hypercalcemia occurs during the diuretic phase of the disease, especially after rhabdomyolysis.[107] Hyperkalemia is exacerbated by extensive muscle injury, accumulation of hematomas in tissue compartments, and gastrointestinal bleeding. Fluid and electrolyte losses should be replaced before surgery. Patients who are already hypervolemic may have to be treated preoperatively with diuretics and/or inotropic agents.

Sometimes the surgery may follow hemodialysis, the most effective treatment for hypervolemia and hyperkalemia. In addition to hypovolemia, arrhythmias may follow dialysis because of abrupt changes in serum electrolytes, particularly potassium; serum electrolytes should be measured immediately after treatment is completed. If the surgery is performed more than 6 hours after dialysis, electrolytes should be measured again as serum $K^+$ may rise rapidly in some patients with ARF.[87,257]

Metabolic acidosis in the septic or hemorrhaging ARF patient has two possible causes: retention of the normally produced acid load and suboptimal tissue perfusion causing the accumulation of lactic acid. If possible, the etiology of this problem should be determined. Metabolic acidosis causes myocardial depression and augments hyperkalemia; thus it should be treated with sodium bicarbonate before surgery. However, overzealous treatment when serum $K^+$ is low may result in cardiac arrhythmias. If time permits, hemodialysis may be considered for treatment of severe metabolic acidosis.

Most patients with ARF are anemic and require transfusion, especially when the contemplated surgery will involve significant blood loss. If possible, the patient should be transfused during dialysis so that fluid overload caused by transfusion can be prevented or treated easily. Patients with ARF may also develop coagulation abnormalities due to reduced platelet adhesiveness,[82] residual heparin effect after dialysis, DIC, or a combination of these factors. Reduced platelet adhesiveness, which results in a prolonged bleeding time, can be partially corrected by preoperative hemodialysis. Residual heparin effect is indicated by prolongation of activated clotting time (ACT) and partial thromboplastin time. This abnormality can be corrected by small doses of protamine sulfate (0.5–1.0 mg/kg). However, preoperative coagulation abnormalities are most commonly treated by transfusion of platelets, fresh-frozen plasma (FFP) and plasma cryoprecipitate, especially when surgery must be performed urgently.[125] When coagulation abnormalities are serious, a hematologist should be consulted.

Gastrointestinal complications—nausea, vomiting, abdominal distention, and hiccups—are common in ARF and may prolong the gastric emptying time. Furthermore, gastrointestinal bleeding, which may occur in 10–30% of these patients,[136] may result in a full stomach, increasing the risk of aspiration pneumonitis. Precautions should be taken to prevent this complication during the induction of anesthesia.

Ischemic coronary artery disease and even acute myocardial infarction may be present in older patients with ARF.[136,175] In addition, cardiac arrhythmias, deep vein thrombosis, and pulmonary emboli may occur.[189] Pericarditis or pericardial effusion should be detected preoperatively by careful history, physical examination, ECG, X-ray, and echocardiography.[27,251]

Septicemia, pneumonia, and urinary tract and wound infections are also common in ARF.[10,175] Preoperative auscultation of the lungs, chest X-ray, and arterial blood gas determinations must be performed routinely to detect pulmonary infections.

Peripheral neuropathy, confusion, stupor, agitation, or coma may be complicating features of ARF.[205,206] It has been suggested that these central nervous system abnormalities may be due to the increased $Ca^{++}$ content of the gray matter.[72] These changes revert to normal upon the recovery of renal function.[56] Many of these problems can be corrected by preoperative hemodialysis.[205,206]

Digitalis, beta-adrenergic blocking and antihypertensive agents, diuretics, antiarrhythmics, and calcium channel blockers are commonly used to treat the complications of ARF. Accumulation of these agents in the presence of renal dysfunction may result in toxicity and interaction with anesthetic agents. The presence of such toxicity should be determined in the preoperative period to avoid intraoperative complications. Although digitalis, clonidine, diazoxide, and methyldopa rely on renal elimination, hydralazine and propranolol do not, and they are not likely to cause significant toxicity in the presence of renal dysfunction (Appendix I).[11]

## PREMEDICATION

Benzodiazepines are considered safe to use in renal failure because they undergo hepatic metabolism. However, the effects of diazepam and chlordiazepoxide (Librium) may be prolonged since excretion of their active metabolites is delayed in ARF (Appendix I).[11] Other benzodiazepines present no problems for patients with ARF because their metabolites are not active.[41]

Only a small fraction (10–15%) of administered morphine and meperidine is excreted in the urine.[32] The terminal elimination half-life and the total body clearance of morphine are similar in patients with chronic renal failure and in those with normal renal function.[4,53,220] These findings suggest that patients with renal dysfunction do not require dosage adjustments of morphine and meperidine. However, potentiation of pharmacologic activity and prolongation of the effects of these drugs have been documented in anecdotal reports.[76] Recent data suggest that these effects are produced by accumulated active metabolites of morphine.[220] The toxic effects of repeated doses of meperidine—irritability, twitching, and seizures—in patients with renal failure may also result from its active metabolite, normeperidine, although there is no conclusive evidence to confirm this suggestion.[158]

Premedication with antacids and/or $H_2$-receptor antagonists has been recommended for prophylaxis of the acid aspiration syndrome.[158,257] However, cimetidine is excreted mainly by the kidney and can cause confusion in patients with renal disease. Its dose should be reduced by 50% when the GFR is less than 10 mL/min.[32] Cimetidine cannot be removed by hemodialysis or peritoneal dialysis.[32] In view of this, the authors do not recommend cimetidine in this group of patients. Ranitidine is also excreted by the kidney, but some degradation occurs in the liver.[32] Its biologic half-life is prolonged in end-stage renal disease from approximately 2 to 7 hours.[32] Like cimetidine, its dose should be reduced by 50% in patients with severe renal dysfunction. Unlike cimetidine, ranitidine can be removed from the body by hemodialysis.[32] Atropine or glycopyrrolate may be given in usual doses to patients in renal failure.[158]

## ANESTHETIC MANAGEMENT

The selection of anesthetic technique and agents is based largely on three considerations: the type of surgery, the effect of anesthetic agents on renal function, and the influence of renal dysfunction on the effect and duration of the anesthetic. Ideally, the technique selected should provide satisfactory surgical conditions, should not produce further deterioration of renal function, and should not be affected by the underlying renal dysfunction. Unfortunately most of the available data on the interactions between anesthetic agents and renal function have been obtained either from patients with normal kidneys or from those with chronic renal failure. These data may not apply to the patient with ARF whose residual renal function is less than normal but usually more than that observed in patients with end-stage chronic renal disease. Nevertheless, familiarity with these data can help guide the anesthetic management of patients with ARF.

### *Regional Anesthesia*

As mentioned earlier, uremic neuropathy may occur during the late stages of ARF,[206] but its presence does not seem to be a contraindication to regional anesthesia.[43,152,158,193,257] A brachial plexus block is particularly useful for creation of an upper extremity arteriovenous fistula since it results in greater blood flow of longer duration through the shunt and less hemodynamic depression than that produced by general anesthesia with halothane or isoflurane.[187] The duration of a supraclavicular brachial plexus block is said to be shorter in patients with renal dysfunction than in those with normal kidneys, probably because the local anesthetic is cleared more rapidly from the perineural site by increased regional blood flow.[43] However, this difference does not seem to be present when an axillary approach is used.[163] Spinal or epidural anesthesia may be used for surgery on the lower extremities, provided the patient does not have coagulation abnormalities.[130] With 0.75% bupivacaine the onset of sensory analgesia in patients with chronic renal failure patients appears to be more rapid than in normal patients.[193] The duration of sensory and motor blockade is also shorter in this group of patients compared to normal individuals.[193] This effect may be caused by a hyperdynamic circulation and rapid washout of the local anesthetic from the site of action.

Early experimental studies demonstrated that spinal or epidural anesthesia (T10 sensory level) did not produce a significant decrease in renal blood flow (RBF). There was, however, a significant reduction in RBF (up to 40%) during high T1 level) spinal or epidural anesthesia.[230,231] At high sensory levels, there was a proportional decrease in mean arterial pressure and cardiac output, suggesting that the decrease in RBF was simply the result of reduced cardiac output, rather than of a direct effect on the renal vasculature. More recent data from animal experiments suggest that spinal anesthesia at a sensory level of T4 or higher causes less reduction of RBF, GFR, renal oxygen consumption, and renal cefoxitin excretion than general anesthesia with thiopental and halothane, if cardiac output is maintained by an infusion of crystalloids before the regional block.[165,213,214] The profound decline in renal function seen with general anesthesia in these studies resulted from the reduction of cardiac output caused by the agents used. Thus, a well-conducted spinal anesthetic appears to have only minimal effects on normal kidney function. Although the effects of spinal anesthesia on the diseased kidney have not yet been elucidated, it is likely that it produces fewer deleterious effects than general anesthesia in this group of patients.

### *General Anesthesia*

General anesthesia may be required for major surgical procedures. All general anesthetic agents cause a reduction of urine flow, GFR, RBF, and water and electrolyte excretion.[60] In the surgical patient without renal disease, anesthetics depress kidney function only temporarily; the function usually returns to normal in the postoperative period.[60] This effect may be more severe in patients with renal disease because of the decreased elimination of some anesthetic and adjunct agents.

Depression of renal function is caused by both direct and indirect effects of anesthetics on the kidneys. These effects are dose dependent and seem to be less severe when extracellular volume is adequate.[60,167] The direct effects are caused primarily by the toxicity of anesthetics and/or their metabolites. With the possible exception of enflurane, which is discussed later, none of the agents used in modern anesthesia appears to have such an effect on the kidneys. Anesthetics depress renal function indirectly by affecting (a) systemic and renal circulation; (b) the sympathetic nervous system; (c) renal autoregulation; and (d) hormones that regulate urine volume, electrolyte excretion, and renal blood flow.[60] Antidiuretic hormone (ADH), adrenaline, noradrenaline, aldosterone, atrial natriuretic factor (ANF), and the renin-angiotensin system are all involved in various functions of the kidney and are all affected by anesthetic agents. Kidney function is further depressed by such factors as stress, anxiety, pain, hypoxemia, and blood loss during surgery. Thus, anesthetic management of the patient with ARF requires adequate knowledge of the renal effects of the various anesthetic agents, adequate perioperative monitoring elimination of all perioperative factors that may adversely effect systemic and renal hemodynamics, and the appropriate use of anesthetic or adjunct drugs.

### *Intravenous Induction Agents*

Thiopental may be used safely as an induction agent in normovolemic ARF patients. In animals with normal renal function, renal blood flow and vascular resistance are maintained reasonably well after the administration of thiopental.[199] The binding of thiopental to plasma proteins is likely to be reduced in patients with renal failure because of decreased albumin levels, acidosis, changes in serum protein structure, and increased levels of nitrogenous end-products that displace the albumin-bound drug.[48,99,267] The blood-brain barrier may be modified in uremic patients and cause an accelerated delivery of thiopental to the brain.[117] The drug should thus be given slowly and the dose titrated to its effects on the central nervous and cardiovascular systems.

In animals diazepam causes a slight reduction of renal blood flow, but renal function remains unaltered.[199] Like thiopental, this drug is bound mainly to serum albumin. Thus, the effects of diazepam should increase in uremic patients with decreased serum albumin concentration.[108] As mentioned, the active metabolite of diazepam (desmethyldiazepam) is excreted by the kidney; thus, a prolonged effect may be noted in patients with renal dysfunction.[158]

Midazolam is metabolized by the liver. Its metabolites, although excreted in the urine, appear to be considerably less active than the parent compound.[211] The unbound plasma fraction of midazolam is increased in patients with renal failure. This results in a decreased onset time and prolonged effect, necessitating reduction in dosage.[250] The elimination half-life, volume of distribution, and renal clearance of midazolam are not changed by ARF.[250]

Ketamine increases the blood pressure, heart rate, and cardiac output of patients with renal failure without changing total peripheral resistance.[119] These effects appear to be mediated by central autonomic stimulation and not by renin-angiotensin hyperactivity.[177,178] In animals, ketamine also increases renal blood flow in a dose-dependent manner.[199] A relatively small fraction (26%) of ketamine is bound to plasma proteins.[69] In patients with normal renal function, less than 4% of the administered drug or its active metabolite (norketamine) can be recovered from the urine.[261,262] Thus, ketamine's effect is not prolonged by decreased renal clearance.[261] In any event, termination of the anesthetic effects of ketamine is primarily caused by redistribution from the brain, rather than by metabolism or excretion.

### *Inhalational Agents*

There is a wide discrepancy in the results of studies on the effects of inhalational agents on renal hemodynamics. Early work using para-aminohippurate (PAH) clearance showed a significant reduction in RBF with inhalational agents.[73] Recently it has become clear that anesthetic agents alter PAH clearance without a proportional change in RBF.[24,60] Experiments in animals with other analytic techniques have demonstrated that, when used alone, inhalational agents do not reduce RBF significantly.[25,26,179,201,248] However, as mentioned above, a significant reduction in cardiac output and thus renal blood flow may be noted if they are used in conjunction with other depressant agents.[165,213,214]

Clinically, the reduction of RBF, GFR, and urine flow with inhalational anesthetics[3,59,169] is mediated by decreased cardiac output.[131] These effects are dose dependent and can be attenuated by preoperative hydration of the patient.[22,25,105,167] Since patients with ARF are prone to hypovolemia, especially shortly after hemodialysis, utmost attention should be given to the proper evaluation of volume status and adequate hydration before using these agents.

Halothane can be used safely in patients with ARF, provided that hemodynamic stability is maintained. Renal autoregulation is preserved with this agent at end-tidal concentrations of up to 0.9%.[25] Supplemental narcotic agents, particularly fentanyl or sufentanil, help keep the halothane concentration below this level.[158] Concomitant use of nitrous oxide also reduces the halothane requirement, although animal studies suggest the augmentation of antidiuresis with this approach.[118]

The renal hemodynamic effects of enflurane are similar to those of halothane.[3] By potentiating the effect of nondepolarizing muscle relaxants, enflurane permits the reduction of muscle relaxant dosage and thereby decreases the risk of prolonged postoperative paralysis in patients with severe renal disease.[158] Enflurane causes a dose-dependent increase in serum inorganic fluoride ($F^-$) concentrations. The peak serum $F^-$ levels reach 22 μM after 2.7 MAC hours exposure to enflurane[59] (Fig 25-5) and 34 μM after 9.6 MAC hours.[170] Although renal function is not altered at serum $F^-$ levels of 22 μM,[59] a level of 34 μM may cause a significant decrease

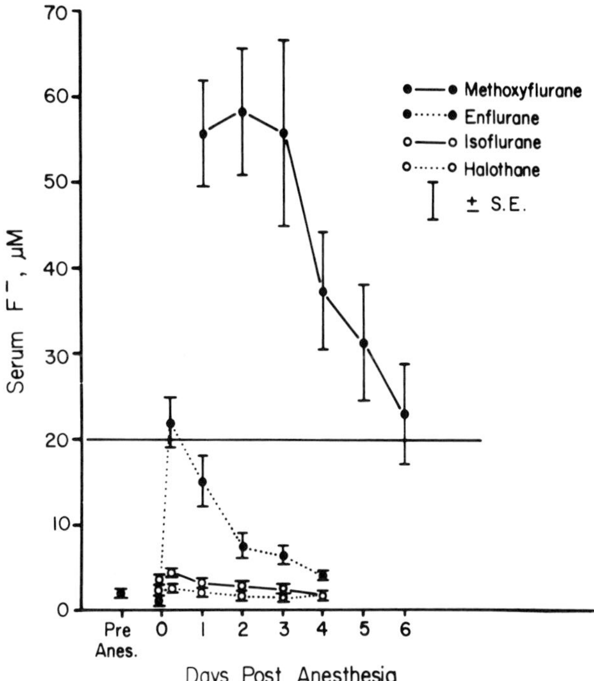


FIG. 25-5. Serum inorganic fluoride ($F^-$) concentrations before and after methoxyflurane, enflurane, isoflurane, and halothane anesthesia. After methoxyflurane anesthesia a sustained increase in serum $F^-$ concentration (55 μM) is noted. After enflurane anesthesia, peak $F^-$ concentration (22 μM) occurs earlier and declines much more rapidly. Only slight increases in $F^-$ occur after isoflurane and halothane anesthesia. (From Cousins et al[59] with permission.)

in maximum urinary osmolality, suggesting a defect in urine concentrating ability.[170] These changes in renal function, however, are brief; serum $F^-$ levels, even after prolonged exposure to enflurane (9.6 MAC hours), remain slightly above 20 μM for approximately 18 hours, and maximum urinary osmolality returns within a few days.[170] Thus, administration of enflurane (less than 5 or 6 MAC hours) to patients with normal kidneys should not adversely affect renal function or fluid homeostasis. It should be remembered that acidification of urine decreases the urinary excretion of $F^-$, resulting in high serum levels; alkalinization has the opposite effect.[117]

The question of whether enflurane should be used in patients with renal failure remains. Several case reports suggest that enflurane may cause further deterioration of renal function in patients with pre-existing renal disease.[80,155] It is possible that the effects of $F^-$ on the renal collecting tubules last longer in these patients than in those with normal kidneys. Experimental studies in rats, in which chronic renal insufficiency was induced either surgically or with gentamicin, demonstrated no further impairment of renal function after enflurane anesthesia.[93,229] Mazze and co-workers[171] administered enflurane for approximately 200 minutes to surgical patients who had moderate renal dysfunction (mean $C_{cr}$ = 35 mL/min). Serum $F^-$ peaked to 20 μM 4 hours after operation, then fell to 17 μM, 11 μM, and 7 μM at 24, 48, and 72 hours after anesthesia, respectively. Postoperative renal function remained unaltered, and in fact, a slight improvement in $C_{cr}$ was noted in patients who received enflurane.

Although urine concentrating ability, the most sensitive test of $F^-$ nephropathy, was not assessed in this study, these results suggest that a relatively short exposure to enflurane does not produce a deterioration of kidney function in patients with moderate renal dysfunction. Even in patients with severe renal insufficiency, enflurane may be without adverse effects. Carter et al.[50] were unable to demonstrate any abnormalities in fluoride kinetics or further postoperative deterioration of renal function in patients with severe renal insufficiency. Normally, 40% of the $F^-$ load is excreted by the kidneys, and the remainder is incorporated into bone. It is likely that in patients with renal dysfunction a greater proportion of $F^-$ enters the bone, preventing exposure of the kidney to more than moderate amounts of this ion. Nevertheless, the combination of preoperative renal dysfunction and high serum $F^-$ levels may potentially result in deterioration of kidney function. Thus, enflurane should probably be avoided in patients with ARF.[166]

Isoflurane provides more hemodynamic stability than either halothane or enflurane, although it produces comparable reductions in RBF, GFR, and urine flow.[169] The minimal hepatic biotransformation of this agent results in a much lower serum $F^-$ concentration (average 4–5 μM) than that produced by enflurane.[169] This agent is also associated with low arrhythmogenicity and enhances the neuromuscular blockade produced by nondepolarizing muscle relaxants, allowing their use in reduced doses.[158] These properties of isoflurane confer distinct advantages in patients with ARF.

### *Narcotic Agents*

Narcotic agents are used for both induction and maintenance of anesthesia. Based on early animal studies, narcotics were thought to stimulate ADH secretion and thereby reduce urine flow.[70] Although there is some evidence in humans that high cerebrospinal fluid concentrations of morphine may result in increased ADH secretion,[141,246] the usual response to normal intravenous doses of narcotics is attenuation of ADH secretion.[139,196] Decreased urine flow, a common finding during surgery, may be caused by increased ADH, but this effect is secondary to surgical stress, rather than to narcotics.[185,245] In fact, the available data suggest that high-dose narcotic agents may be used to attenuate the surgically induced hormonal stress response.[139,196]

Fentanyl undergoes biotransformation in the liver; only a small fraction of this drug is eliminated by the kidney. Priano[200] demonstrated that renal autoregulation is preserved in animals with up to 50 μg/kg fentanyl. The combination of higher doses (100 μg/kg) of fentanyl and $O_2$–$N_2O$ anesthesia improves renal function during major surgery as evidenced by increased urine flow, decreased urine osmolality and $Na^+$, and no change in creatinine clearance.[139] Combined use of droperidol and fentanyl has been recommended for patients with renal failure since renal function is well maintained with these agents.[257] Sufentanil is capable of suppressing hemodynamic and hormonal responses to surgery. However, its safety in renal failure has not yet been established. Prolonged postoperative respiratory depression with elevated plasma sufentanil levels in a patient with chronic renal failure has been described.[263]

The renal effects of high-dose morphine (2 mg/kg) with and without $N_2O$ (60%) were determined by Stanley et al.[236] in patients with normal kidneys undergoing abdominal operations. Morphine alone had little effect on systemic and renal hemodynamics, but the addition of $N_2O$ altered renal function markedly. Meperidine, as mentioned earlier, may cause irritability, twitching, and seizures in patients with renal failure, especially after repeated doses.[79] Thus, caution must be exercised in administering this drug to patients with renal failure.

Although balanced anesthesia appears to maintain reasonably good renal function, sympathetic overactivity may occur more frequently with this technique than with potent inhalational anesthetics. Intraoperative hypertension during balanced anesthesia may have adverse effects on renal blood flow. In these instances, addition of low concentrations of halothane or isoflurane may be desirable.[117]

### *Muscle Relaxants*

Succinylcholine causes a small, transient decrease in renal blood flow in animals.[147] This drug is well known to increase serum $K^+$ by approximately 0.5 mEq/L in normal patients.[106] Although early reports suggested augmentation of this response in renal failure,[198,212] more recent work conclusively demonstrates that the magnitude of serum $K^+$ elevation after succinylcholine is similar to that seen in normal subjects.[55,68,138,182,197] However, succinylcholine should be avoided if serum $K^+$ is greater than 5.5 mEq/L[117,182] or if advanced uremic neuropathy is present.[253] The latter condition may result in an exaggerated hyperkalemic response, although it is extremely rare in adequately dialyzed ARF patients. The duration of action of succinylcholine is not prolonged in patients with renal failure. Early reports suggested decreased serum cholinesterase activity in dialyzed patients. However, this was probably caused by the old cellophane dialysis membranes, which are known to decrease serum cholinesterase. These membranes are no longer in use, and renal failure per se does not decrease serum cholinesterase levels.[215] Thus, prolonged apnea should not occur after succinylcholine in patients with renal failure.

Nondepolarizing muscle relaxants have been studied extensively in patients with kidney dysfunction. Gallamine does not appear to reduce RBF, but its excretion depends primarily on the kidneys. The plasma clearance of this drug is prolonged approximately five times in patients with renal failure, precluding its use.[204,222] d-Tubocurarine in large bolus doses can cause a fall in arterial blood pressure, cardiac output, and renal blood flow.[147] This reduction of RBF may last up to 10 minutes and possibly exacerbate renal failure. Normally, a significant portion of d-tubocurarine is excreted by the kidney. In the presence of renal failure, biliary excretion of this drug is increased, preventing excessive prolongation of muscle paralysis.[180] The plasma clearance rate of d-tubocurarine in renal failure is about half that of normal patients. The elimination half-life of the drug is also prolonged. (Table 25-10).[178] Plasma binding of d-tubocurarine is unchanged in patients with kidney dysfunction.[100] Clinically, renal failure prolongs the effect of d-tubocurarine only slightly at low doses, but significant effects may be seen after a large single dose or multiple doses.[101] Therefore, the drug should be titrated to effect by neuromuscular monitoring. Recurarization after administration of d-tubocurarine to patients with renal failure, although described,[181] is unlikely to occur.

Metocurine has relatively few cardiovascular effects. In normal subjects, 48% of a bolus intravenous dose is excreted unchanged in the urine. In patients with renal failure, the prolonged elimination half-life and decreased clearance of metocurine result in prolonged paralysis. (Table 25-10)[44] The sensitivity of the neuromuscular junction to this drug appears to be less in patients with renal failure than in those with intact kidney function.[44] Generally, metocurine offers no major advantage over the other long-acting nondepolarizing muscle relaxants in patients with renal failure.

Pancuronium has a minimal effect on RBF.[147] Several reports have described prolonged paralysis with pancuronium in patients with renal dysfunction.[98,115] Unlike d-tubocurarine, elimination of pancuronium via the biliary route is not increased in renal failure. Therefore, the decline in plasma pancuronium level is slower than that of d-tubocurarine.[174,180,183] Although the possibility of recurarization after adequate antagonism of pancuronium in patients with renal failure has been suggested,[181] the occurrence of this phenomenon seems unlikely.[36] Nevertheless, when large doses of pancuronium are antagonized with anticholinesterase agents, recovery is often insufficient to ensure normal ventilatory function.

Atracurium is the only nondepolarizing muscle relaxant the effect of which is not prolonged by renal failure.[71,254] Elimination of atracurium does not depend on kidney function; thus it can be used safely in patients with renal failure (Table 25-10). Elevated plasma concentrations of laudanosine have been reported after administration of atracurium to patients with renal failure, but the clinical significance of this finding is uncertain.[90,254]

Early studies demonstrated that vecuronium pharmacokinetics were not altered by renal failure and that the drug could be used safely without prolongation of its action.[30,35] These studies, however, examined single bolus doses and very brief infusions of vecuronium (Table 25-10). When repeated doses are administered or a continuous infusion is used, delayed recovery, sometimes up to 40 hours, has been noted.[234] This prolongation of neuromuscular blockade has been confirmed by a recent pharmacokinetic study that showed that vecuronium's elimination half-life increased and its volume of distribution decreased by about 40% in the presence of renal failure (Table 25-10)[157] Concomitant liver dysfunction, which may be present in some trauma patients with multiorgan failure, may extend the action of vecuronium further. Caution should be exercised when major surgery in a patient with ARF necessitates repeated doses and/or a prolonged infusion of vecuronium.

The effects of nondepolarizing muscle relaxants may be potentiated by respiratory and metabolic acidosis, inhalational anesthetic agents, electrolyte abnormalities, and certain antibiotics, eg, aminoglycosides. Hypothermia may accentuate the already diminished renal excretion of muscle relaxants, thereby causing further prolongation of paralysis. Respiratory depressant drugs should be used judiciously in the postoperative period, as they may result in hypercapnia and acidosis, potentiating any residual paralysis.

Reversal of residual muscle blockade can be achieved by any of the three available anticholinesterase agents.[65,66,186] As with the muscle relaxants, the excretion of edrophonium, neostigmine, and pyridostigmine is prolonged in renal failure. Thus, reversal of residual paralysis does not appear to present a problem. Pharmacokinetic parameters of these agents are shown in Table 25-10.

### *Intraoperative Monitoring*

In addition to routine monitoring (ECG, noninvasive blood pressure, urine output, end-tidal $CO_2$, and pulse oximetry), an arterial catheter and a central venous line may be neces-

TABLE 25-10. Pharmacokinetic Parameters of Nondepolarizing Muscle Relaxants and Reversal Agents in Patients With and Without Renal Failure

| AGENT | Vdss (1/kg) Normal | Vdss (1/kg) Renal Failure | $T_{1/2}$ (min) Normal | $T_{1/2}$ (min) Renal Failure | CLEARANCE (mL/kg/min) Normal | CLEARANCE (mL/kg/min) Renal Failure | REFERENCE |
|---|---|---|---|---|---|---|---|
| Metocurine* | 0.472 | 0.353 | 360 | 684 | 1.2 | 0.38 | Brotherton & Matteo[44] |
| Gallamine* | 0.21 | 0.29 | 131 | 752 | 1.2 | 0.24 | Ramzan et al.[204] |
| d-Tubocurarine* | 0.30 | — | 89 | Increased | 3.0 | Decreased | Fisher et al.[94] |
| | | | | | | | Miller et al.[183] |
| Pancuronium* | 0.26 | 0.30 | 133 | 257 | 1.8 | 0.9 | Somogyi et al.[235] |
| Atracurium* | $V_1$ = 0.6 | $V_1$ = 0.86 | 20.6 | 23.7 | 6.1 | 6.7 | Fahey et al.[89] |
| | $V_d$ area = 182 | $V_d$ area = 224 | | | | | |
| | $V_1$ = 0.05 | $V_1$ = 0.1 | 16.9 | 21.1 | 5.93 | 6.89 | de Bros et al.[71] |
| | $V_d$ area = 142 | $V_d$ area = 211 | | | | | |
| Vecuronium | 0.19 | 0.24 | 79.5 | 97.1 | 3.0 | 2.5 | Fahey et al.[88] |
| Vecuronium+ | 0.51 | 0.47 | 117 | 149 | 3.18 | 2.57 | Bencini et al.[30] |
| Vecuronium* | 0.20 | 0.24 | 53 | 83 | 5.29 | 3.08 | Lynam et al.[157] |
| Edrophonium* | 0.87 | 0.68 | 114 | 206 | 8.2 | 2.7 | Morris et al.[186] |
| Neostigmine* | 1.4 | 1.6 | 79.8 | 181.1 | 16.7 | 7.8 | Cronnelly et al.[66] |
| Pyridostigmine* | 1.1 | 1.0 | 112 | 379 | 8.6 | 2.1 | Cronnelly et al.[65] |

* Renal failure data obtained from anephric patients.
\+ Mixture of anephric and renal insufficiency patients.
Vdss = volume of distribution; $V_1$ clearance volume of central compartment; $V_d$ area = volume of distribution.

sary. The femoral or dorsalis pedis artery should be cannulated, rather than one of the upper limb arteries, because the latter may be needed later for creation of an arteriovenous fistula. Pulmonary artery catheters should be used if the patient is in congestive heart failure or large fluid shifts are expected.

If a Scribner shunt is already in place, the anesthesiologist should protect it by wrapping the arm properly. Doppler monitoring of shunt flow may also be useful since thrombotic occlusion may occur. Intravenous lines must not be started on that arm. Caution must also be exercised in caring for central venous lines since they may be used postoperatively for hyperalimentation.

### *Intraoperative Fluid Management*

Maintenance of adequate blood volume is essential for preventing renal failure in trauma patients. A urinary output of 1 mL/kg/h usually indicates good GFR. Reduction in urine flow can be treated by administering balanced salt solution, 3–5 mL/kg/h. If fluid administration at this rate is not effective, then cardiac filling pressures must be monitored with a central venous line. Guidelines for fluid administration in the anephric patient are presented elsewhere in the chapter. An anuric patient should receive fluid to make up for insensible loss plus any other loss that he or she may incur during surgery. To replace blood loss, washed, frozen RBCs should be used, as they are not associated with isoimmunization by plasma protein or WBC-related antigens.

### *Postoperative Hypertension*

Postoperative hypertension may be a problem in these patients. It usually responds to such vasodilators as sodium nitroprusside. The likelihood of cyanide toxicity may be less in patients in ARF because of diminished renal excretion of thiosulfate, which acts as an endogenous sulfur donor, facilitating the conversion of cyanide to thiocyanate.[243]

## CONCLUSION

Acute renal failure is a serious problem in the trauma patient. The overall mortality is approximately 50%, although intensive therapy may reduce this to 37%.[47] It is important to keep in mind that trauma patients may develop ARF not only because of the initial hypovolemic insult but also, late in their hospital course, from drug- or contrast medium-induced nephrotoxicity. Nonoliguric ARF is very common in this setting.

Improved hyperalimentation, antibiotic therapy, and meticulous attention to drug therapy offer the best chances for survival. Clearly, ARF is only one of the many problems that may exist in a trauma patient. Overall management takes priority over the management of renal failure. In the future synthetic or recombinant proteolytic inhibitors may well be of therapeutic significance in the catabolic, infected, injured patient with acute renal failure.[54a] Promising research on endothelin [91a,267a], endothelium derived relaxing factor, and calcium entry blockers [214a,218a] may have a significant impact on the clinical approach and treatment of future acute renal failure patients.

Any additional insult to the kidneys during the course of ARF carries a poor prognosis. Anesthesia for these patients thus requires extreme care to prevent such unfavorable sequelae. Careful preoperative evaluation and preparation, use of regional anesthetic methods whenever possible, adequate perioperative monitoring, elimination of potential risk factors, and appropriate use of anesthetic and adjunct drugs are some of the important principles of anesthetic management for the patient with ARF.

## REFERENCES

1. Abel RM, Beck CH, Abbott WM, et al. Improved survival from acute renal failure after treatment with intravenous essential L-amino acids and glucose. N Engl J Med 1973;288:695.
2. Acute renal failure (editorial). Br Med J 1980;280:1333.
3. Adams AP. Enflurane in clinical practice. Br J Anaesth 1981;53:27S.
4. Aitkenhead AR, Vater M, Achola K, et al. Pharmacokinetics of single dose I.V. morphine in normal volunteers and patients with end-stage renal failure. Br J Anaesth 1984;56:813.
5. Aizawa Y, Ohmori J, Imai K, et al. Depressant action of acetate upon the human cardiovascular system. Clin Nephrol 1977;8:477.
6. Alwall N. Therapeutic and diagnostic problems in severe renal failure. Copenhagen: Munksgaard, 1963.
7. Anderson CC, Shalvan MBG, Zimmerman JE. The treatment of pulmonary edema in the absence of renal function: a role for sorbitol and furosemide. JAMA 1979;241:1008.
8. Anderson RJ, Schrier RW. Clinical spectrum of oliguric and non-oliguric acute renal failure. In: Brenner BM, Stern JH, eds. Acute renal failure, New York: Churchill Livingstone, 1980:1.
9. Anderson RJ, Schrier RW. Acute renal failure. In: Petersdorf RG, Adams RD, Braunwald E, Isselbacher KJ, Martin JB, Wilson JD, eds. Harrison's principles of internal medicine. 10th ed. New York: McGraw-Hill, 1983:606.
10. Anderson RJ, Linas SL, Berns AS, et al. Non-oliguric acute renal failure. N Engl J Med 1977;296:1134.
11. Anderson RJ, Bennett WM, Gambertoglio JG, et al. Fate of drugs in renal failure. In: Brenner BM, Rector FC, eds. The kidney. 2nd ed. Philadelphia: WB Saunders, 1981:2659.
12. Annest SJ, Scovill WA, Blumenstock PA, et al. Increased creatinine clearance following cryoprecipitate infusion in trauma and surgical patients with decreased renal function. J Trauma 1980;20:276.
13. Anto HR, Chou SY, Porush JG, et al. Mannitol prevention of acute renal failure associated with infusion intravenous pyelography. Clin Res 1979;27:407A.
14. Anto HR, Chou SY, Porush JG, et al. Infusion intravenous pyelography and renal function: effects of hypertonic mannitol in patients with chronic renal failure. Arch Intern Med 1981;141:1652.
15. Antura A. Incidence and prophylaxis of acute postoperative renal failure in obstructive jaundice. Rev Med Chir Soc Med Nat Iasi 1979;83:247.
16. Appel GB, Neu HC. Gentamicin, 1979. Ann Intern Med 1978;89:528.
17. Ardaillou R, Beaufils M, Nevez MP, et al. Increased plasma calcitonin in early acute renal failure. Clin Sci Mol Med 1975;49:301.
18. Arieff AI, Guisado R, Massry SG, Lazarowitz VC. Central nervous system pH in uremia and the effects of hemodialysis. J Clin Invest 1976;58:306.
19. Badr KF, Ichikawa I. Prerenal failure: a deleterious shift from

renal compensation to decompensation. N Engl J Med 1988;319:623.
20. Baek SM, Brown RS, Shoemaker WC. Early prediction of acute renal failure and recovery. I. Sequential measurements of free water clearance. Ann Surg 1973;177:253.
21. Baek SM, Makabali GG, Brown RS, et al. Free-water clearance patterns as predictor and therapeutic guides in acute renal failure. Surgery 1975;77:632.
22. Barry KG, Mazze RI, Schwartz FD. Prevention of surgical oliguria and renal hemodynamic suppression by sustained hydration. N Engl J Med 1964;270:1371.
23. Barsoum RS, Rihan ZEB, Baligh OK, et al. Acute renal failure in the 1973 Middle East war—experience of a specialized base hospital: effect of the site of injury. J Trauma 1980;20:303.
24. Bastron RD, Kaloyanides GJ: Effects of methoxyflurane on PAH uptake by rabbit kidney slices. Am J Physiol 1974;227:460.
25. Bastron RD, Perkins FM, Payne JL. Autoregulation of renal blood flow during halothane anesthetic. Anesthesiology 1977;46:142.
26. Bastron RD, Payne JL, Inagaki M. Halothane-induced renal vasodilation. Anesthesiology 1979;50:126.
27. Beauary C, Nakamoto S, Kolff WJ. Uremic pericarditis and cardiac tamponade in chronic renal failure. Ann Intern Med 1966;64:990.
28. Beaufils M. Glomerular disease complicating abdominal sepsis. (Nephrology Forum) Kidney Int 1981;19:609.
29. Beaufils M, Morel-Maroger L, Sraer JD, et al. Acute renal failure of glomerular origin during visceral abscesses. N Engl J Med 1976;295:185.
30. Bencini AF, Scaf AHJ, Sohn YJ, et al. Disposition and urinary excretion of vecuronium bromide in anesthetized patients with normal renal function and renal failure. Anesth Analg 1986;65:245.
31. Bennett WM. Aminoglycoside nephrotoxicity. Nephron 1983;35:73.
32. Bennett WM. Drug therapy in renal disease. Scientific American Medicine, Nephrology (10) Section 2, Appendix A, 1989.
33. Berksett RD, Kjellstrand C. Radiological contrast-induced nephropathy. Med Clin North Am 1984;68:351.
34. Bertrand YM, Hermant A, Mahieu P, et al. Intracranial pressure changes in patients with head trauma during hemodialysis. Intens Care Med 1983;9:321.
35. Bevan DR, Gyasi H: Vecuronium in renal failure. Can Anaesth Soc J 1984;31:491.
36. Bevan DR, Archer D, Donati F, et al. Antagonism of pancuronium in renal failure: no recurarization. Br J Anaesth 1982;54:63.
37. Bidani A, Churchill P, Fleischmann L. Sodium chloride induced protection of nephrotoxic acute renal failure: independence from renin. Kidney Int 1979;16:481.
38. Bluemle LW, Webster GD, Elkington JR. Acute tubular necrosis. Arch Intern Med 1959;104:18.
39. Board for the Study of the Severely Wounded: The physiologic effects of wounds. In: Mediterranean theater operations. Washington, DC: Office of the Surgeon General, Dept. of the Army, 1952:376.
40. Bolger PM, Eisner GM, Ramwell PW, et al. Renal actions of prostacyclin. Nature 1978;271:467.
41. Breimer DD, Jochemsen R, von Albert HH. Pharmacokinetics of benzodiazepines. Drug Res 1980;30:875.
42. Bristow A, Giesecke AH. Fluid therapy of trauma. Semin Anesth 1985;4:124.
43. Bromage PR, Gertel HM. Brachial plexus anesthesia in chronic renal failure. Anesthesiology 1972;36:488.
44. Brotherton WP, Matteo RS. Pharmacokinetics and pharmacodynamics of metocurine in humans with and without renal failure. Anesthesiology 1981;55:273.
45. Brown R, Babcock R, Talbert J, et al: Renal function in critically ill postoperative patients: sequential assessment of creatinine, osmolar and free water clearance. Crit Care Med 1980;8:68.
46. Brown RS. Renal dysfunction in the surgical patient: maintenance of the high output state with furosemide. Crit Care Med 1979;7:63.
47. Bullock M, Umen A, Findelstein M, et al. The assessment of risk factors in 462 patients with acute renal failure. Am J Kidney Dis 1985;5:2.
48. Burch PG, Stanski DR. Decreased protein binding and thiopental kinetics. Clin Pharmacol Ther 1982;32:212.
49. Bywaters EGL, Beau D. Crush injuries with impairment of renal function. Br Med J 1941;1:427.
50. Carter R, Heerdt M, Acchiardo S. Fluoride kinetics after enflurane anesthesia in healthy and anephric patients and in patients with poor renal function. Clin Pharmacol Ther 1976;20:565.
51. Cattell WR, Fry IK. Urography in acute renal failure. Am Heart J 1975;90:124.
52. Champion H, Sacco W, Long W, et al. Indications for early hemodialysis in multiple trauma. Lancet 1974;1:1125.
53. Chauvin M, Sandouk P, Scherrmann JM, et al. Morphine pharmacokinetics in renal failure. Anesthesiology 1987;66:327.
54. Cockcroft DW, Gault MH. Prediction of creatinine clearance from serum creatinine. Nephron 1975;16:31.
54a. Colman RW. The role of plasma proteases in septic shock. New Engl J Med 1989;320:1207.
55. Cook DR, Cosimi AB, Hammonds MW. Potassium release following administration of succinylcholine in chronically uraemic monkeys. Can Anaesth Soc J 1972;19:634.
56. Cooper JD, Lazarowitz VC, Arieff AI: Neurodiagnostic abnormalities in patients with acute renal failure. J Clin Invest 1978;61:1448.
57. Corcoran AC, Page IH. Renal damage from ferroheme pigments in myoglobin, hemoglobin, hematin. Tex Rep Biol Med 1945;3:528.
57a. Cord JM. Oxygen-derived free radicals in post-ischemic tissue injury. N Engl J Med 1984;312:159.
58. Counts RB, Haisch C, Simon TL, et al. Hemostasis in massively transfused trauma patients. Ann Surg 1979;190:91.
59. Cousins MJ, Greenstein LR, Hitt BA, et al. Metabolism and renal effects of enflurane in man. Anesthesiology 1976;44:44.
60. Cousins MJ, Skowronski G, Plummer JL. Anaesthesia and the kidney. Anaesth Intens Care 1983;11:292.
61. Cox M. Potassium homeostasis. Med Clin North Am 1981;2:363.
62. Craddock P, Fehr J, Brigham K, et al. Complement and leukocyte-mediated pulmonary dysfunction in hemodialysis. N Engl J Med 1977;296:769.
63. Cronin RE. Aminoglycoside nephrotoxicity; pathogenesis and prevention. Clin Nephrol 1979;2:251.
64. Cronin RE. Acute renal failure in the experimental animal. Semin Nephrol 1981;1:5.
65. Cronnelly R, Stanski DR, Miller RD, et al. Pyridostigmine kinetics with and without renal function. Clin Pharmacol Ther 1980;28:78.
66. Cronnelly R, Stanski DR, Miller RD, et al. Renal function and the pharmacokinetics of neostigmine in anesthetized man. Anesthesiology 1981;53:31.
67. Czer LSC, Shoemaker WC. Optimal hematocrit value in critically ill postoperative patients. Surg Gynecol Obstet 1978;147:363.
68. Day S. Plasma potassium changes following suxamethonium and suxethonium in normal patients and in patients in renal failure. Br J Anaesth 1976;48:1011.
69. Dayton PG, Stiller RL, Cook DR, et al. The binding of ketamine to plasma proteins: emphasis on human plasma. Eur J Clin Pharmacol 1983;24:825.

70. De Bodo RC. Antidiuretic action of morphine and its mechanism. J Pharmacol Exp Ther 1944;82:74.
71. de Bros FM, Lai A, Scott R, et al. Pharmacokinetics and pharmacodynamics of atracurium during isoflurane anesthesia in normal and anephric patients. Anesth Analg 1986;65:743.
72. De Torrente A. Acute renal failure. Int Anesthesiol Clin 1984;22:83.
73. Deutsch S, Goldberg M, Martin G, et al. Effects of halothane anesthesia on renal function in normal man. Anesthesiology 1966;27:793.
74. Diamond JR, Yoburn DC. Nonoliguric acute renal failure associated with a low fractional excretion of sodium. Ann Intern Med 1982;96:597.
75. Diskin CJ, Salzsider KH, Solomon RJ, et al. Electrocardiographic changes following dialysis. Nephron 1981;27:94.
76. Don HF, Dieppa RA, Taylor P. Narcotic analgesics in anuric patients. Anesthesiology 1975;42:745.
77. Donohoe JF. Acute bilateral cortical necrosis. In: Brenner BM, Lazarus MS, eds. Acute renal failure. Philadelphia: WB Saunders, 1983:252.
78. Donohoe JF, Ven Katchalam MA, Bernard DB, et al. Tubular leakage and obstruction after renal ischemia: structural functional correlations. Kidney Int 1978;13:208.
79. Drayer DE. Active drug metabolites and renal failure. Am J Med 1977;62:486.
80. Eichhorn JH, Headley-White J, Steinman TI, et al. Renal failure following enflurane anesthesia. Anesthesiology 1976;45:557.
81. Eisenberg RL, Bank WK, Hedgcock MW. Renal failure after major angiography. Am J Med 1980;68:43.
82. Eknoyan G, Wacksman SJ, Glueck HI, et al. Platelet function in renal failure. N Engl J Med 1969;280:677.
83. Eliahou HE, Boichis H, Bott-Kanner G, et al. An epidemiologic study of renal failure. II. Acute renal failure. Am J Epidemiol 1975;101:281.
84. Eneas JF, Schoenfeld PY, Humphreys MH. The effect of infusion of mannitol-sodium bicarbonate on the clinical course of myoglobinuria. Arch Intern Med 1979;139:801.
85. Eriksen C, Sorensen MB, Bille-Brahe NE, et al. Hemodynamic effects of calcium chloride administered intravenously to patients with and without cardiac disease during neuroleptanesthesia. Acta Anaesth Scand 1983;27:13.
86. Espinel CH, Gregory AW. Differential diagnosis of acute renal failure. Clin Nephrol 1980;13:73.
87. Etheredge EE, Hruska KA. Acute renal failure in the surgical patient. In: Zuidema GD, Rutherford RB, Ballinger WF, eds. The management of trauma. 4th ed. Philadelphia: WB Saunders, 1985:169.
88. Fahey MR, Morris RB, Miller RD, et al. Pharmocokinetics of Org NC 45 (Norcuron) in patients with and without renal failure. Br J Anaesth 1981;53:1049.
89. Fahey MR, Rupp SM, Fisher DM, et al. The pharmacokinetics and pharmacodynamics of atracurium in patients with and without renal failure. Anesthesiology 1984;61:699.
90. Fahey MR, Rupp SM, Canfell C, et al. Effect of renal failure on laudanosine excretion in man. Br J Anaesth 1985;57:1049.
91. Finn W. Recovery from acute renal failure. In: Brenner BM, Lazarus MJ eds. Acute renal failure. Philadelphia: WB Saunders, 1983: 753.
91a. Firth JD, Ratcliffe PJ et al. Endothelin: an important factor in acute renal failure. Lancet 1988;2:1179.
92. Fischer RP, Polk HC. Changing etiologic patterns of renal insufficiency in surgical patients. Surg Gynecol Obstet 1975;140:85.
93. Fish K, Sievenpiper T, Rice SA, et al. Renal function in Fischer 344 rats with chronic renal impairment after administration of enflurane and gentamicin. Anesthesiology 1980;53:481.
94. Fisher DM, O'Keefe C, Stanski DR, et al. Pharmacokinetics and pharmocodynamics of d-tubocurarine in infants, children and adults. Anesthesiology 1982;57:203.
95. Flamenbaum W, Gehr M, Gross M, et al. Acute renal failure associated with myoglobinuria and hemoglobinuria. In: Brenner BM, Lazarus MJ, eds. Acute renal failure. Philadelphia: WB Saunders, 1983:269.
96. Fraley DS, Adler S. Isohydric regulation of plasma potassium by bicarbonate in the rat. Kidney Int 1976;9:333.
97. Fry DE. Infection in the trauma patient: the major deterrent to good recovery. Heart Lung 1978;7:257.
98. Geha DG, Blitt CD, Moon BJ. Prolonged neuromuscular blockade with pancuronium in the presence of acute renal failure: a case report. Anesth Analg 1976;55:343.
99. Ghonheim MM, Pandya H. Plasma protein binding of thiopental in patients with impaired renal or hepatic function. Anesthesiology 1975;42:545.
100. Ghonheim MM, Kramer SE, Bannow R, et al. Binding of d-tubocurarine to plasma proteins in normal man and in patients with hepatic or renal disease. Anesthesiology 1973; 39:410.
101. Gibaldi M, Levy G, Hayton WL. Tubocurarine and renal failure. Br J Anaesth 1972;44:163.
102. Gimson AES, Langley PG, Hughes RD, et al. Prostacyclin to prevent platelet activation during charcoal hemoperfusion in fulminant hepatic failure. Lancet 1980;1:173.
103. Glassock RJ, Conen AJ, Bennett CM, et al. Primary glomerular diseases. In: Brenner BM, Rector FC, eds. The kidney. 2nd ed. Philadelphia: WB Saunders, 1981:1351.
104. Gotta AW, Murray D. Sullivan CA, et al. Post-operative renal failure caused by disseminated intravascular coagulation. Can Anaesth Soc J 1975;22:149.
105. Gronert GA. Anesthetic considerations. In: Eknoyan G, Knochel JP, eds. The systemic consequences of renal failure. Orlando, FL: Grune and Stratton, 1984:519.
106. Gronert GA, Theye RA. Pathophysiology of hyperkalemia induced by succinylcholine. Anesthesiology 1975;43:84.
107. Grossman RA, Hamilton RW, Morse BM, et al. Non-traumatic rhabdomyolysis and acute renal failure. N Engl J Med 1974;291:807.
108. Grossman SH, Davis D, Kitchell BB, et al. Diazepam and lidocaine plasma protein binding in renal disease. Clin Pharmacol Ther 1982;31:350.
109. Guerra SMO, Kitabchi AE. Comparison of the effectiveness of various routes on insulin injection: insulin levels and glucose response in normal subjects. J Clin Endocrinol Metab 1976;42:869.
110. Hakim R, Lazarus M. Hemodialysis in acute renal failure. In: Brenner BM, Lazarus MJ, eds. Acute renal failure. Philadelphia: WB Saunders, 1983:643.
111. Halpern M, Bear R, Goldstein MB, et al. Interpretation of the serum potassium concentration in metabolic acidosis. Clin Invest Med 1979;2:55.
112. Handa SP. Acute renal failure in association with hyperuremia: its recovery with ethacrynic acid. South Med J 1971;64:676.
113. Handa SP, Morrin PAF. Diagnostic indices in acute renal failure. Can Med Assoc J 1967;96:78.
114. Hariparsad D, Pather M, Rocke DA, Wesley AG. Renal function in tetanus. Intens Care Med 1984;10:67.
115. Havill JH, Mee AD, Wallace AR, et al. Prolonged curarization in the presence of renal impairment. Anaesth Intens Care 1978;6:234.
116. Henderson IS, Beattie TJ, Kennedy AC. Dopamine hydrochloride in oliguric states. Lancet 1980;2:827.
117. Hilgenberg JC. Renal disease. In: Stoelting RK, Dierdorf SF,

eds. Anesthesia and co-existing disease. New York: Churchill Livingstone, 1983:379.
118. Hill GE, Lunn JK, Hodges MR, et al. $N_2O$ modification of halothane-altered renal function in the dog. Anesth Analg 1977;56:690.
119. Hobika GH, Evers JL, Mostert JW, et al. Comparison of hemodynamic effects of glucagon and ketamine in patients with chronic renal failure. Anesthesiology 1972;37:654.
120. Holland PV, Schmidt PJ. Pathogenesis of acute renal failure associated with incompatible transfusion. Lancet 1967;2:1169.
121. Horowitz HI, Stein IM, Cohen BD. Further studies on the platelet inhibitor effect of guanidinosuccinic acid and its role in uremic bleeding. Am J Med 1970;49:336.
122. Hou SH, Bushinsky DA, Wish JB, et al. Hospital acquired renal insufficiency: a prospective study. Am J Med 1983;74:243.
123. Itagneyik K, Gordon E, Linus L, et al. Glycerol induced hemodialysis with hemoglobinuria and acute renal failure. Lancet 1974;1:75.
124. Jacques T, Lee R. Improvement of renal function after relief of raised intra-abdominal pressure due to traumatic retroperitoneal haematoma. Anaesth Intens Care 1988;16:478.
125. Janson PA, Jubeliker SJ, Weinstein MJ, et al. Treatment of the bleeding tendency in uremia with cryoprecipitate. N Engl J Med 1980;303:1318.
126. Kaplan AA, Longnecker RE, Folkert VW. Continuous arteriovenous hemofiltration. Ann Intern Med 1984;100:358.
127. Kaufman RP, Anner H, Kobzik L, et al. Vasodilator prostaglandins (PG) prevent renal damage after ischemia. Ann Surg 1987;205:195.
128. Kaufman RP, Anner H, Kobzik L, et al. A high plasma prostaglandin to thromboxane ratio protects against renal ischemia. Surg Gynecol Obstet 1987;165:404.
129. Kelton J, Kelley WN, Holmes EW. A rapid method for the diagnosis of acute uric acid nephropathy. Arch Intern Med 1978;138:612.
130. Kennedy WF, Sawyer TK, Gerbershagen HU. Simultaneous systemic, cardiovascular and renal hemodynamic alterations during peridural anesthesia in normal man. Anesthesiology 1969;31:414.
131. Kettler D, Schenk HD. Effects of various anaesthetics on haemodynamics and renal blood flow. Br J Anaesth 1981;53:112P.
132. Kim KE, Onesti G, Osvaldo R, et al. Creatinine clearance in renal disease: a reappraisal. Br Med J 1969;4:11.
133. Kirschbaum BB. Low $FE_{Na}$ acute renal failure. J Trauma 1982;22:511.
134. Kjellstrand CM, Ebben J, Davin T. Time of death, recovery of renal failure, development of chronic renal failure and need for chronic hemodialysis in patients with acute tubular necrosis. Trans Am Soc Artif Intern Organs 1981;27:45.
135. Kjellstrand CM, Pru CE, Jahnke WR, et al. Acute renal failure in replacement of renal function by dialysis. Dordrecht Martinus Nijhoff Publishers, 1983:536.
136. Kleinknecht D, Jungers P, Chanard J, et al. Uremic and nonuremic complications in acute renal failure: evaluation of early and frequent dialysis on prognosis. Kidney Int 1972;1:190.
137. Knochel JP. Rhabdomyolysis and myoglobinuria. Semin Nephrol 1981;1:75.
138. Koide M, Waud BE. Serum potassium concentrations after succinylcholine in patients with renal failure. Anesthesiology 1972;36:142.
139. Kono K, Philbin DM, Coggins CH, et al. Renal function and stress response during halothane and fentanyl anesthesia. Anesth Analg 1981;60:552.
140. Kopple J. Acute renal failure—conservative, nondialytic management. In: Brenner B, Stein OH, eds. Current therapy in nephrology and hypertension. St. Louis: CV Mosby, 1984:236.
141. Korinek AM, Languille M, Bonnet F, et al. Effect of postoperative extradural morphine on ADH secretion. Br J Anaesth 1985;57:407.
142. Kosinski JP, Lucas CE, Ledgerwood AM. Meaning and value of free water clearance in injured patients. J Surg Res 1982;33:184.
143. Koskelo P, Kekki M, Wager O. Kinetic behavior of I-labelled myoglobin in human beings. Clin Chim Acta 1967;17:339.
144. Kumar S, Hull JD, Lathi S, et al. Low incidence of renal failure after angiography. Arch Intern Med 1981;141:1268.
145. Landes RG, Lillehei RC, Lindsay WG, et al. Free-water clearance and the early recognition of acute renal insufficiency after cardiopulmonary bypass. Ann Thorac Surg 1976;22:41.
146. Lee JKT, Baron RL, Meison GL, et al. Can real-time ultrasonography replace static b-scanning in the diagnosis of renal obstruction? Radiology 1981;139:161.
147. Leighton KM, Koth B, Bruce C. Pancuronium and renal perfusion: a comparison of neuromuscular blocking agents. Can Anaesth Soc J 1974;21:131.
148. Levinsky NG. Pathophysiology of acute renal failure. N Engl J Med 1977;296:1453.
149. Levinsky NG, Bernard D, Johnston P. Mannitol and loop diuretics in acute renal failure. In: Brenner BM, Lazarus MJ, eds. Acute renal failure. Philadelphia: WB Saunders, 1983: 712.
150. Lindner A, Sherrand DJ, Shan T, et al. Dopamine plus furosemide diuresis in furosemide resistant oliguric acute renal failure. Tel Aviv Satellite Symposium on Acute Renal Failure 1981:26.
151. Lindseth RE, Hamburger RJ, Szwed JJ, et al. Acute renal failure following trauma. J Bone Joint Surg 1975;57A:830.
152. Linke CL, Merin RG. A regional anesthetic approach to renal transplantation. Anesth Analg 1976;55:69.
153. Linton AL, Clark WF, Driedger AA, et al. Acute interstitial nephritis due to drugs. Ann Intern Med 1980;93:735.
154. Llach F, Felsenfeld AJ, Haussler MR. The pathophysiology of altered calcium metabolism in rhabdomyolysis-induced acute renal failure. Interactions of parathyroid hormone, 25-hydroxycholecalciferol, and 1.25-dihydroxycholecalciferol. N Engl J Med 1981;305:117.
155. Loehning RW, Mazze RI. Possible nephrotoxicity from enflurane in a patient with severe renal disease. Anesthesiology 1974;40:203.
156. Lordon RE, Burton JR. Post-traumatic renal failure in military personnel in Southeast Asia. Am J Med 1972;53:137.
157. Lynam DP, Cronnelly R, Castagnoli KP, et al. The pharmacodynamics and pharmacokinetics of vecuronium in patients anesthetized with isoflurane with normal renal function or with renal failure. Anesthesiology 1988;69:227.
158. Maddern PJ. Anaesthesia for the patient with impaired renal function. Anaesth Intens Care 1983;11:321.
159. Maguire WC, Anderson RJ. Continuous arteriovenous hemofiltration in the intensive care unit. J Crit Care 1986;1:54.
160. Manley CB, Robson AM. Acute renal failure following trauma. In: Ballinger WF, Rutherford RB, Zuidema GB, eds. The management of trauma. 2nd ed. Philadelphia: WB Saunders, 1973;123.
161. Mannucci PM, Remuzzi G, Pusineri F, et al. Deamino-8-D arginine vasopressin shortens the bleeding time in uremia. N Engl J Med 1983;308:8.
162. Marshall V. Secondary surgical intervention in acute renal failure. Aust NZ J Surg 1974;44:96,.
163. Martin R, Beauregard L, Tétrault JP. Brachial plexus blockade and chronic renal failure. Anesthesiology 1988;69:405.
164. Martinez-Maldonado M, Benabe JE, Lopez-Novoa JM. Acute renal failure associated with tubulo-interstitial disease including

papillary necrosis. In: Brenner BM, Lazarus JM, eds, Acute renal failure. Philadelphia: WB Saunders, 1983:434.
165. Mather LE, Runciman WB, Ilsley AH. Anesthesia-induced changes in regional blood flow. Implications for drug disposition. Regional Anesth 1982;7:S24.
166. Mazze RI. Fluorinated anaesthetic nephrotoxicity: an update. Can Anaesth Soc J 1984;31:S16.
167. Mazze RI, Barry KG. Prevention of functional renal failure during anesthesia and surgery by sustained hydration and mannitol infusion. Anesth Analg 1967;46:61.
168. Mazze RI, Escue HM, Houston JB. Hyperkalemia and cardiovascular collapse following administration of succinylcholine to traumatized patients. Anesthesiology 1969;31:540.
169. Mazze RI, Cousins MJ, Barr GA. Renal effects and metabolism of isoflurane in man. Anesthesiology 1974;40:536.
170. Mazze RI, Calverley RK, Smith NT. Inorganic fluoride nephrotoxicity. Prolonged enflurane and halothane anesthesia in volunteers. Anesthesiology 1977;46:265.
171. Mazze RI, Sievenpiper TS, Stevenson J. Renal effects of enflurane and halothane in patients with abnormal renal function. Anesthesiology 1984;60:161.
172. McGoldrick MD. Diagnosis and management of acute renal failure: Part I. Cardiovasc Rev Rep 1984;5:1031.
173. McGoldrick MD. Diagnosis and management of acute renal failure: Part II. Cardiovasc Rev Rep 1984;5:1265.
174. McLeod K, Watson MJ, Rawlins MD. Pharmacokinetics of pancuronium in patients with normal and impaired renal function. Br J Anaesth 1976;48:341.
175. McMurray SD, Luft FC, Maxwell DR, et al. Prevailing patterns and predictor variables in patients with acute tubular necrosis. Arch Intern Med 1978;138:950.
176. Meltz D, Berties J, David D, et al. Delayed hemolytic transfusion reaction with renal failure. Lancet 1971;2:1348.
177. Miller ED, Bailey DR, Kaplan JA, et al. The effect of ketamine on the renin-angiotensin system. Anesthesiology 1975;42:503.
178. Miller ED, Longnecker DE, Peach MJ. The regulatory function of the renin-angiotensin system during general anesthesia. Anesthesiology 1978;48:399.
179. Miller ED, Kistner JR, Epstein RM. Whole-body distribution of radioactively labelled microspheres in the rat during anesthesia with halothane, enflurane, or ketamine. Anesthesiology 1980;52:296.
180. Miller RD. Recent developments with muscle relaxants and their antagonists. Can Anaesth Soc J 1979;26:83.
181. Miller RD, Cullen DJ. Renal failure and postoperative respiratory failure: recurarization? Br J Anaesth 1976;48:253.
182. Miller RD, Way WL, Hamilton WK, et al. Succinylcholine-induced hyperkalemia in patients with renal failure? Anesthesiology 1972;36:138.
183. Miller RD, Matteo RS, Benet LZ, et al. The pharmocokinetics of d-tubocurarine in man with and without renal failure. J Pharmacol Exp Ther 1977;202:1.
184. Miller TR, Anderson RJ, Linas SL, et al. Urinary diagnostic indices in acute renal failure: a prospective study. Ann Intern Med 1978;89:47.
185. Moran WH, Zimmermann B. Mechanisms of antidiuretic hormone (ADH) control of importance to the surgical patient. Surgery 1967;62:639.
186. Morris RB, Cronnelly R, Miller RD, et al. Pharmacokinetics of edrophonium in anephric and renal transplant patients. Br J Anaesth 1981;53:1311.
187. Mouquet C, Bitker MO, Bailliart O, et al. Anesthesia for creation of a forearm fistula in patients with endstage renal failure. Anesthesiology 1989;70:909.
188. Myers BD, Moran SM. Hemodynamically mediated acute renal failure. N Engl J Med 1986;314:97.
189. Myers BD, Hilberman M, Spencer RJ, et al. Glomerular and tubular function in non-oliguric acute renal failure. Am J Med 1982;72:642.
190. Oken DE. Hemodynamic basis for acute renal failure (vasomotor nephropathy). Am J Med 1984;76:702.
191. Oken DE. On the differential diagnosis of acute renal failure. Am J Med 1981;71:916.
192. Olivero JJ, Lozano-Mendez J, Ghafary EM, et al. Mitigation of amphotericin B nephrotoxicity by mannitol. Br Med J 1975;1:550.
193. Orko R, Pitkanen M, Rosenberg H. Subarachnoid anaesthesia with 0.75% bupivacaine in patients with chronic renal failure. Br J Anaesth 1986;58:605.
194. Parfrey PS, Griffiths SM, Barrett BJ, et al. Contrast material-induced renal failure in patients with diabetes mellitus, renal insufficiency, or both. A prospective controlled study. N Engl J Med 1989;320:143.
195. Parker S, Carlon GC, Isaacs M, et al. Dopamine administration in oliguria and oliguric renal failure. Crit Care Med 1981;9:630.
196. Philbin DM, Coggins CH. Plasma antidiuretic hormone levels in cardiac surgical patients during morphine and halothane anesthesia. Anesthesiology 1978;49:95.
197. Powell DR, Miller RD. The effects of repeated doses of succinylcholine on serum potassium in patients with renal failure. Anesth Analg 1975;54:746.
198. Powell JN. Suxamethonium-induced hyperkalemia in a uremic patient. Br J Anaesth 1970;42:806.
199. Priano LL. Alteration of renal hemodynamics by thiopental, diazepam and ketamine in conscious dogs. Anesth Analg 1982;61:853.
200. Priano LL. Effects of high-dose fentanyl on renal haemodynamics in conscious dogs. Can Anaesth Soc J 1983;30:10.
201. Priano LL, Marrone B. Effect of halothane on renal hemodynamics during normovolemia and acute hemorrhagic hypovolemia. Anesthesiology 1985;63:357.
202. Priebe HJ, Skillman JJ, Bushnell LS, et al. Antacid versus cimetidine in preventing acute gastrointestinal bleeding. A randomized trial in 75 critically ill patients. N Engl J Med 1980;302:426.
203. Quebbeman EJ, Maierhofer WJ, Piering WF. Mechanisms producing hypoxemia during hemodialysis. Crit Care Med 1984;12:359.
204. Ramzan MI, Shanks CA, Triggs EJ. Gallamine disposition in surgical patients with chronic renal failure. Br J Clin Pharmacol 1981;12:141.
205. Raskin NH, Fishman RA. Neurologic disorders in renal failure (Part I). N Engl J Med 1976;294:143.
206. Raskin NH, Fishman RA. Neurologic disorders in renal failure (Part II). N Engl J Med 1976;294:204.
207. Rasmussen HH, Ibels LS. Acute renal failure. Multivariate analysis of causes and risk factors. Am J Med 1982;73:211.
208. Reed RL, Ciavarella D, Heimbach DM, et al. Prophylactic platelet administration during massive transfusion. A prospective, randomized, double blind clinical study. Ann Surg 1986;203:40.
209. Relman AS. Metabolic consequences of acid-base disorders. Kidney Int 1972;1:347.
210. Remuzzi G, Livio M, Marchiaro G, et al. Bleeding in renal failure: altered platelet function in chronic uraemia only partially corrected by haemodialysis. Nephron 1978;22:347.
211. Reves JG, Fragen RJ, Vinik R, et al. Midazolam: pharmocology and uses. Anesthesiology 1985;62:310.
212. Roth F, Wuthrich H. The clinical importance of hyperkalemia following suxamethonium administration. Br J Anaesth 1969;41:311.
213. Runciman WB, Mather LE, Ilsley AH, et al. A sheep preparation for studying interactions between blood flow and drug dispos-

tion. III: Effects of general and spinal anaesthesia on regional blood flow and oxygen tensions. Br J Anaesth 1984;56:1247.
214. Runciman WB, Mather LE, Ilsley AH, et al. A sheep preparation for studying interactions between blood flow and drug disposition. IV: The effects of general and spinal anaesthesia on blood flow and cefoxitin disposition. Br J Anaesth 1985;57:1239.
214a. Russell JD, Churchill DN. Calcium antagonists and acute renal failure. Am J Med 1989;87:306.
215. Ryan DW. Preoperative serum cholinesterase concentration in chronic renal failure. Br J Anaesth 1977;49:945.
216. Saba TM. Disturbances in plasma and cell fibronectin: relationship to altered vascular permeability and host defense. J Trauma 1981;21:679.
217. Schimpff SC, Caplan FS. Role of the host in aminoglycoside nephrotoxicity. Curr Opinions: Aminoglycoside Nephrotoxicity 1984;1:16.
218. Schrier RW. Acute renal failure. Kidney Int 1979;15:205.
218a. Schrier RW. Cellular mechanism in ischemic acute renal failure: role of calcium entry blockers. Kidney Int 1987;32:313.
219. Schwab SJ, Hlatky MA, Pieper KS, et al. Contrast nephrotoxicity: a randomized controlled trial of a nonionic and an ionic radiographic contrast agent. N Engl J Med 1989;320:149.
220. Sear JW, Hand CW, Moore RA, McQuay HJ. Studies on morphine disposition: influence of general anaesthesia on plasma concentrations of morphine and its metabolites. Br J Anaesth 1989;62:22.
221. Shafi T, Chou S, Porush JG, et al. Infusion intravenous pyelography and renal function. Arch Intern Med 1978;138:1218.
222. Shanks CA. Muscle relaxants in renal failure patients. In: Katz RL, ed. Muscle relaxants: basic and clinical aspects. Orlando, FL. Grune and Stratton, 1985;171.
223. Sherwood T. Radiology in renal failure. Contrib Nephrol 1977;5:63.
224. Shin B, Isenhower NN, McAslan TC, et al. Early recognition of renal insufficiency in post-anesthetic trauma victims. Anesthesiology 1979;50:262.
225. Shin B, MacKenzie CF, McAslan TC, et al. Postoperative renal failure in trauma patients. Anesthesiology 1979;51:218.
226. Shin B, MacKenzie CF, Helrich M. Creatinine clearance for early detection of post-traumatic renal dysfunction. Anesthesiology 1986;64:605.
227. Shoemaker WC. Fluids and electrolytes in the acutely ill adult. In: Shoemaker WC, Thompson WL, Holbrook PR, eds. Textbook of critical care. Philadelphia: WB Saunders, 1984:614.
228. Shoemaker WC, Bryan-Brown CW, Quigley L, et al. Body fluid shifts in depletion and post-stress states and their correction with adequate nutrition. Surg Gynecol Obstet 1973;136:371.
229. Sievenpiper TS, Rice SA, McClendon F, et al. Renal effects of enflurane anesthesia in Fischer 344 rats with preexisting renal insufficiency. J Pharmacol Exp Ther 1979;211:36.
230. Sivarajan M, Amory DW, Lindbloom LE, et al. Systemic and regional blood flow changes during spinal anesthesia in the rhesus monkey. Anesthesiology 1975;43:78.
231. Sivarajan M, Amory DW, Lindbloom LE. Systemic and regional blood flow during epidural anesthesia without epinephrine in the rhesus monkey. Anesthesiology 1976;45:300.
232. Skillman JJ, Silen W. Stress ulceration in the acutely ill. Annu Rev Med 1976;27:9.
233. Sladen RN, Endo E, Harrison T. Two-hour versus 22-hour creatinine clearance in critically ill patients. Anesthesiology 1987;67:1013.
234. Smith CL, Hunter JM, Jones RS. Vecuronium infusions in patients with renal failure in an ITU. Anaesthesia 1989;42:387.
235. Somogyi AA, Shanks CA, Triggs EJ. The effect of renal failure on the disposition and neuromuscular blocking action of pancuronium bromide. Eur J Clin Pharmacol 1977;12:23.
236. Stanley TH, Gray NH, Bidwai AV, et al. The effect of high dose morphine and morphine plus $N_2O$ on urinary output in man. Can Anaesth Soc J 1974;21:379.
237. Steinman T, Lazarus M. Organ system involvement in acute renal failure. In: Brenner BM, Lazarus MJ, eds. Acute renal failure. Philadelphia: WB Saunders, 1983:586.
237a. Stevens PE, Kox W et al. Practical use of duplex doppler analysis of the renal vasculature in critically ill patients. Lancet 1989;1:240.
238. Summers WK, Jamison RL. The no reflow phenomenon in renal ischemia. Lab Invest 1971;25:635.
239. Talner LB, Scheible W, Ellenbogen PH, et al. How accurate is ultrasonography in detecting hydronephrosis in azotemic patients? Urol Radiol 1981;3:1.
240. Tanner GA, Steinhausen M. Tubular obstruction in ischemia-induced acute renal failure in the rat. Kidney Int 1976;10: S65.
241. Thompson ME, Rault RM, Reddy PS. Uremic pericarditis. Cardiovasc Rev Rep 1981;2:755.
242. Thurau K, Boylan JW. Acute renal success. The unexpected logic of oliguria in acute renal failure. Am J Med 1976;61:308.
243. Tinker JH, Michenfelder JD. Increased resistance to nitroprusside induced cyanide toxicity in anuric dog. Anesthesiology 1980;52:40.
244. Tobimatsu M, Ueda Y, Saito S, et al. Effects of a stable prostacyclin analog on experimental ischemic-acute renal failure. Ann Surg 1988;208:65.
245. Ukai M, Moran WH, Zimmermann B. The role of visceral afferent pathways on vasopressin secretion and urinary excretory patterns during surgical stress. Ann Surg 1968;168:16.
246. Vandeputte-Van Messon G, Peeters G. Effect on intracerebroventricular administration of opioid peptides on urinary function in the conscious goat. Arch Int Pharmacodyn Ther 1980;243:304.
247. Van Ypersele de Strihou C. Acute oliguric interstitial nephritis. Kidney Int 1979;16:751.
248. Vatner SF, Smith NT. Effects of halothane on left ventricular function and distribution of regional blood flow in dogs and primates. Circ Res 1974;34:155.
249. Verney EB. Some aspects of water and electrolyte excretion. Surg Gynecol Obstet 1958;106:441.
250. Vinik HR, Reves JG, Greenblatt DJ, et al. The pharmacokinetics of midazolam in chronic renal failure patients. Anesthesiology 1983;59:390.
251. Wacker W, Merrill JP. Uremic pericarditis in acute renal failure. JAMA 1954;156:764.
252. Walkin KG. The pathophysiology of the dialysis disequilibrium syndrome. Mayo Clin Proc 1969;44:406.
253. Walton JD, Farman JV. Suxamethonium hyperkalaemia in uraemic neuropathy. Anaesthesia 1973;28:66.
254. Ward S, Boheimer N, Weatherley BC, et al. Pharmacokinetics of atracurium and its metabolites in patients with normal renal function, and in patients in renal failure. Br J Anaesth 1987;59:697.
255. Weddington WW, Muelling AE, Moosa HH, et al. Cimetidine toxic reactions masquerading as delirium tremens. JAMA 1981;245:1058.
256. Weinrauch LA, Healy RW, Leland OS, et al. Coronary angiography and acute renal failure in diabetic azotemic nephropathy. Ann Intern Med 1977;86:56.
257. Weir PHC, Chung FF. Anesthesia for patients with chronic renal disease. Can Anaesth Soc J 1984;31:468.
258. Wesson DE, Witch WE, Wilmore DW. Nutritional considerations in the treatment of acute renal failure. In: Brenner BM, Lazarus MJ, eds. Acute renal failure. Philadelphia: WB Saunders, 1983:609.

259. Whelton A. Post-traumatic acute renal failure in Vietnam: a milestone in progress. Conn Med 1974;38:7.
260. Whelton A. Post-traumatic acute renal failure. Bull NY Acad Med 1979;2:150.
261. White PF, Way WL, Trevor AJ. Ketamine—its pharmacology and therapeutic uses. Anesthesiology 1982;56:119.
262. Wieber J, Gugler R, Hengstmann JH, et al. Pharmacokinetics of ketamine in man. Anaesthetist 1975;24:260.
263. Wiggum DC, Cork RC, Weldon ST, et al. Postoperative respiratory depression and elevated sufentanil levels in a patient with chronic renal failure. Anesthesiology 1985;63:708.
264. Wilson RF. Trauma. In: Shoemaker WC, Ayres S, Grenvik A, Holbrook PR, Thompson WL, eds. Textbook of critical care. Philadelphia: WB Saunders, 1989:1258.
265. Wilson RF, Soullier G. The validity of two-hour creatinine clearance studies in critically ill patients. Crit Care Med 1980;8:281.
266. Wing E, Bruns F, Fraley D, et al. Infectious complications with plasmapheresis in rapidly progressive glomerulonephritis. JAMA 1980;244:2423.
267. Wood M. Plasma drug binding: implications for anesthesiologists. Anesth Analg 1986;65:786.
267a. Yanagisawa M, Kurihara H, et al. A novel potent vasoconstrictor peptide produced by vascular endothelial cells. Nature 1988;332:411.
268. Zaske DE. Pharmacokinetics and host factors on dosage requirements and nephrotoxicity. Curr Opinions: Aminoglycoside Nephrotoxicity 1984;16.
269. Zusman RM, Rubin RH, Cato AE, et al. Hemodialysis using prostacyclin instead of heparin as the sole antithrombotic agent. N Engl J Med 1981;204:934.


## APPENDIX 25-1. Guidelines for Drug Therapy in Renal Failure*

| AGENT | $T_{1/2}$ | | SITE OF ELIMINATION AND DEGRADATION | DOSE MODIFICATION IN RENAL FAILURE* | | REMOVAL BY DIALYSIS | COMMENTS |
|---|---|---|---|---|---|---|---|
| | *Normal (h)* | *Anephric (h)* | | *GFR (mL/min) 10–40* | *GFR (mL/min) <10* | | |
| Thiopental | 3.8 | ? | Liver | None | 75% | ? | Hemodialysis preferred to remove the drugs in this group |
| Secobarbital | 20–30 | ? | Liver | None | None | No (H, P) | |
| Phenobarbital | 50–150 | 100–150 | Liver (Renal 25%) | None | None | Yes (H, P) | |
| Pentobarbital | 20–50 | 20–50 | Liver | None | None | No (H) | |
| Hexobarbital | 3–4 | ? | Liver | None | None | No (H) | |
| Lorazepam | 9–16 | 32–70 | Liver | None | 50% | No (H) | All agents in this group may produce excessive sedation or encephalopathy |
| Diazepam | 20–90 | ? | Liver (Renal) | None | None | No (H) | Active metabolite desmethyldiazepam excreted by the kidney |
| Chlordiazepoxide | 5–30 | ? | Liver (Renal) | None | None | No (H) | Active metabolite excreted by the kidney |
| Morphine | 2.5 | ? | Liver (Renal <12%) | None | None | No (H) | All agents in this group may produce excessive sedation and respiratory deperession |
| Meperidine | 3–8 | 3–8 | Liver (Renal <10%) | None | None | No (H) | |
| Methadone | 13–55 | ? | Liver (Renal <21%) | None | 50–75% | No (H, P) | |
| Fentanyl | 5–14 | ? | Liver | None | None | ? | Active metabolite normeperidine may accumulate and may result in seizures |
| Butorphanol | 2.2–3.5 | ? | Liver | None | None | ? | |
| Codeine | 2.5–3.5 | ? | Liver (Renal <16%) | None | None | ? | |
| Naloxone | 1.0–1.5 | ? | Liver | None | None | ? | |
| Clonidine | 6–23 | 39–42 | Renal | None | 50–75% | No (H) | Blood pressure in this group is best guide to dose and interval. Interval between doses should be prolonged. Renal excretion more important with IV drug administration. |
| Methyldopa | Biphasic 1.4 and 5.8 | Biphasic 3–6 and 7–16 | Renal (Hepatic—18–48%) | None | None | Yes (H, P) | |
| Reserpine | Biphasic 4.5 & 50–70 | 87–320 | Liver (GI) | None | Avoid | No (H, P) | |
| Captopril | 1.9 | 21–30 | Renal (Hepatic) | None | 50% | Yes (H) | |
| Amiodarone | 3–100 days | 3–100 days | Liver | None | None | No (H) | |
| Bretylium | 6 (oral) 13.6 (IV) | 16–32 | Renal (Nonrenal 20%) | 25–50% | Avoid | ? | |

*(continued)*

APPENDIX 25-1. Guidelines for Drug Therapy in Renal Failure (*continued*)

| AGENT | $T_{1/2}$ Normal (h) | $T_{1/2}$ Anephric (h) | SITE OF ELIMINATION AND DEGRADATION | DOSE MODIFICATION IN RENAL FAILURE* GFR (mL/min) 10–40 | DOSE MODIFICATION IN RENAL FAILURE* GFR (mL/min) <10 | REMOVAL BY DIALYSIS | COMMENTS |
|---|---|---|---|---|---|---|---|
| Lidocaine | 1.2–2.2 | 1.3–3.0 | Liver (Renal <20%) | None | None | No (H) | $T_{1/2}$ dependent on hepatic blood flow; active metabolite. Excretion enhanced in acid urine |
| Procainamide | 2.5–4.9 | 5.3–5.9 | Renal (Liver 7–24%) | None | None | Yes (H) | Dosage interval to be increased from 6–12 h to 8–24 h. |
| Quinidine | 5.0–7.0 | 4–14 | Liver (Renal 10–50%) | None | None | Yes (H, P) | Active metabolite |
| Propranolol | 3.5–6 | 2.3 | Liver | None | None | No (H) | Metabolites may accmumulate |
| Labetalol | 3–8 | 3–8 | Liver (Renal) | None | None | No (H) | |
| Diltiazem | 2–8 | ? | Liver | None | None | ? | Headache, flushing, or dizziness may occur in patients with renal disease |
| Nifedipine | 4.0–5.5 | ? | Liver | None | None | No (H) | |
| Verapamil | 3–7 | 2.4–4 | Liver | None | 50–75% | No (H) | |
| Digitoxin | 144–200 | 210 | Liver (Renal) | None | 50–75% | No (H, P) | Serum levels should be monitored in renal failure |
| Digoxin | 36–44 | 80–120 | Renal (Nonrenal 15–40%) | 25–75% | 10–25% | No (H, P) | |
| Acetazolamide | 8 | ? | Renal | —— | Avoid | ? | Ineffective when GFR <30 mL/min |
| Ethacrynic Acid | 2–4 | ? | Liver (Renal) | —— | Avoid | No (H) | Ineffective when GFR <30 mL/min |
| Thiazides | 1–2 | 4–6 | Renal | None | Avoid | ? | Ineffective when GFR <30 mL/min |
| Nitroglycerin | 2–4 min | 2–4 min | Liver | None | None | ? | |
| Isosorbide dinitrate | 10–30 min | 10–30 min | Liver | None | None | ? | |
| Diazoxide | 17–31 | >30 | Renal (Liver) | None | None | Yes (H, P) | |
| Hydralazine | 2.0–4.5 | 7–16 | Liver (Nonrenal) | None | None | No (H, P) | Dosage interval to be increased |
| Sodium Nitroprusside | <10 min | <10 min | Nonrenal | None | None | Yes (H, P) | Thiocyanate level to be monitored; $T_{1/2}$ for thiocyanate is 1 week. Thiocyanate is dialyzable. |
| Heparin | 0.3–2.0 | 0.5–3.0 | Nonrenal | None | None | No (H, P) | |
| Warfarin | 42 | 30 | Liver (Renal) | None | None | No (H) | Decreased protein binding in uremia shortens $T_{1/2}$. Metabolites with anticoagulant property excreted renally |
| Cimetidine | 1.5–2.0 | 3.5 | Renal | 75% | 50% | No (H, P) | Can cause confusion in renal failure patients. |
| Ranitidine | 1.5–3 | 6–9 | Renal (Liver) | 75% | 50% | Yes (H) | |
| Metoclopramide | 4 | 14 | Renal (Liver) | 75% | 50% | ? | |
| Terbutaline | 1.0–1.5 | ? | Liver (Renal) | 50% | Avoid | ? | IV or subcutaneous doses cleared by renal excretion. |
| Theophylline | 3–12 | ? | Liver | None | None | Yes (H, P) | Renal gastrointestinal symptoms may be pronounced. |

* Adapted from Bennett.[32]

** Percent of usual dose.

$T_{1/2}$ = biologic half-life; GFR = glomerular filtration rate; H = hemodialysis; P = Peritoneal dialysis; ? = unknown.

# Chapter Twenty-Six

Brian Kaufman

# Infections of the Injured

Postoperative infections occur frequently in patients with multiple trauma. Sepsis is the leading cause of late death after trauma and is second only to severe neurologic injury as the most common cause of death in trauma patients.[7] Sepsis is especially common in patients requiring prolonged intensive care.[3,122] Fry noted life-threatening postoperative septic complications in 34 of 200 traumatized patients. Eleven of the 16 postoperative deaths in this group were due to uncontrolled infection.[43]

Many factors interfere with normal defenses against bacterial contaminants in the injured patient. Blood flow to traumatized, ischemic, or devitalized tissues is poor. Thus, delivery of immunoglobulins and leukocytes to these areas is deficient. The presence of foreign bodies, hematomas, and dead space also promotes the multiplication of bacteria in wounds. In a review of 1,009 patients admitted to the Maryland Institute for Emergency Medical Services, 175 infectious complications were identified.[18] The sites of infection were the urinary tract in 19%, surgical wounds in 11%, the abdomen in 7%, the lower respiratory tract in 13%, the paranasal sinuses in 6%, vascular catheters in 21%, primary bacteremia in 11%, and other sites in 12%.[18] More than 82% of the infections were nosocomial in origin and were related to the various procedures used for monitoring and therapy in these critically ill patients.[18]

Primary bacteremia often occurs within a few hours of traumatic injury. Animal experiments utilizing a hemorrhagic shock model have demonstrated that shocked animals frequently become bacteremic with enteric organisms that escape from the gastrointestinal tract and appear in the bloodstream.[71,127] Fifty-six percent of the patients evaluated by Rush and coworkers,[115] who were admitted with a systolic blood pressure of ≤80 mm Hg, had positive blood cultures within 3 hours of injury. In contrast, only 29% of patients with admission blood pressures of 80–110 mm Hg and 4% of patients with admission blood pressures of ≥110 mm Hg had positive blood cultures. Since enteric organisms were the ones most commonly detected, these findings suggest that one of the important initiating events in the sepsis syndrome and multiple organ failure after hemorrhagic shock is the direct absorption of enteric bacteria and endotoxin into the bloodstream of traumatized, hypotensive patients.[27]

## TYPES OF INFECTIONS

### URINARY TRACT INFECTIONS

One of the most common sites of infection is the urinary tract. The presence of a Foley catheter, used frequently to evaluate urine output, is a major contributor to the high frequency of urinary infection in traumatized patients. Allgöwer and associates[3] noted urinary tract infection in 97 of 300 multiple trauma patients. Clinical evidence of sepsis, however, developed in only three of these patients, suggesting that this infection is not a major contributor to postoperative mortality.

### WOUND INFECTIONS

Wound infections are also very common in the multiple trauma patient. In Allgöwer's series,[3] wound infections occurred in 12.3% of patients. In this group, 45% of traumatic wounds became infected as compared to an infection rate of 4% in surgical wounds. Clinical evidence of sepsis from wound infections was found in less than 1% of their patients. Wound infection rates are related to the amount of bacterial contamination and the mechanism of injury.[144]

## INTRA-ABDOMINAL INFECTIONS

Intra-abdominal sepsis accounts for a significant proportion of late morbidity, prolonged hospitalization, and need for reoperation in major trauma victims.[33,48] The frequency of intra-abdominal infections after trauma is dependent mainly upon the type of injuries incurred. It is probably most common after penetrating abdominal injuries, particularly if the colon is involved.[67] Many other factors increase the likelihood of infection, including the number and type of visceral injuries, the presence of significant hypotension, large transfusion requirements, prolonged operation, advanced age, and the mechanism of injury.[28] Intra-abdominal abscess and peritonitis are by far the most common conditions necessitating abdominal re-exploration. These conditions were present in 58% of reoperations after abdominal trauma.[33] An abscess was detected in 46% of the reoperations, and diffuse peritonitis was found in the remaining 12%. Common causes of these complications were anastomotic leaks and ischemic bowel.

The reported incidence of intra-abdominal infection after penetrating abdominal trauma ranges between 2.4 and 45.7%.[33,47,48,131] Defore et al.[26] noted that 6% of 1,590 patients surviving blunt or penetrating liver trauma developed a subphrenic, intrahepatic, or other intra-abdominal abscess after surgery. Gibson and associates[48] evaluated 2,416 patients after laparotomy for penetrating abdominal trauma. Fifty-seven (2.4%) of these patients developed an intra-abdominal abscess in the postoperative period. The interval between initial injury and operative drainage of the abdominal infection averaged 29 days. Delay of diagnosis appears to be a significant problem in the appropriate treatment of intra-abdominal abscess after trauma. Intra-abdominal abscess after penetrating abdominal wounds may result from breaks in sterile technique due to the urgent nature of the operation, failure to remove feculent material or foreign bodies adequately, undiagnosed gastrointestinal tract injuries, extensive contamination before operative intervention, anastomotic leaks, bowel injury after placement of retention sutures, and postoperative acalculous cholecystitis.

Cholecystitis in the postoperative period is uncommon.[143] However, when it develops in the traumatized patient, stones are usually not found.[36] The diagnosis of acalculous cholecystitis in the critically ill injured patient may be extremely difficult. Physical examination has limited reliability if the patient is sedated or being mechanically ventilated. Unexplained fever may be the initial symptom.[66] Obvious tenderness in the right upper quadrant is a late finding in acalculous cholecystitis and is suggestive of perforation of the gallbladder. Pancreatitis is another potential complication of acalculous cholecystitis.[143] If hemodynamic evidence of sepsis is present without a clearly identifiable source, ultrasonography or an abdominal CT scan should be done to evaluate the gallbladder and other intra-abdominal organs. However, negative results do not exclude the diagnosis of acalculous cholecystitis or intra-abdominal abscess.[17] Localized right upper quadrant exploration of the patient with suspected acalculous cholecystitis may be the most reliable diagnostic approach.[120] Early suspicion, diagnosis, and treatment of this condition are essential as advanced disease (gangrene, empyema, or perforation of the gallbladder) develops rapidly.[66] Johnson reported a 40% incidence (10/26) of gallbladder perforation in patients with a delay greater than 48 hours between the onset of symptoms and operative intervention. Only 8% of patients who underwent surgical treatment within 48 hours of the onset of symptoms had evidence of perforation.

Narcotics may produce spasm of the choledochal and cystic duct sphincters. This may result in biliary stasis, which is conducive to superimposed bacterial growth and the development of cholecystitis.[42,112] However, no controlled study is available to substantiate the clinical importance of this factor in the pathogenesis of acalculous cholecystitis.

Succinylcholine probably should be avoided during the anesthetic management of patients requiring surgery for intra-abdominal infection. Significant increases of serum potassium with this drug in patients undergoing abdominal exploration for peritonitis have been reported.[70]

Animal studies have demonstrated the efficacy of intraoperative peritoneal lavage in reducing the mortality of generalized peritonitis.[76] After surgery, fluid and necrotic debris reaccumulate within the abdomen, and bacteria may continue to proliferate. It therefore seems logical that postoperative peritoneal lavage would have beneficial effects. Leiboff et al.[76] evaluated the treatment of generalized peritonitis with closed postoperative peritoneal lavage (CPPL). After reviewing 39 studies of the clinical application of CPPL, they concluded that there is little hard evidence to recommend CPPL, and its therapeutic value remains to be determined.

Daily reoperation with open lavage has also been used to treat patients with diffuse peritonitis.[134] The use of a zipper allows for easy access to the peritoneal cavity, and the lavage can therefore be done in the operating room or intensive care unit. Teichmann and associates[134] reported a mortality rate of 22.9% when 61 high-risk patients received daily open lavage for treatment of diffuse peritonitis. Controlled prospective studies need to be done to clarify the role of both closed and open abdominal lavage in patients with diffuse peritonitis.

Initiation of antibiotic therapy before surgical intervention decreases the incidence of intra-abdominal and postoperative wound infections compared to starting antibiotics intraoperatively or postoperatively.[44,131] Gram-negative enteric bacilli and anaerobes need to be covered. After penetrating or blunt trauma, cefoxitin alone has a beneficial effect on the intra-abdominal infection rate equivalent to the combination of aminoglycoside and clindamycin or aminoglycoside, clindamycin, and ampicillin.[57,60,67] Mezlocillin, carbenicillin, and moxalactam have all been reported to be as effective as combination therapy when initiated before surgical intervention in these patients.[90,98,109]

The duration of antibiotic therapy after penetrating injury is controversial. A "selective" approach based on operative findings seems rational.[113] Low-risk patients receive antibiotics only in the perioperative period, whereas high-risk patients receive antibiotic therapy for no more than 72 hours postoperatively unless temperature or white blood cell count is elevated when the cessation of therapy is planned.[113] A detailed prophylaxis regimen is provided in Table 2-2.

## RESPIRATORY TRACT INFECTIONS

Acute paranasal sinusitis is a frequent source of infection in head-injured patients.[52] Nineteen of 111 head-injured patients evaluated by Grindlinger and associates developed sinusitis.[52] This infection developed in a majority of patients who were intubated nasotracheally, but was infrequent in those who were intubated orally. The head-injured patient may be at particularly high risk for this complication because of frequent presence of traumatic injury to the sinuses and prolonged intubation of the stomach and trachea via the nares.

The paranasal sinuses can be infected in any critically ill trauma patient with nasal tube(s) in place. The infection is primarily a result of mechanical obstruction of the ostia, which impedes ventilation and drainage of the sinuses. The maxillary sinus is involved most frequently.[52] The paranasal sinuses are frequently missed as the site of infection because the sedated or comatose patient is unable to complain of pain or tenderness over the sinuses. A purulent nasal discharge may be present, or fever and leukocytosis may occur without an obvious source. Paranasal sinusitis is not a benign infection as both local (meningitis, retro-orbital cellulitis, brain abscess) and systemic (sepsis) complications may supervene. The diagnosis can be made on portable sinus films. If the patient is receiving a head CT scan, sinus views should be obtained. Treatment includes surgical drainage and antibiotics. Otitis media can also occur as a complication of nasogastric or nasotracheal tube insertion.

In a series of severely injured patients at the Maryland Institute for Emergency Medical Services, 21% of bacteremic episodes were due to thoracic empyema.[19] Seventy-five percent of these patients had a chest tube placed for hemothorax or pneumothorax before the onset of infection. Thus, it is very likely that this foreign body is a major contributor to the development of infection.

Postoperative pulmonary complications occur frequently. The incidence and severity of pneumonia are dependent on the type and sites of trauma. For instance, 30–50% of patients with severe multiple trauma and up to 70% of patients with severe blunt chest trauma may develop pneumonia. Allgöwer et al.[3] noted that bacterial pneumonia occurred in 54 of 300 patients and progressed to clinical sepsis in 7. All those who developed sepsis subsequently died. They concluded that, although bacterial pneumonia is less common than urinary tract infection, it is much more likely to produce systemic symptoms and to be associated with a fatal outcome.

Most bacterial pneumonias after injury result from aspiration of oropharyngeal contents. Aspiration may occur at the time of injury, especially after head or orofacial trauma. The likelihood of aspiration increases when patients are intoxicated at the time of injury. Pneumonitis may result from aspiration of gastric acid alone without initial bacterial infection. Fever, purulent sputum production, and an infiltrate in a dependent pulmonary segment are the usual findings. The bacteria are usually oropharyngeal in origin. Since the bacterial flora of the oropharyngeal cavity change rapidly after the patient is admitted to an intensive care area, it is important to distinguish between a community- and a hospital-acquired pneumonia. Patients who aspirate outside the hospital setting at the time of injury or shortly thereafter are likely to have Gram-positive cocci (*S. pneumoniae, S. aureus*) involved in the infectious process.[114,132] If nosocomial pneumonia develops postoperatively, the likely pathogens include anaerobic bacteria, aerobic Gram-negative bacilli, and *Staphylococcus aureus*.[132]

The trauma victim is at high risk of aspiration pneumonitis because of depressed mucociliary transport, an increased incidence of aspiration, and alterations in oropharyngeal flora.

### *Depressed Mucociliary Transport*

Mucociliary transport is an important means of keeping the airways clean by moving particles and bacteria deposited on the mucous membrane of the tracheobronchial tree toward the pharynx. Normally, these secretions are subsequently swallowed. This mechanism is depressed by general anesthesia, local anesthesia of the airways, endotracheal intubation, inadequate gas humidification, high inspired oxygen concentration, and airway suctioning.[69,73,117,118] Inflation of the endotracheal tube cuff (whether high or low compliance) decreases tracheal mucous velocity distal to the cuff site.[117] In addition, cuffed endotracheal or tracheostomy tubes can produce measurable tracheal damage.[69] Breathing 90–95% oxygen for as short as 3 hours produces a significant decrease in the mucociliary transport rate. Airway suctioning, often an essential component of postoperative respiratory care, produces erosion and edema of airway mucosa.[73] All these factors, frequently seen in the injured, adversely influence the rate of mucociliary transport, interfere with secretion clearance, and increase the risk of atelectasis and pneumonia.

### *Increased Incidence of Aspiration*

The presence of an endotracheal tube interferes with the ability to prevent aspiration of oropharyngeal contents. Aspiration occurs in 20% of patients intubated with an endotracheal tube with a high-compliance cuff and in as many as 56% of patients intubated using a low-compliance cuff.[128]

Altered consciousness after head injury, shock, the residual effects of general anesthetics, and the use of sedatives and narcotics decrease cough and laryngeal reflexes and increase the likelihood of aspiration. Improper or difficult anesthetic induction, alcohol or drug intoxication at the time of injury, protracted vomiting, presence of a nasogastric tube, and difficulty in swallowing saliva or blood when oral or nasal injuries are present all increase the risk of aspiration.

### *Alterations in Oropharyngeal Flora*

Aspiration of small volumes of oropharyngeal contents occurs frequently in normal subjects during sleep.[62] In the healthy individual, pulmonary defense mechanisms clear the aspirate efficiently. In the critically ill patient, a similar degree of aspiration is much more likely to be associated with the development of pneumonia. Systemic factors that alter defenses against infection may play a substantial role in the increased susceptibility of the traumatized patient to pulmonary and systemic infection.

Within a few days after hospital admission, the endogenous oropharyngeal flora are replaced by a preponderance of virulent Gram-negative rods.[132] Colonization of the respiratory tract with Gram-negative bacilli increases as the severity of illness increases.[65] Bacteria adhere to oropharyngeal epithelial cells. In critically ill patients, the surface binding characteristics of these cells changes and allows the change in flora to occur. The route by which the Gram-negative organisms reach the patient's oropharynx is uncertain, but contamination by fecal-oral transmission, as well as direct patient-to-patient transmission by intensive care unit staff, is likely.[138]

The stomach may be an important source of organisms as well. Normally the acidic environment of the stomach inhibits bacterial growth. The widespread use of prophylactic measures to raise gastric pH may increase the probability that bacteria will survive to be regurgitated and aspirated. Clear evidence of upper airway colonization by gastric micro-organisms in 11 of 60 critically ill patients receiving antacids was shown by Du Moulin.[34] Tracheal colonization from gastric organisms also has been documented in patients with paralytic ileus during intermittent positive pressure ventilation.[5] Johanson and associates[65] demonstrated that 23% of the colonized patients developed pneumonia, but only 3.3% of the patients in whom colonization was not detected developed this complication.

The risk of postoperative pneumonia is increased by a decreased cough response resulting from incisional pain, analgesic drugs, atelectasis, underlying systemic or pulmonary disease, and immunologic abnormalities that frequently follow severe traumatic injuries. When there is clinical or radiologic evidence of pneumonia, the etiologic organisms should be identified. Because the central airways (trachea or mainstem bronchi) are frequently colonized, sputum cultures, even of a specimen obtained by endotracheal suctioning, are unreliable.[13,53,65] A Gram stain is more useful, but is often misleading. Transtracheal aspirates are more reliable, but cannot be done in an intubated patient. Transthoracic needle aspiration is also reliable, but it is usually avoided because of a high frequency of complications. Currently, fiberoptic bronchoscopy to obtain a specimen directly from the involved areas is the safest and most reliable method to obtain specimens for accurate cultures.[21] A protected brush catheter that keeps the sampling brush sterile until it is pushed through a polyethylene glycol plug into the suspicious area is available (No. 1650, Microvasive, Milford, MA).[21] Initially antibiotics should be chosen according to the Gram stain findings and then changed when culture and sensitivity results are available.

Since intubated multiple trauma patients are at high risk for developing both early (<48 hours) primary pneumonia and late nosocomial pneumonia, attempts have been made to modify this risk. The effects of oropharyngeal and intestinal decontamination using topical nonabsorbable antibiotics in intubated multiple trauma patients have been evaluated.[132] There were no episodes of nosocomial Gram-negative pneumonia in patients who had selective decontamination of the intestines and oropharynx compared to a 20% incidence in untreated patients. However, the incidence of early pneumonia (primarily due to Gram-positive cocci) was not reduced as the antibiotics selected were not active against those microorganisms. The incidence of early pneumonia can be reduced significantly with the early use of systemic antibiotics active against Gram-positive cocci.[132]

## VASCULAR CATHETER-RELATED INFECTION

Contaminated arterial, pulmonary artery, central venous, or peripheral venous catheters can be sources of sepsis and occasionally septic shock, especially if breaks in sterile technique occur during insertion or maintenance or if contaminated fluids or devices, such as transducer domes, are used.[108] The frequency of cannula-related septicemia has been estimated to be ten times greater than that caused by the use of extrinsically contaminated fluids.[10] Pulmonary artery catheters are extensively manipulated during routine intensive care. The ports are used for drug and fluid infusion, cardiac output determinations, and sampling for mixed venous gas analysis. Since all of these maneuvers interrupt the integrity of the catheter system, the risk of bacterial colonization and nosocomial infection is substantial. The type of injectate delivery system used for measurement of thermodilution cardiac output determination may also influence the risk of infection. Nelson and associates[97] noted an incidence of microbial colonization of injectate fluid of 35% when an open system was used compared to a 5% incidence when fluid was injected through a closed system.

Many factors affect the colonization rate of intravascular catheters. The insertion site,[104] strictness of the aseptic technique used for catheter insertion[46] and maintenance,[81,82] presence of contaminated infusion fluids,[81,82] the use of total parenteral nutritional therapy,[89] and existing septicemia[83] are all important factors. Thus, a significant and difficult to interpret variation exists in the literature regarding the catheter colonization rate. It appears, however, that even with the use of strict aseptic technique the overall catheter infection rate in a surgical ICU cannot be reduced below 7–8%.[104,119] Pulmonary artery catheters inserted via the internal jugular vein were found to be infected in 29% of patients.[104] From 3 to 20% of central venous catheters, depending on their insertion sites, may be colonized.[104] An increased incidence of central venous catheter sepsis has been reported with triple-lumen catheters (19%) compared with single-lumen catheters (3%).[103] This increase may be secondary to an increased risk of contamination during manipulations involving the three ports. The highest rate of catheter infection occurs with antecubital vein insertion.[104] Arterial catheters, depending on the study, become colonized 4 to 18% of the time.[9,104] The risks are similar for radial and femoral arterial lines.[135] Septicemia has been seen in 3% of patients with arterial catheters in place for a significant length of time.[9] Indwelling vascular catheters should not be left in place for longer than 4 days because of a strong correlation between the duration of catheterization, colonization, and bacteremia.[9,83] Arterial, central venous, or pulmonary artery catheters inserted percutaneously are less likely to become infected than those placed by cutdown.[9]

The most common isolate of catheter infection is *Staphylococcus epidermidis*.[104,119] Although this organism is considered by many authors to be of low virulence,[24] septicemia associated with severe morbidity and resistance to several antibiotics has been reported.[126] Less frequently, *Staphylococcus aureus* is isolated from catheter tips.[104] Other organisms, including *Klebsiella, Streptococcus pneumoniae,* and *Escherichia coli,* have also been isolated.[104] Although the catheter tip may be contaminated by spread from another source, most catheter-related septicemias arise in the cannula tract.[84]

Assessing the probability of catheter-related infection usually requires removal of the suspicious catheter for culturing. Using sterile technique, the catheter tip should be cut off for direct culture after cleaning the surrounding skin with an iodine solution. Maki et al.,[84] described a semiquantitative culturing method that involves rolling the subcutaneous portion of the catheter on an agar culture plate after removal under sterile conditions. Growth of 15 or more colonies per agar plate is strongly associated with local inflammation at the catheter site and catheter-associated bacteremia. Growth of fewer than 15 colonies is considered to represent contamination and does not correlate with catheter-related septicemia.

The major disadvantage of these techniques is that 24 to 48 hours may pass before culture results are available. Cooper and Hopkins[25] diagnosed intravascular catheter-associated infection rapidly by direct Gram staining of catheter segments and examination under an oil immersion lens. The Gram stain was 100% sensitive in detecting the presence of catheter-tip colonization and had a specificity of 96.9%.[25]

Catheter tip cultures are likely to reflect cannula tract infections since the catheter must be withdrawn through the tract. Blood withdrawn through the catheter is more likely to reflect bacteremic spread to the catheter tip or bacteremia. Blood cultures obtained by withdrawing blood from the suspected catheter lack sensitivity in predicting whether a culture of the catheter tip will be positive.[136]

Replacing all central venous catheters in a febrile trauma patient is costly and exposes the patient to an increased risk of pneumothorax. The majority of the catheters removed will be sterile or, if colonized, will prove not to be the source of sepsis. Simultaneous quantitative blood cultures obtained from the central catheter and a peripheral vein may identify reliably, within 24 hours, those infected catheters requiring removal.[91] The central line is left in situ until culture results are available, if the patient's clinical condition permits. A central vein catheter colony count $\geq$ five times the peripheral venous blood colony count is significant and requires removal of the central line.

## IMMUNOLOGIC EFFECTS OF TRAUMA

Impaired neutrophil and monocyte function, deficient T-lymphocyte numbers and responsiveness, depression of cellular immunity, depressed IgG, and complement depletion all occur after traumatic injury, and each correlates with an increased risk of sepsis.[11,56,68,79,80] After trauma, aberrations in host defenses can be detected before clinical signs of sepsis and can be used to identify patients at increased risk for infectious complications.[68] Christou and associates[22,23] noted defects of granulocyte function within 2 hours of injury. The ability of neutrophils to phagocytize bacteria is reduced after trauma. Abnormalities of intrinsic neutrophil function (chemotaxis, adherence, degranulation, superoxide production) have also been described after traumatic injury.[75]

As part of the inflammatory response, circulating monocytes migrate to sites of inflammation and subsequently differentiate into tissue macrophages. Monocytes function as phagocytes and also regulate the lymphocyte response to antigens. Monocyte dysfunction occurs in trauma patients.[4,106] A depression of both chemotaxis and antigen-presenting capacity occurs.[4,107] The latter correlates with the presence or subsequent development of infection.[106]

Profound abnormalities in cellular immunity also appear after injury. Depression of interleukin-2 (IL-2) synthesis is reported consistently in both animal and clinical trauma studies.[1,2,39] Interleukin-2 is a lymphokine released by T-lymphocytes after appropriate stimulation; it is essential for lymphocyte activation and for the development of the proliferative T-cell response to antigenic stimulation. Trauma-induced depression of IL-2 synthesis could be the basis for the defective T-cell function found in these patients[39] and may be caused by excessive prostaglandin-E (PGE) output from inhibitory monocytes.[39] Depressed T-cell function may increase the risk of infectious complications.[23,38,100] The use of cyclooxygenase inhibitors, such as indomethacin (which blocks PGE release), is currently being investigated as immunomodulating therapy to reverse some trauma-induced immunologic abnormalities.[38,39]

Endogenous opioids, such as β-endorphin, may also contribute to the immunosuppression associated with trauma.[78] A temporal association of depressed immune parameters and elevated β-endorphin levels has been shown after traumatic injury, but causality has not been demonstrated.[78]

Patients with skin test anergy on initial evaluation after blunt trauma were more likely to develop sepsis during hospitalization.[23] In this study no patient with a normal initial skin test response became septic or died.

Heideman and coworkers[56] reported rapid depletion of the complement components C3, C4, and C5 in amounts that correlated with the severity of injury. All patients surviving for more than 10 days with a 50% or greater decrease in C3, C4, and C5 levels developed positive blood cultures, suggesting that complement depletion is another possible factor in the increased risk of sepsis.

Reticuloendothelial system dysfunction is implicated in host defense failure and manifests within minutes after trauma. The serum opsonic capacity (ability of the serum to support phagocytosis by normal neutrophils) is reduced in trauma patients. The most marked reductions in serum opsonic capacity are present in patients who ultimately die with infection, suggesting a causal relationship.[107] This form of immunodepression appears to be mediated in part by depletion of the plasma opsonic factor, fibronectin, the levels of which decrease shortly after traumatic injury.[123] Fibronectin normally coats bacteria and particulate matter and helps enhance clearance by the reticuloendothelial system.[116] Its depletion thus decreases resistance to infection.[74,116] In patients surviving severe trauma, fibronectin levels return to normal by 72 hours after injury, whereas in nonsurvivors these levels remain depressed.[123] Cryoprecipitate contains a high concentration of fibronectin, and its infusion increases serum fibronectin levels, restoring reticuloendothelial cell function.[116] Whether this form of prophylactic immunotherapy improves outcome remains to be seen.

Another plasma opsonin is C-reactive protein (CRP). Normally, serum CRP levels are very low (less than 1 mg/dL). Increases of several hundredfold occur after tissue injury caused by trauma, infection, toxins, etc.[8,50] The CRP response to trauma or infection is thus opposite to that of fibronectin. CRP is produced in the liver in response to interleukin-1, which is released from macrophages activated by tissue injury.[61,86] Thus, whenever significant trauma or sepsis exists, CRP levels rise. The function of this substance in host defense includes interaction with the complement system, activation of natural killer cells, and binding to damaged cell membranes as an opsonic substance.[12,95,142] Relatively specific elevations of CRP levels correlating with the severity of injury have been demonstrated.[93,129] Serum levels usually rise by 12 hours and peak at 48 hours after trauma.[129] Patients who develop sepsis after trauma maintain high CRP levels for at least 8 days, whereas in others CRP declines after the fourth postinjury day.[121,129] The use of serial CRP measurements during the posttrauma period has been shown to predict septic complications an average of 2.4 days before their clinical diagnosis.[129] However, further evaluation is needed to determine the accuracy and clinical usefulness of measurement of CRP levels.[93]

Because trauma induces multiple immunologic deficits, attempts have been made to enhance nonspecific host defenses against infection.[105] Muramyl peptides, derived from fragments of mycobacterial cell wall, have been extensively evaluated as immunostimulants in animals. A variety of protective effects have been demonstrated, and clinical evaluation has begun.

Splenectomy, especially in children, may increase the risk of septicemia and death, predominantly from encapsulated organisms, such as *Streptococcus pneumoniae*. Otherwise healthy patients who have undergone splenectomy for trauma have persistent immunologic deficiencies.[32] Such deficiencies are probably responsible for the increased risk of overwhelming postsplenectomy infections (OPSI).[32] The spleen serves several immunologic functions, including mechanical clearance of foreign particles, production of opsonins (important for removal of encapsulated bacteria), and production of IgM antibodies.[77] IgM levels were depressed 36% and T-cell responsiveness to PHA stimulation was depressed 38% compared to controls in 22 trauma patients who had undergone splenectomy an average of 4 years previously.[32] These persistent defects may explain why OPSI may develop years after splenectomy.[51]

The risk of early sepsis (less than 1 month after injury) is not influenced by the splenectomy per se, but rather by the extent of the patient's injuries.[85] Late sepsis after splenectomy for traumatic injuries is seen in 0.5–2.0% of patients.[31,101] This is much lower than the incidence reported in patients after splenectomy for treatment of hematologic disorders. The decreased risk of OPSI after traumatic splenectomy compared to therapeutic splenectomy may be secondary to autotransplantation of splenic tissue (splenosis) resulting from traumatic rupture of the spleen.[102] These splenic implants retain their ability to function; however, it is uncertain whether splenosis protects against OPSI or whether other factors create the risk differential.

Concern about postsplenectomy sepsis syndrome sways many surgeons to salvage the spleen in part or in toto. Although the validity of these concerns is not known, it may be prudent to administer polyvalent pneumococcal vaccine postoperatively if the spleen cannot be salvaged. The vaccine should be administered when the patient is able to develop an antibody response (usually 1 month after surgery). The immunization may then be repeated every 3 years.

General anesthesia may impair the immunologic response directly. A decreased leukocyte accumulation response to intraperitoneal endotoxin occurs in rats anesthetized with halothane.[15] At least in animals, these changes seem to be physiologically significant. Seventy percent of mice anesthetized with halothane died within 7 hours after intraperitoneal injection of live salmonella, whereas all control animals survived.[16] Other anesthetic agents can also impair neutrophil cidal function.[146–148] Halothane and nitrous oxide, enflurane and nitrous oxide, and morphine and nitrous oxide all reduce neutrophil chemotaxis in humans.[130] During phagocytosis neutrophils produce active forms of oxygen (superoxide anions, $O_2^-$; hydrogen peroxide, $H_2O_2^-$; and hydroxyl radicals, $\cdot OH$). Inhalational anesthetics appear to inhibit this function by decreasing intracellular $Ca^{2+}$ mobilization.[94] Although the clinical significance of these findings is uncertain, they represent one additional factor that may predispose traumatized patients to postoperative septic complications.

Because of the failure of numerous host defenses in the trauma patient, attempts have been made to protect the injured patient from infection through enhancement of natural defenses by intravenous infusion of polyvalent immunoglobulins.[35,49] Glinz and associates[49] evaluated the efficacy of a polyclonal polyspecific immunoglobulin preparation in 150 severely injured patients. A significant reduction in the incidence of nosocomial pneumonia and overall number of infections occurred in patients receiving immunoglobulins. However, overall mortality and deaths specifically caused by infection were not decreased by the use of immunotherapy.

The use of intravenous immunoglobulins in association with antibiotics in septic intensive care unit patients was associated with more rapid defervescence compared to patients treated with antibiotics alone, but was not associated with improved survival.[30] Thus, although some favorable effects have been demonstrated with the use of intravenous immunoglobulins, this form of treatment should be considered experimental at this time.

## INFECTIONS SPECIFIC TO INJURED PATIENTS

Infectious complications can obviously be caused by a number of different organisms in the injured patient. There are, however, two infectious disease entities that occur far more often in the injured than the noninjured patient: tetanus and gas gangrene.

### TETANUS

Tetanus has been estimated to cause between 160,000 and 1 million deaths a year worldwide, but only 70 to 100 deaths a year in the United States.[45,139] Tetanus may be a complication of lacerations, open fractures, burns, abrasions, or unrecognized wounds. A patient with a mild injury may be at an enhanced risk for developing tetanus because the routine protective measures employed in severe cases may be omitted. The disease occurs only in patients who have not had adequate immunization or who have not received adequate boosters since their primary immunizations.

#### *Pathogenesis*

The clinical features of tetanus are caused by the production of an extremely potent neurotoxin, tetanospasmin, by *Clostridium tetani* in anaerobic conditions. The toxin acts on four areas of the nervous system[145]: the skeletal muscle motor endplates, the spinal cord, the sympathetic nervous system, and the brain. Tetanospasmin appears to interfere with neuromuscular transmission by inhibiting the nerve terminal release of acetylcholine. It also ascends peripheral nerves and reaches the spinal cord, where it is taken up by presynaptic terminals of inhibitory spinal interneurons, preventing the release of inhibitory transmitter. This results in the excessive motor neuron discharge that is characteristic of tetanus. A similar effect on inhibitory influences in the lateral horn of the spinal cord accounts for the excessive sympathetic activity seen in severe cases of tetanus. Seizures occur in some cases and are probably secondary to fixation of toxin by cerebral gangliosides.

The cardiovascular manifestations of tetanus have been reviewed by Tsueda et al.[141] and are attributed to three mechanisms occurring individually or in combination:

1. *Medullary injury:* Histopathologically, medullary damage has been demonstrated in many cases of tetanus, explaining the wide variation in cardiovascular findings seen in this disease. Pyrexia, sudden and repeated episodes of apnea, gasping respiration, twitching of the tongue, dysphagia, intense diaphoresis, profuse salivation, terminal hypothermia, and muscle flaccidity may also be due to the effects of tetanus toxin on the brainstem.
2. *Toxic myocarditis:* Cardiovascular changes may at least partly be due to a direct effect of the toxin on cardiac muscle. Some clinical observations do not support this mechanism. For instance, many patients with refractory hypotension may have no histologic changes characteristic of myocarditis. In addition, many patients with tetanus have been resuscitated successfully after cardiac arrest without any further signs of cardiac dysfunction. It is not possible to explain how tetanus toxin can reach the myocardium. Long-standing catecholamine stimulation, rather than the toxin itself, may be the cause of myocardial and vascular changes.
3. *Sympathetic nervous system hyperactivity:* Increased sympathetic activity develops rather late and plays an important role in mortality from tetanus. Pharmacologic control of the sympathetic nervous system by continuous central depression, peripheral adrenergic blockade, or both appears to be well justified.

#### *Clinical Features*

After the introduction of clostridial spores, there is an incubation period usually lasting from 3 to 21 days. The further the injury is from the central nervous system, the longer is the incubation period. After the appearance of symptoms, a rapid progression to the full syndrome usually suggests that the disease will be severe.[40] Clinically, the disease can be classified into one of three forms: generalized, local, and cephalic tetanus.

Generalized tetanus is the most common form. Since the transit of the toxin up the peripheral nerves is fairly slow, its effects are first seen in muscle groups with short motor neurons, ie, the head and neck muscles. Later the trunk and limb muscles are involved. Trismus and dysphagia are initial features in most cases. Muscle hypertonicity then spreads to the neck, back, abdomen, and limbs. Superimposed on this background of hypertonicity are acute paroxysmal spasms that are extremely painful, repetitive, and exhausting. Spasms may be so intense that crush fractures of the vertebrae develop. They can precipitate respiratory arrest by causing spasm of the larynx, the intercostal muscles, or the diaphragm.

The majority of patients with generalized tetanus have severe clinical symptoms. Sixty percent of severe cases have signs of cardiovascular instability due to autonomic nervous system overactivity and increased catecholamine secretion. In one series unexpected cardiac arrest that was not preceded by evidence of cardiac arrhythmias, electrolyte imbalance, or hypoxemia accounted for 38% of the deaths.[139] Severe hypertension and/or tachycardia may occur spontaneously or may be precipitated by such manipulations as tracheal suctioning. Other signs of autonomic nervous system instability include hypersalivation and sweating. The mortality rate from generalized tetanus is reported to be from 11 to 60%.[139]

Local tetanus is characterized by persistent rigidity in muscle groups located in close proximity to the site of injury. These symptoms may persist for a few months, but it is in general a mild disorder with a mortality rate of only 1%.[87] Localized tetanus can progress to the generalized form.

Cephalic tetanus is the least common form of tetanus, accounting for 1 to 3% of the total cases reported. It is seen after head injuries and is characterized by dysfunction of the third, fourth, seventh, ninth, tenth, and twelfth cranial nerves.[6] Mortality from cephalic tetanus is a function of generalization of the symptoms and ranges from 15 to 30%.[63]

### *Diagnosis*

The diagnosis of tetanus is based primarily on a history of injury followed by the onset of characteristic symptoms. Laboratory studies are usually nonspecific and thus of little value, with the exception of Gram stain and culture of material obtained from the wound, which may or may not show the characteristic Gram-positive rods.[145]

### *Prevention and Treatment*

Prevention of tetanus is more effective than treatment. Tetanus probably does not occur in patients who have been fully immunized and who have received appropriate booster injections at the time of injury.[40] The production of antibodies to tetanus toxoid renders the patient immune to tetanospasmin. Routine active immunization consists of three spaced doses of absorbed tetanus toxoid. The first and second doses are given 6 weeks apart, and the third injection is given 6 months after the second injection. A routine booster dose should be given thereafter at 10-year intervals.

All traumatized patients with skin wounds should receive 0.5 mL of tetanus toxoid subcutaneously unless they have been completely immunized in the past and have had a booster within the previous 6 months. In patients vaccinated in the past, a single revaccination given immediately after the injury has been generally accepted to provide sufficient protection. However, an evaluation of the kinetics of the antibody response to revaccination against tetanus demonstrated that, in patients who received their primary vaccination 17–20 years earlier, 13% had antibody concentrations just above the "protective" level 4 days after revaccination.[125] Since tetanus has been reported to develop as early as 24 to 48 hours after severe trauma, antibody titers in these patients could be nonprotective.

Therefore, the use of tetanus immune globulin should be considered in patients whose primary vaccination occurred more than 17 years previously and who have sustained injuries judged to favor the rapid development of tetanus.[125] When, as often happens, the immunization history of the patient is unknown, immunization is necessary and should be given a high priority. If the patient has a large or dirty wound, 500 to 1,000 units of human tetanus immune globulin should be administered at a site different from that used for the injection of toxoid. This provides protection until the individual acquires a safe antibody response to the toxoid. Removal of all devitalized tissue and foreign bodies is also an essential part of tetanus prevention. The anesthesiologist should ascertain that the trauma victim has received appropriate tetanus prophylaxis (see Table 2-3).

Successful treatment of generalized tetanus depends on early diagnosis and local wound care.[40] This includes surgical excision of the site at which organisms are producing toxin, neutralization of circulating toxin, intensive nursing care, provision of a quiet environment such that stimulation of the patient is minimized, maintenance of fluid and electrolyte balance, provision of adequate calories, and symptomatic control of the systemic manifestations of the disease.[139] The local infection should be treated by excision and debridement. Penicillin kills the vegetative form of *Clostridium tetani*. One million units of penicillin G should be given parenterally every 6 hours for 10 days. Tetracycline, 2 g/day, can be used in patients allergic to penicillin.[145] Human tetanus immune globulin, 3,000–6,000 units IM, neutralizes circulating toxin effectively, but does not affect the toxin already bound to the nervous tissue.[40]

Recent advances in the management of acute respiratory failure and improvements in intensive care have improved the prognosis of tetanus.[140] Respiratory difficulties and laryngeal spasm are frequently seen. Most patients with severe tetanus should have their airway protected by endotracheal intubation or tracheostomy. Tetanospasms should be controlled by pharmacologic therapy. Diazepam and phenobarbital have been used to control muscle rigidity and spasms, but no sedative reliably prevents the episodes of spasm, and a muscle relaxant is usually necessary. Continuous infusion or intermittent injection of long acting competitive neuromuscular blocking drugs, such as d-tubocurarine or pancuronium, may be regulated to maintain subtotal paralysis. Curare is usually selected if there is tachycardia and hypertension and pancuronium if there is bradycardia and hypotension.[29,37]

Succinylcholine may be given early in tetanus, but should be avoided in later stages as cardiac arrest has been reported after its use in the recovery phase.[37] The dose of relaxant can usually be decreased after 2 weeks and stopped after 3 weeks. However, the duration of relaxant therapy must be individualized.[37] Intravenous sedatives and narcotics must be given continuously to the paralyzed patient. Respiratory support is provided by a volume-controlled ventilator. Maintenance of fluid balance may be difficult as the insensible loss in these patients is often large as a result of profuse sweating and excessive salivation. Therefore, daily measurement of body weight may be more helpful than evaluation of measured fluid input and output. Because of the patient's limited ability to swallow and the presence of a hypermetabolic state, malnutrition may develop rapidly unless nutritional support is started early. Provision of calories through a small-bore nasogastric tube is usually well tolerated.

Treatment of autonomic instability can be difficult. Some success has been achieved by the use of low doses of propranolol.[139] Deep sedation, in addition to muscle paralysis, minimizes the sensory input that may precipitate excessive autonomic activity. Alpha-sympathetic receptor blockade can also be utilized to block the peak increases in blood pressure. When adrenergic blockers are used, abrupt termination of catecholamine discharge may cause a marked decrease in blood pressure. Magnesium sulfate infusions can help control the signs of sympathetic nervous system overactivity and in some instances may be more desirable than alpha blockers.[64] The sympathetic overactivity in severe tetanus has also been controlled successfully with continuous epidural or subarachnoid infusion of bupivacaine. The combination of sympathetic blockade, muscle relaxation, and analgesia provided with continuous epidural blockade or spinal anesthesia benefits selected tetanus patients.[111,124a]

Dantrolene, a direct-acting muscle relaxant with minimal central nervous system depressant effects, may be useful during the convalescent phase of tetanus.[20,137] Dantrolene, IV 100 mg/day, provided excellent relief of muscle spasms in one patient described by Cerda and associates.[20] Muscle contractions that recurred after stopping dantrolene were promptly controlled by restarting the drug. Considerably higher doses were used in another patient reported by Tidyman et al.[137] Since data for treatment of muscle spasms with this agent are limited, specific indications and dosage for dantrolene in the management of tetanus remain uncertain.

Sun et al.[133] described two patients in whom 10 mg of morphine intrathecally resulted in excellent sedation and muscle relaxation for 10–15 hours. Blood pressure and heart rate decreased significantly, however, and apnea was observed in both patients. Smaller doses of intrathecal or epidural morphine may provide adequate sedation and muscle relaxation without these side effects.

Continuous intrathecal infusion of baclofen (an inhibitory neurotransmitter agonist) was completely successful in relieving spasticity in two patients with tetanus.[92] The drug was infused through a subcutaneously tunneled intrathecal catheter. Spinal administration of baclofen or other gamma-aminobutyric acid derivatives may be a significant advance in the treatment of tetanus.

With the widespread use of muscle relaxation and ventilatory support, few patients presently die of respiratory failure. However, cardiac arrest is a common but poorly understood complication of tetanus.[139,140] Pulmonary embolism, pneumonia, and renal failure are also seen.[45,124] Nonoliguric renal failure, ascribed to a reduction in blood flow to the kidney by sympathetic overactivity, is associated with a high mortality rate (65%).[124] Blood urea nitrogen and creatinine levels must be monitored carefully in these patients. Peripheral adrenergic blocking agents may be used to prevent this complication.

Surviving patients are usually able to leave the intensive care unit within 3 to 4 weeks from the onset of illness. Patients who have recovered from tetanus do not develop spontaneous immunity to further attacks; thus, they should be immunized as should anyone else.[145]

Tetanus leaves no residual abnormalities so an all-out therapeutic effort is justified despite its high cost.[145] Psychiatric abnormalities are common after recovery from tetanus, but are usually evanescent. There is little evidence of significant long-term deterioration of lung function.[41]

### *Anesthetic Management*

Surgical debridement should be done using general endotracheal anesthesia and controlled ventilation.[55] Monitoring should include direct measurement of arterial blood pressure and measurement of central venous or pulmonary artery pressure.[55] Excessive sympathetic nervous system activity before induction of anesthesia should be controlled pharmacologically, and this control should be monitored throughout the procedure. Enflurane or isoflurane might be superior to halothane due to halothane's potential for cardiac irritability.

## GAS GANGRENE

Gas gangrene (clostridial myonecrosis) traditionally has been associated with trauma. However, trauma was present only 49% of the time in six large studies of this infection.[54] Traumatic injuries associated with the development of gas gangrene include fractures, lacerations, abrasions, crush injuries, traumatic amputations, penetrating wounds, blunt trauma, and frostbite.[149] Posttraumatic gas gangrene appears to involve the limbs more commonly than the trunk.[96] Estimates of the annual incidence of gas gangrene in the United States has varied from 900 to more than 3,000 cases.[54,59]

### *Etiology and Pathogenesis*

Gas gangrene can develop secondary to soft tissue infection by one or more of several species of Clostridium. The vast majority of cases are due solely to infection by *Clostridium perfringens*. Contamination of tissue with clostridial spores in the absence of low tissue $O_2$ tension does not lead to infection. Under locally hypoxic conditions clostridia multiply and exotoxins are released, producing the syndrome of clostridial myonecrosis. Once started, the pathologic process of gas gangrene can be so fulminating that death often occurs within 30–48 hours. The incubation period of gas gangrene from *Clostridium perfringens* averages 12–24 hours, but may be as short as 1 hour or as long as 6 weeks.

At least 12 exotoxins have been identified as playing a role in producing the local and systemic effects of gas gangrene. The major lethal toxin is lecithinase, which attacks the lecithin component of cell membranes.[72] This toxin produces tissue necrosis and hemolysis; hence, the frequent occurrence of anemia, hemoglobinuria, oliguria, and occasional renal failure. The remaining toxins help liquify the necrotic tissue, causing dissection of the infection into adjacent healthy tissue and producing a rapid spread of the infectious process. Severe edema develops, and if involved tissue is encased in a fascial compartment, pressure in the compartment can increase enough to compromise arterial circulation. This produces tissue hypoxia, enhances further growth of the clostridial organisms, and further threatens tissue viability. Hypotension may develop because of several factors, including translocation of fluid into the involved tissues, increased insensible loss from associated fever, and decreased oral intake.

### *Diagnosis*

The most crucial factor in successful management of gas gangrene is early diagnosis. A high index of suspicion must be maintained since the early signs of infection are subtle. They include a progressive and disproportionate increase in wound or incisional pain, tachycardia out of proportion to fever, apathy, and shiny skin at the infected site indicative of tissue edema. If untreated, signs progress rapidly. The wound begins to drain a thin and watery material that over a few hours changes to a foul-smelling discharge. The wound margins become discolored, and hemorrhagic bullae may be seen. A rapidly extending margin of erythema and palpable crepitations are late findings.

Diagnosis can be confirmed most expeditiously by Gram staining the discharge and identifying the characteristic Gram-positive rods. This diagnostic step is necessary as the combination of gas in the tissues and necrotizing myositis does not always indicate that a clostridial infection is present.[54,99] Although the presence of an intermuscular fascicular gas pattern is characteristically found on X-ray in late infections, gas may not be seen in early infections. Treatment, however, should not be delayed until culture results are available. It should be noted that accurate determination of the extent of muscle damage may not always be possible by physical or radiologic examination. An infection that appears to be isolated may involve more muscle groups than estimated.

### *Treatment*

Antibiotics and surgical debridement remain the cornerstone of treatment of clostridial myonecrosis. Penicillin, 10–24 million units per day, remains the drug of choice. Two to four g/day of tetracycline is suggested for use in penicillin-allergic patients. If the organisms responsible for the wound infection remain uncertain after Gram stain, intravenous broad spectrum antibiotics, such as clindamycin, 40 mg/kg/day, and tobramycin or gentamycin, 5 mg/kg/day, are added to the penicillin until culture results are available. Wide surgical debridement is usually necessary, although debridement alone does not lower the morbidity or mortality of gas gangrene. Antibiotics without adequate surgical debridement will also result in treatment failure. Generous amounts of fluid are usually necessary to compensate for surgical blood loss and exudation into the interstitial space caused by toxin-induced capillary endothelial damage. Blood transfusions may also be necessary if hemolysis is present. In selected patients central venous pressure monitoring may be helpful to guide fluid management.

Hyperbaric oxygen therapy has been demonstrated since 1970 to be a useful adjunctive therapy for treatment of gas gangrene. Several series have reported superior survival rates when hyperbaric oxygen is combined with antibiotic and surgical therapy. However, no controlled study is available to prove the efficacy of this form of treatment.[58,59] Hyperbaric oxygen counteracts the hypoxic environment necessary for clostridial growth and in addition inhibits toxin production. The frequency of complications related to hyperbaric oxygen therapy is low. Since patients can be monitored in the hyperbaric chamber, the existence of cardiorespiratory complications does not present a contraindication to the use of hyperbaric oxygen. Consideration should be given to transferring patients with gas gangrene to a center where a hyperbaric chamber is available, since a combined therapeutic approach with early recognition, aggressive surgical debridement, appropriate antibiotics, and adjunctive hyperbaric oxygen therapy appears to be the most effective method of decreasing the morbidity and mortality associated with gas gangrene.[54]

Hitchcock et al.[59] reported that 94% of patients who developed gas gangrene after trauma survived compared to a 65% survival rate for patients who developed gas gangrene after elective surgery. The authors postulated that this infection is sought with greater diligence in trauma patients and thus is diagnosed and treated at an earlier stage.

### *Anesthetic Management*

Patients with gas gangrene require surgical debridement as a major component of their treatment. Anesthesia is almost always required during this stage of management.[72] Adequate evaluation before surgery should be performed for evidence of hypovolemia or shock, tachycardia, anemia, metabolic acidosis, renal and pulmonary dysfunction, and electrolyte imbalance. Aggressive hemodynamic monitoring with arterial, and central venous or pulmonary artery catheterization may be necessary to assess and optimize fluid status, cardiac function, oxygenation, and acid-base status. Hematocrit should be determined preoperatively since hemolytic anemia may be present. The serum potassium level should be measured as both hemolysis and tissue destruction may result in hyperkalemia. Records documenting urinary output and specific gravity during the hospitalization period may help assess fluid status and kidney function. Arterial blood gases should be measured and base deficit corrected with fluids and sodium bicarbonate as necessary.

It is important to remember that gas gangrene can progress rapidly. Thus, preoperative assessment, fluid resuscitation, and optimization of the patient's status should be done as quickly as possible. In severe cases, resuscitative measures may have to be continued intraoperatively as the infection may not allow satisfactory improvement of the patient's condition, and in fact, delay of surgery may be counterproductive.

Anesthesia should be induced with extreme caution and adequate monitoring. Ketamine, 1–2 mg/kg IV, appears to be an ideal agent for this purpose, but its use in patients with gas gangrene has not been well studied.[72] Sodium thiopental, benzodiazepines, and neuroleptic agents, when used in large doses and administered rapidly, may result in hypotension and decreased tissue perfusion. Morphine sulfate, demerol, and even fentanyl may cause significant reduction of blood pressure in this group of patients. Succinylcholine probably should be avoided as an aid to tracheal intubation because of the possibility of potassium-induced cardiac arrest. Serum potassium elevation in response to succinylcholine may occur because of massive traumatic muscle injury[14] or possibly myonecrosis. Vecuronium has no effect on serum potassium, and its hemodynamic effects are minimal.[88] Thus, it is probably the agent of choice in this group of patients.

Anesthesia can be maintained with halothane, enflurane, isoflurane, or fentanyl titrated to blood pressure and other hemodynamic measurements. Nitrous oxide may be used safely even though it may theoretically expand the gas-containing spaces. Since the infected areas are relatively avascular, it is unlikely that significant amounts of $N_2O$ will diffuse into the affected tissues.[72,110] Azotemia is often present due to both hypovolemia and kidney damage caused by hemoglobinuria. Thus, drugs eliminated by the kidney should be used carefully since their excretion may be delayed.

Spinal or epidural anesthesia in these patients may carry the risk of disseminating the clostridial organisms. Furthermore, in the presence of an unstable cardiovascular system sympathetic blockade may have undesirable hemodynamic effects.[72]

## CONCLUSION

More than half of the postoperative deaths in multiple trauma patients are due to uncontrolled infections. Urinary tract infections secondary to indwelling bladder catheters occur in one-third of victims. However, this type of infection contributes little to postoperative mortality. Infections in traumatized wounds occur at a much greater rate than those in surgical wounds. Peritoneal abscess and peritonitis may develop after abdominal injuries, necessitating repeated anesthetic administrations for abdominal re-exploration. Administration of proper antibiotics before surgery for the initial injury may reduce the rate of this complication. Bacterial pneumonias, especially after chest trauma, may present a real threat to life. Thoracostomy tubes, aspiration of oropharyngeal and occasionally gastric contents, and nosocomial infections also appear to be responsible for this complication.

Infections related to arterial, pulmonary artery, central venous, or peripheral venous catheters may be a source of sepsis and septic shock. Adherence to aseptic technique during catheter insertion and maintenance, keeping catheters in place no longer than 3 to 4 days, periodic inspection of the catheter entry sites during daily dressing changes, Gram staining and culturing of the specimens obtained from these areas and from catheter tips, and appropriate antibiotic therapy may help in reducing the frequency of this complication.

Blunted host defense mechanisms after trauma render the injured patient susceptible to infectious complications. Neutrophil function is impaired, T-lymphocytes are reduced in number and are less responsive, IgG and complement levels are decreased, and reticuloendothelial system function is altered after trauma. Characteristic changes in serum opsonic substance levels (fibronectin, C-reactive protein) occur. These changes may persist for days in patients developing sepsis and may offer some predictive value. Although general anesthesia impairs the immune response, the clinical significance of this impairment in promoting infectious complications in the injured patient is not known.

Tetanus occurs with greater frequency in injured than in noninjured patients. Respiratory muscle spasm and autonomic nervous system hyperactivity require prompt intervention. Tetanospasms can be controlled by diazepam or phenobarbital, but are best treated with long-acting nondepolarizing muscle relaxants. Dantrolene and spinal narcotics may also be used. Deep sedation, alpha-receptor blockade, and magnesium sulfate can be used to control hypertension. Adequate nutritional therapy should be started early to prevent malnutrition. The frequent occurrence of pneumonia and renal failure mandates careful monitoring and preventive measures.

Almost half of the patients who develop gas gangrene are trauma victims. Injuries resulting in significant muscle damage and hypoxic tissue conditions promote this complication. Surgical debridement, proper antibiotic therapy, and hyperbaric oxygen treatment should be instituted early to reduce mortality from this disease. Patients presenting to surgery for debridement of devitalized tissues require aggressive monitoring, adequate fluid resuscitation, and careful anesthetic management.

## REFERENCES


1. Abraham E, Regan RF. The effects of hemorrhage and trauma on interleukin-2 production. Arch Surg 1985;120:1341.
2. Abraham E, Tanaka T, Chang YH. Effects of hemorrhagic serum on interleukin-2 generation and utilization. Crit Care Med 1988;16:307.
3. Allgöwer M, Durig M, Wolff G. Infection and trauma. Surg Clin North Am 1980;60:133.
4. Antrum RM, Solomkin JS. Monocyte dysfunction in severe trauma. Evidence for the role of C5a in deactivation. Surgery 1986;100:29.
5. Atherton ST, White DJ. Stomach as source of bacteria colonizing respiratory tract during artificial ventilation. Lancet 1978;2:968.
6. Bagratuni L. Cephalic tetanus: with report of a case. Br Med J 1952;1:461.
7. Baker CC, Oppenheimer L, Stephens B, et al. Epidemiology of trauma deaths. Am J Surg 1980;140:144.
8. Baltz ML, deBeer FC, Feinstein EA, et al. Phylogenetic aspects of C-reactive protein and related proteins. Ann NY Acad Sci 1982;389:49.
9. Band JD, Maki DG. Infections caused by arterial catheters used for hemodynamic monitoring. Am J Med 1979;67:735.
10. Band JD, Maki DG. Safety of changing intravenous delivery systems at longer than 24-hour intervals. Ann Intern Med 1979;91:173.
11. Bauer AR, McNeil C, Trentelman E, et al. The depression of T lymphocytes after trauma. Am J Surg 1978;136:674.
12. Baum LL, James KK, Glouiano RR, et al. Possible role for C-reactive protein in the human natural killer cell response. J Exp Med 1983;157:301.
13. Berger R, Arango L. Etiologic diagnosis of bacterial nosocomial pneumonia in seriously ill patients. Crit Care Med 1985;13:833.
14. Birch AA, Mitchell GD, Playford GA, et al. Changes in serum potassium response to succinylcholine following trauma. JAMA 1969;210:490.
15. Bruce DL. Effect of halothane anesthesia on extravascular mobilization of neutrophils. J Cell Physiol 1966;68:81.
16. Bruce DL. Effect of halothane on experimental salmonella peritonitis in mice. J Surg Res 1967;7:180.
17. Butler JA, Huang J, Wilson SE. Repeated laparotomy for postoperative intraabdominal sepsis: an analysis of outcome predictors. Arch Surg 1987;122:702.
18. Caplan ES, Hoyt NJ. Identification and treatment of infections in multiply traumatized patients. Am J Med 1985;79(supp):68.
19. Caplan ES, Hoyt N, Cowley RA. Changing patterns of nosocomial infections in severely traumatized patients. Am Surg 1979;45:204.
20. Cerda JJO, Ortiz JMP, Acosta JR. Dentroleno sodico en el tetenos informe de un caso. Rev Invest Clin (Mex) 1981;33:53.
21. Chastre J, Viau F, Brun P, et al. Prospective evaluation of the protected specimen brush for the diagnosis of pulmonary infections in ventilated patients. Am Rev Respir Dis 1984;130:924.
22. Christou NV, Meakins JL. Neutorphil function in anergic surgical patients: Neutrophil adherence and chemotaxis. Ann Surg 1979;190:557.
23. Christou NV, McLean APH, Meakins JL. Host defense in blunt

trauma: interrelationships of kinetics of anergy and depressed neutrophil function, nutritional status, and sepsis. J Trauma 1980;20:833.
24. Cleri DG, Corrado ML, Seligman SJ. Quantitative culture of intravenous catheters and other intravascular inserts. J Infect Dis 1980;141:781.
25. Cooper GL, Hopkins CC. Rapid diagnosis of intravascular catheter-associated infection by direct gram staining of catheter segments. N Engl J Med 1985;312:1142.
26. Defore WW, Mattox KL, Jordan GL, et al. Management of 1,590 consecutive cases of liver trauma. Arch Surg 1976;111:493.
27. Deitch E, Winterton J, Li M, et al. The gut as a portal of entry for bacteremia. Ann Surg 1987;205:681.
28. Dellinger EP, Oreskovich MR, Wertz MJ, et al. Risk of infection following laparotomy for penetrating abdominal injury. Arch Surg 1984;119:20.
29. De Michele DJ, Da Silva T. Cardiovascular findings in a patient with severe tetanus. Crit Care Med 1983;11:828.
30. De Simone C, Delogu G, Corbetta G. Intravenous immunoglobulins in association with antibiotics: a therapeutic trial in septic intensive care unit patients. Crit Care Med 1988;16:23.
31. Dickerman JD. Traumatic asplenia in adults: a defined hazard? Arch Surg 1981;116:361.
32. Downey EC, Shackford SR, Fridlung PH, et al. Long-term depressed immune function in patients splenectomized for trauma. J Trauma 1987;27:661.
33. Driver T, Kelly GL, Biseman B. Reoperation after abdominal trauma. Am J Surg 1978;135:747.
34. Du Moulin GC, Headley-White J, Paterson DG, et al. Aspiration of gastric bacteria in antacid treated patients: a frequent cause of postoperative colonization of the airway. Lancet 1982;1:242.
35. Dunn DL. Vaccines and antibody immunotherapy in surgical patients. Am J Surg 1987;153:409.
36. DuPriest R, Khaneja SC, Cowley RA. Acute cholecystitis complicating trauma. Ann Surg 1979;189:84.
37. Edmondson RS. Tetanus. Br J Hosp Med 1980;25:590.
38. Faist E, Kupper TS, Baker CC, et al. Depression of cellular immunity after major injury: its association with posttraumatic complications and its reversal with immunomodulation. Arch Surg 1986;121:1000.
39. Faist E, Mewes, Baker CC, et al. Prostaglandin $E_2$ ($PGE_2$)-dependent suppression of interleukin-2 (IL-2) production in patients with major trauma. J Trauma 1987;27:837.
40. Faust RA, Vickers OR, Cohn I. Tetanus: 2,449 cases in 68 years at Charity Hospital. J Trauma 1976;16:704.
41. Flowers MW, Edmondson RS. Long-term recovery from tetanus: a study of 50 survivors. Br Med J 1980;2:303.
42. Fox MS, Wilk PJ, Weissman HS, et al. Acute acalculous cholecystitis. Surg Gynec Obstet 1984;159:13.
43. Fry DE. Infection in the trauma patient: the major deterrent to good recovery. Heart Lung 1978;7:257.
44. Fullen WD, Hunt J, Altemeier WA. Prophylactic antibiotics in penetrating wounds of the abdomen. J Trauma 1972;12:282.
45. Furste W. The fifth international conference on tetanus. Ronneby Sweden 1978. J Trauma 1980;20:101.
46. Gardner RM, Schwartz R, Wong HC, et al. Percutaneous indwelling radial artery catheter for monitoring cardiovascular function. N Engl J Med 1974;290:1227.
47. Gentry LO, Feliciano DV, Lea AS, et al. Perioperative antibiotic therapy for penetrating injuries of the abdomen. Ann Surg 1984;200:561.
48. Gibson DM, Feliciano DV, Mattox KL, et al. Intraabdominal abscess after penetrating abdominal trauma. Am J Surg 1981;142:699.
49. Glinz W, Grob PJ, Nydegger VE, et al. Polyvalent immunoglobulins for prophylaxis of bacterial infections in patients following multiple trauma: a randomized, placebo-controlled study. Intens Care Med 1985;11:288.
50. Goester C, Ferrard G, Klumpp T, et al. Interet de la determination de la proteine C reactive en traumatologic cranienne. Clin Chim Acta 1981;117:43.
51. Green JB, Shackford SR, Sise MJ, et al. Late septic complications in adults following splenectomy for trauma: a prospective analysis in 144 patients. J Trauma 1986;26:999.
52. Grindlinger GA, Niehoff J, Hughes L, et al. Acute paranasal sinusitis related to nasotracheal intubation of head-injured patients. Crit Care Med 1987;15:214.
53. Guckien JC, Christensen WD. Quantitative culture and gram stain of sputum in pneumonia. Am Rev Respir Dis 1978;118:997.
54. Hart GB, Lamb RC, Strauss MB. Gas gangrene: a collective review. J Trauma 1983;23:991.
55. Haselby KA. Infectious diseases. In: Stoelting RK, Dierdorf SF, eds. Anesthesia and co-existing diseases. New York: Churchill Livingstone, 1983:605.
56. Heideman M, Saravis C, Clowes GHA. Effect of nonviable tissue and abscesses on complement depletion and the development of bacteremia. J Trauma 1982;22:527.
57. Heseltine PNR, Berne TV, Yellin AE, et al. The efficacy of cefoxitin vs clindamycin/gentamicin in surgically treated stab wounds of the bowel. J Trauma 1986;26:241.
58. Hitchcock CR, Haglin JJ, Arnar O. Treatment of clostridial infections with hyperbaric oxygen. Surgery 1967;62:759.
59. Hitchcock CR, Demello FJ, Haglin JJ. Gangrene infection: new approaches to an old disease. Surg Clin North Am 1975;55:1403.
60. Hofstetter SR, Pachter ML, Bailey AA, et al. A prospective comparison of two regimens of prophylactic antibiotics in abdominal trauma: cefoxitin versus triple drug. J Trauma 1984;24:307.
61. Hurlimann J, Thorbecke GJ, Hochwald GM. The liver as the site of C-reactive protein formation. J Exp Med 1966; 123:365.
62. Huxley EJ, Viroslav J, Gray WR, et al. Pharyngeal aspiration in normal adults and patients with depressed consciousness. Am J Med 1978;64:564.
63. Jagoda A, Riggio S, Burguieres T. Cephalic tetanus: a case report and review of the literature. Am J Emerg Med 1988;6:128.
64. James MFM, Manson T. The use of magnesium sulphate infusions in the management of very severe tetanus. Intens Care Med 1985;11:5.
65. Johanson WG, Pierce AK, Sanford JR, et al. Nosocomial respiratory infections with gram-negative bacilli. Ann Intern Med 1972;77:701.
66. Johnson LB. The importance of early diagnosis of acute acalculous cholecystitis. Surg Gynec Obstet 1987;164:197.
67. Jones RC, Thal BR, Johnson NA, et al. Evaluation of antibiotic therapy following penetrating abdominal trauma. Ann Surg 1985;201:576.
68. Keane RM, Birmingham W, Shatney CM, et al. Prediction of sepsis in the multitraumatic patient by assays of lymphocyte responsiveness. Surg Gynec Obstet 1983;156:163.
69. Klainer AS, Turndorf H, Wu WH, et al. Surface alterations due to endotracheal intubation. Am J Med 1975;58:674.
70. Kohlschutter B, Baur H, Roth F. Suxamethanium induced hyperkalemia in patients with severe intraabdominal infections. Br J Anaesth 1976;48:557.
71. Koziol J, Rush B, Smith S, et al. Occurrence of bacteremia during and after hemorrhagic shock. J Trauma 1988;28:10.
72. Laflin MJ, Tobey RE, Reves JL. Anesthetic considerations in patients with gas gangrene. Anesth Analg 1976;55:247.

73. Landa JF, Kwoka MA, Chapman GA, et al. Effects of suctioning on mucociliary transport. Chest 1980;77:202.
74. Lanser ME, Saba TM. Opsonic fibronectin deficiency and sepsis: cause or effect. Ann Surg 1982;195:340.
75. Lanser ME, Brown GE, Mora R, et al. Trauma serum suppresses superoxide production by normal neutrophils. Arch Surg 1986;121:157.
76. Leiboff AR, Soroff HS. The treatment of generalized peritonitis by closed postoperative peritoneal lavage: a critical review of the literature. Arch Surg 1987;122:1005.
77. Leonard AS, Giebink S, Baesl TJ, et al. The overwhelming postsplenectomy sepsis problem. World J Surg 1980;4:423.
78. Levy EM, McIntosh T, Black PH. Evaluation of circulating β-endorphin levels with concomitant depression of immune parameters after traumatic injury. J Trauma 1986;26:246.
79. MacLean LD, Meakins JL, Taquchi K, et al. Host resistance in sepsis and trauma. Ann Surg 1975;182:207.
80. Maderazo EG, Albano SD, Woronick CL, et al. Polymorphonuclear leukocyte migration abnormalities and their significance in seriously traumatized patients. Ann Surg 1983; 199:736.
81. Maki DG. Nosocomial bacteremia. An epidemiological overview. Am J Med 1981;70:719.
82. Maki DG, Hassemer CA. Endemic rate of fluid contamination and related septicemia in arterial pressure monitors. Am J Med 1981;70:733.
83. Maki DG, Goldman DA, Rhame FS. Infection control in intravenous therapy. Ann Intern Med 1973;79:867.
84. Maki DG, Weise CE, Sarafin HW. A semiquantitative culture method for identifying intravenous-catheter related infection. N Engl J Med 1977;296:1305.
85. Malongoni MA, Dillon LD, Klamer TW, et al. Factors influencing the risk of early and late serious infection in adults after splenectomy for trauma. Surgery 1984;96:775.
86. Merriman CR, Pulliam LA, Kampschmidt RF. The effect of leukocytic endogenous mediator on C-reactive protein in rabbits. Proc Soc Exp Biol Med 1985;149:782.
87. Millard AH. Local tetanus. Lancet 1954;2:844.
88. Miller RD, Rupp SM, Fisher DM, et al. Clinical pharmacology of vecuronium and atracurium. Anesthesiology 1984;61:444.
89. Mogensen VJ, Frederiksen W, Jensen KJ. Subclavian vein catheterization and infection. Scand J Infect Dis 1972;4:31.
90. Moore FA, Moore EE, Mill MR. Preoperative antibiotics for abdominal gunshot wounds. Am J Surg 1983;146:762.
91. Mosca R, Curtas S, Forbes B, et al. The benefits of isolated cultures in the management of suspected catheter sepsis. Surgery 1987;102:718.
92. Müller H, Börner U, Zierski J, et al. Intrathecal baclofen for treatment of tetanus-induced spasticity. Anesthesiology 1987;66:76.
93. Mustard RA, Bohnen JM, Haseeb S, et al. C-reactive protein levels predict postoperative septic complications. Arch Surg 1987;122:69.
94. Nakagawara M, Takeshige K, Takamatsu J, et al. Inhibition of superoxide production and $Ca^{2+}$ mobilization in human neutrophils by halothane, enflurane, and isoflurane. Anesthesiology 1986;64:4.
95. Narkates AJ, Volenekis JE. C-reactive protein binding specificities: artificial and natural phospholipid bilayers. Ann NY Acad Sci 1982;389:172.
96. Neidhardt JH, Kraft FX, Morin A, et al. Actualite persistante de la gangrene gazeuse. Lyon Chirurgicale 1979;75:281.
97. Nelson LD, Martinez OV, Anderson HB. Incidence of microbial colonization in open versus closed delivery systems for thermodilution injectate. Crit Care Med 1986;14:291.
98. Nelson RM, Benitez PR, Newell MA, et al. Single-antibiotic use for penetrating abdominal trauma. Arch Surg 1986;121:153.
99. Nichols RL, Smith JW. Gas in the wound: what does it mean? Surg Clin North Am 1975;55:1289.
100. O'Gorman RB, Feliciano DV, Matthews KS, et al. Correlation of immunologic and nutritional status with infectious complications after major abdominal trauma. Surgery 1986;99:549.
101. O'Neal BJ, McDonald JC. The risk of sepsis in the asplenic adult. Ann Surg 1981;194:775.
102. Pearson HA, Johnston D, Smith KA, et al. The born-again spleen: return of splenic function after splenectomy for trauma. N Engl J Med 1978;298:1389.
103. Pemberton LB, Lyman B, Lander V, et al. Sepsis from triple- vs single-lumen catheters during total parenteral nutrition. Arch Surg 1986;121:591.
104. Pinilla JC, Ross DF, Martin T, et al. Study of the incidence of intravascular catheter infection and associated septicemia in critically ill patients. Crit Care Med 1983;11:21.
105. Polk HC. The enhancement of host defenses against infection—search for the holy grail? Surgery 1986;99:1.
106. Polk HC, George CD, Wellhausen SR, et al. A systematic study of host defense processes in badly injured patients. Ann Surg 1986;204:282.
107. Polk HC, George CD, Hershman M, et al. The capacity of serum to support neutrophil phagocytosis is a vital host defense mechanism in severely injured patients. Ann Surg 1988;207:686.
108. Ponce DeLeon S, Critchley S, Wenzel RP. Polymicrobial bloodstream infections related to prolonged vascular catheterization. Crit Care Med 1984;12:856.
109. Posner MC, Moore EE, Harris LA, et al. Presumptive antibiotics for penetrating abdominal wounds. Surg Gynec Obstet 1987;165:29.
110. Poulton TJ, Haldeman LW, Munson ES. Nitrous oxide administration in the presence of subcutaneous emphysema: an experimental model. Can Anaesth Soc J 1982;29:435.
111. Quintero ML, Ansuategui M, Mederos DL, et al. Epidural anesthesia for sympathetic overactivity in severe tetanus. Crit Care Med 1987;15:801.
112. Rice J, Williams HC, Flint LM, et al. Post-traumatic acalculous cholecystitis. South Med J 1980;73:14.
113. Rowlands BJ, Ericsson CD, Fischer RP. Penetrating abdominal trauma: the use of operative findings to determine length of antibiotic therapy. J Trauma 1987;27:250.
114. Ruiz-Santana S, Jimenez AG, Esteban A, et al. ICU pneumonias. A multi-institutional study. Crit Care Med 1987;15:930.
115. Rush BF, Sori AJ, Murphy TF, et al. Endotoxemia and bacteremia during hemorrhagic shock: the link between trauma and sepsis. Ann Surg 1988;207:549.
116. Saba TM, Blumenstock FA, Scovill WA, et al. Cryoprecipitate reversal of opsonic alpha-2-surface binding glycoprotein deficiency in septic surgical and trauma patients. Science 1978;201:622.
117. Sackner MA, Hirsch J, Epstein S. Effect of cuffed endotracheal tubes on tracheal mucous velocity. Chest 1975;68:774.
118. Sackner MA, Landa J, Hirsch J, et al. Pulmonary effects of oxygen breathing: a 6-hour study in normal men. Ann Intern Med 1975;82:40.
119. Samsoondar W, Freeman JB. Colonization of intravascular monitoring devices. Crit Care Med 1985;13:753.
120. Savino JA, Scalea TM, Del Guercio LRM. Factors encouraging laparotomy in acalculous cholecystitis. Crit Care Med 1985;13:377.
121. Schentag JJ, O'Keeffe D, Marmion M, et al. C-reactive protein as an indicator of infection relapse in patients with abdominal sepsis. Arch Surg 1984;119:300.

122. Schimpff SC, Miller RM, Polakavetz S, et al. Infection in the severely traumatized patient. Ann Surg 1974;179:352.
123. Scovill WA, Saba TM, Kaplin JE, et al. Disturbances in circulatory opsonic activity in man after operative and blunt trauma. J Surg Res 1977;22:709.
124. Seedat YK, Omar MAK, Seedat MA, et al. Renal failure in tetanus. Br Med J 1981;282:360.
124a. Shibuya M, Sugimoto H, Sugimoto T, et al. The use of continuous spinal anesthesia in severe tetanus with autonomic disturbance. J Trauma 1989;29:1423.
125. Simonsen O, Klaerke M, Jensen JE, et al. Revaccination against tetanus 17 to 20 years after primary vaccination: kinetics of antibody response. J Trauma 1987;27:1358.
126. Sitges-Serra A, Puig P, Juarrieta E, et al. Catheter sepsis due to staphylococcus epidermidis during parenteral nutrition. Surg Gynecol Obstet 1980;151:481.
127. Sori A, Rush B, Lysz T, et al. The gut as a source of sepsis following hemorrhagic shock. Am J Surg 1988;155:187.
128. Spray SB, Zuidema GD, Cameron JL. Aspiration pneumonia: incidence of aspiration with endotracheal tubes. Am J Surg 1976;131:701.
129. Stahl W, Sing A, Marcus M. Responses of opsonic substances to major trauma and sepsis. Crit Care Med 1985;13:779.
130. Stanley TH, Hill GE, Portes MR, et al. Neutrophil chemotaxis during and after general anesthesia and operation. Anesth Analg 1976;55:668.
131. Stone JJ, Hester TR. Incisional and peritoneal infection after emergency celiotomy. Ann Surg 1973;177:669.
132. Stoutenbeek CP, Van Saene HK, Miranda DR, et al. The effect of oropharyngeal decontamination using topical nonabsorbable antibiotics on the incidence of nosocomial respiratory tract infections in multiple trauma patients. J Trauma 1987;27:357.
133. Sun S, Dolar D, Ozenc E. Intrathecal morphine in tetanus. Br J Anaesth 1982;54:699.
134. Teichmann W, Wittmann DH, Andreone PA. Scheduled reoperations (Etappenlavage) for diffuse peritonitis. Arch Surg 1986;121:147.
135. Thomas F, Burke JP, Parker J, et al. The risk of infection related to radial vs femoral sites for arterial catheterization. Crit Care Med 1983;11:807.
136. Thomas F, Orme JF, Clemmer TP, et al. A prospective comparison of arterial catheter blood and catheter-tip cultures in critically ill patients. Crit Care Med 1984;12:860.
137. Tidyman M, Prichard JG, Deamer RL, et al. Adjunctive use of dantrolene in severe tetanus. Anesth Analg 1985;64:538.
138. Tobin MJ, Grenvik A. Nosocomial lung infection and its diagnosis. Crit Care Med 1984;12:191.
139. Trujillo MJ, Castillo A, Espana JV, et al. Tetanus in the adult: intensive care and management experience with 233 cases. Crit Care Med 1980;8:419.
140. Trujillo MH, Castillo A, Espana J. Impact of intensive care management on the prognosis of tetanus. Chest 1987;92:63.
141. Tsueda K, Oliver PB, Richter RW. Cardiovascular manifestations of tetanus. Anesthesiology 1974;40:588.
142. Volanakis JE. Complement activation by C-reactive protein complexes. Ann NY Acad Sci 1982;398:235.
143. Wagner DS, Flynn MA. Hemorrhagic acalculous cholecystitis causing acute pancreatitis after trauma. J Trauma 1985;25:253.
144. Weigelt JA, Haley RW, Seibert B. Factors which influence the risk of wound infection in trauma patients. J Trauma 1987;27:774.
145. Weinstein L. Tetanus. N Engl J Med 1973;289:1293.
146. Welch WD. Effect of enflurane, isoflurane and nitrous oxide on the microbicidal activity of human polymorphonuclear leukocytes. Anesthesiology 1984;61:188.
147. Welch WD. Inhibition of neutrophil cidal activity by volatile anesthetics. Anesthesiology 1986;64:1.
148. Welch WD, Zazzari J. Effect of halothane and $N_2O$ on the oxidative activity of human neutrophils. Anesthesiology 1982; 57:172.
149. Werry DG, Meek RN. Clostridial gas gangrene complicating Colles fracture. J Trauma 1986;26:280.

# Chapter Twenty-Seven

Brian Kaufman

# Management of Septic Shock

Bacteremia may develop in the postoperative period as a complication of any of the infections discussed in the preceding chapter. Although some patients may be asymptomatic, the majority demonstrate a systemic response to bacterial pathogens including fever or shaking chills. Approximately 25 to 44% of these patients develop tissue perfusion failure during sepsis.[74,89] Circulatory shock is usually defined as a state characterized by systemic hypotension in which global tissue perfusion and oxygen delivery fall short of metabolic demands. However, there are two problems with such a definition: metabolic imbalance may develop in patients with seemingly normal perfusion pressures, and systemic hypotension may occur without evidence of tissue hypoperfusion. Therefore, shock is better defined on the basis of metabolic indices, rather than absolute blood pressure or cardiac output values. When oxygen transport fails to meet tissue oxygen requirements, anaerobic metabolism develops. This results in increased lactic acid production and elevated blood lactate levels. Serial blood lactate determinations not only help define the severity of the metabolic imbalance in septic shock patients but also serve as a reliable prognostic index.[145,147,153]

In the majority of patients septic shock develops as a complication of infection with Gram-negative enteric bacilli. It has been estimated that up to 300,000 Gram-negative bacteremias occur in the United States each year.[106] McCabe and associates[90] identified Gram-negative bacilli as the responsible pathogens in 780 (81%) of 961 documented cases of bacteremia. *Staphylococcus aureus* was isolated in 58 instances (6%) and *Streptococcus pneumoniae* in 123 (13%). McCabe and coworkers[90] also noted that 42% of their patients with Gram-negative bacteremia had circulatory shock, whereas only 14% of those with *Streptococcus pneumoniae* and 29% of those with *Staphylococcus aureus* bacteremias developed this complication. The frequency of Gram-negative bacteremia and associated deaths has increased over the past 30 years despite the availability of more potent antibiotics and preventive measures.[73] Gram-positive organisms continue to account for a small but significant proportion of septic shock cases. Viruses, fungi, *Rickettsiae,* and protozoa have also been reported to produce the clinical picture of septic shock, but they are not major pathogens in the traumatized patient.

*Escherichia coli* (*E. coli*) continues to be the most frequently isolated pathogen. It is followed by the *Klebsiella-Enterobacter-Serratia* group and then by *Pseudomonas*.[73] The most common source of infection is the genitourinary tract, a result of complications of indwelling catheters in hospitalized patients.[73] Other sources of infection include the respiratory tract, surgical or traumatic wounds, and the gastrointestinal tract. In 10 to 20% of patients with septic shock no definite source of infection can be established.[61] Bacterial pathogens utilize specific portals of entry into the body. For example, in Kreger's series[73] almost 80% of infections due to *E. coli* originated from the genitourinary or gastrointestinal tract, whereas *Bacteroides* almost always gained entry from the gastrointestinal or female reproductive tract.

The trauma victim is predisposed to septicemia and shock, mainly because of immunocompromise induced by the injury (see chapter 26). Pre-existing medical conditions, such as cirrhosis, diabetes mellitus, and neoplastic disease (particularly after chemotherapy or irradiation), and chronic steroid intake also increase the risk of bacteremia. Even in the presence of bacteremia, persons under 40 years of age develop septic shock infrequently. In contrast, elderly patients, patients with congestive heart failure and azotemia, and those who are on immunosuppressive therapy are candidates for developing septic shock after bacteremia.[73] Two special groups of patients, pregnant women and neonates, are also at increased risk of septic shock. The staggering speed with which septic shock develops after septic abortion is well known.

Factors that adversely influence survival of patients with Gram-negative bacteremia include (a) the severity of the underlying disease, (b) the presence of shock, (c) inability to develop a febrile response, (d) the use of inappropriate antibiotics or delayed initiation of appropriate antibiotic therapy, (e) the presence of azotemia at the time of sepsis, and (f) the presence of *Pseudomonas* bacteremia. Shock markedly influences outcome. Kreger and associates[74] reported 7% mortality from Gram-negative bacteremia not complicated by shock compared to a 47% fatality rate when septic shock ensued.

## PATHOPHYSIOLOGY

Although Gram-negative and Gram-positive bacteria induce septic shock by different mechanisms, the clinical picture is the same regardless of the causative organism and the mechanisms involved.[161] Endotoxin is a lipopolysaccharide protein-lipid complex derived from the cell wall of Gram-negative bacteria. It has been suggested that endotoxin plays a major role in the development of septic shock and that the use of antiendotoxin antibodies in humans improves survival.[169] The toxicity of endotoxin is dependent upon the production of endogenous factors by the host.[11]

Endotoxin released from the cell walls of dead bacteria sets in motion a chain reaction that may culminate eventually in septic shock. The lipopolysaccharide portion of bacterial endotoxin plays a major role in the activation of both classic and alternative complement pathways (Fig 27-1). A significant amount of complement consumption occurs in patients with Gram-negative septic shock. McCabe[89] noted that C3 levels in patients with shock induced by Gram-negative bacteria were lower than in those who had bacteremia without shock. Leon and colleagues[80] demonstrated that shock without sepsis does not activate complement, whereas patients in septic shock caused by Gram-negative or Gram-positive bacteria had evidence of complement activation.

Endotoxin directly activates the Hageman factor (factor XII) and thus can initiate intravascular clotting. Activated Hageman factor can also enzymatically activate plasma prekallikrein to form kallikrein, a proteolytic enzyme that is capable in turn of producing bradykinin from plasma kininogen, and of activating plasminogen. Bradykinin, a potent vasodilator, may contribute to the low peripheral vascular resistance seen in many patients with septic shock.[123] Endotoxin also stimulates platelets to release vasoactive amines, such as histamine and serotonin, although the importance of this mechanism in humans is uncertain.

Activation of the endorphin system may also be responsible

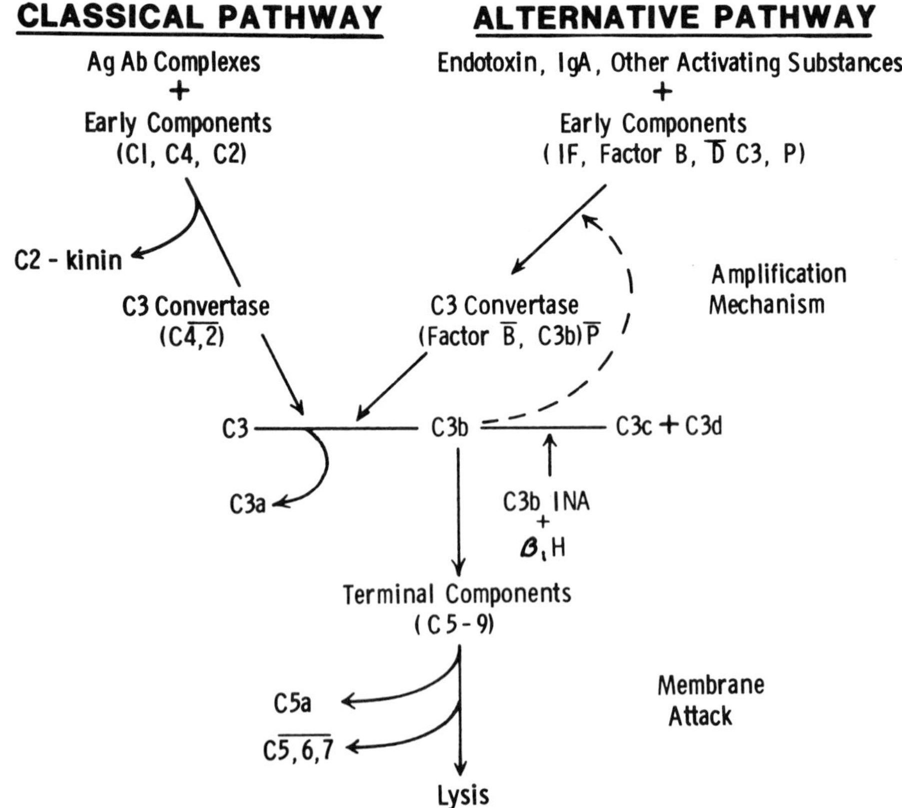


FIG. 27-1. Classical and alternative pathways of complement activation.

for some of the pathophysiologic changes seen in septic shock.[158] However, endorphin release may be a nonspecific stress response, rather than a direct effect of endotoxin. Certain patients with hyperdynamic septic shock demonstrate increased pulmonary vascular resistance despite systemic vasodilation. Prostaglandins may contribute to the development of this state, as the pulmonary vasculature is an important target organ of prostaglandin derivatives. Prostaglandins are derived from arachidonic acid. Endotoxin can activate both pathways of arachidonic acid metabolism (see Fig 24-7).[5] When the cyclo-oxygenase pathway is activated, potent vasoconstrictors, such as $PGF_{2\alpha}$ and thromboxane $A_2$ (TBX), and such vasodilators as prostacyclin are formed. Oettinger et al.[102] demonstrated higher levels of $PGF_{2\alpha}$ in arterial blood than in mixed venous blood of patients with hyperdynamic sepsis and respiratory failure, suggesting pulmonary production of this vasoconstrictor. Increased levels of $PGF_{2\alpha}$ in pulmonary veins of calves exposed to endotoxin parallelled closely the degree of pulmonary hypertension that developed, suggesting a cause-and-effect relationship.[3] Reines et al.[121] reported a tenfold elevation in plasma concentration of thromboxane $B_2$ (the stable metabolite of TBX) in nonsurvivors of sepsis compared to survivors. Plasma concentrations of 6-keto-prostaglandin $F_{1\alpha}$, the stable hydrolysis product of prostacyclin, increase in patients with septic shock.[50] The highest levels have been found in nonsurvivors. It is uncertain at present whether TBX, $PGF_{2\alpha}$, prostacyclin, or other prostanoids contribute directly to the pathogenesis and progression of the sepsis syndrome or represent markers of the severity of cardiopulmonary dysfunction.

There has been much recent interest regarding the role of cachectin (tumor necrosis factor) in the pathogenesis of the sepsis syndrome.[11,12] Cachectin is a polypeptide hormone elaborated by macrophages under a variety of circumstances, including exposure to endotoxin. When cachectin was infused into rats in quantities similar to those produced endogenously in response to endotoxin, physiologic changes occurred that essentially duplicated the effects of endotoxin administration.[12] Mice could be protected from the lethal effects of endotoxin by passive immunization with an antiserum against cachectin.[12] Cachectin may be a proximal mediator of endotoxin effects acting to initiate the sequence of events that result in tissue injury and shock. Corticosteroids administered before macrophage activation inhibit cachectin synthesis completely both by diminishing the quantity of cachectin messenger RNA produced in response to endotoxin and by preventing its translation. However, once macrophages are activated by endotoxin, corticosteroids have no inhibitory effect.[11] This finding may help explain why animal experiments demonstrate beneficial effects of steroids when they are infused before or at the time of bacterial challenge, whereas recent clinical trials have not demonstrated any benefits from steroids given to patients with established sepsis.[14,57]

The initial hemodynamic change in sepsis appears to be mediator-induced peripheral vasodilation (Fig 27-2).[133] Decreased peripheral resistance results in decreased afterload and increased stroke volume and cardiac output. Tachycardia, which is often noted in the septic patient, also causes augmentation of cardiac output. Increased heart rate is caused by fever and increased catecholamine secretion. In this compensated state, which is seen early in the course of a severe septic episode, patients are able to augment their cardiac output in response to the vasodilation. These patients are often febrile and have warm dry skin secondary to cutaneous vasodilation. The increased cardiac output is usually accompanied by widened pulse pressure. Hyperventilation with moderate respiratory alkalosis may also be observed.

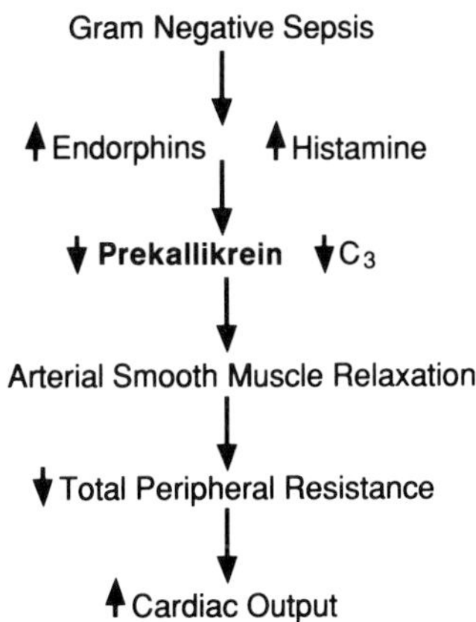


FIG. 27-2. Sequence of events in hyperdynamic septic shock.

With progression of the syndrome, a point is reached where cardiac output is no longer able to compensate for decreased vascular resistance and the systemic blood pressure begins to decline.[166] Peripheral venous pooling and decreased venous return may contribute further to the development of hypotension. This is the so-called warm hyperdynamic phase of septic shock. Circulatory shock is usually recognized by the onset of systemic hypotension, although it can be diagnosed before the development of this sign. Total body oxygen consumption and arterial lactate levels rise early in septic shock. In addition, a narrowed arterial-mixed venous oxygen content difference (a-$vcO_2$) may be observed. These measurements may be used to diagnose shock early when it is treatable. The reduced a-$vcO_2$ may be produced by one or more of the following mechanisms: (a) opening of peripheral arteriovenous shunts, (b) peripheral maldistribution of blood flow, or (c) endotoxin-mediated block of mitochondrial oxygen uptake.[36,41,133,168]

There is little experimental evidence to suggest that in septic shock anatomic shunting occurs through peripheral arteriovenous connections. However, there may be peripheral maldistribution of blood flow such that certain tissues receive blood flow in excess of their metabolic requirements, whereas others receive an inadequate blood supply. Venous blood returning from areas with excessive blood flow tends to have a high oxygen saturation, which may mask the evidence of tissue hypoperfusion in other regions. A normal or even elevated mixed venous oxygen saturation ($S\bar{v}O_2$) thus cannot exclude regional hypoperfusion.

The hypothesis that endotoxin interferes directly with cellular metabolism has not been disproven, but several animal studies have demonstrated normal mitochondrial oxygen utilization during endotoxemia.[62] Clinical studies in patients with fatal septic shock have demonstrated that $\dot{V}O_2$ is main-

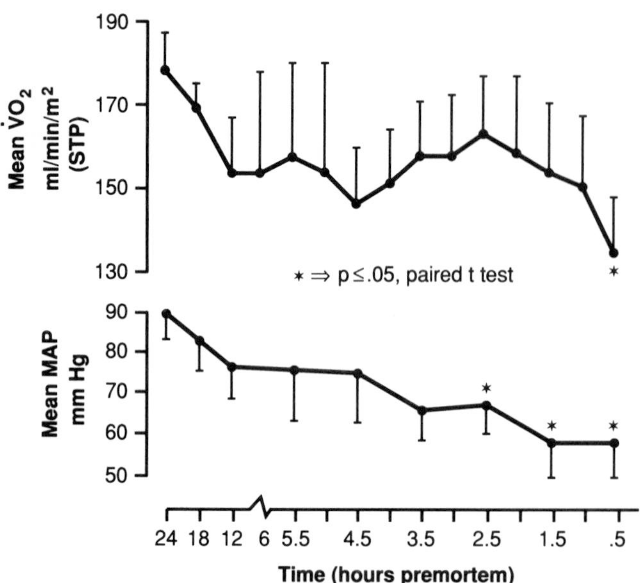


FIG. 27-3. Oxygen consumption ($\dot{V}O_2$) and mean arterial blood pressure in patients with preterminal septic shock. Note that $\dot{V}O_2$ is maintained until 1–1.5 hours before death. (From Houtchens et al[62] with permission.)

tained at above normal levels until a few hours before death (Fig 27-3).[157] The $\dot{V}O_2$ declines only when cardiac output and oxygen delivery decrease. If the hemodynamic deterioration responds to volume resuscitation, $\dot{V}O_2$ is also likely to improve.[52,62] If therapeutic interventions fail to improve cardiac output and oxygen transport, death is likely. A sustained increase in $\dot{V}O_2$ may be an index of the adequacy of therapy, although the optimal value of this parameter in any given patient at a particular stage of the disease is not known.[1,2,62] Thus, measurement of the arterial lactate concentration may provide more useful information than $\dot{V}O_2$ in evaluating the adequacy of resuscitation.[52] Generally, a normal or elevated $S\bar{v}O_2$ in a patient with shock is considered to be caused by sepsis until proven otherwise. In these instances an accumulating oxygen debt causes a moderate elevation in the arterial lactate level.

The sequential hemodynamic and metabolic changes during progression from compensated sepsis to the hyperdynamic phase of septic shock have been described by Abraham and co-workers.[1,2] The hemodynamic pattern during the 24 hours before the hypotensive crisis consists of a high cardiac index, low systemic vascular resistance, and near-normal arterial pressure. During the hypotensive crisis, the mean arterial pressure becomes severely depressed due to a further decrease in systemic vascular resistance and, more importantly, a decrease in cardiac index. Thus, a relative decrease in cardiac output plays a key role in the genesis of shock in patients with severe infections. Many studies have shown that the elevated cardiac index observed during the early phase of septic shock is maintained during the later stages only in survivors. In nonsurvivors cardiac output falls progressively so that just before death low cardiac output and high systemic vascular resistance are usually noted.[85,86,96,100,157,162,163,166] Recently, several authors have demonstrated that nonsurvivors of septic shock frequently maintain an elevated cardiac output to within 24 hours of death.[49,109] Initial hemodynamic measurements were similar in survivors and nonsurvivors in one series,[109] but 24 hours later, survivors had normalized their cardiac output and had a significant decrease in heart rate and a significant increase in systemic vascular resistance compared to nonsurvivors. The patients in this study were relatively young, and the majority were on high doses of catecholamines at the time of "baseline" measurements.

It is difficult to evaluate the hemodynamic features of septic shock because in most studies initial hemodynamic measurements are made after therapeutic interventions have been initiated. Different patient populations and therapeutic interventions may explain the contradictory hemodynamic findings in the above studies. Thus, the hyperdynamic state described in these studies could have been an artifact produced by therapeutic intervention, rather than a naturally occurring phenomenon. In fact, Carroll and Snyder,[20] in a primate model of septic shock, demonstrated that hemodynamic status was dependent upon intravenous fluid administration. When bacterial suspensions were administered without concomitant fluid infusion, the animals had a low cardiac output. The typical "high output state" developed during sepsis only after intravenous fluids were administered.

The author's group has noted that during early septic shock, when hemodynamic measurements are made before significant fluid resuscitation, the mean cardiac index is in the low normal range. Fluid administration during this stage caused the cardiac index to rise to the high normal range.[118] We have also found little evidence of enhanced myocardial contractility in early septic shock. The high cardiac index was produced only by tachycardia, and in fact, left ventricular stroke volume and stroke work index remained depressed even after intravenous volume loading.[118] Our findings are consistent with those of Abraham et al.[2] that hypovolemia appears to be a major contributor to the hypotensive crisis. Hypovolemia is caused by (a) translocation of fluid at the infection site, as observed in peritonitis (third space loss); (b) diffuse capillary exudation[38]; (c) polyuria inappropriate for the effective circulating fluid volume[119]; (d) increase in venous capacitance[85]; and (e) pre-existing blood volume deficit. Nasogastric drainage, blood loss, fever, vomiting, diarrhea, and the use of diuretics are additional factors that contribute to hypovolemia.

During the initial phase of septic shock, cardiac output and arterial lactate concentrations are dependent on plasma volume. In the presence of normal or increased plasma volume the cardiac output is maintained at normal or high levels. This hemodynamic picture is associated with a lower arterial lactate level and a more favorable clinical course.[96,100,151,154] When plasma volume is low, cardiac output decreases, resulting in elevated arterial lactate concentrations. This low flow state (cold shock) is usually associated with a fatal outcome.[75,143] It is characterized by cold and clammy skin, oliguria, arterial vasoconstriction, hypothermia, and a decrease in both pulse pressure and cardiac output. Perfusion failure is clearly evident in this phase of septic shock.

Rather than existing in two distinct stages, septic shock is a continuum. Younger patients may be hyperdynamic and severely vasodilated until shortly before death, whereas elderly patients may have a low cardiac output and vasoconstriction even in the early stages of septicemia. Some patients, however, progress from a hyperdynamic to a hypodynamic state. This transition is influenced by the following factors.

### POOLING OF BLOOD VOLUME

A substantial portion of the blood volume appears to be pooled in the venous capacitance bed, producing relative hypovolemia.[85] The decreased effective circulating volume stimulates increased catecholamine release, sympathetic tone, and peripheral resistance.

### MYOCARDIAL DEPRESSION

Myocardial depression develops early in the course of septic shock,[19,108,117,118] as evidenced by depressed left ventricular ejection fraction and by low left and right ventricular stroke work, despite adequate pulmonary artery wedge pressures and increased left ventricular end-diastolic volume. This depression may be reversible.[39,108,117,157] Parker and associates[108] utilized serial radionucleotide cineangiographic and hemodynamic studies to evaluate cardiac function in 20 patients with septic shock. Survivors demonstrated left ventricular dilation and depressed ejection fractions that were reversible over a period of 7 to 10 days. Dilation of the left ventricle enabled these patients to maintain normal stroke volume and high cardiac index, despite a profound loss of myocardial contractility. Nonsurvivors had normal initial ejection fractions and ventricular volumes, which did not change during serial evaluations. Myocardial depression may be caused by compromised coronary blood flow,[157] myocardial edema,[113] hypoxemia, acidosis, decreased ionized calcium levels,[21,167] circulating myocardial depressant factors,[81] or right ventricular failure.[70] Parillo and associates[106] demonstrated a myocardial depressant factor (MDF) in the serum of patients with septic shock, which appears to be the major etiologic agent in the development of myocardial depression. Myocardial depressant factor may be secreted by the ischemic pancreas during circulatory shock.[81] Cunnion and associates,[29] employing thermodilution coronary sinus catheters, demonstrated that coronary blood flow was not reduced and myocardial lactate extraction was unchanged in a group of patients with septic shock and myocardial depression. Therefore, it is unlikely that myocardial ischemia secondary to decreased coronary blood flow produces myocardial depression in most patients with septic shock.

There is no consensus of opinion regarding the usefulness of cardiac function determination as an outcome predictor in septic shock. Weisel and coworkers[157] noted that myocardial performance curves were better in surviving than in nonsurviving patients. Contrary to this finding, other investigators[105,107] found more profound myocardial depression in survivors than in nonsurvivors. Two-dimensional echocardiograms[104] or radionucleotide cineangiograms can be utilized to assess right and left ventricular function noninvasively at the bedside. Such techniques may provide more accurate data regarding myocardial function in septic shock than the pulmonary artery catheter.[130] Biventricular failure is often evident, and right ventricular failure may precede the development of left ventricular failure,[58,70] a result of increased pulmonary vascular resistance, a common occurrence in progressive septicemia.[132]

### ELEVATION OF PULMONARY VASCULAR RESISTANCE

Pulmonary vascular resistance is often elevated in both animal models and patients with septic shock.[99,132] This elevation is not related to metabolic acidosis or hypoxemia and is thought to result from active vascular constriction mediated by prostaglandins or serotonin released from platelets.[99,132] Ketanserin, a pure serotonin antagonist, prevents platelet aggregation and endotoxin-induced pulmonary vasoconstriction in animal models of sepsis. This agent may eventually have a role in the treatment of severe sepsis and septic shock. Although prostaglandins play a role in increasing pulmonary vascular resistance in animal models of sepsis, their importance as mediators of pulmonary vasoconstriction in human sepsis is uncertain. Thus, a clinical benefit of prostaglandin inhibitors for the therapy of septic shock has not been demonstrated.

Measurement of the pulmonary artery diastolic-pulmonary artery wedge pressure gradient (PAD-PAWP) can be useful for assessing the degree of pulmonary vasoconstriction. Sibbald and associates[132] have reported an 83% mortality in septic patients with an initial PAD-PAWP > 5 mm Hg. Marland and Glauser[88] found that the initial PAD-PAWP was less likely to predict outcome than were serial observations. An elevated gradient that remained stable or increased was associated with 91% mortality. When the initially elevated gradient subsequently returned to normal or when it remained low during the entire clinical course, mortality was only 16%.

## CLINICAL FEATURES

Septicemia is usually suspected when a patient develops shaking chills followed by pyrexia exceeding 38°C. Exotoxins released from Gram-positive bacteria can directly stimulate the hypothalamic thermoregulatory center. Endotoxin released by Gram-negative bacteria stimulates the release from leukocytes or macrophages of endogenous pyrogen (interleukin-1), which acts on the hypothalamus.

Septic shock should be suspected when hyperventilation, alteration in sensorium, and systemic hypotension are present. Hypotension may occur late, after other signs of tissue hypoperfusion are evident. Elderly patients are frequently afebrile or hypothermic rather than hyperthermic at the onset of shock.[47] Altered mental status or tachycardia may be the only symptom present.[59] The absence of a febrile response in Gram-negative septicemia is associated with a poor prognosis.[18] Although some patients may present with warm and dry skin and bounding pulses, the older chronically ill patient usually presents with cold and clammy skin due to reduced cutaneous blood flow caused by sympathetic hyperactivity. Most patients are oliguric or anuric, although an occasional patient may maintain normal urine output.

The most common laboratory abnormalities at the onset of shock include leukocytosis with a WBC count greater than 15,000/$mm^3$ or leukopenia with a WBC count less than 3,500/$mm^3$ with a shift to immature polymorphonuclear cells and thrombocytopenia with a platelet count less than 100,000/$mm^3$. Thrombocytopenia has been reported in 18 to 77% of patients in septic shock.[68,112] Most patients have no laboratory evidence of disseminated intravascular coagulation. The mechanism of the thrombocytopenia appears to be related to the presence of IgG antiplatelet antibodies.[68] It should be emphasized, however, that in acute trauma victims and in operated patients, entirely different hematologic values may be observed. Hyperventilation, which is often present initially, results in respiratory alkalosis, followed by secondary metabolic acidosis. Hyperventilation is caused by direct stimulation of the central nervous system by endotoxin. The blood glucose level is frequently increased due to increased blood levels of glucagon, growth hormone, and catecholamines, which are secreted in response to stress. Hypoglycemia is infrequently seen and suggests a poor prognosis. The arterial lactate level is invariably increased in septic shock because of the diminished tissue oxygen supply in relation to demand. A marked increase in lactate level is usually associated with a fatal outcome.[147,166]

The greater the number of these abnormal clinical and biochemical findings, the greater the likelihood that the patient is in septic shock. When the syndrome is suspected, bacterial cultures should be obtained from blood, urine, tracheal secretions, and other potential sites of infection. Blood cultures are negative in up to 50% of patients in septic shock,[78] since the syndrome may at times be caused by endotoxin released from nonviable bacteria or by vasoactive substances formed in the interaction between bacterial products and white blood cells or platelets. A total and differential WBC and a chest X-ray should be obtained routinely from all patients. The common sites of infection include the chest, urine, abdomen, wounds, and hematomas. When no obvious infective focus can be found, less common sources of infection, such as an indwelling catheter, acalculous cholecystitis, sinusitis, prostatitis, osteomyelitis, and meningitis, should be considered.

Intravascular catheters are important sources of nosocomial sepsis. If catheter sepsis is suspected, the subcutaneous portion and tip of the catheter should be cultured by the semiquantitative solid culture technique described by Maki et al.[87] Culture results, however, will not be available for at least 24 hours. Techniques for making a more rapid diagnosis of catheter-related sepsis have recently been described.[26,27] Cooper et al.[27] directly Gram-stained catheter segments and found that observation of bacteria on the catheter examined under an oil immersion lens correlated with the presence of catheter-related infection. Collignon et al.[26] made impression smears of catheters on a glass slide. The presence of organisms on a subsequent Gram stain of the smear correlated with culture results and the presence of catheter-related bacteremia.

When the patient is hemodynamically stable, further diagnostic studies can be obtained. Sonography of the abdomen followed by a computed tomography scan of any suspicious area may be useful. Occasionally, an exploratory laparotomy may have to be performed to rule out an intra-abdominal infection when persistent evidence of sepsis exists without a diagnosed site of origin.

## COMPLICATIONS OF SEPTIC SHOCK

Despite the fact that reported data suggest a high mortality rate, only a minority of deaths are directly caused by intractable septic shock. In a study by Rackow et al.[116] 17 of 18 patients with severe septic shock could be resuscitated initially, yet only 7 survived. Patients frequently die from one or more complications of sepsis or septic shock. The most devastating of these is multisystem organ failure.

The organs that usually fail are the lungs (falling $PaO_2$ and compliance and increasing intrapulmonary shunt), kidneys (falling creatinine clearance), liver (rising bilirubin and alkaline phosphatase), gastrointestinal tract (stress ulcer bleeding and ileus), heart (biventricular dysfunction), central nervous system (confusion), and vascular system (fluid sequestration into the tissues). Almost every organ is equally at risk for failure during or after an episode of severe sepsis or septic shock. Multiple organ involvement is more common than failure of a single organ.

The onset of organ failure may be precipitous or insidious, and the sequence in which various organs fail is not predictable. However, in the series reported by Fry and associates,[46] the mean time of onset after surgery was 2.3 days for respiratory failure, 5.7 days for liver failure, 9.9 days for stress-induced gastrointestinal bleeding, and 11.6 days for renal failure. They also showed that the mortality rate was 30% when a single organ failed, but this rate increased to 100% with the failure of four or more organ systems.[46]

Although multisystem organ failure can occur postoperatively in the absence of infection, it is now clearly recognized that infection is the most important etiologic factor in the evolution of this complication. In the study of Fry et al.,[46] 90% of the patients who developed multisystem organ failure had sepsis, whereas in a study reported by Faist and colleagues,[40] sepsis could be documented in 56% of injured patients. Almost all the patients in Faist's study had sustained blunt trauma, whereas in Fry's study penetrating trauma had occurred more frequently. In the absence of infection, multisystem organ failure is likely to develop within 24–72 hours of injury and is usually associated with an episode of hemorrhagic shock.

The severely septic patient demonstrates characteristic abnormalities in metabolic substrate utilization.[93] Hyperglycemia resulting from glycogenolysis, gluconeogenesis, and insulin resistance is a prominent finding in early septic shock. Lipolysis is stimulated in adipose tissue by increased catecholamine and glucagon levels. However, the free fatty acids thus formed are not well utilized because of defective transport across the mitochondrial membrane.[13] Increased free fatty acids inhibit pyruvate dehydrogenase, blocking entry of pyruvate into the Krebs cycle and increasing lactic acid formation. Accelerated muscle proteolysis ("autocannibalism") develops, with utilization of branched chain amino acids as an energy source by skeletal muscle.[22] Cachectin and interleukin-1, both of which are macrophage-derived peptides, may mediate proteolysis by inducing the synthesis of prostaglandin $E_2$, which in turn activates various lysosomal hydrolases.[6] These abnormalities result in ineffective energy production, increased protein destruction, and decreased protein synthesis, all of which may play a role in the development of multiple organ failure.[15] Current research is evaluating the utility of various types of nutritional formulations in correcting the metabolic defects of sepsis.

The development of multisystem organ failure may be the first clue to the presence of an otherwise occult intra-abdominal infection in the trauma victim. Because the mortality rate of undrained intra-abdominal abscess approaches 100%, unexplained multisystem organ failure in a trauma victim should alert the physician to the possibility of intra-abdominal abscess, and necessary therapeutic measures should be initiated immediately.[55] Polk and Shields[111] have estimated that exploratory laparotomy will detect intra-abdominal infections in 50% of patients with organ failure and no obvious site of infection. The natural history of multiple organ failure is so dismal without intervention that it is a valid indication for abdominal exploration even in the absence of findings on physical examination, CT scan, ultrasound, etc., if no other source of sepsis is found.[55] Since the mortality rate of urgent reoperation in this setting is between 29 and 82%,[16,55,111] up to 70% of patients who otherwise face an almost certain death may be saved.

Which organs are susceptible to damage in septic shock? The lungs are most vulnerable, and the injury usually presents as adult respiratory distress syndrome (ARDS). Although sepsis without shock can lead to ARDS,[148] this is not usually the case. Acute renal failure often occurs due to renal hypoperfusion in the low output stage of shock and/or to nephrotoxicity caused by aminoglycoside antibiotics if the patient receives them. The development of renal failure complicates the management of fluid and electrolyte balance in the critically ill trauma patient. The diagnosis and treatment of acute renal failure are discussed in Chapter 25. Cholestatic jaundice with elevation of serum bilirubin and alkaline phosphatase is the most common manifestation of hepatic failure. It is essential that an obstructive etiology of the jaundice be excluded by appropriate radiologic testing. Cholestatic jaundice will usually resolve if sepsis is treated adequately. Occasionally, if sepsis is overwhelming, the liver loses its gluconeogenetic ability, resulting in severe hypoglycemia. This condition indicates a poor prognosis and is usually a preterminal event. Gastrointestinal bleeding due to stress is another major complication of septic shock. The incidence of this complication appears to be decreasing due to the widespread use of measures to increase gastric fluid pH. Pseudomembranous colitis and acalculous cholecystitis may occur as a result of septic shock or its therapy with antibiotics.

## TREATMENT OF SEPTIC SHOCK

No clinically useful agent is currently available to reverse the systemic effects of endotoxins, although recent experimental and clinical research holds some promise for the future availability of such agents.[76,169] Presently, the mainstays of septic shock treatment are control of infection and restoration or maintenance of systemic perfusion and tissue oxygen delivery. Infection control can be accomplished by antibiotics and surgical removal or drainage of infected sites. Systemic perfusion and oxygen delivery are optimized by using various means to meet tissue metabolic requirements and thus prevent the development or progression of lactic acidosis.

### INTRAVENOUS FLUID THERAPY

Volume infusion is the most important initial step of resuscitation as relative or absolute hypovolemia plays a major role in the development of the shock state. The primary goal of fluid administration is to restore intravascular volume and hemodynamic stability in order to optimize tissue perfusion. Expansion of the circulating plasma volume alone may correct hypotension and oliguria in almost 50% of patients in septic shock.[138] Increased circulatory volume may increase left ventricular preload, improve cardiac output, and increase oxygen transport. In patients with septic shock, augmentation of oxygen transport results in increased oxygen consumption and decreased lactic acidosis (Fig 27-4).[53,66] Improvement in survival has been reported when stroke volume, cardiac output, and/or oxygen consumption increase in response to fluid administration.[86,143,164]

Hemodynamic monitoring with a pulmonary artery catheter permits rapid fluid infusion while minimizing the risk of circulatory overload. Because patients with septic shock are at risk for both left and right ventricular dysfunction, central venous pressure monitoring alone may provide misleading information regarding the adequacy of resuscitation.[70,105] Although not proven, the use of a strict protocol may also increase the safety of fluid resuscitation (Table 27-1). Serial pulmonary artery wedge pressure measurements help the physician assess the ability of the heart to handle the volume load.[152] An indwelling arterial catheter should also be inserted because auscultatory measurements can severely underestimate true intra-arterial blood pressure.[25] The discrepancy between directly and indirectly measured blood pressures is most marked in patients with low cardiac output and high systemic vascular resistance.[25]

When the hematocrit is less than 30%, packed red blood cells should be transfused to increase blood oxygen-carrying capacity. Controversy still exists regarding the selection of fluids for shock patients. Cost considerations strongly favor the use of crystalloid solutions, such as 0.9% sodium chloride (normal saline) and lactated Ringer's solution. Crystalloid solutions are freely permeable across the capillary membrane and distribute evenly between intravascular and interstitial compartments. When the capillary membrane is intact, three to four times more crystalloid than colloid must be given to replace the intravascular deficit because of the rapid redistribution of these solutions. There is concern that the massive amounts of crystalloid solutions required in some patients may cause pulmonary edema secondary to the reduction of colloid osmotic pressure.[116] In septic shock, the permeability of the pulmonary capillary membrane may be increased. Consequently, the effectiveness of the membrane in maintaining optimal oncotic pressure in the intravascular compartment

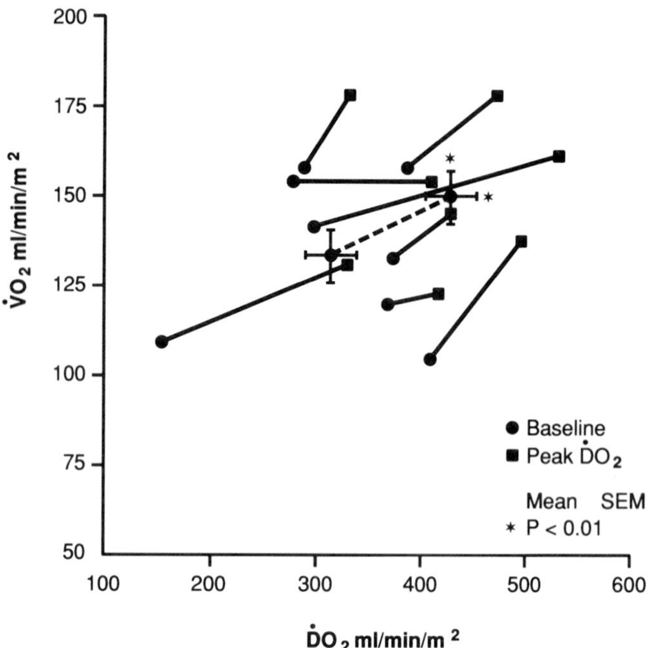


FIG. 27-4. The effects of increasing oxygen delivery ($\dot{D}O_2$) on oxygen consumption ($\dot{V}O_2$) in patients with septic shock. (From Kaufman et al[66] with permission.)

may be diminished. However, there is little clinical evidence to suggest that membrane integrity is lost completely, and rapid equalization of oncotic pressures between intravascular and extravascular compartments occurs. Therefore, the use of colloids may raise plasma oncotic pressure and perhaps decrease the risk of pulmonary edema compared to crystalloids.

Rackow et al.[116] prospectively evaluated 26 non-trauma patients in hypovolemic shock, 75% of whom were septic. Patients were given either 0.9% saline, 5% albumin, or 6% hetastarch at a rate of 250 ml every 15 minutes until a pulmonary artery wedge pressure of 15 mm Hg was reached. The infusion was then maintained at a rate sufficient to keep the

TABLE 27-1. 7/3 Rule for Fluid Challenge

| STEPS | PAWP/PADP | FLUID INFUSION RATE |
|---|---|---|
| Observe PAWP/ PADP (mm Hg) | | |
| For 10 minutes before challenge | <12 | 200 mL × 10 min |
| | <16 | 100 mL × 10 min |
| | ≥16 | 50 mL × 10 min |
| During 10-minute infusion | Change >7* | Stop |
| Immediately after 10-minute infusion | Change ≤3* | Continue infusion without interruption |
| After 10-minute wait | Change >3 ≤7 | Wait 10 minutes |
| | Change >3 | Stop |
| | Change ≤3 | Repeat fluid challenge |

* Note that, during a fluid challenge, an increase of PAWP or PADP greater than 7 mm Hg dictates the cessaton of fluid administration. When the increase is less than 3 mm Hg, additional fluid should be administered.

wedge pressure at 15 mm Hg for the next 24 hours. The initial hemodynamic endpoint was reached by infusion of two to four times more saline than the colloidal solutions (Fig 27-5). Likewise, over the next 24 hours, comparable intravascular pressures could be maintained only by infusion of two to four times more saline than albumin or hetastarch. The lower requirement for colloidal solutions suggests that colloid osmotic pressure plays a role in preventing extravasation of the infused volume. Saline infusion caused a significant decrease in colloid osmotic pressure both at the end of the initial fluid challenge and at 24 hours, whereas colloid osmotic pressure increased after colloid infusion. The colloid osmotic pressure-pulmonary artery wedge pressure gradient, a rough index of transcapillary Starling forces, was decreased by volume resuscitation in all three groups. However, the decrease was much greater in saline-treated patients. This may help explain why six out of eight patients resuscitated with 0.9% saline had radiographic evidence of pulmonary edema 24 hours after completion of resuscitation, whereas only two of nine patients in the 5% albumin and 6% hetastarch groups developed this complication.[114,115,155] Thirty-three percent of the albumin-treated group, 44% of the hetastarch-treated group, and 25% of the saline-treated group survived hospitalization in this study.

On the other hand, several studies have demonstrated that young, otherwise healthy trauma patients can be given crystalloid therapy for shock without an increased risk of pulmonary edema.[82,95] However, most episodes of septic shock in injured patients occur from one to several weeks after the initial injury. These patients may be malnourished, and their vital organ function may be deranged. Their mechanisms for prevention of pulmonary edema may therefore be limited. Nevertheless, there are no current data demonstrating that the use of crystalloid solutions in these patients is associated with an increased risk of pulmonary edema.

Regardless of the type of fluid used, a therapeutic goal must

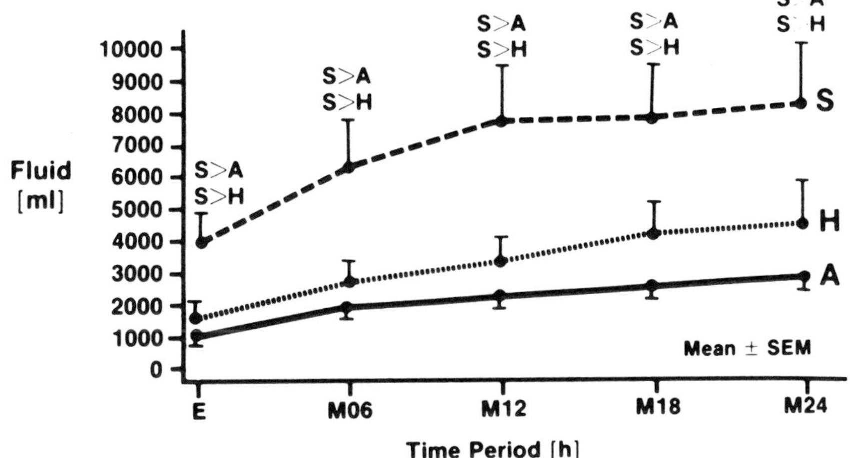


FIG. 27-5. Volumes of 0.9% saline (S), 6% hetastarch (H), and 5% albumin (A) required to resuscitate patients with circulatory shock. (S > A, H; $p < 0.05$ by ANOVA.) (From Rackow et al[116] with permission.)

be defined at the outset. The object of fluid administration to a patient in septic shock is to restore intravascular volume, improve tissue oxygen delivery, and restore hemodynamic stability. Although patients with shock secondary to acute myocardial infarction may achieve maximum cardiac output only at a pulmonary artery wedge pressure of approximately 18 mm Hg, those in septic shock generally maximize output at a considerably lower pressure. For instance, Packman and Rackow[105] showed that, in patients with hypovolemia and septic shock, cardiac output was optimized at a mean filling pressure of 12 mm Hg (Fig 27-6). The difference may be due to lower left ventricular compliance in patients with acute myocardial infarction.

An important consequence of fluid resuscitation with asanguineous solutions is decreased blood oxygen-carrying capacity resulting from hemodilution.[67] Oxygen delivery does not increase during fluid infusion unless the increase in cardiac output resulting from plasma volume expansion adequately offsets the lowered oxygen-carrying capacity. Thus, oxygen delivery and oxygen demand should be monitored carefully. Serial determinations of arterial blood lactate level can thus help determine the adequacy of volume resuscita-

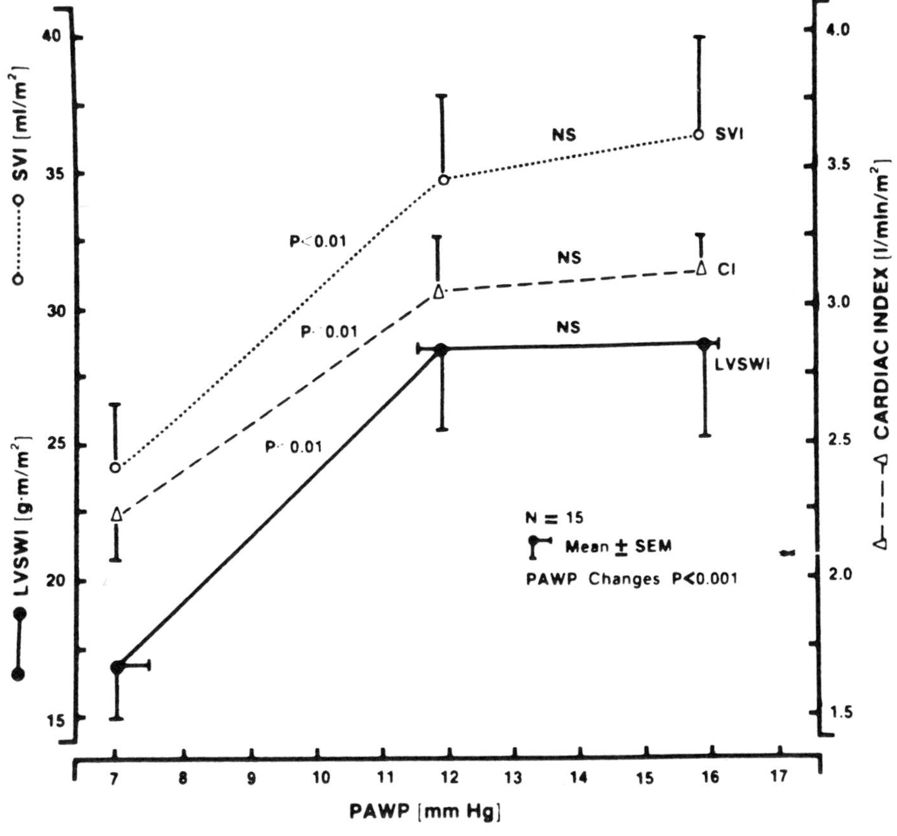


FIG. 27-6. Changes in stroke volume index (SVI), left ventricular stroke work index (LVSWI), and cardiac index (CI) as pulmonary artery wedge pressure (PAWP) is increased during the fluid resuscitation of patients with hypovolemic and septic shock. (From Packman and Rackow[105] with permission.)

tion. If, for example, a reduction in lactate to the normal range occurs at a pulmonary artery wedge pressure of 6 mm Hg and cardiac index of 4 L/min/$m^2$, there is no need to elevate the wedge pressure to 12 mm Hg. Although such a maneuver may increase cardiac output further, the risk of pulmonary edema is also considerably higher.

An exaggerated positive fluid balance is usually present for several days after the onset of septic shock even in successfully resuscitated patients. Because of a fluid shift from the intravascular to the extravascular compartment, fluid requirements are increased. Fluid shift occurs because of increased capillary permeability[38,44] and low colloid osmotic pressure caused by the catabolic state associated with traumatic injury and sepsis. Even when the tissue distribution of fluid returns to normal, fluid requirements may remain high because of the continuing need for intravenous antibiotics and nutritional support. In the presence of acute renal failure this fluid imbalance will be aggravated further.

When patients are refractory to diuretic therapy, hemodialysis or hemofiltration may be used to remove excess fluid. Hemodialysis is poorly tolerated by patients with severe sepsis and has been replaced in many centers by continuous arteriovenous hemofiltration (see Chapter 25). Septic shock patients tolerate hemofiltration without significant changes in blood pressure, cardiac output, or filling pressures, probably because small amounts of fluid are removed slowly.[103]

## ANTIBIOTICS

Before antibiotic therapy is initiated, specimens of blood, urine, and wound exudates should be sent for bacteriologic culture and sensitivity studies. Three blood cultures obtained from different venipuncture sites help distinguish between a contaminated specimen and true bacteremia.

Proper antibiotic therapy decreases both the morbidity and mortality from Gram-negative sepsis and septic shock. Kreger and associates[74] demonstrated that appropriate initial antibiotic therapy reduced the fatality rate of Gram-negative sepsis to one-half of that observed with antibiotics to which the infecting organisms were resistant. Likewise, early initiation of appropriate antibiotics reduced the frequency of shock to one-half of that observed with delayed and inappropriate therapy. Appropriate antibiotic treatment also resulted in a significant decrease in the fatality rate even if the drugs were started after septic shock became evident.

Antibiotic administration should be started during volume resuscitation. The choice of antibiotics is guided by the site of injuries, culture results (if available), and findings of Gram-stained smears of appropriate specimens. If the source of infection cannot be identified, antibiotics must be chosen empirically. As a rule, two or more broad spectrum antibiotics are used initially, and adjustments are made after the results of bacteriologic cultures become available. With the use of two antibiotics, the spectrum of activity is broadened. In addition, the combination of agents may exert synergistic antimicrobial activity. The use of two antibiotics with similar spectrums is not usually warranted if the antibiotic to which the bacteria are sensitive is known.

Antibiotics should be administered intravenously because oral administration may be associated with poor gastrointestinal absorption due to paralytic ileus. The intramuscular route is unreliable because of diminished skeletal muscle perfusion in the shock state. The dosage of antibiotics should be close to the upper limit of the usual range. The first dose should not be reduced in patients with acute renal dysfunction in order to allow rapid achievement of therapeutic plasma levels. Subsequent doses of aminoglycoside antibiotics, which are excreted by the kidney, should be reduced when renal function is compromised. Measuring blood levels of antibiotics minimizes the risk of toxicity. Measurement of serum creatinine concentration and creatinine clearance provides a basis for estimating the intervals required between doses of antibiotics, especially when plasma drug levels cannot be determined.

In septic shock patients the volume of distribution of many antibiotics is increased because of increased extracellular fluid. Summer et al.[139] administered an infusion of tobramycin (aminoglycoside) at a dose of 2 mg/kg to 26 patients in septic shock. Only 41% of these patients had initial peak therapeutic levels above 5 μg/mL. Aminoglycoside levels greater than 5 μ/mL at 15 minutes after drug infusion are associated with a greater survival rate than are lower levels.[94,101]

Empiric antibiotic regimens must be effective against the common strains of enteric Gram-negative bacilli that account for more than 66% of cases of septic shock. Aminoglycosides (gentamicin, tobramycin, amikacin) remain the drugs of choice for initial therapy. The choice of a second antibiotic depends on the suspected source of infection. For example, if a patient has evidence of pneumonia that is possibly due to Gram-positive cocci, a penicillinase-resistant penicillin or first-generation cephalosporin should be added to the aminoglycoside. For a suspected urinary tract infection, ampicillin is added to the aminoglycoside to cover enterococci.

Abdominal infections after penetrating injuries are usually caused by aerobic Gram-negative bacilli and/or anaerobic organisms. It has been demonstrated that *Bacteroides fragilis* and other anaerobic bacteria are responsible for many postoperative intra-abdominal abscesses. Therefore, antibiotics that are effective against anaerobes are preferred for prophylactic therapy of penetrating abdominal wounds.[142] In these situations, clindamycin or cefoxitin should be given in addition to the aminoglycoside. Enterococcus is an occasional cause of abdominal sepsis. Thus in some centers, ampicillin is also added to the antibiotic regimen.[32] Although the incidence of enterococcal infection is low, the trauma patient is at risk for this infection because of immunosuppression. The efficacy of third-generation cephalosporins and the newer broad spectrum penicillins, alone or in combination, as initial therapy of established septic shock has not yet been fully evaluated. The author's current practice of antibiotic treatment is outlined in Table 27-2.

The initial antibiotic coverage should be continued until a definite bacteriologic diagnosis is made. Less toxic antibiotics with a similar spectrum should be substituted, if possible, based on the sensitivity pattern of the identified bacteria. If all cultures are negative and a site of infection has not been identified, antibiotics should be discontinued.

TABLE 27-2. Antibiotic Regimens in Septic Shock

Septic shock of unknown origin
- Aminoglycoside (gentamicin or tobramycin)—2 mg/kg IV initial dose then 1.5 mg/kg every 8 hours; adjust doses if renal dysfunction is present; follow peak and trough drug levels
- Clindamycin—600 mg IV every 6 hours

Septic shock of suspected pulmonary origin
- Aminoglycoside as above
- Nafcillin—1 g IV every 4 hours

Septic shock of suspected intra-abdominal source
- Aminoglycoside as above
- Clindamycin as above

Septic shock of suspected urinary origin
- Aminoglycoside as above
- Ampicillin—1 g IV every 4 hours

Septic shock in leukemic patients
- Aminoglycoside as above
- Ticarcillin—4 g IV every 4 hours

After the initiation of antibiotic therapy, large numbers of bacteria may be killed with resultant massive endotoxin release. For example, fatal vasomotor collapse has occurred shortly after a loading dose of chloramphenicol given to treat typhoid fever.[60] It is possible that hemodynamic deterioration can also occur in other types of Gram-negative infections soon after antibiotic therapy is instituted. Thus, patients should be observed for an adverse hemodynamic response after the initiation of therapy.

## TREATMENT OF ACIDOSIS

Acidosis in septic shock patients is almost always secondary to the accumulation of lactic acid and usually improves with measures that increase tissue perfusion. Sodium bicarbonate is not usually needed. However, an occasional patient with severe acidosis may require this agent to increase cardiovascular responsiveness to endogenous or exogenous catecholamines, although its efficacy is uncertain.[26a]

## TREATMENT OF DISSEMINATED INTRAVASCULAR COAGULATION

Laboratory evidence of disseminated intravascular coagulation (DIC) is found in some patients with septic shock.[74] Gross bleeding due to this disorder is infrequent, but occasionally a bleeding diathesis caused by DIC may develop. These patients may require replacement of clotting factors, including platelets. Successful therapy of shock will itself result in improvement of coagulation.[28] Very rarely heparin may be needed (see also Chapter 7).

## VASOPRESSOR THERAPY

The value of sympathomimetic drugs in the treatment of septic shock is less well established than that of blood volume repletion. Little information is available to support the routine use of vasopressor agents to treat septic shock. In the hypodynamic stage, peripheral vascular resistance is usually increased; drugs with predominant α-adrenergic effects, such as levarterenol or phenylephrine, may actually decrease organ blood flow by further increasing peripheral vascular resistance. As shock progresses, precapillary sphincters dilate in response to increasing hydrogen ion concentration and other locally produced vasoactive mediators. The postcapillary sphincters are resistant to these mediators. Thus, α-adrenergic agents may actually accelerate fluid loss by creating a disproportionate increase in postcapillary venous pressure.

In the hyperdynamic stage of septic shock, peripheral vascular resistance and blood pressure are usually decreased. Under these conditions the use of vasoconstrictor agents seems logical. The systemic pressure should be increased to a level at which coronary blood flow is maintained (90/60 mm Hg). Drugs that can be used for this purpose include levarterenol 0.05–1 μg/kg/min, phenylephrine 0.10–0.50 μg/kg/min, and dopamine 15–30 μg/kg/min (high-dose dopamine). Appropriate fluid infusion will often permit rapid tapering of the vasopressor. The blood pressure at which catecholamine therapy should be initiated must be individualized. A young healthy patient can tolerate a much lower blood pressure than an elderly person with coronary artery disease. Drugs with predominant $\alpha_1$-adrenergic effects, such as phenylephrine, raise systemic blood pressure by increasing vascular resistance and do not necessarily improve tissue perfusion. This explains their limited usefulness in the treatment of septic shock. Isoproterenol, the most potent β-adrenergic agonist, usually produces tachycardia and ventricular arrhythmias and therefore is also rarely considered in the treatment of the syndrome.

Dobutamine or dopamine is commonly used for patients with low cardiac output and high peripheral vascular resistance. Dobutamine hydrochloride is a sympathomimetic agent with predominantly β-adrenergic effects. It increases cardiac output by increasing both myocardial contractility and heart rate. Peripheral vascular resistance usually decreases during its use. At low infusion rates dobutamine is less likely to produce tachycardia than dopamine. However, at higher rates tachycardia and ventricular arrhythmias may develop. Dobutamine is usually infused at a rate between 3 and 15 μg/kg/min; the infusion is adjusted according to the hemodynamic response.

Dopamine hydrochloride is a naturally occurring precursor of norepinephrine. It produces α-adrenergic effects at high doses and β-adrenergic and dopaminergic effects at low doses. Its beta activity produces an increase in cardiac output, which is preferentially channeled to the splanchnic viscera and the kidneys due to a direct vasodilator action on resistance vessels (dopaminergic effect). Dopamine is usually infused at rates of less than 3 μg/kg/min if only its dopaminergic effects are desired and at rates greater than 15 μg/kg/min if a predominant alpha effect is needed. However, depending on the individual, beta and alpha effects may be seen at lower dosage levels. Thus, the dosages mentioned should be used only as guidelines, and therapy should be tailored to suit the individual patient's response.

Dopamine may increase pulmonary artery wedge pressure and can precipitate myocardial ischemia, particularly in older patients with coronary artery disease. ST-T segment elevation has also been described with the use of dopamine in septic shock patients without apparent heart disease.[141] Dopamine can also increase intrapulmonary shunting in patients with adult respiratory distress syndrome.[64] Despite these potential complications, dopamine is often used as an inotropic and vasoconstrictive agent during the treatment of both early hyperdynamic and late hypodynamic stages of septic shock[165,166] and is generally considered the drug of choice for this purpose.

Jardin and colleagues[65] studied dobutamine infusion (12.6 μg/kg/min) in 19 patients with septic shock. They found that cardiac index, stroke index, and mean arterial pressure increased while pulmonary artery wedge pressure decreased. However, a significant increase in heart rate and intrapulmonary shunting was also noted. Regnier and associates[120] noted comparable increases in cardiac index with dopamine and dobutamine. Blood pressure was increased significantly with dopamine, but not with dobutamine. Dobutamine may be useful in the later stages of septic shock in which myocardial failure is likely to occur. Dobutamine infusion in patients with septic shock results in increased cardiac output and oxygen consumption if fluids are given to maintain the pulmonary artery wedge pressure.[146] If increased systemic vascular resistance is desired, another vasoactive agent, such as dopamine or levarterenol, should be chosen.

Levarterenol has mixed α- and β-adrenergic activity. In small doses, a positive inotropic effect accounts for the increase in cardiac output. In large doses, peripheral vascular resistance and systemic blood pressure rise due to its alpha effects. The cardiac output may actually decrease because of increased afterload when this agent is infused at high doses. Levarterenol should not be used to raise the blood pressure to normal. It may result in excessive myocardial oxygen demands that are not balanced by increased coronary blood flow or coronary oxygen supply. Thus, it should be used judiciously to increase blood pressure and cardiac output without causing an undue increase in peripheral vascular resistance.

Levarterenol should be infused when an adequate perfusion pressure cannot be obtained despite volume resuscitation and the use of dobutamine or high-dose dopamine. Peripheral vasoconstriction in response to infusion of α-agonists is less marked in septic than in noninfected patients, most likely secondary to abnormalities in adrenergic receptor function.[23] High-dose levarterenol (0.5–1.0 μg/kg/min) significantly increased mean arterial pressure and systemic vascular resistance without influencing cardiac output in 12 hyperdynamic vasodilated septic shock patients studied by Desjars et al.[31] These patients were all hypotensive despite fluid resuscitation and infusion of high-dose dopamine. Significant increases in urine output were also seen despite the large amounts of levarterenol infused. Seven of the 12 patients survived hospitalization.

Levarterenol-induced vasoconstriction can decrease renal blood flow. Canine studies have demonstrated that addition of low-dose dopamine (4 μg/kg/min) to a high-dose levarterenol infusion did not significantly change systemic hemodynamics, but did result in higher renal blood flow and lower renal vascular resistance than was observed with levarterenol alone.[126] Therefore, use of low-dose dopamine (1–4 μg/kg/min) seems reasonable during the infusion of high-dose levarterenol.

Digitalis may raise cardiac output in patients whose output is low despite a high filling pressure. However, it is a much weaker inotropic agent than dobutamine. The usual dose of digoxin is 0.5 mg, IV bolus, followed by 0.25 mg every 6 hours to a total dose of 1.5 mg. Blood digoxin levels should be monitored periodically to avoid toxicity. Amrinone is a recently released positive inotropic agent with potent vasodilatory effects. It might have a role in the treatment of the hypodynamic stage of septic shock, but clinical trials demonstrating its efficacy in this setting are not available.

Catecholamine infusions are widely used to treat septic shock. However, prospective studies demonstrating the beneficial effects of these agents on the final outcome of septic shock are not available. Retrospective studies have shown a less favorable outcome in patients who received catecholamine infusion than in those who did not.[125] These agents should be administered only when volume therapy fails to restore adequate tissue perfusion, as indicated by increasing arterial lactate concentrations and an imbalance between oxygen delivery and demand.

## VASODILATORS

Vasodilators should theoretically be of value in septic shock since they may enhance microcirculatory flow. However, early clinical trials with phenoxybenzamine, an α-adrenergic blocker, were disappointing.[151,163] Weil suggested that phentolamine might be preferable to phenoxybenzamine for this purpose.[151] Cerra and coworkers[21] more recently used nitroglycerine paste in patients with septic shock and noted decreased vascular resistance and increased cardiac output. Agents that can be continuously infused and titrated (nitroglycerine or nitroprusside) may result in considerable hemodynamic improvement in selected patients. When these agents are used, it is essential that continuous hemodynamic monitoring be available so that cardiac filling pressures and blood pressure can be maintained while afterload is reduced. A combination of a vasodilator and dopamine may be particularly beneficial since dopamine improves myocardial performance and the vasodilator improves peripheral perfusion.

## GLUCOSE-INSULIN-POTASSIUM

Hypertonic solutions of glucose, insulin, and potassium (GIK) (50% glucose, 1 g/kg; insulin, 1.5 unit/kg; potassium chloride, 10 mmol) may improve myocardial contractility and the hemodynamic status of patients in septic shock, particularly if the patient has a low cardiac output.[17,24] Suggested mechanisms for the inotropic effect of GIK include improved energy balance, decreased myocardial edema due to the hyperosmolarity of the solution, and direct effects of insulin on excitation-contraction coupling. The effects of GIK infusions need to be further evaluated before they are acceptable in the therapeutic approach to the patient in septic shock.

## FIBRONECTIN

Fibronectin is a glycoprotein that functions as an opsonin. It may improve the clearance of circulating bacteria and other particulate material by cells of the reticuloendothelial system. After traumatic injury, blood fibronectin levels are decreased at a time when the function of the reticuloendothelial system is depressed.

Cryoprecipitate contains significant quantities of fibronectin and has been used for exogenous repletion of this protein. Uncontrolled trials of cryoprecipitate infusion in septic/traumatized patients demonstrated that normalization of the plasma fibronectin level favorably influenced cardiac, pulmonary, and renal function.[4,129]

Lundsgaard-Hansen and associates[84] demonstrated improved short-term survival in 33 patients with severe abdominal infection who received fibronectin infusions for 5 days. In contrast, a controlled randomized trial of cryoprecipitate infusion in severely septic patients failed to demonstrate either improved organ function or survival.[54] Differences in the amount and activity of infused fibronectin may explain the contrasting results. At the present time, the role of fibronectin infusion for treatment of septic shock remains uncertain.

## INTRA-AORTIC BALLOON COUNTERPULSATION

Patients with septic shock who develop cardiac failure usually die even though the infection itself is controllable. Myocardial failure due to septic shock may be reversible[113,117,118] if myocardial function can be supported until the infective process is brought under control. Unlike catecholamine infusions, intra-aortic balloon counterpulsation does not increase myocardial oxygen demand. Thus, there is little risk of arrhythmias or ischemic episodes. However, the balloon pump can introduce secondary infection into an already contaminated bloodstream.

The use of the balloon pump in the treatment of septic shock was first reported in 1973 by Berger and colleagues.[9] They used the device in two patients with septic shock and pre-existing coronary artery disease. Both patients had low cardiac output and high filling pressures. During counterpulsation, hemodynamic parameters improved dramatically, and the patients survived. Foster and associates[45] reported the use of counterpulsation in five patients with septic shock. Three patients with hyperdynamic shock died, whereas the two patients with low-output shock survived. Mercer and coworkers[92] described an elderly patient in low-output septic shock who benefited from intra-aortic balloon counterpulsation and ultimately survived. The limited data available suggest that there may be a place for intra-aortic balloon counterpulsation in the treatment of patients with septic shock and severe cardiac failure. There is no evidence at present that supports the use of this device in the high-output stage of septic shock.

## CORTICOSTEROIDS

The generalized stress response to sepsis causes an increase in plasma cortisol levels. Sibbald and associates[131] evaluated the adrenocortical response of 26 patients with severe bacterial infections to an intravenous dose of synthetic adrenocorticotrophic hormone (ACTH). Five patients who failed to demonstrate an appropriate increase in plasma cortisol levels after intravenous ACTH administration also had significantly lower basal cortisol levels than the remaining patients. No clinical or laboratory findings were present in these patients to suggest Addison's disease. They thus appeared to have subclinical adrenal insufficiency. Four of these five patients died. The remaining patient, who received a large dose of steroids after the ACTH challenge, survived. The etiology of adrenal insufficiency in these patients was not clear. An autopsy performed in two patients did not reveal adrenal tuberculosis or hemorrhage. Cultures for *Neisseria meningitidis* were negative in all five patients. It was therefore suggested that, when a critically ill patient with sepsis fails to respond to routine fluid and antibiotic therapy, corticosteroids must be administered.

The use of corticosteroids in septic shock has been a subject of controversy since shortly after their introduction. Animal studies have demonstrated that steroids may be effective in high doses and in combination with antibiotics early in the course of shock.[56] Corticosteroids can alleviate the systemic response to endotoxin and help limit nonspecific cellular injury. Other reported effects of steroids include the ability to decrease histamine and serotonin release, stabilize capillary membranes and lysosomes, and inhibit the interaction of endotoxin with complement.[128] Hemodynamic effects of corticosteroids include increased cardiac output and decreased peripheral vascular resistance.

Many of the studies that have assessed the effects of corticosteroids in septic shock are difficult to evaluate because of their poor design. Some used retrospective data, whereas others lacked controls and did not use a random allocation of treatment.[159] Kreger and associates,[74] in a large retrospective series, noted that patients who received hydrocortisone (mean dose, 4,300 mg) on the initial day of shock had a significantly higher fatality rate than those who were not treated with steroids. Animal studies have demonstrated that steroids inhibit complement-induced granulocyte aggregation only when a threshold dose, which is approximately equivalent to 30 mg/kg of methylprednisolone or 150 mg/kg of hydrocortisone, was achieved.[51] The mean dose of steroids given to the patients in Kreger et al.'s study was significantly less than this. Thus, the poor results observed might have been a reflection of an inadequate steroid dose.

Schumer[128] published the first prospective, randomized, well-controlled study of the effects of high-dose corticosteroid therapy in septic shock. He reported that mortality in patients treated with high-dose steroids and antibiotics was only 10.4% compared to 38.4% in a comparable group of patients treated with antibiotics alone. Sprung and associates,[134] in a prospective, randomized, controlled trial, noted that survival was not improved by the use of high-dose corticosteroids in patients with established septic shock. These two studies, however, were not comparable: in Schumer's study,[128] patients were treated at an earlier, more responsive stage, whereas Sprung et al.[134] excluded all patients whose hypotension responded to fluid infusion and withheld steroid administration until a source of infection was confirmed, resulting in a mean delay of 17.5 hours. In addition, 55 of the 59 patients in Sprung et al's.[134] report were dependent on vasopressors for maintenance of blood pressure. Although survival was not improved by the use of steroids, Sprung et al. did note a significantly higher frequency of shock reversal in the steroid group when the agents were infused within 4 hours of the onset of septic shock. The results of these two studies suggest that reversal of septic shock and survival can be improved when large doses of corticosteroids (equivalent to 30 mg/kg of methylprednisolone) are used early in the course of septic shock.

The results of two prospective, randomized multicenter studies evaluating the effects of high-dose corticosteroids in patients with the sepsis syndrome and early septic shock demonstrated no significant differences in overall mortality between steroid and nonsteroid groups.[14,57] In addition, Bone and associates could not demonstrate any beneficial effects of steroids in the prevention or reversal of shock.[14] Based on the results of these studies involving a total of 359 patients, it must be concluded that the use of high-dose corticosteroids as an adjunctive therapy in patients with severe sepsis or septic shock has no proven benefit and therefore cannot be recommended.

## NARCOTIC ANTAGONISTS

The endogenous opiate, β-endorphin, is formed by cleavage of β-lipotropin, a polypeptide derived from the pituitary protein propiocortin, which also contains adrenocorticotrophin (ACTH). Stimuli that initiate the release of ACTH also release β-endorphin. Both factors are released in increased amounts during stress states, including septic shock. The endogenous opiates affect blood pressure control and can produce hypotension. The narcotic antagonist naloxone has been shown to increase blood pressure rapidly in some patients with septic shock.[48,110] However, this effect of naloxone (0.3 mg/kg) is not associated with an increased cardiac index.[48] In addition, nausea and vomiting develop in some patients during this therapy.

Rock et al.[124] studied the efficacy and safety of bolus administration of high-dose naloxone (1.6 mg/kg) in 12 patients in septic shock. As many as 5 doses of naloxone (0.1, 0.2, 0.4, 0.8, and 1.6 mg/kg) were given intravenously at 15-minute intervals. Only four patients had a positive but transient blood pressure response. Of four patients who had significant adverse reactions, one developed pulmonary edema, one had a grand-mal seizure, and two became hypotensive, one of whom had a cardiac arrest.

DeMaria and associates[30] have published a prospective, randomized double-blind study evaluating the effects of naloxone in patients with septic shock. Naloxone (0.4 to 1.2 mg intravenously) was no better than placebo in raising blood pressure or improving survival. Higher doses need to be evaluated similarly before conclusions can be reached regarding the efficacy of this drug.

At the present time naloxone should not be used for treatment of septic shock. There is no evidence that outcome is improved, and in fact, significant adverse effects may develop. An increase in blood pressure alone cannot be considered a beneficial hemodynamic effect.

## IMMUNOTHERAPY

Ziegler et al.[169] have reported the use of a promising therapeutic intervention. In this study, the patient's immunologic system was supported with an infusion of human antiserum to the J5 mutant of *E. coli*. This mutant lacks the oligosaccharide side chain of the lipopolysaccharide to which most antibodies against endotoxin are directed. This side chain varies from one strain of Gram-negative bacteria to another. Thus, antibodies against one strain of bacteria are not protective against others. Antibodies formed after exposure to the J5 mutant strain of *E. coli* are directed against the core polysaccharide, which shows little variation among Gram-negative bacilli. Antiserum to this strain has been effective against the sequelae of infections by other Gram-negative bacilli in laboratory animals. The human study was prospective, randomized, and controlled. Patients in septic shock who received J5 antiserum in addition to the usual intensive management had a mortality rate of 44% (18 out of 44), whereas mortality was 77% (30 out of 39) in the control group. More recently, the same group has demonstrated that J5 antiserum given prophylactically to a group of surgical patients at high risk for developing Gram-negative infections decreased significantly the incidence of postoperative septic shock.[8]

A different approach to immunotherapy was reported by Lachman and associates[76] in septic shock of obstetric or gynecologic origin. These authors used freeze-dried human plasma rich in antilipopolysaccharide immunoglobulin G. Nine out 19 control patients (47.4%) died. Only 1 of the 14 treated patients died.

These observations support the hypothesis that endotoxin is an important factor in the pathophysiology of septic shock and raise expectations that immunologic therapy will improve the outcome of the syndrome in the future.[37] Obviously, this therapy is still experimental. Full exploitation of these findings awaits the development of a large uniform source of antilipopolysaccharide antibody.[7,71]

Animal studies have demonstrated that mice treated with a polyclonal antiserum directed against cachectin become resistant to the lethal effects of endotoxin.[12] It therefore seems possible that neutralizing antibodies directed against human cachectin may be useful in the treatment of the sepsis syndrome.

## PROSTAGLANDIN INHIBITORS

Animal studies with various cyclo-oxygenase inhibitors have demonstrated beneficial effects in endotoxic shock: decreased levels of thromboxane $B_2$, decreased pulmonary vascular resistance, and improved survival.[42] Comparable human studies are not available. The use of a nonspecific cyclo-oxygenase inhibitor could result in shunting of more arachidonic acid to the lipoxygenase pathway with increased leukotriene production, resulting in bronchoconstriction, vasoconstriction, leukocyte aggregation, and increased capillary permeability (see Chapter 24).[5] Whether these agents will prove useful in human septic shock remains for future experiments to demonstrate.

## RESPIRATORY SUPPORT

Respiratory failure is one of the most frequent causes of death in patients with septic shock.[152] Respiratory reserve may already be limited in the trauma patient due to pre-existing chest trauma, upper abdominal surgery, or pneumonia. The increased metabolic cost of sepsis may exceed the capacity of the respiratory system. Respiratory muscle fatigue may develop, followed in a short time by respiratory arrest.[63] Ledingham and associates[78] noted that early use of mechanical ventilation was one of the important factors in improving survival of their patients with septic shock. Mechanical ventilation results in decreased work of breathing and possibly decreases cardiac demand as well. Endotracheal intubation not only protects the airway of the comatose patient but also makes suctioning of secretions easier in the patient with pneumonia. The risk of complications associated with ventilator therapy is increased if adequate sedation and analgesia are not provided (see also Chapter 24).

### SURGERY

Survival is unlikely if the source of infection is not eradicated. Debridement of dead tissue and abscess drainage are the mainstays of infection therapy in the trauma patient. If the infective source is not removed surgically, the patient will develop multisystem organ failure to which he or she will eventually succumb. In patients who have had abdominal trauma, an intra-abdominal abscess may be difficult to diagnose. There may be no clinical evidence other than persistent signs of infection that do not resolve with antibiotic therapy. The most common clinical findings—localized tenderness, fever, and absent bowel sounds—may not be present. Abdominal scans and contrast radiography appear to be the most useful tests, but have only 85% accuracy in diagnosing intra-abdominal abscesses.[55] Sonography and gallium scans are even less accurate (60%).[55] Thus, exploratory laparotomy is indicated when clinical suspicion exists even though these tests are negative. If pus is found and drained, the patient's chance for survival is enhanced greatly.[35] The most common locations of abdominal abscesses are the lesser sac, liver, spleen, pelvis, retroperitoneum, subhepatic and subphrenic areas, and spaces between intestinal loops.[55]

## ANESTHETIC CONSIDERATIONS

Patients with sepsis may present for emergency surgery. A large percentage are hemodynamically stable because they are either in the early compensated phase of septic shock or have been treated vigorously. It is therefore important to obtain information about their clinical course during the hours preceding surgery. Careful review of vital signs; fluid balance; and vasopressor, antibiotic, and other related drug therapy during this period is extremely useful in preoperative evaluation and planning of anesthetic care.

Patients with superficial infections, unless they are hypovolemic, rarely cause difficulties in intraoperative management. The use of sophisticated invasive monitoring techniques is generally unnecessary during the anesthetic management of these patients, although superficial infections caused by clostridial organisms or necrotizing fasciitis may progress rapidly and cause hemodynamic instability before or during surgery (see Chapter 26). Peripheral nerve blocks, performed proximally at an uninfected site, may provide satisfactory operating conditions when the surgical procedure involves drainage or debridement of an infected extremity. Whether spinal or epidural anesthesia can be administered safely to patients with septicemia is not clear. Isolated reports suggest that septic meningitis may occur after lumbar puncture in bacteremic patients.[10,43,83,156] Teele et al.[140] demonstrated an association between lumbar puncture and the subsequent development of septic meningitis in bacteremic children under 1 year old who were not treated with antibiotics. In contrast, children older than 1 year who had been treated with antibiotics at the time of lumbar puncture did not develop this complication. Theoretically, diminished resistance of the blood-brain barrier created by lumbar puncture may allow bacterial contamination and promote meningitis or epidural abscess.[34] There are, however, no solid data available to support this hypothesis. Moreover, a large number of spinal anesthetics have been administered without complication to patients with bacteremia. For instance, bacteremia, although without clinical manifestations, occurs in almost half of patients undergoing urologic procedures.[33] If spinal anesthesia actually predisposed patients to infection, the incidence of postspinal septic meningitis or epidural abscess in this group of patients should be much higher than has been observed. Nevertheless, to err on the safe side, spinal anesthesia should probably be avoided in bacteremic patients, especially those who are not treated with antibiotics.

Surgery may often be indicated for patients who are in severe septic shock or who have had a recent sepsis-induced hypotensive episode. This picture is most commonly seen in patients with an intra-abdominal abscess. Many of these patients are tachypneic, acidotic, and stuporous. Their tracheal reflexes may be depressed, increasing the risk of pulmonary aspiration. They are usually intubated in the intensive care unit. If this has not been done, and depending on the patient's mental status, intubation may be performed either without sedative or hypnotic agents or with small doses of these drugs. If the patient is in shock, surgery should be delayed while measures are taken to optimize hemodynamic and respiratory status, guided by aggressive monitoring of cardiovascular function. Systemic, pulmonary artery, and urinary catheters should be inserted if they are not already in place. Baseline hematocrit, arterial and mixed venous blood gases, and blood lactate levels should be determined. Systemic and pulmonary artery pressures, pulmonary artery wedge pressure, and cardiac output should be measured. Systemic and pulmonary vascular resistances, left ventricular stroke work, oxygen delivery ($\dot{D}O_2$), oxygen consumption ($\dot{V}O_2$), and $O_2$ utilization ratio should be calculated. These measurements should be repeated at frequent intervals while the patient's status is being optimized. By aggressive and well-planned preoperative treatment, the majority of these patients should improve within 2 to 3 hours.

Monitoring should be continued during transportation of the patient to the operating room. In intubated patients, ventilation must be maintained with high inspired oxygen concentrations, using an Ambu bag with PEEP valve, if necessary.

Anesthetic induction of nonintubated patients should be performed with agents that are least likely to cause hemodynamic alteration. Ketamine, 1–2 mg/kg IV, has been used by many clinicians in poor risk patients.[98,160] This drug produces a marked pressor response in normovolemic patients.[160] In acutely hypovolemic patients, the hemodynamic response to ketamine is unpredictable, varying from a slight increase in blood pressure and heart rate to severe depression.[160] Patients with septic shock who have been critically ill for several days may develop marked hypotension after ketamine. Waxman et al.[150] administered ketamine, 24–144 mg IV, to critically ill patients, the majority of whom had sepsis. Significant depression of cardiac performance and of peripheral oxygen transport occurred in about half of the patients. Prolonged stress due to sepsis may result in maximum catecholamine secretion in these patients, which cannot be further enhanced by ketamine; consequently, the myocardial depressant effect of the drug may predominate. Diazepam given in small doses (2.5–5 mg increments) usually induces sleep without significant hemodynamic depression.[135,137] However, in severely hypovolemic septic patients, hypotension may occur. Midazolam administration to normal humans in doses of 0.15 mg/kg may produce a 5–10% reduction in blood pressure, a greater hemodynamic depression than diazepam.[122] Etomidate, once used extensively in hemodynamically compromised trauma patients, produces adrenocortical suppression; therefore, it has been largely abandoned.[149] Sodium thiopental produces hypotension primarily by depressing the myocardium. Thus, it should be used only in small doses and with continuous monitoring of hemodynamic indices.

Both morphine and meperidine may produce hypotension. Fentanyl is devoid of this effect; thus, it is the drug of choice in patients with severe septic shock. A fentanyl-oxygen combination is capable of producing unconsciousness and analgesia without significant hemodynamic alterations.[137] Infusion of fentanyl at a rate of 100–300 μg/min until unconsciousness ensues, followed by an additional 250 μg dose, generally provides satisfactory analgesia without significant cardiovascular depression in septic shock patients.[136] Experience with fentanyl analogs is limited in septic shock, but alfentanil infusion, 1–2 μg/kg/min following a bolus dose of 50–75 μg/kg, may substitute for fentanyl.

The use of succinylcholine in the presence of infection may result in acute, clinically significant elevations of serum $K+$. This has been described in patients with intra-abdominal[72] and peripheral infections (osteomyelitis, limb gangrene).[69] Significant increases in serum potassium were found only in patients whose infection had been present for several days; therefore, this agent should be avoided in patients undergoing reoperation for septic complications of traumatic injury.

Although patients with septic shock may be NPO for a prolonged time and their stomachs may be decompressed by nasogastric suction, they may still be at risk for pulmonary aspiration. Gastrointestinal motility in these patients is diminished as a result of drugs, stress, anxiety, peritonitis, and other problems. Thus, rapid sequence induction may be indicated. Vecuronium, 0.25 mg/kg IV, provides intubating conditions within 60 seconds of injection usually without undue hemodynamic effects.[79]

Inhalation anesthetics depress cardiac function in a dose-dependent manner. They should probably be avoided as primary maintenance agents, although low concentrations of isoflurane (0.5–0.7%) may be combined with narcotics. Halothane, enflurane, and isoflurane can alter the production of superoxide by neutrophils and may therefore interfere with the immune response to sepsis.[97] The clinical importance of this effect, however, is not known.

Significant depression of myocardial function by nitrous oxide has been noted when it is used with opioid or inhalational agents.[91] Nitrous oxide should be discontinued if significant cardiac output reduction occurs. In patients with acute respiratory distress syndrome, nitrous oxide may limit $FIO_2$ and increase pulmonary vascular resistance, which may be detrimental.[77] The level of pre-existing pulmonary vascular resistance (PVR) appears to affect the magnitude of the pulmonary vascular response to nitrous oxide. Patients with markedly elevated PVR due to mitral valve stenosis demonstrated a clinically significant increase in PVR when 50% $N_2O$ was added either to halothane or fentanyl anesthetic.[127] Although the pulmonary vascular response to $N_2O$ has not been evaluated in septic patients with increased PVR, it should be used cautiously in this group of patients.

Mechanical ventilation is continued during the postoperative period. Fluid and electrolyte balance should be monitored carefully as significant sequestration of fluids into the tissues will occur. As in the preoperative and intraoperative period, serial hemodynamic and oxygen transport measurements should be performed to ensure adequate tissue oxygenation. Optimization of tissue perfusion and oxygenation can be achieved by appropriate supportive therapy as described in this chapter.

## CONCLUSION

An increasing number of traumatized patients survive their initial injuries and operative intervention only to succumb in the postoperative period to a septic complication and/or multisystem organ failure. The factors that put the traumatized patient at increased risk for sepsis have been elucidated. Recognition and treatment of this syndrome before the development of refractory hypotension and severe metabolic acidosis may improve the outcome somewhat. Hemodynamic and oxygen transport monitoring have been useful in permitting the rapid resuscitation of the septic shock patient while minimizing the risks of iatrogenic hypervolemia. New advances in antibiotic therapy are barely keeping pace with changes in resistance patterns of invading microbiologic flora. There is now strong evidence that corticosteroid therapy is not beneficial and in fact may increase infectious complications. Early removal of necrotic and purulent material is of paramount importance. Perhaps the only major advance in the therapy of sepsis in the last decade has been the introduction of immunotherapy. This therapeutic option is not yet widely available, but it offers the hope of a dramatic breakthrough in the physicians's battle against the ravages of sepsis and septic shock. Anesthetic management of the patient with septic shock should be individualized. Serial determinations of hemodynamic and oxygen transport indices, including arterial lactate determinations, enable the proper perioperative management of these patients.

## REFERENCES


1. Abraham E, Shoemaker WC, Bland RD, et al. Sequential cardiorespiratory patterns in septic shock. Crit Care Med 1983;11:799.
2. Abraham E, Bland RD, Cobo JC, et al. Sequential cardiorespiratory patterns associated with outcome in septic shock. Chest 1984;85:75.
3. Anderson FL, Tsagaris TJ, Jubiz W, et al. Prostaglandin F and E levels during endotoxin-induced pulmonary hypertension in calves. Am J Physiol 1975;228:1479.
4. Annest SJ, Scovill WA, Blumenstoch FA, et al. Increased creatinine clearance following cryoprecipitate infusion in trauma and surgical patients with decreased renal function. J Trauma 1980;20:726.
5. Ball HA, Cook JA, Wise WC, et al. Role of thromboxane, prostaglandins and leukotrienes in endotoxic and septic shock Intens Care Med 1986;12:116.
6. Baracos V, Rodemann HP, Dinarello CA, Goldberg AL. Stimulation of muscle protein degradation and prostaglandin $E_2$ release by leukocytic pyrogen (interleukin-1): a mechanism for the increased degradation of muscle proteins during fever. N Engl J Med 1983;308:553.
7. Baumgartner JD, Glauser MP. Controversies in the use of passive immunotherapy for bacterial infections in the critically ill patient. Rev Infect Dis 1987;9:194.
8. Baumgartner JD, McCutchan JA, Melle GV, et al. Prevention of gram-negative shock and death in surgical patients by antibody to endotoxin core glycolipid. Lancet 1985;2:59.
9. Berger RL, Saini VK, Long W, et al. The use of diastolic augmentation with intra-aortic balloon in human septic shock with associated coronary artery disease. Surgery 1973;74:601.
10. Berman RS, Eisele JH. Bacteremia, spinal anesthesia and development of meningitis. Anesthesiology 1978;48:376.
11. Beutler B, Cerami AC. Cachectin: more than a tumor necrosis factor. N Engl J Med 1987;316:379.
12. Beutler B, Milsark IW, Cerami AC. Passive immunization against cachectin/tumor necrosis factor protects mice from lethal effects of endotoxin. Science 1985;229:869.
13. Blackburn GL. Lipid metabolism in infection. Am J Clin Nutr 1977;30:1321.
14. Bone RC, Fisher CJ, Clemmer TP, et al. A controlled clinical trial of high-dose methylprednisolone in the treatment of severe sepsis and septic shock. N Engl J Med 1987;317:653.
15. Border JR, Chenier R, McMenamy RH. Multiple systems organ failure: muscle fuel deficit with visceral protein malnutrition. Surg Clin North Am 1976;56:1147.
16. Borzotta AP, Polk HC. Multiple system organ failure. Surg Clin North Am 1983;63:315.
17. Bronsveld W, Van Der Bos GC, Thius LG. Use of glucose-insulin-potassium (GIK) in human septic shock. Crit Care Med 1985;13:566.
18. Bryant RE, Hood AF, Hood CE, et al. Factors affecting mortality of gram-negative rod bacteria. Arch Intern Med 1971;127:120.
19. Calvin JE, Driedger AA, Sibbald WJ. An assessment of myocardial function in human sepsis utilizing ECG gated cardiac scinitigraphy. Chest 1981;80:579.
20. Carroll GC, Snyder JV. Hyperdynamic severe intravascular sepsis depends on fluid administration in cynomolgus monkey. Am J Physiol 1982;243:R131.
21. Cerra FB, Hassett J, Seigel JH. Vasodilator therapy in clinical sepsis with low output syndrome. J Surg Res 1978;25:180.
22. Cerra FB, Siegel JH, Coleman B, et al. Septic autocannibalism: a failure of exogenous nutritional support. Ann Surg 1980;192:570.
23. Chernow B, Roth BL. Pharmacologic manipulation of the peripheral vasculature in shock: clinical and experimental approaches. Circ Shock 1986;18:141.
24. Clowes GHA, O'Donnell TF, Ryan NT, et al. Energy metabolism in sepsis: treatment based on different patterns in shock and high output stage. Ann Surg 1974;179:684.
25. Cohn JN. Blood pressure measurement in shock. Mechanism of inaccuracy in ausculatory and palpatory methods. JAMA 1967;199:118.
26. Collignon P, Chan R, Munro R. Rapid diagnosis of intravascular catheter-related sepsis. Arch Intern Med 1987;147:1609.

26a. Cooper DJ, Walley KR, Wiggs BR, et al. Bicarbonate does not improve hemodynamics in critically ill patients who have lactic acidosis: a prospective, controlled clinical study. Ann Intern Med 1990;112:492.

27. Cooper GL, Hopkins CC. Rapid diagnosis of intravascular catheter-associated infection by direct gram staining of catheter segments. N Engl J Med 1985;313:754.
28. Corrigan JJ. Heparin therapy in bacterial septicemia. J Pediatr 1977;91:695.
29. Cunnion RE, Schaer GL, Parker MM, et al. The coronary circulation in human septic shock. Circulation 1986;73:637.
30. DeMaria A, Heffernan JJ, Grindlinger GA, et al. Naloxone versus placebo in treatment of septic shock. Lancet 1985;1:1363.
31. Desjars P, Pinaud M, Potel G, et al. A reappraisal of norepinephrine therapy in human septic shock. Crit Care Med 1987;15:134.
32. Dougherty SN. Role of enterococcus in intraabdominal sepsis. Am J Surg 1984;148:308.
33. Drach GW, Cox CE. Bladder bacteria: common but unique cause for sepsis. Post-operative endotoxic responses. J Urol 1971;106:67.
34. Dripps RD, Vandam LD. Hazards of lumbar puncture. JAMA 1951;147:1118.
35. Driver T, Kelly GL, Eiseman B. Reoperation after abdominal trauma. Am J Surg 1978;135:747.
36. Duff JH, Groves AC, McLean LPH, et al. Defective oxygen consumption in septic shock. Surg Gynec Obstet 1969;128:1051.
37. Dunn DL, Bogard WC, Cerra FB. Enhanced survival during murine gram-negative bacterial sepsis by use of a murine monoclonal antibody. Arch Surg 1985;120:50.
38. Ellman H. Capillary permeability in septic patients. Crit Care Med 1984;12:629.
39. Ellrodt AG, Riedinger MS, Kimchi A, et al. Left ventricular performance in septic shock: reversible segmental and global abnormalities. Am Heart J 1985;110:402.
40. Faist E, Baue AE, Dittmer H, et al. Multiple organ failure in polytrauma patients. J Trauma 1983;23:775.
41. Finely RJ, Duff JH, Holliday RL, et al. Capillary muscle blood flow in human sepsis. Surgery 1975;78:87.
42. Fink MP, MacVittie TJ, Casey LC. Inhibition of prostaglandin synthesis restores normal hemodynamics in canine hyperdynamic sepsis. Ann Surg 1984;200:619.
43. Fischer GW, Brenz RW, Alden ER, et al. Lumbar punctures and meningitis. Am J Dis Child 1975;129:590.
44. Fleck A, Hawker F, Wallace PI, et al. Increased vascular permeability: a major cause of hypoalbuminaemia in disease and injury. Lancet 1985;1:781.
45. Foster ED, Subramanian VS, Vito L, et al. Response to intraaortic balloon pumping. Am J Surg 1975;129:464.
46. Fry DE, Pearlstein L, Fulton RL, et al. Multiple system organ failure: the role of uncontrolled infection. Arch Surg 1980;115:136.
47. Gleckman R, Hibert D. Afebrile bacteremia: a phenomenon in geriatric patients. JAMA 1982;248:1478.
48. Groeger JS, Carlon GC, Holand WS. Naloxone in septic shock. Crit Care Med 1983;11:650.

49. Groenveld ABJ, Bronsveld W, Thijs LG. Hemodynamic determinants of mortality in human septic shock. Surgery 1986;99:140.
50. Halushka PV, Reines D, Barrow SE, et al. Elevated plasma 6-keto-prostaglandin F1 in patients in septic shock. Crit Care Med 1985;13:451.
51. Hammerschmidt DE, White JG, Craddock PR. Corticosteroids inhibit complement-induced granulocyte aggregation: a possible mechanism for efficacy in shock. J Clin Invest 1979;63:798.
52. Haupt MT, Gilbert EM, Carlson RW. Fluid loading increases oxygen consumption in septic patients with lactic acidosis. Am Rev Respir Dis 1985;131:912.
53. Hauser CJ, Shoemaker WC. Oxygen transport responses to colloids and crystalloids in critically ill surgical patients. Surg Gynec Obstet 1980;150:811.
54. Hesselvik F, Brodin B, Carlsson C, et al. Cryoprecipitate infusion fails to improve organ function in septic shock. Crit Care Med 1987;15:475.
55. Hinsdale JG, Jaffe BM. Re-operation for intra-abdominal sepsis. Indications and results in modern critical care setting. Ann Surg 1984;199:31.
56. Hinshaw LB, Beller-Todd BK, Archer LT. Current management of the septic shock patient: experimental basis for treatment. Circ Shock 1982;9:543.
57. Hinshaw LB, Peduzzi P, Young E, et al. Efficacy of high-dose glucocorticoid therapy on mortality in patients with clinical signs of systemic sepsis. N Engl J Med 1987;317:659.
58. Hoffman MJ, Greenfield LJ, Sugarman HJ, et al. Unsuspected right ventricular dysfunction in shock and sepsis. Ann Surg 1983;198:307.
59. Holloway W. Management of sepsis in the elderly. Am J Med 1986;80(S6B):143.
60. Hopkin DAB. Frapper fort ou frapper docement: a gram-negative dilemma. Lancet 1978;2:1193.
61. Houston MC, Thompson WL, Robertson D. Shock: diagnosis and management. Arch Intern Med 1984;144:1433.
62. Houtchens BA, Westenskow DR. Oxygen consumption in septic shock: collective review. Circ Shock 1984;13:361.
63. Hussain SNR, Simkus G, Roussos CR. Respiratory muscle fatigue: a cause of ventilatory failure in septic shock. J Appl Physiol 1985;58:2033.
64. Jardin F, Gurdjian F, Desfonds P. Effects of dopamine on intrapulmonary shunt fraction and oxygen transport in severe sepsis with circulatory and respiratory failure. Crit Care Med 1979;7:273.
65. Jardin F, Sportiche M, Bazin M, et al. Dobutamine: a hemodynamic evaluation in human septic shock. Crit Care Med 1981;9:329.
66. Kaufman BS, Rackow EC, Falk JL. The relationship between oxygen delivery and consumption during fluid resuscitation of hypovolemic and septic shock. Chest 1984;85:339.
67. Kaufman BS, Rackow EC, Falk JL, et al. Fluid resuscitation in circulatory shock: colloids versus crystalloids. Curr Stud Hematol Blood Trans 1986;53:186.
68. Kelton JG, Neame PB, Gauldie J, et al. Elevated platelet-associated IgG in the thrombocytopenia of septicemia. N Engl J Med 1979;300:760.
69. Khan TZ, Khan RM. Changes in serum potassium following succinylcholine in patients with infections. Anesth Analg 1983;62:327.
70. Kimchi A, Ellrodt G, Berman DS, et al. Right ventricular performance in septic shock: a combined radionuclide and hemodynamic study. J Am Coll Cardiol 1984;4:945.
71. Kirkland TN, Ziegler EJ. An immunoprotective monoclonal antibody to lipopolysaccharide. J Immunol 1984;132:1590.
72. Kohlschustter B, Baur H, Roth F. Suxamethonium-induced hyperkalemia in patients with severe intraabdominal infections. Br J Anaesth 1976;48:557.
73. Kreger BE, Craven DE, McCabe WR, et al. Gram-negative bacteremia. III. Reassessment of etiology, epidemiology and ecology in 612 patients. Am J Med 1980;68:332.
74. Kreger BE, Craven DE, McCabe WR. Gram-negative bacteremia. IV. Re-evaluation of clinical features and treatment in 612 patients. Am J Med 1980;68:344.
75. Kwaan HM, Weil MH. Differences in the mechanisms of shock caused by bacterial infections. Surg Gynec Obstet 1969; 128:37.
76. Lachman E, Pitsoe SB, Gaffin SL. Anti-lipopolysaccharide immunotherapy in management of septic shock of obstetric and gynecological origin. Lancet 1984;1:981.
77. Lappas DG, Lowenstein E, Waller J. Hemodynamic effects of nitroprusside infusion during coronary artery operation in man. Circulation 1976;54:4.
78. Ledingham IM, McArdle CS. Prospective study of the treatment of septic shock. Lancet 1978;1:1194.
79. Lennon RL, Olson RA, Gronert GA. Atracurium or vecurionium for rapid sequence endotracheal intubation. Anesthesiology 1986;64:510.
80. Leon C, Rodrigo MJ, Tomasa A, et al. Complement activation in septic shock due to gram-negative and gram-positive bacteria. Crit Care Med 1982;10:308.
81. Lovett WL, Wangensteen SL, Glenn TM, et al. Presence of a myocardial depressant factor in patients in circulatory shock. Surgery 1971;70:223.
82. Lowe RJ, Moss CS, Jilek J, et al. Crystalloid vs. colloid in the etiology of pulmonary failure after trauma: a randomized trial in man. Surgery 1977;81:676.
83. Lund PC, Cwik JC. Modern trends in spinal anesthesia. Can Anaesth Soc J 1968;15:118.
84. Lundsgaard-Hansen P, Doran JE, Rubli E, et al. Purified fibronectin administration to patients with severe abdominal infections. Ann Surg 1985;202:745.
85. MacLean LD, Duff JH, Scott HN, et al. Treatment of shock in man based on hemodynamic diagnosis. Surg Gynec Obstet 1965;120:1.
86. MacLean LD, Mulligan WG, McLean APH, et al. Patterns of septic shock in man—a detailed study of 56 patients. Ann Surg 1967;166:543.
87. Maki DG, Weise CE, Sarafin HW. A semiquantitative culture method for identifying intravenous-catheter related infection. N Engl J Med 1977;296:1305.
88. Marland AM, Glauser FL. Significance of the pulmonary artery diastolic-pulmonary wedge pressure gradient in sepsis. Crit Care Med 1982;10:658.
89. McCabe WR. Serum complenent levels in bacteremia due to gram-negative organisms. N Engl J Med 1973;288:1.
90. McCabe WR, Treadwell TL, DeMaria A. Pathophysiology of bacteremia. Am J Med 1983;75:7.
91. McDermott R, Stanley TH. The cardiovascular effects of low concentrations of nitrous oxide during anesthesia. Anesthesiology 1974;41:89.
92. Mercer D, Doris P, Salerno TA. Intra-aortic balloon counterpulsation in septic shock. Can J Surg 1981;24:643.
93. Mizock B. Septic shock: a metabolic perspective. Arch Intern Med 1984;144:579.
94. Moore RD, Smith CR, Lietman PS. The association of aminoglycoside plasma levels with mortality in patients with gram-negative bacteremia. J Infect Dis 1984;149:443.
95. Moss GS, Lowe RJ, Jilek J, et al. Colloid or crystalloid in the resuscitation of hemorrhagic shock: a controlled clinical trial. Surgery 1981;89:434.
96. Motsay GJ, Dietzman RH, Resek RA, et al. Hemodynamic al-

terations and results of treatment in patients with gram-negative septic shock. Surgery 1970;67:577.
97. Nakagawara M, Taheshige K, Takamatsu J, et al. Inhibition of superoxide production and $Ca^{2+}$ mobilization in human neutrophils by halothane, enflurane and isoflurane. Anesthesiology 1986;64:4.
98. Nettles DC, Herrin TJ, Mullen JG. Ketamine induction in poor-risk patients. Anesth Analg 1973;52:59.
99. Neuleman TR, Hill DC, Port JD, et al. Ketanserin prevents platelet aggregation and endotoxin-induced pulmonary vasoconstriction. Crit Care Med 1983;14:606.
100. Nishijima H, Weil MH, Shubin H, et al. Hemodynamic and metabolic studies on shock associated with gram-negative bacteremia. Medicine 1973;52:287.
101. Noone P, Parsons TMC, Pattison JR, et al. Experience in monitoring gentamicin therapy during treatment of serious gram-negative sepsis. Br Med J 1974;1:477.
102. Oettinger WK, Walter GO, Jensen UM, et al. Endogenous prostaglandin F2a in the hyperdynamic state of severe sepsis in man. Br J Surg 1983;70:237.
103. Ossenkopplel GJ, Meulen JVD, Bronsveld W, et al. Continuous arteriovenous hemofiltration as adjunctive therapy for septic shock. Crit Care Med 1985;13:102.
104. Ozier Y, Gueret P, Jardin F, et al. Two-dimensional echocardiographic demonstration of acute myocardial depression in septic shock. Crit Care Med 1984;12:596.
105. Packman MI, Rackow EC. Optimum left heart filling pressure during fluid resuscitation of patients with hypovolemic and septic shock. Crit Care Med 1983;11:165.
106. Parillo JE, Burch C, Shelhamer JH, et al. A circulating myocardial depressant substance in humans with septic shock: septic shock patients with a reduced ejection fraction have a circulating factor that depresses in vitro myocardial cell performance. J Clin Invest 1985;76:1539.
107. Parker MM, Parillo JE. Septic shock hemodynamics and pathogenesis. JAMA 1983;250:3324.
108. Parker MM, Shelhamer JH, Bacharach SL, et al. Profound but reversible myocardial depression in patients with septic shock. Ann Intern Med 1984;100:483.
109. Parker MM, Shelhamer JH, Natanson C, et al. Serial cardiovascular variables in survivors and nonsurvivors of human septic shock: heart rate as an early predictor of prognosis. Crit Care Med 1987;15:923.
110. Peters WP, Johnson MW, Freidman PA, et al. Pressor effect of naloxone in septic shock. Lancet 1981;1:529.
111. Polk HC, Shields CL. Remote organ failure. A valid sign of occult intraabdominal infection. Surgery 1977;81:310.
112. Poskitt TR, Poskitt PKF. Thrombocytopenia of sepsis: the role of circulating IgG-containing immune complexes. Arch Intern Med 1985;145:891.
113. Postel J, Schloerb PR. Cardiac depression in bacteremia. Ann Surg 1977;186:74.
114. Rackow EC, Fein IA, Leppo J. Colloid osmotic pressure as a prognostic indicator of pulmonary edema and mortality in the critically ill. Chest 1977;72:709.
115. Rackow EC, Fein IA, Seigel J. The relationship of the colloid osmotic-pulmonary artery wedge pressure gradient to pulmonary edema and mortality in critically ill patients. Chest 1982;82:433.
116. Rackow EC, Falk JL, Fein IA, et al. Fluid resuscitation in circulatory shock: a comparison of the cardiorespiratory effects of albumin, hetastarch and saline solutions in patients with hypovolemic and septic shock. Crit Care Med 1983;11:839.
117. Rackow EC, Kaufman BS, Falk JL, et al. Reversible myocardial dysfunction in patients with septic shock. Clin Res 1985;33:295A.
118. Rackow EC, Kaufman BS, Falk JL, et al. Hemodynamic response to fluid repletion in patients with septic shock: evidence for early depression of cardiac performance. Circ Shock 1987;22:11.
119. Rector F, Goyal S, Rosenberg IK, et al. Sepsis: a mechanism for vasodilatation in the kidney. Ann Surg 1973;178:222.
120. Regnier B, Safran D, Carlet J, et al. Comparative hemodynamic effects of dopamine and dobutamine in septic shock. Intens Care Med 1979;5:115.
121. Reines HD, Halushka PV, Cook JA, et al. Plasma thromboxane concentrations are raised in patients dying with septic shock. Lancet 1982;2:174.
122. Reves JG, Fragen RI, Vinik HR, et al. Midazolam: pharmacology and uses. Anesthesiology 1985;62:310.
123. Robinson JA, Klodnycky ML, Loeb HS, et al. Endotoxin, prekallikrein, complement and systemic vascular resistance. Am J Med 1975;59:61.
124. Rock P, Silverman H, Plump D, et al. Efficacy and safety of naloxone in septic shock. Crit Care Med 1985;13:28.
125. Ruiz CE, Weil MH, Carlson RW. Treatment of circulatory shock with dopamine: studies on survival. JAMA 1979;242:165.
126. Schaer GL, Fink MP, Parrillo JE. Norepinephrine alone versus norepinephrine plus low-dose dopamine: enhanced renal blood flow with combination pressor therapy. Crit Care Med 1985;13:492.
127. Schulte-Sasse V, Hess W, Tarnow J. Pulmonary vascular responses to nitrous oxide in patients with normal and high pulmonary vascular resistance. Anesthesiology 1982;57:9.
128. Schumer W. Steroids in the treatment of clinical septic shock. Ann Surg 1976;184:333.
129. Scovill WA, Annest SJ, Saba TM, et al. Cardiovascular hemodynamics after opsonic alpha-2-surface binding glycoprotein therapy in injured patients. Surgery 1979;86:284.
130. Sibbald WJ. Myocardial function in the critically ill: factors influencing left and right ventricular performance in patients with sepsis and trauma. Surg Clin North Am 1985;65:867.
131. Sibbald WJ, Short A, Cohen MP, et al. Variations in adrenocortical responsiveness during severe bacterial infections: unrecognized adrenocortical insufficiency in severe bacterial infections. Ann Surg 1977;186:29.
132. Sibbald WJ, Paterson NAM, Holliday RL. Pulmonary hypertension in sepsis. Chest 1978;73:583.
133. Siegel JH, Greenspan M, Del Guercio LRM. Abnormal vascular tone, defective oxygen transport and myocardial failure in human septic shock. Ann Surg 1967;165:504.
134. Sprung CL, Caralis PV, Marcial EM, et al. The effects of high-dose corticosteroids in patients with septic shock. N Engl J Med 1984;311:1137.
135. Stanley TH, Webster LR. Anesthetic requirements and cardiovascular effects of fentanyl-oxygen and fentanyl-diazepam-oxygen anesthesia in man. Anesth Analg 1978;57:411.
136. Stanley TH, Reddy P. Fentanyl-oxygen in septic shock. Anesthesiology 1979;51:S100.
137. Stanley TH, Bennett GM, Lowser EA, et al. Cardiovascular effects of diazepam and droperidol during morphine anesthesia. Anesthesiology 1976;44:255.
138. Sugarman HG, Diaco JF, Pollack TW, et al. Physiologic management of septicemic shock in man. Surg Forum 1971;22:3.
139. Summer WR, Michael JR, Lipsky JL. Initial aminoglycoside levels in the critically ill. Crit Care Med 1983;11:948.
140. Teele DW, Dashefsky B, Rakusan T, et al. Meningitis after lumbar puncture in children with bacteremia. N Engl J Med 1981;305:1079.
141. Terradellas JB, Bellot JF, Saris AB, et al. Acute and transient ST segment elevation during bacterial shock in seven patients without apparent heart disease. Chest 1982;81:444.

142. Thadepalli H, Gorbach SL, Broido PW, et al. Abdominal trauma, anaerobes, and antibiotics. Surg Gynec Obstet 1973;137:270.
143. Udhoji VN, Weil MH. Hemodynamic and metabolic studies on shock associated with bacteremia: observations on sixteen patients. Ann Intern Med 1965;62:966.
144. Vincent JL, Weil MH, Puri V, et al. Circulatory shock associated with purulent peritonitis. Am J Surg 1981;142:262.
145. Vincent JL, Durfay P, Berre J, et al. Serial lactate determinations during circulatory shock. Crit Care Med 1983;11:449.
146. Vincent JL, Van der Linden P, Domb M, et al. Dopamine compared with dobutamine in experimental septic shock: relevance to fluid administration. Anesth Analg 1987;66:565.
147. Vitak V, Cowley RA. Blood lactate in the prognosis of various forms of shock. Ann Surg 1971;173:308.
148. Vito L, Dennis RC, Weisel RD, et al. Sepsis presenting as acute respiratory insufficiency. Surg Gynec Obstet 1974;138:896.
149. Wagner RL, White PF, Kan PB, et al. Inhibition of adrenal steroidogenesis by the anesthetic etomidate. N Engl J Med 1984;310:1415.
150. Waxman K, Shoemaker WC, Lippmann M. Cardiovascular effects of anesthetic induction with ketamine. Anesth Analg 1980;59:355.
151. Weil MH. Current understanding of mechanisms and treatment of circulatory shock caused by bacterial infections. Ann Clin Res 1977;9:6.
152. Weil MH, Shubin H. The VIP approach to the bedside management of shock. JAMA 1969;207:337.
153. Weil MH, Afifi AA. Experimental and clinical studies on lactate and pyruvate as indicators of severity of acute circulatory failure. Circulation 1970;41:989.
154. Weil MH, Nishijima H. Cardiac output in bacterial shock. Am J Med 1978;64:920.
155. Weil MH, Henning RJ, Morissette M, et al. Relationship between colloid osmotic pressure and pulmonary artery wedge pressure in patients with acute cardiorespiratory failure. Am J Med 1978;64:643.
156. Weinstein L. Hemophilus infection. In: Harrison TR, ed. Principles of internal medicine. 4th ed. New York: McGraw-Hill, 1962:955.
157. Weisel RD, Vito L, Dennis RC, et al. Myocardial depression during sepsis. Am J Surg 1977;133:512.
158. Weissglas IS. The role of endogenous opiates in shock: experimental and clinical studies in vitro and in vivo. Adv Shock Res 1983;10:87.
159. Weitzman S, Berger S. Clinical trial design in studies of corticosteroids for bacterial infections. Ann Intern Med 1974;81:36.
160. White PF, Way W, Trevor AJ. Ketamine—its pharmacology and therapeutic uses. Anesthesiology 1982;56:119.
161. Wiles JB, Cerra FB, Siegel JH, et al. The systemic septic response: does the organism matter? Crit Care Med 1980;8:55.
162. Wilson RF, Thal AP, Kindling PH, et al. Hemodynamic measurements in septic shock. Arch Surg 1965;91:121.
163. Wilson RF, Chiscano AD, Quadros E, et al. Some observations on 132 patients with septic shock. Anesth Analg 1967;46:751.
164. Wilson RF, Christensen C, Leblanc LP. Oxygen consumption in critically ill surgical patients. Ann Surg 1972;176:801.
165. Wilson RF, Sibbald WJ, Jaanimagi J. Hemodynamic effects of dopamine in critically ill septic patients. J Surg Res 1976;20:163.
166. Winslow EJ, Loeb HS, Rahimtoola SH, et al. Hemodynamic studies and results of therapy in 50 patients with bacteremic shock. Am J Med 1973;54:421.
167. Woo P, Carpenter MA, Trunkey D. Ionized calcium: the effect on septic shock in the human. J Surg Res 1979;26:605.
168. Wright MB, Duff JM, McLean APH, et al. Regional capillary blood flow and oxygen uptake in severe sepsis. Surg Gynec Obstet 1971;132:637.
169. Ziegler BJ, McCutchan JA, Fierer J, et al. Treatment of gram-negative bacteremia and shock with human antiserum to mutant E. Coli. N Engl J Med 1982;307:1225.

# Chapter Twenty-Eight

*Brian Kaufman*

# Deep Vein Thrombosis and Pulmonary Embolism in the Injured Patient

## DEEP VEIN THROMBOSIS

The traumatized patient is prone to develop thromboembolic disease.[41] Although deep vein thrombosis (DVT) and pulmonary embolism (PE) can occur after all types of major trauma, injuries to the lower extremities and in particular to the hips present the greatest risk of these complications.[10,81,185a] Patients with major burns, pelvic fractures, and head and spine injuries are also at high risk of venous thromboembolism.[10,82,140,150a]

Many factors predispose the injured patient to DVT. Posttraumatic or postoperative immobilization is probably the most important factor.[40] Prolonged immobilization may also result in propagation of calf vein thrombi into the veins of the thigh from which emboli may migrate easily to the central circulation.[103] Surgery causes coagulation abnormalities favoring thrombus formation in areas of venous stasis, such as the calf.[40,41,110] The anesthetic technique may also influence the incidence of DVT. Epidural and spinal anesthesia are reported to be associated with a lower incidence of postoperative DVT than is general anesthesia.[128,138,156] Severely traumatized patients demonstrate a significant intraoperative decline in antithrombin III levels, which is not seen in patients with less severe injuries.[185] Antithrombin III is a naturally occurring thrombin inhibitor that combines with and neutralizes the effects of activated clotting factors. Acquired deficiency of antithrombin-III therefore increases the risk for DVT.[185] Other risk factors for the development of DVT include advanced age, presence of congestive heart failure, neoplastic disease, pregnancy, Gram-negative sepsis, obesity, varicose veins, use of oral contraceptives, and a history of previous thromboembolic disease (Table 28-1).[40,41,140]

In injured patients, DVT often develops in both lower extremities even when the injury is unilateral or when the clinical symptoms of thrombosis are present in only one leg.[190] Sevitt and Gallagher[184] noted a 62% incidence of bilateral thrombosis during autopsy examination of trauma victims who sustained unilateral fractures of the femur or tibia; both the injured and the normal legs were involved equally in the DVT process.

As mentioned above, surgery increases the risk of DVT formation. Almost 50% of all new clots develop intraoperatively, and the rest form within a few days after elective surgery.[42] There are no data about the precise timing of DVT formation after trauma, but a similar pattern would be expected. The longer the patient lives after injury, the more likely it is that he or she will develop DVT. In autopsies of injured patients, DVT was demonstrated in 19% of patients who expired within 4 days after the injury, in 47% of patients who died in 4 to 7 days, and in greater than 75% of patients who survived longer than 1 week.[184] Prolonged immobilization may thus be a more important contributing factor to DVT than the type of injury.[58]

Pulmonary embolism is usually caused by migration of a thrombus from the lower extremity veins.[103,140] Emboli arising from the iliofemoral veins are most dangerous because of their size. This is in contrast to thrombi limited to the calf of the leg, which rarely result in emboli and often resolve spontaneously.[103,141]

As mentioned earlier, the incidence of DVT may be influenced by the anesthetic technique used. General anesthesia

TABLE 28-1. Factors Facilitating the Development of Postsurgical or Posttraumatic DVT

| |
|---|
| Immobility |
| Lower extremity injuries or surgery |
| Age |
| Heart failure |
| Varicose veins |
| Use of oral contraceptives |
| Obesity |
| Gram-negative sepsis |
| History of thromboembolic disease |
| Pregnancy |
| Carcinoma |
| General anesthesia |

causes a slowing of the venous blood flow in the lower extremities.[116,156] A 50% reduction in blood velocity in the femoral vein has been reported during induction of anesthesia with thiopental.[156] The venous blood flow may also become less pulsatile during the induction of general anesthesia. The velocity of venous blood flow remains low throughout surgery, facilitating clot formation.[156] In contrast, epidural or spinal anesthesia causes an increase in lower extremity blood flow and thus decreases the likelihood of DVT formation.[136,137,156] In addition, local anesthetic agents reduce platelet aggregation and leukocyte adhesion to the vascular wall.[52,59] The prevention of DVT by regional anesthesia may be dependent upon the type of surgical procedure performed. A lower incidence of DVT with epidural or spinal anesthesia than with general anesthesia has been reported after total hip replacement, retropubic prostatectomy, and open reduction and internal fixation of femoral neck fractures.[78,128,136] On the other hand, the addition of thoracic epidural anesthesia to neurolept anesthesia has been shown not to lower the rate of thromboembolic complications after major abdominal surgery.[129]

In the acutely traumatized patient with significant hypovolemia, epidural and spinal anesthesia produce severe hypotension, precluding their use.[22] However, these anesthetic techniques can be employed safely in injured patients whose hemodynamic status has been stabilized or who require multiple surgical procedures during the course of their hospitalization.

## DIAGNOSIS

The clinical diagnosis of DVT is often uncertain because its signs and symptoms are by no means unique and can be caused by nonthrombotic disorders.[140] Most patients with postoperative DVT are either asymptomatic or have relatively minor signs and symptoms, probably because the thrombi do not obstruct the lower extremity veins completely.[103] In contrast, almost half of the patients with signs and symptoms suggestive of thrombophlebitis do not have actual clots in their calf veins.[140] Thus, a therapeutic decision made only on the basis of clinical findings may place the patient at an unnecessary risk. Both invasive and noninvasive methods of diagnosing DVT are costly and may be associated with complications. However, the overall morbidity associated with diagnostic procedures is considerably less than that associated with unnecessary anticoagulant therapy. This is particularly true in the traumatized patient in whom the risk of anticoagulant-therapy-induced bleeding may be unacceptably high.

Venography is considered the gold standard for diagnosing DVT.[162] Hull and associates[87] documented the safety of withholding anticoagulant therapy in patients with clinically suspected DVT who had negative venograms, providing support for the clinical view that a negative venogram excludes a diagnosis of DVT.[87] In this test, radiocontrast medium is injected into a dorsal pedal vein to outline the deep venous system of the leg. Ascending venography provides adequate visualization of the calf, popliteal, femoral, and iliac veins. The accuracy of venography in diagnosing DVT depends not only upon the quality of the venogram but also the skill of the interpreter.[90] This test is invasive and causes pain in the foot and calf. In addition, a small percentage of patients may develop superficial or deep venous thrombophlebitis resulting from irritation by the contrast medium. Allergic reactions to the radiocontrast dye also may occur.[17]

Noninvasive tests have been used widely in the diagnosis of DVT. These tests can replace venography in the majority of patients. They produce less discomfort than venography and often can be performed at the bedside. Three such methods have received extensive clinical trial: impedance plethysmography, Doppler ultrasonography, and the fibrinogen uptake test.

Impedance plethysmography detects the impedance changes of the leg to externally applied electrical current. The impedance increases when the volume of blood within the leg is decreased, and the opposite occurs with increased blood volume. During the test, deliberate changes in leg blood volume are produced by rapid inflation or deflation of a pneumatic cuff applied around the midthigh. When there is significant venous obstruction, the plethysmogram representing the rate of rise and fall of leg impedance shows a flat pattern compared to normal (Fig 28-1). This technique is highly sensitive and specific for detecting thrombosis in the popliteal, femoral, and iliac veins, but is less satisfactory for diagnosing thrombosis of the calf veins because it detects only those thrombi that produce significant obstruction to venous outflow.[90,91] Since most calf vein thrombi do not obstruct the main outflow tract, they cannot be detected by this technique. In addition, impedance plethysmography cannot distinguish between thrombotic and nonthrombotic venous outflow obstruction. Thus, such factors as inadequate patient relaxation, reduced arterial inflow, and extravascular compression can produce false-positive results. The test must be repeated at least twice before excluding clinically significant DVT (Fig 28-2).[90]

Doppler ultrasonography is another sensitive test recommended for the detection of proximal DVT, but as with the impedance plethysmograph it is not reliable for detecting calf vein thrombosis.[90,186,194] Ultrasound examination is performed by placing a probe over the femoral vein. After the characteristic sound of venous flow is detected, the distal thigh or the calf is compressed. Normally, the accelerated blood flow should produce an augmented sound. In the presence of occlusive proximal DVT, the augmentation of the sound is diminished or absent. The Doppler examination is inexpensive, and the device is more portable than the impedance plethysmograph. However, the interpretation of the re-

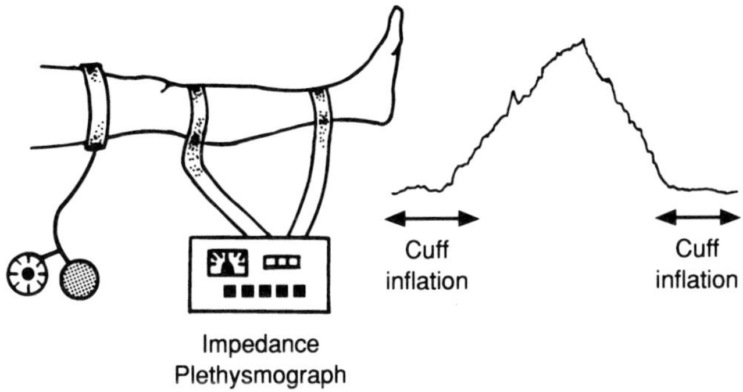


FIG. 28-1. Impedance plethysmography. Left, schematic drawing of the system showing the pressure cuff applied to the midthigh and the sensing electrodes connected to the impedance plethysmograph. Two additional electrodes not shown deliver small electrical currents to the leg. Cuff inflation and deflation produce changes in the volume of the veins of the calf muscles, altering the impedance of the leg to externally delivered electrical current and causing upward and downward deflection of the impedance curve (right). In the presence of venous obstruction, the rate of venous filling and emptying is reduced, causing a decrease in the rates of rise and decline of the impedance curve.

sults is subjective, and thus the accuracy of the test depends on the skill and experience of the investigator.[90]

Duplex B-mode ultrasonic imagers have recently been used as a diagnostic tool for DVT. This instrument provides both real-time ultrasound images of blood flowing through the leg veins and simultaneous auscultation of the flow. The location and extent of clot can be defined noninvasively. It has been suggested that this new diagnostic test may become the most sensitive technique for the diagnosis of DVT.[112]

The fibrinogen uptake test has been used to evaluate the incidence of postoperative DVT. In this test, intravenously injected $^{125}$I-labeled fibrinogen is incorporated into the fresh thrombus, and the increase in surface radioactivity is detected with a gamma scanner.[90] The patient may be scanned as often as required for 5–7 days after a single intravenous injection

FIG. 28-2. Approach to the diagnosis of clinically suspected deep vein thrombosis with serial impedance plethysmography. (From Hull et al[90] with permission.)

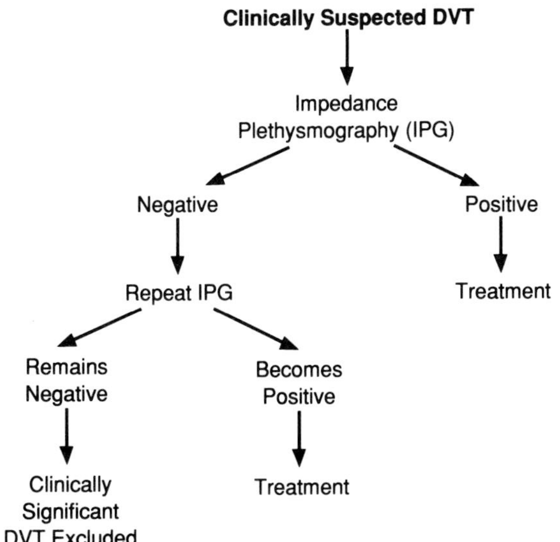


of $^{125}$I-fibrinogen. This test detects over 90% of acute calf vein thrombi, but only 60 to 80% of more proximal thrombi.[90] Fibrinogen uptake is not a reliable test for detecting thrombi in the pelvic and the upper thigh veins because they are in close proximity to the bladder, which accumulates radioactive urine. Since the vast majority of postoperative DVT cases begin in the calf veins, the test is useful in evaluating the efficacy of various prophylactic measures employed to decrease the incidence of DVT.[28] However, the clinical usefulness of a positive fibrinogen scan has been questioned because only a small number of calf vein thrombi go on to cause clinically significant embolic episodes.

The combination of impedance plethysmography and fibrinogen uptake test detects both calf and thigh vein thrombi with an accuracy close to that obtained with venography.[88] Serial determinations using impedance plethysmography also can be an effective strategy for evaluating patients with suspected DVT (Fig 28-2).[91] Nevertheless, in the presence of lower extremity injuries and external fixators impedance plethysmography may be difficult to employ.[150a]

## PREVENTION

Prevention of DVT is of paramount importance because DVT often leads to a dreaded complication, pulmonary embolism (PE). Although innumerable studies have evaluated the efficacy of prophylactic regimens in the prevention of perioperative DVT, no study has yet evaluated their effectiveness in trauma victims. Measures that decrease the risk of perioperative DVT can be divided into two categories: those decreasing the coagulability of the blood and those decreasing venous stasis in the leg veins. Since DVT starts before or during surgery in the majority of patients, prophylactic measures should be initiated preoperatively or in the operating room.

### *Pharmacologic Prophylaxis of Deep Vein Thrombosis*

HEPARIN ANTICOAGULATION. Low-dose heparin administration is the most widely used prophylactic measure in surgical patients. Many studies have demonstrated the efficacy of low-dose heparin prophylaxis during the past decade.[13,101,104,146,147,160,195] This method consists of subcutaneous injection of 5,000 units of heparin every 8 to 12 hours. In electively operated patients, therapy is usually initiated 2 hours before surgery and continued for 7 days after surgery or until the patient is ambulatory.[101]

Low-dose heparin augments the activity of antithrombin III, a potent, naturally occurring inhibitor of activated factor X (Xa) and thrombin, which produces interruption of both the intrinsic and extrinsic clotting pathways. Low-dose heparin causes only minimal changes in conventional clotting tests, such as the activated partial thromboplastin time (APTT). Some authors have reported an increased frequency of perioperative bleeding without any significant decrease in DVT incidence with an 8-hour administration regimen.[108] A 12-hour regimen of heparin is therefore recommended for surgical patients.[13,108]

Most authors believe that low-dose heparin prophylaxis is safe, effective, and well tolerated.[101,160] For patients receiving 5,000 units every 12 hours during the perioperative period, there is a small risk of increased bleeding. Wound hemorrhage is almost invariably minor if the patient is hemostatically competent and has not taken aspirin for 5 days before surgery. Thus, monitoring of clotting parameters is not required in these patients. However, Pachter and Riles[152] using 5,000 units of heparin every 12 hours noted a 27% incidence of bleeding complications (wound hematoma 23%, gross hematuria 4%). The incidence of complications in patients not treated with heparin was only 1.4%. They suggest that low-dose heparin should be reserved for patients over the age of 40 who have additional risk factors for the development of DVT. Van Ooijen,[205] also using 5,000 units of heparin every 12 hours, noted wound hematomas in 32% of heparin-treated patients compared to an incidence of only 15% in the control group. However, no major wound hematomas resulting in wound dehiscence occurred in either group. Concerns regarding hemorrhagic complications of low-dose heparinization led Negus and associates[144] to evaluate the effects of ultra-low-dose intravenous heparin therapy. Patients were given 1 IU/kg/h of heparin intravenously during and after operation for 3–5 days and were compared to patients receiving placebo. The heparin group had a 4% incidence of thrombotic complications, whereas the incidence was 22% in the untreated patients. Whether this approach to DVT prophylaxis is safe or effective in the injured patient remains to be determined.

Heparin is not a homogeneous substance, but is rather a mixture of polysaccharide molecules that vary in molecular weight from 2,000 to 40,000.[175] It has been demonstrated in animals that low-molecular weight fractions are as effective as standard heparin in preventing venous thrombosis, but produce less bleeding.[175] The size of the heparin molecule influences its interaction with platelets: the low molecular weight fraction has less effect.[175] This may decrease the risk of hemorrhagic complications. Clinical trials have demonstrated that low-molecular weight heparin is effective in preventing postoperative DVT, but have not demonstrated a decreased risk of hemorrhagic complications when compared with low-dose heparin.[102,204] Therefore, there is no demonstrated benefit of this new preparation for the trauma patient.

The controversy regarding the safety of low-dose heparin helps explain the reluctance of surgeons to use this prophylactic measure routinely in the traumatized patient.[147] A definite reduction in mortality rate must be demonstrated before this method is widely accepted. Unfortunately, despite a decrease in the incidence of DVT,[101,104,160] to date no clinical trials have demonstrated that prophylactic heparin therapy reduces mortality.[152] The only indirect evidence of the efficacy of prophylactic heparin therapy is a reduced frequency of PE at autopsy.[160] One should remember that most clinical trials have serious limitations and do not therefore prove or disprove the effect of this regimen on the mortality rate.

A trial involving thousands of patients would be necessary to demonstrate a significant reduction in mortality from the use of low-dose heparin, as the clinical endpoint (fatal PE) is an uncommon event. The small numbers of patients in most of the studies that have evaluated low-dose heparin would therefore be unable to demonstrate reduced mortality from PE, even if it was present. A review published in 1988 analyzed the results of all randomized trials of perioperative prophylactic subcutaneous heparin administration.[36] More than 70 trials involving over 16,000 patients were reviewed. The incidence of DVT was reduced approximately 67%, and the incidence of PE was reduced approximately 50%. The incidence of fatal PE was reduced 64% without any apparent increase in deaths ascribed to causes other than PE. A substantial increase in serious bleeding was not found. In patients with traumatic orthopedic injuries in whom the efficacy of low-dose heparin is controversial, a 64% reduction in the incidence of DVT was noted. Perhaps the publication of this extensive review documenting the significant reduction in mortality from PE will overcome to some extent the reluctance of surgeons to use prophylactic heparin.

Patients undergoing elective orthopedic procedures on the lower extremities may not be protected against DVT by low-dose heparin. Williams and associates[213] could not demonstrate a protective effect of this method in patients undergoing hip surgery or amputations of the lower extremity. Hampson et al.[74] also noted that low-dose heparin failed to prevent DVT after hip replacement. The lack of protective effect in these situations may be secondary to factors present only in orthopedic patients. For example, during hip replacement, intermittent compression of the common femoral vein by manipulation of the leg can cause venous stasis, endothelial damage, and release of circulating tissue thromboplastin, counteracting the anticoagulant effect of fixed doses of heparin. Leyvraz and associates[117] showed that heparin prophylaxis was effective in patients undergoing total hip replacement if the dose of heparin was adjusted to keep the APTT between 31.5 and 36.0 seconds. This method achieved maximum DVT protection without a significant increase in hemorrhagic complications.

Another method, which uses the combination of dihydroergotamine (DHE) and low-dose heparin, has been introduced recently in the United States.[82,142] DHE is a vasoconstrictor predominantly affecting the capacitance vessels with minimal effect on resistance vessels. Phlebograms obtained before and after administration of 0.5 mg of DHE demonstrated significant reduction in the diameters of the tibial, soleal, and femoral veins.[105] Allegedly DHE counteracts venous stasis and accelerates venous return from the lower extremities.[82,142] DHE may also work through effects on antithrombin III and by inhibiting platelet aggregation.[105] A multicenter trial compared DHE (0.5 mg) plus heparin (5,000 IU), administered subcutaneously every 12 hours for 5–7 days to heparin 5,000 IU alone at similar intervals.[142] The DHE-heparin combination provided greater prophylaxis against DVT than did the low-dose heparin regimen. Excessive postoperative bleeding or wound hematoma occurred no more frequently in the DHE-heparin group than in the heparin group. However, one patient developed bowel necrosis that was possibly related to the use of DHE. This combination was not more effective than low-dose heparin alone in high-risk patients undergoing post-traumatic hip surgery.[111]

Heparin prophylaxis may be less effective in trauma victims than in patients undergoing elective surgery. Increased concentrations of thromboplastin may be found in the serum of traumatized patients because of tissue injury.[4,5,95] The thrombotic process may thus begin before the initiation of therapy. Under these circumstances low-dose heparin may not be effective, as the coagulation cascade would have already been set in motion.[101] The scarcity of data on efficacy and the risk of bleeding precludes the routine use of low-dose heparin prophylaxis in acutely traumatized patients. However, this treatment may be considered in some patients a few days after the traumatic episode if prolonged immobilization is anticipated.

COUMARIN ANTICOAGULATION. Coumarin derivatives (dicumarol, warfarin) also have been used for prophylaxis against DVT.[139,183] Phenindione, a warfarin-like drug, is effective in patients with femoral neck fractures. Sevitt and Gallagher[183] studied the efficacy of phenindione in 300 patients with femoral neck fractures using a full anticoagulant dose of the drug. Only 2.7% of the phenindione-treated patients had clinical evidence of DVT as compared to 29% of those who did not receive this drug. The mortality rate was 17% in the treated and 28% in the untreated patients. Furthermore, 36% of the untreated patients who died had autopsy evidence of PE that was felt to be the major or sole cause of death; only 8% of the patients who received phenindione died of PE. Although minor hemorrhagic complications occurred more frequently in the phenindione-treated group, the authors did not find an increased incidence of wound bleeding or an increased need for blood transfusion. Similar results were reported by Morris et al.[139] with the use of warfarin in the patients with femoral neck fractures and by Borgström et al.[23] with the use of dicumarol in similar patients.

Warfarin has been shown to be an effective prophylactic antithrombotic agent in traumatized patients.[212] The usual starting dose of warfarin is 10–15 mg. Subsequent daily doses (2.5–10 mg) are adjusted to maintain prothrombin time (PT) at 1.5 to 2.5 times the control. Although this recommendation has been adhered to in North America for the past 30 years, there is little solid evidence to support the need for such high ratios.[85] Keeping the ratio between 1.2 and 1.5 is equally effective, is associated with less hemorrhagic complications, and has been recommended by the participants in the American College of Chest Physicians-National Heart, Lung and Blood Institute National Conference on Antithrombotic Therapy.[83,85] The PT must be measured daily because many drugs and diseases can potentiate or antagonize the action of warfarin (Table 28-2).

TABLE 28-2. Coumarin Interactions*

| ENHANCERS (PROLONGS PROTHROMBIN TIME)** | SUPPRESSORS (DECREASES PROTHOMBIN TIME)† |
|---|---|
| Allopurinol | Adrenal corticosteroids |
| Anabolic steroids | Barbiturates |
| Clofibrate | Cholestyramine |
| Diphenyldydantoin | Diuretics |
| Disulfiram | Griseofulvin |
| Hepatic disease | Haloperidol |
| Hypermetabolic states | Hereditary resistance |
| Low vitamin K diet | High vitamin K diet |
| Metronidazole | Oral contraceptives |
| Phenylbutazole | Rifampin |
| Sallicylates | Uremia |
| Trimethoprim-sulfamethoxazole | |

* Adapted from Hyers[93] with permission.
** Coumarin dose may need to be decreased.
† Coumarin dose may need to be increased.

A two-step warfarin prophylaxis regimen has been proposed for use in orthopedic surgery. This regimen is claimed to minimize the risk of perioperative bleeding.[57] Small doses of warfarin are administered before surgery to prolong the PT by 1.5 to 3 seconds over the control measurement. Doses of this magnitude provide some protection against the development of DVT without increasing the risk of intraoperative bleeding. Postoperatively, the dose of warfarin is increased to prolong the PT to 1.5 times the control.[57] This method cannot be used in acutely traumatized patients undergoing emergency surgery because it takes several days for warfarin to prolong the PT. However, it may be used in selected patients with lower extremity injury whose surgery is delayed for a few days.

Any form of anticoagulation is contraindicated in some patients with multiple trauma. In particular, patients with head injury should not be anticoagulated.[81] Patients with thoracic, intra-abdominal, or limb injuries may be given anticoagulants a few days after surgery if complete hemostasis has been achieved surgically, all related coagulopathies have been corrected fully, and all potential sites of occult bleeding have been evaluated. Although the delay in anticoagulant therapy significantly increases the risk of DVT development, this approach minimizes the potential for massive hemorrhage in a trauma victim.[182] Mechanical methods for prophylaxis of DVT, such as compression boots, can be applied readily in most traumatized patients provided that the presence of orthopedic injuries does not preclude their use. These devices can be used until anticoagulation can be initiated safely. Such delayed use of anticoagulant agents can prevent the propagation of existing thrombi and thereby lessen the risk of fatal embolization.

Certain laboratory tests must be performed before the initiation of anticoagulant prophylaxis. These include a coagulation profile consisting of at least the PT, PTT, and platelet count; measurement of hematocrit; and urine and stool examination for the presence of occult blood. If these tests are normal and surgical bleeding has been well controlled, anticoagulants can be used with a reasonable degree of safety for DVT prophylaxis. Close monitoring for evidence of excessive anticoagulation, heparin-induced thrombocytopenia, and occult bleeding is essential after starting anticoagulation. During heparin therapy the PTT and platelet count should be measured daily. When a warfarin derivative is used, the PT should be measured daily during the first few days and less frequently once a stable state has been achieved.

LIDOCAINE. Lidocaine, 1 mg/kg IV, administered 2 hours before anesthesia and followed by a continuous infusion (2 mg/min) for 6 days decreased the incidence of DVT in patients undergoing elective hip surgery.[39] In this study, mean lidocaine blood levels ranged from 1.4 μg/mL after the initial bolus dose to 4.0 μg/mL on the second postoperative day. Lidocaine can prevent platelet adhesion, aggregation, and release and transendothelial migration of white blood cells.[52,59,150] These actions may minimize progression of endothelial damage and the subsequent initiation of thrombosis.[39] If further studies can substantiate these preliminary findings, lidocaine prophylaxis may become an acceptable treatment in the traumatized patient.

DEXTRAN. Dextrans with average molecular weight of 40,000 (Dextran 40) and 70,000 (Dextran 70) possess significant antithrombotic properties. The antithrombotic effect of dextran is due to (a) reduced platelet aggregation, (b) change in fibrin structure, (c) change in mechanical properties of the fibrin clot, (d) facilitated lysis of fibrin, and (e) increased blood flow due to improved rheology.[70] Some of these properties of dextran might increase the risk of bleeding in the traumatized patient, but this has not been evaluated clinically.

Both dextran 40 and dextran 70 are at least as effective as low-dose heparin in preventing DVT in orthopedic patients.[70,71] However, this form of therapy is less effective than low-dose heparin prophylaxis in patients undergoing nonorthopedic surgery.[7] The usual dose of dextran is 500–1,000 mL every day or every other day for 2–3 days or until the patient is ambulatory. Both dextrans are potent volume expanders. Careful monitoring of central venous pressure or pulmonary artery wedge pressure is recommended to minimize the risk of iatrogenic pulmonary edema.

Minor or major allergic reactions occur in approximately 1% of patients receiving dextrans.[71]

Anaphylactoid reactions occur, with an incidence of 0.013% for dextran 40 and 0.025% for dextran 70.[119] Performed circulating dextran-reactive antibodies have a role in producing severe dextran-induced anaphylaxis. The risk of these uncommon reactions has been markedly reduced, but not eliminated after the introduction of hapten inhibition.[15,131] A monovalent hapten-dextran preparation (Dextran 1) with an average molecular weight of 1,000 infused a few minutes before dextran 40 or 70 combines with dextran-reactive antibodies without producing an anaphylactoid reaction. The reactive antibodies will not then be available to react with the subsequent dextran infusion.

Dextran particles with molecular weight <50,000 are filtered by the glomeruli. These particles are not reabsorbed by the renal tubules, but remain in the filtrate as water is removed. Thus, the highly viscous filtrate contained in the tubule may cause an increase in tubular back pressure, predisposing the patient to renal failure.[33] The possibility of acute renal failure has blunted the enthusiasm for using dextrans in DVT prophylaxis, although this complication is rare (less than one in 140,000).[14,189] In the trauma patient renal dysfunction from various factors may be aggravated by Dextran 40; therefore this agent should be used with caution.

### *Mechanical Methods of Preventing Deep Vein Thrombosis*

In 1856 Virchow enunciated a triad of causes of DVT: (1) stasis or slowing of blood flow, (2) coagulation abnormalities, and (3) vessel wall damage. Of these, venous stasis is felt to be the major predisposing factor in the development of DVT.[140] Enhanced coagulability secondary to a fall in blood fibrinolytic activity is also an important factor in the postoperative trauma victim.[4,5,95] The postoperative decrease in fibrinolytic activity develops within the first 24 hours of surgery and reaches its maximum by the third postoperative day. The necessity for vessel wall damage remains unproven in the genesis of DVT.

Early mobilization, leg elevation, elastic stockings, intermittent pneumatic compression, and administration of low-dose heparin constitute the usual measures taken to prevent DVT after a surgical procedure or extended immobilization. Early ambulation may be a useful method for preventing DVT, although it has not been evaluated rigorously in controlled trials. The benefits of early ambulation are probably related in large part to the restoration of flow in the lower extremity veins after a period of forced immobilization.[115] Leg elevation and the use of elastic stockings are without benefit in the prevention of DVT.[26,169,176] However, individually fitted pressure-gradient stockings increase the venous blood flow velocity in the legs, pelvic veins, and inferior vena cava by producing a pressure differential between the ankles and the knees.[180,215] The use of these stockings decreases significantly the incidence of DVT after abdominal surgery.[180] In addition, the combination of graduated elastic compression stockings with either low-dose heparin or intermittent sequential pneumatic leg compression results in a significantly lower incidence of DVT after major abdominal surgery than when heparin or pneumatic compression is used alone.[181,215] Calf muscle exercises, either in the form of calf motion by a moving pedal strapped to the patient's foot or by application of intermittent pneumatic compression to the calf, have been demonstrated to be as effective as anticoagulant treatment in DVT prevention.[42] Intermittent pneumatic compression, which applies pressure on the legs alternatively, appears to be the most comfortable method and has been studied most extensively (Fig 28-3).

In many clinical trials perioperative application of pneumatic leg compression reduced the incidence of postoperative DVT.[2,42,80,109] In three controlled studies in which the legs were scanned with the $^{125}$I-fibrinogen test for 1 week, this method reduced the incidence of DVT by 60–82%.[80,148] Leg compression with pneumatic devices prevents venous stasis.[176] Peak femoral venous blood flow may increase 240% during intermittent pneumatic leg compression.[148] Devices that sequentially compress the calf and thigh produce higher femoral blood flow velocities than single-chamber devices.[148] However; despite improved hemodynamic effectiveness and superior biologic effects reflected by enhanced fibrinolytic activity, greater antithrombotic effectiveness has not been clearly demonstrated for the more expensive sequential compression device.[177]

The decreased incidence of DVT with pneumatic leg compression may not be caused only by prevention of venous stasis.[80] Intermittent pneumatic compression not only empties the leg veins but also causes venous occlusion.[2] Both venous occlusion and direct compression result in the release of plasminogen activators (found in high concentrations in all layers of the vein wall) into the bloodstream, preventing the usual postoperative decrease in fibrinolytic activity.[2,34,177] Indeed, fibrinolytic activity may remain high for more than 18 hours after discontinuing the compression.[42] Intraoperative compression of the arm veins can also prevent DVT and the postoperative decrease in blood fibrinolytic activity. Knight et al.[109] demonstrated a 50% reduction in DVT incidence in patients receiving intermittent pneumatic arm compression. However, Hills et al.[80] showed that this method had no effect on the incidence of DVT in patients with cancer. Interestingly,

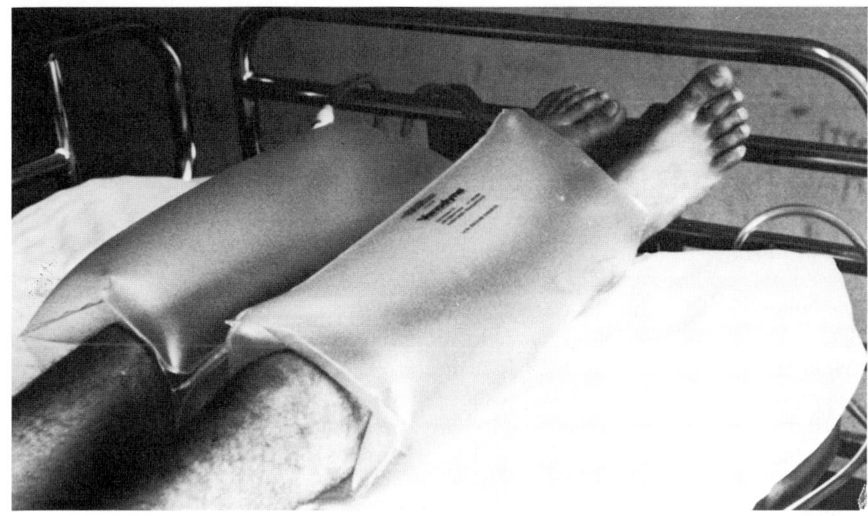

FIG. 28-3. Pneumatic boots applied on the legs of a patient to prevent deep vein thrombosis and pulmonary embolism.

the postoperative decrease in blood fibrinolytic activity also could not be prevented by this method in cancer patients.

The lack of benefit from pneumatic compression in patients with carcinoma supports the contention that it is the release of plasminogen activators that produces the beneficial effects of this therapy. The most pronounced increase in fibrinolytic activity by limb compression occurs locally, rather than systemically.[198] Also, the greater the mass of the compressed tissue, the more the release of fibrinolytic substances.[198] Thus, pneumatic compression of the leg produces the most profound increase in fibrinolytic activity in the blood contained in the lower extremity, which is often a fertile area for development of DVT. Pneumatic leg compression also increases the local generation of prostacyclin, which may act directly to stimulate plasminogen activator, producing hydrolysis of fibrin, in addition to inhibiting platelet aggregation.[73]

Leg compression should be applied at the earliest opportunity. It may be started in the operating room before the induction of anesthesia.[198] If the patient is hospitalized before surgery, the treatment should be applied on admission to the hospital or upon immobilization and then continued throughout the operative and postoperative periods. The use of physical methods to prevent DVT is particularly attractive in traumatized patients because the risks of anticoagulant therapy, such as hemorrhage, can be eliminated. However, in a recent study of patients with major trauma, only 65% of the lower extremities were suitable for pneumatic compression.[185a]

### TREATMENT

Once the diagnosis of DVT is established, heparin should be administered in full doses unless there are specific contraindications to its use. The usual heparin dose for the treatment of DVT is 10,000 units, administered as a single intravenous bolus and followed either by an infusion of 1,000 units per hour or by intermittent injections of 5,000 units every 4 hours. The risk of bleeding complications may be less with the infusion method. The APTT should be maintained between 1.5 and 2 times the control. The duration of intravenous anticoagulant therapy and the subsequent use of oral anticoagulants are discussed in the section on pulmonary embolism.

The fibrinolytic agents, urokinase and streptokinase, are contraindicated in patients with recent traumatic injury. Their use in selected patients is also discussed in the section on pulmonary embolism.

## PULMONARY EMBOLISM

Pulmonary embolism (PE) is a devastating complication of traumatic injury. Coon[40] found a 14.3% incidence of PE during autopsies of 224 patients who died after accidental trauma. Although PE was noted to occur most frequently after hip fractures (60% of patients), the incidence of this complication was not significantly different after injuries involving other sites of the body. The duration of survival after injury and of the associated bedrest appeared to influence the incidence of PE.[40] Only 3.3% of patients who survived less than 24 hours suffered a PE, while the incidence increased to 18.6% in those who lived 1 and 7 days after injury. Pulmonary embolism occurs most commonly between 8 and 12 days after surgery. Autopsy examination of trauma patients who died of PE has shown that the median interval between injury and death was 10 days.[202] Approximately 5% of deaths that occur more than 1 week after blunt trauma are caused by PE.[66] The overall mortality rate of untreated PE ranges between 18 and 35%. With appropriate therapy this rate can be reduced to 5–8%.[6]

In over 85% of patients who develop PE, the sources of emboli are the deep veins of the thigh, including the popliteal, femoral, and iliac veins. In the remainder, the right heart, pelvic veins, and upper limb veins are the sources.[10] Mural thrombi can form in the right heart after myocardial contusion and subsequently produce PE.[201] Thrombosis of the internal jugular or subclavian veins is a frequent complication of pulmonary artery catheterization in critically ill patients.[31] How often these thrombi embolize and what their clinical significance is remain uncertain.[150a] Although numerically minor, these sites of origin above the iliofemoral system are important since they may be occult, cause recurrent emboli, and PE is not prevented by interruption of the inferior vena cava.

Twenty percent of calf vein thrombi propagate into the thigh veins, and 10 percent of these will cause PE with a mortality rate of approximately 10%.

The majority of patients with documented PE do not have clinical evidence of lower extremity DVT. Although PE may be asymptomatic,[214] it is more likely to produce signs and symptoms. However, these are often overlooked or misinterpreted because of their nonspecific nature. Fitts and associates[54] found PE during autopsies in 38% of patients who died after hip fracture. In the same study PE was listed as the primary cause of death in only 2% of patients on whom autopsy was not performed. Cardiovascular complications, such as acute myocardial infarction, were the most frequently listed causes of death in these patients, and it is likely that many of them had actually died of unsuspected PE. Pulmonary embolization should be suspected in injured patients who respond to the initial therapy, but subsequently develop signs of cardiovascular deterioration during convalescence.

## PATHOPHYSIOLOGY

Pulmonary embolization inevitably influences respiratory gas exchange. Arterial hypoxemia occurs in 90 to 100% of patients (Fig 28-4).[44,126,197] When $PaO_2$ is normal, the alveolar-arterial oxygen gradient is almost always increased. Hypocarbia secondary to hyperventilation also occurs in many patients during the acute stage.[197] The mechanism of hyperventilation after PE is not well understood. It cannot be entirely explained by hypoxic stimulation of chemoreceptors, alveolar J receptors, or lung irritant receptors.

FIG. 28-4. The $PaO_2$ values of 54 previously healthy patients with angiographically documented pulmonary embolism. (From Dantzker, Bower[44] with permission.)

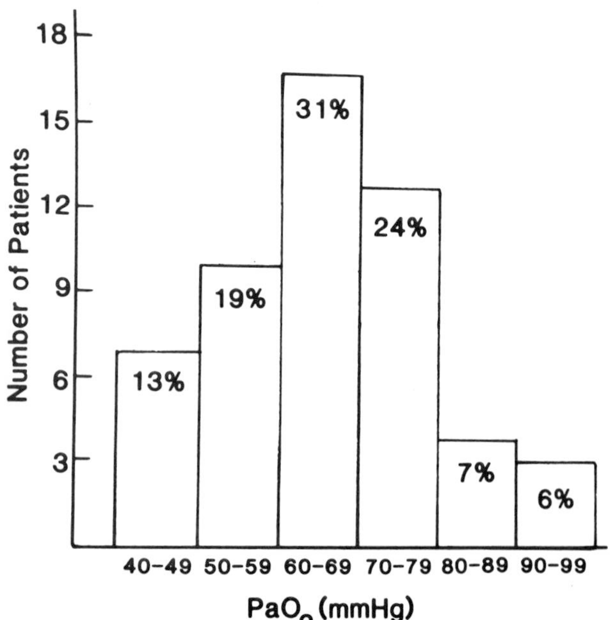


The possible causes of hypoxemia in PE may include hypercarbia, impairment of $O_2$ diffusion, ventilation-perfusion inequality, or intrapulmonary shunting. Hypercarbia does not seem to play a significant role in the development of hypoxemia during pulmonary embolization. Only a few patients with PE have a raised $PaCO_2$, which is probably related to increased dead space.[62]

A decreased $O_2$-diffusing capacity across the pulmonary membrane has been proposed as the mechanism of hypoxemia in acute PE.[167] Theoretically, PE can decrease the diffusing capacity of $O_2$ by decreasing the blood transit time through the reduced pulmonary vascular bed or by reducing the surface area of alveolar capillary membranes. However, even in the presence of massive PE, several studies have demonstrated that the measured $PaO_2$ values were similar to those predicted from the actual $\dot{V}/\dot{Q}$ distribution.[43,86] Thus, impairment of $O_2$ diffusion probably plays little role in the genesis of hypoxemia after PE.

Ventilation-perfusion ($\dot{V}/\dot{Q}$) mismatch has been shown to affect gas exchange in some patients with PE.[86,100] The size and location of the emboli determine how pulmonary blood flow is redistributed.[11,44] If a substantial portion of the right ventricular output flows through poorly ventilated regions of the lung, hypoxemia develops. Animal studies have demonstrated the presence of platelet aggregates on fresh pulmonary thrombi.[200] During degranulation, platelets release serotonin, histamine, catecholamines, prostaglandins, and other neurohumoral substances that cause bronchial smooth muscle constriction and pulmonary arterial vasoconstriction. This may produce not only a $\dot{V}/\dot{Q}$ mismatch but also contribute to the development of pulmonary hypertension.[72]

In some patients, intrapulmonary shunting may be the only causative factor of hypoxemia. D'Alonzo et al.[43] studied $\dot{V}/\dot{Q}$ mismatch and $\dot{Q}s/\dot{Q}t$ ratio in two patients with massive PE. According to these authors, increased intrapulmonary shunting was the only factor responsible for hypoxemia; $\dot{V}/\dot{Q}$ mismatch had little role. Several mechanisms are proposed for the increased $\dot{Q}s/\dot{Q}t$ ratio in PE: (a) the opening of pre-existing pulmonary arterial-venous shunts in response to pulmonary hypertension, (b) the re-establishment of perfusion to embolized areas where alveolar atelectasis may have developed secondary to decreased alveolar surfactant synthesis, and (c) the development of localized areas of pulmonary edema.[94,132] In patients with a patent foramen ovale, a right-to-left intracardiac shunt may also be a contributing factor, especially when acute cor pulmonale is present. A decreased mixed venous oxygen saturation augments arterial hypoxemia when a significant amount of $\dot{V}/\dot{Q}$ mismatch or a $\dot{Q}s/\dot{Q}t$ ratio greater than 0.2 is present.

The hemodynamic response to PE is influenced by the presence of pre-existing cardiopulmonary disease, the extent of embolic occlusion, and the effects of reflex and humoral factors. In previously healthy patients, obstruction of up to 25% of the pulmonary vasculature may be associated with no appreciable change in pulmonary artery pressure.[126] Embolic occlusion of greater than 50% of the pulmonary arterial bed may be necessary before the mean pulmonary artery pressure exceeds 25 mm Hg. When more than 75% of the pulmonary artery circulation is obstructed, the right ventricle must generate a systolic pressure $>$ 50 mm Hg and a mean pulmonary artery pressure > 40 mm Hg in order to maintain adequate pulmonary artery perfusion. These values are at the upper limits of pressures that can be generated by a healthy ventricle. Further embolization will result in right ventricular failure and a fall in cardiac output.[12,126] In a previously healthy patient with suspected pulmonary embolism, a mean pulmonary artery pressure of 30–40 mm Hg suggests severe pulmonary hypertension and massive embolic obstruction, but normal pressures by no means exclude the diagnosis.

In healthy patients the cardiac index is usually normal or increased after PE, probably because of hypoxia-mediated catecholamine secretion. A decrease in the cardiac index usually implies a massive embolus obstructing 40–50% or more of the pulmonary vasculature. Decreased cardiac index is usually associated with elevated pulmonary artery resistance and pressures.[126]

In patients with previous cardiopulmonary disease, there is no correlation between the pulmonary artery pressures and the extent of embolic obstruction. The mean pulmonary artery pressure for a group of such patients studied by McIntyre and Sasahara[127] was 40 mm Hg, a value not seen in patients without underlying cardiopulmonary disease.[127] The cardiac index was reduced by PE in these patients and appeared to be independent of both the magnitude of pulmonary vascular obstruction and the pulmonary artery pressure.

## CLINICAL MANIFESTATIONS

It is difficult to establish the diagnosis of PE on clinical grounds alone.[140,171] No single symptom, sign, or laboratory abnormality is pathognomonic of this potentially lethal condition. The physician who is treating seriously ill trauma victims should always maintain a high degree of suspicion so that diagnostic and therapeutic steps can be taken at the earliest opportunity. The common clinical symptoms and signs of PE include dyspnea, tachypnea, tachycardia, chest pain, apprehension, and hemoptysis. In traumatized patients, these findings may be present after chest or upper abdominal injuries, thus rendering the diagnosis of PE more difficult.[145] The sudden appearance of hypotension, fever, tachycardia, hemoptysis, rales, wheezing, and/or a pleural friction rub is suggestive of PE.

## DIAGNOSTIC TESTS

Diagnostic tests include arterial blood gas and pH measurements, blood enzyme determinations, chest radiograph, electrocardiogram (ECG), $\dot{V}/\dot{Q}$ lung scan, and pulmonary angiograms. Determinations of serum bilirubin, lactic dehydrogenase, and glutamic oxalic transaminase, originally reported to be useful for diagnosing PE,[210] have proven to be of only minimal value. Serial measurements of cardiac isoenzymes may facilitate the differentiation of PE from acute myocardial infarction. Fibrin split products have been used as a screening test to determine the presence of PE,[98] but this test may be too nonspecific to be useful.

As mentioned above, arterial hypoxemia is present in over 90% of patients with PE (Fig 28-4).[44,126,197] However, many conditions that mimic PE are also associated with hypoxemia. A normal $PaO_2$ does not exclude PE, especially in the case of small emboli. Massive emboli are almost always associated with severe hypoxemia.

$PaCO_2$ is usually normal or decreased in acute PE, except in patients with chronic obstructive pulmonary disease.[62,76] A widened arterial-to-end tidal $PCO_2$ gradient may be present because of increased dead-space ventilation.[75] In mechanically ventilated patients who develop PE, an increase in $PaCO_2$ and a concomitant decrease in $PetCO_2$ may occur.[123]

Roentgenographic findings include pleural effusion, pulmonary infiltrates and consolidation, plate-like atelectasis, elevation of the hemidiaphragm, dilated hilar branches of the pulmonary artery, enlarged right ventricle, and transient avascularity of the region of the lung distal to the embolism (Westermark's sign) (Fig 28-5). A wedge-shaped area of atelectasis may develop 24 hours after PE and usually disappears within 6 days. The chest roentgenogram may be normal in up to 40% of patients, including some with massive PE. The combination of a clear chest X-ray and severe dyspnea is thus quite suggestive of PE. Unfortunately, only bedside anterior-posterior films can be obtained in critically ill patients, which limits severely the usefulness of this diagnostic method.

The ECG is abnormal in the majority of patients with PE. Most patients demonstrate only sinus tachycardia and nonspecific ST-T wave changes. Occasionally, the sudden development of atrial fibrillation or flutter may be the first sign of PE.[99] The arrhythmias usually disappear within a few days.[191] Massive pulmonary artery occlusion may be associated with the classic picture of acute cor pulmonale: right axis deviation, a S1-Q3-T3 pattern, and occasionally an incomplete right bundle branch block. The ECG may be helpful in excluding myocardial infarction when PE presents with chest pain, syncope, heart block, or arrhythmia.

Perfusion lung scanning is a simple test that can be used in seriously ill or uncooperative patients. Technetium-99 labeled albumin microspheres are used in this examination. These microspheres transiently embolize fewer than 1% of the pulmonary capillaries without any known harmful effects. Imaging with a gamma scanner then demonstrates the distribution of pulmonary blood flow. The six-view perfusion scan is a sensitive test, and a normal result is deemed by many to virtually exclude PE.[130] However, many clinical conditions, such as chronic obstructive pulmonary disease and pneumonia, may cause perfusion defects. In addition, perfusion abnormalities similar in appearance to PE have been reported to occur in 5% of healthy subjects.[199] Thus, because of the poor specificity of perfusion scan, the diagnosis of PE cannot be definitively established by this test alone. Even when the clinical and lung scan findings strongly suggest the presence of PE, only 66% of patients have angiographically detectable clots in their pulmonary vasculature.[130] Thus, a normal scan usually rules out PE, but an abnormal scan by no means confirms the diagnosis.

The accuracy of a perfusion scan of the lung is enhanced when a simultaneous ventilation scan is obtained using a radioactive inert gas, such as $^{133}$Xenon. This procedure is performed by asking the patient to breath the gas from a closed system until equilibrium is obtained. Elimination of the gas from the lungs is measured for several minutes using surface scanning of the chest wall. The scan is considered to be normal if gas distribution is homogeneous throughout the lung

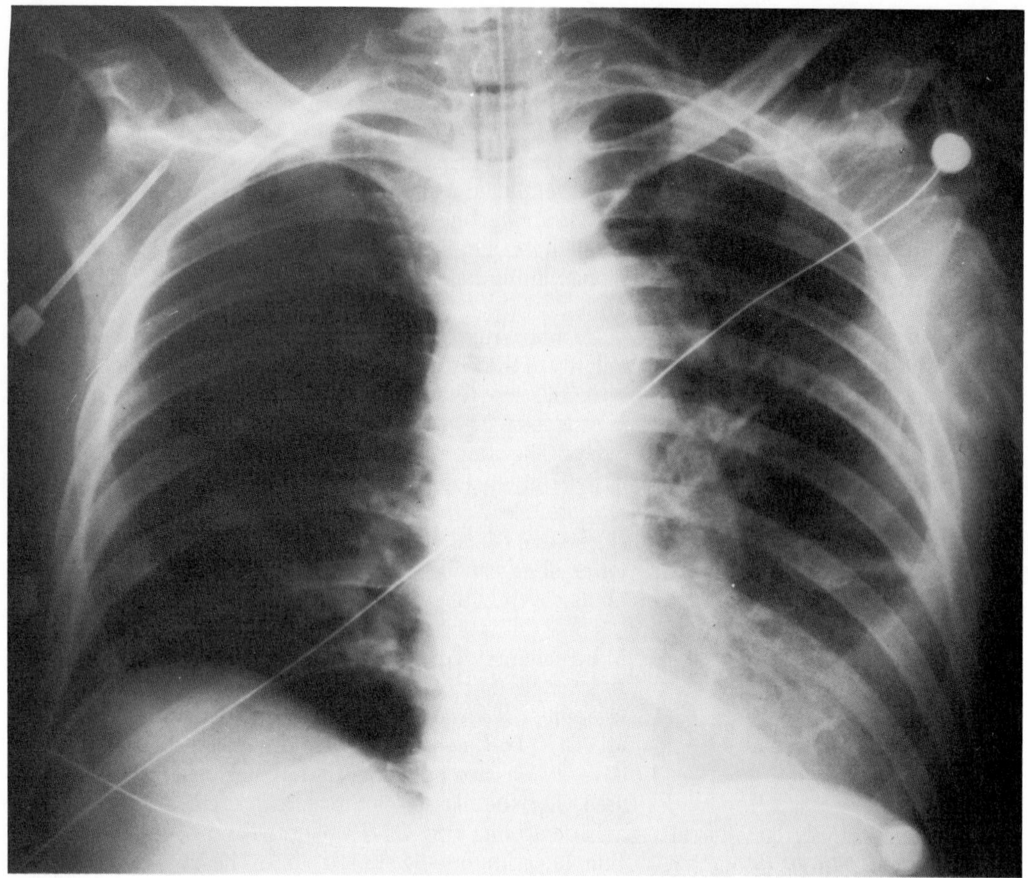

FIG. 28-5. Oligemia of the right lung (Westmark's sign). This patient had pulmonary emboli in the main right pulmonary artery documented by pulmonary angiography.

during both the first breath and the equilibrium phase and gas elimination is uniform. Unfortunately, the need for patient cooperation to obtain the ventilation scan limits somewhat the applicability of this test in critically ill trauma victims.

The classical ventilation-perfusion scan findings in PE are areas of perfusion defects with a normal ventilatory pattern (Fig 28-6). Such conditions as chronic obstructive lung disease produce both perfusion and ventilation defects. When perfusion defects involve two or more segments in the presence of a normal ventilation pattern, PE may be diagnosed with 85–90% accuracy (high-probability scan).[18,92,130] Nevertheless, it has been noted that patients with PE may have matching defects on both ventilation and perfusion scans.[18,89,92,166] The ventilatory abnormality is believed to be caused by bronchoconstriction or atelectasis in the embolized areas. Therefore, the presence of a combined ventilation and perfusion defect does not always rule out pulmonary embolism. In these circumstances, when there is a strong clinical suspicion of PE, a pulmonary angiogram should be obtained for accurate diagnosis.

Pulmonary angiography is the gold standard for diagnosing PE.[65] In most patients, the angiogram remains positive for more than a week following the embolic event, after which spontaneous clot lysis results in restoration of pulmonary blood flow. An angiogram should preferably be obtained within 24 to 72 hours after a PE is first suspected. A positive test shows intraluminal filling defects, vessel cutoffs, or both (Figs 28-7 and 28-8). The pulmonary angiogram may not detect small emboli. This, however, does not reduce the clinical value of the test because when the obstructed vessels are too small to be detected by pulmonary angiography, the patient will have little morbidity from the pulmonary embolism.[149]

Pulmonary angiography is an invasive test causing morbidity in 1–4% and mortality in approximately 0.1% of patients.[134] The presence of cor pulmonale or right ventricular end-diastolic pressures in excess of 20 mm Hg may be associated with increased mortality from this test.[134] However, the complication rates of anticoagulant therapy are greater than those of pulmonary angiography.[8,159] Therefore, pulmonary angiography is recommended for determining the need for anticoagulant therapy in pulmonary thromboembolism.[32]

Heparin treatment of PE may be associated with serious complications.[159] Cheely and associates[32] reported a 30% incidence of hemorrhage and 2% incidence of death associated with anticoagulant therapy of thromboembolic disease. However, in nontraumatized patients whose risk of bleeding is minimal, anticoagulant therapy can be initiated solely on the basis of a highly abnormal $\dot{V}/\dot{Q}$ scan without the need for a pulmonary angiogram. In these patients, the presence of a leg

**PERFUSION** **VENTILATION**

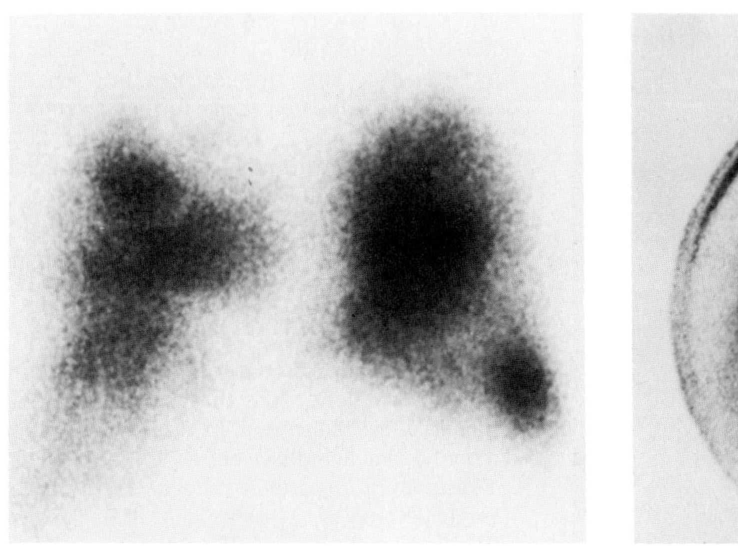

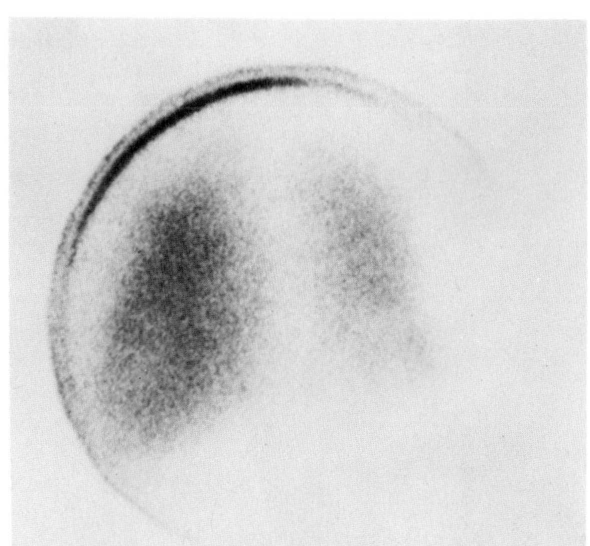

FIG. 28-6. Multiple segmental perfusion defects with normal ventilation. This finding is very suggestive of pulmonary embolism.

FIG. 28-7. Small perfusion defect in the right upper lobe with normal ventilation in a patient with a clinical picture that is highly suggestive of pulmonary embolism.

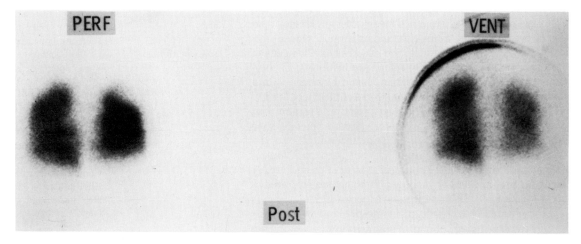

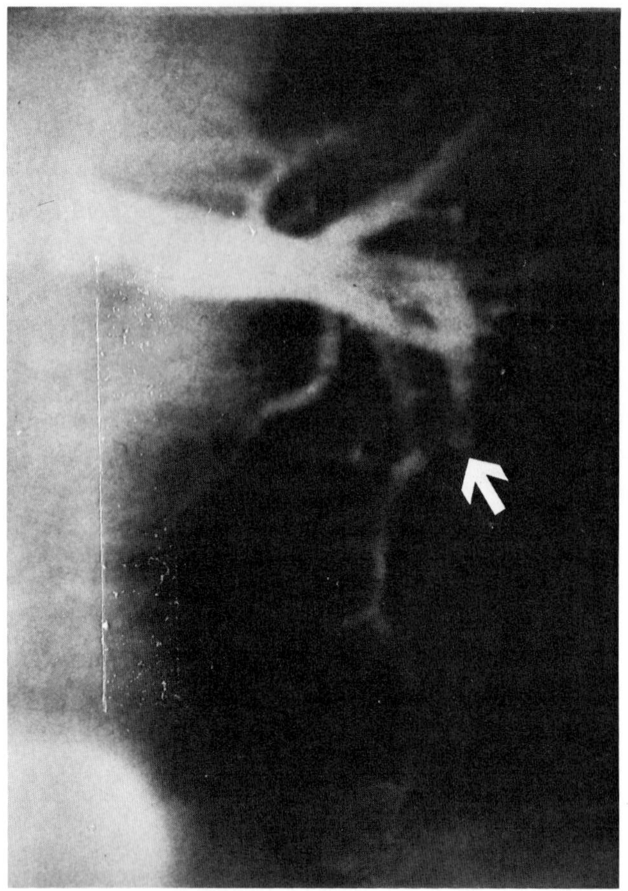

FIG. 28-8. Pulmonary angiogram from the patient with a small perfusion defect shown in Figure 7, demonstrating vessel cutoffs in the right upper lobe.

vein thrombus demonstrated either by venography or impedance plethysmography may further indicate anticoagulation.[89]

Obviously, the risk of anticoagulant-therapy-induced bleeding is increased in patients with recent accidental or surgical trauma. In addition, the options for treating PE in these patients may be limited to invasive and/or surgical procedures. Thus, in most trauma patients the diagnosis of PE needs to be confirmed by angiography before the institution of therapy.[8,10,124] A pulmonary angiogram should be obtained in a trauma patient when (a) PE is suspected clinically but the $\dot{V}/\dot{Q}$ scan is inconclusive; (b) PE is suspected in a patient with pre-existing pulmonary parenchymal disease or congestive heart failure, which renders a $\dot{V}/\dot{Q}$ scan unrewarding; (c) the $\dot{V}/\dot{Q}$ scan is highly suggestive of PE, but the risk of anticoagulation is high because of a recent trauma or surgery; or (d) a surgical or invasive procedure is being contemplated to treat a presumed PE in patients in whom anticoagulation is contraindicated or when PE recurs despite anticoagulation.

Intravenous digital subtraction pulmonary angiography has recently been used to diagnose PE. This method has the advantage (compared to conventional pulmonary angiography) that the dye may be injected into a peripheral vein rather than the pulmonary artery. Although some feel that this technique is as accurate as conventional pulmonary angiography in 85–90% of patients, others conclude that it is not a useful substitute.[65,158] Conventional pulmonary angiography remains the procedure of choice for diagnosing PE.

## TREATMENT

### *Anticoagulant Therapy*

Barrett and Jordon[6] reported that heparin-treated patients with PE had a lower mortality rate (6%) than those who were not anticoagulated (26%). In selected patients, when the diagnosis of PE is strongly suspected, intravenous heparinization should be initiated while further diagnostic evaluation proceeds (Table 28-3). Doing so helps protect the patient against progressive thrombus formation and recurrent embolism, even though heparin does not cause the dissolution of a thromboembolus that is already present. Heparin works by combining with antithrombin III, a circulating anticoagulant protein produced in the liver. This complex rapidly neutralizes the proteolytic actions of activated serine protease clotting factors. The rate of the clotting reaction decreases, and less thrombin becomes available for fibrin formation. Heparin has other actions that may contribute to its antithrombotic effect: adherence to vascular endothelium and reduction of platelet adhesiveness.[155]

Sensitivity to heparin is influenced by the activity of the thrombotic process. A higher dose of heparin is required to achieve a therapeutic APTT in patients with proximal symptomatic DVT and PE because a greater concentration of activated clotting factors is present than is found in patients with smaller peripheral thrombi. The half-life of heparin is also shorter in patients with acute PE than in those with DVT.[84,188] Patients with PE may therefore require larger amounts of heparin during the first 24 hours of therapy. An initial intravenous

TABLE 28-3. Guidelines for Antithrombotic Therapy with Heparin and Warfarin in Venous Thromboembolism

| | |
|---|---|
| Disease suspected | Measure baseline APTT, PT, and platelet count and give heparin bolus (10,000 units) IV. Order diagnostic test, eg, $\dot{V}/\dot{Q}$ scan, pulmonary angiogram, venogram. |
| Disease confirmed | Give additional dose of heparin (5,000 units) and start IV infusion at 1,000 units/h. Monitor APTT at 4- to 6-hour intervals until it is stabilized at between 1.5 and 2.0 times control value. Monitor platelet count while administering heparin. Start oral warfarin by day 2 or 3 with 10 mg followed by a daily maintenance dose (2.5–10 mg). Continue heparin for at least 7–10 days. After at least 4–5 days of joint therapy, stop heparin and check PT 4 hours later. Maintain PT off heparin at 1.2 to 1.5 times control or pretreatment value (using rabbit brain thromboplastin). Continue full-dose anticoagulation for at least 3 months in patients without continuing risk factors and longer in other patients |

dose of 15,000–20,000 units should be administered. A dose of this magnitude is necessary to minimize thrombin-platelet interaction and prevent degranulation of platelets, which releases many neurohumoral substances. For maintenance, an infusion of 1,000–1,200 units heparin per hour may be given, or intermittent intravenous injections of 5,000 units every 4 hours may be administered. In patients with massive PE the maintenance dose may be increased to 10,000 units every 4 hours. The risk of bleeding can be decreased by reducing the total dose of heparin to 20,000–25,000 units per day after the first 48 hours. Pulmonary embolism can also be treated with subcutaneous injections of heparin.[48] An initial dose of 15,000 units is followed by subcutaneous injections every 12 hours, with the dose adjusted to maintain the APTT at 50–70 seconds.[48]

Thrombocytopenia may develop in up to 30% of patients receiving heparin. It is usually mild and transient, has no clinical consequence, and improves with continued heparin administration.[113] The mechanism appears to be related to a heparin-induced release of ADP that produces reversible platelet aggregation, margination, and peripheral sequestration.

A severe, immunologically mediated form of heparin-associated thrombocytopenia occurs in 0.6–10% of patients receiving heparin.[113] Heparin combines with a component of the platelet membrane to form a hapten that stimulates the production of platelet membrane antibodies.[187] Seven to 14 days after initiation of heparin therapy, thrombocytopenia develops along with arterial thrombosis and hemorrhagic phenomena. Thus the platelet count must be measured before the initiation of therapy, daily for the first 2 days, and then once every 2 or 3 days in any patient receiving heparin. Unless the agent is discontinued, a mortality of 18–36% may result, along with significant morbidity in 22–61% of patients.[113,187] If heparin must be discontinued, alternate forms of anticoagulation should be used.[187]

Continuous intravenous infusion of heparin has been used widely for the treatment of PE. Although the risk of recurrent emboli may be slightly greater with this approach, the risk of bleeding may be less than that seen with intermittent injections.[174] Therefore, continuous infusion is preferable in a trauma patient who develops PE in the immediate postoperative period. Activated partial thromboplastin time (APTT) or activated clotting time should be measured several times during the first day of therapy until the desired therapeutic level has been achieved.[93] These measurements may be performed once daily on subsequent days. The APTT should be maintained between 1.5 and 2 times control.[93] Monitoring of the APTT does not decrease the risk of untoward bleeding, but does ensure the adequacy of anticoagulation.

Therapy with heparin is continued for 7–10 days during which time deep venous thrombi undergo resolution or organization. If the risk of a recurrence of PE is high, anticoagulation must be continued until the risk factors no longer exist. Oral coumarin derivatives, such as warfarin, are frequently used for long-term prophylaxis in such patients. For patients with postoperative PE, a 6-week to 6-month course of warfarin therapy is adequate.

After the initiation of warfarin treatment, complete anticoagulant protection is delayed for several days while vitamin K stores and the normal vitamin K-dependent clotting factors are eliminated and subsequently replaced by biologically inactive substances. Since factor VII has the shortest biologic half-life, its depletion results in prolongation of the prothrombin time. However, since this factor is of minor importance in the pathogenesis of DVT, the patient is not yet protected.[155] By the fourth day of warfarin therapy, factors IX and X have been depleted, and the patient is adequately anticoagulated (Table 28-4). Therefore, heparin should be continued for at least 4 days after the initiation of warfarin treatment.[9,10] There may be an increased risk of thrombosis in the first day or two of warfarin use because of the depletion of protein C, a vitamin K-dependent factor with anticoagulant properties and a half-life of 4–6 hours.[155,208] Overlapping heparin and warfarin therapy should minimize this risk. An initial warfarin dose of 10 mg orally followed by daily doses of 5 mg for the next 3 days is the usual regimen. Subsequent doses should be adjusted according to the prothrombin time, which is maintained at 1.2 to 1.5 times the control measurement.[83,85] The optimal time interval between the initiation of heparin therapy and the first dose of warfarin has not been clearly defined. Nevertheless, beginning warfarin administration early in the course of treatment of PE and DVT can decrease the length of hospitalization without adverse effects on efficacy or

TABLE 28-4. Antithrombin Therapy*

| AGENT | MECHANISM OF ACTION | ONSET OF ACTION | APPLICATION | ROUTE OF ADMINISTRATION |
|---|---|---|---|---|
| Heparin 25–35,000 units/day | Prevents extension of established venous thromboembolism by inhibiting thrombin activity via the cofactor antithrombin III | Immediate | Treatment of established DVT or PE | IV |
| Heparin 10–15,000 units/day | Prevents formation of venous thrombi by inhibiting factor Xa activity via the cofactor antithrombin III | Immediate | Prevention of DVT in selected postoperative and other high-risk patients | Subcutaneous |
| Warfarin | Inhibition of synthesis of the vitamin K dependent coagulation factors (II, VII, IX, X) | 4–5 days | Prevention of DVT<br>Long-term treatment of established disease | Oral |
| Pneumatic Leg compression | Prevents venous stasis<br>Activates fibrinolytic system | Immediate | Prevention of DVT in high-risk patient | Local application |

* Adapted from Hyers[93] with permission.

safety.[170] Warfarin interacts with many drugs, and thus it is more difficult to regulate than heparin (Table 28-2). Several aspects of antithrombin therapy are summarized in Table 28-4.

The thrombolytic agents, streptokinase and urokinase, activate the intrinsic fibrinolytic system by converting the normally present proenzyme plasminogen to plasmin,[209] resulting in systemic fibrinolysis. These agents are infused for 24 hours after the onset of PE and are followed by a course of heparin therapy. They produce faster resolution of PE and greater hemodynamic improvement at 24 hours after the initiation of therapy than does heparin alone.[209] However, they do not reduce the mortality from PE when compared to heparin therapy. The fibrinolytic agents are rarely used in patients with a history of recent trauma. The best indication for fibrinolytic therapy is thought to be an acute massive PE causing severe cardiovascular instability. In these instances it is felt that the rate of spontaneous clot resolution may not be fast enough to restore pulmonary blood flow to a degree compatible with survival. Fibrinolytic therapy is an alternative to surgical embolectomy.

Tissue-type plasminogen activator has recently been used in the treatment of acute massive PE.[207] This thrombolytic agent has relative fibrin specificity and usually does not produce systemic fibrinolysis. However, 4 of 11 patients who received this agent an average of 7.5 days after surgery required transfusion of two or more units of blood for puncture site or operative site bleeding.[207] Patients with recent trauma should not receive tissue-type plasminogen activator, although data are not available to determine at what point after traumatic injury thrombolytic therapy is safe to use.

Animal experiments have demonstrated a synergistic effect of heparin with low doses of streptokinase that may result from heparin's ability to retard further fibrin deposition in emboli while the streptokinase produces clot lysis.[29] A preliminary clinical trial evaluated the efficacy of low-dose streptokinase administered directly into the pulmonary artery combined with full doses of systemic heparin as treatment for massive acute PE.[114] Five of the seven patients demonstrated significant clot lysis within 12 to 24 hours of initiation of therapy. Unfortunately, despite infusion of the thrombolytic agent locally and in low doses, a systemic lytic state developed in all patients, and major hemorrhagic complications occurred in two. This regimen therefore cannot be recommended for the recently traumatized patient.

Bleeding is the major complication of fibrinolytic therapy, and in the patient with a recent traumatic injury the risk of hemorrhage is unacceptably high. Active bleeding is an absolute contraindication to the use of these agents. Other contraindications include surgery within the previous 10 days, recent trauma with possible internal injuries, recent external cardiac massage, percutaneous organ biopsies within the preceding 14 days, gastrointestinal ulcerative disease, and a recent cerebrovascular accident, such as an infarction or hemorrhage.[9]

### *Surgical Approaches*

Surgical intervention in pulmonary embolism can be divided into two broad categories: maneuvers designed to prevent further embolization of thrombi to the lungs and procedures to remove clots that are already present in the pulmonary vascular bed. Inferior vena cava interruption prevents transport of thrombi from the deep veins of the legs to the lungs. It is most frequently used in patients in whom anticoagulant therapy is contraindicated or has failed.[68] Techniques for achieving vena cava interruption include surgical ligation or plication with clips and placement of intraluminal filters, such as a vena caval umbrella. Ligation or plication of the vena cava are associated with significant morbidity and mortality. Therefore, these methods have been replaced by percutaneously placed intraluminal devices, such as the Greenfield filter.[68] Unfortunately, randomized trials comparing the efficacy of vena caval clipping to transvenous filter placement are not available.[63] Recurrent embolic incidents are uncommon after placement of a Greenfield filter. Published data on 289 patients disclosed only seven cases of PE after filter insertion (2.4%).[106] Long-term vena caval patency was found in 97%.[106] Complications are infrequent with use of the Greenfield filter. In a series of 198 filter placements in 193 patients, major complications occurred in 4.1% and death due to recurrent PE in 0.5%.[30] Reported complications include filter migration, caval perforation producing retroperitoneal hematoma, incorrect filter position, leg edema, and thrombosis of the inferior vena cava.[30,106]

Pulmonary embolectomy has been reserved for patients with life-threatening embolism. The mortality rate associated with this procedure is usually greater than 50%.[3,35] although with prompt diagnosis and better patient selection mortality rates as low as 23% have been reported.[203] It may be indicated when massive embolism is complicated by cardiopulmonary arrest or in the rare patient who is in circulatory shock after PE and has an absolute contraindication to anticoagulation or fails to improve after 1 hour of nonoperative management.[122] It is not at all clear whether pulmonary embolectomy improves the final outcome when compared to thrombolytic therapy with inotropic support of cardiac function. The majority of patients who die of a massive embolism do so within 1 hour of the event.[61] Thus, in most instances surgery may not be feasible. The use of cardiopulmonary bypass during surgery and the absence of preoperative cardiac arrest are two important factors improving the survival rate from this procedure.[122,133]

A transvenous approach for pulmonary embolectomy has been developed. In this method, a steerable suction catheter is introduced into the femoral vein and advanced to the site of angiographically demonstrated clots under fluoroscopy.[68,192] Greenfield reported a 73% survival rate in 15 critically ill patients who were treated with transvenous embolectomy combined with placement of a Greenfield filter.[69]

### *Supportive Measures and Prognosis*

The initial treatment of PE is aimed at maintaining tissue oxygenation. Thus, the patient should be given supplemental oxygen. Endotracheal intubation and mechanical ventilation are necessary in many patients. Intravenous fluids should be used to maintain right ventricular preload and thus right ventricular output. If circulatory shock or acute cor pulmonale is evident, dopamine, dobutamine, or other inotropic agents may be used to maintain blood pressure and cardiac output.[97] If cardiac arrest occurs, closed chest cardiac massage should be initiated, which may actually fragment an occlusive proximal clot and move it more peripherally to effect a small but critical reduction in right ventricular afterload and restore circulation.

The long-term prognosis of a single episode of PE in previously healthy patients is good. An average 3-year survival rate in excess of 80% has been reported.[153] Chronic pulmonary hypertension rarely develops in such patients,[165] and complete or partial resolution of the emboli usually occurs in the course of time.[153] In contrast, the long-term prognosis of PE in patients with pre-existing heart disease is associated with an average 3-year survival rate of only approximately 18%.[153] Death, however is rarely due to the long-term effects of PE (chronic cor pulmonale with right ventricular failure). The most frequent causes of death are myocardial infarction and congestive heart failure.[153]

## ANESTHETIC CONSIDERATIONS

Trauma victims scheduled for delayed or repeated surgery during their hospitalization are likely to have asymptomatic DVT. Pulmonary embolism may thus occur in these patients during the perioperative period. Operative manipulation of the lower extremity appears to be an important factor in initiating this event. The application of an Esmarch bandage for limb exsanguination,[51,157] inflation of a pneumatic tourniquet on the thigh,[178] elevation of the leg for surgical preparation,[16] and closed reduction of lower extremity fractures[25] have all been described as precipitating sudden pulmonary embolism. These case reports emphasize the importance of assessing patients for the presence of DVT before delayed surgery, especially for procedures involving the lower extremity and pelvis.

The clinical manifestations of intraoperative PE are dependent upon the anesthetic technique. When a regional anesthetic technique is employed, the classical signs and symptoms of PE, including sudden onset of respiratory distress, hyperventilation, and pleuritic chest pain, can be observed.[16,178] During general anesthesia and controlled ventilation, the recognition of PE may be difficult. Under these conditions tachypnea, dyspnea, or chest pain cannot be present. The diagnosis is then based on clinical signs produced by circulatory obstruction and the sympathomimetic response to the PE.

Knowledge of the immediate hemodynamic and respiratory changes of PE in anesthetized patients is based on a few anecdotal reports.[25,46,67,77,121,123,135] In patients monitored with routine techniques, sudden tachycardia and hypotension are the most common clinical findings. In severe cases, tachycardia is followed shortly by bradycardia, electromechanical dissociation, and cardiac arrest.[25,77] Occasionally, cyanosis, ashen gray discoloration of the skin, and jugular venous distension may be observed.[135] If a pulse oximeter is in place, decreased $O_2$ saturation may be noted, especially if $FIO_2$ is in the range of 0.33–0.50. Arterial blood gas measurements reveal hypoxemia or widened A-a $DO_2$, and acidosis is present in almost all patients who develop massive intraoperative PE.[46,77,121] Hypercarbia may occur in some patients, requiring an increase in minute ventilation.[121] In addition, a reduced $CO_2$ concentration in nonperfused alveoli lowers the $CO_2$ concentration in the mixed expired air and results in an increased arterial-to-end tidal $pCO_2$ gradient.[123]

A sudden increase in airway resistance and inspiratory pressures, wheezing, rales, and rhonchi may be clues for diagnosing intraoperative PE.[46,123] However, these signs are not present in all patients.[121] The increased airway resistance is produced by bronchoconstriction, which is caused either by liberation of serotonin from the thrombus or regional hypocapnia in the area of pulmonary vascular occlusion.

If the patient is monitored with CVP, pulmonary artery, and intra-arterial catheters, additional hemodynamic changes may be observed. CVP increases when acute cor pulmonale is produced by PE.[121] However, this may not occur in hemorrhaging or hypovolemic patients.[77] Both systolic and diastolic pulmonary artery pressures increase if the cross-sectional area of the pulmonary arterial bed is reduced by 40% or more.[121,126] Left ventricular function may also be altered in PE. Distension of the right ventricle results in an interventricular septal shift, which encroaches upon the left ventricle and reduces its size.[120,143,193] Thus, an elevated pulmonary artery wedge pressure should be expected. However, caution should be exercised in interpretation of pulmonary artery wedge pressure in massive PE because the pressure measured in an occluded pulmonary vascular zone may not reflect the actual left ventricular end-diastolic pressure.[27,161] Cardiac output is decreased in massive PE; in the presence of hypoxemia this compromises tissue oxygenation. Thus, therapeutic measures should be aimed at improving tissue oxygenation by optimizing both cardiac output and $PaO_2$.

The above clinical signs are not unique for PE, and they may be produced by a variety of conditions in anesthetized patients: hypoventilation, endobronchial intubation, pneumothorax, pulmonary edema, aspiration pneumonitis, air embolus, and administration of vasoconstrictor agents. Thus, a rapid differential diagnosis is necessary before institution of therapeutic measures for PE.

Immediate treatment of intraoperative PE includes increasing $FIO_2$ to 1.0, discontinuation of inhalational anesthetic agents, infusion of fluids, and administration of inotropic agents. Heparin anticoagulation may be initiated at this stage. Closed or open chest cardiac massage in conjunction with other ACLS (Advanced Cardiac Life Support) maneuvers should be started immediately if cardiac arrest occurs. Invasive therapeutic measures, such as emergency pulmonary embolectomy after occlusion of the inferior and superior venae cavae, may be considered.[35,61,77] However, as discussed above, pulmonary embolectomy may be more successful if combined vena cava occlusion and cardiopulmonary bypass are used.[122,133]

Patients who have had a recent PE may require surgery for various conditions related or unrelated to the PE. The extent of monitoring depends upon the cardiovascular and respiratory status of the patient and the type of surgery and anesthesia required. In critically ill patients, an indwelling arterial cannula and a pulmonary artery catheter should be used to monitor blood gases, systemic and pulmonary artery pressures, CVP, and cardiac output. Oxygenation parameters, including blood lactate level, $S\bar{v}O_2$, $\dot{D}O_2$, $\dot{V}O_2$, and tissue oxygen extraction ratio, must be monitored repeatedly to ensure adequate tissue oxygenation. Hypoxemia may be caused by $\dot{V}/\dot{Q}$ mismatch or increased $\dot{Q}S/\dot{Q}T$. Although increasing the $FIO_2$ improves hypoxemia caused by $\dot{V}/\dot{Q}$ mismatch, PEEP therapy is needed in patients with increased $\dot{Q}S/\dot{Q}T$. Invasive monitoring of hemodynamic and oxygenation parameters will simplify the anesthetic management and help in titrating PEEP therapy. A high central venous pressure may be needed to maintain left-sided preload at normal levels as assessed by the pulmonary artery wedge pressure.

Inotropic agents should be available for immediate use during the anesthetic management of the patients with PE. An abrupt increase in pulmonary vascular resistance caused by PE may result in right ventricular failure. Consequently, right ventricular contractility must be augmented pharmacologically to sustain cardiac output. Although isoproterenol improves the contractility of the overloaded right ventricle and has the theoretical advantage of being a pulmonary vasodilator, its chronotropic and arrhythmogenic properties make it an undesirable drug.[96,125] Dobutamine and dopamine are useful alternatives to isoproterenol.[24,97] The doses of these drugs (3–15 μg/kg/min) should be adjusted according to the cardiovascular response. Vasodilators may decrease pulmonary vascular resistance and increase right ventricular ejection. Nitroglycerine appears to be more effective than nitroprusside in patients with pulmonary hypertension.[154]

Patients with recent PE are likely to have pulmonary hypertension with an accompanying increased pulmonary vascular resistance. An increase in right ventricular volume maintains blood flow through the lungs in these patients. However, the right ventricle has only a limited reserve and may easily fail following an additional increase in pulmonary vascular resistance (PVR) or a decrease in myocardial contractility. Thus, factors that augment PVR or cause significant myocardial depression should be avoided during the anesthetic management of patients with PE. Hypoxemia, hypercarbia, acidosis, and alterations in functional residual capacity of the lung increase PVR. Likewise, most anesthetic agents depress the myocardium in a dose-dependent fashion, and some produce pulmonary vasoconstriction.

Another important consideration is the preservation of residual hypoxic pulmonary vasoconstriction (HPV). Experimental data suggest that postembolic hypoxemia is at least partly due to depression of HPV caused by pulmonary hypertension.[53] Since in many patients pulmonary hypertension subsides after the acute episode of PE, it is likely that a concomitant return of HPV also takes place. Thus, depression of the residual HPV during anesthetic management of these patients may result in hypoxemia.

Local anesthesia should be used whenever possible. Placement of inferior vena cava filters can be performed easily with this anesthetic technique. When general anesthesia is required, induction can be accomplished with benzodiazepines.[118] In healthy patients, diazepam causes either no change or a mild decrease in systemic and pulmonary hemodynamics.[55] The cardiovascular effects of this drug in the presence of a recent pulmonary embolism are not known, but similar effects would be expected. Midazolam has a greater negative inotropic and capacitance vessel dilating effect than diazepam, causing a greater decrease in mean arterial pressure.[164] Thiopental is a direct myocardial depressant and causes dilation of capacitance vessels.[55] Thus, it may result in significant hypotension in patients with recent PE, unless it is used in small titrated doses. Ketamine increases the pulmonary vascular resistance, resulting in a secondary increase in right heart work.[64] A transient increase in intrapulmonary shunting may also occur with this agent.[64] Thus, it should not be used in patients with recent PE and compromised right ventricular function. Etomidate is associated with minimal cardiovascular changes.[55] Only a slight reduction in mean arterial pressure and an increase in pulmonary vascular resistance, without an increase in right ventricular work, have been noted with etomidate in patients with aortic and mitral valve disease.[37] However, adrenaocortical depression caused by this agent reduces the stress response to surgery, making it less desirable than diazepam.[56,211]

Anesthesia should be maintained with agents that cause minimal myocardial depression, ie, narcotics. In addition, these agents do not cause pulmonary hypertension or depression of HPV. All inhalational agents produce a dose-dependent depression of myocardial contractility and HPV.[19–21,49,196] Blunting of HPV may result in increased $\dot{V}/\dot{Q}$ mismatch and subsequent reduction of $PaO_2$. Although isoflurane (1 MAC) is shown to depress HPV only minimally and cause a negligible reduction in $PaO_2$,[168,173] direct inhibition of HPV by this agent has been demonstrated experimentally.[47] Isoflurane should be used in small concentrations and $PaO_2$ monitored periodically. Nitrous oxide, barbiturates, and narcotics do not blunt HPV.[19] However, nitrous oxide may increase pulmonary vascular resistance in patients with pre-existing pulmonary hypertension.[79] The magnitude of this increase appears to be related to the baseline pulmonary vascular resistance. The greater the initial pulmonary vascular resistance, the greater the increase with nitrous oxide.[179] Patients with PE may maintain high pulmonary vascular resistance for several days and may thus be adversely affected by nitrous oxide. In addition, this agent may not permit the use of a high $FIO_2$, which is frequently needed in patients with recent PE.

On rare occasions, patients with massive PE require emergency pulmonary embolectomy. These patients arrive in the operating room intubated and ventilated with $O_2$ and varying levels of PEEP. All cardiopulmonary supportive measures must be continued during transportation of these patients. The extracorporeal circulation system must be ready before incision, and inotropic agents (dopamine and dobutamine) and pulmonary vasodilators (nitroglycerine) must be available during the entire perioperative period. The majority of these patients will require only $O_2$, muscle relaxants, and small doses of fentanyl. Potent inhalational agents, nitrous oxide, and ketamine are absolutely contraindicated as the patient is dependent on increased vascular tone to maintain circulation. Right and left ventricular function should be monitored during the perioperative period; acute cor pulmonale is commonly present, resulting in right ventricular dilation and, as discussed earlier, left ventricular dysfunction.[84,120,143] Positive pressure ventilation should be maintained throughout the procedure to optimize arterial oxygenation. It may also facilitate the removal of embolic fragments from the distal pulmonary artery by increasing the resistance of small pulmonary vessels, thereby moving the thrombus proximally. After closure of the chest, surgical interruption of the inferior vena cava should be considered to prevent further embolization of blood clots from the peripheral veins.

The patient with PE or DVT who presents for surgery may be on anticoagulant therapy.[107] The effects of warfarin can be reversed with vitamin $K_1$ (10–15 mg subcutaneously) or fresh-frozen plasma. Heparin should be discontinued 6 hours before surgery and APTT checked 1 hour before the surgery to ensure an adequate reversal of the anticoagulant effect. In urgent situations protamine sulfate (0.5–1.0 mg/kg IV) may be administered to correct the coagulation abnormality. Although data are not available, it seems reasonable to place an inferior vena cava filter before surgery in patients who have been treated for DVT of the legs (with or without PE) for less than 4 days. Doing so should provide protection against perioperative PE. In patients who have been treated with an anticoagulant for more than 2 weeks, the risk of embolization of a leg vein thrombus is minimal, and placement of a filter is probably unnecessary. Clinical judgment must be used when deciding whether patients who have been treated for DVT for less than 2 weeks should receive a filter before surgery. Heparin should be restarted 24 to 48 hours after surgery.

Regional anesthesia should not be administered to patients already receiving anticoagulant therapy.[50,163] Controversy still exists regarding whether epidural or subarachnoid catheters can be inserted in patients before anticoagulation therapy is initiated. There are anecdotal reports describing epidural hematomas in patients anticoagulated after placement of an epidural catheter.[45,60,206] However, large clinical trials have demonstrated that epidural hematoma does not occur in these circumstances if the epidural vessels are not injured during insertion of the needle or catheter.[50,163] Patients who are anticoagulated after lumbar puncture may be at risk of developing extraparenchymal spinal hematoma.[151,172] This risk can be decreased by delaying anticoagulation for at least 1 hour after subarachnoid puncture.[172] A limited number of clinical trials also demonstrated that hemorrhagic complications do not occur after spinal or epidural anesthesia in patients receiving dextran 70 or the combination of heparin and dihydroergotamine (DHE) for prophylaxis of DVT.[1]

Neurologic complications have not been reported after epidural or spinal anesthesia in patients receiving low-dose heparin, but data are not available to document the safety or risk of this approach.[151] Since the anticoagulant response to heparin is unpredictable, therapeutic rather than prophylactic blood levels of heparin can be present after 5,000 units of heparin subcutaneously.[38] Therefore, a conservative approach would be to avoid epidural and spinal anesthesia in patients receiving low-dose heparin.

## CONCLUSION

Thromboembolic complications occur frequently in the traumatized patient. Hypercoagulable blood, immobilization, and venous stasis, which are commonly present in these patients, contribute greatly to the development of deep venous thrombosis (DVT) and pulmonary embolism (PE). Although the pathogenesis and clinical manifestations of these two disorders are different, they are traditionally discussed together because PE is usually a complication of lower extremity DVT.

Venography remains the gold standard for the definitive diagnosis of DVT; however, in the majority of patients noninvasive tests, including impedance plethysmography and Doppler ultrasonography, especially when serial determinations are made, can reliably detect thrombi in the proximal leg veins. DVT may be prevented by pharmacologic and mechanical methods. Low-dose heparin and warfarin are effective prophylactic measures, but they should be used in the trauma patient only after complete hemostasis has been achieved, the coagulation profile is corrected, and potential sites of occult blood loss have been evaluated thoroughly. If used, anticoagulant therapy should continue until the patient is ambulatory. Prophylaxis with anticoagulant agents should not be attempted in head-injured patients; serious bleeding complications may occur. Pneumatic compression boots are effective in preventing DVT formation in most injured patients. DVT is best treated by full-dose anticoagulant therapy unless a contraindication to its use exists. Percutaneous insertion of a inferior vena cava filter should be considered when the potential for bleeding complications precludes the use of anticoagulants.

Pulmonary embolism results in nonspecific symptoms, necessitating the use of radiologic methods for definitive diagnosis. Although a normal perfusion lung scan excludes the possibility of PE, an abnormal scan cannot confirm the diagnosis. An abnormal perfusion scan in multiple lung segments, together with a normal ventilation scan, is highly suggestive but not diagnostic of PE. When both ventilation and perfusion scans of corresponding lung segments are abnormal, there is a low probability of PE. In these circumstances when the clinical suspicion is high, a pulmonary angiogram should be obtained to establish a definitive diagnosis. Although pulmonary angiography is associated with some morbidity, this risk is certainly less than that caused by the therapeutic modalities used for PE. Thus, pulmonary angiography should be obtained to confirm the diagnosis, especially in recently injured patients. Anticoagulant therapy causes a substantial decrease in mortality from PE. If anticoagulants cannot be used, an inferior vena cava filter should be placed to prevent further embolization. Pulmonary embolectomy may be indicated in patients with documented PE associated with cardiac arrest or continued hemodynamic deterioration despite the use of inotropic support and anticoagulants. The thrombolytic agents (streptokinase and urokinase) cause significant bleeding and thus should not be used in the trauma patient.

During anesthetic management of patients with recent PE, myocardial depression, increase in pulmonary vascular resistance, and blunting of hypoxic pulmonary vasoconstriction should be avoided. Serial monitoring of hemodynamic and oxygenation parameters allow for the adequate titration of fluids, anesthetics, inotropes, and vasodilator agents.

## REFERENCES

1. Allemann BH, Gerber H, Gruber UF. Spinal and epidural anesthesia in the presence of s.c. heparin-dihydroergotamine for prevention of thromboembolic complications. Anaesthesist 1983;32:80.

2. Allenby F, Pflug JJ, Boardman L, et al. Effects of external pneumatic intermittent compression on fibrinolysis in man. Lancet 1973;2:1412.
3. Alpert JS, Smith RE, Ockene IS, et al. Treatment of massive pulmonary embolism: the role of pulmonary embolectomy. Am Heart J 1975;89:413.
4. Attar S, Kirby WH, Masaitis C, et al. Coagulation changes in clinical shock. Ann Surg 1966;164:34.
5. Attar S, Boyd D, Layne E, et al. Alterations in coagulation and fibrinolytic mechanisms in acute trauma. J Trauma 1969;9:939.
6. Barrett DW, Jordon SC. Anticoagulant drugs in the treatment of pulmonary embolism: a controlled trial. Lancet 1960;1:1309.
7. Becker J, Schampi D. The incidence of postoperative venous thrombosis of the legs. A comparative study on the prophylactic effect of dextran 70 and electrical calf muscle stimulation. Acta Chir Scand 1973;139:357.
8. Bell WR. Pulmonary embolism: progress and problems. Am J Med 1982;72:181.
9. Bell WR, Meek AG. Guidelines for the use of thrombolytic agents. N Engl J Med 1979;301:1266.
10. Bell WR, Simon TL. Current status of pulmonary thromboembolic disease: pathophysiology, diagnosis, prevention, and treatment. Am Heart J 1982;103:239.
11. Bell WR, Simon TL, DeMets DL. The clinical features of submassive and massive pulmonary embolism. Am J Med 1977;62:355.
12. Benotti JR, Dalen JE. The natural history of pulmonary embolism. Clin Chest Med 1984;1:403.
13. Bergqvist D. Prophylaxis of postoperative thromboembolic complications with low-dose heparin. Acta Chir Scand 1979;145:7.
14. Bergqvist D. Dextran in the prophylaxis of deep-vein thrombosis JAMA 1987;258:324.
15. Bernstein RL, Rosenberg AD, Pada EY, et al. A severe reaction to dextran despite hapten inhibition. Anesthesiology 1987;67:567.
16. Berry AJ. Pulmonary embolism during spinal anesthesia: angiographic diagnosis via a flow-directed pulmonary artery catheter. Anesthesiology 1982;57:57.
17. Bettman MA, Paulin S. Leg phlebography: the incidence, nature and modification of undesirable side effects. Radiology 1977;122:101.
18. Biello DR, Mattar AG, McKnight RC, et al. Ventilation-perfusion studies in suspected pulmonary embolism. Am J Radiol 1979;133:1033.
19. Bjertnaes LJ. Hypoxia-induced vasoconstriction in isolated perfused lungs exposed to injectable or inhalation anesthetics. Acta Anaesth Scand 1977;21:133.
20. Bjertnaes LJ. Hypoxia-induced pulmonary vasoconstriction in man: inhibition due to diethyl ether and halothane anesthesia. Acta Anaesth Scand 1978;22:570.
21. Bjertnaes LJ, Mundal R. The pulmonary vasoconstrictor response to hypoxia during enflurane anesthesia. Acta Anaesth Scand 1980;24:252.
22. Bonica JJ, Kennedy WF, Akamatsu TJ, et al. Circulatory effects of peridural block. III. Effects of acute blood loss. Anesthesiology 1972;30:219.
23. Borgström S, Greitz T, Van Der Linden W, et al. Anticoagulant prophylaxis of venous thrombosis in patients with fractured neck of the femur: a controlled clinical trial using venous phlebography. Acta Chir Scand 1965;129:500.
24. Bourdarias JP, Dubourg O, Gueret P, et al. Inotropic agents in the treatment of cardiogenic shock. Pharmacol Ther 1983;22:53.
25. Browne RA, Catton DV. Massive pulmonary embolism during anaesthesia: a report of two cases. Can Anaesth Soc J 1967;14:413.
26. Browse NL, Jackson BT, Mayo ME et al. The value of mechanical methods of preventing postoperative calf vein thrombosis. Br J Surg 1974;61:219.
27. Butler BD, Drake RE, Hills BA. Effect of bronchial blood flow on pulmonary artery wedge pressure with pulmonary embolism. Crit Care Med 1986;14:495.
28. Cade JF. High risk of the critically ill for venous thromboembolism. Crit Care Med 1982;10:448.
29. Cade JF, Hirsh J, Regoeczi E, et al. Resolution of experimental pulmonary emboli with heparin and streptokinase in different dosage regimens. J Clin Invest 1974;54:782.
30. Carabasi RA, Moritz MJ, Jarrell BE. Complications encountered with the use of the Greenfield filter. Am J Surg 1987;154:163.
31. Chastre J, Cornud F, Bouchama A, et al. Thrombosis as a complication of pulmonary-artery catheterization via the internal jugular vein: Prospective evaluation by phlebography. N Engl J Med 1982;306:278.
32. Cheely R, McCartney WH, Perry JR, et al. The role of noninvasive tests versus pulmonary angiography in the diagnosis of pulmonary embolism. Am J Med 1981;70:17.
33. Chinitz JL, Kim KE, Onesti G, et al. Pathophysiology and prevention of dextran 40 induced anuria. J Lab Clin Med 1981;77:76.
34. Clark RL, Orandi A, Clifton EE. Induction of fibrinolysis by venous obstruction. Angiology 1960;11:367.
35. Clarke DB. Pulmonary embolectomy re-evaluated. Ann R Coll Surg (Engl) 1981;63:18.
36. Collins R, Scrimgeour A, Yusef S, et al. Reduction in fatal pulmonary embolism and venous thrombosis by perioperative administration of subcutaneous heparin: overview of results of randomized trials in general, orthopedic, and urologic surgery. N Engl J Med 1988;318:1162.
37. Colvin MP, Savege TM, Newland PE, et al. Cardiorespiratory changes following induction of anaesthesia with etomidate in patients with cardiac disease. Br J Anaesth 1979;51:551.
38. Cooke ED, Lloyd MJ, Bowcock SA, et al. Monitoring during low-dose heparin prophylaxis. N Engl J Med 1976;294:293.
39. Cooke ED, Lloyd MJ, Bowcock SA, et al. Intravenous lignocaine in prevention of deep venous thrombosis after elective hip surgery. Lancet 1977;2:797.
40. Coon WW. Risk factors of pulmonary embolism. Surg Gynecol Obstet 1976;143:385.
41. Coon WW. Epidemiology of venous thromboembolism. Ann Surg 1977;186:149.
42. Cotton LT, Roberts VC. The prevention of deep venous thrombosis with particular reference to mechanical methods of prevention. Surgery 1977;81:228.
43. D'Alonzo B, Bower JS, DeHart P, et al. The mechanisms of abnormal gas exchange in acute massive pulmonary embolism. Am Rev Respir Dis 1983;128:170.
44. Dantzker DR, Bower JS. Alterations in gas exchange following pulmonary thromboembolism. Chest 1982;81:495.
45. De Angelis J. Hazards of subdural and epidural anesthesia during anticoagulant therapy: a case report and review. Anesth Analg 1972;51:676.
46. Divekar VM, Kamdar BM, Pansare SN. Pulmonary embolism during anaesthesia: case report. Can Anaesth Soc J 1981;28:277.
47. Domino KB, Borowec L, Alexander CM, et al. Influence of isoflurane on hypoxic pulmonary vasoconstriction in dogs. Anesthesiology 1986;64:423.
48. Doyle DJ, Turpie AGG, Hirsh J, et al. Adjusted subcutaneous heparin or continuous intravenous heparin in patients with acute deep vein thrombosis: a randomized trial. Ann Intern Med 1987;107:441.
49. Dueck R, Young, I, Clausen J, et al. Altered distribution of pul-

monary ventilation and blood flow following induction of inhalational anesthesia. Anesthesiology 1980;52:113.
50. Ellison N, Ominsky A. Clinical considerations for the anesthesiologist whose patient is on anticoagulant therapy. Anesthesiology 1973;39:328.
51. Estrera AS, King RP, Platt MR. Massive pulmonary embolism: a complication of the technique of tourniquet ischemia. J Trauma 1982;22:60.
52. Feinstein MB, Fiekers J, Fraser C. An analysis of the mechanism of local anesthetic inhibition of platelet aggregation and secretion. J Pharmacol Exp Ther 1976;197:215.
53. Fisher J, Noble WH, Kay JC. Hypoxemia following pulmonary embolism: a dog model of altering regional perfusion. Anesthesiology 1981;54:204.
54. Fitts WT, Lehr HD, Bitner RL, et al. An analysis of 950 fatal injuries. Surgery 1964;56:663.
55. Fragen RJ, Avram MJ. Comparative pharmacology of drugs used for the induction of anesthesia. In: Stoelting RK, Barash PG, Gallagher TJ, (eds.) Advances in anesthesia vol 3. Chicago: Year Book Medical Publishers, 1986:103.
56. Fragen RJ, Shanks CA, Molteni A, et al. Effects of etomidate on hormonal responses to surgical stress. Anesthesiology 1984;61:652.
57. Francis CW, Marder VJ, Evarts CM, et al. Two-step warfarin therapy: prevention of postoperative venous thrombosis without excessive bleeding. JAMA 1983;249:374.
58. Freeark RJ, Boswick J, Fardin R. Posttraumatic venous thrombosis. Arch Surg 1967;95:567.
59. Giddon DB, Lindhe J. In vivo quantitation of local anesthetic suppression of leukocyte adherence. Am J Pathol 1972;68:327.
60. Gingrich TF. Spinal epidural hematoma following continuous epidural anesthesia. Anesthesiology 1968;29:162.
61. Glassford DM, Alford WC, Burrus GR, et al. Pulmonary embolectomy. Ann Thorac Surg 1981;32:28.
62. Goldberg SK, Lipschutz JB, Fein AM, et al. Hypercapnia complicating massive pulmonary embolism. Crit Care Med 1984;12:686.
63. Goldhaber SZ, Buring JB, Lipnick RJ, et al. Interruption of the inferior vena cava by clip or filter. Am J Med 1984;76:512.
64. Gooding JM, Dimick AR, Tavakoli M, et al. A physiologic analysis of cardiopulmonary responses to ketamine anesthesia in noncardiac patients. Anesth Analg 1977;56:813.
65. Goodman PC. Pulmonary angiography. Clin Chest Med 1984;5:465.
66. Goris RJA, Draaisma J. Causes of death after blunt trauma. J Trauma 1982;22:141.
67. Gotta AW, Sullivan CA. Pulmonary embolism during anesthesia: a case report and review of literature. Anesth Analg 1970;49:73.
68. Greenfield LJ. Vena caval interruption and pulmonary embolectomy. Clin Chest Med 1984;5:495.
69. Greenfield LJ, Zocco JJ. Intraluminal management of acute massive pulmonary thromboembolism. J Thorac Cardiovasc Surg 1979;77:402.
70. Gruber UF. Dextran and prevention of postoperative thromboembolic complications. Surg Clin North Am 1975;55:679.
71. Gruber UF, Sladen T. Incidences of fatal postoperative pulmonary embolism after prophylaxis with dextran 70 and low-dose heparin: an international multicentre study. Br Med J 1980;280:69.
72. Gurewich V, Cohen ML, Thomas DP. Humoral factors in massive pulmonary embolism: an experimental study. Am Heart J 1968;76:784.
73. Guyton DP, Khayat A, Schreiber H. Pneumatic compression stockings and prostaglandin synthesis-A pathway of fibrinolysis. Crit Care Med 1985;13:266.
74. Hampson WGJ, Harris FC, Lucas HK, et al. Failure of low dose heparin to prevent deep vein thrombosis after hip replacement arthroplasty. Lancet 1974;2:795.
75. Hatle L, Rokseth R. The arterial to end-expiratory carbon dioxide tension gradient in acute pulmonary embolism and other cardiopulmonary diseases. Chest 1974;66:352.
76. Haynes JB, Iseman MD. Massive pulmonary embolism. Rocky Mt Med J 1979;77:135.
77. Hecker BR, Lynch C. Intraoperative diagnosis and treatment of massive pulmonary embolism complicating surgery on the abdominal aorta. Br J Anaesth 1983;55:689.
78. Hendolin H, Mattila MAK, Poikolainen E. The effect of lumbar epidural analgesia on the development of deep venous thrombosis of the legs after open prostatectomy. Acta Chir Scand 1981;147:425.
79. Hilgenberg JC, McCammon RL, Stoelting RK. Pulmonary and systemic vascular resistance responses to nitrous oxide in patients with mitral stenosis and pulmonary hypertension. Anesth Analg 1980;59:323.
80. Hills NH, Pflug JJ, Jeyasingh K, et al. Prevention of deep vein thrombosis by intermittent compression of the calf. Br Med J 1972;1:131.
81. Hirsh J. Prevention of deep vein thrombosis. Br J Hosp Med 1981;26:143.
82. Hirsh J. New approaches for deep venous thrombosis occurring after surgery. JAMA 1984;251:2985.
83. Hirsh J, Levine MN. The optimal intensity of oral anticoagulant therapy. JAMA 1987;258:2723.
84. Hirsh J, van Aken WG, Gallus AS. Heparin kinetics in venous thrombosis and pulmonary embolism. Circulation 1976;53:691.
85. Hirsh J, Deykin D, Poller L. "Therapeutic range" for oral anticoagulant therapy. Chest 1986;89:1S.
86. Huet Y, Lemaire F, Brun-Buisson C, et al. Hypoxemia in acute pulmonary embolism. Chest 1985;88:829.
87. Hull R, Hirsh J, Sackett DL, et al. Clinical validity of a negative venogram in patients with clinically suspected venous thrombosis. Circulation 1981;64:622.
88. Hull R, Hirsh J, Sackett DL, et al. Replacement of venography in suspected venous thrombosis by impedance plethysmography and $^{125}$I-fibrinogen leg scanning. A less invasive approach. Ann Intern Med 1981;94:12.
89. Hull RD, Hirsh J, Carter CJ, et al. Pulmonary angiography, ventilation lung scanning, and venography for clinically suspected pulmonary embolism with abnormal perfusion lung scan. Ann Intern Med 1983;98:891.
90. Hull RD, Raskob GE, LeClerc JR, et al. The diagnosis of clinically suspected venous thrombosis. Clin Chest Med 1984;5:439.
91. Hull RD, Hirsh J, Carter CJ, et al. Diagnostic efficacy of impedance plethysmography for clinically suspected deep-vein thrombosis: a randomized trial. Ann Intern Med 1985;102:21.
92. Hull RD, Hirsh J, Carter CJ, et al. Diagnostic value of ventilation-perfusion lung scanning in patients with suspected pulmonary embolism. Chest 1985;88:819.
93. Hyers TM. Antithrombotic therapy for venous thromboembolism. Clin Chest Med 1984;5:479.
94. Hyers TM, Fowler AA, Wicks AB. Focal pulmonary edema after massive pulmonary embolism. Am Rev Respir Dis 1981;123:232.
95. Innes D, Sevitt S. Coagulation and fibrinolysis in injured patients. J Clin Pathol 1964;17:1.
96. Jardin F, Gurdjian F, Margairaz A. Effect deletere de l'isoprenoline au cours d'une embolie pulmonaire massive. Nouv Presse Med 1977;6:1878.
97. Jardin F, Genevray B, Brunney D, et al. Dobutamine: a hemodynamic evaluation in pulmonary embolism shock. Crit Care Med 1985;13:1009.

98. Jareno AJ, De La Serna JL, Corral EE, et al. Fibrinogen/fibrin degradation products in the diagnosis of pulmonary embolism in critically ill patients. Crit Care Med 1980;8:646.
99. Johnson JC, Flowers NC, Horan LG. Unexplained atrial flutter: a frequent herald of pulmonary embolism. Chest 1971;60:29.
100. Kafer ER. Respiratory function in pulmonary thromboembolic disease. Am J Med 1969;47:904.
101. Kakkar VV. The current status of low-dose heparin in the prophylaxis of thrombophlebitis and pulmonary embolism. World J Surg 1978;2:3.
102. Kakkar VV, Murray WJG. Efficacy and safety of low-molecular-weight heparin (C4216) in preventing postoperative venous thrombo-embolism: a co-operative study. Br J Surg 1985;72:786.
103. Kakkar VV, Howe CT, Flanc C, et al. Natural history of postoperative deep vein thrombosis. Lancet 1969;2:230.
104. Kakkar VV, Corrigan TP, Spindler J, et al. Efficacy of low doses of heparin in prevention of deep venous thrombosis after major surgery: a double-blind randomized trial. Lancet 1972;2:101.
105. Kakkar VV, Welzel D, Murray WJG, et al. Possible mechanism of the synergistic effect of heparin and dihydroergotamine. Am J Surg 1985;150(suppl):33.
106. Kanter B, Moser KM. The Greenfield vena cava filter. Chest 1988;93:170.
107. Katholi RE, Nolan SP, McGuire LB. The management of anticoagulation during noncardiac operations in patients with prosthetic heart valves. Am Heart J 1978;96:163.
108. Kiil J, Alexsen F, Kiil J, et al. Prophylaxis against postoperative pulmonary embolism and deep-vein thrombosis by low-dose heparin. Lancet 1978;1:1115.
109. Knight MTN, Dawson R. Effect of intermittent compression of the arms on deep venous thrombosis in the legs. Lancet 1976;2:1265.
110. Knight MTN, Dawson R, Melrose DG. Fibrinolytic response to surgery: labile and stable patterns and their relevance to postoperative deep venous thrombosis. Lancet 1977;2:370.
111. Lahnborg G. Effect of low-dose heparin and dihydroergotamine on frequency of postoperative deep-vein thrombosis in patients undergoing post-traumatic hip surgery. Acta Chir Scand 1980;146:319.
112. Langsfeld M, Hershey FB, Thorpe L, et al. Duplex B-mode imaging for the diagnosis of deep vein thrombosis. Arch Surg 1987;122:587.
113. Laster J, Cikrit D, Walker N, et al. The heparin-induced thrombocytopenia syndrome: an update. Surgery 1987;102:763.
114. Leeper KV, Popovich J, Lesser BA, et al. Treatment of massive acute pulmonary embolism: the use of low doses of intrapulmonary arterial streptokinase combined with full doses of systemic heparin. Chest 1988;93:234.
115. Leithauser DJ, Saraf L, Smyka S, et al. Prevention of embolic complications from venous thrombosis after surgery: standardized regimen of early ambulation. JAMA 1951;147:300.
116. Lewis CE, Mueller C, Edwards WS. Venous stasis on the operating table. Am J Surg 1972;124:780.
117. Leyvraz PP, Richard J, Bachmann F, et al. Adjusted versus fixed-dose subcutaneous heparin in the prevention of deep-vein thrombosis after total hip replacement. N Engl J Med 1983;309:954.
118. LoSasso AM. Pulmonary embolism. In: Stoelting RK, Dierdorf SF, eds. Anesthesia and co-existing disease. New York: Churchill Livingstone, 1983:165.
119. Lungstom KG, Renck H, Strandberg K, et al. Adverse reactions to dextran in Sweden 1970–1979. Acta Chir Scand 1983;149:256.
120. Machida K, Rapaport E. Left ventricular function in experimental pulmonary embolism. Jpn Heart J 1971;12:221.
121. Mangano DT. Immediate hemodynamic and pulmonary changes following pulmonary thromboembolism. Anesthesiology 1980;52:173.
122. Mattox KL, Feldtman RW, Beall AC, et al. Pulmonary embolectomy for acute massive pulmonary embolism. Ann Surg 1982;195:726.
123. Mayrhofer O, Steinbereithner K. Significance of severe respiratory acidosis in pulmonary embolism during anesthesia. Anesth Analg 1966;45:564.
124. McBride K, LaMorte WW, Menzoian JO. Can ventilation-perfusion scans accurately diagnose acute pulmonary embolism? Arch Surg 1986;121:754.
125. McDonald IG, Hirsh J, Male GS, et al. Isoproterenol in massive pulmonary embolism: hemodynamic and clinical effects. Med J Aust 1968;2:201.
126. McIntyre KM, Sasahara AA. The hemodynamic response to pulmonary embolism in patients without prior cardiopulmonary disease. Am J Cardiol 1971;28:288.
127. McIntyre KM, Sasahara AA. Pulmonary angiography, scanning, and hemodynamics in pulmonary embolism: critical review and correlations. Crit Rev Radiol Sci 1972;3:489.
128. McKenzie PJ, Wishart HY, Gray I, et al. Effects of anaesthetic technique on deep vein thrombosis. A comparison of subarachnoid and general anaesthesia. Br J Anaesth 1985;57:853.
129. Mellbring G, Dahlgren S, Reiz S, et al. Thromboembolic complications after major abdominal surgery: effect of thoracic epidural analgesia. Acta Chir Scand 1983;149:263.
130. Menzoian JO, Williams LF. Is pulmonary angiography essential for the diagnosis of acute pulmonary embolism? Am J Surg 1979;137:543.
131. Messmer K, Ljungström KG, Gruber UF, et al. Prevention of dextran-induced anaphylactoid reactions by hapten inhibition. Lancet, 1980;1:975.
132. Meth RF, Tashkin DP, Hansen KS, et al. Pulmonary edema and wheezing after pulmonary embolism. Am Rev Respir Dis 1975;111:693.
133. Miller GA, Hall RJC, Paneth M. Pulmonary embolectomy, heparin and streptokinase: their place in the treatment of acute massive pulmonary embolism. Am Heart J 1977;93:568.
134. Mills SR, Jackson DC, Older RA, et al. The incidence, etiologies, and avoidance of complications of pulmonary angiography in large series. Diagn Radiol 1980;136:295.
135. Minuck M. Massive pulmonary embolism occurring during anaesthesia: report of three cases. Can Anaesth Soc J 1968; 15:297.
136. Modig J, Malmberg P, Karlström G. Effect of epidural versus general anesthesia on calf blood flow. Acta Anesth Scand 1980;24:305.
137. Modig J, Hjelmestedt A, Sahlstedt B, et al. Comparative influences of epidural and general anaesthesia on deep venous thrombosis and pulmonary embolism after total hip replacement. Acta Chir Scand 1981;147:125.
138. Modig J, Borg T, Karlström G, et al. Thromboembolism after total hip replacement: role of epidural and general anesthesia. Anesth Analg 1983;62:174.
139. Morris GK, Mitchell JRA. Warfarin sodium in prevention of deep venous thrombosis and pulmonary embolism in patients with fractured neck of femur. Lancet 1976;2:869.
140. Moser KM. Pulmonary embolism. Am Rev Respir Dis 1977;115:829.
141. Moser KM, LeMoine JR. Is embolic risk conditioned by location of deep vein thrombosis? Ann Intern Med 1981;94:439.
142. Multicenter trial committee. Dihydroergotamine-heparin prophylaxis of postoperative deep venous thrombosis: a multicenter trial. JAMA 1984;251:2960.
143. Myers ML, Calvin JE, Driedger AA, et al. Myocardial dysfunc-

tion associated with massive pulmonary embolus as evaluated by radionuclide angiography. Crit Care Med 1982;10:417.
144. Negus D, Cox SJ, Friedgood A, et al. Ultra-low dose intravenous heparin in the prevention of postoperative deep-vein thrombosis. Lancet 1980;1:891.
145. Neuhaus A, Bentz RR, Weg JG. Pulmonary embolism in respiratory failure. Chest 1978;73:460.
146. Nicolaides AN. Invited commentary. World J Surg 1978;2:13.
147. Nicolaides AN, Dupont PA, Desai S, et al. Small doses of subcutaneous heparin in preventing deep venous thrombosis after major surgery. Lancet 1972;2:890.
148. Nicolaides AN, Fernandes JF, Pollock AV. Intermittent sequential pneumatic compression of the legs in the prevention of venous stasis and postoperative deep venous thrombosis. Surgery 1980;87:69.
149. Nowelline RA, Baltarowich OH, Athanasoulis CA, et al. The clinical course of patients with suspected pulmonary embolism and a negative pulmonary angiogram. Diagn Radiol 1978;126:561.
150. O'Brian JR. The adhesiveness of native platelets and its prevention. J Clin Pathol 1961;14:140.
150a. O'Malley KF, Ross SE. Pulmonary embolism in major trauma patients. J Trauma 1990;30:748.
151. Owens EL, Kasten GW, Hessel EA. Spinal subarachnoid hematoma after lumbar puncture and heparinization: a case report, review of the literature, and discussion of anesthetic implications. Anesth Analg 1986;65:1201.
152. Pachter HL, Riles TS. Low dose heparin: bleeding and wound complications in the surgical patient: a prospective randomized study. Ann Surg 1977;186:669.
153. Paraskos JA, Adelstein SJ, Smith RE, et al. Late prognosis of acute pulmonary embolism. N Engl J Med 1973;289:55.
154. Pearl RG, Rosenthal MH, Ashton JPA. Pulmonary vasodilatory effects of nitroglycerine and sodium nitroprusside in canine oleic acid-induced pulmonary hypertension. Anesthesiology 1983;58:514.
155. Perry MD. Anticoagulation: a surgical perspective. Am J Surg 1988;155:268.
156. Poikolainen E, Hendolin H. Effects of lumbar epidural analgesia and general anesthesia on flow velocity in the femoral vein and postoperative deep venous thrombosis. Acta Chir Scand 1983;149:361.
157. Pollard BJ, Lovelock HA, Jones RM. Fatal pulmonary embolism secondary to limb exsanguination. Anesthesiology 1983;58:373.
158. Pond GD, Ovitt TW, Capp MP. Comparison of conventional pulmonary angiography with intravenous digital subtraction angiography for pulmonary embolic disease. Radiology 1983;147:345.
159. Porter J, Hershel J. Drug related deaths among medical inpatients. JAMA 1977;237:879.
160. Prevention of fatal postoperative pulmonary embolism by low doses of heparin. An international multicentre trial. Lancet 1975;2:45.
161. Quintana E, Sanchez JM, Serra C, et al. Erroneous interpretation of pulmonary capillary wedge pressure in massive pulmonary embolism. Crit Care Med 1983;11:933.
162. Rabinov K, Paulin S. Roentgen diagnosis of venous thrombosis in the leg. Arch Surg 1972;104:134.
163. Rao TLK, El-Etr AA. Anticoagulation following placement of epidural and subarachnoid catheters: an evaluation of neurologic sequelae. Anesthesiology 1981;55:618.
164. Reves JG, Kissin I, Fournier S. Negative inotropic effects of midazolam. Anesthesiology 1984;60:517.
165. Riedel M, Stanek V, Widimsky J, et al. Long-term follow-up of patients with pulmonary thromboembolism: late prognosis and evolution of hemodynamic and respiratory data. Chest 1982;81:151.
166. Robin ED. Overdiagnosis and overtreatment of pulmonary embolism: the emperor may have no clothes. Ann Intern Med 1977;87:775.
167. Robin ED, Forkner CE, Bromberg PA, et al. Alveolar gas exchange in clinical pulmonary embolism. N Engl J Med 1960;262:283.
168. Rogers SN, Benumof JL. Halothane and isoflurane do not decrease $PaO_2$ during one lung ventilation in intravenously anesthetized patients. Anesth Analg 1985;64:946.
169. Rosengarten DS, Laird J, Jeyasingh K, et al. The failure of compression stockings (tubigrip) to prevent deep venous thrombosis after operation. Br J Surg 1970;57:296.
170. Rosiello RA, Chan CK, Tencza F, et al. Timing of oral anticoagulation therapy in the treatment of angiographically proven acute pulmonary embolism. Arch Intern Med 1987;147:1469.
171. Rubenstein I, Murray D, Hoffstein V. Fatal pulmonary emboli in hospitalized patients: an autopsy study. Arch Intern Med 1988;148:1425.
172. Ruff RL, Dougherty JH. Complications of lumbar puncture followed by anticoagulation. Stroke 1981;12:879.
173. Saidman LJ, Trousdale FR. Isoflurane does not inhibit hypoxic pulmonary vasoconstriction. Anesthesiology 1982;57:A472.
174. Salzman EW. Physical methods for prevention of venous thromboembolism. Surgery 1977;81:123.
175. Salzman EW. Low-molecular-weight heparin: is small beautiful? N Engl J Med 1986;315:957.
176. Salzman EW, Deykin D, Shapiro RM, et al. Management of heparin therapy. N Engl J Med 1975;292:1046.
177. Salzman EW, McManama GP, Shapiro AH, et al. Effect of optimization of hemodynamics on fibrinolytic activity and antithrombotic efficacy of external pneumatic calf compression. Ann Surg 1987;206:636.
178. San Juan AC, Stanley TH. Pulmonary embolism after tourniquet inflation. Anesth Analg 1984;63:374.
179. Schulte-Sasse U, Hess W, Tarnow J. Pulmonary vascular responses to nitrous oxide in patients with normal and high pulmonary vascular resistance. Anesthesiology 1982;57:9.
180. Scurr JH, Ibrahim SZ, Faber RG, et al. The efficacy of graduated compression stockings in the prevention of deep vein thrombosis. Br J Surg 1977;64:371.
181. Scurr JH, Coleridge-Smith PD, Hasty JH. Regimen for improved effectiveness of intermittent pneumatic compression in deep venous thrombosis prophylaxis. Surgery 1987;102:816.
182. Sevitt S. Venous thrombosis and pulmonary embolism: their prevention by oral anticoagulants. Am J Med 1962;33:703.
183. Sevitt S, Gallagher NG. Prevention of venous thrombosis and pulmonary embolism in injured patients. Lancet 1959;2:981.
184. Sevitt S, Gallagher NG. Venous thrombosis and pulmonary embolism: a clinico-pathological study in injured and burned patients. Br J Surg 1961;48:475.
185. Seyfer AE, Seaber AV, Dombrose FA, et al. Coagulation changes in elective surgery and trauma. Ann Surg 1981;193:219.
185a. Shackford SR, Davis JW, Hollingsworth-Fridlund P, et al. Venous thromboembolism in patients with major trauma. Am J Surg 1990;159:365.
186. Sigel B, Felix WR, Popky GL, et al. Diagnosis of lower limb venous thrombosis by Doppler ultrasound technique. Arch Surg 1972;104:174.
187. Silver D, Kapsch DN, Tsoi EK. Heparin-induced thrombocytopenia, thrombosis, and hemorrhage. Ann Surg 1983;198:301.
188. Simon TL, Hyers TM, Gaston JP, et al. Heparin pharmacokinetics: increased requirements in pulmonary embolism. Br J Haematol 1978;39:111.
189. Skillman JJ. Postoperative deep venous thrombosis and pul-

monary embolism: a selective review and personal viewpoint. Surgery 1974;75:114.
190. Smyrnis SA, Kolios AS, Agnantis JK. Deep-vein thrombosis in patients with fracture of the upper part of the femur: a phlebographic study. Br J Surg 1973;60:447.
191. Stein PD, Dalen JE, McIntyre KM, et al. The electrocardiogram in acute pulmonary embolism. Prog Cardiovasc Dis 1975;17:247.
192. Stewart JR, Greenfield LJ. Transvenous vena caval filtration and pulmonary embolectomy. Surg Clin North Am 1982;62:411.
193. Stool EW, Mullins CB, Leshin SJ, et al. Dimensional changes of the left ventricle during acute pulmonary arterial hypertension in dogs. Am J Cardiol 1974;33:868.
194. Strandness DE, Sumner DS. Ultrasonic velocity detector in the diagnosis of thrombophlebitis. Arch Surg 1972;104:180.
195. Swann KW, Black PM. Deep vein thrombosis and pulmonary emboli in neurosurgical patients: a review. J Neurosurg 1984;61:1955.
196. Sykes MK. The distribution of pulmonary blood flow. In: Prys-Roberts C, ed. The circulation of anaesthesia. Oxford: Blackwell Scientific Publications, 1980:275.
197. Szucs MM, Brooks HL, Grossman W, et al. Diagnostic sensitivity of laboratory findings in acute pulmonary embolism. Ann Intern Med 1971;74:161.
198. Tarnay TJ, Rohr PR, Davidson AG, et al. Pneumatic calf compression, fibrinolysis, and the prevention of deep venous thrombosis. Surgery 1980;88:489.
199. Tetalman MR, Hoffer PD, Heck LL, et al. Perfusion lung scan in normal volunteers. Radiology 1973;106:593.
200. Thomas DP, Gurewich V, Ashford TP. Platelet adherence to thromboemboli in relation to the pathogenesis and treatment of pulmonary embolism. N Engl J Med 1966;274:953.
201. Timberlake GA, McSwain NE. Thromboembolism as a complication of myocardial contusion: a new capricious syndrome. J Trauma 1988:28:535.
202. Torngran S. Pulmonary embolism and postoperative death. Acta Chir Scand 1983;149:269.
203. Tschirkov A, Krause E, Elert O, et al. Surgical management of massive pulmonary embolism. J Thorac Cardiovasc Surg 1978;75:730.
204. Turpie AG, Levine MN, Hirsh J, et al. A randomized controlled trial of a low-molecular-weight heparin (enoxaparin) to prevent deep-vein thrombosis in patients undergoing elective hip surgery. N Engl J Med 1986;315:925.
205. Van Ooijen B. Subcuraneous heparin and postoperative wound hematomas: a prospective double-blind randomized study. Arch Surg 1986;121:937.
206. Varkey GP, Brindle GF. Peridural anaesthesia and anticoagulant therapy. Can Anaesth Soc J 1974;21:106.
207. Verstraete M, Miller GAH, Bounameaux H, et al. Intravenous and intrapulmonary recombinant tissue-type plasminogen activator in the treatment of acute massive pulmonary embolism. Circulation 1988;77:353.
208. Vigano S, Mannuci PM, Solinas S, et al. Decrease in protein C antigen and formation of an abnormal protein soon after starting anticoagulant therapy. Br J Haematol 1984;57:213.
209. Volgesang GB, Bell WR. Treatment of pulmonary embolism and deep vein thrombosis with thrombolytic therapy. Clin Chest Med 1984;5:487.
210. Wacker WEC, Rosenthal M, Snodgrass P, et al. A triad for the diagnosis of pulmonary embolism and infarction. JAMA 1961;178:8.
211. Wagner RL, White PF. Etomidate inhibits adrenocortical function in surgical patients. Anesthesiology 1984;61:647.
212. Wessler S. The role of antithrombotic prophylaxis among patients subjected to trauma. In: Worth MH, ed. Principles and practice of trauma care. Baltimore: Williams & Wilkins, 1982:415.
213. Williams JW, Eikman EA, Greenberg SH, et al. Failure of low dose heparin to prevent pulmonary embolism after hip surgery or above knee amputation. Ann Surg 1978;188:468.
214. Williams JW, Eikman EA, Greenberg S. Asymptomatic pulmonary embolism: a common event in high risk patients. Ann Surg 1982;195:323.
215. Willie-Jorgensen P, Thorup J, Fischer A, et al. Heparin with and without compression stockings in the prevention of thromboembolic complications of major abdominal surgery: a randomized trial. Br J Surg 1985;72:579.

# Section Four

# Organizational Aspects

# Chapter Twenty-Nine

Paul Mesnick

# Emergency Medical Services, Trauma Care Systems, and Disaster Planning

## EMERGENCY MEDICAL SERVICES SYSTEMS (EMSS)

Medical care of the trauma patient begins with the earliest application of appropriate medical skills. Too often, this application has been unduly delayed because of inadequate planning and coordination of community medical resources. Since the late 1960s there has been a growing effort to develop and improve emergency medical services systems (EMSS) in order to provide coordinated and appropriately structured emergency medical care from the prehospital area into the hospital phase of treatment. The basic components of EMSS include medical director(s), trained personnel, transport vehicles, access and dispatch, communications, and receiving medical facilities. The concept of the domestic EMS program is based largely on military field intervention medicine. The benefits of such a system have been demonstrated in the military sector and have helped in part to reduce military deaths since World War II.[48,66]

The report, "Accidental Death and Disability: The Neglected Disease of Modern Society",[1] is often cited as the landmark document in pointing out the need to improve and better coordinate emergency medical care in the United States. The report identified trauma as the leading cause of death for all persons aged 1 to 38 and overall as the fourth major cause of death in the United States, findings that are still true at the time of this writing.[2] The growing public and medical awareness[89] that the country was dealing rather poorly with acute medical emergencies led to a focus on three central areas of deficiency:

1. An unstructured public and private ambulance system with marked variations in ambulance staffing, design, and equipment
2. A serious lack of appropriately trained and certified ambulance personnel, with no nationally recognized standard of training
3. A lack of appropriate criteria defining hospital capabilities to accept and manage medical emergencies of widely varying types and severity

Public concern with these and related matters resulted in the Federal EMSS Act of 1973.[54] The Act recognized 15 components vital to developing an EMS system: (1) health personnel, (2) training, (3) communications, (4) vehicles, (5) medical facilities, (6) specialized critical care units, (7) public safety personnel, (8) public planning and accessibility to care, (9) hospital transfer agreements, (10) standardized record keeping, (11) public information, (12) public education, (13) system evaluation, (14) disaster planning, and (15) mutual aid agreements between adjacent EMS systems.[55,56] Federal grants were made available for state and local government projects to develop regional plans for the establishment and coordination of these components.

In addition to the federal efforts, a number of leading public and professional agencies began to promote programs in the area of emergency and acute medical care. Such organizations as the National Safety Council, the American National Red Cross, the AMA Commission on Emergency Medical Services, the American Trauma Society, the Committee on Trauma of the American College of Surgeons, the American

Society of Anesthesiologists, the American Heart Association, the American College of Emergency Physicians, and the American Academy of Orthopedic Surgeons helped develop programs and heighten interest in the are of emergency medical care and services.

Unfortunately, these efforts, at least at the state level, have, by and large, been less than successful. A recent survey by West et al.[118] has shown that only two states (Maryland and Virginia) have complete regional trauma services as defined by the American College of Surgeons. Twenty-nine states have not initiated the process of trauma center designation at all, whereas the remaining 19 have incomplete systems in place. Clearly, much political work remains to be done in order to afford optimal care to all seriously injured patients.

This chapter deals primarily with the organizational aspects of trauma management in the United States and the impact of the EMS system on patient care.

## GENERAL EMS SYSTEM DESIGN

Despite progress in developing a general awareness of EMS systems, there is a great deal of variation in the quality and structure of programs throughout the United States. EMS designs differ greatly between rural and urban areas, as well as within each of these areas. In fact, there is no functionally ideal EMS system. Flexibility in design is necessary to optimize the availability of local and regional medical resources to the demographic patterns of a particular region. The system must also be adapted to variations in state and local laws, rules, and procedures.[12,53] Therefore, it is difficult, if not impossible, to describe an EMS design that works well in one area of the country and to predict that it will be successful if adopted in another geographic, demographic, or political setting.[20] However, certain general ingredients need to be in place in any successful EMS system:[21,46]

- The EMS design process should focus on the possible goals of the system in view of the available resources of the region. Once realistic goals are established, relationships among provider, physician, public, and political groups should be determined to tailor the system best to the needs of the community.
- EMS planning, development, and design must use the political process. Enabling legislation to clarify and define areas of responsibility and medical control should be developed as part of this effort. The delivery of emergency medical services is a community service and thereby affects certain public and political realities not usually dealt with by physicians and other health care providers. It is important to remember that the EMS system in its public role is ultimately accountable to state and local governmental authorities.
- The various components of an EMS system need to be interconnected to ensure functional integrity. The EMS system should be a comprehensive and integrated network of medical care. A breakdown at any point may nullify the ability to provide appropriate and definitive treatment for a given medical emergency.
- A high standard for evaluating the various systems components—operational, institutional, and medical—should be developed. All EMS systems require a continuing cycle of assessment and adjustment with time.[46]

The EMS system begins with the identification of a medical emergency, followed by notification of and field treatment by trained personnel acting under medical control.[108] After field evaluation and treatment, the patient is transported to an appropriate medical facility for more definitive evaluation and care. Interhospital transport to a more highly categorized or special care facility is also an integral part of this system.[37,78]

## EMS PERSONNEL AND TRAINING

Fundamental to prehospital care is the training of the "first responders" who are most likely to encounter and treat the accident victim. Levels of training varied greatly across the country in the 1960s, ranging from funeral directors to physicians on city ambulances. Whatever the staffing, however, the basic emphasis seemed to be to expedite transportation of the patient to some medical facility in the area where it was hoped that competent medical care would be available.

The past decade has seen dramatic progress in the development of medical training for prehospital care personnel in the United States. New job titles have been recognized, such as emergency medical technician-intermediate and emergency medical technician-paramedic, to designate levels of training. Certification of such allied health personnel by state and national agencies is also available. The National Registry of Emergency Medical Technicians, located in Columbus, Ohio, is widely recognized and holds regularly scheduled certification examinations for these levels of emergency medical technician performance (Table 29-1).

The anesthesiologist has much to offer in knowledge, background, and training to EMS development and progress. A number of the field medical and monitoring techniques currently employed by paramedical personnel were adapted from the operating room experience of anesthesiologists. It should therefore be no great surprise that a number of anesthesiologists were involved with the development and study of the current mobile intensive prehospital care systems and units.[16,26,87,97] The American Society of Anesthesiologists is a sponsoring member of the Joint Review Committee on Educational Programs for the EMT-Paramedic. The Committee, founded in 1978, operates under the auspices of the Committee on Allied Health Education and Accreditation of the American Medical Association and like its counterparts seeks to accredit qualified programs that train EMS personnel.[4] The Committee is recognized in its accrediting role by the United States Department of Education.

## MEDICAL CONTROL OF EMERGENCY MEDICAL SERVICES

Strong medical control is required to maintain the quality of prehospital care.[8,92,108,109] In addition, such control provides professional and public accountability, particularly in reference to advanced life support programs.[67] The EMT-paramedic essentially acts as "the eyes and ears" of the physician in the field. Thus, physician direction of the EMT's activities, either through written protocols or voice/telemetry commu-

TABLE 29-1. Training, Certification, Capability, and Medical Supervision of the Three Levels of Emergency Medical Technicians

| LEVEL | SYNONYMOUS TITLES | CLASSROOM EDUCATION (hours) | CLINICAL/ HOSPITAL TRAINING (hours) | CERTIFICATION THROUGH | PATIENT CARE ACTIVITIES | MEDICAL SUPERVISION |
|---|---|---|---|---|---|---|
| 1 | Emergency medical technician<br>Emergency medical technician-ambulance<br>EMT/basic<br>EMT-I<br>EMT-A | 81–140 | At least 10 | State agency<br>National boards—optional | Basic life support (BLS)<br>Cardiopulmonary resuscitation (CPR)<br>Extrication techniques | Minimal |
| 2 | Emergency medical technician—intermediate<br>Cardiac technician<br>EMT-II<br>EMT-2<br>CT | 150 | 150 | State agency<br>National boards—optional | Advanced airway management, ECG interpretation, defibrillator/ cardioversion, intravenous fluid therapy | Yes |
| 3 | Emergency medical technician—paramedic<br>Mobile intensive care paramedic<br>MICP<br>EMT-III<br>EMT-3<br>EMT-P<br>Paramedic | 300–400 | 200–300 | State board of medical licensure<br>National boards—optional | All activities of EMT-II plus pharmacologic treatment | Yes |

nication systems, should be provided for the initiation of appropriate medical care. Medical supervision of emergency personnel includes not only monitoring and review of their field activities, but equally important, provision of continuing education and recertification procedures.[80] The lack of physician involvement in the maintenance of advanced life support prehospital care lowers the quality and credibility of the system.[9,106,109] It is important that local medical societies contribute to the development, design, and integrity of the EMS system. Too often such bodies enter the process late, after reacting to members' enquiries about the impact that EMS may have on their practice or patients. The failure of state and local medical bodies to involve themselves in the development of community emergency medical service programs may result in unnecessary conflict and confusion in developing a vital health care delivery system.

In general, the following areas of medical control should be emphasized in an EMS system[8,67,108,109]:

1. *Designation of a supervisory (on-line) medical director for the program:* This is especially important if the program involves the use of advanced life support techniques, drugs, and equipment. Fundamental to this type of medical control is the designation of a medical command linkage between the area resource hospital, which usually houses the hospital-to-field radio and telemetry communications, and the various receiving and participating area hospitals. The resource hospital, under the authority of its medical director, usually holds responsibility for the medical performance of the paramedics in the system, the appropriateness of patient care, and patient distribution to hospitals in the area.
2. *Development and utilization of uniform regional treatment protocols:* These regional protocols, along with the previously mentioned hospital transfer protocols adopted by the area-wide EMS system, allow the paramedic team to operate in the field and secure transport of the patient to an appropriate medical facility in the community.
3. *Appropriate training and medical supervision of EMTs:* The practice of medicine in the prehospital phase of treatment is no less critical than the use of drugs or resuscitative measures in the emergency areas of the hospital and should be treated as such.
4. *Selection of drugs and equipment for utilization in the field and determination of their safety and efficacy:* As new technologic data and treatment methods become available, a medical process must be established to accommodate, audit, review, and update equipment and treatment standards.

The authorization of medical control by appropriate legislation is essential to establish standards of care, fix medical responsibility, and define other pertinent areas of medicolegal concern and responsibility for the regional EMS program.

## TREATMENT PROTOCOLS

Uniform treatment protocols should be developed by the regional medical director(s) in order to permit a structured and clarified approach to the treatment of medical emergencies in the field. These protocols may be of particular benefit should communication with the area resource hospital by radio or voice/telemetry prove impossible in the midst of a serious medical emergency. Specialist input and consensus in the development of such standardized procedures should be enlisted and encouraged.

Some prehospital advanced life support programs operate with little or no communication with the resource or base hospital. These programs rely entirely on standard operating protocols. In this type of system, the lack of physician-paramedic communication may impose a degree of inflexibility since direct medical control over the individual patient's management is restricted. However, legitimate factors, such as system costs, geographic boundaries, system size, etc., may not permit reliable and consistent field-to-hospital communication. In these circumstances, treatment protocols should include carefully and clearly drawn guidelines that allow the paramedic some flexibility in management of the patient.

### ROLE OF THE EMS TECHNICIAN IN PREHOSPITAL TRAUMA CARE

The role of the emergency medical technician-paramedic (EMT-P) is to bring both basic and advanced life support techniques to the field in order to stabilize and minimize deterioration of the patient before transport. Although it is known that prehospital paramedic care can reduce mortality from cardiac arrest,[51,52] its benefits to the severely injured patient remain less clear. Considerable controversy exists regarding the amount of time to be spent in stabilizing the critical trauma patient. Since the time spent on the scene often includes extrication, airway management, stabilization of the spine, splinting of suspected fractures, starting an intravenous line, dressing of wounds, and placement of pneumatic trousers, an average of approximately 25 minutes at the scene is not unusual or necessarily unrealistic.[46]

Whether minimal on-scene intervention (scoop-and-run)[18,105] is preferable to limited or advanced on-scene stabilization[13,69,72,94,96,113] remains a basic and controversial issue for physicians involved in prehospital care of traumatized patients. Unfortunately, data on the efficacy of prehospital care in the management of traumatized patients remain scanty, difficult to interpret, controversial, and inconclusive. However, it is probably reasonable to state that the nature of the injury and the distance from a medical facility should dictate the type and duration of medical care given at the scene.[90,91] The transport of patients with major injuries should not be overly delayed by attempts at field stabilization, especially when a trauma center is nearby. When transportation times of more than 30 minutes are required to reach a capable hospital facility, as may occur in rural areas, on-scene resuscitative efforts of greater intensity may be indicated.[91] It is the author's impression that well-trained paramedical personnel, functioning in a well-designed, medically controlled environment, are able to affect patient outcome favorably by applying skilled and rapid resuscitative techniques in the field. The substantial controversy surrounding this subject may have more to do with the failure to apply such techniques in a proper and expeditious fashion than any other aspect of the debate.[93]

### THE ANESTHESIOLOGIST AND EMS

The anesthesiologist plays a unique and major role in the treatment and medical management of the trauma victim.[65] Frequently, he or she must initiate and maintain stabilization of the acutely injured patient, with little time to spare between the receipt of the patient and the beginning of the operative procedure. Airway management and protection, ventilation, evaluation of the unconscious patient, pain control, resuscitation, and patient monitoring are everyday concerns of the anesthesiologist. His or her expertise in these critical areas should be applied effectively in helping improve and maintain the quality of the community's EMS program.[120] In asking medical directors of EMS programs throughout the United States about which EMT skills require strengthening, the author has found consistently that the most important area is airway management. However, the involvement of anesthesiologists in EMT training remains minimal. Sadly, the teaching of airway management and intubation is often relegated to an EMT instructor with only textbook knowledge of the subject.

Anesthesiologists can and should be involved in studies of prehospital analgesia[107] and resuscitation and need not limit their curiosity and medical interest to the surgical suite and the intensive care unit. It is incumbent upon the practicing anesthesiologist with an interest in acute medicine to become aware of the community's efforts and plans for EMS development and to be involved actively in the process.

The community, its hospitals, and their professional staff should create an environment in which every physician, regardless of specialty, is encouraged and given optimal opportunity to contribute his or her skills, knowledge, and judgment to close the gap between knowledge and its application in acute medicine. This philosophy was stated by the Committee on Acute Medicine of the American Society of Anesthesiologists in its report on Community-Wide Emergency Medical Services in 1968, the early days of EMS.[95] It is surely equally applicable today.

## HOSPITAL CATEGORIZATION AND TRAUMA CARE SYSTEMS

### HOSPITAL CATEGORIZATION

Regional categorization of hospital emergency facilities is the cornerstone upon which any effective EMS system is built. This fact, however, has been overlooked by many localities in their initial rush to obtain large impressive mobile intensive care vehicles and personnel. The best prehospital medical care makes little sense if the hospital emergency department door is locked on the patient's arrival or if the available facilities are inadequate to provide for the patient's medical care.

In recognition of this problem, a joint multidisciplinary conference on Categorization of Hospital Emergency Services, sponsored by the American Medical Association's Commission on Emergency Medical Services and the American Hospital Association, was held in 1971.[11] The conference led to a published report, "Guidelines for Categorization of Hospital Emergency Capabilities." These guidelines served as a basis for evaluating emergency department capabilities for receiving and initially managing general medical and surgical problems.

After this report, the Federal Emergency Medical Services Systems Act of 1973 (P.L. 93–154)[54] and the amended act of 1976 (P.L. 94–573)[55] emphasized hospital categorization and sought to strengthen the concept by the identification of regional critical care capabilities. The term "horizontal categorization" is applied to the general classification of hospital abilities to manage a wide range of medical emergency conditions. A variety of formats have been employed to design and evaluate such capabilities. Most use some variation of the format suggested by the 1971 conference (Table 29-2).[11]

It is, of course, unrealistic to expect that all hospitals in a given geographic area should be equally capable of providing comprehensive medical services.[110] It may be somewhat surprising, then, that no other component of EMS planning has produced such controversy as the development of hospital categorization criteria. However, in most instances, once emergency department categorization is completed, hospitals frequently find they are able to allocate their medical and financial resources more effectively. This system allows certain hospitals to rely on their particular institutional strengths without being distracted by unanticipated medical emergencies that they are not prepared to manage.[15] On the other hand, hospitals with facilities that are adequate to manage acute emergencies are able to provide improved patient care.

Although horizontal categorization is capable of giving a general picture of services provided by each hospital in the region, it is seriously flawed by its lack of precision in identifying capabilities for definitive care of specific types of emergency patients. In addition, horizontal categorization did not entirely meet its intended objectives, probably because hospital participation was usually voluntary and evaluation of the system was empirically based.[64] This led to an additional type of hospital classification now known as vertical categorization or regionalization.

The term "vertical categorization" defines a hospital's capabilities to deal with specific emergent conditions, such as burns, spinal cord injuries, trauma, neonatal and pediatric emergencies, etc. Provisional guidelines for this type of categorization were published by the AMA in 1982 as a result of a second invitational conference co-sponsored by the American Hospital Association in 1975.[10] These guidelines specified eight critical care areas: (1) acute medical, (2) behavioral, (3) burn, (4) cardiac, (5) poisoning/drug, (6) spinal cord, (7) trauma, and (8) neonatal, perinatal, and pediatric. The American College of Surgeons has been especially active in this area in publishing guidelines and inspecting hospital capabilities relative to trauma management.[6,35,38] Vertical categorization, as does horizontal categorization, permits the recognition of medical capability for emergency treatment, but additionally, it identifies institutions capable of treating patients who require specialized care.[6] Systems have been developed to verify the commitment, performance, and capability of regionalized trauma centers in providing care for traumatized patients.[81]

## TRAUMA CARE SYSTEMS

The trauma care system is an integrated structure representing a continuum of care from accident prevention through rehabilitation.[38] Likewise, trauma care is largely a team effort. It requires a group of individuals including emergency medical technicians, nurses, physicians of all disciplines, and all support services to provide optimal care. Commitment, both personal and institutional, is probably the most important ingredient for care of the trauma patient.[47] Capable personnel need to be available immediately, along with so-

TABLE 29-2. Categorization of Hospital Emergency Capabilities (Horizontal Categorization)*

| CATEGORY | SUPPORT SERVICES | | | | | | INTENSIVE CARE UNIT (S) | |
|---|---|---|---|---|---|---|---|---|
| | *Blood Bank* | *Laboratory Services* | *Radiology* | *Angiography* | *Operating Rooms* | *Recovery Room* | *Facility* | *Staff* |
| I Comprehensive emergency service | Bank and storage in ER | Inhospital | Inhospital | Inhospital | Ready and staffed | Ready and staffed | X | X |
| II Major emergency service | Bank and storage in ER | Inhospital | Inhospital | — | Ready and staffed | Ready and staffed | X | X |
| III General emergency service | Storage in hospital | Inhospital or on-call | Inhospital or on-call | — | Readily available | Readily available | X | X |
| IV Basic emergency service | — | Inhospital or on-call | Inhospital or on-call | — | Available | — | — | — |

* Abbreviated format adapted from the AMA: Recommendations of the Conference on the Guidelines for the Categorization of Hospital Emergency Capabilities. Chicago: American Medical Association, 1971.

ER = emergency room; — = not available or not essential; X = essential.

TABLE 29-3. Some Essential (E) and Desirable (D) Characteristics for Level I, II, and III Trauma Centers*

| HOSPITAL ORGANIZATION | LEVELS I | II | III |
|---|---|---|---|
| Trauma service | E | E | E |
| Surgery departments/division/services/sections (each staffed by qualified specialists) | | | |
| *Cardiothoracic surgery | E | D | |
| *General surgery | E | E | E |
| *Neurosurgery | E | E | |
| *Obstetrics-gynecologic surgery | D | D | |
| *Ophthalmic surgery | E | D | |
| *Oral surgery—dental | D | D | |
| *Orthopedic surgery | E | E | |
| *Otorhinolaryngologic surgery | E | D | |
| *Pediatric surgery | E | D | |
| *Plastic and maxillofacial surgery | E | D | |
| *Urologic surgery | E | D | |
| Emergency department/division/service/section | E | E | E |
| Availability of surgical specialties inhospital 24 hours a day | | | |
| *General surgery | E | E | |
| Neurosurgery | E | E | |
| On-call and promptly available from inside or outside hospital | | | |
| *Cardiac surgery | E | D | |
| *General surgery | | | E |
| *Neurologic surgery | | | D |
| *Microsurgery capabilities | E | D | |

| HOSPITAL ORGANIZATION | LEVELS I | II | III |
|---|---|---|---|
| *Gynecologic surgery | E | D | |
| *Hand surgery | E | D | |
| *Ophthalmic surgery | E | E | D |
| *Oral surgery—dental | E | D | |
| *Orthopedic surgery | E | E | D |
| *Otorhinolaryngologic surgery | E | E | D |
| *Pediatric surgery | E | D | |
| *Plastic and maxillofacial surgery | E | E | D |
| *Thoracic surgery | E | E | D |
| *Urologic surgery | E | E | D |
| Nonsurgical specialty availability inhospital 24 hours a day | | | |
| *Emergency medicine | E | E | E |
| *Anesthesiology | E** | E† | E† |
| On-call and promptly available from inside or outside hospital | | | |
| *Cardiology | E | E | D |
| *Chest medicine | E | D | |
| *Gastroenterology | E | D | |
| *Hematology | E | E | D |
| *Infectious diseases | E | D | |
| *Internal medicine | E | E | E |
| *Nephrology | E | E | D |
| *Neuroradiology | D | | |
| *Pathology | E | E | D |
| *Pediatrics | E | E | D |
| *Psychiatry | E | D | |
| *Radiology | E | E | D |

* Complete information on levels of categorization and their essential (E) or desirable (D) characteristics is provided in Committee on Trauma of the American College of Surgeons: Hospital and prehospital resources for optimal care of the injured patient. Bull Am Coll Surg 1986; 71:4.

** Anesthesiology services for Level I trauma centers may be fulfilled by residents capable of assessing and promptly treating emergency conditions, provided the attending staff on call is advised and can be available promptly.

† Anesthesiology services for Level II and III trauma centers may be fulfilled by certified registered nurse anesthetist(s) (CRNA) capable of assessing and promptly treating emergency conditions, if the staff anesthesiologist is in the hospital at the time or shortly after the patient's arrival in the hospital.

phisticated equipment and services that are frequently expensive to purchase and maintain. Priority of access to laboratory facilities, operating room suites, and intensive care units must be ensured. The medical staff must be committed not only to prompt availablity but also to education, audits, and critiques. This commitment must not be limited to the surgical disciplines but should also involve the entire medical staff so that optimal medical care for the trauma patient can be planned and implemented. The anesthesia department has a unique and active role to play in this process. Its efforts in caring for the trauma patient must be on a par with those of the surgical services if excellence in this area is to be achieved.

A matrix designed by the AMA Commission on Emergency Medical Services and the American College of Surgeons Committee on Trauma[35,38] defines the medical staff and specialties requisite for each category of trauma care center (Table 29-3). The Level I trauma center is one that has made a major commitment of personnel and equipment to care for the trauma patient. The ability to manage complicated fractures and head, thoracic, visceral, and vascular injuries requires a high level of experience to ensure maximum benefit to the critically injured.[101] Only a relatively small number of trauma patients (approximately 10%) require the specialized services of a Level I facility.[86] The principal difference between Level I and Level II centers is the availability of staff specialists (Table 29-3). The Level III center is suited to handle minor trauma, which involves almost 80% of injured patients. This hospital therefore has also made a clear commitment to excellence of trauma care.

A similar classification has been proposed by the Trauma Committees of the American Pediatric Surgical Association and the American College of Surgeons.[111] The Level I pediatric trauma center is located in a children's hospital or a large, university-affiliated general hospital with a large pediatric unit and a commitment to trauma care. Such hospitals are capable of treating the most seriously injured children, eg, those with multisystem trauma or severe central nervous system injuries or those requiring care in a pediatric intensive care unit. Less severe injuries may be referred to a Level II facility, a general hospital with limited pediatric medical and surgical personnel and equipment.

Regional hospitals, in concert with the medical community,

should seek consensus on defining and identifying categories of patients who might best benefit from specialized care. Appropriate means of ensuring proper patient selection and distribution for such treatment should also be pursued.[78] It might well be of benefit for a hospital to upgrade to a higher level of categorization in only one or two special care areas that are underserved in its region. High operating costs and limited available resources prevent most facilities from providing highly specialized care for all types of injuries. For instance, the hospital with a Level I burn unit need not be the institution housing a Level I spinal cord injury care capability.

Regionalization ultimately helps ensure appropriate stabilization and transfer of the critically injured patient to a medical institution where a specialized service is ready and waiting.[100] Area-wide transfer protocols should be developed to transfer patients safely between hospitals.[37,78] In addition, these protocols help ensure the appropriate exchange of medical information regarding patient treatment, condition, and supportive care requirements. The regional EMS program is not complete without clear guidelines for patient transfer between medical facilities by air, water, or overland ambulance.[99]

## EFFECT OF TRAUMA CARE SYSTEMS ON OUTCOME

Numerous studies in urban areas show that the number of preventable deaths resulting from an inadequate trauma system varies from 30 to 40%.[41,44,58,79,112] Likewise, substantial data demonstrate that the specialized and sophisticated capabilities provided by categorized and regionalized facilities have a significant bearing on patient morbidity and mortality.[14,25,33,59,101,114] An often-quoted study by West and coworkers[117] comparing two California counties, one served by a Level I trauma center and the other where no such center was identified for the treatment of severely injured patients, showed a dramatic contrast in the intensity of treatment and patient survival between the two systems. The authors suggested that a substantial fraction, perhaps as many as 73% of non-CNS-related deaths and 28% of CNS-related deaths, could have been prevented with the vigorous resuscitation and aggressive surgical intervention offered by a Level I trauma center.

Of equal importance, the utilization of specialized care facilities appears to have a beneficial effect on morbidity, as well as mortality. Meyer et al.[84] have shown the effectiveness of immediate specialized care in decreasing morbidity, length of hospital stay, and medical care costs of spinal cord-injured patients treated within the Illinois trauma and spinal cord injury system as compared to those treated in "nonsystems" or those with delayed entry.

## METHODS FOR TRIAGING PATIENTS TO AN APPROPRIATE FACILITY

The use of clinical scoring systems has been proposed as a means of triaging trauma patients more effectively in the prehospital area.[34,74] Such indices are useful in assisting paramedical personnel to judge the urgency of care, as well as deciding whether a given patient requires the assessment and treatment capabilities of a designated trauma center.[27,86] An example of such a system is the Trauma Score developed by Champion et al. (Table 29-4).[29,30] The trauma score ranges from 1 to 16. The authors suggest that the sophisticated care of a trauma center is beneficial to patients with a score of 12 or less and that a score equal to or less than 3 may predict a fatal outcome even in a level I trauma center.[31] Morris et al.[86] also reported that a trauma score of 14 or less identifies the patient with severe injuries. However, personnel should not rely only on the raw score. Decision rules related to various practical medical judgements should also be utilized to apply the data more effectively to field triage.[29,31,32] In addition to their use in evaluating patient condition in the field, trauma indices may be used to compare the care rendered by a particular institution at different times, as well as by different institutions during a given period. Many variations of the trauma severity index are in use throughout the country, but no single index has won complete endorsement. Further information on trauma indices is offered in Chapter 1.

TABLE 29-4. Trauma Scale Developed by Champion for Field Triage and Evaluation of Care of the Trauma Victim*

| | | |
|---|---|---|
| Trauma Score | | |
| Respirations per minute | >36 | 2 |
| | 25–35 | 3 |
| | 10–24 | 4 |
| | 1–9 | 1 |
| | None | 0 |
| Respiratory expansion | Normal | 1 |
| | Shallow | 0 |
| | Retractive | 0 |
| Systolic blood pressure (mm Hg) | >90 | 4 |
| | 70–89 | 3 |
| | 50–69 | 2 |
| | 0–49 | 1 |
| | No pulse | 0 |
| Capillary return | Normal | 2 |
| | Delayed | 1 |
| | None | 0 |
| Glasgow Coma Scale | | |
| Eye opening | Spontaneous | 4 |
| | To Voice | 3 |
| | To Pain | 2 |
| | None | 1 |
| Verbal response | Oriented | 5 |
| | Confused | 4 |
| | Inappropriate words | 3 |
| | Incomprehensible words | 2 |
| | None | 1 |
| Motor response | Obeys command | 6 |
| | Localizes pain | 5 |
| | Withdraw (pain) | 4 |
| | Flexion (pain) | 3 |
| | Extension (pain) | 2 |
| | None | 1 |
| Contribution of total Glasgow Coma Scale points to Trauma Score | | 14 and 15 = 5 |
| | | 11 to 13 = 4 |
| | | 8 to 10 = 3 |
| | | 5 to 7 = 2 |
| | | 3 to 4 = 1 |
| Total Trauma Score | | 1–16 |

* Adapted from Morris et al[86] with permission.

# DISASTER PLANNING AND MANAGEMENT

The American College of Emergency Physicians defines disaster as "sudden massive disproportion between hostile elements of any kind and the survival resources that are available to counterbalance these in the shortest period of time."[7] What might constitute a disaster in a rural farming area might be routinely managed in a large urban medical center. Thus, except in extreme cases, such as the earthquakes in Mexico City or Armenia or the gas leak that claimed 2,000 lives in Bhopal, India,[116] the number and severity of casualties resulting from an accident may not by themselves always be sufficient data to activate an emergency disaster plan. The capability of the community and the available hospitals to deal with such an emergency must also be considered. Activation of a contingency plan may have serious implications, both in terms of cost and of maintaining existing patient care, necessitating a careful assessment of the situation.

There has been a change in the spectrum of disasters during the last few decades. The frequency of industrial explosions, terrorist attacks,[60,61,96] aircraft or mass ground transportation accidents, nuclear power plant leaks, and war-related injuries appears to have increased,[5,17,23,24,43,57,76,102,103,116] whereas natural disasters–earthquakes, tornados, floods, fires, and volcanic eruptions–continue to occur at a steady rate.[28,83] Therefore, today's contingency plans must include appropriate measures to deal effectively with this wide variety of conditions.

The primary goal of disaster management is to reduce mortality, morbidity, pain, and distress. This goal can be accomplished by thoughtful predisaster preparation, realistic confrontation of the situation, and well-coordinated teamwork among medical and nonmedical personnel at all levels.[61,96,97] All physicians, regardless of their specialization, can have valuable input into the successful management of a mass casualty incident. Thus, a basic knowledge of the principles of disaster management is essential for all physicians. Although very little emphasis is given to this aspect of care in the anesthesia literature, anesthesiologists are by no means exempt from this task. The remainder of this chapter outlines briefly the basic concepts of disaster planning and management.

## GENERAL PRINCIPLES OF DISASTER MANAGEMENT

Although the existing knowledge of disaster management is based on lessons learned from widely varying occurrences in the past and there are significant regional organizational variations in dealing with this type of emergency, certain established principles for civilian disaster management do exist.[115] The most important of these is the requirement for coordination among community and hospital personnel and resources. Emergency medical services systems (EMSS), police and fire departments, news media, clergy, and industrial and volunteer community groups must participate in all phases of disaster planning and management. The EMS system plays a central role in coordinating these groups. Regional EMS systems develop plans to organize the area's medical resources to meet possible contingencies and coordinate plans with those of other areas in order to provide further assistance when required. This coordination may involve linkage with other regional, state, or federal agencies.[85] After preparation of a disaster plan, mock casualty exercises (drills) should be arranged to assess the capacity and readiness of the community and its hospitals to respond and to determine the shortcomings of the plan. Based on these evaluations, necessary improvements and adjustments may be made.

Since civilian disasters occur rarely, the lessons learned from a previous disaster are frequently forgotten by the time the next major incident occurs in the region. It is therefore extremely important that a community's medical contingency plans be reviewed and practiced at least annually, thereby ensuring that they remain current and active. In addition, the changing roster of hospital personnel dictates the need to inform new members of the staff about the hospital and community disaster plan. Disaster planning should be thought of, in part, as a communication exercise in which keeping confusion and error to a minimum is vital.

Although most principles of trauma care remain unchanged during mass casualty incidents, some specific modifications are mandatory if the mortality rate is to be reduced. Treatment should be based on explicit priorities during all phases of management. During the initial sorting of the patients in the field or in the emergency department, two major questions should be answered before attempting treatment. First, how soon is care needed? Second, if treatment is needed, what is the potential for survival? Casualty victims with a low probability of survival will usually not benefit from the time and effort spent in resuscitation, which endangers the lives of those who are less critically injured. Unfortunately, in disaster situations, attempts to provide maximum care to all victims will lead to total paralysis of the medical service, resulting in inadequate care for everyone.[39,122] Certain compromises may also be required in the treatment of casualties in the hospital; the greater the disaster, the greater the compromise.[123] For instance, sophisticated techniques, such as limb replantation, although standard surgical treatment in normal circumstances, may not be appropriate during a major disaster.[22,70,71,123] Likewise, sophisticated radiologic tests may need to be omitted to accelerate patient care. There should be constant evaluation of the number and severity of injuries versus the available manpower and resources before attempting comprehensive and ideal medical or surgical therapy.

The approximate number and types of injuries should be ascertained so that injured victims are distributed according to each hospital's capacity and specialization. Most civilian injuries involve blunt or penetrating multiple trauma, burns, chemical inhalation, exposure to radiation, or combinations of these injuries. Thus, transporting a severely burned patient to a hospital with no specialized burn treatment unit, especially if such a center exists in the area, will result in suboptimal patient care and unnecessary stress on the receiving hospital. Overloading a particular hospital with a large number of casualties will have similar effects. Most modern EMS systems give special consideration to these issues and transport patients to appropriate hospitals.[70] Whenever possible, injured victims should be taken to designated trauma or mass casualty centers where personnel are available with training in handling large numbers of injured patients.

## DISASTER PLANNING

Medical management of disasters involves two areas: prehospital and hospital care. Consequently, plans should be devised for each of these areas emphasizing proper coordination between the two. No universal plan can fit the needs of all hospitals or communities. Thus, each community is responsible for formulating, disseminating, and periodically assessing its own plan.[85,97] Careful consideration should be given to factors that have the potential of limiting the medical management of mass casualties, such as riots or crowds, traffic congestion, communication system failures, floods, weather (snowstorms, torrential rains, extremes of temperature), poor lighting, and difficult terrain.

### *Planning for Prehospital Care of Disasters*

EMSS, fire, and police department personnel are the first responders to a mass casualty. The plan devised for the prehospital care of disaster victims should contain clear guidelines regarding the function of each group during these incidents. In addition to extricating and stabilizing disaster victims, selected paramedical personnel should be in contact with a coordinating medical command center to relay information about the type of accident, the number of injured, the type of injuries, field treatment applied, and the names of regional hospitals to which the victims are being transported. In turn, they should receive physician instruction for further prehospital care. The disaster plan must outline clearly (a) criteria and procedures for declaring a disaster situation, (b) mechanisms for implementation of the disaster plan, (c) triage procedures, (d) means of transportation of the injured, (e) the receiving hospital, (f) available means of communication, and (g) equipment and supply. As the type, place, and magnitude of a mass casualty cannot be predicted, some parts of the plan may not be applicable to the actual situation. Alternative options should be included in each section of the plan to overcome this problem.

Under certain circumstances, medical teams may be required to report to the accident scene to direct the initial triage and stabilization of casualties. These teams are given various titles, such as "Proceed Out Team," "Triage Team," "Go Team," "Mobile Medical Team," or "Mobile Inflatable Treatment Unit." The specialties of the team physicians vary with the geographic location, but a surgeon, an emergency physician, an anesthesiologist, and a nurse are frequently included.[63,124] Prior planning must ensure that these teams are able to function under appropriate medical command and supervision in a relatively secure environment.[124] An effective reporting and communication mechanism to apprise areawide hospitals of the status and numbers of injured being dispatched to them is vital. In turn, hospitals should be able to inform field dispatchers of their current capabilities to handle increased numbers or types of casualties. An effective mechanism to accomplish this type of information linkage can be readily developed with some thought and planning.

In London, Ontario, the activities of the "Mobile Medical Team" are coordinated with a clear plan of their function.[63] This system involves three emergency physicians who represent three active treatment centers in the area. One of these physicians is assigned to the command post. He or she functions as director of all medical personnel at the disaster site and has direct contact with those in charge of other rescue personnel. All communications from medical teams and hospitals go through this coordinator (Fig 29-1). The second physician is assigned to the disaster site to direct triage in this area. The remaining physician is in the casualty collection area to coordinate the evacuation of casualties in order of priority. The responsibilities of each coordinator are shown in Table 29-5. In addition to these coordinators, medical teams are deployed from hospitals as needed to work with rescue personnel.

In Boston, a slightly different system is in operation.[71] Disaster management is coordinated centrally from the Emergency Medical Systems/Regional Trauma Center using online voice and telemetry communication with physicians in the field. "Mobile Medical Teams" are sent to the accident scene along with emergency medical technicians. A triage and collection area is set up in the vicinity of the accident to stabilize and triage patients to regional trauma centers. Little time is spent in stabilization of patients, and emphasis is on the expedited transport of casualties to an appropriate trauma center. Constant communication is maintained through the central EMS/Trauma Center between medical teams on the disaster scene and regional trauma centers or specialized

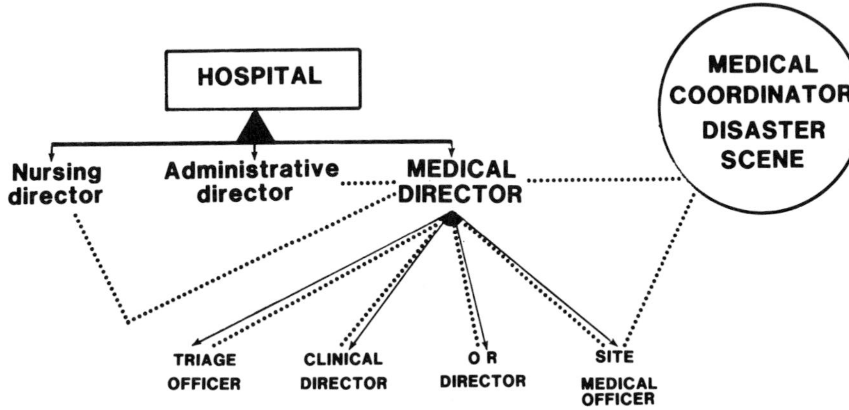


FIG. 29-1. Planned communications and patient flow in a possible mass casualty incident in London, Ontario. (Adapted from Gerace[63] with permission.)

TABLE 29-5. Individual Responsibilities of Members of the Medical On-Site Disaster Coordinating Team in London, Ontario*

Command post (senior)
- Establish authority at scene of disaster.
- Establish command post.
- Establish casualty collection area.
- Ensure communication with disaster site, casualty collection area, and hospitals.
- Coordinate patient transfer.
- Deploy triage team.
- Maintain communication with medical officer of health.
- Coordinate medical care with rescue efforts of nonmedical personnel

Disaster site
- Aid senior coordinator in establishing command post and casualty collection area.
- Establish authority at disaster site.
- Instruct and deploy triage team.
- Coordinate transfer of casualties to casualty collection area.
- Maintain communication with command post.
- Request supplies as needed from senior coordinator.

Casuality collection area
- Aid senior coordinator in establishing command post and casualty collection area.
- Establish authority at casualty collection area.
- Instruct and deploy triage team.
- Indicate priorities in transfer to hospital.
- Maintain communication with command post.
- Request supplies from senior coordinator as needed.

* (From Gerace[63] with permission.)

TABLE 29-6. Categorization of Patients at the Disaster Collection Area

| CATEGORY | COLOR | TYPE OF CASUALTY |
|---|---|---|
| I | Green | Casualties in need of minimal treatment who do not need hospitalization |
| II | Red | Casualties in need of immediate treatment whose probability of recovery is good after such therapy, eg, correctable respiratory obstruction, controllable hemorrhage, compound fractures |
| III | Yellow | Casualties in need of treatment but delay in treatment is not likely to jeoparize recovery, eg, limited thermal injury, closed fractures, mild bleeding |
| IV | Blue or black | Casualties who have poor chance of recovery because of the magnitude of the injury and/or because an excessive commitment of personnel and material would be required; these patients require expectant treatment |

units. All of these activities are based on a well-designed disaster plan.

The disaster plan devised for John F. Kennedy Airport in New York is considerably different from those described above.[45] Physicians from two trauma centers in the city are transported to the accident scene where, in two inflatable hospitals with operating room, ICU, and burn unit facilities, they stabilize patients and then transport them by air ambulances to their medical centers. The effectiveness of this system is unknown, because it has not yet been tested by an actual mass casualty.

In Chicago the chief fire official is responsible for declaring a disaster.[122] Police, paramedics, emergency medical technicians, and medical teams from selected area hospitals reach the disaster scene and function together according to a devised plan. The chief medical officer at the disaster site consults with the chief fire official in selecting a safe casualty collection area. Medical teams and paramedics examine the patients and triage them into four color-coded groups according to the severity of their injuries (Table 29-6). Patients are then moved to the appropriate observation and evacuation areas.

It is obvious that disaster plans vary widely with location. Medical personnel should be familiar with the plans for their area to reduce confusion during a devastating mass casualty.

## *Planning for Hospital Care of Disasters*

Every hospital must be prepared to manage a disaster at any time. The Joint Commission on Accreditation of Hospitals (JCAH) requires a written disaster plan, a semiannual review and hospital-wide rehearsal, and revision of the plan if necessary.[73] These activities should be coordinated by the hospital's disaster committee,[42] which is usually chaired by an emergency department physician. Committee members should include experienced representatives from both medical and nonmedical departments. The plan must be simple, clear, easily understandable, flexible enough to meet the demands of any disaster situation, and adaptable to nights and weekends. In addition, the plan should not include individual names but only designate the holders of relevant positions and should follow normal hospital procedures as much as possible. The hospital disaster committee should be given the responsibility for disseminating the plan throughout the hospital.

Disaster management requires leadership and decision. Consequently, a hierarchical command system should be established. Although the details of the system may be different for each hospital, the basic structure remains the same. An organizational plan described by Williams[123] is shown in Figure 29-2. One senior member each from the surgical or emergency department, nursing, and hospital administration is selected to be in charge of hospital-wide disaster management. The medical director, preferably a senior trauma surgeon or emergency physician with administrative experience, is responsible for organization and coordination. He or she appoints (a) a triage officer to be in charge of patient triage in a designated area of the hospital; (b) a clinical director to supervise patient care and surgical priorities in the ICUs and patient floors; and (c) an operating room director, usually a senior anesthesiologist, to organize operating room activities. In addition, he or she may designate another member of the staff to establish communication with the authorities at the disaster scene and to evaluate the magnitude of the problem. The medical director communicates with nursing and administrative directors, the medical coordinator at the disaster

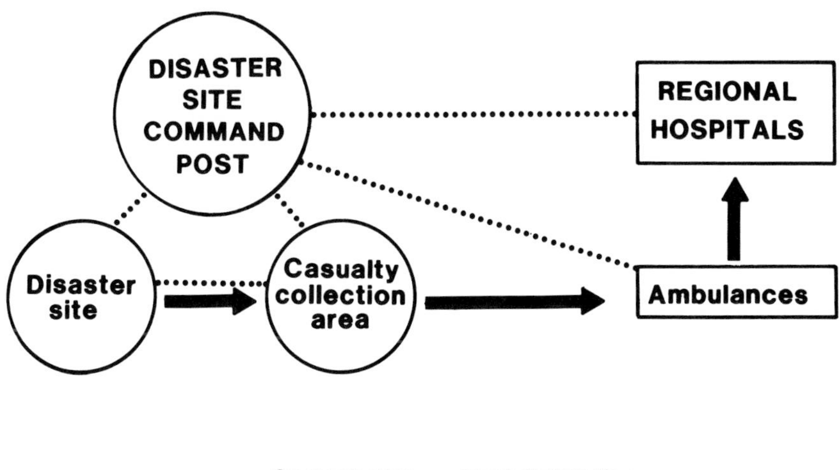


FIG. 29-2. Hospital disaster plan described by Williams.[123]

scene, the triage officer, the clinical director, and the operating room director. In addition, he or she communicates with the directors of various surgical departments if additional manpower is needed. The medical director should not be involved in direct patient care. The director of nursing identifies nursing needs and allocates extra staff to essential areas. The senior hospital administrator manages the nonclinical aspects of the hospital response.

The plan described by Williams[123] may be too simplistic for managing a major disaster. However, it provides a basic structure upon which additional systems may be built according to need and the varying organizational design of different hospitals.

## SPECIFIC ACTIVITIES DURING DISASTER MANAGEMENT

### *Triage*

In Dorland's Medical Dictionary, triage is defined as "the sorting out and classification of casualties of war or other disasters to determine priority of need and proper place of treatment." Thus, triage serves two purposes: to identify those victims who are in the greatest need of immediate medical treatment and with the highest probability of survival and to transport patients to the appropriate medical facility or treatment area. Disaster casualties may be triaged in several locations. Initial triage takes place at the accident site where sorting of victims is usually limited to two categories, the dead and the living. The living injured are then moved to a collection area near the accident site where the victims are divided into four categories and tagged according to the severity of their injury (Table 29-6).[19,22,61,97,122]

In the casualty collection area or in a separate observation area, the patients are observed and treated until they are transported to appropriate hospitals. Constant updating of assessment and categorization is essential in this area since patient condition may change rapidly during the early phase of injury.[97] The use of color-coded tags facilitates the recognition of severity of each patient's injury. Short notes may also be written on these tags to specify the diagnosis and the treatment administered.[63] In the collection area, very little time (15–20 seconds per patient) is spent in evaluating and triaging each victim. Evaluation involves the assessment of general status, estimation of blood pressure (palpable radial pulse = BP> 80 mm Hg, only carotid pulse palpable = BP 60–80 mm Hg, no palpable pulse = BP <60 mm Hg), examination of the airways, ventilation, and consciousness.[122]

A separate triage procedure takes place in the hospital where a specific area is designated for this purpose.[123] Here, those with minor injuries are sent home or to another institution where care can be provided by internists, general physicians, or other nonsurgically trained physicians. Those who require observation are admitted to the ICUs or to patient floors, depending on the severity of their injuries. Patients with minor injuries requiring surgical care are operated on in the emergency department under local anesthesia, whereas those requiring major surgery are sent to the operating room where they are kept in a holding area until the necessary procedure(s) may be performed. Patients requiring radiologic and laboratory examination are sent to appropriate locations or X-rays may be taken with portable units. Resuscitation is carried out in a designated area of the hospital, usually the emergency department.

Interhospital transfer of some patients may be required by hospitals unable to provide further necessary and definitive care due to limited or overburdened resources. The inclusion of transfer protocols into the medical diaster plan expedites greatly the management of this problem.

### *Communications*

A disaster that causes mass casualties may destroy the means of communication as well. A communication system is vital for the operational effectiveness of a disaster plan. Most disaster plans include alternative means of communication, such as two-way radio. With today's advanced technology, communication failures should occur only rarely.

### *Transportation*

Disaster victims should be transported to hospitals capable of managing their specific injuries. The benefits of hospital categorization in identifying the capability of these resources become quite evident under these circumstances.[40] Public and private vehicles should be mobilized as required to expedite the transportation of victims.

### *Operating Room and Recovery Room Management*

Mass casualties have a major impact on the function of operating and recovery rooms. Under normal circumstances, the medical director of this unit, in conjunction with the Operating Room Committee, should devise a comprehensive operational plan for incorporation into the hospital's disaster manual. Potential manpower, supply, and equipment issues and operational problems should be identified, and appropriate responses should be formulated. During a disaster, a physician should be in charge of this unit. His or her responsibility is to ensure that a sufficient number of operating rooms and personnel are available to respond to the additional requirements. In consultation with the clinical director, he or she should arrange a realistic schedule to deal efficiently with the workload and should maintain communication with the triage officer, clinical director, and medical director to plan for further developments. As it is not known when another life-threatening injury will arrive, one or two operating rooms should be kept reserved during the initial stages of a disaster, if possible.[17]

Most operations are performed by residents with one attending surgeon supervising several operating rooms. Likewise, anesthesia is administered by residents and CRNAs under attending supervision. During nights and weekends, anesthesiologists and surgeons should be called in as needed. If the disaster occurs during a time when all operating rooms are busy with elective surgery, special accommodations should be made to provide adequate care for casualties. Frequently, 1 to 2 hours elapse between the occurrence of the disaster and the arrival of patients in the operating room. During this period relatively short surgical operations can be completed and these rooms prepared for emergencies. In addition, most trauma centers reserve one operating room for trauma emergencies. This room can be used, if needed, until the remaining rooms become available.

An experienced surgeon must be in charge to make priority decisions as each operating room becomes available.[50] In general, during the early stages of disaster, surgery is performed only for life- or major function-threatening injuries. Those patients who can tolerate a delay in treatment without significant risk to life or of disability can be operated on after the initial crisis is over. However, in desperate situations, when large numbers of casualty victims are waiting for relatively minor surgery (eg, wound debridements), other available surgical areas, such as delivery suites, may be used.[88] In these circumstances, all surgical staff are expected to function as trauma surgeons.[88,97]

The recovery room treatment of disaster victims may require significant physician input. A sufficient number of anesthesia staff should be assigned to the postanesthetic area to provide adequate care. When the operating room workload does not allow such staffing, physicians from nonsurgical departments may be asked to staff the area under the direction of an anesthesiologist until more anesthesia staff become available.

### *Management of Nuclear Accidents*

Present-day society is under a constant threat of nuclear disaster. Leakage of radioactive substances from nuclear plants[82,116] or explosion of nuclear weapons, either during a war or a terrorist act,[3,49,75] would be the major causes of these incidents. Nuclear disaster victims may present with associated thermal and mechanical injuries caused either by the explosion or by vehicular accidents during the rapid evacuation of the contaminated area.[36] A wide geographic locale including the regional hospitals may be involved.[77] Area-wide evacuation plans must be prepared to deal with such a devastating situation.

Every effort must be made to protect the health care team and to prevent contamination of the hospital. Casualty victims should be handled by trained teams dressed in protective disposable clothing. Triage should be done outside the hospital in an area near the emergency department. Disaster victims should be monitored by Geiger counters for radioactivity. Contaminated clothing should be removed, stored in appropriate containers, and subsequently destroyed by personnel familiar with radiation safety. The area designated for triage should have shower facilities to decontaminate patients.

Triage involves the determination of mechanical and thermal injuries and of the radiation dose received by the patient. The treatment of associated trauma should be given priority because even high doses of radiation do not cause immediate death.[68] In addition, open wounds and burns are excellent portals for entry of infection that, in the radiation-induced immunosuppressed patient, may easily cause sepsis if urgent debridement or antibiotic therapy is not initiated.[62]

The radiation dose received by the patient can be determined by the hospital's radiation safety officers, health physicist, or biologist. Exposure to 5,000 rad or more causes acute central nervous system disorders, such as weakness, disorientation, seizures, and coma. As this type of injury is certainly fatal, such doomed patients are given only supportive care.[68] Doses between 800–1,000 rad also cause death in most victims within 2 weeks after exposure. However, these patients may be treated by intravenous fluids, antibiotics, and blood, platelet and granulocyte transfusions. Bone marrow transplantation may be indicated. The $LD_{50}$ of acute whole body radiation exposure is 450 rad. In the presence of trauma, infections, and malnutrition, this dose may be lower.[75] In any case, disaster victims who receive radiation doses less than 600 rad should be treated aggressively as they may be salvageable. The long-term consequences of radiation exposure include the increased risk of cataracts, cancer, and possibly congenital abnormalities in the offspring of the victim.[68]

## ROLE OF THE ANESTHESIOLOGIST IN DISASTER PLANNING AND MANAGEMENT

The primary medical responsibility for predisaster planning, disaster management, and coordination of the entire system is assumed by emergency physicians.[7] They are involved in planning at all levels: hospital, community, state, and federal government. Anesthesiologists, as well as other surgical and nonsurgical specialists, assist them in this task. On the hospital level, the anesthesia department develops guidelines for departmental procedures to deal with mass emergencies. These guidelines are incorporated into the hospital's disaster manual and disseminated among the staff. Many operating and recovery rooms in the United States and other countries are directed by anesthesia departments. In these centers, anesthesiologists are involved in preparing operational plans to facilitate the effective functioning of the unit in disaster situations. Preparedness requires the effective teaching of appropriate therapy to medical and nonmedical groups who would be utilized in a disaster. Airway management, pain control, and resuscitation are important parts of these instructive sessions. Because of their unique expertise in these areas, anesthesiologists have frequently been requested to participate in these courses.

During an actual disaster, the primary roles of anesthesiologists are (a) to provide anesthetic care in the operating room, (b) to manage immediate postoperative care in the recovery room, and (c) to act as consultants in the management of problems requiring their expertise in other areas of the hospital. In addition, they may take part in prehospital triage and stabilization of disaster victims in any area where expertise in airway management, pain control, and resuscitation may be needed and is not otherwise available. If departmental manpower is sufficient, assignment of anesthesia staff to the emergency department to direct airway management and provide pain relief to disaster victims may be desirable. Regional anesthetic techniques, mainly in the form of peripheral nerve blockade, have been recommended in disaster situations.[119]

## CONCLUSION

Care of the trauma patient is best provided by an integrated system of medical management extending from prevention through rehabilitation and requiring close cooperation among specialists in each phase of care. The EMS system represents a crucial aspect of this approach to improve the quality of care of the injured patient and thus to reduce morbidity and mortality.

Inhospital care of the seriously injured is best provided by facilities with administrations and medical staff that have established a strong commitment to the trauma patient. The anesthesiologist holds a significant position in maintaining that commitment from acute treatment through rehabilitation. It is appropriate therefore for the specialty to encourage interested practitioners to participate and contribute as actively as possible in the design of the EMS trauma system.

Successful management of mass casualties requires adequate preparedness, coordination between community and hospital resources and awareness of the area- and hospital-wide disaster plan by every community and hospital member. All physicians should be familiar with the principles of disaster management. Anesthesiologists can provide valuable input during both the planning and management phases of disasters.

## REFERENCES


1. Accidental death and disability: the neglected disease of modern society. Washington, DC: National Research Council, 1966.
2. Accident facts. Chicago: National Safety Council, 1989;8.
3. Alley EE. Emergency planning in the nuclear age. Practitioner 1981;225:711.
4. Allied health education directory. 14th ed, Chicago: American Medical Association, 1986:35.
5. Allister C, Hamilton GM. Cordowan coal mine explosion: experience of mass burns incident. Br Med J 1983;287:403.
6. American Burn Association. Guidelines for service standards and severity classifications for the treatment of burn injury. Bull Am Coll Surg 1984;69:24.
7. American College of Emergency Physicians. Guidelines for trauma care systems. Ann Emerg Med 1987;16:459.
8. American College of Emergency Physicians. Medical control of pre-hospital emergency medical services. Ann Emerg Med 1982;11:7.
9. American Medical Association Committee on Emergency Medical Services. Proceedings of Emergency Medical Services Futures conference. Chicago: American Medical Association, 1985.
10. American Medical Association Commission on Emergency Medical Services. Provisional guidelines for the optimal categorization of hospital emergency capabilities. Chicago: American Medical Association, 1982.
11. American Medical Association, Commission on Emergency Medical Services. Recommendations of the Conference on the Guidelines for the Categorization of Hospital Emergency Capabilities. Chicago: American Medical Association, 1971:1.
12. Ammons MA, Moore EE, Pons PT, et al. The role of a regional trauma system in the management of a mass disaster: an analysis of the Keystone, Colorado, chairlift accident. J Trauma 1988;28:1468.
13. Aprahamian C, Thompson BM, Towne JB, Darin JC. The effect of a paramedic system on mortality of major open intra-abdominal vascular trauma. J Trauma 1983;23:687.
14. Baker CC, Oppenheimer L, Stephens B, et al. Epidemiology of trauma death. Am J Surg 1980;140:144.
15. Benson DM, Safar P. Categorization and regionalization of hospital emergency facilities. In: Public health aspects of critical care medicine and anesthesiology. Clinical Anesthesia 10/3. Philadelphia: FA Davis, 1974.
16. Benson DM, Esposito MPH, Dirsch J, et al. Mobile intensive care by "unemployable" blacks trained as emergency medical technicians (EMTs) in 1967–1969. J Trauma 1971;12:408.
17. Bliss AR. Major disaster planning. Br Med J 1984;288:1433.
18. Border JR, Lewis FR, Aprahamian C, et al. Pre-hospital trauma care—stabilize or scoop and run. J Trauma 1983;23:708.
19. Bowers WF, Hughes CW. Surgical philosophy in mass casualty management. Springfield, IL: Charles C Thomas, 1960.
20. Boyd DR. Trauma—a controllable disease in the 1980's (Fourth Annual Stone Lecture, American Trauma Society). J Trauma 1980;20:14.
21. Boyd DR. Comprehensive regional trauma and emergency medical service delivery system: a goal of the 1980's. Crit Care Q 1982;5:1.
22. Briggs SE, Flint LM. Mass casualty management. In: Zuidema GD, Rutherford RB, Ballinger WF, eds. The management of trauma. 4th ed. Philadelphia: WB Saunders, 1985:801.
23. Brismar B, Bergenwald L. The terrorist bomb explosion in Bologna, Italy, 1980: an analysis of the effects of the injuries sustained. J Trauma 1982;22:216.
24. Buerk CA, Batdorf JW, Cammack KV, et al. The MGM Grand

Hotel fire. Lessons learned from a major disaster. Arch Surg 1982;117:641.
25. Cales RH, Trunkey DD. Preventable trauma deaths. A review of trauma care systems development. JAMA 1985;254:1059.
26. Caroline NL. Medical care in the streets. JAMA 1977;237:43.
27. Cayten GC. Trauma indices: a critical analysis. Crit Care Q 1972;5:79.
28. Centers for Disease Control. Tornado disaster—North Carolina, South Carolina, March 23, 1984. MMWR 1985;34:205 and 211.
29. Champion HR, Sacco WJ, Hannan DS, et al. Assessment of injury severity: The triage index. Crit Care Med 1980;8:201.
30. Champion HR, Sacco WJ, Carnazzo AJ, et al. Trauma score. Crit Care Med 1981;9:672.
31. Champion HR, Gainer PS, Yackee E. A progress report on the trauma score in predicting a fatal outcome. J Trauma 1986;26:927.
32. Champion HR, Sacco WJ, Gainer, PS, Patow SM. The effect of medical direction on trauma triage. J Trauma 1988;28:235.
33. Clemmer TP, Orme JF, Thomas FO, Brooks KA. Outcome of critically injured patients treated at Level I trauma centers versus full-service community hospitals. Crit Care Med 1985;13:861.
34. Clemmer TP, Orme JF, Thomas F, Brooks KA. Prospective evaluation of the CRAMS scale for triaging major trauma. J Trauma 1985;25:188.
35. Committee on Trauma. Hospital resources for optimal care of the trauma patient. Bull Am Coll Surg 1979;64:11.
36. Committee on Trauma, American College of Surgeons. Disaster planning for mass casualties: In: Walt AJ, ed. Early care of the injured Patient. Philadelphia: WB Saunders, 1982:376.
37. Committee on Trauma. Interhospital transfer of patients. Bull Am Coll Surg 1984;69:29.
38. Committee on Trauma. Hospital and prehospital resources for optimal care of the injured patient. Bull Am Coll Surg 1986;74:4.
39. Cowley RA, Myers RAM, Gretes AJ. EMS response to mass casualties. Emerg Med Clin North Am 1984;2:687.
40. Department of Defense Department of Health and Human Services, F.E.M.A., National Disaster Medical System. Disaster medical assistance team operations manual. Washington, DC: US Government Printing Office, 1984.
41. Detmer DE, Moylan JA, Rose J, et al. Regional categorization and quality of care in major trauma. J Trauma 1980;20:848.
42. Disaster management. A planning guide for hospital administrators. Chicago: American Hospital Association, 1971.
43. District of Columbia Metropolitan Police Department: Post disaster evaluation report: emergency responses to multiple disaster. Washington, DC: University Research Corporation, 1982.
44. Dove DB, Stahl WM, Del Guercio LRM. A five year review of deaths following urban trauma. J Trauma 1980;20:760.
45. Dove DB, Del Guercio LRL, Stahl WM, et al. A metropolitan airport disaster plan—coordination of a multihospital response to provide on-site resuscitation and stabilization before evacuation. J Trauma 1982;22:550.
46. Eastman AB, Lewis FR, Champion HR, Mattox KL. Regional trauma system design: critical concepts. Am J Surg 1987;154:79.
47. Eggold R. Trauma care regionalization: a necessity. J Trauma 1983;23:260.
48. Eiseman B. Combat casualty management in Vietnam. J Trauma 1967;7:53.
49. Eiseman B. Casualty care planning. J Trauma 1979;19:848.
50. Eiseman B. Mass casualties. In: Moore EE, Eiseman B, Van Way CW, Eds. Critical Decisions In trauma. St. Louis: CV Mosby, 1984:16.
51. Eisenberg M, Berger L, Hallstrom A. Paramedic programs and out of hospital cardiac arrest. I. Factors associated with successful resuscitation. Am J Public Health 1979;69:30.
52. Eisenberg M, Berger L, Hallstrom A. Paramedic programs and out of hospital cardiac arrest. II. Impact on community mortality. Am J Public Health 1979;69:39.
53. Emergency medical services at midpassage. A report of the Committee on Emergency Medical Services, Assembly of Life Sciences, National Research Council. Washington, DC: National Academy of Sciences, 1978:15.
54. Emergency Medical Services System Act of 1973. P.L. 93–154, Washington, DC, 1973.
55. Emergency Medical Services System Amendments of 1976. P.L. 94–573, Washington, DC, 1976.
56. Emergency Medical Services Systems program guidelines. DHEW, Public Health Service, Health Services Administration, Bureau of Medical Services. Publication No. (HSA) 75–2013. Revised 1975.
57. Finch P, Nancekievill DG. The role of hospital medical teams at a major accident. Anaesthesia 1975;30:666.
58. Foley RW, Harris LS, Pilcher DB, et al. Abdominal injuries in automobile accidents: review of care in fatally injured patients. J Trauma 1977;17:611.
59. Frey CF, Huelke DF, Gikas PW. Resuscitation and survival in motor vehicle accidents. J Trauma 1969;9:292.
60. Frykberg ER, Tepas JJ: Terrorist bombings: lessons learned from Belfast to Beirut. Ann Surg 1988;208:569.
61. Frykberg ER, Hutton PMJ, Balzer RH. Disaster in Beirut: an application of mass casualty principles. Milit Med 1987;152:563.
62. Gale RP. Immediate medical consequences of nuclear accidents: lessons from Chernobyl. JAMA 1987;258:625.
63. Gerace RV. Role of medical teams in a community disaster plan. Can Med Assoc J 1979;120:923.
64. Gibson G. Categorization of hospital emergency capabilities: some empirical methods to evaluate appropriateness of emergency department utilization. J Trauma 1978;18:94.
65. Giesecke AH. The anesthesiologist and the traumatized patient. Semin Anesth 1985;4:89.
66. Heaton LD. Army medical services activities in Vietnam. Milit Med 1966;131:646.
67. Holroyd BR, Knopp R, Kallsen G. Medical control quality assurance in prehospital care. JAMA 1986;256:1027,
68. Hubner KF, Lushbaugh CC. Radiation injuries. In: Moore EE, Eiseman B, Van Way C, eds. Critical decisions in trauma. St. Louis: CV Mosby, 1984:452.
69. Jacobs LM, Berrizbeitia L. Prehospital trauma care. Emerg Med Clin North Am 1984;2:717.
70. Jacobs LM, Ramp J, Breay J. An emergency medical system approach to disaster planning. J Trauma 1979;19:157.
71. Jacobs LM, Goody MM, Sinclair A. The role of a trauma center in disaster management. J Trauma 1983;23:697.
72. Jacobs LM, Sinclair A, Beiser A, D'Agosinto RB. Prehospital advanced life support. Benefits in trauma. J Trauma 1984;24:8.
73. Joint Commission on Accreditation of Hospitals. Plant, technology and safety management. Accreditation manual for hospitals, Chicago: JCAH 1989;203.
74. Kilberg L, Clemmer TP, Clawson J, et al. Effectiveness of implementing a trauma triage system on outcome: a prospective evaluation. J Trauma 1988;28:1493.
75. Leaf A. New perspectives on the medical consequences of nuclear war. N Engl J Med 1986;315:905.
76. Lewis FR, Trunkey DD, Steele M. Autopsy of a disaster: the Martinez bus accident. J Trauma 1980;20:861.
77. Linnemann RE. Soviet medical response to the Chernobyl nuclear accident. JAMA 1987;258:637.
78. Lockwood BJ. Transport of multisystem trauma patients from rural to urban health care facilities. Crit Care Q 1982;5:22.

79. Lowe DR, Gately HL, Frey CL, et al. Patterns of death, complications and error in the management of motor vehicle accidents. J Trauma 1983;23:503.
80. Luterman A, Ramenofsky M, Berryman C, et al. Evaluation of prehospital emergency medical service (EMS): defining areas for improvement. J Trauma 1983;23:702.
81. Maull KI, Schwab W, McHenry SD, et al. Trauma center verification. J Trauma 1986;26:521.
82. Maxwell C. Hospital organizational response to the nuclear accident at Three Mile Island: implications for future-oriented disaster planning. Am J Public Health 1982;72:275.
83. Merchant JA. Preparing for disaster. Am J Public Health 1986;76:233.
84. Meyer P, Rosen HB Hall W. Fracture dislocations of the cervical spine: transportation, assessment and immediate management. Instructional course lecture series, Am Acad Orthop Surg 1976;25:171.
85. Moritsugu KP, Reutershan TP. The National Disaster Medical System: a concept in large-scale emergency medical care. Ann Emerg Med 1986;15:1496.
86. Morris JA, Auerbach PS, Marshall GA, et al. The trauma score as a triage tool in the prehospital setting. JAMA 1986;256:1319.
87. Nagel EL. Improving emergency medical care. N Engl J Med 1980;302;1416.
88. Nissan S, Eldar R. Organization of surgical care of mass casualties in a civilian hospital. J Trauma 1971;11:974.
89. Ogilvie RB. Special message on health care. Springfield, IL: State of Illinois Printing Office, April 1, 1971.
90. O'Gorman M, Trabulsy P Pilcher DB. Zero time prehospital IV. J Trauma 1989;29:84.
91. Ornato J, Craren E, Nelson NM, Kimball KF. Impact of improved emergency medical services and emergency trauma care on the reduction in mortality from trauma. J Trauma 1985;25:575.
92. Pepe PE, Stewart RD. Role of the physician in the prehospital setting. Ann Emerg Med 1986;15:1480.
93. Pepe PE, Stewart RD, Copass MK. Prehospital management of trauma: a tale of three cities. Ann Emerg Med 1986;15:1484.
94. Pons PT, Honigman B, Moore EE, et al. Prehospital advanced trauma life support for critical penetrating wounds to the thorax and abdomen. J Trauma 1985;25:828.
95. Recommendations by the Committee on Acute Medicine of the American Society of Anesthesiologists. Community-wide emergency medical services. JAMA 1968;204:133.
96. Rignault DP, Deligny MC. The 1986 terrorist bombing experience in Paris. Ann Surg 1989;209:368.
97. Rodning CB. Disaster preparedness. South Med J 1983;76:229.
98. Safar P, Esposito G, Benson DM. Ambulance design and equipment for mobile intensive care. Arch Surg 1971;102:163.
99. Schwab WC, Teclet M, Zackowski WS, et al. The impact of an air ambulance system on an established trauma center. J Trauma 1985;25:580.
100. Shackford RS Hollingsworth-Friedland P, Cooper FG, Eastman BA. The effect of regionalization upon the quality of trauma care as assessed by concurrent audit before and after institution of a trauma system—a preliminary report. J Trauma 1986;26:812.
101. Shackford RS, MacKersie RC, Hoyt DB, et al. Impact of a trauma system on outcome of severely injured patients. Arch Surg 1987;122:523.
102. Sharpe DT, Roberts AHN, Barclay TL, et al. Treatment of burn casualties after fire at Bradford City football ground. Br Med J 1985;291:945.
103. Shehadi SI. Anatomy of a hospital in distress. The story of the American University of Beirut Hospital during the Lebanese civil war. Middle East J Anaesthesiol 1983;7:23.
104. Sherman M, Rath G. Threats to the validity of emergency medical services evaluation: a case study of mobile intensive care units. Med Care 1979;17:127.
105. Smith JP, Bodai BI, Hill AS, Frey CF. Prehospital stabilization of critically injured patients: a failed concept. J Trauma 1985;25:65.
106. Stewart RD. EMS in the 1980s: NY State Med J 1986;86:405.
107. Stewart RD, Paris PM, Stoy WA, Cannon G. Patient-controlled inhalational analgesia in prehospital care: a study of side-effects and feasibility. Crit Care Med 1983;11:851.
108. Subcommittee on Emergency Medical Services, Assembly of Life Sciences, National Research Council. Medical control in emergency medical services systems. Washington, DC: National Academy Press, 1981.
109. Subcommittee on Medical Control, Committee on EMS, Assembly of Life Sciences, National Research Council. Medical control in emergency medical services systems: subcommittee report conclusions and recommendations. Washington, DC: National Academy Press, 1981.
110. Tell R. Categorization: a community based approach. JACEP 1975;4:152.
111. Trauma Committee of the American Pediatric Surgical Association and the Committee on Trauma of the American College of Surgeons. Appendix J to hospital resources document: planning pediatric trauma care. Bull Am Coll Surg 1986;72:12.
112. Trunkey DD. Bay area trauma care. San Francisco Med Soc Bull 1982;55:22.
113. Trunkey DD. Is A.L.S. necessary for pre-hospital trauma care? J Trauma 1984;24:86.
114. Trunkey DD, Lim RC. Analysis of 425 consecutive trauma fatalities. An autopsy study. JACEP 1974;3:368.
115. United States Department of Transportation, National Highway Traffic Safety Administration. Mass casualties: A lessons learned approach. Proceedings of First International Assembly on EMS. June 13–17, 1982.
116. Waldholz M. Bhopal death toll, survivor problems still being debated. Wall Street J 1985;March 21:19.
117. West JG, Trunkey DD, Lim RC. Systems of trauma care: a study of two counties. Arch Surg 1979;114:455.
118. West JG, Williams MJ, Trunkey DD, Wolferth CC Jr. Trauma systems. JAMA 1988;259:3597.
119. Whiffler K, Leiman BC. The application of regional anesthesia in a disaster situation. S Afr Med J 1983;63:409.
120. White RD. The role of the anesthesiologist in emergency medical services. Semin Anesth 1985;4:102.
121. White RD, O'Donovan TPB. Prehospital life-support systems in traumatic and cardiac emergencies. Anesth Analg 1974;53:734.
122. Wiener SL, Barrett J. Mass casualties and triage. In: Wiener SL, Barrett J, eds. Trauma management for civilian and military physicians. Philadelphia: WB Saunders, 1986:536.
123. Williams DJ. Major disasters. Disaster planning in hospitals. Br J Hosp Med 1979;22:308.
124. Yates DW. Major disasters. Surgical triage. Br J Hosp Med 1979;22:323.

# Index

Note: Page numbers followed by f indicate figures; those followed by t indicate tables.